COLORADO MOUNTAIN COLLEGE
1 03 0003565484

D1571695

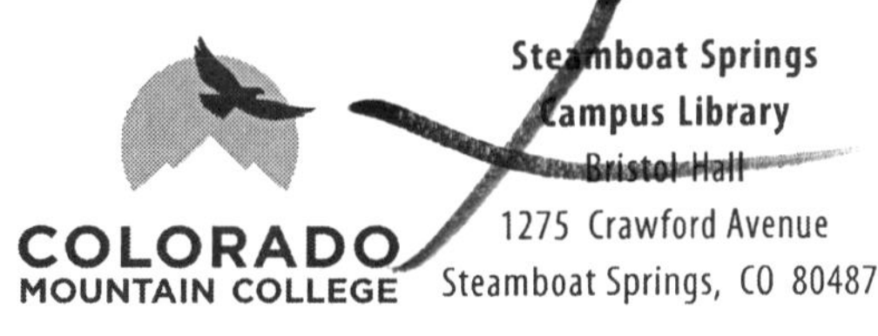
COLORADO
MOUNTAIN COLLEGE
Steamboat Springs
Campus Library
Bristol Hall
1275 Crawford Avenue
Steamboat Springs, CO 80487

THE COLOR ATLAS OF PHYSICAL THERAPY

THE COLOR ATLAS OF PHYSICAL THERAPY

EDITOR

Eric Shamus, PhD, DPT, PT, CSCS

Chair and Associate Professor, Department of Physical Therapy and Human Performance
College of Health Professions and Social Work
Florida Gulf Coast University
Fort Myers, Florida

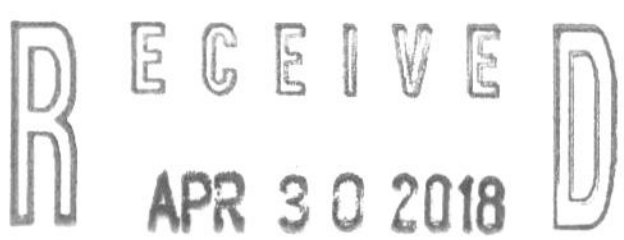

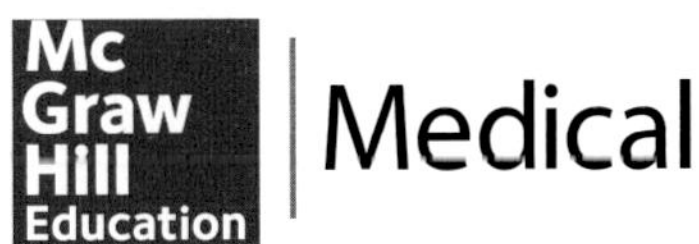

New York Chicago San Francisco Athens London Madrid Mexico City
Milan New Delhi Singapore Sydney Toronto

The Color Atlas of Physical Therapy

1 2 3 4 5 6 7 8 9 0 CTP/CTP 19 18 17 16 15 14

ISBN 978-0-07-181351-8
MHID 0-07-181351-9

This book was set in Adobe Garamond Pro by Aptara, Inc.
The editor was Michael Weitz.
The production supervisor was Richard Ruzycka.
Project management was provided by Abhishan Sharma of Aptara, Inc.
China Translation & Printing Services, Ltd. was printer and binder.
This book is printed on acid-free paper.

Library of Congress Cataloging-in-Publication Data

The color atlas of physical therapy / editor, Eric Shamus.
p. ; cm.
Includes bibliographical references and index.
ISBN 978-0-07-181351-8 (hardback : alk. paper) –
ISBN 0-07-181351-9 (hardback : alk. paper)
I. Shamus, Eric, editor.
[DNLM: 1. Physical Therapy Modalities–Atlases. 2. Physical Therapy Modalities–Case Reports. 3. Diagnosis, Differential–Atlases. 4. Diagnosis, Differential–Case Reports. 5. Rehabilitation–methods–Atlases. 6. Rehabilitation–methods–Case Reports. WB 17]
RM725
615.8'20222–dc23

2014010426

DEDICATION

This book is dedicated to my mother, Judy Shamus. Our thoughts and love will always be with her.

CONTENTS

PART 5

PEDIATRIC DISORDERS

Erika Albertini, DPT, PT, ATC
Director of Rehabilitation
Nurse on Call, Inc.
Coral Springs, Florida

Steven B. Ambler, DPT, PT, OCS
Assistant Clinical Professor
School of Physical Therapy and Rehabilitation Sciences
USF Health Morsani College of Medicine
University of South Florida
Tampa, Florida

Stephanie Boren Baker, MS, PT, CSCS
Clinic Director
Envision Physical Therapy
Lake Mary, Florida

Josh A. Barabas, MPT, OCS, CSCS
Staff Physical Therapist
UF Health Rehab Center-Magnolia Parke
Gainesville, Florida

Tiffany M. Barber, DPT
Physical Therapist
Select Physical Therapy
Hollywood, Florida

Sharon Irish Bevins, PhD, PT
Associate Professor
Department of Physical Therapy and Human Performance
College of Health Professions and Social Work
Florida Gulf Coast University
Fort Myers, Florida

Thomas Bevins, MS, PT
Assistant Professor
Department of Physical Therapy and Human Performance
College of Health Professions and Social Work
Florida Gulf Coast University
Fort Myers, Florida

Stephen A. Black, DSc, MEd, PT, ATC, CSCS
Assistant Professor
Department of Physical Therapy and Human Performance
College of Health Professions and Social Work
Florida Gulf Coast University
Fort Myers, Florida

Martha Henao Bloyer, DPT, PT, PCS
Clinical Assistant Professor, Director of Clinical Education
Department of Physical Therapy
Nicole Wertheim College of Nursing and Health Sciences
Florida International University
Miami, Florida

David Boesler, DO, MS
Associate Professor and Chairman, Department of Neuromusculoskeletal Medicine
College of Osteopathic Medicine
Nova Southeastern University
Fort Lauderdale, Florida

Colin Brooks, MBA
Adjunct Professor, Department of Management
University of New Orleans
New Orleans, Louisiana

Annie Burke-Doe, PhD, MPT, PT
Professor, Department of Physical Therapy
University of St. Augustine for Health Sciences
San Marcos, California

Stephanie Bush, DPT, MEd, WCS
Women's Health Program Coordinator
Center Manager, Amelia Island Clinic
Brooks Rehabilitation
Fernandina Beach, Florida

Jennifer Cabrera, DPT, GCS
Senior Physical Therapist
Geriatric Residency Admissions Coordinator
St. Catherine's West Rehabilitation Hospital
Villa Maria West Skilled Nursing Facility
Miami, Florida

Kristie Centner, DPT
Miami, Florida

Eric J. Chaconas, DPT, PT, FAAOMPT
Assistant Professor, Department of Physical Therapy
University of St. Augustine
St. Augustine, Florida

Mitchell L. Cordova, PhD, ATC, FNATA, FACSM
Professor and Dean
College of Health Professions and Social Work
Florida Gulf Coast University
Fort Myers, Florida

Jason C. Craddock, EdD, ATC, CSCS
Assistant Professor, Program Director-Athletic Training Program
Department of Physical Therapy and Human Performance
College of Health Professions and Social Work
Florida Gulf Coast University
Fort Myers, Florida

Daniel Curtis, DPT, PT, MTC
Outpatient Supervisor, Health Central Hospital
Adjunct Faculty, University of Central Florida
Orlando, Florida

Matthew Daugherty, DPT, MOT, OCS, FAAOMPT
Assistant Professor, Department of Physical Therapy
University of St. Augustine for Health Sciences
St. Augustine, Florida

Elizabeth E. Demarse, DPT, MTC
Physical Therapist
H. Lee Moffitt Cancer Center and Research Institute
Tampa, Florida

Christopher S. Ellis, DPT
Advanced Physical Therapy and Rehabilitation
Cape Coral, Florida

Reuben Escorpizo, DPT, MSc, PT
Assistant Professor, Department of Physical Therapy
Louisiana State University Health Sciences Center
New Orleans, Louisiana
ICF Research Branch
Nottwil, Switzerland

Christopher C. Felton, DO, ATC
Family Medicine
New Hanover Regional Medical Center
Wilmington, North Carolina

Shawn D. Felton, EdD, ATC
Assistant Professor, Department of Physical Therapy and Human Performance
College of Health Professions and Social Work
Florida Gulf Coast University
Fort Myers, Florida

Shallen (McClain) Flory, DPT
Chicago, Illinois

Stacey L. Frazee, DPT
Fort Myers, Florida

Angela S. Garcia, PharmD, MPH, CPh
Assistant Professor, Public Health
College of Osteopathic Medicine
Nova Southeastern University
Fort Lauderdale, Florida

Ben Greenberg, PhD
Department of Psychiatry and Psychology
Cleveland Clinic Foundation
Cleveland, Ohio

George Hanbury, PhD
President
Nova Southeastern University
Fort Lauderdale, Florida

Greg W. Hartley, DPT, PT, GCS, CEEAA
Director of Rehabilitation, St. Catherine's Rehabilitation Hospitals
Voluntary Assistant Professor, Department of Physical Therapy
University of Miami, Miller School of Medicine
Miami, Florida

Kelley Henderson, MEd, ATC
Instructor, Department of Physical Therapy and Human Performance
College of Health Science and Social Work
Florida Gulf Coast University
Fort Myers, Florida

Lindsey (Davis) Hornecke, DPT
Fort Myers, Florida

Dennis Hunt, EdD, CSCS
Assistant Professor and Program Director, Exercise Science
Department of Physical Therapy and Human Performance
College of Health Professions and Social Work
Florida Gulf Coast University
Fort Myers, Florida

W. Justin Jones, DPT, PT, OCS
Associate Professor of Practice and Associate Chair
School of Nursing and Health Sciences
Physical Therapy Department
Simmons College
Boston, Massachusetts

Patricia M. King, PhD, PT, OCS, MTC
Professor and Chair
Department of Physical Therapy
East Tennessee State University
Johnson City, Tennessee

Kenneth Lee, DPT, PT
Chairperson, School of Health Sciences
Miami Dade College
Miami, Florida

John Leschitz, DPT, PT, OCS
Board-Certified Orthopaedic Clinical Specialist
Brooks Rehabilitation-UNF Orthopaedic OMPT Fellow in Training
Brooks Rehabilitation
Jacksonville, Florida

Abby Lopez, LMT, CT, NCTMB
Staten Island, New York

Jennie Q. Lou, MD, MSc
Professor and Director of Medical Informatics
Professor of Public Health/Internal Medicine
Nova Southeastern University College of Osteopathic Medicine
Biomedical Informatics Program
Fort Lauderdale, Florida

Christina Machuca, DPT, CSCS
Siskin Hospital for Physical Rehabilitation
Chattanooga, Tennessee

David W. Mandel, PhD, PT
Assistant Professor, Department of Physical Therapy
University of Miami Miller School of Medicine
Coral Gables, Florida

Mila Marhovich, DPT
Fort Myers, Florida

Linda M. Martin, PhD, OTR/L, FAOTA
Chair and Professor, Department of Occupational Therapy and Community Health
College of Health Professions and Social Work
Florida Gulf Coast University
Fort Myers, Florida

B. James Massey, DPT, OCS, FAAOMPT
Assistant Professor of Physical Therapy, Doctor of Physical Therapy Program
Wingate University
Wingate, North Carolina
Former Residency
Brooks Rehabilitation and the University of Northern Florida
Jacksonville, Florida

Lisa Ward McVey, DPT, PT, CCS
School of Health Professions
Shenandoah University

Gina DiBagno-Moreno, DPT, CSCS
Fort Myers, Florida

Ana Marcelina Moura, PT (Brazil)
Coordinator, Pain Management Clinic Physical Therapy Department
Physios - Clínica de Saúde Funcional Ltda.
Teresina, Piauí, Brazil

Oseas Florencio de Moura Filho, PT (Brazil), MSc
Director, Physical Therapy Department
Physios - Clínica de Saúde Funcional Ltda.
Teresina, Piauí, Brazil

Tasha Mouton, DPT, MOT, OCS, FAAOMPT, MTC
Staff Physical Therapist
Brooks Rehabilitation
Jacksonville, Florida

Kevin Murdoch, DPT, PT, OCS
Assistant Professor, School of Physical Therapy and Rehabilitation Sciences
USF Health Morsani College of Medicine
University of South Florida
Tampa, Florida

Cynthia E. Neville, DPT, PT, WCS
Jacksonville, Florida

Doris Newman, DO, PT, FAAO
Associate Professor
Director of Rural Medicine
College of Osteopathic Medicine
Nova Southeastern University
Fort Lauderdale, Florida

Elizabeth R. Northrop, DPT, PT
McIver Women's Center for Urogynecology and Pelvic Floor Health
Jacksonville, Florida

Marangela Obispo, MSPT, GCS
Program Director
Physical Therapist Assistant Program
Keiser University Miami Campus
Miami, Florida

Jacqueline Osborne, DPT, PT, GCS, CEEAA
Geriatric Residency Coordinator
Brooks Institute of Higher Learning
Brooks Rehabilitation
Jacksonville, Florida

Raine Osborne, DPT, PT, OCS, FAAOMPT
Coordinator, Brooks/UNF Orthopaedic Residency Program
Brooks Institute of Higher Learning
Jacksonville, Florida

Patrick S. Pabian, DPT, PT, SCS, OCS, CSCS
Clinical Associate Professor
Program Director
Program in Physical Therapy, Department of Health Professions
University of Central Florida
Orlando, Florida

Erin N. Pauley, DPT, MS, ATC, CSCS
Fort Myers, Florida

Christina L. Pettie, MHA, PT
Site Manager
UF Health Rehab Center-Magnolia Parke
UF Health Shands Hospital
Gainesville, Florida

E. Thomas Pitney, DPT, PT, SCS, ATC
Adjunct Professor
Florida Gulf Coast University
Fort Myers, Florida

Yasmin Qureshi, DPT, MPT, MHS (Osteo)
Assistant Professor
Osteopathic Principles and Practice
College of Osteopathic Medicine
Nova Southeastern University
Fort Lauderdale, Florida

Shari Rone-Adams, DBA, MHSA, PT
Director, Entry Level Doctor of Physical Therapy Programs
Associate Professor, College of Health Care Sciences
Nova Southeastern University
Fort Lauderdale, Florida

Megan Samantha Rosga, DPT, MSPT, NCS
Physical Therapist, RIC River North Day Rehab
Rehabilitation Institute of Chicago
Chicago, Illinois

Stephen A. Russo, PhD
Assistant Professor, Center for Psychological Studies
Director of Sport Psychology, College of Osteopathic Medicine
Nova Southeastern University
Fort Lauderdale, Florida

Daphne Ryan, DPT, MS, PT
Therapist, St. Joseph Therapy and Spine Clinic
Peacehealth Medical Center
Bellingham, Washington

Ariel Diana Schumer, DPT
Traveling Physical Therapist
Bala Cynwyd, Pennsylvania

Eric Shamus, PhD, DPT, PT, CSCS
Chair and Associate Professor, Department of Physical Therapy and Human Performance
College of Health Professions and Social Work
Florida Gulf Coast University
Fort Myers, Florida

Ilan Shamus, DDS
Private Practice, Orthodontics
Armonk and White Plains, New York

Jennifer Shamus, PhD, DPT, COMT, CSCS
Market Manager
Select Physical Therapy
Pembroke Pines, Florida

Erika Simmerman-Mabes, DO
General Surgery Resident
Georgia Regents University
Augusta, Georgia

Jesse Solotoff, DPT
Physical Therapist
Select Physical Therapy
Pembroke Pines, Miramar, Florida

Wendy Song, DO
Family Medicine Resident
Beth Israel Medical Center
New York, New York

Debra F. Stern, DPT, DBA, MSM, PT
Associate Professor
Physical Therapy Department
College of Health Care Sciences
Nova Southeastern University
Fort Lauderdale, Florida

Kathy Swanick, DPT, PT, OCS
Instructor
Department of Physical Therapy and Human Performance
College of Health Professions and Social Work
Florida Gulf Coast University
Fort Myers, Florida

Melissa Tabor, DO
Team Physician
Sports and Non-Surgical Orthopedic Medicine
Assistant Professor, Sports Medicine Clinic
College of Osteopathic Medicine
Nova Southeastern University
Fort Lauderdale, Florida

Kay Tasso, PhD, PT, PCS
Independent Contractor
Ponte Vedra, Florida

Adrian Taylor, DPT
Lee Center for Sports Medicine and Rehab
Cape Coral, Florida

Brady L. Tripp, PhD, ATC
Clinical Associate Professor and Director
Graduate Athletic Training Program
College of Health and Human Performance
University of Florida
Gainesville, Florida

Patricia M. Tripp, PhD, ATC, CSCS
Clinical Associate Professor and Director
Undergraduate Athletic Training Program
College of Health and Human Performance
University of Florida
Gainesville, Florida

Arie J. Van Duijn, EdD, MSc, PT, OCS
Associate Professor and Program Director, Doctor of Physical Therapy Program
Department of Physical Therapy and Human Performance
Florida Gulf Coast University
Fort Myers, Florida

Jacqueline van Duijn, DPT, PT, OCS
Director of Clinical Education
Doctor of Physical Therapy Program
Department of Physical Therapy and Human Performance
Florida Gulf Coast University
Fort Myers, Florida

Mollie Venglar, DSc, MSPT, NCS
Assistant Professor
Department of Physical Therapy and Human Performance
College of Health Professions and Social Work
Florida Gulf Coast University
Fort Myers, Florida

Jennifer Volz, DPT
Fort Myers, Florida

Sean M. Wells, DPT, PT, OCS, ATC, CSCS
Naples Personal Training, LLC
Naples, Florida

Natalie V. Wessel, DO, MPH
Resident Physician, Department of Obstetrics and Gynecology
Maimonides Medical Center
Brooklyn, New York

Stanley Wilson, EdD, PT, CAES
Dean and Associate Professor
College of Health Care Sciences
Nova Southeastern University
Fort Lauderdale, Florida

Stephanie N. Wright, MOT, OTR/L
Occupational Therapist
H. Lee Moffitt Cancer Center and Research Institute
Tampa, Florida

Mae L. Yahara, MS, PT, ATC
Director of the Physical Therapist Assistant Program
Keiser University
West Palm Beach, Florida

Amber Yampolsky, MPT, ATP
Physical Therapist
Arnold Palmer Hospital for Children
Orlando, Florida

Thomas S. Zeller, MPT
Founder, Advanced Physical Therapy and Rehabilitation
Fort Myers and Cape Coral, Florida

Today's evolving health care environment demands efficiency and effectiveness. In response to these demands and growth of the physical therapy profession through the beginning of the twenty-first century, the APTA has developed "Vision 2020".[1] "By 2020, physical therapy will be provided by physical therapists (PTs) who are doctors of physical therapy, recognized by consumers and other health care professionals as the practitioners of choice to whom consumers have direct access for the diagnosis of, interventions for, and prevention of impairments, functional limitations, and disabilities related to movement, function, and health … with all privileges of autonomous practice."[1] The implications of autonomy increase the emphasis on collaboration with other health professionals, requiring competency in diagnosis as well as recommendations for follow-up, referral, and intervention. Even though PTs can functionally diagnose, the need to determine if a client or individual requires diagnostic testing and subsequent medical diagnosis is paramount to best practice. If a consumer is able to have direct access to a physical therapist or direct access into the medical system through physical therapy, the physical therapist needs to determine the appropriateness of that access during the initial encounter, regardless of setting or venue. One tool to facilitate clinical decision making is the process or act of "screening," which is acknowledged as a skill needed by PTs by the American Physical Therapy Association.

Screening is an accepted and expected practice in all health professions. Screens are historically performed in a variety of settings for individuals or groups. In the APTA Guide to Physical Therapist Practice, it states that PTs "… conduct screening to determine the need for primary, secondary or tertiary prevention services for further examination, intervention, or consultation; or for referral to another health care practitioner. … Screening is based on a problem focused, systematic collection and analysis of data."[2]

DEFINITIONS

Most definitions of screening are medically oriented. Merriam-Webster defines screening as "the act of examining people or things in order to decide if they are suitable for a particular purpose."[3] David Eddy, MD, PhD defines screening as "the application of a test to detect a potential disease or condition in a person who has no known symptoms of that disease or condition."[4] He further states, "There are two main purposes for screening. One is to detect a disease early in its natural history when treatment might be more effective, less expensive, or both. The other purpose is to detect risk factors that put a person at a higher than average risk for developing disease, with the goal of modifying the risk factor or factors to prevent the disease."[4]

WHO SHOULD SCREEN?

The PT is identified as the physical therapy professional skilled to perform screens according to The Guide to Physical Therapist Practice.[2] However, based on physical therapist assistant (PTA) education and the Guide for the Conduct of the Affiliate Member, using the Standards of Ethical Conduct for the Physical Therapist Assistant,[5] there may be venues in which it may be appropriate for a PTA to perform components of a screen. The appropriateness is dependent on the practice venue, the state in which one practices or is licensed, and internal policies and procedures. If one looks globally at the issue of screening in the general population, there are many health care professionals as well as non-healthcare professionals who screen individuals for identification of need for further medical evaluation. In determining whether a PTA can perform a screen in a specific venue, consideration of the education of the PTA should be considered. Examples of situations in which it may be appropriate for PTAs to screen include: public school screening for scoliosis, body mass screening at a health fair, and solicitation of history. Venues in which it may be inappropriate include: athletic venues in which preperformance athletic screens are performed to determine if an athlete can participate and pre-employment screens in which the decision as to whether an individual is capable of physical work is made. However, as PTA education includes training in performing specific assessment and examination, such as range of motion and strength determinations, there may also be a role for PTAs to perform components of certain screens, with the PT as the ultimate decision maker regarding the plan of care or referral elsewhere.

Although the literature supports the need for screening by PTs, screening in the context of physical therapy is primarily contextual and unclear. Essentially, however, screening is the performance of history taking (oral or written), systems review, observation and brief general tests, in individuals or groups of individuals to identify risk factors that may be present or absent, associated with functional or medical problems and or variations in findings from normative values in context appropriate for PTs. Findings may identify the need for physical therapy, the need for referral to another healthcare professional (i.e. physician) or the presence or absence of problems that may be contributing to, causative of or be present exclusive of and in addition to, the primary client complaint.

PTs are expected to provide quality examination, evaluation, diagnosis, prognosis, referral determination and evidenced based approaches whenever possible. Increased productivity demands in recent decades have necessitated more time efficient and cost-effective approaches to data gathering and provision of care including screening. The move to doctoral entry level education has necessitated expansion of knowledge and clinical expertise to differential diagnosis, which includes screening of all body systems. These changes are evidence of the changing role of the physical therapist in an evolving healthcare system. Screening in a variety of venues and situations is beneficial for all PTs as well students during entry level education to facilitate and sustain the transition to a doctoring profession. It will facilitate the adoption of functional screening protocols that can be easily incorporated into any practice model that evolves in the future.

IMPLICATIONS OF SCREENING

The cost benefits of risk identification with subsequent behavioral changes that can minimize or eliminate the risks have significant implications for health cost containment and quality of life. Examples of screening activities that PTs commonly engage in according to the APTA Guide to Practice,[2] "include:

- identifying lifestyle factors (e.g., amount of exercise, stress, weight) that may lead to increased risk for serious health problems
- identifying children who may need an examination for idiopathic scoliosis
- identifying elderly individuals in a community center or nursing home who are at risk for slipping, tripping, or falling

- identifying risk factors in the workplace
- pre-performance testing of individuals who are active in sports
- conducting pre-work screening programs."[2]

These examples illustrate that screens are performed in multiple venues, from shopping mall health fairs and schools, to hospitals, extended care facilities and other clinical settings across the lifespan.

In the context of health and wellness, screening may be performed in the presence or absence of any pre-identified signs, symptoms or individual concerns. Most of the screens performed by PTs do not require testing equipment that bears significant cost. Generally speaking, if there is cost associated with screening in the short term, it is warranted in the wellness and prevention arena to minimize costs and maximize health and quality of life in the long term. In reality, much of the screening performed by PTs may be performed at no cost to the client as in venues such as health fairs, or as included components of initial examinations and evaluations that include the screens. There is however, the cost of time that should be considered.

Many conditions, benign and/or malignant, may be potentially identified by appropriate screens.With identification of certain "markers," the need for further evaluation of a potential pathology by the appropriate skilled healthcare professional can be obtained as needed. Although the Guide to Physical Therapist Practice states "Candidates for screening generally are not patients/clients currently receiving physical therapy services,"[2] that is not necessarily the case, as a variety of circumstances may exist in which the physical therapist may be performing screening procedures. Circumstances include clients who self-refer in direct consumer access situations, clients referred to PT by physicians or others, and those in the general population who may be participating in screening activities offered to the public or in pre-arranged situations such as pre-employment or pre-performance athletic screens. Depending on the circumstances and venue, there may or may not be information available to the "screener" about the patient or client. In venues such as a skilled nursing facility or extended care facility, information is available in the form of the medical record and from the caretakers; professional and nonprofessional, for example, family. In public venues, where there is no information available, the "screener" must elicit appropriate information by history, interview and or observation and assessment only as appropriate and in accordance with HIPAA. It should be noted that when screens are performed in public venues, such as health fairs, the PT should be careful not to establish a PT/patient relationship in order to prevent potential liability issues. Screens performed should be general and reproducible with essentially objective findings noted and given to the "client" with recommendations for "follow up" if the client chooses to, on a form that expressly states such. Any PT that plans to engage in community screening or screening as a marketing tool in a community, should check with their attorney or liability provider about their risk and coverage. In some instances, if a PT is screening under the auspices of a county public health department, there may be immunity status granted for the screening process, thereby precluding liability concerns. It should be noted that even if a referral with a diagnosis comes from a physician, a physician extender such as a physician assistant (PA), or other practice act acceptable referral source, screening may be needed to determine the accuracy or appropriateness of the diagnosis or referral. In this case, the liability would be consistent, the regular course of PT care. In the educational setting, the types of screening that can be done in public with physical therapy students under the supervision of licensed PTs should be sanctioned by both the legal department and consultants for the college or university as well as the professional liability carrier.

Clients, who self-refer to physical therapy, require screening, examination, and evaluation to determine if their primary complaint is appropriate for physical therapy or is indicative of a medical condition that warrants referral to another health professional. They may have multiple conditions that require the attention of a PT in addition to another health professional such as a physician. Clients referred to physical therapy by physicians, in spite of the referrals, may have conditions that require further medical assessment based on the results of the PT screening, examination, and evaluation. Those individuals in the general population screened in public venues may demonstrate signs and or symptoms or history that warrant referral to a physician or other health care professional, such as identification of a suspicious skin growth. If a client is referred for PT by a physician for a specific problem or diagnosis, areas other than that of the primary problem area, should be screened to determine if they are causal or contributing to the problem, or if other problems coexist. For example, if a patient is referred with a hand or wrist problem, the PT would screen the cervical and shoulder area to rule out pathology proximal to the regions of primary complaint. The PT should also confirm that it is not a problem related to body system that is not neuromuscular or musculoskeletal in nature that is "referring pain" to the area. "Screening examinations allow the therapist to quickly scan through the data from the body systems, noting areas of deficit. Screening examinations indicate areas where more detailed assessments are warranted. More definitive assessments are then used to provide objective data to accurately determine the degree of specific function and dysfunction, for example, manual muscle tests, range of motion tests, oxygen consumption."[6]

In the context of current societal cultural demand, it is assumed that all health care professionals will practice screening, as they do in all interactions, with cultural competence. "Cultural competence initiatives may even help control costs, by making care more efficient and effective."[7] To effectively screen, a PT must be able to communicate effectively with any group of individuals regardless of cultural or ethnic background. It is also imperative to be aware of the healthcare disparities inherent in the US healthcare system, and being aware of the same, emphasize the need for cultural sensitivity and competence for equality of service provision. There are also pathologies that may be more prevalent in some ethnicities than others. In today's world, many communities are more culturally integrated than in the past, although pockets of ethnic groups may choose to live in enclaves within a larger geographic area. There may also be groups living in more isolated geographic areas that may or not be rural. There are six primary dimensions of culture to be considered in all client encounters: age, ethnicity, gender, physical ability race, and sexual orientation. Socioeconomic status, education, religion, marital status, parental status, personal habits, recreational habits, appearance, and work experience, and work status or student status must also be considered in the context of culture. With the high incidence of unemployment in the current decade, sensitivity to the lack of health insurance should also be considered. Community offered screening may be the only healthcare services an individual has access to.

Therefore, it is in the best interest of the PT or healthcare professional to be able to appropriately solicit information from all cultural groups in a competent manner. As it is impossible to be familiar with the behaviors of all cultural groups and subgroups, it is more practical to become skilled in open-ended culturally sensitive questions. An example of this is in the context of a fall screen: Why are you here today? What is the reason you may have had a steadiness problem? Are you doing anything for the problem you're having at home?

The LEARN model is applicable in all client encounters to facilitate communication in broad categories.[8]

(L) Listen to patient
(E) Elicit patients' health beliefs
(A) Assess potential problems that may have impact on health behaviors
(R) Recommend a treatment plan
(N) Negotiate a mutually agreed-on treatment plan

The LEARN model, may be found by the physical therapist to be more contextually relevant in a longer history or initial encounter included in an initial examination and evaluation.

THE ETHNIC MODEL[9]

The ETHNIC mnemonic is another example of simple framework for practicing culturally competent care, without any pre-judgment or cultural assumptions. It includes the following guiding principles.

E Explanation (How do you explain your illness?)
T Treatment (What treatment have you tried?)
H Healers (Have you sought any advice from folk healers?)
N Negotiate (mutually acceptable options)
I (Agree on) Intervention
C Collaboration (with patient, family, and healers)

As with the LEARN model, the EHTNIC model may be more indicated in the history component of an initial examination and evaluation, but is presented here as a guiding concept.

Encompassing cultural factors in the screening process should facilitate the process of appropriate decision making following completion of the screening process. Decades of data from the United States Census Bureau[10] indicate that as the nation's population grows, there is an increasingly more diversity in the United States. The bureau projects that the population of the United States will grow from 282 million in 2000 to 420 million in 2050, with an almost 50% increase of minorities accounting for nearly 90% of this increase. The US population of non-whites is projected to grow from approximately 31% in 2000 to approximately 52% in 2050 representing the majority of the population by the middle of the century. These statistics emphasize the need for cultural competence not only in the process of screening, but all aspects of PT/patient/client management to ensure effective, efficient, and quality healthcare.

SUMMARY

Although there is disagreement in the rehabilitation literature as to what constitutes screening, there is no debate that screening as a process is a useful tool in prevention, wellness, and identification of risk factors, pathological conditions or illness. Media attention, do-it-yourself-health care trends, access to the internet, millions of underinsured, and an estimated 45+ million of currently uninsured Americans (proposed to decrease to ~10,000,000 as a result of healthcare reform) have created a market for "quick" screening identification of potential problems that merit referral to appropriate healthcare professionals. The human body is made up of multiple systems that work synergistically to achieve function. As there is a vague line in some respects between screening and tests and measures or examination, a combination may actually be considered examinations that ultimately can combine to result in physical therapy evaluation. However, all of the contexts for screening previously identified are expected to continue and are included in the American Physical Therapy Associations basic competencies for physical therapist graduates.

As the reader progresses through an evaluation, it is important to fully screen all systems of the body and not stop secondary to pattern recognition. Even the best clinician will occasionally fail to recognize additional contributing factors. It is our goal that this textbook will provide insight regarding contributing factors with the hope that outstanding patient care will be delivered consistently.

REFERENCES

1. *APTA Vision 2020*. http://www.apta.org/Vision2020/. Accessed February 14, 2014.
2. *APTA Guide to PT Practice*, 2nd ed, Revised 2003. Interactive Guide to Physical Therapist Practice by American Physical Therapy Association. ISBN: 978-1-887759-87-8. doi : 10.2522/ptguide.978-1-931369-64-0. http://guidetoptpractice.apta.org. Accessed February 2, 2014.
3. Screening. *Merriam-Webster*. An Encyclopedia Britannica Company. 2014. http://www.merriam-webster.com/dictionary/screening. Accessed February 28, 2014.
4. Eddy DM, (Ed). *Common Screening Tests*. American College of Physicians. Philadelphia, PA, 1991, page 1.
5. *Standards of Ethical Conduct for the Physical Therapist Assistant*. http://www.apta.org/uploadedFiles/APTAorg/About_Us/Policies/Ethics/StandardsEthicalConductPTA.pdf#search=%22Standards of Ethical Conduct for the Physical Therapist Assistant%22. Accessed February 2, 2014.
6. O'Sullivan SB, Schmitz TJ, Fulk GD. *Physical Rehabilitation*, 6th ed. FA Davis. Philadelphia, PA, 2014, page 5.
7. Betancourt JR, Green AR, Carrillo JE, Park ER. Cultural Competence and Health Care Disparities: Key Perspectives and Trends. *Health Affairs*. March/April 2005;24(2):499–505.
8. Berlin EA, Fowkes WC, Jr. A teaching framework for cross-cultural healthcare-application in family practice. *The Western Journal of Medicine*. 1983;139(6):934–938.
9. Levin SJ, Like RC, Gottlieb JE. ETHNIC: a framework for culturally competent clinical practice. In: Appendix: Useful clinical interviewing mnemonics. *Patient Care*. 2000;34(9)188–189.
10. *US Interim Projections by Age, Sex, Race, and Hispanic Origin*. Washington, DC: U.S. Census Bureau; 2004: Table 1a.

Stanley Wilson, EdD, PT, CAES
Debra F. Stern, DPT, DBA, MSM, PT

ACKNOWLEDGMENTS

Special thanks to the McGraw-Hill staff, Deborah Cruz, Michael Weitz, and Kim Davis for their help and guidance throughout the process. I would like to thank my family, Jennifer, Grant, Lexie, and my dad Stuart for allowing me the time and support to work on this book. Also, to the administration, faculty, staff and Dean Cordova at Florida Gulf Coast University for providing the time and support needed for this project. With everyone's contribution this book was taken from a vision to a reality.

THE COLOR ATLAS OF PHYSICAL THERAPY

PART 1

INTRODUCTION

PART 1
INTRODUCTION

The Color Atlas of Physical Therapy textbook provides images and detailed information about a wide variety of diagnoses. There are 280 of the more common diagnoses that are seen by physical therapists and physical therapist assistants. The book provides quick and easy detailed information that is all in one place: from etiology, differential diagnosis, impairments, functional goals, references, and patient resources. Each diagnosis is broken out into six sections and outlined with the same format.

The first group of information includes the name of the diagnosis, contributing authors, Conditions/Synonyms, ICD 9 and ICD 10 codes, American Physical Therapy Association: *Guide to Physical Therapy Practice Patterns* and a patient presentation. Many diagnoses are known by similar names or have diagnoses that are closely related. The ICD 9 and ICD 10 information is provided and as practitioners switch this information is easy to find. The *Guide to Physical Therapy Practice* lays out a framework of patterns for examination and treatment categories. The patient presentation is included to help the clinician identify common patterns to combine with the images that are imbedded within the chapter.

The second group of information is under the category Key Features. Under key features of the diagnosis are the description, essentials of diagnosis, general considerations, and demographics. The description provides details about what the diagnosis is and information that describes the diagnosis. The essentials of diagnosis section describe the information that is needed to assist in making the diagnosis. Under general considerations, information is provided about implications in rehabilitation, possible secondary effects, and complications that may occur. The demographics are provided to get a better sense of the population that is usually affected. Incidence rates are provided when possible.

The third group of information is under the category Clinical Findings. Under clinical findings are the signs and symptoms, functional implications, possible contributing causes, and differentials diagnoses. The signs and symptoms are helpful in recognizing other potential problems and can be used to identify a grouping of signs and symptoms. Many practitioners use the signs and symptoms to determine severity or to rule in or out other differential diagnoses. The section of functional implications are important as this information is not always readily available and can assist the practitioner in considering functional activities that maybe limited. Possible contributing causes provides information on the causes if known and may also help in future patient education in limiting further progression or prevention of the dysfunction.

The fourth group of information is under the heading of Medical Interventions. Under the medical interventions section, one finds the means of confirming a diagnosis that can include imaging, medical tests, and interventional diagnosis techniques along with the findings and interpretations of these tests. It also includes medical treatments such as surgical procedures and common medications. This provides very good information and other options that maybe available for the patient. The group ends with referral/admittance that is a list of some of the providers that may be used for a consultation or referral source.

The fifth group covers the physical therapy specific information. The categories include impairments, physical therapy tests and measures, intervention, functional goals, and prognosis. With greater details needed in documentation and functional outcome reporting being aware of the functional limitations and impairments have become and important component. Many of the documentation books like *Effective Documentation for Physical Therapy* provide the framework for writing goals and identifying impairments. Interventions and prognosis help the therapist with the plan of care and setting the timeframes for goals. It also helps in the discussion with the patient regarding realistic goals.

The sixth category is provided for reference material. The categories included are patient resources, references, and additional resources. Patients are often looking for support group information and links to websites and organizations that provide medical information about their condition or disorder. The references and additional resources are from scientific journals and textbooks and provide good information for further investigation.

The Color Atlas of Physical Therapy goes beyond color images and anatomical drawings. The information provided on impairments, functional goals, and patient resources are often contents that are not easily found in other resources. The compilation of information about the diagnosis provides great details for students and practitioners alike.

Happy reading.

Eric Shamus

PART 2

ASSOCIATED MEDICAL DISORDERS

SECTION A AMPUTATION

1 TRANSFEMORAL AMPUTATION

Jacqueline Osborne, DPT, PT, GCS, CEEAA

CONDITION/DISORDER SYNONYM

- Above-knee amputation

ICD-9-CM CODE

- V49.76 Above-knee amputation status

ICD-10-CM CODE

- Z89.619 Acquired absence of unspecified leg above knee

PREFERRED PRACTICE PATTERN

- 4J: Impaired Motor Function, Muscle Performance, Range of Motion, Gait, Locomotion, and Balance Associated With Amputation

PATIENT PRESENTATION

A 22-year-old male with a right above the knee amputation presents in a manual wheelchair with his prosthetic leg in his lap. He notes that he picked up his prosthesis from his prosthetist earlier that day and is eager to see if the adjustments made to the socket will improve his gait mechanics. When you assessed him last week you found that he was not achieving full hip extension at terminal stance on the right and that he was circumducting on the right in the swing period of gait. You discovered that he has an 8-degree hip flexion contracture on the right and a 4/5 strength of the right adductor magnus. His gluteus medius strength is 3/5 on the right and 4/5 on the left.

KEY FEATURES

Description

- Result of ultimate loss of tissue perfusion from the surrounding circulation at any level proximal to the femoral condyles.
- A transfemoral amputation is an amputation of the lower limb between the knee and the hip.

Essentials of Diagnosis[1]

- A surgeon makes diagnosis after surgery.
- A transfemoral amputation is made between the femur at the level of the greater trochanter and proximal to the level of the femoral condyles.
- Efforts are made to preserve the attachment of the adductor magnus at the medial distal third of the femur to maintain the normal biomechanical alignment of the femur.

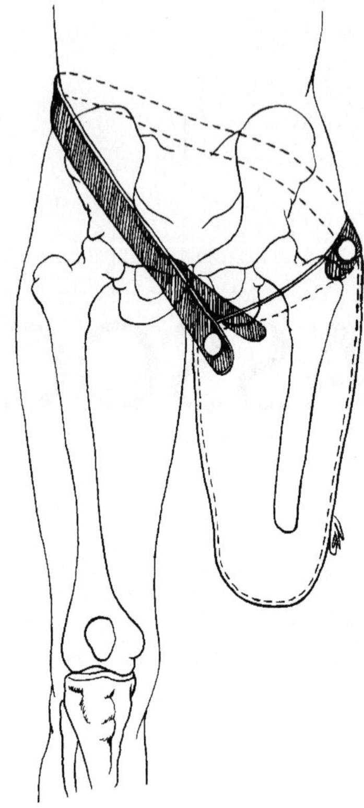

FIGURE 1-1 Silesian band suspension of a transfemoral prosthesis. (From Skinner HB. *Current Diagnosis & Treatment in Orthopedics*, 4th ed. http://www.accessmedicine.com. Copyright © The McGraw-Hill Companies, Inc. All rights reserved.)

- An amputation at the level proximal to the greater trochanter of the femur is called a hip disarticulation.
- The amputation of the entire lower extremity (LE) and half of the ipsilateral pelvis is called a hemipelvectomy.

General Considerations[1–3]

- Loss of a limb above the knee results in widespread impairments in body structure and function as well as significant activity limitations and participation restrictions that will ultimately affect the individual's participation in family and home life as well as reintegration into the society.
- Emotional support and education must infiltrate postoperative rehabilitation beginning on postoperative day 1 to assist the individual with repossessing life roles.
- The total recovery period is consistently 12 to 18 months and includes activity recovery, reintegration, prosthetic training, and prosthetic management.
- The acute hospital stay ranges from 5 to 14 days, and the post-acute hospital stay could range from 2 to 8 weeks.

- This period includes surgery recovery, wound healing, early rehabilitation, and determination of prosthetic readiness.
- The immediate recovery stage begins with the healing of the wound and could extend up to 6 months.
  - This stage ends with stabilization of limb volume after accommodating to prosthetic use with ambulation.
- The last stage of recovery is widely variable. During this time, limb volumes continue to stabilize but are no longer rapidly changing.
  - Prosthetic adjustments can be made as the limb continues to stabilize.
  - When the prosthesis is worn full time for a period of at least 6 months and the limb volume has stabilized to a point that socket fit remains relatively consistent for at least 2 to 3 weeks, a definitive prosthesis may be indicated.
  - Higher-level functional training and social reintegration mark the end of this stage.
- Promotion of independence can start as early as postoperative day 1 with quadriceps and gluteus medius and maximus strengthening of the contralateral limb.
- Exercises that promote muscle control of the residual limb depend on the patient's pain tolerance, the surgical procedure, and the healing response. Clear communication among the care team is warranted.
- Trunk stability will assist with mobility activities and provide the foundation for prosthetic control, sitting posture, standing posture, and gait training.
- As the level of the amputation moves proximally, gait speed decreases and oxygen consumption increases, effectively increasing the energy expenditure for ambulation.
- The PT is responsible for ensuring that the patient reaches his or her maximum activity level with or without prosthesis for at least the first 12 to 18 months after amputation.

Demographics[1,4]

- Susceptibility to transfemoral amputation depends on the etiology of the amputation.
- Most amputations occur secondary to ischemic disease.
- Patients with diabetes mellitus, complications of diabetes mellitus, or peripheral artery disease are at a much higher risk of lower-limb amputation.
- Young individuals without comorbidity are at greater risk of lower-limb amputation secondary to trauma, tumors, or congenital defects.

CLINICAL FINDINGS

SIGNS AND SYMPTOMS

- Swelling and edema around the amputation site
- Phantom limb pain
- Decreased ability to inspect the sound limb and/or residual limb for skin breakdown
- Hip flexion contracture
- Scar adhesion
- Decreased ROM at the hip
- Decreased muscle strength, power, and endurance in the LEs and trunk
- Poor static and dynamic balance (sitting)
- Poor static and dynamic balance (standing)
- Decreased ability to don/doff compression garments, prosthetic limb
- Gait dysfunction
- Decreased ability with transfers and bed mobility
- Decreased aerobic capacity

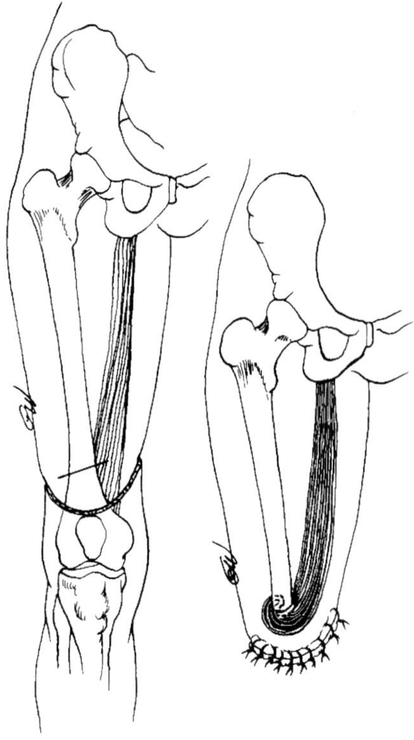

FIGURE 1-2 Transfemoral amputation with adductor myodesis. (From Skinner HB. *Current Diagnosis & Treatment in Orthopedics*, 4th ed. http://www.accessmedicine.com. Copyright © The McGraw-Hill Companies, Inc. All rights reserved.)

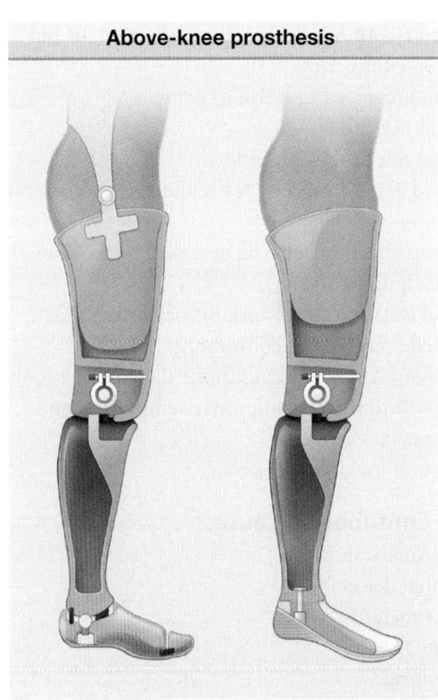

FIGURE 1-3 Above-knee prosthesis. Suction-socket prosthesis. (From Goldsmith LA, Katz SI, Gilchrest BA, et al., eds. *Fitzpatrick's Dermatology in General Medicine*, 8th ed. http://www.accessmedicine.com. Copyright © The McGraw-Hill Companies, Inc. All rights reserved.)

TABLE 1-1 Implications of Various Knee, Foot, and Ankle Designs

Component	Characteristic	Outcome
Knee joint (above-knee prosthesis)	TKA line position	The more posterior the joint to the TKA line, the more knee extension is maintained. This creates a more stable leg during stance, but is harder to initiate knee flexion for the swing phase.
	Internal rotation position	Too much internal rotation creates a lateral heel whip on heel raise.
	External rotation position	Too much external rotation creates a medial heel with heel raise.
	Friction	Less friction makes it easier to bend the knee at heel raise, but permits more terminal swing impact at heel strike.
Heel	Too soft	Forces knee into extension at heel strike (can be advantageous with an above-knee socket as it speeds knee extension up). Causes premature foot slap at heel strike.
	Too hard	Forces knee into flexion at heel strike (can be advantageous with below-knee socket with patellar-bearing prosthesis).
Toe break	Too posterior	Creates early knee flexion in midstance.
	Too anterior	Creates delayed knee flexion in midstance.
Ankle moment	Dorsiflexed	Encourages excessive knee flexion in early stance as amputee attempts to achieve foot flat.
	Plantarflexed	Encourages excessive knee extension throughout stance. Creates a "hill climbing" sensation of premature heel rise at the end of stance.
	Inverted or everted	Does not affect the knee. Prosthetic foot is matched to uninvolved foot.
Foot placement	Anterior	Creates a moment which increases knee extension.
	Posterior	Creates a moment which increases knee flexion.
	Lateral	Creates a valgus moment at the knee.
	Medial	Creates a varus moment at the knee.

Source: Dutton M: *McGraw-Hill's National Physical Therapy Examination*, 2nd ed. New York, NY: McGraw-Hill; 2012.

Functional Implications[2,3]

- Delayed ambulation because of the potential need for secondary wound healing
- Difficulty with ADLs and instrumental ADLs until fully healed and proficient with prosthesis
- Increased risk of hip flexion, hip abduction, or hip adduction contracture
- Potential presence of persistent pain
- Increased risk of falling
- Increased risk of skin breakdown
- Decreased aerobic capacity for household and community ambulation
- Home modifications may be necessary to accommodate adaptive equipment
- Potential isolation from work or social situations
- Decreased access to the community
- High risk of comorbid conditions such as pneumonia, deep vein thrombosis, pulmonary embolism, and cardiovascular events
- High risk of long-term disability

Possible Contributing Causes[4,5]

- African American race
- Congenital defect
- Diabetes mellitus
- Frostbite
- Increasing age
- Infection
- Loss of protective sensation
- Male gender
- Participation in high-risk occupation
- Peripheral neuropathy
- Peripheral vascular disease
- Previous amputation (toes, foot)
- Previous ulceration
- Trauma
- Tumor

Differential Diagnosis

- Since this is a surgical technique, there are no differential medical diagnoses.
- Differential diagnoses are associated with complications.

MEANS OF CONFIRMATION OR DIAGNOSIS[6]

Laboratory Tests

- C-reactive protein (CRP): This inflammatory marker is an indicator of infection
- Hemoglobin
- Absolute lymphocyte count
- Serum albumin level

Imaging

- Anteroposterior and lateral radiography of the involved extremity is obtained.
- CT scanning and MRI are performed for the patient's tumor workup or for osteomyelitis to ensure that the surgical margins are appropriate.
- Technetium-99m (^{99m}Tc) pyrophosphate bone scanning has been used to predict the need for amputation in persons with electrical burns and frostbite.
- Doppler ultrasonography is used to measure arterial pressure and to predict wound healing.

TABLE 1-2 Gait Deviations According to Prosthetic Causes and Amputee Causes

Deviation	Prosthetic Causes	Amputee Causes
Lateral bending of the trunk	Prosthesis may be too short Improperly shaped lateral wall High medial wall Prosthesis aligned in abduction	Poor balance Abduction contracture Improper training Short residual limb Weak hip abductors on prosthetic side Hypersensitive and painful residual limb
Abducted gait	Prosthesis may be too long High medial wall Improperly shaped lateral wall Prosthesis positioned in too much abduction Inadequate suspension Excessive knee friction	Abduction contracture Improper training Adductor roll Weak hip flexors and adductors Pain over lateral residual limb
Circumducted gait (this is different from above in that the foot returns to the proper position at heel strike)	Prosthesis may be too long Too much friction in the knee Socket is too small Excessive plantar flexion of prosthetic foot	Abduction contracture Improper training Weak hip flexors Lacks confidence to flex the knee Painful anterior distal stump Inability to initiate prosthetic knee flexion
Excessive knee flexion during stance	Socket set forward in relation to foot Foot set in excessive dorsiflexion Stiff heel Prosthesis too long	Knee flexion contracture Hip flexion contracture Pain anteriorly in residual limb Decrease in quadriceps strength Poor balance
Vaulting	Prosthesis may be too long Inadequate socket suspension Excessive alignment stability Foot in excess plantar flexion	Residual limb discomfort Improper training Fear of stubbing toe Short residual limb Painful hip/residual limb
Rotation of forefoot at heel strike (usually external rotation)	Excessive toe-out built-in Loose-fitting socket Inadequate suspension Rigid SACH heel cushion	Poor muscle control Improper training Weak medial rotators Short residual limb
Forward trunk flexion	Socket too big Poor suspension Knee instability	Hip flexion contracture Weak hip extensors Pain with ischial weight bearing Inability to initiate prosthetic knee flexion
Medial or lateral whip	Excessive rotation of the knee Tight socket fit Valgus in the prosthetic knee Improper alignment of toe break	Improper training Weak hip rotators Knee instability
Foot drag (one of the most common problems of swing phase)	Inadequate suspension of the prosthesis A prosthesis that is too long	Weakness in the hip abductors or ankle plantarflexors on the contralateral side
Uneven arm swing (characterized by the arm on the prosthetic side held close to the body during locomotion)	An improperly fitting socket may cause limb discomfort	Inadequate balance Fear and insecurity accompanied by uneven timing

Source: Dutton M: *McGraw-Hill's National Physical Therapy Examination*, 2nd ed. New York, NY: McGraw-Hill, 2012.

FINDINGS AND INTERPRETATION

- CRP: This inflammatory marker is an indicator of infection.
  - A level less than 1 mg/L indicates no infection; a level greater than 8 mg/L indicates significant infection.
- Hemoglobin: A measurement greater than 10 g/dL is required. Oxygenated blood is necessary for wound healing.
- Absolute lymphocyte count: Less than 1500 μ/L indicates immune deficiency and increases the possibility of infection.
- Serum albumin level: A level of 3.5 g/dL or less indicates malnutrition and a diminished ability to heal the wound.

TREATMENT

Medication

- Medications are directly related to the individual's comorbid conditions.
  - Care should be taken to avoid adverse drug reactions that are common in older adults taking multiple medications.

TABLE 1-3 Levels of Amputation

Level of Amputation	Description
Partial toe	Excision of any part of one or more toes
Toe disarticulation	Disarticulation of one or more toes at the metatarsophalangeal joint
Partial foot/ray resection	Resection of the third, fourth, fifth metatarsals, and digits
Tarsometatarsal (LisFranc) disarticulation	The disarticulation of all five metatarsals and the digits
Transmetatarsal (Chopart)	Amputation through the midsection of all metatarsals leaving only the calcaneus and talus
Syme's	Ankle disarticulation which may include removal of the malleoli and distal tibial/fibular flares to create a smooth bony distal end with the attachment of the heel pad to the distal end of the tibia
Long transtibial (below knee)	More than 50% of tibial length
Transtibial (below knee)	Between 20% and 50% of tibial length
Short transtibial (below knee)	Less than 20% of tibial length
Knee disarticulation	Amputation through the knee joint with shaping of the distal femur, squaring the condyles for an even weight-bearing surface. The knee disarticulation is most often used in children and young adults, but is nearly always avoided in the elderly and patients with ischemic disease. Several advantages of the knee disarticulation include: • A large distal end covered by skin and soft tissues that is naturally suited for weight bearing. • A long lever arm controlled by strong muscles. • Increased stability of the patient's prosthesis. A main disadvantage of the knee disarticulation is cosmetic—the patient's prosthetic leg will have a knee that extends far beyond his own knee in the sitting position.
Long transfemoral (above knee)	More than 60% of the femoral length
Transfemoral (above knee)	Between 35% and 60% of the femoral length
Short transfemoral (above knee)	Less than 35% of the femoral length
Hip disarticulation	An amputation through the hip joint capsule that removes the entire lower extremity, with closure of the remaining musculature over the exposed acetabulum. Hip disarticulation is generally performed as a result of failed vascular procedures following multiple lower-level amputations, or for massive trauma with crush injuries to the lower extremity.
Hemipelvectomy (HP)	Generally, the leg, hip joint, and half of the pelvis are removed, and the remaining gluteal muscles are brought around and attached to the oblique abdominal muscles. The most common reason for HP is a rare form of connective tissue cancer known as sarcoma. There are various types of sarcomas such as fibrosarcoma, osteosarcoma, and chondrosarcoma.
Hemicorporectomy	Involves removal of the bony pelvis below the L4–L5 level, both lower limbs, the external genitalia, the bladder, rectum, and anus. Necessary life functions are maintained in the upper torso. Hemicorporectomy has been performed for a variety of indications including locally invasive pelvic cancer without metastatic spread, benign spinal tumors, intractable decubitus ulcers with malignant change, paraplegia in association with intractable pelvic osteomyelitis and decubitus ulceration, and crushing trauma to the pelvis. Given the high mortality following this procedure, especially when performed for visceral malignancy, the indications for its use are very restrictive.

Source: Dutton M: *McGraw-Hill's National Physical Therapy Examination*, 2nd ed. New York, McGraw-Hill, 2012.

REFERRALS/ADMITTANCE

- The multidisciplinary care team includes:
  - Patient
  - Family
  - Surgeon
  - Physiatrist
  - Physical Therapist
  - Wound care specialist
  - Occupational therapist
  - Cognitive therapist
  - Prosthetist
  - Nurse
  - Social worker
  - Psychologist
  - Dietician
  - Peer support
  - Case manager

IMPAIRMENTS

- Edema
- Altered sensation
- Altered coordination
- Hip flexion contracture
- Hip abduction contracture
- Hip adduction contracture
- Phantom/residual limb pain
- ADL limitations (bed mobility, transfers)
- Decreased flexibility
- Altered muscle performance

TABLE 1-4 Energy Expenditure for Amputation

Amputation Level	Energy Above Baseline (%)	Speed (m/min)	Oxygen Cost (mL/kg/m)
Long transtibial	10	70	0.17
Average transtibial	25	60	0.20
Short transtibial	40	50	0.20
Bilateral transtibial	41	50	0.20
Transfemoral	65	40	0.28
Wheelchair	0–8	70	0.16

Source: Wu YJ, Chen SY, Lin MC, et al. Energy expenditure of wheeling and walking during prosthetic rehabilitation in a woman with bilateral transfemoral amputations. *Arch Phys Med Rehabil.* 2001;82:265–269.; Traugh GH, Corcoran PJ, Reyes RL. Energy expenditure of ambulation in patients with above-knee amputations. *Arch Phys Med Rehabil.* 1975;56:67–71.

- Decreased aerobic capacity
- Balance dysfunction
- Gait dysfunction
- Fall risk
- Fear of falling

TESTS AND MEASURES

- Self-report condition-specific measures of health-related quality of life[3]
  - Prosthetic evaluation questionnaire (PEQ): Modified version
  - Orthotic and Prosthetic Users Survey (OPUS)
- Self-report patient-specific measures of health-related quality of life[3]
  - Patient-specific functional scale (PSFS)
- Performance-based measures[7]
  - 2-minute walk test
  - 6-minute walk test
  - Timed up and go test
  - Amputee mobility predictor (AMP)
  - Participants in validation studies were allowed to walk with a mobility aid of their choice, stop and rest if needed, and resume walking if time allowed
- Age-specific measures[3]
  - American Academy of Orthopedic Surgeons/Pediatric Orthopedic Society of North America (AAOS/POSNA) Pediatric Questionnaire
  - Child Health Questionnaire (CHQ)
  - Functional Disability Inventory-Child Version (FDI-Child)
  - Functional Independence Measure for Children (WeeFIM)
  - Functional status questionnaire (for children)
  - Gross Motor Function Measure (GMFM)
- Pain, visual analog scale (VAS)
  - 24-hour pain
  - Worst average pain
  - Best average pain
- Functional independence measure
  - Bed mobility
  - Transfers
  - Locomotion
- Medication review (identify potential for adverse drug reactions)
- Cardiovascular integrity
  - Blood pressure at rest and after activity
  - Blood pressure in response to position changes
  - Heart rate at rest and after activity
  - Oxygen saturation
  - Presence of LE pulses on contralateral limb
- Skin Integrity
  - Scar
    - Approximation
    - Mobility/pliability
  - Associated skin assessment
    - Edema (linear girth measurements, palpation)
    - Color
    - Signs of infection
    - Mobility/turgor
    - Hair growth
    - Temperature
    - Sensation
    - Presence of skin breakdown
- Neurologic Examination
  - Sensation
    - Light touch
    - Pin prick
    - Protective sensation (5.07 monofilament at varied locations on the residual limb)
  - LE deep tendon reflexes at contralateral limb
  - Proprioception at the hip of residual limb
  - Kinesthetic awareness at the hip of residual limb
  - Coordination
- Trunk active and passive ROM
- Hip and knee active and passive ROM of residual limb
- Flexibility testing of residual limb
  - Hamstrings
  - Iliopsoas
  - Quadriceps
  - Iliotibial band
  - Abductors
  - Adductors
- Joint integrity of the spine
- Sacroiliac joint integrity
- Hip joint integrity of residual limb
  - Hip scour
  - Flexion abduction external rotation (FABER) test
  - Flexion adduction internal rotation (FAIR) test
  - Flexion adduction internal rotation impingement (FADDIR) test
- Residual limb strength
  - Functional strength testing
    - Five times sit-to-stand test
  - Manual muscle test (MMT)
    - Hamstrings
    - Quadriceps

    - Iliopsoas
    - Gluteus maximus
    - Gluteus medius
    - Gluteus minimus
    - Adductors
    - Abdominals
    - Multifidus
- LE contralateral limb strength
- Upper extremity (UE) Strength
  - Ability to assist with transfers and bed mobility
  - Ability to don/doff residual limb shrinkers and prosthesis
  - Ability to use assistive device
- Balance
  - Static and dynamic sitting
    - Sitting functional reach
  - Static single-leg standing (eyes open, eyes closed)
    - Residual limb with prosthesis
    - Contralateral LE
  - Dynamic standing (with prosthesis)
    - Berg Balance Scale
    - Functional gait assessment
- Gait assessment (with appropriate assistive device and/or prosthesis)
  - Observational analysis
  - Timed up and go test
  - Gait speed via the 10-m walk test
  - 2-minute walk test
  - 6-minute walk test
  - Dual task assessment
    - Timed up and go: Manual, cognitive
    - Walking while talking test: Simple, complex
- Fall risk
  - Dynamic gait assessment
  - Functional gait assessment
- Fear of falling
  - Activities-specific balance confidence scale
  - Falls Efficacy Scale

INTERVENTIONS

- Preoperative care[2,3]
  - Level selection based on a thorough assessment by medical and surgical teams
  - Education
  - Emotional support
  - PT
  - Conditioning
  - Nutritional support
  - Pain management
- Postoperative care
  - Wound healing
    - It is not uncommon for an individual with a lower-limb amputation to require secondary healing with active wound care, given the high likelihood of comorbid conditions that may have led to the amputation
    - Categories of wound healing
      - I: Primary: Heals without open areas, infection, or wound complications
      - II: Secondary: Small open areas that can be managed with dressing strategies and wound care
      - III: Requires minor surgical revision of skin and subcutaneous tissue
      - IV: Requires major surgical revision of muscle or bone; original amputation level is maintained
      - V: Requires revision to a higher amputation level
    - Weight-bearing activities
      - Dependent upon clear communication among the care team
      - Weight-bearing activities with a prosthetic in the presence of a wound may help to control edema and facilitate wound healing
  - Scar management
    - Soft tissue mobilization
  - Limb volume management[2,3]
    - Soft dressings
      - Soft gauze alone (not recommended)
      - Soft gauze with adjunctive mechanism to obtain limb compression
        - ACE wrap
        - Tubular compressive gauze
        - Traditional shrinker socks
        - Gel liners
        - Unna paste wraps
    - Nonremovable rigid dressings without an immediate prosthetic attachment
      - Custom-molded thigh-high device (fiberglass, plaster, combination)
        - Preformed brim
        - Soft or rigid spica component around the waist
    - Nonremovable rigid dressings with an immediate postoperative prosthesis (IPOP)
      - Traditional thigh-level cast (fiberglass, plaster, or combination)
        - Pylon
        - Foot attachment
        - Proximal socket style brim
        - Soft or rigid spica component around the waist
      - Nonremovable rigid dressings result in significantly less edema compared with soft gauze dressings
      - Nonremovable rigid dressings result in significantly accelerated rehabilitation times compared with soft gauze dressings
    - Removable rigid plaster dressings
      - Made of casting material (fiberglass, plaster, or combination)
      - Can be used with or without a prosthetic attachment
        - Allows for easy access to inspect the incision or manage small wounds after amputation
    - Prefabricated postoperative prosthetic systems
      - Designed for early management and prosthetic fitting of the limb after surgery
      - Easily removed and replaced for wound evaluation
      - Prefabricated postoperative prosthetic systems were found to have significantly fewer postoperative complications compared with soft gauze dressings
      - Prefabricated postoperative prosthetic systems lead to fewer higher-level revisions compared with soft gauze dressings
  - Contracture prevention
    - Positioning
    - ROM
    - Flexibility
    - Joint mobilization
  - Pain management[2,3]
    - Desensitization techniques

        - Distal-end residual limb loading
        - Weight-bearing activities
    - Joint integrity
        - Hip
        - Lumbar spine
    - Bed mobility training
        - Without prosthesis
        - With prosthesis
    - Transfer training (including floor-to-chair transfers)
        - Without prosthesis
        - With prosthesis
    - Contralateral lower-limb preservation
        - Use of appropriate liners with and without the prosthesis
        - Foot inspections prior to and after ambulation (in those with altered sensation)
    - Strengthening
        - Trunk and core control
        - UE
        - Progressive resistance exercise bilaterally
        - Muscular endurance training bilaterally
    - Aerobic conditioning
    - Wheelchair management (when appropriate)
    - Gait training[2,3]
        - Nonpedal: Wheelchair ambulation
        - Unipedal: Contralateral limb with assistive device
        - Bipedal: Prosthetic with and/or without assistive device
    - Balance training
    - Fall prevention
    - Proper lifting and body mechanics
    - Pressure ulcer prevention (when altered sensation is present)
    - Lifestyle education
        - Habitual home exercise program
        - Activity level
        - Nutritional intake
        - Promotion of health and wellness
        - Participation in sports

FUNCTIONAL GOALS

- Patient will verbalize signs and symptoms of abnormal pressures and signs of infection of residual limb to prevent future injury/complication at residual limb.
- Patient will demonstrate the ability to independently manage residual limb shape with the use of compression garments to prevent complications and so that ambulation with prosthesis is feasible.
- Patient will independently perform residual limb and contralateral foot assessment before and after weight-bearing exercise to prevent future injury/complications.
- Patient will demonstrate neutral knee positioning while sitting without prosthesis and when sleeping for prevention of knee flexion contracture at residual limb so that ambulation with prosthesis is feasible.
- Patient will demonstrate ability to achieve supine, side-lying, and prone positions with and without prosthesis for independence with bed mobility and to demonstrate ability to manage prosthesis in the event of a fall.
- Patient will demonstrate safe sit-to-stand commode transfer with and without prosthesis using appropriate assistive device.
- Patient will perform sit-to-stand with prosthesis 10 times from average height surface without UE assistance to demonstrate independence with chair transfers.
- Patient will demonstrate ability to independently don/doff residual limb for optimal positioning of residual limb in prosthesis and for safe ambulation.
- Patient will demonstrate safe dynamic standing with prosthesis for at least 20 minutes for meal preparation.
- Patient will demonstrate the ability to ambulate household distances over even surfaces with prosthesis and appropriate assistive device with safety and independence.
- Patient will demonstrate the ability to ambulate over uneven surfaces such as the transition from tile to carpet or up and down a ramp with prosthesis and appropriate assistive device with safety and independence.
- Patient will demonstrate the ability to ascend/descend a standard height curb with prosthesis and appropriate assistive device.
- Patient will demonstrate a gait speed of at least 1 m/s which indicates increasing health status.[8]

PROGNOSIS

- Good for individuals who have the support of a multidisciplinary care team throughout the recovery process.
- Dependent on several contextual factors such as premorbid status, etiology, postsurgical complications, family support, motivational status, and ability to obtain early and on-going rehabilitation.
- Functional status among amputees can range from those who utilize wheelchair ambulation as the primary means of mobility to high-level competitive athletes.

PATIENT RESOURCES

- Disabled Sports USA. http://www.dsusa.org. Accessed March 17, 2013.
- National Amputation Foundation. http://www.nationalamputation.org. Accessed March 17, 2013.
- United States Paralympics. http://www.usparalympics.org. Accessed March 17, 2013.

REFERENCES

1. Gottschalk F. Chapter 20A: Transfemoral amputation: surgical procedures. In: *Atlas of Limb Prosthetics: Surgical, Prosthetic, and Rehabilitation Principles*. http://www.oandplibrary.org/alp/chap20-01.asp. Accessed March 17, 2013.
2. Smith DG, McFarland LV, Sangeorzan BJ, Reiber GE, Czerniecki JM. Postoperative dressing and management strategies for transtibial amputation: a critical review. *J Rehabil Res Dev*. 2003;40(3):213-224.
3. Overview: The Clinical Standards of Practice (CSOP) consensus conference. *JPO*. 2004;16(3S):2-5. http://www.oandp.org/jpo/library/2004_03S_002.asp. Accessed March 17, 2013.
4. Deshpande AD, Harris-Hayes M, Schootman M. Epidemiology of diabetes and diabetes-related complications. *Phys Ther*. 2008;88(11):1254-1264. doi: 10.2522/ptj.20080020.
5. Birke JA, Patout CA, Foto JG. Factors associated with ulceration and amputation in the neuropathic foot. *JOSPT*. 2000;30(2):91-97.
6. Ertl J, Choun J, Ertl W, et al. Amputations of the lower extremity: workup. *Medscape*. http://emedicine.medscape.com/article/1232102-workup#a0719. Accessed March 17, 2013.
7. Resnik L, Borgia M. Reliability of outcome measures for people with lower limb amputations: distinguishing true change from statistical error. *Phys Ther*. 2011;91(4):555-565.

8. Studenski S, Perera S, Wallace D, et al. Physical performance measures in the clinical setting. *J Am Geriatr Soc.* 2003;51(3):314-322. doi: 10.1046/j.1532-5415.2003.51104.x.

ADDITIONAL REFERENCES

- Edelstein JE. Prosthetics. In: O'Sullivan SB, Schmitz TJ, eds. *Physical Rehabilitation.* 5th ed. Philadelphia, PA: FA Davis; 2007:1251-1286.
- Gailey RS. Orthotics in rehabilitation. In: Prentice WE, Voight ML, eds. *Techniques in Musculoskeletal Rehabilitation*. New York, NY: McGraw-Hill; 2001:325-346.
- Pattern 4J: Impaired motor function, muscle performance, range of motion, gait, locomotion, and balance associated with amputation. In: *Guide to Physical Therapist Practice*. 2nd ed. Alexandria, VA: American Physical Therapy Association; 2001. Revised 2003.

2 TRANSTIBIAL AMPUTATION

Jacqueline Osborne, DPT, PT, GCS, CEEAA

CONDITION/DISORDER SYNONYM

- Below-knee amputation

ICD-9-CM CODE

- V49.75 Below-knee amputation status

ICD-10-CM CODE

- Z89.519 Acquired absence of unspecified leg below knee

PREFERRED PRACTICE PATTERN

- 4J: Impaired Motor Function, Muscle Performance, Range of Motion, Gait, Locomotion, and Balance Associated With Amputation

PATIENT PRESENTATION

Your patient is a 72-year-old male with a left transtibial amputation. His surgery was done 3 days before. He has an 18-year history of insulin-dependent diabetes mellitus (IDDM). He was diagnosed with Chronic Obstructive Pulmonary Disorder (COPD) 2 years ago. He presents in a semi-recumbent position in the hospital bed with his left limb supported on three pillows. His limb is wrapped, but you can see drainage on the outer layer of the bandage distal to the knee. He is receiving IV antibiotics and pain medication. He is also receiving supplemental oxygen via a nasal cannula.

KEY FEATURES

Description

- Result of ultimate loss of tissue perfusion from the surrounding circulation at any level distal to the tibial plateau

Essentials of Diagnosis

- A surgeon makes diagnosis after surgery.
- A transtibial amputation is an amputation of the lower limb between the ankle and the knee where the knee joint is retained.
  - The superior tibiofibular joint is preserved; however, the tibia and the fibula are no longer joined distally.
- A transtibial amputation is made between the area of the tibial plateau and the junction of the middle and lower third of the tibia.
  - Amputations distal to the lower third of the leg are avoided because of the lack of soft tissue to pad the distal end of the residual limb.
- An amputation that preserves the femur and the patella is called a knee disarticulation.
- An amputation at the level of the talocrural joint that leaves the distal end of tibia and fibula intact is called an ankle disarticulation.

General Considerations[1,2]

- Loss of a limb below the knee results in widespread impairments in body structure and function, as well as significant activity limitations and participation restrictions that will ultimately affect the individual's participation in family and home life as well as reintegration into society.
- Emotional support and education must infiltrate postoperative rehabilitation beginning on postoperative day 1 to assist the individual with repossessing life roles.

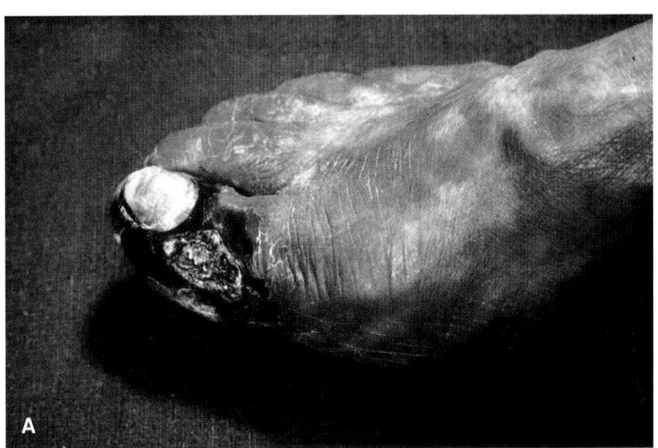

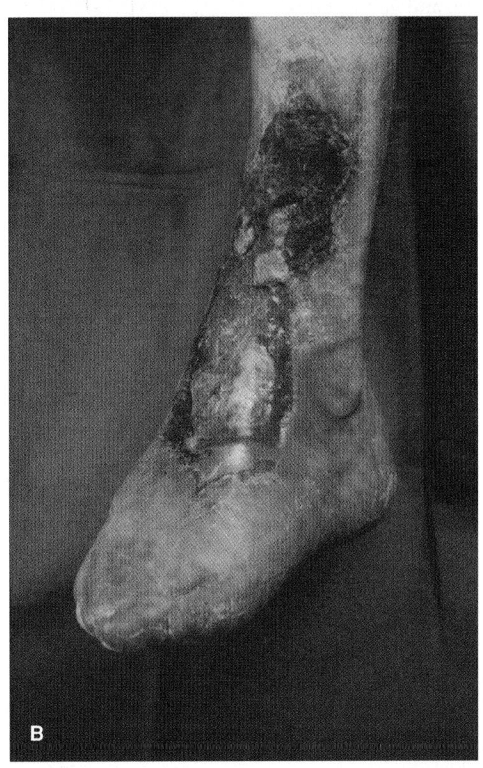

FIGURE 2-1 Patient with vasculitis resulting in ischemia (**A**) that required amputation (**B–C**). This recurred on the amputation stump (**D–E**) but fortunately responded to systemic therapy. (From Goldsmith LA, Katz SI, Gilchrest BA, et al., eds. *Fitzpatrick's Dermatology in General Medicine*, 8th ed. http://www.accessmedicine.com. Copyright © The McGraw-Hill Companies, Inc. All rights reserved.) *(continued)*

CHAPTER 2

- The total recovery period is consistently 12 to 18 months and includes activity recovery, reintegration, prosthetic training, and prosthetic management.
- The acute hospital stay ranges from 5 to 14 days, and the postacute hospital stay could range from 2 to 8 weeks.
  - This period includes surgery recovery, wound healing, early rehabilitation, and determination of prosthetic readiness.
- The immediate recovery stage begins with the healing of the wound and could extend up to 6 months.
  - This stage ends with stabilization of limb volume after accommodating to prosthetic use with ambulation.
- The last stage of recovery is widely variable.
  - During this time, limb volumes continue to stabilize but are no longer rapidly changing.
  - Prosthetic adjustments can be made as the limb continues to stabilize.
  - When the prosthesis is worn full time for a period of at least 6 months and the limb volume has stabilized to a point that socket fit remains relatively consistent for at least 2 to 3 weeks, a definitive prosthesis may be indicated.
  - Higher-level functional training and social reintegration mark the end of this stage.
- Promoting independence can start as early as postoperative day 1 with quadriceps, and gluteus medius and maximus strengthening of the contralateral limb.
- Exercises that promote muscle control of the residual limb depend on the patient's pain tolerance, the surgical procedure, and the healing response. Clear communication among the care team is warranted.
- Trunk stability will assist with mobility activities and provide the foundation for prosthetic control, sitting posture, standing posture, and gait training.
- The PT is responsible for ensuring that the patient reaches their maximum activity level with or without a prosthesis for at least the first 12 to 18 months after amputation.

Demographics[3,4]

- Susceptibility to transtibial amputation depends on the etiology of the amputation.
- Most amputations occur secondary to ischemic disease.
- Patients with diabetes mellitus, complications of diabetes mellitus, or peripheral artery disease are at a much higher risk of lower-limb amputation.
- Amputations can occur in older and younger individuals secondary to trauma, tumors, infection, or congenital defects.

CLINICAL FINDINGS

SIGNS AND SYMPTOMS

- Swelling and edema around the amputation site
- Phantom limb pain
- Decreased ability to inspect the sound limb and/or residual limb for skin breakdown
- Hip flexion and knee flexion contracture
- Scar adhesion
- Decreased ROM at the hip and knee
- Decreased muscle strength, power, and endurance in the lower extremities (LEs) and trunk
- Poor static and dynamic balance (sitting)
- Poor static and dynamic balance (standing)
- Decreased ability to don/doff compression garments, prosthetic limb
- Gait dysfunction
- Decreased ability with transfers and bed mobility
- Decreased aerobic capacity

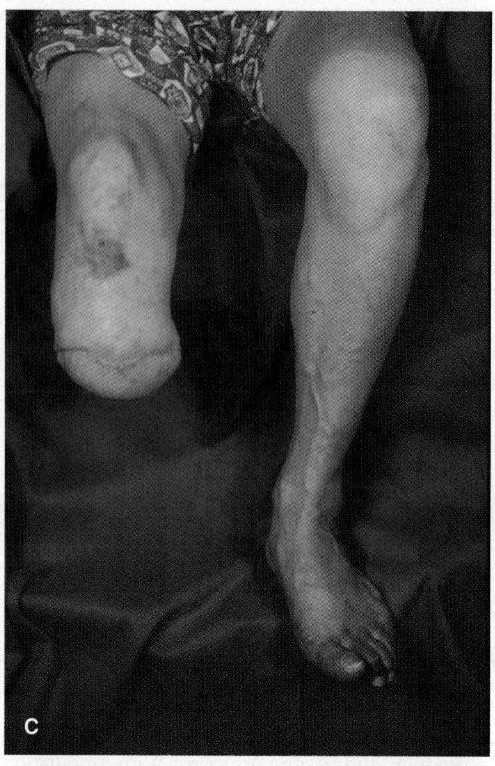

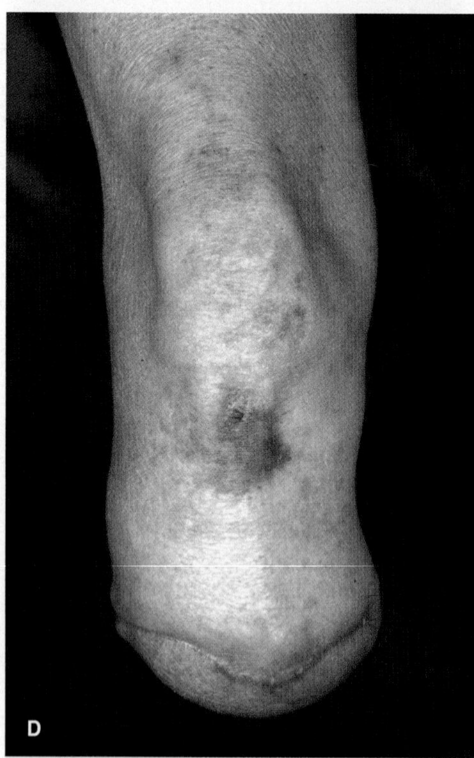

FIGURE 2-1 *(Continued)*

Functional Implications[1,2]

- Delayed ambulation because of the potential need for secondary wound healing
- Difficulty with basic ADLs and instrumental ADLs until fully healed and proficient with prosthesis
- Increased risk of knee flexion or hip flexion contracture
- Potential presence of persistent pain
- Increased risk of falling
- Increased risk of skin breakdown
- Decreased aerobic capacity for household and community ambulation
- Home modifications may be necessary to accommodate adaptive equipment
- Potential isolation from work or social situations
- Decreased access to the community
- High risk of comorbid conditions such as pneumonia, deep vein thrombosis, pulmonary embolism, and cardiovascular events
- High risk of long-term disability

Possible Contributing Causes[3,5]

- Increasing age
- Male gender
- African American race
- Diabetes mellitus
- Previous ulceration
- Previous amputation (toes, foot)
- Peripheral vascular disease
- Peripheral neuropathy
- Loss of protective sensation
- Participation in high-risk occupation
- Infection
- Tumor
- Trauma
- Frostbite
- Congenital defect

Differential Diagnosis

- Since this is a surgical technique, there are no differential medical diagnoses.
- Differential diagnoses are associated with complications.

MEANS OF CONFIRMATION OR DIAGNOSIS[6]

Laboratory Tests

- C-reactive protein (CRP)
- Hemoglobin
- Absolute lymphocyte count
- Serum albumin level

Imaging

- Anteroposterior and lateral radiography of the involved extremity is obtained.
- CT scanning and MRI are performed for the patient's tumor workup or for osteomyelitis to ensure that the surgical margins are appropriate.
- Technetium-99m (^{99m}Tc) pyrophosphate bone scanning has been used to predict the need for amputation in persons with electrical burns and frostbite.
- Doppler ultrasonography is used to measure arterial pressure and to predict wound healing.

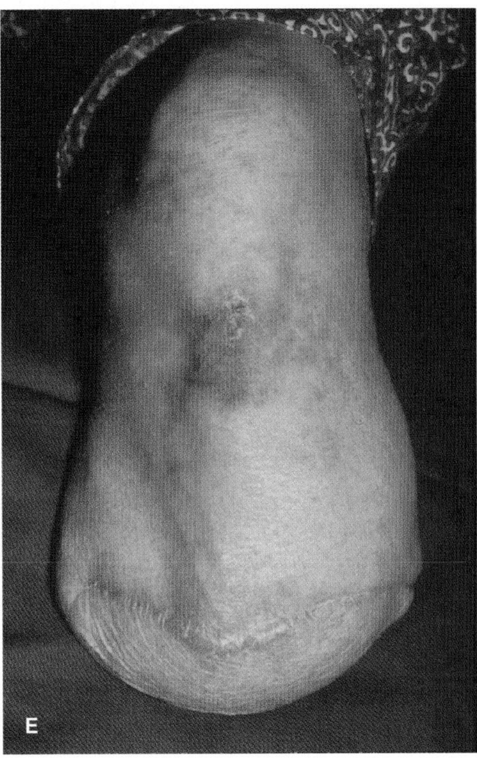

FIGURE 2-1 *(Continued)*

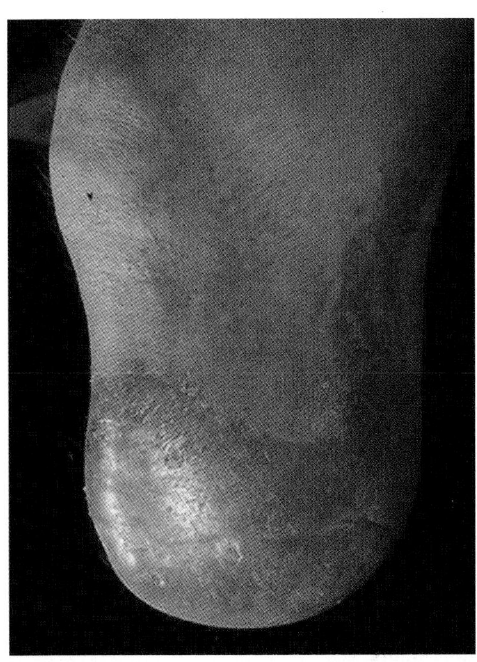

FIGURE 2-2 Atopic eczema in a patient with a below-knee prosthesis. With this modular appliance, the socket shown is placed over the stump and the whole then fitted into the prosthetic leg. (From Goldsmith LA, Katz SI, Gilchrest BA, et al., eds. *Fitzpatrick's Dermatology in General Medicine*, 8th ed. http://www.accessmedicine.com.)

FINDINGS AND INTERPRETATION

- CRP: This inflammatory marker is an indicator of infection.
  - A level less than 1 mg/L indicates no infection; a level greater than 8 mg/L indicates significant infection.
- Hemoglobin: A measurement greater than 10 g/dL is required. Oxygenated blood is necessary for wound healing.
- Absolute lymphocyte count: Less than 1500 μ/L indicates immune deficiency and increases the possibility of infection.
- Serum albumin level: A level of 3.5 g/dL or less indicates malnutrition and a diminished ability to heal the wound.

TREATMENT

Medication

- Medications are directly related to the individual's comorbid conditions.
  - Care should be taken to avoid adverse drug reactions, which are common in older adults taking multiple medications.

REFERRALS/ADMITTANCE

- The multidisciplinary care team includes:
  - Patient
  - Family
  - Surgeon
  - Physiatrist
  - PT
  - Wound care specialist
  - Occupational therapist
  - Cognitive therapist
  - Prosthetist
  - Nurse
  - Social worker
  - Psychologist
  - Dietician
  - Peer support
  - Case manger
  - Physical therapist

IMPAIRMENTS

- Edema
- Altered sensation
- Altered coordination
- Knee flexion contracture
- Phantom/residual limb pain
- ADL limitations (bed mobility, transfers)
- Decreased flexibility
- Altered muscle performance
- Decreased aerobic capacity
- Balance dysfunction
- Gait dysfunction
- Fall risk
- Fear of falling

TESTS AND MEASURES

- Self-report condition-specific measures of health-related quality of life[2]
  - Prosthetic evaluation questionnaire (PEQ): Modified version
  - Orthotic and Prosthetic Users Survey (OPUS)
- Self-report patient-specific measures of health-related quality of life[2]
  - Patient-specific functional scale (PSFS)
- Performance-based measures[7]
  - 2-minute walk test
  - 6-minute walk test
  - Timed up and go test
  - Amputee mobility predictor (AMP)
  - Participants in validation studies were allowed to walk with a mobility aid of their choice, stop and rest if needed, and resume walking if time allowed

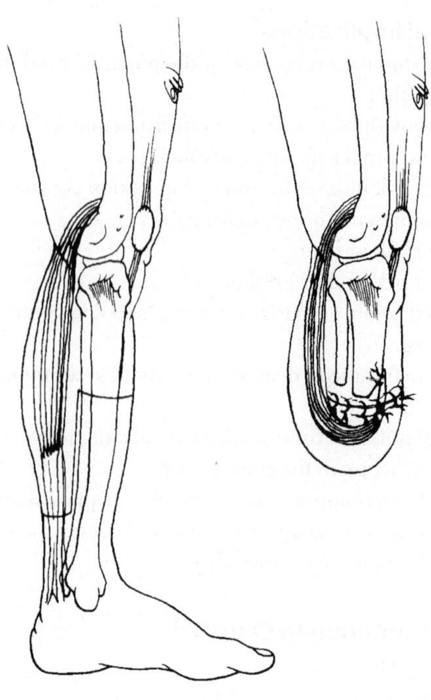

FIGURE 2-3 Transtibial amputation with long posterior flap technique. (From Skinner HB. *Current Diagnosis & Treatment in Orthopedics*, 4th ed. http://www.accessmedicine.com. Copyright © The McGraw-Hill Companies, Inc. All rights reserved.)

- Age-specific measures[2]
  - American Academy of Orthopedic Surgeons/Pediatric Orthopedic Society of North America (AAOS/POSNA) Pediatric Questionnaire
  - Child Health Questionnaire (CHQ)
  - Functional Disability Inventory-Child Version (FDI-Child)
  - Functional Independence Measure for Children (WeeFIM)

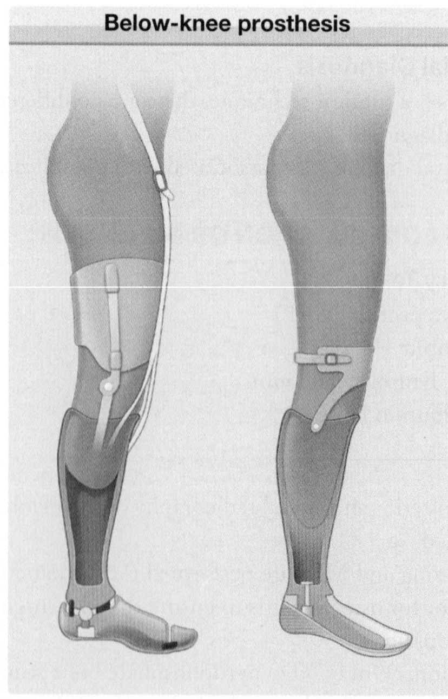

FIGURE 2-4 Below-knee prosthesis. Patellar tendon-bearing cuff suspension. (From Goldsmith LA, Katz SI, Gilchrest BA, et al., eds. *Fitzpatrick's Dermatology in General Medicine*, 8th ed. http://www.accessmedicine.com. Copyright © The McGraw-Hill Companies, Inc. All rights reserved.)

TABLE 2-1 Gait Analysis of the Below-Knee Amputee

Problem	Cause	Solution
Delayed, abrupt, and limited knee flexion after initial contact	Heel wedge is too soft; the foot is too far anterior	Stiffen the heel wedge; move the foot posterior
Toe stays off floor after initial contact	Heel wedge is too stiff; the foot is too anterior; there is too much dorsiflexion	Soften heel wedge; move the foot posterior; plantarflex the foot
Extended knee throughout stance phase	There is too much plantar flexion	Dorsiflex the foot
"Hillclimbing" sensation toward end of stance phase	The foot is too far anterior; there is too much plantar flexion	Move the foot posterior; dorsiflex the foot
Knee is too forcefully and rapidly flexed after initial contact; high pressure against anterior-distal tibia at initial contact and/or prolonged discomfort at this point	Heel wedge is too stiff; the foot is too dorsiflexed	Soften the heel; move the foot anterior; plantarflex the foot
Hip level, but prosthesis appears short	The foot is too far posterior; the foot is too dorsiflexed	Move the foot anterior; plantarflex the foot
Toe off floor as patient stands or knee flexed too much	The foot is too dorsiflexed	Plantarflex the foot
Uneven heel rise	Knee joint may have insufficient friction; there may be an inadequate extension aid	Modify accordingly
The foot slaps	Plantar flexion resistance is usually too soft	Increase plantar flexion resistance

Source: Dutton M: *McGraw-Hill's National Physical Therapy Examination*, 2nd ed. New York, NY: McGraw-Hill; 2012.

- Functional Independence Measure (FIM™)
- Functional status questionnaire (for children)
- Gross Motor Function Measure (GMFM)

- Pain, visual analog scale (VAS)
  - 24-hour pain
  - Worst average pain
  - Best average pain
- FIM
  - Bed mobility
  - Transfers
  - Locomotion
- Medication review (identify potential for adverse drug reactions)
- Cardiovascular integrity
  - Blood pressure at rest and after activity
  - Blood pressure in response to position changes
  - Heart rate at rest and after activity
  - Oxygen saturation
  - Presence of popliteal pulse on residual limb and LE pulses on contralateral limb
- Skin integrity
  - Scar
    - Approximation
    - Mobility/pliability
  - Associated skin assessment
    - Edema (linear girth measurements, palpation)
    - Color
    - Signs of infection
    - Mobility/turgor
    - Hair growth
    - Temperature
    - Sensation
    - Presence of skin breakdown
- Neurologic examination
  - Sensation
    - Light touch
    - Pin prick
    - Protective sensation (5.07 monofilament at varied locations on the residual limb)
  - Patellar tendon reflex bilaterally
  - Proprioception at the knee and hip of residual limb
  - Kinesthetic awareness at the knee and hip of residual limb
  - Coordination
- Trunk active and passive ROM
- Hip and knee active and passive ROM of residual limb
- Flexibility testing of residual limb
  - 90/90 hamstring length
  - Thomas test
  - Ober's test
  - Ely's test
  - Straight leg raise test
- Joint integrity of the spine
- Sacroiliac joint integrity
- Hip joint integrity of the residual limb
  - Hip scour test
  - Flexion abduction external rotation (FABER) test
  - Flexion adduction internal rotation (FAIR) test
  - Flexion adduction internal rotation impingement (FADDIR) test
- Knee joint integrity of the residual limb
  - Varus/valgus stress tests
  - Lachman's test
  - Patellar mobility
- Residual limb strength
  - Functional strength testing
    - Five times sit-to-stand test
  - Manual muscle test (MMT)
    - Hamstrings
    - Quadriceps
    - Sartorius

    - Iliopsoas
    - Gluteus maximus
    - Gluteus medius
    - Gluteus minimus
    - Adductors
    - Abdominals
    - Multifidus
- LE contralateral limb strength
- Upper Extremity (UE) strength
  - Ability to assist with transfers and bed mobility
  - Ability to don/doff residual limb shrinkers and prosthesis
  - Ability to use assistive device
- Balance
  - Static and dynamic sitting
    - Sitting functional reach
  - Static single-leg standing (eyes open, eyes closed)
    - Residual limb with prosthesis
    - Contralateral LE
  - Dynamic standing (with prosthesis)
    - Berg Balance Scale
    - Gait Assessment Rating Score
    - Rancho Los Amigo observational gait analysis
    - Multi-directional reach test (MDRT)
- Gait assessment (with appropriate assistive device and/or prosthesis)
  - Observational analysis
  - Timed up and go test
  - Gait speed via the 10-m walk test
  - 2-minute walk test
  - 6-minute walk test
  - Dual task assessment
    - Timed up and go: Manual, cognitive
    - Walking while talking test: Simple, complex
- Fall risk
  - Dynamic gait assessment
  - Functional gait assessment
- Fear of falling
  - Activity-specific balance confidence scale
  - Falls Efficacy Scale

INTERVENTIONS

- Preoperative care[1,2]
  - Level selection based on a thorough assessment by medical and surgical teams
  - Education
  - Emotional support
  - PT
  - Conditioning
  - Nutritional support
  - Pain management
- Postoperative care
  - Wound healing[1,2]
  - It is not uncommon for an individual with a lower-limb amputation to require secondary healing with active wound care, given the high likelihood of comorbid conditions that may have led to the amputation
  - Categories of wound healing
    - I Primary: Heals without open areas, infection, or wound complications
    - II Secondary: Small open areas that can be managed with dressing strategies and wound care
    - III: Requires minor surgical revision of skin and subcutaneous tissue
    - IV: Requires major surgical revision of muscle or bone; original amputation level is maintained
    - V: Requires revision to a higher amputation level
  - Dependent upon clear communication within the care team
  - Weight-bearing activities with a prosthetic in the presence of a wound may help to control edema and facilitate wound healing
- Scar management
  - Soft tissue mobilization
- Limb volume management[1,2]
  - Soft dressings
    - Soft gauze alone (not recommended)
    - Soft gauze with adjunctive mechanism to obtain limb compression
      - ACE wrap
      - Tubular compressive gauze
      - Traditional shrinker socks
      - Gel liners
      - Unna paste wraps
    - Supplemental devices (no evidence to support effectiveness for preventing knee flexion contractures or allowing limb maturation)
      - Knee immobilizers
      - Low-temperature thermoplastic protective shells
  - Nonremovable rigid dressings without an immediate prosthetic attachment
    - Custom molded thigh-high device (fiberglass, plaster, or combination)
  - Nonremovable rigid dressings with an immediate postoperative prosthesis (IPOP)
    - Traditional thigh-level cast (fiberglass, plaster, combination)
      - Pylon
      - Foot attachment
    - Nonremovable rigid dressings result in significantly less edema compared with soft gauze dressings
    - Nonremovable rigid dressings result in significantly accelerated rehabilitation times compared with soft gauze dressings
  - Removable rigid plaster dressings
    - Made of casting material (fiberglass, plaster, or combination)
    - Can be used with or without a prosthetic attachment
    - Allows for easy access to inspect the incision or manage small wounds after amputation
  - Prefabricated postoperative prosthetic systems
    - Designed for early management and prosthetic fitting of the limb after surgery
    - Easily removed and replaced for wound evaluation
    - Prefabricated postoperative prosthetic systems were found to have significantly fewer postoperative complications compared with soft gauze dressings
    - Prefabricated postoperative prosthetic systems lead to fewer higher-level revisions compared with soft gauze dressings
- Contracture prevention
  - Positioning
  - Range of motion (ROM)
  - Flexibility
  - Joint mobilization
- Pain management[1,2]
  - Desensitization techniques
  - Distal-end residual limb loading
  - Weight-bearing activities

- Joint integrity
  - Hip
  - Knee
  - Lumbar spine
- Bed mobility training
  - Without prosthesis
  - With prosthesis
- Transfer training (including floor-to-chair transfers)
  - Without prosthesis
  - With prosthesis
- Contralateral lower-limb preservation
  - Use of appropriate liners with and without the prosthesis
  - Foot inspections before and after ambulation (in those with altered sensation)
- Strengthening
  - Trunk and core control
  - UE
  - Progressive resistance exercise bilaterally
  - Muscular endurance training bilaterally
  - Hip abduction strengthening
- Aerobic conditioning
- Wheelchair management (when appropriate)
- Gait training[1,2]
  - Nonpedal: Wheelchair ambulation
  - Unipedal: Contralateral limb with assistive device
  - Bipedal: Prosthetic with and/or without assistive device
- Balance training
- Fall prevention
- Proper lifting and body mechanics
- Pressure ulcer prevention (when altered sensation is present)
- Lifestyle education
  - Habitual home exercise program
  - Activity level
  - Nutritional intake
  - Promotion of health and wellness
  - Participation in sports

FUNCTIONAL GOALS

- Patient will verbalize signs and symptoms of abnormal pressures and signs of infection of residual limb to prevent future injury/complication at residual limb.
- Patient will demonstrate the ability to independently manage residual limb shape with the use of compression garments to prevent complications and so that ambulation with prosthesis is feasible.
- Patient will independently perform residual limb and contralateral foot assessment before and after weight-bearing exercise to prevent future injury/complications.
- Patient will demonstrate neutral knee positioning while sitting without prosthesis and when sleeping for prevention of knee flexion contracture at residual limb, so that ambulation with prosthesis is feasible.
- Patient will demonstrate ability to achieve supine, side-lying, and prone positions with and without prosthesis for independence with bed mobility and to demonstrate ability to manage prosthesis in the event of a fall.
- Patient will demonstrate safe sit-to-stand commode transfer with and without prosthesis using appropriate assistive device.
- Patient will perform sit-to-stand with prosthesis 10 times from average height surface without UE assistance to demonstrate independence with chair transfers.
- Patient will demonstrate ability to independently don/doff residual limb for optimal positioning of residual limb in prosthesis and for safe ambulation.
- Patient will demonstrate safe dynamic standing with prosthesis for at least 20 minutes for meal preparation.
- Patient will demonstrate the ability to ambulate household distances over even surfaces with prosthesis and appropriate assistive device with safety and independence.
- Patient will demonstrate the ability to ambulate over uneven surfaces such as the transition from tile to carpet or up and down a ramp with prosthesis and appropriate assistive device with safety and independence.
- Patient will demonstrate the ability to ascend/descend a standard height curb with prosthesis and appropriate assistive device.
- Patient will demonstrate a gait speed of at least 1 m/s which indicates increasing health status.[8]

PROGNOSIS

- Good for individuals who have the support of a multidisciplinary care team throughout the recovery process.
- Dependent on several contextual factors such as premorbid status, etiology, postsurgical complications, family support, motivational status, and ability to obtain early and on-going rehabilitation.
- Functional status among amputees can range from those who utilize wheelchair ambulation as the primary means of mobility to high-level competitive athletes.

PATIENT RESOURCES

- Disabled Sports USA. http://www.dsusa.org. Accessed March 17, 2013.
- National Amputation Foundation. http://www.nationalamputation.org. Accessed March 17, 2013.
- United States Paralympics. http://www.usparalympics.org. Accessed March 17, 2013.

REFERENCES

1. Smith DG, McFarland LV, Sangeorzan BJ, Reiber GE, Czerniecki JM. Postoperative dressing and management strategies for transtibial amputation: a critical review. *J Rehabil Res Dev.* 2003;40(3):213-224.
2. Overview: The Clinical Standards of Practice (CSOP) consensus conference. *JPO.* 2004;16(3S):2-5. http://www.oandp.org/jpo/library/2004_03S_002.asp. Accessed March 13, 2013.
3. Deshpande AD, Harris-Hayes M, Schootman M. Epidemiology of diabetes and diabetes-related complications. *Phys Ther.* 2008;88(11):1254-1264. doi: 10.2522/ptj.20080020.
4. Lipsky BA, Berendt AR, Deery HG, et al. Diagnosis and treatment of diabetic foot infections. *Clin Infect Dis.* 2004;39(7):885-910. doi: 10.1086/424846.
5. Birke JA, Patout CA, Foto JG. Factors associated with ulceration and amputation in the neuropathic foot. *JOSPT.* 2000;30(2):91-97.
6. Ertl J, Choun J, Ertl W, et al. Amputations of the lower extremity: workup. *Medscape.* http://emedicine.medscape.com/article/1232102-workup#a0719. Accessed March 28, 2012.
7. Resnik L, Borgia M. Reliability of outcome measures for people with lower limb amputations: distinguishing true change from statistical error. *Phys Ther.* 2011;91(4):555-65. doi: 10.2522/ptj.20100287.

8. Studenski S, Perera S, Wallace D, et al. Physical performance measures in the clinical setting. *J Am Geriatr Soc*. 2003; 51(3):314-322. doi: 10.1046/j.1532-5415.2003.51104.x.

ADDITIONAL REFERENCES

- Components of the Gait Assessment Rating Score (GARS). University of Missouri. http://geriatrictoolkit.missouri.edu/gars/index.htm. Accessed March 23, 2014.
- Dutton M. *Orthopaedic Examination, Evaluation, and Intervention*. 2nd ed. New York, NY: McGraw-Hill; 2008. http://www.accessphysiotherapy.com/resource/612. Accessed March 17, 2013.
- Dutton M. Chapter 8. The hip joint. In: Dutton M, ed. *Dutton's Orthopedic Survival Guide: Managing Common Conditions*. New York, NY: McGraw-Hill; 2011. http://www.accessphysiotherapy.com/content/8653838. Accessed March 17, 2013.
- Multidirectional Reach Test. Temple University. Gait Study Center. Temple University. http://podiatry.temple.edu/gaitlab/facilities/mdrt.html. Accessed March 17, 2013.
- Observational Gait Analysis. University of Oklahoma Health Sciences Center. http://moon.ouhsc.edu/dthompso/gait/knmatics/oga.htm. Accessed March 17, 2013.
- Pattern 4J: Impaired motor function, muscle performance, range of motion, gait, locomotion, and balance associated with amputation. *Guide to Physical Therapist Practice*. 2nd ed. Alexandria, VA: American Physical Therapy Association;2001. Revised 2003.
- Shamus E, Stern DF. *Effective Documentation for Physical Therapy Professionals*. 2nd ed. New York, NY: McGraw-Hill; 2011. http://www.accessphysiotherapy.com/resource/696. Accessed March 17, 2013.
- Six-minute Walk Test (6MWT). StrokEngine. http://www.aadep.org/documents/filelibrary/presentations/pmd_evaluationmartin_and_pilley_aafp/Appendix_E__6MWT_Instructions_055C0C5AD9774.pdf. Accessed March 26, 2014.

SECTION B ARTHRITIS DISORDERS

3 OSTEOARTHRITIS

Eric Shamus, PhD, DPT, PT, CSCS
Reuben Escorpizo, DPT, MSc, PT

CONDITION/DISORDER SYNONYM

- Osteoarthrosis

ICD-9-CM CODES

- 715 Osteoarthrosis and allied disorders
- 715.0 Osteoarthrosis generalized
- 715.00 Osteoarthrosis generalized involving unspecified site
- 715.04 Osteoarthrosis generalized involving hand
- 715.09 Osteoarthrosis generalized involving multiple sites
- 715.1 Osteoarthrosis localized primary
- 715.10 Osteoarthrosis localized primary involving unspecified site
- 715.11 Osteoarthrosis localized primary involving shoulder region
- 715.12 Osteoarthrosis localized primary involving upper arm
- 715.13 Osteoarthrosis localized primary involving forearm
- 715.14 Osteoarthrosis localized primary involving hand
- 715.15 Osteoarthrosis localized primary involving pelvic region and thigh
- 715.16 Osteoarthrosis localized primary involving lower leg
- 715.17 Osteoarthrosis localized primary involving ankle and foot
- 715.18 Osteoarthrosis localized primary involving other specified sites
- 715.2 Osteoarthrosis localized secondary
- 715.20 Osteoarthrosis localized secondary involving unspecified site
- 715.21 Osteoarthrosis localized secondary involving shoulder region
- 715.22 Osteoarthrosis localized secondary involving upper arm
- 715.23 Osteoarthrosis localized secondary involving forearm
- 715.24 Osteoarthrosis localized secondary involving hand
- 715.25 Osteoarthrosis localized secondary involving pelvic region and thigh
- 715.26 Osteoarthrosis localized secondary involving lower leg
- 715.27 Osteoarthrosis localized secondary involving ankle and foot
- 715.28 Osteoarthrosis localized secondary involving other specified sites
- 715.3 Osteoarthrosis localized not specified whether primary or secondary
- 715.30 Osteoarthrosis localized not specified whether primary or secondary involving unspecified site
- 715.31 Osteoarthrosis localized not specified whether primary or secondary involving shoulder region
- 715.32 Osteoarthrosis localized not specified whether primary or secondary involving upper arm
- 715.33 Osteoarthrosis localized not specified whether primary or secondary involving forearm
- 715.34 Osteoarthrosis localized not specified whether primary or secondary involving hand
- 715.35 Osteoarthrosis localized not specified whether primary or secondary involving pelvic region and thigh
- 715.36 Osteoarthrosis localized not specified whether primary or secondary involving lower leg
- 715.37 Osteoarthrosis localized not specified whether primary or secondary involving ankle and foot
- 715.38 Osteoarthrosis localized not specified whether primary or secondary involving other specified sites

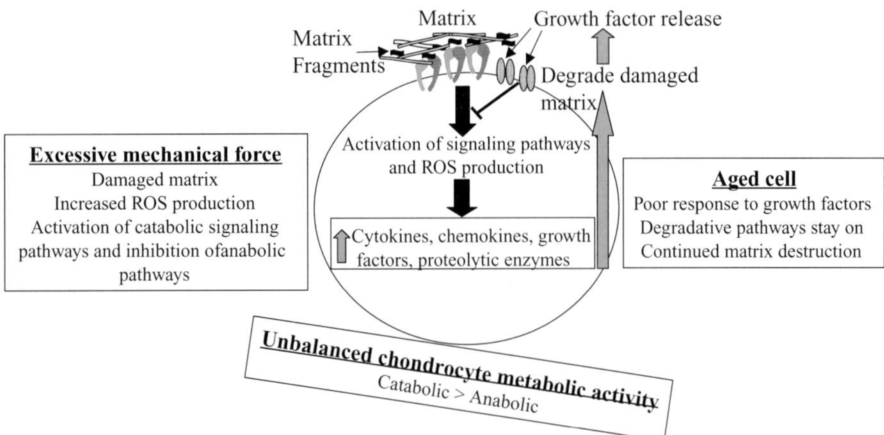

FIGURE 3-1 Theoretical model for pathways involved in cartilage destruction during the development of *osteoarthritis*. Excessive mechanical forces stimulate the chondrocyte directly or indirectly through signals generated by matrix damage including generation of matrix fragments. The resultant activation of signaling pathways, including ROS generation, results in increased production of cytokines, chemokines, and proteolytic enzymes. This catabolic response to injury serves to degrade the damaged matrix. Matrix degradation results in release of growth factors stored in the matrix, which would normally feedback on the cell and shut down the catabolic pathways. But aged chondrocytes have an insufficient response to growth factor stimulation resulting in continued matrix destruction from unbalanced catabolic and anabolic activity. (Reproduced with permission from Loeser RF. Molecular mechanisms of cartilage destruction: mechanics, inflammatory mediators and aging collide. *Arthritis Rheum.* 2006;54:1357.)

- 715.8 Osteoarthrosis involving or with mention of more than one site but not specified as generalized
- 715.80 Osteoarthrosis involving or with more than one site but not specified as generalized and involving unspecified site
- 715.89 Osteoarthrosis involving or with multiple sites but not specified as generalized
- 715.9 Osteoarthrosis unspecified whether generalized or localized
- 715.90 Osteoarthrosis unspecified whether generalized or localized involving unspecified site
- 715.91 Osteoarthrosis unspecified whether generalized or localized involving shoulder region
- 715.92 Osteoarthrosis unspecified whether generalized or localized involving upper arm
- 715.93 Osteoarthrosis unspecified whether generalized or localized involving forearm
- 715.94 Osteoarthrosis unspecified whether generalized or localized involving hand
- 715.95 Osteoarthrosis unspecified whether generalized or localized involving pelvic region and thigh
- 715.96 Osteoarthrosis unspecified whether generalized or localized involving lower leg
- 715.97 Osteoarthrosis unspecified whether generalized or localized involving ankle and foot
- 715.98 Osteoarthrosis unspecified whether generalized or localized involving other specified sites

ICD-10-CM CODES

- M15 Polyarthrosis
- M19 Other arthrosis
- M47 Spondylosis

PREFERRED PRACTICE PATTERNS

- 4D: Impaired Joint Mobility, Motor Function, Muscle Performance, and Range of Motion Associated With Connective Tissue Dysfunction
- 4F: Impaired Joint Mobility, Motor Function, Muscle Performance, Range of Motion, and Reflex Integrity Associated With Spinal Disorders
- 4H: Impaired Joint Mobility, Motor Function, Muscle Performance, and Range of Motion Associated With Joint Arthroplasty
- 4I: Impaired Joint Mobility, Motor Function, Muscle Performance, and Range of Motion Associated With Bony or Soft Tissue Surgery

PATIENT PRESENTATION

A 64-year-old male was referred to your OP PT clinic. He has been having difficulty walking because of pain in his left great toe. The patient had blood work done to rule out RA and gout. The patient states that when he wakes up the toe is very stiff and painful. If he massages it for a few minutes, he is able to walk. He has a decreased step length and cannot push off on that foot. X-rays show osteophytes and decreased joint space. The patient has talked with his orthopedic surgeon and they have discussed a joint replacement if he is unable to get good relief with physical therapy.

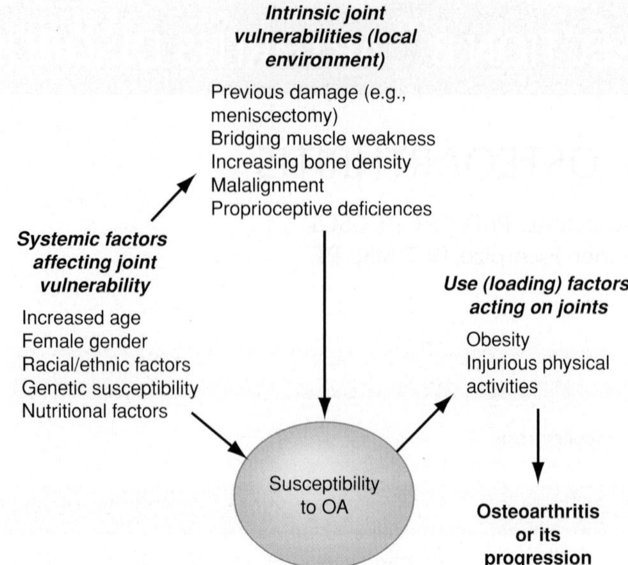

FIGURE 3-2 Risk factors for osteoarthritis either contribute to the susceptibility of the joint (systemic factors or factors in the local joint environment) or increase risk by the load they put on the joint. Usually a combination of loading and susceptibility factors is required to cause disease or its progression. (From Longo DL et al [eds]: *Harrison's Principles of Internal Medicine,* 18th ed. New York, McGraw-Hill, 2012. Copyright © The McGraw-Hill Companies, Inc. All rights reserved.)

KEY FEATURES

▶ Description

- Most common form of arthritis
- Degenerative joint disease
- Commonly affects

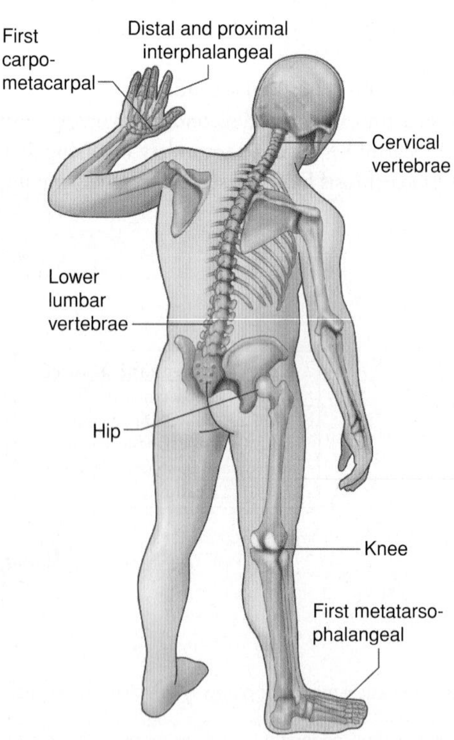

FIGURE 3-3 Joints affected by osteoarthritis. (From Longo DL et al [eds]: *Harrison's Principles of Internal Medicine,* 18th ed. New York, McGraw-Hill, 2012. Copyright © The McGraw-Hill Companies, Inc. All rights reserved.)

- Weight-bearing joints (e.g., hand, hip, knee)
- Interphalangeal joints, first metatarsophalangeal joint, and spinal facet joints

- Associated with increasing age, obesity, females, and race/ethnicity
- Associated with abnormal loading of the joints
- Joint pain

Essentials of Diagnosis

- X-ray
- Kellgren and Lawrence (KL) grade ≥2 (definite radiographic osteoarthritis [OA])[1]
- Osteophytes, joint-space narrowing, sclerosis
- Cartilage lesions, bone marrow lesions, synovitis, effusion, and subchondral bone attrition/sclerosis
- Erosion of articular cartilage
- Synovial hyperplasia
- Fibrosis
- Inflammatory cell infiltration with or without OA symptoms
- OA is a clinical diagnosis which can be based on
  - Persistent usage-related pain in joint or joints
  - Age usually ≥45 years[2]
  - Morning stiffness equal or less than 30 minutes[2]

General Considerations

- Low bone mineral density (BMD)
- Secondary problems
  - Muscle atrophy and weakness
  - Bony protrusion/prominence
  - Joint deformity
  - Walking difficulty
  - Difficulty with ADLs

Demographics

- Prevalent in middle-to-older age groups
- Women are more affected than men
- Predominantly affects African Americans and Caucasians
- May affect about 12% of the population (United States and other developed countries)[2]

CLINICAL FINDINGS

SIGNS AND SYMPTOMS

- Joint pain
- Aching joint
- Joint stiffness
- Morning stiffness
- Muscle weakness
- Muscle atrophy
- Repetitive joint use or loading
- Poor joint alignment
- Leg-length discrepancy (LLD)/inequality
- Bone or joint morphology
- Calcification (e.g., of the knee meniscus)
- Bone formation, cyst formation
- Thickening of subchondral bone plate (osteosclerosis)
- Overall joint dysfunction
- Joint swelling and inflammation (in certain severe cases)
- Long-term disease
- Crepitus
- Bony enlargement
- Limited joint ROM
- Joint line tenderness
- Joint deformity in severe cases
- Heberden's nodes

Functional Implications

- Limited mobility
- Activity limitation
- Household and work-related activity limitations/restrictions
- Decreased overall activity and participation

Possible Contributing Causes

- Chronic factors affecting the joint such as obesity, BMD, LLD
- Aging
- Chronic and vigorous joint loading
- Previous chronic joint injury (e.g., accident, trauma); hence, secondary OA

Differential Diagnoses

- Rheumatoid arthritis
- Gout
- Fibromyalgia
- Spondyloarthropathy
- Ankylosing spondylitis

MEANS OF CONFIRMATION OR DIAGNOSIS

Laboratory Tests

- Synovial fluid examination
- Other laboratory tests can be done to rule out other conditions

Imaging

- X-ray of the joint
- MRI of the joint

Diagnostic Procedures

- Ultrasound of the joint and synovium

FINDINGS AND INTERPRETATION

- Osteophytes, joint-space narrowing, sclerosis
- Cartilage and/or bone marrow lesions, synovitis, effusion, and subchondral bone attrition/sclerosis
- Erosion of articular cartilage
- Kellgren and Lawrence (KL) grade ≥2 (definite radiographic OA)[1]

TREATMENT

Medication

- NSAIDs (including topical NSAIDs, e.g., capsaicin)
- Acetaminophen
- Opioids
- Glucosamine and chondroitin sulfate
- Glucocorticoids or corticosteroids
- Intra-articular injections
  - Corticosteroids
  - Viscosupplementation: Hyaluronic acid (Synvisc)
- Emerging drugs, for example, anti-tumor necrosis factors (anti-TNFs), calcitonin, growth factors, nerve growth factor antibodies

MEDICAL PROCEDURES

- Total joint replacements
- Joint lavage
- Debridement

REFERRALS/ADMITTANCE

- To rheumatologist to assess underlying complications
- To internal medicine specialist
- To orthopedist for surgical consultation
- To physical and rehabilitation medicine specialist
- To dietician/nutritionist

IMPAIRMENTS

- Mobility
- Self-care
- Role at home and in the community
- School and work
- Recreation, leisure, and sports

TESTS AND MEASURES

- Limb strength
  - Functional strength testing
    - Five times sit-to-stand test
  - Manual muscle test (MMT)
    - Hamstrings
    - Quadriceps
    - Iliopsoas
    - Gluteus maximus
    - Gluteus medius
    - Gluteus minimus
    - Adductors
- Balance
  - Static single-leg standing (eyes open, eyes closed)
    - Contralateral LE
  - Dynamic standing
    - Berg Balance Scale
    - Functional gait assessment
- Gait assessment
  - Observational analysis
  - Gait speed via the 10-m walk test
  - 2-minute walk test
  - 6-minute walk test
- Range of motion
- Joint mobility

INTERVENTION

- Exercises
  - Aquatic exercises
  - Resistance
  - Endurance
  - Flexibility
- ADL training
- Use of assistive or adaptive devices
- Heat therapy
- Weight management; diet
- Rest
- Orthoses; splints; footwear
- Walking aids
- Ice
- Acupuncture
- Pain management
- Energy conservation techniques
- Joint protection
- Psychosocial support
- Ultrasound
- Electric stimulation
- Patient education

FUNCTIONAL GOALS

- Improve joint mobility and stability for balance.
- Improve muscle strength to climb stairs.
- Improve muscle and general (aerobic) endurance.
- Improve activity and participation at home, at work, and in the community.
- Walk 0.5 mile pain free without assistive device.
- Walk 1 mile pain free with assistive device.
- Pain-free ADLs (e.g., sweeping, mopping).
- Turn a key or door knob pain free.
- Lift baby from crib without pain and maintain a neutral wrist posture.

PROGNOSIS

- No definite cure for OA; It is a chronic, long-term disease.
- Joint damage is irreversible.
- Treatment is for symptoms, but emerging drugs may modify OA disease management.
- Recovery or relief depends on disease duration and timely intervention.
- Prognosis can be affected by:
  - Demographics.
  - Severity and natural history of the disease.
  - Medical and behavioral comorbidities (e.g., fear avoidance, catastrophization, central sensitization.
- Positive prognosticating factors: Competent general endurance, good muscle strength, and joint mobility.
- PT treatment outcomes improved by motivation and compliance with physical therapy intervention (e.g., home exercise program), and family and environmental support.

PATIENT RESOURCE

Osteoarthritis Research Society International. OARSI Primer; 2010 (last updated 2011). http://primer.oarsi.org. Accessed June 1, 2013.

REFERENCES

1. Kellgren JH. *Atlas of standard radiographs of arthritis*. Vol. II. Oxford: Blackwell Scientific; 1963.
2. Osteoarthritis: National clinical guideline for care and management in adults. In: *NICE Clinical Guidelines*, No. 59. London: Royal College of Physicians (UK); 2008.

ADDITIONAL REFERENCES

- Chandrasoma P, Taylor CR. Disorders of Joints. In: Chandrasoma P, Taylor CR, eds. *Concise Pathology*. 3rd ed. New York, NY: McGraw-Hill; 2011. http://www.accessphysiotherapy.com/content/193719. Accessed June 10, 2013.
- Dutton M. Musculoskeletal disorders and diseases. In: Dutton M, ed. *McGraw-Hill's NPTE (National Physical Therapy Examination), 2e*. New York, NY: McGraw-Hill; 2012. http://www.accessphysiotherapy.com/content/5403488. Accessed June 10, 2013.

- Hall SJ. Chapter 5. The biomechanics of human skeletal articulations. In: Hall SJ, ed. *Basic Biomechanics*. 5th ed. New York, NY: McGraw-Hill; 2007. http://www.accessphysiotherapy.com/content/6061046. Accessed June 10, 2013.
- ICD9DATA. http://www.icd9data.com. Accessed June 6, 2013.
- ICD10DATA. http://www.icd10data.com. Accessed June 1, 2013.
- Malone TR, Hazle C, Grey ML. Shoulder: standard plain radiographs. In: Malone TR, Hazle C, Grey ML, eds. *Imaging in Rehabilitation*. New York, NY: McGraw-Hill; 2008. http://www.accessphysiotherapy.com/content/5940767. Accessed June 10, 2013.
- The American Physical Therapy Association. *Interactive Guide to Physical Therapist Practice 2003*. doi: 10.2522/ptguide.3.1_5. http://guidetoptpractice.apta.org/. Accessed June 1, 2013.

4 RHEUMATOID ARTHRITIS

Reuben Escorpizo, DPT, MSc, PT
Eric Shamus, PhD, DPT, PT, CSCS

CONDITION/DISORDER SYNONYM

- Rheumatoid arthritis (RA)

ICD-9-CM CODES

- 714.0 Rheumatoid arthritis
- 714.1 Felty's syndrome
- 714.2 Other rheumatoid arthritis with visceral or systemic involvement
- 714.4 Chronic postrheumatic arthropathy
- 714.8 Other specified inflammatory polyarthropathies
- 714.81 Rheumatoid lung
- 714.9 Unspecified inflammatory polyarthropathy

ICD-10-CM CODES

- M05.6 Rheumatoid arthritis with involvement of other organs and systems
- M05.60 Rheumatoid arthritis of unspecified site with involvement of other organs and systems
- M05.61 Rheumatoid arthritis of shoulder with involvement of other organs and systems
- M05.611 Rheumatoid arthritis of right shoulder with involvement of other organs and systems
- M05.612 Rheumatoid arthritis of left shoulder with involvement of other organs and systems

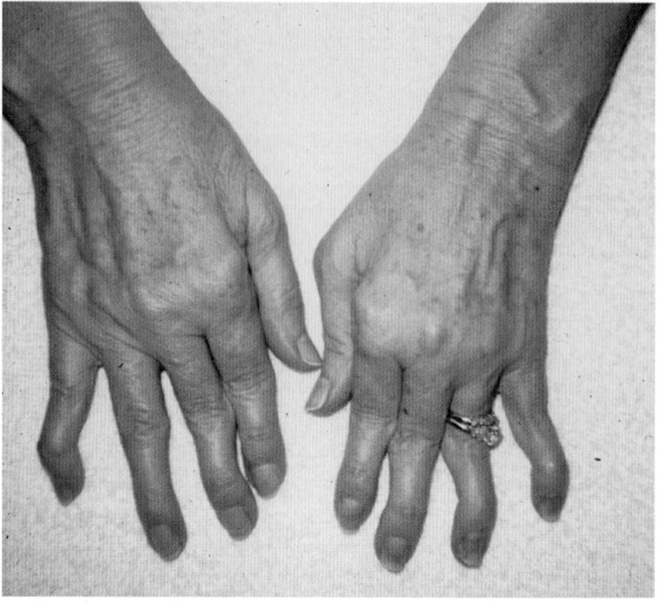

FIGURE 4-1 Rheumatoid arthritis with ulnar deviation of the fingers and flexion of the distal interphalangeal joints with hyperextension of the proximal interphalangeal joints. (From Fuster V, Walsh RA, Harrigton RA. *Hurst's The Heart*, 13th ed.)

- M05.619 Rheumatoid arthritis of unspecified shoulder with involvement of other organs and systems
- M05.62 Rheumatoid arthritis of elbow with involvement of other organs and systems

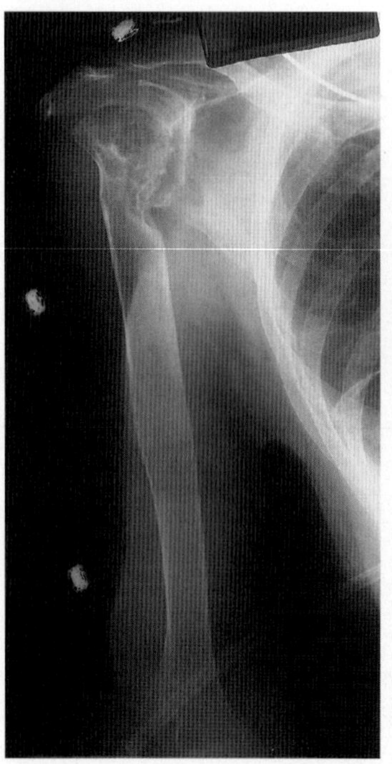
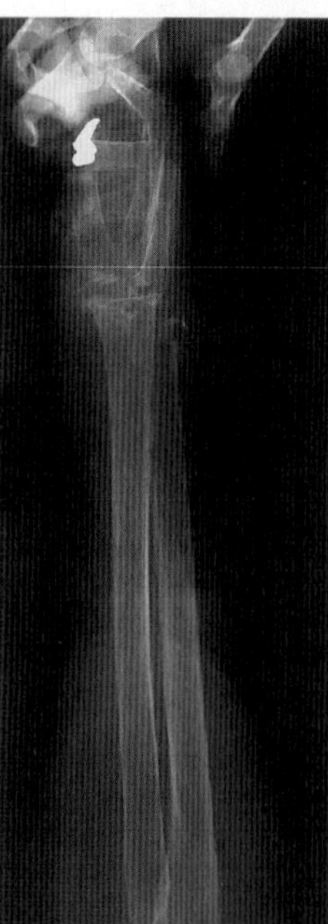
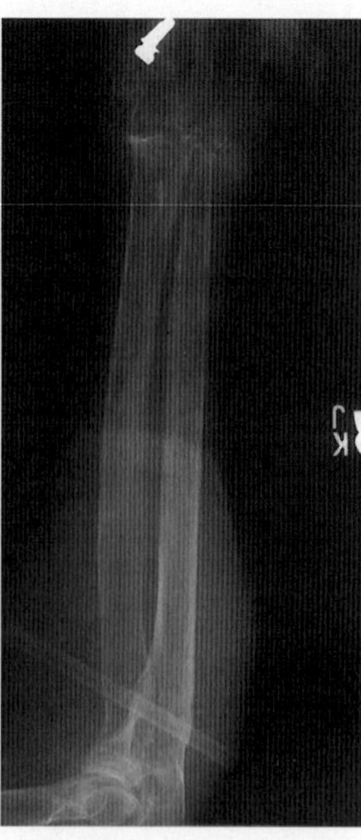

FIGURE 4-2 Rheumatoid arthritis of the wrist, elbow, and shoulder. (From Simon RR, Sherman SC: *Emergency Orthopedics*, 6th edition. www.accessemergencymedicine.com.)

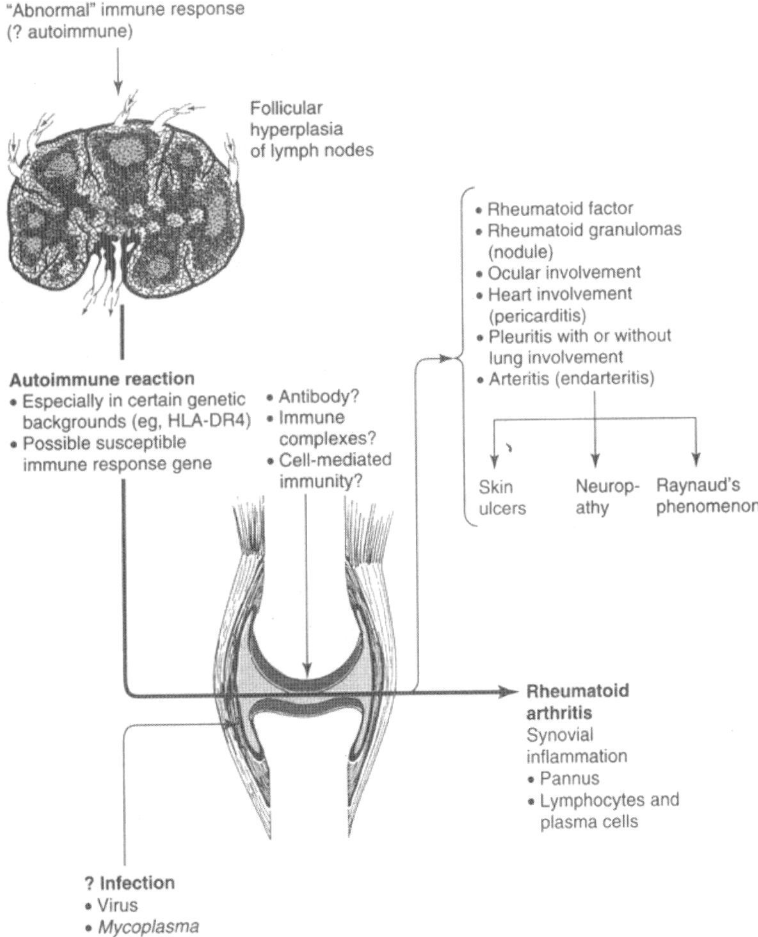

FIGURE 4-3 Proposed etiologic factors and pathologic effects of rheumatoid arthritis. (From Chandrasoma P, Taylor CR: *Concise Pathology*, 3rd edition. www.accessmedicine.com.)

- M05.621 Rheumatoid arthritis of right elbow with involvement of other organs and systems
- M05.622 Rheumatoid arthritis of left elbow with involvement of other organs and systems
- M05.629 Rheumatoid arthritis of unspecified elbow with involvement of other organs and systems
- M05.63 Rheumatoid arthritis of wrist with involvement of other organs and systems
- M05.631 Rheumatoid arthritis of right wrist with involvement of other organs and systems
- M05.632 Rheumatoid arthritis of left wrist with involvement of other organs and systems
- M05.639 Rheumatoid arthritis of unspecified wrist with involvement of other organs and systems
- M05.64 Rheumatoid arthritis of hand with involvement of other organs and systems
- M05.641 Rheumatoid arthritis of right hand with involvement of other organs and systems
- M05.642 Rheumatoid arthritis of left hand with involvement of other organs and systems
- M05.649 Rheumatoid arthritis of unspecified hand with involvement of other organs and systems
- M05.65 Rheumatoid arthritis of hip with involvement of other organs and systems
- M05.651 Rheumatoid arthritis of right hip with involvement of other organs and systems
- M05.652 Rheumatoid arthritis of left hip with involvement of other organs and systems
- M05.659 Rheumatoid arthritis of unspecified hip with involvement of other organs and systems
- M05.66 Rheumatoid arthritis of knee with involvement of other organs and systems
- M05.661 Rheumatoid arthritis of right knee with involvement of other organs and systems
- M05.662 Rheumatoid arthritis of left knee with involvement of other organs and systems
- M05.669 Rheumatoid arthritis of unspecified knee with involvement of other organs and systems
- M05.67 Rheumatoid arthritis of ankle and foot with involvement of other organs and systems
- M05.671 Rheumatoid arthritis of right ankle and foot with involvement of other organs and systems
- M05.672 Rheumatoid arthritis of left ankle and foot with involvement of other organs and systems
- M05.679 Rheumatoid arthritis of unspecified ankle and foot with involvement of other organs and systems
- M05.69 Rheumatoid arthritis of multiple sites with involvement of other organs and systems
- M05.7 Rheumatoid arthritis with rheumatoid factor without organ or systems involvement
- M05.70 Rheumatoid arthritis with rheumatoid factor of unspecified site without organ or systems involvement

- M05.71 Rheumatoid arthritis with rheumatoid factor of shoulder without organ or systems involvement
- M05.711 Rheumatoid arthritis with rheumatoid factor of right shoulder without organ or systems involvement
- M05.712 Rheumatoid arthritis with rheumatoid factor of left shoulder without organ or systems involvement
- M05.719 Rheumatoid arthritis with rheumatoid factor of unspecified shoulder without organ or systems involvement
- M05.72 Rheumatoid arthritis with rheumatoid factor of elbow without organ or systems involvement
- M05.721 Rheumatoid arthritis with rheumatoid factor of right elbow without organ or systems involvement
- M05.722 Rheumatoid arthritis with rheumatoid factor of left elbow without organ or systems involvement
- M05.729 Rheumatoid arthritis with rheumatoid factor of unspecified elbow without organ or systems involvement
- M05.73 Rheumatoid arthritis with rheumatoid factor of wrist without organ or systems involvement
- M05.731 Rheumatoid arthritis with rheumatoid factor of right wrist without organ or systems involvement
- M05.732 Rheumatoid arthritis with rheumatoid factor of left wrist without organ or systems involvement
- M05.739 Rheumatoid arthritis with rheumatoid factor of unspecified wrist without organ or systems involvement
- M05.74 Rheumatoid arthritis with rheumatoid factor of hand without organ or systems involvement
- M05.741 Rheumatoid arthritis with rheumatoid factor of right hand without organ or systems involvement
- M05.742 Rheumatoid arthritis with rheumatoid factor of left hand without organ or systems involvement
- M05.749 Rheumatoid arthritis with rheumatoid factor of unspecified hand without organ or systems involvement
- M05.75 Rheumatoid arthritis with rheumatoid factor of hip without organ or systems involvement
- M05.751 Rheumatoid arthritis with rheumatoid factor of right hip without organ or systems involvement
- M05.752 Rheumatoid arthritis with rheumatoid factor of left hip without organ or systems involvement
- M05.759 Rheumatoid arthritis with rheumatoid factor of unspecified hip without organ or systems involvement
- M05.76 Rheumatoid arthritis with rheumatoid factor of knee without organ or systems involvement
- M05.761 Rheumatoid arthritis with rheumatoid factor of right knee without organ or systems involvement
- M05.762 Rheumatoid arthritis with rheumatoid factor of left knee without organ or systems involvement
- M05.769 Rheumatoid arthritis with rheumatoid factor of unspecified knee without organ or systems involvement
- M05.77 Rheumatoid arthritis with rheumatoid factor of ankle and foot without organ or systems involvement
- M05.771 Rheumatoid arthritis with rheumatoid factor of right ankle and foot without organ or systems involvement
- M05.772 Rheumatoid arthritis with rheumatoid factor of left ankle and foot without organ or systems involvement
- M05.779 Rheumatoid arthritis with rheumatoid factor of unspecified ankle and foot without organ or systems involvement
- M05.79 Rheumatoid arthritis with rheumatoid factor of multiple sites without organ or systems involvement
- M05.8 Other rheumatoid arthritis with rheumatoid factor

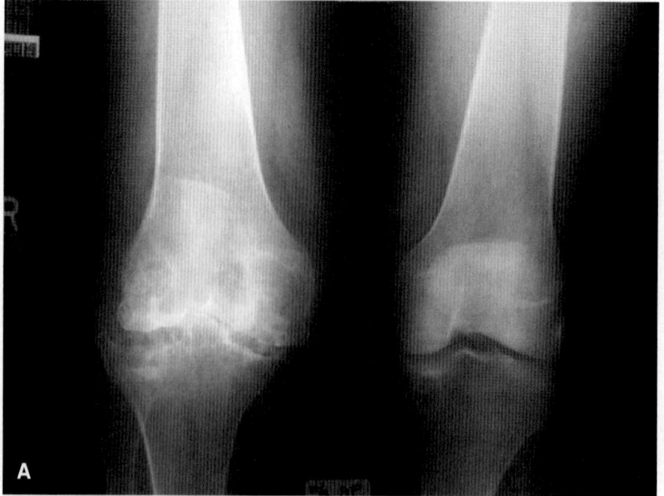

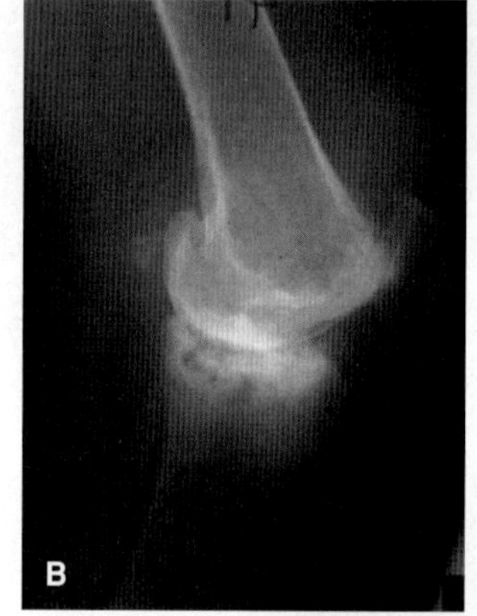

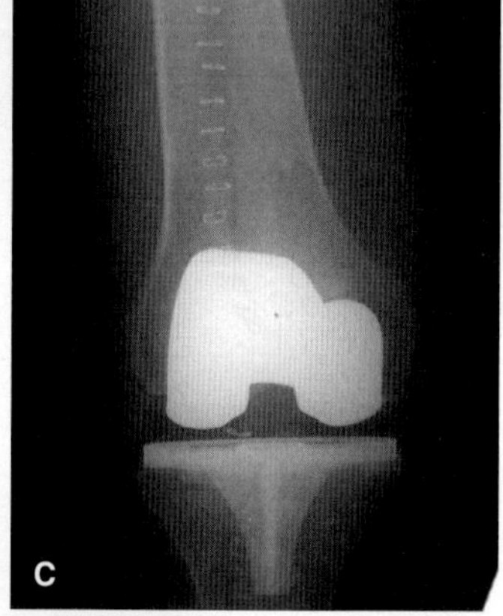

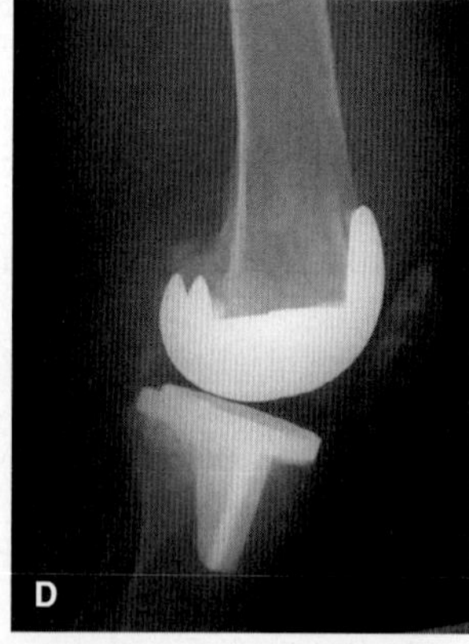

FIGURE 4-4 (**A–B**). Patient with rheumatoid arthritis and severe joint destruction of the right knee. (**C–D**). Patient was treated with a cemented right total knee replacement. (From Doherty GM. *Current Diagnosis & Treatment: Surgery*, 13th ed. Copyright © The McGraw-Hill Companies, Inc. All rights reserved.

- M05.80 Other rheumatoid arthritis with rheumatoid factor of unspecified site
- M05.81 Other rheumatoid arthritis with rheumatoid factor of shoulder
- M05.811 Other rheumatoid arthritis with rheumatoid factor of right shoulder
- M05.812 Other rheumatoid arthritis with rheumatoid factor of left shoulder

- M05.819 Other rheumatoid arthritis with rheumatoid factor of unspecified shoulder
- M05.82 Other rheumatoid arthritis with rheumatoid factor of elbow
- M05.821 Other rheumatoid arthritis with rheumatoid factor of right elbow
- M05.822 Other rheumatoid arthritis with rheumatoid factor of left elbow
- M05.829 Other rheumatoid arthritis with rheumatoid factor of unspecified elbow
- M05.83 Other rheumatoid arthritis with rheumatoid factor of wrist
- M05.831 Other rheumatoid arthritis with rheumatoid factor of right wrist
- M05.832 Other rheumatoid arthritis with rheumatoid factor of left wrist
- M05.839 Other rheumatoid arthritis with rheumatoid factor of unspecified wrist
- M05.84 Other rheumatoid arthritis with rheumatoid factor of hand
- M05.841 Other rheumatoid arthritis with rheumatoid factor of right hand
- M05.842 Other rheumatoid arthritis with rheumatoid factor of left hand
- M05.849 Other rheumatoid arthritis with rheumatoid factor of unspecified hand
- M05.85 Other rheumatoid arthritis with rheumatoid factor of hip
- M05.851 Other rheumatoid arthritis with rheumatoid factor of right hip
- M05.852 Other rheumatoid arthritis with rheumatoid factor of left hip
- M05.859 Other rheumatoid arthritis with rheumatoid factor of unspecified hip
- M05.86 Other rheumatoid arthritis with rheumatoid factor of knee
- M05.861 Other rheumatoid arthritis with rheumatoid factor of right knee
- M05.862 Other rheumatoid arthritis with rheumatoid factor of left knee
- M05.869 Other rheumatoid arthritis with rheumatoid factor of unspecified knee
- M05.87 Other rheumatoid arthritis with rheumatoid factor of ankle and foot
- M05.871 Other rheumatoid arthritis with rheumatoid factor of right ankle and foot
- M05.872 Other rheumatoid arthritis with rheumatoid factor of left ankle and foot
- M05.879 Other rheumatoid arthritis with rheumatoid factor of unspecified ankle and foot
- M05.89 Other rheumatoid arthritis with rheumatoid factor of multiple sites
- M05.9 Rheumatoid arthritis with rheumatoid factor, unspecified

PREFERRED PRACTICE PATTERNS

- 4D: Impaired Joint Mobility, Motor Function, Muscle Performance, and Range of motion (ROM) Associated with Connective Tissue Dysfunction
- 4E: Impaired Joint Mobility, Motor Function, Muscle Performance, and ROM Associated with Localized Inflammation

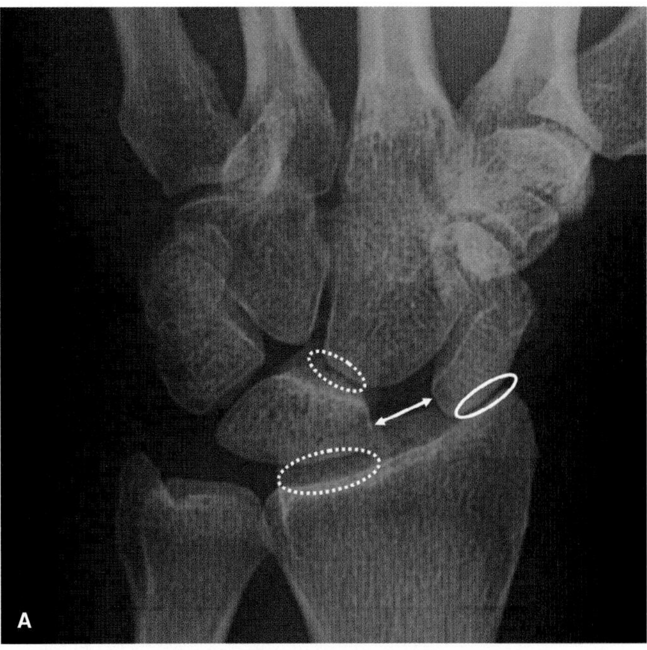

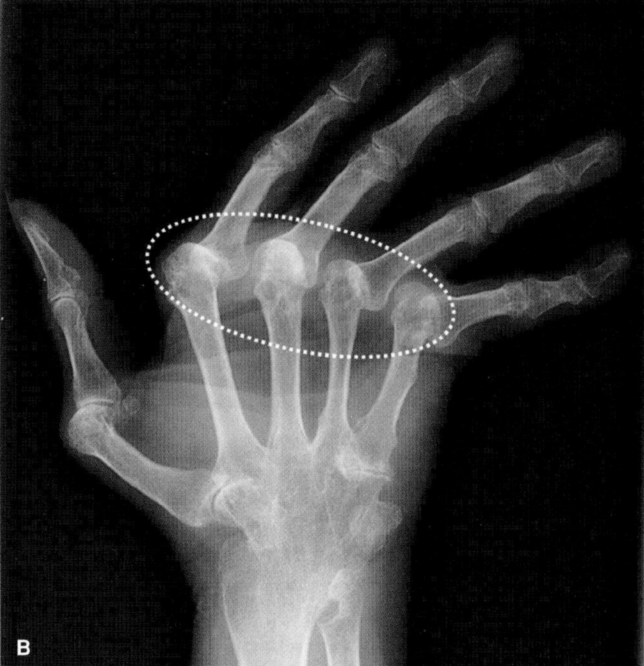

FIGURE 4-5 Arthritis of the hand and wrist. **A.** This patient injured her scapholunate ligament years before presentation. The scapholunate interval is widened (*double arrow*), and the radioscaphoid joint is degenerated (*solid oval*), but the radiolunate and lunocapitate joint spaces are well preserved (*dashed ovals*). **B.** This patient has had rheumatoid arthritis for decades. The classic volar subluxation of the metacarpophalangeal joints of the fingers (*dashed oval*) and radial deviation of the fingers are apparent. (From Brunicardi FC, Andersen D, Billiar T, et al. *Schwartz's Principles of Surgery*, 9th ed. Copyright © The McGraw-Hill Companies, Inc. All rights reserved.)

PATIENT PRESENTATION

A 32-year-old nurse presents to your office with a complaint of intermittent episodes of pain, stiffness, and swelling in both hands and wrists for approximately 1 year. The episodes last for several weeks and then resolve. More recently, she noticed similar symptoms in her knees and ankles. Joint pain and stiffness are making it harder for her to get out of bed in the morning and are interfering with her ability to perform her duties at work. The joint stiffness usually lasts for several hours before improving. She also reports malaise and easy fatigability for the past few months, but she denies having fever, chills, skin rashes, and weight loss. Physical examination reveals a well-developed woman, with blood pressure 120/70 mm Hg, heart rate 82 bpm, and respiratory rate 14 breaths per minute. Her skin does not reveal any rashes. Head, neck, cardiovascular, chest, and abdominal examinations are normal. There is no hepatosplenomegaly. The joint examination reveals the presence of bilateral swelling, redness, and tenderness of most proximal interphalangeal (PIP) joints, metacarpophalangeal (MCP) joints, the wrists, and the knees. Laboratory studies show a mild anemia with hemoglobin 11.2 g/dL, hematocrit 32.5%, mean corpuscular volume (MCV) 85.7 fL, white blood cell (WBC) count 7.9/mm^3 with a normal differential, and platelet count 300,000/mm. The urinalysis is clear with no protein and no red blood cells (RBCs). The erythrocyte sedimentation rate (ESR) is 75 mm/h, and the kidney and liver function tests are normal.[1]

KEY FEATURES

Description

- Autoimmune disease
- Chronic and systemic inflammatory disease
- Unknown etiology
- Usually affects diarthrodial joints, synovial membranes
- Affects muscles, joints, and extra-articular structures of the body
- Fibrinoid degeneration of the collagen fibers in mesenchymal tissues
- Arthropathy
- Synovitis
- Polyarthritis

Essentials of Diagnosis[2]

- Begins between ages 20 and 40.[2]
- RA is part of a broad spectrum of rheumatic disorders characterized as autoimmune.
- Conventional radiograph is the most commonly used tool in RA.[2]
- Diagnosis is made based on taking a careful history, physical examination, imaging studies, laboratory examination, and exclusion of other possible diseases.
- 2010 ACR-EULAR classification criteria for RA: A score of ≥6/10 is needed for classification of a patient as having definite RA.
- Joint involvement (0 = large joint, 1 = 2–10 large joints, 2 = 1–3 small joints [with or without involvement of large joints], 3 = 4–10 small joints [with or without involvement of large joints], 5 = >10 joints [at least one small joint]).
- Serology (0 = negative rheumatoid factor [RF] and negative anti-citrullinated protein antibody [ACPA], 2 = low-positive RF or ACPA, 3 = high-positive RF or ACPA).
- Acute-phase reactants (0 = normal C-reactive protein [CRP] and normal ESR, 1 = abnormal CRP or abnormal ESR).
- Duration of symptoms (0 = <6 weeks, 1 = ≥6 weeks).

General Considerations

- Overall joint dysfunction
- Joint swelling and inflammation
- Joint pain
- Morning stiffness
- Episodes of flares and remission
- Long-term disease
- Joint instability or ankylosis
- Joint deformity
- Secondary problems include extra-articular manifestations such as:
  - Rheumatoid nodules
  - Retinitis
  - Vasculitis
  - Pericarditis
  - Myocarditis
  - Distal sensory neuropathy
  - Cervical spine instability

Demographics

- Women are more affected than men
- Adult: Begins between ages 20 and 40[2]
- RA of children: Juvenile chronic polyarthritis

CLINICAL FINDINGS

SIGNS AND SYMPTOMS

- Unexplained weight loss, fever, or weakness with joint pain
- Loss of ROM and joint play
- Joint stiffness
- Joint pain and swelling of small joints of the hands and feet
- Inflamed joints
- Flexion contracture
- Neuropathies (such as ulnar nerve)
- Joint deformities (such as hammer toe, swan neck, boutonniere, ulnar drift)

Functional Implications

- Limited mobility
- Aerobic endurance limitation
- Decreased activity and participation

Possible Contributing Causes

- Various risk factors are possible such as tobacco use, oral contraceptives, hormone replacement, low live birth history, genetics, and breastfeeding, but no definitive link is established.[2]
- Genetic and environmental factors are associated.[3]
- RF (antibodies) has long been pinpointed as a major contributing factor because it reacts with immunoglobulin antibodies in the blood, leading to inflammation.

Differential Diagnosis

- Ankylosing spondylitis
- Fibromyalgia syndrome
- Lyme disease
- Osteoarthritis
- Psoriatic arthritis
- Reiter's syndrome
- Rheumatism
- Scleroderma
- Spondyloarthropathy
- Systemic lupus erythematosus

MEANS OF CONFIRMATION

Laboratory Tests

- Negative or positive RF (serology)
- Negative or positive ACPA (serology)
- Normal or abnormal CRP (acute-phase reactant)
- Normal or abnormal ESR (acute-phase reactant)

Imaging

- Conventional radiograph of the joint
- MRI of the joint
- Diagnostic ultrasound of the joint and synovium

FINDINGS AND INTERPRETATION

- For imaging, the following are radiographic features of RA[4]
  - Earliest signs: Fusiform periarticular swelling (joint effusion, tenosynovitis, and edema
  - Radiolucent defects, subchondral bone restoration, synovial cysts
  - Rarefaction, diminished bone density in periarticular regions
  - Joint space narrowing
  - Joint deformities, subluxations, dislocations (such as flexion contracture)

TREATMENT

Medication

- NSAIDs
- Cortisone injection
- Glucocorticoids or corticosteroids
- Disease-modifying antirheumatic drugs (DMARDs)
- Anti-TNF
- Anti-bone resorption agents like osteoprotegerin
- Antibiotics like minocycline
- Methotrexate (most commonly used)

MEDICAL PROCEDURES

- Surgery: Synovectomy (common in the wrist), total joint replacements, and tenosynovectomy.

REFERRALS/ADMITTANCE

- Rheumatologist to assess underlying complications
- Internal medicine specialist
- Physical and rehabilitation medicine specialist
- Surgical consult

IMPAIRMENTS

- Mobility
- Self-care
- Role at home and in the community
- School and work
- Recreation, leisure, and sports

TESTS AND MEASURES

- Straight leg raise limited secondary to muscle tightness
- Gait assessment (with appropriate assistive device and/or prosthesis)
  - Observational analysis
  - Gait speed via the 10-m walk test
  - 2-minute walk test
  - 6-minute walk test
- Balance
  - Static single-leg standing (eyes open, eyes closed)
  - Dynamic standing (with prosthesis)
    - Berg Balance Scale
    - Gait Assessment Rating Score
    - Rancho Los Amigo observational gait analysis
    - Multi-directional reach test (MDRT)
- Pain with resistance
- Functional Strength/Strength Testing
  - Five times sit-to-stand test
  - Manual muscle test (MMT)

INTERVENTION

- Exercises (resistance, endurance, and flexibility)
  - Aquatic exercises
- Training on ADLs
- Use of assistive or adaptive devices
- Heat therapy
- Weight management
- Rest
- Orthoses, splints
- Ice
- Dietary components such as fish oil, gamma-linolenic acid, and foods rich in antioxidants
- Acupuncture
- Balneotherapy
- Diets
- Pain management
- Energy conservation techniques
- Joint protection
- Orthotics and footwear
- Psychosocial support
- Low-level cold laser
- Ultrasound
- Electric stimulation
- Patient education

FUNCTIONAL GOALS

- Improve joint mobility and stability to improve balance.
- Improve muscle strength to climb stairs.
- Improve muscle and general (aerobic) endurance.
- Improve activity and participation related to the role at home and the community.
- Patient will be able to:
  - Grasp a gallon of milk pain free with two hands.
  - Turn a key or door knob pain free.
  - Lift baby crib without pain and maintain a neutral wrist posture.
- Return patient to pain-free ADL, sweeping, mopping.

PROGNOSIS

- No definite cure for RA.
- Joint damage is irreversible.
- Recovery or relief from symptoms may depend on disease duration and timely intervention.
- Complications associated with RA could lead to death.
- May affect prognosis: Demographics, severity and natural history of the disease, medical comorbidities, and behavioral comorbidities such as fear avoidance, expectations, and self-efficacy.[5]
- Competent general endurance, good muscle strength, and mobile joints are good prognosticating factors.

- Motivation and compliance with PT intervention (e.g., home exercise program) and family and environmental support could also improve PT treatment outcomes especially during flare.

PATIENT RESOURCES

- American College of Rheumatology. http://www.rheumatology.org. Accessed June 17, 2013.
- Rheumatoid Arthritis, Arthritis Foundation. http://www.arthritis.org/conditions-treatments/disease-center/rheumatoid-arthritis. Accessed June 17, 2013.

REFERENCES

1. Toy EC. Rheumatoid Arthritis, Case 79. LANGE Case Files. http://www.accessmedicine.com/casecontent.aspx?aid=510023770&tabid=1. Accessed June 17, 2013.
2. Rheumatoid Arthritis. http://www.cdc.gov/arthritis/basics/rheumatoid.htm. Accessed June 17, 2013.
3. Goodman CC, Fuller KS. *Pathology Implications for the Physical Therapist.* 3rd ed. St. Louis, MO: Saunders Elsevier; 2009.
4. McKinnis LN. *Fundamentals of Musculoskeletal Imaging.* 2nd ed. Philadelphia, PA: F.A. Davis Company; 2005.
5. Beattie PF, Nelson RM. Evaluating research studies that address prognosis for patients receiving physical therapy care: a clinical update. *Phys Ther.* 2007;87(11):1527–1535. doi: 10.2522/ptj.20060284.

ADDITIONAL REFERENCES

- Diokno E. Introduction to bracing, splinting, and casting. In: Patel DR, Greydanus DE, Baker RJ, eds. *Pediatric Practice: Sports Medicine.* New York, NY: McGraw-Hill; 2009: Appendix A. http://www.accessphysiotherapy.com/content/6983252#6983256. Accessed June 17, 2013.
- Dutton M. Adjunctive interventions. In: Dutton M, ed. *McGraw-Hill's NPTE (National Physical Therapy Examination).* 2nd ed. New York, NY: McGraw-Hill; 2012: Chapter 18. http://www.accessphysiotherapy.com/content/5405918. Accessed June 17, 2013.
- Dutton M. Imaging studies in orthopaedics. In: Dutton M, ed. *Orthopaedic Examination, Evaluation, and Intervention.* 2nd ed. New York, NY: McGraw-Hill; 2008. http://www.accessphysiotherapy.com/content/55601056. Accessed June 17, 2013.
- ICD9Data.com.http://www.icd9data.com. Accessed June 17, 2013
- ICD10Data.com.http://www.icd10data.com. Accessed June 17, 2013.
- The American Physical Therapy Association. *Guide to Physical Therapist Practice.* 2nd ed. Alexandria, VA: The American Physical Therapy Association; 2001. Revised 2003.
- Verhagen AP, Bierma-Zeinstra SMA, Cardoso JR, de Bie R, Boers M, de Vet HCW. Balneotherapy for rheumatoid arthritis. *Cochrane Database Syst Rev.* 2003;(4):CD000518.

SECTION C CARDIOVASCULAR DISORDERS

5 ACQUIRED COAGULATION DISORDERS

Kay Tasso, PhD, PT, PCS
Eric Shamus, PhD, DPT, PT, CSCS
Wendy Song, DO

CONDITION/DISORDER SYNONYMS

- Coagulation defects
- Disorders of blood coagulation

ICD-9-CM CODES[1]

- 286.5 Hemorrhagic disorder due to intrinsic circulating anticoagulants
- 286.52 Acquired hemophilia
- 286.53 Antiphospholipid antibody with hemorrhagic disorder
- 286.59 Other hemorrhagic disorder due to intrinsic circulating anticoagulants, antibodies, or inhibitors

ICD-10-CM CODES[2]

- D68.311 Acquired hemophilia
- D68.312 Antiphospholipid antibody with hemorrhagic disorder
- D68.318 Other hemorrhagic disorder due to intrinsic circulating anticoagulants, antibodies, or inhibitors

PREFERRED PRACTICE PATTERNS

- 4D: Impaired Joint Mobility, Motor Function, Muscle Performance, and Range of Motion Associated With Connective Tissue Dysfunction[3]

PATIENT PRESENTATION

A 52-year-old male presents with a deep thigh bruise and knee pain from a fall 1 week ago. The patient has a history of celiac disease has noticed increased bruising and prolonged gum bleeding after brushing his teeth for the past week. He has not adhered to his gluten-free diet due to hectic work hours as a police officer. Vitals are: Temperature: 98.2 °F, Pulse: 84, Respirations: 16, Blood Pressure: 130/86, and SpO_2% of 98%. Physical examination shows diffuse small ecchymosis on his upper and lower extremities with gingival petechiae. Laboratory tests show a normal hemoglobin and platelet count with a prolonged prothrombin time (PT) and mildly elevated partial PT.

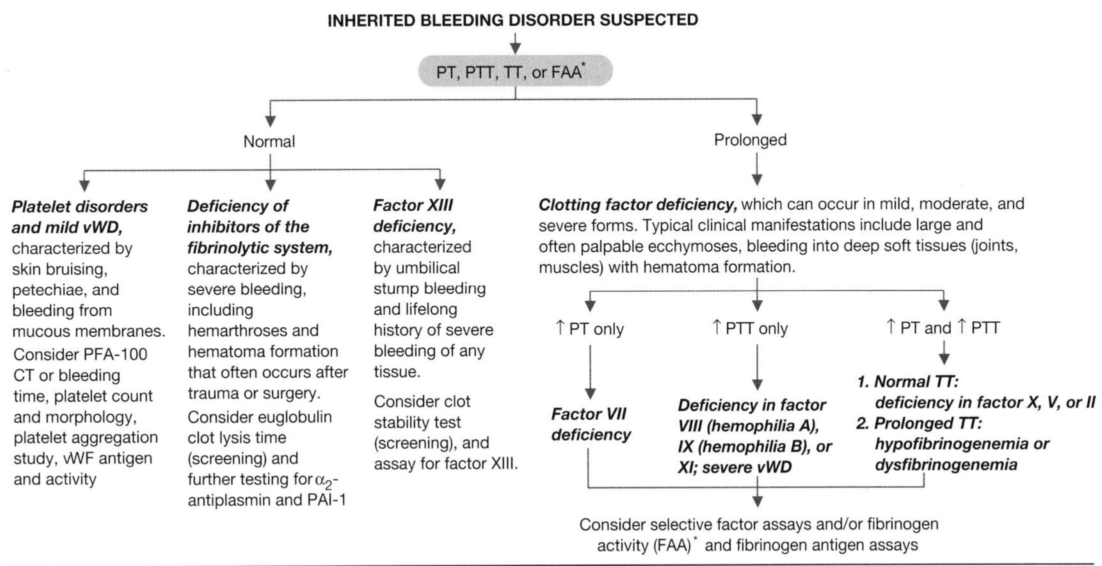

*FAA (fibrinogen activity assay) is now routinely available in clinical laboratories and has largely replaced the need for TT for evaluation of fibrinogen activity (function).

FIGURE 5-1 Bleeding disorders, inherited: Evaluation of suspected inherited bleeding disorders. PAI-1, plasminogen activator inhibitor 1; PFA-100 CT, platelet function analyzer-100 closure time; PT, prothrombin time; PTT, partial thromboplastin time; TT, thrombin time; vWD, von Willebrand disease; vWF, von Willebrand factor. (From Nicoll D, Mark Lu C, Pignone M, Mcphee SJ. *Pocket Guide to Diagnostic Tests*, 6th ed. www.accessmedicine.com. Copyright © The McGraw-Hill Companies, Inc. All rights reserved.)

KEY FEATURES

Description

- Disorders involving slower than normal blood clotting
- Occurs spontaneously or as an excessive response to injury leading to bleeding into joints (termed hemarthrosis) or tissues

Essentials of Diagnosis

- Classification
  - Hepatic disease
  - Vitamin K deficiency
  - Renal disease
- Laboratory values
- Identifying the underlying cause

General Considerations

- Vitamin K deficiency can be a result of malabsorption disorders
- Liver disorders
  - Decreased synthesis of coagulation
  - Impaired clearance of activated hemostatic components

Demographics

- Acquired or hereditary.
- Factor V Leiden mutation in 5% of Caucasian population.
- Vitamin K deficiency can occur in a newborn or later stages in life where there is intestinal malabsorption.[4]

CLINICAL FINDINGS

SIGNS AND SYMPTOMS[4]

- Shock including end-organ dysfunction
- Diffuse bleeding
  - Hematuria
  - Melena
  - Purpura
  - Petechiae
- Thrombotic lesions
  - Major vessel thrombosis
  - Purpura fulminans

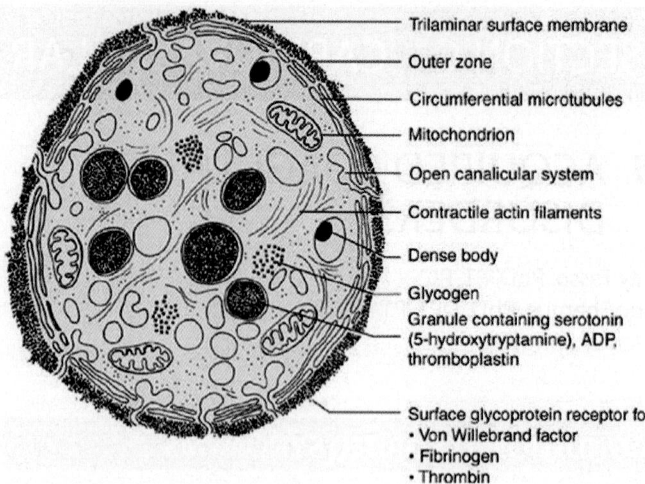

FIGURE 5-2 Structure of a normal platelet. ADP, adenosine diphosphate. (From Chandrasoma P, Taylor CR. *Concise Pathology*, 3rd ed. www.accessmedicine.com. Copyright © The McGraw-Hill Companies, Inc. All rights reserved.)

Functional Implications

- Bleeding episodes
- Excessive bruising

Possible Contributing Causes[5]

- Hemophilia
- Endothelial damage from endotoxin or virus
- Tissue necrosis from burns
- Diffuse ischemic injury from shock or hypoxia acidosis
- Systemic release of tissue procoagulants from cancer and placental disorders
- Liver disease
- Vitamin K deficiency
- von Willebrand disease
- Broad-spectrum antibiotics
- Fulminant hepatitis
- Acute fatty liver from pregnancy

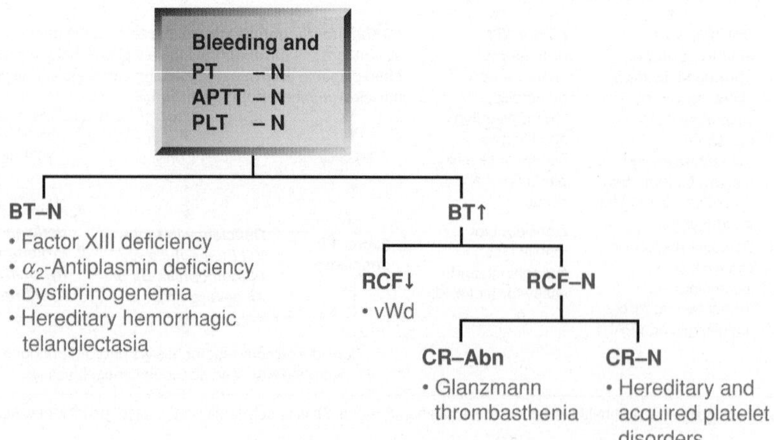

FIGURE 5-3 Tentative diagnoses in patients with bleeding manifestations and normal primary hemostatic tests using secondary tests. Abn, abnormal; aPTT, activated partial thromboplastin time; BT, bleeding time; CR, clot retraction; N, normal; PK, prekallikrein; PLT, platelets; PT, prothrombin time; RCF, ristocetin cofactor activity; vWd, von Willebrand disease. (From Kaushansky K, Lichtman M, Beutler E, Kipps T, Prchal J, Seligsohn U. *Williams Hematology*, 8th ed. www.accessmedicine.com. Copyright © The McGraw-Hill Companies, Inc. All rights reserved.)

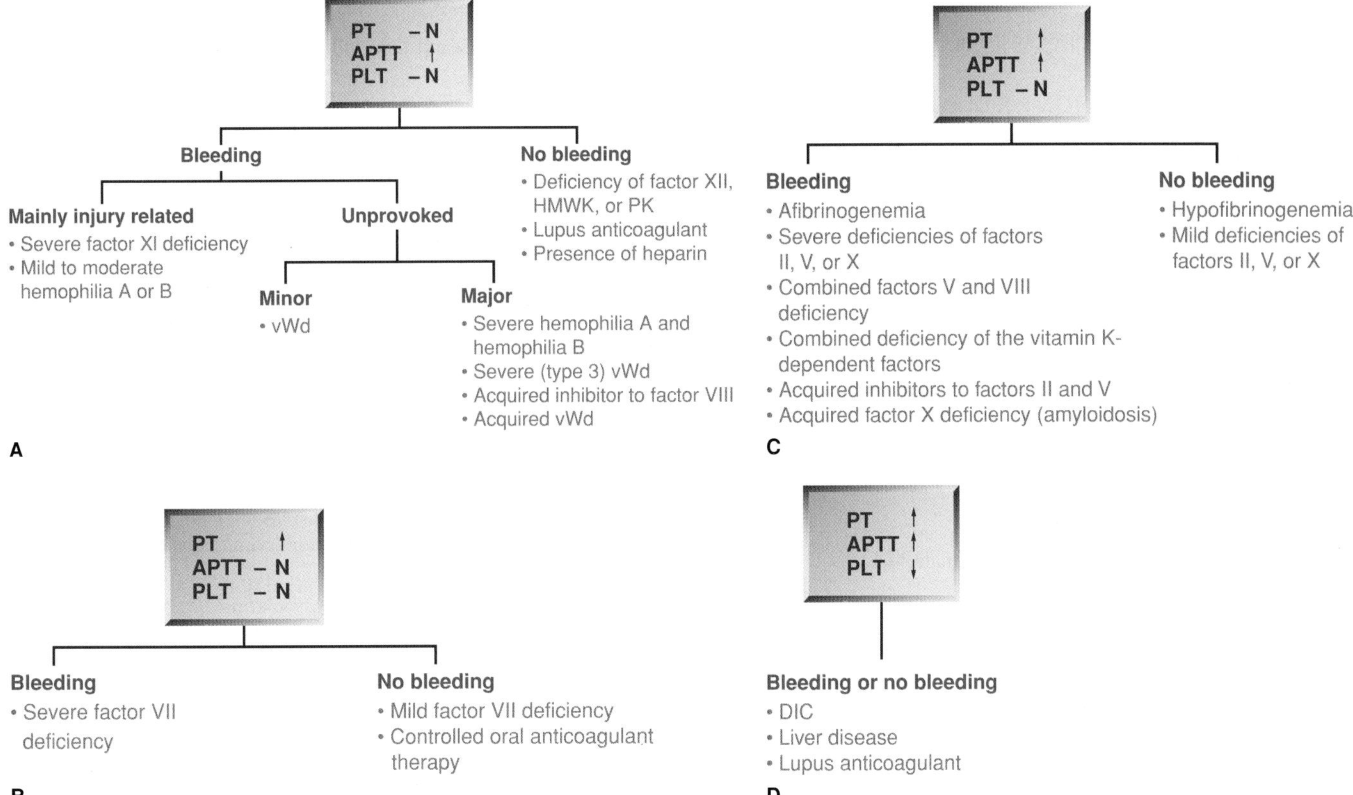

FIGURE 5-4 Measures for establishing a tentative diagnosis of a hemostatic disorder using basic tests of hemostasis and the patient's history of bleeding. aPTT, activated partial thromboplastin time; BT, bleeding time; DIC, disseminated intravascular coagulation; HK, high-molecular-weight kininogen; N, normal; PK, prekallikrein; PLT, platelets; PT, prothrombin time; vWd, von Willebrand disease. (From Kaushansky K, Lichtman M, Beutler E, Kipps T, Prchal J, Seligsohn U. *Williams Hematology*, 8th edition. www.accessmedicine.com. Copyright © The McGraw-Hill Companies, Inc. All rights reserved.)

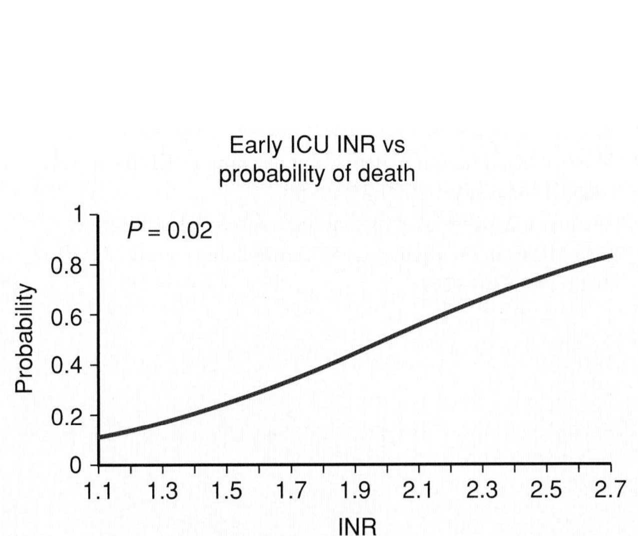

FIGURE 5-5 The relationship between coagulopathy and mortality in trauma patients. Civilian trauma data show that severity of coagulopathy as determined by an increasing International Normalized Ratio (INR) early after intensive care unit (ICU) admission is predictive of mortality. (From Gonzalez EA, Moore FA, Holcomb JB, et al. Fresh frozen plasma should be given earlier to patients requiring massive transfusion. *J Trauma*. 2007;62:112–119, with permission.)

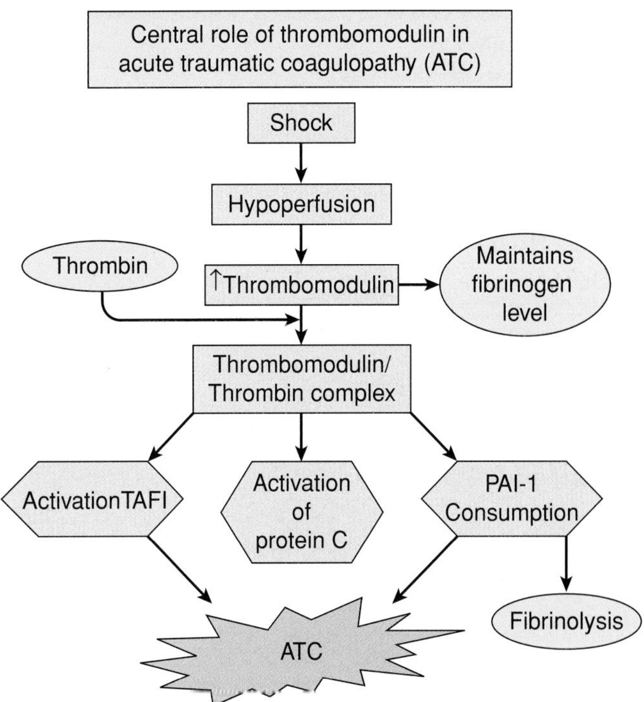

FIGURE 5-6 Illustration of the pathophysiologic mechanism responsible for the acute coagulopathy of trauma. PAI-1, plasminogen activator inhibitor 1; TAFI, thrombin-activatable fibrinolysis inhibitor. (From Brunicardi FC, Andersen D, Billiar T, et al. *Schwartz's Principles of Surgery*, 9th ed. www.accessmedicine.com. Copyright © The McGraw-Hill Companies, Inc. All rights reserved.)

Differential Diagnosis

- Coagulopathy of liver disease (hepatic synthetic dysfunction)

MEANS OF CONFIRMATION OR DIAGNOSIS

Laboratory Tests

- CBC
- Coagulation tests
- Platelet count
- Clotting time
- Bleeding time (BT)
- PT
- Partial thromboplastin time (PPT)
- Thrombin time (TT)

FINDINGS AND INTERPRETATION[5]

- Consumptive coagulopathy
  - Prolonged
    - Activated partial thromboplastin time (aPTT)
    - PT
    - TT
- Increase in fibrin–fibrinogen split products (FSP)
- Elevated levels of plasma *D*-dimer
- Decreased plasma fibrinogen or platelets

TREATMENT

Medications

- Replacement therapy for consumptive coagulopathy
- Anticoagulant therapy for coagulation activation
- Specific factor concentrates

REFERRALS/ADMITTANCE

- Genetic counselor
- Physician for laboratory tests

IMPAIRMENTS

- Unable to participate in contact sports

TESTS AND MEASURES

- Skin observation

INTERVENTION

- Mostly medical interventions
- Modalities to slow or decreased bleeding, compression
- Education on refraining from activities that can cause injury, like contact sports

FUNCTIONAL GOALS

- Patient will understand risks of bleeding.

PROGNOSIS

- If the pathogenic process underlying is reversed, often no other therapy is needed.[6]

PATIENT RESOURCE

- Overview of Coagulation Disorders. The Merk Manual for Health Professionals. http:/www.merckmanuals.com/professional/hematology_and_oncology/coagulation_disorders/overview_of_coagulation_disorders.html. Accessed January 20, 2013.

REFERENCES

1. ICD9DATA. http://www.icd9data.com. Accessed January 19, 2013.
2. ICD10DATA. http://www.icd10data.com. Accessed January 20, 2013.
3. The American Physical Therapy Association. *Interactive Guide to Physical Therapist Practice.* Alexandria, VA: The American Physical Therapy Association; 2003. http://guidetoptpractice.apta.org/. Accessed March 20, 2013.
4. Prentice CR. Acquired coagulation disorders. *Clin Haematol.* 1985;14(2):413–442.
5. Hay WW, Levin MJ, Deterding RR, Abzug MJ, Sondheimer JM. Bleeding disorders. In: Hay WW, Levin MJ, Deterding RR, Abzug MJ, Sondheimer JM, eds. *CURRENT Diagnosis & Treatment: Pediatrics.* 21st ed. New York, NY: McGraw-Hill; 2012. http://www.accessphysiotherapy.com/content/56826831. Accessed January 31, 2013.
6. Chandrasoma P, Taylor CR. Blood Coagulation. In: Chandrasoma P, Taylor CR, eds. *Concise Pathology.* 3rd ed. New York, NY: McGraw-Hill; 2011. http://www.accessphysiotherapy.com/content/187371. Accessed January 20, 2013.

ADDITIONAL REFERENCES

- Levi M. Guidelines for the diagnosis and management of disseminated intravascular coagulation. British Committee for Standards in Haematology. *Br J Haematol.* 2009;145:24–33.
- Shearer MJ. Vitamin K deficiency bleeding (VKDB) in early infancy. *Blood Rev.* 2009;23:49–59.
- Witmer CM. Off-label recombinant factor VIIa use and thrombosis in children: a multi-center cohort study. *J Pediatr.* 2011;158:820–825.

6 AORTIC REGURGITATION

Natalie V. Wessel, DO, MPH
Eric Shamus, PhD, DPT, PT, CSCS

CONDITION/DISORDER SYNONYMS

- Aortic insufficiency (AI)
- Aortic valve regurgitation

ICD-9-CM CODES

- 395.1 Rheumatic AI
- 746.4 Congenital insufficiency of aortic valve

ICD-10-CM CODES

- I06.1 Rheumatic AI
- I35 Nonrheumatic aortic valve disorders
- Q23.1 Congenital insufficiency of aortic valve

PREFERRED PRACTICE PATTERN

- 6D: Impaired Aerobic Capacity/Endurance Associated With Cardiovascular Pump Dysfunction or Failure[1]

PATIENT PRESENTATION

A 68-year old male presents with a "pounding" heartbeat when lying down, particularly on his left side. He reports intermittent chest pain that does not seem to be correlated with exercise and frequent episodes of palpitations. Vitals are: Pulse: 96, Respirations: 18, Blood Pressure: 140/50, and SpO_2% of 98%. On physical examination, the patient has a "water hammer" pulse in the brachial and radial arteries bilaterally. You notice a head bob occurring with each heart beat and audible systolic and diastolic sounds over the femoral arteries. On auscultation, there is a diastolic murmur in the second right intercostal space.

KEY FEATURES

Description

- Aortic valve does not close tightly
- Inadequacy of the aortic valve or the aortic root
- Leaking of the aortic valve
- Blood flow in reverse direction: Some blood pumped out of the heart leaks back in
- Diastolic flow of blood from aorta into left ventricle
- Acute
  - No compensatory mechanism
  - Occurs suddenly
  - Shortness of breath
  - Pulmonary edema
  - Left-sided heart failure
- Chronic
  - Heart adapts to increased volume load early in disease process

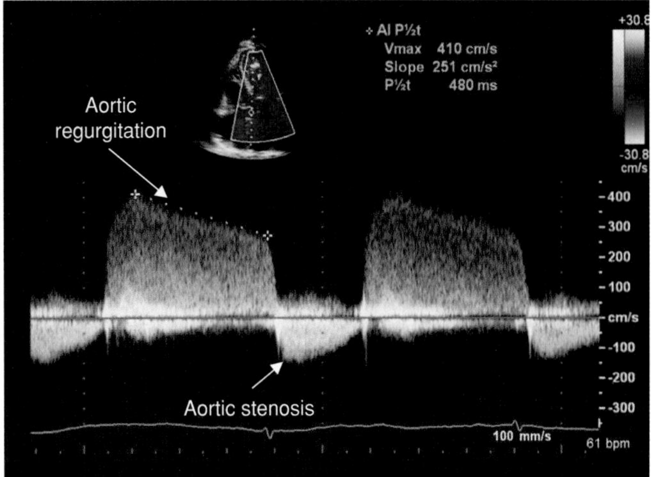

FIGURE 6-1 Aortic regurgitation. Apical five-chamber Doppler display of aortic valve regurgitation with a pressure half-time of 480 ms. P½t, pressure half-time. (From Pahlm O, Wagner GS. *Multimodal Cardiovascular Imaging: Principles and Clinical Applications*. www.accessmedicine.com. Copyright © The McGraw-Hill Companies, Inc. All rights reserved.)

  - Progresses to left-sided heart failure
  - Fatigue
- Increased diastolic pressure
- Increased volume of left ventricle of the heart
- Sites of aortic regurgitation (AR)[2]
  - Valvular
    - Cusp abnormalities
  - Aortic
    - Dilation

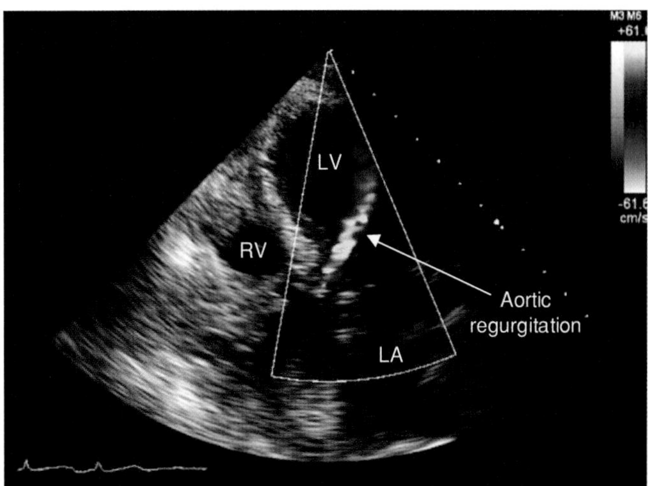

FIGURE 6-2 Aortic regurgitation. Apical five-chamber color flow image of aortic valve regurgitation. LA, left atrium; LV, left ventricle; RV, right ventricle. (From Pahlm O, Wagner GS. *Multimodal Cardiovascular Imaging: Principles and Clinical Applications*. www.accessmedicine.com. Copyright © The McGraw-Hill Companies, Inc. All rights reserved.)

- Inflammation
- Tears

Essentials of Diagnosis

- Stethoscope for auscultation provides a high pitched decrescendo diastolic murmur: Three murmurs can be heard
- EKG/ECG[3]
- Transthoracic echocardiogram
- Cardiac catheterization
- Chest X-ray
- Exercise stress test

General Considerations

- Education on disease management reduces hospitalization
- Strenuous activity should be limited
- Signs and symptoms should be monitored
- Emphasis on wellness and prevention

Demographics

- Chronic form begins after age 50 years; most severe after age 80 years

CLINICAL FINDINGS

SIGNS AND SYMPTOMS

- Increased stroke volume
- Cyanosis
- Hyperdynamic pulses[2]
- Third heart sound[2]
- Pulmonary edema
- Dyspnea on exertion
- Nocturnal dyspnea
- Diaphoresis
- Apical impulse[2]
- Angina pectoris[2]
- Syncope[2]
- Congestive heart failure[2]
- Dyspnea on exertion
- Shortness of breath[2]
- Anginal chest pain that increases with exercise
- Orthopnea[2]
- Fatigue, weakness[2]
- Fainting, dizziness with activity
- Palpitations
- Palpable heaves or thrills over precordium
- Audible diastolic murmur in midclavicular fifth intercostal space[2]
- Swelling of feet and ankles

Functional Implications

- Symptoms depend on the degree of valve regurgitation.
- Patients may be unaware of their reduced cardiovascular capacity.
- Patients at higher risk of atrial arrhythmias and embolic events.
- Fatigue from pulmonary edema.

Possible Contributing Causes

- Causes of AR[2]
  - Endocarditis
  - Infectious illness
  - Ankylosing spondylitis
  - Marfan syndrome
  - Ehler–Danlos syndrome
  - Aortitis
  - High blood pressure
  - Aortic root disease
  - Dilation of ascending aorta
  - Syphilis
  - Reiter syndrome
  - Trauma
  - Congenital valve dysfunction
  - Rheumatic fever
  - Coronary artery disease

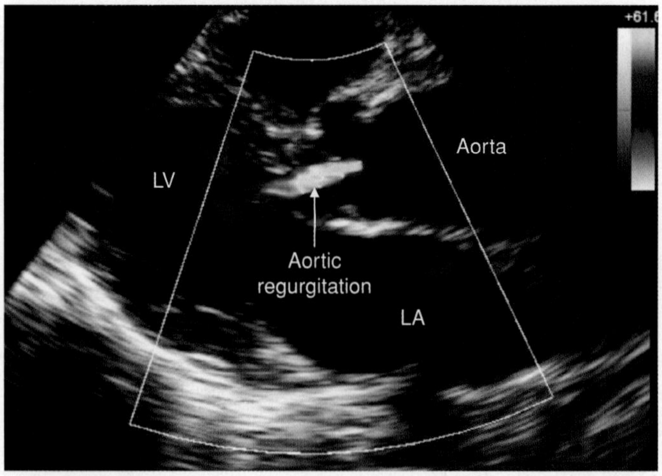

FIGURE 6-3 Aortic regurgitation. Parasternal long axis color flow image of aortic valve regurgitation. LA, left atrium; LV, left ventricle. (From Pahlm O, Wagner GS. *Multimodal Cardiovascular Imaging: Principles and Clinical Applications*. www.accessmedicine.com.)

  - Hyperlipoproteinemia
  - Hypertension
  - Diabetes mellitus
  - Older age

Differential Diagnosis

- Acute coronary syndrome
- Aortic stenosis
- Cardiac pump dysfunction
  - Cardiac muscle dysfunction produces slight-to-moderate reduction in cardiac output (CO).
  - Mild-to-moderate activity limitation
  - Functional capacity of ≤5 to 6 metabolic equivalents (METS)

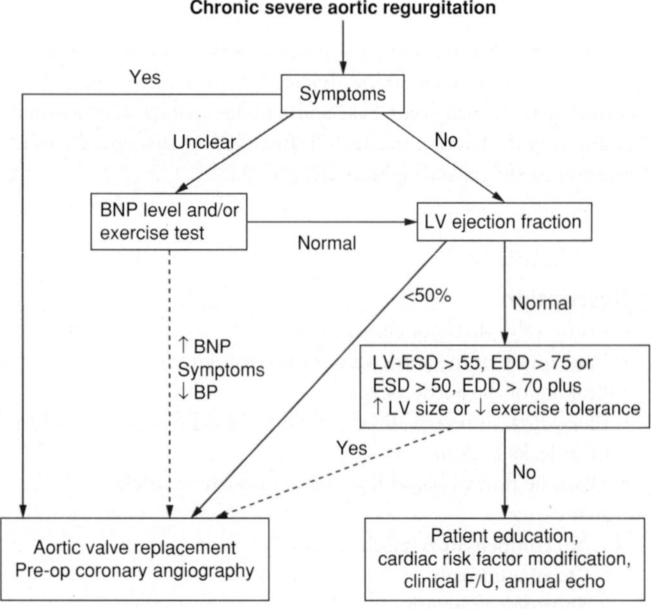

FIGURE 6-4 Suggested algorithm for management of adults with severe chronic aortic regurgitation.[92] BNP, brain natriuretic peptide; BP, blood pressure; EDD, end-diastolic diameter; ESD, end-systolic diameter; F/U, follow-up; LV, left ventricular. (From Fuster V, Walsh RA, Harrington RA. *Hurst's The Heart*, 13th ed. www.accessmedicine.com.)

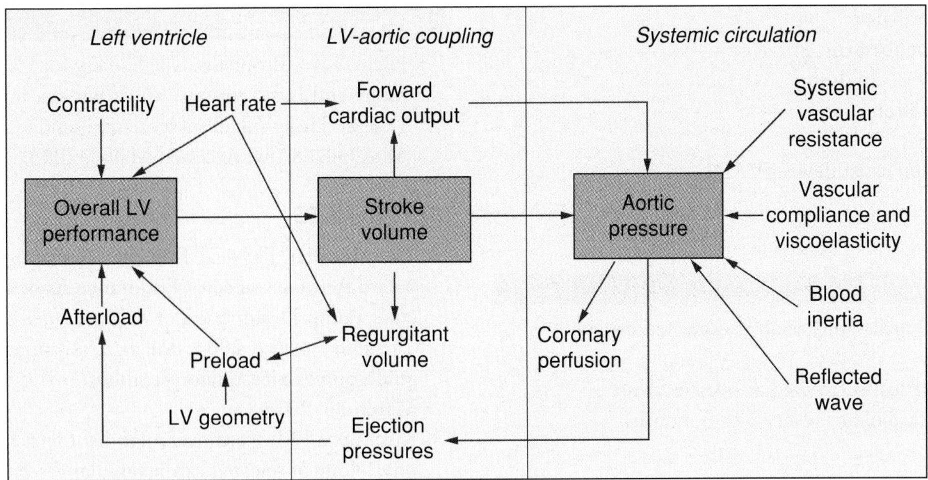

FIGURE 6-5 Pathophysiology of chronic aortic regurgitation. Left ventricular (LV) stroke volume includes forward cardiac output and regurgitant volume. Although increased stroke volume increases systemic systolic ejection pressure and aortic pressure, increased regurgitant volume lowers systemic diastolic pressures and, as a result, coronary perfusion. Compensatory mechanisms of the LV to maintain cardiac output despite increased regurgitant volume include dilation and remodeling of the LV. When compensatory mechanisms fail, there is adverse effect on LV contractility. The volume of regurgitant flow is determined by the diastolic pressure difference between the aorta and LV, the size of the regurgitant orifice, the duration of diastole, and the relative compliance of the aorta and LV. (Modified with permission from Borow KM, Marcus RH. Aortic regurgitation: the need for an integrated physiologic approach. *J Am Coll Cardiol*. 1991;17(4):898–900.)

- Cardiac pump failure
  - Cardiac muscle dysfunction produces moderate-to-severe reduction in CO
  - Marked activity limitation
  - Functional capacity of ≤4 to 5 METS
- Mitral regurgitation
- Mitral valve stenosis/prolapse
- Myocardial infarction
- Shock, hypovolemia

MEANS OF CONFIRMATION OR DIAGNOSIS

Imaging

- Transesophageal echocardiography (TEE)
  - Aortic leaflets thickened and calcified
  - Presence of congenital bicuspid aortic valve
  - Hypertrophic left ventricular wall
  - Doppler flow will show increased jet velocity across the valve
  - Increased pulmonary artery pressure
- Angiogram/Aortogram
- Radionuclide ventriculogram
- MRI of the heart
- Chest X-ray
  - Left atrial enlargement
  - Pulmonary edema from valvular-induced heart failure
- Electrocardiogram ECG/EKG
  - Left atrial hypertrophy
  - ST–T wave changes
  - Possible left ventricular hypertrophy

Diagnostic Procedures

- Elevated left atrial pressure
  - Indirect measure of elevated pulmonary vein pressure
- Cardiac catheterization
  - Assessment of coronary artery disease, ejection fraction (EF), pulmonary artery wedge pressure, and mitral valve function
  - Phonocardiogram[2]

FINDINGS AND INTERPRETATION

- Use an electronically amplified stethoscope
  - Murmur difficult to hear and rarely detected
- Can lead to sudden cardiac death, arrhythmias, increased risk of bleeding, embolic events, coronary disease
- Characteristics of heart failure
  - Chest X-ray evidence of pulmonary edema
  - Signs and symptoms of right and left heart failure
  - Markedly decreased exercise tolerance
  - Decreased systolic BP during exercise
  - EF <30 to 40%
  - Disability
  - Markedly decreased quality of life
- 12-lead EKG/ECG that may be observed
  - Notched P wave
  - Associated ST-T wave changes
- Echocardiogram
  - Congenital anatomic abnormalities
  - Pulmonary vein pressure
  - Fluid overload
- Cardiac catheterization
  - Pulmonary vein pressure

TREATMENT

Medication

- For heart failure induced by AR
  - Diuretics
  - Beta-blockers
  - Positive inotropic agents
  - Angiotensin-converting enzyme (ACE)
  - Aldosterone antagonists
  - Antibiotics for patients with history of rheumatic fever
  - Inpatient pharmacologic management[4]

MEDICAL PROCEDURES

- Dietary instruction
  - Sodium restriction
  - May require limited fluid intake

- Internal cardiac defibrillator
- Aortic valve replacement/repair
- Balloon valvuloplasty in children
- Cardiac resynchronization
- Coronary artery bypass
- Left or right ventricular assist device (VAD)
- Cardiac transplant

REFERRALS/ADMITTANCE

- To primary care or cardiac physician if suspected cardiac muscle dysfunction
- To ER or call 911 if suspected cardiac muscle failure
- Patient must see a cardiologist every 3 to 6 months

IMPAIRMENTS

- Significant morbidity from pulmonary edema
- Shortness of breath
- Dyspnea on exertion
- Limited activity tolerance
- Limited functional capacity

TEST AND MEASURES

- 6-minute walk test
  - For mild or nonsymptomatic cases
- Borg Rating of Perceived Exertion (RPE)
- Monitor vital signs to include lung auscultations
- Short-Form 36
- New York Heart Association Functional Classification Scale

INTERVENTION

- Risk-factor modification
- Cardiac rehabilitation[5]
  - Decreases morbidity and mortality
  - Three phases[5]
- Education on signs and symptoms
- Aerobic exercise training as tolerated
- Resistance exercise training

FUNCTIONAL GOALS

- Patient will be able to
  - State the signs and symptoms of AR.
  - Tolerate 30 minutes of continuous exercise while maintaining stable vital signs and RPE of 13.
- Short-term goals[5]
  - "Reconditioning" sufficient for resuming normal activities.
  - Limiting physiologic and psychological effects of AR.
  - Reduced risk of sudden cardiac arrest or myocardial infarction.
  - Controlling symptoms of cardiac disease.
- Long-term goals[5]
  - Identification and treatment of risk factors.
  - Stabilizing or reversing atherosclerotic processes.
  - Improve patient's psychological status.

PROGNOSIS

- Depends on severity and cause of AR

PATIENT RESOURCE

- Heart Valve Problems. The Society for Cardiovascular Angiography and Interventions. http://www.scai.org/SecondsCount/Disease/HeartValveProblem.aspx?gclid=CIXO1Mrg2rUCFQ4FnQodz28Ajw. Accessed May 6, 2013.

REFERENCES

1. The American Physical Therapy Association. Pattern 6D: Impaired Aerobic Capacity/Endurance Associated With Cardiovascular Pump Dysfunction or Failure. *Interactive Guide to Physical Therapist Practice*. 2003. doi: 10.2522/ptguide.3.3_4. http://guidetoptpractice.apta.org/content/1/SEC30.extract. Accessed March 13, 2013.
2. Kusumoto FM. Cardiovascular disorders: Heart disease: pathophysiology of selected cardiovascular disorders. In: *Pathophysiology of Disease*. New York, NY: McGraw-Hill; 2009: Chapter 10. http://www.accessphysiotherapy.com/abstract/5367685#5367687. Accessed March 13, 2013.
3. Cassady SL, Cahalin LP. Cardiovascular pathophysiology. In: DeTurk WE, Cahalin LP, eds. *Cardiovascular and Pulmonary Physical Therapy*. New York, NY; McGraw-Hill: 2011: Chapter 6. http://www.accessphysiotherapy.com/abstract/6872858. Accessed March 13, 2013.
4. Miyamoto SD, Sondheimer HM, Fagan TE, Collins KK. Cardiovascular diseases. In: Hay W, Levin MJ, Sondheimer JM, Detering RR, eds. *CURRENT Diagnosis & Treatment: Pediatrics*. New York, NY: McGraw-Hill; 2011: Chapter 19. http://www.accessphysiotherapy.com/abstract/6583154#6583208. Accessed March 13, 2013.
5. Dutton M. *McGraw-Hill's NPTE (National Physical Therapy Examination)*, 2nd ed. New York, NY: McGraw-Hill; 2012. http://www.accessphysiotherapy.com/content/5401905. Accessed March 13, 2013.

ADDITIONAL REFERENCES

- Blume ED, Naftel DC, Bastardi HJ, Duncan BW, Kirklin JK, Webber SA. Outcomes of children bridged to heart transplantation with ventricular assist devices: a multi-institutional study. *Circulation*. 2006;113(19):2313–2319.
- Dubin D. *Rapid Interpretation of EKG's*. Fort Myers, FL: COVER Inc.; 2000.
- ICD9DATA. http://www.icd9data.com. Accessed March 13, 2013.
- ICD10DATA. http://www.icd10data.com. Accessed March 13, 2013.
- Kutryk M, Fitchett D. Hill's sign in aortic regurgitation: enhanced pressure wave transmission or artefact?. *Can J Cardiol*. 1997;13(3):237–240.
- McPhee SJ, Hammer GD. Valvular heart disease. In: McPhee SJ, Hammer GD, eds. *Pathophysiology of Disease*. 6th ed. New York, NY: McGraw-Hill; 2010. http://www.accessphysiotherapy.com/content/5367782. Accessed March 13, 2013.
- Panus PC, Jobst EE, Masters SB, Katzung B, Tinsley SL, Trevor AJ. *Pharmacology for the Physical Therapist*. New York, NY: McGraw-Hill; 2009. http://www.accessphysiotherapy.com/resource/615. Accessed March 13, 2013.
- Rosenthal D, Chrisant MR, Edens E, et al. International Society for Heart and Lung Transplantation: practice guidelines for management of heart failure in children. *J Heart Lung Transplant*. 2004;23(12):1313–1333.

7 AORTIC STENOSIS

Natalie V. Wessel, DO, MPH
Eric Shamus, PhD, DPT, PT, CSCS

CONDITION/DISORDER SYNONYMS

- Aortic valve stenosis
- Left ventricular outflow tract obstruction
- Rheumatic aortic stenosis
- Calcium aortic stenosis

ICD-9-CM CODES

- 395.0 Rheumatic aortic stenosis
- 396.0 Mitral valve stenosis and aortic valve stenosis
- 746.3 Congenital stenosis of aortic valve

ICD-10-CM CODES

- I06.0 Rheumatic aortic valve diseases
- I35.0 Aortic (valve) stenosis
- I35.2 Aortic (valve) stenosis with insufficiency
- Q23.0 Congenital stenosis of aortic valve

PREFERRED PRACTICE PATTERN

- 6D: Impaired aerobic capacity/endurance associated with cardiovascular pump dysfunction or failure[1]

PATIENT PRESENTATION

An 80-year-old male becomes short of breath while playing with his grandchildren at a family picnic. The patient states that he is dizzy and has chest pain. Vitals are: Pulse: 98, Respirations: 22, Blood pressure: 142/86, and SpO_2% of 96%. On physical examination, the patient has a slow rate of rise in the carotid pulse, a systolic ejection murmur at the right second intercostal space and a reduced intensity of the second heart sound. The EKG reveals left ventricular hypertrophy, but no ST-T wave changes and a chest X-ray shows a rounding of the left ventricular apex.

KEY FEATURES

Description

- Aortic valve does not open fully[2]
- Narrowing of the aortic valve causing left ventricular outflow tract obstruction[2]
- Causes decreased blood flow from left ventricle into the ascending aorta
- Decreases blood flow from heart to rest of the body and brain
- Decreased flow can cause lightheadedness, fainting, chest pain
- Three types[2]
  - Congenital
  - Rheumatic
  - Degenerative

Essentials of Diagnosis

- Stethoscope auscultation for ejection murmur at right second intercostal space
- EKG/ECG[3]
- Echocardiogram
- Cardiac catheterization
- Chest X-ray
- Exercise stress test

General Considerations

- Education on disease management reduces hospitalization
- Patients with significant aortic stenosis (AS) should not participate in competitive sports, even without symptoms
- Strenuous activity should be limited for symptomatic AS
- Signs and symptoms should be monitored
- Emphasis on wellness and prevention
- Can lead to sudden cardiac death, arrhythmias, increased risk of bleeding, embolic events, coronary disease
- Children can develop bacterial endocarditis
- Can cause syncope, chest pain, heart failure if untreated

Demographics

- Can be congenital, present from birth
- More commonly develops later in life as a result of calcification of the valve or previous rheumatic fever
- More common in men than women

CLINICAL FINDINGS

SIGNS AND SYMPTOMS

- Symptoms depend on the degree of valve stenosis
- Patient may have no symptoms until stenosis progresses
- Audible systolic ejection murmur at right second intercostal space
- Angina pectoris[2]
- Syncope[2]
- Congestive heart failure[2]
- Dyspnea on exertion
- Shortness of breath[2]
- Anginal chest pain that increases with exercise
- Orthopnea[2]
- Fatigue, weakness[2]
- Fainting, dizziness with activity
- Palpitations
- Palpable heaves/thrills over precordium
- *Pulsus parvus et tardus:* Faint pulse or altered quality of pulse in the neck
- Arrhythmias
- Endocarditis

Functional Implications

- Mild-to-moderate stenosis generally does not cause symptoms
- Severe AS causes progressive shortness of breath, may be subtle
- Patients may be unaware of reduced cardiovascular capacity

Possible Contributing Causes

- Causes of AS include[2]
  - Individuals with a two-leaflet aortic valve instead of three-leaflet

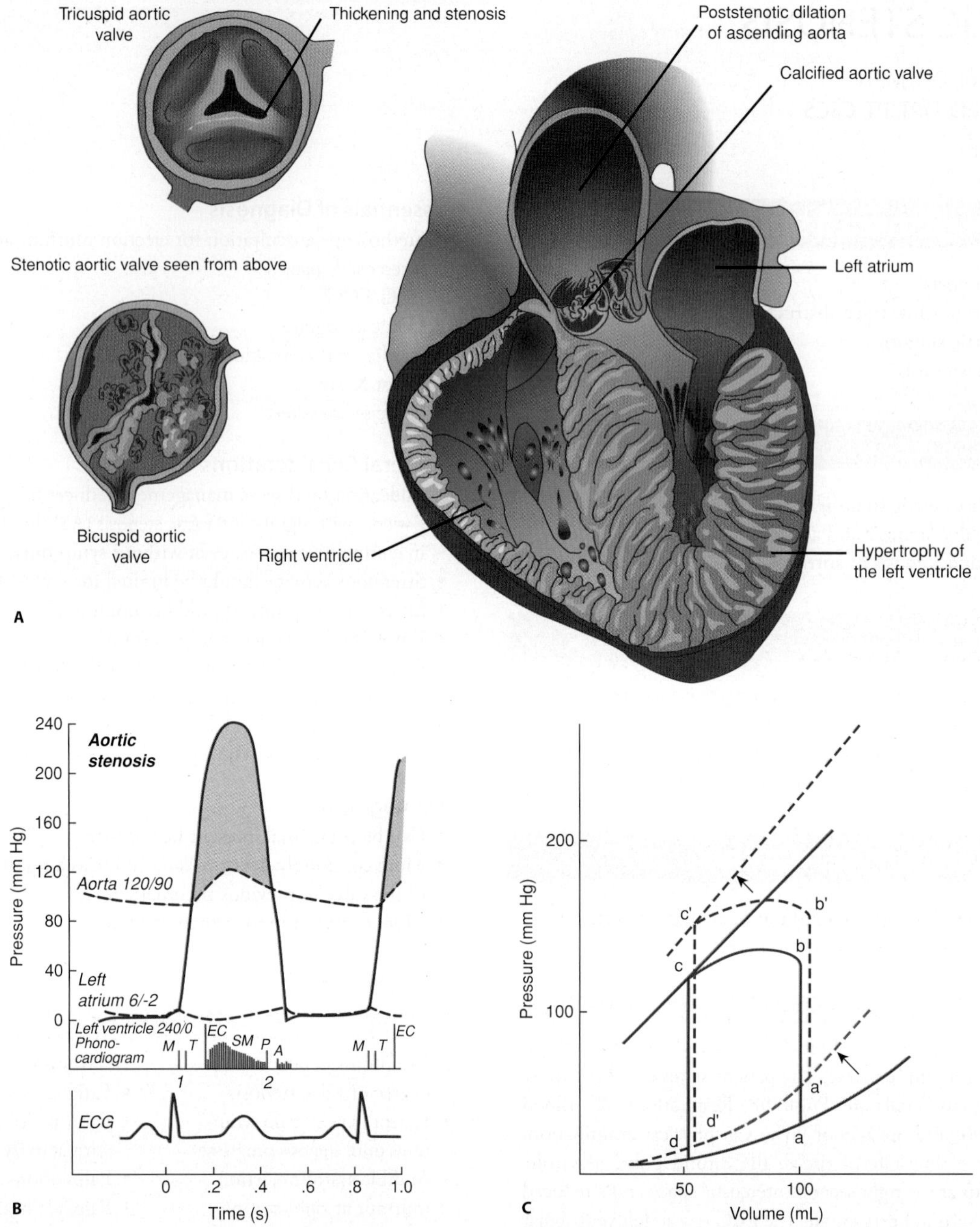

FIGURE 7-1 **A.** Drawing of the left heart in left anterior oblique view showing anatomic features of aortic stenosis. Note the structures enlarged: left ventricle (thickened); poststenotic dilation of the aorta. **B.** Drawing showing auscultatory and hemodynamic features of predominant aortic stenosis. Cardinal features include left ventricular hypertrophy; systolic ejection murmur. EC, ejection click; SM, systolic murmur; P, pulmonary valve; A, aortic valve. (Redrawn, with permission, from Cheitlin MD, Sokolow M, McIlroy MB. *Clinical Cardiology*, 6th ed. Originally published by Appleton & Lange. Copyright © 1993 by the McGraw-Hill Companies, Inc.) **C.** Pressure–volume loop in aortic stenosis. The left ventricle becomes thickened and less compliant, forcing the diastolic pressure–volume curve upward, which results in elevated left ventricular end-diastolic pressure (**a'**). Because the left ventricle must pump against a fixed gradient (increased afterload), b increases to **b'**. Finally, the hypertrophy of the ventricle results in increased inotropic force, which shifts the isovolumic pressure curve leftward. (From McPhee SJ, Hammer GD. *Pathophysiology of Disease: An Introduction to Clinical Medicine*, 6th ed. www.accessmedicine.com. Copyright © The McGraw-Hill Companies, Inc. All rights reserved.)

- Age-related progressive calcification
- Calcification of congenital bicuspid aortic valve
- Acute rheumatic fever
- Coronary artery disease
- Diabetes mellitus
- Hyperlipoproteinemia
- Hypertension
- Uremia
- Older age

Differential Diagnosis

- Acute coronary syndrome
- Cardiac pump dysfunction
  - Cardiac muscle dysfunction produces slight-to-moderate reduction in cardiac output (CO)
  - Mild-to-moderate activity limitation
  - Functional capacity of ≤5 to 6 metabolic equivalents (METS)
- Cardiac pump failure

- Cardiac muscle dysfunction produces moderate-to-severe reduction in CO
- Marked activity limitation
- Functional capacity of ≤4 to 5 METS

- Mitral regurgitation
- Mitral stenosis
- Mitral valve prolapse
- Myocardial infarction
- Shock, hypovolemia

MEANS OF CONFIRMATION OR DIAGNOSIS

Imaging

- Echocardiography
  - Aortic leaflets thickened and calcified
  - Presence of congenital bicuspid aortic valve
  - Hypertrophic left ventricular wall
  - Doppler flow will show increased jet velocity across the valve
  - Increased pulmonary artery pressure
- MRI of the heart
- Chest X-ray
  - Left ventricular hypertrophy
  - Possible calcification of aortic leaflets and aortic root
- EKG
  - Left ventricular hypertrophy
  - ST–T wave changes
  - Possible left atrial hypertrophy

Diagnostic Procedures

- Elevated pulmonary artery pressure
  - Indirect measure of elevated left ventricular pressure
- Left cardiac catheterization
  - Assessment of coronary artery disease, ejection fraction (EF), pulmonary artery wedge pressure
  - Phonocardiogram[2]

FINDINGS AND INTERPRETATION

- Crescendo–decrescendo systolic ejection murmur in right second intercostal space
- Slow rate of rise in carotid pulse
- Reduced intensity of second heart sound
- Precordial palpitations
- Characteristics of heart failure
  - Chest X-ray evidence of pulmonary edema
  - Signs and symptoms of right and left heart failure
  - Markedly decreased exercise tolerance
  - Decreased systolic BP during exercise
  - EF <30 to 40%
  - Disability
  - Markedly decreased quality of life
- 12-lead EKG/ECG that may be observed
  - Voltage of QRS complex markedly increased
  - Often associated ST–T wave changes
- Echocardiogram
  - Thickened and calcified aortic leaflets
  - Possible congenital bicuspid valve
  - Hypertrophied left ventricular wall
  - Increased pulmonary artery pressure
- Cardiac catheterization

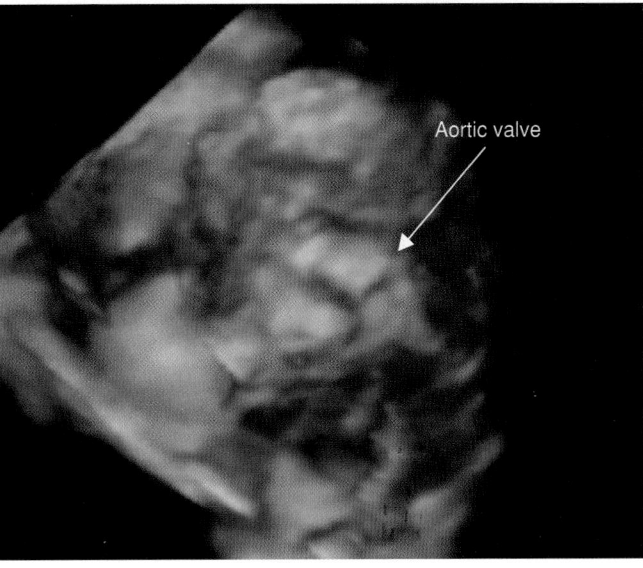

FIGURE 7-2 Aortic stenosis. Three-dimensional illustration of calcific aortic stenosis. (From Pahlm O, Wagner GS. *Multimodal Cardiovascular Imaging: Principles and Clinical Applications*. www.accessmedicine.com. Copyright © The McGraw-Hill Companies, Inc. All rights reserved.)

- Elevated pulmonary artery pressure
- Elevated pressure around the aortic valve

TREATMENT

Medication

- For heart failure induced by AS
  - Diuretics
  - Beta-blockers
  - Positive inotropic agents
  - Angiotensin-converting enzyme
  - Aldosterone antagonists
  - Antibiotics for patients with history of rheumatic fever
  - Inpatient pharmacologic management[4]

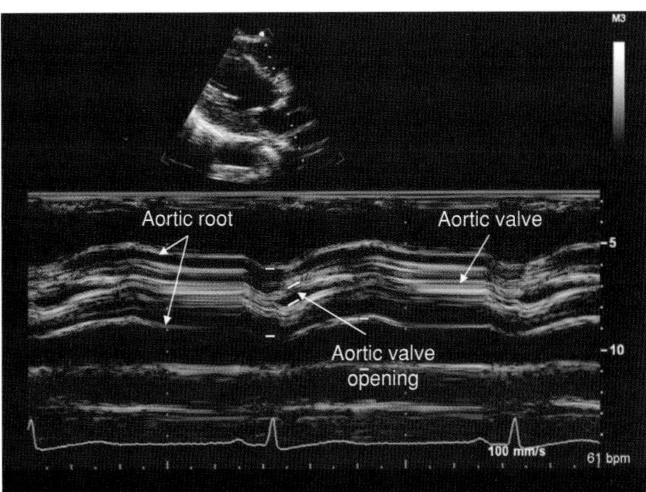

FIGURE 7-3 Aortic stenosis. Parasternal long axis M-mode image demonstrating thickened aortic valve leaflets with diminished systolic opening. (From Pahlm O, Wagner GS. *Multimodal Cardiovascular Imaging: Principles and Clinical Applications*. www.accessmedicine.com. Copyright © The McGraw-Hill Companies, Inc. All rights reserved.)

MEDICAL PROCEDURES

- Dietary instruction
  - Sodium restriction
  - May require limited fluid intake
- Internal cardiac defibrillator
- Aortic valve replacement/repair
- Balloon valvuloplasty in children
- Cardiac resynchronization
- Coronary artery bypass
- Left or right ventricular assist device (VAD)
- Cardiac transplant

REFERRALS/ADMITTANCE

- To primary care or cardiac physician if suspected cardiac muscle dysfunction
- To ER or call 911 if suspected cardiac muscle failure
- Patient must see a cardiologist every 3 to 6 months

IMPAIRMENTS

- Shortness of breath
- Dyspnea on exertion
- Limited activity tolerance
- Limited functional capacity

TEST AND MEASURES

- 6-minute walk test for mild or nonsymptomatic cases
- Borg Rating of Perceived Exertion (RPE)
- Monitor vital signs to include lung auscultations
- Short-Form 36
- New York Heart Association Functional Classification scale

TABLE 7-1 Rating of Perceived Exertion

Scale	Verbal Rating
6	
7	Very, very light
8	
9	Very light
10	
11	Fairly light
12	
13	Somewhat hard
14	
15	Hard
16	
17	Very hard
18	
19	Very, very hard
20	

Source: Borg GAV: Psychophysical basis of perceived exertion. *Med Sci Sports Exerc.* 1992;14:377–381.

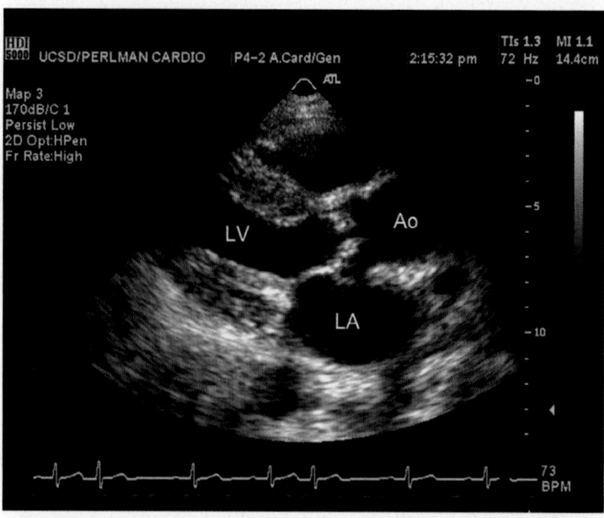

FIGURE 7-4 Parasternal long-axis plane demonstrating a thickened, stenotic aortic valve. Ao, aorta; LA, left atrium; LV, left ventricle. (Reproduced with permission from Fuster V, O'Rourke RA, Walsh RA, Poole-Wilson P, eds. *Hurst's The Heart*, 12th ed. Copyright © 2008, McGraw-Hill, New York.)

INTERVENTION

- Risk-factor modification
- Cardiac rehabilitation[5]
  - Decreases morbidity and mortality
  - Three phases[5]
- Education on signs and symptoms
- Nonaerobic resistance training

FIGURE 7-5 Pathologic variations in the heart sounds. Pulmonary hypertension causes an increased P2. Right bundle branch block delays right ventricular emptying, increasing the normal split and accentuating P2. Pulmonic stenosis also delays P2, but decreases its intensity. In left bundle branch block and aortic stenosis, LV ejection is delayed so A2 coincides with P2 and the normal expiratory movement of P2 causes paradoxic splitting during expiration. (From LeBlond RF, DeGowin RL, Brown DD. *DeGowin's Diagnostic Examination*, 9th ed. www.accessmedicine.com. Copyright © The McGraw-Hill Companies, Inc. All rights reserved.)

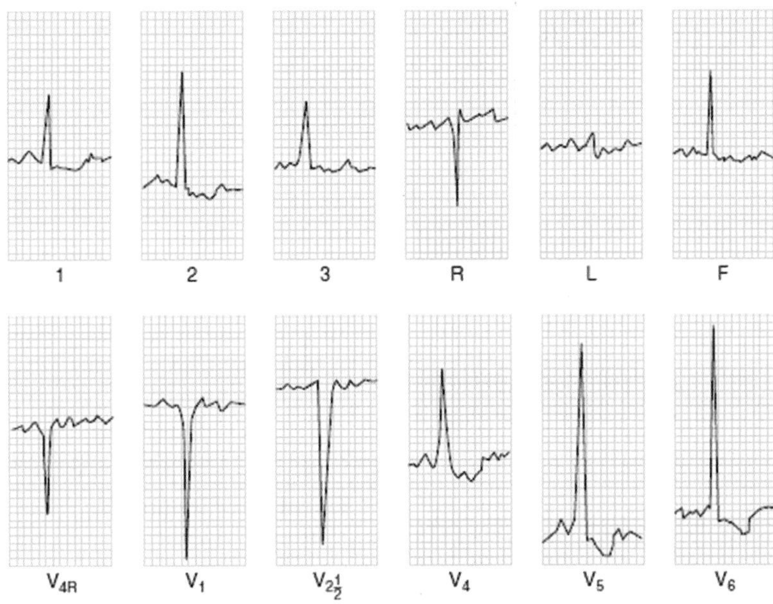

FIGURE 7-6 ECG of a patient with aortic stenosis is consistent with severe left ventricular hypertrophy. (Reproduced, with permission, from Fuster V, O'Rourke RA, Walsh RA, et al. *Hurst's the Heart.* 12th ed. New York, NY: McGraw-Hill, 2008. Fig. 82–23.)

FUNCTIONAL GOALS

- Patient will be able to
  - State the signs and symptoms of AS.
  - Tolerate 30 minutes of continuous exercise while maintaining stable vital signs and RPE of 13.
- Short-term goals[5]
  - "Reconditioning" sufficient for resuming normal activities.
  - Limiting physiologic and psychological effects of AS.
  - Reduced risk of sudden cardiac arrest or myocardial infarction.
  - Controlling symptoms of cardiac disease.
- Long-term goals[5]
  - Identification and treatment of risk factors.
  - Stabilizing or reversing atherosclerotic processes.
  - Improving patient's psychological status.

PROGNOSIS

- Depends on severity and cause of AS.
- Valve problems can develop 5 to 10 years after episode of rheumatic fever.

PATIENT RESOURCE

- Aortic Valve Stenosis (AVS). American Heart Association. http://www.heart.org/HEARTORG/Conditions/CongenitalHeartDefects/AboutCongenitalHeartDefects/Aortic-Valve-Stenosis-AVS_UCM_307020_Article.jsp. Accessed June 16, 2013.

REFERENCES

1. The American Physical Therapy Association. Pattern 6D: Impaired aerobic capacity/endurance associated with cardiovascular pump dysfunction or failure. *Interactive Guide to Physical Therapist Practice*. 2003. doi: 10.2522/ptguide.3.3_4. Accessed June 16, 2013.
2. Kusumoto FM. Cardiovascular disorders: heart disease. In: McPhee SJ, Hammer GD, eds. *Pathophysiology of Disease*. 6th ed. New York, NY: McGraw-Hill; 2010. http://www.accessphysiotherapy.com/content/5367631. Accessed June 16, 2013.
3. Cassady SL, Cahalin LP. Cardiovascular pathophysiology. In: DeTurk WE, Cahalin LP, eds. *Cardiovascular and Pulmonary Physical Therapy: An Evidence-Based Approach*. 2nd ed. New York, NY: McGraw-Hill; 2011. http://www.accessphysiotherapy.com/abstract/6872858. Accessed June 16, 2013.
4. Miyamoto SD, Sondheimer HM, Fagan TE, Collins KK. Cardiovascular diseases. In: Hay WW, Levin MJ, Sondheimer JM, Deterding RR. *CURRENT Diagnosis & Treatment: Pediatrics*. 20th ed. New York, NY: McGraw-Hill; 2011. http://www.accessphysiotherapy.com/content/6583757. Accessed June 16, 2013.
5. Dutton M. Cardiovascular physical therapy. In: Dutton M, ed. *McGraw-Hill's NPTE (National Physical Therapy Examination), 2e*. New York, NY: McGraw-Hill; 2012. http://www.accessphysiotherapy.com/content/5401905. Accessed June 16, 2013.

ADDITIONAL REFERENCES

- Blume ED, Naftel DC, Bastardi HJ, Duncan BW, Kirklin JK, Webber SA. Outcomes of children bridged to heart transplantation with ventricular assist devices: a multi-institutional study. *Circulation*. 2006;113(19):2313–2319.
- Dubin D. *Rapid Interpretation of EKG's*. Fort Myers, FL: COVER Publishing Co.; 2000.
- Dutton M. Valvular disease. In: Dutton M, ed. *McGraw-Hill's NPTE (National Physical Therapy Examination), 2e*. New York, NY: McGraw-Hill; 2012. http://www.accessphysiotherapy.com/content/5401838. Accessed June 16, 2013.
- Panus PC, Jobst EE, Masters SB, Katzung B, Tinsley SL, Trevor AJ. *Pharmacology for the Physical Therapist*. New York, NY: McGraw-Hill; 2009. http://www.accessphysiotherapy.com/resource/615. Accessed June 16, 2013.
- Rosenthal D, Chrisant MR, Edens E, et al. International Society for Heart and Lung Transplantation: practice guidelines for management of heart failure in children. *J Heart Lung Transplant*. 2004;23(12):1313–1333.

8 CAROTID ARTERY DISEASE

Eric Shamus, PhD, DPT, PT, CSCS
Natalie V. Wessel, DO, MPH

CONDITION/DISORDER SYNONYM

- Carotid stenosis

ICD-9-CM CODE

- 433.1 Occlusion and stenosis of carotid artery

ICD-10-CM CODE

- I65.29 Occlusion and stenosis of unspecified carotid artery

PREFERRED PRACTICE PATTERN

- 5D: Impaired motor function and sensory integrity associated with nonprogressive disorders of the central nervous system—acquired in adolescence or adulthood[1]

PATIENT PRESENTATION

A 78-year-old male, with a history of TIA, presents for a general physical examination. He is on 81 mg of Aspirin, 40 mg of Lovastatin, and 50 mg of Hydrochlorothiazide. Vitals are: Pulse: 80 Respirations: 16, Blood Pressure: 132/88, Temperature: 98.2°F, and SpO_2% of 99%. On physical examination, the physician hears a bruit in the left side of the neck. The patient is sent for carotid ultrasound which reveals 70% blockage of the left carotid and 35% blockage of the right carotid.

KEY FEATURES

Description

- Carotid arteries become blocked or receive limited blood flow
- Carotid stenosis: Narrowing of the artery
- Plaque builds up in the artery
- Plaque can be stable and asymptomatic
- Clots can lead to a stroke
- Can result in a sudden, specific neurological deficit

Essentials of Diagnosis

- Stethoscope on carotid artery, bruit sound
- Lipid profile
- Triglycerides test
- Cerebrovascular accident (CVA) symptoms

General Considerations

- Ischemic (two types)
  - Thrombotic: Atherosclerotic plaques that form at the branching and curves of arteries in the brain can be large vessel thrombosis or small-vessel thrombosis.
  - Embolic: An embolus that forms somewhere other than in the brain, often the heart, and then travels to the brain and restricts or blocks blood flow to the brain.
    - Branches of the middle cerebral artery (MCA) are most commonly affected.

Demographics

- About four million Americans suffer physical impairments and disability from stroke.
- Two-thirds of all CVAs occur in individuals older than 65 years of age.
  - After age 55, risk of stroke doubles every 10 years.

(A) Hyperkinetic pulse

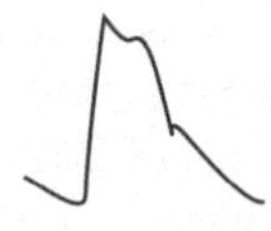

Normal

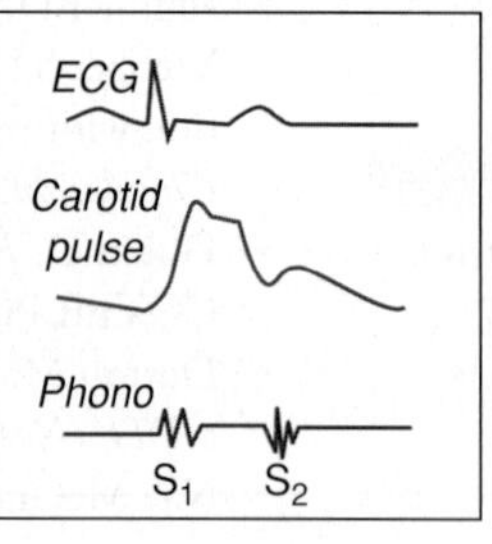

(B) Bisferiens pulse

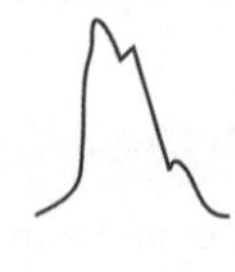

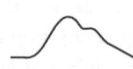

(C) Hypokinetic pulse

(D) Parvus et tardus pulse

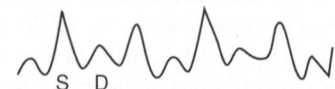

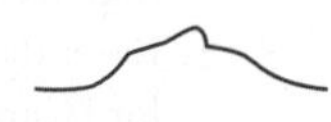

(E) Dicrotic pulse + alternans

S D

FIGURE 8-1 Schematic representation of the normal carotid arterial pulse, five types of abnormal pulses, and pulsus alternans. D, diastole; ECG, electrocardiogram; phono, phonocardiogram; S, systole; S_1, first heart sound; S_2, second heart sound. (From Fuster V, Walsh RA, Harrington RA. *Hurst's The Heart*, 13th ed. www.accessmedicine.com. Copyright © The McGraw-Hill Companies, Inc. All rights reserved.)

- Incidence is greater in men than in women and twice as high in Blacks as in Whites.
- Cerebral infarction (thrombosis or embolism) is the most common form, accounting for 70% of all strokes, followed by hemorrhages at 20%, and 10% unspecified.

CLINICAL FINDINGS

SIGNS AND SYMPTOMS

- Unlikely to have any narrowing or blockage of arteries
- Palpable pulse under the jaw line
- Headaches
- Blurred vision
- Memory loss
- Signs and symptoms are dependent on the part(s) of the brain affected by the CVA as well as the amount of damage to the tissues from obstruction or hemorrhage
- Weakness in a region, motor planning deficits
- Symptoms of CVA include
  - Aphasia
  - Autonomic dysfunction
  - Changes in consciousness
  - Cognitive impairment
  - Communication difficulties/ dysphagia
  - Dysarthria
  - Hemiplegia (most commonly) motor loss
  - Perceptual changes
  - Personality and behavioral changes
  - Sensory loss/dysfunction
  - Spasticity or hypertonicity
  - Visual field defects

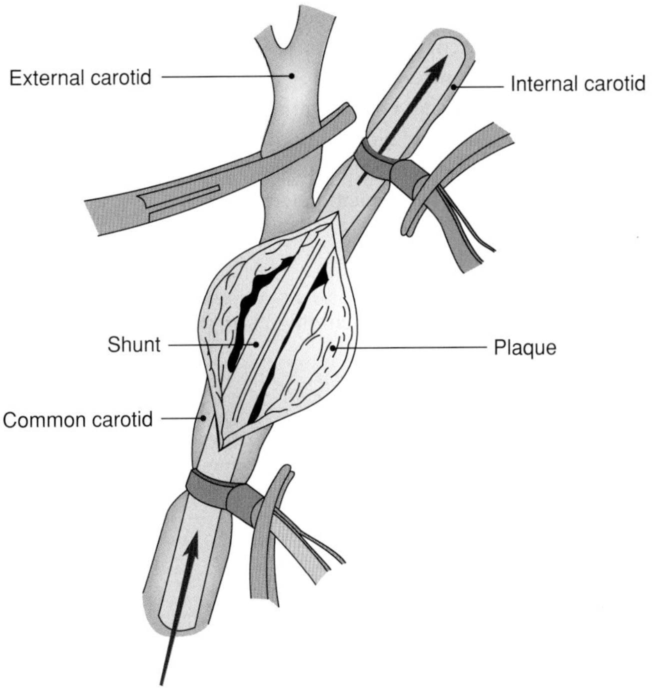

FIGURE 8-2 Indwelling shunt in place to preserve internal carotid flow during the endarterectomy. (From Fuster V, Walsh RA, Harrington RA. *Hurst's The Heart*, 13th ed. www.accessmedicine.com. Copyright © The McGraw-Hill Companies, Inc. All rights reserved.)

▶ Functional Implications

- CVA
  - Loss of independence with all aspects of mobility, ADLs, self-care
  - Loss of ability to interact with others effectively
  - Difficulty with cognitive processing, particularly executive function

▶ Possible Contributing Causes

- Alcohol abuse
- Arteriovenous malformation (AVM)
- Cardiovascular disease, coronary artery disease, atrial fibrillation
- Diabetes
- Family history of stroke or transient ischemic attack (TIA)
- Fibromuscular dysplasia
- HTN
- Hyperlipidemia
- Marfan syndrome
- Obesity
- Patent foramen ovale
- Peripheral vascular disease
- Pulmonary insufficiency
- Sedentary lifestyle
- Smoking

▶ Differential Diagnosis

- Hydrocephalus
- Hypertensive encephalopathy
- Meningitis
- TIA

MEANS OF CONFIRMATION OR DIAGNOSIS

▶ Laboratory Tests

- Vital signs
- Stethoscope on carotid artery, bruit sound

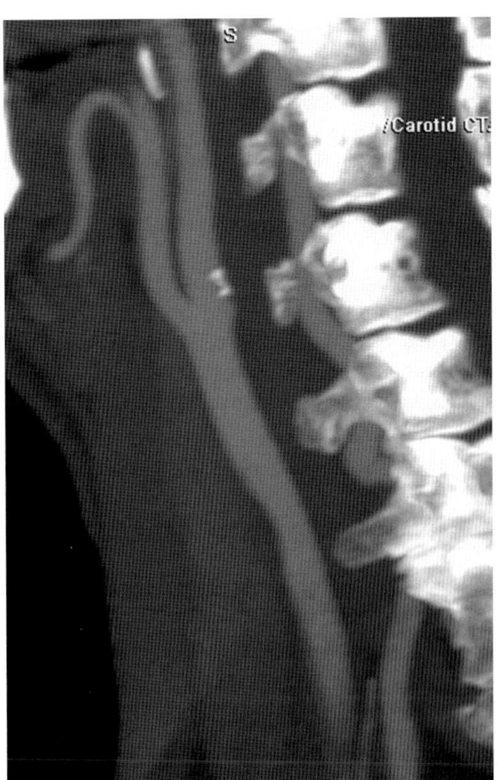

FIGURE 8-3 Small calcified plaque at the right carotid bulb. (From Pahlm O, Wagner GS. *Multimodal Cardiovascular Imaging: Principles and Clinical Applications*. www.accessmedicine.com. Copyright © The McGraw-Hill Companies, Inc. All rights reserved.)

- Neurovascular tests: Neck flexion for meningeal irritation, palpation of arteries, auscultation of heart and blood vessels, ophthalmic pressures
- Profile of the timing: Look for pattern of onset, speed of onset, and initial neurologic symptoms; thrombosis
- Blood analysis: Complete blood count, platelet count, prothrombin time, erythrocyte sedimentation rate
- Lipid profile
- Triglyceride test
- Thyroid function
- Full cardiac evaluation including radiographs, electrocardiogram

▶ Imaging

- Carotid or cerebral angiography
- CT
- MRI

FINDINGS AND INTERPRETATION

- CT: Most commonly used with contrast to enhance the density of intravascular blood; inaccurate in the acute phase of an ischemic stroke but often used to rule out other brain lesions (such as tumor, abscess), accurate for a hemorrhagic stroke
- MRI: More sensitive than CT for the acute ischemic stroke (within 2 to 6 hours)

TREATMENT

▶ Medication

- Medication to control cholesterol
- Antihypertensive medication
- CVA
  - Antidepressant medication
  - Gabapentin for intractable neurogenic pain or seizure
  - Seizure medications
  - Thrombolytics (in ischemic stroke only)
  - Antiplatelet (in ischemic stroke only)
  - Anticoagulants (in ischemic stroke only)

REFERRALS/ADMITTANCE

- Vascular surgeon to access blockage
- Emergency-room physician if signs of stroke
- Neurologist or neurosurgeon as needed, based on location and severity of injury, management of medications, and management of future needs

IMPAIRMENTS

- For a CVA
  - Aerobic capacity
  - Arousal
  - Attention
  - Balance
  - Behavior
  - Cognition
  - Coordination
  - Cranial nerve integrity
  - Dynamic sit
  - Dynamic stand
  - Endurance
  - Fine motor
  - Gait
  - Home management
  - Motor planning
  - Moving base of support (BOS)
  - Muscle recruitment
  - Muscle strength
  - Muscle tone (common synergy patterns after stroke)
  - Neglect/inattention to a single side of the body
  - Neurogenic pain
  - Peripheral nerve integrity, possibly from a comorbid diagnosis

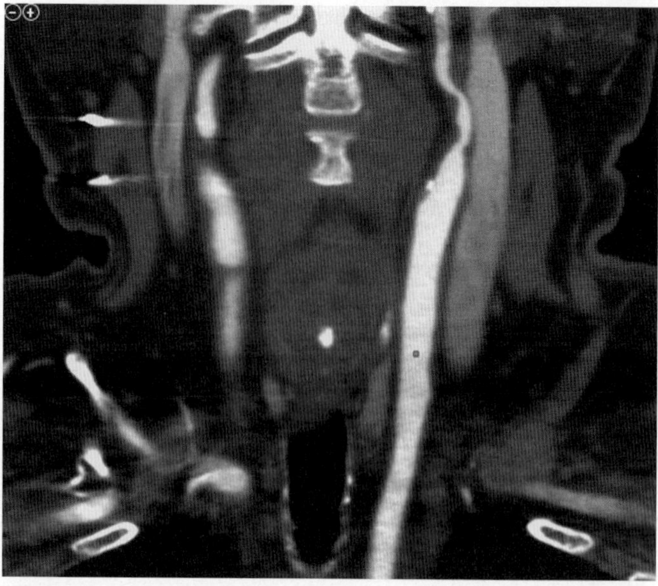

FIGURE 8-4 Axial view before carotid endarterectomy. (From Pahlm O, Wagner GS. *Multimodal Cardiovascular Imaging: Principles and Clinical Applications*. www.accessmedicine.com. Copyright © The McGraw-Hill Companies, Inc. All rights reserved.)

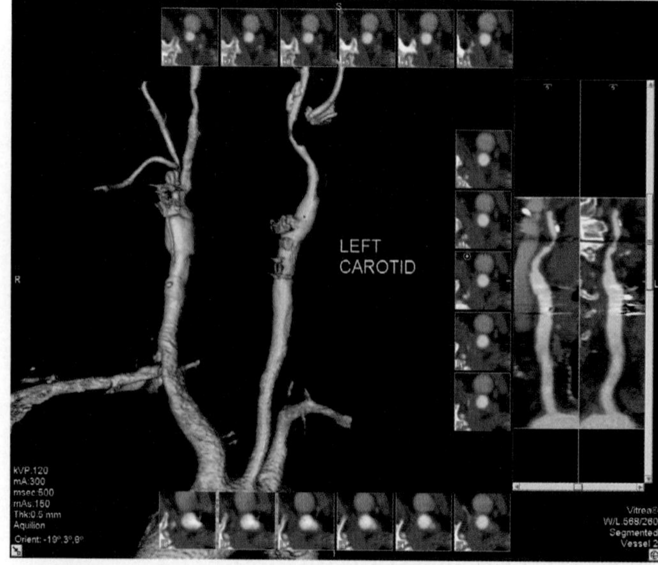

FIGURE 8-5 Volume-rendered image before stenting indicating severe stenosis of the left internal carotid artery. (From Pahlm O, Wagner GS. *Multimodal Cardiovascular Imaging: Principles and Clinical Applications*. www.accessmedicine.com. Copyright © The McGraw-Hill Companies, Inc. All rights reserved.)

- Postural control
- Posture
- Respiratory compromise
- Self-care
- Sensation
- Static sit
- Static stand

TESTS AND MEASURES

- The StrokEDGE Taskforce of the Neurology Section of the American Physical Therapy Association completed a detailed study of outcome measures for patients with strokes.
  - A compendium of the outcome tools is provided on the Neurology Section website.
- NIH stroke scale
- Glasgow coma scale
- Modified Ashworth scale
- Functional measures
  - Barthel index
  - Functional independence measure
- Gait and balance measures
  - Tinetti performance-oriented mobility assessment
  - Berg Balance Scale (BBS)
  - Motor assessment scale
  - Gait assessment rating scale
  - Rancho los amigo observational gait analysis
  - 6-minute walk test (6MWT)
  - Timed up and go (TUG)
  - 10-m walk test
  - Romberg
  - Dynamic gait index (DGI)
  - Functional gait assessment (FGA)
  - Multidirectional reach test
  - Physical performance test
  - High-level mobility assessment tool (HiMAT), if appropriate, for patients who have appropriate scores on BBS and DGI
- Cognitive testing
- Sensory testing: May be limited by cognition, consciousness, and aphasias
- Strength testing: Include speed of force production and ability to change force production
- Active and passive ROM, flexibility, muscle length
- Transfers from bed to chair and chair to floor
- Cranial nerves—particularly vision
- Vestibular assessment
- Cardiovascular assessment (include the Borg scale)
- Pulmonary assessment

INTERVENTION

- For CVA
  - Balance training
  - Bed mobility training
  - Cardiovascular and pulmonary endurance
  - Gait training (appropriate bracing and assistive devices), body-weight–supported treadmill training
  - Orthotics management
  - Postural re-training, shoulder subluxation management
  - ROM/stretching/positioning
  - Specific approaches: Neuro-developmental treatment (NDT), motor learning, and motor control (including constraint-induced movement therapy, forced use), proprioceptive neuromuscular facilitation
  - Strengthening (including biofeedback, functional electrical stimulation)
  - Tone management
  - Transfer training
  - Wheelchair mobility training

FUNCTIONAL GOALS

- CVA goals
  - The patient will increase 6-minute walk test to greater than or equal to 1500 feet with supervision and appropriate assistive device indoors, over level surfaces.
  - Patient will perform static tandem standing without upper extremity (UE) support for 30 seconds with supervision.
  - The patient will improve BBS score to greater than or equal to 53/56.
  - The patient will ambulate on a variety of indoor/outdoor surfaces, with distant supervision and assistive devices as needed.

PROGNOSIS

- Very good if diagnosed prior to the artery being blocked or clot being thrown

PATIENT RESOURCE

- Screening for Carotid Artery Stenosis. U.S. Preventive Services Task Force. Agency for Healthcare Research and Quality. http://www.uspreventiveservicestaskforce.org/uspstf/uspsacas.htm#summary. Release date: December 2007. Accessed May 6, 2013.

REFERENCE

1. The American Physical Therapy Association. Pattern 5D: impaired motor function and sensory integrity associated with nonprogressive disorders of the central nervous system—acquired in adolescence or adulthood. *Interactive Guide to Physical Therapist Practice.* doi: 10.2522/ptguide.3.2_4. Accessed May 6, 2013.

ADDITIONAL REFERENCES

- Balance Training. StrokEngine. http://strokengine.ca/intervention/index.php?page=topic&id=30. Accessed May 6, 2013.
- Body Weight Supported Treadmill Training. StrokEngine. http://strokengine.ca/intervention/index.php?page=topic&id=33. Accessed May 6, 2013.
- Chandrasoma P, Taylor CR. The central nervous system: III. Traumatic, vascular, degenerative, & metabolic diseases. In: Chandrasoma P, Taylor CR, eds. *Concise Pathology.* 3rd ed. New York, NY: McGraw-Hill; 1998. http://www.accessphysiotherapy.com/content/193097. Accessed May 6, 2013.
- Constraint-Induced Movement Therapy—Upper Extremity. StrokEngine. http://strokengine.ca/intervention/index.php?page=topic&id=52. Accessed May 6, 2013.
- Dutton M. Neuromuscular physical therapy. In: Dutton M, ed. *McGraw-Hill's NPTE (National Physical Therapy Examination), 2e.* New York, NY: McGraw-Hill; 2012. http://www.accessphysiotherapy.com/content/5399379. Accessed May 6, 2013.

- Geriatric Examination Toolkit. University of Missouri. http://web.missouri.edu/~proste/tool. Accessed May 6, 2013.
- ICD9Data.com. http://www.icd9data.com. Accessed May 6, 2013.
- ICD10Data.com. http://www.icd10data.com/ICD10CM/Codes. Accessed May 6, 2013.
- Naylor AR. The asymptomatic carotid surgery trial: bigger study, better evidence. *Br J Surg*. 2004;91(7):787–789. doi: 10.1002/bjs.4552.
- O'Sullivan SB. Stroke. In: O'Sullivan SB, Schmitz TJ, eds. *Physical Rehabilitation: Assessment and Treatment*. 5th ed. Philadelphia, PA: F.A. Davis; 2007.
- Panus PC, Jobst EE, Masters SB, Katzung B, Tinsley SL, Trevor AJ, eds. *Pharmacology for the Physical Therapist*. New York, NY: McGraw-Hill; 2009. http://www.accessphysiotherapy.com/resource/615. Accessed May 6, 2013.
- Ryerson SD. Hemiplegia. In: Umphred DA, ed. *Neurological Rehabilitation*. 5th ed. St. Louis, MO: Mosby; 2007.
- Sisto S. Cardiopulmonary concerns in the patient with neurological deficits: an evidence-based approach. In: DeTurk WE, Cahalin LP, eds. *Cardiovascular and Pulmonary Physical Therapy: An Evidence-Based Approach*. 2nd ed. New York, NY: McGraw-Hill; 2011. http://www.accessphysiotherapy.com/content/6879511. Accessed May 6, 2013.
- Strength Training—Lower Extremity. StrokEngine. http://strokengine.ca/intervention/index.php?page=topic&id=50. Accessed May 6, 2013.
- StrokEDGE Task Force. Neurology Section of the American Physical Therapy Association. http://www.rehabmeasures.org/lists/rehabmeasures/admin.aspx. Accessed April 8, 2014.

9 CONGESTIVE HEART FAILURE

Eric Shamus, PhD, DPT, PT, CSCS
Natalie V. Wessel, DO, MPH
Lisa Ward McVey, DPT, PT, CCS

CONDITION/DISORDER SYNONYMS

- Heart failure (HF)
- Systolic heart failure
- Diastolic heart failure

ICD-9-CM CODE

- 428 Heart failure

ICD-10-CM CODES

- I50 Heart failure
- I50.2 Systolic (congestive) heart failure
- I50.3 Diastolic (congestive) heart failure
- I50.9 Heart failure, unspecified

PREFERRED PRACTICE PATTERN

- Pattern 6D: Impaired Aerobic Capacity/Endurance Associated With Cardiovascular Pump Dysfunction or Failure[1]

PATIENT PRESENTATION

An 80-year-old female presents with shortness of breath and chest pain with exertion and cough. She states that she has to sleep with four pillows at night or she gets short of breath. She has a history of long-standing hypertension and noncompliance with her medication. Vitals are: Pulse: 120, Respiration: 22, Temperature: 97.8° F, Blood Pressure: 150/80, and SpO_2% of 94%. The patient appears diaphoretic with cool pale extremities. There are audible rales in the lungs bilaterally and +2 edema of the legs bilaterally. There is an audible S_3 gallop. EKG shows some left ventricular strain. Chest X-ray shows fluid in the bases of the lungs bilaterally and enlargement of the heart. Brain natriuretic peptide (BNP) level in the blood is 500 pg/mL.

KEY FEATURES

Description

- Heart is unable to produce sufficient cardiac output (CO) to meet demands of the body.
- HF is a syndrome caused by several pathophysiologic conditions, resulting in left ventricular and/or right ventricular dysfunction (cardiac pump dysfunction).

Essentials of Diagnosis

- EKG/ECG[2]
- Echocardiogram
- Chest X-ray
- Elevated BNP levels
- Elevated pulmonary artery catheter readings

General Considerations

- HF is a result of cardiac muscle dysfunction or damage.
- Education on disease management reduces hospitalization.
- Vital signs should be monitored before, during, and after exercise.
- Both aerobic and resistive exercises have shown positive benefits.
- Signs and symptoms should be monitored.
- Emphasis on wellness and prevention.
- Physiologic changes associated with HF.[3]

Demographics

- Affects three million people in the United States[3]
- 400,000 new cases annually[3]

CLINICAL FINDINGS

SIGNS AND SYMPTOMS

- Left-sided HF
  - Dyspnea on exertion
  - Shortness of breath[3]
  - Paroxysmal nocturnal dyspnea[3]
  - Orthopnea[3]
  - Fatigue, weakness[3]
  - Crackles
  - S_3 heart sound
  - Cold, pale, cyanotic extremities
- Right-sided HF
  - Weight gain
  - Peripheral edema
  - Jugular venous distention[3]
  - Hepatomegaly
  - Ascites
  - Fatigue[3]
  - Cyanosis

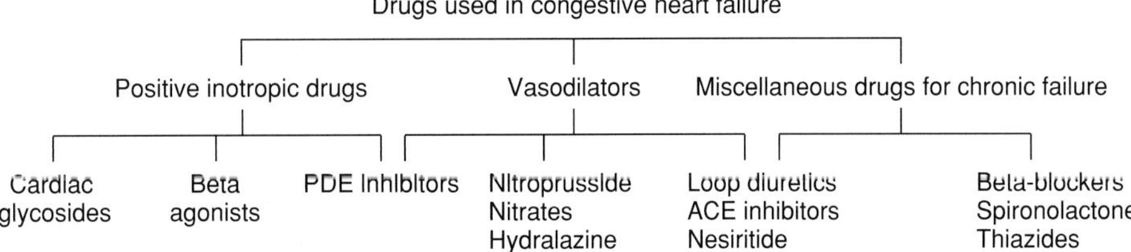

FIGURE 9-1 Drugs used in the treatment of heart failure. Several pharmacologic classes have a combination of physiologic effects and do not fall into a single category. ACE, angiotensin-converting enzyme inhibitors; PDE, phosphodiesterase. Spironolactone is a potassium-sparing diuretic that inhibits the aldosterone receptor in the collecting tubes of the kidney and nonrenal tissue sites. (From Panus PC, Jobst EE, Masters SB, Katzung B, Tinsley SL, Trevor AJ, . *Pharmacology for the Physical Therapist*. New York, NY: McGraw-Hill; 2009.)

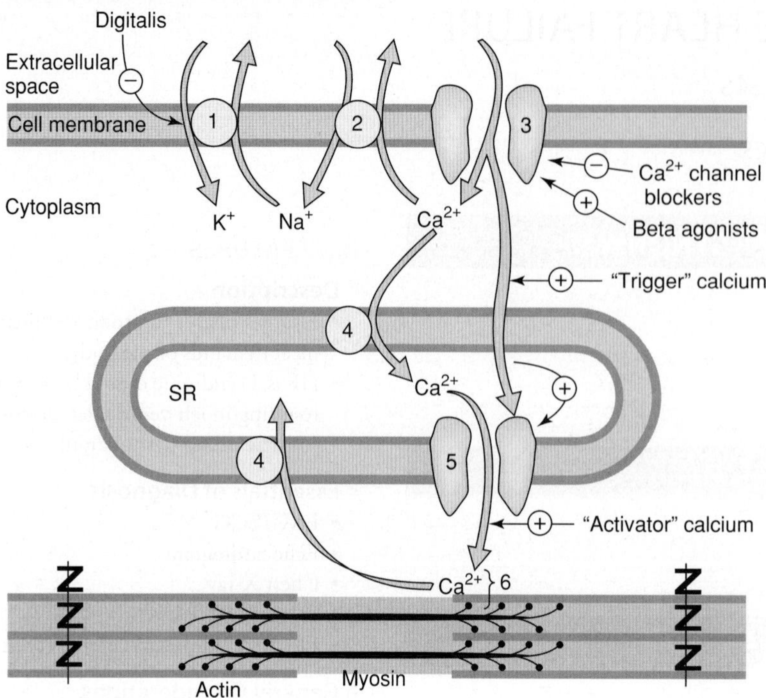

FIGURE 9-2 Schematic diagram of a cardiac muscle sarcomere, with the sites of action of several drug classes that alter contractility (numbered structures). Site 1 is Na^+/K^+-ATPase, the sodium pump. Site 2 is the Na-Ca^{2+} exchanger. Site 3 is the voltage-gated calcium channel. Site 4 is a calcium transporter that pumps calcium into the sarcoplasmic reticulum (SR). Site 5 is a calcium channel in the membrane of the SR that is activated to release stored calcium by an influx of calcium that enters the cell through calcium channels; that is, "trigger" calcium. Site 6 is the actin-troponin-tropomyosin complex at which "activator" calcium is released from the sarcoplasmic reticulum brings about contractile interaction of actin and myosin. (From Panus PC, Jobst EE, Masters SB, Katzung B, Tinsley SL, Trevor AJ. *Pharmacology for the Physical Therapist*. New York, NY: McGraw-Hill; 2009.)

Functional Implications

- New York Heart Association functional status[4]
  - Class I: Normal physical activity not limited by symptoms
  - Class II: Ordinary physical activity results in fatigue, dyspnea, other symptoms
  - Class III: Marked limitation in normal physical activity
  - Class IV: Symptoms present at rest or with any physical activity
- Depending on the severity of HF
  - Decreased activity tolerance
  - Decreased exercise tolerance
  - Dyspnea on exertion
  - Hypoxia
  - Muscle weakness
  - Cardiac arrhythmia

Possible Contributing Causes

- Causes of left ventricular failure[3]
- Causes of right ventricular failure[3]
- Myocardial damage
- Coronary artery disease (CAD)
- Autoimmune diseases
- Alcohol abuse
- Cardiac arrhythmias
- Fluid overload
- Cardiogenic shock
- Hypertension
- Cor pulmonale
- Cardiac valve abnormalities
- Pulmonary hypertension
- Renal insufficiency

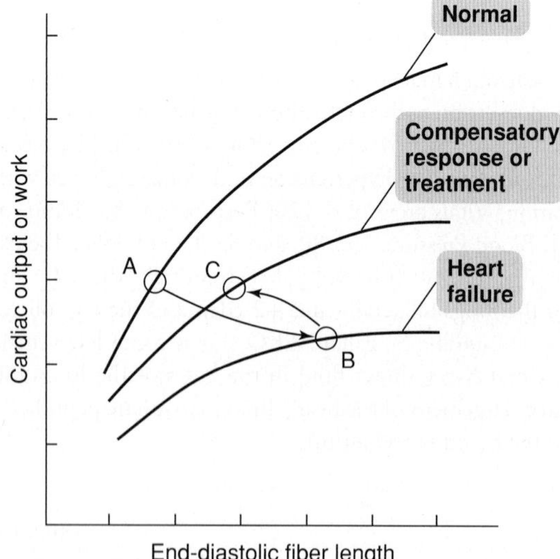

FIGURE 9-3 Ventricular function (Frank–Starling) curves. The abscissa can be any measure of preload-fiber length, filling pressure, or pulmonary capillary wedge pressure. The ordinate is a measure of useful external cardiac work, stroke volume, or CO. In heart failure, output is reduced at all fiber lengths and the heart dilates because ejection fraction is decreased. As a result, the heart moves from point A to point B. Compensatory sympathetic discharge or effective clinical treatment allows the heart to eject more blood, and the heart moves to point C on the middle curve. (From Panus PC, Jobst EE, Masters SB, Katzung B, Tinsley SL, Trevor AJ. *Pharmacology for the Physical Therapist*. New York, NY: McGraw-Hill; 2009.)

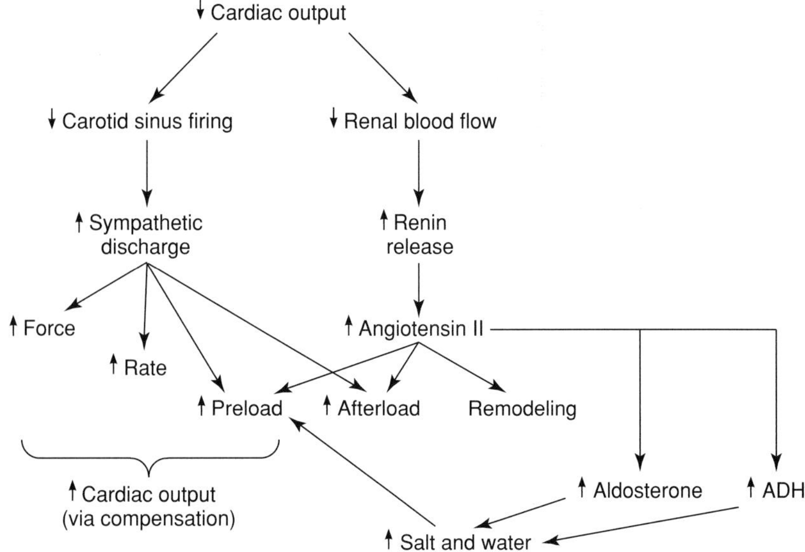

FIGURE 9-4 Some compensatory responses that occur during congestive heart failure. These responses play an important role in the progression of the disease. Responses include increased sympathetic activity and increases in renin-angiotensin-aldosterone and antidiuretic hormone (ADH). (From Panus PC, Jobst EE, Masters SB, Katzung B, Tinsley SL, Trevor AJ. *Pharmacology for the Physical Therapist*. New York, NY: McGraw-Hill; 2009.)

- Myocarditis
- Spinal cord injury
- Pulmonary embolism
- Older age

Differential Diagnosis

- Cardiac pump dysfunction
  - Cardiac muscle dysfunction produces slight-to-moderate reduction in CO
  - Mild-to-moderate activity limitation
  - Functional capacity of ≤5 to 6 metabolic equivalents (METS)
- Cardiac pump failure
  - Cardiac muscle dysfunction produces moderate-to-severe reduction in CO
  - Marked activity limitation
  - Functional capacity of ≤4 to 5 METS

MEANS OF CONFIRMATION OR DIAGNOSIS

Laboratory Tests

- Elevated BNP
  - Hormone is released with stretch on the myocardium

Imaging

- Chest X-ray
  - Cardiomegaly
  - Acute pulmonary edema resulting in ventricular failure[3]
- EKG
  - Left ventricular hypertrophy

Diagnostic Procedures

- Elevated pulmonary artery pressure
  - Indirect measure of elevated left ventricular pressure
- Echocardiogram
  - Assessment of valves and ejection fraction (EF)
- Cardiac catheterization
  - Assessment of CAD, EF, pulmonary artery wedge pressure
  - Phonocardiogram[3]

FINDINGS AND INTERPRETATION

- Characteristics of cardiac pump dysfunction
  - EF >30% to 40%
  - Myocardial ischemia
  - Cardiac arrhythmias
  - Myocardial infarction
  - Hypertension
  - Decreased systolic BP during controlled expiratory maneuver
  - Mild-to-moderate decrease in exercise tolerance, functional abilities
  - Disability
  - Decreased quality of life
- Characteristics of cardiac pump failure
  - Chest X-ray evidence of pulmonary edema
  - Signs and symptoms of right and left HF
  - Markedly decreased exercise tolerance
  - Decreased systolic BP during exercise
  - EF <30 to 40%
  - Disability
  - Markedly decreased quality of life
- 12-lead EKG/ECG that may be observed
  - Large R wave in lead V_1 becoming progressively smaller in the chest leads V_2, V_3, V_4
  - Exaggerated amplitude of QRS complexes in the chest leads
  - Inverted T wave
- Elevated BNP
  - Normal values 0 to 125 pg/mL
- Echocardiogram
  - Decreased EF or left ventricular dysfunction
  - Valve disease
- Cardiac catheterization
  - Decreased EF or left ventricular dysfunction
  - Noted CAD

TREATMENT

Medication

- Diuretics
- Beta-blockers

- Positive inotropic agents
- Angiotensin-converting enzyme
- Aldosterone antagonists
- Inpatient pharmacologic management[5]

MEDICAL PROCEDURES

- Dietary instruction
  - Sodium restriction
  - May require limited fluid intake
- Internal cardiac defibrillator
- Cardiac resynchronization
- Coronary artery bypass
- Left or right ventricular assisting device
- Cardiac transplant

REFERRALS/ADMITTANCE

- To primary care or cardiac physician if suspected cardiac muscle dysfunction
- To ER or call 911 if suspected cardiac muscle failure

IMPAIRMENTS

- Shortness of breath
- Dyspnea on exertion
- Limited activity tolerance
- Limited functional capacity

TEST AND MEASURES

- 6-minute walk test
- BORG Rating of Perceived Exertion
- Monitor vital signs to include lung auscultations
- SF-36 health survey
- New York Heart Association Functional Classification scale

INTERVENTION

- Risk factor modification
- Cardiac rehabilitation[4]
  - Decreases morbidity and mortality
  - Three phases[4]
- Education on signs and symptoms
- Aerobic exercise training
- Resisted exercise training

FUNCTIONAL GOALS

- Patient will be able to state the signs and symptoms of HF.
- Patient will be able to tolerate 30 minutes of continuous aerobic exercise while maintaining stable vital signs and rating of perceived exertion (RPE) of 13.
- Short-term goals[4]
  - Reconditioning sufficient for resuming normal activities.
  - Limiting physiologic and psychological effects of heart disease.
  - Decreased risk of sudden cardiac arrest or reinfarction.
  - Controlling symptoms of cardiac disease.
- Long-term goals[4]
  - Identification and treatment of risk factors.
  - Stabilizing or reversing atherosclerotic processes.
  - Improve patient's psychological status.

PROGNOSIS

- Depends on the severity and cause of HF

PATIENT RESOURCES

- Get with the guidelines-heart failure. American Heart Association. http://www.heart.org/HEARTORG/HealthcareResearch/GetWithTheGuidelinesHFStroke/GetWithTheGuidelines-HeartFailureHomePage/Get-With-The-Guidelines-Heart-Failure-Home-Page_UCM_306087_SubHomePage.jsp. Accessed May 6, 2013.
- Heart Failure. American Family Physician. http://www.aafp.org/afp/topicModules/viewTopicModule.htm?topicModuleId=26. Accessed May 6, 2013.

REFERENCES

1. The American Physical Therapy Association. Pattern 6D: impaired aerobic capacity/endurance associated with cardiovascular pump dysfunction or failure. *Interactive Guide to Physical Therapist Practice.* 2003. doi: 10.2522/ptguide.3.3_4. http://guidetoptpractice.apta.org/content/1/SEC30.extract. Accessed April 8, 2014.
2. Cassady SL, Cahalin LP. Cardiovascular pathophysiology. In: DeTurk WE, Cahalin LP, eds. *Cardiovascular and Pulmonary Physical Therapy: An Evidence-Based Approach.* 2nd ed. New York, NY: McGraw-Hill; 2011. http://www.accessphysiotherapy.com/abstract/6872858. Accessed May 6, 2013.
3. Kusumoto FM. Cardiovascular disorders: heart disease: pathophysiology of selected cardiovascular disorders. In: Kusumoto FM, ed. *Pathophysiology of Disease: An Introduction to Clinical Medicine.* 6th ed. New York, NY: McGraw-Hill; 2010. http://www.accessphysiotherapy.com/abstract/5367685#5367687. Accessed May 6, 2013.
4. Dutton M. Cardiovascular physical therapy. In: Dutton M, ed. *McGraw-Hill's NPTE (National Physical Therapy Examination).* New York, NY: McGraw-Hill; 2009. http://www.accessphysiotherapy.com/content/5401905. Accessed May 6, 2013.
5. Miyamoto SD, Sondheimer HM, Fagan TE, Collins KK. Cardiovascular diseases. In: Hay WW, Levin MJ, Sondheimer JM, Detering RR. *CURRENT Diagnosis & Treatment: Pediatrics.* 20th ed. New York, NY: McGraw-Hill; 2011. http://www.accessphysiotherapy.com/abstract/6583154#6583208. Accessed May 6, 2013.

ADDITIONAL REFERENCES

- Blume ED, Naftel DC, Bastardi HJ, Duncan BW, Kirklin JK, Webber SA. Outcomes of children bridged to heart transplantation with ventricular assist devices: a multi-institutional study. *Circulation.* 2006;113(19):2313–2319.
- Dubin D. *Rapid Interpretation of EKG's.* Fort Myers, FL: COVER Publishing Co.; 2000.
- Panus PC, Jobst EE, Masters SB, Katzung B, Tinsley SL, Trevor AJ. Drugs used in heart failure. In: Panus PC, Jobst EE, Masters SB, Katzung B, Tinsley SL, Trevor AJ, eds. *Pharmacology for the Physical Therapist.* New York, NY: McGraw-Hill; 2009. http://www.accessphysiotherapy.com/content/6091371. Accessed May 6, 2013.
- Rosenthal D, Chrisant MR, Edens E, et al. International Society for Heart and Lung Transplantation: practice guidelines for management of heart failure in children. *J Heart Lung Transplant.* 2004;23(12):1313–1333.

10 DEEP VEIN THROMBOSIS

Thomas S. Zeller, MPT
Mila Marhovich, DPT
Eric Shamus, PhD, DPT, PT, CSCS

CONDITION/DISORDER SYNONYMS

- Blood clot
- Deep vein thrombophlebitis
- Venous thrombosis
- Venous thromboembolism

ICD-9-CM CODES[1]

- 453.4 Acute venous embolism and thrombosis of deep vessels of the lower extremity
- 453.5 Chronic venous embolism and thrombosis of deep vessels of lower extremity

ICD-10-CM CODES[2]

- I74.9 Embolism and thrombosis of unspecified artery
- I82.4 Acute embolism and thrombosis of deep veins of lower extremity
- I82.90 Acute embolism and thrombosis of unspecified vein

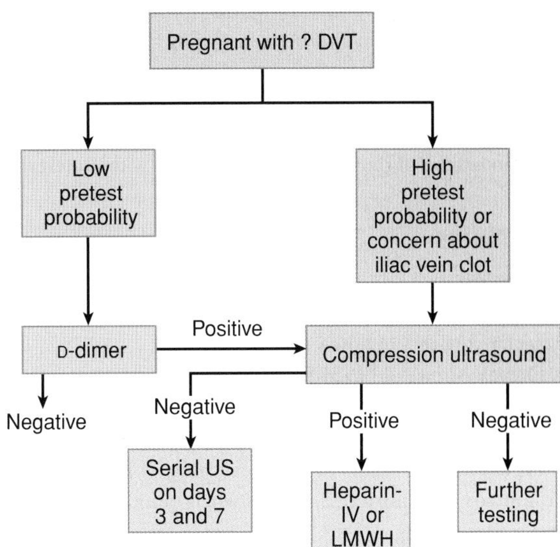

FIGURE 10-1 Algorithm for diagnosis of deep venous thrombosis (DVT) in pregnancy with D-dimer as the first decision node. LMWH, low-molecular-weight heparin. (From Tintinalli JE, Stapczynski J, John Ma O, Cline D, Cydulka R, Meckler G *Tintinalli's Emergency Medicine: A Comprehensive Study Guide*, 7th ed. www.accessmedicine.com. Copyright © The McGraw-Hill Companies, Inc. All rights reserved.)

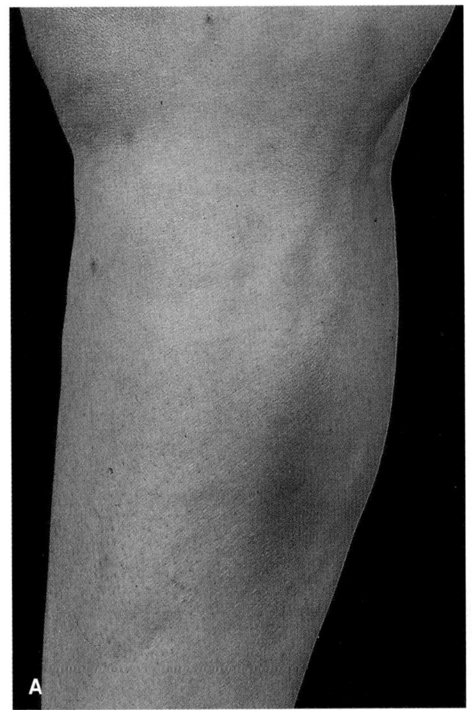

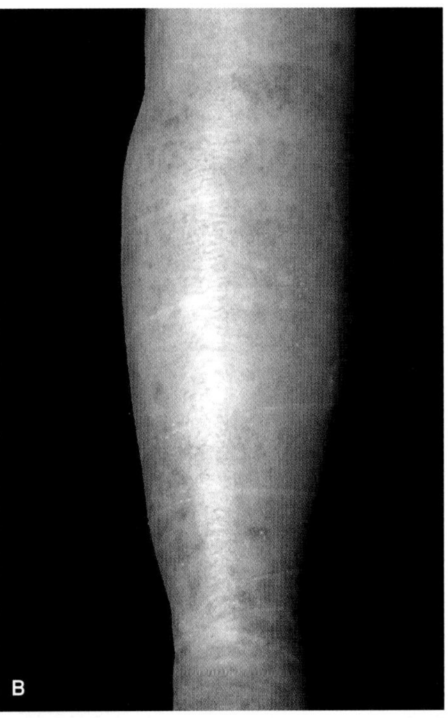

FIGURE 10-2 Superficial phlebitis and deep venous thrombosis. **A.** A linear painful erythematous cord extending from the popliteal fossa to the mid-calf in a 35-year-old man who had moderate varicosities. Phlebitis occurred after a 15-hour flight. **B.** The leg is swollen, pale, with a blotchy cyanotic discoloration, and is painful. The episode occurred after abdominal surgery (the circular marks are from a compression bandage). (From Wolff K, Johnson RA. *Fitzpatrick's Color Atlas and Synopsis of Clinical Dermatology*, 6th ed. www.accessmedicine.com. Copyright © The McGraw-Hill Companies, Inc. All rights reserved.)

PREFERRED PRACTICE PATTERN

- Pattern 6A: Primary Prevention/Risk Reduction for Cardiovascular/Pulmonary Disorders[3]

PATIENT PRESENTATION

A 42-year-old diabetic woman complains of soreness of the left leg. She is moderately obese and has been recovering from surgical removal of her gallbladder (cholecystectomy) performed 2 weeks ago. On examination, she has obvious swelling in the left lower leg and some tenderness of the calf that increases when the calf is gently squeezed. There is no redness of the leg, and she is afebrile (without fever).[4]

KEY FEATURES

Description

- Clot formation and acute inflammation of deep vein
- Associated with Virchow's triad:[5]
  - Decreased rate of blood flow (venous stasis)
  - Damage to blood vessel
  - Hypercoagulation
- Most commonly occurs in lower extremity (LE)
- Pulmonary embolism (PE) occurs when blood clot breaks off and settles in lung

Essentials of Diagnosis

- Clinical decision rule for outpatients suspected of having a proximal deep vein thrombosis (DVT)[6]
- History: Family history, recent trauma, cancer, oral contraceptives
- Subjective report of pain
- Visual examination
- Reproduction of symptoms with dorsiflexion of the ankle (Homan's sign) and palpation[5]
- Diagnostic ultrasound of affected veins
- Ankle-brachial index
- D-dimer test
- Well's score or criteria: Possible scores range from −2 to 9
  - Active cancer (treatment within last 6 months or palliative): +1 point
  - Calf swelling ≥3 cm compared to asymptomatic calf (measured 10 cm below tibial tuberosity): +1 point

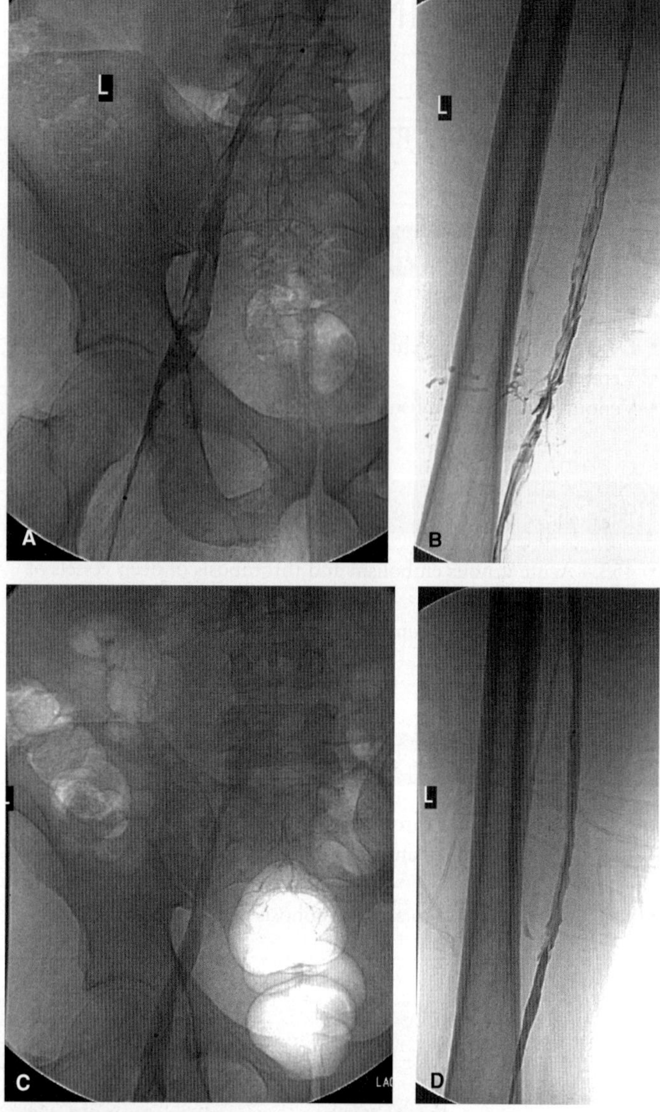

FIGURE 10-3 This series of panels demonstrates an acute left iliac vein thrombosis (**A**) with extension into the femoral vein (**B**). Following 48 hours of catheter-directed thrombolysis, the thrombus is essentially resolved at the iliac (**C**) with slight residual narrowing at the left femoral vein (**D**). (From Fuster V, Walsh RA, Harrington RA. *Hurst's The Heart*, 13th ed. www.accessmedicine.com. Copyright © The McGraw-Hill Companies, Inc. All rights reserved.)

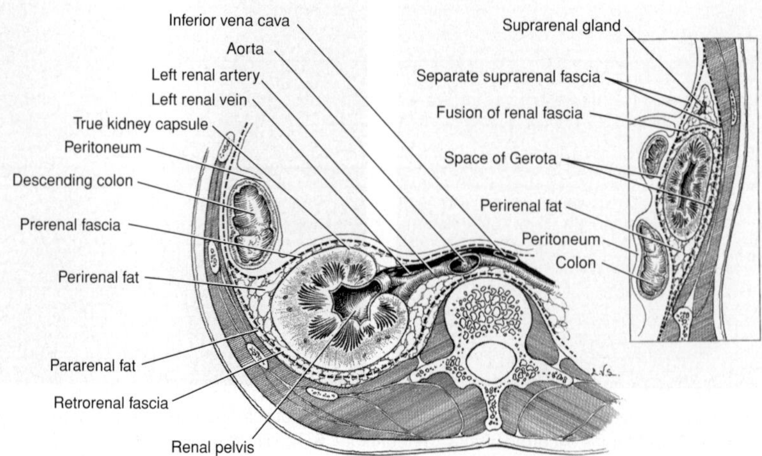

FIGURE 10-4 Arterial supply to the leg. (Reproduced, with permission, from Lindner HH. *Clinical Anatomy*. East Norwalk, CT: Appleton & Lange, 1989:602.)

- Swollen unilateral superficial veins (nonvaricose) in symptomatic leg: +1 point
- Unilateral pitting edema in symptomatic leg: +1 point
- Previous documented DVT: +1 point
- Swelling of entire leg: +1 point
- Localized tenderness along deep venous system: +1 point
- Paralysis, paresis, or recent cast immobilization of LEs: +1 point
- Recently bedridden ≥3 days, or major surgery requiring regional or general anesthetic in past 12 weeks: +1 point
- Alternative diagnosis equally or more likely: −2 points

General Considerations

- DVT may result in a PE, a life-threatening medical emergency.
- DVT and PE are the two manifestations of venous thromboembolism (VTE).
- Late complication of DVT is post-thrombotic syndrome: Results in limb edema, pain, swelling.
- Virchow's triad is primary mechanism of DVT onset.[5]

Demographics

- Individuals subjected to prolonged hospitalization or immobilization (orthopedic cast, long airplane flight, bed rest).
- Prevalence increases with age.
- Women at increased risk while taking oral contraceptives and during pregnancy.

CLINICAL FINDINGS

SIGNS AND SYMPTOMS

- May be asymptomatic in early stage
- Sudden unilateral leg symptoms including
  - Edema
  - Swelling, inflammation
  - Skin discoloration, redness
  - Warmth
  - Tenderness
- Low-grade fever
- Tachycardia
- Pain exacerbated with exercise but still present at rest

Functional Implications

- If DVT suspected, initiate therapeutic interventions
- PE
- Cerebrovascular accident
- Death

Possible Contributing Causes

- Family history of DVT
- Older age
- Protein C or S deficiencies
- Oncology treatment
- Recent surgery
- Postoperative[7]
- Post-pregnancy up to 6 weeks
- Obesity
- Prolonged bed rest
- Smoking
- Trauma
- Recent fracture
- Immobilization
- Oral contraceptives
- Hormone therapy

Differential Diagnosis

- LE tumor
- Musculoskeletal injury
- Cellulitis
- Baker's cyst
- Lymphedema

MEANS OF CONFIRMATION OR DIAGNOSIS

Imaging

- Doppler ultrasound to examine vascular function
- CT venography
- MRI venography
- MRI of thrombosis
- Contrast venography (gold standard)
- D-dimer test

FINDINGS AND INTERPRETATION

- Positive Homan's sign[5]
- Presence of pain
- Swelling
- Warmth and discoloration are indications for referral to primary care physician

TREATMENT

Medication

- Blood thinners (anticoagulants)
  - Warfarin or Heparin
  - Laboratory tests required to monitor anticoagulant therapy[8]

MEDICAL PROCEDURES

- Vena cava filter
- Compression stockings

REFERRALS/ADMITTANCE

- To hospital for imaging
- To primary care physician for medical diagnosis, medication

IMPAIRMENTS

- Primary complications
  - Immobility
  - Pain
- Secondary complications
  - PE
  - Stroke
  - Death

INTERVENTION

- Prevention
- Early and frequent ambulation
- Graduated compression stockings (GCS)
- Intermittent pneumatic compression (IPC)

FUNCTIONAL GOALS

- Prevent secondary complications (PE, stroke, death) through timely diagnosis and treatment of DVT.

- Relieve pain and discomfort through use of mechanical devices, elevation of extremity, adherence to medication.
- Patient education on clot prevention through appropriate exercise, diet, smoking cessation.

PROGNOSIS

- Varies based on
    - Age
    - Blood composition
    - Timely administration of anticoagulation therapy
    - Adherence to prevention strategies

PATIENT RESOURCES

- Deep vein thrombosis. American Academy of Orthopeadic Surgeons. http://orthoinfo.aaos.org/topic.cfm?topic=a00219. Accessed August 8, 2014.
- Deep vein thrombosis. American Academy of Family Physicians. http://familydoctor.org/familydoctor/en/diseases-conditions/deep-vein-thrombosis.html. Accessed August 8, 2014.

REFERENCES

1. ICD-9-CM. http://www.icd9data.com. Accessed March 1, 2013.
2. ICD-10-CM. http://www.icd10data.com. Accessed March 1, 2013.
3. The American Physical Therapy Association. Pattern 6A: primary prevention/risk reduction for cardiovascular/pulmonary disorders. *Interactive Guide to Physical Therapist Practice*. 2003. doi: 10.2522/ptguide.3.3_1. http://guidetoptpractice.apta.org/content/1/SEC27.extract. Accessed April 8, 2014.
4. Toy EC. Deep vein thrombosis, Case 25. LANGE Case Files. http://www.accessmedicine.com/casecontent.aspx?aid=8650502&tabid=1. Accessed February 25, 2013.
5. Dutton M. *McGraw Hill's NPTE (National Physical Therapy Examination)*.2nd ed. New York, NY: McGraw-Hill; 2012. http://www.accessphysiotherapy.com/resource/611. Accessed April 3, 2013.
6. Dutton M. *Orthopaedic Examination, Evaluation, and Intervention*. New York, NY: McGraw-Hill; 2008. http://www.accessphysiotherapy.com/resource/612. Accessed April 3, 2013.
7. Prendergast TJ, Ruoss SJ, Seeley EJ. Pulmonary disease: pathophysiology of selected lung diseases. In: McPhee SJ, Hammer GD, eds. *Pathophysiology of Disease*. New York, NY: McGraw-Hill; 2009: Chapter 9. http://www.accessphysiotherapy.com/abstract/5369340. Accessed April 3, 2013.
8. Ciesla ND, Kuramoto JD. Physical therapy associated with respiratory failure. In: DeTurk WE, Cahalin LP, eds. *Cardiovascular and Pulmonary Physical Therapy*. New York, NY: McGraw-Hill; 2011: Chapter 19. http://www.accessphysiotherapy.com/abstract/6884973. Accessed April 3, 2013.

ADDITIONAL REFERENCE

- Hay WW, Levin MJ, Sondheimer JM, Deterding RR. Special clinical problems associated with spinal cord injury. In: Hay WW, Levin MJ, Sondheimer JM, Deterding RR, eds. *CURRENT Diagnosis & Treatment: Pediatrics*. 20th ed. New York, NY: McGraw-Hill; 2011. http://www.accessphysiotherapy.com/content/6586454. Accessed April 3, 2013.

11 MARFAN SYNDROME

Jacqueline van Duijn, DPT, PT, OCS
Eric Shamus, PhD, DPT, PT, CSCS
Arie J. Van Duijn, EdD, MSc, PT, OCS

CONDITION/DISORDER SYNONYM

- Marfan's syndrome

ICD-9-CM CODE

- 759.82 Marfan syndrome

ICD-10-CM CODES

- Q87.4 Marfan syndrome
- Q87.40 Marfan syndrome, unspecified
- Q87.41 Marfan syndrome with cardiovascular manifestations
- Q87.410 Marfan syndrome with aortic dilation
- Q87.418 Marfan syndrome with other cardiovascular manifestations
- Q87.42 Marfan syndrome with ocular manifestations
- Q87.43 Marfan syndrome with skeletal manifestation

PREFERRED PRACTICE PATTERN

- 4D: Impaired Joint Mobility, Motor Function, Muscle Performance, and Range of motion Associated With Connective-Tissue Dysfunction[1]

PATIENT PRESENTATION

A 38-year-old woman presents with increasing complaints of fatigue, nearsightedness, and increasing joint pain, especially in the morning. She has an ectomorphic body type, with long and thin extremities and fingers. Her joints are generally hypermobile, and she has a moderate kyphosis of the thoracic spine. She complains of foot pain due to low arches, which is relieved by foot orthoses. She was previously diagnosed with mitral valve prolapse (MVP). Patient states she is having difficulty with when she is carrying her groceries from the car.

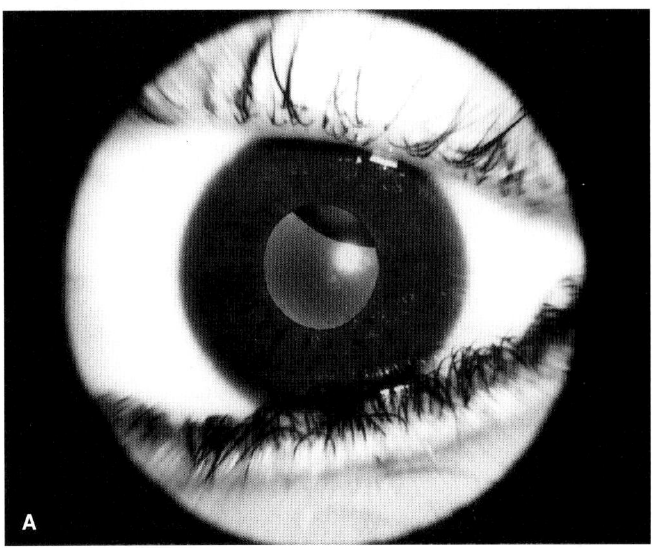

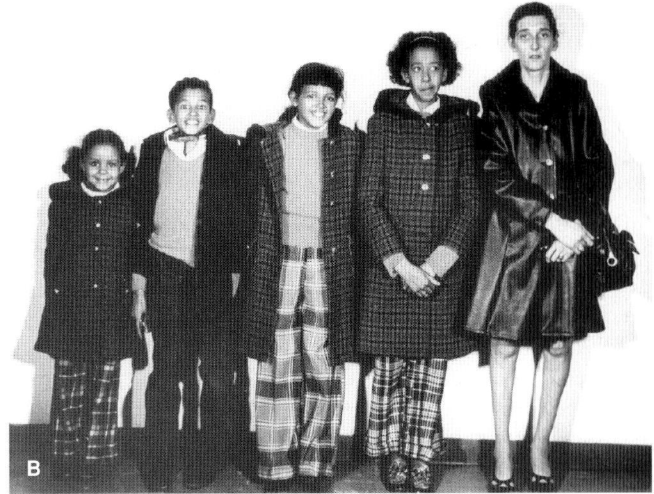

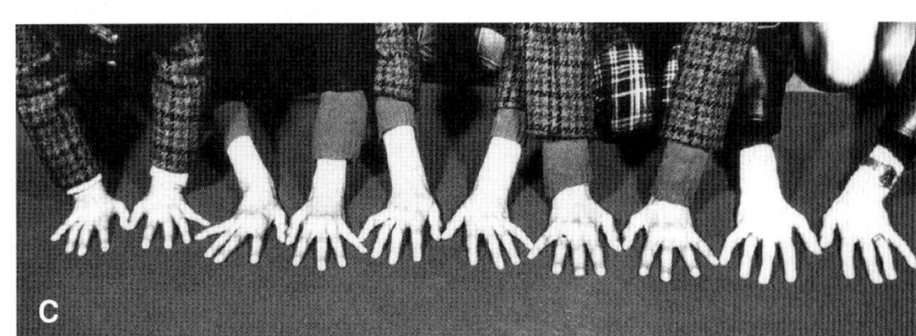

FIGURE 11-1 Marfan syndrome. Familial expression of upward dislocation of the lens (**A, B**) and arachnodactyly (**C**). (From Riordan-Eva P, Cunningham Jr ET. *Vaughan & Asbury's General Ophthalmology*, 18th ed. http://www.accessmedicine.com. Copyright © The McGraw-Hill Companies, Inc. All rights reserved.)

KEY FEATURES

Description

- Connective-tissue disorder characterized by long fingers and toes (arachnodactyly)[2,3]
- Dominant inherited trait
- Defect in fibrillin-1 gene
- Excessive growth of long bones
- Individuals are tall with elongated extremities
- Elongated face
- Pectus Carinatum (pigeon chest)

Essentials of Diagnosis

- Diagnostic criteria defined in the Ghent nosology

General Considerations

- Associated cardiac disorders
  - Heart failure
  - MVP
  - Aortic dissection and disruption, which may cause sudden death

▶ Demographics

- Inherited as an autosomal trait
- Rare cases of spontaneous gene defect
- Incidence: 1 in 5000 people[2]
- Men and women equally affected

CLINICAL FINDINGS

SIGNS AND SYMPTOMS

- Vision changes with possible retinal dysfunction
  - Detached retina
  - Cataracts
  - Subluxation of the lens
- Joint hypermobility
- Spiderlike fingers (arachnodactyly)[3]
- Wing span exceeds body height
- Morning stiffness
- Joint instability
- Joint deformity
- Pes planus (Flat feet)
- Pectus excavatum
- Scoliosis
- Learning disability
- Connective-tissue disorder
- High arch palate
- Collapsed lung
- Arrhythmia
- Sleep apnea
- Secondary problems
  - Aneurysm
  - Dilatation of the ascending aorta
  - Scoliosis

▶ Functional Implications

- Limited mobility
- Aerobic endurance limitation
- Visual deficiency
- Decreased activity participation

▶ Possible Contributing Causes

- Gene mutation

▶ Differential Diagnosis

- Osteoarthritis
- Rheumatoid arthritis
- Ehlers–Danlos syndrome
- Stickler syndrome
- Loeys–Dietz syndrome
  - Mutation in the transforming growth factor B-receptor
- Aortic aneurysm
- Marfanoid habitus
- Systemic lupus erythematosus
- Fibromyalgia syndrome
- Scleroderma
- Homocystinuria
- Lujan syndrome
- Spondyloarthropathy
- Ankylosing spondylitis
- Reiter syndrome
- Psoriatic arthritis
- Lyme disease

MEANS OF CONFIRMATION OR DIAGNOSIS

▶ Imaging

- Conventional radiograph of the joints and long bones
- Diagnostic ultrasound of the aorta for possible aneurysm
- Echocardiogram
- EKG

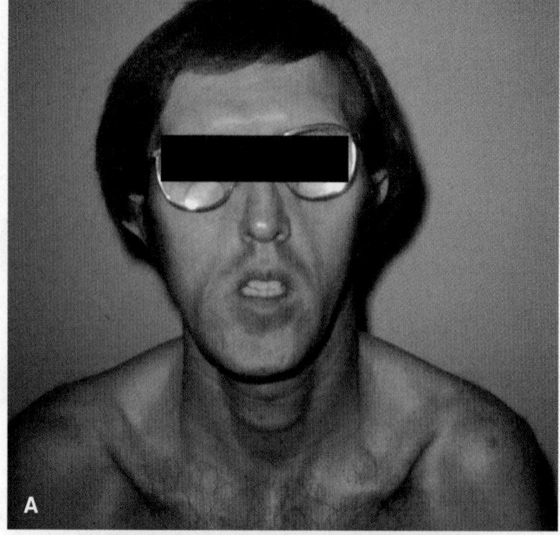

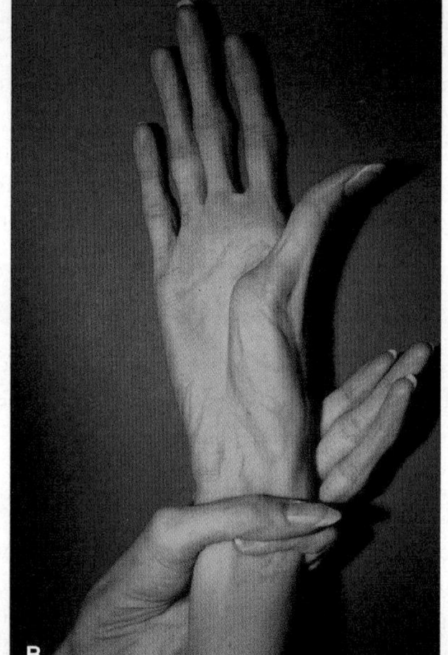

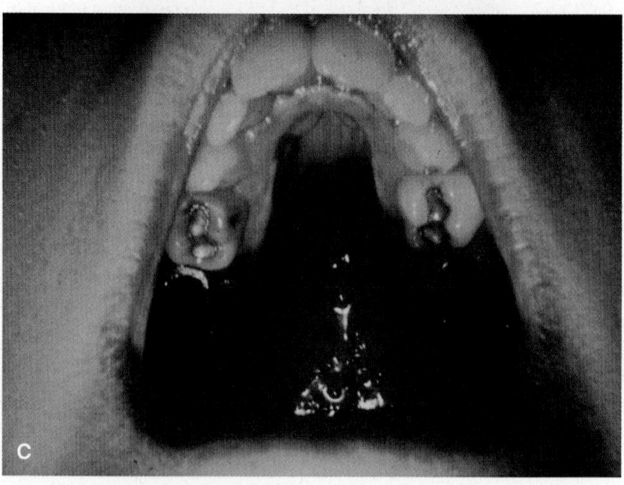

FIGURE 11-2 Marfan syndrome. **A.** Long, narrow face. **B.** Arachnodactyly and positive wrist sign. **C.** High-arched palate. (From Fuster V, Walsh RA, Harrington RA. *Hurst's The Heart*, 13th ed. http://www.accessmedicine.com. Copyright © The McGraw-Hill Companies, Inc. All rights reserved.)

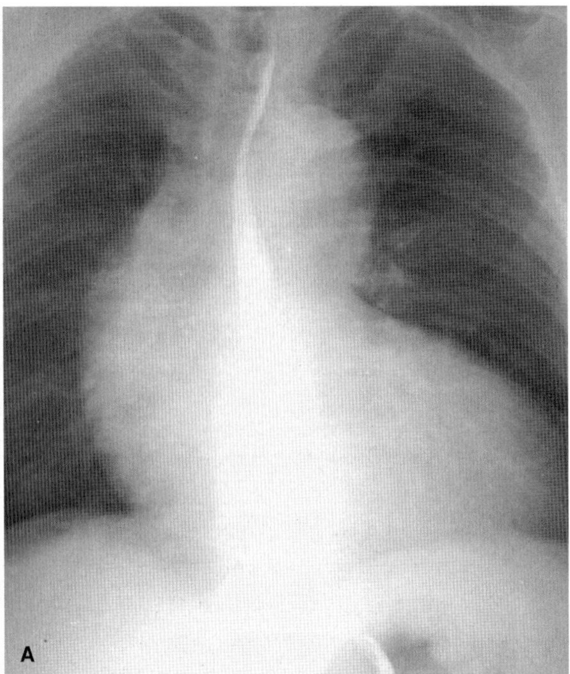

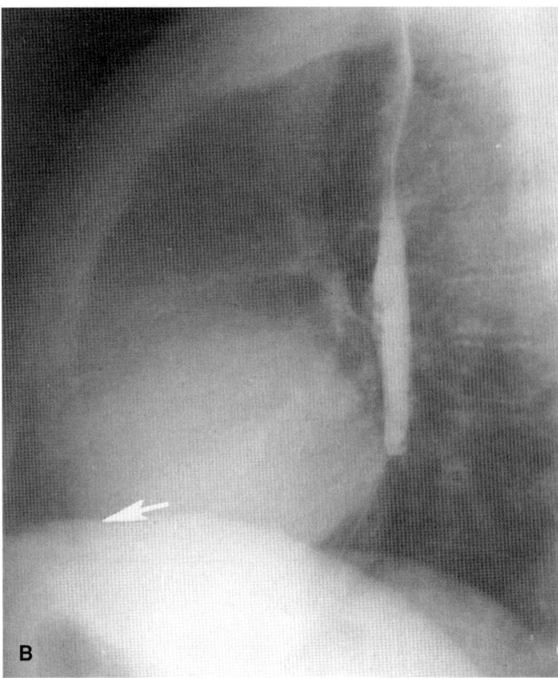

FIGURE 11-3 Radiograph of a 45-year-old man with Marfan syndrome, severe aortic regurgitation, and proximal aortic dissection into the pericardial cavity. **A.** The posteroanterior view shows a huge left ventricle and aneurysmal dilatation of the ascending aorta. There is no sign of heart failure. **B.** The lateral view shows a small pericardial effusion (*arrow*). (From Fuster V, Walsh RA, Harrington RA. *Hurst's The Heart,* 13th ed. http://www.accessmedicine.com.)

▶ Diagnostic Procedures

- Genetic testing for fibrillin-1
- Vision, annual eye examination
- Pulmonary function test

FINDINGS AND INTERPRETATION

- Joint deformities, subluxations, dislocations on plain radiograph
- Aortic dilation or aneurysm on echocardiogram
- Heart-valve dysfunction on echocardiogram

TREATMENT

▶ Medication

- NSAIDs
- Cortisone injection
- Glucocorticoids or corticosteroids
- Antibiotics

MEDICAL PROCEDURES

- Surgery for aortic aneurysm, heart valve, detached retina

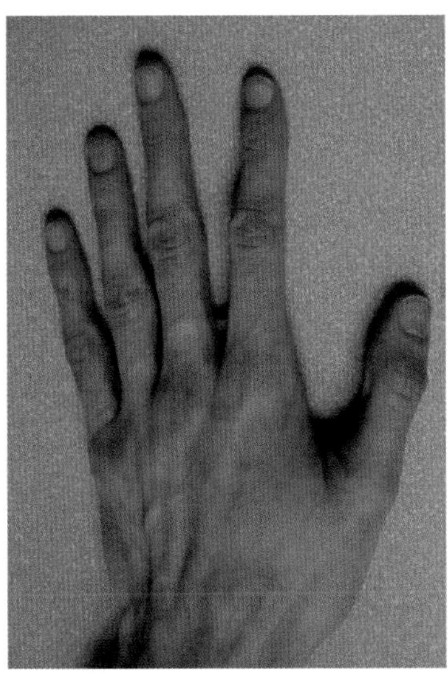

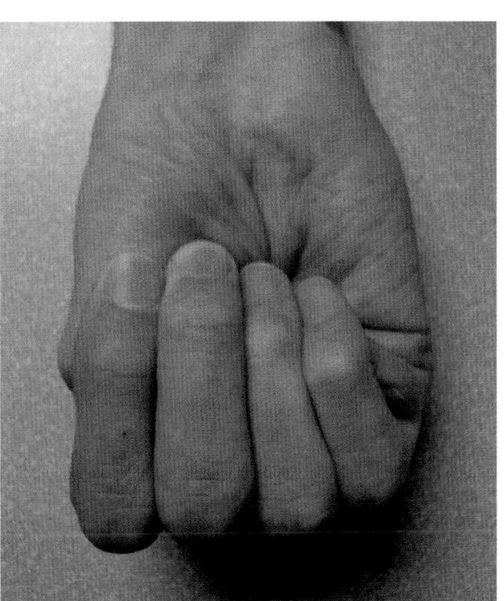

FIGURE 11-4 Marfan syndrome: Arachnodactyly and positive thumb sign. These are signs of Marfan syndrome. The long thin fingers are notable and the tip of the thumb extends beyond the fifth finger when bent into the palm of the hand. (From LeBlond RF, DeGowin RL, Brown DD. *DeGowin's Diagnostic Examination,* 9th ed. http://www.accessmedicine.com.)

REFERRALS/ADMITTANCE

- To rheumatologist for assessment of underlying complications
- To internal medicine specialist
- To optometrist, for an annual eye examination
- To cardiologist
- To pulmonologist
- To physical and rehabilitation medicine specialist
- To geneticist for genetic testing

IMPAIRMENTS

- Mobility
- Self-care
- Role at home and in community
- School and work
- Recreation, leisure, sports
- Should avoid contact sports due to weakness of blood vessels and possible retinal detachment

TESTS AND MEASURES

- Pain, visual analog scale (VAS)
  - 24-hour pain
  - Worst average pain
  - Best average pain
- Functional independence measure
  - Locomotion
- Neurologic examination
  - Sensation
    - Light touch
    - Pin prick
  - Lower-extremity deep tendon reflexes
  - Proprioception
  - Kinesthetic awareness
  - Coordination
- Gait assessment
  - Observational analysis
  - Gait speed via the 10-m walk test
  - 2-minute walk test
  - 6-minute walk test
- Cardiovascular integrity
  - Blood pressure at rest and after activity
  - Heart rate at rest and after activity

INTERVENTION

- Exercises (resistance, endurance)
  - Aquatic exercises
- Training on ADLs
- Use of assistive or adaptive devices
- Weight management, muscle gain
- Energy conservation
- Orthoses, splints for pes planus, and scoliosis
- Breathing exercises
- Diet
- Pain management
- Joint protection
- Orthotics and footwear
- Psychosocial support
- Patient education

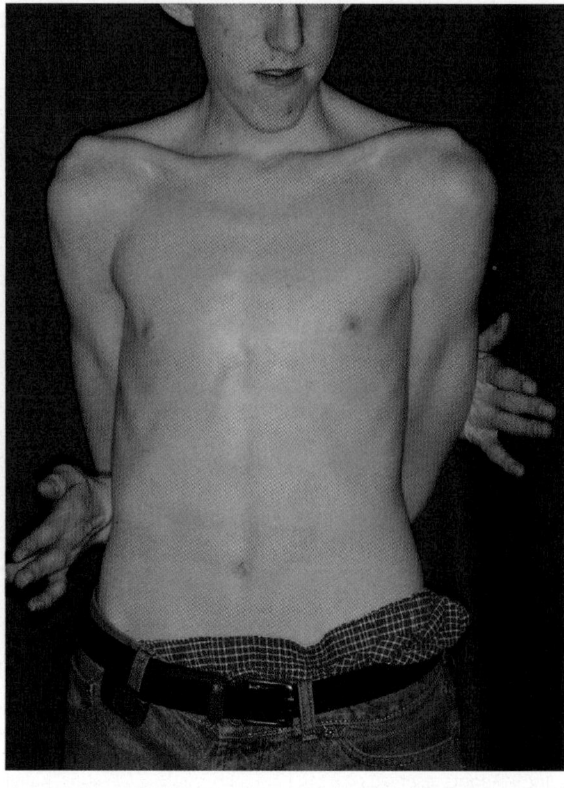

FIGURE 11-5 Marfan syndrome: Frontal view of teenage boy with Marfan syndrome. Note the tall stature, arachnodactyly, abnormally low ratio of the upper segment to lower segment, and long arms. (From Goldsmith LA, Katz SI, Gilchrest BA, et al. *Fitzpatrick's Dermatology in General Medicine,* 8th ed. http://www.accessmedicine.com. Copyright © The McGraw-Hill Companies, Inc. All rights reserved.)

FUNCTIONAL GOALS

- Patient will have improved joint stability so as to improve balance.
- Patient will have improved lower-extremity muscle strength so as to climb stairs.
- Patient will have improved muscle and aerobic endurance so as to go grocery shopping.
- Patient will have improved activity and participation related to roles at home and the community.
- Patient will be able to resume ADLs (e.g., sweeping, mopping) pain free.
- Patient will be able to lift baby from crib without pain, maintaining neutral wrist posture.

PROGNOSIS

- Cardiac complications result in decreased life expectancy; annual evaluation of aortic base advised.
- Long-term prognosis has improved with better treatment for aortic aneurysms.[3]
- No definite cure.
- Demographics, severity, natural history of the disease, medical comorbidities, and behavioral comorbidities (such as fear-avoidance, expectations, and self-efficacy) may affect prognosis.
- General endurance, muscle strength, and stable joints are good prognosticating factors.
- Motivation and compliance with physical therapy intervention (e.g., home exercise program), along with family and environmental support may improve PT treatment outcomes, especially during flare-ups.

PATIENT RESOURCES

- Marfan Syndrome. NIH, National Institute of Arthritis and Musculoskeletal and Skin Diseases. http://www.niams.nih.gov/health_info/Marfan_Syndrome/default.asp. Accessed July 1, 2013.
- National Marfan Foundation. www.marfan.org. Accessed July 5, 2013.

REFERENCES

1. The American Physical Therapy Association. Pattern 4D: impaired joint mobility, motor function, muscle performance, and range of motion associated with connective tissue dysfunction. *Interactive Guide to Physical Therapist Practice*. 2003. doi: 10.2522/ptguide.3.1_4. http://guidetoptpractice.apta.org/content/1/SEC11.extract.
2. National Marfan Foundation. www.marfan.org. Accessed July 5, 2013.
3. Hay WW, Levin MJ, Sondheimer JM, Deterding RR. Generalized disorders of skeletal or mesodermal tissues. In: Hay WW, Levin MJ, Sondheimer JM, Deterding RR, eds. *CURRENT Diagnosis & Treatment: Pediatrics*. 20th ed. New York, NY: McGraw-Hill; 2011. http://www.accessphysiotherapy.com/content/6585856. Accessed July 5, 2013.

ADDITIONAL REFERENCES

- Diokno E. Appendix A. Introduction to bracing, splinting, and casting. In: Patel DR, Greydanus DE, Baker RJ, eds. *Pediatric Practice: Sports Medicine*. New York, NY: McGraw-Hill; 2009. http://www.accessphysiotherapy.com/abstract/6983252#6983252. Accessed July 5, 2013.
- Dutton M. *Dutton's Orthopaedic Examination, Evaluation, and Intervention,* 3rd ed. New York, NY: McGraw-Hill; 2012. http://www.accessphysiotherapy.com/resource/612. Accessed July 5, 2013.
- Goodman CC, Fuller KS, Boissonnault WG. *Pathology Implications for the Physical Therapist*. 2nd ed. Philadelphia, PA: Saunders; 2003.
- McKinnis LN. *Fundamentals of Musculoskeletal Imaging*. 2nd ed. Philadelphia, PA: F.A. Davis Company; 2005.
- Medeiros WM, Peres PA, Carvalho AC, Gun C, De Luca FA. Effect of a physical exercise program in a patient with marfan syndrome and ventricular dysfunction. *Arq Bras Cardiol.* 2012;98(4):e70–e73.
- Williams AM, Crabbe DCG. Pectus deformities of the anterior chest wall. *Paediatr Respir Rev*. 2003;4(3):237–242.

12 MITRAL VALVE PROLAPSE

Natalie V. Wessel, DO, MPH
Eric Shamus, PhD, DPT, PT, CSCS

CONDITION/DISORDER SYNONYMS

- Barlow syndrome
- Floppy mitral valve
- Mitral-click murmur syndrome
- Systolic-click murmur syndrome

ICD-9-CM CODE

- 424.0 Mitral valve disorders

ICD-10-CM CODE

- I34.1 Nonrheumatic mitral (valve) prolapse

PREFERRED PRACTICE PATTERN

- 6D: Impaired Aerobic Capacity/Endurance Associated With Cardiovascular Pump Dysfunction or Failure[1]

PATIENT PRESENTATION

A 38-year-old woman presents with palpitations, anxiety, and dizziness. She states that nothing in particular has been causing her stress lately, but she feels her "heart racing." Vitals are: Pulse: 84, Respirations: 18, Blood Pressure: 110/70, and SpO_2% of 99%. On examination, there is an audible non-ejection click and a faint, late systolic murmur. On the musculoskeletal examination, there is a narrow anteroposterior chest diameter and a mild scoliosis. On echocardiogram, there is a 2.5-mm displacement of the mitral valve leaflet.

KEY FEATURES

Description

- Abnormally thickened mitral valve that becomes displaced into left atrium during systolic contraction
- Classic and nonclassic
  - Nonclassic carries low risk of complications
  - Complications of classic mitral valve prolapse (MVP) include mitral valve regurgitation, endocarditis, congestive heart failure, cardiac arrest

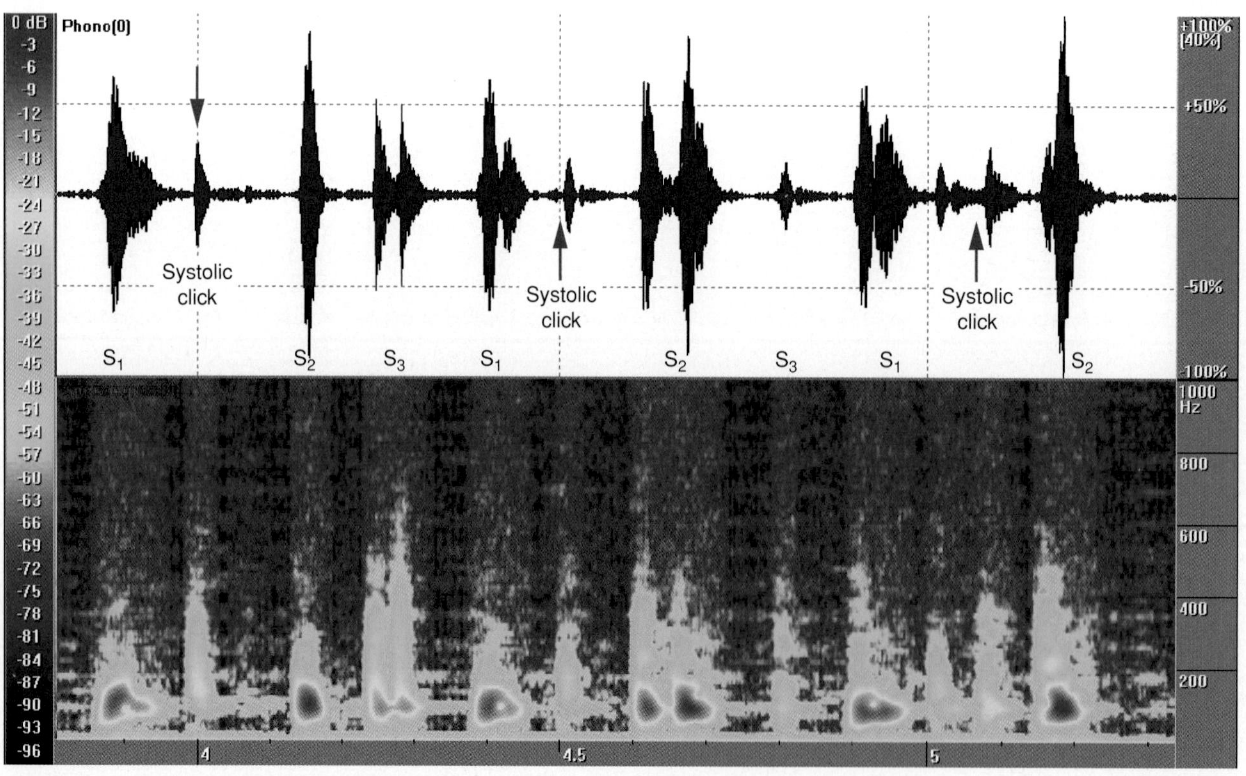

FIGURE 12-1 Mitral valve prolapse in an asymptomatic 8-year-old child. The cardiac echo demonstrated a mitral prolapse without regurgitation. Both the phonogram and spectrogram show a systolic mitral click and a diastolic S_3 prominent during inspiration. (From Pahlm O, Wagner GS. *Multimodal Cardiovascular Imaging: Principles and Clinical Applications.* www.accessmedicine.com. Copyright © The McGraw-Hill Companies, Inc. All rights reserved.)

Essentials of Diagnosis

- Stethoscope for auscultation systolic click in the mitral position, possible late systolic murmur
- EKG/ECG[2]
- Echocardiography
- Exercise stress test

General Considerations

- Education on disease management reduces hospitalization.
- Patients with significant prolapse may show signs and symptoms of congestive heart failure.
- Strenuous activity should be limited for symptomatic mitral prolapse.
- Can lead to sudden cardiac death, arrhythmias, embolic events, and coronary disease.
- Patients can develop bacterial endocarditis.
- Mild-to-moderate prolapse generally does not cause symptoms.

Demographics

- Prevalent in 2% of thin female adolescents[3]
- Equal incidence of classic and nonclassic
- Equal incidence between genders and age groups
- More common in patients with underlying genetic disease

CLINICAL FINDINGS

SIGNS AND SYMPTOMS

- Murmur accentuated with standing, hand-grip maneuver, Valsalva maneuver, and diminished with squatting
- Cardiovascular collapse or shock
- Angina pectoris[4]
- Syncope[4]
- Congestive heart failure[4]
- Dyspnea on exertion
- Shortness of breath[4]
- Anginal chest pain that increases with exercise
- Orthopnea[4]
- Fatigue, weakness[4]
- Fainting, dizziness with activity
- Palpitations
- Palpable heaves/thrills over precordium
- Arrhythmias, particularly atrial fibrillation
- Endocarditis

Functional Implications

- Symptoms depend on degree of valvular dysfunction.
- Severe mitral prolapse causes progressive shortness of breath and signs of congestive heart failure.
- Patients may be unaware of reduced cardiovascular capacity.
- MVP can cause syncope, chest pain, heart failure if severe.

Possible Contributing Causes

- Excessive connective tissue in valve leaflets
- Ehlers–Danlos syndrome
- Marfan syndrome
- Polycystic kidney disease
- Graves disease
- Pectus excavatum

Differential Diagnosis

- Acute coronary syndrome
- Aortic regurgitation
- Aortic stenosis

FIGURE 12-2 Mitral valve prolapse. Parasternal long-axis image demonstrating systolic ballooning of the posterior mitral valve leaflet approximately 7 mm beyond the plane of the mitral annulus into the left atrium. LA, left atrium; LV, left ventricle. (From Pahlm O, Wagner GS. *Multimodal Cardiovascular Imaging: Principles and Clinical Applications.* www.accessmedicine.com. Copyright © The McGraw-Hill Companies, Inc. All rights reserved.)

- Mitral valve regurgitation
- Mitral stenosis
- Myocardial infarction complication
- Shock, hypovolemia
- Cardiac pump dysfunction
  - Muscle dysfunction produces slight-to-moderate reduction in cardiac output (CO)
  - Mild-to-moderate activity limitation
  - Functional capacity of ≤5 to 6 metabolic equivalents (METS)
- Cardiac pump failure
  - Muscle dysfunction produces moderate-to-severe reduction in CO
  - Marked activity limitation
  - Functional capacity of ≤4 to 5 METS

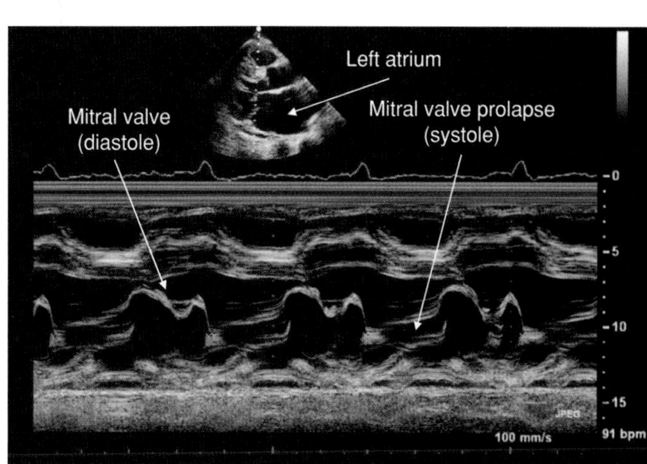

FIGURE 12-3 Mitral valve prolapse. Parasternal long-axis M-mode image demonstrating pansystolic posterior ballooning of the posterior mitral valve leaflet. (From Pahlm O, Wagner GS. *Multimodal Cardiovascular Imaging: Principles and Clinical Applications.* www.accessmedicine.com. Copyright © The McGraw-Hill Companies, Inc. All rights reserved.)

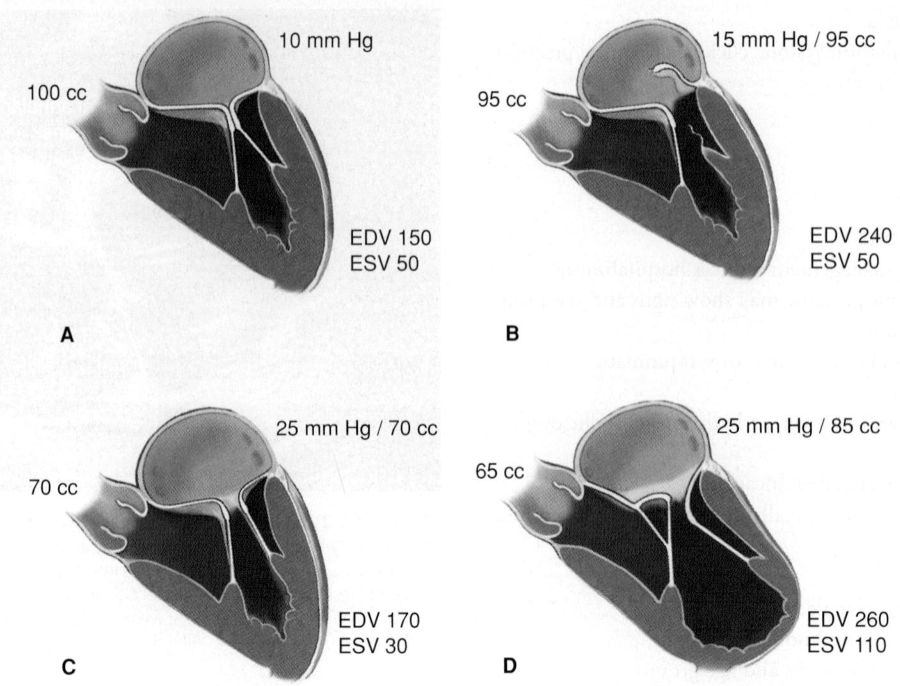

	Preload (SL)	Afterload (ESS)	Contractile function	Ejection fraction	Regurgitant fraction	Stroke volume (cc)
Control (A)	2.07	90	N	0.67	0.0	100
Acute MR (B)	2.25	60	N	0.82	0.5	70
Compensated MR (C)	2.19	90	N	0.79	0.5	95
Decompensated MR (D)	2.19	100	↓	0.58	0.7	65

FIGURE 12-4 Normal physiology (control) is compared with that of acute mitral regurgitation (chordal rupture), compensated mitral regurgitation, and decompensated chronic mitral regurgitation starting with the upper left hand panel and going counterclockwise. The sudden opening of a new pathway for regurgitant flow into the left atrium increases left atrial pressure and preload (sarcomere length), in turn mildly increasing end-diastolic volume because resting sarcomere length is still 90% of maximum length. Afterload (end-systolic stress) is decreased, allowing more complete left ventricular (LV) ejection fraction and reducing end-systolic volume. These changes in loading increase ejection fraction and total stroke volume, but because 50% of the total stroke volume is lost to regurgitation (regurgitant fraction), forward stroke volume is decreased; therefore, despite normal contractile fraction and increased ejection fraction, the patient presents with the hemodynamics of congestive heart failure. In chronic compensated mitral regurgitation (upper right), eccentric hypertrophy leads to substantial LV enlargement allowing it to pump extra volume, in turn resetting forward stroke volume toward normal. Enlargement of the left atrium allows it to accommodate the regurgitant volume at lower filling pressure. In the presence of decompensated chronic mitral regurgitation, muscle damage caused by prolonged severe volume overload reduces the effectiveness of ventricular ejection, and end-systolic volume increases. There is a further increase in diastolic volume, which is not compensatory, resulting in a decrease in total and forward stroke volumes. EDV, end-diastolic volume; ESS, end-systolic stress; ESV, end-systolic volume; MR, mitral regurgitation; SL, sarcomere length. (Adapted from O'Gara P, Sugeng L, Lang R, et al. The role of imaging in chronic degenerative mitral regurgitation. *JACC Cardiovasc Imaging.* 2008;1(2):221–237.)

MEANS OF CONFIRMATION OR DIAGNOSIS

Imaging[2]

- Echocardiography
  - Visualization of enlarged mitral leaflets
  - Displacement of leaflets into left atrium during systolic contraction
  - Mitral valve leaflets >5 mm, displacement >2 mm indicates classic MVP
- Chest x-ray
  - Possible enlargement of left atrium or ventricle is concomitant mitral regurgitation (MR)
- ECG
  - Results usually normal
- Possible biphasic T waves
  - Possible signs of arrhythmias: Fibrillation, tachycardia

Diagnostic Procedures

- Left cardiac catheterization: Generally for severe cases with MR
  - Assessment of coronary artery disease, ejection fraction (EF), pulmonary artery wedge pressure
  - Exercise stress test
  - Stethoscope for auscultation of mid-systolic click and late systolic murmur in the fourth intercostal space, midclavicular line
  - Phonocardiogram[4]

FINDINGS AND INTERPRETATION

- Mid-systolic click and late systolic murmur at the fourth intercostal space midclavicular line
- Precordial palpitations
- Characteristics of heart failure
  - Pulmonary edema (evident in chest x-ray)

- Signs and symptoms of right-sided and left-sided heart failure
- Markedly decreased exercise tolerance
- Decreased systolic blood pressure during exercise
- EF <30% to 40%
- Disability

- 12-lead EKG/ECG that may be observed
  - Findings: Biphasic T waves
  - Interpretation: Arrhythmias and/or tachycardia
- Echocardiogram
  - Findings
    - Enlarged valve leaflets
    - Displacement of leaflet into left atrium during systole
  - Interpretation
    - Possible MR
    - Possible emboli
- Cardiac catheterization
  - Elevated left-atrial pressure if MR present

TREATMENT

Medication[5]

- Beta-blockers
  - Atenolol (Tenormin)
  - Metoprolol (Lopressor)
  - Propranolol (Inderal)
- Aspirin
- Anticoagulants
  - Warfarin (Coumadin)

MEDICAL PROCEDURES

- Surgery
  - Valve repair
  - Valve replacement

REFERRALS/ADMITTANCE

- To primary care or cardiac physician if suspected cardiac muscle dysfunction
- To ER or call 911 if suspected cardiac muscle failure
- Monitoring sufficient if asymptomatic, no need for further treatment
- To cardiologist if symptomatic

IMPAIRMENTS

- Shortness of breath
- Dyspnea on exertion
- Limited activity tolerance
- Limited functional capacity

TEST AND MEASURES

- 6-minute walk test for mild or nonsymptomatic cases
- BORG Rating of Perceived Exertion (RPE)
- Monitor vital signs to include lung auscultations
- Short-Form 36 Health Survey (SF-36)
- New York Heart Association Functional Classification scale

INTERVENTION

- Risk-factor modification
- Cardiac rehabilitation[6]
  - Decreases morbidity and mortality

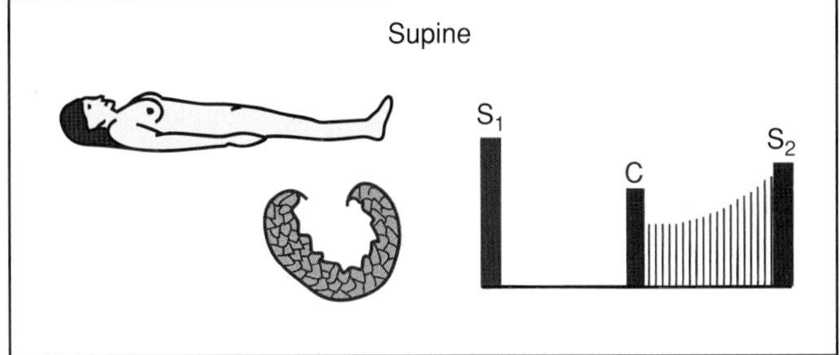

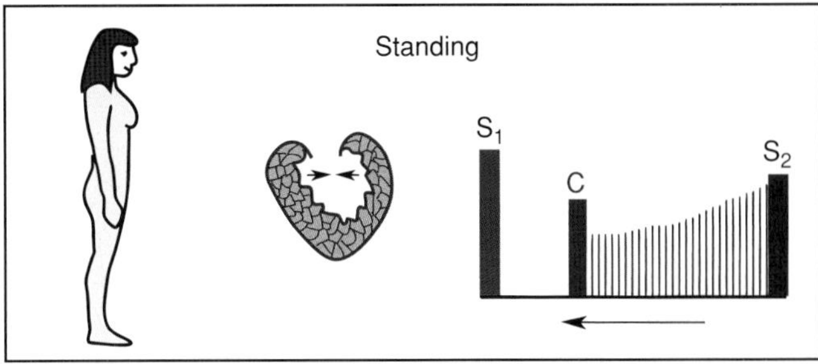

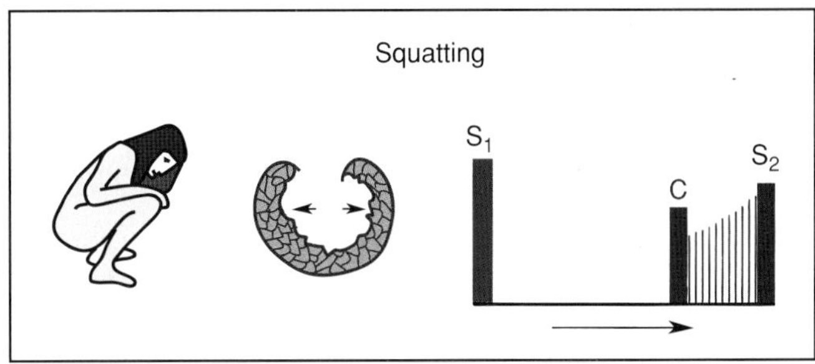

FIGURE 12-5 A midsystolic nonejection sound (C) occurs in mitral valve prolapse and is followed by a late systolic murmur that crescendos to a first heart sound (S_1). With assumption of the upright posture, venous return decreases, the heart becomes smaller, the C moves closer to S_1, and the mitral regurgitant murmur has an earlier onset. With prompt squatting, both venous return and afterload increase, the heart becomes larger, the C moves toward a second heart sound (S_2), and the duration of the murmur shortens. (From Fuster V, Walsh RA, Harrington RA, eds. In: *Hurst's The Heart*. 13th ed. http://www.accessmedicine.com. Copyright © The McGraw-Hill Companies, Inc. All rights reserved.)

  - Three phases[6]
  - Emphasis on wellness and prevention
- Aerobic training as tolerated
- Education on signs and symptoms
- Dietary instruction
  - Avoid excess caffeine, cigarettes, alcohol
- Good dental hygiene to prevent endocarditis along with antibiotic prophylaxis

FUNCTIONAL GOALS

- Patient will be able to
  - State signs and symptoms of MVP
  - Tolerate 30 minutes of continuous exercise while maintaining stable vital signs and RPE of 13.
- Short-term goals[6]
  - To recondition sufficiently in order to resume normal activities.
  - To limit physiologic and psychological effects of aortic stenosis.
  - To decrease risk of sudden cardiac arrest or myocardial infarction.
  - Controlling symptoms of cardiac disease.

- Long-term goals[6]
  - To identify and treat risk factors.
  - To stabilize or reverse atherosclerotic processes.
  - To improve psychological status.

PROGNOSIS

- Depends on the severity of MVP
- Generally no adverse outcome unless progression to MR occurs

PATIENT RESOURCE

- Society for Mitral Valve Prolapse Syndrome. http://www.mitralvalveprolapse.com. Accessed July 6, 2013.

REFERENCES

1. The American Physical Therapy Association. Pattern 6D: impaired aerobic capacity/endurance associated with cardiovascular pump dysfunction or failure. *Interactive Guide to Physical Therapist Practice.* 2003. doi: 10.2522/ptguide.3.3_4. http://guidetoptpractice.apta.org/content/1/SEC30.extract. Accessed July 6, 2013.
2. Cassady SL, Cahalin LP. Cardiovascular pathophysiology. In: DeTurk WE, Cahalin LP, eds. *Cardiovascular and Pulmonary Physical Therapy: An Evidence-Based Approach.* 2nd ed. New York, NY: McGraw-Hill; 2011. http://www.accessphysiotherapy.com/abstract/6872858. Accessed July 6, 2013.
3. Miyamoto SD, Sondheimer HM, Fagan TE, Collins KK. Cardiovascular diseases. In: Hay WW, Levin MJ, Sondheimer JM, Deterding RR. *CURRENT Diagnosis & Treatment: Pediatrics.* 20th ed. New York, NY: McGraw-Hill; 2011. http://www.accessphysiotherapy. com/abstract/6583154#6583208. Accessed July 6, 2013.
4. Kusumoto FM. Cardiovascular disorders: heart disease: pathophysiology of selected cardiovascular disorders. In: *Pathophysiology of Disease: An Introduction to Clinical Medicine.* 6th ed. New York, NY: McGraw-Hill; 2010. http://www.accessphysiotherapy.com/abstract/5367685#5367687. Accessed July 6, 2013.
5. Panus PC, Jobst EE, Masters SB, Katzung B, Tinsley SL, Trevor AJ. *Pharmacology for the Physical Therapist.* New York, NY: McGraw-Hill; 2009. http://www.accessphysiotherapy.com/resource/615. Accessed July 6, 2013.
6. Dutton M. Cardiovascular physical therapy. In: Dutton M, ed. *McGraw-Hill's NPTE (National Physical Therapy Examination).* 2nd ed. New York, NY: McGraw-Hill; 2012. http://www.accessphysiotherapy.com/content/5401905. Accessed July 6, 2013.

ADDITIONAL REFERENCES

- Blume ED, Naftel DC, Bastardi HJ, Duncan BW, Kirklin JK, Webber SA. Outcomes of children bridged to heart transplantation with ventricular assist devices: a multi-institutional study. *Circulation.* 2006;113(19):2313–2319.
- Dubin D. *Rapid Interpretation of EKG's.* Fort Myers, FL: COVER Publishing Co.; 2000.
- ICD9Data.com. http://www.icd9data.com. Accessed July 6, 2013.
- ICD10Data.com. http://www.icd10data.com. Accessed July 6, 2013.
- Knackstedt C, Mischke K, Schimpf T, Neef P, Schauerte P. Ventricular fibrillation due to severe mitral valve prolapse. *Int J Cardiol.* 2007;116:e101–e102.
- Mechleb BK, Kasasbeh ES, Iskandar SB, Schoondyke JW, Garcia ID. Mitral valve prolapse: relationship of echocardiography characteristics to natural history. *Echocardiography.* 2006;23(5):434–437.
- Rosenthal D, Chrisant MR, Edens E, et al. International Society for Heart and Lung Transplantation: practice guidelines for management of heart failure in children. *J Heart Lung Transplant.* 2004;23(12):1313–1333.

13 MITRAL REGURGITATION

Natalie V. Wessel, DO, MPH
Eric Shamus, PhD, DPT, PT, CSCS

CONDITION/DISORDER SYNONYMS

- Left atrial overload
- Mitral valve regurgitation
- Mitral valve insufficiency

ICD-9-CM CODES

- 394.1 Rheumatic mitral insufficiency
- 424.0 Mitral valve disorders
- 746.6 Congenital mitral insufficiency

ICD-10-CM CODES

- I05.1 Rheumatic mitral insufficiency
- I34.0 Nonrheumatic mitral (valve) insufficiency
- Q23.3 Congenital mitral insufficiency

PREFERRED PRACTICE PATTERN

- 6D: Impaired Aerobic Capacity/Endurance Associated With Cardiovascular Pump Dysfunction or Failure[1]

PATIENT PRESENTATION

A 65-year-old female, with a history of mitral valve prolapse (MVP) and an irregular heartbeat, presents with shortness of breath on walking. Vitals are: Pulse: 92, Respirations: 24, Blood Pressure: 132/80, and SpO_2% of 97%. On physical examination there are bounding arterial pulses bilaterally and a leftward displacement of the apical impulse. Cardiac auscultation reveals a holosystolic murmur over the apex of the heart. EKG readings are nonspecific and the echocardiogram shows an enlarged left ventricle, enlarged left atria, and a regurgitant volume into the left atria of 65 mL.

KEY FEATURES

Description

- Mitral valve does not close properly during systolic contraction of left ventricle.
  - Causes backflow and fluid overload in left atrium.
- Fluid overload in left atrium can lead to weakening of left atrial wall.
- Fluid overload in left atrium can also cause pooling and clotting in left atrium.
- Mitral regurgitation (MR) is the most common type of valvular heart disease.

Essentials of Diagnosis

- Stethoscope for auscultation systolic murmur in mitral position
- EKG/ECG[2]
- Echocardiogram

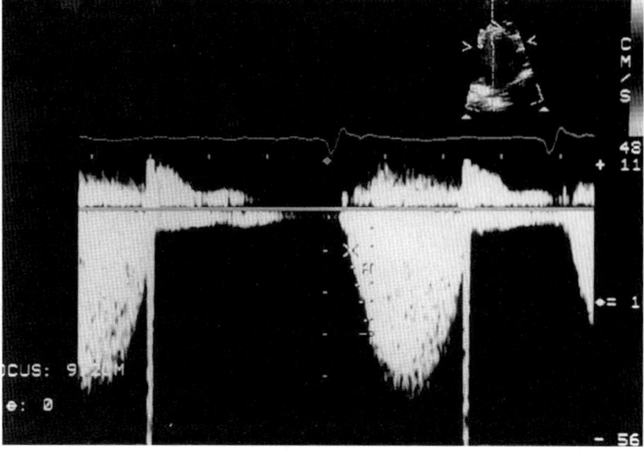

FIGURE 13-1 Continuous wave tracing of mitral regurgitation with calculation of dP/dt (apical transducer position). The time period between velocities of 1 and 3 m/s is 0.07 second, the calculated dP/dt is approximately 460 mm Hg/s. (From Fuster V, Walsh RA, Harrington RA. *Hurst's The Heart*, 13th ed. www.accessmedicine.com. Copyright © The McGraw-Hill Companies, Inc. All rights reserved.)

General Considerations

- Patients with significant MR can show signs and symptoms of congestive heart failure.
- Strenuous activity should be limited for symptomatic MR.
- Signs and symptoms should be monitored.
- Can lead to sudden cardiac death, arrhythmias, embolic events, and coronary disease.
- Patients can develop bacterial endocarditis.
- Valve problems can develop 5 to 10 years after rheumatic fever.
- Ischemic heart disease, rheumatic fever, and Marfan syndrome are also associated with MR.

Demographics

- MR can be congenital, present from birth.
- More common in women and with advanced age.

CLINICAL FINDINGS

SIGNS AND SYMPTOMS

- Symptoms depend on the degree of valvular dysfunction
- Mild-to-moderate regurgitation generally does not cause symptoms
- Deviation of heartbeat or point of maximal impulse (PMI)
- Cardiovascular collapse or shock
- Audible systolic murmur at left fourth intercostal space, midclavicular line
- Angina pectoris
- Syncope
- Congestive heart failure
- Dyspnea on exertion
- Shortness of breath
- Anginal chest pain that increases with exercise
- Orthopnea
- Fatigue, weakness
- Fainting, dizziness with activity
- Palpitations
- Palpable heaves/thrills over precordium
- Arrhythmias, particularly atrial fibrillation
- Endocarditis

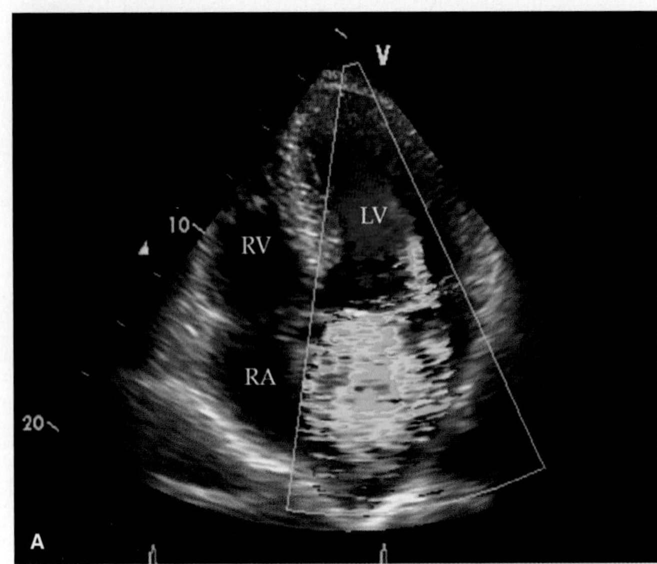

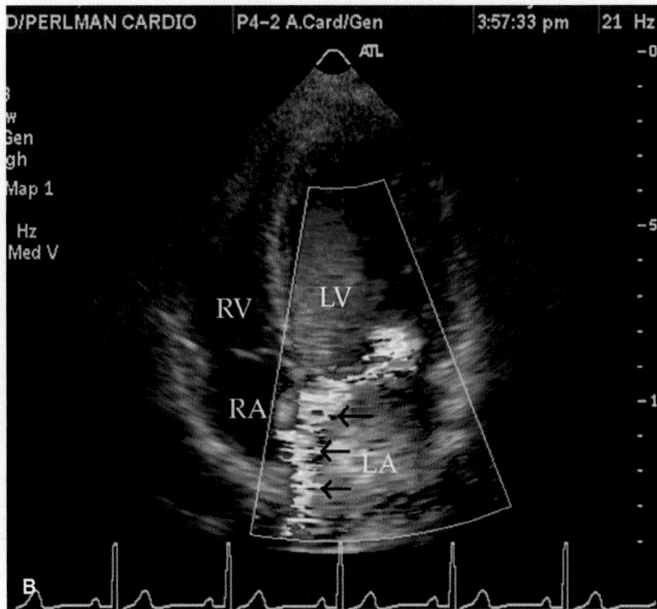

FIGURE 13-2 **A.** Mitral regurgitation. In this apical four-chamber image, a large central jet of severe mitral regurgitation fills the left atrium. **B.** Apical four-chamber view from a patient with angiographically proven severe mitral regurgitation. The color Doppler jet in this case is eccentric and directed medially (*black arrows*). The jet hugs the wall of the interatrial septum and wraps around to the right upper pulmonary vein. LA, left atrium; LV, left ventricle; RA, right atrium; RV, right ventricle. (From Fuster V, Walsh RA, Harrington RA. *Hurst's The Heart,* 13th ed. www.accessmedicine.com. Copyright © The McGraw-Hill Companies, Inc. All rights reserved.)

Functional Implications

- Severe MR causes progressive shortness of breath and signs of congestive heart failure.
- Minimal functional implications, and patients may be unaware of reduced cardiovascular capacity until it becomes severe.
- MR can cause syncope, chest pain, and heart failure if untreated.

Possible Contributing Causes

- Acute rheumatic fever
- MVP: Most common cause of MR is MVP due to weakening of connective tissue
- Coronary artery disease
- Diabetes mellitus
- Hyperlipoproteinemia
- Hypertension
- Marfan syndrome
- Older age
- Congenital heart defects
- Endocarditis
- Prior heart attack

Differential Diagnosis

- Acute coronary syndrome
- Aortic regurgitation
- Aortic stenosis
- MVP
- Mitral stenosis
- Myocardial infarction dysfunction
- Shock, hypovolemia
- Heart failure
  - Chest X-ray evidence of pulmonary edema
  - Signs and symptoms of right and left heart failure
  - Markedly decreased exercise tolerance
  - Decreased systolic BP during exercise
  - Ejection fraction (EF) <30 to 40%
  - Disability

MEANS OF CONFIRMATION OR DIAGNOSIS

Imaging

- Echocardiography
- MRI of the heart
- Chest X-ray
- ECG

Diagnostic Procedures

- Exercise stress test
- Left cardiac catheterization
  - Assessment of coronary artery disease, EF, pulmonary artery wedge pressure
  - Phonocardiogram[3]

FINDINGS AND INTERPRETATION

- Holosystolic murmur at fourth intercostal space, midclavicular line
- Palpable heave of precordium and over apex

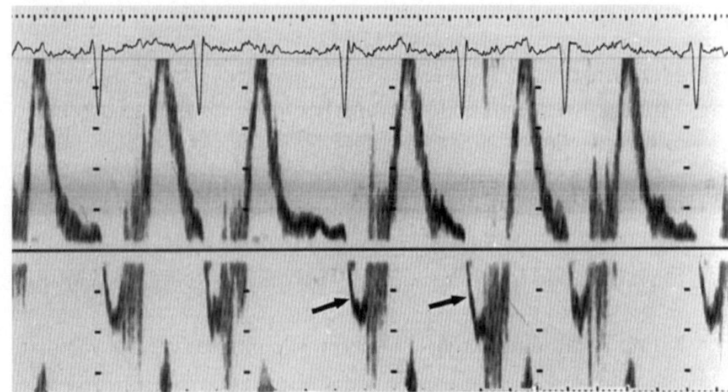

FIGURE 13-3 Pulmonary venous pulsed-wave Doppler in severe mitral regurgitation. Systolic flow reversal (i.e., systolic flow into the pulmonary vein) is present (*arrows*). (From Fuster V, Walsh RA, Harrington RA. *Hurst's The Heart,* 13th ed. www.accessmedicine.com. Copyright © The McGraw-Hill Companies, Inc. All rights reserved.)

Dysfunction	Lesions	Etiology
Type I		
Normal leaflet motion 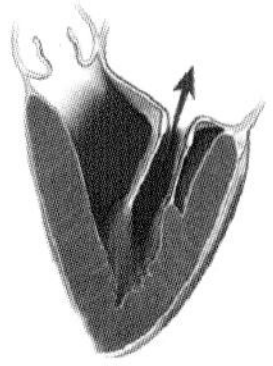	Annular dilatation Annular deformation Leaflet perforation Leaflet cleft	Ischemic cardiomyopathy Dilated cardiomyopathy Endocarditis Congenital
Type II		
Increased leaflet motion (leaflet prolapse) 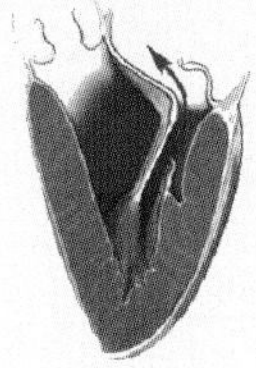	Myxomatous degeneration Chordal elongation Chordal rupture Papillary muscle elongation Papillary muscle rupture	Degenerative disease Fibroelastic deficiency Marfan syndrome Forme fruste Barlow Barlow disease Endocarditis Rheumatic disease Trauma Ischemic cardiomyopathy Ehlers–Danlos syndrome
Type IIIA		
Restricted leaflet motion (restricted opening) 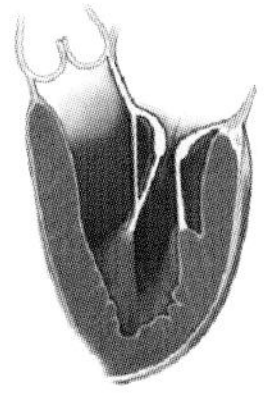	Leaflet thickening Leaflet retraction Chordal thickening Chordal retraction Chordal fusion Calcification Commissural fusion Ventricular fibrosis	Rheumatic disease Carcinoid disease Radiation Lupus eythematosus Ergotamine use Hypereosinophilic syndrome Mucopolysaccharidosis
Type IIIB		
Restricted leaflet motion (restricted closure) 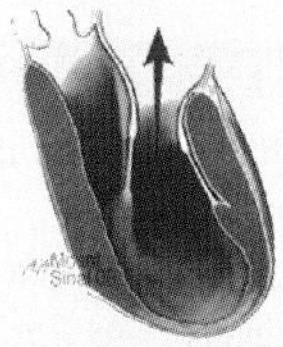	Leaflet tethering Papillary muscle displacement Ventricular dilatation Ventricular aneurysm Ventricular fibrosis	Ischemic cardiomyopathy Dilated cardiomyopathy

FIGURE 13-4 Pathophysiologic triad of mitral valve regurgitation composed of etiology, valve lesions, and leaflet dysfunction. (From Fuster V, Walsh RA, Harrington RA. *Hurst's The Heart,* 13th ed. www.accessmedicine.com. Copyright © The McGraw-Hill Companies, Inc. All rights reserved.)

- Lateral deviation of PMI
- Precordial palpitations
- Echocardiography
  - Jet stream of blood into the left atrium during systole
  - Dilated left atrium with possible left atrial clot
  - Decreased left ventricular function
  - Systolic backflow in pulmonary veins
- 12-lead EKG/ECG that may be observed
  - Broad notched P waves a sign of left atrial overload
  - Negative component of P wave in V_1 a sign of left atrial overload
  - Can be associated with ST-T wave changes and Q waves if associated with ischemic heart disease
- Echocardiogram
  - Enlarged left atrium
  - Backflow of blood into left atrium during systole
  - Left ventricular dysfunction
  - Possible increase in left pulmonary venous pressure
- Cardiac catheterization

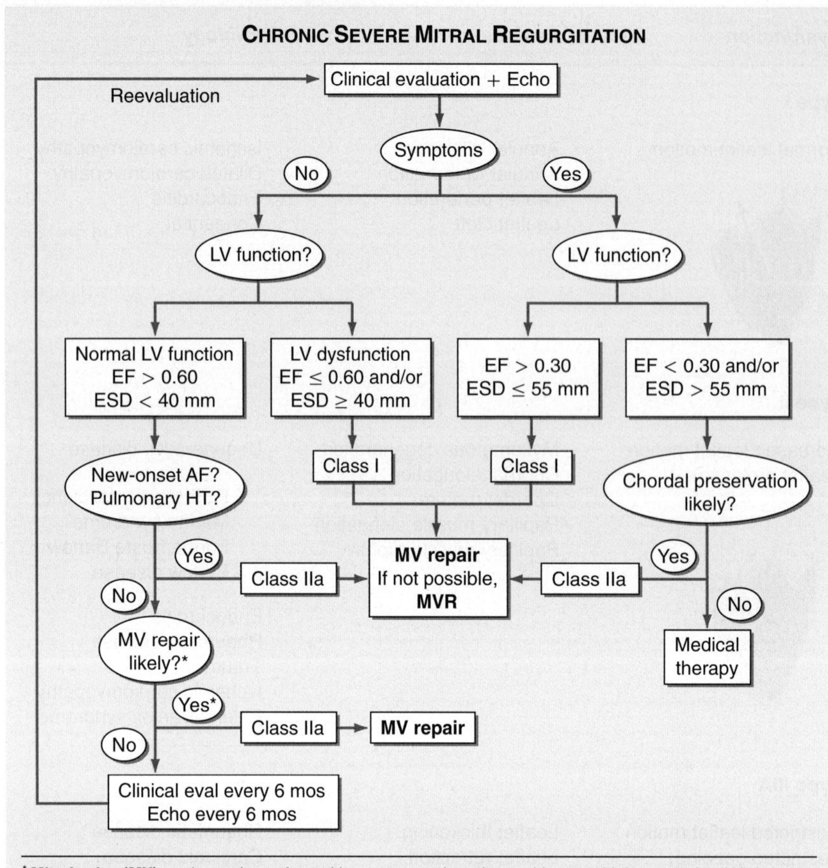

FIGURE 13-5 Management strategy for patients with chronic severe nonischemic mitral regurgitation. AF, atrial fibrillation; Echo, echocardiography; EF, ejection fraction; ESD, end-systolic dimension; eval, evaluation; HT, hypertension; MVR, mitral valve replacement. (From RO Bonow, Carabello BA, Chatterjee K, et al. *J Am Coll Cardiol.* 2006;48:e1–e148., with permission.)

- Elevated left atrial pressure
- Elevated pressure around pulmonary veins (may not be detectable)

TREATMENT

▶ Medications

- For heart failure induced by MR
  - Diuretics
  - Beta-blockers
    - Atenolol (Tenormin)
    - Metoprolol (Lopressor)
    - Propranolol (Inderal)
  - Positive inotropic agents
  - Angiotensin-converting enzyme (ACE)
  - Aldosterone antagonists
  - Antibiotics for patients with a history of rheumatic fever
  - Vasodilators such as nitroprusside and hydralazine to decrease afterload
  - Anticoagulation with associated MVP or atrial fibrillation
  - Inpatient pharmacologic management[4]

MEDICAL PROCEDURES

- Internal cardiac defibrillator
- Mitral valve replacement/repair
- Noninvasive clip repair of mitral valve
- Intra-aortic balloon pump
- Cardiac resynchronization
- Coronary artery bypass
- Left or right ventricular assisting device
- Cardiac transplant

REFERRALS/ADMITTANCE

- To primary care or cardiac physician if suspected cardiac muscle dysfunction
- To ER or call 911 if suspected cardiac muscle failure
- Must see a cardiologist every 3 to 6 months

IMPAIRMENTS

- Shortness of breath
- Dyspnea on exertion
- Limited activity tolerance
- Limited functional capacity

TEST AND MEASURES

- 6-minute walk test for mild or nonsymptomatic cases
- BORG Rating of Perceived Exertion (RPE)
- Monitor vital signs to include lung auscultations
- Short-Form 36 Health Survey (SF-36)
- New York Heart Association Functional Classification scale

INTERVENTION

- Risk-factor modification
- Cardiac rehabilitation[5]
  - Decreases morbidity and mortality
  - Three phases[5]
    - Phase 1: Inpatient rehabilitation
    - Phase 1.5: Postdischarge phase
    - Phase 2: Supervised exercise
    - Phase 3: Maintenance phase
  - Emphasis on wellness and prevention
- Education on signs and symptoms
- Education on disease management reduces hospitalization
- Dietary instruction
  - Sodium restriction
  - May require limited fluid intake
- Nonaerobic resistance training

FUNCTIONAL GOALS

- Patient will be able to
  - State the signs and symptoms of MR.
  - Tolerate 30 minutes of continuous exercise while maintaining stable vital signs and rate of perceived exertion (RPE) of 13.
- Short-term goals[5]
  - To recondition sufficiently for resuming normal activities.
  - To limit physiologic and psychological effects of MR.
  - To decrease the risk of sudden cardiac arrest or myocardial infarction.
  - To control symptoms of cardiac disease.
- Long-term goals[5]
  - To identify and treat risk factors.
  - To stabilize or reverse atherosclerotic processes.
  - To improve patient's psychological status.

PROGNOSIS

- Depends on severity and cause of aortic stenosis

PATIENT RESOURCE

- Mitral Valve Regurgitation. CardioSmart. American College of Cardiology. https://www.cardiosmart.org/Healthwise/aa14/3442/aa143442. Accessed July 4, 2013.

REFERENCES

1. The American Physical Therapy Association. *Interactive Guide to Physical Therapist Practice*. Alexandria, VA: The American Physical Therapy Association; 2003. http://guidetoptpractice.apta.org. Accessed July 4, 2013.
2. Cassady SL, Cahalin LP. Cardiovascular pathophysiology. In: DeTurk WE, Cahalin LP, eds. *Cardiovascular and Pulmonary Physical Therapy*. 2nd ed. New York, NY: McGraw-Hill; 2011. http://www.accessphysiotherapy.com/abstract/6872858. Accessed July 4, 2013.
3. Kusumoto FM. Cardiovascular disorders: heart disease. In: McPhee SJ, Hammer GD, eds. *Pathophysiology of Disease: An Introduction to Clinical Medicine*. 6th ed. New York, NY: McGraw-Hill; 2010. http://www.accessphysiotherapy.com/abstract/5367685. Accessed July 4, 2013.
4. Miyamoto SD, Sondheimer HM, Fagan TE, Collins KK. Cardiovascular diseases. In: Hay WW, Levin MJ, Sondheimer JM, Deterding RR,eds. *CURRENT Diagnosis & Treatment: Pediatrics*. 20th ed. New York, NY: McGraw-Hill; 2011. http://www.accessphysiotherapy.com/abstract/6583154#6583208. Accessed July 4, 2013.
5. Dutton M. Cardiovascular physical therapy. In: Dutton M, ed. *McGraw-Hill's NPTE (National Physical Therapy Examination)*. New York, NY: McGraw-Hill; 2009. http://www.accessphysiotherapy.com/content/5401373. Accessed July 4, 2013.

ADDITIONAL REFERENCES

- Blume ED, Naftel DC, Bastardi HJ, Duncan BW, Kirklin JK, Webber SA. Outcomes of children bridged to heart transplantation with ventricular assist devices: a multi-institutional study. *Circulation*. 2006;113(19):2313–2319.
- Dubin D. *Rapid Interpretation of EKG's*. Fort Myers, FL: COVER Publishing Co.; 2000.
- Dutton M. Cardiovascular physical therapy. In: Dutton M, ed. *McGraw-Hill's NPTE (National Physical Therapy Examination)*. 2nd ed. New York, NY: McGraw-Hill; 2012. http://www.accessphysiotherapy.com/abstract/5401746. Accessed July 4, 2013.
- ICD9DATA. http://www.icd9data.com. Accessed July 4, 2013.
- ICD10DATA. http://www.icd10data.com. Accessed July 4, 2013.
- Panus PC, Jobst EE, Masters SB, Katzung B, Tinsley SL, Trevor AJ. *Pharmacology for the Physical Therapist*. New York, NY: McGraw-Hill; 2009. http://www.accessphysiotherapy.com/resource/615. Accessed July 4, 2013.
- Rosenthal D, Chrisant MR, Edens E, et al. International Society for Heart and Lung Transplantation: practice guidelines for management of heart failure in children. *J Heart Lung Transplant*. 2004;23(12):1313–1333.

14 MITRAL STENOSIS

Natalie V. Wessel, DO, MPH
Eric Shamus, PhD, DPT, PT, CSCS

CONDITION/DISORDER SYNONYM

- Mitral valve stenosis

ICD-9-CM CODES

- 394.0 Mitral stenosis
- 394.2 Mitral stenosis with insufficiency
- 396.0 Mitral valve stenosis and aortic valve stenosis
- 396.1 Mitral valve stenosis and aortic valve insufficiency
- 746.5 Congenital mitral stenosis

ICD-10-CM CODES

- I05.0 Rheumatic mitral stenosis
- I05.2 Rheumatic mitral stenosis with insufficiency
- I34.2 Nonrheumatic mitral (valve) stenosis
- Q23.2 Congenital mitral stenosis

PREFERRED PRACTICE PATTERN

- 6D: Impaired Aerobic Capacity/Endurance Associated With Cardiovascular Pump Dysfunction or Failure[1]

PATIENT PRESENTATION

A 55-year-old male, originally from Guatemala, is preparing to run his first 5K. He states that while training his heart was racing and he coughed up a little bit of blood. He states that he had rheumatic fever as a child, but has been very healthy ever since. Vitals are: Pulse: 80, Respirations: 16, Blood Pressure: 126/80, and SpO_2% of 99%. On physical examination there is an opening snap and a faint diastolic murmur over the cardiac apex. A chest X-ray and EKG are within normal limits and the cardiac echo reveals a narrowing of the mitral valve.

KEY FEATURES

Description

- Narrowing of the mitral valve[2]
- Causes reduced blood flow
- Limited blood flow between left atrium and left ventricle
- Increased volume and pressure of left ventricle
- Atrial fibrillation and dysrhythmia-induced thrombi
- Decreased blood flow can cause decreased cardiac output (CO) leading to lightheadedness, fainting, chest pain
- Decreased blood flow to the rest of the body and brain
- Four types[2]
  - Rheumatic
  - Calcific
  - Congenital
  - Collagen vascular disease

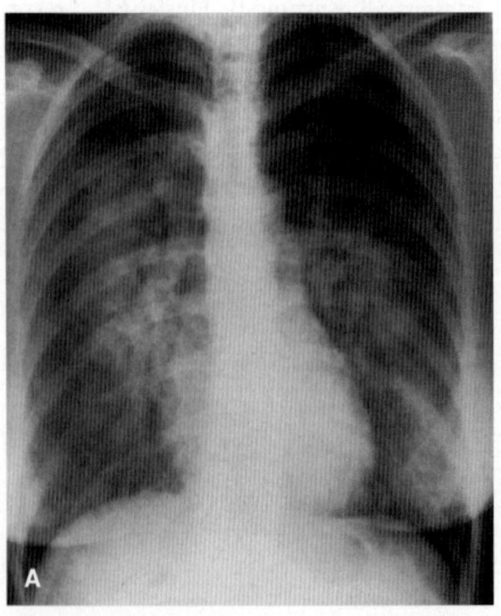

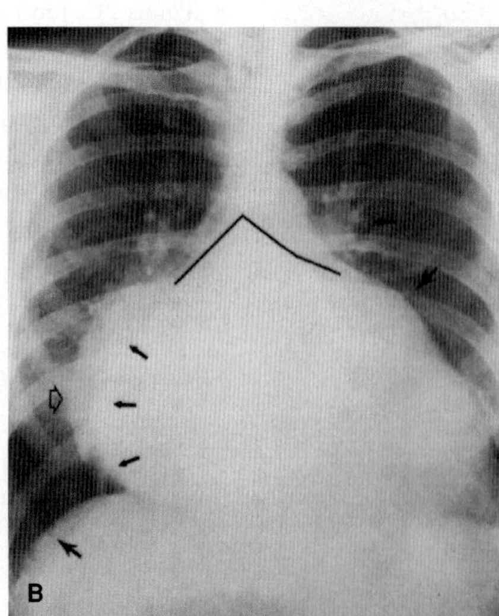

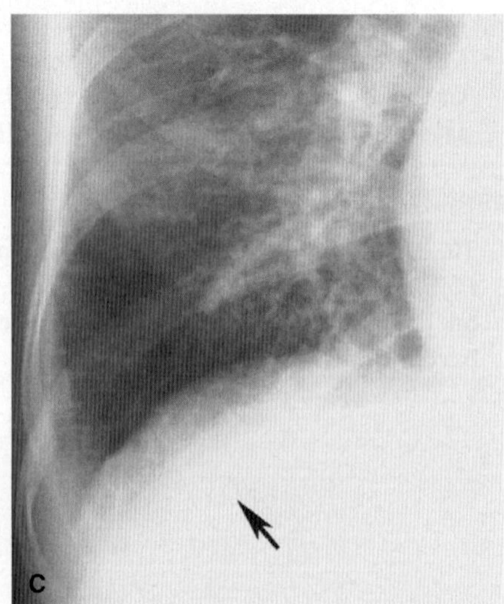

FIGURE 14-1 Radiographic appearance of left heart failure. **A.** Acute. Patient with acute mitral regurgitation because of the rupture of chordae tendineae showing the "bat-wings" appearance of a severe alveolar type of pulmonary edema and a normal-sized heart. **B.** Chronic. Patient with severe mitral and tricuspid regurgitation and mild aortic regurgitation. This is a predominantly left-sided failure pattern. Note the gross cardiomegaly with striking cephalization and interstitial pulmonary edema. The giant left atrium forms the right cardiac border (*open arrow*), makes its appendage bulge outward on the left side (*upper large arrow*), and splays the mainstem bronchi wide apart (*solid lines*). The huge right atrium forms a double density within the right cardiac border (*three small arrows*). The *small upper arrow* marks the peribronchial cuffing of edema fluid. The *large lower arrow* points to multiple Kerley B lines. **C.** Magnified view of right costophrenic sulcus showing multiple Kerley B lines (*arrow*). (*continued*)

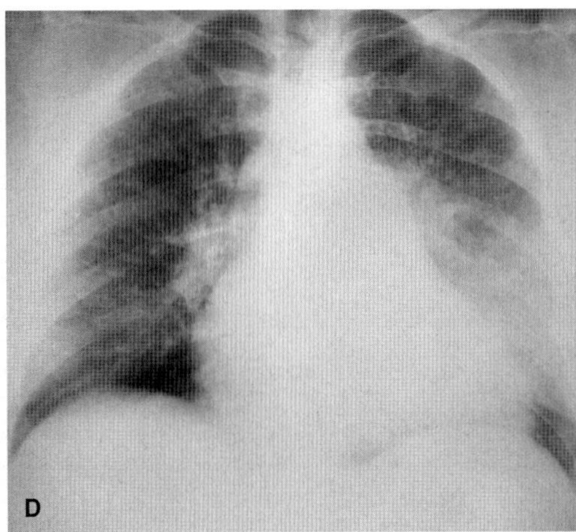

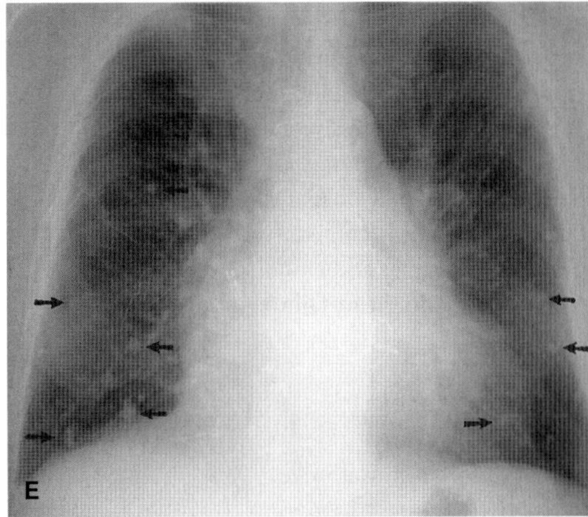

FIGURE 14-1 (*Continued*) **D.** A 44-year-old woman with severe mitral stenosis (MS). The radiograph shows a diffuse stippling with fine nodules representing hemosiderosis. Hemosiderin-laden macrophages were found in her sputa. **E.** Posteroanterior radiograph of a 63-year-old man with severe MS, status post–mitral-valve replacement, shows multiple scattered bony nodules (*arrows*) 2 to 10 mm in diameter throughout the lower two-thirds of both lungs, compatible with pulmonary ossification. (From Fuster V, Walsh RA, Harrington RA. *Hurst's The Heart,* 13th ed. www.accessmedicine.com. Copyright © The McGraw-Hill Companies, Inc. All rights reserved.)

Essentials of Diagnosis

- Stethoscope auscultation for murmur on carotid artery; bruit sound
- EKG/ECG[2]
- Echocardiogram
- Cardiac catheterization
- Chest X-ray
- Exercise stress test

General Considerations

- Worsens over time, neither exercise or diet improves the stenosis.
- Education on disease management reduces hospitalization.
- Patients with significant mitral stenosis should not participate in competitive sports.
- Strenuous activity should be limited for symptomatic mitral valve stenosis.
- Signs and symptoms should be monitored.
- Emphasis on wellness and prevention.

Demographics

- Affects women twice as often as men.
- Occurs in only 40% of all rheumatic heart disease cases.
- Can be congenital, present from birth.
- Can be caused by age-induced dysfunction of the valve from calcification or atherosclerosis.
- More common in patients with history of rheumatic fever.

CLINICAL FINDINGS

SIGNS AND SYMPTOMS

- Pulmonary hypertension
- Pulmonary edema
- Right ventricular failure
- Decreased CO
- Peripheral edema
- Cough with pink, frothy sputum
- Dyspnea on exertion
- Hemoptysis
- Shortness of breath[2]
- Anginal chest pain that increases with exercise
- Orthopnea[2]
- Fatigue, weakness[2]
- Fainting, dizziness with activity
- Palpitations
- Dysphagia
- Hoarseness

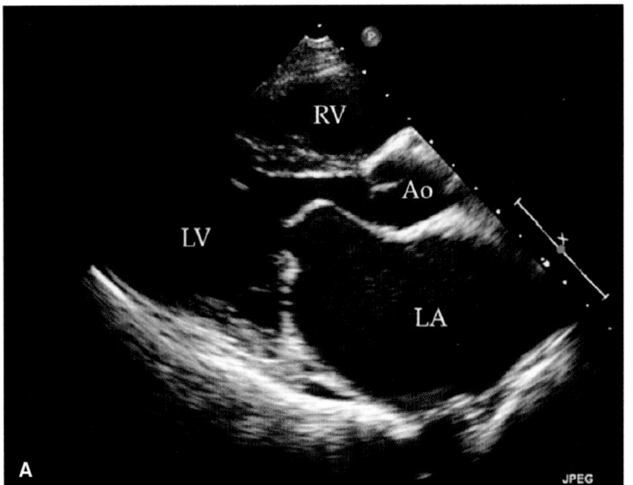

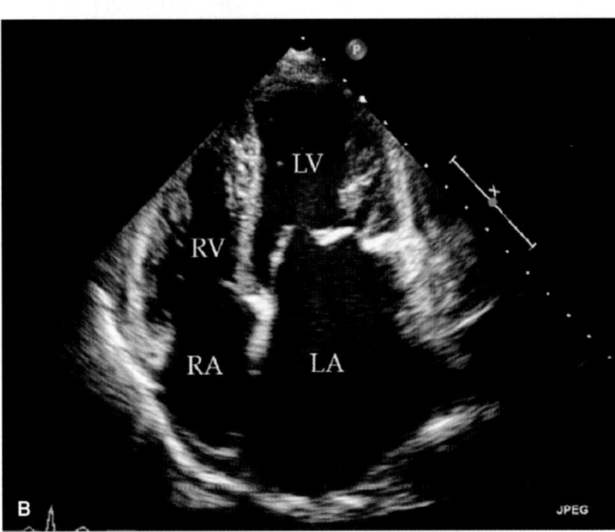

FIGURE 14-2 **A.** Parasternal long-axis view of mitral stenosis. The LA is enlarged, mitral opening is limited, and *doming* of the anterior mitral leaflet is present. **B.** Apical four-chamber view in mitral stenosis. The LA is markedly dilated. (From Fuster V, Walsh RA, Harrington RA. *Hurst's The Heart,* 13th ed. www.accessmedicine.com. Copyright © The McGraw-Hill Companies, Inc. All rights reserved.)

Functional Implications

- Symptoms depend on degree of stenosis.
- Mild-to-moderate stenosis generally does not cause symptoms.
- Severe mitral stenosis causes progressive shortness of breath and increased risk of left atrial overload.
- Minimal at first and patients may be unaware of reduced cardiovascular capacity until it becomes severe.
- Higher risk of atrial arrhythmias and embolic events.
- Can cause syncope, chest pain, heart failure, deadly cardiac arrhythmias if untreated.

Possible Contributing Causes

- Causes of mitral stenosis[2]
  - Age-related calcification of mitral valve
  - Congenital valve dysfunction
  - Rheumatic fever
  - Recurrent strep infections
  - Use of medications such as ergot preparation
  - Congenital heart defect
  - Blood clots or tumor can block mitral valve
  - Radiation exposure to chest
  - Systemic lupus erythematosus
  - Rheumatoid arthritis

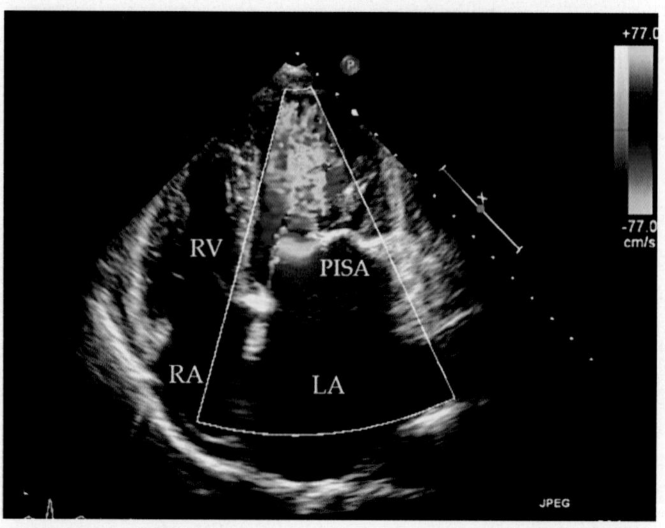

FIGURE 14-3 Apical four-chamber plane in mitral stenosis. Color flow imaging in the mitral valve region shows flow convergence (*PISA*) proximal to the valve during diastole. LA, left atrium; RA, right atrium; RV, right ventricle. (From Fuster V, Walsh RA, Harrington RA. *Hurst's The Heart,* 13th ed. www.accessmedicine.com. Copyright © The McGraw-Hill Companies, Inc. All rights reserved.)

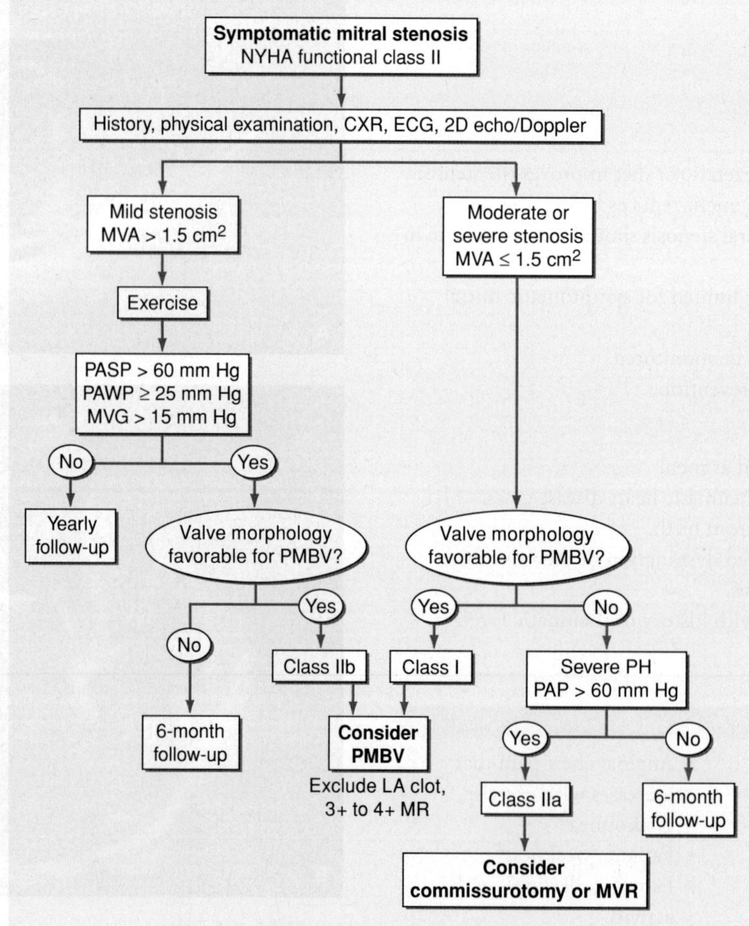

FIGURE 14-4 Management Strategy for patients with mitral stenosis (MS) and mild symptoms. There is controversy as to whether patients with severe MS (MVA <1 cm)[2] and severe pulmonary hypertension (PH) (PASP >60 mm Hg) should undergo percutaneous mitral balloon valvotomy (PMBV) or mitral valve replacement (MVR) to prevent right ventricular failure. CXR, chest X-ray; ECG, electrocardiogram; echo, echocardiography; LA, left atrial; MR, mitral regurgitation; MVA, mitral valve area; MVG, mean mitral valve pressure gradient; NYHA, New York Heart Association; PASP, pulmonary artery systolic pressure; PAWP, pulmonary artery wedge pressure; 2D, 2-dimensional. (From Bonow RO, Carabello BA, Chatterjee K, et al. *J Am Coll Cardiol.* 2006;48:e1–e148, with permission.)

- Coronary artery disease
- Hyperlipoproteinemia
- Hypertension
- Diabetes mellitus
- Older age

Differential Diagnosis[3]

- Acute coronary syndrome
- Mitral regurgitation
- Aortic stenosis
- Cor triatriatum (triatrial heart)
- Aortic regurgitation
- Idiopathic pulmonary atrial hypertension (IPAH)
- Mitral valve prolapse
- Myocardial infarction
- Shock, hypovolemia
- Cardiac pump dysfunction
  - Cardiac muscle dysfunction produces slight-to-moderate reduction in CO
  - Mild-to-moderate activity limitation
  - Functional capacity of ≤5 to 6 metabolic equivalents (METS)
- Cardiac pump failure
  - Cardiac muscle dysfunction produces moderate-to-severe reduction in CO
  - Marked activity limitation
  - Functional capacity of ≤4 to 5 METS

MEANS OF CONFIRMATION OR DIAGNOSIS

Laboratory Tests

- Lipid profile
- Triglycerides test
- Blood analysis: Complete blood count, platelet count, prothrombin time, erythrocyte sedimentation rate
- Rheumatic heart disease: C-reactive protein, sedimentation rate, and antistreptolysin O (ASLO) antibodies
- Levels of antibody to streptococcal group A carbohydrate (chronic rheumatic mitral valve disease)
- Lupus erythematosus cells, antinuclear antibodies, and antibodies to double-stranded DNA (systemic lupus erythematosus)

Imaging

- Echocardiography
  - Best to watch stenosis (narrowing of the valve) over time
  - Transesophageal echocardiography
  - Mitral leaflets with narrowing, calcification
  - Congenital deformities of mitral valve
  - Enlarged left atrium
  - Doppler flow will show increased jet velocity across the valve
  - Increased left atrial pressure
- Chest X-ray
  - Left atrial enlargement
  - Pulmonary edema from valvular-induced heart failure
- ECG
  - Left atrial hypertrophy
  - ST–T wave changes
  - Possible left ventricular hypertrophy

Diagnostic Procedures

- Elevated left atrial pressure
  - Indirect measure of elevated pulmonary vein pressure

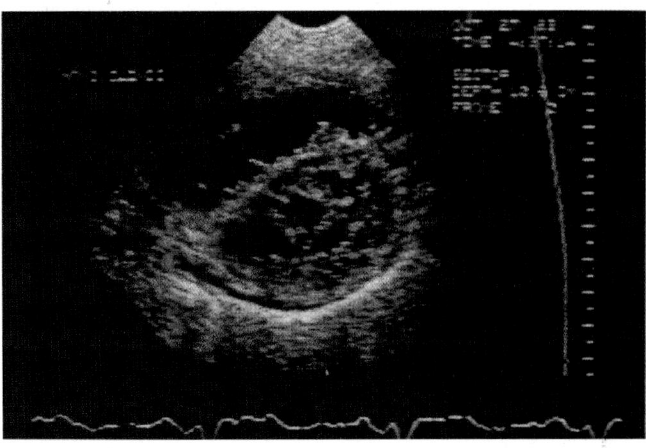

FIGURE 14-5 An echocardiogram from a patient with mitral stenosis. (From Fuster V, Walsh RA, Harrington RA. *Hurst's The Heart,* 13th ed. www.accessmedicine.com. Copyright © The McGraw-Hill Companies, Inc. All rights reserved.)

- Cardiac catheterization
  - Assessment of coronary artery disease, ejection fraction (EF), pulmonary artery wedge pressure, mitral valve function
  - Phonocardiogram[2]

FINDINGS AND INTERPRETATION

- Diastolic ejection murmur in the fifth left intercostal space, midclavicular
- Can lead to sudden cardiac death, arrhythmias, increased risk of bleeding, embolic events, coronary disease
- Characteristics of heart failure
  - Chest X-ray evidence of pulmonary edema
  - Signs and symptoms of right and left heart failure
  - Markedly decreased exercise tolerance
  - Decreased systolic BP during exercise
  - EF <30% to 40%
  - Disability
  - Markedly decreased quality of life
- 12-lead EKG/ECG that may be observed
  - Notched P wave
  - Often associated ST–T wave changes
- Echocardiogram
  - Thickened, narrowed mitral leaflets
  - Possible congenital anatomic abnormalities of valve
  - Enlarged left atrium
  - Increased pulmonary vein pressure
  - Fluid overload in left atrium
- Cardiac catheterization
  - Elevated pulmonary vein pressure
  - Increased pressure across the mitral valve

TREATMENT

Medication

- For heart failure induced by mitral valve stenosis
  - Diuretic drugs for congestive heart failure (CHF)
  - Anti-arrhythmic drugs, class I and class III medications
  - Beta-blockers, digoxin and calcium-channel blockers for rapid atrioventricular (AV) conduction
  - Anti-coagulants (in thromboembolic complication)
  - Positive inotropic agents
  - Angiotensin-converting enzyme (ACE)

- Aldosterone antagonists
- Antibiotics for patients with an history of rheumatic fever
- Inpatient pharmacologic management[4]

MEDICAL PROCEDURES

- Percutaneous mitral balloon valvotomy to replace or repair
- Dietary instruction
  - Sodium restriction
  - May require limited fluid intake
- Internal cardiac defibrillator
- Cardiac resynchronization
- Coronary artery bypass
- Left or right ventricular assist device (VAD)
- Cardiac transplant

REFERRALS/ADMITTANCE

- To cardiovascular surgeon to asses valve blockage
- To cardiologist to asses atrial arrhythmias and atrial/ventricular function
- To primary care or cardiac physician if suspected cardiac muscle dysfunction
- To ER or call 911 if suspected cardiac muscle failure
- Patient must see a cardiologist every 3 to 6 months

IMPAIRMENTS

- Shortness of breath
- Dyspnea on exertion
- Limited activity tolerance
- Limited functional capacity

TEST AND MEASURES

- 6-minute walk test for mild or nonsymptomatic cases
- Borg Rating of Perceived Exertion (RPE)
- Monitor vital signs to include lung auscultations
- Short-Form 36
- New York Heart Association Functional Classification scale

INTERVENTION

- Risk-factor modification
- Neither exercise nor diet will improve mitral valve stenosis
- Cardiac rehabilitation[5]
  - Decreases morbidity and mortality
  - Three phases[5]
- Education on signs and symptoms
- Aerobic exercise training as tolerated
- Resistance exercise training

FUNCTIONAL GOALS

- Patient will be able to
  - State the signs and symptoms of mitral valve stenosis.
  - Tolerate 30 minutes of continuous exercise while maintaining stable vital signs and RPE of 13.
- Short-term goals[5]
  - "Reconditioning" sufficient for resuming normal activities.
  - Limiting physiologic and psychological effects of mitral valve stenosis.
  - Reduced risk of sudden cardiac arrest or myocardial infarction.
  - Controlling symptoms of cardiac disease.
- Long-term goals[5]
  - Identification and treatment of risk factors
  - Stabilizing or reversing atherosclerotic processes
  - Improve patient's psychological status

PROGNOSIS

- Depends on severity and cause of mitral valve stenosis
- Surgery may be needed if valve narrows

PATIENT RESOURCE

- Mitral Valve Stenosis. CardioSmart. American College of Cardiology. https://www.cardiosmart.org/Heart-Conditions/Mitral-Valve-Stenosis. Accessed May 3, 2013.

REFERENCES

1. The American Physical Therapy Association. Pattern 6D: impaired aerobic capacity/endurance associated with cardiovascular pump dysfunction or failure. *Interactive Guide to Physical Therapist Practice*. 2003. doi: 10.2522/ptguide.3.3_4. Accessed May 3, 2013.
2. Kusumoto FM. Cardiovascular disorders: heart disease. In: McPhee SJ, Hammer GD, eds. *Pathophysiology of Disease: An Introduction to Clinical Medicine*. 6th ed. New York, NY: McGraw-Hill; 2010. http://www.accessphysiotherapy.com/abstract/5367685. Accessed May 3, 2013.
3. Cassady SL, Cahalin LP. Cardiovascular pathophysiology. In: DeTurk WE, Cahalin LP, eds. *Cardiovascular and Pulmonary Physical Therapy*. 2nd ed. New York, NY: McGraw-Hill; 2011. http://www.accessphysiotherapy.com/abstract/6872858. Accessed May 3, 2013.
4. Miyamoto SD, Sondheimer HM, Fagan TE, Collins KK. Cardiovascular diseases. In: Hay WW, Levin MJ, Sondheimer JM, Deterding RR. *CURRENT Diagnosis & Treatment: Pediatrics*. 20th ed. New York, NY: McGraw-Hill; 2011. http://www.accessphysiotherapy.com/abstract/6583154#6583208. Accessed May 3, 2013.
5. Dutton M. Cardiovascular physical therapy. In: Dutton M, ed. *McGraw-Hill's NPTE (National Physical Therapy Examination)*. 2nd ed. New York, NY: McGraw-Hill; 2012. http://www.accessphysiotherapy.com/content/5401373. Accessed May 3, 2013.

ADDITIONAL REFERENCES

- Blume ED, Naftel DC, Bastardi HJ, Duncan BW, Kirklin JK, Webber SA. Outcomes of children bridged to heart transplantation with ventricular assist devices: a multi-institutional study. *Circulation*. 2006;113(19):2313–2319.
- Dubin D. *Rapid Interpretation of EKG's*. Fort Myers, FL: COVER Publishing Co.; 2000.
- Dutton M. Cardiovascular physical therapy. In: Dutton M, ed. *McGraw-Hill's NPTE (National Physical Therapy Examination)*. 2nd ed. New York, NY: McGraw-Hill; 2012. http://www.accessphysiotherapy.com/abstract/5401746. Accessed May 3, 2013.
- ICD9DATA. http://www.icd9data.com. Accessed May 3, 2013.
- ICD10DATA. http://www.icd10data.com. Accessed May 3, 2013.
- Panus PC, Jobst EE, Masters SB, Katzung B, Tinsley SL, Trevor AJ. *Pharmacology for the Physical Therapist*. New York, NY: McGraw-Hill; 2009. http://www.accessphysiotherapy.com/resource/615. Accessed January 3, 2013.
- Rosenthal D, Chrisant MR, Edens E, et al. International Society for Heart and Lung Transplantation: practice guidelines for management of heart failure in children. *J Heart Lung Transplant*. 2004;23(12):1313–1333.

15 MYOCARDIAL INFARCTION

Eric Shamus, PhD, DPT, PT, CSCS
Lisa Ward McVey, DPT, PT, CCS

CONDITION/DISORDER SYNONYMS

- Non-ST-elevation myocardial infarction (NSTEMI)
- ST-elevation myocardial infarction (STEMI)
- Subendocardial myocardial infarction (SEMI)
- Non–Q-wave myocardial infarction
- Acute coronary syndrome (ACS)

ICD-9-CM CODES

- 410 Acute myocardial infarction
  - See entire list under 410
- 412 Old myocardial infarction
  - See entire list under 412

ICD-10-CM CODES

- I21.09 ST-elevation (STEMI) myocardial infarction involving other coronary artery of anterior wall
- I21.11 ST-elevation (STEMI) myocardial infarction involving right coronary artery
- I21.19 ST-elevation (STEMI) myocardial infarction involving other coronary artery of inferior wall
- I21.29 ST-elevation (STEMI) myocardial infarction involving other sites
- I21.3 ST-elevation (STEMI) myocardial infarction of unspecified site
- I21.4 Non–ST-elevation (NSTEMI) myocardial infarction
- I25.2 Old myocardial infarction

PREFERRED PRACTICE PATTERNS[1]

- 6A: Primary Prevention/Risk Reduction for Cardiovascular/Pulmonary Disorders
- 6B: Impaired Aerobic Capacity/Endurance Associated with Deconditioning
- 6D: Impaired Aerobic Capacity/Endurance Associated With Cardiovascular Pump Dysfunction or Failure
- 6E: Impaired Ventilation and Respiration/Gas Exchange Associated With Ventilatory Pump Dysfunction or Failure
- 6F: Impaired Ventilation and Respiration/Gas Exchange Associated With Respiratory Failure
- 6G: Impaired Ventilation, Respiration/Gas Exchange, and Aerobic Capacity/Endurance Associated With Respiratory Failure in the Neonate

PATIENT PRESENTATION

A 51-year-old male presents to the emergency center with chest pain. He states that he has had chest discomfort or pressure intermittently over the last year especially with increased activity. He describes the chest pain as a pressure behind his breastbone that spreads to the left side of his neck. Unlike previous episodes, he was lying down, watching television. The chest pain lasted approximately 15 minutes then subsided on its own. He also noticed that he was nauseated and sweating during the pain episode. He has no medical problems that he is aware of and has not been to a physician for several years. On examination, he is in no acute distress with normal vital signs. His lungs were clear to auscultation bilaterally, and his heart had a regular rate and rhythm with no murmurs. An electrocardiogram (ECG) revealed ST-segment elevation and peaked T waves in leads II, III, and aVF. Serum troponin I and T levels are elevated.[2]

KEY FEATURES

Description

- Blood flow to a region of the heart is blocked.
- Supply does not equal demand, resulting in myocardial ischemia.
- Coronary arteries supply oxygen.
- Without oxygen, heart cells die.
- Chest pain with or without left shoulder, jaw, neck, and teeth pain.

Essentials of Diagnosis

- Acute myocardial infarction (MI)
  - Amount and time of blockage
    - Within 18 to 24 hours after MI: Inflammatory response occurs because of necrosis
    - Visible necrosis is present in 2 to 4 days
  - EKG/ECG[3]
  - Cardiac enzymes
- Old MI
  - EKG/ECG[3]
  - Echocardiogram to assess left ventricular function and ejection fraction (EF)
  - Cardiolite to assess for myocardial perfusion
  - Cardiac catheterization to assess for EF

General Considerations

- MI can result in
  - Sudden death
  - Permanent myocardium damage
  - Valve dysfunction
  - Cardiac arrhythmias
  - Respiratory failure
  - Heart failure
  - Cardiogenic shock.
  - Minimal to no myocardium damage.
- Stratification for risk of event (not specific solely to exercise).
- Patients may have an MI without experiencing signs or symptoms (silent MI may be seen in patients who have diabetes).
- Vital signs should be monitored before, during, and after exercise.
- Greater emphasis has been placed on wellness and prevention.

Demographics

- Heart disease is the number one cause of death in both women and men.
- Women are more likely to present with atypical symptoms compared to men.

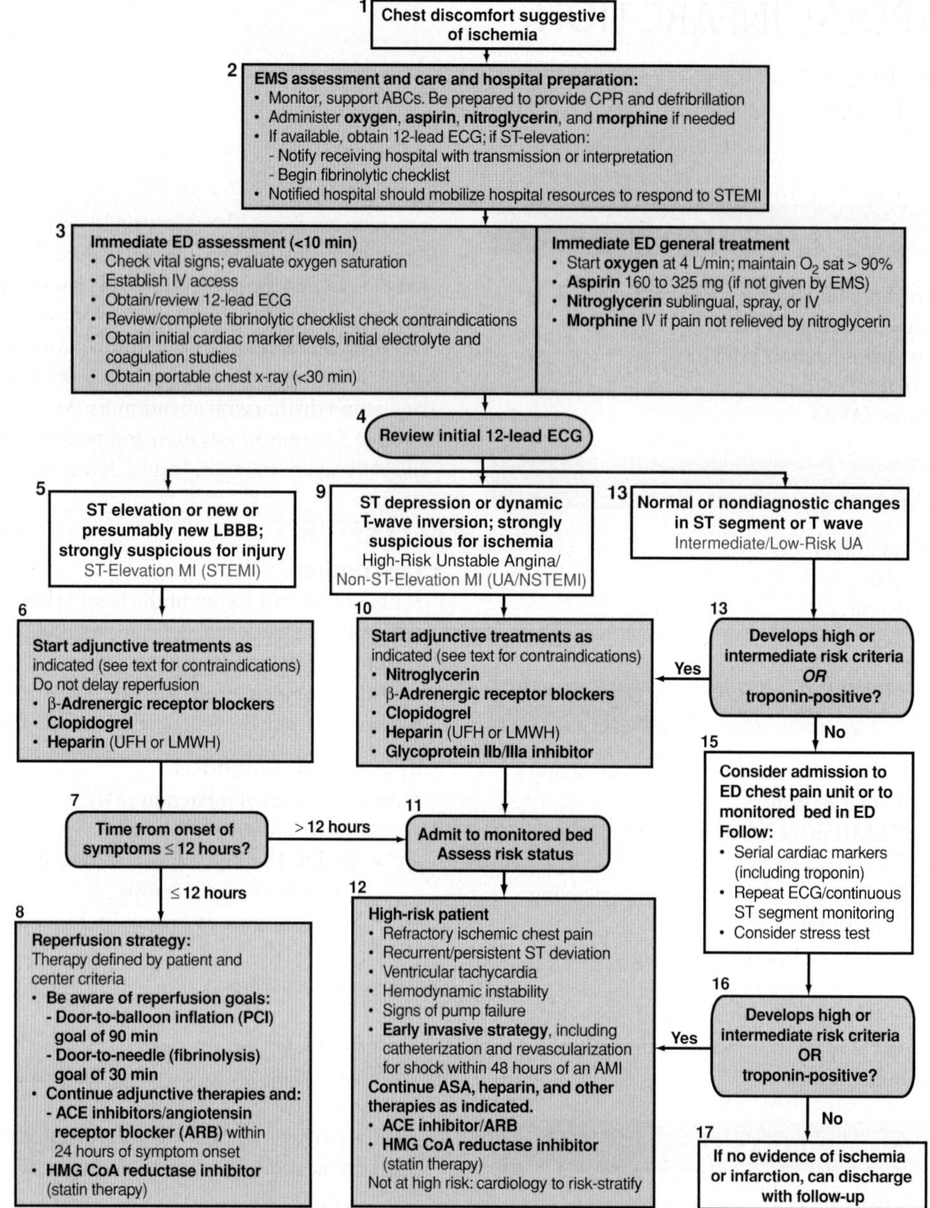

FIGURE 15-1 Acute coronary syndromes algorithm. STEMI, ST-elevation myocardial infarction; ED, emergency department; UFH, unfractionated heparin; PCI, percutaneous coronary intervention. (Reproduced with permission from *Circulation*. 2005;112:IV-89–IV-110.)

CLINICAL FINDINGS

SIGNS AND SYMPTOMS

- Acute MI
  - Chest pain, discomfort, pressure, tightness, or squeezing
  - Radiating pain, discomfort, pressure, tightness, or squeezing to the neck, throat, jaw, back, or right or left upper extremity
  - Shortness of breath
  - Excessive fatigue
  - Diaphoresis
  - Nausea/vomiting
  - Anxiety
  - Fainting
  - Wheezing
  - Abdominal bloating
  - Palpitations
  - Cough
  - Lightheadedness
  - Sweating, cold feeling
  - Rapid pulse
  - Complications associated following MI

Functional Implications

- Depending on the amount of myocardial damage
  - Decreased activity tolerance
  - Decreased exercise tolerance
  - Dyspnea on exertion

Possible Contributing Causes

- Coronary artery disease
- Cardiac arrhythmias
- Vasoconstriction of the coronary arteries
- Blood clot from slow build up
- Postsurgical acute blood clot
- Drug use (i.e., cocaine)
- Decreased perfusion
- Traditional risk factors

  - Smoking
  - Family history
  - Hypertension
  - Diabetes
  - Hyperlipidemia
  - Sedentary lifestyle
  - Obesity
  - Stress
- Nontraditional risk factors
  - C-reactive protein
  - Homocysteine
  - Thrombogenesis

Differential Diagnosis

- Pneumothorax
- Pericarditis
- Esophageal rupture
- Aortic dissection
- Angina
  - Stable angina
    - Transient myocardial ischemia, which occurs with activity and dissipates with rest
  - Unstable angina
    - Transient myocardial ischemia, which occurs at rest

MEANS OF CONFIRMATION OR DIAGNOSIS

Imaging

- Imaging for an acute MI
  - EKG
  - Elevated cardiac enzymes
  - Serum markers, see evolution of serum markers following an MI
- Imaging for an old MI
  - EKG
  - Echocardiogram (assessing left ventricular function)
  - Cardiolite (assessing myocardial perfusion)
  - Cardiac catheterization (assessing coronary artery disease [CAD] and/or EF)
  - Chest radiograph looking for congestive heart failure

Diagnostic Procedures

- Cardiac catheterization
  - Assessment of coronary artery disease, EF
  - Phonocardiogram[3]

Laboratory Tests[4]

- Lipid profile
- Triglycerides test
- Blood analysis: Complete blood count, platelet count, prothrombin time, erythrocyte sedimentation rate

FINDINGS AND INTERPRETATION

- Acute MI
  - 12-lead EKG that may be observed
    - ST-segment elevation
    - Hyperacute T waves
    - Q-wave development
    - T-wave inversion
    - Poor R-wave progression

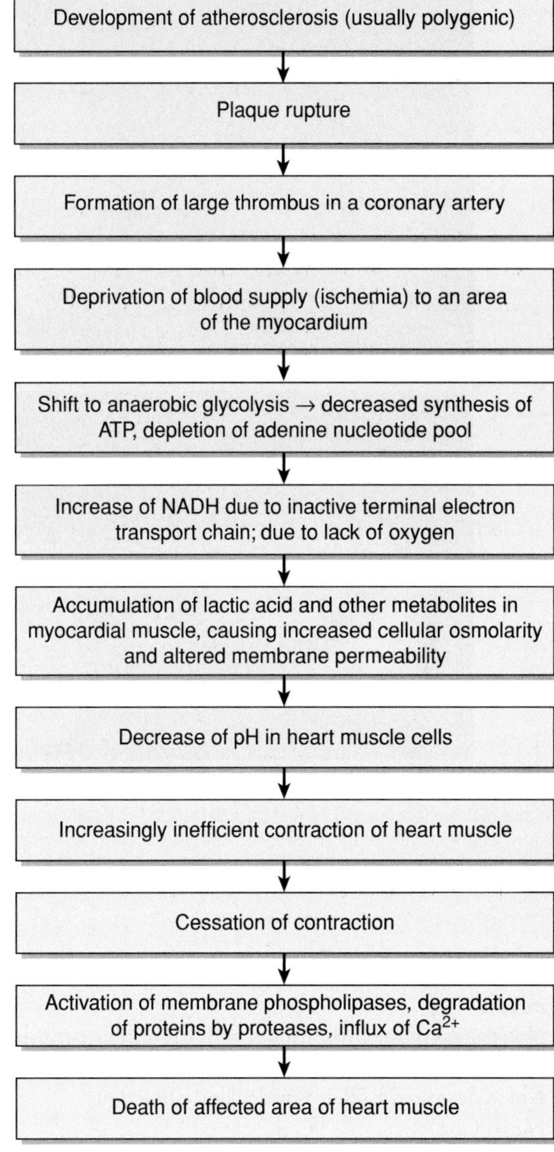

FIGURE 15-2 Summary of mechanisms involved in the causation of an acute myocardial infarction. The arrows do not in all cases imply a strict causal relationship. (From Murray RK, Bender DA, Botham KM, et al. *Harper's Illustrated Biochemistry.* 29th ed. www.accessmedicine.com. Copyright © The McGraw-Hill Companies, Inc. All rights reserved.)

    - If the patient has ST segment depression or T-wave inversion along with cardiac enzymes, a non–ST-elevation MI is suspected
    - ECG changes associated with the three zones of infarction
  - Cardiac enzymes: Noted rise with myocardial cell death
    - Creatine kinase (CK)
    - Creatine kinase MB (CK-MB)
    - Troponin: Blood levels rise with 4 to 6 hours after a heart attack, reach the highest within 10 to 24 hours and fall to normal after 10 days[3]
- Old MI
  - EKG
    - Noted permanent Q wave
  - Cardiac enzymes
    - Troponin may be elevated several days following MI
  - Echocardiogram

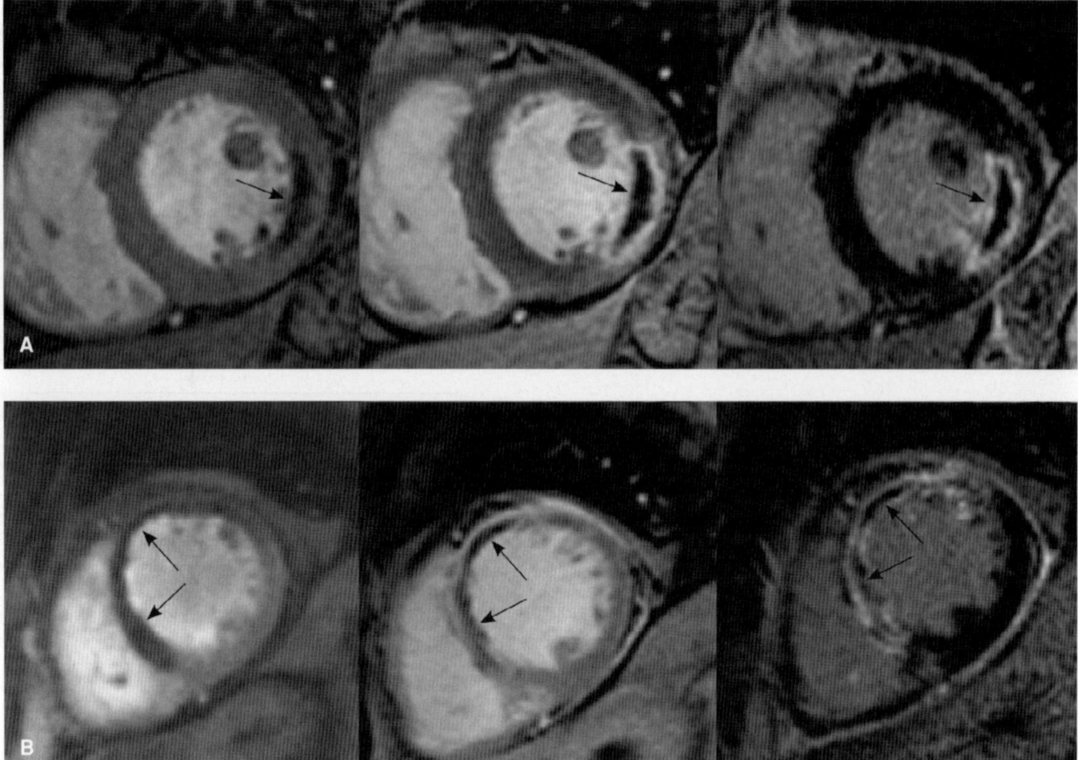

FIGURE 15-3 **A.** Cardiac magnetic resonance (CMR) images from a patient with acute lateral myocardial infarction. *Arrows* point to microvascular obstruction (MO; areas of hypoenhancement) on first-pass perfusion (left), early gadolinium enhancement (EGE; middle), and late gadolinium enhancement (LGE; right). **B.** CMR images from a patient with acute anterior myocardial infarction. *Arrows* point to MO on (areas of hypoenhancement) first-pass perfusion (left), EGE (middle), and LGE (right). (Reproduced from Mather AN, Lockie T, Nagel E, et al. Appearance of microvascular obstruction on high resolution first-pass perfusion, early and late gadolinium enhancement CMR in patients with acute myocardial infarction. *J Cardiovasc Magn Reson*. 2009;11:33.)

    - Noted decreased EF/left ventricular dysfunction
  - Cardiolite
    - Noted areas of the myocardium with irreversible perfusion
  - Cardiac catheterization
    - Noted decreased EF/left ventricular dysfunction
    - Noted CAD

TREATMENT

▶ Medication

- Acute MI
  - MONA
    - Morphine
    - Oxygen
    - Nitroglycerin
    - Aspirin
- Medications that may be used following MI
  - Beta-blockers
  - Calcium channel blockers
  - Aspirin
  - ACE inhibitors
  - Cholesterol medications (statins)
  - Blood thinners
  - Nitroglycerin
  - Diuretics

MEDICAL PROCEDURES

- Current treatment of myocardial infarction
- Surgery
  - Angioplasty/CAD stenting
  - Coronary artery bypass

REFERRALS/ADMITTANCE

- Suspected acute MI: 911 should be contacted
- Suspected old MI: Referral to a cardiologist

IMPAIRMENTS

- Shortness of breath
- Dyspnea on exertion
- Limited activity tolerance
- Limited functional capacity

TEST AND MEASURES

- 6-minute walk test
- Borg Scale of Perceived Exertion
- Vital sign monitoring
- Short-Form 36 Health Survey (SF-36)
- New York Heart Association Functional Classification scale

INTERVENTION

- Risk-factor modification
- Education on signs and symptoms
- Cardiac rehabilitation[5]
  - Decreases mortality and morbidity

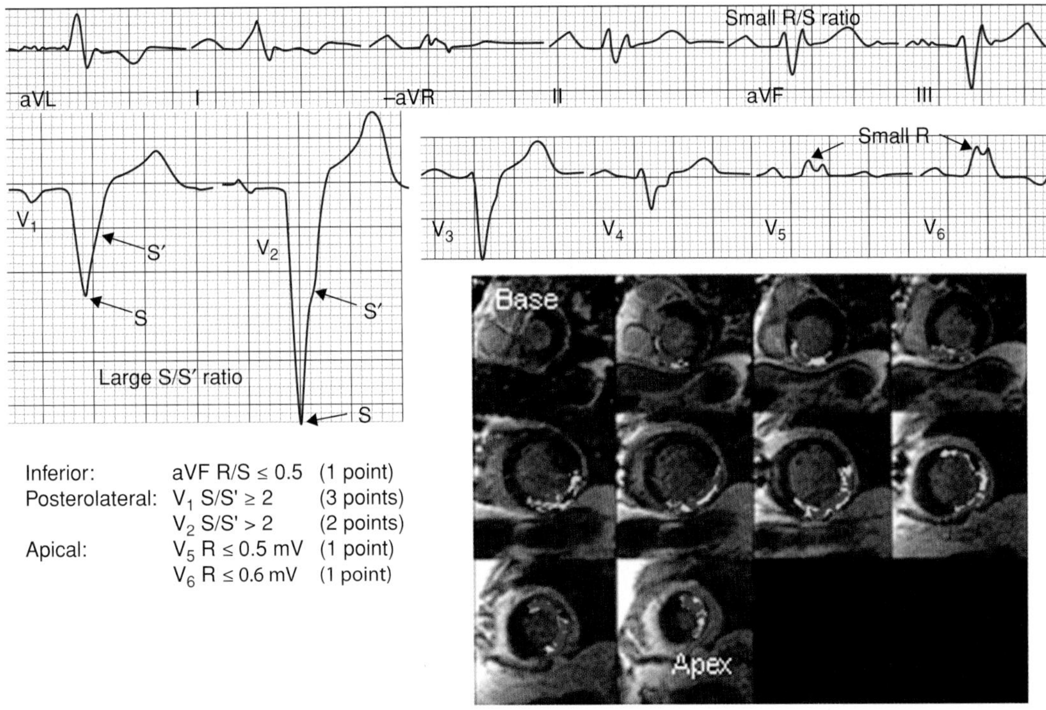

FIGURE 15-4 Electrocardiogram (ECG) and short-axis cardiovascular magnetic resonance (CMR) images from a patient with left bundle branch block and ischemic cardiomyopathy due to inferior and posterolateral infarcts comprising 23% of the left ventricle (LV) by CMR and that received 8 QRS points (ECG-estimated scar = 24%). Note the large S/S′ ratio in V_1 and V_2, which reflects posterolateral scar. For the CMR images, the regions with solid scar (core) are shown in red, and the regions with heterogeneous scar and live myocardium (gray zone) are shown in yellow. For comparison with the QRS score, total CMR scar was defined as core + 1/2 gray. (Reproduced with permission from Strauss DG, Selvester RH, Lima JA, et al. ECG quantification of myocardial scar in cardiomyopathy patients with or without conduction defects: correlation with cardiac magnetic resonance and arrhythmogenesis. *Circ Arrhythm Electrophysiol.* 2008;1:327–336.)

FUNCTIONAL GOALS

- The patient will be able to
  - State the signs and symptoms of MI.
  - State the risk factors for MI.
  - Reduce his/her body mass index (BMI) by———.
  - Tolerate 30 minutes of continuous aerobic exercise while maintaining a rated perceived exertion (RPE) of 13 with stable vital signs.

PROGNOSIS

- Depends on the size of the MI along with complications.
  - Smaller MIs have good prognosis.
- Larger MIs may have poor prognosis or death.

PATIENT RESOURCE

- Heart Attack Risk Assessment. http://www.heart.org/HEARTORG/Conditions/HeartAttack/HeartAttackToolsResources/Heart-Attack-Risk-Assessment_UCM_303944_Article.jsp. Accessed April 14, 2014.

REFERENCES

1. APTA. Guide to Physical Therapy Practice. Atlanta: American Physical Therapy Association; 2003. http://guidetoptpractice.apta.org. Accessed July 2, 2013.
2. Toy EC. Myocardial Infarction, Case 45. LANGE Case Files. http://www.accessmedicine.com/casecontent.aspx?aid=8651245&tabid=1. Accessed July 2, 2103.
3. Kusumoto FM. Cardiovascular disorders: heart disease. In: McPhee SJ, Hammer GD, eds. *Pathophysiology of Disease: An Introduction to Clinical Medicine.* 6th ed. New York, NY: McGraw-Hill; 2010. http://www.accessphysiotherapy.com/abstract/5367685. Accessed July 2, 2013.
4. Dutton M. Laboratory tests and values. In: Dutton M, ed. *McGraw-Hill's NPTE (National Physical Therapy Examination).* 2nd ed. New York, NY: McGraw-Hill; 2012. http://www.accessphysiotherapy.com/content/56516355. Accessed July 2, 2013.
5. Dutton M. Cardiovascular physical therapy. In: Dutton M, ed. *McGraw-Hill's NPTE (National Physical Therapy Examination).*. 2nd ed. New York, NY: McGraw-Hill; 2012. http://www.accessphysiotherapy.com/content/5401373. Accessed July 2, 2013.

ADDITIONAL REFERENCES

- Cassady S, Cahalin LP. Cardiovascular pathophysiology. In DeTurk WE, Cahalin LP, eds. *Cardiovascular and Pulmonary Physical Therapy: An Evidence-Based Approach.* 2nd ed. New York, NY: McGraw-Hill; 2011. http://www.accessphysiotherapy.com/content/6872740. Accessed July 2, 2013.
- Chen SF, El-Bialy A, Matthews R, Clavijo L. Use of drug-eluting versus bare-metal stents in ST-segment elevation myocardial infarction. *J Invasive Cardiol.* 2009;21(11):E206–E212.

- Dagenais GR, Poque J, Fox K, Simoons ML, Yusuf S. Angiotensin-converting-enzyme inhibitors in stable vascular disease without left ventricular systolic dysfunction or heart failure: a combined analysis of three trials. *Lancet.* 2006;368(9535):581–588. doi:10.1016/S0140–6736(06)69201–5.
- Kumar A, Cannon CP. Acute coronary syndromes: diagnosis and management, part II. *Mayo Clin Proc.* 2009;84(11):1021–1036. doi: 10.4065/84.11.1021.
- Kushner FG, Hand M, Smith SC Jr, et al. 2009 focused updates: ACC/AHA guidelines for the management of patients with ST-elevation myocardial infarction (updating the 2004 guideline and 2007 focused update) and ACC/AHA/SCAI guidelines on percutaneous coronary intervention (updating the 2005 guideline and 2007 focused update): a report of the American College of Cardiology Foundation/American Heart Association Task Force on Practice Guidelines. *Circulation.* 2009;120(22):2271–2306.
- Mehta S, Alfonso CE, Oliveros E, et al. Adjunct therapy in STEMI intervention. *Cardiol Clin.* 2010;28(1):107–125. doi:10.1016/j.ccl.2009.09.005.
- Task Force on Myocardial Revascularization of the European Society of Cardiology (ESC) and the European Association for Cardio-Thoracic Surgery (EACTS); European Association for Percutaneous Cardiovascular Interventions (EAPCI), Wijns W, et al. Guidelines on myocardial revascularization. *Eur Heart J.* 2010;31(20):2501–2555. doi: 10.1093/eurheartj/ehq277.
- Thygesen K, Alpert JS, White HD; Joint ESC/ACCF/AHA/WHF Task Force for the Redefinition of Myocardial Infarction, et al. Universal definition of myocardial infarction. *Circulation.* 2007;116(22):2634–2653. doi: 10.1161/CIRCULATIONAHA.107.187397.
- Torpy JM, Lynm C, Glass RM. JAMA patient page. Myocardial infarction. *JAMA.* 2008;299(4):476. doi: 10.1001/jama.299.4.476.

16 RAYNAUD SYNDROME

Eric Shamus, PhD, DPT, PT, CSCS
Oseas Florencio de Moura Filho, PT (Brazil), MSc

CONDITION/DISORDER SYNONYMS

- Raynaud phenomenon
- Raynaud's
- Primary Raynaud's

ICD-9-CM CODE

- 443.0 Raynaud syndrome

ICD-10-CM CODES

- I73.00 Raynaud syndrome without gangrene
- I73.01 Raynaud syndrome with gangrene

PREFERRED PRACTICE PATTERN

- 7A: Primary Prevention/Risk Reduction for Integumentary Disorders
- 7E: Impaired Integumentary Integrity Associated with Skin Involvement Extending into Fascia, Muscle, or Bone, and Scar Formation[1]

PATIENT PRESENTATION

A 56-year-old female presents with bilateral hand and finger pain. She states that her hands and fingers are always cold. She especially has difficulty in the supermarket when reaching for frozen foods. She notices her fingers go blue and then white. She states the pain occurs when they start to warm up. She carries gloves with her even during the summer months.

KEY FEATURES

Description

- Vasospasm of the arteries to the distal extremities
- Most common in the fingers and toes, can affect the nose, ears, and lips
- Sensitivity to cold

Essentials of Diagnosis

- Primary Raynaud's, the etiology is unknown, more common
  - Criteria for primary Raynaud phenomenon (see table)[2]
- Secondary Raynaud's has a known etiology from another disease or cause
  - Criteria for secondary Raynaud phenomenon (See table)
    - Connective tissue disease
    - Obstructive arterial disease
    - Neurologic disorders
    - Drugs and toxins
    - Occupational/environmental exposure
    - Hyperviscosity

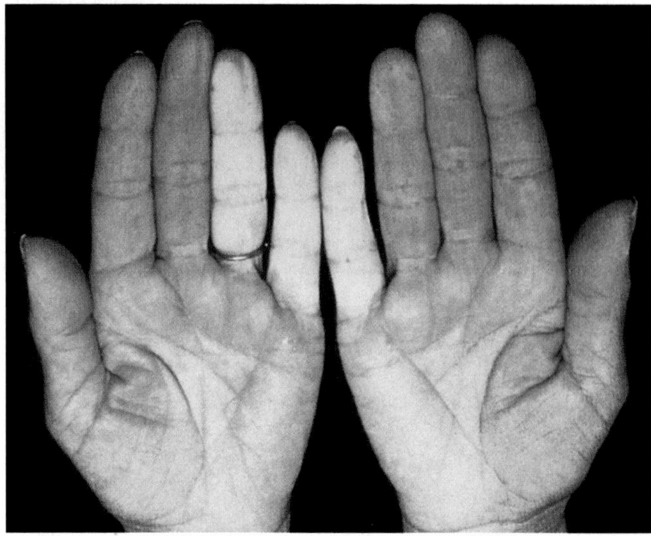

FIGURE 16-1 Ischemic phase of attack of Raynaud phenomenon with marked pallor of the ring and little fingers of the left hand and little finger of the right hand. (From Goldsmith LA, Katz SI, Gilchrest BA, et al. *Fitzpatrick's Dermatology in General Medicine.* 8th ed. www.accessmedicine.com. Copyright © The McGraw-Hill Companies, Inc. All rights reserved.)

General Considerations

- Cold temperature can cause a Raynaud attack where there is a brief period of little-to-no blood flow.
- Brief temperature changes can cause an attack
- Can cause skin sores or gangrene

Demographics

- Affects 10% of the population
- Primary Raynaud's usually begins before age 30
- Secondary Raynaud's usually begins after age 30

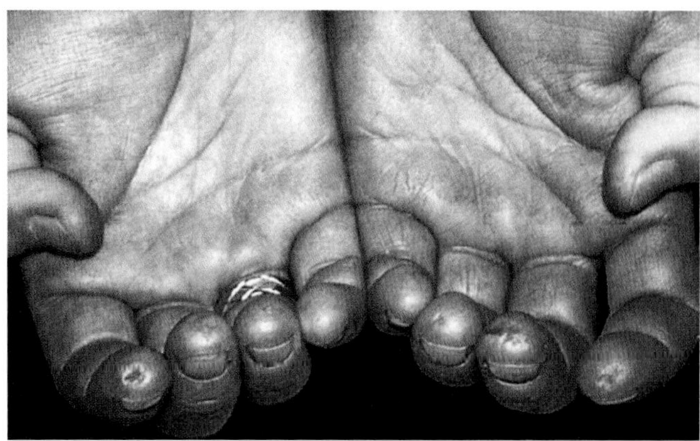

FIGURE 16-2 Loss of pulp of the pad of the digit with pitting scars and ulcerations from chronic, severe Raynaud phenomenon. (From Goldsmith LA, Katz SI, Gilchrest BA, et al. *Fitzpatrick's Dermatology in General Medicine.* 8th ed. www.accessmedicine.com. Copyright © The McGraw-Hill Companies, Inc. All rights reserved.)

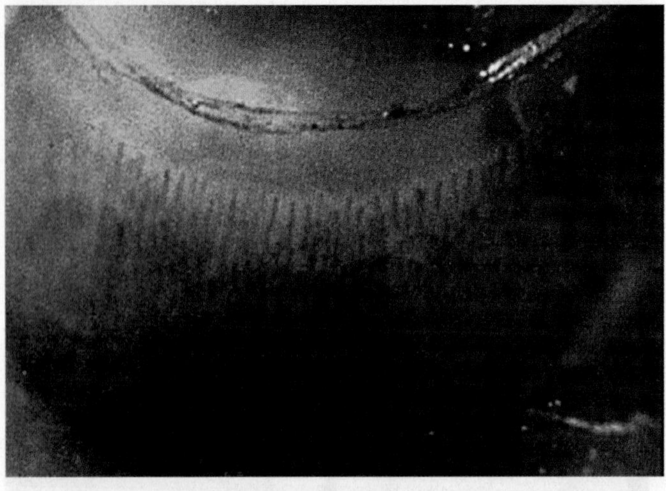
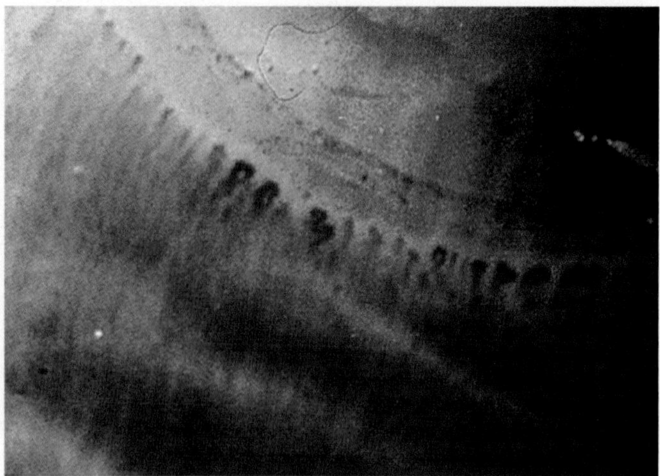
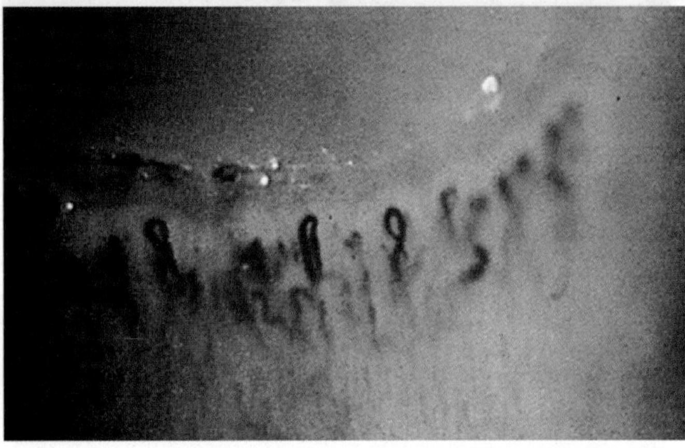
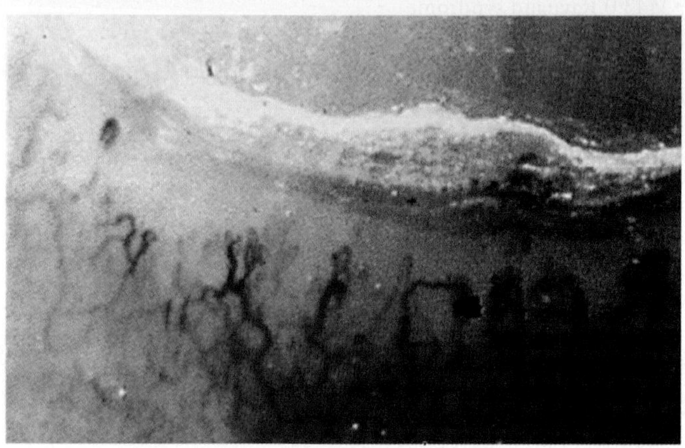

FIGURE 16-3 Nailfold capillary microscopy, in a patient with scleroderma, showing capillary drop out with enlarged, dilated, tortuous capillary loops. (From Goldsmith LA, Katz SI, Gilchrest BA, et al. *Fitzpatrick's Dermatology in General Medicine*. 8th ed. www.accessmedicine.com. Copyright © The McGraw-Hill Companies, Inc. All rights reserved.)

- Women are more likely than men, 4:1 ratio
- Family history
- Living in cold regions

CLINICAL FINDINGS

SIGNS AND SYMPTOMS

- Throbbing
- Tingling
- Burning
- Decreased sensation
- Circulation changes: White or redness
- Rare occasions: Skin sore and gangrene
- Dry skin

Functional Implications

- Severe symptoms may cause inability to leave home in the winter
- Limit fine finger dexterity
- Limited ROM, ADLs, IADLs
- Lifestyle changes secondary to pain and fatigue

Possible Contributing Causes

- Physical or emotional stress, anxiety
- Systemic immunological condition (inflammatory autoimmune disease)
- Medication side effects that cause constriction
- Toxin or chemical exposure
- Diseases that damage arteries or the nerves that control the arteries
- Rheumatoid arthritis
- Atherosclerosis
- Cryoglobulinemia
- Sjögren syndrome

TABLE 16-1 Criteria for Primary Raynaud Phenomenon

- Vasospastic attacks precipitated by exposure to cold or emotional stimuli
- Bilateral involvement of extremities
- Normal vascular examination with symmetric peripheral pulses and normal nailfold capillary microscopy
- Absence of gangrene or, if present, limited to the skin of the fingertips
- No evidence of an underlying disease, drug, or occupational exposure that could be responsible for vasospastic attacks
- Negative antinuclear antibody test
- Normal erythrocyte sedimentation rate
- History of symptoms for at least 2 yrs

Source: Combined criteria of Allen EV, Brown GE. Raynaud's disease: A critical review of minimal prerequisites for diagnosis. *Am J Med Sci*. 1932;183:187–200.; LeRoy EC, Medsger TA Jr. Raynaud's phenomenon: A proposal for classification. *Clin Exp Rheumatol*. 1992;10:485–488.

- Thyroid problems
- Work hazards like excessive vibration
- Frostbite

▶ Differential Diagnosis

- Carpal tunnel syndrome
- Thoracic outlet syndrome
- Chronic fatigue syndrome
- Sjögren syndrome
- Vasculitis
- Rheumatoid arthritis

MEANS OF CONFIRMATION OR DIAGNOSIS

▶ Laboratory Tests

- Blood tests, complete blood count (CBC)
- Chemistry panel (kidney function, liver, electrolytes, blood sugar, cholesterol, triglycerides)
  - Erythrocyte sedimentation rate (ESR)
  - Antinuclear antibody (ANA)
  - C-reactive protein (CRP)

▶ Imaging

- MRI
- Doppler ultrasound

▶ Diagnostic Procedures

- Cold stimulation test
- Nailfold capillaroscopy

FINDINGS AND INTERPRETATION

- Decreased blood flow with cold temperature

TREATMENT

▶ Medication (See table for medical management)

- Vasodilators
- Alpha-blockers
- Calcium channel blockers
- Nifedipine
- Epoprostenol

MEDICAL PROCEDURES

- Protective clothing
- Surgery
  - Block nerve signals
- Dietary modifications

REFERRALS/ADMITTANCE

- Rheumatologist

IMPAIRMENTS

- Muscle weakness
- Joint pain
- Diffuse soft tissue pain
- Soft tissue and or joint deformity with biomechanical malalignment
- Inability to perform self-care
- Limited aerobic endurance
- Functional decline; decrease in functional abilities
- Coordination deficits

TABLE 16-2 Secondary Raynaud Phenomenon

- Connective tissue disease
  - Scleroderma
  - Systemic lupus erythematosus
  - Dermatomyositis and polymyositis
  - Undifferentiated connective tissue disease
  - Systemic vasculitis
  - Sjögren syndrome
  - Eosinophilic fasciitis
- Obstructive arterial disease
  - Atherosclerosis
  - Thromboangiitis obliterans (Buerger disease)
  - Thromboembolism
  - Thoracic outlet syndrome
- Neurologic disorders
  - Carpal tunnel syndrome
  - Reflex sympathetic dystrophy
  - Hemiplegia
  - Poliomyelitis
  - Multiple sclerosis
  - Syringomyelia
- Drugs and toxins
  - Beta-Adrenergic blockers
  - Ergotamines
  - Oral contraceptives
  - Methysergide
  - Bleomycin and vinblastine
  - Clonidine
  - Bromocriptine
  - Cyclosporine
  - Amphetamines
  - Fluoxetine
  - Interferon-alpha
- Occupation/environmental exposure
  - Vibration injury (lumberjacks, pneumatic hammer operators)
  - Post-traumatic injury (hypothenar hammer syndrome, crutch pressure)
  - Vinyl chloride disease
  - Cold injury
- Hyperviscosity disorders
  - Cryoproteins
  - Cold agglutinins
  - Macroglobulins
  - Polycythemia
  - Thrombocytosis
- Miscellaneous
  - Hypothyroidism
  - Infections (bacterial endocarditis, Lyme disease, viral hepatitis)
  - Neoplasms
  - Primary pulmonary hypertension
  - Arteriovenous fistula
  - Intra-arterial injections

Source: Goldsmith LA, Katz SI, Gilchrest BA, et al. *Fitzpatrick's Dermatology in General Medicine*. 8th ed. www.accessmedicine.com.

TESTS AND MEASURES

- Edema measurements
- Integumentary
- Joint integrity, mobility
- Medical history
- Muscle performance
- Pain
- Palpation
- Peripheral nerve integrity
- Range of motion (ROM)
- Reflex integrity
- Self-care and home management
- Sensory integrity
- Vital signs

INTERVENTION

- Physical therapy intervention consistent with movement-related problems occurring from the effects of decreased circulation
- Therapeutic exercise: All relevant categories, energy conservation, aerobic capacity related, stretching
- Neuromuscular re-education
- Self-care management, including the use of adaptive equipment or home modification
- Physical agents for management of pain, inflammation, edema
  - Heat
  - Electrical stimulation
  - Laser
  - Soft tissue mobilization
- Biofeedback to facilitate vasodilatation in fingers
- Lifestyle changes limiting alcohol and caffeine

FUNCTIONAL GOALS

- Patient will be able to
  - Demonstrate volitional vasodilatation in fingers to avoid vaso-constriction and minimize/eliminate response to cold and finger ulcerations.
  - Reduce edema from _____ to or by ____in (body part) in order to (state function, such as ability to wear shoes or protect skin on feet).
  - Increase muscle performance in (body part; specify muscle group or functional activity) from ____ to ____ in order to (state function).
  - Achieve functional aerobic capacity, ability to talk during activity so as to achieve functional gait and activity tolerance for ADLs/IADLs.
  - Tolerate 30 minutes of continuous, moderate exercise three times a week in ______weeks, and five times a week in ___________weeks, depending on disease severity.

PROGNOSIS

- Patients should be able to lead an active lifestyle with appropriate medical management
- Most patient have no long-term disabilities

PATIENT RESOURCES

- Raynaud's and Scleroderma Association. http://www.raynauds.org.uk. Accessed June 11, 2013.
- Scleroderma Foundation. http://www.scleroderma.org/site/PageServer. Accessed June 11, 2013.

TABLE 16-3 Management of Raynaud Phenomenon

Infrequent or mild attacks	Preventive measures Cessation of smoking
Frequent or severe attacks	Calcium channel blockers (nifedipine, diltiazem) Antiadrenergic drugs (prazosin, reserpine) Topical nitroglycerin
Acute, severe ischemia	Intravenous prostaglandin E_1 or prostacyclin Digital sympathectomy Microvascular surgery
Digital ulcers	Antiseptic soaks, antibiotic ointments, occlusive dressing Calcium channel blockers (maximal doses) Intravenous prostaglandin E_1 or prostacyclin
Gangrenous, infected ulcers	Analgesics Antibiotics Surgical debridement Amputation

Source: Goldsmith LA, Katz SI, Gilchrest BA, et al. *Fitzpatrick's Dermatology in General Medicine.* 8th ed. www.accessmedicine.com.

REFERENCES

1. The American Physical Therapy Association. Pattern 7E: impaired integumentary integrity associated with skin involvement extending into fascia, muscle, or bone and scar formation. *Interactive Guide to Physical Therapist Practice.* 2003. doi: 10.2522/ptguide.3.4_5. Accessed June 10, 2013.
2. Klippel JH. Raynaud phenomenon. In: Goldsmith LA, Katz SI, Gilchrest BA, Paller AS, Leffell DJ, Dallas NA, eds. *Fitzpatrick's Dermatology in General Medicine.* 8th ed. New York, NY: McGraw-Hill; 2012: Chapter 170, Table 170-1. http://www.accessmedicine.com/popup.aspx?aID=56080131. Accessed June 16, 2013.

ADDITIONAL REFERENCES

- Barreett ME, Heller MM, Stone FF, Murase JE. Raynaud phenomenon of the nipple in breastfeeding mothers: an under diagnosed cause of nipple pain. *JAMA Dermatol.* 2013;149 (3):300–306.
- Bulpitt KJ, Clements PJ, Lachenbruch PA, et al. Early undifferentiated connective tissue disease: III. Outcome and prognostic indicators in early scleroderma (systemic sclerosis). *Ann Intern Med.* 1993;118(8):602–609.
- Chen GS, Yu HS, Yang SA, Chen SS. Responses of cutaneous microcirculation to cold exposure and neuropathy in vibration-induced white finger. *Microvasc Res.* 1994;47(1):21–30.
- Dutton M. Integumentary physical therapy. In: Dutton M. *McGraw-Hill's NPTE (National Physical Therapy Examination).* 2nd ed. New York, NY: McGraw-Hill; 2012. http://www.accessphysiotherapy.com/content/5403118. Accessed June 10, 2013.
- Goodman CC, Fuller KS. *Pathology: Implications for the Physical Therapist.* 3rd ed. Philadelphia, PA: Saunders Elsevier; 2009.
- Goodman CC, Snyder TK. *Differential Diagnosis for Physical Therapists: Screening for Referral.* 4th ed. St. Louis, MO: Saunders Elsevier; 2007.

- Herrick AL, Illingworth K, Blann A, Hay CR, Hollis S, Jayson MI. Von Willebrand factor, thrombomodulin, thromboxane, beta-thromboglobulin and markers of fibrinolysis in primary Raynaud's phenomenon and systemic sclerosis. *Ann Rheum Dis.* 1996;55(2):122–127.
- LeRoy EC, Medsger TA Jr. Raynaud's phenomenon: a proposal for classification. *Clin Exp Rheumatol.* 1992;10(5):485–488.
- Minai OA, Dweik RA, Arroliga AC. Manifestations of scleroderma pulmonary disease. *Clin Chest Med.* 1998;19(4):713–731.
- Raynaud's phenomenon. NIH National Institute of Arthritis and Musculoskeletal and Skin Diseases. http://www.niams.nih.gov/Health_Info/Raynauds_Phenomenon/default.asp. Accessed June 11, 2013.
- Rodgers M. Images in clinical medicine. Primary Raynaud's phenomenon. *N Engl J Med.* 2013;368(14):1344. doi:10.1056/NEJMicm1209600.

17 TRICUSPID REGURGITATION

Eric Shamus, PhD, DPT, PT, CSCS
Natalie V. Wessel, DO, MPH

CONDITION/DISORDER SYNONYMS

- Tricuspid (valve) regurgitation (TR)
- Tricuspid (valve) insufficiency (TI)

ICD-9-CM CODE

- 397.0 Diseases of tricuspid valve

ICD-10-CM CODES

- I07.1 Rheumatic tricuspid insufficiency
- I36.1 Nonrheumatic tricuspid (valve) insufficiency

PREFERRED PRACTICE PATTERN

- 6D: Impaired Aerobic Capacity/Endurance Associated with Cardiovascular Pump Dysfunction or Failure[1]

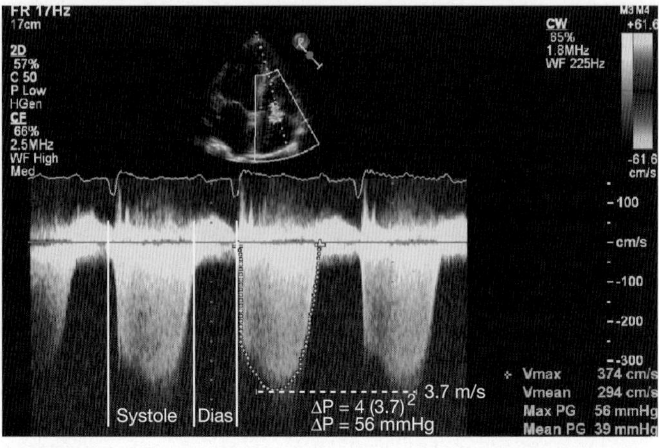

FIGURE 17-1 A Doppler signal due to the severe tricuspid regurgitation. In tricuspid regurgitation, the high-velocity flow is recorded during systole and not in diastole (Dias). Because the jet of tricuspid regurgitation is flowing away from the transducer, a negative signal is recorded. The simplified Bernoulli equation can be used to estimate the pressure difference between the right ventricle and the right atrium from the peak velocity recorded from the tricuspid regurgitation signal (3.74 m/s or 374 cm/s). (From Nicoll D, Lu CM, Pignone M, et al. *Pocket Guide to Diagnostic Tests*. 6th ed. www.accessmedicine.com. Copyright © The McGraw-Hill Companies, Inc. All rights reserved.)

PATIENT PRESENTATION

A 65-year-old male presents to physical therapy for weakness, pulsations in the neck, and fatigue. He has a history of mild hypertension that is well controlled on lisinopril. Vitals are: Pulse: 70, Respirations: 14, Blood Pressure: 124/84, Temperature: 97.9°F, and SpO_2% of 96%. On physical examination, there is mild distension of the jugular veins on the right side of the neck and a palpable right ventricular heave. On auscultation, there is a holosystolic murmur at the right mid-sternal border. With leg raising the murmur gets louder. The patient was referred to the cardiologist. ECG and chest X-ray show signs of right atrial and ventricular enlargement. Echocardiography reveals a vena contracta of 0.8 cm and a dilated tricuspid annulus.

KEY FEATURES

Description

- Tricuspid valve does not close properly during systole
- Causes a backflow and fluid overload in the right atrium
- Fluid overload in the right atrium can lead to weakening of the right atrial wall
- Usually asymptomatic
- Irregular heartbeat

Essentials of Diagnosis

- Stethoscope for auscultation of a pansystolic heart murmur at lower left sternal border
- Echocardiography
- EKG/ECG
- CT/MRI for enlargement of the right side of the heart
- Cardiac catheterization
- Chest X-ray
- Exercise stress test

General Considerations

- Signs and symptoms should be monitored
- Mild-to-moderate regurgitation generally does not cause symptoms
- Symptoms are often weakness and fatigue
- Patients can develop bacterial endocarditis

Demographics

- Seen in individuals with Ebstein anomaly (congenital heart disease)

CLINICAL FINDINGS

SIGNS AND SYMPTOMS

- Jugular venous distension
- Weakness
- Fatigue
- Endocarditis
- Cirrhosis
- Weight loss
- Swelling
  - Abdomen
  - Liver
  - Spleen
  - Peripheral edema
  - Feet
  - Ankles
- Decreased urine output
- Heart murmur

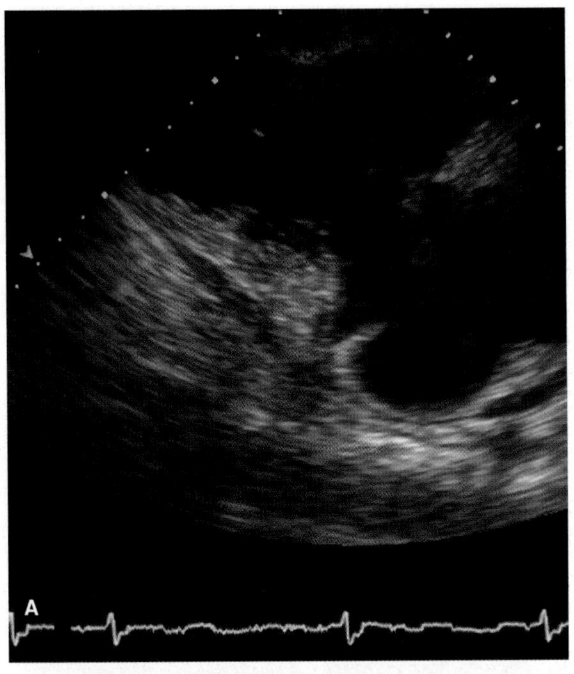

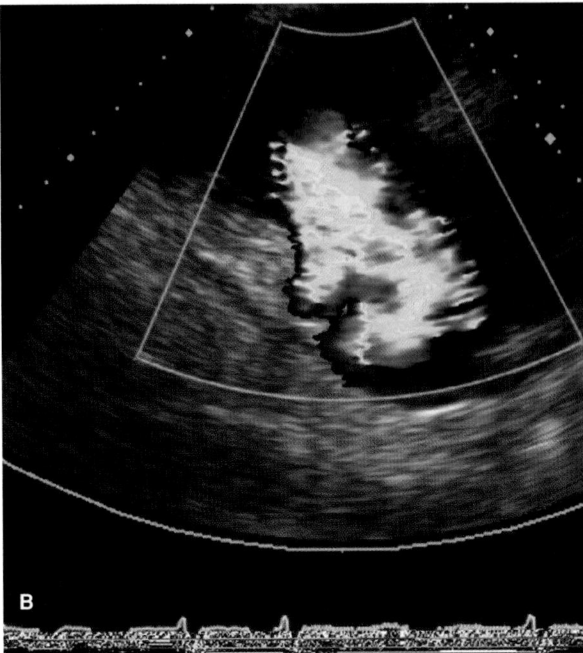

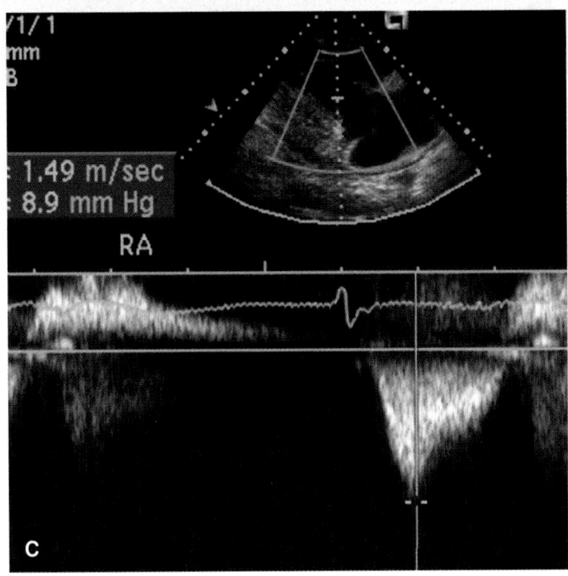

FIGURE 17-2 Severe secondary tricuspid regurgitation caused by extreme tethering of the tricuspid valve without intrinsic leaflet pathology. **A.** The right ventricular inflow view from parasternal transducer location shows a markedly tethered valve in late systole. **B.** The color Doppler image shows flow accelerating and severe tricuspid regurgitation jet without turbulence. **C.** Continuous-wave Doppler shows early peaking systolic profile associated with high right atrial pressure, which was estimated to be 25 mm Hg. The peak tricuspid regurgitation velocity is measured at 9 mm Hg and thus indicates the right ventricular systolic pressure to be 34 mm Hg (9 + 25). (From Fuster V, Walsh RA, Harrington RA, eds. In: *Hurst's The Heart*. 13th ed. http://www.accessmedicine.com.)

▶ Functional Implications

- Symptoms depend on degree of valvular dysfunction.
- Mild-to-moderate regurgitation generally does not cause symptoms.
- Severe regurgitation causes fatigue, weakness, and signs of congestive heart failure.
- Patients may be unaware of their reduced cardiovascular capacity.
- Can cause syncope, chest pain, and heart failure if untreated.

▶ Possible Contributing Causes

- Bacteria in the blood stream
- Blunt trauma
- Carcinoid disease
- Chronic lung disease
- Cor pulmonale
- Diet medication: Phentermine and fenfluramine
- Drug abuse
- Ebstein anomaly (congenital heart disease)
- Endomyocardial fibrosis
- Enlargement of the right ventricle
- Infective endocarditis
- Inferior myocardial infarction
- Marfan syndrome
- Myxomatous
- Pulmonary hypertension
- Rheumatic fever
- Rheumatoid arthritis
- Right ventricular infarction
- Systemic lupus erythematosus
- Tricuspid valve prolapse

Differential Diagnosis

- Acute coronary syndrome
- Aortic regurgitation
- Aortic stenosis
- Mitral valve prolapse
- Mitral stenosis
- Myocardial infarction complication
- Shock, hypovolemia
- Cardiac pump dysfunction
- Cardiac muscle dysfunction
- Cardiac pump failure

MEANS OF CONFIRMATION OR DIAGNOSIS

Imaging

- Echocardiography to measure blood pressure inside the heart and lungs
- MRI of the heart
- Chest X-ray
  - Enlarged left atrium
  - Enlarged left ventricle
- EKG

Diagnostic Procedures

- Cardiac catheterization
  - Assessment of coronary artery disease, EF, pulmonary artery wedge pressure
- Phonocardiogram

FINDINGS AND INTERPRETATION

- Elevated jugular venous pressure
- Backflow of blood into the left atrium during systole
- Left ventricular dysfunction
- Possible increase in left pulmonary venous pressure
- Pansystolic murmur at the lower left sternal border

TREATMENT

Medication

- Medications for heart failure induced by tricuspid regurgitation
  - Diuretics
  - Beta-blockers
  - Positive inotropic agents
  - Angiotensin-converting enzyme (ACE)
  - Aldosterone antagonists
  - Antibiotics for patients with a history of rheumatic fever
  - Vasodilators like nitroprusside and hydralazine to decrease afterload
  - Inpatient pharmacologic management

MEDICAL PROCEDURES

- Internal cardiac defibrillator
- Tricuspid valve replacement/repair
- Cardiac resynchronization
- Coronary artery bypass
- Left or right ventricular assisting device
- Cardiac transplant

REFERRALS/ADMITTANCE

- To primary care or cardiac physician if suspected cardiac muscle dysfunction

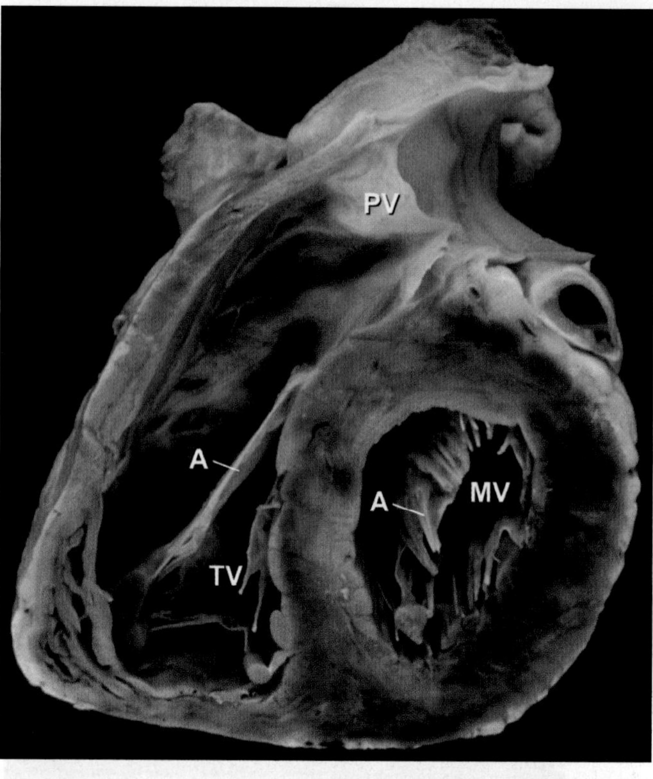

FIGURE 17-3 This oblique short-axis view of the heart shows the triangular-shaped tricuspid orifice (TV) and the elliptical mitral orifice (MV) at mid-leaflet level. The anterior tricuspid and anterior mitral leaflets (A) separate the inflow and outflow tracts of the right and left ventricles, respectively, and are parallel to one another. PV, pulmonary valve. (From Fuster V, Walsh RA, Harrington RA. *Hurst's The Heart*. 13th ed. www.accessmedicine.com. Copyright © The McGraw-Hill Companies, Inc. All rights reserved.)

- To ER or call 911 if suspected cardiac muscle failure
- Must see a cardiologist every 3 to 6 months

IMPAIRMENTS

- Shortness of breath
- Dyspnea on exertion
- Limited activity tolerance
- Limited functional capacity

TEST AND MEASURES

- 6-minute walk test for mild/non-symptomatic cases
- BORG rating of perceived exertion
- Monitor vital signs to include lung auscultations
- Short-Form 36 health survey
- New York Heart Association Functional Classification scale

INTERVENTION

- Risk-factor modification
- Cardiac rehabilitation
  - Decreases morbidity and mortality
- Education on signs and symptoms
- Nonaerobic resistance training
- Emphasis on wellness and prevention

FUNCTIONAL GOALS

- Patient will be able to state the signs and symptoms of tricuspid regurgitation.

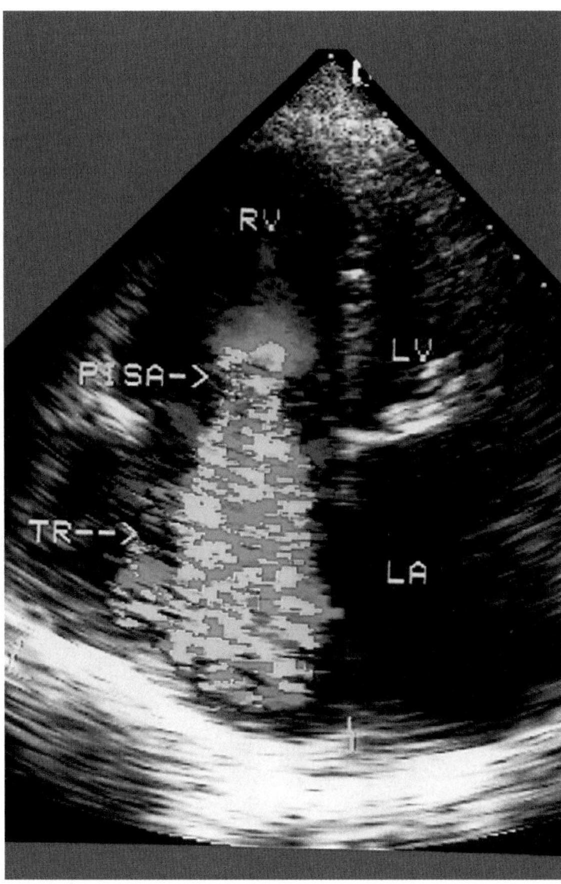

FIGURE 17-4 Apical four-chamber view of severe tricuspid regurgitation. The Doppler color jet fills the tricuspid regurgitation. LA, left atrium; LV, left ventricle; PISA, proximal isovelocity surface area; RV, right ventricle; TR, tricuspid regurgitation. (From Fuster V, Walsh RA, Harrington RA. *Hurst's The Heart.* 13th ed. www.accessmedicine.com. Copyright © The McGraw-Hill Companies, Inc. All rights reserved.)

- Patient will be able to tolerate 30 minutes of continuous exercise while maintaining stable vital signs and a rate of perceived exertion (RPE) of 13.
- Short-term goals
  - Reconditioning, sufficient for resuming normal activities.
  - Limit physiologic and psychological effects.
  - Decreasing the risk of sudden cardiac arrest or myocardial infarction.
  - Controlling symptoms of cardiac disease.
- Long-term goals
  - Identification and treatment of risk factors.
  - Stabilizing or reversing atherosclerotic processes.
  - Improve psychological status.

PROGNOSIS

- Valve repair or replacement usually solves the problem.
- Valve problems can develop 5 to 10 years after rheumatic fever.

PATIENT RESOURCE

- Heart Valve Problems. The Society for Cardiovascular Angiography and Interventions. http://www.scai.org/SecondsCount/Disease/HeartValveProblem.aspx?gclid=CIXO1Mrg2rUCFQ4FnQodz28Ajw. Accessed May 6, 2013.

REFERENCE

1. The American Physical Therapy Association. Pattern 6D: impaired aerobic capacity/endurance associated with cardiovascular pump dysfunction or failure. *Interactive Guide to Physical Therapist Practice.* http://guidetoptpractice.apta.org/. Accessed May 6, 2013.

ADDITIONAL REFERENCES

- Blume ED, Naftel DC, Bastardi HJ, Duncan BW, Kirklin JK, Webber SA. Outcomes of children bridged to heart transplantation with ventricular assist devices: a multi-institutional study. *Circulation.* 2006;113(19):2313–2319.
- Cassady SL, Cahalin LP. Cardiovascular pathophysiology. In: DeTurk WE, Cahalin LP, eds. *Cardiovascular and Pulmonary Physical Therapy: An Evidence-Based Approach.* 2nd ed. New York, NY: McGraw-Hill; 2011. http://www.accessphysiotherapy.com/abstract/6872858. Accessed May 6, 2013.
- Dubin D. *Rapid Interpretation of EKG's.* Fort Myers, FL: COVER Publishing Co.; 2000.
- Dutton M. Cardiovascular physical therapy. In: Dutton M, ed. *McGraw-Hill's NPTE (National Physical Therapy Examination).* 2nd ed. New York, NY: McGraw-Hill; 2012. http://www.accessphysiotherapy.com/content/5401905. Accessed May 6, 2013.
- Ewy G. Tricuspid valve disease. In: Alpert JS, Dalen JE, Rahimtoola SH, eds. *Valvular Heart Disease.* 3rd ed. Philadelphia, PA: Lippincott Williams &Wilkins; 2000: 377–392.
- ICD9Data.com. http://www.icd9data.com. Accessed May 6, 2013.
- ICD10Data.com. http://www.icd10data.com. Accessed May 6, 2013.
- Kusumoto FM.. Cardiovascular disorders: heart disease: pathophysiology of selected cardiovascular disorders. In: Kusumoto FM, ed. *Pathophysiology of Disease.* 6th ed. New York, NY: McGraw-Hill; 2010: Chapter 10. http://www.accessphysiotherapy.com/abstract/5367685#5367687. Accessed May 6, 2013.
- Miyamoto SD, Sondheimer HM, Fagan TE, Collins KK. Cardiovascular diseases. In: Hay WW, Levin MJ, Sondheimer JM, Detering RR. *CURRENT Diagnosis & Treatment: Pediatrics.* 20th ed. New York, NY: McGraw-Hill; 2011. http://www.accessphysiotherapy.com/abstract/6583154#6583208. Accessed May 6, 2013.
- Panus PC, Jobst EE, Masters SB, Katzung B, Tinsley SL, Trevor AJ. *Pharmacology for the Physical Therapist.* New York, NY: McGraw-Hill; 2009. http://www.accessphysiotherapy.com/resource/615. Accessed May 6, 2013.
- Rosenthal D, Chrisant MR, Edens E, et al. International Society for Heart and Lung Transplantation: practice guidelines for management of heart failure in children. *J Heart Lung Transplant.* 2004;23(12):1313–1333.

18 PERICARDITIS

Eric Shamus, PhD, DPT, PT, CSCS
Christopher C. Felton, DO, ATC

CONDITION/DISORDER SYNONYM

- Dressler syndrome

ICD-9-CM CODES

- 420 Acute pericarditis
- 420.0 Acute pericarditis in diseases classified elsewhere
- 420.90 Acute pericarditis, unspecified
- 420.91 Acute idiopathic pericarditis
- 420.99 Other acute pericarditis
- 423 Other diseases of pericardium
- 423.0 Hemopericardium
- 423.1 Adhesive pericarditis
- 423.2 Constrictive pericarditis
- 423.3 Cardiac tamponade
- 423.8 Other specified diseases of pericardium
- 423.9 Unspecified disease of pericardium

ICD-10-CM CODES

- I30 Acute pericarditis
- I30.0 Acute nonspecific idiopathic pericarditis
- I30.1 Infective pericarditis
- I30.8 Other forms of acute pericarditis
- I30.9 Acute pericarditis, unspecified
- I31 Other diseases of pericardium
- I31.0 Chronic adhesive pericarditis
- I31.1 Chronic constrictive pericarditis
- I31.4 Cardiac tamponade
- I31.8 Other specified diseases of pericardium
- I31.9 Disease of pericardium, unspecified
- I32 Pericarditis in diseases classified elsewhere

PREFERRED PRACTICE PATTERN

- 6D: Impaired Aerobic Capacity/Endurance Associated with Cardiovascular Pump Dysfunction or Failure

PATIENT PRESENTATION

A 70-year-old male presents with a recent onset of substernal chest pain. The pain is sharp and pleuritic and has started to radiate to the left trapezius muscle. Inspiration causes the pain to become more severe, but sitting up and leaning forward helps to relieve it. This patient's review of systems reveals a recent viral illness, including "flu-like" symptoms and low-grade fever for 1 week. His past medical history is otherwise unremarkable. His current temperature is 100.9°F, BP is 130/84 mm Hg, HR is 95 bpm, RR is 24 breaths/min, and O_2 Saturation is 99% in room air. Heart auscultation reveals a scratchy, rubbing sound at the lower left sternal border. Lungs are clear, but breathing is shallow. The patient is referred to the emergency room. ECG reveals widespread ST-segment elevation and chest X-ray (CXR) is normal.

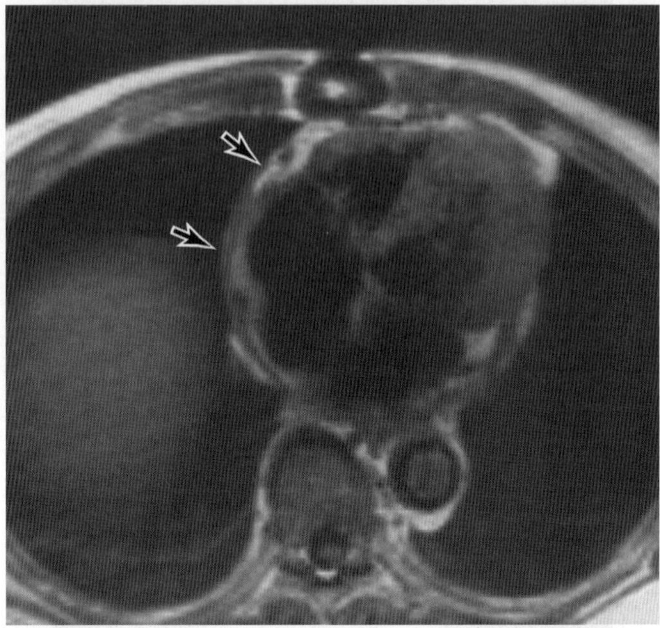

FIGURE 18-1 Magnetic resonance image of cross-section of thorax showing pericardial thickening (*arrows*) in a patient with constrictive pericarditis. (Courtesy of C Higgins. Reproduced with permission from Sokolow M, McIlroy MB. *Clinical Cardiology*. 6th ed. Originally published by Appleton & Lange. Copyright © 1993 by the McGraw-Hill Companies, Inc.)

KEY FEATURES

Description

- Inflammation of the pericardium (fibrous sac surrounding the heart)
- Can be acute or chronic

Essentials of Diagnosis

- Chest pain can be relieved by sitting up and leaning forward
- Stethoscope: Pericardial rub sound
- Bacterial infection: Mycobacterium tuberculosis
- Acute to chronic
  - Acute <6 weeks
  - Subacute 6 weeks to 6 months
  - Chronic >6 months
- Classification secondary to type of fluid
  - Serous
  - Purulent
  - Fibrinous
  - Caseous
  - Hemorrhagic
  - Post infarction (from a heart attack)

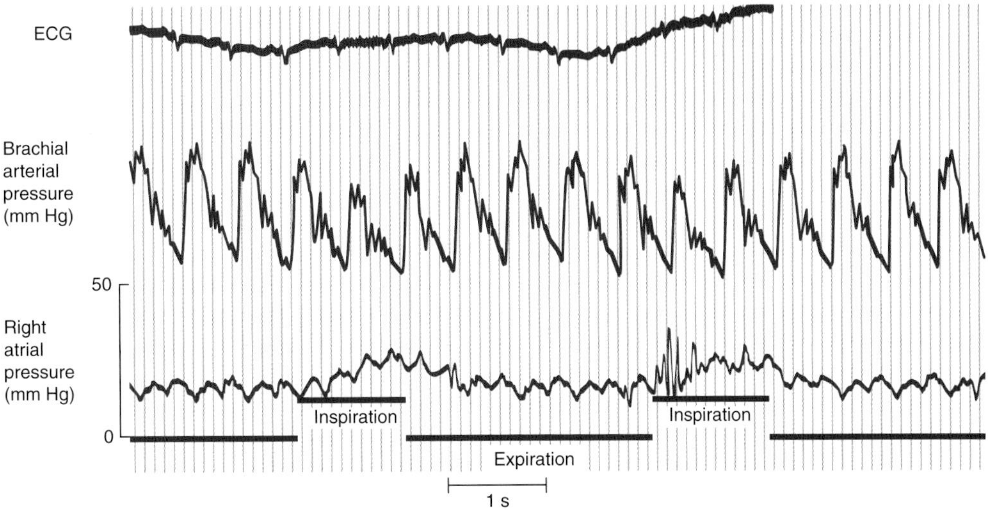

FIGURE 18-2 Brachial arterial and right atrial pressures showing pulsus paradoxus in a patient with constrictive pericarditis and an increase in right atrial pressure on inspiration (Kussmaul sign). Both the systolic and diastolic atrial pressures rise with inspiration. (Redrawn with permission from Cheitlin MD, Sokolow M, McIlroy MB. *Clinical Cardiology*. 6th ed. Originally published by Appleton & Lange. Copyright © 1993 by the McGraw-Hill Companies, Inc.)

General Considerations

- Can be misdiagnosed as a heart attack
- Often the result of an infection
- No change with exertion
- Often unknown etiology

Demographics

- Mostly men aged 20 to 50 years of age

CLINICAL FINDINGS

SIGNS AND SYMPTOMS

- Cardiac tamponade
- Sharp stabbing chest pain
- Pain can radiate into the upper trapezius muscle
- Shortness of breath
- Fatigue, weakness
- Swelling in the lower extremities
- Anxiety
- Diaphoresis
- Dry cough
- Fever
- Crackles in the lungs
- Heart sounds
  - Decreased breath sounds
  - Pericardial rub sound

Functional Implications

- New York Heart Association functional status
  - Class I: A patient who is not limited with normal physical activity by symptoms
  - Class II: Occurs when ordinary physical activity results in fatigue, dyspnea, or other symptoms
  - Class III: Characterized by a marked limitation in normal physical activity
  - Class IV: Defined by symptoms at rest or with any physical activity
- Depending on the severity
  - Decreased activity tolerance
  - Decreased exercise tolerance
  - Dyspnea on exertion
  - Hypoxia
  - Muscle weakness
  - Cardiac arrhythmia

Possible Contributing Causes[1]

- Infections
  - Viral infection: Coxsackievirus
  - Bacterial infection: Tuberculosis, purulent (staphylococcal, pneumococcal)
  - Fungal infection
  - Protozoal: Amebiasis
  - Mycotic: Actinomycosis, coccidioidomycosis

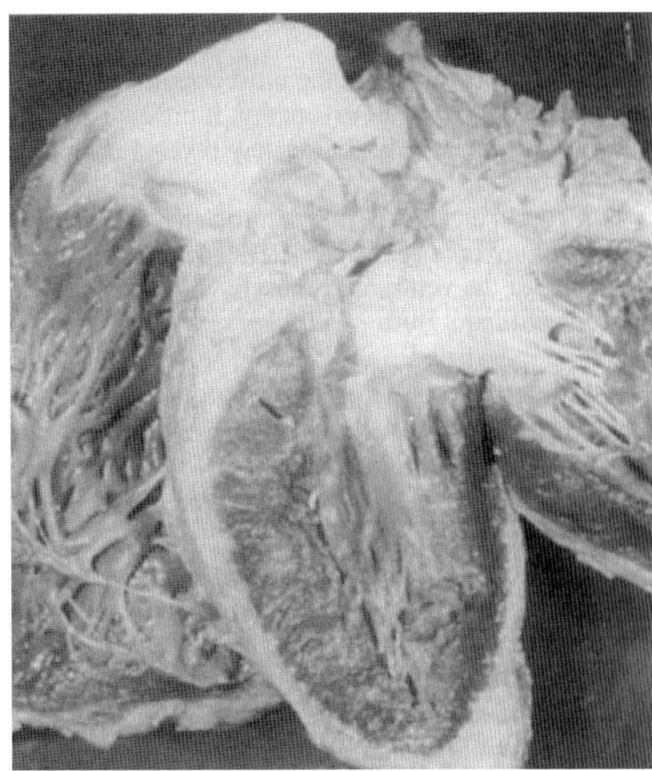

FIGURE 18-3 Chronic constrictive pericarditis caused by tuberculous pericarditis. The heart is encased by a thickened fibrous pericardium, and the ventricular luminal size is decreased as a result of restriction of filling. (From Chandrasoma P, Taylor CR. *Concise Pathology*. 3rd ed. www.accessmedicine.com. Copyright © The McGraw-Hill Companies, Inc. All rights reserved.)

- Collagen vascular disease
  - Systemic lupus erythematosus
  - Scleroderma
  - Rheumatoid arthritis
- Heart attack
- Medications: Tetracyclines
- Radiation
- Trauma
- Rheumatic fever
- Metabolic
  - Kidney failure
- Neoplasm: Cancer
- HIV infection
- Idiopathic
- Auto-immune (Dressler syndrome)

Differential Diagnosis

- Cardiac pump dysfunction
- Angina pectoris
- Aortic dissection
- Aortic stenosis
- Gastritis
- Gastroesophageal reflux disease (GERD)
- Myocardial infarction
- Myocardial ischemia
- Pulmonary embolism

MEANS OF CONFIRMATION OR DIAGNOSIS

Laboratory Tests

- Antinuclear antibody (ANA)
- Complete blood count (CBC)
- C-reactive protein

Imaging

- Chest x-ray
- EKG
- Echocardiogram
- Radionuclide scanning
- Phonocardiogram
- Chest/heart MRI

FINDINGS AND INTERPRETATION

- Increased urea (BUN)
- ECG with elevated ST segments

TREATMENT

Medication

- Antibiotics if bacterial infection
- Antifungal if fungal pericarditis
- Corticosteroids (prednisone)
- Diuretics for fluid buildup

REFERRALS

- Suspected cardiac muscle dysfunction: Call primary care and/or cardiologist.
- Suspected cardiac muscle failure: Call 911.

IMPAIRMENTS

- Shortness of breath
- Dyspnea on exertion
- Limited activity tolerance
- Limited functional capacity

TESTS AND MEASURES

- 6-minute walk test
- BORG rate of perceived exertion
- Vital sign monitoring to include lung auscultations
- Short-Form 36 Health Survey

INTERVENTION

- Risk-factor modification
- Cardiac rehabilitation
- Education on signs and symptoms
- Aerobic exercise training to improve efficiency in oxygen consumption

FUNCTIONAL GOALS

- The patient will be able to tolerate 30 minutes of continuous aerobic exercise while maintaining an RPE of 13, with stable vital signs.
- Short-term goals
  - Reconditioning sufficient for resumption of customary activities.
  - Limiting the physiologic and psychological effects of heart disease.
    - Decreasing the risk of sudden cardiac arrest or infarction.
    - Controlling the symptoms of cardiac disease.
- Long-term goals
  - Identification and treatment of risk factors.
  - Stabilizing or even reversing the atherosclerotic process.
  - Enhancing the psychological status of the patients.

PROGNOSIS

- Mild to life-threatening
- Recovery in weeks to 3 months, depending on severity

PATIENT RESOURCE

- What is Pericarditis? American Heart Association. http://www.heart.org/HEARTORG/Conditions/More/What-is-Pericarditis_UCM_444931_Article.jsp. Accessed August 8, 2014.

REFERENCE

1. Kusumoto FM. Pericardial disease. In: McPhee SJ, Hammer GD, eds. *Pathophysiology of Disease: An Introduction to Clinical Medicine.* 6th ed. New York, NY: McGraw-Hill; 2010. http://www.accessphysiotherapy.com/content/5367913. Accessed July 7, 2013.

ADDITIONAL REFERENCES

- Cassady SL, Cahalin LP. Cardiovascular pathophysiology. In: DeTurk WE, Cahalin LP, eds. *Cardiovascular and Pulmonary Physical Therapy: An Evidence-Based Approach.* 2nd ed. New York, NY: McGraw-Hill; 2011. http://www.accessphysiotherapy.com/content/6872740. Accessed July 7, 2013.
- Demmler GJ. Infectious pericarditis in children. *Pediatr Infect Dis J.* 2006;25(2):165–166.
- Dubin D. *Rapid Interpretation of EKG's.* Fort Myers, FL: COVER Publishing Company. http://www.emergencyekg.com/Reference_Sheets.pdf. Accessed July 7, 2013.

- Dutton M. Cardiovascular physical therapy. In: Dutton M, ed. *McGraw-Hill's NPTE (National Physical Therapy Examination).* 2nd ed. New York, NY: McGraw-Hill; 2009. http://www.accessphysiotherapy.com/content/5401905. Accessed July 7, 2013.
- Goodman CC. The cardiovascular system. In: Goodman CC, Boissonnault WG, Fuller KS, eds. *Pathology: Implications for the Physical Therapist.* 2nd ed. Philadelphia, PA: Saunders; 2003: 367–476.
- Kusumoto FM. Cardiovascular disorders: heart disease. In: McPhee SJ, Hammer GD, eds. *Pathophysiology of Disease: An Introduction to Clinical Medicine.* 6th ed. New York, NY: McGraw-Hill; 2010. http://www.accessphysiotherapy.com/content/5367684. Accessed July 7, 2013.
- LeWinter MM, Tischler MD. Pericardial diseases. In: Bonow RO, Mann DL, Zipes DP, Libby P, eds. *Braunwald's Heart Disease: A Textbook of Cardiovascular Medicine.* 9th ed. Philadelphia, PA: Saunders Elsevier; 2011: Chapter 75.
- Maisch B, Seferović PM, Ristić AD, et al. Guidelines on the diagnosis and management of pericardial diseases executive summary; The Task force on the diagnosis and management of pericardial diseases of the European society of cardiology. *Eur Heart J April.* 2004;25(7):587–610. doi:10.1016/j.ehj.2004.02.002.
- McPhee SJ, Hammer GD. Pericardial disease. In: McPhee SJ, Hammer GD, eds. *Pathophysiology of Disease.* 6th ed. New York, NY: McGraw-Hill; 2010.
- Miyamoto SD, Sondheimer HM, Fagan TE, Collins KK. Cardiovascular diseases. In: Hay WW, Levin MJ, Sondheimer JM, Deterding RR, eds. *CURRENT Diagnosis & Treatment: Pediatrics.* 20th ed. New York, NY: McGraw-Hill; 2011. http://www.accessphysiotherapy.com/content/6583435. Accessed July 7, 2013.
- The American Physical Therapy Association. *Guide to Physical Therapist Practice.* Alexandria, VA: APTA. 2003. http://guidetoptpractice.apta.org/. Accessed July 7, 2013.

SECTION D ENDOCRINE DISORDERS

19 ADDISON DISEASE

Debra F. Stern, DPT, DBA, MSM, PT
Eric Shamus, PhD, DPT, PT, CSCS

CONDITION/DISORDER SYNONYMS

- Chronic renal insufficiency[1]
- Hypocortisolism[1]

ICD-9-CM CODES[2]

- 255.41 Glucocorticoid deficiency
- PT diagnoses/treatment diagnoses that may be secondary adrenal gland disorders
  - 315.4 Developmental coordination disorder
  - 719.70 Difficulty in walking involving joint site, unspecified
  - 728.2 Muscular wasting and disuse atrophy, not elsewhere
  - 728.89 Other disorders of muscle, ligament, and fascia classified
  - 729.9 Other and unspecified disorders of soft tissue
  - 780.7 Malaise and fatigue
  - 781.2 Abnormality of gait
  - 782.3 Edema
  - 786.0 Dyspnea and respiratory abnormalities
  - 786.05 Shortness of breath

ICD-10-CM CODES[3]

- E27.1 Primary adrenocortical insufficiency
- E27.2 Addisonian crisis
- E27.40 Unspecified adrenocortical insufficiency

PREFERRED PRACTICE PATTERNS[4]

- 4B: Impaired Posture
- 4C: Impaired Muscle Performance

PATIENT PRESENTATION

A 25-year-old female referred with significant sarcopenia and a BMI of 16. Her gait is unstable and she demonstrates coordination deficits. She is mildly short of breath on exertion. She describes little interest in food, but does have self-described craving for potato chips at times. Of late, she is too tired to exercise and she thinks it is because she is depressed. Her history reveals that she menstruates infrequently over the past year and that her skin tone has changed.

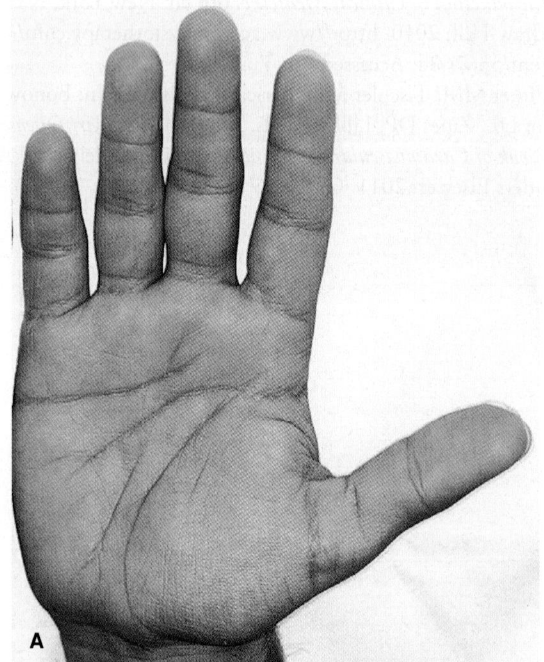

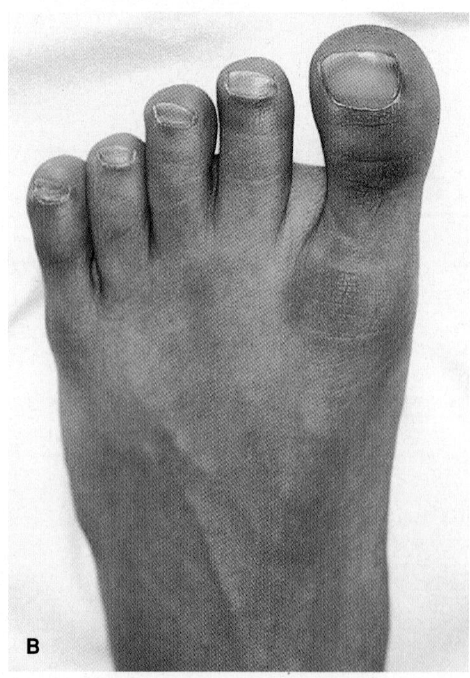

FIGURE 19-1 Clinical features of *Addison disease.* Note the hyperpigmentation in areas of increased friction including (**A**) palmar creases, (**B**) dorsal foot, *(continued)*

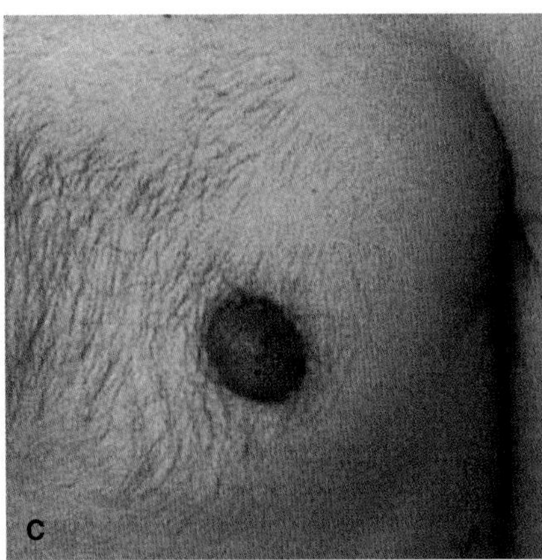

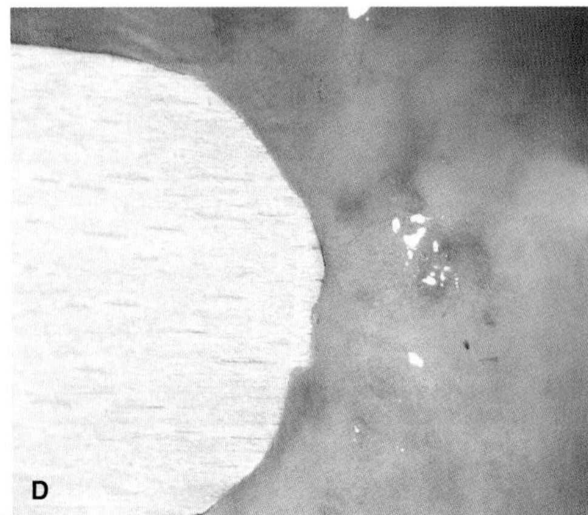

FIGURE 19-1 *(Continued)* (**C**) nipples and axillary region, and (**D**) patchy hyperpigmentation of the oral mucosa. (From Longo DL, Fauci A, Kasper D, et al., eds. *Harrison's Principles of Internal Medicine*. 18th ed. New York, NY: McGraw-Hill; 2012.)

KEY FEATURES

Description

- Insufficient production or release of glucocorticoids (cortisol),[1] androgens, and mineralocorticoids from the adrenal glands
- These hormones play a role in
  - Conversion of food to energy
  - Inflammatory response
  - Response to stress
  - Maintaining sodium–potassium balance for blood pressure regulation and production of androgens in males and women, involved in maintaining libido

Essentials of Diagnosis

- May be insidious onset or sudden onset as in Addisonian crisis
- May cause pathology in multiple organ systems or be caused by pathology in other organ systems
  - Cardiovascular: Heart, peripheral circulation, blood pressure
  - Integumentary system
- Confirmation of suspected disease through blood testing

General Considerations

- Clinic should have carbohydrates available if needed for drop in blood sugar
  - Orange juice, sugar packets, or similar
- May result in secondary problems such as
  - Aerobic capacity and muscle endurance impairment
  - Sarcopenia
  - Weakness/impaired muscle performance
  - Musculoskeletal problems

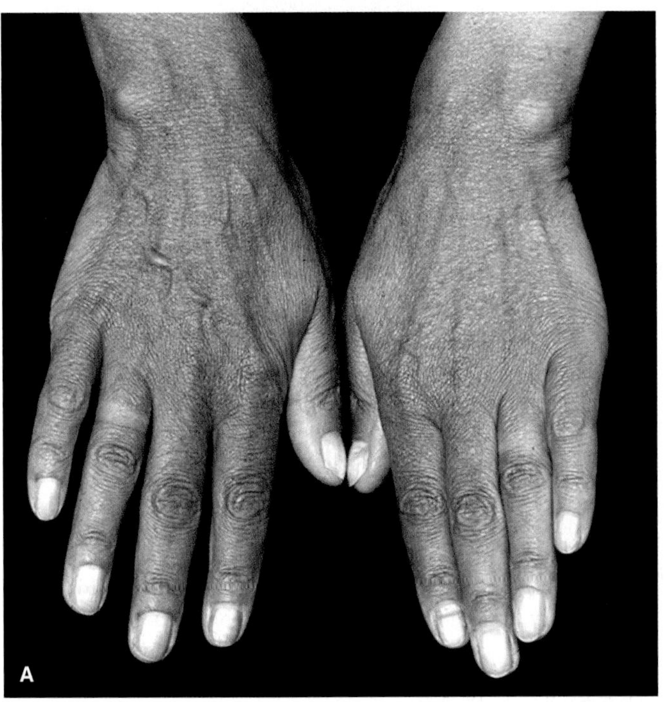

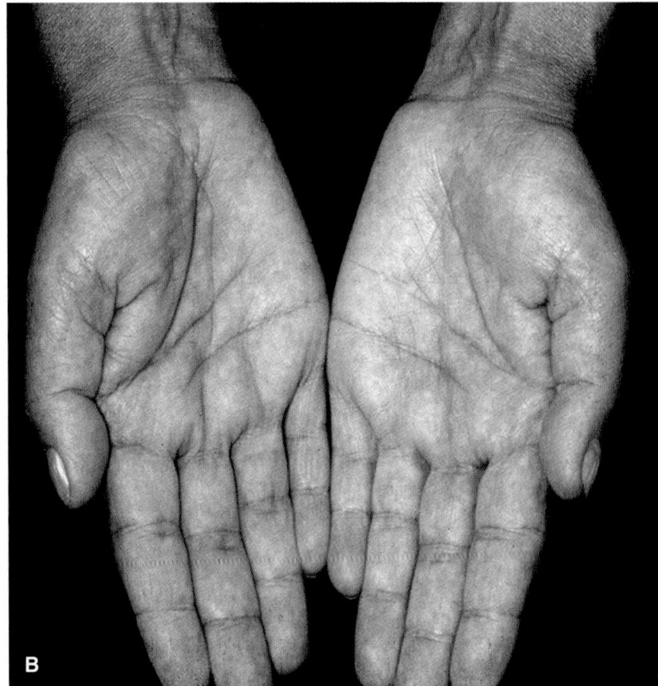

FIGURE 19-2 Addison disease **A.** Hyperpigmentation representing an accentuation of normal pigmentation of the hand of a patient with Addison disease. **B.** Note the accentuated pigmentation in the palmar creases. (From Wolff K, Johnson RA. *Fitzpatrick's Color Atlas and Synopsis of Clinical Dermatology.* 6th ed. http://www.accessmedicine.com. Copyright © The McGraw-Hill Companies, Inc. All rights reserved.)

- Neuromuscular problems
- Weight loss indicating the need for PT intervention depending on severity

Demographics
- Males and females equally
- Can develop at any age
- May be familial[5]

CLINICAL FINDINGS

SIGNS AND SYMPTOMS
- It is not the purview of a PT to medically diagnose hypothyroid, but rather to recognize the possibility in the differential diagnosis process, especially when the findings are not consistent with conditions commonly treated such as musculoskeletal, neuromuscular, integumentary, and cardiopulmonary.
  - PTs may, however, treat conditions caused by adrenal disorders or treat patients with Addison disease for other pathologies that are unrelated.
- Hypotension
- Fatigue
- Weight loss,[1] loss of appetite
- Decreased activity tolerance
- Fainting/loss of consciousness
- Headaches
- Sweating
- Anorexia
- Muscle weakness[1]
- Darkening/hyperpigmentation of skin
- Craving for salt
- Hypoglycemia
- Nausea
- Diarrhea
- Vomiting
- Irritability
- Depression
- Pain
- Joint pain
- Low back pain
- Abdominal pain
- Leg pain
- Hyperkalemia
- Loss of libido
- Oral lesions
- Metabolic acidosis
- Personality changes
- Amenorrhea
- Sparseness of hair in axilla

Functional Implications
- Severe symptoms such as immediacy of need to defecate and diarrhea may be disabling and result in the inability to leave home.
- Decreasing weight with inability to exercise or move well.
- Sarcopenia resulting in weakness, muscle mass loss, inability to ambulate or perform self-care, and aerobic capacity limitation secondary to inactivity.
- Decreased exercise tolerance.
- Limitations in ADLs, or IADLs.

Possible Contributing Causes
- Damage to the adrenal glands
- Autoimmune dysfunction
- Tuberculosis
- Infections of the adrenal glands
- Metastatic cancer
- Adrenal tumors
- Surgery
- Bleeding into the adrenals, as in trauma
- Illness
- Systemic infection
- Hypoparathyroidism

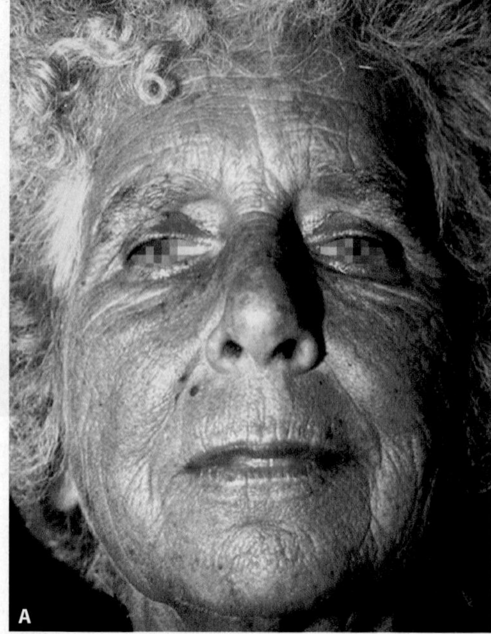

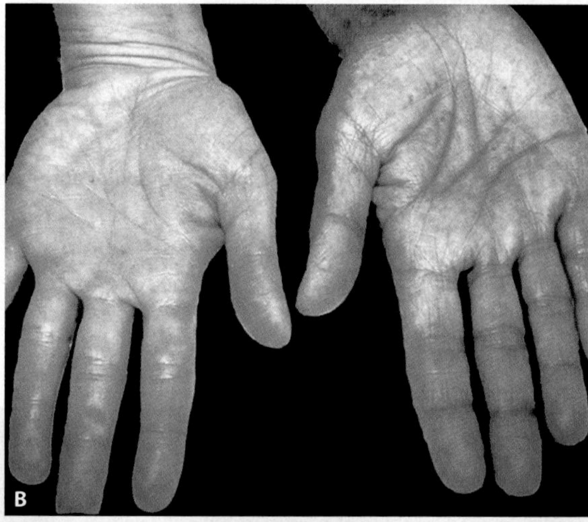

FIGURE 19-3 A. This patient with Addison disease demonstrates the characteristic hyperpigmentation of the skin with accentuation in sun-exposed areas. **B.** Palmar creases are also hyperpigmented compared with a normal hand. (Goldsmith LA, Katz SI, Gilchrest BA, et al. *Fitzpatrick's Dermatology in General Medicine*. 8th ed. http://www.accessmedicine.com. Copyright © The McGraw-Hill Companies, Inc. All rights reserved.)

- Type 1 diabetes mellitus
- Celiac sprue
- Primary ovarian failure
- Testicular failure
- Pernicious anemia
- Trauma
- Anticoagulation therapy
- Heredity
  - Such as polyglandular syndrome, familial glucocorticoid deficiency, congenital adrenal hypoplasia or hyperplasia, X-linked adrenal leukodystrophy
- Secondary adrenal disease may be caused by
  - Pituitary disease, inadequate adrenocorticotropic hormone (ACTH) production which leads to inadequate production of adrenal hormones

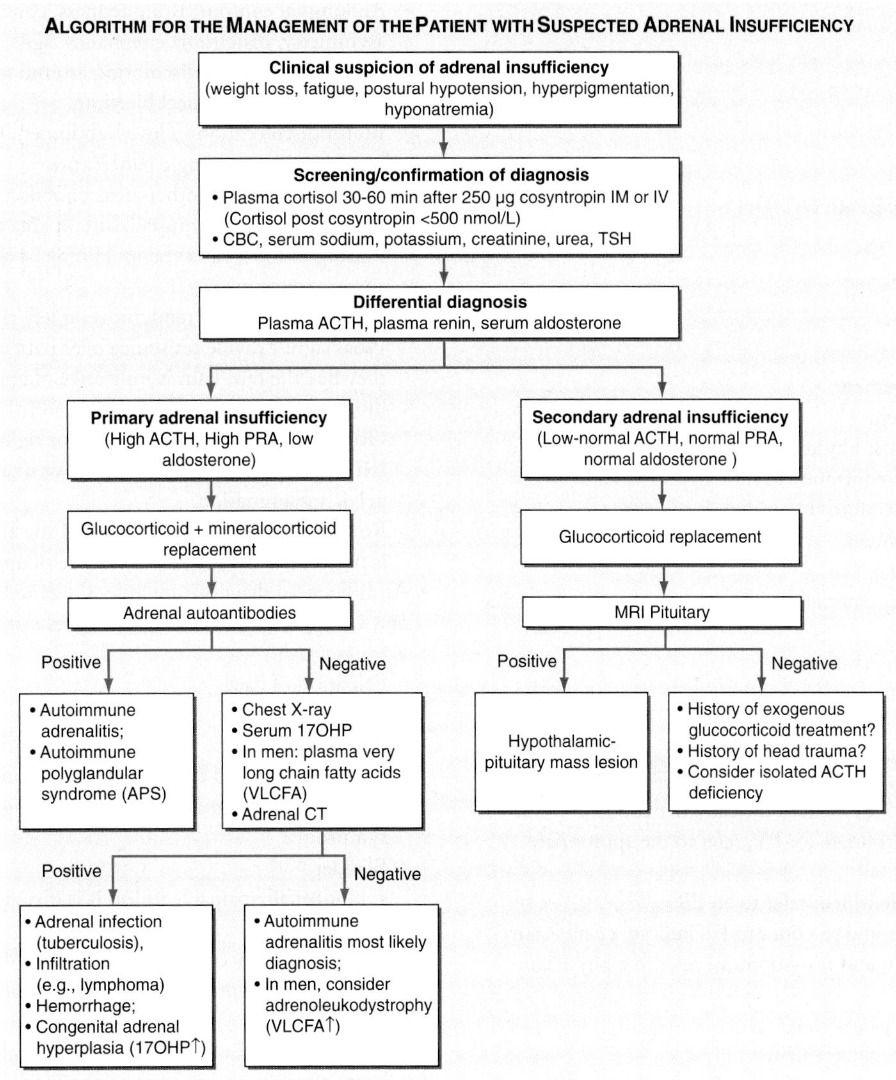

FIGURE 19-4 Management of the patient with suspected adrenal insufficiency. PRA, plasma renin activity. (From Longo DL, Fauci A, Kasper D, et al., eds. *Harrison's Principles of Internal Medicine.* 18th ed. New York, NY: McGraw-Hill; 2012.)

  - Abrupt stopping of corticosteroids, which may be taken for a variety of conditions including, but not limited to, asthma, arthritis, and inflammatory conditions

Differential Diagnosis

- Anorexia nervosa
- Appendicitis
- Benign prostatic hypertrophy
- Bladder infections, urinary tract infections, kidney pathology
- Bowel disorders
- Celiac disease
- Endocrine disorders
- Gastroenteritis
- Gynecologic problems in females such as
  - Endometriosis
  - Menses, amenorrhea
  - Ovarian cysts, ovarian dysfunction, or ovarian disease
  - Fibroids
  - Menopause
- Hyperpigmentation from other causes
- Hypoaldosteronism
- Hypotension from other causes
- Infections in the abdomen
- Kidney disease
- Nonmalignant tumors in the abdomen or organs
- Organ dysfunction as a result of cancer or malignancy
- Pelvic inflammatory disease
- Perforated ulcers anywhere in GI system
- Peritonitis
- Pituitary dysfunction
- Prostatitis

MEANS OF CONFIRMATION OR DIAGNOSIS

Laboratory Tests

- Blood tests/lab tests: Complete blood count (CBC)
  - Levels of: Sodium, potassium, antibodies associated with Addison disease
  - Cortisol levels
  - ACTH levels
- ACTH stimulation test
- Insulin-induced hypoglycemia test

▸ **Imaging**
- Ultrasound
- Chest X-rays
- CT scans
- MRIs

FINDINGS AND INTERPRETATION

- Low cortisol levels
- Elevated ACTH levels

TREATMENT

- Pharmacologic management
  - Hormone replacement
    - Oral corticosteroids: Fludrocortisones for aldosterone, hydrocortisone, prednisone
    - Corticosteroid injections if vomiting is present
    - Androgen replacement
- Other
  - Sodium supplements especially with exercise or during episodes of stress
  - Sugar (if Addisonian crisis)
  - Saline (if Addisonian crisis)

REFERRALS/ADMITTANCE

- If a patient is referred for PT and the causative problem is not considered to be appropriate for PT, refer to the appropriate physician.
- If an emergency is identified, refer to an ER.
- If the patient's history and reactions to PT indicate possible adrenal gland dysfunction and or symptoms, refer to a physician.
- Interprofessional
  - Physician: Smoking cessation
  - Physician: Weight management
  - Nutritionist: Dietary counseling
  - Optometry
  - Ophthalmology
  - Audiology
  - Psychological intervention
  - Occupational therapy

IMPAIRMENTS

- Muscle weakness
- Muscle atrophy, sarcopenia
- Gait abnormality/difficulty walking
- Shortness of breath, fatigue
- Inability to perform self-care
- Balance impairment
- Impaired skin integrity

TESTS AND MEASURES

- Observation
  - Scars may indicate adhesions or abdominal surgeries that may be causative of diverticula.
  - Striae pink or purplish may be indicative of Cushing syndrome, and dilated veins may indicate hepatic pathology or inferior vena cava obstruction, not diverticulitis.
  - Abdominal contour: Roundedness, concavity/hollowness, asymmetry, distension, pregnancy signs.
  - Cullen sign: Bluish discoloring around umbilicus, which may be a sign of retroperitoneal bleeding.
  - Bluish discoloration in lower abdomen; Grey Turner sign which is a sign of hemorrhagic pancreatitis.
  - Bulging in groin or other areas of abdomen especially apparent with contraction of musculature in area may be hernia.
  - Pulsing in the area of the navel may be abdominal aortic aneurysm.
  - Palpable abdominal tenderness on left/right or generalized.
  - Psoas sign: Provide resistance over patient's right knee as they flex the hip. Pain is indicative of appendicitis or possible inflammation of the abdomen.
  - Obturator sign: Internal rotation of right lower extremity (RLE) and flexion may be indicative of appendicitis or pelvic inflammation.
  - Rovsing sign: Pain on right side of the abdomen when pressure is put on the left may be indicative of appendicitis.
- As differential diagnosis includes GI as well as other endocrine and UG pathologies, the following tests and measures are presented:
  - Palpation of back
  - Skin changes: Turgor, dryness, hairlessness, pigmentation
  - Kidneys: In supine, place one hand under client between ribs and iliac crest and other hand on abdomen below ribs pointing in opposite direction: +/− tenderness or reproduction of symptoms.
  - Bladder
    - Not usually palpable unless it is distended and rises above pubic bone.
    - In supine, place hand above pubis and press down: + = tenderness, reproduction of pain, or ability to feel the bladder: __+ __−.
  - Appendix (McBurney's): Apply vertical pressure halfway between right anterior superior iliac spine (ASIS) and umbilicus.
  - Liver: In supine, with left hand under trunk parallel to 11th and 12th rib, lift upward; right hand lateral to rectus and press in and up: + = reproduction of symptoms with deep breath.
  - Ascites: With the fingers, percuss outward from center, if sound is dull, ascites may be present.
  - Spleen: It is not recommended for PT to palpate an enlarged spleen (only palpable if enlarged) because of the potential of rupture.
  - Gallbladder (Murphy's): Place fingers right of rectus abdominus below rib cage: + = sudden pain and muscle tensing with deep breath.

INTERVENTION

- Carbohydrates, available if needed for drop in blood sugar
  - Orange juice, sugar packets, or similar
- PT intervention is consistent with the movement-related problems that may occur secondary to weakness and hormone deficiencies
- Gait training
- Therapeutic exercise: All relevant categories, energy conservation
  - Assess for orthostasis, hypotension
  - As hypoglycemia may occur, ensure blood sugar levels are in appropriate ranges

  - May require supplemental sodium during exercise, as sodium deficiency is characteristic, and cramping, nausea should be prevented
  - PT should inquire about medications taken
- Self-care management training, including skin care/moisturizing, lifestyle management
- Neuromuscular re-education: Balance and postural training
- Wound management as indicated

FUNCTIONAL GOALS

- Patient will be able to
  - Achieve adequate functional aerobic capacity and the ability to talk during activity in order to achieve functional gait and activity tolerance for work, play, school, self-care; ADLs and IADLs.
  - Functional gait in the home and community (with or without a device), allowing for work, play, self-care; ADLs and IADLS; up to ___ feet based on patient need and prior functional level.
  - Achieve 600 m or greater in a 6-minute walk test for initiation of safe functional gait in the community.
  - Perform active verbalization with increasing taxonomy for safety during gait, including negotiation of even and uneven surfaces, opening and closing doors, and transferring in and out of a car.
  - Tolerate 30 minutes of continuous moderate exercise three times a week in ___ weeks, and five times a week in ___ weeks, depending on the severity of disease.

PROGNOSIS

- As this pathology is primarily medical in nature, the physician establishes the medical prognosis. Most are able to maintain active lifestyles with normal life expectancy. It can, however, be life threatening, especially in sudden onset as in an Addisonian crisis.
- PT prognosis should be good to return to premorbid function if condition is adequately managed.

PATIENT RESOURCE

- Adrenal Insufficiency and Addison's Disease. National Institute of Diabetes and Digestive and Kidney Diseases. NIH Publication No. 09-3054. National Endocrine and Metabolic Diseases Information Service. http://www.endocrine.niddk.nih.gov/pubs/addison/addison.aspx#symptoms. Accessed March 13, 2013.

REFERENCES

1. Dutton M. Adrenal disorders. In: Dutton M, ed. *McGraw-Hill's NPTE (National Physical Therapy Examination)*. 2nd ed. New York, NY: McGraw-Hill; 2012. http://www.accessphysiotherapy.com/content/56510071. Accessed January 25, 2013.
2. ICD9Data.com. http://www.icd9data.com. Accessed March 13, 2013.
3. ICD10Data.com. http://www.icd10data.com. Accessed March 13, 2013.
4. The American Physical Therapy Association. *Interactive Guide to Physical Therapist Practice*. Alexandria, VA: The American Physical Therapy Association; 2003. http://guidetoptpractice.apta.org/. Accessed March 13, 2013.
5. Hay WW, Levin MJ, Deterding RR, Abzug MJ, Sondheimer JM. Adrenal cortex. In: Hay WW, Levin MJ, Deterding RR, Abzug MJ, Sondheimer JM, eds. *CURRENT Diagnosis & Treatment: Pediatrics*. 21st ed. New York, NY: McGraw-Hill; 2012. http://www.accessphysiotherapy.com/content/56829956. Accessed January 25, 2013.

ADDITIONAL REFERENCES

- Adams R, Hinkebein MK, McQuillen M, Sutherland S, El Asyouty S, Lippmann S. Prompt differentiation of Addison's disease from anorexia nervosa during weight loss and vomiting. *South Med J.* 1998;91(2):208–211.
- Baskin HJ, Cobin RH, Duick DS, et al. American Association of Clinical Endocrinologists medical guidelines for clinical practice for the evaluation and treatment of hyperthyroidism and hypothyroidism. *Endocr Pract.* 2002;8(6):457–469.
- de Herder WW, van der Lely AJ. Addisonian crisis and relative adrenal failure. *Rev Endocr Metab Disord.* 2003;4(2):143–147. doi:10.1023/A:1022938019091.
- Nieman LK, Chanco Turner ML. Addison's disease. *Clin Dermatol.* 2006;24(4):276–280. doi:10.1016/j.clindermatol.2006.04.006.
- Reisch N, Arlt W. Fine tuning for quality of life: 21st century approach to treatment of Addison's disease. *Endocrinol Metab Clin North Am.* 2009;38(2):407–418, ix–x. doi: 10.1016/j.ecl.2009.01.008.
- Ten S, New M, Maclaren N. Clinical review 130: Addison's disease 2001. *J Clin Endocrinol Metab.* 2001;86(7):2909–2922. doi: 10.1210/jc.86.7.2909.
- Winqvist O, Karlsson FA, Kämpe O. 21-Hydroxylase, a major autoantigen in idiopathic Addison's disease. *Lancet.* 1992;339(8809): 1559–1562. doi: 10.1016/0140-6736(92)91829-W.

20 ADRENAL GLAND HYPERFUNCTION

Debra F. Stern, DPT, DBA, MSM, PT
Eric Shamus, PhD, DPT, PT, CSCS

CONDITION/DISORDER SYNONYMS

- Hyperadrenalism
- Hyperadrenocorticism
- Adrencorticalhyperfunction

ICD-9-CM CODES

- 255.0 Cushing syndrome
- 255.3 Other corticoadrenal overactivity
- 255.6 Medulloadrenal hyperfunction
- Associated physical therapy diagnoses
  - 315.4 Coordination disorder (clumsiness, dyspraxia and/or specific motor development disorder)
  - 718.45 Contracture of joint, pelvic region, and thigh
  - 719.70 Difficulty in walking
  - 728.2 Muscular wasting and disuse atrophy
  - 728.89 Disorders of muscle, ligament, and fascia
  - 729.9 Other disorders of soft tissue
  - 780.7 Malaise and fatigue
  - 781.2 Abnormality of gait: Ataxic, paralytic, spastic, staggering
  - 782.3 Edema
  - 786.0 Dyspnea and respiratory abnormalities
  - 786.05 Shortness of breath

ICD-10-CM CODES

- E24.0 Pituitary-dependent Cushing disease
- E24.2 Drug-induced Cushing syndrome
- E24.3 Ectopic ACTH syndrome
- E24.8 Other Cushing syndrome
- E24.9 Cushing syndrome, unspecified
- E27.5 Adrenomedullary hyperfunction

PREFERRED PRACTICE PATTERNS

- 4D: Impaired Joint Mobility, Motor Function, Muscle Performance, and Range of Motion Associated with Connective Tissue Dysfunction[1]
- 4E: Impaired Joint Mobility, Motor Function, Muscle Performance, and Range of Motion Associated with Localized Inflammation[2]
- 6B: Impaired Aerobic Capacity/Endurance Associated with Deconditioning[3]
- 7B: Impaired Integumentary Integrity Secondary to Superficial Skin Involvement[4]

PATIENT PRESENTATION

A 60-year-old male is referred to PT for generalized muscle weakness, back pain, and complaints of fatigue. His history reveals type 2 diabetes, hypertension, and illegal drug use in his somewhat remote past. He complains of being sweaty most of the time, even without exertion, and is drinking a lot of water. The back pain is constant and he describes it as dull. His lower back is tender to touch, and the pain is not relieved with rest or change in activity. He states his wife is complaining about his decreased libido. Although he used to be an avid exerciser, he complains of being too tired and his legs are getting "skinny."

KEY FEATURES

Description

- Excessive production and release of adrenal hormones, glucocorticoids (cortisol), androgens, mineralocorticoids from the adrenal glands
- Adrenal glands are critical in regulating inflammation and cardiovascular function
- Insidious or sudden onset
- High cortisol levels

Essentials of Diagnosis

- Fatigue
- Weight gain
- Decreased activity tolerance
- Hypertension
- Confirmation of suspected disease through blood testing

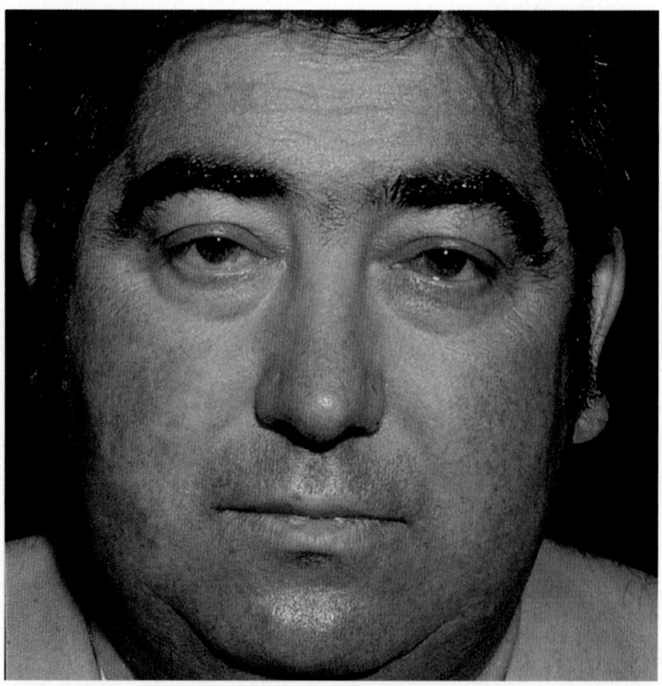

FIGURE 20-1 Moon (round, full, puffy) facies and facial flushing in Cushing syndrome. (From Wolff K, Johnson RA. *Fitzpatrick's Color Atlas and Synopsis of Clinical Dermatology.* 6th ed. New York, NY: McGraw-Hill; 2009.)

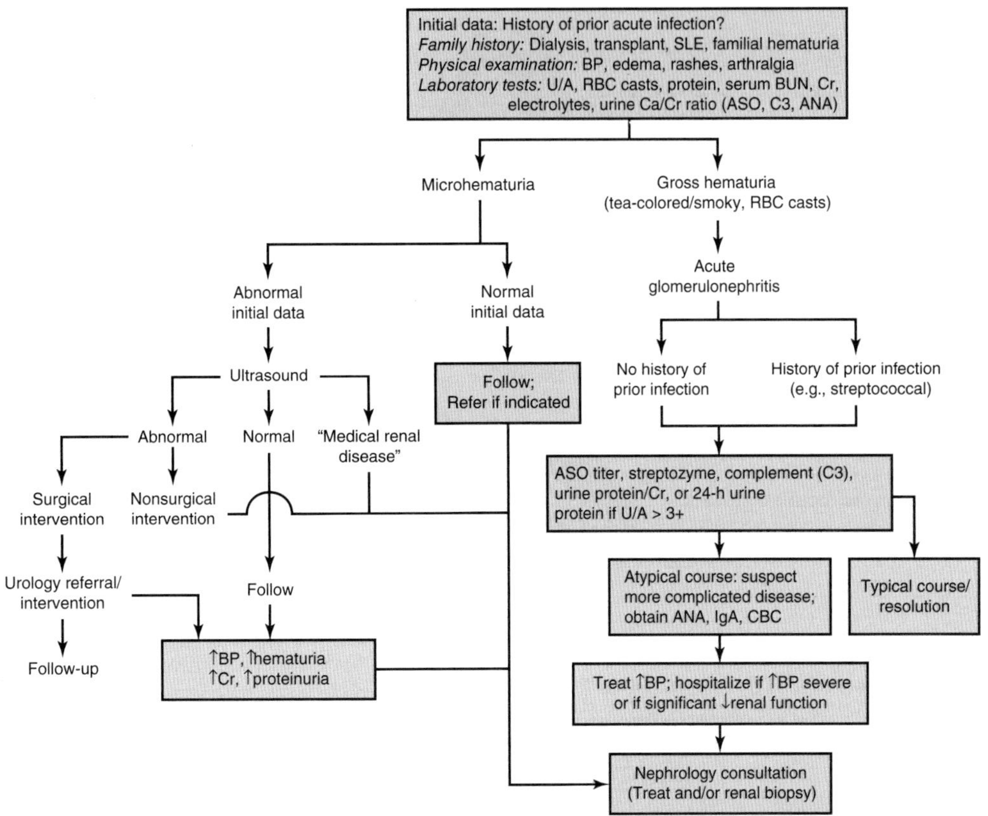

FIGURE 20-2 Approach to the renal workup of hematuria. (Exclude UTI, lithiasis, trauma, bleeding disorders, sickle cell disease.) Complement is depressed in acute poststreptococcal type of glomerulonephritis (about 30 days), chronic glomerulonephritis (persistent), and lupus. ANA, antinuclear antibody; ASO, antistreptolysin antibody; BP, blood pressure; BUN, blood urea nitrogen; C3, complement; Ca, calcium; CBC, complete blood count; Cr, creatinine; IgA, immunoglobulin A; RBC, red blood cell; SLE, systemic lupus erythematosus; U/A, urinalysis. (From Hay WM, Levin MJ, Deterding RR, et al. *Current Diagnosis & Treatment: Pediatrics.* 21st ed. www.accessmedicine.com. Copyright © The McGraw-Hill Companies, Inc. All rights reserved.)

General Considerations

- Diagnosis for more occult problems may take time and require intensive diagnostic testing
- May cause or be caused by pathology in multiple organ systems
  - Cardiovascular: Heart, peripheral circulation, blood pressure
  - Integumentary
- May result in secondary problems needing physical therapy intervention depending on severity: Such as aerobic capacity/muscle endurance impairment, weakness/impaired muscle performance, musculoskeletal problems, neuromuscular problems, weight gain

Demographics

- Males and females equally affected
- Can develop at any age

CLINICAL FINDINGS

SIGNS AND SYMPTOMS

- Fatigue
- Weight loss or gain
- Libido changes
- Pallor
- Flushed face
- Chest pain
- Rapid breathing
- Tachycardia
- Palpitations
- Hypertension
- Excessive thirst
- Sweating
- Increased heat sensitivity
- Headaches
- Decreased gastrointestinal motility
- Tingling
- Increased or decreased muscle bulk
- Muscle weakness
- Paralysis
- Increased frequency of urination
- Increased bowel frequency
- Darkening/hyperpigmentation of skin
- Stretch marks
- Acne
- Hyperglycemia or diabetes
- Inability to absorb calcium
- Water retention, edema
- Thinning of skin
- Easy bruising
- Poor wound healing
- Abdominal pain
- Diarrhea
- Vomiting
- Nausea
- Depression, irritability, personality changes
- Tremors
- Low-back pain in area of kidneys
- Hypokalemia
- Increased sodium levels
- Hallucinations
- Amenorrhea, menstrual irregularities
- Reduced uterus or breast size
- Infertility
- Increased body or facial hair
- Deepened voice
- Baldness
- Growth deficiency, short stature
- Round face, moon face
- Increased excess body fat in trunk and thoracic back
- Osteoporosis
- Increased infection risk
- Kidney stones
- Goiter
- Sleep disturbances
- Cushing syndrome
- Adrenal crisis
  - Coma
  - Shock
  - Seizures
  - Death

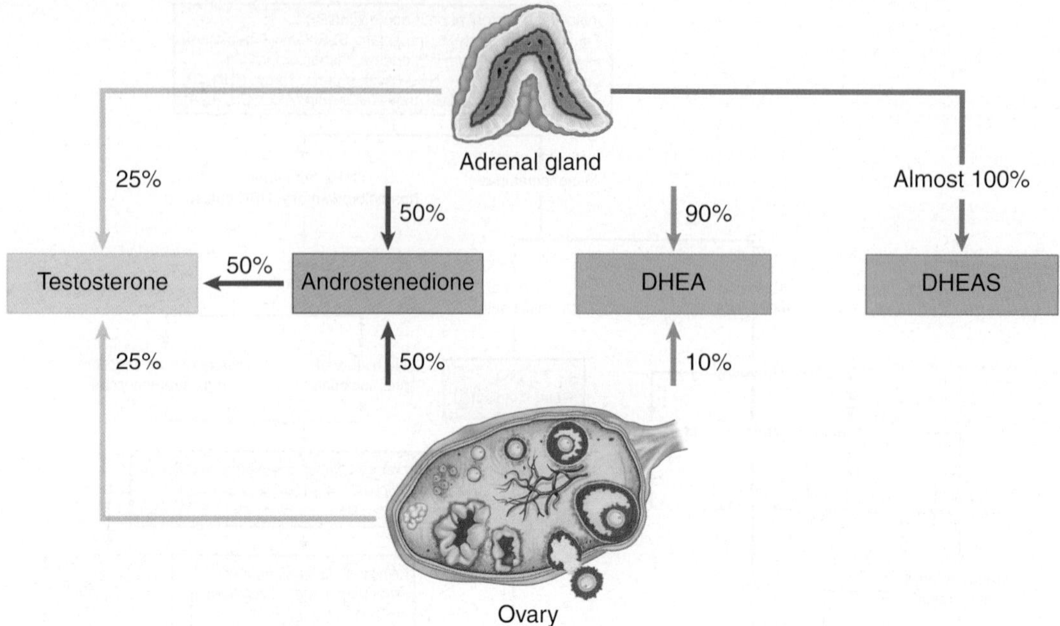

FIGURE 20-3 Diagram depicts the approximate contribution of the adrenal glands and ovaries to levels of androgens, dehydroepiandrosterone (DHEA), and DHEA sulfate (DHEAS). (From Hoffman BL et al. *Williams Gynecology*. 2nd ed. New York: McGraw-Hill, 2012.)

Functional Implications

- Decreased libido in males
- Eating disorders
- Fatigue, weakness, muscle-mass loss
- Inability to ambulate or perform self-care
- Infertility
- Limited ADLs, IADLs
- Limited aerobic capacity or decreased exercise tolerance secondary to inactivity
- Onset of diabetes
- Psychological changes, anxiety, depression, irritability
- Severe symptoms may be disabling, causing inability to leave home
- Sleep disturbances

Possible Contributing Causes

- Adrenal tumor (pheochromocytoma)
- Alcohol
- Autoimmune dysfunction
- Bleeding into the adrenals (i.e., from trauma)
- Cancer of adrenal glands
- Cushing syndrome
- Damage to adrenal glands
- Diabetes mellitus type 1
- Dietary stimulants such as caffeine
- Excessive production of pituitary hormones (causing over stimulation of adrenal glands)
- Excessive stimulation of adrenal glands
- Heredity
- Hyperparathyroidism
- Hypothalamic disorders
- Illegal drugs: Cocaine, heroin
- Illness
- Impending adrenal failure
- Infection of adrenal glands
- Medications: Prescription stimulants, ephedrine
- Metastatic cancer
- Obesity
- Oral corticosteroids
- Pituitary gland pathology/disorder
- Systemic infection

Differential Diagnosis

- Autoimmune disease affecting upper and lower GI tracts or cardiovascular system (involve multiple organs and have fatigue component)
  - Crohn disease or irritable bowel syndrome
  - Rheumatoid arthritis
- Cardiovascular disease
- Celiac disease
- Cushing syndrome
- Endocrine disorder
- Gynecologic problems in females
- Hyperaldosteronism
- Hyperpigmentation from other cause
- Hypertension from other cause
- Kidney disease
- Nonmalignant tumor in abdomen or organs
- Organ dysfunction from cancer or malignancy
- Pituitary dysfunction

MEANS OF CONFIRMATION OR DIAGNOSIS

Laboratory Tests

- Complete blood count (CBC)
- Levels of sodium, potassium, cortisol, adrenocorticotropic hormone (ACTH), antibodies
- Dexamethasone suppression test
- Corticotropin-releasing hormone (CRH) stimulation test to determine adrenal versus pituitary cause

- Urinalysis
- 24-hour urine test
- Saliva tests
- Biopsy

▶ Imaging

- CT
- MRI
- X-ray

FINDINGS AND INTERPRETATION

- Excessive production and release of adrenal hormones
  - Glucocorticoids (cortisol)
  - Androgens
  - Mineralocorticoids

TREATMENT

▶ Medication

- Diabetes medication as indicated
- Cardiac medications as indicated
- Management of hypertension as indicated (Diuretics, Vasodilators, Ace inhibitors, etc.)
- Drug therapy: Nizoral (Ketoconazole), Lysodren (Mitotane), Metopirone (Metyrapone)
- Hormone-replacement therapy

MEDICAL PROCEDURES

- Surgery: Tumor removal as indicated from adrenal glands, pancreas, pituitary, lungs
- Radiation therapy: Gamma knife or small doses over several weeks

REFERRALS/ADMITTANCE

- If the patient history, symptoms, reactions to PT indicate possible adrenal gland dysfunction, refer to physician
- If causative problem is not considered appropriate for PT intervention, refer to appropriate physician
- Refer to ER if emergency identified

IMPAIRMENTS

- Muscle weakness
- Gait abnormality, difficulty walking
- Balance impairment
- Shortness of breath, fatigue
- Inability to perform self-care
- Impaired skin integrity

TESTS AND MEASURES

- Observation
  - Scars may indicate adhesions or abdominal surgeries causative of diverticula.
  - Pink or purplish striae may be indicative of Cushing syndrome.
  - Dilated veins may indicate hepatic pathology or inferior vena cava obstruction, not diverticulitis.
  - Contour: Roundness, concavity, asymmetry, distension, pregnancy signs.
  - Cullen sign: Bluish discoloring around umbilicus may be a sign of retroperitoneal bleeding.
  - Bluish discoloration in lower abdomen: Grey Turner sign, signals hemorrhagic pancreatitis.
  - Bulging in groin and abdomen especially apparent with contraction of musculature in area may be hernia.
  - Pulsing in navel area may be abdominal aortic aneurysm.
  - Left lower quadrant pain, often following a meal.
  - Palpable abdominal tenderness: On left side or generalized.
  - Psoas sign: Provide resistance over patient's right knee as they flex the hip; pain indicates appendicitis, possible inflammation of abdomen.
  - Obturator sign: Internal rotation and flexion of right lower extremity may indicate appendicitis, pelvic inflammation.
  - Rovsing sign: Pain on right side of abdomen when pressure applied to left may indicate appendicitis.
- Palpation
  - Appendix (McBurney's): Apply vertical pressure halfway between right ASIS and umbilicus; −/+ may indicate appendicitis.
  - Liver: In supine, with left hand under trunk parallel to 11th and 12th ribs, lift upward; right hand lateral to rectus, press in and up: +/= reproduction of symptoms with deep breath, indicates liver involvement.
  - Ascites: Percuss outward from center with fingers; if sound is dull, ascites may be present.
  - Spleen: Not recommended for PT to palpate enlarged spleen secondary to possible rupture (only palpable if enlarged).
  - Gallbladder (Murphy's): Place fingers right of rectus abdominus below rib cage: +/= sudden pain and muscle tensing with deep breath.
  - Kidneys: In supine, place one hand under client between ribs and iliac crest, other hand on abdomen below ribs and ribs pointing in opposite direction; +/− tenderness or reproduction of symptoms.
  - Bladder: Not usually palpable unless distended and raised above pubic bone; in supine, place hand above pubis and press down; +/= tenderness, reproduction of pain, ability to feel the bladder: __+ ___−.

INTERVENTION

- Gait training
- Therapeutic exercise: All relevant categories, energy conservation
  - If stoma from a colostomy or ileostomy, PT must avoid activities that cause retraction.
  - If insulin pump, take care not to interfere in any way.
  - As hypoglycemia may occur, ensure blood sugar levels in appropriate range.
  - May require supplemental sodium during exercise; cramping, nausea should be prevented.
  - PT should inquire about medications taken.
- Therapeutic activities for bed mobility, transfer and transitional movement.
- Wheelchair management.
- Self-care training, including skin care and moisturizing, lifestyle management.
- Neuromuscular re-education: Balance and postural training.
- Wound management as indicated; skin inspection.

FUNCTIONAL GOALS

- Patient will be able to
  - Achieve functional aerobic capacity, ability to talk during activity so as to achieve functional gait and activity tolerance for ADLs/IADLs.

- Achieve 600 m or greater in a 6-minute walk test for initiation of safe, functional gait in the community.
- Tolerate 30 minutes of continuous, moderate exercise three times a week in ______weeks, and five times a week in ____________weeks, depending on the severity of the disease.

PROGNOSIS

- Most patients respond to treatment and can maintain active lifestyles.
- Poor prognosis if condition is caused by cancerous tumor or metastatic disease.
- Physician establishes the medical prognosis, as pathology is primarily medical in nature.
- Prognosis from a PT perspective is good if condition is adequately managed; patient should return to premorbid level of function.

PATIENT RESOURCE

- Hyperfunction of the adrenal cortex and social security disability. http://www.disabilitybenefitscenter.org/social-security-disabling-conditions/hyperfunction-of-adrenal-cortex. Accessed April 14, 2014.

REFERENCES

1. The American Physical Therapy Association. Pattern 4D: impaired joint mobility, motor function, muscle performance, and range of motion associated with connective tissue dysfunction. *Interactive Guide to Physical Therapist Practice*. 2003. doi: 10.2522/ptguide.3.1_4. http://guidetoptpractice.apta.org/content/1/SEC11.short. Accessed January 20, 2013.
2. The American Physical Therapy Association. Pattern 4E: impaired joint mobility, motor function, muscle performance, and range of motion associated with localized inflammation. *Interactive Guide to Physical Therapist Practice*. 2003. doi: 10.2522/ptguide.3.1_5. http://guidetoptpractice.apta.org/content/1/SEC12.short. Accessed January 20, 2013.
3. The American Physical Therapy Association. Pattern 6B: impaired aerobic capacity/endurance associated with deconditioning. *Interactive Guide to Physical Therapist Practice*. 2003. doi: 10.2522/ptguide.3.3_2. http://guidetoptpractice.apta.org/content/1/SEC28.extract?sid=16923df1-6a2d-4480-a71c-6f9e6453b9ad. Accessed January 20, 2013.
4. The American Physical Therapy Association. Pattern 7B: impaired integumentary integrity associated with superficial skin involvement. *Interactive Guide to Physical Therapist Practice*. 2003. doi: 10.2522/ptguide.3.4_2. http://guidetoptpractice.apta.org/content/1/SEC36.extract?sid=ec1eaf5a-4c10-4b04-ae93-465180eb5e64. Accessed January 20, 2013.

ADDITIONAL REFERENCES

- Baskin HJ, Cobin RH, Duick DS, et al. American Association of Clinical Endocrinologists medical guidelines for clinical practice for the evaluation and treatment of hyperthyroidism and hypothyroidism. *Endocr Pract*. 2002;8(6):457–469.
- David RR. Adrenal virilism in childhood. *Ann N Y Acad Sci*. 1967;142(3):787–793.
- Dutton M. Adrenal disorders. In: Dutton M, ed. *McGraw-Hill's NPTE (National Physical Therapy Examination)*. 2nd ed. New York, NY: McGraw-Hill; 2012. http://www.accessphysiotherapy.com/content/5402409. Accessed January 20, 2013.
- Elte JW. Diagnosis of Cushing's syndrome. *Eur J Intern Med*. 2006;17(5):311–312.
- Goodman CC, Fuller KS. *Pathology Implications for the Physical Therapist*. 3rd ed. St. Louis, MO: Saunders Elsevier; 2009.
- Goodman CC, Snyder TE. *Differential Diagnosis for Physical Therapists Screening for Referral*. 4th ed. St. Louis, MO: Saunders Elsevier; 2007.
- Hay WW, Levin MJ, Sondheimer JM, Deterding RR. Adrenal cortex. In: Hay WW, Levin MJ, Sondheimer JM, Deterding RR, eds. *CURRENT Diagnosis & Treatment: Pediatrics*. 20th ed. New York, NY: McGraw-Hill; 2011. http://www.accessphysiotherapy.com/content/6588287. Accessed January 20, 2013.
- ICD9DATA. http://www.icd9data.com. Accessed January 20, 2013.
- ICD10DATA. http://www.icd10data.com. Accessed January 20, 2013.
- Makras P, Toloumis G, Papadogias D, Kaltas GA, Besser M. The diagnosis and differential diagnosis of endogenous Cushing's syndrome. *Hormones (Athens)*. 2006;5(4):231–250.
- Magiakou MA, Smyrnaki P, Chrousos GP. Hypertension in Cushing's syndrome. *Best Pract Res Clin Endocrinol Metab*. 2006;20(3):467–482.
- Newell-Price J, Bertagna X, Grossman AB, Nieman LK. Cushing's syndrome. *Lancet*. 2006;367(9522):1605–1617.
- Quinkler M, Lepenies J, Diederich S. Primary hyperaldosteronism. *Exp Clin Endocrinol Diabetes*. 2002;110(6):263–271.
- Riddick DH, Hammond CB. Adrenal virilism due to 21-hydroxylase deficiency in the postmenarchial female. *Obstet Gynecol*. 1975;45(1):21–24.
- Shibli-Rahhal A, Van Beek M, Schlechte JA. Cushing's syndrome. *Clin Dermatol*. 2006;24(4):260–265.
- Storr HL, Chan LF, Grossman AB, Savage MO. Paediatric Cushing's syndrome: epidemiology, investigation and therapeutic advances. *Trends Endocrinol Metab*. 2007;18(4):167–174.

21 CUSHING SYNDROME

Eric Shamus, PhD, DPT, PT, CSCS
Debra F. Stern, DPT, DBA, MSM, PT
Marangela Obispo, MSPT, GCS

CONDITION/DISORDER SYNONYMS

- Hyperadrenocorticalism
- Hypercortisolism

ICD-9-CM CODES

- 255.0 Cushing syndrome
- Associated physical therapy diagnoses
  - 315.4 Developmental coordination disorder
  - 718.45 Contracture of joint, pelvic region, and thigh
  - 719.70 Difficulty in walking involving joint site unspecified
  - 728.2 Muscular wasting and disuse atrophy, not elsewhere classified
  - 728.89 Other disorders of muscle, ligament, and fascia
  - 729.9 Other and unspecified disorders of soft tissue
  - 780.7 Malaise and fatigue
  - 781.2 Abnormality of gait
  - 782.3 Edema
  - 786.0 Dyspnea and respiratory abnormalities
  - 786.05 Shortness of breath

ICD-10-CM CODES

- E24.0 Pituitary-dependent Cushing disease
- E24.2 Drug-induced Cushing syndrome
- E24.3 Ectopic ACTH syndrome
- E24.8 Other Cushing syndrome
- E24.9 Cushing syndrome, unspecified

APTA PRACTICE PATTERNS

- 4D: Impaired Joint Mobility, Motor Function, Muscle Performance, and Range of Motion Associated with Connective Tissue Dysfunction[1]
- 4E: Impaired Joint Mobility, Motor Function, Muscle Performance, and Range of Motion Associated with Localized Inflammation
- 6B: Impaired Aerobic Capacity/Endurance Associated with Deconditioning
- 7B: Impaired Integumentary Integrity Associated with Superficial Skin Involvement

PREFERRED PRACTICE PATTERN

- 5F: Impaired Peripheral Nerve Integrity and Muscle Performance Associated with Peripheral Nerve Injury

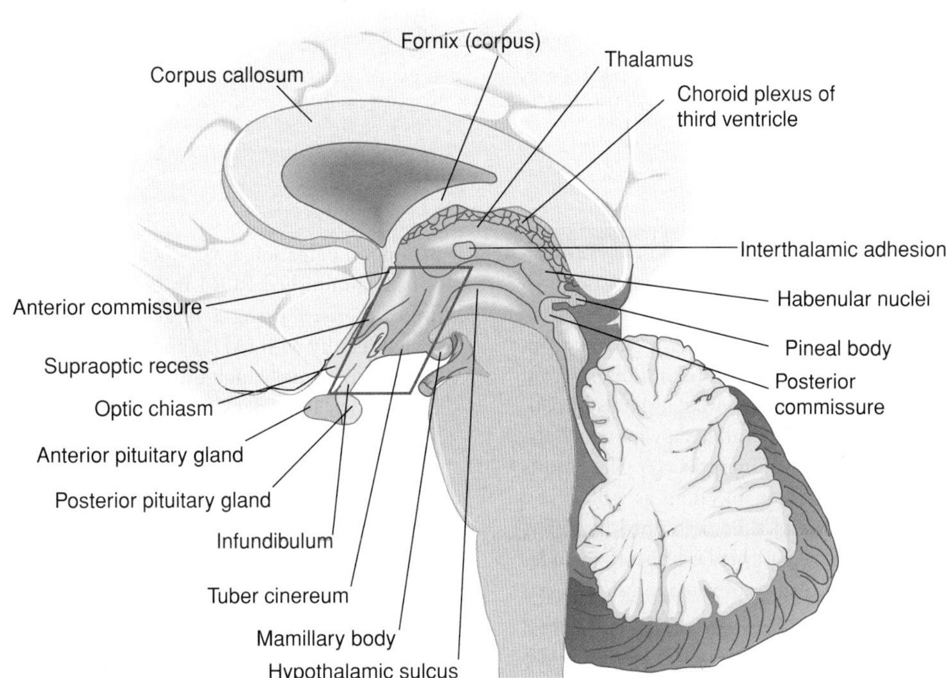

FIGURE 21-1 Typical findings in Cushing syndrome. (From McPhee SJ, Hammer GD. *Pathophysiology of Disease: An Introduction to Clinical Medicine.* 6th ed. http://www.accessmedicine.com. Copyright © The McGraw-Hill Companies, Inc. All rights reserved.)

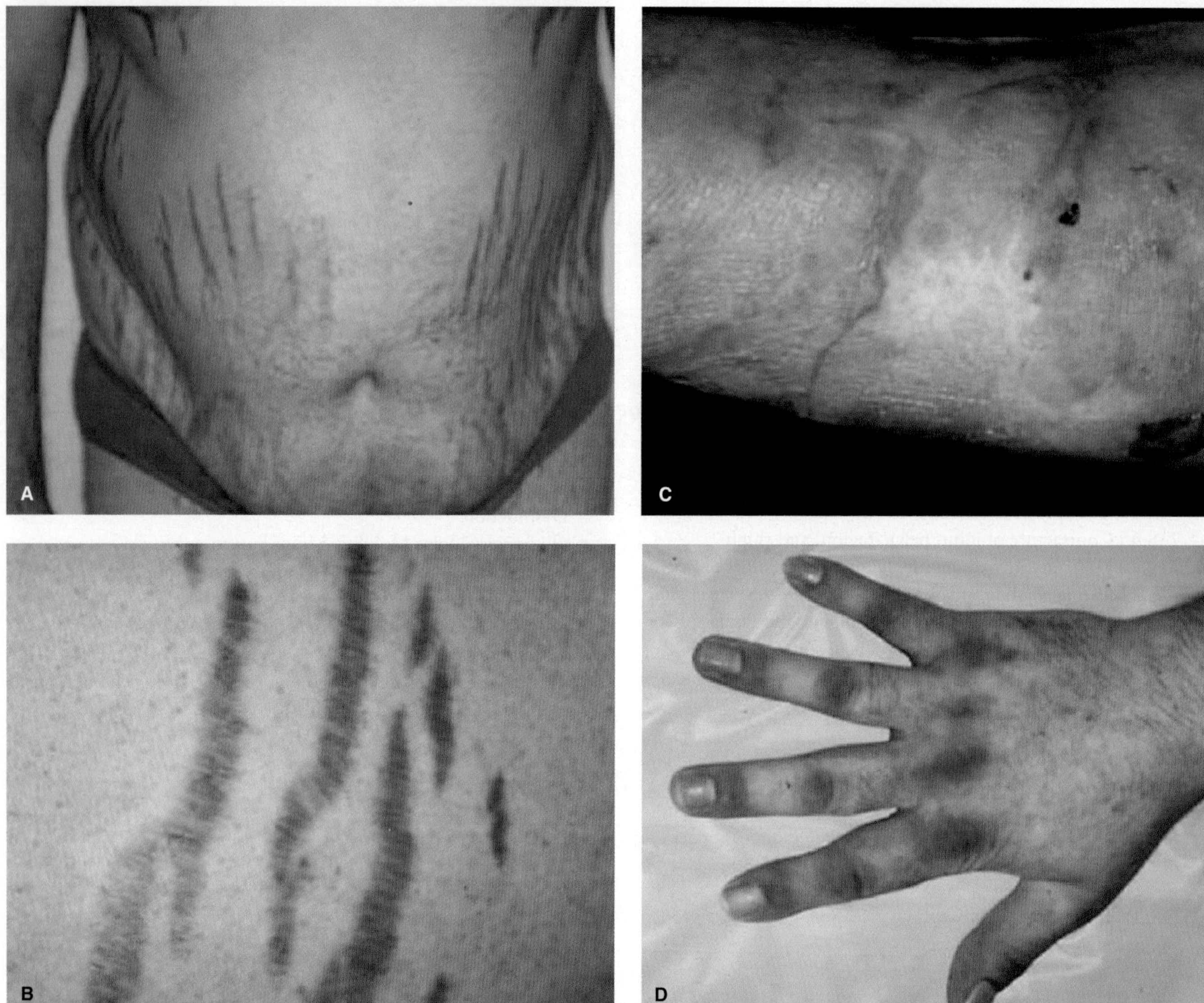

FIGURE 21-2 Clinical features of Cushing syndrome. **A.** Note central obesity and broad, purple stretch marks (**B** close-up). **C.** Note thin and brittle skin in an elderly patient with Cushing. **D.** Hyperpigmentation of the knuckles in a patient with ectopic ACTH excess. (From Longo DL, Fauci A, Kasper D, et al., eds. *Harrison's Principles of Internal Medicine*. 18th ed. New York, NY: McGraw-Hill; 2012.)

PATIENT PRESENTATION

A 38-year-old female who works as a certified nurse assistant in a nursing home arrived complaining of upper and lower back pain which started 3 years ago after transferring a patient from wheelchair to bed. Patient reports that she has been suffering from back pain since then for which she has received all kinds of conservative treatment, including prior physical therapy for which she specifies hot packs and massage about 8 months ago. She reports having received multiple corticosteroids injections as well as oral corticosteroids for multiple periods of time prescribed by different physicians for pain control. The past medical history includes hypertension. Patient denies any history of osteoporosis and has never received a bone density test. In addition, patient reported that she feels very depressed because she has been unable to get pregnant. Upon observation, patient appears with central obesity and thin extremities (all four), kyphotic posture, thick neck, and round moon like face. During examination, patient presents pain upon palpation at C7-T2 and L3-S1 paraspinals with tender points, diminished ROM in the lumbar and cervical spines, and mild decreased strength in all four extremities. Patient presents with difficulty with IADLs and job related duties. Laboratory tests showed abnormally high urine cortisol levels. CT scan of the brain was normal. Bone density test showed osteopenia.

KEY FEATURES

Description

- Pituitary gland releases excessive adrenocorticotropic hormone (ACTH)
- The adrenals play a critical role in regulating inflammation and cardiovascular function
- High cortisol levels
- Tumor or increased growth of the pituitary gland
- Can be drug induced

Essentials of Diagnosis

- Noniatrogenic[1]
  - ACTH dependent
    - Cushing disease (ACTH-secreting pituitary adenoma
    - Ectopic ACTH syndrome
  - ACTH independent
    - Functional adrenocortical tumor
- Iatrogenic[1]
  - Exogenous glucocorticoid administration in high doses
- Round, full face (moon face)[1]
- 24-hour urine cortisol test
- Confirmation of suspected disease through blood testing, blood-ACTH level

General Considerations

- May cause pathology in multiple organ systems or be caused by pathology in other organ systems
  - Cardiovascular: Heart, peripheral circulation, blood pressure
  - Integumentary system
- Mnemonic for each letter of CUSHING
- May result in secondary problems such as
  - Aerobic capacity and muscle endurance impairment
  - Weakness/impaired muscle performance
  - Musculoskeletal problems
  - Neuromuscular problems
  - Weight gain
- May indicate a need for physical therapy intervention depending on severity

Demographics

- Cushing disease (ACTH-secreting pituitary adenoma[1]
  - More common in women (female–male ratio of approximately 8:1)
  - Age at diagnosis, 20 to 40 years
- Ectopic ACTH syndrome[1]
  - More common in men (male–female ratio of approximately 3:1)
  - Age at diagnosis, 40 to 60 years
- Functional adrenocortical tumor[1]
  - More common in women
  - Adrenal carcinoma occurs in about two per million population per year
  - Age at diagnosis, usually 35 to 40 years.

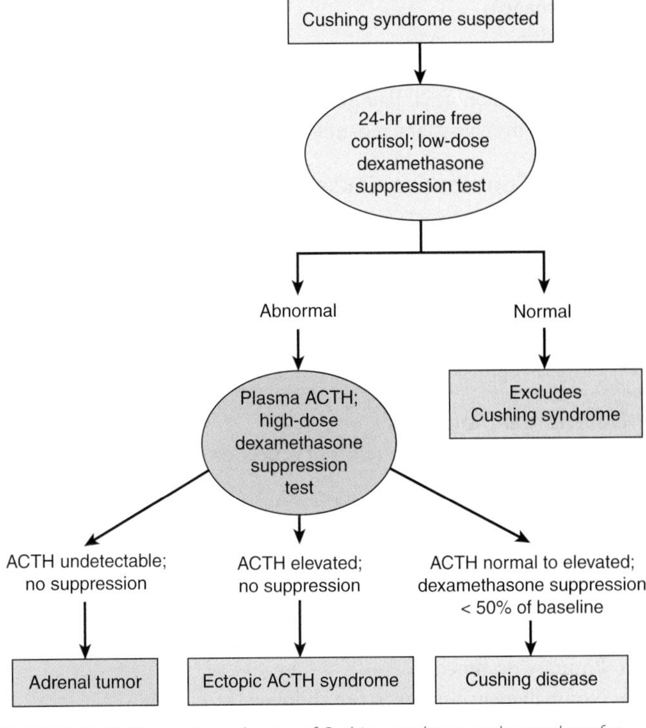

FIGURE 21-3 Diagnostic evaluation of Cushing syndrome and procedures for determining the cause. Boxes enclose clinical diagnoses, and ovals enclose diagnostic tests. (Redrawn with permission from Baxter JD, Tyrrell JB. The adrenal cortex. In: Felig P, Baxter JD, eds. *Endocrinology and Metabolism.* 2nd ed. McGraw-Hill; 1987.)

CLINICAL FINDINGS

SIGNS AND SYMPTOMS

- Growth retardation in children (85%)[1]
- Psychiatric effects: Depression (50% to 80%)[1]
- Round face: Moon face (80%)[1]
- Thick neck (80%)[1]
- Thin extremities (80%)[1]
- Atrophy of skin and dermal connective tissue (70%)[1]
- Easy bruising (50%)[1]
- Muscle wasting and weakness (70%)[1]
- Weight gain: Increased body fat in trunk and thoracic back (80%)[1]
- Pallor
- Flushed face
- Chest pain
- Fatigue
- Rapid breathing
- Tachycardia
- Palpitations
- Hypertension
- Skin changes: Striae on the abdomen and chest
- Darkening/hyperpigmentation of skin
- Stretch marks
- Acne
- Excessive thirst
- Sweating
- Increased heat sensitivity
- Decreased gastrointestinal motility
- Increased frequency of urination
- Increased bowel movement frequency
- Poor healing of wounds
- Abdominal pain
- Irritability
- Low back pain in kidney area
- Decreased libido
- Infertility
- Increased body and facial hair
- Growth deficiencies: Short stature
- Osteoporosis
- Increased infection risk
- Sleep disturbances
- Adrenal crisis
  - Coma
  - Shock
  - Seizures
  - Death

Functional Implications

- Severe symptoms such as immediacy of need to urinate may be disabling, resulting in an inability to leave home
- Ability/inability to afford testing and medications or other treatment
- Fatigue
- Weakness, muscle-mass loss, inability to ambulate or perform self-care, aerobic capacity limitation, secondary to inactivity
- Decreased exercise tolerance
- Sleep disturbances
- Changes in lifestyle
- Psychological changes
- Eating disorders
- Inappropriate self-medication
- Anxiety and depression
- Irritability
- Limitations in ADLs or IADLs

- Skin changes
- Infertility
- Decreased libido in males
- In females, abnormal hair growth
- Increase in male characteristics for females

Possible Contributing Causes

- Adrenal tumors
- Cancer of the adrenal glands
- Excessive stimulation of the adrenal glands
- Excessive production of pituitary hormones, which stimulate the adrenals
- Drug use; glucocorticoids[2]

Differential Diagnosis

- Organ dysfunction as a result of cancer or malignancy
- Kidney disease
- Cardiovascular disease
- Hypertension from other causes
- Hyperaldosteronism
- Hyperpigmentation from other causes
- Celiac disease
- Pituitary dysfunction
- Nonmalignant tumors in the abdomen or organs
- Malignancies in other organs/systems
- Type 1 diabetes mellitus
- Endocrine disorders
- Bleeding into the adrenals, often due to trauma
- Systemic infection
- Medications: Prescription stimulants, ephedrine
- Alcohol
- Illegal drugs: Cocaine, heroin
- Gynecologic problems in females
- Autoimmune diseases that affect the upper and lower gastrointestinal tracts as well as the cardiovascular system
  - Crohn or irritable bowel syndrome
  - Rheumatoid arthritis RA

MEANS OF CONFIRMATION OR DIAGNOSIS

Laboratory Tests

- Complete blood count (CBC)
- Levels of: Sodium, potassium, cortisol, ACTH, antibodies
- ACTH (Cosyntropin test) stimulation test
- Dexamethasone suppression test
- Corticotropin-releasing hormone (CRH) stimulation test to determine adrenal versus pituitary
- Urinalysis: Urinary free cortisol and 17-hydroxycorticosteroid excretion
- 24-hour urine test
- Saliva tests
- Biopsy

Imaging

- CT scans
- MRI of the brain
- X-ray of rib and spine to check for thinning of the bones

FINDINGS AND INTERPRETATION

- Confirmation of suspected disease through blood testing, blood-ACTH level
- Excessive production and release of adrenal hormones
  - Glucocorticoids (cortisol)[2]
  - Androgens

TREATMENT

Medications

- Cardiac medications as indicated
- Medications for management of hypertension as indicated
- Cortisol replacement therapy

MEDICAL PROCEDURES

- Surgery: Tumor removal as indicated from adrenals, pancreas, pituitary, lungs
- Radiation therapy: Small doses over several weeks or gamma knife

REFERRAL/ADMITTANCE

- If the patient's history and reactions to PT indicate possible adrenal gland dysfunction and or symptoms, referral to a physician should be made.

IMPAIRMENTS

- Muscle weakness
- Gait abnormality/difficulty walking
- Shortness of breath/fatigue
- Inability to perform self-care
- Balance impairment
- Impaired skin integrity

TESTS AND MEASURES

- Observation
  - Scars may indicate adhesions or abdominal surgeries causative of diverticula.
  - Pink or purplish striae may be indicative of Cushing syndrome.
  - Dilated veins may indicate hepatic pathology or inferior vena cava obstruction, not diverticulitis.
  - Contour: Roundness, concavity, asymmetry, distension, pregnancy signs.
  - Cullen sign: Bluish discoloring around umbilicus may be a sign of retroperitoneal bleeding.
  - Bluish discoloration in lower abdomen: Grey Turner sign, signals hemorrhagic pancreatitis.
  - Bulging in groin and/or abdomen especially apparent with contraction of musculature in area; may be hernia.
  - Pulsing in navel area; may be abdominal aortic aneurysm.
  - Left lower quadrant pain, often following a meal.
  - Palpable abdominal tenderness on left side or generalized.
  - Psoas sign: Provide resistance over patient's right knee as they flex the hip; pain indicates appendicitis, possible inflammation of abdomen.
  - Obturator sign: Internal rotation and flexion of right lower extremity; may indicate appendicitis, pelvic inflammation.
  - Rovsing sign: Pain on right side of abdomen when pressure applied to left may indicate appendicitis.
- Palpation
  - Appendix (McBurney's): Apply vertical pressure halfway between right ASIS and umbilicus; −/+ may indicate appendicitis.
  - Liver: In supine, with left hand under trunk parallel to 11th and 12th ribs, lift upward; right hand lateral to rectus, press in and

up: +/= reproduction of symptoms with deep breath, indicates liver involvement.
- ○ Ascites: Percuss outward from center with fingers; if sound is dull, ascites may be present.
- ○ Spleen: Not recommended for PT to palpate enlarged spleen secondary to rupture (only palpable if enlarged).
- ○ Gallbladder (Murphy's): Place fingers right of rectus abdominus below rib cage: +/= sudden pain and muscle tensing with deep breath.
- ○ Kidneys: In supine, place one hand under client between ribs and iliac crest, other hand on abdomen below ribs and ribs pointing in opposite direction; +/− tenderness or reproduction of symptoms.
- ○ Bladder: Not usually palpable unless distended and raised above pubic bone; in supine, place hand above pubis and press down; +/= tenderness, reproduction of pain, ability to feel the bladder: __+ ___−.

INTERVENTION

- Gait training
- Therapeutic exercise: All relevant categories, energy conservation
- Therapeutic activities for bed mobility training, transfer and transitional movement training
- Self-care management training including skin care/moisturizing, lifestyle management
- Neuromuscular re-education; balance and postural training
- Wound management as indicated; skin inspection

FUNCTIONAL GOALS

- Patient will be able to
  - ○ Achieve adequate functional aerobic capacity and the ability to talk during activity, in order to achieve functional gait and activity tolerance for work, play, school, and self-care; ADLs and IADLS.
  - ○ Functional gait in the home and community (with or without a device), allowing for work, play, and self-care; ADLs and IADLS, up to __________ feet based on patient need and prior functional level.
  - ○ Achieve 600 m or greater in a 6-minute walk test for initiation of safe functional gait in the community.
  - ○ Tolerate 30 minutes of continuous moderate exercise three times a week in ______weeks, and five times a week in ____________, depending on the severity of the disease.
- Increase score levels of a standardized balance test (Berg, Tinetti's, etc.) from _____ to _____, depending on the severity of the patient's balance.

PROGNOSIS

- As this pathology is primarily medical in nature, it is the physician who establishes the medical prognosis.
- Most are able to maintain active lifestyles and respond to treatment.
- The prognosis is not as good if tumors are cancerous or a result of metastatic disease and are not treated.
- PT prognosis if condition is adequately managed; patient should be good to return to premorbid functioning with tumor removal.

PATIENT RESOURCES

- Cushing's Support & Research Foundation. http://csrf.net/. Accessed May 6, 2013.
- Cushing's Understanding Support & Help Organization. http://www.cush.org. Accessed May 6, 2013.

REFERENCES

1. McPhee SJ, Hammer GD. Pathophysiology of selected adrenocortical disorders. In: McPhee SJ, Hammer GD, eds. *Pathophysiology of Disease.* 6th ed. New York, NY: McGraw-Hill; 2010. http://www.accessphysiotherapy.com/content/5371816. Accessed May 6, 2013.
2. Panus PC, Jobst EE, Masters SB, Katzung B, Tinsley SL, Trevor AJ. Immunosuppressive agents. In: Panus PC, Jobst EE, Masters SB, Katzung B, Tinsley SL, Trevor AJ, eds. *Pharmacology for the Physical Therapist.* New York, NY: McGraw-Hill; 2009. http://www.accessphysiotherapy.com/content/6095411. Accessed May 6, 2013.

ADDITIONAL REFERENCES

- Baskin HJ, Cobin RH, Duick DS, et al. American Association of Clinical Endocrinologists medical guidelines for clinical practice for the evaluation and treatment of hyperthyroidism and hypothyroidism. *Endocr Pract.* 2002;8(6):457–469.
- David RR. Adrenal virilism in childhood. *Ann NY Acad Sci.* 1967;142(3):787–793.
- Dutton M. Pathology, gynecology, and psychology. In: Dutton M, ed. *McGraw-Hill's NPTE (National Physical Therapy Examination).* 2nd ed. New York, NY: McGraw-Hill; 2012. http://www.accessphysiotherapy.com/content/5402409. Accessed January 26, 2013.
- Elte JW. Diagnosis of Cushing's syndrome. *Eur J Intern Med.* 2006;17:311–312.
- Goodman CC, Fuller KS. *Pathology: Implications for the Physical Therapist.* 3rd ed. St. Louis, MO: Saunders Elsevier; 2009.
- Goodman CC, Snyder TE. *Differential Diagnosis for Physical Therapists: Screening for Referral.* 4th ed. St. Louis, MO: Saunders Elsevier; 2007.
- Kita M, Sakalidou M, Saratzis A, Ioannis S, Avramidis A. Cushing's syndrome in pregnancy: report of a case and review of the literature. *Hormones (Athens).* 2007;6(3):242–246.
- Makras P, Toloumis G, Papadogias D, Kaltsas GA, Besser M. The diagnosis and differential diagnosis of endogenous Cushing's syndrome. *Hormones (Athens).* 2006;5(4):231–250.
- Magiakou MA, Smyrnaki P, Chrousos GP. Hypertension in Cushing's syndrome. *Best Pract Res Clin Endocrinol Metab.* 2006;20(3):467–482.
- Newell-Price J, Bertagna X, Grossman AB, Nieman LK. Cushing's syndrome. *Lancet.* 2006;367(9522):1605–1617.
- Quinkler M, Lepenies J, Diederich S. Primary hyperaldosteronism. *Exp Clin Endocrinol Diabetes.* 2002;110(6):263–271.
- Riddick DH, Hammond CB. Adrenal virilism due to 21-hydroxylase deficiency in the postmenarchial female. *Obstet Gynecol.* 1975;45(1):21–24.
- Shibli-Rahhal A, Van Beek M, Schlechte JA. Cushing's syndrome. *Clin Dermatol.* 2006;24(4):260–265.
- Storr HL, Chan LF, Grossman AB, Savage MO. Paediatric Cushing's syndrome: epidemiology, investigation and therapeutic advances. *Trend Endocrinol Metab.* 2007;18(4):167–174.
- Zeitler PS, Travers SH, Nadeau K, Barker J, Kelsey MM, Kappy MS. Endocrine disorders. In: Hay WW, Levin MJ, Sondheimer JM, Deterding RR, eds. *CURRENT Diagnosis & Treatment: Pediatrics.* 20th ed. New York, NY: McGraw-Hill; 2011. http://www.accessphysiotherapy.com/content/6588287. Accessed January 26, 2013.

22 DIABETES MELLITUS

Debra F. Stern, DPT, DBA, MSM, PT
Eric Shamus, PhD, DPT, PT, CSCS

CONDITION/DISORDER SYNONYMS

- Juvenile diabetes
- Diabetes type 1
- Diabetes type 1.5
- Diabetes type 2
- Gestational diabetes

ICD-9-CM CODES

- 249.91 Secondary diabetes mellitus with unspecified complication, uncontrolled
- 250 Diabetes mellitus

ICD-10-CM CODES

- E08.65 Diabetes mellitus due to underlying condition with hyperglycemia
- E08.8 Diabetes mellitus due to underlying condition with unspecified complications
- E09.8 Drug or chemical-induced diabetes mellitus with unspecified complications

PREFERRED PRACTICE PATTERNS

- As of June, 2014, the APTA *Guide to Physical Therapist Practice* does not include practice patterns for organ system pathology; therefore, the associated or secondary musculoskeletal, cardiovascular/pulmonary, or potential neuromuscular patterns would be indicated.

PATIENT PRESENTATION

A 30-year-old woman presents to the physician's office with the chief complaint of a "yeast infection that I can't seem to shake." She also has noticed that she has been urinating more frequently, but thinks that it is related to her yeast infection. Over the last several years she has noticed that she has gained more than 40 lb. She has tried numerous diets, most recently a low-carbohydrate, high-fat diet. The patient's only other pertinent history is that she was told to watch her diet during pregnancy because of excessive weight gain. Her baby had to be delivered by cesarean because he weighed more than 9 lb. Her family history is not known, as she was adopted. On physical examination, her blood pressure is 138/88 mm Hg, her pulse is 72 beats/min, and her respiratory rate is 16 breaths/min. Her height is 65 in and her weight is 190 lb (body mass index [BMI] = 31.6). Her physical examination reveals darkened skin that appears to be thickened on the back of her neck and moist, reddened skin beneath her breasts. Her

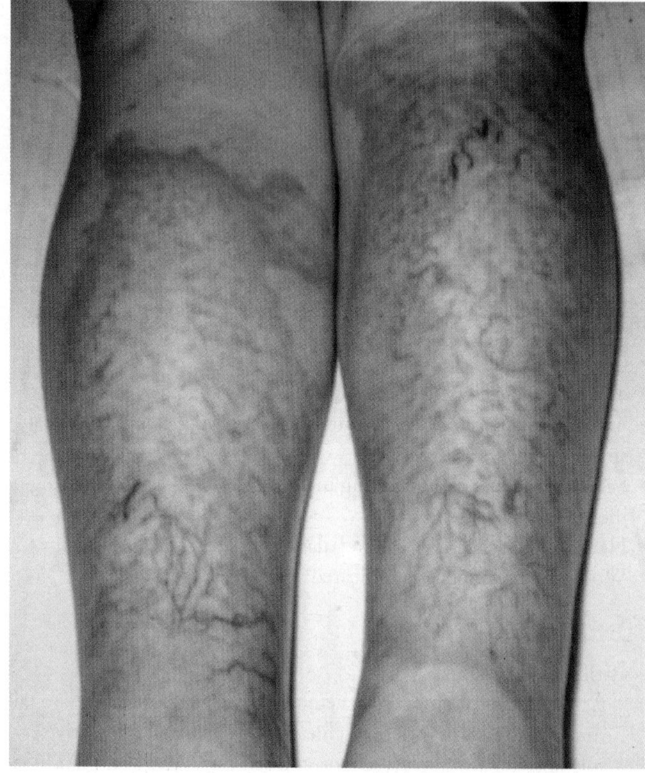

FIGURE 22-1 Diabetes mellitus: atrophy of skin (necrobiosis diabeticorum) of legs with coronary disease. (From Fuster V, Walsh RA, Harrington RA. *Hurst's The Heart.* 13th ed. www.accessmedicine.com.)

pelvic examination reveals a thick, white, vaginal discharge. A wet preparation from the vaginal discharge reveals branching hyphae consistent with *Candida*. A urine dipstick is performed that is negative for leukocyte esterase, nitrites, protein, and glucose.[1]

KEY FEATURES

Description

- Diabetes mellitus
  - Primary diabetes mellitus
    - Type 1: Inability of the body to produce insulin, formerly referred to as juvenile diabetes
    - Type 1.5: Latent autoimmune diabetes in adults (LADA), signs of both type 1 and type 2 diabetes where the body can initially produce some insulin but ultimately cannot
    - Type 2: Insulin resistance; inability of the body to produce adequate insulin or inability for adequate insulin uptake by the body to sufficiently regulate insulin/glucose, some insulin is produced by the pancreas
    - Impaired glucose tolerance (IGT)
    - Gestational diabetes mellitus

- Secondary diabetes mellitus
  - Destructive pancreatic disease
  - Endocrine diseases
  - Drug-induced diabetes
  - Stress diabetes

Essentials of Diagnosis

- Frequent urination
- Unexplained weight loss, especially with Type 1
- Excessive thirst
- Increased hunger
- Inappropriate sweating
- Dizziness
- Nausea
- Decreased activity tolerance
- Hyperosmolar Hyperglycemic Nonketotic Syndrome
  - Rare condition in which blood sugar is 600 mg/dL or above and can result in death; in those who may have diagnosed or undiagnosed diabetes can result in coma and death.

General Considerations

- May cause pathology in multiple organ systems
  - Kidney and urinary tract
  - GI: Liver, pancreas
  - Cardiovascular: Heart, peripheral circulation
  - Neuromuscular: Neuropathy
  - Integumentary
  - Vision
  - Reproductive system
- May result in secondary problems, such as aerobic capacity and muscle endurance impairment, sarcopenia, weakness/impaired muscle performance, musculoskeletal problems, neuromuscular problems, weight loss or weight gain—indicating the need for physical therapy intervention depending on severity
- Increased incidence of tendonitis
- Increased incidence of frozen shoulder
- Exercise may cause hypoglycemia
- Exercise may interfere with timed insulin uptake if performed in the area of injection site soon after injecting
- Metabolic syndrome: Presence of
  - High blood pressure
  - High cholesterol
  - Belly fat
  - Elevated blood sugar
- Hyperlipidemia

Demographics

- Occurs in males and females.
- Higher incidence in African Americans and Hispanics.
- Type 2 is more common in individuals who are obese, and is on the rise in children secondary to sedentary lifestyle and obesity.
- During 2002 to 2005, 15,600 children were newly diagnosed with type 1 diabetes annually, and 3600 youth were newly diagnosed with type 2 diabetes annually.[2]
- Among children younger than 10 years, the rate of new cases was 19.7 per 100,000 each year for type 1 diabetes and 0.4 per 100,000 for type 2 diabetes. Among children ages 10 years or older, the rate of new cases was 18.6 per 100,000 each year for type 1 diabetes and 8.5 per 100,000 for type 2 diabetes.[2]

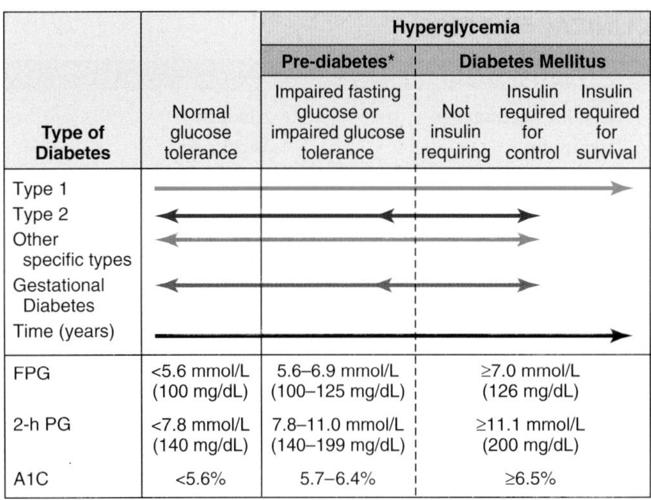

Hyperglycemia
Pre-diabetes*
Diabetes Mellitus
Type of Diabetes
Normal glucose tolerance
Impaired fasting glucose or impaired glucose tolerance
Not insulin requiring
Insulin required for control
Insulin required for survival
Type 1
Type 2
Other specific types
Gestational Diabetes
Time (years)
FPG
<5.6 mmol/L (100 mg/dL)
5.6–6.9 mmol/L (100–125 mg/dL)
≥7.0 mmol/L (126 mg/dL)
2-h PG
<7.8 mmol/L (140 mg/dL)
7.8–11.0 mmol/L (140–199 mg/dL)
≥11.1 mmol/L (200 mg/dL)
A1C
<5.6%
5.7–6.4%
≥6.5%

FIGURE 22-2 Spectrum of glucose homeostasis and diabetes mellitus (DM). The spectrum from normal glucose tolerance to diabetes in type 1 DM, type 2 DM, other specific types of diabetes, and gestational DM is shown from left to right. In most types of DM, the individual traverses from normal glucose tolerance to impaired glucose tolerance to overt diabetes (these should be viewed not as abrupt categories but as a spectrum). *Arrows* indicate that changes in glucose tolerance may be bidirectional in some types of diabetes. For example, individuals with type 2 DM may return to the impaired glucose tolerance category with weight loss; in gestational DM, diabetes may revert to impaired glucose tolerance or even normal glucose tolerance after delivery. The fasting plasma glucose (FPG), the 2-hour plasma glucose (PG) after a glucose challenge, and the A1C for the different categories of glucose tolerance are shown at the lower part of the figure. These values do not apply to the diagnosis of gestational DM. The World Health Organization uses an FPG of 110 to 125 mg/dL for the prediabetes category. Some types of DM may or may not require insulin for survival. *Some use the term "increased risk for diabetes" (ADA) or "intermediate hyperglycemia" (WHO) rather than "prediabetes." (Adapted from the American Diabetes Association: Clinical Practice Recommendations 2007. *Diabetes Care.* 2007;30:S4.)

- Non-Hispanic White youth had the highest rate of new cases of type 1 diabetes: 24.8 per 100,000 per year among those younger than 10 years and 22.6 per 100,000 per year among those ages 10 to 19 years.[2]
- Type 2 diabetes was extremely rare among youth ages younger than 10 years. Although still infrequent, rates were greater among youth ages 10 to 19 years than in younger children, with higher rates among US minority populations than in non-Hispanic Whites.[2]
- Among non-Hispanic White youth ages 10 to 19 years, the rate of new cases was higher for type 1 than for type 2 diabetes.
- For Asian/Pacific Islander Americans and American Indian youth ages 10 to 19 years, the opposite was true; the rate of new cases was greater for type 2 than for type 1 diabetes.
- Among non-Hispanic Black and Hispanic/Latino youth ages 10 to 19 years, the rates of new cases of type 1 and type 2 diabetes were similar.[2]
- There is a 4% incidence rate during pregnancy.[2]
- In people under the age of 20 years, 0.22% have diabetes.[2]
- In people over the age of 20 years, 10.7% have diabetes.[3]
- In people over the age of 60 years, 23.1% have diabetes.[3]
- Twelve million men in the United States over the age of 20 years have diabetes.[3]
- In the United States 11.5 million women aged 20 years or older have diabetes.[3]
- African Americans have a 70% higher chance of getting diabetes than Caucasian Americans.[3]

CLINICAL FINDINGS

SIGNS AND SYMPTOMS

- Insulin necessary in treatment
  - Type I: Almost always
  - Type 2: Sometimes
- Abnormal metabolism
- Lethargy after consuming large amounts of carbohydrates
- Nausea
- Emesis
- Frequent urination
- Increased hunger
- Thirst
  - Type 1: Common
  - Type 2: Rare
- Weight loss
  - Type 1: Common
  - Type 2: Rare
- Irritability
- Shakiness following physical activity
- Unexplained weight loss
- Peripheral neuropathy
- Fever
- Skin infections
- Skin tags
- UTIs
- Gum infections
- Heart disease
- Chronic complications with the organ systems
- Circulatory problems that may lead to amputation (i.e., peripheral artery disease)
- Sudden changes in mental status or behavior
- Sweet smelling or alcohol-like smelling breath
- Vision impairment: Retinopathy, blurred vision
- Hearing impairment
- Kidney disease: Nephropathy
- Hypoglycemia: When awake
  - Hunger
  - Shakiness
  - Nervousness
  - Sweating
  - Dizziness or light headedness
  - Sleepiness
  - Confusion
  - Difficulty speaking
  - Anxiety
  - Weakness
- Hypoglycemia: When asleep
  - Crying out
  - Nightmares
  - Damp sleep clothing from perspiration
  - Tiredness, irritability or confusion upon wakening
- Hyperglycemia early signs
  - Frequent urination
  - Increased thirst
  - Blurred vision
  - Fatigue
  - Headache
- Hyperglycemia (later signs): Medical emergency; persistent blood sugar 240+
  - Toxic acids (ketones) build up in blood and urine
  - Fruity-smelling breath
  - Nausea and vomiting
  - Abdominal pain
  - Shortness of breath
  - Dry mouth
  - Weakness
  - Confusion
  - Coma
- Ketoacidosis
  - Common in type 1 diabetes
  - Rare in type 2 diabetes
  - Condition in which there is too little insulin
  - Body produces very high levels of blood acids (ketones), in which the body is breaking down fats
  - Blood sugar 300+, medical emergency
  - Excessive thirst
  - Frequent urination
  - Nausea and vomiting
  - Abdominal pain
  - Loss of appetite
  - Weakness or fatigue
  - Shortness of breath
  - Fruity-scented breath
  - Confusion
  - High blood sugar level
  - High ketone levels in urine (home test)

Functional Implications

- Severe symptoms such as immediacy of need to urinate, may be disabling and result in the inability to leave home
- Need to check blood sugar levels on regular basis and appropriately discard needles
- Challenges with travel relative to managing medication, especially insulin; time changes, possible need for refrigeration
- Sarcopenia, resulting in weakness, muscle-mass loss, inability to ambulate or perform self-care, as well as aerobic capacity limitation secondary to inactivity
- Decreased exercise tolerance although indicated for management of type 2 and health lifestyle for type 1
- Sleep disturbances
- Changes in lifestyle to accommodate dietary changes such as counting carbohydrates and medication regiments: Oral, injected, or pump
- Eating disorders
- Fatigue
- Inappropriate self-medication
- Noncompliance with dietary recommendations or medication regiments
- Possible management of insulin pump
- Anxiety and depression
- Can be indicative of serious medical conditions such as pancreatitis, cancer of the pancreas
- Limitations in ADLs, or IADLs
- Infection; systemic
- Skin lesions
- Neuropathy; increased risk for falls
- Vision impairment; most often retinal
- Prone to infections (i.e., bacteria in the skin, fungal, UTIs, kidney)
- Potential for kidney problems
- Gastroparesis

Possible Contributing Causes

- Type 1: Body stops production of insulin; autoimmune
  - Not usually associated with obesity
- Type 1.5: Most probably a genetic type of slowly progressing Type 1
- Type 2
  - Obesity
  - Lack of exercise
  - Pancreatic disease
- Secondary effect of other illnesses such as pancreatitis, cancer of the pancreas
- Genetic disposition
  - Type 1: Weak, polygenic
  - Type 2: Strong, polygenic
- Pregnancy (gestational diabetes)
  - 4% incidence
  - May disappear following the pregnancy
  - Increased chance for development of diabetes later in life with a history of gestational diabetes
- Metastatic cancer
- Cushing syndrome
- Infections (i.e., congenital rubella and cytomegalovirus
- Cystic fibrosis
- Down syndrome

- Prader–Willi syndrome
- Leprechaunism
- Chemical inducement

Differential Diagnosis

- Organ dysfunction as a result of cancer or malignancy, especially the pancreas
- Non-malignant tumors in the abdomen or organs
- Endocrine disorders
- Gastroparesis
- Gynecologic problems in females
- Autoimmune diseases that affect the upper and lower gastrointestinal tracts
  - Crohn or irritable bowel syndrome
  - SLE
  - Rheumatoid arthritis (RA)
- Appendicitis
- Peritonitis
- Prostitis
- Benign prostatic hypertrophy
- Pelvic inflammatory disease
- Gastroenteritis
- Perforated ulcers anywhere in GI system
- Bladder infections, urinary tract infections, kidney pathology
- Infections in the abdomen
- Bowel disorders

MEANS OF CONFIRMATION OR DIAGNOSIS

Laboratory Tests

- Blood tests, complete blood test
- Kidney function: Creatinine, protein
- Screening for microalbuminuria
- Blood glucose levels: HbA1C; average over 3 months, not fasting, fructosamine; average over 1 month
- Glucose tolerance testing
- Fasting plasma glucose (FPG) test
- Random plasma glucose test: Based on when last food was taken

Imaging

- Ultrasound
- Intravenous urinary pyelogram using dye for kidneys
- CT scans
- MRIs

FINDINGS AND INTERPRETATION

- Glucose
  - Before meals: Between 70 and 130 mg/dL (4 and 7 mmol/L)
  - 1 to 2 hours after meals: Lower than 180 mg/dL (10 mmol/L)
  - Type 1: Severe intolerance
  - Type 2: Mild glucose intolerance
- Serum insulin level
  - Type 1: Reduced
  - Type 2: Normal to high
- Fasting plasma glucose test
  - 99 or below: Normal
  - 100 to 125: Prediabetes
  - 126 or above: Diabetes
- Hemoglobin AIC >6.5
  - 5.7 to 6.4 = prediabetes

TREATMENT

Medication

- Pharmacologic management
  - Sulfonylureas: Glyburide (DiaBeta®), glipizide (Glucotrol®), and glimepiride (Amaryl®)
    - Increases insulin production
  - Biguanides: Metformin
    - Decreases liver glucose production
  - Thiazolidinediones
    - Mostly removed from market, stimulate insulin receptors
  - Alpha-glucosidase inhibitors: **Acarbose (Precose®) and miglitol (Glyset®)**
    - Blocks the action of alpha-glucosidase enzymes at the brush border of the intestine. The inhibition slows the breakdown of dietary oligosaccharides and disaccharides.
  - Meglitinides: **Repaglinide (Prandin®) and nateglinide (Starlix®) are**
    - Rapid lowering of postprandial glucose
  - Insulin
    - Type 1 is managed strictly with insulin and diet
    - Type 2 may be managed with or without a combination of diet, oral medications, and insulin
    - Insulin: Short acting, medium acting, long acting

MEDICAL PROCEDURES

- Hospitalization if severe, with IV insulin if glucose is high and not controlled with regular medication
- Insertion of insulin pumps
- Bariatric surgery: Gastric bypass, lap bands, sleeves for weight loss for management of type 2

REFERRALS/ADMITTANCE

- If a patient is referred for PT and the causative problem is not considered to be appropriate for PT, referral to the appropriate physician must be made.
- If an emergency is identified, referral to an ER may be necessary.
- If the patient's history and reactions to PT indicate possible diabetes signs and/or symptoms, referral to a physician should be made immediately.

IMPAIRMENTS

- Muscle weakness
- Muscle atrophy
- Gait abnormality/difficulty walking
- Shortness of breath
- Inability to perform self-care
- Peripheral neuropathy
- Balance impairment
- Impaired skin integrity
- Vision impairment

TESTS AND MEASURES

- Palpation
- Hemosiderin in lower extremities
- Open skin lesions, especially distally
- Skin changes: Turgor, dryness, flakiness, redness, shininess, hairlessness
- Increase capillary refill >3 seconds for fingers and toes

INTERVENTION

- Physical therapy intervention is consistent with the movement-related problems that occur secondary to diabetes and includes (as indicated).
  - Gait training.
  - Therapeutic exercise: All relevant categories, energy conservation.
  - Therapeutic exercise: Aerobic, strengthening, flexibility.
    - If there is an insulin pump, care must be taken not to interfere with it in any way.
    - PT should inquire if medication is taken, when, and where (if insulin is injected) to avoid facilitating rapid uptake if patient has eaten appropriately; if patient has glucose testing monitor with them for monitoring.
    - If glucose >300, exercise should be avoided.
    - If glucose 250 to 300, exercise should be performed with caution.
    - Patients with diabetes should be instructed in alternative methods of monitoring exertion as they may not experience chest pain or other pain secondary to neuropathy.
    - Snacks high in carbs, juice, or sugar cubes should be available for patients in care of blood sugar lows during PT.
  - Therapeutic activities: Bed-mobility training, transfer- and transitional-movement training.
  - Therapeutic activities: Posture, breathing, functional training, pelvic floor retraining as applicable.
- Self-care management training including skin care, lifestyle management.
- Neuromuscular re-education: Balance and postural training.
- Wound management.
- Shoe wear training.
- Relaxation training.
- Lifestyle modification.
- Smoking cessation.
- Weight management.
- Dietary counseling.
- Support group participation.
- Psychological intervention.
- Surgical management.
- Spiritual support.
- Palliative care or instruction to caretakers in end stages of kidney disease.

FUNCTIONAL GOALS

- Patient will be able to
  - Achieve adequate functional aerobic capacity, and the ability to talk during activity, in order to achieve functional gait and activity tolerance for work, play, school, self-care; ADLs and IADLs.
  - Functional gait in the home and community, (with or without a device) allowing for work, play, self-care; ADLs and IADLs, up to __________ feet based on patient need and prior functional level.
  - Achieve 600 m or greater in a 6-minute walk test for initiation of safe functional gait in the community.
  - Perform active verbalization with increasing taxonomy for safety during gait, including negotiation of even and uneven surfaces, opening and closing doors, transferring in and out of a car.
  - Determine location, if patient has an insulin pump.
  - Determine time and injection site, if patient has taken insulin.
  - Determine when patient last ate and if medication is taken as directed.
  - Clinics should have carbohydrates available if needed for drop in blood sugar.
    - Orange juice, sugar packets, or similar.
  - Tolerate 30 minutes of continuous moderate exercise three times a week in ______ weeks, and five times a week in ____________ weeks, depending on the severity of the disease.

PROGNOSIS

- As this pathology is primarily medical in nature, it is the physician who establishes the medical prognosis.
- If untreated or poorly managed, the prognosis is poor, resulting in limb amputation, stroke, heart disease, skin infections/ulcers, chronic infections, vision and hearing loss, and kidney failure.
- If type 2 can be managed with dietary changes and weight loss, the prognosis is good.
- PTs do not specifically manage diabetes, but may be managing conditions secondary to diabetes in which compensatory behaviors are being taught, as in proprioceptive loss.
- If the individual can effectively learn compensatory behaviors, the prognosis would be good.
- PTs may be involved in teaching foot care, skin inspection, and exercise programs for which the prognosis should be good.

PATIENT RESOURCE

- American Diabetes Association. Diagnosis and classification of diabetes mellitus. *Diabetes Care.* 2010;33(suppl 1):S62–S69.

REFERENCES

1. Toy EC. Diabetes Mellitus, Case 72. LANGE Case Files. http://www.accessmedicine.com/casecontent.aspx?aid=510023498&tabid=1. Accessed June 20, 2013.
2. National Diabetes Statistics, 2011. National Diabetes Information Clearinghouse (NDIC); a service of the National Institute of Diabetes and Digestive and Kidney Diseases (NIDDK) and the National Institutes of Health (NIH). http://diabetes.niddk.nih.gov/dm/pubs/statistics. Accessed June 20, 2013.
3. Demographics of Diabetes in America. DefeatingDiabetes.com. http://www.defeatingdiabetes.com/diabetes-demographics.htm. Accessed June 20, 2013.

ADDITIONAL REFERENCES

- Chandrasoma P, Taylor CR. The endocrine pancreas (islets of Langerhans). In: Chandrasoma P, Taylor CR, eds. *Concise Pathology.* 3rd ed. New York, NY: McGraw-Hill; 1998. http://www.accessphysiotherapy.com/content/190198. Accessed June 20, 2013.
- Chase HP, Eisenbarth GS. Diabetes mellitus. In: Hay WW, Levin MJ, Sondheimer JM, Deterding RR, eds. *CURRENT Diagnosis & Treatment: Pediatrics.* 20th ed. New York, NY: McGraw-Hill; 2011. http://www.accessphysiotherapy.com/content/6588451. Accessed June 20, 2013.
- Colcher A, Hurtig HI. Endocrine disorders. In: Watts RL, Standaertt DG, Obeso JA, eds. *Movement Disorders.* 3rd ed. New York, NY: McGraw-Hill; 2012. http://www.accessphysiotherapy.com/content/55806123. Accessed June 20, 2013.
- Dutton M. Pharmacology for the physical therapist. In: Dutton M, ed. *McGraw-Hill's NPTE (National Physical Therapy Examination).*

2nd ed. New York, NY: McGraw-Hill; 2012. http://www.accessphysiotherapy.com/content/5406725. Accessed June 20, 2013.
- Fainardi V, Scarabello C, Cangelosi A, et al. Physical activity and sedentary lifestyle in children with type 1 diabetes: a multicentre Italian study. *Acta Biomed.* 2011;82(2):124–131.
- Goodman CC, Fuller KS. *Pathology: Implications for the Physical Therapist.* 3rd ed. St. Louis, MO: Saunders; 2009.
- Goodman CC, Snyder TE. *Differential Diagnosis for Physical Therapists: Screening for Referral.* 4th ed. St. Louis, MO: Saunders; 2007.
- Kamboj MK, Draznin MB. Diabetes mellitus. In: Patel DR, Greydanus DE, Baker RJ, eds. *Pediatric Practice: Sports Medicine.* New York, NY: McGraw-Hill; 2009. http://www.accessphysiotherapy. com/content/6975753. Accessed June 20, 2013.
- Panus PC, Jobst EE, Masters SB, Katzung B, Tinsley SL, Trevor AJ. Pancreatic hormones and antidiabetic drugs: introduction. In: Panus PC, Jobst EE, Masters SB, Katzung B, Tinsley SL, Trevor AJ, eds. *Pharmacology for the Physical Therapist.* New York, NY: McGraw-Hill; 2009. http://www.accessphysiotherapy.com/content/6093568. Accessed June 20, 2013.
- Patel P, Macerollo A. Diabetes mellitus: diagnosis and screening. *Am Fam Physician.* 2010;81(7):863–870.
- Sakurai T, Iimuro S, Sakamaki K, et al. Risk factors for a 6-year decline in physical disability and functional limitations among elderly people with type 2 diabetes in the Japanese Elderly Diabetes Intervention Trial. *Geriatr Gerontol Int.* 2012;12 (Suppl 1):117–126. doi: 10.1111/j.1447–0594.2011.00819.x.

23 DIABETIC NEUROPATHY

Mollie Venglar, DSc, MSPT, NCS

CONDITION/DISORDER SYNONYMS

- Diabetic polyneuropathy
- Metabolic polyneuropathy

ICD-9-CM CODES

- 250.60 Diabetes mellitus with neurological manifestations type 2 or unspecified type not stated as controlled
- 357.2 Polyneuropathy in diabetes

ICD-10-CM CODE

- E13.40 Diabetes, diabetic (mellitus) with neuropathy

PREFERRED PRACTICE PATTERN

- 5G: Impaired Motor Function and Sensory Integrity Associated with Acute or Chronic Polyneuropathies[1]

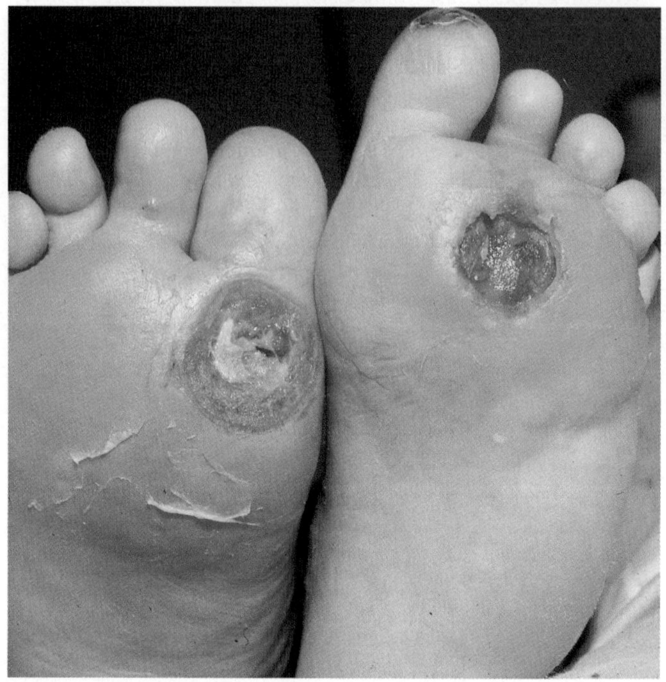

FIGURE 23-1 Diabetic foot and diabetic neuropathy. Data from Physical activity/exercise in diabetes. Diabetes Care. 2004;27(suppl 1):S58–S62.

PATIENT PRESENTATION

A 59-year-old man was brought begrudgingly to outpatient physical therapy by his wife. She reports that he has been complaining that his ankle hurts. She also reports noticing that he constantly holds on to the wall, furniture, or other objects whenever he is walking. The man reports having fallen about 2 weeks ago when his toe caught the edge of the sidewalk, and his right ankle has hurt since then. On examination, the right ankle is discolored and demonstrates excessive inversion on passive testing. Grossly, manual muscle testing of the upper and lower extremities is within normal limits. The man does not have two-point discrimination in his feet, ankles, and up to mid-calf bilaterally. Proprioception is impaired in bilateral feet and ankles. Balance testing reveals loss of balance with feet together and eyes closed on a stable surface and with feet together and eyes open on a compliant surface. He is able to maintain single-leg stance on the left for 2 seconds with eyes open. His right ankle is too painful to perform single-leg stance. Past medical history includes: diabetes mellitus, morbid obesity, and coronary artery disease.

KEY FEATURES

Description

- Damage to peripheral sensory (most common) and/or motor neurons
- Three major types
  - Distal, primarily sensory, symmetric polyneuropathy (most common)
  - Autonomic neuropathy
  - Transient asymmetric neuropathies
- Most likely due to demyelination, inflammation, ischemia, or infarction from as yet poorly understood metabolic abnormality

Essentials of Diagnosis

- Distinct clinical syndromes include
  - Distal, symmetrical, primarily sensory polyneuropathy affecting feet and legs in a chronic, slowly progressive manner (most common)
    - Usually unnoticed by patient until fairly progressed
    - Most common complaint is persistent numbness or tingling, worse at night
  - Acute ophthalmoplegia affecting cranial nerve III (oculomotor) and less often cranial nerve VI (abducens) on one side
  - Acute mononeuropathy of limbs or trunk, including painful thoracolumbar radiculopathy
  - Acute or subacute painful, asymmetrical, predominantly motor multiple neuropathy affecting upper lumbar roots and proximal leg muscles (diabetic amyotrophy)
  - Symmetrical, proximal motor weakness and wasting, usually without pain, with variable sensory loss, pursing subacute or chronic course
  - Autonomic neuropathy involving bowel, bladder, sweating, circulatory reflexes

General Considerations

- Sensory loss puts patient at risk for skin tears, skin breakdown
- Sensory and motor loss can result in loss of normal forces on joints, particularly foot and ankle, causing joint deformity over time
- Sensory and motor loss puts patient at higher risk for injury, acute and repetitive
- Peripheral nerve damage most common in lower extremities, but may occur in the upper extremities

Demographics

- In patients with diabetes, 15% have symptoms of polyneuropathy
- In cross-sectional sample of people with diabetes, 50% have evidence of peripheral nerve damage on nerve conduction velocity testing
- Less than 10% have clinical neuropathy on diagnosis of diabetes
- Infrequent in people under 30 years of age

CLINICAL FINDINGS

SIGNS AND SYMPTOMS

- Numbness
- Tingling
- Weakness, muscle atrophy
- Loss or impairment of deep tendon reflexes, vibration, proprioception
- Pain, burning, stabbing
- Impaired balance
- Altered gait
- Impaired vision
- Orthostatic hypotension

Functional Implications

- Fall risk with mobility on uneven or unpredictable surfaces
- Injury risk with items of unknown sharpness or temperature
- Impaired driving due to lower-extremity neuropathy or ophthalmoplegia
- Difficulty with fine motor tasks (writing, grooming, cooking, feeding, bathing)
- Difficulty with gross motor tasks (transfers, gait, stair climbing, dressing)

Possible Contributing Causes

- Cardiovascular risk factors associated with "metabolic syndrome" thought to be risk factors for diabetic polyneuropathy: Triglyceride levels, body mass, hypertension
- Poorly controlled diabetes results in higher likelihood of developing polyneuropathy

Differential Diagnosis

- Spinal cord injury
- Guillain–Barré syndrome (GBS)
- Tabes dorsalis
- Lumbar radiculopathy
- Peripheral vascular disease
- Lyme disease
- Leprosy
- HIV-related neuropathy
- Lupus erythematosus
- Sarcoidosis
- Polyarteritis nodosa
- Rheumatoid arthritis

TABLE 23-1 General Guidelines for Exercise Based on Preexercise Blood Glucose

Preexercise Blood Glucose	Recommended Action
Less than 100 mg/dL	Ingest 15 g of carbohydrates snack with protein
Between 250 and 300 mg/dL	Test urine for ketones Exercise if urine negative for ketones If urine positive for ketones, delay exercise until negative
More than 300 mg/dL	May exercise with caution if urine negative for ketones If urine positive for ketone, delay exercise until negative

Source: Data from Physical activity/exercise in diabetes. *Diabetes Care.* 2004;27(suppl 1):S58–S62

MEANS OF CONFIRMATION OR DIAGNOSIS

Laboratory Tests

- CSF

Imaging

- Nerve conduction velocity testing
- Electromyography

FINDINGS AND INTERPRETATION

- CSF: Elevated protein concentration

TREATMENT

Medication

- Pharmacologic management
  - Sulfonylureas: Glyburide (DiaBeta®), glipizide (Glucotrol®), and glimepiride (Amaryl®)
    - Increase insulin production
  - Biguanides: Metformin
    - Decreases liver glucose production

TABLE 23-2 Onset, Peak, and Duration of Action of Insulin Preparations

Insulin	Onset of Action (hours)	Peak of Action (hours)	Duration of Action (hours)
Rapid acting			
• Lispro	0.25–0.5	0.5–2.5	≤5
• Aspart	≤0.20	1–3	3–5
• Glulisine	Rapid	0.9	Not listed
Short acting			
• Regular	0.5–1	2–3	3–6
Intermediate acting			
• NPH (Isophane)	2–4	4–10	10–16
Long acting			
• Glargine	2–4	Peakless	20–24

Source: American Diabetes Association. Tools of therapy: Exercise. In: BW Bode, ed. *Medical Management of Type I Diabetes Mellitus.* 4th ed. Alexandria, VA; American Diabetes Association. LEVEMIR Insulin detemir [rDNA origin] injection; Product insert; Robinson, DM, Wellington, K. Insulin glulisine. *Drugs.* 2006;66(6):861–869.

- Thiazolidinediones
  - Mostly removed from market, stimulate insulin receptors
- Alpha-glucosidase inhibitors: **Acarbose (Precose®) and miglitol (Glyset®)**
  - Blocks the action of alpha-glucosidase enzymes at the brush border of the intestine. The inhibition slows the breakdown of dietary oligosaccharides and disaccharides.
- Meglitinides: **Repaglinide (Prandin®) and nateglinide (Starlix®) are**
  - Rapid lowering of postprandial glucose
- Insulin
  - Type 1 is managed strictly with insulin and diet
  - Type 2 may be managed with or without a combination of diet, oral medications, and insulin
  - Insulin: Short acting, medium acting, long acting

MEDICAL PROCEDURES

- Hospitalization if severe, with IV insulin if glucose is high and not controlled with regular medication
- Insertion of insulin pumps

REFERRALS/ADMITTANCE

- To endocrinologist for regular management of diabetes
- To neuroendocrinologist for management of more severe neuropathy
- To occupational therapist for fine motor compensation, ADL modification
- To orthotist for appropriate footwear, custom bracing as needed
- To wound care specialist for foot ulcers if needed

IMPAIRMENTS

- Peripheral nerve integrity
- Cranial nerve integrity
- Gait training
- Balance
  - Static standing
  - Dynamic standing
  - Moving base of support
- Muscle strength
- Muscle recruitment
- Coordination
- Posture, postural control
- ROM
- Reflexes: Deep tendon reflexes reduced or absent
- Muscle tone
- Bed mobility
- Transfers
- Endurance
- Aerobic capacity
- Self-care
- Home management
- Decreased fine motor control in people who have upper-extremity involvement

TESTS AND MEASURES

- Blood pressure (test specifically for orthostatic hypotension)
- Vascular examination (particularly blood flow to feet)
- Heart rate

TABLE 23-3 Chronic Complications of Diabetes Mellitus

Microvascular disease
Nephropathy
Neuropathy
Sensorimotor distal symmetric neuropathy
Autonomic neuropathy
Focal and multifocal neuropathies
Vascular
Nonvascular (entrapment)
Macrovascular disease
Coronary artery disease
Cerebrovascular disease
Peripheral vascular disease
Associated complications
Foot ulcers
Infections

Source: McPhee SJ, Hammer GD. *Pathophysiology of Disease: An Introduction to Clinical Medicine.* 6th ed. www.accessmedicine.com.

- Sensory testing
- Reflex testing
- Cranial nerve testing
- Manual muscle test
- Active and passive ROM testing, muscle length testing
- Functional assessment (assist, device, environment)
  - Bed mobility
  - Transitions
  - Sitting balance
  - Standing balance
  - Transfers
  - Gait
  - Stairs
- Pain assessment
- Postural assessment
- Cardiovascular endurance

INTERVENTION

- Lifestyle modification
- Postural correction
- Mobility: Walking or wheelchair
  - Include devices, bracing, shoe selection
- Balance strategies
- Compensatory strategies for lost sensory feedback
- Pain management
- Diet modifications to control weight gain, glycemic index, hydration
- Cardiovascular exercise with glucose monitoring
- Orthotic or bracing as needed for joint support/deformity
- Total contact casting for patients with significant or chronic diabetic foot ulcers

FUNCTIONAL GOALS

- Specific to individual's lifestyle, glycemic control, type of neuropathy.
- Geared toward individuals with lower-extremity sensory neuropathy.

- Patient will show written evidence of appropriate insulin use in conjunction with home exercise program for 2 weeks.
- Patient will demonstrate accurate, consistent stepping strategy with unanticipated balance perturbations from all directions with eyes open, feet shoulder-width apart.
- Patient will tolerate 15 minutes of aerobic exercise at 65% to 80% maximum heart rate with appropriate blood pressure response.

PROGNOSIS

- Life expectancy reduced by 7 to 9 years for those who control diabetes appropriately; reduced further for those who do not appropriately control the disease.
- Causes of death related to diabetes include: Myocardial infarction, renal failure, cerebrovascular accident, infection, ketoacidosis, hyperosmolar coma, hypoglycemia.

PATIENT RESOURCES

- Neuropathy. American Diabetes Association. http://www.diabetes.org/living-with-diabetes/complications/neuropathy. Accessed June 19, 2013.
- Peripheral Neuropathy. The Neuropathy Association. http://www.neuropathy.org/site/PageServer?pagename=Type_Diabetic. Accessed April 28, 2014.

REFERENCE

1. The American Physical Therapy Association. Pattern 5G: impaired motor function and sensory integrity associated with acute or chronic polyneuropathies. *Interactive Guide to Physical Therapist Practice*. 2003. http://guidetoptpractice.apta.org/content/1/SEC24.extract. Accessed April 28, 2014.

ADDITIONAL REFERENCES

- Chandrasoma P, Taylor CR. Chronic complications. In: Chandrasoma P, Taylor CR, eds. *Concise Pathology*. 3rd ed. New York, NY: McGraw-Hill; 2011. http://www.accessphysiotherapy.com/content/190262. Accessed June 19, 2013.
- Dutton M. Signs and symptoms of DM. In: Dutton M, ed. *McGraw-Hill's NPTE (National Physical Therapy Examination)*. 2nd ed. New York, NY: McGraw-Hill; 2012. http://www.accessphysiotherapy.com/content/5402380. Accessed June 19, 2013.
- ICD9DATA. http://www.icd9data.com. Accessed June 19, 2013.
- ICD10DATA. http://www.icd10data.com. Accessed June 19, 2013.
- McPhee SJ, Hammer GD. Microvascular complications. In: McPhee SJ, Hammer GD, eds. *Pathophysiology of Disease*. 6th ed. New York, NY: McGraw-Hill; 2010. http://www.accessphysiotherapy.com/content/5371165. Accessed June 19, 2013.
- Ropper AL, Samuels MA. *Adams and Victor's Principles of Neurology*. 9th ed. New York, NY: McGraw-Hill; 2009:1277–1280.

24 GOITER

Debra F. Stern, DPT, DBA, MSM, PT
Eric Shamus, PhD, DPT, PT, CSCS
Wendy Song, DO

CONDITION/DISORDER SYNONYM

- Enlarged thyroid

ICD-9-CM CODES

- 240.9 Goiter, unspecified
- 241.0 Nontoxic uninodular goiter
- 241.1 Nontoxic multinodular goiter
- 241.9 Unspecified nontoxic nodular goiter
- 242 Thyrotoxicosis with or without goiter
- 242.0 Toxic diffuse goiter
- 242.00 Toxic diffuse goiter without mention of thyrotoxic crisis or storm
- 242.01 Toxic diffuse goiter with mention of thyrotoxic crisis or storm
- 242.1 Toxic uninodular goiter
- 242.10 Toxic uninodular goiter without mention of thyrotoxic crisis or storm
- 242.11 Toxic uninodular goiter with mention of thyrotoxic crisis or storm
- 242.2 Toxic multinodular goiter
- 242.20 Toxic multinodular goiter without mention of thyrotoxic crisis or storm
- 242.21 Toxic multinodular goiter with mention of thyrotoxic crisis or storm
- 242.3 Toxic nodular goiter unspecified type
- 242.30 Toxic nodular goiter, unspecified type, without mention of thyrotoxic crisis or storm
- 242.31 Toxic nodular goiter, unspecified type, with mention of thyrotoxic crisis or storm
- 242.40 Thyrotoxicosis from ectopic thyroid nodule without mention of thyrotoxic crisis or storm

ICD-10-CM CODES

- E01.1 Iodine-deficiency related multinodular (endemic) goiter
- E01.2 Iodine-deficiency related (endemic) goiter, unspecified
- E03.0 Congenital hypothyroidism with diffuse goiter
- E03.1 Congenital hypothyroidism without goiter
- E04 Other nontoxic goiter
- E04.0 Nontoxic diffuse goiter
- E04.2 Nontoxic multinodular goiter
- E04.8 Other specified nontoxic goiter
- E04.9 Nontoxic goiter, unspecified
- E05.00 Thyrotoxicosis with diffuse goiter without thyrotoxic crisis or storm
- E05.0 Thyrotoxicosis with diffuse goiter
- E05.2 Thyrotoxicosis with toxic multinodular goiter
- E07.1 Dyshormogenetic goiter
- P72.0 Neonatal goiter, not elsewhere classified

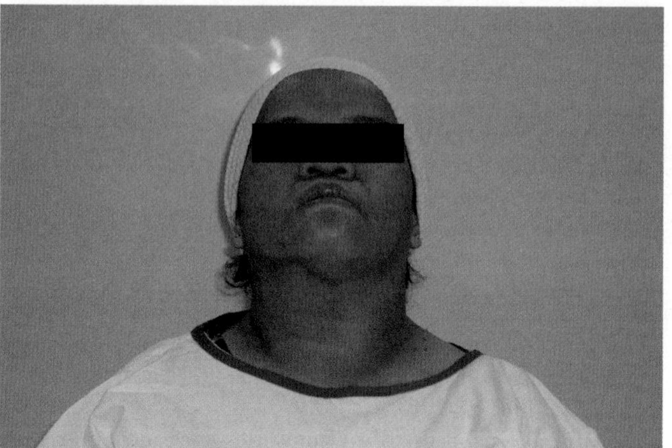

FIGURE 24-1 Goiter with hyperthyroidism symptoms: Patient has large solitary toxic adenoma on the left lobe. (From Tintinalli JE, Stapczynski JS, Ma JA, Cline DM, Cydulka RK, Meckler GD. *Tintinalli's Emergency Medicine: A Comprehensive Study Guide.* 7th ed. http://www.accessmedicine.com. Copyright © The McGraw-Hill Companies, Inc. All rights reserved.)

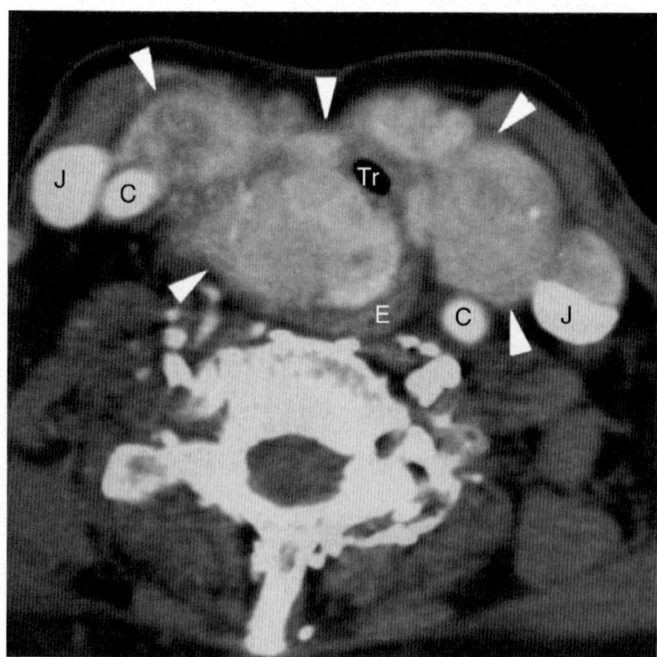

FIGURE 24-2 Axial contrast-enhanced CT scan of the neck in an elderly woman with a gradually enlarging neck mass demonstrates massive enlargement of a heterogeneously enhancing thyroid gland (*arrowheads*). There is maintenance of a smooth margin; however, no evidence of any invasion of adjacent structures. No abnormal lymph nodes are identified. Adjacent structures are displaced and compressed by this large mass, notably, the trachea (Tr), esophagus (E), and carotid (C) and jugular (J) vessels. The surgical pathology confirmed diffuse goiter. (From Lalwani AK. *Current Diagnosis & Treatment in Otolaryngology-Head & Neck Surgery.* 3rd ed. www.accesssurgery.com. Copyright © The McGraw-Hill Companies, Inc. All rights reserved.)

PREFERRED PRACTICE PATTERNS

- 4E: Impaired Joint Mobility, Motor Function, Muscle Performance, and Range of Motion Associated with Localized Inflammation[1]
- 6A: Primary Prevention/Risk Reduction for Cardiovascular/Pulmonary Disorders[2]
- 6B: Impaired Aerobic Capacity/Endurance Associated with Deconditioning[3]

PATIENT PRESENTATION

A 35-year-old female presents with low back pain and fatigue from standing at work for 4 hours. The patient reports feeling fatigue despite of getting 9 hours of sleep daily. She also experiences constipation, a 15 lb weight gain over the last year and a "lump" above her Adam's apple. Family history is positive for a "thyroid problem" in her mother. Vitals are: Temperature: 97.8°F, Pulse: 64, Respirations: 16, Blood pressure: 136/78, and SpO_2% of 97%. Physical examination shows an overweight woman with dry flaky skin. Her thyroid gland is uniformly enlarged, but nontender to palpation. A blood test for thyroid stimulating hormone (TSH) is elevated at 17.4.

KEY FEATURES

Description

- Enlarged thyroid gland, can result in decreased production of thyroid hormone
- Prolonged elevation of TSH
- Weight gain or loss
- May range from single or small nodules to significant enlargement
- Multinodular goiter[4]
- Enlargement can limit neck mobility and swallowing

Essentials of Diagnosis

- Fatigue
- Decreased activity tolerance
- Sensitivity to cold
- Abnormal thyroid function tests
- Thyroid enlargement

General Considerations

- Diagnosis for more occult problems may take time and require intensive diagnostic testing, inability to afford testing and medications, noncompliance with medication regimen
- May cause pathology in multiple organ systems
  - GI: Liver
  - Cardiovascular: Heart, peripheral circulation, blood pressure
  - Integumentary
- May result in secondary problems indicating need for PT intervention: Aerobic capacity and muscle endurance impairment, sarcopenia, weakness, musculoskeletal problems, neuromuscular problems, weight gain
- Hyperlipidemia
- Can result in hyperthyroidism

Demographics

- Can occur in anyone throughout lifespan, beginning at birth (1 in 4000 infants affected)
- Estimated five million people affected in the United States, and an equal number undiagnosed
- Higher incidence in women and people aged 60 years and older

CLINICAL FINDINGS

SIGNS AND SYMPTOMS

- Nausea
- Vomiting
- Diarrhea
- Coughing
- Sweating
- Shaking agitation
- Hoarseness
- Dizziness with arms overhead
- Difficulty swallowing
- Sensitivity to cold
- Slowed or rapid heart rate
- Constipation
- Joint or muscle pain
- Paleness
- Dry skin
- Thinning hair, including eyebrows
- Brittle fingernails
- Weakness
- Unexplained weight gain
- Depression
- Heavy menstruation
- Decreased sense of smell or taste
- Swollen hands, feet, face
- Slowed speech
- Thickened skin
- Liver dysfunction
- Heart disease
- In severe cases
  - Below-normal body temperature
  - Depressed breathing
  - Low blood pressure
  - Low blood sugar
  - Unresponsiveness

Functional Implications

- Severe symptoms, such as immediacy of need to urinate, may cause inability to leave home
- Swelling in throat
- Fatigue
- Infertility, miscarriage
- Heart disease
- Weight gain from inability to exercise or move well
- Sarcopenia resulting in weakness, muscle-mass loss, inability to ambulate or perform self-care, limited aerobic capacity secondary to inactivity
- Decreased exercise tolerance
- Sleep disturbance
- Lifestyle changes
- Eating disorders
- Difficulty swallowing
- Dizziness with neck extension
- Limited ROM in neck
- Inappropriate self-medication
- Anxiety, depression
- Liver problems
- Limited ADLs, IADLs
- Infection (systemic)
- Skin lesions from dryness
- Neuropathy, increased risk for falls
- Vision impairment (most often retinal)
- Risk for infection (bacterial, fungal) of skin, urinary tract, kidney

Possible Contributing Causes

- Autoimmune or Hashimoto thyroiditis[5]
- Viral thyroiditis
- Congenital
- Grave disease

- Overexposure to radiation, as in CT scan or radiation therapy to neck or brain
- Inflammation of thyroid
- Pregnancy
- Cancer, metastatic
- Chemical inducement
- Radioactive iodine to treat hyperthyroidism
- Surgical removal of part or whole thyroid gland to treat other thyroid problems
- Drugs: Amiodarone, drugs to treat hyperthyroidism, lithium
- Low or excess iodine[4]
- Pituitary dysfunction

Differential Diagnosis

- Organ dysfunction from cancer or malignancy, especially the liver
- Pituitary dysfunction
- Non-malignant tumor in the abdomen, organs, or thyroid
- Endocrine disorder
- Thyroiditis
- Hashimoto thyroiditis
- Grave disease
- Hypo- or hyperthyroidism
- Autoimmune disease, causing bowel inflammation or dysfunction
- Gastroparesis
- Autoimmune disease affecting upper and lower GI tracts
- Appendicitis
- Peritonitis
- Prostatitis
- Benign prostatic hypertrophy
- Pelvic inflammatory disease
- Gastroenteritis
- Perforated ulcer in GI system
- Bladder or urinary tract infection, kidney pathology
- Throat infection
- Bowel disorders

MEANS OF CONFIRMATION OR DIAGNOSIS

Laboratory Tests

- Blood tests, complete blood count (CBC)
- Thyroid function test: TSH and T4
- Cholesterol
- Liver enzymes
- Prolactin, normal value: 1.6 to 18.8 ng/mL
- Sodium levels

Imaging

- Ultrasound
- Chest x-ray
- CT
- Thyroid scan
- MRI

Diagnostic Procedure

- Biopsy

FINDINGS AND INTERPRETATION

- Prolactin (may be elevated in women)
- Sodium levels (low in hypothyroidism)
  - Normal range: 135 to 145 milliequivalents per liter (mEq/L)

TREATMENT

Medication

- If hyperthyroid
  - Thyroid hormone replacement : Levothyroxine
  - Lifelong, with levels checked annually at least
- If hyperthyroid: Methimazol (Tapazole) or propylthiouracil
- If inflammation: Aspirin
- If iodine deficiency: Iodine

MEDICAL PROCEDURES

- Surgical removal may be indicated if hyperthyroidism results
- Surgical removal (full or partial) may also be indicated if vessel or esophageal compression
- Surgery may also be considered for cosmesis

REFERRALS/ADMITTANCE

- If patient history and reactions to PT indicate possible hypo- or hyperthyroidism, refer to appropriate physician
- If causative problem is not considered appropriate for PT intervention, refer to appropriate physician
- Refer to ER if emergency identified

IMPAIRMENTS

- Muscle weakness
- Muscle atrophy
- Gait abnormality, difficulty walking
- Shortness of breath, fatigue
- Inability to perform self-care
- Balance impairment, dizziness with neck extension
- Impaired skin integrity

TESTS AND MEASURES

- Palpation
  - Appendix (McBurney's): Apply vertical pressure halfway between right ASIS and umbilicus: −/+ may indicate appendicitis.
  - Liver: In supine, with left hand under trunk parallel to 11th and 12th ribs, lift upward; right hand lateral to rectus, press in and up: +/= reproduction of symptoms with deep breath, indicates liver involvement.
  - Ascites: Percuss outward from center with fingers; if sound is dull, ascites may be present.
  - Spleen: Not recommended for PT to palpate enlarged spleen secondary to ease of rupture (only palpable if enlarged).
  - Gallbladder (Murphy's): Place fingers right of rectus abdominus below rib cage: +/= sudden pain and muscle tensing with deep breath.
  - Kidneys: In supine, place one hand under client, between ribs and iliac crest, other hand on abdomen below ribs and ribs pointing in opposite direction: +/− tenderness or reproduction of symptoms.
  - Bladder: Not usually palpable unless distended and raised above pubic bone; in supine, place hand above pubis and press down: +/= tenderness, reproduction of pain, ability to feel the bladder: __+ ___−.

INTERVENTION

- Gait training
- Therapeutic exercise: All relevant categories, energy conservation

- Self-care training: Skin care, moisturizing, lifestyle management
- Neuromuscular re-education: Balance and postural training

FUNCTIONAL GOALS

- Patient will be able to
  - Achieve functional aerobic capacity, ability to talk during activity so as to achieve functional gait and activity tolerance for ADLs/IADLs.
  - Achieve 600 m or greater in a 6-minute walk test for initiation of safe functional gait in the community.
  - Perform active verbalization with increasing taxonomy for safety during gait, including negotiation of even and uneven surfaces, opening and closing doors, transferring in and out of car.
  - Tolerate 30 minutes of continuous, moderate exercise three times a week in ______ weeks, and five times a week in ____________ weeks, depending on disease severity.

PROGNOSIS

- Physician establishes the medical prognosis, as pathology is primarily medical in nature.
- May be lifelong condition unless viral, transient type.
- Asymptomatic in some cases.
- Can usually be managed with medication.
- If thyroid hormones get too low, myxedema coma and ensuing death may result.
- Prognosis for return to premorbid function is good with adequate medical management.

PATIENT RESOURCE

- American Thyroid Association. Goiter. http://www.thyroid.org/what-is-a-goiter. Accessed June 12, 2013.

REFERENCES

1. The American Physical Therapy Association. Pattern 4E: impaired joint mobility, motor function, muscle performance, and range of motion associated with localized inflammation. *Interactive Guide to Physical Therapist Practice.* 2003. doi: 10.2522/ptguide.3.1_5. http://guidetoptpractice.apta.org/content/1/SEC12.extract?sid=108e960a-5e95-419c-90f2-4a47ca50d8f4. Accessed April 28, 2014.
2. The American Physical Therapy Association. Pattern 6A: primary prevention/risk reduction for cardiovascular/pulmonary disorders. *Interactive Guide to Physical Therapist Practice.* 2003. doi: 10.2522/ptguide.3.3_1. http://guidetoptpractice.apta.org/content/1/SEC27.extract?sid=e04b1cce-7657-4a83-80cb-fa2d2d550f4a. Accessed April 28, 2014.
3. The American Physical Therapy Association. Pattern 6B: impaired aerobic capacity/endurance associated with deconditioning. *Interactive Guide to Physical Therapist Practice.* 2003. doi: 10.2522/ptguide.3.3_2. http://guidetoptpractice.apta.org/content/1/SEC28.extract?sid=52429ec2-d21c-46d5-90f7-038735671158. Accessed April 28, 2014.
4. Bauer DC, McPhee SJ. Thyroid disease: introduction. In: McPhee SJ, Hammer GD, eds. *Pathophysiology of Disease.* 6th ed. New York, NY: McGraw-Hill; 2010. http://www.accessphysiotherapy. com/content/5371499. Accessed June 12, 2013.
5. Chronic thyroiditis (Hashimoto's disease). NIH National Institutes of Health. MedlinePlus. http://www.nlm.nih.gov/medlineplus/ency/article/000371.htm. Online June 4, 2012. Accessed June 12, 2013.

ADDITIONAL REFERENCES

- Baskin HJ, Cobin RH, Duick DS,et al. American Association of Clinical Endocrinologists medical guidelines for clinical practice for the evaluation and treatment of hyperthyroidism and hypothyroidism. *Endocr Pract.* 2002;8(6):457–469.
- Bauer DC, McPhee SJ. Thyroid diseases. In: McPhee SJ, Hammer GD, eds. *Pathophysiology of Disease: An Introduction to Clinical Medicine.* 6th ed. New York, NY: McGraw-Hill; 2010. http://www.accessphysiotherapy.com/content/5371561. Accessed June 12, 2013.
- Goodman CC, Fuller KS. *Pathology: Implications for the Physical Therapist.* 3rd ed. Philadelphia, PA: Saunders Elsevier; 2009.
- Goodman CC, Snyder TK. *Differential Diagnosis for Physical Therapists: Screening for Referral.* 4th ed. St. Louis, MO: Saunders Elsevier; 2007.
- Reid JR, Wheeler SF. Hyperthyroidism: diagnosis and treatment. *Am Fam Physician.* 2005;72(4):623–630.

25 HASHIMOTO THYROIDITIS

Debra F. Stern, DPT, DBA, MSM, PT
Eric Shamus, PhD, DPT, PT, CSCS

CONDITION/DISORDER SYNONYMS

- Chronic lymphocytic thyroiditis
- Autoimmune thyroiditis

ICD-9-CM CODES

- 244.0 Postsurgical hypothyroidism
- 244.1 Other postablative hypothyroidism
- 244.2 Iodine hypothyroidism
- 244.3 Other iatrogenic hypothyroidism
- 244.8 Other specified acquired hypothyroidism
- 244.9 Unspecified acquired hypothyroidism
- 245.0 Acute thyroiditis
- 245.2 Chronic lymphocytic thyroiditis
- Associated ICD-9-CM PT diagnoses/treatment diagnoses that may be directly related
  - 315.4 Developmental coordination disorder
  - 718.45 Contracture of joints of pelvic region and thigh
  - 719.70 Difficulty in walking involving joint site unspecified
  - 728.2 Muscular wasting and disuse atrophy, not elsewhere specified
  - 728.89 Other disorders of muscle, ligament, and fascia
  - 729.9 Other and unspecified disorders of soft tissue
  - 780.7 Malaise and fatigue
  - 781.2 Abnormality of gait
  - 782.3 Edema
  - 786.0 Dyspnea and respiratory abnormalities
  - 786.05 Shortness of breath

ICD-10-CM CODES

- E06.0 Acute thyroiditis
- E06.3 Autoimmune thyroiditis
- E89.0 Postprocedural hypothyroidism

PREFERRED PRACTICE PATTERNS[1]

- 4E: Impaired Joint Mobility, Motor Function, Muscle Performance, and Range of Motion Associated with Localized Inflammation
- 6A: Primary Prevention/Risk Reduction for Cardiovascular/Pulmonary Disorders
- 6B: Impaired Aerobic Capacity/Endurance Associated with Deconditioning

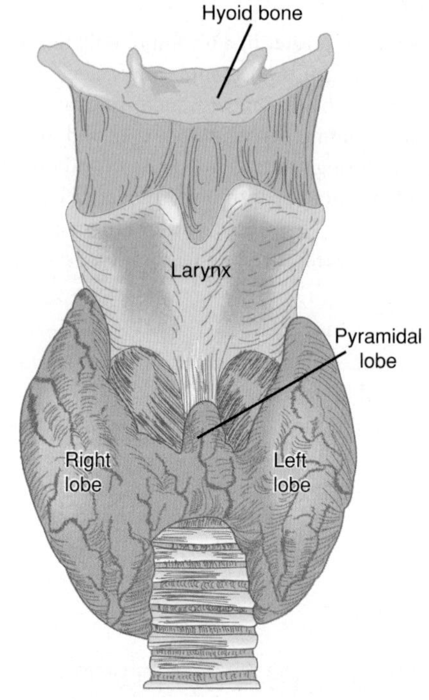

FIGURE 25-1 The human thyroid. (Redrawn with permission from Ganong WF. *Review of Medical Physiology*. 22nd ed. McGraw-Hill; 2005.)

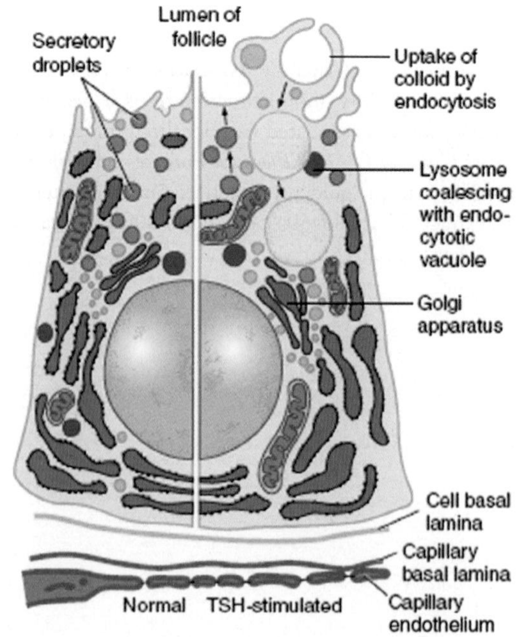

FIGURE 25-2 Thyroid cell. Left: normal pattern. Right: after TSH stimulation. The *arrows* on the right show the secretion of thyroglobulin into the colloid. On the right, endocytosis of the colloid and merging of a colloid-containing vacuole with a lysosome are also shown. The cell rests on a capillary with gaps (fenestrations) in the endothelial wall. (From Barrett KE, Barman SM, Boitano S, Brooks HL. *Ganong's Review of Medical Physiology.* www.accessmedicine.com. Copyright © The McGraw-Hill Companies, Inc. All rights reserved.)

PATIENT PRESENTATION

A 46-year-old female has been referred to PT for sarcopenia and fatigue. She is a high school teacher, and describes barely being able to get through a day. She complains of generalized achiness and has been treated for depression over the past 3 months but has not seen any improvement. Up until about a year ago she was an avid walker, and walked with colleagues at least three to four times a week. Her history indicates weight gain without change in diet. During postural assessment, the PT notes what appears to be a swelling in her neck, which she attributes to the weight gain. There is a nontender palpable mass in her neck. When tested, her muscle performance demonstrated extremity and core weakness, with easy fatigability.

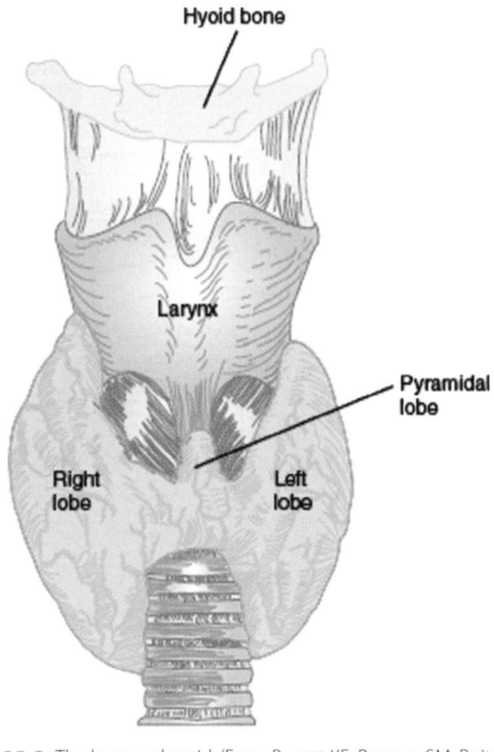

FIGURE 25-3 The human thyroid. (From Barrett KE, Barman SM, Boitano S, Brooks HL. *Ganong's Review of Medical Physiology*. www.accessmedicine.com. Copyright © The McGraw-Hill Companies, Inc. All rights reserved.)

KEY FEATURES

Description

- Autoimmune disease
- Thyroid gland is gradually destroyed
- Results in hypothyroidism
- Enlargement of the thyroid

Essentials of Diagnosis

- Thyroid gland becomes lobulated
- Decreased activity tolerance
- Sensitivity to cold
- Abnormal thyroid function tests
- Often misdiagnosed as fibromyalgia and depression

General Considerations

- Diagnosis for more occult problems may take time and require intensive medical diagnostic testing
- May cause pathology in multiple organ systems
  - Cardiovascular: Heart, peripheral circulation, blood pressure
  - Integumentary
- May result in secondary problems indicating the need for PT intervention depending on severity
  - Aerobic capacity and muscle endurance impairment
  - Sarcopenia
  - Weakness/impaired muscle performance
  - Musculoskeletal problems
  - Neuromuscular problems
  - Weight gain, indicating the need for physical therapy intervention depending on severity
- Gradual onset
- Hyperlipidemia

Demographics

- Can occur in anyone
- Higher incidence in women, primarily middle aged
- Tends to run in families
- Between 0.1% and 5% of all adults

CLINICAL FINDINGS

SIGNS AND SYMPTOMS

- Asymptomatic in some cases
- Clinical findings for hypothyroidism
- Constipation
- Hair loss
- Fatigue
- Weight gain
- Slowed heart rate
- Dry skin
- Depression
- Infertility
- Goiter
- Panic attacks
- Memory loss
- Joint stiffness
- Facial swelling (lion mask)

Functional Implications

- Severe symptoms such as immediacy of need to urinate may be disabling, resulting in the inability to leave home
- Inability to afford testing and medications
- Fatigue
- Drowsiness
- Infertility
- Miscarriage
- Heart disease
- Decreased sex drive
- Increasing weight with inability to exercise or move well
- Sarcopenia resulting in
  - Weakness
  - Muscle-mass loss
  - Inability to ambulate or perform self-care
  - Aerobic capacity limitation secondary to inactivity
- Decreased exercise tolerance
- Sleep disturbances
- Changes in lifestyle
- Eating disorders
- Anxiety and depression
- Can lead to problems with liver
- Limitations in ADLs or IADLs
- Systemic infection
- Skin lesions from dryness
- Neuropathy, increased risk for falls

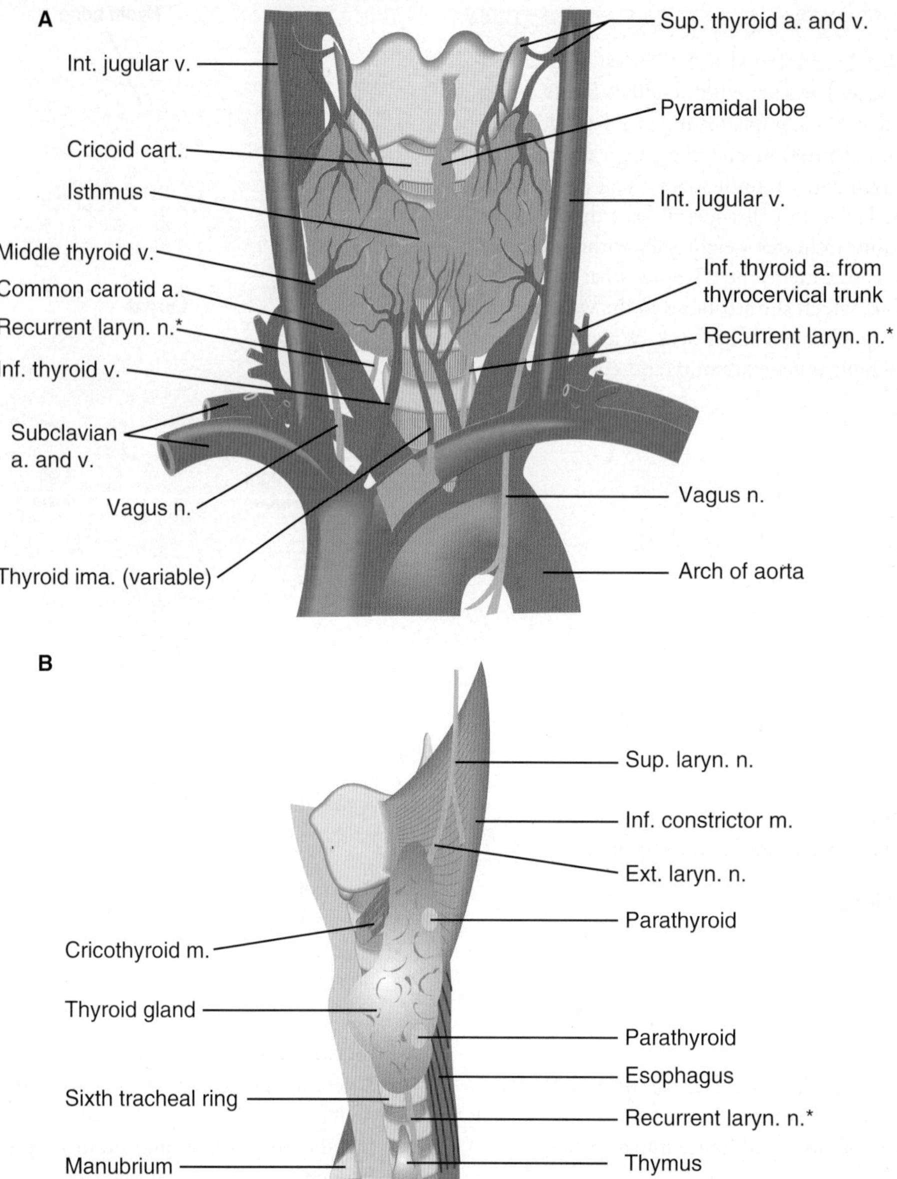

FIGURE 25-4 Thyroid anatomy. **A.** Anterior view **B.** Lateral view. *The recurrent laryngeal nerve runs in the tracheoesophageal groove on the left and has a slightly more oblique course on the right before it enters the larynx just posterior to the cricothyroid muscle at the level of the cricoid cartilage. (From Doherty GM. *Current Diagnosis & Treatment: Surgery*. 13th ed. www.accessmedicine.com. Copyright © The McGraw-Hill Companies, Inc. All rights reserved.)

- Vision impairment, most often retinal
- Prone to infections such as bacterial and fungal in the skin, urinary tract (UT), kidney
- Potential for liver problems
- Difficulty thinking clearly
- Birth defects in newborns of mothers with Hashimoto
- In severe cases
  - Below-normal body temperature
  - Depressed breathing
  - Low blood pressure
  - Low blood sugar
  - Unresponsiveness: Myxedema coma

▶ Possible Contributing Causes

- Inappropriate self-medication
- Noncompliance with medication regiments/inability to pay

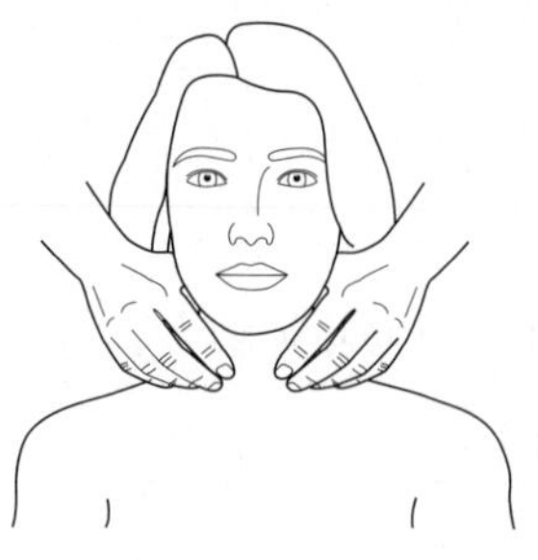

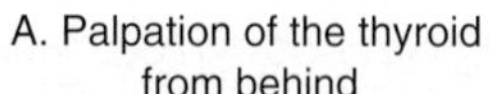

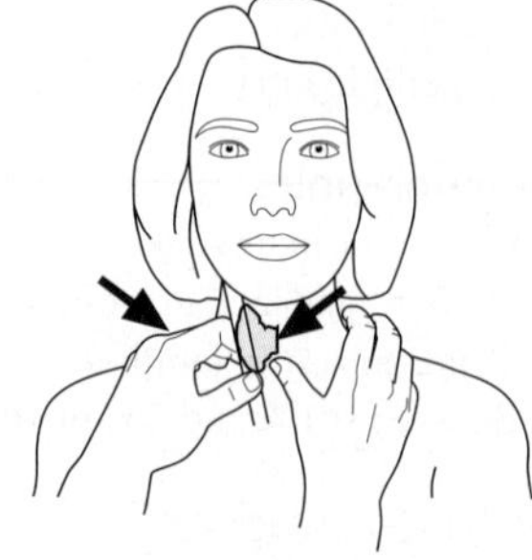

FIGURE 25-5 Palpation of the thyroid gland and adjacent structures. **A.** Palpation from behind. **B.** Frontal palpation of the thyroid gland. (From LeBlond RF, DeGowin RL, Brown DD. *DeGowin's Diagnostic Examination*. 9th ed. www.accessmedicine.com. Copyright © The McGraw-Hill Companies, Inc. All rights reserved.)

- Inflammation of the thyroid
- Family history
- Hypoparathyroidism
- Adrenal insufficiency
- Fungal infections, mouth and nails
- Goiters
- Environmental
- Pregnancy
- Cancer
- Metastatic cancer
- Other autoimmune disorders
- Chemical inducement
- Radiation treatments to the neck
- Viral thyroiditis
- Older than age 50
- Being female
- Congenital birth defects
- Low iodine
- Pituitary dysfunction as the pituitary signals production of thyroid-stimulating hormone (TSH)

Differential Diagnosis

- Organ dysfunction as a result of cancer or malignancy, especially the liver
- Goiter
- Euthyroid sick syndrome
- Fibromyalgia
- Pituitary dysfunction
- Thyroid lymphoma
- Non-malignant tumors in the abdomen or organs
- Other forms of thyroiditis
- Endocrine disorders, diabetes
- Cardiac disorders
- Gynecologic problems in females
- Autoimmune diseases that affect the upper and lower GI tracts
- Crohn disease
- Irritable bowel syndrome
- Bladder infections
- UTIs
- Kidney pathology
- Fatigue syndromes such as Epstein–Barr
- Infections in the abdomen
- Bowel disorders

MEANS OF CONFIRMATION OR DIAGNOSIS

Laboratory Tests

- Complete blood count (CBC)
- Total cholesterol
- Thyroid function: TSH, T3, and Free T4[2]
- Serum prolactin
- Sodium levels, low in hypothyroid
- Cell pathology
- Thyroid autoantibodies
  - Antithyroid peroxidase antibody
  - Antithyroglobulin antibody

Imaging

- Ultrasound
- Chest X-ray
- CT scans
- MRIs
- Radioactive iodine uptake

FINDINGS AND INTERPRETATION

- Thyroid function: TSH and free T4 (low)[2]
- T3 (low or normal)[2]

TREATMENT

Medication

- Thyroid hormone replacement therapy, most commonly levothyroxine, lifelong, with levels checked at least annually
- Bone density monitoring required when on levothyroxine

REFERRALS/ADMITTANCE

- If a patient is referred for PT and the causative problem is not appropriate for PT, refer to the appropriate physician.
- If an emergency is identified, refer to an ER.
- If the patient's history and reactions to PT indicate possible hypothyroidism and/or symptoms, refer to a physician.

IMPAIRMENTS

- Muscle weakness/cramps
- Muscle atrophy
- Gait abnormality/difficulty walking
- Shortness of breath, fatigue
- Inability to perform self-care
- Balance impairment
- Impaired skin integrity

TESTS AND MEASURES

- Observation
  - Scars may indicate adhesions or abdominal surgeries causative of diverticula.
  - Pink or purplish striae may be indicative of Cushing syndrome.
  - Dilated veins may indicate hepatic pathology or inferior vena cava obstruction, not diverticulitis.
  - Contour: Roundness, concavity, asymmetry, distension, pregnancy signs.
  - Cullen sign: Bluish discoloring around umbilicus may be a sign of retroperitoneal bleeding.
  - Bluish discoloration in lower abdomen: Grey Turner sign, signals hemorrhagic pancreatitis.
  - Bulging in groin and abdomen especially apparent with contraction of musculature in area may be hernia.
  - Pulsing in navel area may be abdominal aortic aneurysm.
  - Left lower quadrant pain, often following a meal.
  - Palpable abdominal tenderness on left side or generalized.
  - Psoas sign: Provides resistance over patient's right knee as they flex the hip; pain indicates appendicitis, possible inflammation of abdomen.
  - Obturator sign: Internal rotation and flexion of right lower extremity may indicate appendicitis, pelvic inflammation.
  - Rovsing sign: Pain on right side of abdomen when pressure applied to left may indicate appendicitis.
- Palpation
  - Appendix (McBurney's): Apply vertical pressure halfway between right anterior superior iliac spine (ASIS) and umbilicus: –/+ may indicate appendicitis.

- Liver: In supine, with left hand under trunk parallel to 11th and 12th ribs, lift upward; right hand lateral to rectus, press in and up: +/= reproduction of symptoms with deep breath, indicates liver involvement.
- Ascites: Percuss outward from center with fingers.
  - If sound is dull, ascites may be present.
- Spleen: It is not recommended for PT to palpate enlarged spleen secondary to rupture issues (only palpable if enlarged).
- Gallbladder (Murphy's): Place fingers right of rectus abdominus below rib cage: +/= sudden pain and muscle tensing with deep breath.
- Kidneys: In supine, place one hand under client between ribs and iliac crest, other hand on abdomen below ribs pointing in opposite direction: +/− tenderness or reproduction of symptoms.
- Bladder
  - Not usually palpable unless distended and raised above pubic bone.
  - In supine, place hand above pubis and press down: +/= tenderness, reproduction of pain, ability to feel the bladder: ____ + ____ −.

INTERVENTION

- PT intervention is consistent with the movement-related problems that occur secondary to diabetes.
- Therapeutic exercise, all relevant categories, energy conservation
  - If there is a stoma from a colostomy or ileostomy, PT must be aware that activities are avoided if they cause retraction.
  - If there is an insulin pump, take care not to interfere with it in any way.
  - PT should inquire if medication is taken.
    - If glucose >300, exercise should be avoided.
  - Monitor heart rate.
    - Cardiac monitoring with possible MET calculation if history of angina.
- Therapeutic activities for bed-mobility training, transfer-, and transitional-movement training.
- Wheelchair management (in severe cases).
- Self-care management training including skin care/moisturizing, lifestyle management.
- Neuromuscular re-education: Balance and postural training.

FUNCTIONAL GOALS

- Patient will be able to
  - Achieve adequate functional aerobic capacity and the ability to talk during activity in order to achieve functional gait and activity tolerance for work, play, school, self-care, ADLs, and IADLs.
  - Achieve functional gait in the home and community (with or without a device), allowing for work, play, self-care ADLs, and IADLs, up to _____ feet based on patient's need and prior functional level.
  - Achieve 600 m or greater in a 6-minute walk test for initiation of safe functional gait in the community.
  - Perform active verbalization with increasing taxonomy for safety during gait, including negotiation of even and uneven surfaces, opening and closing doors, transferring in and out of a car.
  - Determine when patient last ate and if medication taken as directed.
  - Tolerate 30 minutes of continuous moderate exercise three times a week in _____ weeks, and five times a week in _____ weeks, depending on disease severity.

PROGNOSIS

- As this pathology is primarily medical in nature, the physician establishes the medical prognosis.
- Prognosis is usually good and the condition may be asymptomatic.
- From a PT perspective, the prognosis to return to premorbid functional status is good.
- Outcome is usually very good.

PATIENT RESOURCE

- Hashimoto's disease. National Endocrine and Metabolic Diseases Information Service. http://www.endocrine.niddk.nih.gov/pubs/hashimoto. Accessed July 5, 2013.

REFERENCES

1. APTA. *Guide to Physical Therapy Practice*. Atlanta, GA: American Physical Therapy Association; 2003. http://guidetoptpractice.apta.org. Accessed July 5, 2013.
2. McPhee SJ, Hammer GD. Formation & secretion of thyroid hormones. In: McPhee SJ, Hammer GD, eds. *Pathophysiology of Disease*. 6th ed. New York, NY: McGraw-Hill; 2010. http://www.accessphysiotherapy.com/content/5371509. Accessed July 5, 2013.

ADDITIONAL REFERENCES

- Baskin HJ, Cobin RH, Duick DS,et al. American Association of Clinical Endocrinologists medical guidelines for clinical practice for the evaluation and treatment of hyperthyroidism and hypothyroidism. *Endocr Pract*. 2002;8(6):457–469.
- Bauer DC, McPhee SJ. Thyroid disease. In: McPhee SJ, Hammer GD, eds. *Pathophysiology of Disease*. 6th ed. New York, NY: McGraw-Hill; 2010. http://www.accessphysiotherapy.com/content/5371611. Accessed July 5, 2013.
- Chandrasoma P, Taylor CR. The thyroid gland. In: Chandrasoma P, Taylor CR, eds. *Concise Pathology*. 3rd ed. New York, NY: McGraw-Hill; 1998. http://www.accessphysiotherapy.com/content/192117. Accessed July 5, 2013.
- Fazio S, Palmieri EA, Lombardi G, Biondi B. Effects of thyroid hormone on the cardiovascular system. *Recent Prog Horm Res*. 2004;59:31–50.
- Goodman CC, Fuller KS. *Pathology: Implications for the Physical Therapist*. 3rd ed. Philadelphia, PA: Saunders Elsevier; 2009.
- Goodman CC, Snyder TK. *Differential Diagnosis for Physical Therapists: Screening for Referral*. 4th ed. St. Louis, MO: Saunders Elsevier; 2007.
- Reid JR, Wheeler SF. Hyperthyroidism: diagnosis and treatment. *Am Fam Physician*. 2005;72(4):623–630.
- Staii A, Mirocha S, Todorova-Koteva K, Glinberg S, Jaume JC. Hashimoto thyroiditis is more frequent than expected when diagnosed by cytology which uncovers a pre-clinical state. *Thyroid Res*. 2010;3(1):11. doi:10.1186/1756–6614–3–11.
- Wémeau JL. Hashimoto's thyroiditis (hypertrophic chronic lymphocytic thyroiditis): the centennial of a discovery. *Presse Med*. 2012;41(12 P 2):e609–e610. doi: 10.1016/j.lpm.2012.10.004.
- Zeitler PS, Travers SH, Nadeau K, Barker J, Kelsey MM, Kappy MS. Endocrine disorders. In: Hay WW, Levin MJ, Sondheimer JM, Deterding RR, eds. *CURRENT Diagnosis & Treatment: Pediatrics*. 20th ed. New York, NY: McGraw-Hill; 2011. http://www.accessphysiotherapy.com/content/6588008. Accessed March 5, 2013.

26 HYPERPARATHYROIDISM

Debra F. Stern, DPT, DBA, MSM, PT
Eric Shamus, PhD, DPT, PT, CSCS

CONDITION/DISORDER SYNONYM

- Primary Hyperparathyroidism

ICD-9-CM CODES

- 252.0 Hyperparathyroidism
- 252.00 Hyperparathyroidism, unspecified
- 252.01 Primary hyperparathyroidism
- 252.08 Other hyperparathyroidism
- 252.02 Secondary hyperparathyroidism, nonrenal
- 588.81 Secondary hyperparathyroidism (of renal origin)
- Associated ICD-9-CM PT diagnoses/treatment diagnoses that may be directly related
    - 315.4 Developmental coordination disorder
    - 718.45 Contracture of joint, pelvic region and thigh
    - 719.70 Difficulty in walking involving joint site unspecified
    - 728.2 Muscular wasting and disuse atrophy not elsewhere classified
    - 728.89 Other disorders of muscle, ligament, and fascia
    - 729.9 Other and unspecified disorders of soft tissue
    - 780.7 Malaise and fatigue
    - 781.2 Abnormality of gait
    - 782.3 Edema
    - 786.0 Dyspnea and respiratory abnormalities
    - 786.05 Shortness of breath

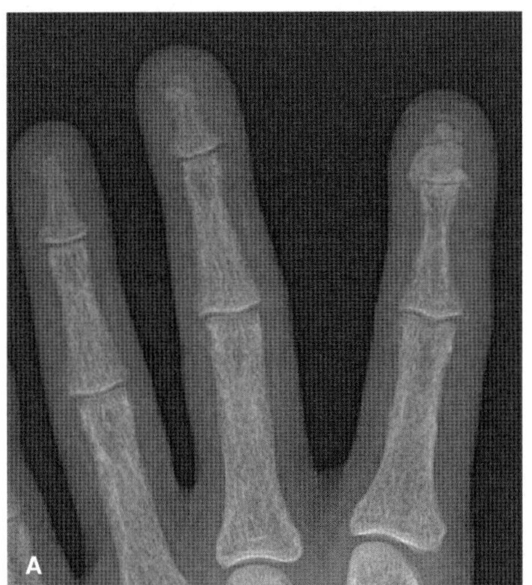

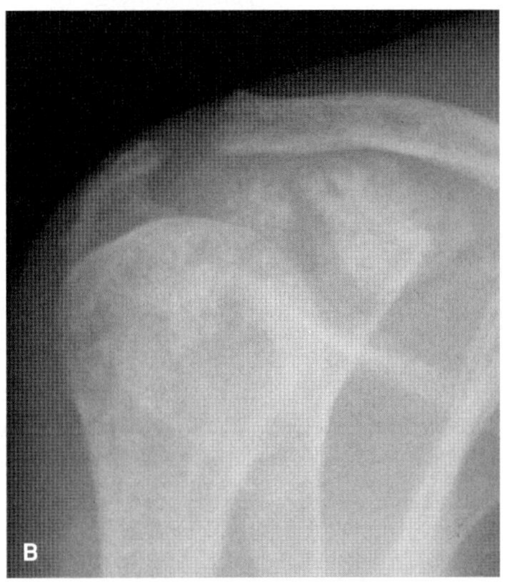

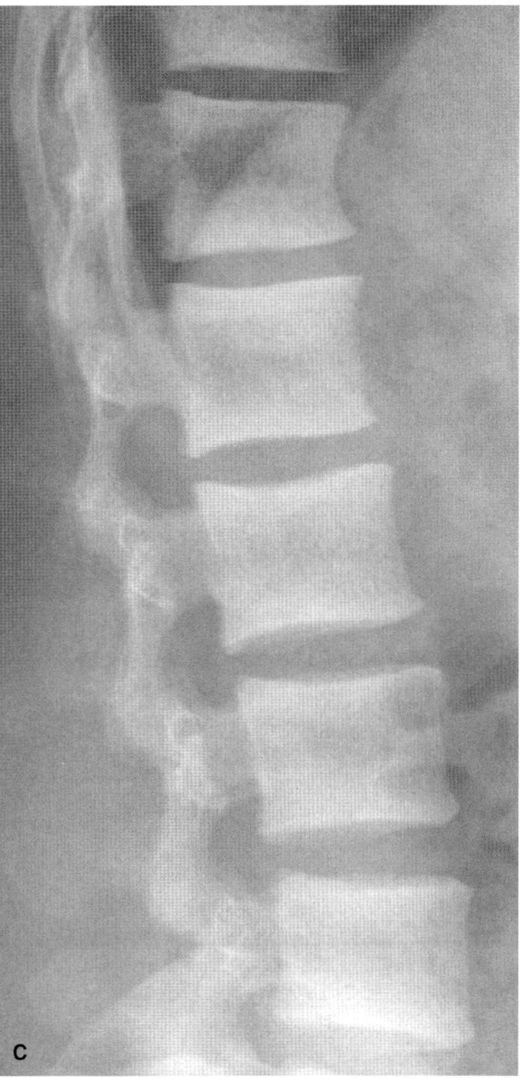

FIGURE 26-1 Skeletal changes of hyperparathyroidism. **A.** Subperiosteal resorption of the phalanges and calcification of the digital arteries. **B.** Erosion of the distal clavicle and soft tissue calcification. **C.** "Rugger jersey" spine. (From Imboden J, Hellmann DB, Stone JH. *Current Rheumatology Diagnosis & Treatment*. 2nd ed. http://www.accessmedicine.com.)

ICD-10-CM CODES

- E21 Hyperparathyroidism and other disorders of parathyroid gland
- E21.0 Primary hyperparathyroidism
- E21.1 Secondary hyperparathyroidism, not elsewhere classified
- E21.2 Other hyperparathyroidism
- E21.3 Hyperparathyroidism, unspecified
- N25.81 Secondary hyperparathyroidism of renal origin
- R19.2 Hyperperistalsis

PREFERRED PRACTICE PATTERNS[1]

- 4D: Impaired Joint Mobility, Motor Function, Muscle Performance, and Range of Motion Associated with Connective Tissue Dysfunction
- 4E: Impaired Joint Mobility, Motor Function, Muscle Performance, and Range of Motion Associated with Localized Inflammation
- 6B: Impaired Aerobic Capacity/Endurance Associated with Deconditioning

PATIENT PRESENTATION

A 66-year-old male referred to physical therapy with cervical pain. In his history, he stated that he was recently diagnosed with low Vitamin D and was put on a supplement. His doctor told him his circulating calcium levels were a bit elevated, but that he was not concerned and would check it again in 6 months. He complains of some mild loss of appetite, but is happy about it because he needs to lose a few pounds. Most surprising to him was when his bone density was tested at a recent health fair and he was told he had osteopenia. He also complains of recent onset of constipation. Cervical assessment demonstrated mild limitation in ROM and muscles pulling especially with forward flexion. In addition, when actively forward flexing, he described feeling like "maybe there was lump in his throat."

KEY FEATURES

Description

- Excess of systemic hyperparathyroid hormone (PTH) (hypersecretion) from one or more of the four parathyroid glands
  - Hormone regulates calcium in the bloodstream, producing hypercalcemia and hyperphosphatemia
- May be primary or secondary to another disease process
- Primary hyperparathyroidism (HPT) (most common)
  - Enlargement of one of the glands
  - Excess production of the hormone
  - Increased calcium in the blood/hypercalcemia
- Secondary hyperthyroidism
  - Secondary disease causing low levels of calcium in the body
  - Chromic renal insufficiency
  - Calcium malabsorption
  - Osteomalacia
- Tertiary hyperparathyroidism
  - Glandular hyperfunction and hypersecretion even after correction of abnormality

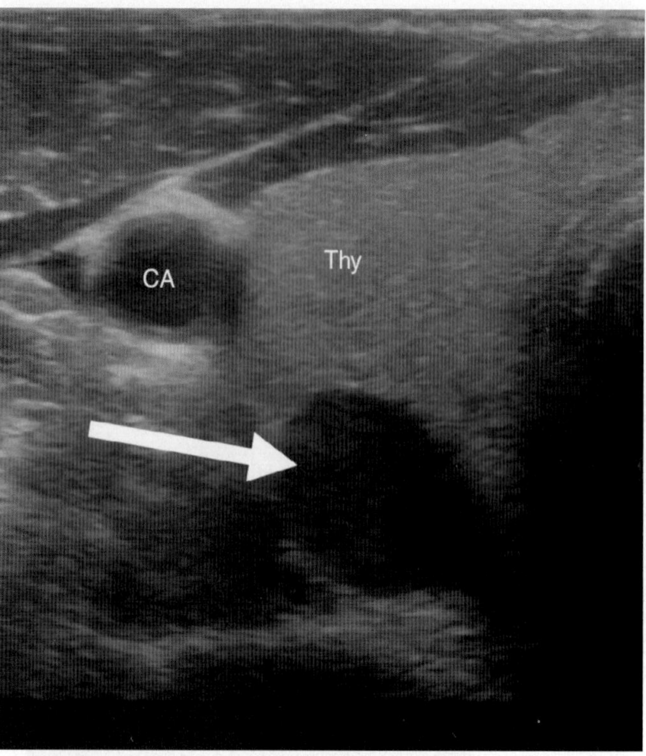

FIGURE 26-2 Transverse image from a B-mode ultrasound image of the thyroid bed demonstrating a large, ovoid hypoechoic lesion consistent with a parathyroid adenoma (*white arrow*). Also seen are the carotid artery (CA) and the thyroid gland (Thy). (From Lalwani AK. *Current Diagnosis & Treatment in Otolaryngology-Head & Neck Surgery*. 3rd ed. www.accesssurgery.com. Copyright © The McGraw-Hill Companies, Inc. All rights reserved.)

  - Caused by chronic renal failure
- Quartary hyperthyroidism
  - After surgical removal of primary hyperparathyroidism
- Familial hypocalciuric hypercalcemia (FHH)
  - Autosomal inheritance

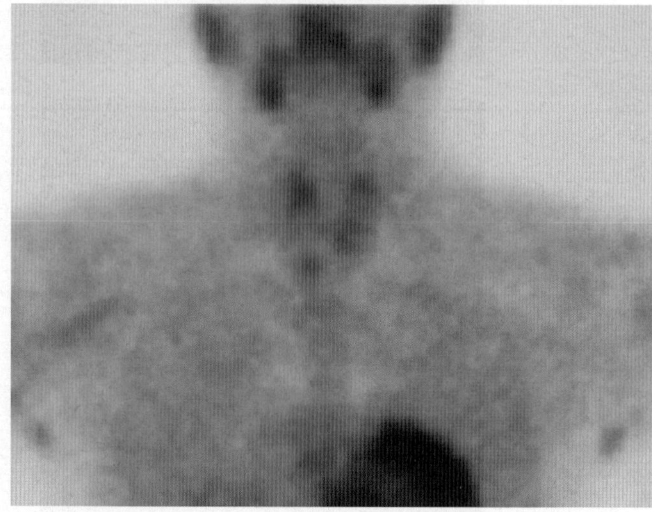

FIGURE 26-3 Images from a ^{99m}technetium-sestamibi scan 2 hours after injection in a patient with renal hyperparathyroidism showing uptake in each of four hyperplastic parathyroid glands. Note that the right inferior parathyroid gland has descended into an ectopic location in the anterior mediastinum. (From Lalwani AK. *Current Diagnosis & Treatment in Otolaryngology-Head & Neck Surgery*. 3rd ed. www.accesssurgery.com. Copyright © The McGraw-Hill Companies, Inc. All rights reserved.)

Essentials of Diagnosis

- Usually diagnosed before symptoms occur via complete blood count (CBC) test
- Elevated calcium in the blood
- Elevated parathyroid hormone
- Decreased phosphorus in the blood
- Vitamin D deficiency

General Considerations

- May cause pathology in multiple organ systems
  - Gastrointestinal (GI): Liver
  - Cardiovascular: Heart, peripheral circulation, blood pressure
  - Integument
- Decreased calcium in the bones
- May result in secondary problems such as aerobic capacity and muscle endurance impairment, sarcopenia, weakness/impaired muscle performance, musculoskeletal problems, neuromuscular problems, indicating the need for physical therapy intervention depending on severity

Demographics

- Primary type in adults: 1:1000 in the Unites States[2]
- More common in individuals with Columbia descent
- More common over age 50
- More common in females after menopause[2]

CLINICAL FINDINGS

SIGNS AND SYMPTOMS

- Signs and symptoms of primary hyperparathyroidism
- Abdominal pain
- Abdominal pain
- Blood in urine
- Bone cysts
- Bone pain
- Cardiovascular disease (usually as a result of high calcium): Small-vessel necrosis
- Depression
- Excessive urination
- Fatigue
- Forgetfulness
- Frequent complaints of illness, unknown etiology
- Hypercalcemia
- Hypertension
- Impaired muscle function
- Joint pain
- Kidney stones
- Loss of appetite/anorexia
- Mental changes, confusion
- Nausea
- Osteoporosis/osteomalacia
- Pancreatitis (rare)
- Pseudogout
- Skin necrosis
- Urinary tract infections (UTIs)
- Vomiting
- Weakness
- Weight loss

Functional Implications

- Anxiety and irritability
- Decreased exercise tolerance
- Fatigue
- Inability or reluctance to leave home secondary to excessive urination, not feeling well
- Inability to focus
- Kidney disease
- Limitations in activities of daily living (ADLs) or instrumental activities of daily living (IADLs)
- Muscle performance deficits, inability to ambulate or perform self-care as well as aerobic capacity limitation secondary to inactivity
- Neuropathy, increased risk for falls
- Osteoporosis
- Pathological fractures
- Shortness of breath
- Sleep disturbances
- Systemic infection
- Untreated hyperparathyroidism in pregnant women may cause dangerously low levels of calcium in newborns

Possible Contributing Causes

- Solitary adenomas causes primary hyperparathyroidism 85%[2]
- Parathyroid hyperplasia causes primary hyperparathyroidism 10%[2]
- Parathyroid Carcinoma causes primary hyperparathyroidism 2% to 5%[2]
- Multiple adenomas causes primary hyperparathyroidism 2%[2]
- Noncompliance with medication regiments/inability to pay
- Changes in lifestyle
- Inappropriate self-medication
- Vitamin D deficiency
- Benign parathyroid tumors
- Enlargement of two or more parathyroid glands
- Heredity, genetic disorder
  - Multiple endocrine neoplasia: Type 1
- Calcium deficiency
- Chronic kidney/renal failure
- Menopause
- Multiple endocrine neoplasia
- Radiation to the neck
- Lithium use

Differential Diagnosis

- Autoimmune diseases (i.e., sarcoidosis)
- Bladder infections, UTIs, kidney pathology
- Bowel disorders
- Corticosteroid therapy
- Differential diagnosis of hypercalcemia
- Endocrine disorders
- Hypercalcemia
- Hypercalcemia
- Hyperthyroidism
- Infections in the abdomen
- Multiple myeloma
- Non-malignant tumors in the abdomen or organs
- Prolonged bed rest
- Renal dysfunction as result of cancer or malignancy
- Tuberculosis
- Vitamin D deficiency
- Vitamin D toxicity

MEANS OF CONFIRMATION OR DIAGNOSIS

Laboratory Tests

- CBC
- 24-hour urine collection
- Urinalysis
- Thyroid function test

Imaging

- Ultrasound
- X-rays
- CT scans
  - Sestamibi scan (CT scan with radioactive compound)

- MRI
  - Imaging of kidneys
- Bone mineral density test
- ECG

FINDINGS AND INTERPRETATION

- Laboratory findings in hypercalcemia from various causes
- Elevated calcium in the blood
- Elevated parathyroid hormone
- Decreased phosphorus in the blood
- Vitamin D deficiency

TREATMENT

▸ Medication

- Hormone replacement therapy
- Bisphosphonates
- Calcimimetic agents
- Calcium supplements
- Vitamin D supplements

MEDICAL PROCEDURES

- Surgery, removal of one to three glands

REFERRALS/ADMITTANCE

- If patient is referred for PT and causative problem is not considered appropriate for PT, refer to appropriate physician.
- If an emergency is identified, refer to ER.
- If patient's history and reactions to PT indicate possible hyperthyroid and/or symptoms, refer to a physician.

IMPAIRMENTS

- Muscle weakness
- Muscle spasm
- Gait abnormality/difficulty walking
- Shortness of breath, fatigue
- Limited aerobic capacity
- Inability to perform self-care
- Balance impairment
- Impaired skin integrity

TESTS AND MEASURES

- Observation
  - Scars may indicate adhesions or abdominal surgeries.
  - Pink or purplish striae may be indicative of Cushing syndrome.
  - Dilated veins may indicate hepatic pathology or inferior vena cava obstruction, not diverticulitis.
  - Contour: Roundedness, concavity/hollowness, asymmetry, distension, pregnancy signs.
  - Cullen sign: Bluish discoloring around umbilicus, which may be a sign of retroperitoneal bleeding.
  - Bluish discoloration in lower abdomen: Grey Turner sign, a sign of hemorrhagic pancreatitis.
  - Bulging in groin or other area of abdomen especially apparent with contraction of musculature in area may be hernia.
  - Pulsing in area of the navel may be abdominal aortic aneurysm.
  - Palpable abdominal tenderness: On left/right or generalized.
  - Psoas sign: Provides resistance over patient's right knee as patient flexes hip.
  - Pain is indicative of appendicitis or possible inflammation of abdomen.
  - Obturator sign: Internal rotation of right lower extremity and flexion may be indicative of appendicitis or pelvic inflammation.
  - Rovsing sign: Pain on right side of abdomen when pressure is put on the left may be indicative of appendicitis.
- Because there may be GI signs associated with hypoparathyroidism, the following tests and measures are necessary:
- Palpation of thyroid/neck
  - Test for enlargement of thyroid or any abnormalities
  - Skin changes
  - Vital signs
  - Chvostek sign: Tap on the face at a point just anterior to the ear and just below the zygomatic bone; positive response in hypoparathyroid; twitching of the ipsilateral facial muscles, suggests neuromuscular excitability caused by hypocalcemia.
  - Trousseau sign: Inflate a sphygmomanometer cuff above systolic blood pressure for several minutes; positive response in hypoparathyroid, muscular contraction including flexion of the wrist and metacarpophalangeal joints, hyperextension of the fingers, and flexion of the thumb on the palm, suggesting neuromuscular excitability.
  - Abdominal palpation, may be enlargement of ovaries.
  - Kidneys: In supine position, place one hand under patient between ribs and iliac crest, other hand on abdomen below ribs and pointing in opposite direction: +/− tenderness or reproduction of symptoms.
  - Bladder: Not usually palpable unless it is distended and rises above pubic bone; in supine position, place hand above pubis and press down: +/= tenderness, reproduction of pain, or ability to feel the bladder: __ + __ −.
  - Appendix (McBurney's): Apply vertical pressure halfway between right anterior superior iliac spine (ASIS) and umbilicus.
  - Liver: In supine position, with left hand under trunk parallel to 11th and 12th rib, lift upward; right hand lateral to rectus and press in and up: +/= reproduction of symptoms with deep breath.
  - Ascites: With the fingers, percuss outward from center; if sound is dull, ascites may be present.
  - Spleen: It is not recommended for PT to palpate an enlarged spleen (only palpable if enlarged) because of the potential of rupture.
  - Gallbladder (Murphy's): Place fingers right of rectus abdominus below rib cage: +/= sudden pain and muscle tensing with deep breath.

INTERVENTION

- PT intervention is consistent with movement-related problems that occur secondary to hypoparathyroidism and include
  - Gait training
  - Therapeutic exercise: All relevant categories, energy conservation
    - Stretching if contractures present in neck postsurgery
  - Therapeutic activities for bed mobility, transfer-, and transitional-movement training
  - Self-care management training including skin care/moisturizing, lifestyle management
  - Neuromuscular re-education: Balance and postural training
  - Soft tissue mobilization if contractures present in neck postsurgery

FUNCTIONAL GOALS

- Patient will be able to
  - Extend and rotate head and neck left and right with adequate functional range in all directions to safely use mirrors while driving (if postsurgical).
  - Achieve adequate functional aerobic capacity and ability to talk during activity to achieve functional gait and activity tolerance for work, play, school, self-care; ADLs, and IADLs.
  - Achieve functional gait in the home and community (with or without a device), allowing for work, play, self-care; ADLs, and IADLs, up to _____ feet, based on patient's need and prior functional level.
  - Achieve 600 m or greater in a 6-minute walk test for initiation of safe functional gait in the community.
  - Perform active verbalization with increasing taxonomy for safety during gait, including negotiation of even and uneven surfaces, opening and closing doors, and transferring in and out of a car.
  - Tolerate 30 minutes of continuous moderate exercise three times a week in _____ weeks, and five times a week in _____ weeks, depending on disease severity.

PROGNOSIS

- As this pathology is primarily medical, physician establishes medical prognosis.
- Prognosis from a PT perspective is based on effective medical management to return to healthy level of function, prior to onset of disease, if individual is receiving care secondary to problems related to hyperparathyroidism.

PATIENT RESOURCE

- American Thyroid Association. http://www.thyroid.org. Accessed August 8, 2014.

REFERENCES

1. The American Physical Therapy Association. *Interactive Guide to Physical Therapist Practice*. Alexandria, VA: The American Physical Therapy Association; 2003. http://guidetoptpractice.apta.org/. Accessed July 5, 2013.
2. Shoback DM, Sellmeyer DE. Disorders of the parathyroids & calcium & phosphorus metabolism. In: McPhee SJ, Hammer GD, eds. *Pathophysiology of Disease*. 6th ed. New York, NY: McGraw-Hill; 2010. http://www.accessphysiotherapy.com/content/5370820. Accessed July 5, 2013.

ADDITIONAL REFERENCES

- Baskin HJ, Cobin RH, Duick DS, et al. American Association of Clinical Endocrinologists medical guidelines for clinical practice for the evaluation and treatment of hyperthyroidism and hypothyroidism. *Endocr Pract*. 2002;8(6):457–469.
- Bryant LR, Wulsin JH, Altemeier WA. Hyperparathyroidism and hypoparathyroidism. *Ann Surg*. 1964;159:411–415.
- Colcher A, Hurtig HI. Systemic illnesses that cause movement disorders. In: Watts RL, Standaert DG, Obeso JA, eds. *Movement Disorders*. 3rd ed. New York, NY: McGraw-Hill; 2012. http://www.accessphysiotherapy.com/content/55806123. Accessed July 5, 2013.
- Dutton M. Parathyroid disorders. In: Dutton M, ed. *McGraw-Hill's NPTE (National Physical Therapy Examination)*. 2nd ed. New York, NY: McGraw-Hill; 2012. http://www.accessphysiotherapy.com/content/56510065#56510065. Accessed July 5, 2013.
- Goodman CC, Fuller KS. *Pathology: Implications for the Physical Therapist*. 3rd ed. Philadelphia, PA: Saunders Elsevier; 2009.
- Goodman CC, Snyder TK. *Differential Diagnosis for Physical Therapists: Screening for Referral*. 4th ed. St. Louis, MO: Saunders Elsevier; 2007.
- Habib Z, Camacho P. Primary hyperparathyroidism: an update. *Curr Opin Endocrinol Diabetes Obes*. 2010;17(6):554–560.
- Hay WW, Levin MJ, Sondheimer JM, Deterding RR, eds. *CURRENT Diagnosis & Treatment: Pediatrics*. 20th ed. New York, NY: McGraw-Hill; 2011. http://www.accessphysiotherapy.com/resource/14. Accessed July 5, 2013.
- Ng SM, Anand D, Weindling AM. High versus low dose of initial thyroid hormone replacement for congenital hypothyroidism. *Cochrane Database Syst Rev*. 2009;21:CD006972. doi: 10.1002/14651858.CD006972.pub2.
- Parathyroid.com. Norman Parathyroid Center. *Hyperparathyroidism: Disease of the parathyroid glands*. http://www.parathyroid.com/parathyroid-disease.htm. Accessed July 5, 2013.
- Panus PC, Jobst EE, Masters SB, Katzung B, Tinsley SL, Trevor AJ. Growth, thyroid, and gonadal pharmacology. In: Panus PC, Jobst EE, Masters SB, Katzung B, Tinsley SL, Trevor AJ, eds. *Pharmacology for the Physical Therapist*. New York, NY: McGraw-Hill; 2009. http://www.accessphysiotherapy.com/content/6093102. Accessed July 5, 2013.
- Reid JR, Wheeler SF. Hyperthyroidism: diagnosis and treatment. *Am Fam Physician*. 2005;72(4):623–630.
- Tahmi AS, Saunders J, Sinha P. A parathyroid adenoma: benign disease presenting with hyperthyroid crisis. *Case Report Med*. 2010:596185. doi: 10.1155/2010/596185.

27 HYPERTHYROIDISM

Debra F. Stern, DPT, DBA, MSM, PT
Eric Shamus, PhD, DPT, PT, CSCS
Marangela Obispo, MSPT, GCS

CONDITION/DISORDER SYNONYM

- Overactive thyroid

ICD-9-CM CODES

- 242.20 Toxic multinodular goiter without mention of thyrotoxic crisis or storm
- 242.90 Thyrotoxicosis without mention of goiter or other cause, and without mention of thyrotoxic crisis or storm
- PT diagnosis codes that may be secondary to thyroid disorders
  - 315.4 Developmental coordination disorder
  - 709.2 Scar conditions and fibrosis of the skin
  - 719.70 Difficulty in walking involving joint site unspecified
  - 728.2 Muscular wasting and disuse atrophy, not elsewhere classified
  - 728.89 Other disorders of muscle, ligament, and fascia
  - 729.9 Other and unspecified disorders of soft tissue
  - 780.7 Malaise and fatigue
  - 781.2 Abnormality of gait
  - 782.3 Edema
  - 786.0 Dyspnea and respiratory abnormalities
  - 786.05 Shortness of breath

ICD-10-CM CODES

- E05.20 Thyrotoxicosis with toxic multinodular goiter without thyrotoxic crisis or storm
- E05.90 Thyrotoxicosis, unspecified without thyrotoxic crisis or storm

PREFERRED PRACTICE PATTERNS[1]

- 4D: Impaired Joint Mobility, Motor Function, Muscle Performance, and Range of Motion Associated with Connective Tissue Dysfunction
- 6B: Impaired Aerobic Capacity/Endurance Associated with Deconditioning

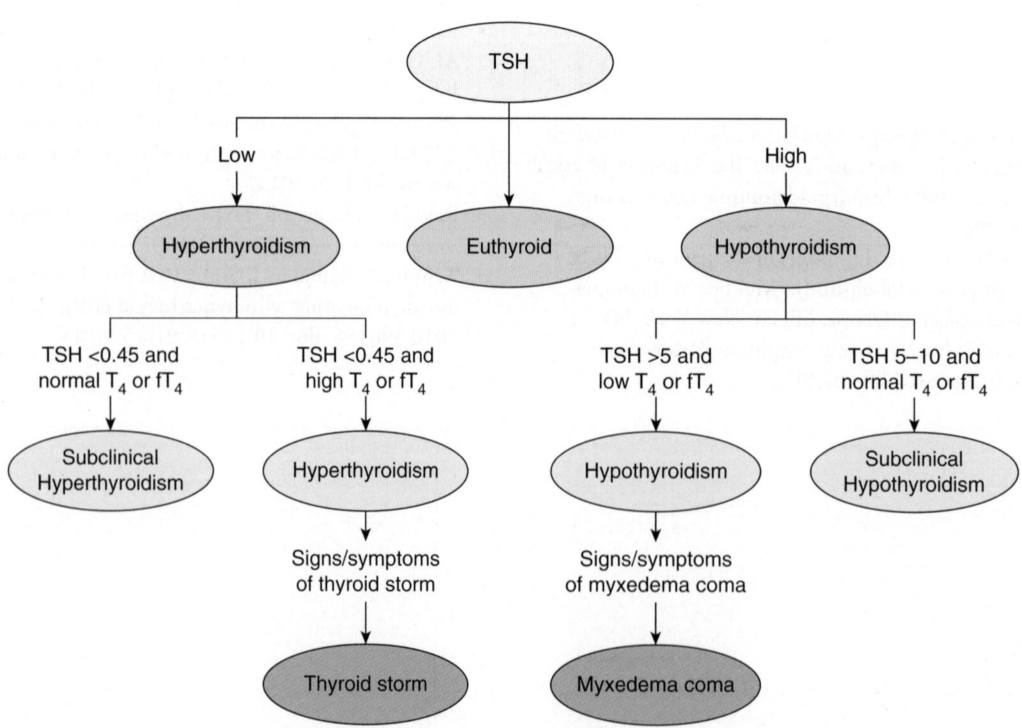

FIGURE 27-1 Algorithm for thyroid function tests. This algorithm does not apply in patients with hypothalamic–pituitary disease, serious illness, or those who are taking certain medications such as amiodarone, glucocorticoids, and dopamine. (From McKean SC, Ross JJ, Dressler DD, Brotman DJ, Ginsberg JS. *Principles and Practice of Hospital Medicine*. www.accessmedicine.com. Copyright © The McGraw-Hill Companies, Inc. All rights reserved.)

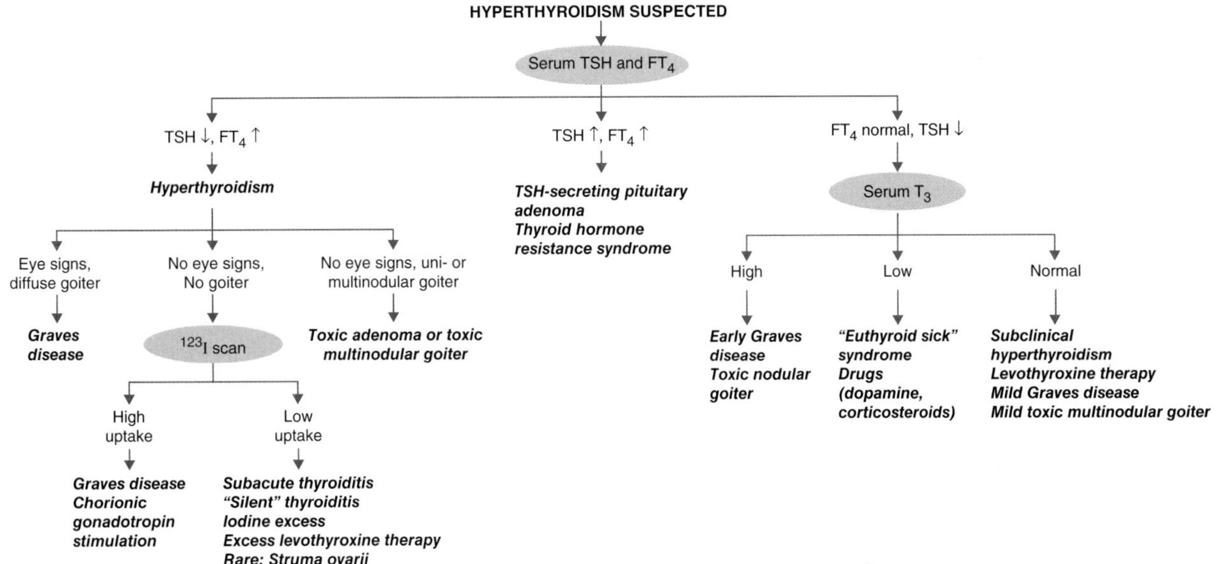

FIGURE 27-2 Hyperthyroidism: laboratory evaluation. **FT_4**, free thyroxine; **T_3**, 3,5,3′-triiodothyronine; **TSH**, thyroid-stimulating hormone. (Modified with permission from Gardner DG, Shoback D, eds. *Greenspan's Basic & Clinical Endocrinology*. 9th ed. Originally published by Appleton & Lange. Copyright © 2011 by the McGraw-Hill Companies, Inc.)

PATIENT PRESENTATION

A 47-year-old female has been suffering from bilateral shoulder pain for the last 2 months, which increases with dressing her upper body and washing her head. She reports a decreased ability to perform her job as an administrative assistant for a lawyer's firm because of pain, difficulty in concentrating which she attributes to being concerned about her shoulder pain, and increased frequency of urination requiring her to leave her workstation several times during the day. She reports that she enjoys running; however, was unable to finish her last 5K because of heat intolerance and palpitations. She has noticed weight loss, however, reports feeling hungry at all times. Upon examination patient presents with clammy skin and mild exophthalmos. Vital signs were normal except heart rate of 110 bpm at rest. ROM was limited in bilateral shoulders. MMT was decreased in bilateral shoulders and bilateral hip flexors. Gait was normal. Endurance was impaired by demonstrating abnormally increased vitals after a gait assessment on short distance. Patient presents with limited ability to perform ADLs, specifically dressing and showering.

KEY FEATURES

Description

- Increased thyroid gland activity
- Characterized by increased basal metabolic rate
- The thyroid regulates metabolism and produces thyroid hormones (thyroxine [T4] and triiodothyronine [T3])
- Hyperthyroidism is a cause of thyrotoxicosis[2]

Essentials of Diagnosis

- It is not the purview of a PT to medically diagnose hypothyroid but rather to recognize the possibility in the differential diagnosis process, especially when findings are not consistent with conditions commonly treated such as musculoskeletal, neuromuscular, integumentary, and cardiopulmonary.
- PTs may treat conditions caused by hyperthyroid or treat patients with hyperthyroidism for other unrelated pathologies.

General Considerations

- May cause pathology in multiple organ systems
  - GI: Liver
  - Cardiovascular: Heart, peripheral circulation, blood pressure
- Integumentary
- May result in secondary problems
  - Aerobic capacity and muscle endurance impairment
  - Sarcopenia
  - Weakness/impaired muscle performance
  - Musculoskeletal problems
  - Neuromuscular problems
  - Weight gain, indicating the need for PT intervention depending on severity

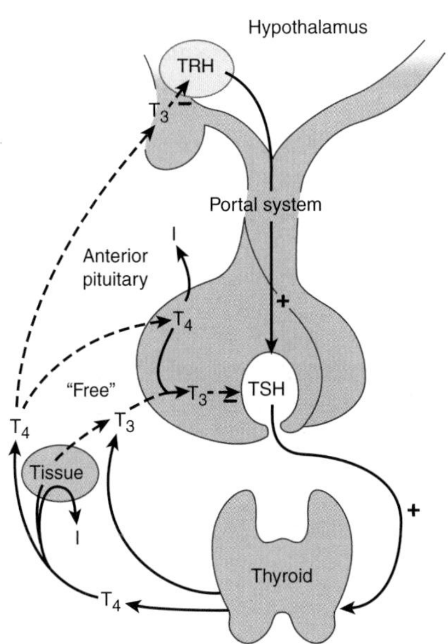

FIGURE 27-3 Hypothalamic–pituitary-thyroid axis. T_4, thyroxine; T_3, triiodothyronine; TRH, thyrotropin-releasing hormone; TSH, thyroid-stimulating hormone. (Redrawn and modified with permission from Greenspan FS, Gardner DG, eds. *Basic and Clinical Endocrinology*. 8th ed. McGraw-Hill; 2007.)

Demographics

- Higher incidence in women[2]
- More difficult to diagnose in the elderly

CLINICAL FINDINGS

SIGNS AND SYMPTOMS

- Graves ophthalmopathy, red or swollen eyes, bulging or protruding eyeballs, impaired vision, inflammation, light sensitivity
- Tachycardia
- Cardiac: Atrial fibrillation, arrhythmias, palpitations
- Heart disease
- Racing/rapid pulse
- High blood pressure
- Hyperactivity
- Difficulty concentrating and focusing
- Heat intolerance
- Sweating, clammy skin
- Confusion, disorientation
- Diuresis
- Weakness
- Tremors
- Neck pain
- Unexplained weight loss with inability to gain weight
- Difficulty swallowing
- Change in voice
- Fatigue[2]
- Decreased activity tolerance
- Sensitivity to cold
- Dyspnea, shortness of breath
- Airway obstruction
- Enlarged thyroid
- Increased appetite
- Menstrual disturbance, irregularity[2]
- Increased bowel frequency
- Breast development in men
- Clammy skin
- Diarrhea
- Hair loss
- Hand tremor
- Itching
- Nausea and vomiting
- Skin blushing or flushing
- Difficulty sleeping
- Osteoporosis

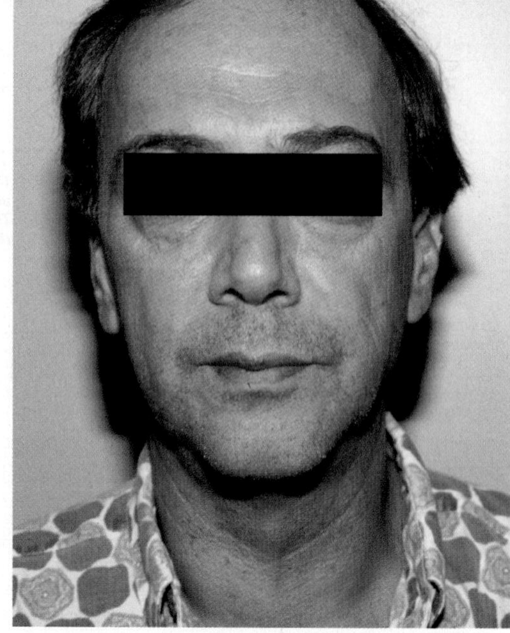

FIGURE 27-4 Hyperthyroidism: exophthalmos and atrial fibrillation manifestations of hyperthyroidism. (From Fuster V, Walsh RA, Harrington RA. *Hurst's The Heart*. 13th ed. www.accessmedicine.com. Copyright © The McGraw-Hill Companies, Inc. All rights reserved.)

Functional Implications

- Severe symptoms such as immediacy of need to urinate, increased volume of urine, and an increase in bowel frequency may be disabling and result in the inability or reluctance to leave home.
- Sarcopenia resulting in weakness, muscle-mass loss, inability to ambulate or perform self-care as well as aerobic capacity limitation secondary to inactivity.

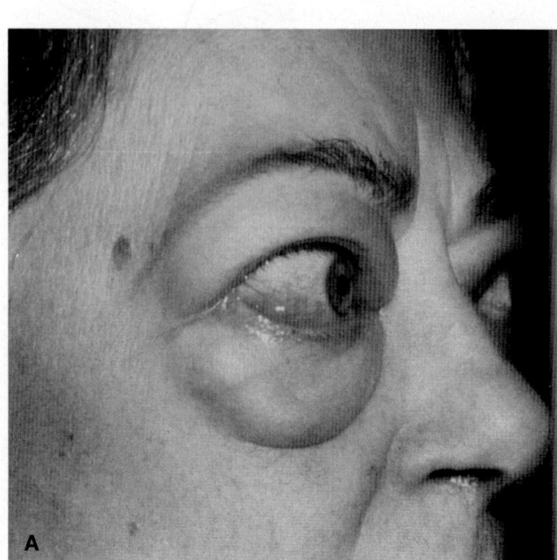

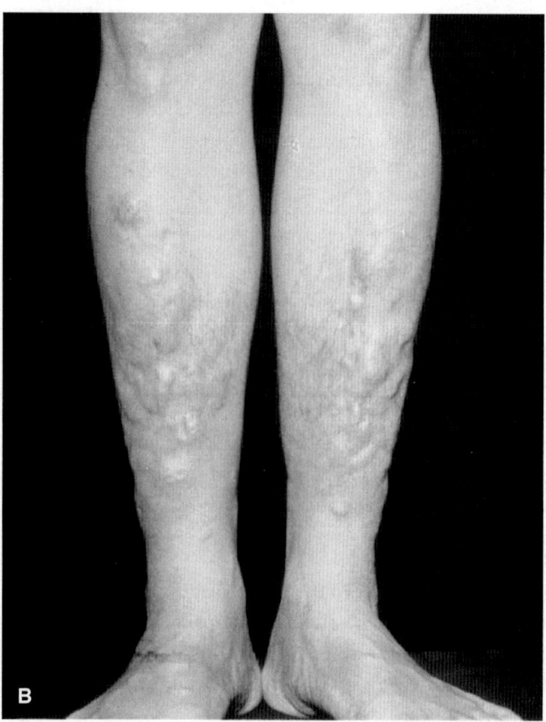

FIGURE 27-5 Clinical features of hyperthyroidism. The patient shows (**A**) ophthalmopathy with exophthalmos (proptosis), and (**B**) pretibial myxedema. (From Brunicardi CF, Andersen DK, Billiar TR, et al. *Schwartz's Principles of Surgery*. 9th ed. New York, NY: McGraw Hill; 2009.)

- Decreased exercise tolerance
- Limitations in ADLs or IADLs
- Neuropathy, increased risk for falls
- Vision impairment, driving issues
- Voice changes, hoarseness

Possible Contributing Causes

- Autoimmune or Hashimoto thyroiditis
- Body production of too much thyroid hormone
- Cancer
- Chemical inducement
- Congenital birth defects
- Female
- Getting too much iodine
- Graves disease
- Older than age 50
- Growths/tumor of the thyroid or pituitary gland
- Heredity
- Inflammation of the thyroid
- Metastatic cancer
- Pituitary dysfunction/tumors as the pituitary signals production of thyroid stimulating hormone (TSH)
- Plummer disease (toxic multinodular goiter)
- Radiation to the brain
- Radiation treatments to the neck
- Taking large amounts or overdoses of thyroid hormone
- Testicular or ovarian tumors
- Thyroiditis
- Toxic adenoma
- Viral thyroiditis

Differential Diagnosis

- Organ dysfunction as a result of cancer or malignancy, especially the liver
- Severe anemia[2]
- Pituitary dysfunction
- Non-malignant tumors in the abdomen or organs
- Pheochromocytoma[2]
- Testicular tumors
- Endocrine disorders
- Gastroparesis
- Gynecologic problems in females
- Autoimmune diseases that affect the upper and lower GI tracts, Crohn or irritable bowel syndrome, systemic lupus erythematosus, rheumatoid arthritis (as they involve organs and have a fatigue component)
- Bladder infections, urinary tract infections, kidney pathology
- Chronic infections in the abdomen[2]
- Bowel disorders

MEANS OF CONFIRMATION OR DIAGNOSIS

Laboratory Tests

- Blood tests/lab tests: Complete blood count (CBC)
- Thyroid function: TSH, T3, T4 (usually high)
- Abnormal thyroid function tests[2]
- Cholesterol
- Liver enzymes
- Prolactin
- Sodium levels low (normal range: 135 to 145 mEq/L)

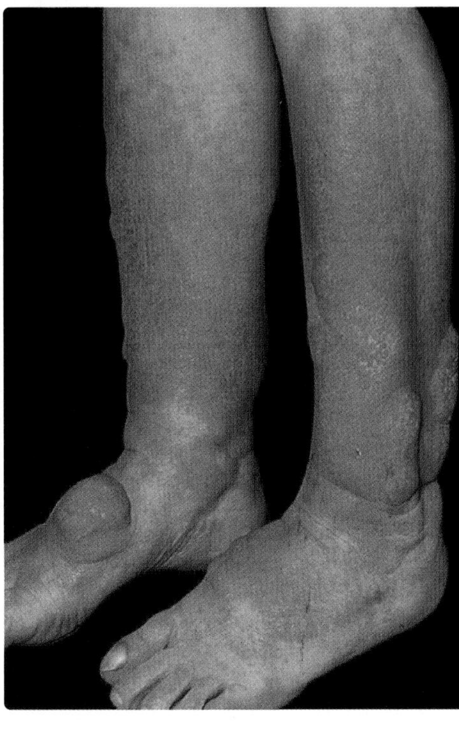

FIGURE 27-6 Hyperthyroidism with thyroid dermopathy in a classic location on the anterior shins. Note that infiltrated plaques extend to the calf and are partially hyperkeratotic. An isolated nodule is also present on the dorsum of the foot. (From Goldsmith LA, Katz S, Gilchrest B, Paller A, Leffell DJ, Wolff K. *Fitzpatrick's Dermatology in General Medicine*. 8th ed. www.accessmedicine.com. Copyright © The McGraw-Hill Companies, Inc. All rights reserved.)

Imaging

- Ultrasound
- Chest X-ray
- CT scans
- MRIs

FINDINGS AND INTERPRETATION

- Thyroid function: TSH (usually low) and T3 and T4 (usually high)
- Abnormal thyroid function tests
- Prolactin (may be elevated in women)
- Sodium levels low in hypothyroid
- Radioactive iodine uptake by the thyroid is increased[2]

TREATMENT

Medication

- Antithyroid medications
  - Methimazole (tapazole)
  - Propylthiouracil (PTU)
- Beta-blockers (to control the cardiac symptoms and anxiety)
- Other
  - Radioactive iodine to destroy the thyroid
  - Surgical removal of thyroid (making thyroid hormone a lifelong necessity)
  - Newer treatment options under investigation include
    - Endoscopic subtotal thyroidectomy
    - Embolization of the thyroid arteries
    - Plasmapheresis
    - Percutaneous ethanol injection of toxic thyroid nodules
    - Autotransplantation of cryopreserved thyroid
  - Nutritional supplementation with L-carnitine

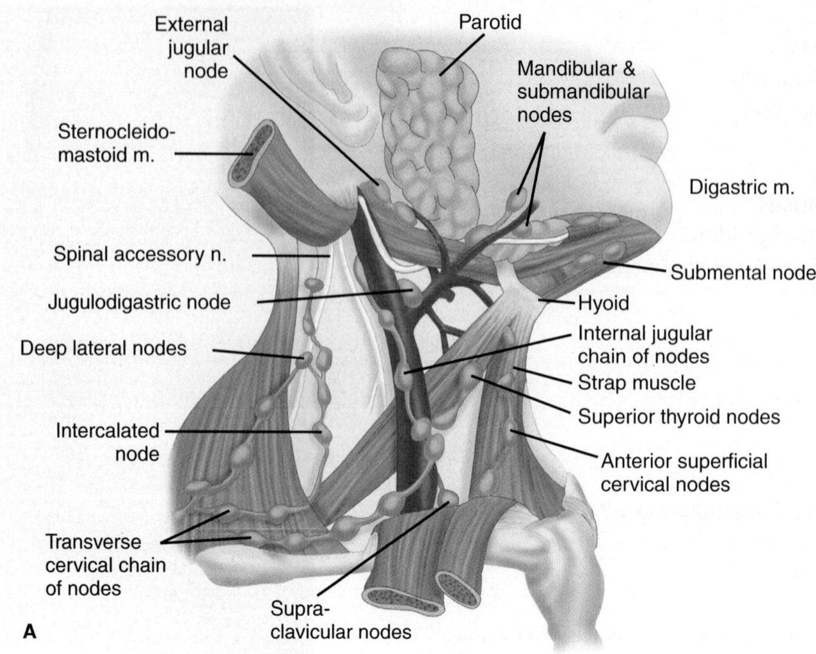

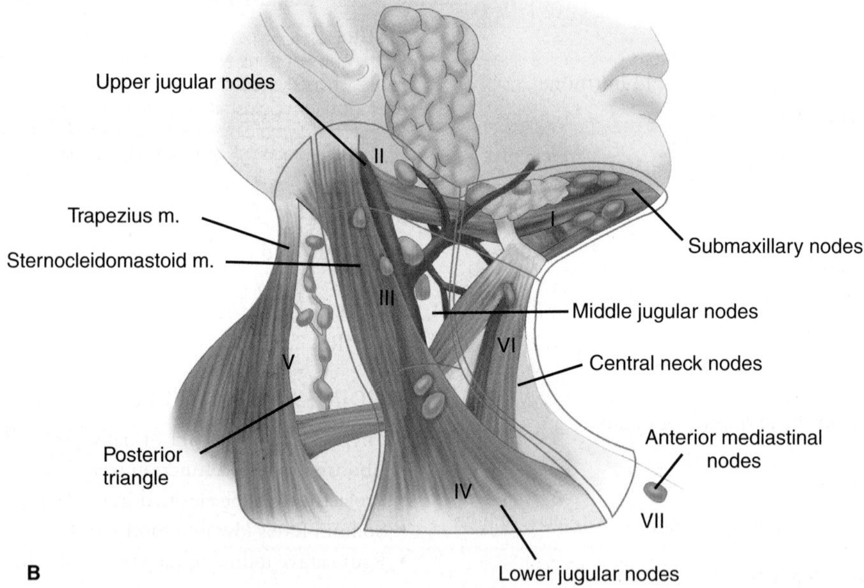

FIGURE 27-7 **A.** and **B.** Lymph nodes in the neck can be divided into six regions. Upper mediastinal nodes constitute level VII. m., muscle; n., nerve. (From Brunicardi CF, Andersen DK, Billiar TR, et al. *Schwartz's Principles of Surgery*. 9th ed. New York, NY: McGraw Hill; 2009.)

REFERRALS/ADMITTANCE

- If a patient is referred for PT and the causative problem is not considered appropriate for PT, refer to the appropriate physician.
- If an emergency is identified, refer to ER.
- If the patient's history and reactions to PT indicate possible hyperthyroidism and or symptoms, refer to a physician.
- Lifestyle modification
- Physician: Smoking cessation
- Physician/nutritionist for weight management
- Nutritionist for dietary counseling
- Optometry
- Ophthalmology
- Audiology
- Psychological intervention
- Occupational therapy
- Speech language pathology

IMPAIRMENTS

- Balance impairment
- Gait abnormality/difficulty walking
- Impaired skin integrity
- Inability to perform self-care
- Limited aerobic capacity
- Muscle atrophy
- Muscle weakness
- Shortness of breath, fatigue

TESTS AND MEASURES

- Observation
  - Scars may indicate adhesions or abdominal surgeries.

- Pink or purplish striae may be indicative of Cushing syndrome.
- Dilated veins may indicate hepatic pathology or inferior vena cava obstruction, not diverticulitis.
- Abdominal contour: Roundedness, concavity/hollowness, asymmetry, distension, pregnancy signs.
- Cullen sign: Bluish discoloring around umbilicus, which may be a sign of retroperitoneal bleeding.
- Bluish discoloration in lower abdomen: Grey Turner sign, which is a sign of hemorrhagic pancreatitis.
- Bulging in groin or other areas of abdomen especially apparent with contraction of musculature in area may be hernia.
- Pulsing in the area of the navel may be abdominal aortic aneurysm.
- Palpable abdominal tenderness on left/right or generalized.
- Psoas sign: Provides resistance over patient's right knee as they flex the hip; pain is indicative of appendicitis or possible inflammation of the abdomen.
- Obturator sign: Internal rotation of right lower extremity and flexion may be indicative of appendicitis or pelvic inflammation.
- Rovsing sign: Pain on the right side of abdomen when pressure is put on the left may be indicative of appendicitis.

- Because there may be GI signs associated with hyperthyroid, GI tests and measures are included in this section.
- Palpation of thyroid/neck for enlargement of thyroid or any abnormalities.
  - Skin changes: Turgor, dryness, hairlessness with hyperthyroid, sweaty, clammy.
  - Abdominal palpation, may be enlargement of ovaries.
  - Kidneys: In supine, place one hand under client between ribs and iliac crest, and other hand on abdomen below ribs and pointing in opposite direction: +/− tenderness or reproduction of symptoms.
  - Bladder
    - Not usually palpable unless it is distended and rises above pubic bone.
    - In supine, place hand above pubis and press down: +/= t enderness, reproduction of pain, or ability to feel the bladder: __+ __−.
  - Appendix (McBurney's): Apply vertical pressure halfway between right anterior superior iliac spine (ASIS) and umbilicus.
  - Liver: In supine, with left hand under trunk parallel to 11th and 12th rib, lift upward; right hand lateral to rectus and press in and up: +/= reproduction of symptoms with deep breath.
  - Ascites: With the fingers, percuss outward from center; if sound is dull, ascites may be present.
  - Spleen: It is not recommended for PT to palpate an enlarged spleen (only palpable if enlarged) because of the potential of rupture.
  - Gallbladder (Murphy's): Place fingers right of rectus abdominus below rib cage: +/= sudden pain and muscle tensing with deep breath.

INTERVENTION

- PT intervention is consistent with the movement-related problems that occur secondary to diabetes and include
  - Gait training.
  - Therapeutic exercise: All relevant categories, energy conservation.
    - Stretching if contractures present in neck postsurgery.
    - PT should inquire about the medication taken. If glucose >300, exercise should be avoided.
  - Therapeutic activities for bed mobility training, transfer, and transitional movement training.
  - Self-care management training including skin care/moisturizing, lifestyle management.
  - Neuromuscular re-education; balance and postural training.
  - Soft tissue mobilization if contractures present in neck postsurgery.

FUNCTIONAL GOALS

- Patient will be able to
  - Extend and rotate head and neck left/right with adequate functional range in all directions to safely use mirrors while driving (if postsurgery).
  - Achieve adequate functional aerobic capacity, and the ability to talk during activity, in order to achieve functional gait and activity tolerance for work, play, school, and self-care as well as ADLs and IADLs.
  - Functional gait in the home and community (with or without a device), allowing for work, play, and self-care as well as ADLs and IADLs, up to __ feet, based on patient's need and prior functional level.
  - Achieve 600 m or greater in a 6-minute walk test for initiation of safe functional gait in the community.
  - Perform active verbalization with increasing taxonomy for safety during gait, including negotiation of even and uneven surfaces, opening and closing doors, and transferring in and out of a car.
  - Tolerate 30 minutes of continuous moderate exercise three times a week in __ weeks, and five times a week in __ weeks, depending on disease severity.

PROGNOSIS

- As this pathology is primarily medical in nature, the physician establishes the medical prognosis.
- The condition is lifelong unless it is the viral transient type.
- It can usually be managed with medication.
- In general, medical prognosis is good unless there is a surgical complication or inappropriate medication management.
- Hyperthyroidism spontaneously disappears in some cases, but the disease does carry a risk of thyrotoxicosis.
- If the hyperthyroidism is caused by Graves disease, the prognosis is not as good.
- Prognosis from a PT perspective: Based on effective medical management, patient is good to return to a healthy level of functioning before onset of disease if individual receives care secondary to the problems related to hyperthyroid.

PATIENT RESOURCE

- American Thyroid Association. http://www.thyroid.org. Accessed July 5, 2013.

REFERENCES

1. APTA. *Guide to Physical Therapy Practice.* Atlanta, GA: American Physical Therapy Association; 2003. http://guidetoptpractice.apta.org. Accessed July 5, 2013.
2. Hay WW, Levin MJ, Sondheimer JM, Deterding RR. Thyroid gland. In: Hay WW, Levin MJ, Sondheimer JM, Deterding RR, eds. *CURRENT Diagnosis & Treatment: Pediatrics.* 20th ed. New

York, NY: McGraw-Hill; 2011. http://www.accessphysiotherapy.com/content/6588008. Accessed July 5, 2013.

ADDITIONAL REFERENCES

- Baskin HJ, Cobin RH, Duick DS, et al. American Association of Clinical Endocrinologists medical guidelines for clinical practice for the evaluation and treatment of hyperthyroidism and hypothyroidism. *Endocr Pract.* 2002;8(6):457–469.
- Dutton M. Thyroid disorders. In: Dutton M, ed. *McGraw-Hill's NPTE (National Physical Therapy Examination)*. 2nd ed. New York, NY: McGraw-Hill; 2012. http://www.accessphysiotherapy.com/content/56510055. Accessed July 5, 2013.
- Goodman CC, Fuller KS. *Pathology: Implications for the Physical Therapist.* 3rd ed. Philadelphia, PA: Saunders Elsevier; 2009.
- Goodman CC, Snyder TK. *Differential Diagnosis for Physical Therapists: Screening for Referral.* 4th ed. St. Louis, MO: Saunders Elsevier; 2007.
- Reid JR, Wheeler SF. Hyperthyroidism: diagnosis and treatment. *Am Fam Physician.* 2005;72(4):623–630.
- Watts RL, Standaert D, Obeso JA. Other neurological and systemic diseases. In: Watts RL, Standaert D, Obeso JA, eds. *Movement Disorders.* 3rd ed. New York, NY: McGraw-Hill; 2012. http://www.accessphysiotherapy.com/content/55801578. Accessed July 5, 2013.

28 HYPOPARATHYROIDISM

Debra F. Stern, DPT, DBA, MSM, PT
Eric Shamus, PhD, DPT, PT, CSCS

CONDITION/DISORDER SYNONYMS

- Acquired Hypoparathyroidism
- Autoimmune Hypoparathyroidism
- Congenital Hypoparathyroidism
- Idiopathic Hypoparathyroidism
- Familial isolated hypoparathyroidism (FIH)

ICD-9-CM CODES

- 252.1 Hypoparathyroidism
- Associated ICD-9-CM PT diagnoses/treatment diagnoses that may be directly related
  - 315.4 Developmental coordination disorder
  - 718.45 Contracture of joint, pelvic region and thigh
  - 719.70 Difficulty in walking involving joint site unspecified
  - 728.2 Muscular wasting and disuse atrophy not elsewhere classified
  - 728.89 Other disorders of muscle, ligament, and fascia
  - 729.9 Other and unspecified disorders of soft tissue
  - 780.7 Malaise and fatigue
  - 781.2 Abnormality of gait
  - 782.3 Edema
  - 786.0 Dyspnea and respiratory abnormalities
  - 786.05 Shortness of breath

ICD-10-CM CODES

- E20.0 Idiopathic hypoparathyroidism
- E20.1 Pseudohypoparathyroidism
- E20.8 Other hypoparathyroidism
- E20.9 Hypoparathyroidism, unspecified
- E89.2 Postprocedural hypoparathyroidism
- P71.4 Transitory neonatal hypoparathyroidism

PREFERRED PRACTICE PATTERNS[1]

- 4D: Impaired Joint Mobility, Motor Function, Muscle Performance, and Range of Motion Associated With Connective Tissue Dysfunction
- 4E: Impaired Joint Mobility, Motor Function, Muscle Performance, and Range of Motion Associated With Localized Inflammation
- 6B: Impaired Aerobic Capacity/Endurance Associated With Deconditioning

PATIENT PRESENTATION

A 30-year-old female marathon runner referred to physical therapy with complaints of lower extremity (LE) cramping and tingling in her feet, limiting her ability to compete. She also described feeling short of breath as she struggles to increase distances again. There is no history of injury. In the course of casual conversation, she also complains of her nails breaking more than usual with her manicures not lasting more than a few days. Her boyfriend told her that her "legs were looking skinny" and observation reveals sarcopenia in her calves. The skin on her feet is dry and pealing, but she stated

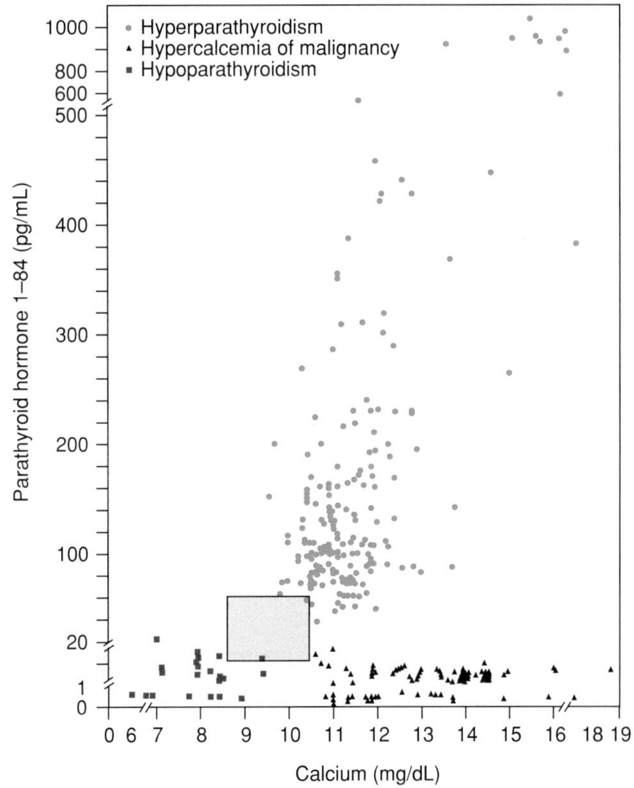

FIGURE 28-1 Levels of immunoreactive parathyroid hormone (PTH) detected in patients with primary hyperparathyroidism, hypercalcemia of malignancy, and hypoparathyroidism. Boxed area represents the upper and normal limits of blood calcium and/or immunoreactive PTH. (From SR Nussbaum, JT Potts, Jr, in L DeGroot, JL Jameson, eds. *Endocrinology*. 4th ed. Philadelphia, PA: Saunders; 2001, with permission.)

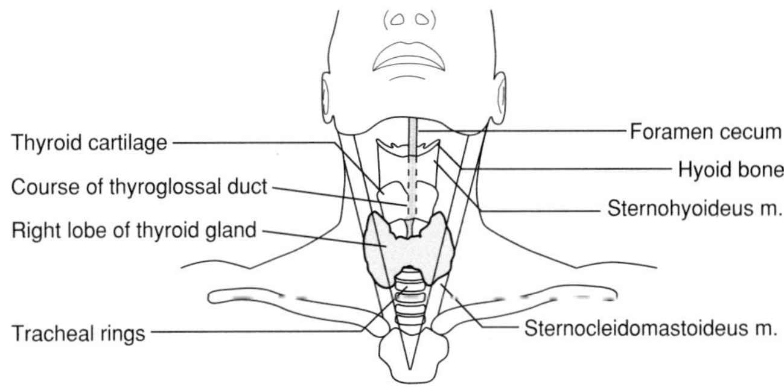

FIGURE 28-2 Anatomic relations of the thyroid gland, anterior view. The blue structures are the thyroid gland and the course of the obliterated thyroglossal duct. (From LeBlond RF, DeGowin RL, Brown DD. *DeGowin's Diagnostic Examination*. 9th ed. http://www.accessmedicine.com. Copyright © The McGraw-Hill Companies, Inc. All rights reserved.)

they have a tendency to be dry. She has started a reconditioning program in PT which is not responding well. Although referred by an orthopedist to PT, she is scheduled for an annual physical with her primary doctor in the next few weeks. The PT has suggested discussing her signs and symptoms with her physician and has offered to give her a summary of her PT to be brought to him.

KEY FEATURES

Description

- Insufficient hyperparathyroid hormone from four parathyroid glands resulting in low calcium and high phosphorus
- Muscle cramps
- Low calcium

Essentials of Diagnosis

- Muscle spasms as severe as tetany
- Abdominal cramps
- Low calcium
- High phosphorus levels
- Decreased calcium in urine
- Positive Chvostek sign
- Positive Trousseau phenomenon

General Considerations

- Can be congenital or acquired[2]
- Can have autoimmune bias[2]
- Diagnosis for more occult problems may take time and require intensive medical diagnostic testing
- May cause pathology in multiple organ systems
  - GI: Liver
  - Cardiovascular: Heart, peripheral circulation, blood pressure
  - Integumentary
- May result in secondary problems indicating the need for PT intervention depending on severity
  - Aerobic capacity and muscle endurance impairment
  - Sarcopenia
  - Weakness/impaired muscle performance
  - Musculoskeletal problems
  - Neuromuscular problems

Demographics

- Considered rare
- Lifespan

CLINICAL FINDINGS

SIGNS AND SYMPTOMS

- Abdominal pain
- Anxiety
- Arrhythmias
- Breathing difficulties secondary to throat spasms
- Brittle nails
- Calcium deposits in the brain
- Depression, mood swings
- Dry, coarse, scaly skin
- Fatigue
- Headaches
- Heart failure
- Hyperphosphatemia[2]
- Kidney disease
- Loss of consciousness, fainting
- Malformations of teeth
- Memory problems
- Muscle aches/pain
- Muscle cramps in LEs, abdomen, or face
- Nervousness
- Painful menstruation
- Paresthesias in lips
- Patchy hair loss (e.g., eyebrows)
- Peripheral paresthesias
- Seizures
- Short stature
- Signs and symptoms of hypocalcemia[2]
- Slow mental development in children
- Twitching or spasms in muscles and throat
- Vision impairment, cataracts
- Weakness

Functional Implications

- Inability or reluctance to leave home secondary to not feeling well or impaired mental status
- Fatigue
- Inability to focus
- Kidney disease
- Shortness of breath
- Muscle performance deficits, inability to ambulate or perform self-care, and aerobic capacity limitation secondary to inactivity
- Decreased exercise tolerance
- Sleep disturbances
- Changes in lifestyle
- Inappropriate self-medication
- Anxiety and irritability
- Limitations in ADLs or IADLs
- Neuropathy, increased risk for falls
- Low mentation, need for special schooling considerations

Possible Contributing Causes

- Inability to afford testing and medications and noncompliance with medication regiments/inability to pay
- Damage/trauma to the parathyroid glands
- Heredity
- Autoimmune disease
- Radiation for cancer
- Low magnesium levels
- Recent neck surgery
- Addison disease
- Removal of the parathyroid glands

Differential Diagnosis

- Autoimmune diseases
- Bladder infections, urinary tract infections, kidney pathology
- Bowel disorders
- Brain tumor
- Candidiasis
- Differential diagnosis of hypocalcemia
- Endocrine disorders
- Hypermagnesemia
- Hyperphosphatemia
- Hyperthyroidism
- Hyperventilation syndrome
- Hypocalcemia secondary to other pathology
- Hypomagnesemia
- Hypoparathyroidism
- Infections in the abdomen
- Malignant tumors in the neck
- Metabolic alkalosis
- Non-malignant tumors in neck

- Organ dysfunction as a result of cancer or malignancy
- Renal failure

MEANS OF CONFIRMATION OR DIAGNOSIS

▶ Laboratory Tests

- Complete blood count (CBC)
- 24-hour urine collection
- Urinalysis
- Thyroid function test, T-cell dysfunction[2]

▶ Imaging

- Ultrasound
- X-rays
- CT scans
- MRIs
- Bone mineral density test
- Other
  - ECG

FINDINGS AND INTERPRETATION

- Hypocalcemia
  - Laboratory findings of hypocalcemia
- Hypophosphatemia
- Hypomagnesemia
  - Laboratory findings of magnesium depletion

TREATMENT

▶ Medication

- Calcium carbonate
- Vitamin D
- Other
  - Low-phosphorus diet
  - Diet rich in calcium

REFERRALS/ADMITTANCE

- If a patient is referred for PT and the causative problem is not considered appropriate for PT, refer to the appropriate physician.
- If an emergency is identified, refer to an ER.
- If the patient's history and reactions to PT indicate possible hyperthyroidism and or symptoms, refer to a physician.

IMPAIRMENTS

- Muscle weakness
- Muscle spasm
- Gait abnormality/difficulty walking
- Shortness of breath, fatigue
- Limited aerobic capacity
- Inability to perform self-care
- Balance impairment
- Impaired skin integrity

TESTS AND MEASURES

- Observation
  - Scars may indicate adhesions or abdominal surgeries.
  - Pink or purplish striae may be indicative of Cushing syndrome.
    - Dilated veins may indicate hepatic pathology or inferior vena cava obstruction, not diverticulitis.
  - Contour: Roundedness, concavity/hollowness, asymmetry, distension, pregnancy signs.
  - Cullen sign: Bluish discoloring around umbilicus, which may be a sign of retroperitoneal bleeding.
  - Bluish discoloration in lower abdomen: Grey Turner sign, which is a sign of hemorrhagic pancreatitis.
  - Bulging in groin or other areas of abdomen especially apparent with contraction of musculature in area may be hernia.
  - Pulsing in the area of the navel may be abdominal aortic aneurysm.
  - Palpable abdominal tenderness: On left/right or generalized.
  - Psoas sign: Provides resistance over patient's right knee as they flex the hip.
  - Pain is indicative of appendicitis or possible inflammation of the abdomen.
  - Obturator sign: Internal rotation of right LE and flexion may be indicative of appendicitis or pelvic inflammation.
  - Rovsing sign: Pain on the right side of abdomen when pressure is put on the left may be indicative of appendicitis.
- Because there may be GI signs associated with hypoparathyroidism, the tests and measures listed here are included.
- Palpation of thyroid/neck
  - For enlargement of thyroid or any abnormalities
  - Skin changes
  - Vital signs
  - Chvostek sign: Tap on the face at a point just anterior to the ear and just below the zygomatic bone.
    - Positive response in hypoparathyroidism: Twitching of the ipsilateral facial muscles suggestive of neuromuscular excitability caused by hypocalcemia.
  - Trousseau sign: Inflate a sphygmomanometer cuff above systolic blood pressure for several minutes.
    - Positive response in hypoparathyroidism: Muscular contraction including flexion of the wrist and metacarpophalangeal joints, hyperextension of the fingers, and flexion of the thumb on the palm, suggestive of neuromuscular excitability.
  - Abdominal palpation, may be enlargement of ovaries.
  - Kidneys: In supine, place one hand under client between ribs and iliac crest, and other hand on abdomen below ribs and pointing in opposite direction: +/− tenderness or reproduction of symptoms.
  - Bladder
    - Not usually palpable unless it is distended and rises above pubic bone.
    - In supine, place hand above pubis and press down: +/= tenderness, reproduction of pain, or ability to feel the bladder: __ + __ −.
  - Appendix (McBurney's): Apply vertical pressure halfway between right anterior superior iliac spine (ASIS) and umbilicus.
  - Liver: In supine, with left hand under trunk parallel to 11th and 12th rib, lift upward; right hand lateral to rectus and press in and up: +/= reproduction of symptoms with deep breath.
  - Ascites: With the fingers, percuss outward from center, if sound is dull, ascites may be present.
  - Spleen: It is not recommended for PT to palpate an enlarged spleen (only palpable if enlarged) because of the potential of rupture.
  - Gallbladder (Murphy's): Place fingers to the right of rectus abdominus below rib cage: +/= sudden pain and muscle tensing with deep breath.

INTERVENTION

- PT intervention is consistent with the movement-related problems that occur secondary to hypoparathyroidism and include
  - Gait training

- Therapeutic exercise: All relevant categories, energy conservation
  - Stretching if contractures present in neck postsurgery
- Therapeutic activities for bed mobility, transfer-, and transitional-movement training
- Self-care management training including skin care/moisturizing, lifestyle management
- Neuromuscular re-education: Balance and postural training
- Soft tissue mobilization if contractures present in neck postsurgery

FUNCTIONAL GOALS

- Patient will be able to
  - Extend and rotate head and neck left and right with adequate functional range in all directions to safely use mirrors while driving (if postsurgical).
  - Achieve adequate functional aerobic capacity and the ability to talk during activity in order to achieve functional gait and activity tolerance for work, play, school, self-care; ADLs, and IADLs.
  - Achieve functional gait in the home and community (with or without a device), allowing for work, play, self-care; ADLs, and IADLs, up to _____ feet based on patient's need and prior functional level.
  - Achieve 600 m or greater in a 6-minute walk test for initiation of safe functional gait in the community.
  - Perform active verbalization with increasing taxonomy for safety during gait, including negotiation of even and uneven surfaces, opening and closing doors, and transferring in and out of a car.
  - Tolerate 30 minutes of continuous moderate exercise three times a week in _____ weeks, and five times a week in _____ weeks, depending on disease severity.

PROGNOSIS

- As this pathology is primarily medical in nature, the physician establishes the medical prognosis.
- It can usually be kept under control, although changes in dentition, cataracts, and calcium deposits in the brain are not reversible.
- Prognosis from a PT perspective, based on effective medical management, to return to prior level of function is good if individual is receiving care secondary to the problems related to hypoparathyroidism.

PATIENT RESOURCES

- American Thyroid Association. http://www.thyroid.org. Accessed August 8, 2014.
- The National Academy of Hypothyroidism. http://nahypothyroidism.org. Accessed August 8, 2014.

REFERENCES

1. APTA. *Guide to Physical Therapy Practice*. Alexandria, VA: American Physical Therapy Association; 2003. http://guidetoptpractice.apta.org. Accessed July 2, 2013.
2. Dutton M. Thyroid disorders. In: Dutton M, ed. *McGraw-Hill's NPTE (National Physical Therapy Examination)*. 2nd ed. New York, NY: McGraw-Hill; 2012. http://www.accessphysiotherapy.com/content/56510055. Accessed July 2, 2013.

ADDITIONAL REFERENCES

- American Academy of Pediatrics, et al. Update of newborn screening and therapy for congenital hypothyroidism. *Pediatrics*. 2006;117:2290–2303. doi: 10.1542/peds.2006-0915.
- Baskin HJ, Cobin RH, Duick DS, et al. American Association of Clinical Endocrinologists medical guidelines for clinical practice for the evaluation and treatment of hyperthyroidism and hypothyroidism. *Endocr Pract*. 2002;8(6):457–469.
- Colcher A, Hurtig HI. Systemic illnesses that cause movement Disorders. In: Watts RL, Standaert DG, Obeso JA, eds. *Movement Disorders*. 3rd ed. New York, NY: McGraw-Hill; 2012. http://www.accessphysiotherapy.com/content/55806123. Accessed July 2, 2013.
- Goodman CC, Fuller KS. *Pathology: Implications for the Physical Therapist*. 3rd ed. Philadelphia, PA: Saunders Elsevier; 2009.
- Goodman CC, Snyder TK. *Differential Diagnosis for Physical Therapists: Screening for Referral*. 4th ed. St. Louis, MO: Saunders Elsevier; 2007.
- Hay WW, Levin MJ, Sondheimer JM, Deterding RR, eds. *CURRENT Diagnosis & Treatment: Pediatrics*. 20th ed. New York, NY: McGraw-Hill; 2011. http://www.accessphysiotherapy.com/resource/14. Accessed July 2, 2013.
- LaFranchi SH, Austin J. How should we be treating children with congenital hypothyroidism? *J Pediatr Endocrinol Metab*. 2007;20(5):559–578.
- Ng SM, Anand D, Weindling AM. High versus low dose of initial thyroid hormone replacement for congenital hypothyroidism. *Cochrane Database Syst Rev*. 2009;21:CD006972. doi: 10.1002/14651858.CD006972.pub2.
- Panus PC, Jobst EE, Masters SB, Katzung B, Tinsley SL, Trevor AJ. Growth, thyroid, and gonadal pharmacology. In: Panus PC, Jobst EE, Masters SB, Katzung B, Tinsley SL, Trevor AJ, eds. *Pharmacology for the Physical Therapist*. New York, NY: McGraw-Hill; 2009. http://www.accessphysiotherapy.com/content/6093102. Accessed July 2, 2013.
- Powers J, Joy K, Ruscio A, Lagast H. Prevalence and incidence of hypoparathyroidism in the USA using a large claims database. *J Bone Miner Res*. 2013;28:2570–2576. doi: 10.1002/jbmr.2004.
- Rovet JF. Children with congenital hypothyroidism and their siblings: do they really differ? *Pediatrics*. 2005;115:e52–e57. doi: 10.1542/peds.2004-149.
- Shoback DM, Sellmeyer DE. Disorders of the parathyroids & calcium & phosphorus metabolism. In: McPhee SJ, Hammer GD, eds. *Pathophysiology of Disease: An Introduction to Clinical Medicine*. 6th ed. New York, NY: McGraw-Hill; 2010. http://www.accessphysiotherapy.com/content/5370820. Accessed July 2, 2013.

29 HYPOTHYROIDISM

Debra F. Stern, DPT, DBA, MSM, PT
Eric Shamus, PhD, DPT, PT, CSCS

CONDITION/DISORDER SYNONYMS

- Hypothyreosis
- Underactive thyroid

ICD-9-CM CODES

- 244 Acquired hypothyroidism
- 244.0 Postsurgical hypothyroidism
- 244.1 Other postablative hypothyroidism
- 244.2 Iodine hypothyroidism
- 244.3 Other iatrogenic hypothyroidism
- 244.8 Other specified acquired hypothyroidism
- 244.9 Unspecified acquired hypothyroidism
- Associated ICD-9-CM PT diagnoses/treatment diagnoses that may be directly related
  - 315.4 Developmental coordination disorder
  - 718.45 Contracture of joint, pelvic region and thigh
  - 719.70 Difficulty in walking involving joint site unspecified
  - 728.2 Muscular wasting and disuse atrophy not elsewhere classified
  - 728.89 Other disorders of muscle, ligament, and fascia
  - 729.9 Other and unspecified disorders of soft tissue
  - 780.7 Malaise and fatigue
  - 781.2 Abnormality of gait
  - 782.3 Edema
  - 786.0 Dyspnea and respiratory abnormalities
  - 786.05 Shortness of breath

ICD-10-CM CODES

- E03.9 Hypothyroidism, unspecified
- E89.0 Postprocedural hypothyroidism

PREFERRED PRACTICE PATTERNS[1]

- 4D: Impaired Joint Mobility, Motor Function, Muscle Performance, and Range of Motion Associated with Connective Tissue Dysfunction
- 4E: Impaired Joint Mobility, Motor Function, Muscle Performance, and Range of Motion Associated with Localized Inflammation
- 6B: Impaired Aerobic Capacity/Endurance Associated with Deconditioning

PATIENT PRESENTATION

A 65-year-old female presents to the clinic feeling tired and fatigued all the time. She has also noticed an increasing problem of constipation despite adequate fiber intake. She is frequently cold when others are hot. Her skin has become dry, and she has noticed a swelling sensation in her neck area. On examination she is afebrile with a pulse of 60 beats per minute. She is in no acute distress and appears in good health. She has an enlarged, nontender thyroid noted on her neck. Her reflexes are diminished, and her skin is dry to the touch.[2]

KEY FEATURES

Description

- A deficiency of thyroid gland activity

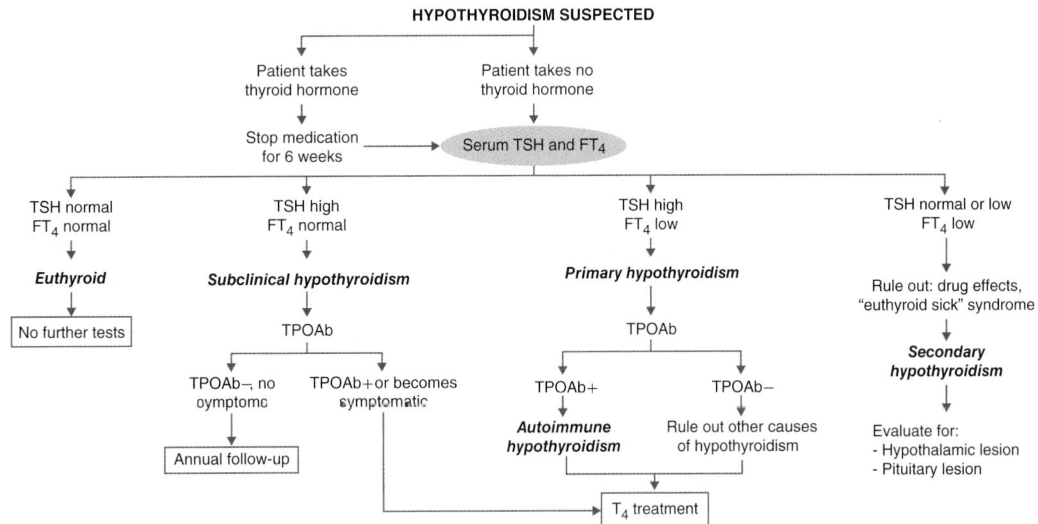

FIGURE 29-1 Hypothyroidism: diagnostic approach. FT_4, free thyroxine; TPOAb+, thyroid peroxidase antibodies positive; TPOAb–, thyroid peroxidase antibodies negative; TSH, thyroid-stimulating hormone. (From Nicoll D, Lu CM, Pignone M, Mcphee SJ. *Pocket Guide to Diagnostic Tests*. 6th ed. www.accessmedicine.com.

- Characterized by decreased basal metabolic rate, fatigue and lethargy, sensitivity to cold, and menstrual disturbances
- In infants, severe hypothyroidism leads to cretinism
- Thyroid regulates metabolism and produces three types of thyroid hormone[3]

Essentials of Diagnosis

- Gradual onset
- Palpation of thyroid/neck for enlargement of thyroid or any abnormalities
- Thyroid function test
- Three types of hypothyroidism
  - Primary: Thyroid gland dysfunction
  - Secondary: Pituitary gland dysfunction
  - Tertiary: Hypothalamus dysfunction

General Considerations

- Can progress to myxedema if untreated
- Thyroid needs iodine as a critical element[3]
- May cause pathology in multiple organ systems
  - GI: Liver
  - Cardiovascular: Heart, peripheral circulation, blood pressure
  - Integumentary
- May result in secondary problems indicating the need for PT intervention depending on severity
  - Aerobic capacity and muscle endurance impairment
  - Sarcopenia
  - Weakness/impaired muscle performance
  - Musculoskeletal problems
  - Neuromuscular problems
  - Weight gain, indicating the need for PT intervention depending on severity
- Hyperlipidemia

Demographics

- Affects individuals throughout the lifespan, starting at birth (1 in 4000 infants)
- Estimated five million in the United States and possibly double that are undiagnosed
- Higher incidence in women
- Higher incidence in those older than age 60

CLINICAL FINDINGS

SIGNS AND SYMPTOMS

- Cold sensitivity
- Fatigue
- Weight gain
- Slowed heart rate
- Constipation
- Joint pain
- Muscle pain
- Muscle cramps
- Paleness
- Dry skin
- Hair thinning, including eyebrows
- Brittleness of fingernails
- Weakness
- Unexplained weight gain with inability to lose it
- Depression
- Heavier menstrual periods
- Decreased ability to smell
- Decreased taste
- Puffiness of hands, feet, and face
- Peripheral neuropathy/numbness
- Slowness of speech
- Thickening of skin
- Liver dysfunction
- Heart disease
- Worsening of angina if history of angina
- Anemia
- In severe cases

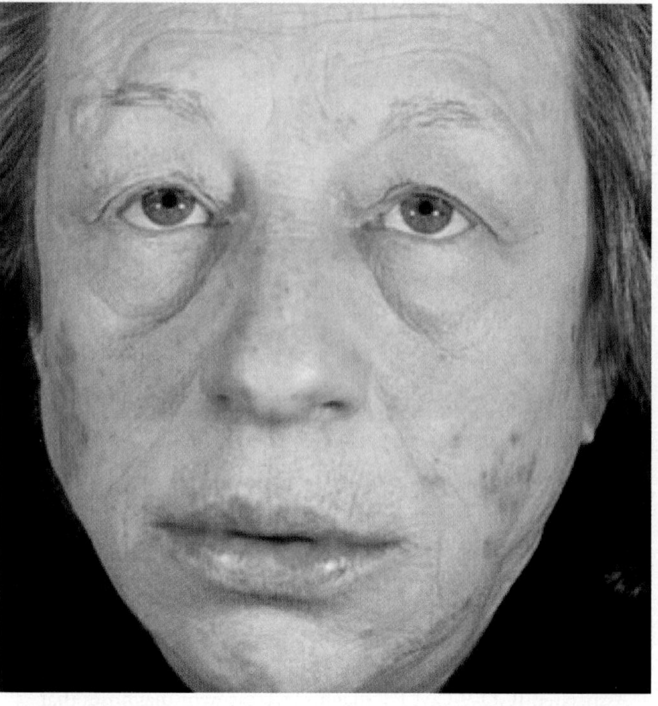

FIGURE 29-2 Clinical features of hypothyroidism. The patient shows a lack of facial expression, together with pallor, dry skin, loss of hair in the lateral eyebrows, facial puffiness, broadening of the nose, and drooping eyelids. (From Wolff K, Goldsmith LA, Katz, Gilchrest BA, Paller A, Leffel DJ. *Fitzpatrick's Dermatology in General Medicine*. 7th ed. New York, NY: McGraw-Hill; 2007.)

  - Below normal body temperature
  - Depressed breathing
  - Low blood pressure
  - Low blood sugar
  - Unresponsiveness

Functional Implications

- Severe symptoms such as immediacy of need to urinate may be disabling, resulting in the inability to leave home
- Fatigue
- Infertility
- Miscarriage
- Heart disease
- Decreased sex drive
- Increasing weight with inability to exercise or move well
- Sarcopenia resulting in
  - Weakness
  - Muscle-mass loss
  - Inability to ambulate or perform self-care
  - Aerobic capacity limitation secondary to inactivity
- Decreased exercise tolerance
- Sleep disturbances
- Changes in lifestyle
- Eating disorders
- Inappropriate self-medication
- Anxiety and depression
- Can lead to problems with liver
- Limitations in ADLs or IADLs
- Infection (systemic)
- Skin lesions from dryness
- Neuropathy, increased risk for falls
- Vision impairment, most often retinal

- Prone to infections such as bacterial or fungal in the skin, urinary tract (UT), kidney
- Potential for liver problems
- Difficulty in thinking clearly

Possible Contributing Causes

- Acquired (juvenile hypothyroidism) causes
- Autoimmune or Hashimoto thyroiditis
- Cancer
- Chemical inducement
- Congenital birth defects
- Congenital causes
- Drugs: Amiodarone, drugs used for hyperthyroidism, lithium
- Female
- Goiters
- Older than age 50
- Inflammation of the thyroid
- Iodine deficiency
- Low iodine
- Metastatic cancer
- Pituitary dysfunction as the pituitary signals production of thyroid stimulating hormone (TSH)
- Pregnancy
- Radiation to the brain
- Radiation treatments to the neck
- Radioactive iodine to treat hyperthyroidism
- Surgical removal of part or all of the thyroid gland to treat other thyroid problems
- Viral thyroiditis

Differential Diagnosis

- Autoimmune diseases that affect the upper and lower GI tracts
- Bladder infections, UTIs, kidney pathology
- Bowel disorders
- Cardiac disorders
- Crohn or irritable bowel syndrome
- Endocrine disorders, diabetes
- Gastroparesis
- Gynecologic problems in females
- Infections in the abdomen
- Non-malignant tumors in the abdomen or organs
- Organ dysfunction as the result of cancer or malignancy, especially the liver
- Pituitary dysfunction

MEANS OF CONFIRMATION OR DIAGNOSIS

Laboratory Tests

- Complete blood count (CBC)
- Thyroid function: TSH, T3, T4[3]
- Cholesterol
- Liver enzymes
- Prolactin
- Sodium levels

Imaging

- Ultrasound
- Chest X-ray
- CT scans
- MRIs

FINDINGS AND INTERPRETATION

- Prolactin (may be elevated in women and men)

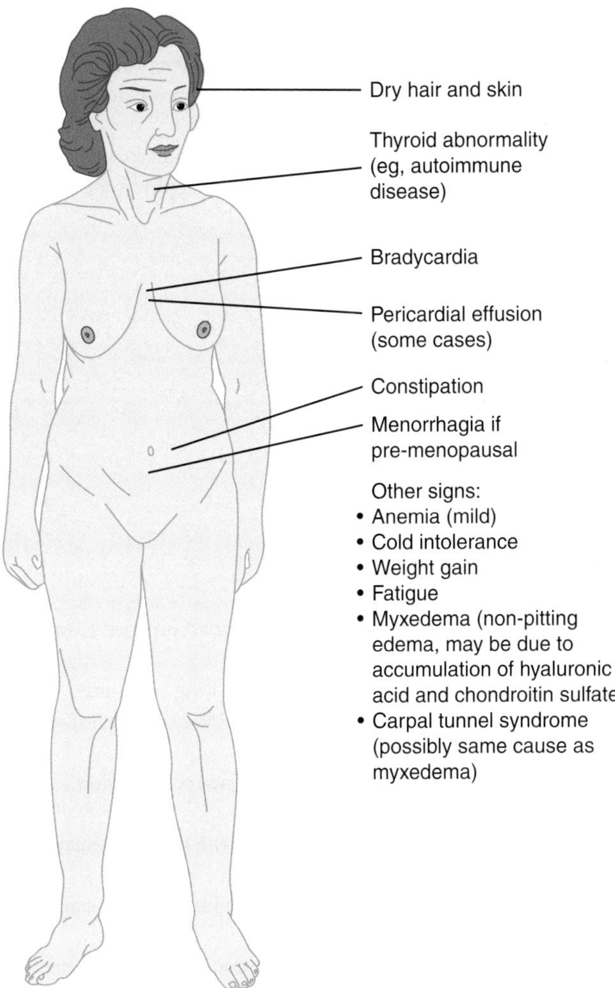

FIGURE 29-3 Some of the major signs of hypothyroidism. (From Murray RK, Bender DA, Botham KM, Kennelly PJ, Rodwell V, Weil PA. *Harper's Illustrated Biochemistry*. 29th ed. www.accessmedicine.com. Copyright © The McGraw-Hill Companies, Inc. All rights reserved.)

- Sodium levels, low in hypothyroidism
  - The normal range: 135 to 145 milliequivalents per liter (mEq/L)

TREATMENT

Medication

- Thyroid hormone replacement therapy, most commonly levothyroxine, lifelong, with levels checked at least annually
- Bone density monitoring is required on levothyroxine

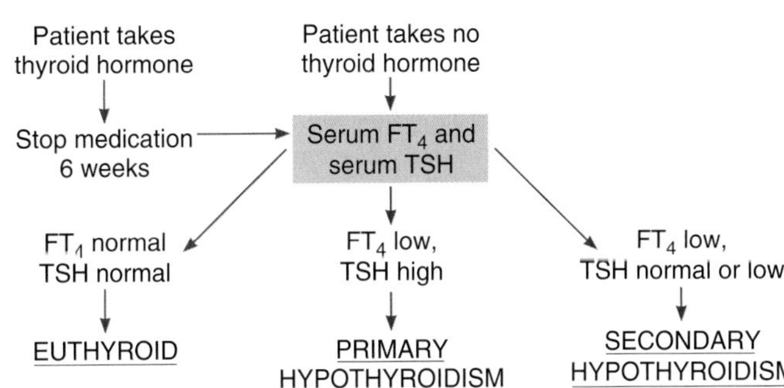

FIGURE 29-4 Diagnosis of hypothyroidism. (From Gardner DG, Shoback D. *Greenspan's Basic & Clinical Endocrinology*. 9th ed. www.accessmedicine.com. Copyright © The McGraw-Hill Companies, Inc. All rights reserved.)

REFERRALS/ADMITTANCE

- If a patient is referred for PT and the causative problem is not considered appropriate for PT, refer to the appropriate physician.
- If an emergency is identified, refer to an ER.
- If the patient's history and reactions to PT indicate possible hypothyroidism and/or symptoms, refer to a physician.

IMPAIRMENTS

- Muscle weakness/cramps
- Muscle atrophy
- Gait abnormality/difficulty walking
- Shortness of breath, fatigue
- Inability to perform self-care
- Balance impairment
- Impaired skin integrity

TESTS AND MEASURES

- Observation
  - Scars may indicate adhesions or abdominal surgeries causative of diverticula.
  - Pink or purplish striae may indicate Cushing syndrome.
  - Dilated veins may indicate hepatic pathology or inferior vena cava obstruction, not diverticulitis.
  - Contour: Roundness, concavity, asymmetry, distension, pregnancy signs.
  - Cullen sign: Bluish discoloring around the umbilicus may be a sign of retroperitoneal bleeding.
  - Bluish discoloration in lower abdomen: Grey Turner sign, signals hemorrhagic pancreatitis.
  - Bulging in groin/abdomen especially apparent with contraction of musculature in area may be hernia.
  - Pulsing in navel area may be abdominal aortic aneurysm.
  - Left lower quadrant pain, often following a meal.
  - Palpable abdominal tenderness on left side or generalized.
  - Psoas sign: Provides resistance over patient's right knee as they flex the hip.
    - Pain indicates appendicitis, possible inflammation of abdomen.
  - Obturator sign: Internal rotation and flexion of right lower extremity (LE) may indicate appendicitis, pelvic inflammation.
  - Rovsing sign: Pain on the right side of abdomen when pressure applied to the left may indicate appendicitis.
- The following list of tests and measures are included for a variety of pathology from a differential diagnosis perspective.
- Palpation of thyroid/neck
  - For enlargement of thyroid or any abnormalities.
  - Skin changes: Turgor, dryness, hairlessness.
  - Kidneys: In supine, place one hand under client between ribs and iliac crest and other hand on abdomen below ribs and pointing in opposite direction: +/− tenderness or reproduction of symptoms.
  - Bladder
    - Not usually palpable unless it is distended and rises above pubic bone.
    - In supine, place hand above pubis and press down: +/= tenderness, reproduction of pain, or ability to feel the bladder: __ + __ −.
  - Appendix (McBurney's): Apply vertical pressure halfway between right anterior superior iliac spine (ASIS) and umbilicus.

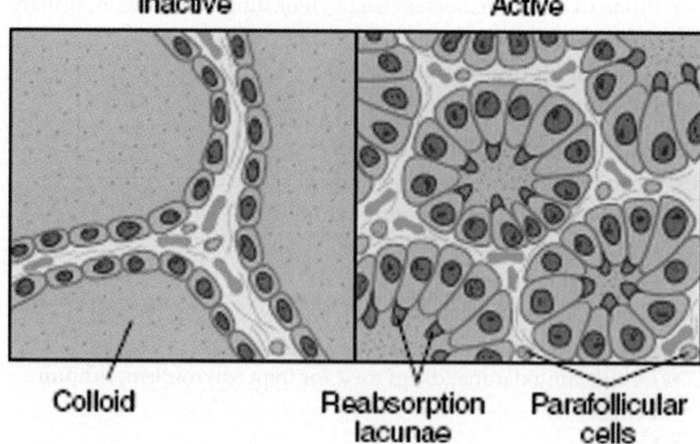

FIGURE 29-5 Thyroid histology. The appearance of the gland when it is inactive (left) and actively secreting (right) is shown. Note the small, punched-out "reabsorption lacunae" in the colloid next to the cells in the active gland. (From Barrett KE, Barman SM, Boitano S, Brooks HL. *Ganong's Review of Medical Physiology*. www.accessmedicine.com. Copyright © The McGraw-Hill Companies, Inc. All rights reserved.)

  - Liver: In supine, with left hand under trunk parallel to 11th and 12th rib, lift upward; right hand lateral to rectus and press in and up: +/= reproduction of symptoms with deep breath.
  - Ascites: With the fingers, percuss outward from center, if sound is dull, ascites may be present.
  - Spleen: It is not recommended for PT to palpate an enlarged spleen (only palpable if enlarged) because of the potential of rupture.
  - Gallbladder (Murphy's): Place fingers to the right of rectus abdominus below rib cage: +/= sudden pain and muscle tensing with deep breath.

INTERVENTION

- PT intervention is consistent with the movement-related problems that occur secondary to diabetes and include
  - Gait training
  - Therapeutic exercise: All relevant categories, energy conservation
    - If there is an insulin pump, take care not to interfere with it in any way.
    - PT should inquire about medication taken; if glucose >300, exercise should be avoided.
    - Monitoring heart rate.
    - Cardiac monitoring with possible metabolic equivalent (MET) calculation if history of angina.
  - Therapeutic activities for bed-mobility training, transfer-, and transitional-movement training.
  - Self-care management training including skin care/moisturizing, lifestyle management.
  - Neuromuscular re-education: Balance and postural training.
  - Wound management.

FUNCTIONAL GOALS

- Patient will be able to
  - Achieve adequate functional aerobic capacity and the ability to talk during activity in order to achieve functional gait and activity tolerance for work, play, school, self-care, ADLs, and IADLs.
  - Achieve functional gait in the home and community (with or without a device), allowing for work, play, self-care, ADLs, and IADLs, up to _____ feet based on patient's need and prior functional level.

- Achieve 600 m or greater in a 6-minute walk test for initiation of safe functional gait in the community.
- Perform active verbalization with increasing taxonomy for safety during gait, including negotiation of even and uneven surfaces, opening and closing doors, and transferring in and out of a car.
- Tolerate 30 minutes of continuous moderate exercise three times a week in _____ weeks, and five times a week in _____ weeks, depending on disease severity.

PROGNOSIS

- As this pathology is primarily medical in nature, the physician establishes the medical prognosis.
- The condition is lifelong, unless it is the viral transient type.
- It can usually be managed with medication.
- If thyroid hormones are too low, myxedema coma can result with ensuing death.

ADDITIONAL INFORMATION

- See problem-oriented patient study on AccessPhysiotherapy.com for more information.

PATIENT RESOURCES

- American Thyroid Association. http://www.thyroid.org. Accessed August 8, 2014.
- The National Academy of Hypothyroidism. http://nahypothyroidism.org. Accessed August 8, 2014.

REFERENCES

1. The American Physical Therapy Association. *Interactive Guide to Physical Therapist Practice*. Alexandria, VA: The American Physical Therapy Association; 2003. http://guidetoptpractice.apta.org/. Accessed July 5, 2013.
2. Toy EC. Hypothyroidism, Case 48. LANGE Case Files. http://www.accessmedicine.com/casecontent.aspx?aid=8651335&tabid=1. Accessed July 3, 2013.
3. McPhee SJ, Hammer GD. Formation & secretion of thyroid hormones. In: McPhee SJ, Hammer GD, eds. *Pathophysiology of Disease*. 6th ed. New York, NY: McGraw-Hill; 2010. http://www.accessphysiotherapy.com/content/5371509. Accessed July 5, 2013.

ADDITIONAL REFERENCES

- American Academy of Pediatrics, et al. Update of newborn screening and therapy for congenital hypothyroidism. *Pediatrics*. 2006;117:2290–2303. doi: 10.1542/peds.2006–0915.
- Baskin HJ, Cobin RH, Duick DS, et al. American Association of Clinical Endocrinologists medical guidelines for clinical practice for the evaluation and treatment of hyperthyroidism and hypothyroidism. *Endocr Pract*. 2002;8(6):457–469.
- Colcher A, Hurtig HI. Systemic illnesses that cause movement disorders. In: Watts RL, Standaert DG, Obeso JA, eds. *Movement Disorders*. 3rd ed. New York, NY: McGraw-Hill; 2012. http://www.accessphysiotherapy.com/content/55806123. Accessed July 5, 2013.
- Goodman CC, Fuller KS. *Pathology: Implications for the Physical Therapist*. 3rd ed. Philadelphia, PA: Saunders Elsevier; 2009.
- Goodman CC, Snyder TK. *Differential Diagnosis for Physical Therapists: Screening for Referral*. 4th ed. St. Louis, MO: Saunders Elsevier; 2007.
- Hay WW, Levin MJ, Sondheimer JM, Deterding RR, eds. *CURRENT Diagnosis & Treatment: Pediatrics*. 20th ed. New York, NY: McGraw-Hill; 2011. http://www.accessphysiotherapy.com/resource/14. Accessed March 5, 2013.
- LaFranchi SH, Austin J. How should we be treating children with congenital hypothyroidism? *J Pediatr Endocrinol Metab*. 2007;20(5):559–578.
- Ng SM, Anand D, Weindling AM. High versus low dose of initial thyroid hormone replacement for congenital hypothyroidism. *Cochrane Database Syst Rev*. 2009;21:CD006972. doi: 10.1002/14651858.CD006972.pub2.
- Panus PC, Jobst EE, Masters SB, Katzung B, Tinsley SL, Trevor AJ. Growth, thyroid, and gonadal pharmacology. In: Panus PC, Jobst EE, Masters SB, Katzung B, Tinsley SL, Trevor AJ, eds. *Pharmacology for the Physical Therapist*. New York, NY: McGraw-Hill; 2009. http://www.accessphysiotherapy.com/content/6093102. Accessed July 5, 2013.
- Rovet JF. Children with congenital hypothyroidism and their siblings: do they really differ? *Pediatrics*. 2005;115:e52–e57. doi: 10.1542/peds.2004–149.

SECTION E GASTROINTESTINAL DISORDERS

30 APPENDICITIS

Eric Shamus, PhD, DPT, PT, CSCS
Natalie V. Wessel, DO, MPH

ICD-9-CM CODES

- 540 Acute appendicitis
- 540.0 Acute appendicitis with generalized peritonitis
- 540.1 Acute appendicitis with peritoneal abscess
- 540.9 Acute appendicitis without mention of peritonitis
- 541 Appendicitis, unqualified
- 542 Other appendicitis
- 543.0 Hyperplasia of appendix (lymphoid)
- 543.9 Other and unspecified diseases of appendix
- Associated physical therapy diagnoses
  - 315.4 Developmental coordination disorder (clumsiness, dyspraxia and/or specific motor development disorder)
  - 718.45 Contracture of joint, pelvic region and thigh
  - 719.70 Difficulty in walking involving joint site unspecified
  - 728.2 Muscular wasting and disuse atrophy, not elsewhere classified
  - 728.89 Other disorders of muscle, ligament, and fascia
  - 729.9 Other and unspecified disorders of soft tissue
  - 780.70 Other malaise and fatigue
  - 781.2 Abnormality of gait
  - 782.3 Edema
  - 786.0 Dyspnea and respiratory abnormalities

ICD-10-CM CODES

- K35.2 Acute appendicitis with generalized peritonitis
- K35.3 Acute appendicitis with localized peritonitis
- K35.80 Unspecified acute appendicitis
- K35.89 Other acute appendicitis
- K36 Other appendicitis
- K37 Unspecified appendicitis
- K38.0 Hyperplasia of appendix
- K38.1 Appendicular concretions
- K38.2 Diverticulum of appendix
- K38.3 Fistula of appendix
- K38.8 Other specified diseases of appendix
- K38.9 Disease of appendix, unspecified

PREFERRED PRACTICE PATTERN

- As of June, 2014, the APTA *Guide to Physical Therapist Practice* does not include practice patterns for organ system pathology; therefore, the associated or secondary musculoskeletal, cardiovascular/pulmonary, or potential neuromuscular patterns would be indicated.

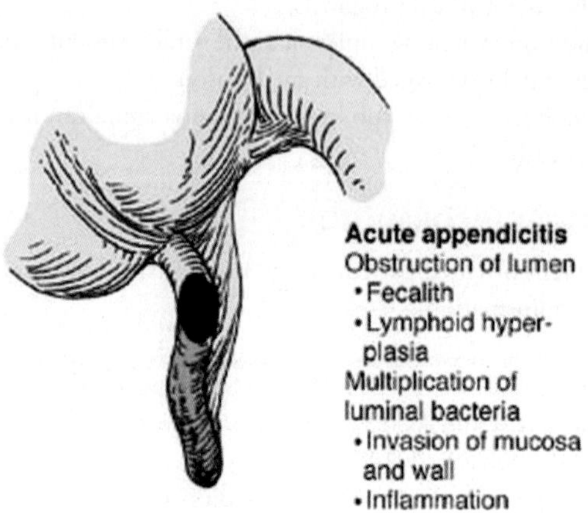

Acute appendicitis
Obstruction of lumen
• Fecalith
• Lymphoid hyper-plasia
Multiplication of luminal bacteria
• Invasion of mucosa and wall
• Inflammation

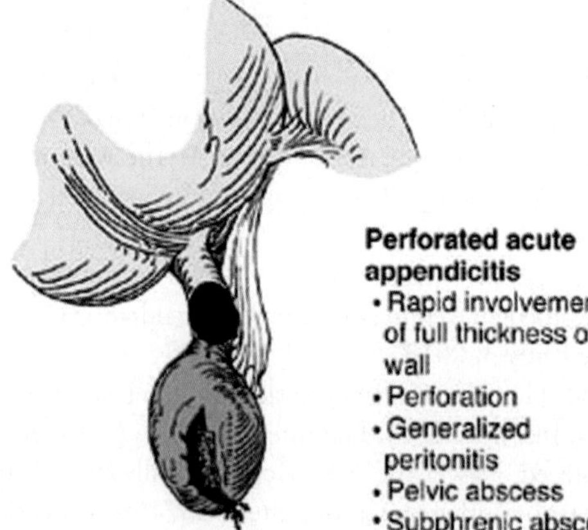

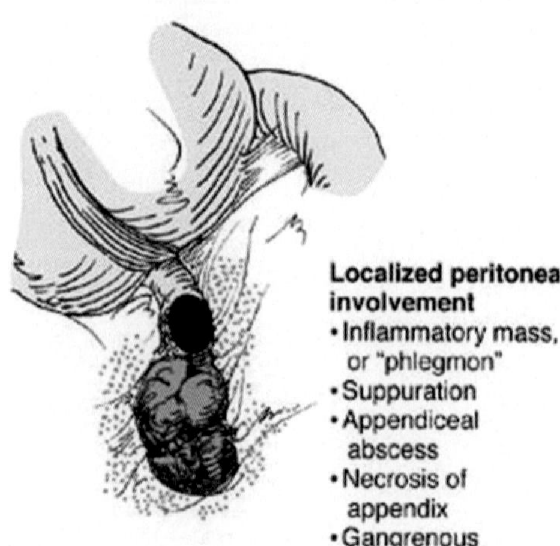

• Rapid involvement of full thickness of wall

• Subphrenic abscess

FIGURE 30-1 Pathogenesis and complications of acute appendicitis. (From Chandrasoma P, Taylor CR. *Concise Pathology*. 3rd ed. www.accessmedicine.com. Copyright © The McGraw-Hill Companies, Inc. All rights reserved.)

PATIENT PRESENTATION

A 23-year-old male college student presents with severe abdominal pain for 3 hours that woke him up from sleep. Pain is sharp, 9/10 and in the right lower quadrant. Laying still helps the pain and movement makes it worse. He took two 250 mg ibuprofen, but the pain has been constant and getting worse. Vitals are Pulse: 120, Respirations: 24 , Blood Pressure: 134/78, Temperature: 100°F, and SpO_2% of 99%. On exam the patient is alert and oriented, but visibly uncomfortable. Abdominal exam reveals guarding in the right lower quadrant with rebound tenderness. A STAT CBC shows a mildly elevated WBC count and a CT scan shows inflammation of the appendix.

KEY FEATURES

Description

- Inflammation of the appendix
- Pain in the lower abdominal region on the right side
- Appendix can rupture when blocked by an object, tumor, or feces
- Appendix is a tube of tissue off of the large intestine with an unknown function

Essentials of Diagnosis

- Right abdominal and side (flank) pain
- Positive cultures
- McBurney point, tip of right 12th rib tenderness
- Palpation over appendix
- Lab tests

General Considerations

- If untreated can possibly rupture
- Possible referred pain to back, pelvic region, or rectal area (in men)
- Possible secondary problems that may, depending on severity, indicate the need for physical therapy intervention
  - Impairment of aerobic capacity and muscle endurance
  - Sarcopenia
  - Musculoskeletal problems
  - Neuromuscular problems
  - Weight loss
- May mimic colon cancer or tumors, irritable bowel, colitis or, in females, gynecological problems such as endometriosis, uterine fibroids, or ectopic pregnancies
- Symptoms are frequently referred to the back and abdominal areas, so it may be common to have patients inappropriately referred to PT
- Pseudoappendicitis: *Yersinia enterocolitica*

Demographics

- Can occur across the lifespan, from 2 years old and up[1]
- Most common in individuals between 15 and 30 years of age[1]

CLINICAL FINDINGS

SIGNS AND SYMPTOMS

- High fever
- Diarrhea
- Shaking
- Chills
- Nausea
- Vomiting
- Discomfort or sharp pain in the right lower quadrant of the abdominal area
- Abdominal tenderness and guarding of the right lower quadrant
- McBurney point, tip of right 12th rib tenderness
- Pain in the belly button region without trauma
- Right, low back pain without trauma, insidious onset
- Difficulty standing up straight
- Psoas sign
- Obturator sign
- Rovsing sign
- Increased heart rate and temperature may indicate perforation
- Tenderness on the right side of the rectum

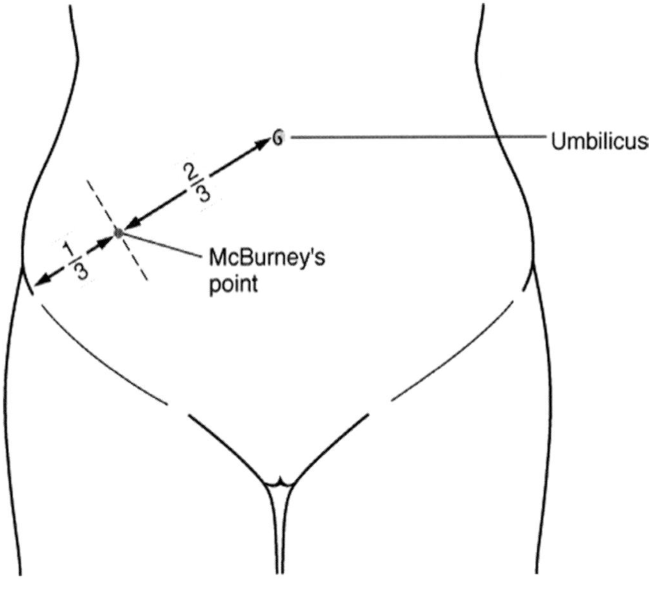

FIGURE 30-2 McBurney point. (From Sanders MJ, Toy EC, Yetman R, et al. *Case Files: Pediatrics*. 3rd ed. www.accesspediatrics.com. Copyright © The McGraw-Hill Companies, Inc. All rights reserved.)

Functional Implications

- Chronic problems
  - Changes in lifestyle, limiting physical activity
  - Eating disorders, anorexia

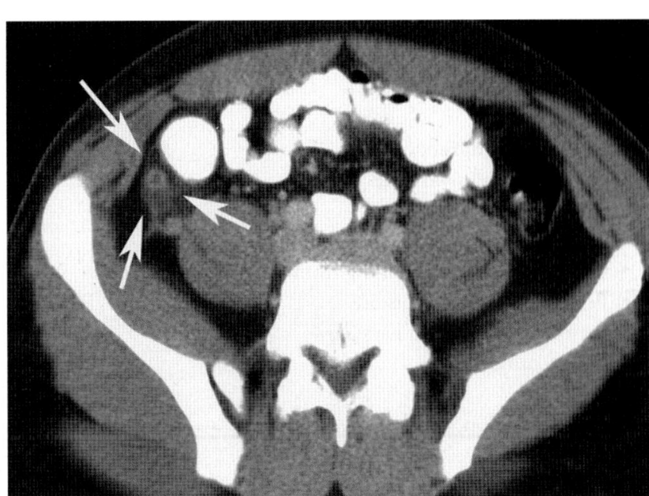

FIGURE 30-3 Appendicitis. Axial MDCT image shows hyperenhancement of the wall of the appendix and periappendiceal fat stranding (*arrows*). (From Greenberger NJ, Blumberg RS, Burakoff R. *Current Diagnosis & Treatment: Gastroenterology, Hepatology, & Endoscopy*. 2nd ed. www.accessmedicine.com. Copyright © The McGraw-Hill Companies, Inc. All rights reserved.)

- Fatigue
- Diarrhea
- Inappropriate self medication
- Anxiety and depression
- Can be indicative of serious medical conditions
- Limitations in ADLs or IADLs

- Acute problems
  - May need rapid attention to prevent serious complications
  - Death
  - Acute appendicitis
  - Rupture
  - Infection

Possible Contributing Causes

- Blockage in the appendix
  - Feces
  - Tumor
  - Foreign object
- Infection
- Trauma

Differential Diagnoses

- Appendicitis
- Autoimmune diseases that affect the upper and lower gastrointestinal (GI) tracts
- Benign prostatic hypertrophy
- Bowel disorders
  - Constipation or diarrhea
  - Inflammation of the abdominal or organ linings
  - Obstructions
  - Torsions
- Cholecystitis
- Crohn disease
- Cystitis of bladder
- Endocrine disorders
- Gastroenteritis
- Gynecologic problems in females
  - Endometriosis
  - Menses
  - Ectopic pregnancies
  - Ovarian cysts
  - Fibroids
  - Menopause
- Infections in the abdomen
- Irritable bowel syndrome
- Kidney pathology
- Non-malignant tumors in the abdomen or organs
- Organ dysfunction resulting from cancer or malignancy
- Pelvic inflammatory disease
- Perforated ulcers in GI system
- Perihepatitis
- Peritonitis
- Pleural effusion
- Pneumonia
- Prostatitis
- Urethritis
- Urinary tract infection
- Referred pain from heart, spine, or hip
- Post bariatric surgery complications

MEANS OF CONFIRMATION OR DIAGNOSIS

Laboratory Tests

- Blood tests (CBC)
- Urinalysis

Imaging

- Abdominal ultrasound
- Abdominal computed tomography (CT)

Diagnostic Procedures

- Rectal exam with right-sided rectal tenderness
- Manual palpation for tenderness

FINDINGS AND INTERPRETATION

- Blood tests (CBC) looking for raised white blood cells
- Urinalysis to determine if it is a urinary tract infection

TREATMENT

Medication

- Antibiotics

MEDICAL PROCEDURES

- Hospitalization with IV antibiotics if severe
- Appendectomy

REFERRALS/ADMITTANCE

- If a patient is referred for PT and the causative problem is not considered to be appropriate for PT, referral to the appropriate physician must be made.
- Individuals may be referred to PT with complaints of back pain, or lower or upper or anterior chest and shoulder pain, which is not attributable to the structures in that anatomical area.
- If findings are negative for primary patient complaint area, the pain may be referred from the abdomen or elsewhere in the body.
- Referral to the appropriate health professional is necessary to determine the root cause and facilitate appropriate medical treatment.
- If appropriate for PT, referral or treatment for UG pathology is usually performed by PT specialists in women's and men's health.
- If an emergency is identified, refer to emergency room (ER).
- Nutritionist for diet of high fiber, fresh fruits, and vegetables.

IMPAIRMENTS

- Muscle weakness in the pelvic floor
- Muscle atrophy
- Gait abnormality or difficulty walking
- Contractures of soft tissue (i.e., fascia, muscle)
- Muscle impairment in the pelvic floor
- Inability to perform self-care

TESTS AND MEASURES

- Observation
  - Scars may indicate adhesions or abdominal surgeries that may be causative of diverticula.
  - Striae, pink or purplish, may be indicative of Cushing syndrome.

- Dilated veins may indicate hepatic pathology or inferior vena cava obstruction, not diverticulitis.
- Contour: Roundedness, concavity/hollowness, asymmetry, distension, pregnancy signs.
- Cullen sign: Bluish discoloration around the umbilicus, which may be a sign of retroperitoneal bleeding.
- Grey Turner sign: Bluish discoloration in lower abdomen, which is a sign of hemorrhagic pancreatitis.
- Bulging in groin or other areas of abdomen, especially apparent with contraction of musculature in area may be hernia.
- Pulsing in the area of the navel may be abdominal aortic aneurysm.
- Left lower quadrant pain, often following a meal.
- Palpable abdominal tenderness on left/right side or generalized.
- Psoas sign: Provides resistance over patient's right knee as they flex the hip; pain would be indicative of appendicitis or possible inflammation of the abdomen.
- Obturator sign: Internal rotation of RLE and flexion may be indicative of appendicitis or pelvic inflammation.
- Rovsing sign: Pain on right side of abdomen when pressure is put on the left may be indicative of appendicitis.

- Palpation
  - Kidneys: In supine position, place one hand under client between ribs and iliac crest; other hand on abdomen below ribs pointing in opposite direction: +/− tenderness or reproduction of symptoms.
  - Bladder: Not usually palpable unless it is distended and rises above pubic bone; in supine, place hand above pubis and press down: +/= tenderness, reproduction of pain, or ability to feel the bladder: __+ ___−.
  - Appendix (McBurney's): Apply vertical pressure halfway between right ASIS and umbilicus.
  - Liver: In supine, with left hand under trunk parallel to 11th and 12th rib, lift upward; right hand lateral to rectus and press in and up: +/= reproduction of symptoms with deep breath.
  - Ascites: With the fingers, percuss outward from center; if sound is dull, ascites may be present.
  - Spleen: Not recommended for PT to palpate an enlarged spleen (only palpable if enlarged) because of the potential of rupture.
  - Gallbladder (Murphy's): Place fingers to the right of rectus abdominus below rib cage: +/= sudden pain and muscle tensing with deep breath.

INTERVENTION

- Physical therapy intervention is indicated for movement-related problems that occur.
  - Gait training
  - Therapeutic exercise: All relevant categories, energy conservation
    - If there is a stoma from a colostomy or ileostomy, PT must be aware that activities should be avoided if they cause retraction.
  - Therapeutic activities for bed-mobility training, transfer- and transitional-movement training, and pelvic floor retraining
- Self-care management training
  - If a male has an external catheter, ensure it is secure to prevent accidental loss.
  - For indwelling catheters, ensure they are not pulled out and that drainage clamps are locked.
  - Determine if a leg bag or tube and hanging bag are in use.
  - Bag should be below waist/bladder level at all times and should not touch the floor.
  - If full, bag should be emptied to prevent backflow.
  - Neuromuscular re-education
  - Electrical stimulation
  - Interprofessional
    - Lifestyle modification
    - Smoking cessation
    - Weight management
    - Dietary counseling
    - Psychological intervention
- Massaging of the abdominal area is contraindicated in appendicitis

FUNCTIONAL GOALS

- Patient will be able to
  - Achieve adequate functional aerobic capacity and ability to talk during activity in order to achieve functional gait and activity tolerance for work, play, school, self-care; ADLs and IADLs.
  - Functional independent gait in the home and community (with or without a device), allowing for work, play, self-care; ADLs and IADLs, up to __________ feet based on patient's need and prior functional level.
  - Achieve 600 m or greater in a 6-minute walk test for initiation of safe functional gait in the community.
  - Perform active verbalization with increasing taxonomy for safety during gait, including negotiation of even and uneven surfaces, opening and closing doors, transferring in and out of a car.
  - Tolerate 30 minutes of continuous moderate exercise three times a week in ______weeks, and five times a week in ____________ weeks, depending on disease severity.

PROGNOSIS

- As this pathology is primarily medical in nature, it is the physician who establishes the medical prognosis.
- If treated promptly and effectively with antibiotics, should resolve.
- Surgery prior to rupture heals quickly.
- If left untreated, a rupture can create a peritonitis infection in the region; can be fatal.
- Unless the medical condition is unstable or the goals unrealistic, the prognosis from a physical therapy perspective should be good.

PATIENT RESOURCE

- Antibiotics may be a safe alternative to surgery for appendicitis. Association of PeriOperative Registered Nurses AORN. http://www.aorn.org/News.aspx?id=22710. Accessed August 8, 2014.

REFERENCE

1. Hay WW, Levin MJ, Sondheimer JM, Deterding RR. Disorders of the small intestine. In: Hay WW, Levin MJ, Sondheimer JM, Deterding RR, eds. *CURRENT Diagnosis & Treatment: Pediatrics*. 20th ed. New York, NY: McGraw-Hill; 2011. http://www.accessphysiotherapy.com/content/6583860. Accessed June 16, 2013.

ADDITIONAL REFERENCES

- Bundy DG, Byerley JS, Liles EA, Perrin EM, Katznelson J, Rice H. Does this child have appendicitis? *JAMA*. 2007;298(4):438–451.
- Chandrasoma P, Taylor CR. Miscellaneous diseases of the intestine. In: Chandrasoma P, Taylor CR, eds. *Concise Pathology*. 3rd ed. New York, NY: McGraw-Hill; 2011. http://www.accessphysiotherapy.com/content/189241. Accessed June 16, 2013.

- Chandrasoma P, Taylor CR. The Intestines: I. Structure & function; malabsorption syndrome; intestinal obstruction. In: Chandrasoma P, Taylor CR, eds. *Concise Pathology*. 3rd ed. New York, NY: McGraw-Hill; 2011. http://www.accessphysiotherapy.com/content/189094. Accessed June 16, 2013.
- Dutton M. Chapter 9, Differential diagnosis. In: Dutton M, ed. *Orthopaedic Examination, Evaluation, and Intervention*. 3rd ed. New York, NY: McGraw-Hill; 2012. http://www.accessphysiotherapy.com/content/5547528. Accessed June 16, 2013.
- Dutton M. Imaging studies in orthopaedics. In: Dutton M, ed. *Orthopaedic Examination, Evaluation, and Intervention*. 3rd ed. New York, NY: McGraw-Hill; 2012. http://www.accessphysiotherapy.com/content/55601056. Accessed June 16, 2013.
- Garcia K, Hernanz-Schulman M, Bennett DL, Morrow SE, Yu C, Kan JH. Suspected appendicitis in children: diagnostic importance of normal abdominopelvic CT findings with nonvisualized appendix. *Radiology*. 2009;250(2):531–537.
- Wan MJ, Krahn M, Ungar WJ, et al. Acute appendicitis in young children: cost-effectiveness of US versus CT in diagnosis—a Markov decision analytic model. *Radiology*. 2009;250(2):378–386.
- Whyte C, Levin T, Harris BH. Early decisions in perforated appendicitis in children: lessons from a study of nonoperative management. *J Pediatr Surg*. 2008;43(8):1459–1463.
- Zheng H, Sun Y, Lin S, Mao Z, Jiang B. Yersinia enterocolitica infection in diarrheal patients. *Eur J Clin Microbiol Infect Dis*. 2008;27(8):741–752.

31 BOWEL INCONTINENCE

Debra F. Stern, DPT, DBA, MSM, PT
Eric Shamus, PhD, DPT, PT, CSCS

CONDITION/DISORDER SYNONYM

- Fecal incontinence (FI)

ICD-9-CM CODES

- 315.4 Coordination disorder (clumsiness, dyspraxia and/or specific motor development disorder)
- 718.45 Contracture of joint, pelvic region and thigh
- 719.70 Difficulty in walking
- 728.2 Muscular wasting and disuse atrophy
- 728.89 Other disorders of muscle, ligament, and fascia
- 729.9 Other disorders of soft tissue
- 780.7 Malaise and fatigue
- 781.2 Abnormality of gait: Ataxic, paralytic, spastic, staggering
- 782.3 Edema
- 786.0 Dyspnea and respiratory abnormalities
- 786.05 Shortness of breath
- 787.6 Incontinence of feces

ICD-10-CM CODE

- R15.9 Full incontinence of feces

PREFERRED PRACTICE PATTERN

As of July, 2014, the APTA Guide to Physical Therapist Practice does not include practice patterns for organ systems pathology; therefore, the associated or secondary musculoskeletal, cardiovascular/pulmonary, or potential neuromuscular patterns would be indicated.

PATIENT PRESENTATION

A 75-year-old male is referred to home health for PT after a 23-hour-observation hospital stay for dehydration and cachexia. He received IV fluids and was discharged home; a friend had brought him to the hospital and took him home. The patient is referred for functional decline and muscle atrophy. His history reveals that over the past 6 months he went out less and less, as he had "occasional accidents" soiling himself and was getting increasingly depressed. He describes little or no appetite, but likes to drink tea. Initial exam reveals limited endurance, fatiguing after 10 minutes of continuous low-level activity, muscle wasting in both of the lower extremities, and difficulty rising from a standard height chair. Throughout the 45 minutes, he is almost continuously expelling gas, and there is a distinct odor of feces.

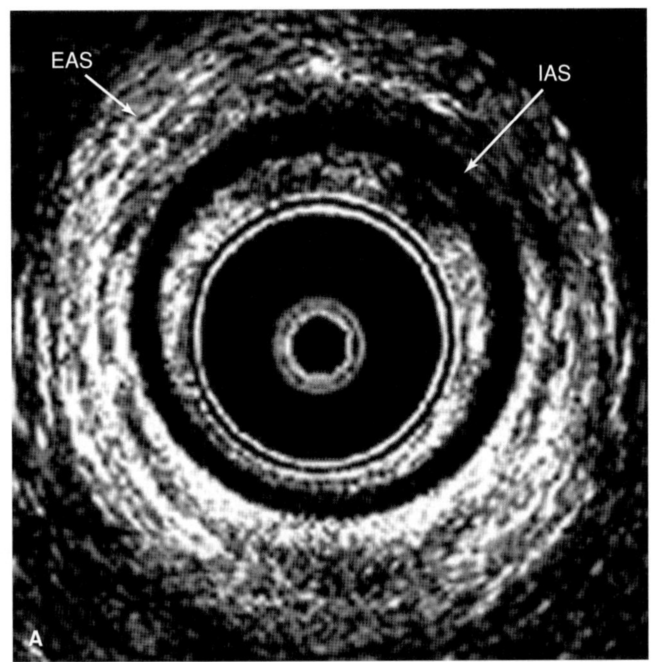

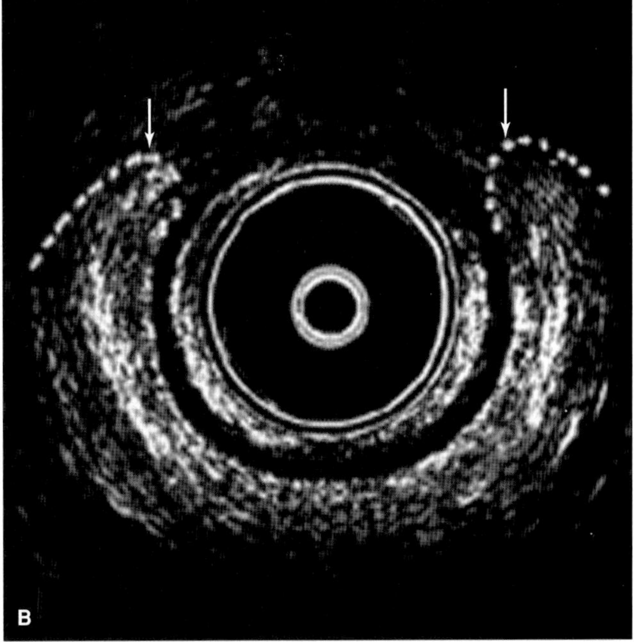

FIGURE 31-1 Anal endosonography. **A.** A woman with normal anal sphincters. **B.** Anterior defects of the external and internal anal sphincter muscles. EAS, external anal sphincter; IAS, internal anal sphincter. *Dashed lines* and *arrows* in **B** illustrate the ends of the torn EAS. (From Hoffman BL, Schorge J, Schaffer J, Halvorson L, Bradshaw K, Cunningham F. *Williams Gynecology*. 2nd ed. New York, NY: McGraw-Hill; 2012.)

KEY FEATURES

Description

- Loss of bowel control, complete or occasional.
- There is a broad array of gastrointestinal (GI) disorders that may be encountered, though not managed specifically, by physical therapists.
- Patients with GI pathology may receive care as a result of secondary problems such as weakness, gait abnormalities, and limited aerobic endurance.
- Symptoms may be acute, postoperative, chronic, viral, bacterially related, or congenital/hereditary.
- Complaints often include changes in bowel habits: Constipation, diarrhea, bowel urgency, incontinence, and cramping.
- Pain is frequently referred to the low back.

Essentials of Diagnosis

- Must be made by a physician and confirmed by medical diagnostic testing
- Complaints of
  - Abdominal pain: Constant or intermittent
  - Abdominal tenderness
  - Nausea
  - Vomiting
  - Diarrhea or constipation: Changes in bowel habits
  - Bloating
  - Possible rectal bleeding
  - Rectal/anal irritation
  - Acute drops in blood pressure, which may result in decreased blood flow to intestines
  - Inability to swallow
  - Lack of appetite
  - Unexplained weight loss
  - Abdominal pain upon ingesting food
  - Possible joint pains
  - Dark stool or bright red blood in stool
  - Malaise/fatigue
- Description by individual
  - Recent illness (bacterial, viral)
  - Ingestion of spoiled food

General Considerations

- PTs should recognize the possibility of GI pathology in differential diagnosis, especially when findings are not consistent with conditions commonly treated: Musculoskeletal, neuromuscular, integumentary, cardiopulmonary, functional, and mobility dysfunction secondary to medical pathology.
- As GI symptoms are frequently referred to the back and shoulders, patients may be inappropriately referred to PT.
- Diagnosis for more occult problems may take time and require intensive medical diagnostic testing.
- GI disorders occur throughout the lifespan (birth through geriatric).
- May result in secondary problems indicating the need for physical therapy intervention: Impairment of aerobic capacity and muscle endurance, sarcopenia, weakness, impaired muscle performance, musculoskeletal problems, neuromuscular problems, weight loss, or weight gain.
- Symptoms may include chronic diarrhea, episodic diarrhea, loss of bowel control (incontinence or urgency), blood in stool.

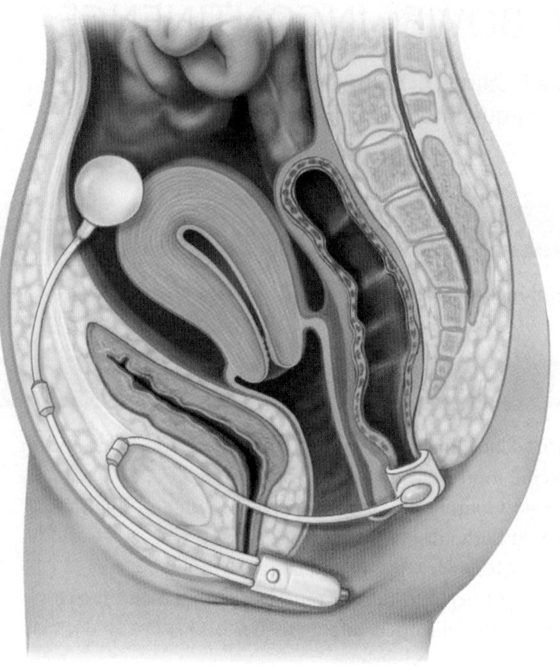

FIGURE 31-2 Artificial anal sphincter. The inflated cuff occludes the anal canal. When defecation is desired, the control pump in the labia is squeezed to remove fluid from the anal cuff into the reservoir balloon. Once emptied, the cuff relieves pressure around the anus and permits defecation. After several minutes, the fluid within the reservoir returns to the anal cuff to restore circumferential pressure and continence. (From Hoffman BL, Schorge J, Schaffer J, Halvorson L, Bradshaw K, Cunningham F. *Williams Gynecology*. 2nd ed. New York, NY: McGraw-Hill; 2012.)

- Because GI disorders frequently refer pain to other body areas, individuals may be referred to PT inappropriately.
- GI problems may be commonly related to stress, constipation, more serious problems such as autoimmune conditions (Crohn disease), or acute pain from appendicitis.
- In adults females, GI complaints may be .. indicative of cancer or tumors in the reproductive organs, or gynecological problems such as endometriosis, uterine fibroids, ectopic pregnancies.
- In males and females, GI problems may be related to inguinal or umbilical hernias.
- History of heartburn or indigestion may be indicative of GI or cardiac problems.

Demographics

- Equal occurrence in males and females
- No difference based on race or ethnicity
- Estimated 8.3% of noninstitutionalized adults[1]
- Risk increases with age
- Higher incidence associated with childbirth complications in females.

CLINICAL FINDINGS

SIGNS AND SYMPTOMS

- May be characteristic of multiple GI disorders, often confounding medical diagnosis
- Bowel changes
  - Diarrhea (acute, chronic)
  - Constipation (acute, chronic)
  - Change in odor or color

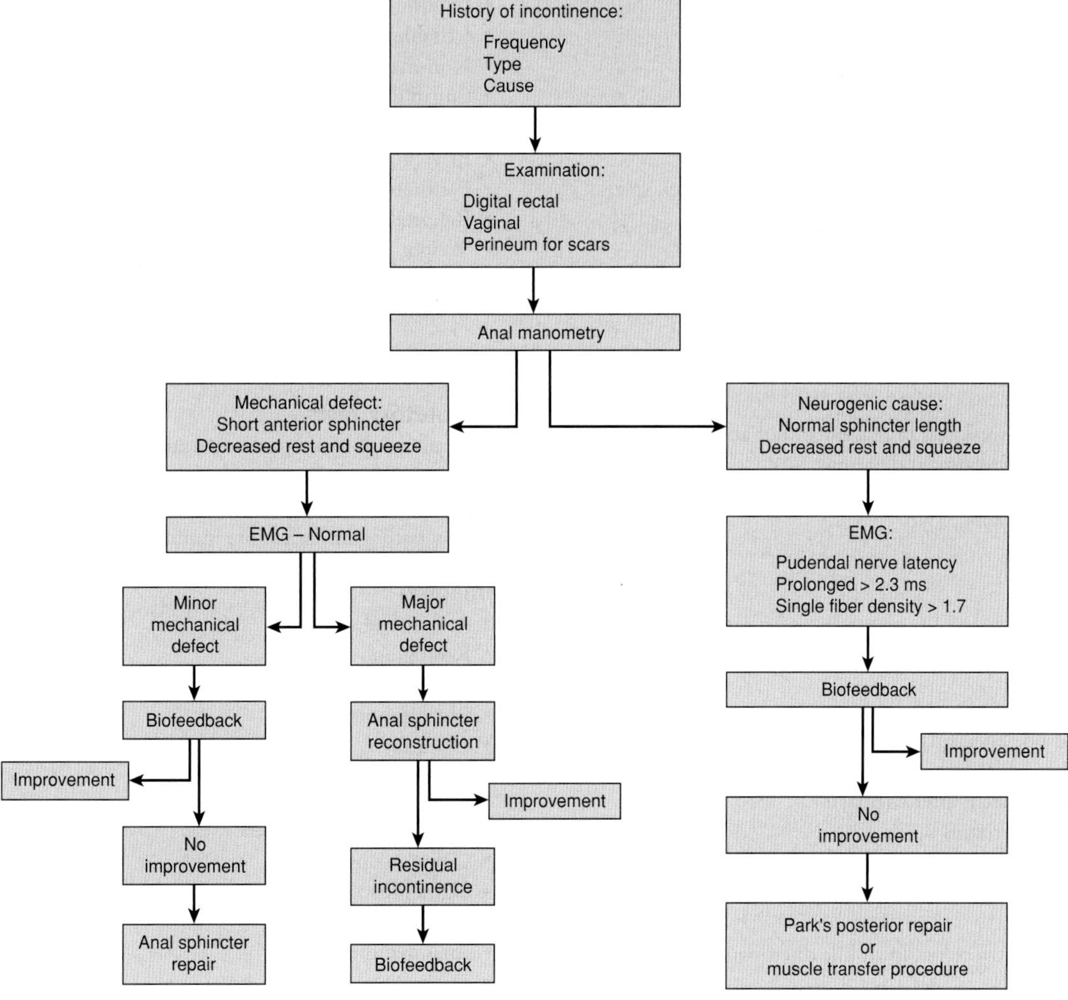

FIGURE 31-3 Algorithm for workup and treatment of fecal incontinence. (Reproduced with permission from Grendel JH, McQuaid KR, Friedman SL. *Current Diagnosis & Treatment in Gastroenterology.* Originally published by Appleton & Lange. Copyright © 1996 by The McGraw-Hill Companies, Inc.)

  - Blood in stool (dark or bright), rectal bleeding (fresh blood vs. darkened stool color)
  - Pain with defecation
  - Changes in bowel habits
  - Mucous in stool or mucous discharge
  - Feeling of having to move bowels constantly
- Changes in appetite
  - Loss of appetite, cachexia
  - Unexplained weight loss
  - Complaints of "feeling full" regardless of having ingested food
- Pain
  - Abdominal/stomach pain or cramping (constant or intermittent and severe)
  - Abdominal pain upon ingesting food or liquid
    - May be cardiac in nature
  - Lower abdominal pain
  - Pain after ingesting fatty foods (gallbladder sign)
  - Abdominal muscle spasm, guarding
- Bloated or swollen abdomen, abdominal distention
- Fever
- Chills
- Fatigue
- Anemia
- Skin irritation
- Flatulence
- Ascites
- Difficulty swallowing (related to esophageal or oral problems rather than neuromuscular)
- Intestinal necrosis

Functional Implications

- Severe symptoms associated with immediacy of defecation, such as diarrhea, may be disabling and result in the inability to leave home
- Chronic constipation, resulting in severe pain or fecal material backing up through the esophagus, requiring manual extraction, surgery, bowel retraining, and leakage of fecal material
- Dehydration caused by severe diarrhea, emesis, loss of appetite, inability to drink or eat secondary to nausea, or inability to swallow
- Eating disorders/anorexia secondary to fear of pain associated with ingesting food, bulimia, binge eating
- Anemia
- Sarcopenia resulting in weakness, loss of muscle mass, inability to ambulate, or perform self-care as well as aerobic capacity limitation secondary to inactivity
- Need for colostomies or ileostomies, temporary or permanent (usually with intestinal problems vs. upper GI)
  - May present a problem with stoma retraction associated with abdominal contraction
- Decreased exercise tolerance
- Lifestyle changes limiting physical activity
- Reluctance to leave home

- Fatigue
- Inappropriate self-medication
- Anxiety and depression
- Limitations in ADLs or IADLs
- Infection
- Osteoporosis
- Dietary restrictions: Consistency, types of food (dairy, spices, wheat/gluten in celiac disease)
- Psychological challenges
- Need to wear protective undergarments: Adult "briefs"

Possible Contributing Causes

- Constipation
- Diarrhea
- Muscle damage, weakness in rectum and or anus
- Nerve damage of rectum and or anus
- Complications of childbirth
- Infections: Bacterial or viral
  - Food poisoning
  - Parasites
- Stress, anxiety
- Obstruction in colon decreasing blood supply and causing inflammation
- Inflammatory: Autoimmune disease
- Medication side effects: Diarrhea, GI "upset," constipation, GI bleeding, rectal bleeding, blood in stool
- Chemical (may occur after enemas)
- Environmental irritants
- Allergy (gluten/wheat, dairy)
- Food intolerance (lactose, prurines)
- Diet
- Cancer: Esophagus, colon, liver, bile duct, pancreatic, metastatic, anal/rectal
- Systemic rheumatologic disorders (scleroderma, rheumatoid arthritis [RA])
- Systemic immunological condition
- Medical error (nicked/cut vessels or tissues unidentified at time of surgery, pharmacological errors)
- Endocrine dysfunction

Differential Diagnosis

- Autoimmune diseases affecting upper and lower GI tracts
- Appendicitis
- Bladder infections, urinary tract infections, kidney pathology
- Bowel disorders including
  - Constipation or diarrhea
  - Inflammation of abdominal or organ linings
  - Obstructions or torsions
- Celiac disease/gluten intolerance
- Colitis (ulcerative, non-ulcerative)
- Crohn disease
- Endocrine disorders
- Gastroenteritis
- Gynecologic problems in females such as
  - Endometriosis
  - Menses
  - Ectopic pregnancies
  - Ovarian cysts
  - Fibroids
- Infections in the abdomen
- Inflammatory bowel disease
- Irritable bowel syndrome
- Non-malignant tumors in abdomen or organs
- Organ dysfunction as a result of cancer or malignancy (colon cancer, ovarian cancer)
- Pelvic inflammatory disease
- Perforated ulcers anywhere in GI system
- Referred pain from heart, spine, hip
- Weight–loss/bariatric-surgery complications (intestinal and liver nicks, leaking between sutures); side effects may mimic diverticulitis or cause flare-up

MEANS OF CONFIRMATION OR DIAGNOSIS

Laboratory Tests

- Fecal occult blood tests/stool samples
- Blood tests
- Hemoglobin and hematocrit (H & H) for signs of bleeding, anemia, pathogens, infection, immune status, vitamin deficiencies

Imaging

- Abdominal scans
- Radiography
- Barium enemas
- Proctography
- CT scans
- Anorectal ultrasonography

Diagnostic Procedures

- Colonoscopy
- Sigmoidoscopy
- Proctosigmoidoscopy
- Anal manometry
- Digital rectal exam
- Manual palpation for tenderness
- Anal electromyography

FINDINGS AND INTERPRETATION

- Chronic diarrhea, episodic diarrhea, loss of bowel control (incontinence or urgency), blood in stool may be symptomatic of inflammatory disease, precancerous conditions, or cancer.

TREATMENT

Medication

- Antidiarrheals
- Laxatives
- Stool softeners
- Drugs that decrease bowel motility

MEDICAL PROCEDURES

- Bowel resection, with or without colostomy or ileostomy
- Removal of tumors/growths
- Release of adhesions
- Stomach resections
- Ulcer repairs
- Nasogastric (NG) tubes
- Percutaneous endoscopic gastrostomy (PEG) tubes/feeding
- Total parental nutrition (TPN)/peripheral parenteral nutrition (PPN)
- IV for hydration

REFERRALS/ADMITTANCE

- If patient is referred for PT but causative problem is not appropriate for PT, refer to appropriate physician
- If emergency is identified, refer to ER

IMPAIRMENTS

- Muscle weakness
- Muscle atrophy
- Gait abnormality, difficulty walking
- Contractures of soft tissue (fascia, muscle), joint limitations
- Shortness of breath
- Possible rectal muscle impairment
- Inability to perform self-care
- Limited aerobic endurance
- Functional decline

TESTS AND MEASURES

- Observation
  - Scars may indicate adhesions or abdominal surgeries that may be causative of diverticula.
  - Pink or purplish striae may be indicative of Cushing syndrome; dilated veins may indicate hepatic pathology or inferior vena cava obstruction, not diverticulitis.
  - Contour: Roundedness, concavity/hollowness, asymmetry, distension, pregnancy signs.
  - Cullen sign: Bluish discoloring around umbilicus, may be a sign of retroperitoneal bleeding.
  - Bluish discoloration in lower abdomen: Grey Turner sign indicates hemorrhagic pancreatitis.
  - Bulging in groin or other areas of abdomen especially apparent with contraction of musculature may be hernia.
  - Pulsing in the area of the navel may be abdominal aortic aneurysm.
  - Left lower quadrant pain, often following a meal.
  - Palpable abdominal tenderness, generalized.
  - Psoas sign: Provides resistance over patient's right knee as they flex the hip, pain indicative of appendicitis or possible inflammation of the abdomen.
  - Obturator sign: Pain with internal rotation of the thigh with the right hip flexed and flexion may be indicative of appendicitis or pelvic inflammation.
  - Rovsing sign: Pain on the right side of abdomen when pressure is put on the left may be indicative of appendicitis.
- Palpation
  - Appendix (McBurney's): Apply vertical pressure halfway between right ASIS and umbilicus: −/+ may be indicative of appendicitis.
  - Liver: In supine, with left hand under trunk parallel to 11th and 12th rib, lift upward; right hand lateral to rectus, press in and up: +/= reproduction of symptoms with deep breath indicates liver involvement.
  - Ascites: With the fingers, percuss outward from center; ascites may be present if sound is dull.
  - Spleen: It is not recommended for PT to palpate an enlarged spleen secondary to rupture issues (only palpable if enlarged).
  - Gallbladder (Murphy's): Place fingers to the right of rectus abdominus below rib cage: +/= sudden pain and muscle tensing with deep breath.
  - Kidneys: In supine, place one hand under client between ribs and iliac crest, other hand on abdomen below ribs and pointing in opposite direction: +/− tenderness or reproduction of symptoms.
  - Bladder: Not usually palpable unless it is distended and rises above pubic bone; in supine, place hand above pubis and press down: +/= tenderness, reproduction of pain, or ability to feel the bladder: __+ ___−.

INTERVENTION

- If there is a stoma from colostomy or ileostomy, PT must be aware that activities should be avoided if they cause retraction.
- Physical therapy intervention is consistent with movement-related problems occurring secondary to GI problem and include
  - Gait training.
  - Therapeutic exercise: All relevant categories, energy conservation
  - Therapeutic activities for bed-mobility training, transfer- and transitional-movement training.
  - Neuromuscular re-education, biofeedback for muscle re-education
  - Self-care management training.
  - Electrical stimulation of rectus/anus in cases of incontinence, muscle control, coordination.
  - Manual therapy.
  - Massage.
  - Lifestyle-modification training.
- Weight management.
- Dietary counseling.
- Psychological intervention.

FUNCTIONAL GOALS

- Patient will be able to
  - A achieve adequate functional aerobic capacity, and the ability to talk during activity in order to achieve functional gait and activity tolerance for work, play, school, self-care; ADLs and IADLs.
  - Have functional gait in the home and community (with or without a device) allowing for work, play, self-care; ADLs and IADLs.
  - A achieve 600 m or greater in a 6-minute walk test for initiation of safe functional gait in the community.
  - Perform active verbalization with increasing taxonomy for safety during gait, including negotiation of even and uneven surfaces, opening and closing doors, transferring in and out of a car.
  - Perform activities requiring abdominals with appropriate muscle splinting/guarding to prevent retraction of stoma, if patient has a colostomy or ileostomy.
  - Tolerate 30 minutes of continuous moderate exercise three times a week in ______weeks, and five times a week in ___________ weeks, depending on disease severity.

PROGNOSIS

- Physician who establishes the medical prognosis, as pathology is primarily medical in nature.
- For PT prognosis, goals should be established based on the patient's overall condition.
- Prognosis from a PT perspective should be good unless medical condition is unstable or the goals unrealistic.

PATIENT RESOURCE

- Bowel Incontinence. American Society of Colon and Rectal Surgeons. http://www.fascrs.org/patients/conditions/bowel_incontinence. Accessed August 8, 2014.

REFERENCE

1. Whitehead WE, Borrud L, Goode PS, et al. Fecal incontinence in U.S. adults: epidemiology and risk factors. *Gastroenterology.* 2009;137(2):512–517.e2. doi: 10.1053/j.gastro.2009.04.054.

ADDITIONAL REFERENCES

- Chandrasoma P, Taylor CR. Idiopathic inflammatory bowel disease. In: Chandrasoma P, Taylor CR, eds. *Concise Pathology.* 3rd ed. New York, NY: McGraw-Hill; 2011. http://www.accessphysiotherapy.com/content/189377, Accessed June 9, 2013.
- Goodman CC, Fuller KS. *Pathology Implications for the Physical Therapist.* 3rd ed. St. Louis, MO: Saunders Elsevier; 2009.
- Goodman CC, Snyder TE. *Differential Diagnosis for Physical Therapists Screening for Referral.* 4th ed. St. Louis, MO: Saunders Elsevier; 2007.
- Hay WW, Levin MJ, Sondheimer JM, Deterding RR. Biliary tract disease. In: Hay WW, Levin MJ, Sondheimer JM, Deterding RR, eds. *CURRENT Diagnosis & Treatment: Pediatrics.* 20th ed. New York, NY: McGraw-Hill; 2011. http://www.accessphysiotherapy.com/content/6584598. Accessed June 9, 2013.
- ICD9DATA. http://www.icd9data.com. Accessed June 9, 2013.
- ICD10DATA. http://www.icd10data.com. Accessed June 9, 2013.
- McOmber M, Shulman RJ. Pediatric functional gastrointestinal disorders. *Nutr Clin Prac.* 2008;23(3):268–274.
- McPhee SJ, Hammer GD. Disorders of the gallbladder. In: McPhee SJ, Hammer GD, eds. *Pathophysiology of Disease.* 6th ed. New York, NY: McGraw-Hill; 2010. http://www.accessphysiotherapy.com/content/5369694. Accessed June 9, 2013.
- Nelson H. Diseases of the rectum and anus. In: Goldman L, Ausiello D, eds. *Cecil Medicine.* 23rd ed. Philadelphia, PA: Saunders Elsevier; 2007.
- Rao SSC. Fecal incontinence. In: Feldman M, Friedman LS, Brandt LJ, eds. *Sleisenger and Fordtran's Gastrointestinal and Liver Disease.* 9th ed. Philadelphia, PA: Saunders Elsevier; 2010.
- Suleiman S, Johnston DE. The abdominal wall: an overlooked source of pain. *Am Fam Physician.* 2001;64(3):431–439.

32 CELIAC DISEASE

Debra F. Stern, DPT, DBA, MSM, PT
Eric Shamus, PhD, DPT, PT, CSCS
David W. Mandel, PhD, PT

ICD-9-CM CODE[1]

- 579.0 Celiac disease
- Associated physical therapy diagnosis
  - 718.45 Contracture of joint, pelvic region and thigh
  - 719.70 Difficulty in walking
  - 728.2 Muscular wasting and disuse atrophy
  - 728.89 Other disorders of muscle, ligament, and fascia
  - 729.9 Other disorders of soft tissue
  - 780.7 Malaise and fatigue
  - 781.2 Abnormality of gait: Ataxic, paralytic, spastic, staggering
  - 782.3 Edema
  - 786.0 Dyspnea and respiratory abnormalities
  - 786.05 Shortness of breath

ICD-10-CM CODE[2]

- K90.0 Celiac disease

PREFERRED PRACTICE PATTERN[3]

As of July, 2014, the APTA Guide to Physical Therapist Practice does not include practice patterns for organ system pathology; therefore, the associated or secondary musculoskeletal, cardiovascular/pulmonary, or potential neuromuscular patterns would be indicated.

PATIENT PRESENTATION

Patient is a 28-year-old male who presents to the outpatient physical therapy department by referral from his primary physician for general strengthening and endurance training. The patient appears very cachectic and muscle wasted. He reports malaise and fatigue with minimal activity. He reports frequent achy joint pain throughout his body. The patient states his symptoms increase with the types of food he eats, and that his physician has stressed he needs to eat a "gluten-free" diet. In addition, the patient reports occasional abdominal bloating and loose bowel movements.

Upon physical therapy examination, the patient's mobility status is modified independent because of decreased speed and general joint discomfort. Bilateral upper extremity and lower extremity strength is 4/5 but with decreased muscle endurance. Joint range of motion is full with inconsistent discomfort. Sensory is fully intact. Performance on the functional strength and endurance tests (30-second chair stand and the 6-minute walk) results are in below-average scores for his age. Heart rate at rest was 72 bpm but was elevated to 140 during the 6-minute walk. During pulmonary testing the patient demonstrated poor maximal inspiratory and expiratory pressures revealing weakness of his diaphragmatic and respiratory musculature.

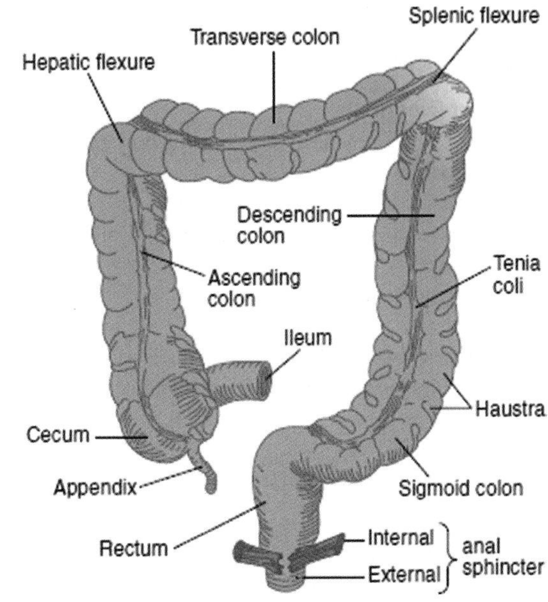

FIGURE 32-1 The human colon. (From Barrett KE, Barman SM, Boitano S, Brooks HL. *Ganong's Review of Medical Physiology*. www.accessmedicine.com. Copyright © The McGraw-Hill Companies, Inc. All rights reserved.)

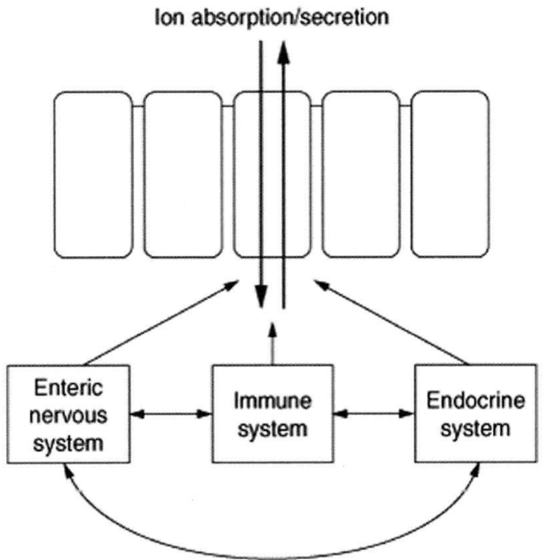

FIGURE 32-2 Regulation of intestinal ion transport. The balance between fluid and electrolyte absorption and secretion across the intestinal epithelium is regulated by an interplay between endocrine, neurocrine, and immune cell factors. (From Barrett K. *Gastrointestinal Physiology*. www.accessmedicine.com. Copyright © The McGraw-Hill Companies, Inc. All rights reserved.)

KEY FEATURES

Description

- Intolerance of the protein gluten, found in wheat, rye, and barley products
- Clients may have GI pathology and be receiving physical therapy for secondary problems, such as weakness, gait abnormalities, limited aerobic endurance
- Changes in bowel habits: Constipation, diarrhea, bowel urgency, incontinence, abdominal cramping
- Pain frequently referred to the low back

Essentials of Diagnosis

- Must be made by a physician and confirmed by medical diagnostic testing
- Abdominal pain, constant or intermittent
- Abdominal pain upon ingesting food, especially meals containing gluten products
- Abdominal tenderness
- Vomiting
- Changes in bowel habits: Diarrhea or constipation
- Acute drop in blood pressure, may result in decreased blood flow to intestines
- Lack of appetite
- Dark stool or bright red blood in stool
- Malaise/fatigue

General Considerations

- GI disorders occur across the lifespan (birth through geriatric).
- Depending on severity, secondary problems may indicate the need for physical therapy, such as aerobic capacity, muscle endurance impairment, sarcopenia, weakness, impaired muscle performance, musculoskeletal problems, neuromuscular problems, weight loss, or weight gain.
- Symptoms include chronic diarrhea, episodic diarrhea, loss of bowel control (incontinence or urgency), blood in stool, which may also be symptomatic of inflammatory disease, precancerous conditions, or cancer.
- Diagnosis for more occult problems may take time and required intensive medical diagnostic testing.
- GI disorders often refer pain to other body areas; individuals may be referred to PT inappropriately.
- In adult females, GI complaints may indicate cancer/tumors in the reproductive organs or gynecological problems such as endometriosis, uterine fibroids, ectopic pregnancies.
- May indicate inguinal or umbilical hernias in males or females.
- History of heartburn or indigestion may indicate GI or cardiac problems.
- Iron deficiency anemia.
- Early onset osteoporosis or osteopenia.
- Vitamin K deficiency associated with hemorrhaging risk.
- Vitamin and mineral deficiencies.
- Central and peripheral nervous system disorders: Usually due to unsuspected nutrient deficiencies.
- Pancreatic insufficiency.
- Intestinal lymphomas and other GI cancers (malignancies).
- Gall bladder malfunction.
- Neurological manifestations.

Demographics

- Can occur at any age
- Men and women equally affected

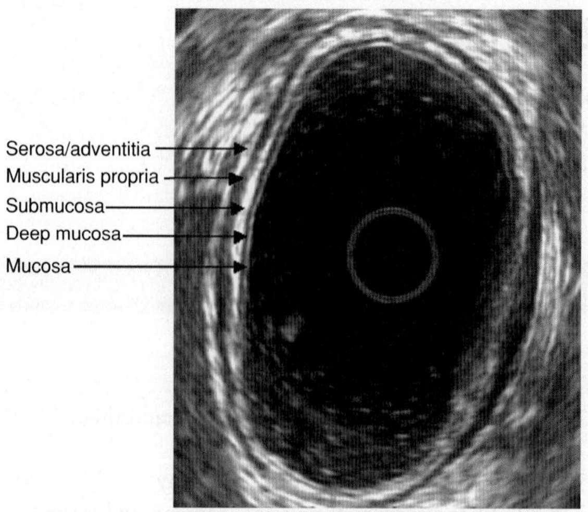

FIGURE 32-3 EUS image of normal gastrointestinal wall layers. (From Greenberger NJ, Blumberg RS, Burakoff R. *Current Diagnosis & Treatment: Gastroenterology, Hepatology, & Endoscopy.* 2nd ed. www.accessmedicine.com. Copyright © The McGraw-Hill Companies, Inc. All rights reserved.)

- Familial
- Higher incidence in people of White European descent
- Overall incidence unknown, underdiagnosed
- Estimated incidence: 1 in 5000 to 1 in 100[4]

CLINICAL FINDINGS

SIGNS AND SYMPTOMS

- Signs and symptoms indicated below may be characteristic of multiple GI disorders, often confounding medical diagnosis.
- Physical therapists should recognize the possibility of GI pathology in the differential diagnosis process, especially when findings are not consistent with conditions commonly treated: Musculoskeletal, neuromuscular, integumentary, cardiopulmonary, functional/mobility dysfunction secondary to medical pathology.
- GI symptoms frequently referred to back and shoulders; patients may be inappropriately referred to PT.
- Bowel Changes
  - Change in odor or color
  - Diarrhea (acute, chronic)
  - Constipation (acute, chronic)
  - Blood in stool: Dark or bright (fresh bleeding), rectal bleeding, fatty stools
  - Rectal bleeding (fresh blood rather than darkened stool)
  - Mucous in stool or mucous discharge
- Pain
  - Abdominal/stomach pain or cramping; severe, may be constant or intermittent
  - Abdominal pain after ingesting food or liquid (may be cardiac in nature)
  - Lower abdominal pain
  - Pain associated with defecation
  - Pain after ingesting fatty foods (gallbladder sign)
- Bloated or swollen abdomen, abdominal distention
- Unexplained weight loss or gain
- Abdominal muscle spasm, guarding
- Fatigue
- Anemia
- Loss of appetite, cachexia
- Joint pain
- Osteoporosis/osteopenia
- Flatulence

- Gastroesophageal reflux (GERD), heartburn
- Nausea
- Complaints of "feeling full" regardless of having ingested food
- Skin rash
- Migraine headaches
- Delayed puberty
- Mouth ulcers
- Numbness and or tingling in stocking glove pattern
- Defects in tooth enamel
- Failure to thrive in infants
- Muscle cramps
- Amenorrhea

Functional Implications

- Severe symptoms associated with immediacy of defecation may be disabling and result in the inability to leave home.
- Chronic constipation may cause severe pain and, in severe forms, may result in fecal material backing up through the esophagus, require manual extraction, surgery, in some cases bowel retraining
- Dehydration from severe diarrhea, emesis, loss of appetite, inability to drink or eat, nausea, inability to swallow
- Eating disorders or anorexia secondary to fear of pain associated with ingesting food
- Anemia
- Sarcopenia resulting in weakness, muscle-mass loss, inability to ambulate or perform self-care, and limited aerobic capacity secondary to inactivity
- Need for colostomies or ileostomies, temporary or permanent (usually with intestinal problems rather than upper GI)
  - May present a problem with stoma retraction associated with abdominal contraction
  - Decreased exercise tolerance
- Changes in lifestyle limiting physical activity
- Fatigue
- Inappropriate self-medication
- Anxiety, depression
- Irritability
- May indicate serious medical conditions
- Limitations in ADLs, IADLs
- Osteoporosis
- Dietary restrictions: Consistency, food types (wheat, barley, rye)
- Infertility (males and females)
- Depression

Possible Contributing Causes

- Causes unknown in most cases
- Heredity
- Autoimmune
- Systemic immunological condition

Differential Diagnosis

- Organ dysfunction as a result of cancer or malignancy
- Non-malignant tumors in the abdomen or organs
- Endocrine disorders
- Gynecologic problems in females such as
  - Endometriosis
  - Menses
  - Ectopic pregnancies
  - Ovarian cysts
  - Fibroids
- Autoimmune diseases that affect upper and lower GI tracts
- Appendicitis

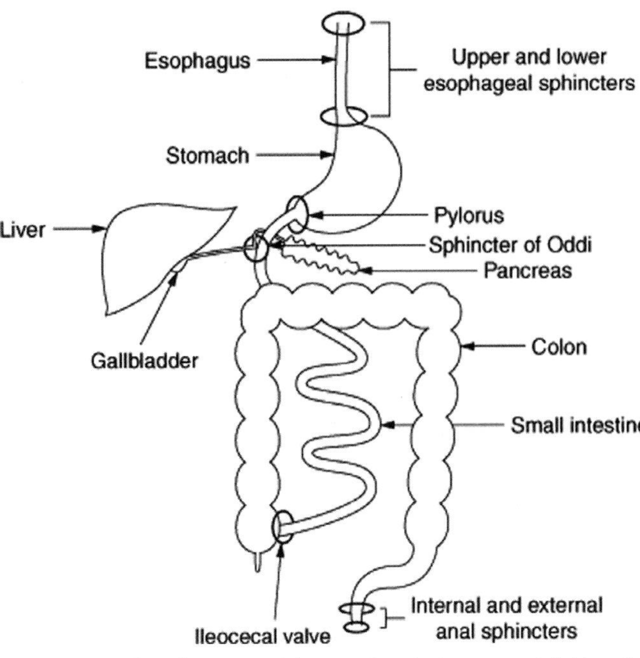

FIGURE 32-4 Overall anatomy of the gastrointestinal system and division of the GI tract into functional segments by sphincters and valves. (From Barrett K. *Gastrointestinal Physiology*. www.accessmedicine.com. Copyright © The McGraw-Hill Companies, Inc. All rights reserved.)

- Irritable bowel syndrome
- Crohn disease
- Colitis (ulcerative, non-ulcerative)
- Colon cancer
- Ovarian cancer
- Inflammatory bowel disease
- Pelvic inflammatory disease
- Gastroenteritis
- Perforated ulcers in GI system
- Bladder infections, urinary tract infections, kidney pathology
- Abdominal infections
- Bowel disorders, including constipation or diarrhea
- Referred pain from heart, spine, hip
- Weight loss–surgery complications: Side effects may mimic celiac disease or cause a flare-up

MEANS OF CONFIRMATION OR DIAGNOSIS

Laboratory Tests

- Fecal occult blood tests/stool samples
- Blood tests
- H & H for signs of bleeding, anemia, pathogens, immune status, vitamin deficiencies, infection

Imaging

- Abdominal scans
- Radiography
- Barium enemas
- CT scans

Diagnostic Procedures

- Upper endoscopy
- Colonoscopy
- Sigmoidoscopy
- Manual palpation for tenderness

FINDINGS AND INTERPRETATION

- Anti-tissue transglutaminase antibody (tTG–IgA and IgG) or anti-endomysial antibody (EMA-IgA) are highly specific markers for celiac disease
- Anti-deamidated gliadin peptide (DGP–IgA and IgG) or total serum IgA anti-gliadin antibody (AgA–IgG and IgA) in children under age 12

TREATMENT

- Dietary management: Gluten is removed from the diet

REFERRAL/ADMITTANCE

- If causative problem is not considered appropriate for PT, referral to appropriate physician must be made.
- If emergency is identified, refer to ER.

IMPAIRMENTS

- Muscle weakness
- Muscle atrophy
- Gait abnormality, difficulty walking
- Contractures of soft tissue (fascia, muscle) or joint limitations
- Possible rectal muscle impairment
- Inability to perform self-care
- Limited aerobic endurance
- Functional decline or decrease

TESTS AND MEASURES

- Observation
  - Scars may indicate adhesions or abdominal surgeries that may be causative of diverticula.
  - Pink or purplish striae may be indicative of Cushing syndrome, dilated veins may indicate hepatic pathology or inferior vena cava obstruction, not diverticulitis.
  - Contour: Roundedness, concavity/hollowness, asymmetry, distension, pregnancy signs.
  - Cullen Sign: Bluish discoloring around umbilicus may be the sign of retroperitoneal bleeding.
  - Bluish discoloration in lower abdomen (Grey Turner sign) is a sign of hemorrhagic pancreatitis.
  - Bulging in groin or other areas of abdomen especially apparent with contraction of musculature may be hernia.
  - Pulsing in navel area may be abdominal aortic aneurysm.
  - Abdominal pain, following ingestion of gluten.
  - Palpable abdominal tenderness.
  - Psoas sign: Provides resistance over patient's right knee as they flex the hip; pain would be indicative of appendicitis or possible inflammation of the abdomen.
  - Obturator sign: Internal rotation of RLE and flexion may be indicative of appendicitis or pelvic inflammation.
  - Rovsing sign: Pain on the right side of abdomen when pressure is put on the left may be indicative of appendicitis.
- Palpation
  - Appendix (McBurney's): Apply vertical pressure halfway between right ASIS and umbilicus: −/+ may be indicative of appendicitis.
  - Liver: In supine, with left hand under trunk parallel to 11th and 12th rib, lift upward; right hand lateral to rectus, press in and up: +/= reproduction of symptoms with deep breath indicates liver involvement.
  - Ascites: Percuss outward from center; if sound is dull, ascites may be present.
  - Spleen: Not recommended for PT to palpate enlarged spleen secondary to rupture issues.
  - Gallbladder (Murphy's): Place fingers to the right of rectus abdominus below rib cage: +/= sudden pain and muscle tensing with deep breath.
  - Kidneys: In supine, place one hand under client between ribs and iliac crest, other hand on abdomen below ribs pointing in opposite direction: +/− tenderness or reproduction of symptoms.
  - Bladder: Not usually palpable unless distended and rises above pubic bone; in supine, place hand above pubis and press down: +/= tenderness, reproduction of pain, ability to feel the bladder.

INTERVENTION

- Physical therapy intervention is consistent with movement-related problems that occur secondary to the GI problem
- Therapeutic exercise: All relevant categories, energy conservation
- Neuromuscular re-education
- Self-care training
- Manual therapy
- Abdominal massage
- Interprofessional
  - Lifestyle modification
  - Smoking cessation
  - Weight management
  - Dietary counseling
  - Psychological intervention
  - Pastoral counseling
  - Surgical management
  - Occupational therapy
  - Speech-language pathology (swallowing deficits, speech impairment)

FUNCTIONAL GOALS

- Patient will be able to
  - Achieve functional gait and activity tolerance for ADLs and IADLs.
  - Achieve functional gait in the home and community (with or without a device) allowing for ADLs and IADLs based on patient's need and prior functional level.
  - Achieve 600 m or greater in a 6-minute walk test for initiation of safe functional gait in the community.
  - Perform active verbalization with increasing taxonomy for safety during gait, including negotiation of even and uneven surfaces, opening and closing doors, transferring in and out of car.
- Patient will perform activities requiring abdominals with appropriate muscle splinting/guarding to prevent retraction of stoma, if patient has colostomy or ileostomy.
- Tolerate 30 minutes of continuous moderate exercise three times a week in ______ weeks, and five times a week in ____________ weeks, depending on disease severity.

PROGNOSIS

- Physician establishes medical prognosis, as this pathology is primarily medical in nature.

- For PT prognosis, goals should be established based on patient's overall condition.
- Prognosis good from PT perspective, unless the medical condition is unstable or goals unrealistic.
- Once on a gluten-free diet it takes 3 to 6 months for healing to take place.

PATIENT RESOURCE

- Celiac Disease Foundation. *Celiac Disease.* http://www.celiac.org. Accessed August 8, 2014.

REFERENCES

1. ICD-9-CM. http://www.icd9data.com. Accessed January 20, 2013.
2. ICD-10-CM. http://www.icd10data.com. Accessed January 20, 2013.
3. APTA Guide to Physical Therapist Practice. http://guidetoptpractice.apta.org./ Accessed January 20, 2013.
4. Hay WW, Levin MJ, Deterding RR, Abzug MJ, Sondheimer JM. Malabsorption syndromes. In: Hay WW, Levin MJ, Deterding RR, Abzug MJ, Sondheimer JM, eds. *CURRENT Diagnosis & Treatment: Pediatrics.* 21st ed. New York, NY: McGraw-Hill; 2012. http://www.accessphysiotherapy.com/content/56821435. Accessed March 13, 2013.

ADDITIONAL REFERENCES

- Goodman CC, Fuller KS. *Pathology Implications for the Physical Therapist.* 3rd ed. St. Louis, MO: Saunders Elsevier; 2009.
- Goodman CC, Snyder TE. *Differential Diagnosis for Physical Therapists Screening for Referral.* 4th ed. St. Louis, MO: Saunders Elsevier; 2007.
- Green PH, Cellier C. Celiac disease. *N Engl J Med.* 2007;357(17):1731–1743.
- McOmber MA, Shulman RJ. Pediatric functional gastrointestinal disorders. *Nutr Clin Prac.* 2008;23(3):268–274.
- McPhee SJ, Hammer GD. Pathophysiology of disorders of the esophagus. In: McPhee SJ, Hammer GD, eds. *Pathophysiology of Disease.* 6th ed. New York, NY: McGraw-Hill; 2010. http://www.accessphysiotherapy.com/content/5369615. Accessed May 13, 2013.
- Mills JC, Stappenbeck TS, Bunnett N. Gastrointestinal disease. In: McPhee SJ, Hammer GD, eds. *Pathophysiology of Disease: An Introduction to Clinical Medicine.* 6th ed. New York, NY: McGraw-Hill; 2010. http://www.accessphysiotherapy.com/content/5369615. Accessed May 13, 2013.
- Suleiman S, Johnston DE. The abdominal wall: an overlooked source of pain. *Am Fam Physician.* 2001;64(3):431–439. http://www.aafp.org/afp/2001/0801/p431.html.
- Ulcerative Colitis. NIH National Institute of Heath. National Digestive Diseases Information Clearinghouse (NDDIC0). US Department of Health and Human Services. NIH *Publication No. 12–1597.* October 2011. http://digestive.niddk.nih.gov/ddiseases/pubs/colitis/. Accessed March 13, 2013.
- Wang KK, Sampliner RE. Updated guidelines 2008 for the diagnosis, surveillance and therapy of Barrett's esophagus. *Am J Gastroenterol.* 2008;103(3):788–797.

33 CHOLELITHIASIS

Debra F. Stern, DPT, DBA, MSM, PT
Eric Shamus, PhD, DPT, PT, CSCS

CONDITION/DISORDER SYNONYM

- Gallstones

ICD-9-CM CODES

- 574 Cholelithiasis
- 574.0 Calculus of gallbladder with acute cholecystitis
- 574.00 Calculus of gallbladder with acute cholecystitis without obstruction
- 574.01 Calculus of gallbladder with acute cholecystitis with obstruction
- 574.1 Calculus of gallbladder with other cholecystitis
- 574.10 Calculus of gallbladder with other cholecystitis without obstruction
- 574.11 Calculus of gallbladder with other cholecystitis with obstruction
- 574.2 Calculus of gallbladder without mention of cholecystitis
- 574.20 Calculus of gallbladder without cholecystitis without obstruction
- 574.21 Calculus of gallbladder without cholecystitis with obstruction
- 574. Calculus of bile duct with acute cholecystitis
- 574.30 Calculus of bile duct with acute cholecystitis without obstruction
- 574.31 Calculus of bile duct with acute cholecystitis with obstruction
- 574.4 Calculus of bile duct with other cholecystitis
- 574.40 Calculus of bile duct with other cholecystitis without obstruction
- 574.41 Calculus of bile duct with other cholecystitis with obstruction
- 574.5 Calculus of bile duct without mention of cholecystitis
- 574.50 Calculus of bile duct without cholecystitis without obstruction
- 574.51 Calculus of bile duct without cholecystitis with obstruction
- 574.6 Calculus of gallbladder and bile duct with acute cholecystitis
- 574.60 Calculus of gallbladder and bile duct with acute cholecystitis without obstruction
- 574.61 Calculus of gallbladder and bile duct with acute cholecystitis with obstruction
- 574.7 Calculus of gallbladder and bile duct with other cholecystitis
- 574.70 Calculus of gallbladder and bile duct with other cholecystitis without obstruction
- 574.71 Calculus of gallbladder and bile duct with other cholecystitis with obstruction

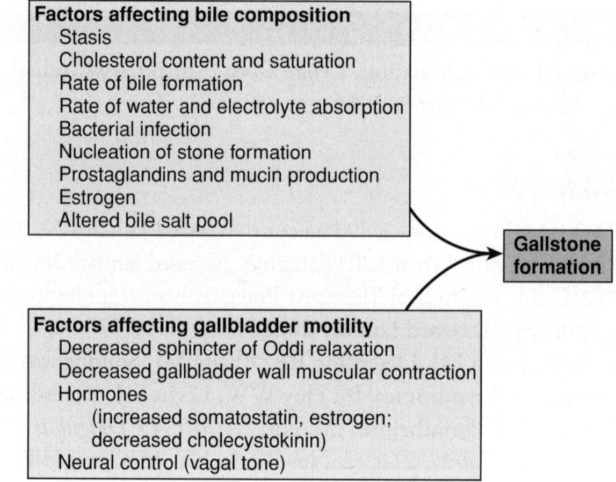

FIGURE 33-1 Pathophysiology of cholelithiasis. (From McPhee SJ, Hammer GD. *Pathophysiology of Disease: An Introduction to Clinical Medicine.* 6th ed. www.accessmedicine.com. Copyright © The McGraw-Hill Companies, Inc. All rights reserved.)

- 574.8 Calculus of gallbladder and bile duct with acute and chronic cholecystitis
- 574.80 Calculus of gallbladder and bile duct with acute and chronic cholecystitis without obstruction
- 574.81 Calculus of gallbladder and bile duct with acute and chronic cholecystitis with obstruction
- 574.9 Calculus of gallbladder and bile duct without cholecystitis
- 574.90 Calculus of gallbladder and bile duct without cholecystitis without obstruction
- 574.91 Calculus of gallbladder and bile duct without cholecystitis with obstruction
- Associated physical therapy diagnoses
  - 315.4 Coordination disorder (clumsiness, dyspraxia and/or specific motor development disorder)
  - 718.45 Contracture of joint, pelvic region and thigh
  - 719.70 Difficulty in walking
  - 728.2 Muscular wasting and disuse atrophy
  - 728.89 Other disorders of muscle, ligament, and fascia
  - 729.9 Other disorders of soft tissue
  - 780.7 Malaise and fatigue
  - 781.2 Abnormality of gait: Ataxic, paralytic, spastic, staggering
  - 782.3 Edema
  - 786.0 Dyspnea and respiratory abnormalities
  - 786.05 Shortness of breath

ICD-10-CM CODE

- K80.00 Calculus of gallbladder with acute cholecystitis without obstruction

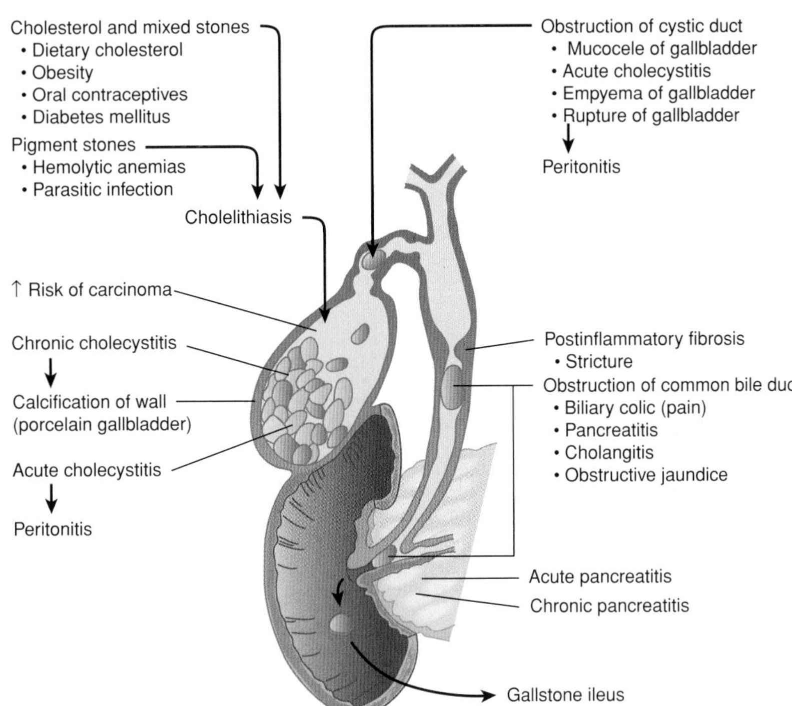

FIGURE 33-2 Clinical and pathologic effects of cholelithiasis. (Redrawn with permission from Chandrasoma P, Taylor CE. *Concise Pathology*. 3rd ed. Originally published by Appleton & Lange. Copyright © 1998 by The McGraw-Hill Companies, Inc.)

PREFERRED PRACTICE PATTERN

As of June, 2014, the APTA Guide to Physical Therapist Practice does not include practice patterns for organ system pathology; therefore, the associated or secondary musculoskeletal, cardiovascular/pulmonary, or potential neuromuscular patterns would be indicated.

PATIENT PRESENTATION

A 50-year-old slightly obese female is complaining of low back pain for about 6 weeks. The pain is constant, but has both exacerbated and remitted since its onset. She has had some mild joint pain in her hips and lower extremities (LEs) that has responded to NSAIDS. Her nights are restless and she is having trouble sleeping and wakes up several times because of discomfort. She is having episodes of nausea and some vomiting with loss of appetite, so she has decreased the NSAIDS to morning only before going to work. She has also had increasing episodes of diarrhea and complains of some abdominal tenderness. She has been referred to PT for the back and hip pain.

KEY FEATURES

Description

- Stones made of cholesterol are the most common type
- Not related to blood cholesterol levels
- Stones made of bilirubin (pigment stones) may occur when red blood cells are destroyed (hemolysis[1]), causing excess bilirubin in the bile
- Complaints include change in bowel habits: Constipation, diarrhea, bowel urgency, incontinence, cramping
- Pain frequently referred to low back

Essentials of Diagnosis

- Abdominal pain in right upper quadrant (constant or intermittent)
- Abdominal tenderness
- Elevated bilirubin nausea
- Vomiting
- Change in bowel habits: Diarrhea, constipation
- Bloating
- Rectal bleeding possible
- Rectal/anal irritation

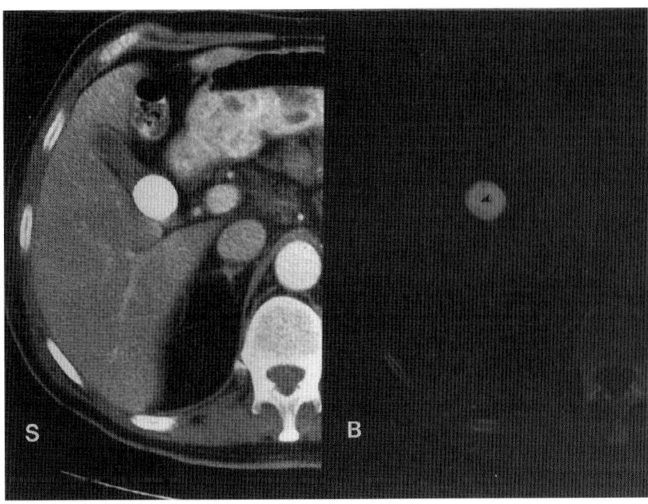

FIGURE 33-3 CT in cholelithiasis using both soft tissue windows (S) and bone windows (B) showing an extremely dense structure lying in the gallbladder. Note the laminated architecture of the gallstone on the bone windows (*arrowhead*). (From Chen MYM, Pope TL, Ott DJ. *Basic Radiology*. 2nd ed. www.accessmedicine.com. Copyright © The McGraw-Hill Companies, Inc. All rights reserved.)

- Acute drop in blood pressure, resulting in decreased blood flow to intestines
- Inability to swallow
- Lack of appetite
- Unexplained weight loss
- Abdominal pain upon ingesting food
- Joint pain possible
- Dark stool or bright red blood in stool
- Malaise, fatigue

General Considerations

- Broad array of GI disorders may be encountered by physical therapists
- Diagnosis for occult problems may take time and require intensive diagnostic testing
- Although PT may not manage GI disorders specifically, clients may receive care for secondary problems: Weakness, gait abnormalities, limited aerobic endurance, sarcopenia, musculoskeletal problems, neuromuscular problems, weight loss, or weight gain
  - May be acute, postoperative, chronic, viral, bacterial, congenital/hereditary
- GI disorders frequently refer pain to other body areas; individuals may be inappropriately referred to PT
- GI problems commonly related to stress or constipation
- More serious problems include autoimmune conditions like Crohn syndrome
- Acute pain indicative of appendicitis
- GI complaints in females may indicate cancer/tumors in reproductive organs, or gynecological problems: Endometriosis, uterine fibroids, ectopic pregnancies
- GI complaints may indicate inguinal or umbilical hernias
- History of heartburn/indigestion may indicate GI or cardiac problems
- Chronic diarrhea, episodic diarrhea, loss of bowel control, blood in stool may indicate inflammatory disease, precancerous condition, cancer

Demographics

- GI disorders occur throughout the lifespan (birth through geriatric)
- More common in females than males
- Higher incidence among Native Americans, Hispanics
- More common in people aged 40 years or older

CLINICAL FINDINGS

SIGNS AND SYMPTOMS

- Symptoms may be characteristic of multiple GI disorders, confounding medical diagnosis.
- PT should recognize the possibility of GI pathology in differential diagnosis, especially when findings are not consistent with conditions commonly treated.
- Pain
  - Abdominal/stomach pain, cramping (constant or intermittent, severe)
  - Pain upon ingesting food or liquid
    - May be cardiac in nature
  - Lower abdominal pain
  - Pain with defecation
  - Pain after ingesting fatty foods (gallbladder sign)
  - Joint pain
  - Pain secondary to hernias
    - Palpable bulging with or without muscle contraction
    - Commonly in the groin, umbilical area or abdomen (especially after pregnancy or any surgery in the abdominal region)
    - Sports hernias
  - Acute, severe pain in right lower quadrant
    - Appendicitis or ectopic pregnancy
- Bowel changes
  - Diarrhea (acute, chronic)
  - Constipation (acute, chronic)
  - Blood in stool, dark or fresh bleeding
  - Rectal bleeding
  - Change in stool odor or color, clay-colored stool
  - Feeling of having to move bowels constantly
  - Mucous in stool or mucous discharge
- Abdominal distention
- Abdominal muscle spasm, guarding
- Unexplained weight loss
- Fever
- Chills
- Fatigue
- Anemia
- Loss of appetite, cachexia
- Skin lesions
- Failure to grow if onset at early age
- Flatulence
- Gastroesophageal reflux (GERD), heartburn
- Nausea
- Emesis
- Ascites
- Difficulty swallowing (related to esophageal or oral problems, not neuromuscular)
- Intestinal necrosis
- Dietary restrictions: Consistency, food types (dairy, spices, wheat/gluten)
- Complaints of "feeling full" regardless of having ingested food
- Jaundice

Functional Implications

- Severe symptoms associated with immediacy of defecation may be disabling, causing inability to leave home
- Chronic constipation may cause severe pain, result in fecal material backing up through the esophagus, require manual extraction, surgery, bowel retraining

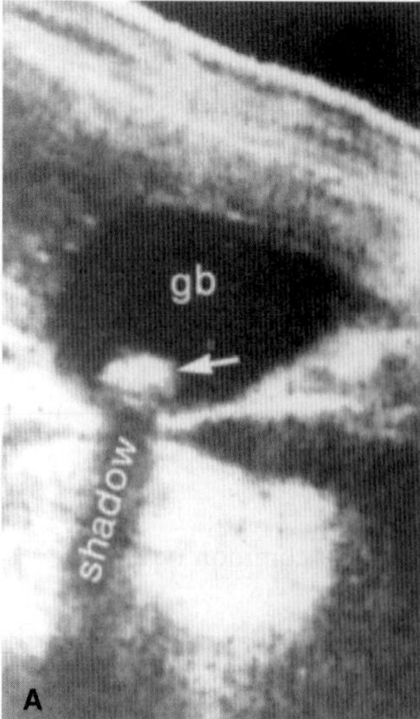

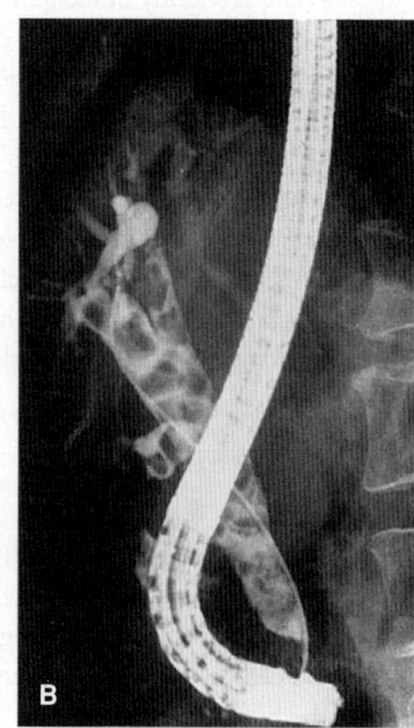

FIGURE 33-4 Gallstones. **A.** Visualization of a lone large gallstone by sonography. Note acoustic shadowing. **B.** Endoscopic retrograde cholangiopancreatogram (ERCP) showing multiple common-duct stones. (From Greenberger NJ, Paumgartner G. Diseases of the gallbladder and bile ducts. In: Fauci AS, Braunwald E, Kasper DL, et al., eds. *Harrison's Principles of Internal Medicine*. 17th ed. New York, NY: McGraw-Hill; 2008: p. 1991, with permission.)

- Dehydration secondary to diarrhea, emesis, appetite loss, nausea, inability to swallow
- Eating disorder/anorexia secondary to fear of pain upon ingesting food
- Anemia
- Sarcopenia resulting in weakness, decreased muscle mass, inability to ambulate or perform self-care, limited aerobic capacity secondary to inactivity
- Decreased exercise tolerance
- Limited physical activity
- Reluctance to leave home
- Fatigue
- Inappropriate self-medication
- Psychological symptoms
  - Anxiety, depression
  - Fear of pain
- Limited ADLs/IADLs
- Infection
- Jaundice of the eye, liver disease
- Dietary restrictions

Possible Contributing Causes

- Infections of biliary tract
- Chronic hemolytic anemia
- Sickle cell anemia
- Inflammatory: Autoimmune disease
- Environmental irritants
- Obesity
- Lack of exercise
- Heredity
- Diet
- Cancer: Esophageal, colon, liver, bile duct, pancreatic, metastatic, anal/rectal
- Medication side effects: Diarrhea, GI upset, constipation, bleeding
- Endocrine dysfunction
- Cholecystitis (acute, chronic)
- Cholangitis
- Choledocholithiasis
- Pancreatitis
- Additional risk factors include
  - Bone marrow or organ transplant[2]
  - Diabetes[3]
  - Failure of gallbladder to empty bile properly (more likely during pregnancy)
  - Liver cirrhosis,[4] biliary tract infections (pigmented stones)
  - Chronic hemolytic anemia and sickle cell anemia can cause the liver to produced excess from low-calorie diet, after bariatric surgery
  - Prolonged intravenous feeding bilirubin[5,6]
  - Rapid weight loss

Differential Diagnosis

- Organ dysfunction from cancer or malignancy
  - Colon cancer
  - Ovarian cancer
- Non-malignant tumor in abdomen or organs
- Endocrine disorder
- Gynecologic problems
  - Endometriosis
  - Menses
  - Ectopic pregnancies
  - Ovarian cysts
  - Fibroids
- Autoimmune diseases affecting upper and lower GI tracts
  - Irritable bowel syndrome (IBS)
  - Systemic lupus erythematosus (SLE)
  - Rheumatoid arthritis (RA)
- Appendicitis
- Crohn disease
- Colitis (ulcerative, non-ulcerative)
- Inflammatory bowel disease (IBD)
- Pancreatic pathology
- Pelvic inflammatory disease
- Celiac disease, gluten intolerance
- Gastroenteritis
- Perforated ulcer in GI system
- Bladder or urinary tract infection, kidney pathology
- Abdominal infection

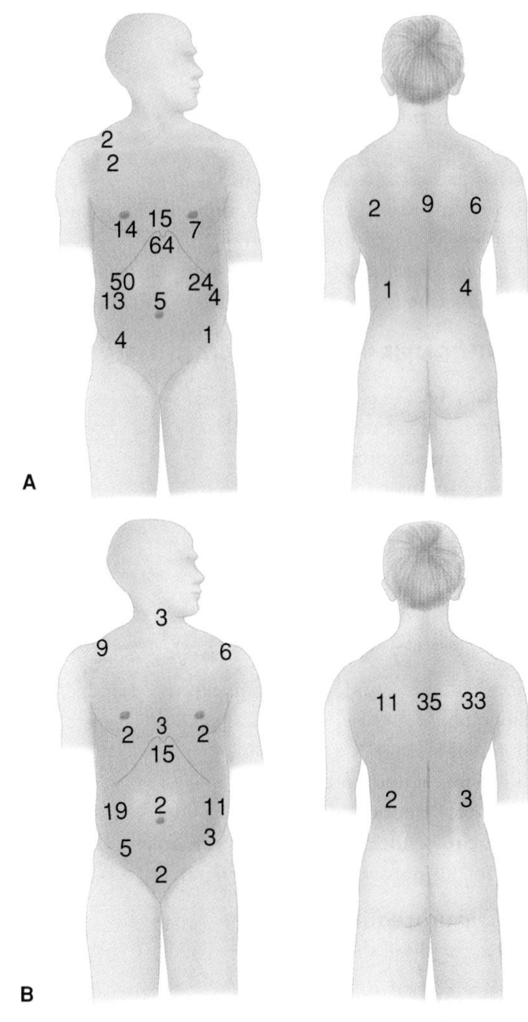

FIGURE 33-5 **A.** Sites of the most severe pain during an episode of biliary pain in 107 patients with gallstones (% values add up to >100% because of multiple responses). The subxiphoid and right subcostal areas were the most common sites; note that the left subcostal area was not an unusual site of pain. **B.** Sites of pain radiation (%) during an episode of biliary pain in the same group of patients. (Reprinted from Gunn A, Keddie N. Some clinical observations on patients with gallstones. *The Lancet*. 1972;300(7771):239–241, Copyright 1972, with permission from Elsevier.)

- Bowel disorder including
  - Constipation, diarrhea
  - Inflamed lining of abdomen
  - Organs obstruction
  - Torsion
- Referred pain from heart, spine, hip
- Post–weight-loss surgery complications: Bariatric surgeries for weight loss are increasingly common
- Post–weight-loss (bariatric) surgery complications
  - Side effects may mimic diverticulitis or cause a flare-up

MEANS OF CONFIRMATION OR DIAGNOSIS

Laboratory Tests

- Fecal occult blood tests/stool samples
- Complete blood count (CBC)
- Amylase and lipase
- H & H
- Bilirubin
- Liver function
- Pancreatic enzymes

Imaging

- Abdominal ultrasound, can identify stones or sludge
- Radiography
- Abdominal CT
- Gallbladder radionuclide scan
- Endoscopic ultrasound
- Magnetic resonance cholangiopancreatography (MRCP)
- Percutaneous transhepatic cholangiogram

Diagnostic procedures

- History and physical
- Colonoscopy
  - Virtual
  - Procedural
- Sigmoidoscopy
- Manual palpation for tenderness

FINDINGS AND INTERPRETATION

- CBC for high white blood cells
- H & H for signs of bleeding, anemia, pathogens, immune status, vitamin deficiencies, white blood cell count

TREATMENT

Medication

- Chenodeoxycholic acids (CDCA)
- Ursodeoxycholic acid (UDCA, ursodiol)

MEDICAL PROCEDURES

- Surgical removal of gallbladder
- Lithotripsy

REFERRALS/ADMITTANCE

- If causative problem is not considered appropriate for PT intervention, refer to appropriate physician.
- If emergency identified, refer to ER.

IMPAIRMENTS

- Muscle weakness
- Muscle atrophy
- Gait abnormality, difficulty walking
- Contractures of soft tissue (fascia, muscle); joint limitations
- Shortness of breath
- Possible rectal muscle impairment
- Inability to perform self-care
- Limited aerobic endurance
- Functional decline

TESTS AND MEASURES

- Observation
  - Scars may indicate adhesions or abdominal surgeries causative of diverticula.
  - Pink or purplish striae may be indicative of Cushing syndrome.
  - Dilated veins may indicate hepatic pathology or inferior vena cava obstruction, not diverticulitis.
  - Contour: Roundness, concavity, asymmetry, distension, pregnancy signs.
  - Cullen sign: Bluish discoloring around the umbilicus may be a sign of retroperitoneal bleeding.
  - Bluish discoloration in lower abdomen: Grey Turner sign, signals hemorrhagic pancreatitis.
  - Bulging in groin or abdomen especially apparent with contraction of musculature in area may be hernia.
  - Pulsing in navel area may be abdominal aortic aneurysm.
  - Left lower quadrant pain, often following a meal.
  - Palpable abdominal tenderness: On left side or generalized.
  - Psoas sign: Provides resistance over patient's right knee as they flex the hip; pain indicates appendicitis, possible inflammation of abdomen.
  - Obturator sign: Internal rotation and flexion of right LE may indicate appendicitis, pelvic inflammation.
  - Rovsing sign: Pain on the right side of abdomen when pressure applied to the left may indicate appendicitis.
- Palpation
  - Appendix (McBurney's): Apply vertical pressure halfway between right ASIS and umbilicus: −/+ may indicate appendicitis.
  - Liver: In supine, with left hand under trunk parallel to 11th and 12th ribs, lift upward; right hand lateral to rectus, press in and up: +/= reproduction of symptoms with deep breath, indicates liver involvement.
  - Ascites: Percuss outward from center with fingers; if sound is dull, ascites may be present.
  - Spleen: Not recommended for PT to palpate enlarged spleen (only palpable if enlarged).
  - Gallbladder (Murphy's): Place fingers to the right of rectus abdominus below rib cage: +/= sudden pain and muscle tensing with deep breath.
  - Kidneys: In supine, place one hand under client between ribs and iliac crest, other hand on abdomen below ribs and ribs pointing in opposite direction: +/− tenderness or reproduction of symptoms.
  - Bladder: Not usually palpable unless distended and raised above pubic bone; in supine, place hand above pubis and press down: +/= tenderness, reproduction of pain, ability to feel the bladder: __+ ___−.

INTERVENTION

- PT intervention is consistent with movement-related problems secondary to GI disorder and includes
  - Therapeutic exercise: All relevant categories, energy conservation

- Therapeutic activities for bed-mobility training, transfer- and transitional-movement training
- Wheelchair management
- Neuromuscular re-education
- Self-care management training
- Electrical stimulation of rectus/anus in cases of incontinence or lost muscle control/coordination
- Manual therapy
- Interprofessional
  - Lifestyle modification
  - Smoking cessation
  - Weight management
  - Dietary counseling
  - Restriction of fatty foods
  - Psychological intervention
  - Surgical management

FUNCTIONAL GOALS

- Patient will be able to
  - Achieve functional aerobic capacity, ability to talk during activity so as to achieve functional gait and activity tolerance for ADLs/IADLs.
  - Achieve 600 m or greater in a 6-minute walk test for initiation of safe, functional gait in the community.
  - Perform active verbalization with increasing taxonomy for safety during gait, including negotiation of even and uneven surfaces, opening and closing doors, transferring in and out of car.
  - Perform activities requiring abdominals with appropriate muscle splinting/guarding to prevent retraction of stoma, if patient has colostomy or ileostomy.
  - Patient will tolerate 30 minutes of continuous, moderate exercise three times a week in _______ weeks, and five times a week in _____________ weeks, depending on the severity of the disease.

PROGNOSIS

- Physician establishes the medical prognosis, as pathology is primarily medical in nature.
- Patients are usually symptom-free once the gallbladder is removed.
- For PT prognosis, goals should be established that the patient can achieve based on their overall condition.
- Prognosis from a PT perspective should be good, unless medical condition is unstable or goals unrealistic.

PATIENT RESOURCE

- Treatment of Gallstone and Gallbladder Disease. The Society for Surgery of the Alimentary Tract. http://www.ssat.com/cgi-bin/chole7.cgi. Accessed August 8, 2014.

REFERENCES

1. Gersten T. Hemolysis. *MedlinePlus*. http://www.nlm.nih.gov/medlineplus/ency/article/002372.htm. Accessed March 14, 2013.
2. Chen Y. Bone marrow transplant. *MedlinePlus*. http://www.nlm.nih.gov/medlineplus/ency/article/003009.htm. Accessed March 14, 2013.
3. A.D.A.M. Diabetes. *MedlinePlus*. http://www.nlm.nih.gov/medlineplus/ency/article/001214.htm. Accessed March 14, 2013.
4. Longstreth GF. Cirrhosis. *MedlinePlus*. http://www.nlm.nih.gov/medlineplus/ency/article/000255.htm. Accessed March 14, 2013.
5. Vorvick L. Hemolytic anemia. *MedlinePlus*. http://www.nlm.nih.gov/medlineplus/ency/article/000571.htm. Accessed March 14, 2013.
6. Zieve D. Sickle cell anemia. *MedlinePlus*. http://www.nlm.nih.gov/medlineplus/ency/article/000527.htm. Accessed March 14, 2013.

ADDITIONAL REFERENCES

- Banim PJ, Luben RN, Wareham NJ, Sharp SJ, Khaw KT, Hart AR. Physical activity reduces the risk of symptomatic gallstones: a prospective cohort study. *Eur J Gastroenterol Hepatol.* 2010;22(8):983–988. doi: 10.1097/MEG.0b013e32833732c3.
- Goodman CC, Fuller KS. *Pathology Implications for the Physical Therapist.* 3rd ed. St. Louis, MO: Saunders Elsevier; 2009.
- Goodman CC, Snyder TE. *Differential Diagnosis for Physical Therapists Screening for Referral.* 4th ed. St. Louis, MO: Saunders Elsevier; 2007.
- Hay WW, Levin MJ, Sondheimer JM, Deterding RR. Biliary tract disease. In: Hay WW, Levin MJ, Sondheimer JM, Deterding RR, eds. *CURRENT Diagnosis & Treatment: Pediatrics.* 20th ed. New York, NY: McGraw-Hill; 2011. http://www.accessphysiotherapy.com/content/6584598. Accessed January 18, 2013.
- ICD9DATA. http://www.icd9data.com. Accessed March 6, 2013.
- ICD10DATA. http://www.icd10data.com. Accessed March 6, 2013.
- McOmber M, Shulman RJ. Pediatric functional gastrointestinal disorders. Nutr Clin Prac. 2008;23:268–274.
- McPhee SJ, Hammer GD. Disorders of the gallbladder. In: McPhee SJ, Hammer GD, eds. *Pathophysiology of Disease.* 6th ed. New York, NY: McGraw-Hill; 2010. http://www.accessphysiotherapy.com/content/5369694. Accessed January 18, 2013.
- Suleiman S, Johnston DE. The abdominal wall: an overlooked source of pain. *Am Fam Physician.* 2001;64(3):431–439.
- Ulcerative Colitis. National Digestive Diseases Information Clearinghouse (NDDIC0). US Department of Health and Human Services. *NIH Publication No. 12–1597.* October 2011. http://digestive.niddk.nih.gov/ddiseases/pubs/colitis/. Accessed January 2, 2013.

34 CIRRHOSIS

Debra F. Stern, DPT, DBA, MSM, PT
Eric Shamus, PhD, DPT, PT, CSCS

CONDITION/DISORDER SYNONYM

- Cirrhosis of the liver

ICD-9-CM CODES

- 571.5 Cirrhosis of liver without mention of alcohol
- Associated physical therapy diagnoses
  - 315.4 Developmental coordination disorder
  - 718.45 Contracture of joint, pelvic region and thigh
  - 719.70 Difficulty in walking involving joint site unspecified
  - 728.2 Muscular wasting and disuse atrophy, not elsewhere classified
  - 728.89 Other disorders of muscle, ligament, and fascia
  - 729.9 Other and unspecified disorders of soft tissue
  - 780.7 Malaise and fatigue
  - 781.2 Abnormality of gait
  - 782.3 Edema
  - 786.0 Dyspnea and respiratory abnormalities
  - 786.05 Shortness of breath

ICD-10-CM CODES

- K74.0 Hepatic fibrosis
- K74.60 Unspecified cirrhosis of liver
- K74.69 Other cirrhosis of liver

PREFERRED PRACTICE PATTERN

- As of June, 2014, the APTA *Guide to Physical Therapist Practice* does not include practice patterns for organ system pathology; therefore, the associated or secondary musculoskeletal, cardiovascular/pulmonary, or potential neuromuscular patterns would be indicated.

PATIENT PRESENTATION

A 38-year-old man comes into the emergency department presenting with fatigue and abdominal swelling. For several months, he has noticed that his abdomen has been growing larger and that his skin has turned yellow. He denies any medical problems but admits to drinking alcohol almost every day. On examination, his skin clearly has a yellow hue indicative of icterus. His palms have some redness. His abdomen is markedly distended and tense, and a fluid wave is present. On the surface of the abdomen there are prominent vascular markings.

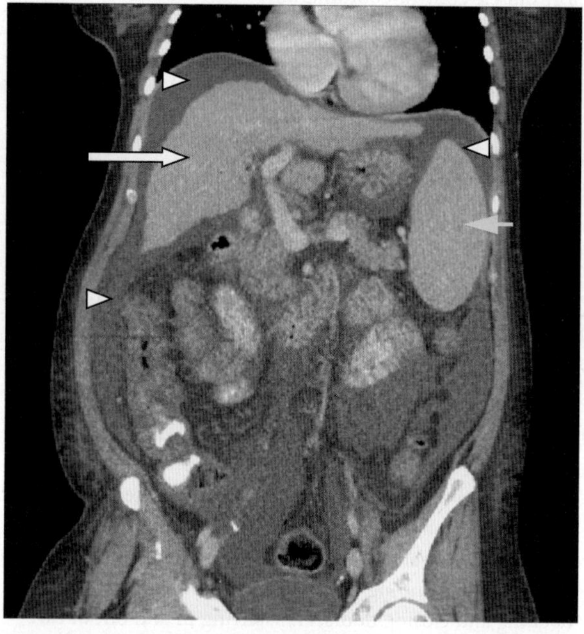

FIGURE 34-1 CT of a patient with a cirrhotic, nodular liver (*white arrow*), splenomegaly (*yellow arrow*), and ascites (*arrowheads*). (From Longo DL, et al., [eds.]. *Harrison's Principles of Internal Medicine*. 18th ed. New York, NY: McGraw-Hill, 2012.)

KEY FEATURES

Description

- Destruction of liver, liver disease
- May result from excessive alcohol use over time
- Complaints often include changes in bowel habits: Constipation, diarrhea, urgency, incontinence, cramping
- Pain is frequently referred to lower back

Essentials of Diagnosis

- Abdominal pain or tenderness (constant, intermittent)
- Nausea, vomiting
- Changes in bowel habits: Diarrhea, constipation
- Bloating
- Acute drop in blood pressure, may cause decreased blood flow to intestines
- Lack of appetite, unexplained weight loss
- Abdominal pain upon ingesting food
- Joint pain possible
- Malaise, fatigue

General Considerations

- While PT may not manage GI disorders specifically, clients may receive care for secondary problems: Weakness, gait abnormalities, limited aerobic endurance, sarcopenia, musculoskeletal/neuromuscular problems, weight loss/gain.
- Symptoms may be characteristic of multiple GI disorders, confounding medical diagnosis.

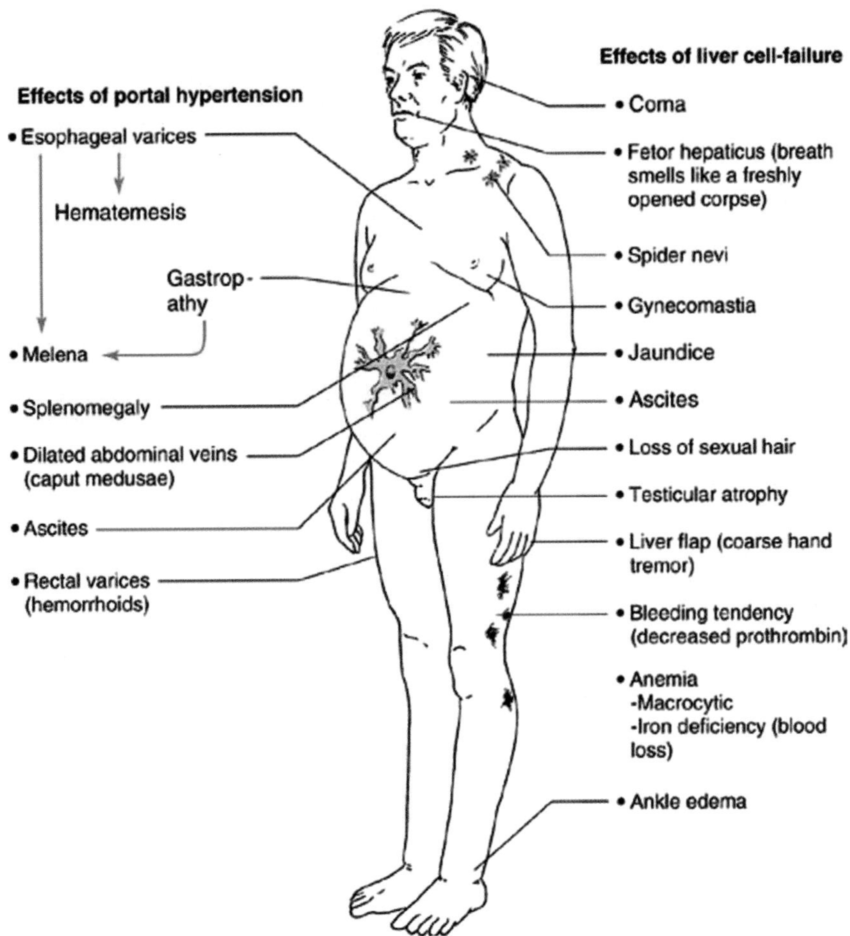

FIGURE 34-2 Clinical effects of cirrhosis of the liver. (Reproduced with permission from Chandrasoma P, Taylor CE. *Concise Pathology*. 3rd ed. Originally published by Appleton & Lange. Copyright © 1998 by The McGraw-Hill Companies, Inc.)

- PT should recognize possible GI pathology in differential diagnosis, especially when findings are inconsistent with conditions commonly treated.
- Diagnosis for occult problems may take time, require intensive diagnostic testing.
- GI disorders frequently refer pain to other body areas; individuals may be inappropriately referred to PT.
- GI problems commonly related to stress, constipation.
- More serious problems include autoimmune conditions: Crohn's, appendicitis (acute pain).
- May indicate inguinal or umbilical hernia.
- In females, GI complaints may indicate gynecological problems: Cancer/tumors in reproductive organs, endometriosis, uterine fibroids, ectopic pregnancies.
- History of heartburn or indigestion may indicate GI or cardiac problems.
- Chronic or episodic diarrhea, loss of bowel control (incontinence or urgency), blood in stool may be symptomatic of inflammatory disease, precancerous condition, or cancer.

Demographics

- Affects adults; higher rate among alcoholics
- Familial

CLINICAL FINDINGS

SIGNS AND SYMPTOMS[1]

- Jaundice
- Itching
- Spider-like vessels on the skin
- Extremity edema
- Splenomegaly
- Hepatic encephalopathy
- Sensitivity to medications
- Insulin resistance
- Pain
  - Abdominal/stomach pain, cramping (constant or intermittent, severe)
  - Pain upon ingesting food or liquid
    - May be cardiac in nature
  - Lower abdominal pain
  - Pain with defecation
  - Pain after ingesting fatty foods (gallbladder sign)
  - Joint pain
- Bowel changes
  - Diarrhea (acute, chronic)
  - Constipation (acute, chronic)
  - Blood in stool, dark or fresh bleeding
  - Rectal bleeding
  - Change in stool odor or color
  - Feeling of having to move bowels constantly
  - Mucous in stool or mucous discharge
- Unexplained weight loss
- Nausea, loss of appetite, cachexia
- Fever, chills

- Abdominal muscle spasm, guarding
- Fatigue
- Anemia
- Skin lesions
- Flatulence
- Gastroesophageal reflux (GERD), heartburn
- Emesis
- Ascites
- Bruising
- Infection
- Osteoporosis

Functional Implications

- Intolerance to medications
- Encephalopathy
- Severe symptoms associated with immediacy of defecation may be disabling, and cause inability to leave home
- Dehydration secondary to diarrhea, emesis, appetite loss, nausea, inability to swallow
- Sarcopenia resulting in weakness, muscle-mass loss, inability to ambulate and perform self-care
- Limited aerobic activity, decreased exercise tolerance, limited physical activity
- Psychological challenges
  - Reluctance to leave home
  - Anxiety, depression
  - Inappropriate self-medication
- Fatigue
- Limited ADLs, IADLs
- Dietary restrictions

Possible Contributing Causes

- Heavy alcohol consumption
- Chronic hepatitis C
- Obesity, lack of exercise, poor diet
- Infection: Bacterial or viral
- Nonalcoholic fatty liver disease (NAFLD)
- Ischemic
  - Atherosclerosis, impaired blood supply to any structure
- Stress, anxiety
- Inflammatory: Autoimmune disease
- Chemical toxicity
- Environmental irritants
- Heredity
- Cancer: Esophageal, colon, liver, bile duct, pancreatic, metastatic, anal/rectal
- Systemic rheumatologic disorders: Scleroderma, rheumatoid arthritis
- Systemic immunological condition
- Effects of medication
- Endocrine dysfunction

Differential Diagnosis

- Organ dysfunction from cancer or malignancy
  - Colon cancer
  - Ovarian cancer
- Non-malignant tumor in abdomen or organs
- Endocrine disorder
- Autoimmune diseases affecting upper and lower GI tracts
- Appendicitis
- Irritable bowel syndrome
- Crohn disease
- Colitis (ulcerative, non-ulcerative)

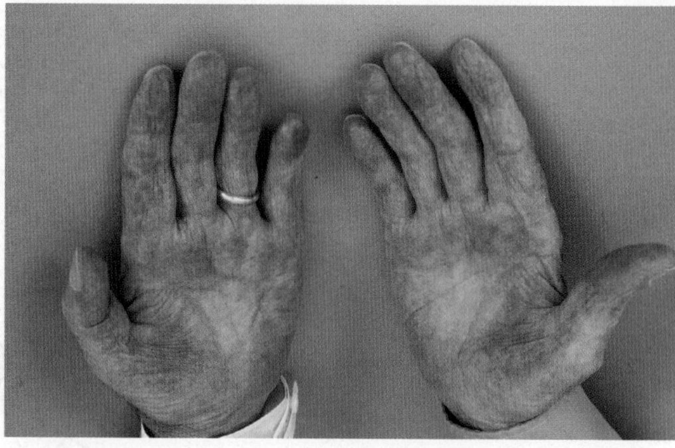

FIGURE 34-3 Palmar erythema. This figure shows palmar erythema in a patient with alcoholic cirrhosis. The erythema is peripheral over the palm with central pallor. (From Longo DL, et al., [eds.]. *Harrison's Principles of Internal Medicine*. 18th ed. New York, NY: McGraw-Hill, 2012.)

- Inflammatory bowel disease
- Pelvic inflammatory disease
- Celiac disease
- Gastroenteritis
- Perforated ulcers in GI system
- Bladder or urinary tract infection, kidney pathology
- Abdominal infection
- Bowel disorder
- Referred pain from heart, spine, hip
- Post–weight-loss (bariatric) surgery complications/side effects

MEANS OF CONFIRMATION OR DIAGNOSIS

Laboratory Tests

- Fecal occult blood test/stool sample
- Blood tests
- H & H

Imaging

- Liver scan
- Abdominal scan
- Radiography
- CT
- Ultrasound

Diagnostic Procedures

- Medical history
- Upper endoscopy
- Manual palpation
- Laparoscopy

FINDINGS AND INTERPRETATION

- H & H for signs of bleeding, anemia, pathogens, immune status, vitamin deficiencies, white blood cell count

TREATMENT

Medication

- Beta-blocker or nitrates
  - For hepatic hypertension
- Laxatives
- Antibiotics

MEDICAL PROCEDURES

- Biopsy
- Liver transplants
- Nasogastric tube
- Feeding tube
- Total/peripheral parenteral nutrition (TPN/PPN)
- IV for hydration

REFERRALS/ADMITTANCE

- If causative problem is not considered appropriate for PT intervention, refer to appropriate physician.
- If emergency identified, refer to ER.

IMPAIRMENTS

- Muscle weakness, atrophy
- Gait abnormality, difficulty walking
- Contractures of soft tissue (fascia, muscle); joint limitations
- Shortness of breath
- Inability to perform self-care
- Limited aerobic endurance
- Functional decline

TESTS AND MEASURES

- Observation
  - Scars may indicate adhesions or abdominal surgeries causative of diverticula.
  - Pink or purplish striae may be indicative of Cushing syndrome.
  - Dilated veins may indicate hepatic pathology or inferior vena cava obstruction, not diverticulitis.
  - Contour: Roundness, concavity, asymmetry, distension, pregnancy signs.
  - Cullen sign: Bluish discoloring around the umbilicus may be a sign of retroperitoneal bleeding.
  - Bluish discoloration in lower abdomen: Grey Turner sign, signals hemorrhagic pancreatitis.
  - Bulging in groin and/or abdomen especially apparent with contraction of musculature in area, may be hernia.
  - Pulsing in navel area may be abdominal aortic aneurysm.
  - Left lower quadrant pain, often following a meal.
  - Palpable abdominal tenderness, on left side or generalized.
  - Psoas sign: Provides resistance over patient's right knee as they flex the hip; pain indicates appendicitis, possible inflammation of abdomen.
  - Obturator sign: Internal rotation and flexion of right lower extremity may indicate appendicitis, pelvic inflammation.
  - Rovsing sign: Pain on the right side of abdomen when pressure applied to the left may indicate appendicitis.
- Palpation
  - Appendix (McBurney's): Apply vertical pressure halfway between right ASIS and umbilicus: –/+ may indicate appendicitis.
  - Liver: In supine, with left hand under trunk parallel to 11th and 12th ribs, lift upward; right hand lateral to rectus, press in and up: +/= reproduction of symptoms with deep breath indicates liver involvement.
  - Ascites: Percuss outward from center with fingers; if sound is dull, ascites may be present.
  - Spleen: Not recommended for PT to palpate enlarged spleen secondary to ease of rupture (only palpable if enlarged).
  - Gallbladder (Murphy's): Place fingers to the right of rectus abdominus below rib cage: +/= sudden pain and muscle tensing with deep breath.
  - Kidneys: In supine, place one hand under client between ribs and iliac crest, other hand on abdomen below ribs and ribs pointing in opposite direction: +/– tenderness or reproduction of symptoms.
  - Bladder: Not usually palpable unless distended and raised above pubic bone; in supine, place hand above pubis and press down: +/= tenderness, reproduction of pain, ability to feel the bladder: __+ ___–.

INTERVENTION

- PT intervention is consistent with movement-related problems secondary to GI disorder
- Gait training
- Therapeutic exercise: All relevant categories, energy conservation
- Therapeutic activities for bed mobility, transfers, transitional movement
- Neuromuscular re-education
- Self-care training
- Manual therapy
- Healthy diet; avoidance of shellfish
- Interprofessional
  - Lifestyle modification
  - Smoking cessation
  - Alcohol control
  - Weight management
  - Dietary counseling
  - Psychological intervention
  - Pastoral counseling
  - Surgical management

FUNCTIONAL GOALS

- Patient will be able to
  - Achieve functional aerobic capacity, ability to talk during activity so as to achieve functional gait and activity tolerance for ADLs/IADLs.
  - Achieve 600 m or greater in a 6-minute walk test for initiation of safe, functional gait in the community.
  - Perform active verbalization with increasing taxonomy for safety during gait, including negotiation of even and uneven surfaces, opening and closing doors, transferring in and out of car.
  - Tolerate 30 minutes of continuous, moderate exercise three times a week in ______ weeks, and five times a week in ____________ weeks, depending on disease severity, depending on disease severity.

PROGNOSIS

- May be curable in some cases, depending on cause.
- Generally progressive, symptoms do not usually appear until disease is advanced.
- Liver transplant may prevent severe complications and death.
- Physician should establish medical prognosis, as pathology is primarily medical in nature.
- For PT prognosis, goals should be established that the patient can achieve based on their overall condition.
- Prognosis from a PT perspective should be good, unless medical condition is unstable or goals unrealistic.

PATIENTS RESOURCES

- American Liver Foundation. http://www.liverfoundation.org/. Accessed August 8, 2014.
- Centers for Disease Control and Prevention. *Chronic Liver Disease or Cirrhosis.* http://www.cdc.gov/nchs/fastats/liverdis.htm. Accessed August 8, 2014.

REFERENCE

1. Toy EC. Cirrhosis. *Lange Case Files.* http://www.accessmedicine.com/casecontent.aspx?aid=8650604&tabid=1. Access May 6, 2013.

ADDITIONAL REFERENCES

- Goodman CC, Fuller KS. *Pathology: Implications for the Physical Therapist.* 3rd ed. St. Louis, MO: Saunders; 2009.
- Goodman CC, Snyder TK. *Differential Diagnosis for Physical Therapists Screening for Referral.* 4th ed. St. Louis, MO: Saunders; 2007.
- McOmber MA, Shulman RJ. Pediatric functional gastrointestinal disorders. *Nutr Clin Pract.* 2008;23(3):268–274.
- Mills JC, Stappenbeck TS, Bunnett N. Gastrointestinal disease. In: McPhee SJ, Hammer GD, eds. *Pathophysiology of Disease: An Introduction to Clinical Medicine.* 6th ed. New York, NY: McGraw-Hill; 2010. http://www.accessphysiotherapy.com/content/5369615. Accessed May 6, 2013.
- Suleiman S, Johnston DE. The abdominal wall: an overlooked source of pain. *Am Fam Physician.* 2001;64(3):431–438.
- Wang KK, Sampliner RE. Updated guidelines 2008 for the diagnosis, surveillance and therapy of Barrett's esophagus. *Am J Gastroenterol.* 2008;103(3):788–797.

35 COLITIS

Debra F. Stern, DPT, DBA, MSM, PT
Eric Shamus, PhD, DPT, PT, CSCS
Erika Simmerman-Mabes, DO

CONDITION/DISORDER SYNONYM

- Ulcerative colitis

ICD-9-CM CODES

- 009.1 Colitis, enteritis, and gastroenteritis of presumed infectious origin
- 556.9 Ulcerative colitis, unspecified
- Associated physical therapy diagnoses
  - 315.4 Developmental coordination disorder
  - 718.45 Contracture of joint, pelvic region and thigh
  - 719.70 Difficulty in walking involving joint site unspecified
  - 728.2 Muscular wasting and disuse atrophy, not elsewhere classified
  - 728.89 Disorders of muscle, ligament, and fascia
  - 729.9 Other and unspecified disorders of soft tissue
  - 780.7 Malaise and fatigue
  - 781.2 Abnormality of gait
  - 782.3 Edema
  - 786.0 Dyspnea and respiratory abnormalities
  - 786.05 Shortness of breath

ICD-10-CM CODES

- A09 Infectious gastroenteritis and colitis, unspecified
- K51.90 Ulcerative colitis, unspecified, without complications

PREFERRED PRACTICE PATTERN

- As of June, 2014, the APTA *Guide to Physical Therapist Practice* does not include practice patterns for organ system pathology; therefore, the associated or secondary musculoskeletal, cardiovascular/pulmonary, or potential neuromuscular patterns would be indicated.

PATIENT PRESENTATION

A 40-year-old male presents with abdominal discomfort and low back spasms. The back pain was insidious. Special tests were negative for straight leg raise (SLR) and slump tests. Bilateral lower extremity (LE) strength, reflexes, and sensation were within normal limits. Pain was not reproducible. Review of the systems reveals a 2-month history of decreased appetite, a 10 lb unintentional weight loss, and occasional bright red blood in his stools. He denies recent use of antibiotics, recent travel, or exposure to sick people. He does report a history of "some sort of irritable bowel problems" ailing his father and uncle for years. Physical examination is unremarkable except for minimal lower abdominal tenderness to deep palpation. The patient was referred to his primary care physician with a 3-month history of back pain, abdominal bloating, pain, cramping, and diarrhea. The physician did a digital rectal examination revealing hemoccult positive stool, so the patient was referred to a gastroenterologist for further evaluation. Colonoscopy revealed colonic mucosal erythema with occasional areas of bleeding.

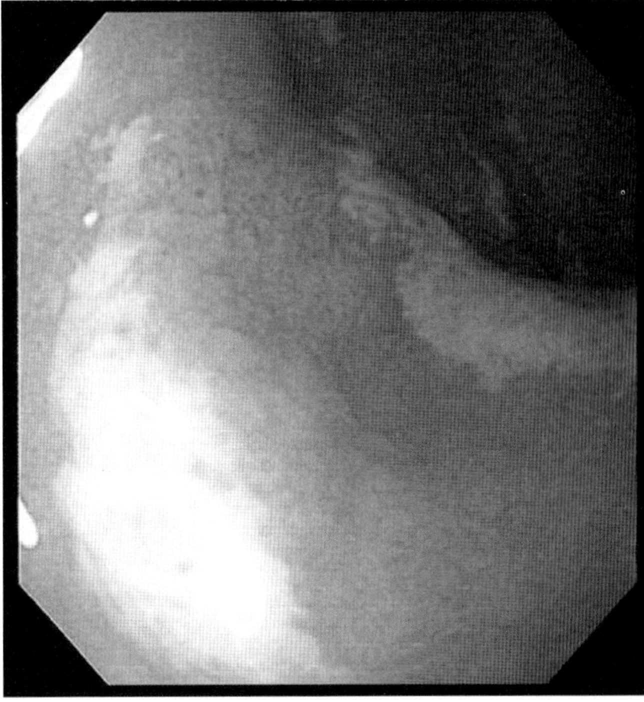

FIGURE 35-1 Ulcerative colitis. White exudate is present overlying an abnormal colonic mucosa that has lost its typical vascular pattern. (From Hay WM, Levin MJ, Deterding RR, Abzug MJ. *Current Diagnosis & Treatment: Pediatrics*. 21st ed. www.accessmedicine.com. Copyright © The McGraw-Hill Companies, Inc. All rights reserved.)

KEY FEATURES

Description

- Inflammation of large intestine and bowel
- Ulcer formation may cause some constipation
- Frequent diarrhea associated with bowel urgency and cramping
- Pathologic features[1]
- Involves mainly mucosa

Essentials of Diagnosis

- Unknown etiology
- Abdominal pain, tenderness
- Nausea, vomiting
- Diarrhea: Watery, may be bloody
- Bloating

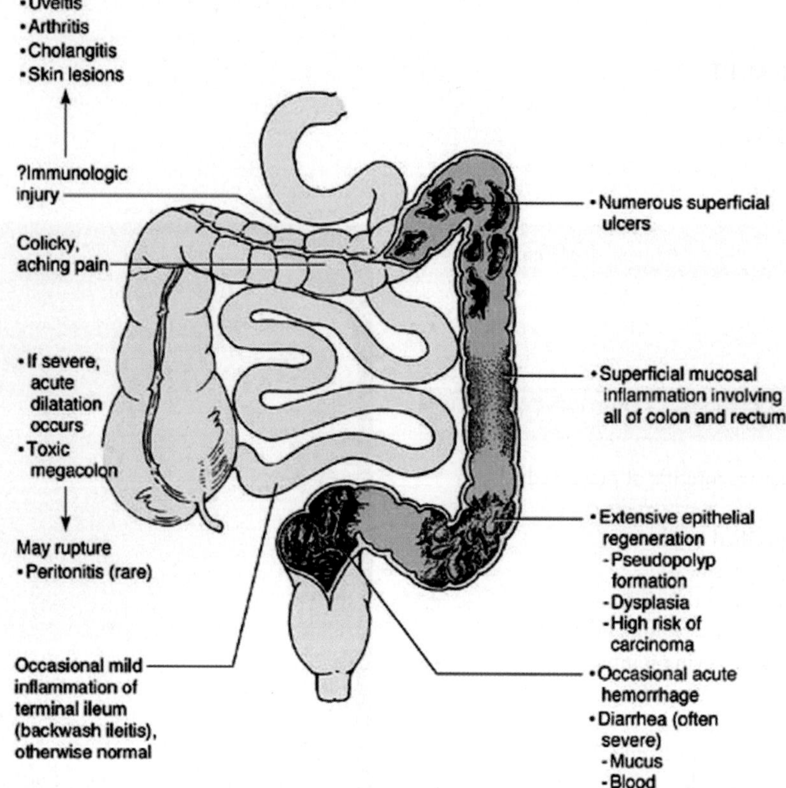

FIGURE 35-2 Pathologic features of ulcerative colitis. (From Chandrasoma P, Taylor CR. *Concise Pathology*. 3rd ed. www.accessmedicine.com. Copyright © The McGraw-Hill Companies, Inc. All rights reserved.)

- Rectal bleeding possible
- Acute drop in blood pressure may cause decreased blood flow to intestines

General Considerations

- Various types of colitis
  - Short-term: Resolves quickly
  - Lifelong: Chronic, recurrent
- Broad array of GI disorders may be encountered by physical therapists
- While PT may not manage GI disorders specifically, clients may receive care for secondary problems: Weakness, gait abnormalities, limited aerobic endurance, sarcopenia, musculoskeletal/neuromuscular problems, weight loss/gain
- Symptoms may be characteristic of multiple GI disorders, confounding medical diagnosis
- PT should recognize possible GI pathology in differential diagnosis, especially when findings are inconsistent with conditions commonly treated
- Diagnosis for occult problems may take time and require intensive diagnostic testing
- Referred pain to back possible
- May mimic colon cancer, tumors, irritable bowel
- Chronic or episodic diarrhea, loss of bowel control, and/or blood in stool may indicate inflammatory disease, precancerous condition, or cancer

Demographics

- Higher incidence in Caucasians and Jews of European descent
- May occur at any age: Onset most common between ages 15 and 30 years, less common between ages 50 and 70 years

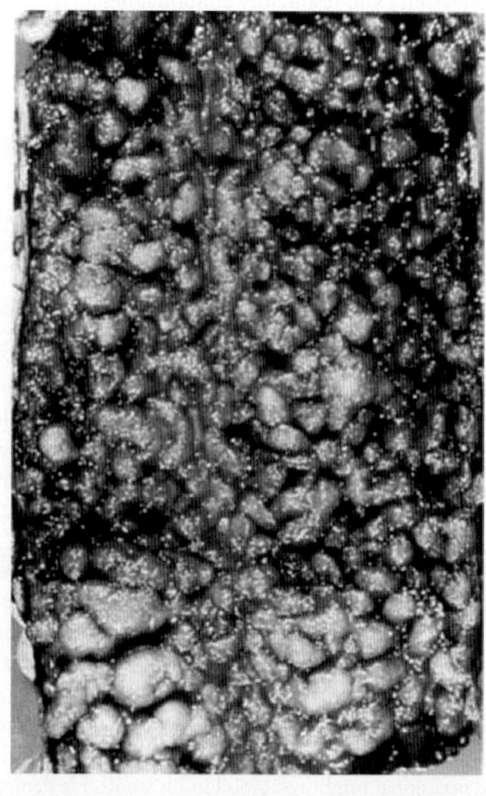

FIGURE 35-3 Acute ulcerative colitis, showing diffuse erythema and edema of the colonic mucosa. The extensive ulceration of the mucosa is masked by the pseudopolypoid appearance of the inflamed surviving mucosa. (From Chandrasoma P, Taylor CR. *Concise Pathology*. 3rd ed. www.accessmedicine.com. Copyright © The McGraw-Hill Companies, Inc. All rights reserved.)

- Mostly 10% of cases develop before age 18
- Affects men and women equally
- Familial
- Estimated incidence in United States: 1.4 in 100,000

CLINICAL FINDINGS

SIGNS AND SYMPTOMS

- Pain
  - Abdominal/stomach pain, cramping (constant or intermittent, severe)
  - Pain upon ingesting food or liquid
    - May be cardiac in nature
  - Lower abdominal pain
  - Pain with defecation
  - Joint pain
- Bowel changes
  - Diarrhea (acute, chronic)
  - Constipation (acute, chronic)
  - Blood in stool, dark or fresh bleeding
  - Rectal bleeding
  - Change in stool odor or color
  - Feeling of having to move bowels constantly
- Intestinal hemorrhage
- Abdominal distention
- Abdominal muscle spasm, guarding
- Fever, chills
- Dysplasia
- Pseudopolyps
- Crypt abscesses
- Fatigue
- Anemia
- Weight loss, loss of appetite
- Skin lesions
- Failure to grow if onset at early age

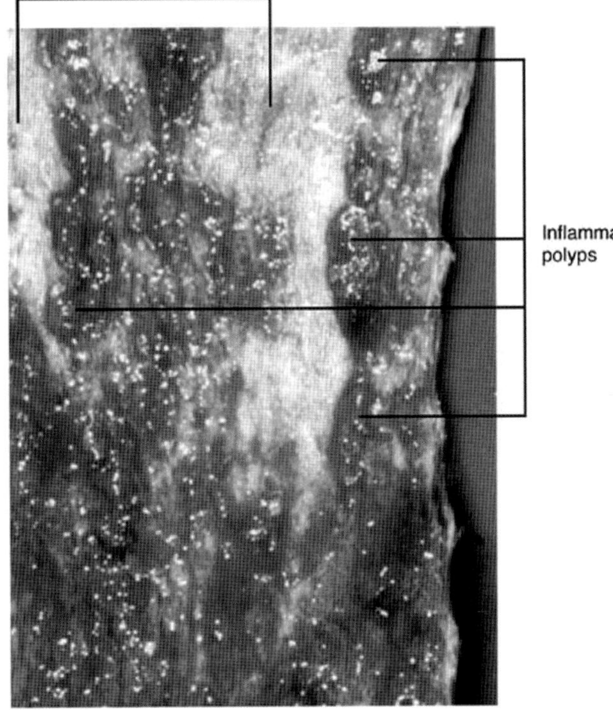

FIGURE 35-4 Chronic ulcerative colitis, showing flat areas of atrophic mucosa in which numerous inflammatory polyps are seen. (From Chandrasoma P, Taylor CR. *Concise Pathology*. 3rd ed. www.accessmedicine.com. Copyright © The McGraw-Hill Companies, Inc. All rights reserved.)

▶ Functional Implications

- Severe symptoms associated with immediacy of defecation may be disabling, causing inability to leave home
- Dehydration secondary to diarrhea, emesis, appetite loss, nausea, inability to swallow

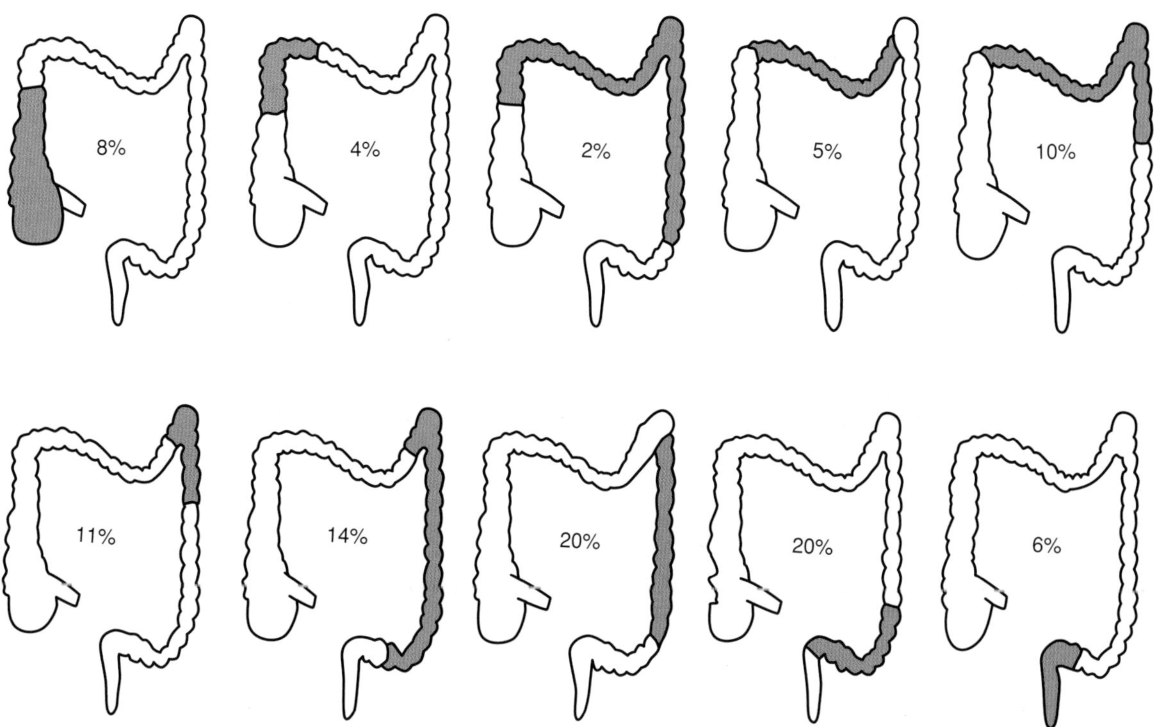

FIGURE 35-5 Distribution of colonic ischemia in 250 cases. (Reproduced with permission from Brandt L, Boley SJ. Colonic ischemia. *Surg Clin North Am.* 1992;72:212. Copyright Elsevier.)

- Anemia
- Sarcopenia resulting in weakness, decreased muscle mass, inability to ambulate or perform self-care, limited aerobic capacity secondary to inactivity
- Need for temporary or permanent colostomies/ileostomies (usually with intestinal problems vs. upper GI)
  - May present problems with stoma retraction associated with abdominal contraction
- Decreased exercise tolerance, limited physical activity
- Eating disorder/anorexia secondary to fear of pain upon ingesting food
- Fatigue
- Inappropriate self-medication
- Anxiety, depression
- May indicate serious medical conditions
- Limited ADLs, IADLs
- Infection
- Arthritis
- Inflammation of eye, liver disease, skin lesions
- Osteoporosis

Possible Contributing Causes

- Infection: Bacterial, viral
  - Food poisoning
  - Parasites
- Ischemic
  - Atherosclerosis, impaired blood supply
- Idiopathic
- Stress, anxiety
- Obstruction in colon decreasing blood supply, causing inflammation
- Inflammatory: Autoimmune disease
- Chemical
  - May occur after enemas
- Heredity
- Environmental irritant
- Obesity, lack of exercise

Differential Diagnosis

- Organ dysfunction from cancer or malignancy
  - Colon cancer
  - Ovarian cancer

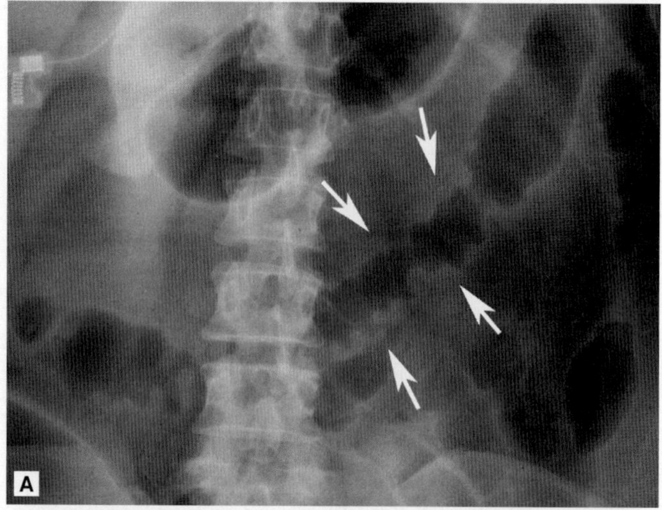

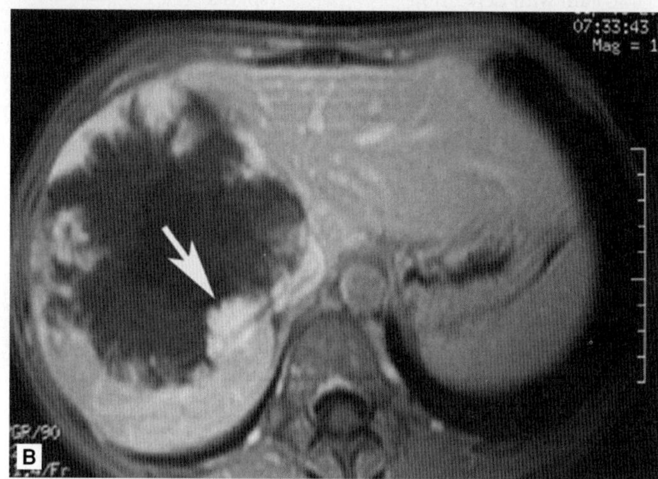

FIGURE 35-6 Ischemic colitis. **A.** KUB (kidney, ureter, bladder) image shows wall thickening (*arrows*) of the transverse colon with thumbprinting. **B.** Axial MDCT image shows thickening of the wall of the left colon (*arrow*) with lack of wall enhancement. (From Greenberger NJ, Blumberg RS, Burakoff R. *Current Diagnosis & Treatment: Gastroenterology, Hepatology, & Endoscopy*. 2nd ed. www.accessmedicine.com. Copyright © The McGraw-Hill Companies, Inc. All rights reserved.)

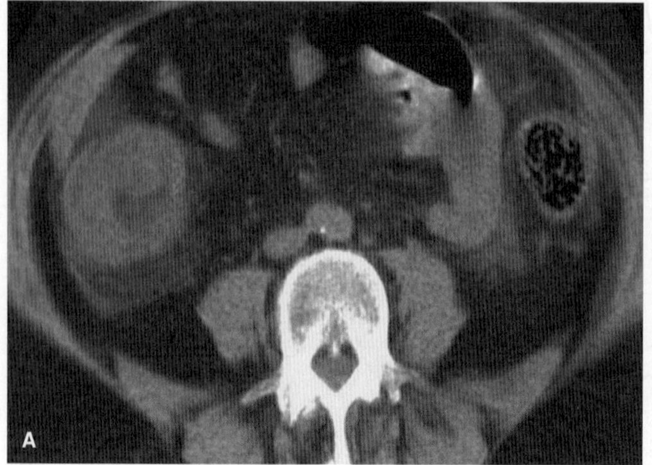

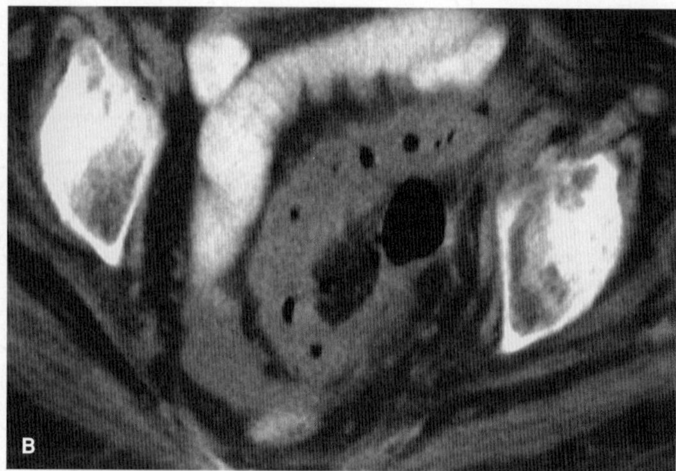

FIGURE 35-7 CT scans demonstrating findings in colonic ischemia. **A.** Colonic thickening. **B.** Pneumatosis. (Used with permission from Koenraad Mortele, MD.)

- Non-malignant tumor in abdomen or organs
- Endocrine disorder
- Gynecologic problems in females
  - Endometriosis
  - Menses
  - Ectopic pregnancies
  - Ovarian cysts
  - Fibroids
- Autoimmune diseases affecting upper and lower GI tracts
  - Crohn's or irritable bowel syndrome (IBS)[1]
  - Systemic lupus erythematosus (SLE)
  - Rheumatoid arthritis (RA)
- Appendicitis
- Inflammatory bowel disease
- Pelvic inflammatory disease
- Celiac disease
- Gastroenteritis
- Perforated ulcer in GI system
- Bladder or urinary tract infection, kidney pathology
- Abdominal infection
- Bowel disorders including
  - Constipation, diarrhea
  - Inflamed lining of abdomen or organ obstruction
  - Torsions
- Referred pain from heart, spine, hip
- Post–weight-loss (bariatric) surgery complications
  - Side effects may result in liver problems

MEANS OF CONFIRMATION

Laboratory Tests

- Fecal occult blood test/stool samples
- Blood tests
- H & H

Imaging

- Abdominal scan
- Radiography
- Barium enemas
- CT

Diagnostic Procedures

- Colonoscopy
- Sigmoidoscopy
- Manual palpation for tenderness

FINDINGS AND INTERPRETATION

- H & H for signs of bleeding, anemia, pathogens, immune status, vitamin deficiencies, white blood cell count

TREATMENT

Medication

- Aminosalicylates
- Corticosteroids
- Immunomodulators
- Antidiarrheals

MEDICAL PROCEDURES

- Bowel resection
- Bowel resection with colostomy/ileostomy
  - PTs must be sure not to cause retraction of ostomies

REFERRALS/ADMITTANCE

- If causative problem is not considered appropriate for PT intervention, refer to appropriate physician.
- If emergency identified, refer to ER.

IMPAIRMENTS

- Muscle weakness, atrophy
- Gait abnormality, difficulty walking
- Contractures of soft tissue (fascia, muscle); joint limitations
- Shortness of breath
- Possible impairment of rectal muscle
- Inability to perform self-care

TESTS AND MEASURES

- Observation
  - Scars may indicate adhesions or abdominal surgeries causative of diverticula.
  - Pink or purplish striae may be indicative of Cushing syndrome.
  - Dilated veins may indicate hepatic pathology or inferior vena cava obstruction, not diverticulitis.
  - Contour: Roundness, concavity, asymmetry, distension, pregnancy signs.
  - Cullen sign: Bluish discoloring around the umbilicus may be a sign of retroperitoneal bleeding.
  - Bluish discoloration in lower abdomen: Grey Turner sign, signals hemorrhagic pancreatitis.
  - Bulging in groin and abdomen especially apparent with contraction of musculature in area may be hernia.
  - Pulsing in navel area may be abdominal aortic aneurysm.
  - Left lower quadrant pain, often following a meal.
  - Palpable abdominal tenderness: On left side or generalized.
  - Psoas sign: Provides resistance over patient's right knee as they flex the hip; pain indicates appendicitis, possible inflammation of abdomen.
  - Obturator sign: Internal rotation and flexion of right LE may indicate appendicitis, pelvic inflammation.
  - Rovsing sign: Pain on the right side of abdomen when pressure applied to the left may indicate appendicitis.
- Palpation
  - Appendix (McBurney's): Apply vertical pressure halfway between right ASIS and umbilicus: –/+ may indicate appendicitis.
  - Liver: In supine, with left hand under trunk parallel to 11th and 12th ribs, lift upward; right hand lateral to rectus, press in and up: +/= reproduction of symptoms with deep breath, indicates liver involvement.
  - Ascites: Percuss outward from center with fingers; if sound is dull, ascites may be present.
  - Spleen: Not recommended for PT to palpate enlarged spleen secondary to rupture issues (only palpable if enlarged).
  - Gallbladder (Murphy's): Place fingers to the right of rectus abdominus below rib cage: +/= sudden pain and muscle tensing with deep breath.
  - Kidneys: In supine, place one hand under client between ribs and iliac crest, other hand on abdomen below ribs and pointing in opposite direction: +/– tenderness or reproduction of symptoms.
  - Bladder: Not usually palpable unless distended and raised above pubic bone; in supine, place hand above pubis and press down: +/= tenderness, reproduction of pain, ability to feel the bladder: __+ ___–.

INTERVENTION

- Psychological intervention
- PT intervention is consistent with movement-related problems secondary to GI disorder
- Therapeutic exercise: All relevant categories, energy conservation
  - If stoma from colostomy or ileostomy, PT must avoid activities that may cause retraction
- Therapeutic activities for bed mobility, transfers, transitional movement
- Neuromuscular re-education: Rectal/anal biofeedback
- Self-care training
- Electrical stimulation of rectus/anus in cases of incontinence or poor muscle control/coordination
- Lifestyle modification
- Smoking cessation
- Weight management
- Dietary modification
  - Nasogastric tube
  - Feeding tube
  - Total/peripheral parenteral nutrition (TPN/PPN)
- Dietary counseling
- Surgical management

FUNCTIONAL GOALS

- Patient will be able to
  - Achieve functional aerobic capacity, ability to talk during activity so as to achieve functional gait and activity tolerance for ADLs/IADLs.
  - Achieve 600 m or greater in a 6-minute walk test for initiation of safe, functional gait in the community.
  - Perform active verbalization with increasing taxonomy for safety during gait, including negotiation of even and uneven surfaces, opening and closing doors, transferring in and out of car.
  - Perform activities requiring abdominals with appropriate muscle splinting/guarding to prevent retraction of stoma, if patient has colostomy or ileostomy.
  - Tolerate 30 minutes of continuous, moderate exercise three times a week in ______ weeks, and five times a week in ____________ weeks, depending on disease severity.

PROGNOSIS

- Increased risk of colon cancer.
- Physician establishes the medical prognosis, as pathology is primarily medical in nature.
- For PT prognosis, goals should be established that the patient can achieve based on their overall condition.
- Prognosis from a PT perspective should be good, unless medical condition is unstable or goals unrealistic.

PATIENT RESOURCES

- Crohn's & Colitis Foundation of America (CCFA). http://www.ccfa.org. Accessed August 8, 2014.
- Crohn's and Colitis UK. http://www.nacc.org.uk/content/home.asp. Accessed August 8, 2014.
- Ulcerative Colitis. American Society of Colon and Rectal Surgeons. http://www.fascrs.org/patients/conditions/ulcerative_ colitis. Accessed August 8, 2014.
- Ulcerative Colitis. National Digestive Diseases Information Clearinghouse (NDDIC). U.S. Department of Health and Human Services. *NIH Publication No. 12–1597.* October 2011. http://digestive.niddk.nih.gov/ ddiseases/pubs/colitis/. Accessed August 8, 2014.

REFERENCE

1. Chandrasoma P, Taylor CR. *Concise Pathology.* 3rd ed. New York, NY: McGraw-Hill; 1998. http://www.accessphysiotherapy.com/resource/7. Accessed March 15, 2013.

ADDITIONAL REFERENCES

- Goodman CC, Fuller KS. *Pathology: Implications for the Physical Therapist.* 3rd ed. Philadelphia, PA: Saunders Elsevier; 2009.
- Goodman CC, Snyder TK. *Differential Diagnosis for Physical Therapists: Screening for Referral.* 4th ed. St. Louis, MO: Saunders Elsevier; 2007.
- McOmber MA, Shulman RJ. Pediatric functional gastrointestinal disorders. *Nutr Clin Prac.* 2008;23(3):268–274.
- Mills JC, Stappenbeck TS, Bunnett N. Gastrointestinal disease. In: McPhee SJ, Hammer GD, eds. *Pathophysiology of Disease.* 6th ed. New York, NY: McGraw-Hill; 2010. http://www.accessphysiotherapy.com/content/5369694. Accessed March 15, 2013.
- Sokol RJ, Narkewicz MR. Liver & pancreas. In: Hay WW, Levin MJ, Sondheimer JM, Deterding RR, eds. *CURRENT Diagnosis & Treatment: Pediatrics.* 20th ed. New York, NY: McGraw-Hill; 2011. http://www.accessphysiotherapy.com/content/6584598. Accessed March 15, 2013.
- Suleiman S, Johnston DE. The abdominal wall: an overlooked source of pain. *Am Fam Physician.* 2001;64(3):431–438.

36 CONSTIPATION

Cynthia E. Neville, DPT, PT, WCS

CONDITION/DISORDER SYNONYMS

- Obstructed defecation
- Pelvic floor dyssynergia
- Paradoxical puborectalis syndrome
- Anismus

ICD-9-CM CODES

- 564 Constipation
- 564.02 Outlet obstruction constipation

ICD-10-CM CODES

- K59 Constipation
- K59.02 Outlet obstruction constipation
- R32 Unspecified urinary incontinence

PREFERRED PRACTICE PATTERN

- As of June, 2014, the APTA Guide to Physical Therapist Practice does not include practice patterns for organ system pathology; therefore, the associated or secondary musculoskeletal, cardiovascular/pulmonary, or potential neuromuscular patterns would be indicated.
- 4C: Impaired Muscle Performance[1]

PATIENT PRESENTATION

A 40-year-old mother of three reports difficulty passing bowel movements (BMs). Symptoms have gradually worsened over the past 5 years since the birth of her third child. During that vaginal delivery, she suffered a fourth degree perineal tear which extended into the anal sphincter and rectal mucosa. She is now having BMs once every 3 to 4 days, as compared to daily just a few years ago. She reports that she has to "splint" her perineum with her hand, in order to evacuate her bowels.

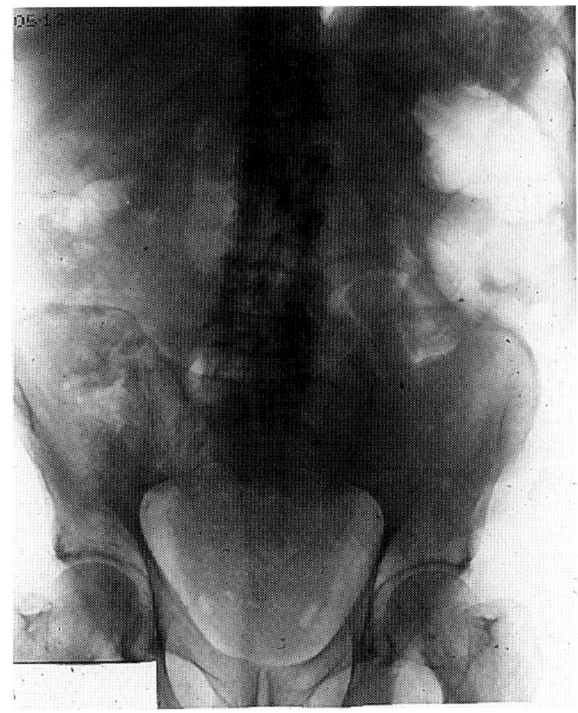

FIGURE 36-1 Abdominal radiograph of an 83-year-old man with Parkinson disease and long-standing symptoms of continuous fecal leakage. As his caregiver at home, his wife was changing his clothing up to six times a day. The rectosigmoid colon is completely impacted, and the dilated bowel loop implies obstruction. He was briefly hospitalized for disimpaction with enemas and laxatives, resulting in complete resolution of incontinence. He and his wife were educated in regular use of laxatives and suppositories, as well as in lifestyle measures. (From Halter JB, Ouslander J, Tinetti M, Studenski S, High K, Asthana S. *Hazzard's Geriatric Medicine and Gerontology*. 6th ed. www.accessmedicine.com. Copyright © The McGraw-Hill Companies, Inc. All rights reserved.)

KEY FEATURES

Description

- Difficulty passing feces
- Obstructed defecation is also known as anismus, sphincter dyssynergia, nonrelaxing puborectalis
  - Pelvic floor muscles (PFMs) and external anal sphincter inappropriately contract instead of relaxing during defecation

General Considerations

- Constipation is a symptom, and is not a disease
- Constipation is the most common digestive complaint
- The chief cause of constipation is inadequate alimentary fiber content

Demographics[2]

- In the United States, estimates are between 2% and 34%
  - 16.7% (1 in 6 people)
  - 6% of children
  - 80% of nursing home residents
  - In children: More common in males than females
  - In adults: More common in females than males
  - Very common during pregnancy and postpartum
  - In elders: Equally as common in males and females
  - More common in non-Whites than Whites
- More than three million prescriptions per year for laxatives; over $725 million on over-the-counter laxatives
- In patients with constipation, 15% to 38% have obstructed defecation[3]

CLINICAL FINDINGS

SIGNS AND SYMPTOMS[4,5]

- ROME-III criteria for constipation: In a patient who does not take laxatives or have irritable bowel syndrome (IBS), patient has at least two of the following in any 12 weeks of the last 6 months:
  - Straining more than 25% of BMs
  - Fewer than three BMs/week
  - Sensation of incomplete evacuation/anorectal blockage for more than 25% of BMs
  - Lumpy or hard stool in more than 25% of BMs
  - The necessity of digital manipulation to facilitate evacuation for more than 25% of BMs

Functional Implications

- Headache
- Decreased energy
- Bad breath
- Difficulty concentrating
- Decreased appetite
- Coating on the tongue
- Abdominal bloating
- Gas/flatulence
- Skin problems
- Depression

Possible Contributing Causes

- Underactive, overactive, or nonfunctioning Pelvic floor muscle
- Medications: Multiple medicines can cause constipation
- Hormonal fluctuations: Pregnancy, lactation, menopause
- Neurological conditions: Parkinson disease, multiple sclerosis.
- Diabetes Mellitus
- Scleroderma
- Anorexia nervosa
- Thyroid disease
- Hyperparathyroidism
- Hysterectomy
- Dietary: Inadequate fiber, fluid, weight loss
- Poor defecation patterns, ignoring urge to defecate
- Travel: Change in food, time zones, stress
- Change in routine: Exercise, sleep, new job
- Admission to hospital or nursing home
- Decreased activity, bed rest

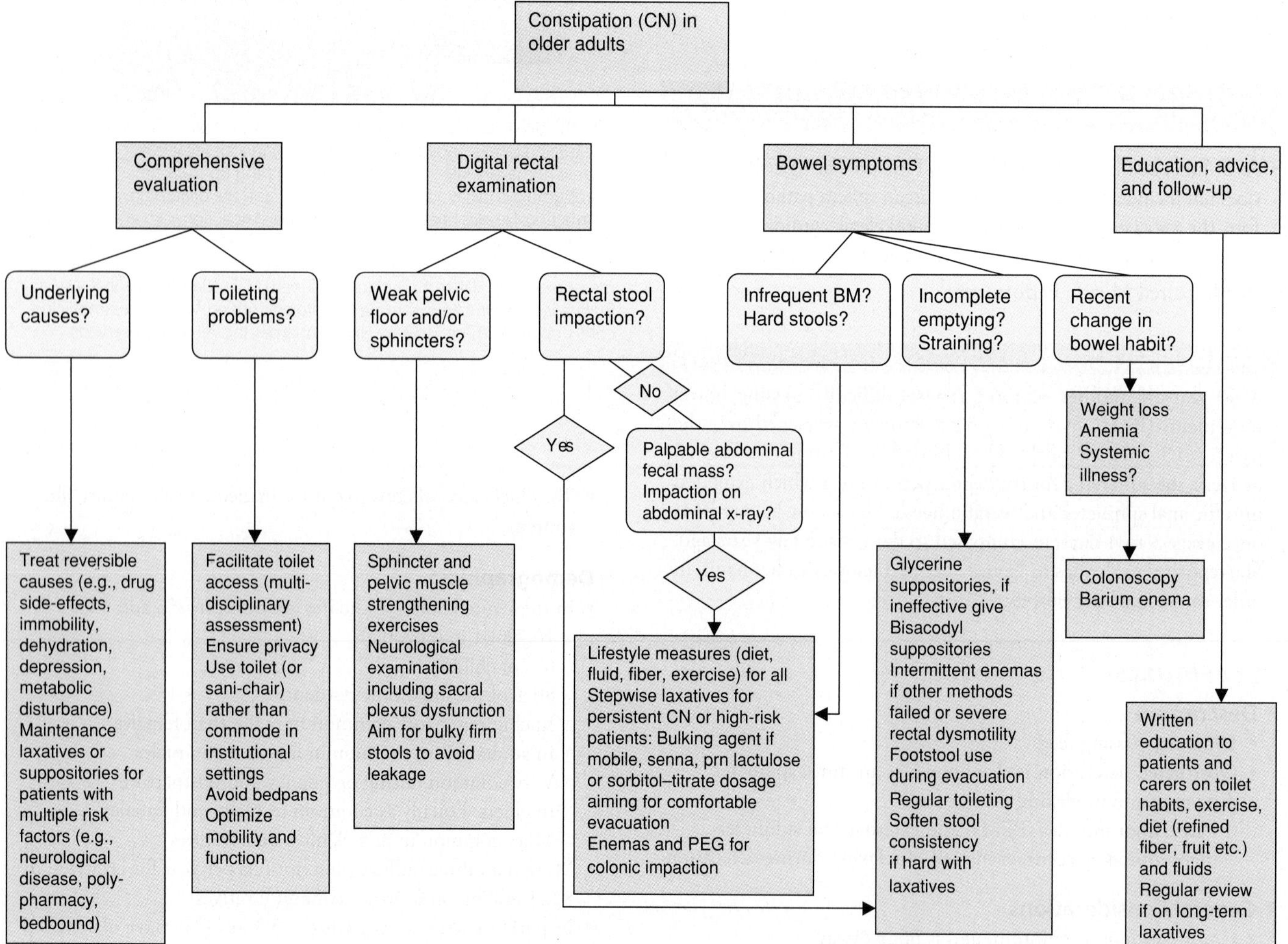

FIGURE 36-2 Practical approach to assessment and treatment of constipation in older people. (From Halter JB, Ouslander J, Tinetti M, Studenski S, High K, Asthana S. *Hazzard's Geriatric Medicine and Gerontology*. 6th ed. www.accessmedicine.com.

Differential Diagnosis

- Hirschsprung disease: Aganglionosis
- Colorectal neoplasm
- Colorectal stricture, scaring
- Diverticular disease
- Irritable bowel syndrome (IBS)
- Anorectal fissure, hemorrhoids, episiotomy, scar
- Pelvic organ prolapse: Cystocele, rectocele, descended perineum
- Rectal prolapse
- Referred pain from the gut
- Abdominal pain or tenderness: Constant or intermittent, possibly related to ingesting food
- Nausea, vomiting
- Changes in bowel habits
- Inability to swallow
- Lack of appetite
- Unexplained weight loss
- Dark stool or bright red blood in stool
- Malaise/fatigue

MEANS OF CONFIRMATION OR DIAGNOSIS

- See ROME-III criteria in "Signs and Symptoms" earlier.

Imaging[6]

- Endoanal ultrasound
- Dynamic proctography, defecography
- Dynamic pelvic MRI
- Colonic transit time: Marker study
- Flexible sigmoidoscopy
- Colonoscopy

Diagnostic Procedures

- Anal manometry
  - Anal canal pressure
  - Rectal sensation
  - Rectal compliance
- Rectal balloon expulsion
- Pudendal nerve terminal motor latency (PNTML)
- Needle EMG of external anal sphincter
- Barium Enema

FINDINGS AND INTERPRETATION[7]

- There is a lack of evidence to support the routine use of blood tests, endoscopy, and radiography in constipation evaluation.
- Colonic transit, anal manometry, and balloon expulsion tests have shown utility in selected patients with constipation.
- No single test defines pathophysiology.

TREATMENT

Medication[8]

- Chloride channel activators (lubiprostone: Amitiza) increases fluid content of stool
- Bulking agents, fiber supplements (Metamucil)
- Stimulants: Causes contraction of intestines, can cause dependency (Ex-Lax, caffeine, Dulcolax, Senikot)
- Osmotics: Increase water in intestines (Milk of Magnesia, Miralax)
- Stool softeners: Moisture to stool (Colace)

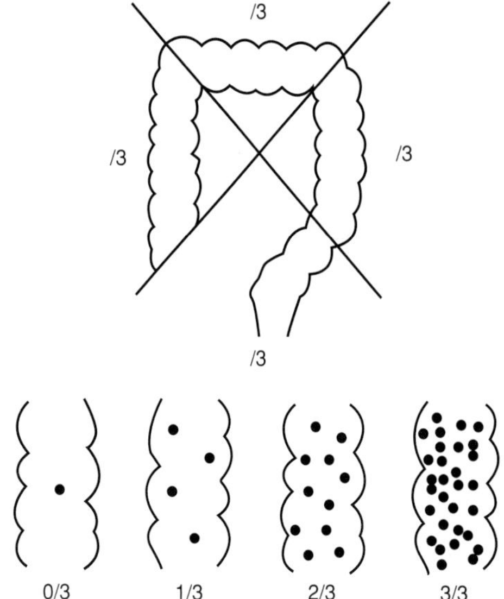

*On a flat abdominal x-ray, draw two diagonal lines intersecting at the umbilicus as shown here. This transects the abdomen into four quadrants corresponding to the ascending, transverse, descending, and rectosigmoid colons. Then, assess the amount of stool in each of the four quadrants using the following scoring system: 0 = no stool; 1 = stool occupying <50% of the lumen of colon; 2 = stool occupying >50% of the lumen; 3 = stool completely occupying the lumen. The total score will therefore range from 0 to 12. A score of 7 indicates severe constipation and requires immediate intervention.

FIGURE 36-3 How to calculate a "constipation score" using a flat abdominal x-ray. (From Kantarjian HM, Wolff RA, Koller CA. *The MD Anderson Manual of Medical Oncology*. 2nd ed. www.accessmedicine.com. Copyright © The McGraw-Hill Companies, Inc. All rights reserved.)

- Lubricants: Grease stool for ease of expulsion (mineral oil); lubricants may decrease absorption of other medications and/or nutrients
- 5-HT-4 agonists: Are not available in the United States (Prucalopride), increase fluid secretion in the intestines and decrease colonic transit time

Dietary Supplements[9]

- Aloe vera, aloe vera juice
- Dandelion
- Dong Quai
- Fiber
- Flaxseed
- Grape seed
- Psylium

MEDICAL PROCEDURES

- Manual disimpaction
- Botulism toxin injections for anal sphincter muscle spasm
- Surgical repair of anal fissure, hemorrhoids
- Colon resection in cases of severe symptoms
- Pessary device inserted vaginally to support pelvic organ prolapse

REFERRALS/ADMITTANCE

- Pelvic floor physical therapist
- Primary care physicians
- Gastroenterologists
- Colorectal surgeon
- Gynecologists
  - Women: Pelvic exam
- Urogynecologists
- Acupuncture

IMPAIRMENTS

- Pelvic floor muscle dysfunction: Overactive, underactive, nonrelaxing, noncontracting
- Abdominal muscle weakness, incoordination

- Sacrococcygeal joint dysfunction
- Pelvic girdle pain
- Pelvic pain
- Pelvic organ prolapse

TESTS AND MEASURES

- Pelvic floor muscle examination and assessment
  - sEMG biofeedback assessment of the pelvic floor muscles
  - Pressure manometry of the pelvic floor muscles
- Bowel diary to assess patient's behaviors related to defecation including fluid and food intake, voiding habits, symptoms
- Sacrococcygeal joint position and mobility assessment

INTERVENTION

- Pelvic floor muscle exercises/training
  - Contraction: "Kegel" exercises
  - Relaxation/"bulging": Necessary for defecation
  - Motor control, coordination
  - Endurance
  - Power
  - sEMG biofeedback: Assess behavior of pelvic floor muscle while sitting on toilet to simulate defecation, provide feedback for pelvic floor muscle exercise training
  - Pressure manometry
- Manual therapy: Mobilize sacrococcygeal joint, release pain, and trigger points in pelvic floor and coccygeus muscles
- Abdominal muscle coordination training: Bulging lateral walls during defecation
- US imaging to facilitate pelvic floor muscle training
- Bowel training: Defecation posture instruction
- Abdominal massage
- Patient education
  - Fluid management: Drink enough water
  - Dietary management: Optimize fiber intake
  - Daily physical activity

FUNCTIONAL GOALS

- Patient will be able to
  - Restore PFM function to perform voluntary contraction and relaxation to promote normal coordination during defecation.
  - Independently assumes optimal posture on toilet for defecation.
  - Verbalize understanding of fluid and fiber intake, recommended daily requirements (fluid intake at least 48 oz per day, and increase dietary fiber intake to at least 25 g per day).
  - Increase frequency of BMs from ____ times per week to at least four times per week.
  - Independence with long-term pelvic floor muscle training program, as appropriate, to manage bowel symptoms.

PROGNOSIS

- In patients with pelvic floor muscle dysfunction and constipation, symptom severity decreased after physical therapy (2.1 +/− 0.7 vs. 1.3 +/− 0.9, P = 0.007).[10]
  - Quality of life also improved significantly (2.6 +/− 0.8 vs. 1.5 +/− 1.0, P = 0.007).
  - Patients reported less physical discomfort, fewer worries/concerns, and indicated satisfaction with treatment.
  - The difference in symptom severity was highly correlated with improvement in quality of life (r = 0.7, P = .005).
- Following biofeedback treatment for puborectalis syndrome, patients with constipation showed improvement in all subcategories of the SF-36, except general health, surpassing pretreatment baseline values and equaling those for normals.[11]

PATIENT RESOURCE

- Constipation. NDDIC; National Digestive Diseases Information Clearinghouse.http://digestive.niddk.nih.gov/ddiseases/pubs/constipation/index.htm. Accessed August 8, 2014.

REFERENCES

1. The American Physical Therapy Association. Pattern 4C: impaired muscle performance. *Guide to Physical Therapist Practice*. Alexandria, VA: The American Physical Therapy Association; 2003. http://guidetoptpractice.apta.org/content/1/SEC10.extract?sid=9af82a7e-5fc3–41d2–86ab-b8336a9655e9. Accessed June 21, 2013.
2. Constipation. National Digestive Diseases Information Clearinghouse (NDDIC). http://digestive.niddk.nih.gov/ddiseases/pubs/constipation/index.htm. Accessed June 21, 2013.
3. Varma MD, Hart SL, Brown JS, Creasman JM, Van Den Eeden SK, Thom DH. Obstructive defecation in middle–aged women. *Dig Dis Sci*. 2008;53(10):2702–2709.
4. ROME Criteria. http://www.romecriteria.org/assets/pdf/19_RomeIII_apA_885–898.pdf. http://www.romecriteria.org/. Accessed May 3, 2014.
5. Thompson WG, Longstreth GF, Drossman DA, Heaton KW, Irwin EJ, Müller-Lissner SA. Functional bowel disorders and functional abdominal pain. *Gut*. 1999;45:1143–1147.
6. Bharucha AE. Update of tests of colon and rectal structure and function. *J Clin Gastroenterol*. 2006;40(2):96–103.
7. Rao SS, Ozturk R, Laine L. Clinical utility of diagnostic tests for constipation in adults: a systematic review. *Am J Gastroenterolo*. 2005;100(7):1605–1615.
8. Constipation: Treatment and Drugs. http://www.mayoclinic.com/health/constipation/DS00063/DSECTION=treatments-and-drugs. Accessed June 21, 2013.
9. Herbs and Supplements for Constipation. University of Maryland Medical Center. http://www.umm.edu/altmed/articles/constipation-002441.htm. http://umm.edu/health/medical/altmed/lookup/herbs-and-supplements-for-constipation. Accessed May 3, 2014.
10. Lewicky-Gaupp C, Morgan D, Chey WD, Muellerleile P, Fenner DE. Successful physical therapy for constipation related to puborectalis dyssynergia improves symptom severity and quality of life. *Dis Colon Rectum*. 2008;51(11):1686–1691.
11. Zhu FF, Lin Z, Lin L, Wang MF. Changes in quality of life during biofeedback for people with puborectalis dyssynergia: generic and disease-specific measures. *J Adv Nurs*. 2011;67(6):1285–1293.

ADDITIONAL REFERENCE

- Dutton M. Pathology, gynecology, and psychology. In: Dutton M, ed. *McGraw-Hill's NPTE (National Physical Therapy Examination)*. 2nd ed. New York, NY: McGraw-Hill; 2012. http://www.accessphysiotherapy.com/content/5402334. Accessed June 21, 2013.

37 DIVERTICULITIS

Debra F. Stern, DPT, DBA, MSM, PT
Eric Shamus, PhD, DPT, PT, CSCS
David W. Mandel, PhD, PT

CONDITION/DISORDER SYNONYM

- Diverticulosis

ICD-9-CM CODES

- 562 Diverticula of intestine
- 562.01 Diverticulitis of small intestine (without mention of hemorrhage)
- 562.11 Diverticulitis of colon (without mention of hemorrhage)
- Associated physical therapy diagnoses
  - 718.45 Contracture of joint, pelvic region and thigh
  - 781.2 Abnormality of gait
  - 728.89 Other disorders of muscle, ligament, and fascia
  - 728.2 Muscular wasting and disuse atrophy, not elsewhere classified
  - 729.9 Other and unspecified disorders of soft tissue
  - 719.70 Difficulty in walking involving joint site unspecified
  - 782.3 Edema
  - 315.4 Developmental coordination disorder
  - 786.05 Shortness of breath
  - 780.7 Malaise and fatigue
  - 786.0 Dyspnea and respiratory abnormalities

ICD-10-CM CODES

- K57.12 Diverticulitis of small intestine without perforation or abscess without bleeding
- K57.32 Diverticulitis of large intestine without perforation or abscess without bleeding

PREFERRED PRACTICE PATTERN

- As of June, 2014, the APTA *Guide to Physical Therapist Practice* does not include practice patterns for organ system pathology. Therefore, the associated or secondary musculoskeletal, cardiovascular/pulmonary, or potential neuromuscular patterns would be indicated.

PATIENT PRESENTATION

Patient is a 46-year-old female who presents to your clinic with dull left lower back and pelvic pain. She denies any movements that make the pain worse or better. The patient also reports a crampy lower abdominal pain that increases after eating. Further interview of the patient reveals she frequents the restroom with urgency and that her stools are dark. In addition, the patient states that she has trouble getting through her day as she has felt more fatigued recently.

Patient is a direct access, self-pay, without a physician's referral. During the initial physical therapy examination, palpation of the thoraco-lumbar musculature does not reveal pain. Active and passive movements at trunk rotation, side bending, and forward flexion do not increase low back pain but result in increased abdominal discomfort. Hip flexion also does not reveal increased pelvic discomfort. Special tests such as palpation of McBurney point and the Pinch-an-inch test are positive for increased abdominal tenderness. Palpation of the left iliopsoas muscle and resisted left hip flexion does not increase low back pain; however, the tests do reproduce abdominal tenderness.

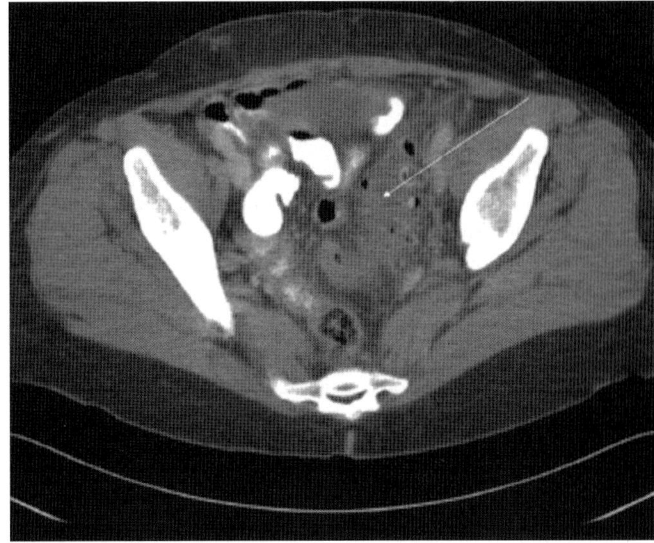

FIGURE 37-1 CT of abdomen in a 60-year-old female presenting with left lower quadrant abdominal pain showing sigmoid colon mural thickening, several colonic diverticula, and associated mesocolic fat infiltration, findings consistent with acute diverticulitis. (From McKean S, Ross JJ, Dressler DD, Brotman DJ, Ginsberg JS. *Principles and Practice of Hospital Medicine*. www.accessmedicine.com. Copyright © The McGraw-Hill Companies, Inc. All rights reserved.)

KEY FEATURES

Description

- Focal inflammation of the diverticula (sacs) in any part of the digestive tract but most commonly in the large intestine[1]
- Secondary problems such as weakness, gait abnormalities, and limited aerobic endurance
- May be acute, postoperative, chronic, viral or bacterially related, or congenital/hereditary
- Diverticulosis are pouches in the wall of the colon, when inflamed called diverticulitis

Essentials of Diagnosis

- Individuals may be referred to PT with complaints of back pain, or anterior chest and shoulder pain, which is not attributable to the structures in that anatomical area.
- Diagnosis for more occult problems may take time and require intensive medical diagnostic testing.

- Sudden onset may mimic colon cancer or tumors, irritable bowel syndrome, colitis, or gynecological problems in females such as endometriosis, uterine fibroids, or ectopic pregnancies.
- Abdominal pain often on the left side of abdomen (may start slow and worsen over days, but this is less common).
- It is not the purview of a physical therapist to medically diagnose a gastrointestinal (GI) pathology, but rather to recognize the possibility in the differential diagnosis process, especially when the findings are not consistent with conditions commonly treated (musculoskeletal, neuromuscular, integumentary, cardiopulmonary).

General Considerations

- May result in secondary problems such as aerobic capacity and muscle-endurance impairment, sarcopenia, weakness/impaired muscle performance, musculoskeletal problems, neuromuscular problems, weight loss, or weight gain, indicating the need for physical therapy intervention depending on severity
- Chronic diarrhea, episodic diarrhea, loss of bowel control (incontinence or urgency), and blood in stool may be symptomatic of diverticulitis

Demographics

- Most common after 40 years of age
- Low-fiber diets
- Those who lack exercise
- Obesity
- Uncommon in third world or developing countries

CLINICAL FINDINGS

SIGNS AND SYMPTOMS

- Left lower quadrant pain
- Constipation: Chronic, acute
- Abdominal or stomach pain or cramping, often left sided with sudden onset
- Abdominal (stomach or intestinal) pain after ingesting food or liquid
- Difficulty swallowing (related to esophageal diverticulitis)
- Abdominal tenderness
- Fever
- Nausea and vomiting
- Changes in bowel habits: Constipation, diarrhea, frequency
- Diarrhea: Acute, chronic
- Bloating
- Rectal bleeding, but this is uncommon
- Emesis
- Flatulence (gas)
- Blood in stool: Dark or bright (fresh bleeding)
- Pain associated with defecation
- Changes in bowel habits
- Flatulence
- Urinary tract infection
- Abdominal muscle spasm, guarding
- Abdominal distention
- Palpable abdominal mass
- Bloated or swollen abdomen
- Unexplained weight loss
- Abdominal bloating
- Fistulas
- General abdominal pain
- Abdominal muscle spasm, guarding
- As the symptoms are frequently related to the back and shoulders, it may be more common than previously identified to have patients inappropriately referred to PT

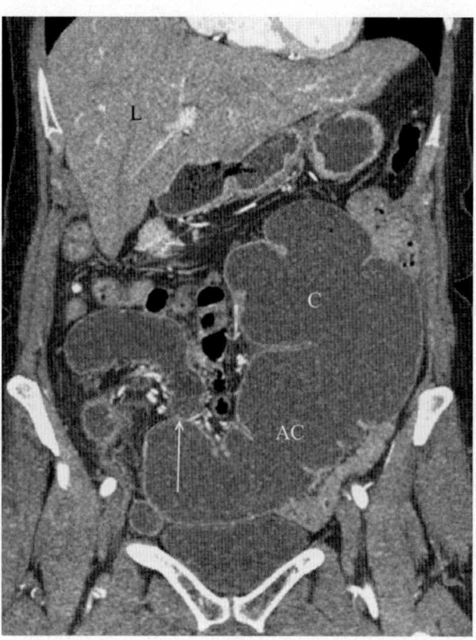

FIGURE 37-2 Coronal CT image showing a right colon volvulus with the twist in the ascending colon (*arrow*) causing marked distention of a portion of the ascending colon (AC) and the cecum (C). L, liver. (From Chen MYM, Pope TL, Ott DJ. *Basic Radiology*. 2nd ed. www.accessmedicine.com. Copyright © The McGraw-Hill Companies, Inc. All rights reserved.)

Functional Implications

- Severe symptoms such as diarrhea associated with immediacy of defecation may be disabling, resulting in the inability to leave home
- Chronic constipation can result in severe pain, and in its severe forms can result in fecal material backing up through the esophagus, requiring manual extraction or surgery, and in some cases, bowel retraining
- Dehydration with severe diarrhea, emesis, loss of appetite, inability to drink or eat secondary to nausea, or inability to swallow
- Sarcopenia, resulting in weakness, muscle-mass loss, inability to ambulate or perform self-care, as well as aerobic capacity limitation secondary to inactivity
- Need for colostomies or ileostomies: Temporary or permanent
    - Presence of same may present a problem with stoma retraction associated with abdominal contraction
- Eating disorders/anorexia secondary to fear of pain associated with ingesting food
- Fatigue
- Limitations in ADLs or IADLs from fatigue
- Decreased exercise tolerance
- Changes in lifestyle limiting physical activity

Possible Contributing Causes

- Abdominal mass
- Stress and anxiety
- Pressure against weak areas in colon causing diverticula
- Trapping of fecal matter in diverticula
- Obstruction of the diverticulum, decreasing blood supply, and causing inflammation
- The narrow openings of diverticula may trap fecal matter, which can lead to infection

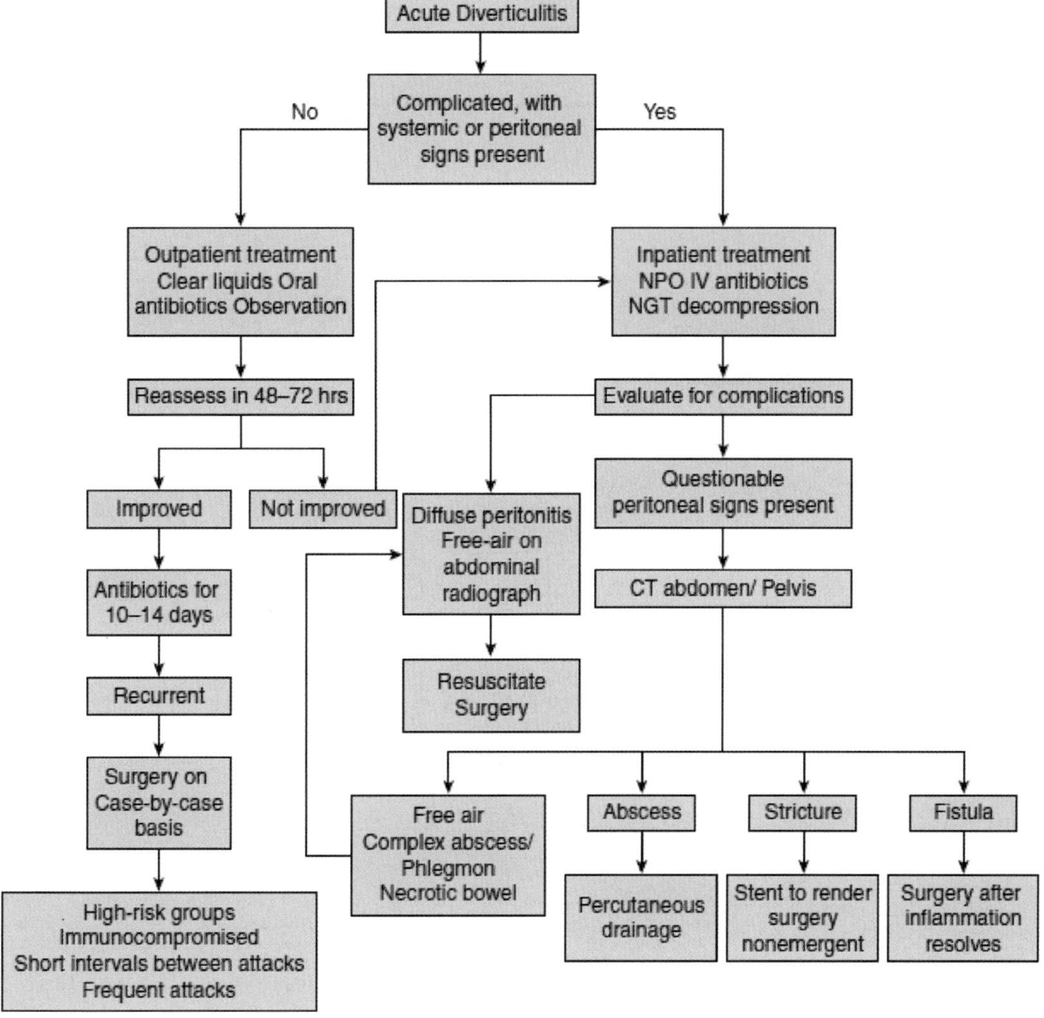

FIGURE 37-3 An algorithm for the management of acute diverticulitis, depending on severity and presence of complications. IV, intravenous; NGT, nasogastric tube; NPO, nothing per os. (From McKean S, Ross JJ, Dressler DD, Brotman DJ, Ginsberg JS. *Principles and Practice of Hospital Medicine*. www.accessmedicine.com. Copyright © The McGraw-Hill Companies, Inc. All rights reserved.)

- Diet: It is no longer believed that seeds or nuts getting caught are causative, but lack of fiber is considered contributory
- Heredity
- Environmental irritant
- Infection: Bacterial or viral including food poisoning
- Obesity
- Lack of exercise
- Ehlers–Danlos syndrome
- Marfan syndrome
- Scleroderma
- Kidney transplant

Differential Diagnosis

- Organ dysfunction as a result of cancer or malignancy
- Inflammatory bowel disease
- Atherosclerosis
- Non-malignant tumors in the abdomen or organs
- Endocrine disorders
- Gynecologic problems in females such as
  - Menses
  - Endometriosis
  - Ectopic pregnancies
  - Ovarian cysts
  - Fibroids
- Autoimmune diseases that affect the upper and lower GI tracts: Crohn disease, SLE, rheumatoid arthritis
- Appendicitis
- Irritable bowel syndrome
- Colon cancer
- Ovarian cancer
- Colitis
- Pelvic inflammatory disease
- Celiac disease
- Ovarian cysts
- Ectopic pregnancy
- Endometriosis
- Gastroenteritis
- Perforated ulcers anywhere in GI system
- Heart disease
- Bladder infections, urinary tract infections, kidney pathology
- Infections in the abdomen
- Bowel disorders including
  - Constipation or diarrhea
  - Inflammation of the lining of the abdomen

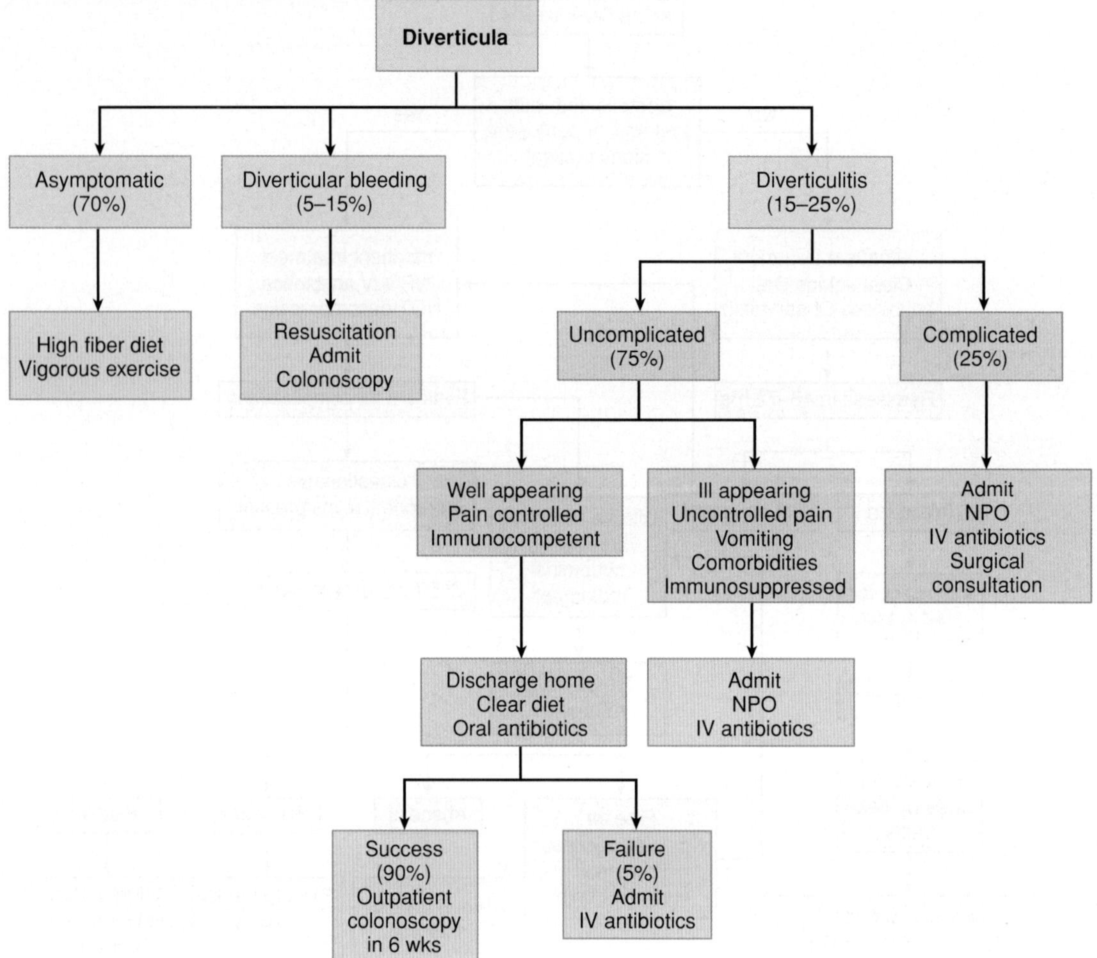

FIGURE 37-4 Algorithm for treatment of diverticulitis. ((Figure created using data from Parks TG. Natural history of diverticular disease of the colon: a review of 521 cases. *Br Med J.* 1969; 4: 639–642.)

- Organ obstructions
- Torsions
- Referred pain from heart, spine, hip
- Post–weight-loss surgery complications
  - Bariatric surgeries for weight loss
  - Some of the side effects of bariatric surgeries such as gastric bypass, lap bands, and sleeves, while considered safe and medically indicated may mimic diverticulitis or possibly be causative of a flare-up

MEANS OF CONFIRMATION OR DIAGNOSIS

Laboratory Tests

- Fecal occult blood tests
- Blood tests/lab tests

Imaging

- Abdominal scans
- Radiography of the abdomen
- Ultrasound of the abdomen
- Computed tomography (CT)

Diagnostic Procedures

- Upper GI series
- Lower GI series
- Endoscopy
- Colonoscopy: Virtual or invasive
- Manual palpation for tenderness

FINDINGS AND INTERPRETATION

- Blood tests/lab tests: To determine hemoglobin and hematocrit (H & H) for signs of bleeding, anemia, pathogens, immune status, and/or vitamin deficiencies, check white blood cell count for infection

TREATMENT

Medication

- Antibiotics
- Anticholinergics

MEDICAL PROCEDURES

- Bowel resection
- Bowel resection with colostomy

TESTS AND MEASURES

- Observation
  - Scars may indicate adhesions or abdominal surgeries that may be causative of diverticula.
  - Striae: Pink or purplish may be indicative of Cushing syndrome, dilated veins may indicate hepatic pathology or inferior vena cava obstruction, not diverticulitis.

- Contour: Roundedness, concavity/hollowness, asymmetry, distension, pregnancy signs.
- Cullen sign: Bluish discoloring around the umbilicus, which may be a sign of retroperitoneal bleeding.
- Bluish discoloration in lower abdomen: Grey Turner sign, which is a sign of hemorrhagic pancreatitis.
- Bulging in groin or other areas of abdomen especially apparent with contraction of musculature in area may be hernia.
- Pulsing in the area of the navel may be abdominal aortic aneurysm.
- Left lower quadrant pain, often following a meal.
- Palpable abdominal tenderness: On left or generalized.
- Psoas sign: Provides resistance over patient's right knee as they flex the hip; pain would be indicative of appendicitis or possible inflammation of the abdomen.
- Obturator sign: Internal rotation of right lower extremity (RLE) and flexion may be indicative of appendicitis or pelvic inflammation.
- Rovsing sign: Pain on the right side of abdomen when pressure is put on the left may be indicative of appendicitis.

- Palpation
  - Appendix (McBurney's): Apply vertical pressure halfway between right ASIS and umbilicus.
  - Liver: In supine, with left hand under trunk parallel to 11th and 12th rib, lift upward; right hand lateral to rectus and press in and up: +/= reproduction of symptoms with deep breath.
  - Ascites: With the fingers, percuss outward from center, if sound is dull, ascites may be present.
  - Spleen: It is not recommended for PT to palpate an enlarged spleen (only palpable if enlarged) because of the potential of rupture.
  - Gallbladder (Murphy's): Place fingers right of rectus abdominus, below rib cage: +/= sudden pain and muscle tensing with deep breath.
  - Kidneys: In supine, place one hand under client between ribs and iliac crest, and other hand on abdomen below ribs and ribs pointing in opposite direction: +/− tenderness or reproduction of symptoms.
  - Bladder: Not usually palpable unless it is distended and rises above pubic bone; in supine, place hand above pubis and press down: +/= tenderness, reproduction of pain, or ability to feel the bladder: __+ ___−.

REFERRALS/ADMITTANCE

- If an emergency is identified, refer to emergency room.
  - Blood in the stool
  - Fever that does not go away
  - Severe back pain
- Smoking cessation
- Weight management
- Dietary counseling
- Psychological intervention
- Surgical management
- Occupational therapy

IMPAIRMENTS

- Muscle weakness
- Muscle atrophy
- Gait abnormality/difficulty walking
- Contractures of soft tissue, fascia, muscle
- Shortness of breath
- Possible rectal muscle impairment
- Inability to perform self-care

INTERVENTION

- Physical therapy intervention is consistent with the movement-related problems that occur secondary to the GI problem and include as indicated.
  - Gait training
  - Therapeutic exercise: All relevant categories, energy conservation
- If there is a stoma from a colostomy or ileostomy, PT must be aware that activities are avoided if they cause retraction.
  - Therapeutic exercise: Aerobic, strength, flexibility
  - Therapeutic activities for bed-mobility training, posture, breathing, functional training, transfer-, and transitional-movement training
  - Neuromuscular re-education
  - Self-care management training
  - Electrical stimulation: Rectal/anal in cases of incontinence or muscle control or coordination
  - Lifestyle modification
  - Soft tissue mobilization for scar management

FUNCTIONAL GOALS

- Patient will be able to
- Achieve adequate functional aerobic capacity, and the ability to talk during activity, in order to achieve functional gait and activity tolerance for work, play, school, self-care; ADLs and IADLs.
- Achieve functional gait in the home and community (with or without a device), allowing for work, play, self-care; ADLs and IADLs, up to __________ feet, based on patient's need and prior functional level
- Achieve 600 m or greater in a 6-minute walk test for initiation of safe functional gait in the community.
- Perform active verbalization with increasing taxonomy for safety during gait, including negotiation of even and uneven surfaces, opening and closing doors, transferring in and out of a car.
  - Perform activities requiring abdominals with appropriate muscle splinting/guarding to prevent retraction of stoma, if patient has a colostomy or ileostomy.
- Tolerate 30 minutes of continuous moderate exercise three times a week in ______ weeks, and five times a week in ____________ weeks, depending on the severity of the disease.

PROGNOSIS

- It is common to see a repeated attack of diverticulitis.
- Prognosis differs based on the pathology.
- Most GI pathologies do not affect lifespan, but may impact lifestyle.
- As this pathology is primarily medical in nature, it is the physician who establishes the medical prognosis.
- For the physical therapy prognosis, goals should be established that the patient can achieve based on their overall condition.
- Unless the medical condition is unstable or the goals unrealistic, the prognosis from a physical therapy perspective should be good; good refers only to the realistic functional goals established.

ADDITIONAL RESOURCES

- Case 64 In: *Pathophysiology of disease*. 6th ed. www.accessphysiotherapy.com. Accessed May 22, 2013.

PATIENT RESOURCE

- Diverticular Disease. American Society of Colon and Rectal Surgeons. http://www.fascrs.org/patients/conditions/diverticular_disease/. Accessed August 8, 2014.

REFERENCE

1. McPhee SJ, Hammer GD. Pathology & pathogenesis. In: McPhee SJ, Hammer GD, eds. *Pathophysiology of Disease*. 6th ed. New York, NY: McGraw-Hill; 2010. http://www.accessphysiotherapy. com/content/5369771. Accessed May 22, 2013.

ADDITIONAL REFERENCES

- Bacon HE, Berkley JL. The surgical management of diverticulitis of the colon with particular reference to rehabilitation. *Arch Surg*. 1960;80(4):646–649.
- Fox JM, Stollman NH. Diverticular disease of the colon. In: Feldman M, Friedman LS, Brandt LJ, eds. *Sleisenger and Fordtran's Gastrointestinal and Liver Disease*. 9th ed. Philadelphia, PA: Saunders Elsevier; 2010:Chapter 117.
- Goodman CC, Fuller KS. *Pathology Implications for the Physical Therapist*. 3rd ed. Philadelphia, PA: Saunders Elsevier; 2009.
- Goodman CC, Snyder TK. *Differential Diagnosis for Physical Therapists: Screening for Referral*. 4th ed. St. Louis, MO: Saunders; 2007.
- Larson DW, Batdorf NJ, Touzios JG, et al. A fast-track recovery protocol improves outcomes in elective laparoscopic colectomy for diverticulitis. *J Am Coll Surg*. 2012;211(4):485–489. http://dx.doi.org/10.1016/j.jamcollsurg.2010.05.007. Accessed May 3, 2014.
- McOmber MA, Shulman RJ. Pediatric functional gastrointestinal disorders. *Nutr Clin Pract*. 2008;23(3):268–274. doi: 10.1177/0884533608318671. http://www.ncbi.nlm.nih.gov/pmc/articles/PMC2821593/Accessed May 3, 2014.
- Suleiman S, Johnston DE. The abdominal wall: an overlooked source of pain. *Am Fam Physician*. 2001;64(3):431–439. http://www.aafp.org/afp/2001/0801/p431.html. Accessed May 3, 2014.

38 GASTRITIS

Debra F. Stern, DPT, DBA, MSM, PT
Eric Shamus, PhD, DPT, PT, CSCS

ICD-9-CM CODES

- 535 Gastritis and duodenitis
- 535.0 Acute gastritis
- 535.00 Acute gastritis, without mention of hemorrhage
- 535.01 Acute gastritis, with hemorrhage
- 535.1 Atrophic gastritis
- 535.10 Atrophic gastritis, without mention of hemorrhage
- 535.11 Atrophic gastritis, with hemorrhage
- 535.3 Alcoholic gastritis
- 535.30 Alcoholic gastritis, without mention of hemorrhage
- 535.31 Alcoholic gastritis, with hemorrhage
- 535.4 Other specified gastritis
- 535.40 Other specified gastritis, without mention of hemorrhage
- 535.41 Other specified gastritis, with hemorrhage
- 535.5 Unspecified gastritis and gastroduodenitis
- 535.50 Unspecified gastritis and gastroduodenitis, without mention of hemorrhage
- 535.51 Unspecified gastritis and gastroduodenitis, with hemorrhage
- 535.6 Duodenitis
- 535.60 Duodenitis, without mention of hemorrhage
- 535.61 Duodenitis, with hemorrhage
- 535.7 Eosinophilic gastritis
- 535.70 Eosinophilic gastritis, without mention of hemorrhage
- 535.71 Eosinophilic gastritis, with hemorrhage
- Associated physical therapy diagnoses
  - 315.4 Developmental coordination disorder
  - 718.45 Contracture of joint, pelvic region and thigh
  - 719.70 Difficulty in walking involving joint site unspecified
  - 728.2 Muscular wasting and disuse atrophy, not elsewhere classified
  - 728.89 Other disorders of muscle, ligament, and fascia
  - 729.9 Other and unspecified disorders of soft tissue
  - 780.7 Malaise and fatigue
  - 781.2 Abnormality of gait
  - 782.3 Edema
  - 786.0 Dyspnea and respiratory abnormalities
  - 786.05 Shortness of breath

ICD-10-CM CODE

- K29.00 Acute gastritis without bleeding

PREFERRED PRACTICE PATTERN

- 6B: Impaired Aerobic Capacity/Endurance Associated with Deconditioning[1]

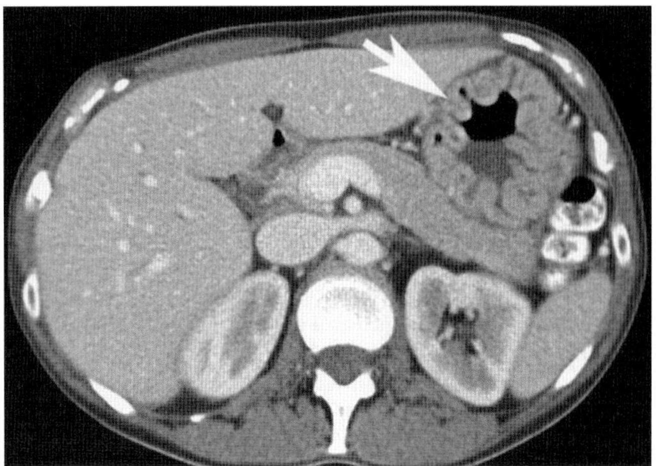

FIGURE 38-1 Gastritis. Axial MDCT image shows severe thickening of the gastric folds (*arrow*). (From Greenberger NJ, Blumberg R, Burakoff R. *Current Diagnosis & Treatment: Gastroenterology, Hepatology, & Endoscopy.* 2nd ed. www.accessmedicine.com. Copyright © The McGraw-Hill Companies, Inc. All rights reserved.)

PATIENT PRESENTATION

A 50-year-old male referred for OP PT for left shoulder bursitis. He has a history of degenerative joint disease (DJD) of both shoulders attributed to years of playing tennis and other sports. He is left hand dominant. When asked about medicines at the time of initial examination and evaluation, he reported that he was taking metoprolol for hypertension that was under control, and a variety of dietary supplements and occasional antacids for heartburn. It is his second week of therapy to which he is responding with a decrease in pain and an increase in ability to use the left upper extremity

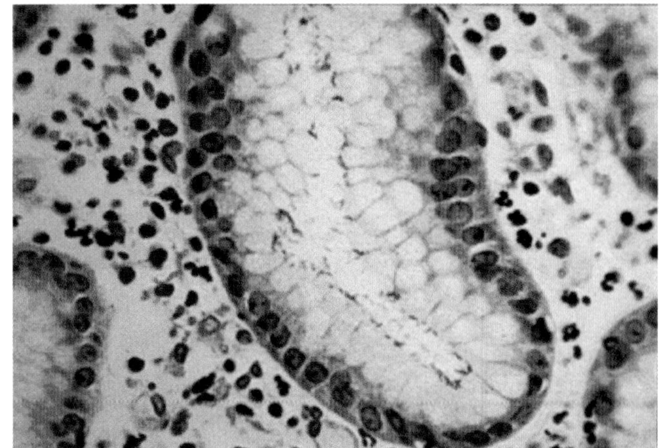

FIGURE 38-2 Chronic gastritis and *H. pylori* organisms. Steiner silver stain of superficial gastric mucosa, showing abundant darkly stained microorganisms layered over the apical portion of the surface epithelium. Note that there is no tissue invasion. (From Longo DL, Fauci AS, Kasper DL, Hauser SL, Jameson JL, Loscalzo J, eds. *Harrison's Principles of Internal Medicine.* 18th ed. New York, NY: McGraw-Hill; 2012.)

(LUE) functionally. You notice however, since the evaluation, that he has persistent bad breath, belching that increases with slouching posture, and that he intermittently rubs his chest. When asked if he is experiencing chest pain, he describes indigestion, states he ran out of antacids, and has some abdominal tenderness.

KEY FEATURES

Description

- Inflammation of stomach lining
- May be transient or chronic
- Stomach or upper-abdominal pain
- Dark stool

Essentials of Diagnosis

- Heartburn that responds to antacids
- Positive findings on biopsy or endoscopy and upper GI series
- Chronic gastritis is an increased number of lymphocytes and plasma cells in the gastric mucosa

General Considerations

- Diagnosis for more occult problems may take time and require intensive diagnostic testing
- May cause stomach cancer
- May indicate more serious problem, such as an autoimmune disease
- May result in secondary problems indicating need for PT intervention: Aerobic capacity and muscle endurance impairment, sarcopenia, weakness, musculoskeletal problems, neuromuscular problems, weight loss

Demographics

- Can occur in anyone throughout the lifespan
- Approximately one-third of US population is infected with *Helicobacter pylori*
- Incidence increases with age
- In United States, overall age-related incidence is 20% in people younger than 30 years, 50% in people older than 60 years
- Equally common in males and females

CLINICAL FINDINGS

SIGNS AND SYMPTOMS

- Indigestion
- Heartburn
- Hiccups
- Pain in abdomen or stomach
- Black stool
- Blood in stool
- Loss of appetite
- Nausea
- Vomiting: Blood or coffee ground-type substance
- Belching
- Feeling of fullness
- Halitosis
- Tachycardia (if GI bleeding)
- Pallor (if GI bleeding)

Functional Implications

- Severe symptoms such as immediacy of need to urinate or defecate may cause inability to leave home
- Inability to afford testing and medications, noncompliance with medication regimen
- Fatigue
- Drowsiness
- Nausea
- Vomiting

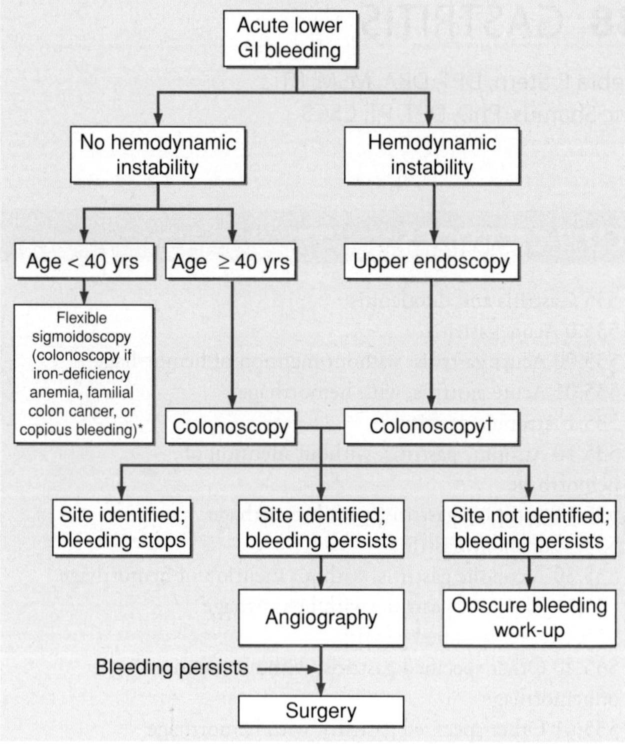

FIGURE 38-3 Suggested algorithm for patients with acute lower gastrointestinal bleeding. *Some suggest colonoscopy for any degree of rectal bleeding in patients <40 years as well. †If massive bleeding does not allow time for colonic lavage, proceed to angiography. (From Longo DL, Fauci AS, Kasper DL, Hauser SL, Jameson JL, Loscalzo J, eds. *Harrison's Principles of Internal Medicine.* 18th ed. New York, NY: McGraw-Hill; 2012.)

- Severe stomach pain with or without eating
- Heart disease
- Weight loss from inability to tolerate food, inability to exercise or move well
- Sarcopenia resulting in weakness, muscle-mass loss, inability to ambulate or perform self-care, limited aerobic capacity secondary to inactivity
- Decreased exercise tolerance
- Sleep disturbances
- Changes in lifestyle and diet
- Eating disorders, as eating becomes painful
- Inappropriate self-medication
- Anxiety, depression
- Esophageal problems or worn tooth enamel from persistent vomiting
- Limited ADLs, IADLs
- Infection (systemic)
- Difficulty with clear thinking
- Potential for blood clots, cardiac problems if aspirin cannot be taken prophylactically
- Gastric polyps
- Gastric tumors (benign or malignant)
- Peptic ulcers

Possible Contributing Causes[2]

- NSAIDs, especially aspirin, ibuprofen, naproxen sodium
- Excesses alcohol consumption
- *H. pylori* infection in stomach
- Autoimmune disorders

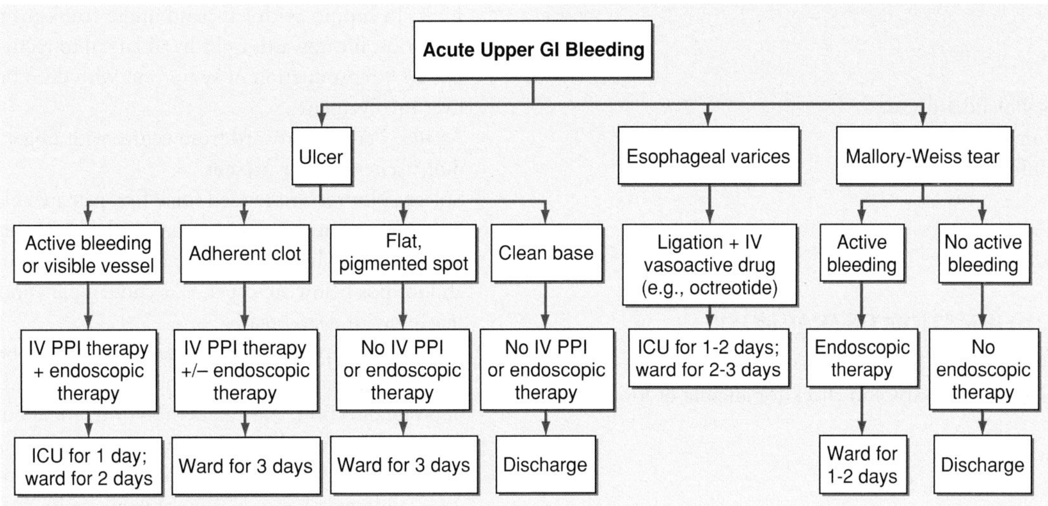

FIGURE 38-4 Suggested algorithm for patients with acute upper gastrointestinal bleeding. Recommendations on level of care and time of discharge assume that patient is stabilized without further bleeding or other concomitant medical problems. ICU, intensive care unit; PPI, proton-pump inhibitor. (From Longo DL, Fauci AS, Kasper DL, Hauser SL, Jameson JL, Loscalzo J, eds. *Harrison's Principles of Internal Medicine.* 18th ed. New York, NY: McGraw-Hill; 2012.)

- Pernicious anemia
- Bile reflux into stomach
- Illegal substance abuse, especially cocaine
- Ingestion of poisons
- Stress
- Viral or fungal infections
- Parasites
- Radiation
- Trauma
- Sudden or critical illness
- Severe body burns
- Surgery
- Kidney failure
- Ventilator dependence
- Food intolerance or allergy
- Malabsorption syndromes, such as celiac
- Smoking
- Chronic vomiting
- Sarcoidosis
- Systemic diseases
- Environmental irritants
- Dental disease, plaque
- Mother-to-child transmission
- Person-to-person transmission of *H. pylori* in crowded conditions with poor hygiene
- Working in endoscopy suites

Differential Diagnosis

- Organ dysfunction from cancer or malignancy
- Stomach cancer
- Colorectal cancer
- Ulcers: Stomach, peptic, esophageal, duodenal
- Non-malignant tumor in the abdomen or organs
- Internal hemorrhage
- Endocrine disorder, diabetes
- Cardiac disorder (may be secondary to GI bleeding)
- Gynecologic problems
- Autoimmune disease affecting upper and lower GI tracts
- Crohn disease
- Irritable bowel syndrome
- Rheumatoid arthritis (RA)
- Bladder or urinary tract infection, kidney pathology
- Diverticulitis
- Gastroparesis
- Intestinal paresis
- Inflammatory bowel disease
- Anemia
- Lymphoma

TABLE 38-1 Classification of Gastritis

I. Acute gastritis
  A. Acute *H. pylori* infection
  B. Other acute infectious gastritides
    1. Bacterial (other than *H. pylori*)
    2. *H. heilmannii*
    3. Phlegmonous
    4. Mycobacterial
    5. Syphilitic
    6. Viral
    7. Parasitic
    8. Fungal

II. Chronic atrophic gastritis
  A. Type A: Autoimmune, body-predominant
  B. Type B: *H. pylori*–related, antral-predominant
  C. Indeterminant

III. Uncommon forms of gastritis
  A. Lymphocytic
  B. Eosinophilic
  C. Crohn disease
  D. Sarcoidosis
  E. Isolated granulomatous gastritis

Source: Longo DL, Fauci AS, Kasper DL, Hauser SL, Jameson JL, Loscalzo J, eds. *Harrison's Principles of Internal Medicine.* 18th ed. New York, NY: McGraw-Hill; 2012.

- Ascites
- Cirrhosis
- Pancreatitis
- Gallstones, gallbladder disease
- Malabsorption, celiac
- Abdominal infection
- Pregnancy
- Hemorrhoids
- Bowel disorder

MEANS OF CONFIRMATION OR DIAGNOSIS

Laboratory Tests

- Complete blood count (CBC) to check for anemia or low blood cell count[3,4]
- *H. pylori* tests
- Stool sample to check for blood

Imaging

- Ultrasound
- Chest x-ray
- CT
- MRI
- Upper GI series
- Lower GI series
- Colonoscopy
- Endoscopy with stomach biopsy

FINDINGS AND INTERPRETATION

- Imaging not generally needed; may help rule out differential diagnosis
- Positive findings on biopsy, endoscopy, or upper GI series

TREATMENT

Medication

- Antacids
- H2 antagonists: Famotidine, cimetidine, ranitidine, rabeprazole, lansoprazole
- Antibiotics

REFERRALS/ADMITTANCE

- If causative problem is not considered appropriate for PT intervention, refer to appropriate physician
- If emergency is identified, refer to ER.

IMPAIRMENTS

- Muscle weakness, cramping
- Muscle atrophy
- Gait abnormality, difficulty walking
- Shortness of breath, fatigue
- Inability to perform self-care
- Balance impairment
- Impaired skin integrity

TESTS AND MEASURES

- Palpation
  - Appendix (McBurney's): Apply vertical pressure halfway between right ASIS and umbilicus: −/+ may indicate appendicitis.
  - Liver: In supine, with left hand under trunk parallel to 11th and 12th ribs, lift upward; right hand lateral to rectus, press in and up: +/= reproduction of symptoms with deep breath, indicates liver involvement.
  - Ascites: Percuss outward from center with fingers; if sound is dull, ascites may be present.
  - Spleen: Not recommended for PT to palpate enlarged spleen secondary to ease of rupture (only palpable if enlarged).
  - Gallbladder (Murphy's): Place fingers to the right of rectus abdominus below rib cage: +/= sudden pain and muscle tensing with deep breath.
  - Kidneys: In supine, place one hand under client between ribs and iliac crest, other hand on abdomen below ribs and ribs pointing in opposite direction: +/− tenderness or reproduction of symptoms.
  - Bladder: Not usually palpable unless distended and raised above pubic bone; in supine, place hand above pubis and press down: +/= tenderness, reproduction of pain, ability to feel the bladder: __+ ___−.

INTERVENTION

- Dietary counseling: Avoiding inflammatory foods (i.e., rice); elimination of alcohol, drugs, food irritants[5]
- Physical therapy intervention is consistent with the movement-related problems occurring secondary to gastritis, including
  - Gait training
  - Therapeutic exercise: All relevant categories, energy conservation
  - Bed-mobility training, transfer- and transitional-movement training
  - Self-care training: Skin care, moisturizing, lifestyle management
  - Neuromuscular re-education: Balance and postural training

FUNCTIONAL GOALS

- Patient will be able to
  - Perform active verbalization with increasing taxonomy for safety during gait, including negotiation of even and uneven surfaces, opening and closing doors, transferring in and out of car
  - Tolerate 30 minutes of continuous, moderate exercise three times a week in ______ weeks, and five times a week in ____________ weeks, depending on disease severity.

PROGNOSIS

- Physician establishes the medical prognosis, as pathology is primarily medical in nature.
- For PT prognosis, goals should be established that the patient can achieve based on their overall condition.
- Prognosis from a PT perspective should be good, unless medical condition is unstable or goals unrealistic.

PATIENT RESOURCE

- Gastritis. National Digestive Diseases Information Clearinghouse (NDDIC). http://digestive.niddk.nih.gov/ddiseases/pubs/gastritis/. Accessed August 8, 2014.

REFERENCES

1. The American Physical Therapy Association. Pattern 6B: impaired aerobic capacity/endurance associated with deconditioning. *Interactive Guide to Physical Therapist Practice.* 2003. doi: 10.2522/ptguide.3.3_2. http://guidetoptpractice.apta.org/content/1/SEC28.extract. Accessed May 3, 2014

2. Chandrasoma P, Taylor CR. Blood: II. Hemolytic anemias; polycythemia. In: Chandrasoma P, Taylor CR, eds. *Concise Pathology.* 3rd ed. Stamford, CT: Appleton & Lang; 1998. http://www.accessphysiotherapy.com/content/187050. Accessed June 12, 2013.
3. U.S. National Library of Medicine. CBC Complete blood count. PubMed Health. http://www.ncbi.nlm.nih.gov/pubmedhealth/PMH0004108/. Accessed June 12, 2013.
4. Chandrasoma P, Taylor CR. Blood: I. Structure & function; anemias due to decreased erythropoiesis. In: Chandrasoma P, Taylor CR, eds. *Concise Pathology.* 3rd ed. Stamford, CT: Appleton & Lang; 1998. http://www.accessphysiotherapy.com/content/186793. Accessed June 12, 2013.
5. Reinagel M. *The Inflammation Free Diet Plan.* New York, NY: McGraw-Hill; 2007. ISBN 0071510524. http://www.mhprofessional.com/product.php?isbn=0071510524. Accessed June 12, 2013.

ADDITIONAL REFERENCES

- Goodman CC, Fuller KS. *Pathology: Implications for the Physical Therapist.* 3rd ed. Philadelphia, PA: Saunders Elsevier; 2009.
- Goodman CC, Snyder TK. *Differential Diagnosis for Physical Therapists: Screening for Referral.* 4th ed. St. Louis, MO: Saunders Elsevier; 2007.
- McColl KE. Clinical practice. *Helicobacter pylori* infection. *N Engl J Med.* 2010;362(17):1597–604.
- McOmber MA, Shulman RJ. Pediatric functional gastrointestinal disorders. *Nutr Clin Pract.* 2008;23(3):268–274.
- Mills JC, Stappenbeck TS, Bunnett N. Gastrointestinal disease. In: McPhee SJ, Hammer GD, eds. *Pathophysiology of Disease.* 6th ed. New York, NY: McGraw-Hill; 2010. http://www.accessphysiotherapy.com/content/5369694. Accessed June 12, 2013.
- Sokol RJ, Narkewicz MR. Liver & Pancreas. In: Hay WW, Levin MJ, Sondheimer JM, Deterding RR, eds. *CURRENT Diagnosis & Treatment: Pediatrics.* 20th ed. New York, NY: McGraw-Hill; 2011. http://www.accessphysiotherapy.com/content/6584598. Accessed June 12, 2013.
- Suleiman S, Johnston DE. The abdominal wall: an overlooked source of pain. *Am Fam Physician.* 2001;64(3):431–438.
- Ulcerative Colitis. National Digestive Diseases Information Clearinghouse (NDDIC). U.S. Department of Health and Human Services. *NIH Publication No. 12–1597.* October 2011. http://digestive.niddk.nih.gov/ddiseases/pubs/colitis/. Accessed June 12, 2013.

39 GASTROESOPHAGEAL REFLUX DISEASE

Debra F. Stern, DPT, DBA, MSM, PT
Eric Shamus, PhD, DPT, PT, CSCS

CONDITION/DISORDER SYNONYMS

- Gastroesophageal reflux disease (GERD)
- Reflux esophagitis

ICD-9-CM CODES

- 530.81 Esophageal reflux
- Associated physical therapy diagnoses
  - 315.4 Developmental coordination disorder
  - 718.45 Contracture of joint, pelvic region and thigh
  - 719.70 Difficulty in walking
  - 728.2 Muscular wasting and disuse atrophy, not elsewhere classified
  - 728.89 Disorders of muscle, ligament, and fascia
  - 729.9 Other and unspecified disorders of soft tissue
  - 780.7 Malaise and fatigue
  - 781.2 Abnormality of gait
  - 782.3 Edema
  - 786.0 Dyspnea and respiratory abnormalities
  - 786.05 Shortness of breath

ICD-10-CM CODE

- K21.9 Gastroesophageal reflux disease without esophagitis

PREFERRED PRACTICE PATTERN

- As of June, 2014, the APTA *Guide to Physical Therapist Practice* does not include practice patterns for organ system pathology; therefore, the associated or secondary musculoskeletal, cardiovascular/pulmonary, or potential neuromuscular patterns would be indicated.

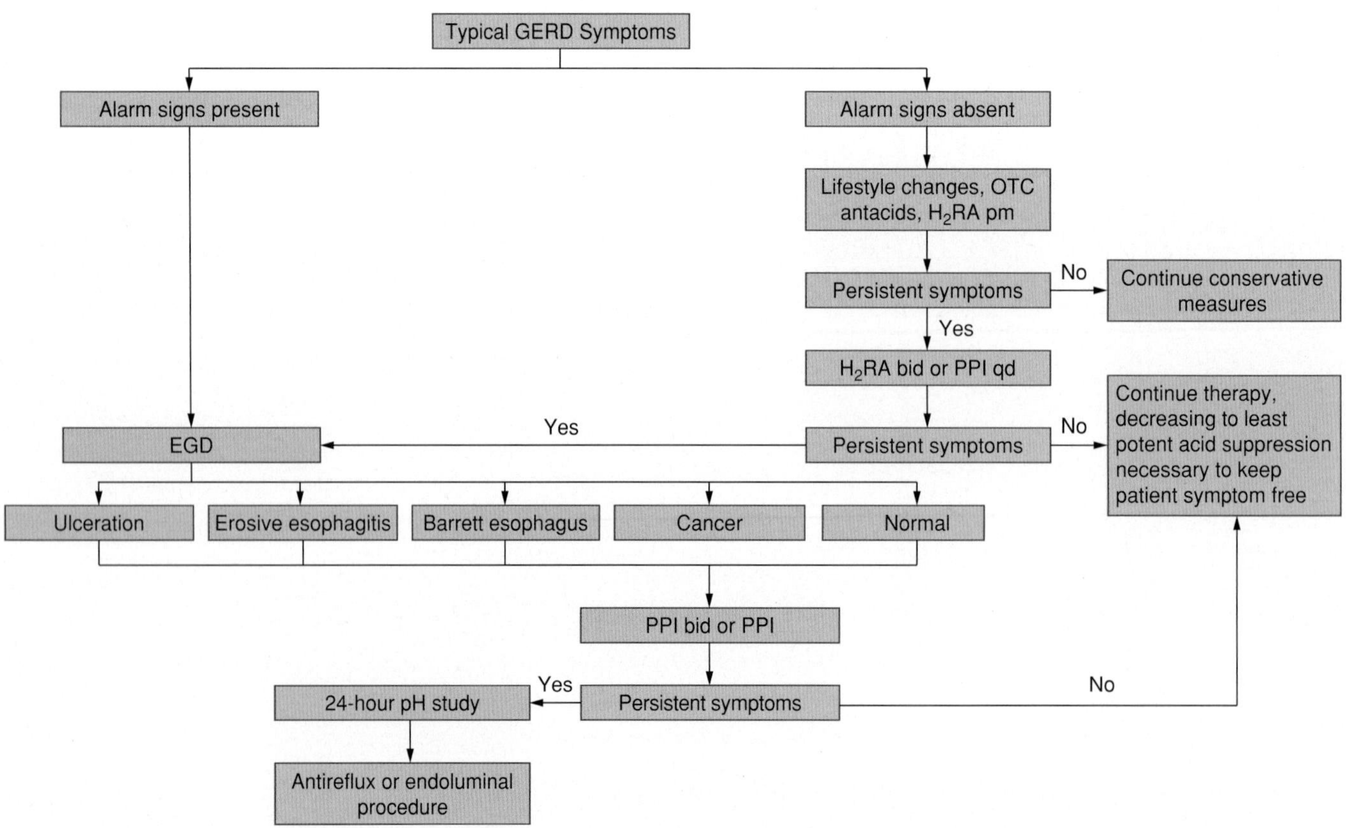

FIGURE 39-1 Algorithm for the diagnosis and treatment of gastroesophageal reflux (GERD). bid, twice daily; EGD, esophagogastroduodenoscopy; H_2RA, H_2-receptor antagonist; OTC, over-the-counter; prn, as needed; qd, daily. (From Greenberger NJ, Blumberg RS, Burakoff R. *Current Diagnosis & Treatment: Gastroenterology, Hepatology, & Endoscopy,* 2nd ed. www.accessmedicine.com. Copyright © The McGraw-Hill Companies, Inc. All rights reserved.)

PATIENT PRESENTATION

A 60-year-old patient is referred to PT with general shoulder pain. He plays softball in a senior league and somehow injured his shoulder. Although he cannot be specific about any single event or injury, he plays first base and occasionally fills in for the pitcher. He is moderately obese, but does go regularly to the gym to work out. His medications include an ace inhibitor for high blood pressure and occasional antacids for heartburn. During the initial examination he is rubbing the front of his shoulder and pectoralis area on the right. Hiccups and occasional coughing interfere with conversation at times, and he complains that he suffers from them more and more often. He is anxious to get better as his team is in the playoffs. Physical examination reveals bursitis and soreness in both shoulders.

KEY FEATURES

Description

- Condition in which stomach acid backs up into esophagus
- Patients experience burning feeling in abdominal, chest, or throat areas
- Common symptom and complaint is "heartburn"

Essentials of Diagnosis

- Acid reflux or indigestion, minimum twice weekly[1]
- Inability to or difficulty with swallowing
- Burning in chest
- Hoarseness
- Sore throat
- Regurgitation of food or sour liquid (acid reflux)
- Complaint of lump in throat
- Cough without mucous production or congestion
- Chest pain
- Nausea, vomiting

General Considerations

- Broad array of GI disorders may be encountered by physical therapists
- While PT may not manage GI disorders specifically, clients may receive care for secondary problems: Weakness, gait abnormalities, limited aerobic endurance, sarcopenia, musculoskeletal/neuromuscular problems, weight loss/gain
  - Problems may be acute, postoperative, chronic, viral, bacterial, or congenital/hereditary
- PT should recognize possible GI pathology in differential diagnosis, especially when findings are inconsistent with conditions commonly treated
- GI disorders frequently refer pain to other body areas; individuals may be inappropriately referred to PT
- History of heartburn or indigestion may indicate GI or cardiac problems
- May lead to more serious conditions such as Barrett esophagus
- May increase risk of cancer or ulcer

Demographics

- GI disorders occur throughout the lifespan (birth through geriatric)
- 55% to 60% of general population suffer from occasional symptoms of GERD[2]
- Some indication of genetic tendency

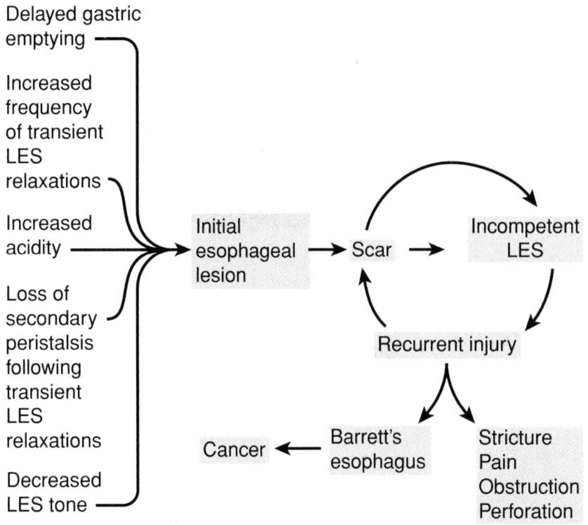

FIGURE 39-2 Pathophysiology of esophageal reflux disease. LES, lower esophageal sphincter.(From McPhee SJ, Hammer GD. *Pathophysiology of Disease: An Introduction to Clinical Medicine,* 6th ed. www.accessmedicine.com. Copyright © The McGraw-Hill Companies, Inc. All rights reserved.)

- Depending on the pathology, occurrence rates may differ based on ethnicity, diet, lifestyle, gender, age
- High incidence in general population due to potential for lifespan occurrence

CLINICAL FINDINGS

SIGNS AND SYMPTOMS

- Chronic indigestion
- Burning in throat, heartburn
- Relief with antacids
- Indigestion at least twice weekly
- Symptoms worsen when lying flat
- Wheezing
- Hiccups
- Difficulty in swallowing (related to esophageal or oral problems rather than neuromuscular)
- Pain
  - Abdominal/stomach pain, cramping (constant or intermittent, severe)
  - Chest pain
  - Pain upon ingesting food or liquid
    - May be cardiac in nature
  - Pain after ingesting fatty foods (gallbladder sign)
- Bowel changes
  - Diarrhea (acute, chronic)
  - Constipation (acute, chronic), especially with antacid ingestion
  - Occult blood in stool
  - Change in stool odor or color
  - Mucous in stool or mucous discharge
- Unexplained weight loss
- Abdominal muscle spasm, guarding
- Fatigue
- Loss of appetite, cachexia, complaints of "feeling full" regardless of having ingested food
- Nausea
- Emesis
- Dietary restrictions
- Headaches
- Dental problems

Functional Implications

- Severe symptoms may be disabling or cause inability to leave home
- Sleep disturbance, inability to lie flat

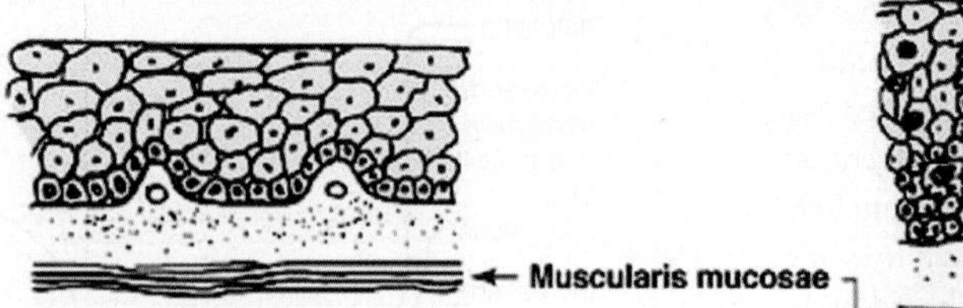

A. Normal

- Thin mucosa
- Single layer of basal cells <15% of mucosal thickness

B. Reflux esophagitis

- Thickened mucosa
- Basal cell hyperplasia > 15% of mucosa
- Increased height of lamina propria papillae > 70% of mucosa
- Marked congestion of papillary tips
- Neutrophil and eosinophil infiltration
- Lamina propria congestion, edema, and inflammation

FIGURE 39-3 Histologic changes in reflux esophagitis (**B**) compared with normal squamous epithelium lining the esophagus (**A**). (From Chandrasoma P, Taylor CR. *Concise Pathology,* 3rd ed. www.accessmedicine.com. Copyright © The McGraw-Hill Companies, Inc. All rights reserved.)

- Dietary restrictions (e.g., dairy, spices)
- Need to eat smaller meals
- Dehydration secondary to diarrhea, emesis, appetite loss, nausea, inability to swallow
- Eating disorder/anorexia secondary to fear of pain upon ingesting food
- Sarcopenia resulting in weakness, decreased muscle mass, inability to ambulate, perform self-care
- Limited aerobic capacity, limitation secondary to inactivity, deceased exercise tolerance, limited physical activity
- Limited ADLs, IADLs
- Fatigue
- Inappropriate self-medication
- Psychological challenges: Anxiety, depression
- May indicate serious medical condition

Possible Contributing Causes

- Lower esophageal pressure[3]
- Diabetes, endocrine dysfunction
- Alcohol
- Infection (bacterial, viral)
  - Food poisoning
  - Parasite
- Stress, anxiety
- Asthma
- Obesity, lack of exercise, diet

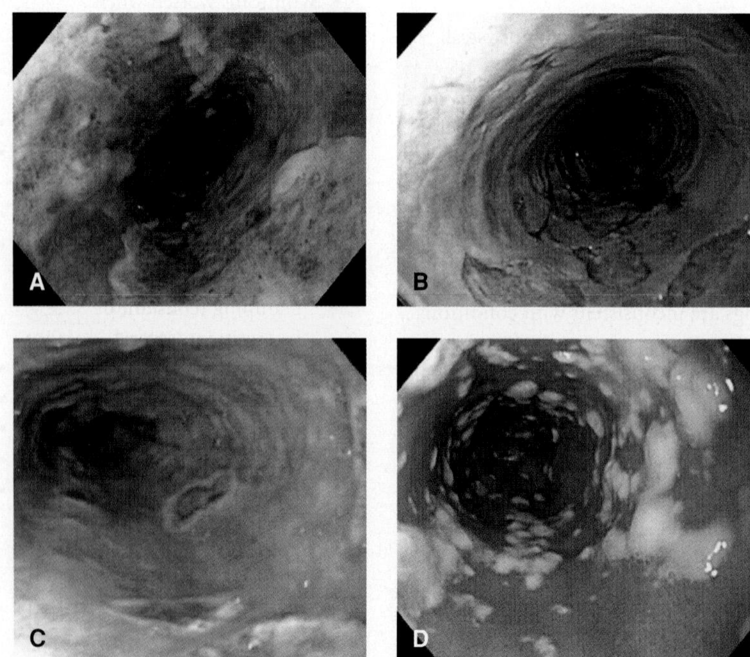

FIGURE 39-4 Causes of esophagitis. **A.** Severe reflux esophagitis with mucosal ulceration and friability. **B.** Cytomegalovirus esophagitis. **C.** Herpes simplex virus esophagitis with target-type shallow ulcerations. **D.** Candida esophagitis with white plaques adherent to the esophageal mucosa. (From Longo DL, Fauci AS, Kasper DL, et al., eds. *Harrison's Principles of Internal Medicine,* 18th ed. New York, NY: McGraw-Hill; 2012.)

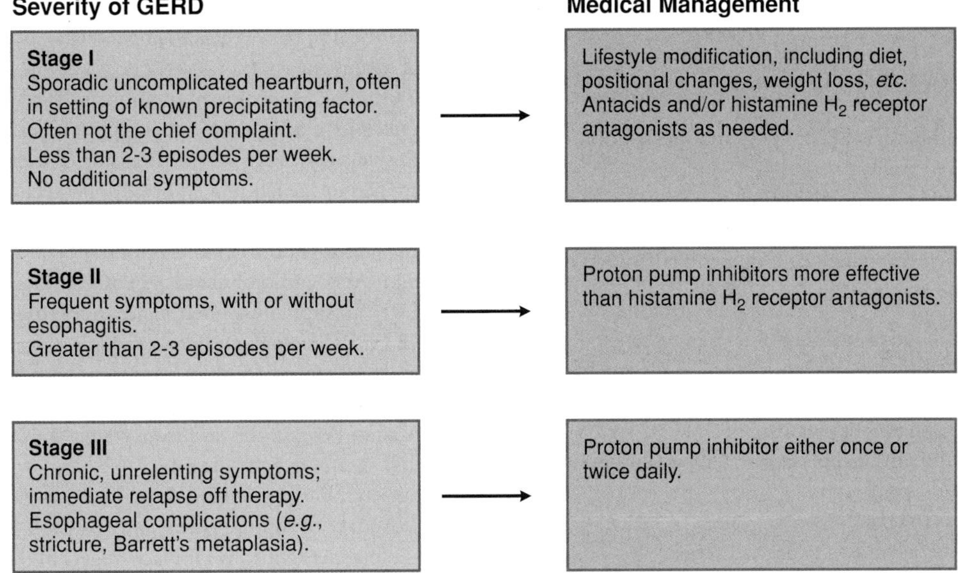

Severity of GERD
Medical Management
Stage I
Sporadic uncomplicated heartburn, often in setting of known precipitating factor.
Often not the chief complaint.
Less than 2-3 episodes per week.
No additional symptoms.
Lifestyle modification, including diet, positional changes, weight loss, etc.
Antacids and/or histamine H2 receptor antagonists as needed.
Stage II
Frequent symptoms, with or without esophagitis.
Greater than 2-3 episodes per week.
Proton pump inhibitors more effective than histamine H2 receptor antagonists.
Stage III
Chronic, unrelenting symptoms; immediate relapse off therapy.
Esophageal complications (e.g., stricture, Barrett's metaplasia).
Proton pump inhibitor either once or twice daily.

FIGURE 39-5 General guidelines for the medical management of gastroesophageal reflux disease (GERD). Only medications that suppress acid production or that neutralize acid are shown. (Adapted from Wolfe MM, Sachs G. Acid suppression: optimizing therapy for gastroduodenal ulcer healing, gastroesophageal reflux disease, and stress-related erosive syndrome. *Gastroenterology.* 2000; 118:S9–S31., with permission from Elsevier. Copyright © Elsevier.)

- Heredity, family history
- Food allergy or intolerance (gluten/wheat, dairy)
- Dry mouth (i.e., Sjögren syndrome)
- Cancer: Esophageal, colon, liver, bile duct, pancreatic, metastatic, anal/rectal
- Systemic rheumatologic disorders: Scleroderma, rheumatoid arthritis
- Delayed stomach emptying
- Systemic immunological condition, inflammatory or autoimmune disease
- Postsurgical scarring, adhesions
- Pregnancy
- Smoking
- Medication side effects
    - Anticholinergics (for seasickness)
    - Beta-blockers
    - Bronchodilators for asthma
    - Calcium-channel blockers for high blood pressure
    - Dopaminergic drugs for Parkinson disease
    - Progestin for abnormal menstrual bleeding or birth control
    - Sedatives for insomnia or anxiety
    - Tricyclic antidepressants
    - Salicylates
    - Anti-inflammatories
- Zollinger–Ellison syndrome
    - Gastrinomas (tumors) in small intestine, pancreas, lymph nodes, secrete gastrin hormone, cause excess production of stomach acid

Differential Diagnosis

- Organ dysfunction, from cancer or malignancy
- Non-malignant tumor in abdomen or organs
- Endocrine disorder
- Hiatal hernia
- Autoimmune/inflammatory disease affecting upper and lower GI tracts
- Irritable bowel syndrome, inflammatory bowel disease
- Rheumatoid arthritis
- Crohn disease
- Esophageal ulcer, perforated ulcer in GI system
- Esophageal cancer
- Barrett esophagus
- Gastric paresis
- Stomach ulcers
- Celiac disease, gluten intolerance
- Gastroenteritis
- Stomach disorder
- Referred pain from heart, spine, hip
- Post–weight-loss (bariatric) surgery complications
    - Side effects may cause reflux

MEANS OF CONFIRMATION OR DIAGNOSIS

Laboratory Tests

- Blood tests
    - Sedimentation rate
    - H & H

Imaging

- Radiography
    - Upper GI series
- CT

Diagnostic Procedures

- Medical history
- Endoscopy
- Acid measurement
- Esophageal motility

FINDINGS AND INTERPRETATION

- H & H for signs of bleeding, anemia, pathogens, immune status, vitamin deficiencies, white blood cell count

TREATMENT

Medication

- Antacids to neutralize stomach acid[4]
- Acid blockers[4]
  - Proton pump inhibitors (PPIs): OTC and prescription
- Acid reducers[4]
  - H-2 receptors: OTC and prescription
- Prokinetic agents[4]
  - Facilitate stomach emptying, valve tightening between the stomach and the esophagus

MEDICAL PROCEDURES

- Hernia repair (if hiatal or other hernia identified)
- Reinforcement of esophageal sphincter
- EndoCinch (endoluminal gastroplication): Creates barrier between stomach and esophagus
- Removal of tumors, growths
- Creation of scar tissue/adhesions to prevent reflux
- Stomach resection
- Ulcer repair
- Nasogastric tube
- Feeding tube
- Total/peripheral parenteral nutrition (TPN/PPN)
- IV for hydration

REFERRALS/ADMITTANCE

- If causative problem is not considered appropriate for PT intervention, refer to appropriate physician
- Refer to ER if emergency identified

IMPAIRMENTS

- Muscle weakness, atrophy
- Gait abnormality, difficulty in walking
- Contractures of soft tissue (fascia, muscle), joint limitations
- Shortness of breath
- Inability to perform self-care
- Limited aerobic endurance
- Functional decline

TESTS AND MEASURES

- Observation
  - Scars may indicate adhesions or abdominal surgeries causative of diverticula.
  - Pink or purplish striae may be indicative of Cushing syndrome.
  - Dilated veins may indicate hepatic pathology or inferior vena cava obstruction, not diverticulitis.
  - Contour: Roundness, concavity, asymmetry, distension, pregnancy signs.
  - Cullen sign: Bluish discoloring around umbilicus may be a sign of retroperitoneal bleeding.
  - Bluish discoloration in lower abdomen: Gary Turner sign, signals hemorrhagic pancreatitis.
  - Bulging in groin/abdomen especially apparent with contraction of musculature in area may be hernia.
  - Pulsing in navel area may be abdominal aortic aneurysm.
  - Left lower quadrant pain, often following a meal.
  - Palpable abdominal tenderness: On left side or generalized.
  - Psoas sign: Provide resistance over patient's right knee as they flex the hip; pain indicates appendicitis, possible inflammation of abdomen.
  - Obturator sign: Internal rotation and flexion of right lower extremity may indicate appendicitis, pelvic inflammation.
  - Rovsing sign: Pain on the right side of abdomen when pressure applied to the left may indicate appendicitis.
- Palpation
  - Appendix (McBurney's): Apply vertical pressure halfway between right ASIS and umbilicus: −/+ may indicate appendicitis.
  - Liver: In supine, with left hand under trunk parallel to 11th and 12th ribs, lift upward; right hand lateral to rectus, press in and up: +/= reproduction of symptoms with deep breath, indicates liver involvement.
  - Ascites: Percuss outward from center with fingers; if sound is dull, ascites may be present.
  - Spleen: Not recommended for PT to palpate enlarged spleen secondary to rupture issues (only palpable if enlarged).
  - Gallbladder (Murphy's): Place fingers to the right of rectus abdominus below rib cage: +/= sudden pain and muscle tensing with deep breath.
  - Kidneys: In supine, place one hand under client between ribs and iliac crest, other hand on abdomen below ribs and pointing in opposite direction: +/− tenderness or reproduction of symptoms
  - Bladder: Not usually palpable unless distended and raised above pubic bone; in supine, place hand above pubis and press down: +/= tenderness, reproduction of pain, ability to feel the bladder: __+ ___−.

INTERVENTION

- PT intervention is consistent with movement-related problems secondary to GI disorder.
- If there is a stoma from a colostomy or ileostomy, PT should avoid activities that may cause retraction.
- Gait training
- Therapeutic exercise: All relevant categories, energy conservation
- Therapeutic activities for bed mobility, transfers, transitional movement
- Neuromuscular re-education
- Self-care management
- Interprofessional
  - Lifestyle modification
  - Smoking cessation
  - Weight management
  - Dietary counseling
  - Psychological intervention
  - Pastoral counseling
  - Surgical management
  - Pharmacologic management[4]
  - Medical management
  - Occupational therapy
  - Speech-language pathology
    - Swallowing deficits
    - Speech impairment

FUNCTIONAL GOALS

- Patient will be able to
  - Achieve functional aerobic capacity, ability to talk during activity so as to achieve functional gait and activity tolerance for ADLs/IADLs

- ○ Achieve 600 m or greater in a 6-minute walk test for initiation of safe, functional gait in the community
- ○ Perform active verbalization with increasing taxonomy for safety during gait, including negotiation of even and uneven surfaces, opening and closing doors, transferring in and out of car
- ○ Perform activities requiring abdominals with appropriate muscle splinting/guarding to prevent retraction of stoma, if patient has colostomy or ileostomy.
- ○ Tolerate 30 minutes of continuous, moderate exercise three times a week in ______weeks, and five times a week in ____________weeks, depending on the severity of the disease.

PROGNOSIS

- Prognosis for GERD is generally good with appropriate medical intervention, medication, dietary modification.
- Physician should establish medical prognosis, as pathology is primarily medical in nature.
- For PT prognosis, goals should be established that the patient can achieve based on their overall condition.
- Prognosis from a PT perspective should be good, unless medical condition is unstable or goals unrealistic.

PATIENT RESOURCES

- GERD. American Gastoenterological Association (AGA). http://www.gastro.org/practice/resource-library/hot-topics/gerd. Accessed August 8, 2014.
- GERD. The Society of Thoracic Surgeons. http://www.sts.org/patient-information/esophageal-surgery/gastroesophageal-reflux-disease. Accessed August 8, 2014.

REFERENCES

1. Mayo Clinic. GERD. http://www.mayoclinic.com/health/gerd/DS00967. Accessed June 20, 2013.
2. Locke GR III. EGJ and GER disease. In Giuli R, Galmiche JP, Jamieson GG, Scarpignato C. *The Esopagogastric Junction*. Oeso; 1998. https://www.hon.ch/OESO/books/Vol_5_Eso_Junction/Articles/art126.html. Accessed June 20, 2013.
3. Mills JC, Stappenbeck TS, Bunnett N. Gastrointestinal disease. In: McPhee SJ, Hammer GD, eds. *Pathophysiology of Disease*. 6th ed. New York, NY: McGraw-Hill; 2010. http://www.accessphysiotherapy.com/abstract/5369632. Accessed June 20, 2013.
4. Panus PC, Jobst EE, Masters SB, Katzung B, Tinsley SL, Trevor AJ. *Pharmacology for the Physical Therapist*. New York, NY: McGraw-Hill; 2009. http://www.accessphysiotherapy.com/resource/615. Accessed June 20, 2013.

ADDITIONAL REFERENCES

- Goodman CC, Fuller KS. *Pathology: Implications for the Physical Therapist*. 3rd ed. Philadelphia, PA: Saunders Elsevier; 2009.
- Goodman CC, Snyder TK. *Differential Diagnosis for Physical Therapists: Screening for Referral*. 4th ed. St. Louis, MO: Saunders Elsevier; 2007.
- McOmber MA, Shulman RJ. Pediatric functional gastrointestinal disorders. *Nutr Clin Pract*. 2008;23(3):268–274.
- McPhee SJ, Hammer GD. Pathophysiology of disorders of the esophagus. In: McPhee SJ, Hammer GD, eds. *Pathophysiology of Disease*. 6th ed. New York, NY: McGraw-Hill; 2010. http://www.accessphysiotherapy.com/content/5369615. Accessed June 20, 2013.
- Suleiman S, Johnston DE. The abdominal wall: an overlooked source of pain. *Am Fam Physician*. 2001;64(3):431–438.
- Ulcerative Colitis. National Digestive Diseases Information Clearinghouse (NDDIC). U.S. Department of Health and Human Services. *NIH Publication No. 12–1597*. October 2011. http://digestive.niddk.nih.gov/ddiseases/pubs/colitis/. Accessed June 20, 2013.
- Wang KK, Sampliner RE. Updated guidelines 2008 for the diagnosis, surveillance and therapy of Barrett's esophagus. *Am J Gastroenterol*. 2008;103(3):788–797.

40 HEPATITIS

Debra F. Stern, DPT, DBA, MSM, PT
Eric Shamus, PhD, DPT, PT, CSCS

CONDITION/DISORDER SYNONYMS

- Hepatitis A
- Hepatitis B
- Hepatitis C

ICD-9-CM CODES

- 573.3 Hepatitis, unspecified
- Associated physical therapy diagnoses
  - 315.4 Developmental coordination disorder
  - 718.45 Contracture of joint, pelvic region and thigh
  - 719.70 Difficulty in walking
  - 728.2 Muscular wasting and disuse atrophy
  - 728.89 Disorders of muscle, ligament, and fascia
  - 729.9 Other disorders of soft tissue
  - 780.7 Malaise and fatigue
  - 781.2 Abnormality of gait
  - 782.3 Edema
  - 786.0 Dyspnea and respiratory abnormalities
  - 786.05 Shortness of breath

ICD-10-CM CODE

- K75.9 Inflammatory liver disease, unspecified

PREFERRED PRACTICE PATTERN

- As of July, 2014, the APTA *Guide to Physical Therapist Practice* does not include practice patterns for organ system pathology; therefore, the associated or secondary musculoskeletal, cardiovascular/pulmonary, or potential neuromuscular patterns would be indicated.

PATIENT PRESENTATION

A 62-year-old male is presented to the physician's office for follow- up of some abnormal blood test results. Blood tests revealed that his liver enzymes were elevated by approximately three times the upper limits of normal. The patient says that to his knowledge he has never had abnormal liver tests before, and he has not been to a doctor in several years. He denies alcohol or drug use and is not taking any medications. He gives no history of jaundice. His past medical history is significant only for hospitalization at the age of 45 for a bleeding stomach ulcer. He required surgery and had transfusion of 4 units of blood. He recovered from this episode without further complication and has had no recurrences. Your completed physical examination 2 weeks ago was normal, and a focused physical examination on the day shows no signs of jaundice, no hepatosplenomegaly, and no physical examination findings suggestive of portal hypertension. You diagnose an infectious etiology for the laboratory findings (elevated liver enzymes).[1]

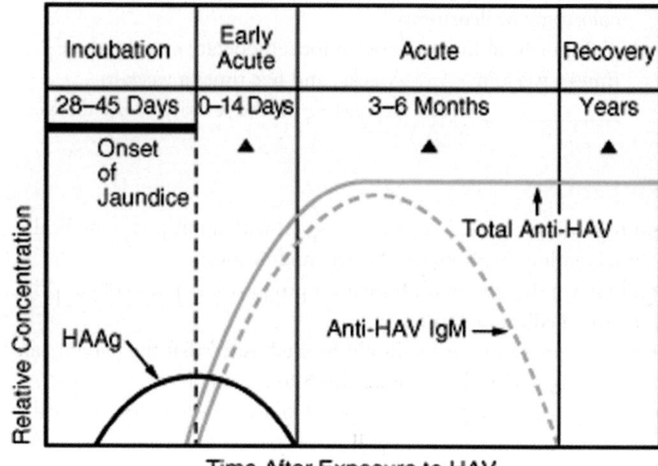

FIGURE 40-1 Hepatitis A diagnostic profile. (Based on data from Abbott Laboratories, Diagnostic Division, North Chicago, IL.)

KEY FEATURES

Description

- Inflammation of the liver
- Complaints include changes in bowel habits: Constipation, diarrhea, bowel urgency, incontinence, cramping
- Pain, frequently referred to low back
- May be viral or secondary to toxic agents
  - Types: A, B, C (D and E are rare forms)
- Hepatitis A[2]
  - RNA enterovirus
  - Spread by contact with fecal matter or blood, often through ingestion of contaminated food
  - Rarely fatal
  - Treated with bed rest for 1 to 4 weeks, no alcohol consumption during that time
- Hepatitis B[2]
  - Spread through blood, semen, vaginal secretions, saliva approximately 4 to 6 weeks after symptoms develop
  - May heal slowly
  - Leading cause of chronic liver disease and cirrhosis
- Hepatitis C[2]
  - Remains in blood for years
  - Accounts for large percentage of cirrhosis, liver failure, liver cancer cases
  - Transmitted through blood transfusion, possibly sexual intercourse
- Hepatitis D and Hepatitis E: Not commonly seen

Essentials of Diagnosis

- Abdominal pain (constant or intermittent)
- Abdominal pain upon ingesting food
- Abdominal tenderness

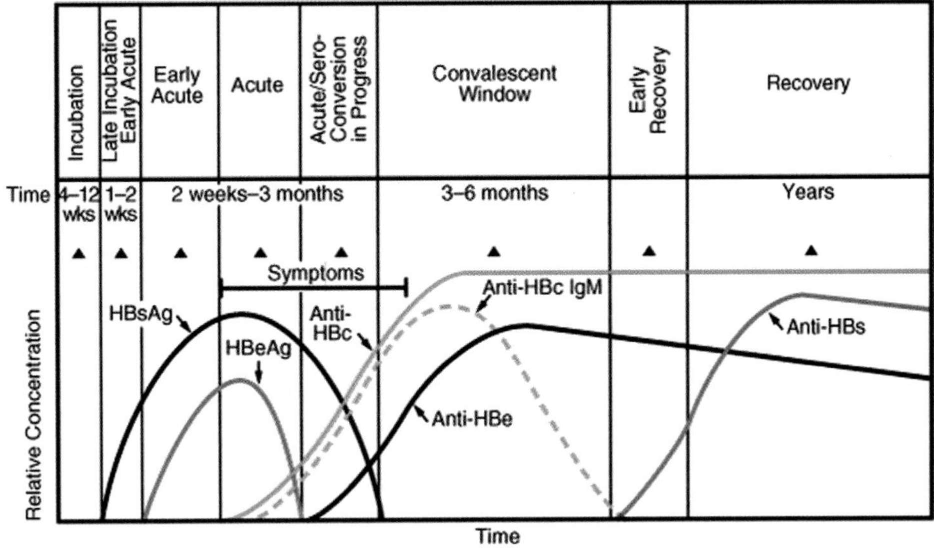

FIGURE 40-2 Hepatitis B diagnostic profile. (Based on data from Abbott Laboratories, Diagnostic Division, North Chicago, IL.)

- Acute drop in blood pressure causing decreased blood flow to intestines
- Bloating
- Change in skin color and eyes (yellow)
- Change in urine color (dark urine)
- Changes in bowel habits: Diarrhea, constipation
- Dark stool or bright red blood in stool
- Inability to swallow
- Joint pain possible
- Lack of appetite
- Malaise, fatigue
- Nausea
- Rectal bleeding possible
- Rectal/anal irritation
- Unexplained weight loss
- Vomiting

General Considerations

- GI disorders may be acute, postoperative, chronic, viral, bacterial, or congenital/hereditary
- Although PT may not manage GI disorders specifically, clients may receive care for secondary problems: Weakness, gait abnormalities, limited aerobic endurance, sarcopenia, musculoskeletal problems, neuromuscular problems, weight loss, or weight gain
- Diagnosis for occult problems may take time and require intensive diagnostic testing
- Symptoms may be characteristic of multiple GI disorders, confounding medical diagnosis
- PT should recognize possible GI pathology in differential diagnosis, especially when findings are inconsistent with conditions commonly treated
- GI disorders frequently refer pain to other body areas; individuals may be inappropriately referred to PT
- GI problems may be related to stress, constipation
- More serious problems include autoimmune conditions, such as Crohn disease
- Acute pain indicative of appendicitis
- GI complaints in females may indicate cancer/tumors in reproductive organs, or gynecological problems: Endometriosis, uterine fibroids, ectopic pregnancies
- May indicate inguinal or umbilical hernia
- History of heartburn/indigestion may indicate GI or cardiac problems
- Chronic diarrhea, episodic diarrhea, loss of bowel control, blood in stool may indicate inflammatory disease, precancerous condition, or cancer
- Possible breast development in males with hepatitis

Demographics

- GI disorders occur throughout the lifespan (birth through geriatric)
- Incidence between 1.2 and 1.6 per 100,000[3]
- Vaccinations have resulted in decreased incidence of hepatitis B and hepatitis A in children
- Hepatitis C incidence stabilized around 2005, increasing only slightly[3]

CLINICAL FINDINGS

SIGNS AND SYMPTOMS

- Darkened urine color
- Skin yellowing, lesions
- Pain
  - Abdominal/stomach pain, cramping (constant or intermittent, severe)
  - Pain upon ingesting food or liquid
    - May be cardiac in nature
  - Pain with defecation
  - Joint pain
- Bowel changes
  - Diarrhea (acute, chronic)
  - Constipation (acute, chronic)
  - Blood in stool
- Abdominal distention
- Unexplained weight loss
- Fever
- Chills
- Abdominal muscle spasm, guarding
- Fatigue
- Loss of appetite, cachexia
- Nausea
- Emesis
- Ascites

- Difficulty swallowing (related to esophageal or oral problems rather than neuromuscular)
- Fever
- Chills
- Complaints of "feeling full" regardless of having ingested food
- Osteoporosis
- Intestinal necrosis

▶ Functional Implications

- Severe symptoms associated with immediacy of defecation may be disabling, cause inability to leave home.
- Chronic constipation may cause severe pain, result in fecal material backing up through the esophagus, requiring manual extraction, surgery, bowel retraining.

Recommended Immunization Schedule for Persons Aged 0 Through 6 Years—United States • 20

For those who fall behind or start late, see the catch-up schedule

Vaccine ▼ Age ►	Birth	1 month	2 months	4 months	6 months	12 months	15 months	18 months	19–23 months	2–3 years	4–6 years
Hepatitis B[1]	HepB	HepB					HepB				
Rotavirus[2]			RV	RV	RV[2]						
Diphtheria, Tetanus, Pertussis[3]			DTaP	DTaP	DTaP	see footnote[3]	DTaP				DTaP
Haemophilus influenzae type b[4]			Hib	Hib	Hib[4]	Hib					
Pneumococcal[5]			PCV	PCV	PCV	PCV				PPSV	
Inactivated Poliovirus[6]			IPV	IPV			IPV				IPV
Influenza[7]							Influenza (Yearly)				
Measles, Mumps, Rubella[8]						MMR		see footnote[8]			MMR
Varicella[9]						Varicella		see footnote[9]			Varicella
Hepatitis A[10]							HepA (2 doses)			HepA Series	
Meningococcal[11]										MCV	

Range of recommended ages for all children except certain high-risk groups

Range of recommended ages for certain high-risk groups

This schedule includes recommendations in effect as of December 15, 2009. Any dose not administered at the recommended age should be administered at a subsequent visit, when indicated and feasible. The use of a combination vaccine generally is preferred over separate injections of its equivalent component vaccines. Considerations should include provider assessment, patient preference, and the potential for adverse events. Providers should consult the relevant Advisory Committee on Immunization Practices statement for detailed recommendat **http://www.cdc.gov/vaccines/pubs/acip-list.htm**. Clinically significant adv events that follow immunization should be reported to the Vaccine Adverse E Reporting System (VAERS) at **http://www.vaers.hhs.gov** or by teleph **800-822-7967**.

1. **Hepatitis B vaccine (HepB).** (Minimum age: birth)
   At birth:
   - Administer monovalent HepB to all newborns before hospital discharge.
   - If mother is hepatitis B surface antigen (HBsAg)-positive, administer HepB and 0.5 mL of hepatitis B immune globulin (HBIG) within 12 hours of birth.
   - If mother's HBsAg status is unknown, administer HepB within 12 hours of birth. Determine mother's HBsAg status as soon as possible and, if HBsAg-positive, administer HBIG (no later than age 1 week).

   After the birth dose:
   - The HepB series should be completed with either monovalent HepB or a combination vaccine containing HepB. The second dose should be administered at age 1 or 2 months. Monovalent HepB vaccine should be used for doses administered before age 6 weeks. The final dose should be administered no earlier than age 24 weeks.
   - Infants born to HBsAg-positive mothers should be tested for HBsAg and antibody to HBsAg 1 to 2 months after completion of at least 3 doses of the HepB series, at age 9 through 18 months (generally at the next well-child visit).
   - Administration of 4 doses of HepB to infants is permissible when a combination vaccine containing HepB is administered after the birth dose. The fourth dose should be administered no earlier than age 24 weeks.
2. **Rotavirus vaccine (RV).** (Minimum age: 6 weeks)
   - Administer the first dose at age 6 through 14 weeks (maximum age: 14 weeks 6 days). Vaccination should not be initiated for infants aged 15 weeks 0 days or older.
   - The maximum age for the final dose in the series is 8 months 0 days
   - If Rotarix is administered at ages 2 and 4 months, a dose at 6 months is not indicated.
3. **Diphtheria and tetanus toxoids and acellular pertussis vaccine (DTaP).** (Minimum age: 6 weeks)
   - The fourth dose may be administered as early as age 12 months, provided at least 6 months have elapsed since the third dose.
   - Administer the final dose in the series at age 4 through 6 years.
4. ***Haemophilus influenzae* type b conjugate vaccine (Hib).** (Minimum age: 6 weeks)
   - If PRP-OMP (PedvaxHIB or Comvax [HepB-Hib]) is administered at ages 2 and 4 months, a dose at age 6 months is not indicated.
   - TriHiBit (DTaP/Hib) and Hiberix (PRP-T) should not be used for doses at ages 2, 4, or 6 months for the primary series but can be used as the final dose in children aged 12 months through 4 years.
5. **Pneumococcal vaccine.** (Minimum age: 6 weeks for pneumococcal conjugate vaccine [PCV]; 2 years for pneumococcal polysaccharide vaccine [PPSV])
   - PCV is recommended for all children aged younger than 5 years. Administer 1 dose of PCV to all healthy children aged 24 through 59 months who are not completely vaccinated for their age.
   - Administer PPSV 2 or more months after last dose of PCV to children aged 2 years or older with certain underlying medical conditions, including a cochlear implant. See *MMWR* 1997;46(No. RR-8).
6. **Inactivated poliovirus vaccine (IPV)** (Minimum age: 6 weeks)
   - The final dose in the series should be administered on or after the fo birthday and at least 6 months following the previous dose.
   - If 4 doses are administered prior to age 4 years a fifth dose should be ad istered at age 4 through 6 years. See *MMWR* 2009;58(30):829–30.
7. **Influenza vaccine (seasonal).** (Minimum age: 6 months for trivalent inac vated influenza vaccine [TIV]; 2 years for live, attenuated influenza vaccin [LAIV])
   - Administer annually to children aged 6 months through 18 years.
   - For healthy children aged 2 through 6 years (i.e., those who do not have un lying medical conditions that predispose them to influenza complicatio either LAIV or TIV may be used, except LAIV should not be given to chil aged 2 through 4 years who have had wheezing in the past 12 months.
   - Children receiving TIV should receive 0.25 mL if aged 6 through 35 mo or 0.5 mL if aged 3 years or older.
   - Administer 2 doses (separated by at least 4 weeks) to children aged you than 9 years who are receiving influenza vaccine for the first time or who vaccinated for the first time during the previous influenza season but received 1 dose.
   - For recommendations for use of influenza A (H1N1) 2009 monovalent vac see *MMWR* 2009;58(No. RR-10).
8. **Measles, mumps, and rubella vaccine (MMR).** (Minimum age: 12 mont
   - Administer the second dose routinely at age 4 through 6 years. However second dose may be administered before age 4, provided at least 28 have elapsed since the first dose.
9. **Varicella vaccine.** (Minimum age: 12 months)
   - Administer the second dose routinely at age 4 through 6 years. However second dose may be administered before age 4, provided at least 3 mo have elapsed since the first dose.
   - For children aged 12 months through 12 years the minimum interval betw doses is 3 months. However, if the second dose was administered at 28 days after the first dose, it can be accepted as valid.
10. **Hepatitis A vaccine (HepA).** (Minimum age: 12 months)
    - Administer to all children aged 1 year (i.e., aged 12 through 23 mon Administer 2 doses at least 6 months apart.
    - Children not fully vaccinated by age 2 years can be vaccinated at subseq visits
    - HepA also is recommended for older children who live in areas where cination programs target older children, who are at increased risk for infec or for whom immunity against hepatitis A is desired.
11. **Meningococcal vaccine.** (Minimum age: 2 years for meningococcal conju vaccine [MCV4] and for meningococcal polysaccharide vaccine [MPSV4])
    - Administer MCV4 to children aged 2 through 10 years with persistent com ment component deficiency, anatomic or functional asplenia, and certain o conditions placing tham at high risk.
    - Administer MCV4 to children previously vaccinated with MCV4 or MP after 3 years if first dose administered at age 2 through 6 years. See *MM* 2009;58:1042–3.

The Recommended Immunization Schedules for Persons Aged 0 through 18 Years are approved by the Advisory Committee on Immunization Practices

FIGURE 40-3 Recommended childhood immunization schedule, 2010, United States. (See the Age 7–18 and Catch-UP schedules at http://www.cdc.gov/vaccines/recs/schedules/default.htm.)

- Dehydration secondary to diarrhea, emesis, appetite loss, nausea, inability to swallow
- Eating disorder/anorexia secondary to fear of pain upon ingesting food
- Anemia
- Sarcopenia resulting in weakness, decreased muscle mass, inability to ambulate or perform self-care, limited aerobic capacity secondary to inactivity
- Decreased exercise tolerance, limited physical activity; ADLs, IADLs
- Fatigue
- Psychological challenges: Anxiety, depression, reluctance to leave home
- Dietary restrictions
- Infection
- Arthritis
- Inflammation of eye, liver disease

Possible Contributing Causes

- Contact with fecal matter
- Infection: Bacterial or viral
  - Food poisoning
  - Parasites
- Medication side effects, toxicity
- Endocrine dysfunction
- Intravenous drug use; contaminated needles
- Inappropriate self-medication
- Ischemic
  - Atherosclerosis, impaired blood supply to any structure
- Stress, anxiety
- Obstruction in colon decreasing blood supply, causing inflammation
- Autoimmune disease
- Chemical
- Environmental irritants
- Obesity
- Lack of exercise
- Heredity
- Food allergy or intolerance (gluten/wheat, dairy)
- Diet
- Cancer: Esophageal, colon, liver, bile duct, pancreatic, metastatic, anal/rectal
- Systemic rheumatologic disorders (scleroderma, rheumatoid arthritis)
- Systemic immunological condition

Differential Diagnosis

- Organ dysfunction from cancer or malignancy
  - Colon cancer
  - Ovarian cancer
- Non-malignant tumor in abdomen or organs
- Endocrine disorder
- Gynecologic problem in females
- Autoimmune disease affecting upper and lower GI tracts
- Appendicitis
- Irritable bowel syndrome
- Crohn disease
- Colitis (ulcerative, non-ulcerative)
- Inflammatory bowel disease
- Pelvic inflammatory disease
- Celiac disease, gluten intolerance
- Gastroenteritis

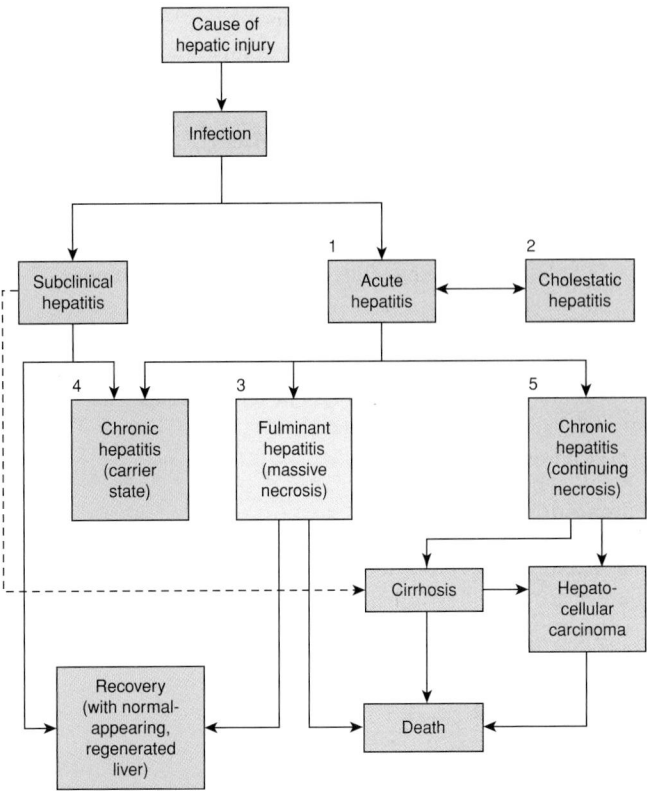

FIGURE 40-4 Clinical syndromes associated with hepatitis: acute hepatitis (1), which is sometimes associated with intrahepatic cholestasis (2). Fulminant hepatitis (3) is associated with massive necrosis and has a high mortality rate. Chronic viral hepatitis may lead to a carrier state without (4) or with (5) continuing hepatocyte necrosis. Chronic hepatitis associated with continuing necrosis often progresses to cirrhosis, whereas that associated simply with a carrier state does not. (Redrawn with permission from Chandrasoma P, Taylor CE. *Concise Pathology*. 3rd ed. Originally published by Appleton & Lange. Copyright © 1998 by The McGraw-Hill Companies, Inc.)

- Perforated ulcer in GI system
- Bladder or urinary tract infection, kidney pathology
- Abdominal infection
- Bowel disorder
  - Constipation, diarrhea
  - Inflammation of abdominal lining or organ obstruction

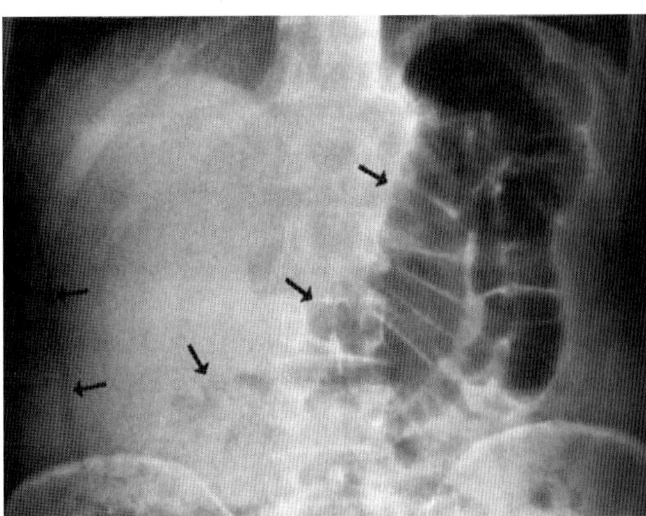

FIGURE 40-5 A 57-year-old man presents with history of hepatitis. (From Chen MYM, Pope TL, Ott DJ: Basic Radiology, 2nd edition. www.accessmedicine.com. Copyright © The McGraw-Hill Companies, Inc. All rights reserved.)

- Referred pain from heart, spine, hip
- Post–weight-loss (bariatric) surgery complications
  - Side effects may result in liver problems

MEANS OF CONFIRMATION OR DIAGNOSIS

Laboratory Tests

- Fecal occult blood test/stool sample
- Blood tests[2]
- H & H for signs of bleeding, anemia, pathogens, immune status, vitamin deficiencies, white blood cell count
- Liver function test, liver enzymes
- Bilirubin
- Alkaline phosphatase (ALP) for bile-duct blockage
- Serum albumin for low protein levels
- Prothrombin time

Imaging

- Abdominal scans
- Radiography
- CT
- MRI

Diagnostic Procedures

- Liver biopsy
- Paracentesis
- Manual palpation for tenderness in liver

FINDINGS AND INTERPRETATION

- Blood tests[2]
  - Identification of IgM anti-HAV antibodies for hepatitis A
  - Surface antigen (HBsAg) for hepatitis B
  - Antibody to hepatitis B core antigen (anti-HBc)
  - Antibody to HBsAg (anti-HBs)
  - Hepatitis E surface antigen (HBeAg) indicates someone with chronic infection and is more contagious
  - Hepatitis C RNA assays

TREATMENT

Medication

- Hepatitis B: Blocks replication of virus
  - Peginterferon alfa-2a (Pegasys)
  - Interferon alfa-2b (Intron A)
  - Lamivudine (Epivir-HBV)
  - Entecavir (Baraclude)
  - Telbivudine (Tyzeka)
  - Adefovir (Hepsera)
  - Tenofovir (Viread)
- Hepatitis C
  - Pegylated interferon
  - Ribavirin (Copegus)

MEDICAL PROCEDURES

- No treatment for hepatitis B
  - Preventative vaccine
- Liver transplant
- Nasogastric tube
- Feeding tube
- Total/peripheral parenteral nutrition (TPN/PPN)
- IV for hydration

REFERRALS/ADMITTANCE

- If causative problem is not considered appropriate for PT intervention, refer to appropriate physician
- Refer to ER if emergency identified

IMPAIRMENTS

- Muscle weakness, atrophy
- Gait abnormality, difficulty walking
- Contractures of soft tissue (fascia, muscle), joint limitations
- Shortness of breath
- Possible impairment of rectal muscle
- Inability to perform self-care
- Limited aerobic endurance
- Functional decline

TESTS AND MEASURES

- Observation
  - Scars may indicate adhesions or abdominal surgeries causative of diverticula.
  - Pink or purplish striae may be indicative of Cushing syndrome.
  - Dilated veins may indicate hepatic pathology or inferior vena cava obstruction, not diverticulitis.
  - Contour: Roundness, concavity, asymmetry, distension, pregnancy signs.
  - Cullen sign: Bluish discoloring around the umbilicus may be a sign of retroperitoneal bleeding.
  - Bluish discoloration in lower abdomen: Grey Turner sign, signals hemorrhagic pancreatitis.
  - Bulging in groin/abdomen especially apparent with contraction of musculature in area may be hernia.
  - Pulsing in navel area may be abdominal aortic aneurysm.
  - Left lower quadrant pain, often following a meal.
  - Palpable abdominal tenderness: On left side or generalized.
  - Psoas sign: Provides resistance over patient's right knee as they flex the hip; pain indicates appendicitis, possible inflammation of abdomen.
  - Obturator sign: Internal rotation and flexion of right lower extremity may indicate appendicitis, pelvic inflammation.
  - Rovsing sign: Pain on the right side of abdomen when pressure applied to the left may indicate appendicitis.
- Palpation
  - Appendix (McBurney's): Apply vertical pressure halfway between right ASIS and umbilicus: −/+ may indicate appendicitis.
  - Liver: In supine, with left hand under trunk parallel to 11th and 12th ribs, lift upward; right hand lateral to rectus, press in and up: +/= reproduction of symptoms with deep breath, indicates liver involvement.
  - Ascites: Percuss outward from center with fingers; if sound is dull, ascites may be present.
  - Spleen: Not recommended for PT to palpate enlarged spleen secondary to rupture issues (only palpable if enlarged).
  - Gallbladder (Murphy's): Place fingers to the right of rectus abdominus below rib cage: +/= sudden pain and muscle tensing with deep breath.
  - Kidneys: In supine, place one hand under client between ribs and iliac crest, other hand on abdomen below ribs and pointing in opposite direction: +/− tenderness or reproduction of symptoms.

- Bladder: Not usually palpable unless distended and raised above pubic bone; in supine, place hand above pubis and press down: +/= tenderness, reproduction of pain, ability to feel the bladder: __+ ___–.

INTERVENTION

- PT intervention is consistent with movement-related problems secondary to GI disorder
- Gait training
- Therapeutic exercise: All relevant categories, energy conservation
- Therapeutic activities for bed mobility, transfers, transitional movement
- Neuromuscular re-education
- Self-care training
- Manual therapy
- Massage
- Interprofessional
  - Lifestyle modification
  - Smoking cessation
  - Weight management
  - Dietary counseling
  - Psychological intervention
  - Spiritual counseling
  - Surgical management

FUNCTIONAL GOALS

- Patient will be able to
  - Achieve functional aerobic capacity, ability to talk during activity so as to achieve functional gait and activity tolerance for ADLs/IADLs.
  - Achieve 600 m or greater in a 6-minute walk test for initiation of safe, functional gait in the community.
  - Perform active verbalization with increasing taxonomy for safety during gait, including negotiation of even and uneven surfaces, opening and closing doors, transferring in and out of car.
  - Perform activities requiring abdominals with appropriate muscle splinting/guarding to prevent retraction of stoma, if patient has colostomy or ileostomy.
  - Tolerate 30 minutes of continuous, moderate exercise three times a week in ______ weeks, and five times a week in ___________ weeks, depending on the severity of the disease.

PROGNOSIS

- Physician establishes the medical prognosis, as pathology is primarily medical in nature.
- Hepatitis A
  - Least serious
  - Usually resolved within 6 months
  - Rarely causes liver failure
  - Results in immunity
- Hepatitis B
  - No cure
  - Preventative vaccine
  - Acute or chronic; most patients recover
  - Increased risk for cancer, cirrhosis
  - Liver disease is a primary cause of death
- Hepatitis C
  - Chronic in most cases
  - High risk for liver cancer, cirrhosis
  - Causes other conditions
    - Porphyria
    - Inflammatory kidney disease
    - Lymphoma
    - Cryoglobulinemia: Protein-clumping disorder
- For PT prognosis, goals should be established that the patient can achieve based on their overall condition.
- Prognosis from a PT perspective should be good, unless medical condition is unstable or goals unrealistic.

PATIENT RESOURCES

- Hepatitis A. American Liver Foundation. http://www.liverfoundation.org/abouttheliver/info/hepatitisa/. Accessed August 8, 2014.
- Hepatitis B Foundation. www.hepb.org. Accessed July 4, 2013.
- Hepatitis Foundation International. www.hepfi.org. Accessed July 4, 2013.

REFERENCES

1. Toy EC. Hepatitis, Case 86. LANGE Case Files. http://www.accessmedicine.com/casecontent.aspx?aid=510023995&tabid=1. Accessed July 4, 2013.
2. Sokol RJ, Narkewicz MR. Liver disorders. In: Hay WW, Levin MJ, Sondheimer JM, Deterding RR, eds. *CURRENT Diagnosis & Treatment: Pediatrics*. 20th ed. New York, NY: McGraw-Hill; 2011. http://www.accessphysiotherapy.com/content/6584227. Accessed July 4, 2013.
3. Centers for Disease Control and Prevention. Hepatitis C Information for Health Professionals: Statistics and Surveillance. http://www.cdc.gov/hepatitis/HCV/StatisticsHCV.htm. Accessed July 4, 2013.

ADDITIONAL REFERENCES

- Belongia EA, Costa J, Gareen IF, et al. National Institutes of Health Consensus Development Conference Statement: management of hepatitis B. *Ann Intern Med.* 2009;150:104–110. http://consensus.nih.gov/2008/hepbstatement.pdf. Accessed July 4, 2013.
- Lok ASF, McMahon BJ. Chronic hepatitis B. *Hepatology.* 2007;45(2):507–539.
- National Institute of Diabetes and Digestive and Kidney Diseases. www2.niddk.nih.gov. Accessed July 4, 2013.
- Scott JD, Gretch DR. Molecular diagnostics of hepatitis C virus infection: a systematic review. *JAMA*. 2007;297(7):724–732.

41 INFLAMMATORY BOWEL DISEASE

Debra F. Stern, DPT, DBA, MSM, PT
Eric Shamus, PhD, DPT, PT, CSCS
David W. Mandel, PhD, PT

CONDITION/DISORDER SYNONYMS

- Crohn disease
- Ulcerative colitis (UC)
- Regional enteritis

ICD-9-CM CODES

- 555 Regional enteritis
- 555.0 Regional enteritis of small intestine
- 555.1 Regional enteritis of large intestine
- 555.2 Regional enteritis of small intestine with large intestine
- 555.9 Regional enteritis of unspecified site
- Associated physical therapy diagnoses
  - 315.4 Developmental coordination disorder
  - 718.45 Contracture of joint, pelvic region and thigh
  - 719.70 Difficulty in walking involving joint site unspecified
  - 728.2 Muscular wasting and disuse atrophy, not elsewhere classified
  - 728.89 Other disorders of muscle, ligament, and fascia
  - 729.9 Other and unspecified disorders of soft tissue
  - 780.7 Malaise and fatigue
  - 782.3 Edema
  - 786.0 Dyspnea and respiratory abnormalities

ICD-10-CM CODES

- K50.00 Crohn disease of small intestine without complications
- K50.10 Crohn disease of large intestine without complications
- K50.80 Crohn disease of both small and large intestine without complications
- K50.90 Crohn disease, unspecified, without complications

PREFERRED PRACTICE PATTERN

- As of July, 2014, the APTA Guide to Physical Therapist Practice does not include practice patterns for organ system pathology; therefore, the associated or secondary musculoskeletal, cardiovascular/pulmonary, or potential neuromuscular patterns would be indicated.

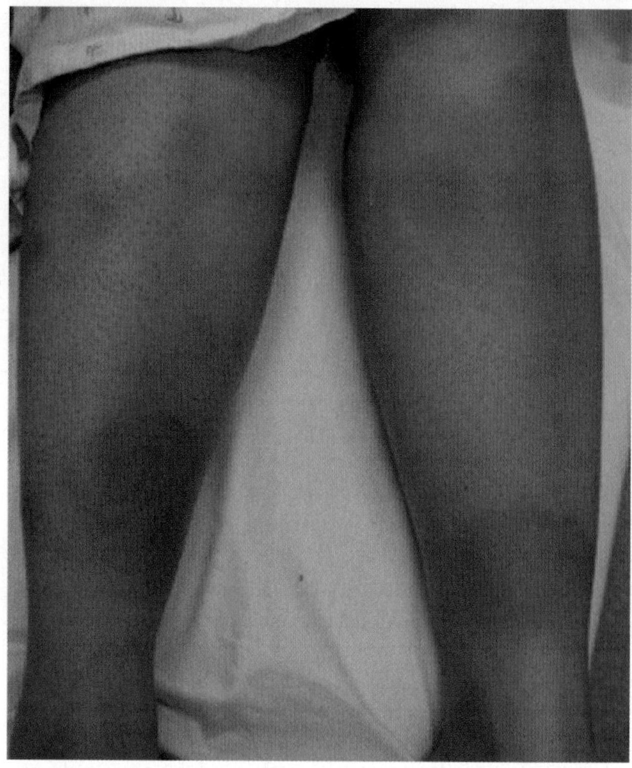

FIGURE 41-1 Erythema nodosum: typical erythematous, tender nodules involving the pretibial region. (From McKean SC, Ross JJ, Dressler DD, Brotman DJ, Ginsberg JS. *Principles and Practice of Hospital Medicine*. www.accessmedicine.com. Copyright © The McGraw-Hill Companies, Inc. All rights reserved.)

PATIENT PRESENTATION

The patient is a 19-year-old female who presents to the clinic with antalgic gait and deconditioning. She presents as very thin and petite. She reports all her family is much taller but her growth has been limited by the inflammatory bowel disease (IBD). The patient states she has moderate pain in her low back, hips, and knees during walking. She reports abdominal cramping pain and it is exacerbated by her diet that is limited to nonfibrous foods. In addition, she frequently has upper respiratory colds due to the immune suppressant medication she takes for her IBD.

Upon physical therapy examination, the patient's mobility status is modified independent because of pain during gait. Strength testing is 4/5 for bilateral upper extremities and lower extremities. Palpation of the thoracolumbar musculature does not reproduce pain. Active and passive movements of trunk rotation, side bending, and forward flexion mildly increase her low back pain and result in increased abdominal discomfort. She has full range of motion in her hips and knees but they are also mildly painful throughout the entire range. The patient is observed to have a healed vertical incision just below her umbilicus resulting from a previous abdominal surgery. Patient reports she required a small bowel resection 5 years ago resulting from her IBD. Special tests such as palpation of McBurney point and the Pinch-an-inch test are positive for increased abdominal tenderness and you feel some firmness proximal to the incision which is indicative of adhesions. Performance on the functional strength and endurance tests (30-second chair stand and the 6-minute walk) result in below-average scores for her age.

KEY FEATURES

Description

- Chronic inflammation of the gastrointestinal (GI) track.
- Crohn can affect any part of the GI tract, all or part of the GI system from the mouth to the anus.
- Ulcerative colitis affects somewhere from the colon to the rectum.
- Complaints often include changes in bowel habits such as constipation, diarrhea, bowel urgency, incontinence, and cramping
- Pain is frequently referred to the lower back.

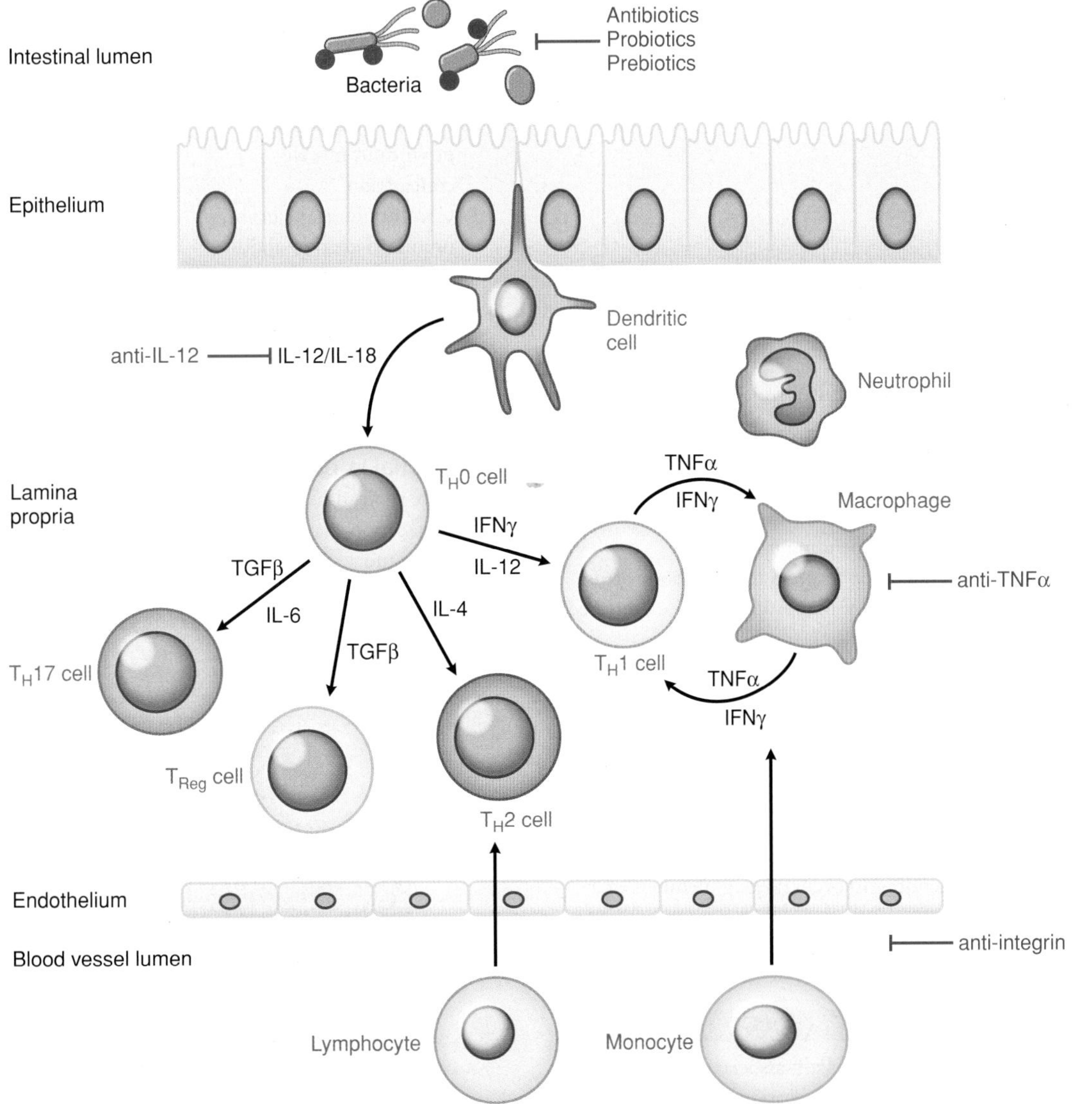

FIGURE 41-2 Proposed pathogenesis of inflammatory bowel disease and target sites for pharmacological intervention. Shown are the interactions among bacterial antigens in the intestinal lumen and immune cells in the intestinal wall. If the epithelial barrier is impaired, bacterial antigens can gain access to antigen-presenting cells (APC) such as dendritic cells in the lamina propria. These cells then present the antigen(s) to $CD4^+$ lymphocytes and also secrete cytokines such interleukin (IL)-12 and IL-18, thereby inducing the differentiation of T_H1 cells in Crohn disease (or, under the control of IL-4, type 2 helper T cells [T_H2] in ulcerative colitis). The balance of pro-inflammatory and anti-inflammatory events is also governed by regulatory T_H17 and T_{Reg} cells, both of which serve to limit immune and inflammatory responses in the GI tract. Transforming growth factor (TGF)β and IL-6 are important cytokines that drive the expansion of the regulatory T cell subsets. The T_H1 cells produce a characteristic array of cytokines, including interferon (IFN)γ and TNFα, which in turn activate macrophages. Macrophages positively regulate T_H1 cells by secreting additional cytokines, including IFNγ and TNFα. Recruitment of a variety of leukocytes is mediated by activation of resident immune cells including neutrophils. Cell adhesion molecules such as integrins are important in the infiltration of leukocytes and novel biological therapeutic strategies aimed at blocking leukocyte recruitment are effective at reducing inflammation. General immunosuppressants (e.g., glucocorticoids, thioguanine derivatives, methotrexate, and cyclosporine) affect multiple sites of inflammation. More site-specific intervention involves intestinal bacteria (antibiotics, prebiotics, and probiotics) and therapy directed at TNFα or IL-12. (From Brunton LL, Chabner BA, Knollmann RC. *Goodman & Gilman's The Pharmacological Basis of Therapeutics*. 12th ed. www.accessmedicine.com.)

- IBD describes disorders with chronic or recurring immune response and inflammation of the GI tract.
- A common IBD.
- There is a broad array of GI disorders that may be encountered by physical therapists.
- Many clients with GI pathology may be receiving physical therapy as a result of secondary problems such as weakness, gait abnormalities, and limited aerobic endurance.

Essentials of Diagnosis[1]

- Normal healthy bowel between patches of diseased bowel
- Abdominal pain: Constant or intermittent
- Abdominal tenderness
- Nausea
- Vomiting
- Diarrhea or constipation
- Changes in bowel habits
- Bloating
- Possible rectal bleeding
- Rectal/anal irritation
- Acute drops in blood pressure, which may result in decreased blood flow to intestines

General Considerations

- Crohn disease commonly involves the terminal ileum[2]
- May result in secondary problems such as aerobic capacity and muscle-endurance impairment, sarcopenia, weakness/impaired muscle performance, musculoskeletal problems, neuromuscular problems, weight loss, or weight gain, indicating the need for physical therapy intervention depending on severity
- Because GI disorders frequently refer pain to other body areas, individuals may get referred to PT inappropriately (i.e., referred for low back pain)
- Chronic diarrhea, episodic diarrhea, loss of bowel control (incontinence or urgency), and blood in stool may be symptomatic of inflammatory disease, precancerous conditions, or cancer

Demographics

- Higher incidence in Jews of European descent
- Women may have slightly higher incidence than males
- Familial: Occurring or tending to occur among members of a family, usually by heredity

CLINICAL FINDINGS

SIGNS AND SYMPTOMS

- Diarrhea: Acute, chronic
- Abdominal or stomach pain or cramping: Constant or intermittent and severe
- Abdominal (stomach or intestinal) pain after ingesting food or liquid
  - May be cardiac in nature
- Lower abdominal pain
- Blood in stool, dark or bright (fresh bleeding): Rectal bleeding
- Pain associated with defecation
- Pain after ingesting fatty foods
- Changes in bowel habits
- Bloated or swollen abdomen: Abdominal distention
- Unexplained weight loss
- Fever
- Chills
- Abdominal muscle spasm, guarding
- Feeling of having to move bowels constantly
- Anemia
- Weight loss
- Infection
- Loss of appetite, cachexia
- Skin lesions
- Eye problems
- Liver impairment
- Failure to grow if onset at early age
- Flatulence
- Gastroesophageal reflux (GERD), heartburn
- Pain secondary to hernias
  - Palpable bulging with or without muscle contraction
  - Commonly in the groin, umbilical area, or abdomen (especially after pregnancy or any surgery in the abdominal region)
  - Sports hernias
- Nausea
- Emesis
- Ascites
- Mucous in the stool or just mucous discharge
- Change in bowel odor or color
- Acute, severe pain regionally located in right lower quadrant
  - Appendicitis or ectopic pregnancy
- Intestinal necrosis
- Dietary restrictions in consistency and/or foods (i.e., dairy, spices, wheat/gluten as in celiac disease)
- Anxiety and depression
- Arthritis
- Osteoporosis
- Lack of appetite
- Unexplained weight loss
- Possible joint pain
- Malaise/fatigue

Functional Implications

- Severe symptoms such as diarrhea associated with immediacy of defecation may be disabling and result in the inability to leave home
- Dehydration with severe diarrhea, emesis, loss of appetite, inability to drink or eat secondary to nausea or inability to swallow

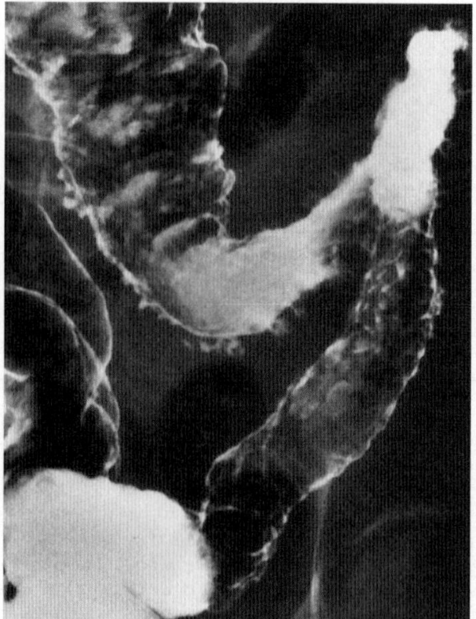

FIGURE 41-3 Segmental Crohn disease of the transverse and descending portions of the colon, showing multiple deep ulcers projecting from the margins of the affected colon and small "aphthoid" ulcers appearing like erosions seen in the upper gastrointestinal tract. (From Chen MYM, Pope TL, Ott DJ. *Basic Radiology*. 2nd ed. www.accessmedicine.com. Copyright © The McGraw-Hill Companies, Inc. All rights reserved.)

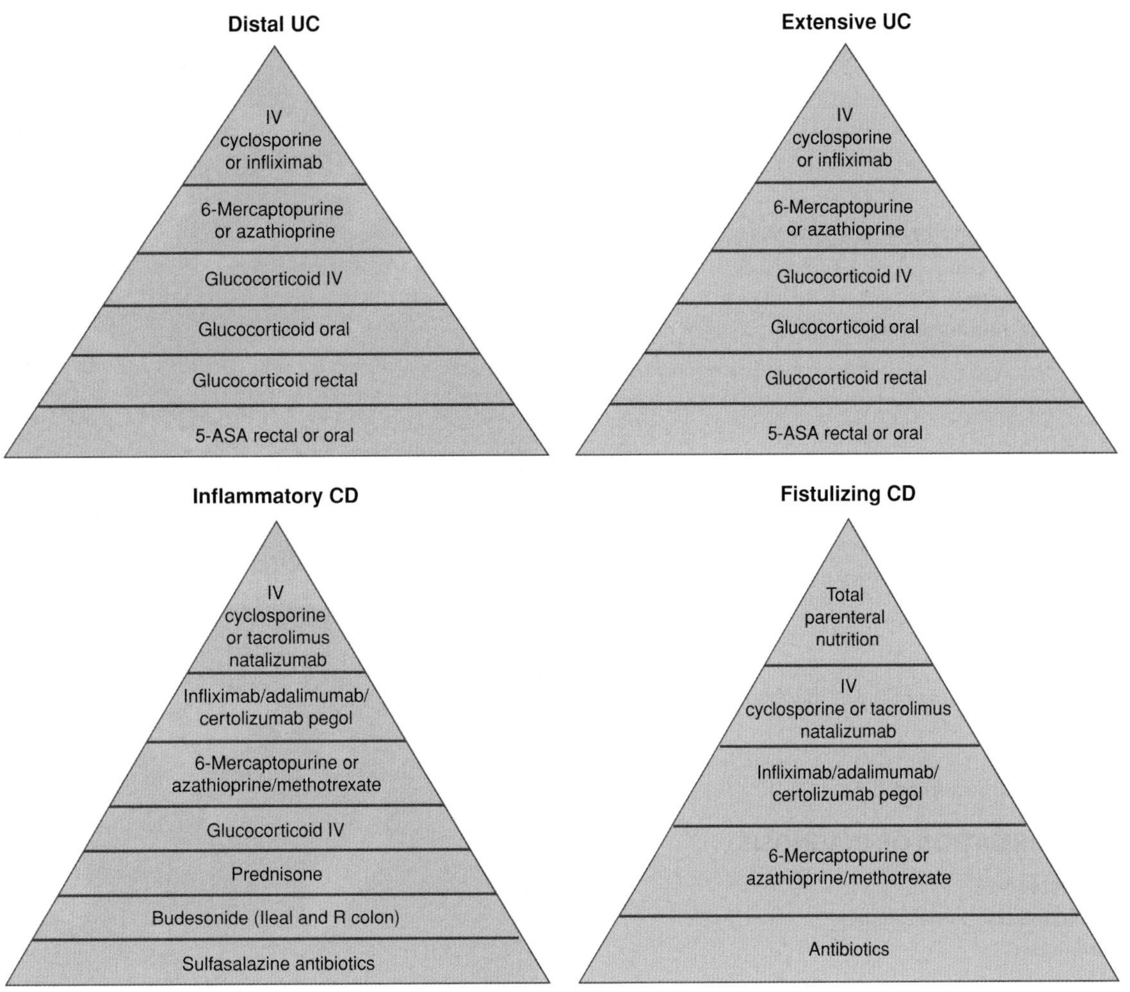

FIGURE 41-4 Medical management of IBD. 5-ASA, 5-aminosalicylic acid; CD, Crohn disease; UC, ulcerative colitis. (From Longo DL, Fauci AS, Kasper DL, Hauser SL, Jameson JL, Loscalzo J, eds. *Harrison's Principles of Internal Medicine*. 18th ed. New York, NY: McGraw-Hill; 2012.)

- Eating disorders secondary to fear of pain associated with ingesting food
- Anemia
- Sarcopenia resulting in weakness, muscle-mass loss, inability to ambulate or perform self-care
- Aerobic capacity limitation secondary to inactivity
- Need for colostomies or ileostomies: Temporary or permanent (usually with intestinal problems vs. upper GI)
  - Presence of same may present a problem with stoma retraction associated with abdominal contraction
- Decreased exercise tolerance
- Changes in lifestyle limiting physical activity
- Fatigue
- Limitations in ADLs and/or IADLs
- Dietary restrictions affecting lifestyle

Possible Contributing Causes[3]

- Infection: Bacterial or viral including food poisoning
  - Food poisoning
  - Parasites
- Atherosclerosis, impaired blood supply to any structure(s)
- Stress and anxiety
- Obstruction in the colon decreasing blood supply and causing inflammation
- Autoimmune disease
- May occur after enemas
- Environmental irritants
- Obesity
- Lack of exercise
- Heredity
- Allergy (i.e., gluten/wheat, dairy)
- Food intolerance (i.e., lactose, purines)
- Diet
- Cancer: Esophagus, colon, liver, bile duct, pancreatic, metastatic, anal/rectal
- Systemic rheumatologic disorders such as scleroderma, rheumatoid arthritis (RA)
- Genetic predisposition
- Systemic immunological condition
- Effects of medications: Diarrhea, GI upset, constipation, GI bleeding, rectal bleeding, blood in stool
- Postsurgical scarring/adhesions
- Medical error (i.e., postsurgical instrumentation left in abdomen, inadequately sutured tissue, nicked or cut vessels or tissues unidentified at the time of surgery before closure, pharmacological errors
- Endocrine dysfunction

Differential Diagnosis[4–6]

- Organ dysfunction as a result of cancer or malignancy
- Non-malignant tumors in the abdomen or organs

- Endocrine disorders
- Gynecologic problems in females such as
  - Endometriosis
  - Menses
  - Ectopic pregnancies
  - Ovarian cysts
  - Fibroids
- Autoimmune diseases that affect the upper and lower GI tracts
- Appendicitis
- Irritable bowel syndrome
- Colitis: Ulcerative, non-ulcerative
- Colon cancer
- Ovarian cancer
- IBD
- Pelvic inflammatory disease
- Celiac disease
- Gastroenteritis
- Perforated ulcers anywhere in GI system
- Bladder infections, urinary tract infections, kidney pathology
- Infections in the abdomen
- Bowel disorders including
  - Constipation or diarrhea
  - Inflammation of the lining of the of the abdomen or organs
  - Obstructions
  - Torsions
- Referred pain from heart, spine, hip

MEANS OF CONFIRMATION OR DIAGNOSIS

Laboratory Tests

- Fecal occult blood tests/stool samples
- Blood tests/lab tests
  - H & H

Imaging

- Abdominal scans
- Radiography
- Barium enemas
- CT scans

Diagnostic Procedures

- Colonoscopy
  - Virtual
  - Procedural
- Sigmoidoscopy
- Manual palpation for tenderness

FINDINGS AND INTERPRETATION

- H & H for signs of bleeding, anemia, pathogens, immune status, vitamin deficiencies; check white blood cell count for infection

TREATMENT

Medication

- Aminosalicylates
- Corticosteroids
- Immunomodulators
- Antacids

MEDICAL PROCEDURES

- Bowel resection
- Bowel resection with colostomy or ileostomy

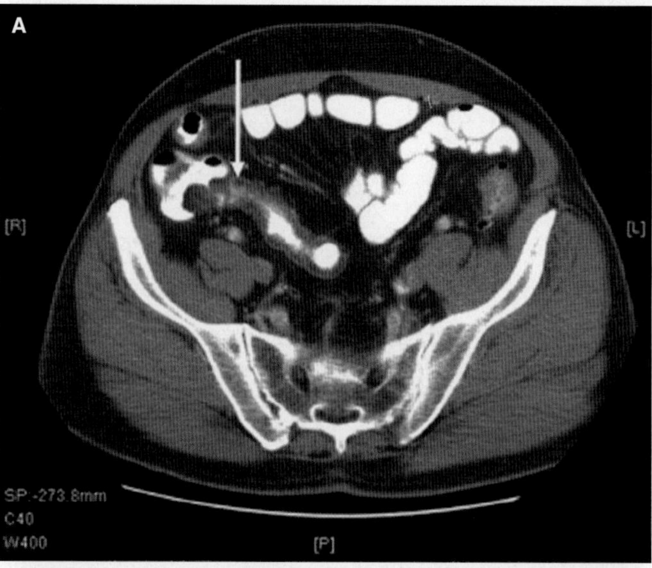

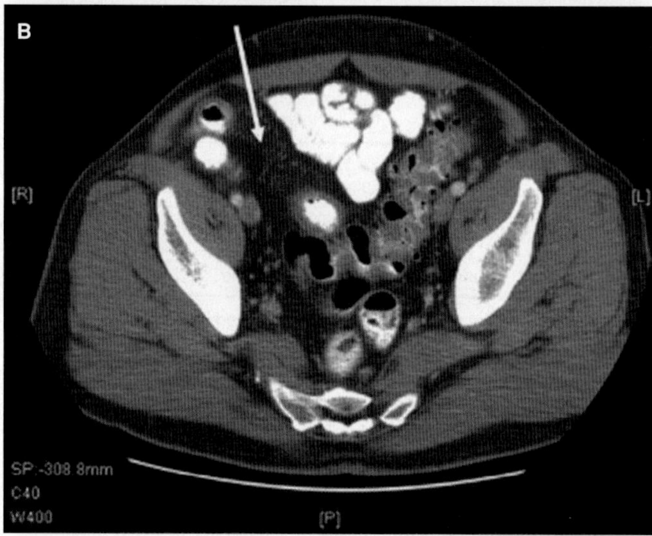

FIGURE 41-5 Characteristic CT manifestations of CD involving the terminal ileum. **A.** Inflamed terminal ileum and ileocecal valve resulting in irregular contrast enhancement and bowel wall thickening (*arrow*). **B.** Encasement of terminal ileum by fat tissue, termed "creeping fat." (From McKean SC, Ross JJ, Dressler DD, Brotman DJ, Ginsberg JS. *Principles and Practice of Hospital Medicine*. www.accessmedicine.com. Copyright © The McGraw-Hill Companies, Inc. All rights reserved.)

- Removal of tumors/growths
- Release of adhesions
- Stomach resections
- Ulcer repairs
- NG tubes
- PEG tubes/feeding
- TPN/PPN
- IV for hydration

REFERRALS/ADMITTANCE

- If a patient is referred for PT and the causative problem is not considered appropriate, referral to appropriate physician must be made.
- If an emergency is identified, referral to an ER may be necessary.

IMPAIRMENTS

- Muscle weakness
- Muscle atrophy
- Gait abnormality/difficulty walking
- Contractures of soft tissue: Fascia, muscle; joint limitations
- Shortness of breath
- Possible rectal muscle impairment
- Inability to perform self-care
- Limited aerobic endurance
- Functional decline: Decrease in functional abilities

TESTS AND MEASURES[7,8]

- Rome II criteria
- Bristol Stool Form Scale
- Observation
  - Scars may indicate adhesions or abdominal surgeries that may be causative of diverticula.
  - Striae, pink or purplish, may be indicative of Cushing syndrome.
  - Dilated veins may indicate hepatic pathology or inferior vena cava obstruction, not diverticulitis.
  - Contour: Roundedness, concavity/hollowness, asymmetry, distension, pregnancy signs.
  - Cullen sign: Bluish discoloring around the umbilicus may be a sign of retroperitoneal bleeding.
  - Bluish discoloration in lower abdomen: Grey Turner sign, which is a sign of hemorrhagic pancreatitis.
  - Bulging in groin or other areas of abdomen, especially apparent with contraction of musculature in area, may be hernia.
  - Pulsing in the area of the navel may be abdominal aortic aneurysm.
  - Left lower quadrant pain, often following a meal.
  - Palpable abdominal tenderness: On left or generalized.
  - Psoas sign: Provides resistance over patient's right knee as they flex the hip; pain would be indicative of appendicitis or possible inflammation of the abdomen.
  - Obturator sign: Internal rotation of RLE and flexion may be indicative of appendicitis or pelvic inflammation.
  - Rovsing sign: Pain on the right side of abdomen when pressure is put on the left may be indicative of appendicitis.
- Palpation
  - Appendix (McBurney's): Apply vertical pressure halfway between right ASIS and umbilicus: −/+ may be indicative of appendicitis.
  - Liver: In supine, with left hand under trunk parallel to 11th and 12th rib, lift upward; right hand lateral to rectus and press in and up: +/= reproduction of symptoms with deep breath indicates liver involvement.
  - Ascites: With the fingers, percuss outward from center; if sound is dull, ascites may be present.
  - Spleen: It is not recommended for PT to palpate an enlarged spleen (only palpable if enlarged) because of the potential of rupture.
  - Gallbladder (Murphy's): Place fingers to the right of rectus abdominus below rib cage: +/= sudden pain and muscle tensing with deep breath.
  - Kidneys: In supine, place one hand under client between ribs and iliac crest, and other hand on abdomen below ribs and ribs pointing in opposite direction: +/− tenderness or reproduction of symptoms.
  - Bladder: Not usually palpable unless it is distended and rises above pubic bone; in supine, place hand above pubis and press down: +/= tenderness, reproduction of pain, or ability to feel the bladder: __+ __−.

INTERVENTION

- Therapeutic exercise: All relevant categories, energy conservation
- Therapeutic activities for bed-mobility training, transfer- and transitional-movement training
- Neuromuscular re-education
- Self-care management training
- Electrical stimulation (rectal/anal) in cases of incontinence or muscle control or coordination
- Manual therapy
- Massage
- Lifestyle modification
- Smoking cessation
- Weight management
- Dietary counseling
- Psychological intervention
- Speech-language pathology
  - Swallowing deficits
  - Speech impairment

FUNCTIONAL GOALS

- Patient will be able to
  - Achieve adequate functional aerobic capacity, and the ability to talk during activity in order to achieve functional gait and activity tolerance for work, play, school, self-care; ADLs and IADLs.
  - Functional I gait in the home and community (with or without a device), allowing for work, play, self-care; ADLs and IADLs, up to ___ feet based on patient's need and prior functional level.
  - Achieve 600 m or greater in a 6-minute walk test for initiation of safe functional gait in the community.
  - Perform active verbalization with increasing taxonomy for safety during gait, including negotiation of even and uneven surfaces, opening and closing doors, transferring in and out of a car.
  - Perform activities requiring abdominals with appropriate muscle splinting/guarding to prevent retraction of stoma, if patient has a colostomy or ileostomy.
  - Tolerate 30 minutes of continuous moderate exercise three times a week in ___ weeks, and five times a week in ____ weeks, depending on the severity of the disease.

PROGNOSIS

- As this pathology is primarily medical in nature, it is the physician who establishes the medical prognosis.
- Crohn disease can cause inflammation or changes in bowel tissue or increase your risk of colorectal cancer.
- Unless the medical condition is unstable or the goals unrealistic, the prognosis from a physical therapy perspective should be good (refers only to the realistic functional goals established).

PATIENT RESOURCES

- Chron's. Chron's & Colitis Foundation of America. www.ccfa.org. Accessed June 12, 2013.
- Inflammatory bowel disease. American Gastroenterological Association. http://www.gastro.org/patient-center/digestive-conditions/inflammatory-bowel-disease. Accessed August 8, 2014.

REFERENCES

1. Chandrasoma P, Taylor CR. The intestines: II. Infections; inflammatory bowel diseases. In: Chandrasoma P, Taylor CR, eds. *Concise Pathology*. 3rd ed. New York, NY: McGraw-Hill; 1998. http://www.accessphysiotherapy.com/content/189377. Accessed June 12, 2013.
2. Crohn's Disease. American Society of Colon and Rectal Surgeons. http://www.fascrs.org/patients/conditions/crohns_disease. Accessed June 12, 2013.
3. Goodman CC, Fuller KS. *Pathology: Implications for the Physical Therapist*. 3rd ed. St. Louis, MO: Saunders; 2009.
4. Goodman CC, Snyder TK. *Differential Diagnosis for Physical Therapists: Screening for Referral*. 4th ed. St. Louis, MO: Saunders Elsevier; 2007.
5. Sokol RJ, Narkewicz MR. Liver & pancreas. In: Hay WW, Levin MJ, Sondheimer JM, Deterding RR, eds. *CURRENT Diagnosis & Treatment: Pediatrics*. 20th ed. New York, NY: McGraw-Hill; 2011. http://www.accessphysiotherapy.com/content/6584598. Accessed June 12, 2013.
6. McOmber M, Shulman RJ. Pediatric functional gastrointestinal disorders. *Nutr Clin Prac*. 2008;23:268–274.
7. Mills JC, Stappenbeck TS, Bunnett N. Gastrointestinal disease. In: McPhee SJ, Hammer GD, eds. *Pathophysiology of Disease: An Introduction to Clinical Medicine*. 6th ed. New York, NY: McGraw-Hill; 2010. http://www.accessphysiotherapy.com/content/5369694. Accessed June 12, 2013.
8. Suleiman S, Johnston DE. The abdominal wall: an overlooked source of pain. *Am Fam Physician*. 2001;64(3):431–439. http://www.aafp.org/afp/2001/0801/p431.html. Accessed May 3, 2014.

ADDITIONAL REFERENCE

- Ballard AE. Traditional and complementary therapies used together in the treatment, relief and control of Chron's disease and polyarthritis. *Complement Ther Nurs Midwifery*. 1996;2(2):52–54.

42 IRRITABLE BOWEL SYNDROME

Debra F. Stern, DPT, DBA, MSM, PT
Eric Shamus, PhD, DPT, PT, CSCS

CONDITION/DISORDER SYNONYMS

- Spastic colon
- Irritable colon
- Mucous colitis
- Spastic colitis

ICD-9-CM CODES

- 564.1 Irritable bowel syndrome
- Associated physical therapy diagnoses
  - 315.4 Developmental coordination disorder
  - 718.45 Contracture of joint, pelvic region and thigh
  - 719.70 Difficulty in walking
  - 728.2 Muscular wasting and disuse atrophy
  - 728.89 Disorders of muscle, ligament, and fascia
  - 729.9 Other disorders of soft tissue
  - 780.7 Malaise and fatigue
  - 782.3 Edema
  - 786.0 Dyspnea and respiratory abnormalities

ICD-10-CM CODE

- K58.9 Irritable bowel syndrome without diarrhea

PREFERRED PRACTICE PATTERN

- As of July, 2014, the APTA *Guide to Physical Therapist Practice* does not include practice patterns for organ system pathology; therefore, the associated or secondary musculoskeletal, cardiovascular/pulmonary, or potential neuromuscular patterns would be indicated.

PATIENT PRESENTATION

A 28-year-old White woman presents to your office with a chief complaint of constipation and abdominal pain. On further questioning, she reports she has had this problem since beginning college at the age of 18 years. Her symptoms have waxed and waned since this time, but never have worsened. She describes her abdominal pain as dull, crampy, and nonfocal but more prominent in the left lower quadrant, and sometimes relieved with defecation. She denies radiation of pain, nausea, vomiting, fever, chills, weight loss, heartburn, or bloody or dark stool. She reports having a bowel movement every 1 to 2 days that is hard and feels incomplete.

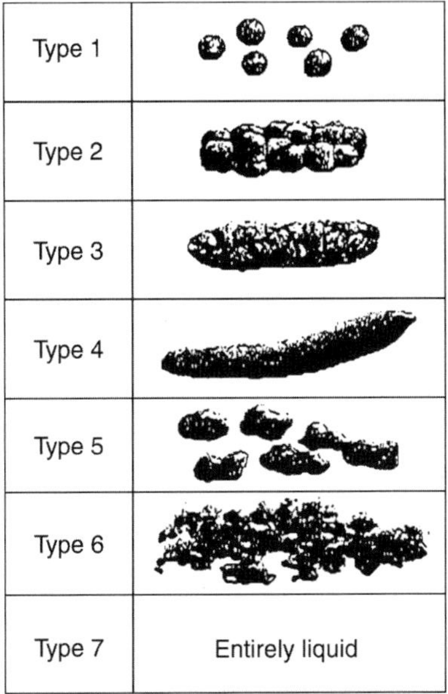

FIGURE 42-1 Bristol Stool Form Scale. (From South-Paul JE, Matheny SC, Lewis EL. *Current Diagnosis & Treatment in Family Medicine*. 3rd ed. www.accessmedicine.com. Copyright © The McGraw-Hill Companies, Inc. All rights reserved.)

She has tried over-the-counter remedies, including stool softeners and antacids, but experienced only minimal improvement in her symptoms. She takes only birth control pills and denies any use of herbs or laxatives. Her family history is negative, including for colorectal cancer and inflammatory bowel disease, and she reports that her parents and siblings are healthy. She is currently engaged

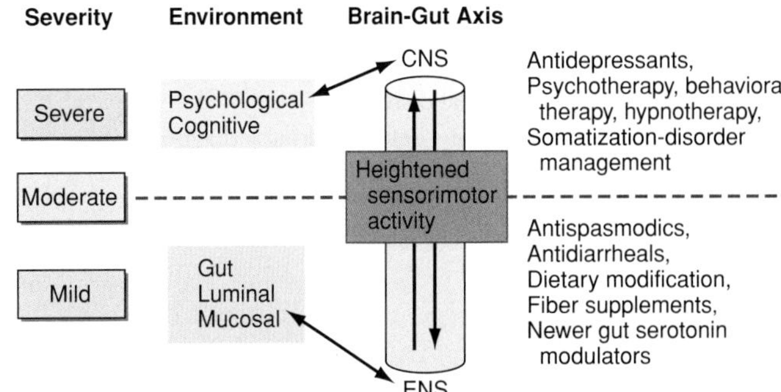

FIGURE 42-2 Therapeutic targets for irritable bowel syndrome. Patients with mild-to-moderate symptoms usually have intermittent symptoms that correlate with altered gut physiology. Treatments include gut-acting pharmacologic agents such as antispasmodics, antidiarrheals, fiber supplements, and gut serotonin modulators. Patients who have severe symptoms usually have constant pain and psychosocial difficulties. This group of patients is best managed with antidepressants and other psychosocial treatments. CNS, central nervous system; ENS, enteric nervous system. (From Longo DL, Fauci AS, Kasper DL, Hauser SL, Jameson JL, Loscalzo J, eds. *Harrison's Principles of Internal Medicine*. 18th ed. New York, NY: McGraw-Hill; 2012.)

and reports significant stress in preparing for the wedding. On physical examination, you note her to be somewhat anxious, but otherwise in no apparent distress. Her vital signs and general physical examinations are normal. Her abdomen has normal bowel sounds, no tenderness on superficial and deep palpation, and no rebound, rigidity, or guarding. Liver and spleen size are within normal limits and no masses are palpable. Pelvic examination is normal. Rectal examination shows normal sphincter tone, no masses, and brown stool that is occult blood negative. [1]

KEY FEATURES

Description

- There is a broad array of gastrointestinal (GI) disorders that may be encountered by physical therapists.
- While physical therapists may not manage GI disorders specifically, many clients may have GI pathology and be receiving care as a result of secondary problems such as weakness, gait abnormalities, and limited aerobic endurance.
- They may be acute, postoperative, chronic, viral, bacterially related, or congenital/hereditary.
- Abdominal pain and altered bowel habits without pathology.
- Considered a disorder and not a disease.
- Complaints often include changes in bowel habits such as constipation, diarrhea, bowel urgency, bloating, incontinence, and cramping.
- Pain is frequently referred to the low back.
- Does not result in permanent damage to colon and is not inflammatory.
- Symptoms may come and go or, in some cases, disappear.

Essentials of Diagnosis

Abdominal pain, constant or intermittent history

- ROME criteria
  - Abdominal pain over a course of 12 weeks, not necessarily continuous weeks
  - At least two of the following:
    - A change in the frequency or consistency of the bowels
    - Straining, urgency or a feeling that the bowels will not completely empty
    - Mucus in the stool
    - Bloating or abdominal distension
- Rule out red flag symptoms before making a diagnosis of irritable bowel syndrome (IBS)
- Bristol Stool Form Scale
- Diarrhea or constipation
- Bloating
- Possible rectal bleeding
- Rectal/anal irritation
- Acute falls in blood pressure, which may result in decreased blood flow to intestines
- Inability to swallow
- Lack of appetite
- Unexplained weight loss
- Abdominal pain related to ingesting food
- Possible joint pains
- Dark stool or bright red blood in stool
- Malaise/fatigue
- Cramping

TABLE 42-1 Diagnostic Criteria for Irritable Bowel Syndrome[a]

Recurrent Abdominal Pain or Discomfort[b] At Least 3 Days Per Month in the Last 3 Months Associated With *Two Or More* of the Following:
1. Improvement with defecation
2. Onset associated with a change in frequency of stool
3. Onset associated with a change in form (appearance) of stool

[a]Criteria fulfilled for the last 3 months with symptom onset at least 6 months before diagnosis.
[b]Discomfort means an uncomfortable sensation not described as pain. In pathophysiology research and clinical trials, a pain/discomfort frequency of at least 2 days a week during screening evaluation is required for subject eligibility.
Source: Longstreth GF, Thompson WG, Chey WD, Houghton LA, Mearin F, Spiller RC. Functional bowel disorders. *Gastroenterology.* 2006;130:1480–1491.

General Considerations

- Diagnosis for more occult problems may take time and require intensive medical diagnostic testing.
- GI disorders occur across the lifespan; birth through geriatric.
- May result in secondary problems such as aerobic capacity and muscle-endurance impairment, sarcopenia, weakness/impaired muscle performance, musculoskeletal problems, neuromuscular problems, weight loss, or weight gain, indicating the need for physical therapy intervention depending on severity.
- Because GI disorders frequently refer pain to other body areas, individuals may get referred to PT inappropriately, such as when referred to the low back.
- GI problems may be commonly related to stress or constipation, more serious problems such as autoimmune conditions like Crohn, or acute pain may be indicative of appendicitis.
- In adults females, GI complaints may actually be related or indicative of cancer or tumors in the reproductive organs, or gynecological problems such as endometriosis, uterine fibroids, ectopic pregnancies, and inguinal or umbilical hernias in males or females.
- History of heartburn or indigestion may be indicative of GI or cardiac problems.
- Chronic diarrhea, episodic diarrhea, loss of bowel control (incontinence or urgency), blood in stool may be symptomatic of inflammatory disease, precancerous conditions, or cancer.

Demographics

- Women may have slightly higher incidence than males according to the CDC in the United States
- 8% to 20% of adults, or 1 in 6
- Often occurs in teens or young adults

CLINICAL FINDINGS

SIGNS AND SYMPTOMS

- The signs and symptoms indicated here may be characteristic of multiple GI disorders (vs. one, often confounding medical diagnosis).
- As GI symptoms are frequently referred to the back and shoulders, it may be more common than previously identified to have patients inappropriately referred to PT.
- Diarrhea: Acute, chronic[2]
- Constipation[2]
- Bowel urgency
- Incontinence

- Abdominal or stomach pain or cramping: Constant or intermittent and severe[2]
- Abdominal (stomach or intestinal) pain after ingesting food or liquid[2]
  - May be cardiac in nature
- Lower abdominal pain
- Blood in stool: Dark or bright (fresh bleeding); rectal bleeding
- Pain associated with defecation
- Pain after ingesting fatty foods (gallbladder sign)
- Changes in bowel habits
- Bloated or swollen abdomen: Abdominal distention
- Unexplained weight loss
- Fever
- Chills
- Abdominal muscle spasm, guarding
- Feeling of having to move bowels constantly
- Fatigue
- Anemia
- Weight loss
- Loss of appetite, cachexia
- Skin lesions
- Joint pain
- Eye problems
- Liver impairment
- Failure to grow if onset at early age
- Flatulence
- Gastroesophageal reflux (GERD), heartburn
- Pain secondary to hernias
  - Palpable bulging with or without muscle contraction
  - Commonly in the groin, umbilical area, or abdomen (especially after pregnancy or any surgery in the abdominal region)
  - Sports hernias
- Nausea
- Emesis
- Rectal bleeding: Fresh blood versus darkened stool
- Ascites
- Difficulty swallowing
  - Related to esophageal or oral problems rather than neuromuscular issues
- Pain associated with defecation
- Any changes in bowel habits
- Mucous in the stool or mucous discharge
- Change in bowel odor or color
- Fever
- Chills
- Acute, severe pain regionally located (as in right lower quadrant)
  - Appendicitis or ectopic pregnancy
- General abdominal pain
- Intestinal necrosis
- Dietary restrictions: Consistency, foods (i.e., dairy, spices, wheat/gluten for celiac disease)
- Abdominal muscle spasm, guarding

Functional Implications

- Severe symptoms such as diarrhea associated with immediacy of defecation, may be disabling and result in the inability to leave home
- Dehydration with severe diarrhea, emesis, loss of appetite, inability to drink or eat secondary to nausea, or inability to swallow
- Eating disorders/anorexia secondary to fear of pain associated with ingesting food, bulimia, binge eating
- Anemia
- Sarcopenia resulting in weakness, muscle-mass loss, inability to ambulate or perform self-care as well as aerobic capacity limitation secondary to inactivity
- Need for colostomies or ileostomies: Temporary or permanent (usually with intestinal problems vs. upper GI)
- Decreased exercise tolerance
- Changes in lifestyle limiting physical activity
- Self-limiting of sex secondary to pain
- Reluctance to leave the home
- Fatigue
- Anxiety and depression
- Can be indicative of serious medical conditions
- Limitations in ADLs or IADLs
- Infection
- Arthritis
- Inflammation of the eye
- Liver disease
- Osteoporosis
- Intestinal necrosis
- Dietary restrictions: Consistency, foods, that is, dairy, spices, wheat/gluten as in celiac disease
- Dietary changes: Increasing fiber, water

Possible Contributing Causes

- Abnormal serotonin levels
- Bacteria imbalance
- Hormones
- Infections: Bacterial or viral
  - Food poisoning
  - Parasites
- Ischemic
  - Atherosclerosis, impaired blood supply to any structure(s)
- Stress and anxiety
- Obstruction in the colon, decreasing blood supply and causing inflammation
- Inflammatory: Autoimmune disease
- Chemical
  - May occur after enemas
- Environmental irritants
- Obesity
- Lack of exercise
- Heredity
- Allergy (i.e., celiac: Gluten/wheat, dairy)
- Food intolerance (i.e., dairy, lactose, chocolate)
- Diet
- Fibromyalgia
- Interstitial cystitis
- Temporomandibular joint disorder
- Sjögren syndrome
- Cancer: Esophagus, colon, liver, bile duct, pancreatic, metastatic, anal/rectal
- Systemic rheumatologic disorders such as scleroderma, rheumatoid Arthritis (RA)
- Genetic predisposition
- Systemic immunological condition
- Effects of medications: Diarrhea, GI upset, constipation, GI bleeding, rectal bleeding, blood in stool
- Postsurgical scarring/adhesions
- Endocrine dysfunction

Differential Diagnosis

- Symptom onset after age 50
- Organ dysfunction as the result of cancer or malignancy
- Non-malignant tumors in the abdomen or organs
- Endocrine disorders
- Gynecologic problems in females such as
  - Endometriosis
  - Menses
  - Ectopic pregnancies
  - Ovarian cysts
  - Fibroids

- Autoimmune diseases that affect the upper and lower GI tracts
  - SLE
  - RA
- Appendicitis
- IBS
- Crohn disease
- Colitis: Ulcerative, non-ulcerative
- Colon cancer
- Ovarian cancer
- Inflammatory bowel disease
- Pelvic inflammatory disease
- Celiac disease/gluten intolerance
- Gastroenteritis
- Perforated ulcers anywhere in GI system
- Bladder infections, urinary tract infections, kidney pathology
- Infections in the abdomen
- Bowel disorders
  - Constipation or diarrhea
  - Inflammation of the lining of the of the abdomen or organs
  - Obstructions or torsions
- Referred pain from heart, spine, hip

MEANS OF CONFIRMATION OR DIAGNOSIS

Laboratory Tests

- Fecal occult blood tests/stool samples
- Blood tests/lab tests
  - H & H
- Lactose intolerance
- Rule out possible celiac
  - Anti-tissue transglutaminase antibody (tTG–IgA and IgG), anti-endomysial antibody (EMA-IgA): Highly specific marker for celiac disease
  - Anti-deamidated gliadin peptide (DGP–IgA and IgG), total serum IgA anti-gliadin antibody (AgA–IgG and IgA)

Imaging

- Abdominal scans
- Radiography
- Barium enemas
- CT scans

Diagnostic Procedures

- Colonoscopy
  - Virtual
  - Procedural
- Sigmoidoscopy
- Endoscopic biopsy
- Manual palpation for tenderness

FINDINGS AND INTERPRETATION

- H & H for signs of bleeding, anemia, pathogens, immune status, vitamin deficiencies, check white blood cell count for infection

TREATMENT

Medication

- Antidiarrheals
- Anticholinergics
- Antidepressants
- Antibiotics
- Alosetron (Lotronex)
- Lubiprostone (Amitiza)

MEDICAL PROCEDURES

- Ulcer repairs
- NG tubes
- PEG tubes/feeding
- TPN/PPN
- IV for hydration

REFERRALS/ADMITTANCE

- If a patient is referred for PT and the causative problem is not considered to be appropriate for PT, referral to the appropriate physician must be made
- If an emergency is identified, referral to an emergency room (ER) may be necessary

IMPAIRMENTS

- Muscle weakness
- Muscle atrophy
- Gait abnormality/difficulty walking
- Contractures of soft tissue (fascia, muscle), joint limitations
- Shortness of breath
- Possible rectal muscle impairment
- Inability to perform self-care
- Limited aerobic endurance
- Functional decline: Decrease in functional abilities[3]

TESTS AND MEASURES

- Bristol Stool Form Scale
- Observation
  - Scars may indicate adhesions or abdominal surgeries that may be causative of diverticula.
  - Striae: Pink or purplish may be indicative of Cushing syndrome; dilated veins may indicate hepatic pathology or inferior vena cava obstruction, not diverticulitis.
  - Contour: Roundedness, concavity/hollowness, asymmetry, distension, pregnancy signs.
  - Cullen sign: Bluish discoloring around the umbilicus, which may be a sign of retroperitoneal bleeding.
  - Bluish discoloration in lower abdomen: Grey Turner sign, which is a sign of hemorrhagic pancreatitis.
  - Bulging in groin or other areas of abdomen, especially apparent with contraction of musculature in area, may be hernia.
  - Pulsing in the area of the navel may be abdominal aortic aneurysm.
  - Left lower quadrant pain, often following a meal.
  - Palpable abdominal tenderness: On left or generalized.
  - Psoas sign: Provides resistance over patient's right knee as they flex the hip; pain would be indicative of appendicitis or possible inflammation of the abdomen.
  - Obturator sign: Internal rotation of RLE and flexion may be indicative of appendicitis or pelvic inflammation.
  - Rovsing sign: Pain on the right side of abdomen when pressure is put on the left may be indicative of appendicitis.
- Palpation
  - Appendix (McBurney's): Apply vertical pressure halfway between right ASIS and umbilicus: −/+ may be indicative of appendicitis.

- Liver: In supine, with left hand under trunk parallel to 11th and 12th rib, lift upward; right hand lateral to rectus and press in and up: +/= reproduction of symptoms with deep breath indicates liver involvement.
- Ascites: With the fingers, percuss outward from center; if sound is dull, ascites may be present.
- Spleen: It is not recommended for PT to palpate an enlarged spleen (only palpable if enlarged) because of the potential of rupture.
- Gallbladder (Murphy's): Place fingers to the right of rectus abdominus below rib cage: +/= sudden pain and muscle tensing with deep breath.
- Kidneys: In supine, place one hand under client between ribs and iliac crest, and other hand on abdomen below ribs and ribs pointing in opposite direction: +/− tenderness or reproduction of symptoms.
- Bladder: Not usually palpable unless it is distended and rises above pubic bone; in supine, place hand above pubis and press down: +/= tenderness, reproduction of pain, or ability to feel the bladder: __+ ___−.

INTERVENTION

- Therapeutic exercise: All relevant categories, energy conservation
  - If there is a stoma from a colostomy or ileostomy, PT must be aware that activities are avoided if they cause retraction.
  - Deep breathing
  - Progressive relaxation
- Therapeutic activities for bed-mobility training, transfer- and transitional-movement training
- Neuromuscular re-education
- Self-care management training
- Rectal/anal electrical stimulation in cases of incontinence or muscle control or coordination
- Biofeedback
- Manual therapy
- Massage
- Interprofessional
  - Lifestyle modification
  - Smoking cessation
  - Weight management
  - Dietary counseling
  - Psychological intervention

FUNCTIONAL GOALS

- Patient will be able to
  - Achieve adequate functional aerobic capacity, and the ability to talk during activity, in order to achieve functional gait and activity tolerance for work, play, school, self-care; ADLs and IADLs.
  - Functional gait in the home and community (with or without a device), allowing for work, play, self-care; ADLs and IADLs, up to __________ feet based on patient's need and prior functional level.
  - Achieve 600 m or greater in a 6-minute walk test for initiation of safe functional gait in the community.
  - Perform active verbalization with increasing taxonomy for safety during gait, including negotiation of even and uneven surfaces, opening and closing doors, transferring in and out of a car
  - Perform activities requiring abdominals with appropriate muscle splinting/guarding to prevent retraction of stoma, if patient has a colostomy or ileostomy.
  - Tolerate 30 minutes of continuous moderate exercise three times a week in ______ weeks, and five times a week in ____________ weeks, depending on the severity of the disease.

PROGNOSIS

- As this pathology is primarily medical in nature, it is the physician who establishes the medical prognosis.
- Most people with IBS find that symptoms improve as they learn to control their condition; only a small number of people with IBS have disabling signs and symptoms.
- Fortunately, unlike more serious intestinal diseases such as ulcerative colitis and Crohn disease, IBS does not cause inflammation or changes in bowel tissue or increase your risk of colorectal cancer.
- In many cases, you can control IBS by managing your diet, lifestyle, and stress.
- For a physical therapy prognosis, goals should be established that the patient can achieve based on their overall condition.
- Unless the medical condition is unstable or the goals unrealistic, the prognosis from a physical therapy perspective should be good (referring only to the realistic functional goals established).

ADDITIONAL INFORMATION

See Case study 65. In: *Pathophysiology of Disease*. 6th ed. New York, NY: McGraw-Hill; 2010.

PATIENT RESOURCES

- IBS Network. http://www.theibsnetwork.org. Accessed August 8, 2014.
- Irritable Bowel Syndrome Association. www.ibsassociation.org. Accessed August 8, 2014.

REFERENCES

1. Toy EC. Irritable Bowel Syndrome (IBS), Case 65. LANGE Case Files. http://www.accessmedicine.com/casecontent.aspx?aid=510023164&tabid=1. Accessed July 2, 2013.
2. McPhee SJ, Hammer GD. Pathophysiology of disorders of the small intestine & colon. In: McPhee SJ, Hammer GD, eds. *Pathophysiology of Disease*. 6th ed. New York, NY: McGraw-Hill; 2010. http://www.accessphysiotherapy.com/content/5369710. Accessed July 2, 2013.
3. Patel DR, Greydanus DE, Baker RJ. Dismotility or "runner's trots". In: Patel DR, Greydanus DE, Baker RJ, eds. *Pediatric Practice: Sports Medicine*. New York, NY: McGraw-Hill; 2009. http://www.accessphysiotherapy.com/content/6976909. Accessed July 2, 2013.

ADDITIONAL REFERENCES

- Chandrasoma P, Taylor CR. The Intestines: II. Infections; inflammatory bowel diseases. In: Chandrasoma P, Taylor CR, eds. *Concise Pathology*. 3rd ed. New York, NY: McGraw-Hill; 1998. http://www.accessphysiotherapy.com/content/189377. Accessed July 2, 2013.

- Goodman CC, Fuller KS. *Pathology: Implications for the Physical Therapist.* 3rd ed. St. Louis, MO: Saunders; 2009.
- Goodman CC, Snyder TK. *Differential Diagnosis for Physical Therapists: Screening for Referral.* 4th ed. St. Louis, MO: Saunders Elsevier; 2007.
- Houghton LA, Lea R, Agrawal A, et al. Relationship of abdominal bloating to distention in irritable bowel syndrome and effect of bowel habit. *Gastroenterology.* 2006;131:1003–1010.
- McOmber MA, Shulman RJ. Pediatric functional gastrointestinal disorders. *Nutr Clin Prac.* 2008;23(3):268--274.
- Sokol RJ, Narkewicz MR. Liver & pancreas. In: Hay WW, Levin MJ, Sondheimer JM, Deterding RR, eds. *CURRENT Diagnosis & Treatment: Pediatrics.* 20th ed. New York, NY: McGraw-Hill; 2011. http://www.accessphysiotherapy.com/content/6584598. Accessed July 2, 2013.
- Suleiman S, Johnston DE. The abdominal wall: an overlooked source of pain. *Am Fam Physician.* 2001;64(3);431–439. http://www.aafp.org/afp/2001/0801/p431.html. Accessed July 2, 2013.
- Ulcerative Colitis. National Digestive Diseases Information Clearinghouse (NDDIC). U.S. Department of Health and Human Services. *NIH Publication No. 12–1597.* October 2011. http://digestive.niddk.nih.gov/ddiseases/pubs/colitis/. Accessed July 2, 2013.

43 MALABSORPTION SYNDROMES

Debra F. Stern, DPT, DBA, MSM, PT
Eric Shamus, PhD, DPT, PT, CSCS
David W. Mandel, PhD, PT

ICD-9-CM CODES

- 579 Intestinal malabsorption
- 579.0 Celiac disease
- 579.1 Tropical sprue
- 579.2 Blind loop syndrome
- 579.3 Other and unspecified postsurgical nonabsorption
- 579.4 Pancreatic steatorrhea
- 579.8 Other specified intestinal malabsorption
- 579.9 Unspecified intestinal malabsorption
- Associated physical therapy diagnoses
  - 315.4 Developmental coordination disorder
  - 718.45 Contracture of joint, pelvic region and thigh
  - 719.70 Difficulty in walking
  - 728.2 Muscular wasting and disuse atrophy
  - 728.89 Disorders of muscle, ligament, and fascia
  - 729.9 Other and unspecified disorders of soft tissue
  - 780.7 Malaise and fatigue
  - 781.2 Abnormality of gait
  - 782.3 Edema
  - 786.0 Dyspnea and respiratory abnormalities
  - 786.05 Shortness of breath

ICD-10-CM CODES

- K90.1 Tropical sprue
- K90.2 Blind loop syndrome, not elsewhere classified
- K90.3 Pancreatic steatorrhea
- K90.4 Malabsorption due to intolerance, not elsewhere classified
- K90.89 Other intestinal malabsorption
- K90.9 Intestinal malabsorption, unspecified
- K91.2 Postsurgical malabsorption, not elsewhere classified

PREFERRED PRACTICE PATTERN

As of July, 2014, the APTA Guide to Physical Therapist Practice does not include practice patterns for organ system pathology. Therefore, the associated or secondary musculoskeletal, cardiovascular/pulmonary, or potential neuromuscular patterns would be indicated.

PATIENT PRESENTATION

The patient is a 47-year-old male who presents to the clinic with increasing difficulty in ambulating and poor tolerance for activity. He presents to the outpatient facility with a referral from his primary care physician for gait training and conditioning. The patient appears very cachectic with pale skin and sunken eyes. The patient stands and sits with a slumped kyphotic posture. He reports malaise and fatigue with small bouts of activity and appears to be depressed. In addition, the patient reports he has no appetite, and when he does eat he feels bloated and nauseous.

Upon physical therapy examination, the patient's mobility status is modified independent due to decreased speed and general joint discomfort. He can only ambulate for 45 m before he needs to sit and rest. Bilateral upper extremity and lower extremity strength is 3+/5 proximally and 4/5 distally. Joint range of motion is full with inconsistent achy discomfort. Sensory is fully intact. Performance on the functional strength and endurance tests (30-second chair stand and the 6-minute walk) results in significantly below-average scores for his age. The patient requires several sitting rest periods during the 6-minute walk test. His Borg scale perceived exertion grade during the 6-minute walk is "very hard." During pulmonary testing the patient demonstrated poor maximal inspiratory and expiratory pressures and a weak cough ability revealing weakness of his diaphragmatic and respiratory musculature.

KEY FEATURES

Description

- Malabsorption: Decreased absorption of fat and other nutrients caused by liver, biliary, pancreatic, or intestinal disease[1]
- Impaired absorption of nutrients in gastrointestinal (GI) tract
- Symptoms such as gas, bloating, abdominal pain, diarrhea resulting from malabsorption
- May be acute, postoperative, chronic, viral, bacterial, congenital/hereditary
- Complaints of change in bowel habits (constipation, urgency, incontinence, cramping)
- Referred pain in low back
- Inflammatory bowel diseases (IBD): Chronic or recurring immune response, inflammation of GI tract
  - Ulcerative colitis
  - Crohn disease

Essentials of Diagnosis

- Intraluminal abnormalities[1]
- Mucosal abnormalities[1]
- Vascular abnormalities[1]
- Metabolic genetic disease[1]
- Abdominal pain (constant or intermittent)
- Abdominal tenderness
- Nausea
- Vomiting[1]
- Changes in bowel habits: Diarrhea, constipation

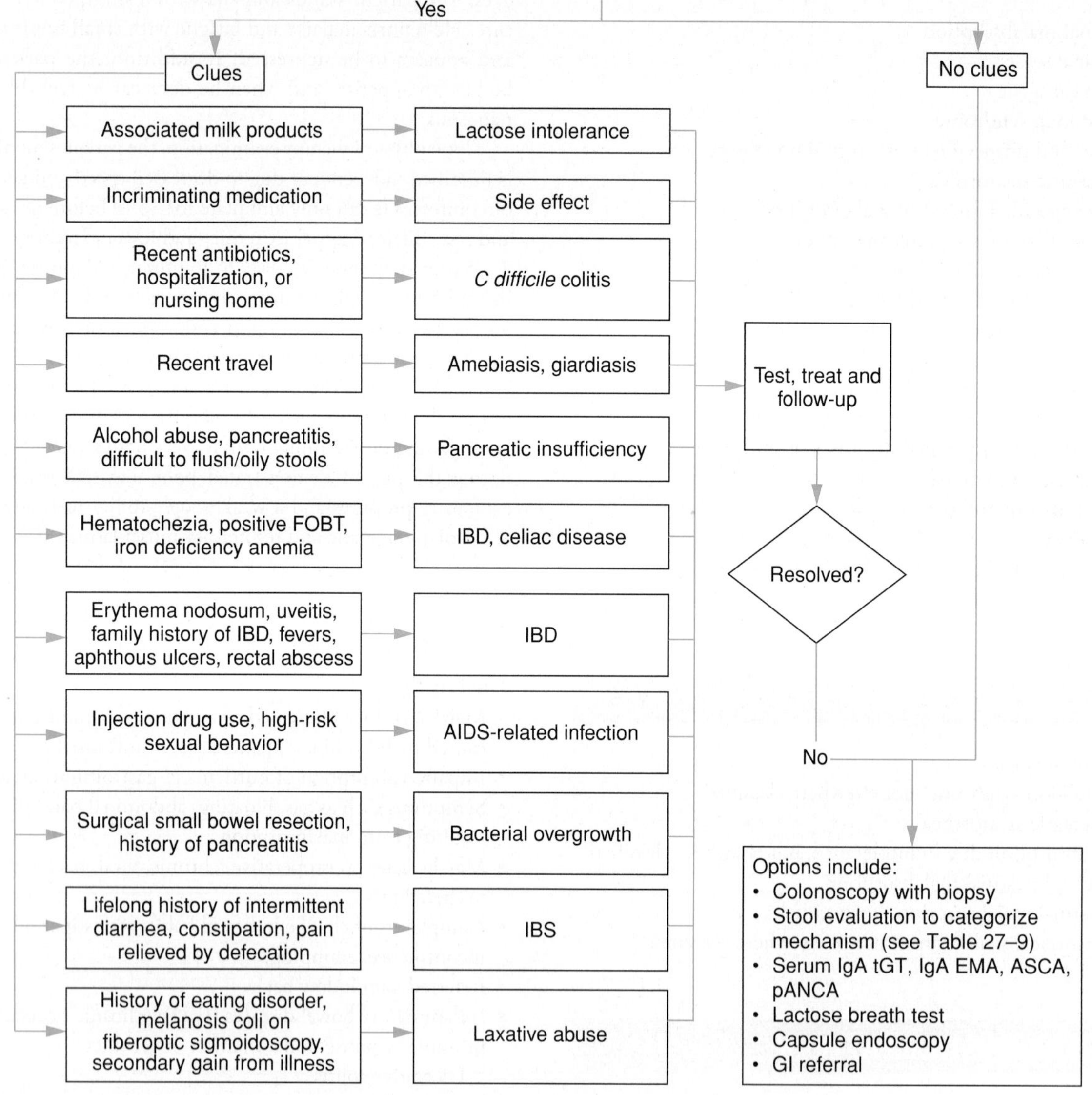
History
Dietary history: Association with milk products, sorbitol-containing mints or gums, caffeine, ruffage
Medication history: Including over-the-counter medications, antacids, recent antibiotics, metformin
Social history: Recent travel, alcohol use, risk factors for HIV
Family history: Jewish descent, family history of IBD or celiac disease
Clinical clues: Weight loss, stool appearance (bloody, oily), history of pancreatitis, alcohol use, manifestations of IBD (hematochezia, erythema nodosum, uveitis, aphthous ulcers, rectal abscess, fever);
Past medical history: Prior small bowel or gastric resection, cholecystectomy, radiation
Physical exam: Include comprehensive exam, weight, thyroid and abdominal exam, FOBT. Pallor, edema, easy bruisability
Laboratory studies: CBC with differential, stool cultures, O & P (or stool Giardia antigen), stool C difficile toxin, TSH, LFTs, BMP, serum albumin, cholesterol, HIV if appropriate
Yes
Clues
No clues
Associated milk products
Lactose intolerance
Incriminating medication
Side effect
Recent antibiotics, hospitalization, or nursing home
C difficile colitis
Recent travel
Amebiasis, giardiasis
Alcohol abuse, pancreatitis, difficult to flush/oily stools
Pancreatic insufficiency
Hematochezia, positive FOBT, iron deficiency anemia
IBD, celiac disease
Erythema nodosum, uveitis, family history of IBD, fevers, aphthous ulcers, rectal abscess
IBD
Injection drug use, high-risk sexual behavior
AIDS-related infection
Surgical small bowel resection, history of pancreatitis
Bacterial overgrowth
Lifelong history of intermittent diarrhea, constipation, pain relieved by defecation
IBS
History of eating disorder, melanosis coli on fiberoptic sigmoidoscopy, secondary gain from illness
Laxative abuse
Test, treat and follow-up
Resolved?
No
Options include:
• Colonoscopy with biopsy
• Stool evaluation to categorize mechanism (see Table 27–9)
• Serum IgA tGT, IgA EMA, ASCA, pANCA
• Lactose breath test
• Capsule endoscopy
• GI referral
BMP, basic metabolic panel; FOBT, fecal occult blood test; IBD, inflammatory bowel disease; IBS, irritable bowel syndrome; LFTs, liver function tests; O & P, ova and parasite.

FIGURE 43-1 Diagnostic approach: malabsorption and diarrhea. (From Stern SDC, Cifu AS, Aitkorn D. *Symptom to Diagnosis: An Evidence-Based Guide*. 2nd ed. www.accessmedicine.com.)

- Bloating
- Possible rectal bleeding
- Rectal irritation
- Acute drop in blood pressure, may result in decreased blood flow to intestines
- Inability to swallow
- Lack of appetite
- Unexplained weight loss
- Abdominal pain upon ingesting food
- Possible joint pain
- Dark stool or bright red blood in stool
- Malaise, fatigue

General Considerations

- Broad array of GI disorders may be encountered by physical therapists.
- Although PT may not manage GI disorders specifically, clients may receive care for secondary problems: Weakness, gait abnormalities, limited aerobic endurance, musculoskeletal problems, neuromuscular problems, weight loss, or weight gain.
- Diagnosis for occult problems may take time and require intensive diagnostic testing.
- GI disorders frequently refer pain to other body areas; individuals may be inappropriately referred to PT.
- GI problems commonly related to stress or constipation.
- More serious problems include autoimmune conditions like Crohn's.
- Acute pain may be indicative of appendicitis.
- GI complaints in females may indicate cancer/tumors in reproductive organs, or gynecological problems: Endometriosis, uterine fibroids, ectopic pregnancies.
- May indicate inguinal or umbilical hernia.
- History of heartburn/indigestion may indicate GI or cardiac problems.

Demographics

- GI disorders occur throughout the lifespan (birth through geriatric)
- Higher incidence of colitis in Caucasians
- Higher incidence of Crohn and irritable bowel syndrome (IBS) in individuals of Jewish European descent
- Colitis may occur at any age: More common between ages 15 and 30 years, less frequent between ages 50 and 70 years
- Men and women equally affected
- Familial

CLINICAL FINDINGS

SIGNS AND SYMPTOMS

- PT should recognize the possibility of GI pathology in differential diagnosis, especially when findings are not consistent with conditions commonly treated
- Protein loss
  - Muscle wasting[2]
  - Hyoproteinemia[2]
- Calcium loss
  - Hypocalcemia[2]
  - Osteomalacia[2]
  - Bone pain[2]
- Magnesium loss
  - Hypomagnesemia[2]
- Iron loss
  - Glossitis[2]
  - Hypochromic microcytic anemia[2]
- Folic acid loss
  - Macrocytic megaloblastic anemia[2]
- Vitamin B12 loss
  - Macrocytic megaloblastic anemia[2]
- Vitamin K loss
  - Hemorrhagic diathesis[2]
  - Hypoprothrombinemia[2]
- Vitamin D loss
  - Hypocalcemia[2]
  - Osteomalacia[2]
- Vitamin A loss
  - Night blindness[2]
  - Bitot spots[2]
- Pain
  - Abdominal/stomach pain, cramping (constant or intermittent, severe)
  - Pain upon ingesting food or liquid
  - Lower abdominal pain
  - Pain with defecation
  - Pain after ingesting fatty foods (gallbladder sign)
  - Joint pain
  - Pain secondary to hernias
    - Palpable bulging with or without muscle contraction
    - Commonly in the groin, umbilical area, or abdomen (especially after pregnancy or any surgery in the abdominal region)
    - Sports hernias
  - Acute, severe pain in right lower quadrant
    - Appendicitis or ectopic pregnancy
- Bowel changes
  - Diarrhea (acute, chronic)
  - Constipation (acute, chronic)
  - Blood in stool, dark or fresh bleeding
  - Rectal bleeding
  - Change in stool odor or color
  - Feeling of having to move bowels constantly
  - Abdominal distention
  - Abdominal muscle spasm, guarding
  - Unexplained weight loss
  - Fever
  - Chills
  - Fatigue
  - Anemia
  - Loss of appetite, cachexia
  - Skin lesions
  - Failure to grow if onset at early age
  - Flatulence
  - Gastroesophageal reflux (GERD), heartburn
  - Mucous in stool or mucous discharge
- Nausea
- Emesis
- Ascites
- Difficulty swallowing (related to esophageal or oral problems, not neuromuscular)
- Intestinal necrosis
- Dietary restrictions: Consistency, food types (dairy, spices, wheat/gluten)
- Complaints of "feeling full" regardless of having ingested food

Functional Implications

- Severe symptoms associated with immediacy of defecation may be disabling, causing inability to leave home
- Chronic constipation may cause severe pain, results in fecal material backing up through the esophagus, require manual extraction, surgery, bowel retraining

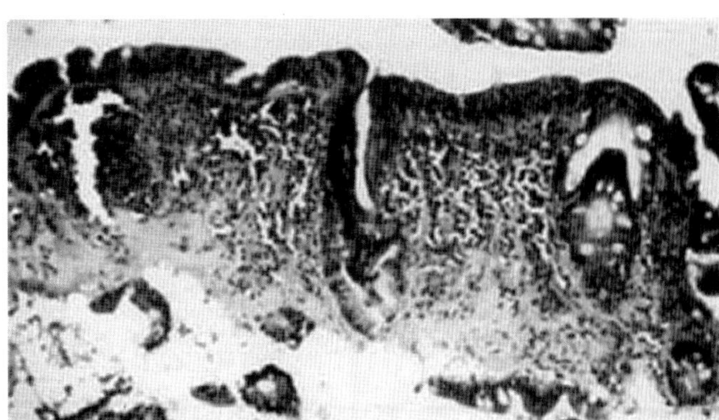

FIGURE 43-2 Total villous atrophy in a case of celiac disease. Note the flat surface epithelium without villi. The surface epithelium also appears more cuboidal, with less cytoplasmic mucin than is normal. The hypercellular appearance of the surface epithelium is caused by the presence of numerous intraepithelial lymphocytes (visible only at higher magnification). (From Chandrasoma P, Taylor CR. *Concise Pathology*. 3rd ed. www.accessmedicine.com. Copyright © The McGraw-Hill Companies, Inc. All rights reserved.)

- Dehydration secondary to diarrhea, emesis, appetite loss, nausea, inability to swallow
- Eating disorder/anorexia secondary to fear of pain upon ingesting food
- Anemia
- Sarcopenia resulting in weakness, decreased muscle mass, inability to ambulate or perform self-care, limited aerobic capacity secondary to inactivity
- Need for temporary or permanent colostomies/ileostomies (usually with intestinal problems vs. upper GI)
  - May present problem with stoma retraction associated with abdominal contraction
- Decreased exercise tolerance
- Limited physical activity
- Reluctance to leave the home
- Fatigue
- Inappropriate self-medication
- Anxiety, depression, psychological symptoms
- Limitations in ADLs/IADLs
- Infection
- Arthritis
- Inflammation of the eye, liver disease
- Osteoporosis
- Intestinal necrosis
- Dietary restrictions

Possible Contributing Causes

- Infections: Bacterial, viral, food poisoning, parasites
- Ischemic
  - Atherosclerosis, impaired blood supply to structures
- Stress, anxiety
- Obstruction in colon decreasing blood supply, causing inflammation
- Inflammatory: Autoimmune disease
- Chemical
  - May occur after enemas
- Environmental irritants
- Obesity
- Lack of exercise
- Heredity
- Food allergy/intolerance (gluten, lactose, purines)
- Excessive dieting
- Cancer: Esophagus, colon, liver, bile duct, pancreatic, metastatic, anal/rectal
- Systemic rheumatologic disorders (scleroderma, RA)
- Genetic predisposition
- Whipple disease
- Systemic immunological condition
- Medication side effects: Diarrhea, GI upset, constipation, bleeding
- Postsurgical scarring, adhesions
- Surgical error: Instrument left in abdomen, inadequately sutured tissue, cut vessels or tissues, pharmacological errors
- Endocrine dysfunction

Differential Diagnosis

- Organ dysfunction from cancer or malignancy
  - Colon cancer
  - Ovarian cancer
- Non-malignant tumors in abdomen or organs
- Endocrine disorders

TABLE 43-1 Malabsorption Syndrome

Intraluminal Abnormalities
Acid hypersecretion (e.g., Zollinger–Ellison syndrome)
Exocrine pancreatic insufficiency
Cystic fibrosis
Shwachman syndrome
Malnutrition
Enzyme deficiency
Enterokinase deficiency
Trypsinogen deficiency
Co-lipase deficiency
Decreased intraluminal bile acids
Chronic parenchymal liver disease
Biliary obstruction
Bile acid loss (short gut, ileal disease)
Bile acid deconjugation by bacterial overgrowth
Mucosal Abnormalities
Infection (e.g., Giardia, cryptosporidium)
Graft versus host disease
Mucosal injury
Celiac disease
Allergic enteropathy
IBD
Radiation enteritis
Enzyme deficiency
Lactase deficiency
Sucrase-isomaltase deficiency
Short bowel syndrome
Vascular Abnormalities
Ischemic bowel
Vasculitis: Lupus, mixed connective tissue disorder
Congestive heart failure
Intestinal lymphangiectasia
Metabolic Genetic Disease
Abetalipoproteinemia
Congenital secretory diarrheas
Lysinuric protein intolerance
Cystinosis

Source: Hay WW, Levin MJ, Deterding RR, Abzug M. *Current Diagnosis & Treatment: Pediatrics.* 21st ed. www.accessmedicine.com.

- Gynecologic problems
- Autoimmune disease affecting upper and lower GI tracts
- Appendicitis
- IBS, IBD
- Crohn disease
- Colitis (ulcerative, non-ulcerative)
- Pelvic inflammatory disease
- Celiac disease or gluten intolerance
- Gastroenteritis
- Perforated ulcer in GI system
- Bladder or urinary tract infection, kidney pathology
- Abdominal infection
  - Bowel disorders
- Referred pain from heart, spine, hip
- Post–weight-loss (bariatric) surgery complications
  - Side effects may mimic diverticulitis or cause a flare-up

MEANS OF CONFIRMATION OR DIAGNOSIS

Laboratory Tests

- 72-hour fecal fat determination
- Fecal occult blood test/stool sample
- Blood test
- H & H for signs of bleeding, anemia, pathogens, immune status, vitamin deficiencies, white blood cell count

Imaging

- Abdominal scans
- Barium enemas
- CT
- Radiography

Diagnostic Procedures

- Colonoscopy
- History of eating/dietary habits
- Manual palpation for tenderness
- Sigmoidoscopy

FINDINGS AND INTERPRETATION

- Chronic diarrhea, episodic diarrhea, loss of bowel control, blood in stool may indicate inflammatory disease, precancerous condition, or cancer

TREATMENT

Medication

- Aminosalicylates (ASA)
- Antacids
- Corticosteroids
- Immunomodulators

MEDICAL PROCEDURES

- Bowel resection with colostomy or ileostomy
- IV for hydration
- Nasogastric feeding tube
- Release of adhesions
- Removal of tumors or growths
- Stomach resection
- Total/peripheral parenteral nutrition (TPN/PPN)
- Ulcer repair

REFERRALS/ADMITTANCE

- If causative problem is not considered appropriate for PT intervention, refer to appropriate physician
- If emergency is identified, refer to ER.

IMPAIRMENTS

- Contractures of soft tissue (fascia, muscle); joint limitations
- Functional decline, decreased functional abilities
- Gait abnormality, difficulty walking
- Inability to perform self-care
- Limited aerobic endurance
- Muscle atrophy
- Muscle wasting/weakness

TESTS AND MEASURES

- Observation
  - Scars may indicate adhesions or abdominal surgeries causative of diverticula.
  - Pink or purplish striae may be indicative of Cushing syndrome.
  - Dilated veins may indicate hepatic pathology or inferior vena cava obstruction, not diverticulitis
  - Contour: Roundness, concavity, asymmetry, distension, pregnancy signs.
  - Cullen sign: Bluish discoloring around the umbilicus may be a sign of retroperitoneal bleeding.
  - Bluish discoloration in lower abdomen: Grey Turner sign, signals hemorrhagic pancreatitis.
  - Bulging in groin and abdomen especially apparent with contraction of musculature in area may be hernia.
  - Pulsing in navel area may be abdominal aortic aneurysm.
  - Left lower quadrant pain, often following a meal.
  - Palpable abdominal tenderness: On left side or generalized.
  - Psoas sign: Provides resistance over patient's right knee as they flex the hip; pain indicates appendicitis, possible inflammation of abdomen.
  - Obturator sign: Internal rotation and flexion of right lower extremity may indicate appendicitis, pelvic inflammation.
  - Rovsing sign: Pain on the right side of abdomen when pressure applied to the left may indicate appendicitis.
- Palpation
  - Appendix (McBurney's): Apply vertical pressure halfway between right ASIS and umbilicus: −/+ may indicate appendicitis.
  - Liver: In supine, with left hand under trunk parallel to 11th and 12th ribs, lift upward; right hand lateral to rectus, press in and up: +/= reproduction of symptoms with deep breath, indicates liver involvement.
  - Ascites: Percuss outward from center with fingers; if sound is dull, ascites may be present.
  - Spleen: Not recommended for PT to palpate enlarged spleen (only palpable if enlarged).
  - Gallbladder (Murphy's): Place fingers to the right of rectus abdominus below rib cage: +/= sudden pain and muscle tensing with deep breath.
  - Kidneys: In supine, place one hand under client between ribs and iliac crest, other hand on abdomen below ribs and ribs pointing in opposite direction: +/− tenderness or reproduction of symptoms.
  - Bladder: Not usually palpable unless distended and raised above pubic bone; in supine, place hand above pubis and press down: +/= tenderness, reproduction of pain, ability to feel the bladder: __+ ___−.

INTERVENTION

- PT intervention is consistent with movement-related problems secondary to GI disorder.
  - Gait training
  - Therapeutic exercise: All relevant categories, energy conservation
    - If stoma from colostomy or ileostomy, avoid activities that cause retraction.
  - Therapeutic activities for bed-mobility training, transfer- and transitional-movement training
  - Neuromuscular re-education

- Self-care training
- Electrical stimulation of rectus/anus in cases of incontinence or lost muscle control/coordination
- Manual therapy
- Massage
- Interprofessional
  - Lifestyle modification
  - Smoking cessation
  - Weight management
  - Dietary counseling
  - Psychological intervention
  - Surgical management
  - Medical management

FUNCTIONAL GOALS

- Patient will be able to
  - Achieve functional aerobic capacity, ability to talk during activity so as to achieve functional gait and activity tolerance for ADLs/IADLs.
  - Achieve 600 m or greater in a 6-minute walk test for initiation of safe, functional gait in the community.
  - Perform active verbalization with increasing taxonomy for safety during gait, including negotiation of even and uneven surfaces, opening and closing doors, transferring in and out of car.
  - Perform activities requiring abdominals with appropriate muscle splinting/guarding to prevent retraction of stoma, if patient has colostomy or ileostomy.
  - Tolerate 30 minutes of continuous, moderate exercise three times a week in ______ weeks, and five times a week in ____________ weeks, depending on the severity of the disease.

PROGNOSIS

- Physician establishes the medical prognosis, as pathology is primarily medical in nature.
- For PT prognosis, goals should be established that the patient can achieve based on their overall condition.
- Prognosis from a PT perspective should be good, unless medical condition is unstable or goals unrealistic.

PATIENT RESOURCE

- Malabsorption syndromes. MedlinePlus, NIH National Institutes of Health. http://www.nlm.nih.gov/medlineplus/malabsorptionsyndromes.html. Accessed August 8, 2014.

REFERENCES

1. Sundaram S, Hoffenberg E, Kramer R, Sondheimer JM, Furuta GT. Gastrointestinal tract. In: Hay WW, Levin MJ, Sondheimer JM, Deterding RR, eds. *CURRENT Diagnosis & Treatment: Pediatrics*. 20th ed. New York, NY: McGraw-Hill; 2011: Chapter 20. http://www.accessphysiotherapy.com/content/6583755. Accessed June 12, 2013.
2. Chandrasoma P, Taylor CR. The Intestines: I. Structure & function; malabsorption syndrome; intestinal obstruction. In: Chandrasoma P, Taylor CR, eds. *Concise Pathology*. 3rd ed. New York, NY: McGraw-Hill; 2011: Chapter 39. http://www.accessphysiotherapy.com/content/189094. Accessed June 12, 2013.

ADDITIONAL REFERENCES

- APTA. *Interactive Guide to Physical Therapist Practice*. http://guidetoptpractice.apta.org/. Accessed June 12, 2013.
- Goodman CC, Fuller KS. *Pathology: Implications for the Physical Therapist*. 3rd ed. St. Louis, MO: Saunders; 2009.
- Goodman CC, Snyder TK. *Differential Diagnosis for Physical Therapists: Screening for Referral*. 4th ed. St. Louis, MO: Saunders Elsevier; 2007.
- McOmber MA, Shulman RJ. Pediatric functional gastrointestinal disorders. *Nutr Clin Prac*. 2008;23(3):268–274.
- Mills JC, Stappenbeck TS, Bunnett N. Gastrointestinal disease. In: McPhee SJ, Hammer GD, eds. *Pathophysiology of Disease: An Introduction to Clinical Medicine*. 6th ed. New York, NY: McGraw-Hill; 2010. http://www.accessphysiotherapy.com/content/5369694. Accessed June 12, 2013.
- Suleiman S, Johnston DE. The abdominal wall: an overlooked source of pain. *Am Fam Physician*. 2001;64(3);431--438. http://www.aafp.org/afp/2001/0801/p431.html
- Ulcerative Colitis. National Digestive Diseases Information Clearinghouse (NDDIC). U.S. Department of Health and Human Services, *NIH Publication No. 12–1597*. Accessed June 12, 2013.
- Watts RL, Standaert D, Obeso JA. Metabolic/nutritional disorders. In: Watts RL, Standaert D, Obeso JA, eds. *Movement Disorders*. 3rd ed. New York, NY: McGraw-Hill; 2012. http://www.accessphysiotherapy.com/content/55806135. Accessed June 12, 2013.

SECTION F GENITOURINARY DISORDERS

44 ERECTILE DYSFUNCTION

Debra F. Stern, DPT, DBA, MSM, PT
Eric Shamus, PhD, DPT, PT, CSCS

CONDITION/DISORDER SYNONYM

- Impotence

ICD-9-CM CODE

- 607.84 Impotence of organic origin

ICD-10-CM CODE

- N52.9 Male erectile dysfunction, unspecified

PREFERRED PRACTICE PATTERN

- As of June, 2014, the *APTA Guide to Physical Therapist Practice* does not include practice patterns for organ system pathology; therefore, associated or secondary musculoskeletal, cardiovascular/pulmonary, or potential neuromuscular patterns are indicated.

PATIENT PRESENTATION

A 60-year-old male patient with a history of type 2 diabetes, hypertension, and recent bilateral lower extremity weakness secondary to a motor vehicle accident, presents as increasingly withdrawn and without enthusiastic participation in his therapy. He is talking less and less, although he is complying with all instructions. When you address the changes observed, he states that his wife is unhappy with his sexual performance, complains that he does not find her attractive and he feels increasingly depressed. He loves his wife and finds her very sexy, but no matter how much he tries, he cannot always maintain an erection and at times is unable to get an erection at all.

KEY FEATURES

Description

- Inability to perform sexually: Inability to form an erection
- Loss of erection from arterial, venous, neurogenic, or psychological reasons
- Physical therapists treat secondary problems: Weakness, gait abnormalities, limited aerobic endurance
- May be acute, postoperative, chronic, or congenital/hereditary; related to medication or other pathology

Essentials of Diagnosis

- Diagnosis is usually based on history; a need for targeted diagnostic procedures if neurogenic causes suspected
- Can have organic or psychosocial basis
  - Organic basis may be an early sign of cardiovascular disease

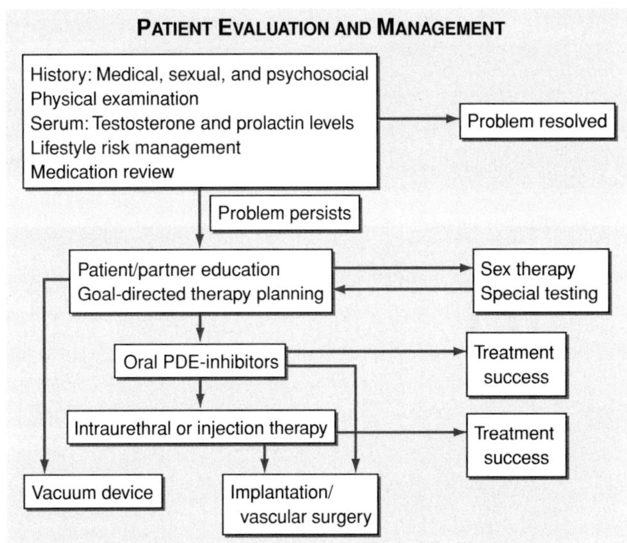

FIGURE 44-1 Algorithm for the evaluation and management of patients with ED. PDE, phosphodiesterase. (From Longo DL, Fauci AS, Kasper DL, Hauser SL, Jameson JL, Loscalzo J, eds. *Harrison's Principles of Internal Medicine.* 18th ed. New York, NY: McGraw-Hill; 2012.)

General Considerations

- Can result from spinal cord injury
- Incidence increases with age
- Psychological pathology

Demographics

- Chronic erectile dysfunction (ED) affects[1]
  - Approximately 4% of men in their 50s
  - Approximately 17% of men in their 60s
  - Approximately 47% of men over the age of 75 years
- Transient ED and inadequate erection
  - Affects approximately 50% of men between the ages of 40 and 70 years

CLINICAL FINDINGS

SIGNS AND SYMPTOMS

- ED: Inability to form or maintain an erection
- Premature ejaculation
- Prostatic enlargement
- Hypertension
- Penile discharge

Functional Implications

- Inability to procreate
- Inability to have an erection, sexual dysfunction

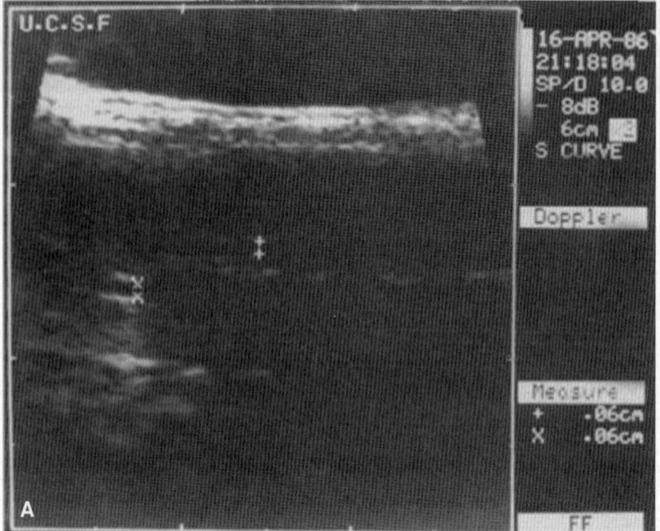

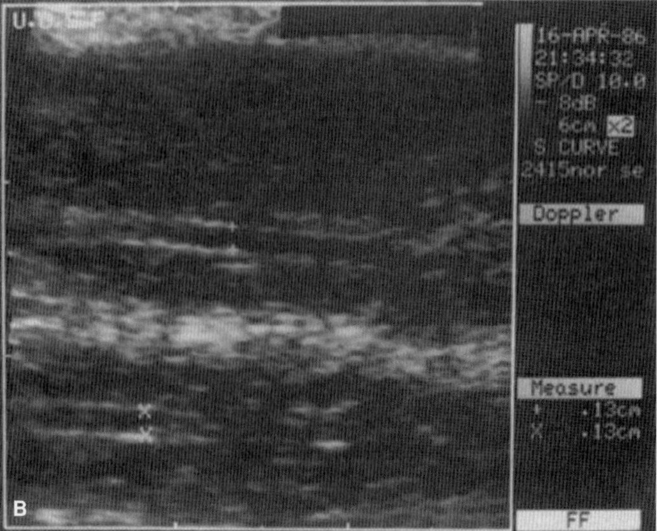

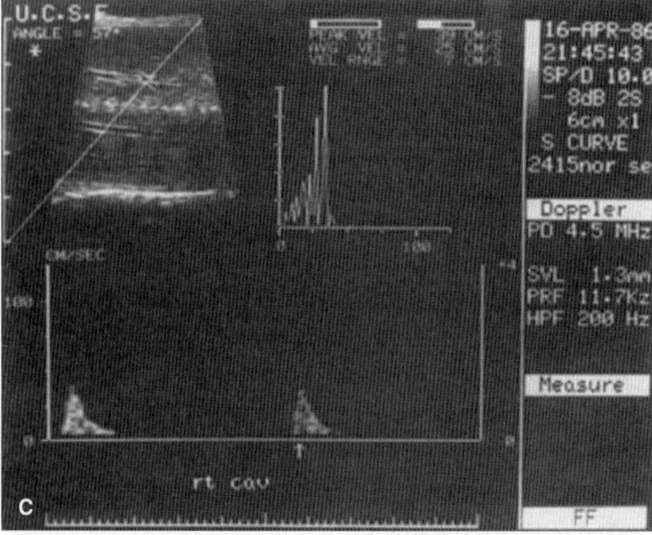

FIGURE 44-2 Duplex ultrasonography and Doppler analysis of the arterial response to intracavernous papaverine injection. In the flaccid state (**A**), the luminal diameter of the cavernous artery is 0.06 cm; after papaverine injection (**B**), this increases to 0.13 cm. Wave analysis (**C**) shows normal flow in the cavernous artery (peak velocity, 39 cm/s). (From Tanagho EA, McAninch WJ. *Smith's General Urology*. 17th ed. www.accessmedicine.com. Copyright © The McGraw-Hill Companies, Inc. All rights reserved.)

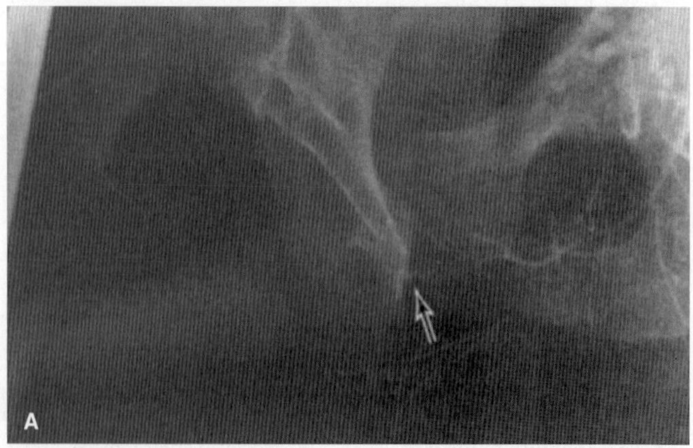

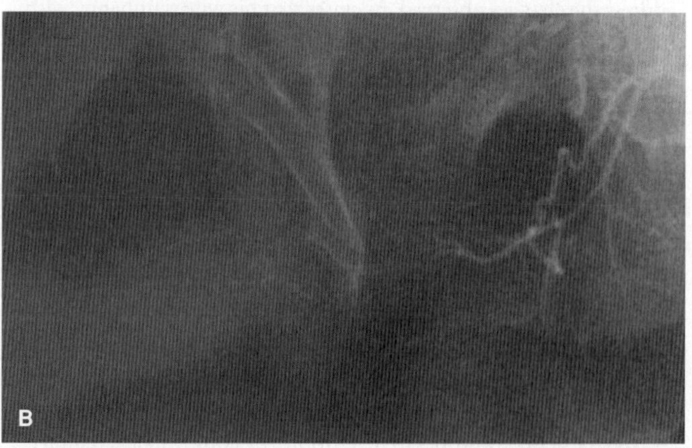

FIGURE 44-3 Internal iliac arteriogram in the flaccid penis (**A**) shows poor visualization of penile arteries, simulating occlusion (*arrow*). After intracavernous injection of 60 mg of papaverine (**B**), all the branches of the penile artery are well visualized. (From Tanagho EA, McAninch WJ. *Smith's General Urology*. 17th ed. www.accessmedicine.com. Copyright © The McGraw-Hill Companies, Inc. All rights reserved.)

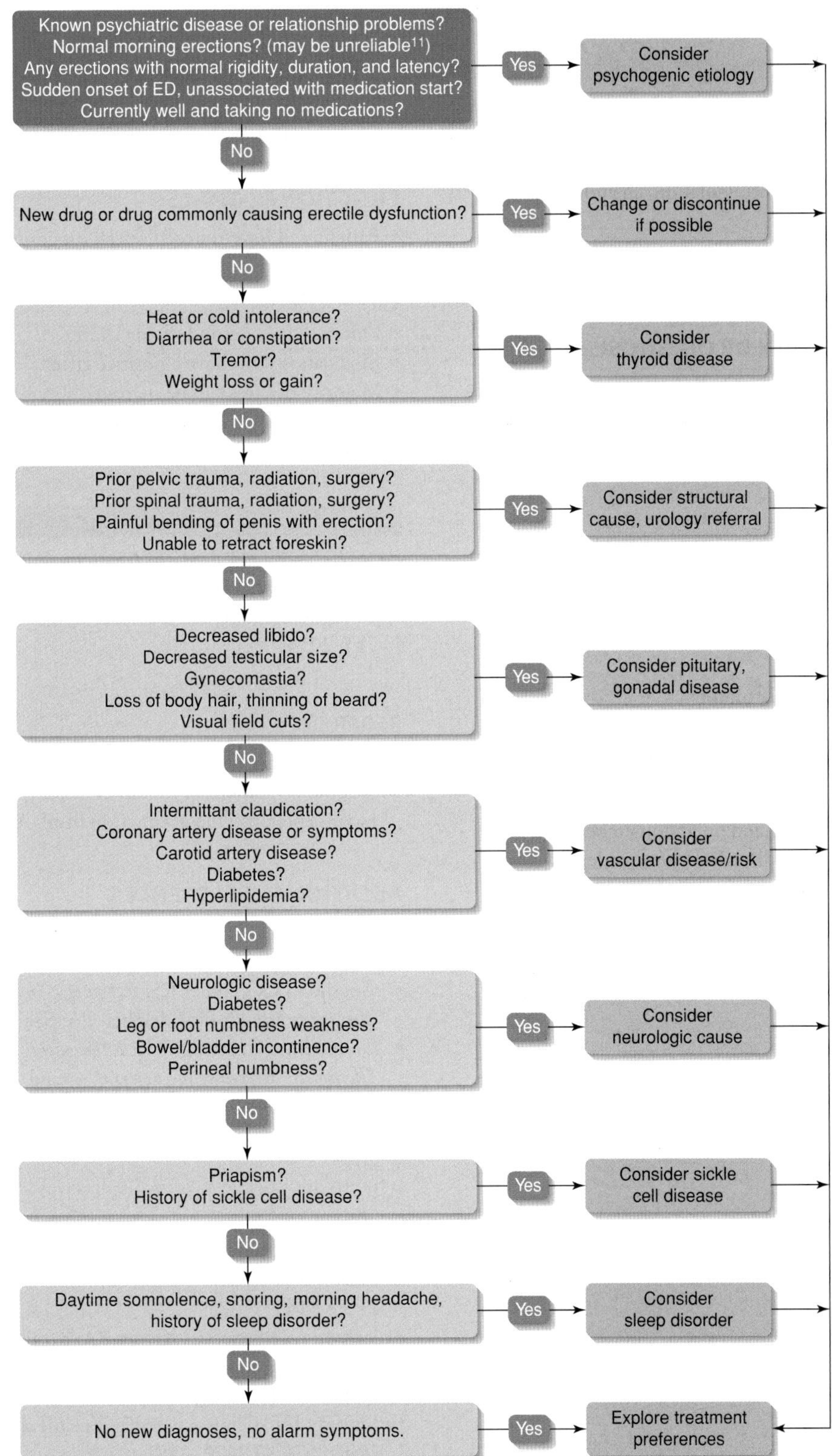

FIGURE 44-4 Diagnostic approach: erectile dysfunction (ED). (Adapted from O'Keefe M, Hunt DK. Assessment and treatment of impotence. *Med Clin North Am.* 1995,79.415–434.)

▸ Possible Contributing Causes

- Urinary tract infection (bacterial or viral)
- Diabetes (type I or II) and associated medications
- Enlarged prostate
- Cardiac and hypertension medications
- Antihypertensive and antidepressant medications
- Damage to nerves, such as with multiple sclerosis, Parkinson's, trauma
- Weak pelvic floor muscles
- Smoking (cancer related)

- Occupational exposures
- Tumors (benign or metastatic)
- Metastases
- Age
- Spinal cord injury or neuromuscular pathology, such as stroke
- Neuropathy
- Postsurgical scarring or adhesions
- Side effect of cancer treatment: Radiation, chemotherapy, surgery

Differential Diagnosis

- Cancer
- Enlarged prostate

MEANS OF CONFIRMATION OR DIAGNOSIS

Laboratory Tests

- Pathogen identification
- Complete blood count
- Urinalysis
- Lipid profile

Imaging

- Radiography
- CT
- MRI
- Ultrasound
- Abdominal scans for possible tumor

Diagnostic Procedures

- Palpation for differential diagnosis
  - Kidneys: In supine, place one hand under client between ribs and iliac crest, other hand on abdomen below ribs and ribs pointing in opposite direction: +/− tenderness or reproduction of symptoms.
  - Bladder (not usually palpable unless distended and raised above pubic bone): In supine, place hand above pubis, press down: +/= tenderness, reproduction of pain, or ability to feel the bladder: __+ __−.
- Electromyography

FINDINGS AND INTERPRETATION

- Radiography for spine involvement
- CT and MRI for spinal involvement, tumor, neurologic

TREATMENT

Medication

- Discontinue medications that may be causal

MEDICAL PROCEDURES

- Penile surgical implants
- Surgical management

IMPAIRMENTS

- Potential depression
- Anxiety
- Inability to perform sexually

INTERVENTION

- Interprofessional
  - Biofeedback
  - Lifestyle modification
  - Smoking cessation
  - Support group
  - Psychological intervention
    - Anxiety or depression
  - Spiritual support

FUNCTIONAL GOALS

- Patient will have restored sexual function

PROGNOSIS

- Differs, based on underlying cause.
- Medications can have a positive effect.
- Majority of cases can be managed successfully.
- Surgical intervention for implantation is highly effective in some cases.

PATIENT RESOURCE

- U.S. National Library of Medicine, National Institute of Health. *Erectile Dysfunction.* MedlinePlus. http://www.nlm.nih.gov/medlineplus/erectiledysfunction.html. Accessed June 13, 2013.

REFERENCE

1. U.S. National Library of Medicine, National Institute of Health. Erectile Dysfunction. MedlinePlus. http://www.nlm.nih.gov/medlineplus/erectiledysfunction.html. Accessed June 13, 2013.

ADDITIONAL REFERENCES

- Basson R, Schultz WW. Sexual sequelae of general medical disorders. *Lancet.* 2007;369(9559):409–424.
- Goodman CC, Fuller KS. *Pathology: Implications for the Physical Therapist.* 3rd ed. Philadelphia, PA: Saunders Elsevier; 2009.
- Goodman CC, Snyder TK. *Differential Diagnosis for Physical Therapists: Screening for Referral.* 4th ed. St. Louis, MO: Saunders Elsevier; 2007.
- ICD9Data.com. http://www.icd9data.com. Accessed June 13, 2013.
- ICD10Data.com. http://www.icd10data.com. Accessed June 13, 2013.
- Jackson G. Prevention of cardiovascular disease by the early identification of erectile dysfunction. *Int J Impot Res.* 2008;20(Suppl 2):S9–S14.
- Jackson G, Rosen RC, Kloner RA, Kostis JB. The second Princeton consensus on sexual dysfunction and cardiac risk: new guidelines for sexual medicine. *J Sex Med.* 2006;3(1):28–36.
- McVary KT. Clinical practice. Erectile dysfunction. *N Engl J Med.* 2007;357(24):2472–2481.
- Smith JF, Caan BJ, Sternfeld B, et al. Racial disparities in erectile dysfunction among participants in the California Men's Health Study. *J Sex Med.* 2009;6(12):3433–3439.
- Tsertsvadze A, Fink HA, Yazdi F, et al. Oral phosphodiesterase-5 inhibitors and hormonal treatments for erectile dysfunction: a systematic review and meta-analysis. *Ann Intern Med.* 2009;151(9):650–661.

SECTION G HEMATOLOGICAL

45 HEMOPHILIA

Kay Tasso, PhD, PT, PCS
Wendy Song, DO

CONDITION/DISORDER SYNONYMS

- Christmas disease
- Classic hemophilia
- Coagulation defects
- Disorders of blood coagulation
- Hemophilia A
- Hemophilia B
- von Willebrand disease

ICD-9-CM CODES[1]

- 286.0 Congenital factor VIII disorder
- 286.1 Congenital factor IX disorder
- 286.2 Congenital factor XI deficiency
- 286.3 Congenital deficiency of other clotting factors
- 286.4 von Willebrand disease

ICD-10-CM CODES[2]

- D66 Hereditary factor VIII deficiency
- D67 Hereditary factor IX deficiency
- D68.0 von Willebrand disease
- D68.1 Hereditary factor XI deficiency
- D86.2 Hereditary deficiency of other clotting factors

PREFERRED PRACTICE PATTERN[3]

- 4D: Impaired Joint Mobility, Motor Function, Muscle Performance, and Range of Motion Associated with Connective Tissue Dysfunction

PATIENT PRESENTATION

A 12-year-old male presents with right knee pain and swelling after being tackled with a planted right leg during a youth league football game. Family history is significant for a bleeding disorder in his paternal uncle. Vitals are Temperature: 98.4°F, Pulse: 87, Respirations: 20, Blood Pressure: 110/72, and SpO_2% of 98%. Physical examination of the right knee demonstrates swelling, tenderness along the medial joint line, pain with valgus deviation. Lab tests show a prolonged partial prothrombin time, normal prothrombin time, normal bleeding time, and decreased factor VIII.

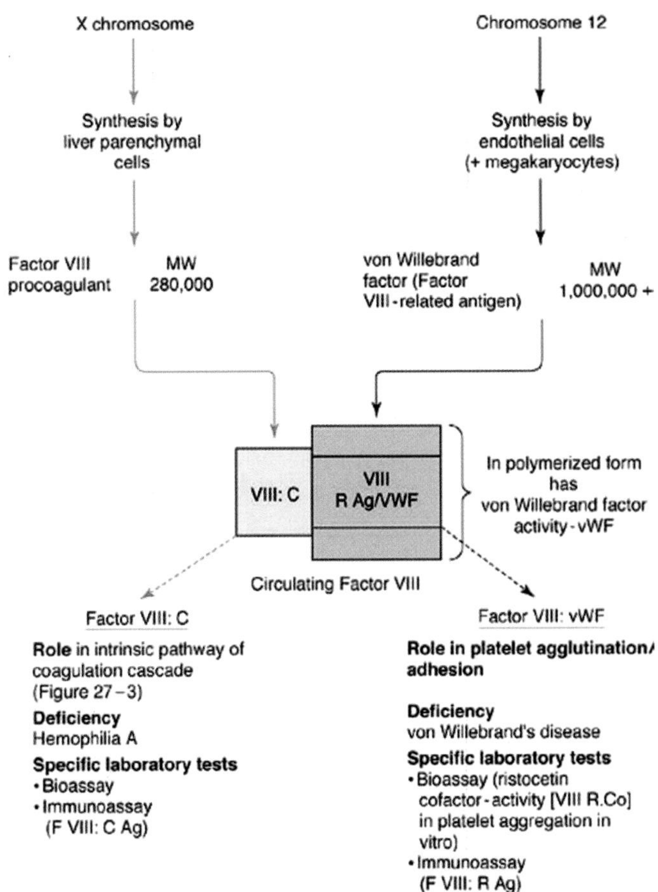

FIGURE 45-1 Structure and inheritance of the factor VIII molecule. The function, the result of deficiency, and the method of testing of the various components are also shown. (From Chandrasoma P, Taylor CR. *Concise Pathology*, 3rd ed. http://www.accessmedicine.com. Copyright © The McGraw-Hill Companies, Inc. All rights reserved.)

KEY FEATURES

Description

- Disorders involving slower than normal blood clotting that occurs spontaneously or as an excessive response to injury leading to bleeding into joints (termed hemarthrosis) or tissues

Essentials of Diagnosis

- Factor VIII deficiency is the most common clotting deficiency
- Severity of hemophilia, plasma level of factor VIII or IX
  - Mild: More than 5%
  - Moderate: Between 1% and 5%
  - Severe: Less than 1%

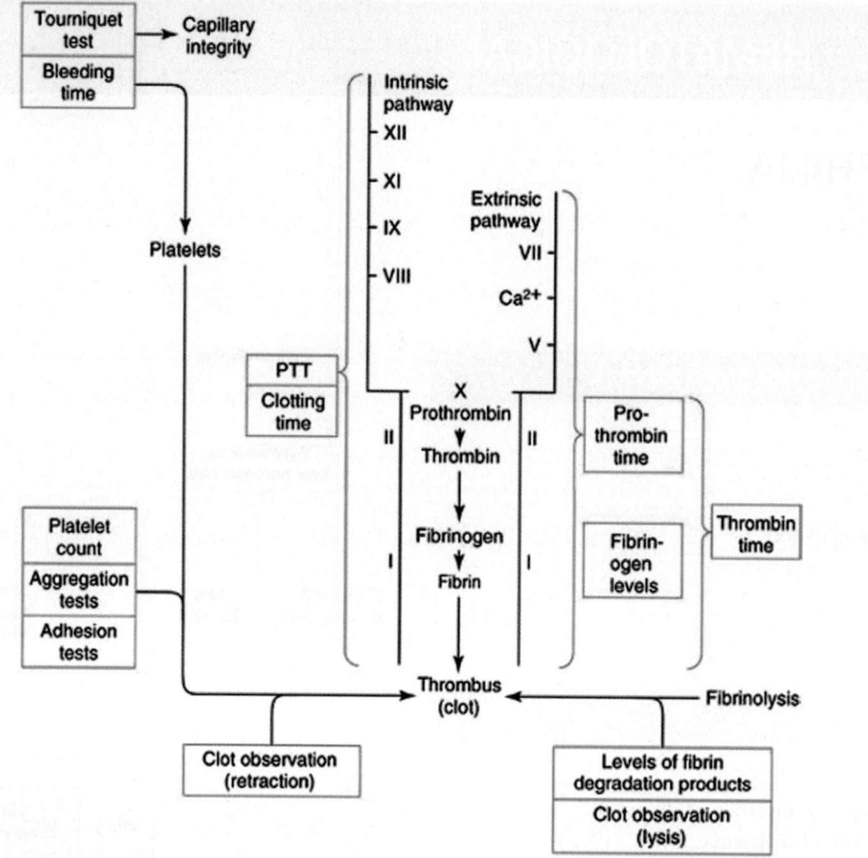

FIGURE 45-2 Tests used clinically to detect abnormalities in the blood coagulation and fibrinolytic systems. PTT, partial thromboplastin time. (From Chandrasoma P, Taylor CR. *Concise Pathology*, 3rd ed. http://www.accessmedicine.com. Copyright © The McGraw-Hill Companies, Inc. All rights reserved.)

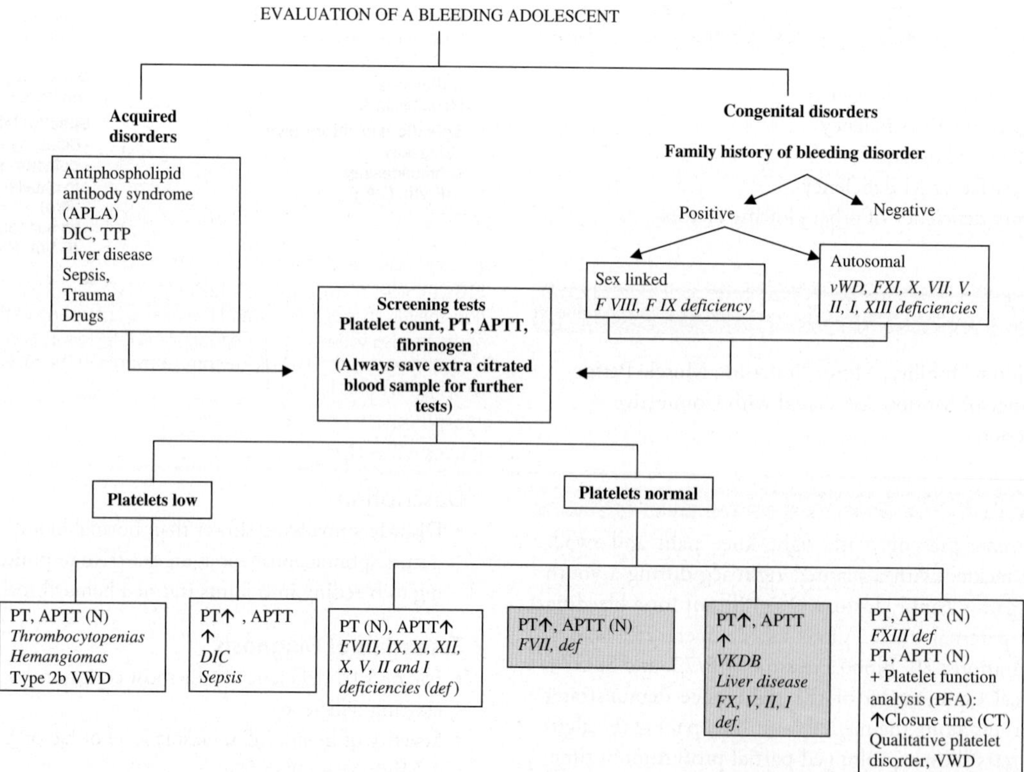

FIGURE 45-3 Evaluation of bleeding patient. Screening tests assess the degree of hemorrhage and the adequacy of hemostasis in a bleeding patient. (Used with permission from Kulkarni R, Gera R, Scott-Emuakpor AB. Adolescent hematology. In: Greydanus DE, Patel DR, Pratt HD, eds. *Essential Adolescent Medicine*. New York, NY: McGraw Hill; 2006:371–390.)

General Considerations

- Genetic factor deficiencies occur almost exclusively in males with females as asymptomatic carriers
- Hemophilia classified as mild (asymptomatic), moderate (excessive bleeding after minor injury), or severe
- Bleeding into joint results in fibrosis
- von Willebrand disease results in bleeding into skin or mucous membranes rather than joints or muscles

Demographics

- Inheritance
- Factor VIII deficiency occurs in 1 of every 5000 to 10,000 males
- Factor IX deficiency occurs in 1 of every 50,000 people[4]
- von Willebrand disease is the most common bleeding disorder in Caucasians[5]
- von Willebrand disease is seen in both males and females[6]

CLINICAL FINDINGS

SIGNS AND SYMPTOMS

- Pain
- Erythema
- Edema
- Bruises easily
- Bleeding into joints or muscles without a history of injury
- Excessive bleeding that results from injury

Functional Implications

- Joint contractures
- Hematoma of muscles can cause compartment syndrome[5]

Possible Contributing Causes

- Genetic x-linked recessive (such as factor VIII, or IX deficiencies) or autosomal dominant disorder (such as von Willebrand disease)
- Multiple episodes of bleeding in the same joint can cause hemophilic arthritis (hemarthropathy)[6]

Differential Diagnosis

- Platelet disorder

TABLE 45-1 Blood Coagulation Factors[a]

Factor	Name	Source
Factor I	Fibrinogen	Liver
Factor II	Prothrombin	Liver[b]
Factor III	Tissue thromboplastin	
Factor IV	Calcium	
Factor V	Proaccelerin; labile factor	Liver
Factor VI	Obsolete; activated factor V	
Factor VII	Proconvertin; stable factor	Liver[b]
Factor VIII	Antihemophilic globulin (AHG)	Vascular endothelial cell
Factor IX	Plasma thromboplastin; component (PTC); Christmas factor	Liver[b]
Factor X	Stuart–Prower factor	Liver[b]
Factor XI	Plasma thromboplastin antecedent (PTA)	Liver
Factor XII	Hageman factor	Uncertain
Factor XIII	Fibrin-stabilizing factor	Platelets

[a]These factors occur in an inactive form in plasma. When they are activated, they are designated by the letter "a" after the Roman numeral (eg, VIII and VIIIa).
[b]The synthesis of factors VII, IX, X, and prothrombin in the liver is dependent on the presence of vitamin K.
Source: Chandrasoma P, Taylor CR. *Concise Pathology*, 3rd ed. http://www.accessmedicine.com.

MEANS OF CONFIRMATION OR DIAGNOSIS

Laboratory Tests

- Platelet count
- Clotting time
- Bleeding time
- Prothrombin time

TABLE 45-2 Diseases Resulting from an Inherited Coagulation Factor Deficiency

Deficient Factor	Disease	Inheritance	Frequency[a]	Disease Severity
Fibrinogen	Afibrinogenemia	AR	Rare	Variable
	Congenital dysfibrinogenemia	AD	Rare	Variable
Prothrombin	. . .	. . .	Very rare	Variable
Factor V	Parahemophilia	AR	Very rare	Moderate to severe
Factor VII	. . .	AR	Very rare	Moderate to severe
Factor VIII	Hemophilia A	XR	Common	Mild to severe
	von Willebrand disease	AD	Common	Mild to moderate
Factor IX	Hemophilia B	XR	Uncommon	Mild to severe
Factor X	. . .	AR	Rare	Variable
Factor XI	Rosenthal syndrome	AR	Uncommon	Mild
Factor XII	Hageman trait	AR/AD	Rare	Asymptomatic
Factor XIII	. . .	AR	Rare	Severe

AR, autosomal recessive; AD, autosomal dominant; XR, X–linked recessive.
[a]Frequency: Very rare, fewer than 100 reported cases; compare to hemophilia A, with a frequency of 1:10,000 males.
Source: Chandrasoma P, Taylor CR. *Concise Pathology*, 3rd ed. http://www.accessmedicine.com.

TABLE 45-3 Major Bleeding Disorders: Differential Laboratory Features

	Tourniquet Test	Bleeding Time	Whole Blood Clotting Time	Platelet Count	Partial Thromboplastin Time (PTT)	Prothrombin Time (PT)	Comments
Vascular Defects	+	↑ or N	N	N	N	N	
Platelet Defects							
Thrombocytopenia	+	↑	N	↓	N	N	Abnormal clot retraction.
Platelet function defects	+	↑	N	N	N	N	See Table 27-4.
Coagulation Defects							
Hemophilia A	N	N	↑	N	↑	N	VIII:C ↓ VIII:RAg and VIII:vWF normal.
von Willebrand disease	+ or N	↑	↑ or N	N	↑	N	VIII:C ↓VIII:RAg ↓ VIII:vWF ↓abnormal ristocetin test.
Christmas disease (hemophilia B)	N	N	↑	N	↑	N	IX ↓
Deficiency of vitamin K-dependent factors (II, VII, IX, X)	N	N	↑ or N	N	↑	↑	Corrected by vitamin K therapy.
Liver diseases	N	N	↑ or N	N	↑	↑	Not corrected by vitamin K.
Disorders of Fibrinolysis							
Disseminated intravascular coagulation	+ or N	↑	↑	↓	↑	↑	Presence of fibrin degradation products; positive protamine sulfate test.
Primary fibrinolysis	N	N	↑	N	↑	↑	

Source: Chandrasoma P, Taylor CR. *Concise Pathology,* 3rd ed. http://www.accessmedicine.com.

- Partial thromboplastin time
- Thrombin time
- DNA analysis
- Factor assays
- Fibrinogen test

▶ Imaging

- Standard radiograph for hemarthropathy
- Magnetic resonance imaging (MRI) or computerized axial tomography (CT scan) for head trauma or organ involvement

FINDINGS AND INTERPRETATION

- Factor VIII deficiency: Prolonged partial thromboplastin time, normal prothrombin, and bleeding times
- von Willebrand disease: Prolonged partial thromboplastin and bleeding times, normal prothrombin time

TREATMENT

▶ Medications

- Injection or infusion of blood concentrate of the deficient factor
- Desmopressin acetate for von Willebrand disease[5] or factor VIII deficiency[7]
- Amicar

MEDICAL PROCEDURES[6]

- Synovectomy
- Arthroscopy
- Arthrodesis

REFERRALS/ADMITTANCE

- Admission due to uncontrolled bleeding or bleeding involving head trauma or organs
- Geneticist
- Hematologist

IMPAIRMENTS

- Pain
- Edema
- Decreased range of motion
- Decreased strength

TESTS AND MEASURES

- Goniometer
- Circumferential measurements
- Manual muscle testing
- Dynamometer
- 6-minute walk test

INTERVENTION

- Avoid passive range of motion[7]
- Therapeutic exercises
  - Active range of motion
  - Strengthening
  - Isometrics
  - Gentle stretching
- Modalities to treat pain and inflammation
- Cardiovascular exercise or non-contact sports such as swimming, golf, ice skating, or bicycling
- Splints or braces

TABLE 45-4 Tests Used to Evaluate Hemorrhagic (Bleeding) Disorders. (See Also Figure 45-2.)

Platelet Count And Morphology

Clotting Time

(Whole blood coagulation time): The time taken for the patient's blood to clot in a test tube (normal, 5–10 minutes). Very insensitive test; even severe abnormalities may be missed.

Clot Observation

The formed clot is observed for 24 hours; failure of clot retraction in 1–4 hours indicates thrombocytopenia or abnormal platelet function. Clot fragmentation or lysis indicates excessive fibrinolysis.

Bleeding Time

(Normal, 3–8 minutes): The time taken for a standardized skin puncture to stop bleeding. It is not a test of coagulation. Rather, it tests the ability of the vessels to vasoconstrict and the platelets to form a hemostatic plug.

Tourniquet Test

Inflation of blood pressure cuff above diastolic pressure for 5 minutes produces scattered petechiae in some normal persons, but the presence of numerous (100 or more) petechiae indicates capillary fragility, thrombocytopenia, or platelet abnormalities.

Prothrombin Time[a] (PT)

The time taken for clotting to occur when tissue thromboplastin (brain extract) and calcium are added to the patient's plasma (normal, approximately 12 s; 100% when expressed as a percentage of control). Tests for adequate amounts of factors V, VII, X, prothrombin and fibrinogen, that is, the extrinsic pathway (see Figure 46-2).

Partial Thromboplastin Time[a]

(PTT; also known as the kaolin-cephalin clotting time [KCCT]): The time taken for clotting when surface activation of factor XII is effected by Kaolin (cephalin provides platelet factors; normal, 40–50 s). Tests the adequacy of the intrinsic pathway (factors XII, XI, IX, VIII, X, V, prothrombin, and fibrinogen; see Figure 46-2).

Thrombin Time (TT)

The time taken for clotting to occur when thrombin is added to the patient's plasma (normal, <15 s). It tests the conversion of fibrinogen to fibrin and depends on adequate fibrinogen levels.

Tests for Circulating Anticoagulants

Should be performed if PT or PTT is abnormal.

Tests for Specific Factors

Measure levels of factor VIII, factor IX, etc.

Measurements of Fibrinogen Levels and Fibrin Degradation Products

Assesses fibrinolysis and disseminated intravascular coagulation.

Protamine Sulfate Test

Detects fibrin monomer and is good evidence for the presence of disseminated intravascular coagulation.

[a]The prothrombin time and the partial thromboplastin time are the two tests used most extensively for screening purposes.

Source: Chandrasoma P, Taylor CR. *Concise Pathology,* 3rd ed. http://www.accessmedicine.com.

TABLE 45-5 Characteristics and Differences between Hemophilias and von Willebrand Disease

	Hemophilia A	Hemophilia B	von Willebrand Disease
Incidence	1:5,000	1:30,000	1%–3% of US population
Abnormality	Factor (F) VIII deficiency. Normal levels: 50%–150%	F IX deficiency Normal levels: 50%–150%	vWF abnormality
Inheritance	X-linked, affects males Gene at the tip of X-chromosome	X-linked, affects males	Autosomal dominant (gene on chromosome 12). Affects males and females
Site of production	Unknown	Liver, vitamin K-depended protein	Megakaryocytes and endothelial cells
Function of protein	Cofactor; forms "tenase" complex with FIX and activate FX	Clotting protein (zymogen). Activated by F XI or VIIa and forms a "tenase" complex with FVIII and activates FX	Platelet adhesion, protection of F VIII
Classification (normal plasma levels of FIII and IX = 50%–150%)	Mild (>5%) Moderate (1%–5%) Severe (<1%)	Mild (>5%) Moderate (1%–5%) Severe (<1%)	Types 1 Type 2 (2A, 2B, 2M, 2N) Type 3
Clinical manifestations	Positive family history (30% new mutation). Hemarthroses, hematomas, intracranial hemorrhages, hematuria, gastrointestinal hemorrhage, and so forth	Positive family history (30% new mutation). Milder disease, though identical hemorrhage sites as hemophilia A	Positive family history Mucocutaneous (epistaxis, menorrhagia, postdental bleeding). Type 3 may present as hemophilia A
PFA/Bleeding time	Normal	Normal	May be prolonged
PT	Normal	Normal	Normal
APTT	Prolonged	Prolonged	Prolonged or normal
F VIII assay	Decreased or absent	Normal	↓ or Normal
F IX assay	Normal	Decreased or absent	Normal
vWF: antigen	Normal	Normal	Decreased or absent (type 3)
vWF R: Co	Normal	Normal	Decreased or abnormal
vWF multimers	Normal	Normal	Normal or abnormal
Specific treatment	Recombinant (r) F VIII (preferred), virally safe plasma derived concentrates	Recombinant F IX, virally safe plasma derived concentrates	DDAVP (intranasal or intravenous) vWF concentrates (plasma derived)
Inhibitor patients	rFVIIa, FEIBA	rFVIIa	Rare
Adjunct treatment	Antifibrinolytics	Antifibrinolytics	Oral contraceptives, antifibrinolytics

Source: Kulkarni R, Gera R, Scott-Emuakpor AB. Adolescent hematology. In: Greydanus DE, Patel DR, Pratt HD, eds. *Essential Adolescent Medicine*. New York, NY: McGraw Hill; 2006:371–390.

FUNCTIONAL GOALS

- Patient will be able to
  - Increase active knee flexion to 120 degrees for independent stair climbing within 2 months.
  - Decrease pain in elbow to less than 3 out of 10 to allow sleeping through the night within 2 weeks.
  - Increase shoulder strength to 4/5 so that patient can shampoo and brush own hair within 6 weeks.
  - Decrease edema in knee to allow for independent transfer from sitting to standing within 4 weeks.
  - Increase cardiovascular fitness by riding stationary bike 20 minutes at 75% target heart rate.

TABLE 45-6 Severity of Hemophilia

Severity	Plasma Level of Factor VIII or IX
Mild	More than 5%
Moderate	Between 1% and 5%
Severe	Less than 1%

Source: Patel DR, Greydanus DE, Baker RJ. *Pediatric Practice: Sports Medicine*. www.accesspediatrics.com.

TABLE 45-7 Canadian Hemophilia Society Guidelines for Sport Participation

Sport	Risk of Sport	Joints Involved (Ranked in Descending Order of Involvement)	Degree of Stress to Joints	Recommended Equipment	Additional Comments
Swimming	Very low	Shoulders	+	None	Swimming is a low-risk sport assuming no diving is involved.
□	□	□	□	□	Stress to joints is directly related to intensity and duration of swimming.
□	□	□	□	□	Whipkick may irritate knees.
Waterskiing	High	Knees	+++	Life jacket	Very stressful on muscles.
□	□	Shoulders	++	□	□
□	□	Elbows	++	□	The overall risk is high because of outside forces over which skier has no control (e.g., speed at which he hits the water, being hit by a ski).
Windsurfing	Medium	Spine	++	Life jacket	Lessons useful initially to learn proper technique. High winds increase risk especially if inexperienced.
□	□	Shoulders	++	□	□
□	□	Elbows	+	□	□
Golf	Low	Shoulders	+	Appropriate footwear	□
□	□	Elbows	+	□	□
□	□	Knees	+	□	□
Tennis	Low	Knees	++	Tennis shoes	□
□	□	Ankles	++	□	□
□	□	Elbows	+	□	□
Squash/Racquetball	Medium	Knees	+++	Appropriate footwear	Protective eyeglasses. Contact with ball, racquet could be harmful.
□	□	Ankles	+++	□	□
□	□	Elbows	++	□	□
□	□	Shoulders	++	□	□
Volleyball	Low/Medium	Knees	++	Knee pads	Increased risk with higher level of competition.
□	□	Hands (fingers/wrists)	++	High-top running shoes	□
□	□	Ankles	+	□	□
Basketball	Low/Medium	Knees	+++	High-top running shoes	High-top running shoes may prevent ankle sprains. Knee pads provide some form of cushioning when falling on knees.
□	□	Ankles	+++	□	□
□	□	Fingers	++	Knee pads	□
Baseball	Medium	Shoulders	++	Knee pads	Higher risk of soft tissue injuries

(continued)

TABLE 45-7 Canadian Hemophilia Society Guidelines for Sport Participation (*Continued*)

Sport	Risk of Sport	Joints Involved (Ranked in Descending Order of Involvement)	Degree of Stress to Joints	Recommended Equipment	Additional Comments
□	□	Knees	++	Appropriate footwear	□
□	□	Elbows	++	□	□
□	□	Ankles	++	Helmet (batting)	□
Soccer	Medium	Ankles	+++	Appropriate footwear	Higher risk of soft tissue injuries
□	□	Knees	++	□	□
□	□	Hips	++	Shin pads	□
Football (tackle)	High	Knees	+++	Helmet	High risk of head injuries and traumatic bleeds because of repeated heavy physical contact in tackle football.
□	□	Ankles	+++	Protective pads	□
□	□	Shoulders	+++	□	□
Rugby	High	Knees	+++	Generally not used in this sport	Harmful because of high risk of physical contact.
□	□	Ankles	+++	□	□
□	□	Shoulders	+++	□	□
□	□	□	□	□	Increased risk of head injury and jarring injury to the spine.
Weight lifting	Medium	Elbows	+++	□	Proper lifting techniques can lessen risk of injury.
□	□	Shoulders	+++	□	□
□	□	Back	+++	□	□
□	□	□	□	□	Recommended lifting through mid-range only. Increase number of repetitions rather than weight. Train regularly. Not recommended for young children.
Skating	Low	Knees	++	Proper fitting skates with good ankle support.	Helmet is advisable during initial learning period. Knee pads or snow pants.
□	□	Ankles	++	□	□
Skateboarding	High	Knees	+++	Helmet	Risk of fracture and head injury owing to falling.
□	□	Ankles	+++	Knee and elbow pads	□
Roller skating/Roller blading	High	Spine	Stress on joints related to falling.	Helmet	Risk of injury is high owing to risk of falling on hard surfaces. Rough surfaces, hills, and ramps increase risk.
□	□	□	□	Knee, elbow and shin pads	□
Road hockey	Medium	Knees	++	Helmet and knee pads may be beneficial.	Contact with stick and other players could be harmful.
□	□	Ankles	++	□	□

Ice hockey	High	Knees	+++	Proper fitting skates with good ankle support.	Contact with puck, stick, boards, other players could be harmful.
□	□	Shoulders	+++	□	□
□	□	Ankles	++	□	□
□	□	□	□	Protective padding (shoulder, elbows, knees).	□
□	□	□	□	Helmet	□
Nordic skiing (cross-country)	Low/Medium	Knees	++	Skis and poles of appropriate length.	The difficulty of the course will directly affect the degree of stress on joints and overall risk such as risk of falling.
□	□	Ankles	++	□	□
□	□	Shoulders	+	□	□
□	□	□	□	Boots with good support.	□
Alpine skiing (downhill)	High	Knees	+++	Helmet	Appropriate length of skis and poles. The risk of head injury is high owing to the inherent risk of falling at high speeds.
□	□	□	□	Ski boots	□
Horseback riding	High	Spine	++	Helmet	The risk of head injury and serious muscle or joint injury is high owing to the possibility of falling off or being thrown from the horse. Jumping should be avoided.
Bicycling	Low	Knees	+	Properly adjusted bike with seat at proper height.	To minimize stress on knees: □□1.□□□ Keep seat high. □□2.□□□ Avoid hills. □□3.□□□ Stay in lower gears. □□4.□□□ Pedal at high revolution (80–100/min).
□	□	□	□	Bicycle helmet.	□
□	□	□	□	Toe straps.	□
Running	Low/Medium	Ankles	++	Appropriate footwear (need good shock absorption, firm heel-counter, arch support).	Running surface (e.g., concrete or uneven ground) will affect risk. Intensity of running (such as distance, speed, frequency) will also affect risk.
□	□	Knees	□	□	□
Karate/Judo	Medium/High	Knees	++	□	None. If there is contact, the risk of injury is high. Without contact, the training can be good for improving muscle flexibility, coordination, and balance.
□	□	Elbow	++	□	□
□	□	Ankles	+	□	□

Scale: +, Low degree of stress; ++, Moderate degree of stress; +++, High degree of stress.
Source: Canadian Hemophilia Society. http://www.hemophila.ca.

TABLE 45-8 When to Refer

When to Consult Hematologist
Bleeding disorders
Sickle cell disease and other hemoglobinopathies
Thrombotic disorders and thrombophilia
Thrombocytopenias
Severe iron deficiency anemia with complications
Chronic anemia not responding to treatment
Hemolytic anemias
Aplastic anemias

Source: Patel DR, Greydanus DE, Baker RJ. *Pediatric Practice: Sports Medicine.* www.accesspediatrics.com.

PROGNOSIS

- Death can occur due to intracranial hemorrhage.
- von Willebrand disease: Normal life expectancy.

PATIENT RESOURCES

- Hemophilia. Centers for Disease Control and Prevention. http://www.cdc.gov/ncbddd/hemophilia/treatment.html. Accessed June 21, 2013.
- Pediatric Von Willebrand Disease. Medscape. http://emedicine.medscape.com/article/959825-overview#a0199. Accessed June 21, 2013.

REFERENCES

1. ICD9DATA. http://www.icd9data.com. Accessed June 19, 2013.
2. ICD10DATA. http://www.icd10data.com/ICD10CM/Codes/D50-D89/D65-D69. Accessed June 20, 2013.
3. The American Physical Therapy Association. *Interactive Guide to Physical Therapist Practice*. Alexandria, VA: The American Physical Therapy Association; 2003. http://guidetoptpractice.apta.org/. Accessed June 20, 2013.
4. Chandrasoma P, Taylor CR. Blood coagulation. In: Chandrasoma P, Taylor CR, eds. *Concise Pathology*. 3rd ed. New York, NY: McGraw-Hill; 2011. http://www.accessphysiotherapy.com/content/187371. Accessed June 20, 2013.
5. Hay WW, Levin MJ, Deterding RR, Abzug MJ, Sondheimer JM. Bleeding disorders. In: Hay WW, Levin MJ, Deterding RR, Abzug MJ, Sondheimer JM, eds. *CURRENT Diagnosis & Treatment: Pediatrics*. 21st ed. New York, NY: McGraw-Hill; 2012. http://www.accessphysiotherapy.com/content/56826831. Accessed June 20, 2013.
6. Mulvaney R, Zucker-Levin AR, Jeng M, et al. Effects of 6-week individualized, supervised exercise program for people with bleeding disorders and hemophiliac arthritis. *Physical Therapy*. 2010;90(4):509–526. http://ptjournal.apta.org./content/90/4/509.full.pdf+html?sid=2ef7785a-7a68-425a-b7e9-adc8d8de52cd. Accessed May 4, 2014.
7. Patel DR. Chapter 16. Hematologic conditions. In: Patel DR, Greydanus DE, Baker RJ, eds. *Pediatric Practice: Sports Medicine*. New York, NY: McGraw-Hill; 2009. http://www.accessphysiotherapy.com/content/6976199. Accessed June 20, 2013.

ADDITIONAL REFERENCE

- Dutton M. Physical therapy roles for specific pediatric pathologies. In: Dutton M, ed. *McGraw-Hill's NPTE (National Physical Therapy Examination)*. 2nd ed. New York, NY: McGraw-Hill; 2012. http://www.accessphysiotherapy.com/content/56513738. Accessed June 20, 2013.

SECTION H IMMUNOLOGICAL DISORDERS

46 GOUT

Debra F. Stern, DPT, DBA, MSM, PT
Eric Shamus, PhD, DPT, PT, CSCS
Greg W. Hartley, DPT, PT, GCS, CEEAA

CONDITION/DISORDER SYNONYMS

- Hyperuricemia
- Tophaceous gout
- Gouty arthritis

ICD-9-CM CODES

- 274.9 Gout, unspecified
- 315.4 Coordination disorder (clumsiness, dyspraxia and/or specific motor development disorder)
- 718.03 Articular cartilage disorder, forearm
- 718.04 Articular cartilage disorder, hand
- 718.07 Articular cartilage disorder, ankle and foot
- 719.39 Palindromic rheumatism involving multiple sites
- 719.4 Pain in joint
- 729.1 Myalgia and myositis, unspecified
- 736.9 Acquired deformity of limb
- Physical therapy diagnoses/treatment diagnoses that may be associated with Rheumatologic disorders affecting movement
  - 718.45 Contracture of joint; pelvic region and thigh
  - 719.70 Difficulty in Walking
  - 728.89 Other disorders of muscle, ligament, and fascia
  - 728.2 Muscular wasting and disuse atrophy
  - 729.9 Other disorders of soft tissue
  - 781.2 Abnormality of gait: Ataxic, paralytic, spastic, staggering
  - 782.3 Edema

ICD-10-CM CODE

- M10.9 Gout, unspecified

PREFERRED PRACTICE PATTERNS

- 4D: Impaired Joint Mobility, Motor Function, Muscle Performance, and Range of Motion Associated with Connective Tissue Dysfunction[1]
- 4E: Impaired Joint Mobility, Motor Function, Muscle Performance, and Range of Motion Associated with Localized Inflammation
- 7B: Impaired Integumentary Integrity Associated with Superficial Skin Involvement

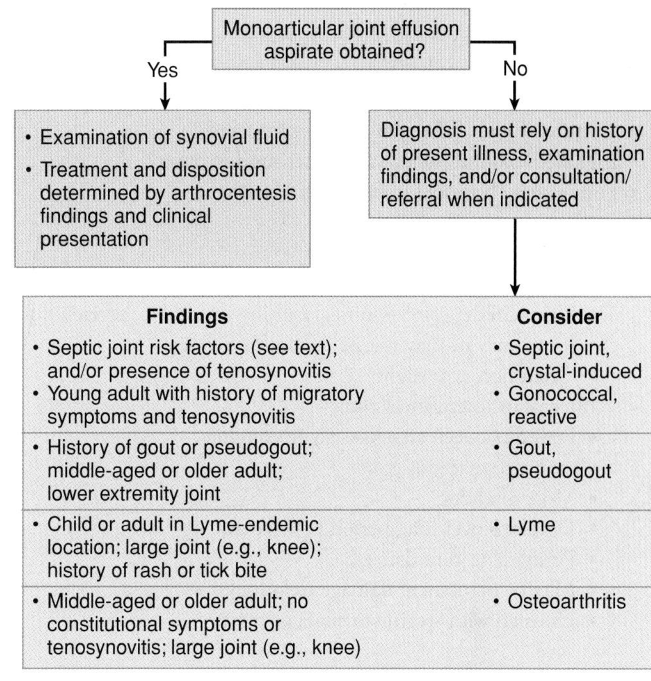

FIGURE 46-1 Diagnostic algorithm for the nontraumatic, acute monoarticular arthritis patient. Common, acute diagnoses and disease presentations are included in this algorithm. Patients may have uncommon disease presentation, overlapping diagnoses (e.g., gout and septic joint), or illnesses not included in the algorithm. (From Tintinalli JE, Stapczynski JS, Ma OJ, et al. *Tintinalli's Emergency Medicine: A Comprehensive Study Guide*, 7th ed. www.accessmedicine.com. Copyright © The McGraw-Hill Companies, Inc. All rights reserved.)

PATIENT PRESENTATION

A 69-year-old male presents to the outpatient physical therapy clinic with complaints of pain (8/10) in the right great toe. The pain appeared suddenly over the past 2 days. Upon examination, you find redness and erythema of the right great toe, pain localized to the great toe, especially in the metatarsal–phalangeal joint, which is worse at night. He has a clear difficulty in walking due to the pain. The patient is moderately obese, diabetic, has sleep apnea, and reports he consumes two alcoholic beverages per day. No lab values are available and other historical information is noncontributory.

KEY FEATURES

Description

- Gout is a form of arthritis that is caused by uric acid (sodium urate) buildup in the blood, resulting in crystal formation that can inflame the joints.

- Considered a rheumatic condition because it involves the joints
- Joint pain: Often in great toe, knee or ankle; episodic but may last for long periods of time
- Sudden onset: May be over a course of a day, and frequently with severe pain at night
- Edema
- Soft tissue pain surrounding affected joints
- Kidney dysfunction

Essentials of Diagnosis

- Must be made by a physician and confirmed by medical diagnostic testing
- Acute or chronic
- Elevated uric acid levels (hyperuricemia) based on lab values
- Synovial fluid samples from inflamed joints with presence of uric acid
- Culture of joint fluid if infections suspected
- Inflamed, painful joints with rather sudden onset
- Four stages (National Institutes of Health)
  - Asymptomatic hyperuricemia
    - Elevated uric acid levels only
  - Acute gout or acute gouty arthritis
    - Uric acid deposits in joints resulting in sudden, severe pain
    - Joints may or may not be red and or tender
    - Often occurs at night
  - Interval or intercritical gout
    - Period between attacks—asymptomatic
  - Chronic tophaceous gout
    - Most disabling
    - Develops over long period (~10 years)
    - Permanent joint damage
    - May be permanent damage to kidneys
    - Unusual with treatment/management

General Considerations

- Differential diagnosis may take time and require intensive medical diagnostic testing as gout must be differentiated from other conditions that present similarly.
- May be misdiagnosed or confused with pseudogout, which presents similarly but deposits are phosphate crystals in pseudogout.
- May result in secondary problems such as aerobic capacity and muscle-endurance impairment, sarcopenia, weakness/impaired muscle performance, musculoskeletal problems, neuromuscular problems, indicating the need for physical therapy intervention depending on severity of attack over time.
- Can be disabling.
- May occur once, episodically or become chronic.
- Presence of tophi under the skin especially around joints and ear rim.
- Often presents in a single joint: Great toe, ankle, or knee with sudden onset.

Demographics

- Males more likely than females (more rare in women before menopause)
- Estimates are six million adults
- Most common inflammatory arthritis in males between 40 and 50
- Can affect individuals of all ages, although rare in children
- Some indication of genetic familial tendency

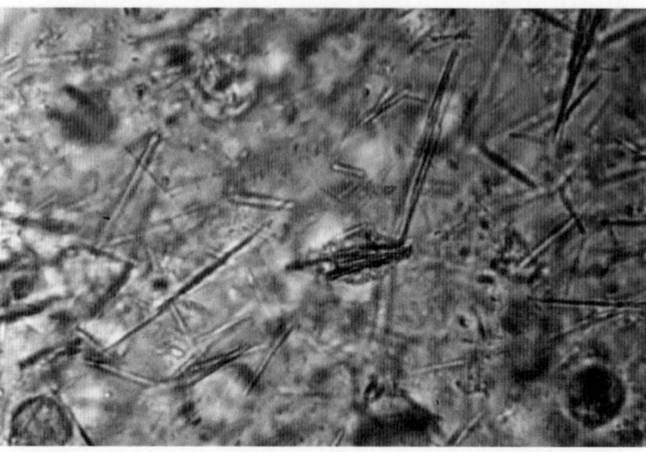

FIGURE 46-2 Extracellular and intracellular monosodium urate crystals, as seen in a fresh preparation of synovial fluid, illustrate needle- and rod-shaped crystals. These crystals are strongly negative birefringent crystals under compensated polarized light microscopy; 400×. (From Longo DL, Fauci AS, Kasper DL, Hauser SL, Jameson JL, Loscalzo J, eds. *Harrison's Principles of Internal Medicine*, 18th ed. New York, NY: McGraw-Hill, 2012.)

CLINICAL FINDINGS

SIGNS AND SYMPTOMS

- The signs and symptoms indicated below may be characteristic of multiple rheumatic disorders, often confounding medical diagnosis, especially with less common presentation.
- It is not the purview of a physical therapist to medically diagnose a rheumatic disease, but rather to recognize the possibility in the differential diagnosis process.
- Severe pain in the great toe(podagra) but can affect anywhere in the feet, ankles, wrists, fingers, elbows; not necessarily in joints, but rather in soft tissue (painful to touch)
- Pain starting at night
- Mid-foot pain and/or edema
- Sudden onset of pain
- Inflammation of involved joint(s)

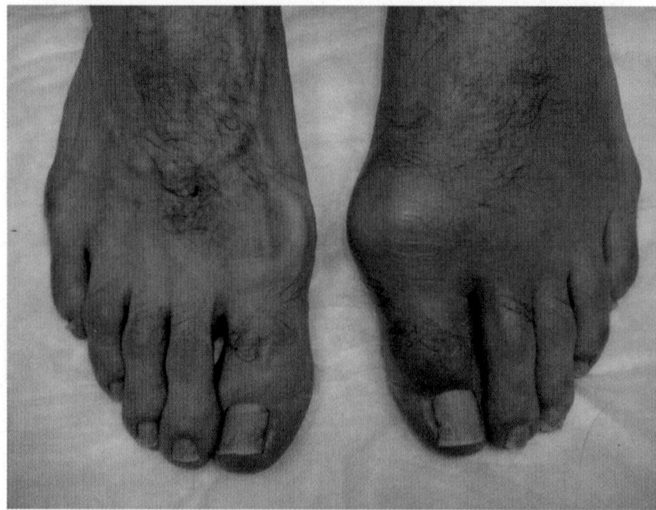

FIGURE 46-3 Podagra: gout. The left first MTP joint is swollen and exquisitely tender; the entire forefoot is erythematous and warm. Note also the bunions (L > R). (From LeBlond RF, DeGowin RL, Brown DD. *DeGowin's Diagnostic Examination*, 9th ed. www.accessmedicine.com. Copyright © The McGraw-Hill Companies, Inc. All rights reserved.)

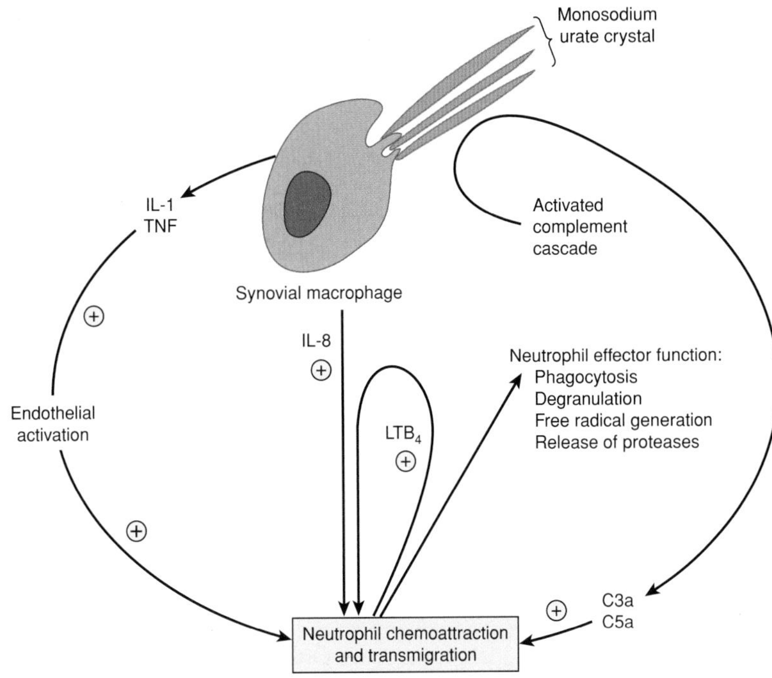

FIGURE 46-4 Mechanisms in initiation and amplification of the acute inflammatory response in gout involve both cytokines and humoral mediators. (McPhee SJ, Hammer GD. *Pathophysiology of Disease: An Introduction to Clinical Medicine*, 6th ed. www.accessmedicine.com. Copyright © The McGraw-Hill Companies, Inc. All rights reserved.)

- Redness of involved joint(s)
- Presence of tophi under the skin especially around joints and ear rim
- Possible kidney stones at the same time or a history of
- Joint pain: Frequently in single joints
- Muscle pain
- Fatigue
- Weakness in extremities secondary to pain or disuse over time
- Anxiety: Secondary to pain and dysfunction
- Depression
- Kidney dysfunction: Disease, nephritis
- Edema in extremities: Feet, hands
- Leukocytosis
- Persistent pain after acute episode diminishes
- Fever
- Decreased exercise tolerance
- Changes in lifestyle secondary to pain and fatigue limiting physical activity
- Inappropriate self-medication
- Anxiety and depression
- Limitations in ADLs, or IADLs
- Psychological challenges
- Impotence in males secondary to medication side effects
- Need for weight management

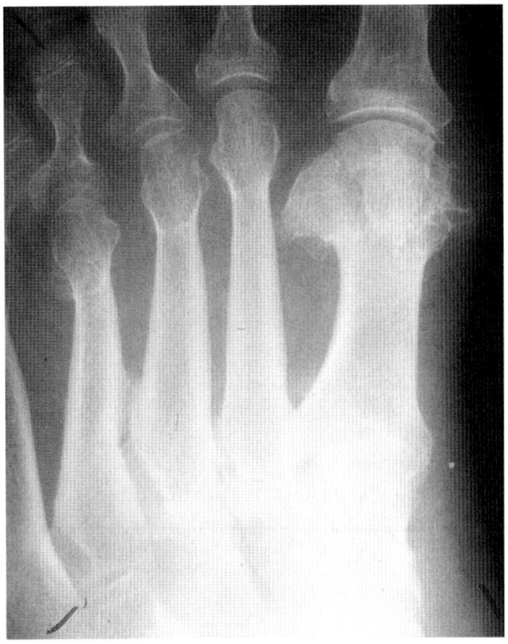

Functional Implications

- Severe symptoms may be disabling resulting in the inability to leave home
- Inability to concentrate
- Inability to ambulate secondary to joint deformity and or pain, or soft tissue/connective tissue involvement
- Joint deformity
- Joint pain in one or more joints
- Soft tissue pain
- Edema: Limiting ability to wear shoes or certain clothing or causing secondary problems such as sensory impairment
- Activity limiting fatigue
- Sleep disturbances; sleeplessness
- Frequent urination from recommended large quantities of fluid intake
- GI upset, diarrhea from medications
- Sarcopenia resulting in weakness, muscle-mass loss, inability to ambulate or perform self-care as well as aerobic capacity limitation secondary to inactivity, edema

FIGURE 46-5 Radiographic changes of gout. (From Imboden J, Hellmann DB, Stone JH. *Current Rheumatology Diagnosis & Treatment*, 2nd ed. www.accessmedicine.com. Copyright © The McGraw-Hill Companies, Inc. All rights reserved.)

Possible Contributing Causes

- Diabetes
- Kidney Disease
- Obesity
- Sickle cell anemia
- Leukemia
- Radical diet changes
- Diet high in purines
- Uric acid buildup in blood
- Fructose consumption (high fructose corn syrup)
- Dehydration
- Very low calorie diets
- Surgery
- Joint injury
- Side effects of medications such as diuretics, that is, furosemide, Lasix
- Infections: Bacterial or viral diseases
- Side effect of rapid uric acid lowering medications
- Excessive alcohol consumption, especially beer
- Exposure to lead
- Renal insufficiency
- High blood pressure
- Hypothyroidism
- Any condition that causes rapid cell turnover, that is, cancer, psoriasis, hemolytic anemia
- Gender: More in males than females
- Heredity
- Diuretics
- Aspirin or other salicylate containing drugs
- Niacin
- Cyclosporine
- Levodopa
- Organ transplants
- Physical stress
- Stress and anxiety
- Systemic immunological conditions: Inflammatory conditions; autoimmune diseases
- Postsurgical
- Smoking

Differential Diagnosis

- Pseudogout
- Fibromyalgia
- Cellulitis
- Bursitis
- Traumatic arthritis
- Psoriatic arthritis
- Rheumatoid arthritis
- Organ dysfunction as a result of cancer or malignancy
- Peripheral neuropathy
- Endocrine disorders
- Autoimmune/inflammatory diseases that cause joint pain and or edema
- Synovitis
- Tendinitis
- Septic arthritis
- Reactive arthritis
- Sarcoidosis
- Scleroderma
- Glomerulonephritis

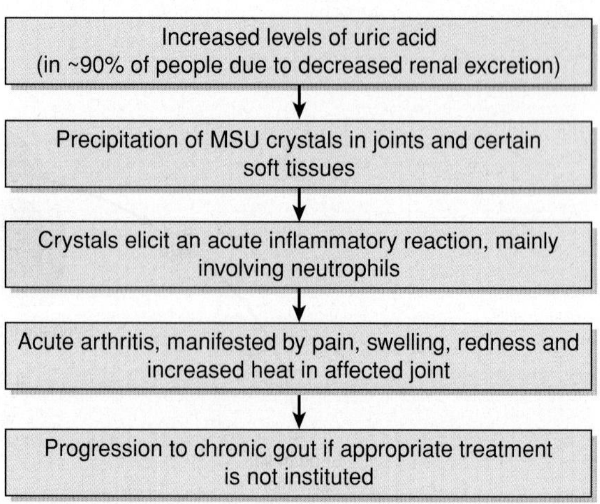

FIGURE 46-6 Simplified scheme of some of the events involved in the causation of gout. (From Murray RK, Bender DA, Botham KM, Kennelly PJ, Rodwell VW, Weil PA. *Harper's Illustrated Biochemistry*, 29th ed. www.accessmedicine.com. Copyright © The McGraw-Hill Companies, Inc. All rights reserved.)

- Osteomyelitis
- Dislocated joints
- Osteoarthritis
- Sjögren syndrome
- Vasculitis
- Irritable bowel syndrome
- Crohn disease
- Inflammatory bowel disease
- Celiac disease
- Kidney failure/disease
- Food allergies
- Referred pain from heart, spine, hip

MEANS OF CONFIRMATION OR DIAGNOSIS

Laboratory Tests

- Blood tests/Lab tests
  - CBC, chemistry panel (kidney function, liver, electrolytes, blood sugar, cholesterol, triglycerides)
  - Synovial fluid test
  - Erythrocyte sedimentation rate (ESR)
  - Antinuclear antibody (ANA)
  - Antiphospholipid antibodies (APLs)
  - Anti-Sm
  - Anti-dsDNA
  - Anti-Ro(SSA) and anti-La(SSB)
  - C-reactive protein (CRP)
  - Uric acid levels, blood and urine tests
  - Blood urea nitrogen (BUN)

Imaging

- Dual-energy computed tomography (DECT)
- CT scan
- Radiography of affected areas
- MRIs

Diagnostic Procedures

- Removal of crystals for analysis
- Analysis of synovial fluid

FINDINGS AND INTERPRETATION

- Radiography sensitivity 31%, specificity 93%
- Ultrasonography sensitivity 96%, specificity 73%
- Radiographic imaging usually does not appear until more than 1 year of uncontrolled disease
- Chronic gout: Tophus deposits
- Identification of uric acid crystals in joints
- Keeping uric acid levels <6 mg/dL, normal 4 to 5 mg/dL
- Glomerular filtration rate and proteinuria for kidney function
- Protein/Creatinine ratio for kidney function: Protein loss
- Urinalysis for kidney disease/infection

TREATMENT

Medication

- Xanthine oxidase inhibitors
  - Medications that decrease uric acid production
  - Allopurinol (Aloprim, Lopurin, Zyloprim)
  - Febuxostat (Uloric)
- Uricosuric agents
  - Medications that facilitate the kidneys to get rid of excess uric acid
- Colchicine
  - Anti-inflammatory used short term or long term, which prevents flare ups and is used to manage acute onsets
- NSAIDs for pain management
  - Oral or injected
- Corticosteroids
- Cardiac medications as indicated
- Antihypertensives as indicated
  - Losartan (Cozaar): Angiotensin II receptor antagonist that may help lower uric acid levels
- Cholesterol lowering medications
- If GI symptoms present secondary to medications:
  - Acid blockers
    - Proton pump inhibitors: Available over the counter and prescription for GI symptoms
  - Acid reducers
    - H-2 receptors: Available over the counter and prescription
  - Prokinetic agents
    - Facilitate stomach emptying and valve tightening between stomach and esophagus

MEDICAL PROCEDURES

- Surgical removal

REFERRALS/ADMITTANCE

- Rheumatologist
- If a patient is referred for PT and the causative problem is not considered to be appropriate for PT, referral to the appropriate physician must be made.
- If PT management is not resulting in improvement, referral is indicated.

IMPAIRMENTS

- Muscle weakness
- Joint pain
- Diffuse soft tissue pain
- Soft tissue and or joint contracture
- Soft tissue and or joint deformity with biomechanical malalignment
- Muscle atrophy
- Gait abnormality/difficulty in walking
- Contractures of soft tissue (fascia, muscle), joint limitations
- Inability to perform self-care
- Limited aerobic endurance
- Functional decline: Decrease in functional abilities
- Coordination deficits
- Balance dysfunction
- Postural abnormalities

TESTS AND MEASURES

- According to Guide for Physical Therapist Practice
  - History
  - Palpation
  - Vital signs
  - Muscle performance testing
  - Range of motion measurements
  - Joint integrity and mobility
  - Edema measurements
  - Gait
  - Balance
  - Locomotion
  - Motor function
  - Orthotic: Protective and supportive device
  - Pain scales
  - Posture
  - Reflex integrity
  - Self-care and home management
  - Sensory integrity
  - Integument, skin
  - Ventilation and respiration (deconditioning or comorbidity)
  - Work/Community and leisure integration including ADLs
- As gout may be misdiagnosed, the tests and measures given next are included to assist in differential diagnosis from other rheumatologic disorders that may affect joints.
- Palpation
  - Liver: In supine, with left hand under trunk parallel to 11th and 12th rib, lift upward; right hand lateral to rectus and press in and up: +/= reproduction of symptoms with deep breath, indicates liver involvement.
  - Ascites: With the fingers, percuss outward from center, if sound is dull, ascites may be present.
  - Spleen: It is not recommended for PT to palpate an enlarged spleen (only palpable if enlarged) because of the potential of rupture.
  - Gallbladder (Murphy's): Place fingers to the right of rectus abdominus below rib cage: +/= sudden pain and muscle tensing with deep breath.
  - Kidneys: In supine, place one hand under client between ribs and iliac crest, and other hand on abdomen below ribs and ribs pointing in opposite direction: +/− tenderness or reproduction of symptoms.
  - Bladder: Not usually palpable unless it is distended and rises above pubic bone. In supine, place hand above pubis and press down: +/= tenderness, reproduction of pain, or ability to feel the bladder.

INTERVENTION

- Physical therapy intervention is consistent with the movement related problems that occur.

- Gait training with use of an assistive device to offset weight bearing/pain
- Therapeutic exercise: All relevant categories, energy conservation, aerobic capacity related
- Therapeutic activities for bed-mobility training, transfer- and transitional-movement training
- Neuromuscular re-education
- Wheelchair management
- Self-care management training including use of adaptive equipment/home-modification assessment, energy conservation
- Ability to don/doff compression garments or compression wraps to involved extremities
- Physical agents for management of pain and inflammation
  - Heat, cold
  - Electrical stimulation
  - Transcutaneous electrical nerve stimulation (TENS)
  - Laser
  - Soft tissue mobilization
  - Compression—intermittent
- Orthotic instruction/management—check out for the same for feet/hands
- Weight management
- Dietary management: There is evidence that certain foods may trigger gout attacks
  - High fluid intake, especially water or other non-alcoholic beverages
  - Diet that includes low-fat dairy products
  - Intake of dark cherry juice
  - Fluid intake: Six to eight glasses of water plus additional fluids
  - Some evidence that coffee or caffeine intake may be a benefit
  - Vitamin C supplements
  - Avoidance of ketosis, which results from low carbohydrate intake
  - Evidence that modifying diets to reduce purine intake, reduction in:
    - Beef, pork, lamb, meat-based gravies
    - Avoidance of organ meats
    - Shellfish: Shrimp, lobster, scallops, dark fishes, that is, mackerel, sardines
    - Although purines can be found in vegetables such as asparagus, cauliflower, spinach, peas, and mushrooms, there is less evidence in the literature that eliminating them will improve uric acid levels. The ACR recommendations do not limit vegetables.
    - Oatmeal
    - Beer
    - Fructose (high-fructose corn syrup)

FUNCTIONAL GOALS

Note: As of 2014, CMS has modified documentation requirements for OP to include functional assessment based on tests and measures with goals linked to the same.

- Patient will be able to:
  - Demonstrate reduction in pain from ___ to ___ in (body part) in order to ________ (state function) or use sleep; that is, in order to facilitate continuous sleep up to ______ hours to enable alertness during waking hours required for work.
  - Demonstrate safe, independent gait with ________________ (insert device name) with the ability to appropriately compensate for pain/immobility in ________________ in order to safely "ambulate" with appropriate LE unweighting.
  - Increase muscle performance in (body part; specify muscle group or functional activity) from ____ to ____ in order to ____ (state function).
  - Achieve adequate functional aerobic capacity, and the ability to talk during activity in order to achieve functional gait and activity tolerance for work, play, school, self-care; ADLs and IADLs
  - Have functional independent gait in the home and community, (with or without a device) allowing for work, play, self-care; ADLs and IADLs, up to __________ feet based on patient's need and prior functional level.
  - Achieve 600 m or greater in a 6-minute walk test for initiation of safe functional gait in the community.
  - Perform active verbalization with increasing taxonomy for safety during gait, including negotiation of even and uneven surfaces, opening and closing doors, transferring in and out of a car.
  - Tolerate 30 minutes of continuous moderate exercise three times a week in ______ weeks, and 5 times a week in order to sustain functional aerobic capacity and muscle endurance for ______________ weeks, depending on the severity of the disease.
  - Independently don/doff compression garments (or compression bandages) ensuring adequate pressure and care of the garments to maintain the integrity of the compression.

PROGNOSIS

- As this pathology is medical in nature, it is the physician who establishes the medical prognosis.
- It is a chronic disease but with appropriate medical management, individuals should be able to lead an active lifestyle and it is considered one of the most treatable forms of arthritis.
- For the physical therapy prognosis, goals should be established that the patient can achieve based on their overall condition.
- Unless the medical condition is unstable or the goals unrealistic, the prognosis from a physical therapy perspective should be good.
- "Good" refers only to the realistic functional goals established.

PATIENT RESOURCES

- Davis J. The latest gout research. Arthritis Today. http://www.arthritistoday.org/conditions/gout/all-about-gout/gout-research.php. Accessed June 20, 2013.
- Gout. American College of Rheumatology. http://www.rheumatology.org/practice/clinical/patients/diseases_and_conditions/gout.asp. Accessed June 20, 2013.
- Gout. Takeda Pharmaceuticals. http://www.gout.com. Accessed June 20, 2013.
- Gout Medications. About.com http://arthritis.about.com/od/goutmeds/Gout_Medications_Gout_Medicines_Gout_Drug_Information.htm. Accessed June 20, 2013.

REFERENCE

1. Rettenbacher T, Ennemoser S, Weirich H, et al. Diagnostic imaging of gout: comparison of high-resolution US versus conventional X-ray. *Eur Radiol.* 2008;18(3):621–630.

ADDITIONAL REFERENCES

- Chandrasoma P, Taylor CR. Metabolic diseases of joints. In: Chandrasoma P, Taylor CR, eds. *Concise Pathology.* 3rd ed.

New York, NY: McGraw-Hill; 2011. http://www.accessphysiotherapy.com/citepopup.aspx?aid=193823&citeType=1. Accessed February 15, 2013.

- Choi HK, Atkinson K, Karlson EW, Willett W, Curhan G. Purine-rich foods, dairy and protein intake, and the risk of gout in men. *N Engl J Med.* 2004;350(11):1093–1103.
- Cronstein BN, Terkeltaub R. The inflammatory process of gout and its treatment. *Arthritis Res Ther.* 2006;8(Suppl 1):S3.
- Dutton M. Juvenile rheumatoid arthritis. In: Dutton M, ed. *McGraw-Hill's NPTE (National Physical Therapy Examination).* 2nd ed. New York, NY: McGraw-Hill; 2012. http://www.accessphysiotherapy.com/content/56505040. Accessed February 15, 2013.
- Goodman CC, Fuller KS. *Pathology Implications for the Physical Therapist.* 3rd ed. St. Louis, MO: Saunders Elsevier; 2009.
- Goodman CC, Snyder TE. *Differential Diagnosis for Physical Therapists Screening for Referral.* 4th ed. St. Louis, MO: Saunders Elsevier; 2007.
- Hunt J, McTigue J, Edwards NL. Diagnosis and management of gout in 2011. *J Muscoskel Med.* 2011;28(10). http://www.musculoskeletalnetwork.com/gout/content/article/1145622/1973052. Accessed February 15, 2013.
- Khanna D, Fitzgerald JD, Khanna PP, et al. 2012 American College of Rheumatology guidelines for management of gout. Part 1: Systematic nonpharmacologic and pharmacologic therapeutic approaches to hyperuricemia. *Arthritis Care Res.* 2012;64(10):1431–1446. doi 10.1002/acr.21772. http://www.rheumatology.org/practice/clinical/guidelines/Gout_Part_1_ACR-12–0014.pdf#toolbar=1. Accessed February 15, 2013.
- Khanna D, Fitzgerald JD, Khanna PP, et al. American College of Rheumatology guidelines for management of gout. Part 2: Therapy and antiinflammatory prophylaxis of acute gouty arthritis. *Arthritis Care Res.* 2012;64(10):1447–1461. doi 10.1002/acr.21773. http://www.rheumatology.org/practice/clinical/guidelines/Gout_Part_2_ACR-12–0013.pdf#toolbar=1.
- McPhee SJ, Hammer GD. Pathophysiology of Selected Rheumatic Diseases. In: McPhee SJ, Hammer GD, eds. *Pathophysiology of Disease.* 6th ed. New York, NY: McGraw-Hill; 2010. http://www.accessphysiotherapy.com/content/5372636. Accessed June 20, 2013.
- Panus PC, Jobst EE, Masters SB, Katzung B, Tinsley SL, Trevor AJ. Drugs affecting eicosanoid metabolism, disease-modifying antirheumatic drugs, and drugs used in gout. In: Panus PC, Jobst EE, Masters SB, Katzung B, Tinsley SL, Trevor AJ, eds. *Pharmacology for the Physical Therapist.* New York, NY: McGraw-Hill; 2009: Chapter 34. http://www.accessphysiotherapy.com/content/6095707. Accessed June 20, 2013.
- Richette P, Bardin T. Gout. *Lancet.* 2010;375(9711):318–328. doi: 10.1016/S0140–6736(09)60883–7.
- Schlesinger N. Management of acute and chronic gouty arthritis: present state-of-the-art. *Drugs.* 2004;64(21):2399–2416.
- Wilson JF. In the clinic. *Gout. Ann Intern Med.* 2010;152(3): ITC21. doi: 10.1059/0003–4819–152–3–201002020–01002.

47 GRAVES DISEASE

Debra F. Stern, DPT, DBA, MSM, PT
Eric Shamus, PhD, DPT, PT, CSCS
Erika Simmerman-Mabes, DO

CONDITION/DISORDER SYNONYM

- Diffuse thyrotoxic goiter

ICD-9-CM CODES

- 242.0 Toxic diffuse goiter
- PT diagnoses codes that may be secondary to thyroid disorders
  - 315.4 Developmental coordination disorder
  - 709.2 Scar conditions and fibrosis of the skin
  - 719.70 Difficulty in walking involving joint site unspecified
  - 728.2 Muscular wasting and disuse atrophy, not elsewhere classified
  - 728.89 Other disorders of muscle, ligament, and fascia
  - 729.9 Other and unspecified disorders of soft tissue
  - 781.2 Abnormality of gait
  - 782.3 Edema
  - 786.0 Dyspnea and respiratory abnormalities
  - 786.05 Shortness of breath

ICD-10-CM CODES

- E05 Thyrotoxicosis (hyperthyroidism)
- E05.0 Thyrotoxicosis with diffuse goiter

PREFERRED PRACTICE PATTERNS[1]

- 4D: Impaired Joint Mobility, Motor Function, Muscle Performance, and Range of Motion Associated with Connective Tissue Dysfunction
- 4E: Impaired Joint Mobility, Motor Function, Muscle Performance, and Range of Motion Associated with Localized Inflammation
- 6B: Impaired Aerobic Capacity/Endurance Associated with Deconditioning

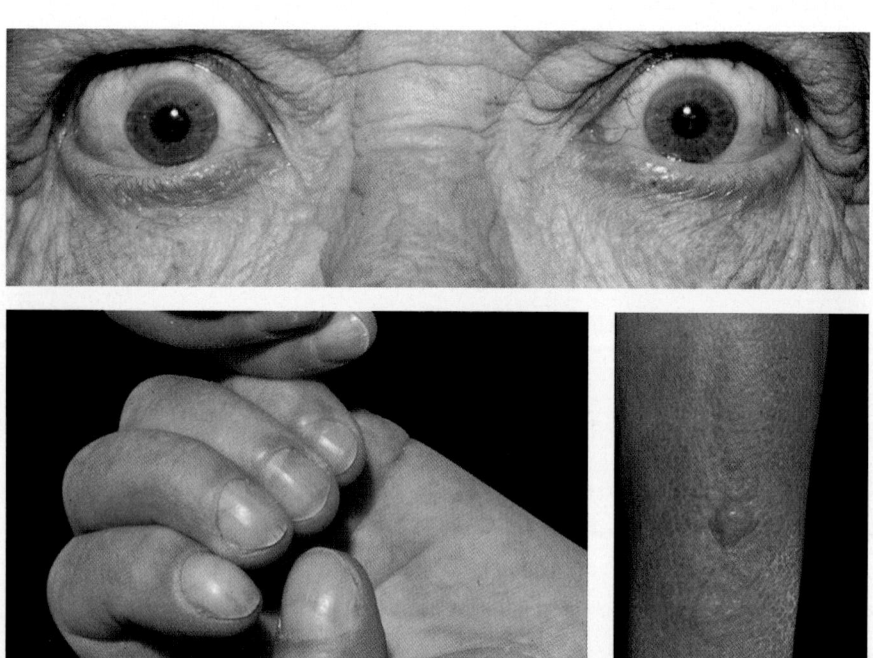

FIGURE 47-1 Graves disease. Note the proptosis of the eyes, thyroid acropachy, and the thyroid dermopathy on the pretibial region. (From Goldsmith LA, Katze S, Gilchrest B, Paller A, Leffel D, Wolff K. *Fitzpatrick's Dermatology in General Medicine*, 8th ed. www.accessmedicine.com. Copyright © The McGraw-Hill Companies, Inc. All rights reserved.)

PATIENT PRESENTATION

A 35-year-old female presents with complaints of a rapid heartbeat, excessive sweating, difficulty sleeping, irritability, and weight loss of 25 lb in the last 4 months despite having an increased appetite. Upon further questioning, she reports frequently feeling hot, having increased loose stools or diarrhea, and thinning of her hair. She has no other past medical history. Family history reveals a history of maternal "thyroid issues" and paternal hypertension. Past routine physical examinations document heart rates in the 70s and blood pressures around 110/70, but today her blood pressure is 135/90 and heart rate is 110 beats per minute. On examination, you note a fine tremor in her hands, bulging eyes, pretibial myxedema (PTM), and a diffusely enlarged thyroid.

KEY FEATURES

Description

- Graves disease is an autoimmune disorder
- Overactivity of the thyroid gland (hyperthyroidism)
- Produces excessive amount of thyroid hormone
- Enlargement of the thyroid gland

Essentials of Diagnosis

- Diagnosis is made by the symptoms
- Thyroid hormone test
- Onset of symptoms is often insidious
- Symptoms build over a period of time, which can delay diagnosis

General Considerations

- Diagnosis for more occult problems may take time and require intensive medical diagnostic testing
- May cause pathology in multiple organ systems
  - GI: Liver
  - Cardiovascular: Heart, peripheral circulation, blood pressure
  - Integumentary
- May result in secondary problems
  - Aerobic capacity and muscle endurance impairment
  - Sarcopenia
  - Weakness/impaired muscle performance
  - Musculoskeletal problems
  - Neuromuscular problems
  - Weight gain indicating the need for PT intervention, depending on severity

Demographics

- Higher incidence in young women: 5 to 10 times more common
- Most common form of hyperthyroidism in children
- Presents during early adolescence
- Less common in Blacks
- Gender: Females at greater risk

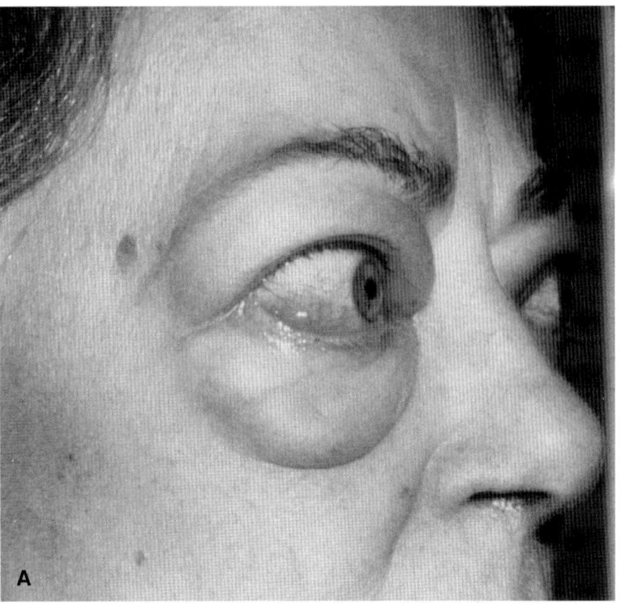

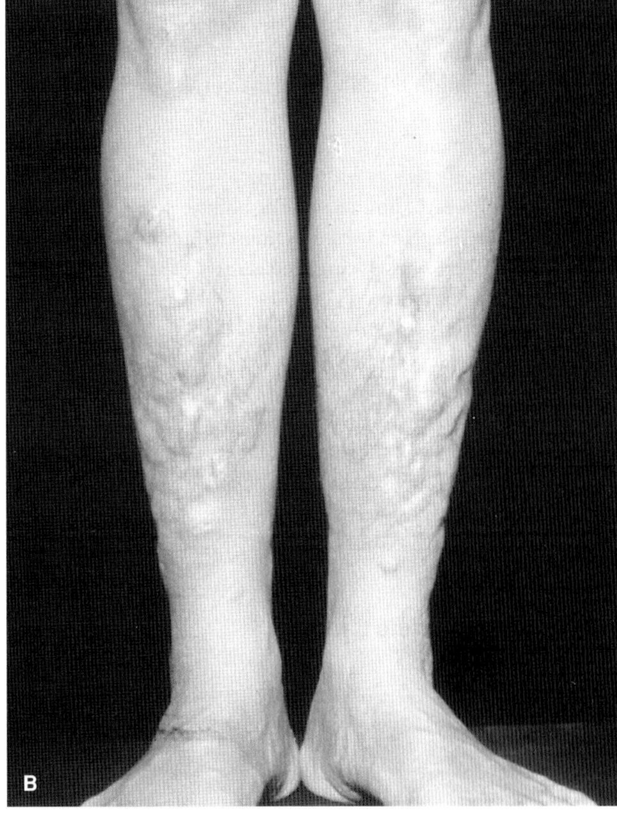

FIGURE 47-2 Graves ophthalmopathy (**A**) and (**B**) pretibial myxedema. This patient demonstrates exophthalmos, proptosis, periorbital swelling, congestion, and edema of the conjunctiva. (From Brunicardi FC, Andersen D, Billiar T, et al: *Schwartz's Principles of Surgery*, 9th ed. www.accessmedicine.com. Copyright © The McGraw-Hill Companies, Inc. All rights reserved.)

CLINICAL FINDINGS

SIGNS AND SYMPTOMS

- PTs may treat conditions caused by hyperthyroid or treat patients with hyperthyroidism for other pathologies that are unrelated.
  - Graves ophthalmopathy: Red or swollen eyes, bulging or protruding eyeballs, impaired vision, inflammation, light sensitivity
  - Eye irritation
  - Double vision
  - Enlarged thyroid
  - Fatigue
  - Weight loss
  - Bulging of eyes
  - PTM
  - Possible goiter
  - Tachycardia
  - Cardiac: Atrial fibrillation, arrhythmias, palpitations
  - Racing/rapid pulse

- High blood pressure
- Hyperactivity
- Difficulty in concentrating and focusing
- Heat intolerance
- Sweating, clammy skin
- Confusion, disorientation
- Diuresis
- Muscle weakness
- Tremors
- Neck pain
- Unexplained weight loss with inability to gain weight
- Difficulty swallowing
- Change in voice
- Heart disease
- Dyspnea, shortness of breath with exertion
- Airway obstruction
- Increased appetite
- Menstrual disturbance, irregularity
- Increased bowel frequency
- Breast development in men
- Clammy skin
- Diarrhea
- Hair loss
- Hand tremor
- Itching
- Nausea and vomiting
- Skin blushing or flushing
- Difficulty sleeping
- Osteoporosis
- Nervousness/anxiety

Functional Implications

- Severe symptoms such as immediacy of need to urinate, increased volume of urine, and increase in bowel frequency may be disabling and result in the inability or reluctance to leave home
- Vision impairment
- Inability to focus, issues with driving
- Shortness of breath, limited walking ability
- Sarcopenia resulting in weakness, muscle-mass loss, inability to ambulate or perform self-care, and aerobic capacity limitation secondary to inactivity
- Decreased exercise tolerance
- Sleep disturbances
- Changes in lifestyle
- Eating disorders, overeating
- Noncompliance with medication regiments/inability to pay attention
- Limitations in ADLs or IADLs
- Neuropathy, increased risk for falls
- Voice changes, hoarseness

Possible Contributing Causes

- Heredity
- Toxic adenoma
- Plummer disease (toxic multinodular goiter)
- Thyroiditis
- Inflammation of the thyroid
- Autoimmune or Hashimoto thyroiditis
- Cancer
- Metastatic cancer
- Chemical inducement
- Radiation treatments to the neck
- Viral thyroiditis
- Radiation to the brain
- Congenital birth defects
- Pituitary dysfunction/tumors as the pituitary signals production of thyroid stimulating hormone (TSH)
- Getting too much iodine
- Growths/tumors of the thyroid or pituitary gland
- Body production of too much thyroid hormone

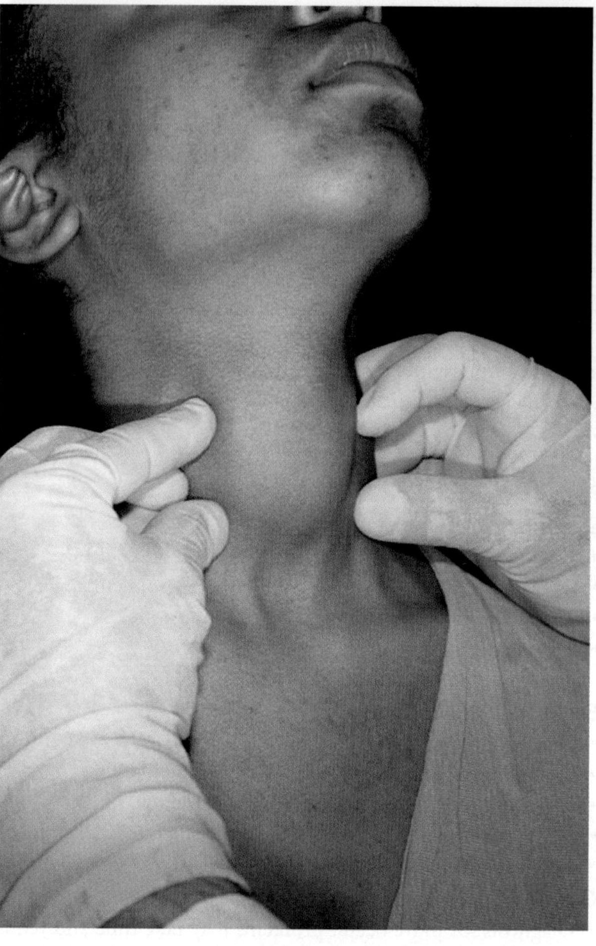

FIGURE 47-3 Goiter resulting from Graves disease in a 16-year-old girl. (Reproduced with permission from Shah BR, Lucchesi M. *Atlas of Pediatric Emergency Medicine*. New York, NY: McGraw-Hill;2006: Figure 14-3, © 2006.)

- Testicular or ovarian tumors
- Immune dysfunction
- Increased risk associated with other immune disorders such as type 1 diabetes or rheumatoid arthritis (RA)
- Stress
- Pregnancy
- Smoking

Differential Diagnosis

- Organ dysfunction as a result of cancer or malignancy, especially the liver
- Pituitary dysfunction
- Non-malignant tumors in the abdomen or organs
- Testicular tumors
- Endocrine disorders
- Gastroparesis
- Gynecologic problems in females
  - Endometriosis
  - Menses
  - Ectopic pregnancies
  - Ovarian cysts: Tumors
  - Fibroids
  - Menopause
- Autoimmune diseases that affect the upper and lower GI tracts such as Crohn disease or irritable bowel syndrome, systemic

lupus erythematosus (SLE), RA; as they involve organs and have a fatigue component
- Bladder infections, urinary tract infections, kidney pathology
- Infections in the abdomen
- Bowel disorders

MEANS OF CONFIRMATION OR DIAGNOSIS

Laboratory Tests

- Blood tests/lab tests: Complete blood count (CBC)
- Thyroid function: TSH, T3, and T4
- Radioactive iodine uptake
- Cholesterol
- Liver enzymes
- Prolactin
- Thyroid-stimulating immunoglobulin test
- Abnormal thyroid function tests

Imaging

- Ultrasound
- Chest x-ray
- CT scans: Orbit CT scan
- MRIs

FINDINGS AND INTERPRETATION

- Prolactin (may be elevated in women)
- Thyroid function: TSH (usually low), and T3 and T4 (usually high)

TREATMENT

Medication

- Antithyroid medication
  - Methimazole (Tapazole)
  - Propylthiouracil (PropylThyracil or PTU)
- Beta-blockers (to control cardiac symptoms and anxiety)
- Prednisone for eye irritation
- Eye drops for eye irritation
- Other
  - Radioactive iodine to destroy the thyroid

MEDICAL PROCEDURES

- Surgical removal of thyroid (thyroid hormone then a lifelong necessity)
  - Surgery is not a treatment of choice with the exception of
    - Pregnant women, who cannot tolerate antithyroid drugs, or those with cancer
    - When other treatments fail
- Taping eyes shut at night to prevent eye dryness
- Sleeping with head elevated to minimize eye discomfort
- Radiation of eyes
- Surgery for repositioning of eyes
  - Orbital decompression
  - Eye muscle repositioning
  - Prism glasses

REFERRALS/ADMITTANCE

- If a patient is referred for PT and the causative problem is not considered appropriate for PT, refer to the appropriate physician
- If an emergency is identified, refer to an ER
- If the patient's history and reactions to PT indicate possible hyperthyroidism and or symptoms, refer to a physician
- Occupational therapy
- Speech-language pathology
  - Swallowing deficits
  - Speech impairment

IMPAIRMENTS

- Muscle weakness
- Muscle atrophy
- Gait abnormality/difficulty walking
- Shortness of breath/fatigue
- Limited aerobic capacity
- Inability to perform self-care
- Balance impairment
- Impaired skin integrity
- Vision impairment

TESTS AND MEASURES

- Because there may be GI signs associated with hyperthyroidism, GI tests and measures are included in this section.
- Palpation
  - Palpation of thyroid/neck for enlargement of thyroid or any abnormalities
  - Skin changes: Turgor, dryness, hairlessness with hyperthyroid, sweaty, clammy
  - Identification of PTM
  - Abdominal palpation: May be enlargement of ovaries.
  - Kidneys: In supine, place one hand under client between ribs and iliac crest, and other hand on abdomen below ribs and pointing in opposite direction: +/– tenderness or reproduction of symptoms.
  - Bladder
    - Not usually palpable unless it is distended and rises above pubic bone.
    - In supine, place hand above pubis and press down: +/= tenderness, reproduction of pain, or ability to feel the bladder: __+ __–.
  - Appendix (McBurney's): Apply vertical pressure halfway between right anterior superior iliac spine (ASIS) and umbilicus.
  - Liver: In supine, with left hand under trunk parallel to 11th and 12th rib, lift upward; right hand lateral to rectus and press in and up: +/= reproduction of symptoms with deep breath.
  - Ascites: With the fingers, percuss outward from center; if sound is dull, ascites may be present.
  - Spleen: It is not recommended for PT to palpate an enlarged spleen (only palpable if enlarged) because of the potential of rupture
  - Gallbladder (Murphy's): Place fingers right of rectus abdominus below rib cage: +/= sudden pain and muscle tensing with deep breath.
- Observation
  - Scars may indicate adhesions after surgery.
  - Pink or purplish striae may be indicative of Cushing syndrome, and dilated veins may indicate hepatic pathology or inferior vena cava obstruction, not diverticulitis.
  - Abdominal contour: Roundedness, concavity/hollowness, asymmetry, distension, pregnancy signs.
  - Cullen sign: Bluish discoloring around umbilicus, which may be a sign of retroperitoneal bleeding.
  - Bluish discoloration in lower abdomen, Grey Turner sign, which is a sign of hemorrhagic pancreatitis.

- Bulging in groin or other areas of abdomen especially apparent with contraction of musculature in area may be hernia.
- Pulsing in the area of the navel may be abdominal aortic aneurysm.
- Palpable abdominal tenderness on left/right or generalized.
- Psoas sign: Provide resistance over patient's right knee as they flex the hip; pain is indicative of appendicitis or possible inflammation of the abdomen.
- Obturator sign: Internal rotation of right lower extremity and flexion may be indicative of appendicitis or pelvic inflammation.
- Rovsing sign: Pain on the right side of abdomen when pressure is put on the left may be indicative of appendicitis.

INTERVENTION

- No cure
- Physical therapy intervention is consistent with movement-related problems that occur secondary to diabetes and include.
  - Gait training
  - Therapeutic exercise: All relevant categories, energy conservation
    - Stretching if contractures present in neck postsurgery
    - If there is an insulin pump, take care not to interfere with it in any way.
    - PT should inquire about medication taken; if glucose >300, exercise should be avoided.
  - Therapeutic activities for bed-mobility training, transfer-, and transitional-movement training
  - Wheelchair management
  - Self-care management training including skin care/moisturizing, lifestyle management
  - Neuromuscular re-education: Balance, and postural training
  - Soft tissue mobilization if contractures present in neck postsurgery
  - Wound management
  - Interprofessional
    - Lifestyle modification
    - Smoking cessation
    - Weight management
    - Dietary counseling
    - Dentistry
    - Optometry
    - Ophthalmology
    - Audiology

FUNCTIONAL GOALS

- Patient will be able to
  - Extend and rotate head and neck left/right with adequate functional range in all directions to safely use mirrors while driving (if postsurgical).
  - Achieve adequate functional aerobic capacity and the ability to talk during activity, in order to achieve functional gait and activity tolerance for work, play, school, and self-care, as well as ADLs and IADLs.
  - Functional gait in the home and community (with or without a device) that allows for work, play, self-care as well as ADLs and IADLs, up to __ feet, based on patient's need and prior functional level.
  - Achieve 600 m or greater in a 6-minute walk test for initiation of safe functional gait in the community.
  - Perform active verbalization with increasing taxonomy for safety during gait, including negotiation of even and uneven surfaces, opening and closing doors, transferring in and out of a car.
  - Tolerate 30 minutes of continuous moderate exercise three times a week in __ weeks, and five times a week in __ weeks, depending on disease severity.

PROGNOSIS

- As this pathology is primarily medical in nature, the physician establishes the medical prognosis.
- In general, although it commonly responds well to treatment, surgery results in hypothyroidism, which must be well managed with thyroid hormone.
- There can be problems postsurgery with low calcium from parathyroid damage as a result of thyroid surgery.
- Thyroid crisis, severe hyperthyroidism is a possibility.
- In children, the disease is serious and can result in death.
- Prognosis from a PT perspective, based on effective medical management, is good to return to healthy level of function before onset of disease if individual receives care secondary to the problems related to hyperthyroid.

PATIENT RESOURCE

- American Thyroid Association. www.thyroid.org. Accessed August 8, 2014.

REFERENCE

1. APTA. *Guide to Physical Therapy Practice*. Atlanta, GA: American Physical Therapy Association; 2003. http://guidetoptpractice.apta.org. Accessed June 12, 2013.

ADDITIONAL REFERENCES

- Baskin HJ, Cobin RH, Duick DS, et al. American Association of Clinical Endocrinologists medical guidelines for clinical practice for the evaluation and treatment of hyperthyroidism and hypothyroidism. *Endocr Pract*. 2002;8(6):457–469.
- Davidson A, Diamond B. Autoimmune diseases. *N Engl J Med*. 2001,345(5):340–350.
- Goodman CC, Fuller KS. *Pathology: Implications for the Physical Therapist*. 3rd ed. Philadelphia, PA: Saunders Elsevier; 2009.
- Goodman CC, Snyder TK. *Differential Diagnosis for Physical Therapists: Screening for Referral*. 4th ed. St. Louis, MO: Saunders Elsevier; 2007.
- Graves' Disease and Thyroid Foundation. www.ngdf.org. Accessed June 12, 2013.
- Patel P, Macerollo A. Diabetes mellitus: diagnosis and screening. *Am Fam Physician*. 2010;81(7):863–870.
- Sloka JS, Phillips PW, Stefanelli M, Joyce C. Co-occurrence of autoimmune thyroid disease in a multiple sclerosis cohort. *J Autoimmune Dis*. 2005;2:9.doi:10.1186/1740–2557–2–9.

48 PRIMARY IMMUNODEFICIENCY

Debra F. Stern, DPT, DBA, MSM, PT
Mila Marhovich, DPT

CONDITION/DISORDER SYNONYM

- Severe combined immunodeficiency (SCID)

ICD-9-CM CODES

- 279.06 Common variable immunodeficiency
- 279.2 Combined immunity deficiency
- Associated ICD-9-CM PT diagnoses/treatment diagnosis that may be directly related
  - 315.4 Developmental coordination disorder
  - 718.45 Contracture of joint, pelvic region and thigh
  - 719.70 Difficulty in walking involving joint site unspecified
  - 728.2 Muscular wasting and disuse atrophy, not elsewhere classified
  - 728.89 Other disorders of muscle, ligament, and fascia
  - 729.9 Other and unspecified disorders of soft tissue
  - 780.7 Malaise and fatigue
  - 781.2 Abnormality of gait
  - 782.3 Edema
  - 786.0 Dyspnea and respiratory abnormalities
  - 786.05 Shortness of breath

ICD-10-CM CODES

- D81.0 Severe combined immunodeficiency (SCID) with reticular dysgenesis
- D81.1 Severe combined immunodeficiency (SCID) with low T- and B-cell numbers
- D81.2 Severe combined immunodeficiency (SCID) with low or normal B-cell numbers
- D81.89 Other combined immunodeficiencies
- D81.9 Combined immunodeficiency, unspecified
- D83.8 Other common variable immunodeficiencies
- D83.9 Common variable immunodeficiency, unspecified

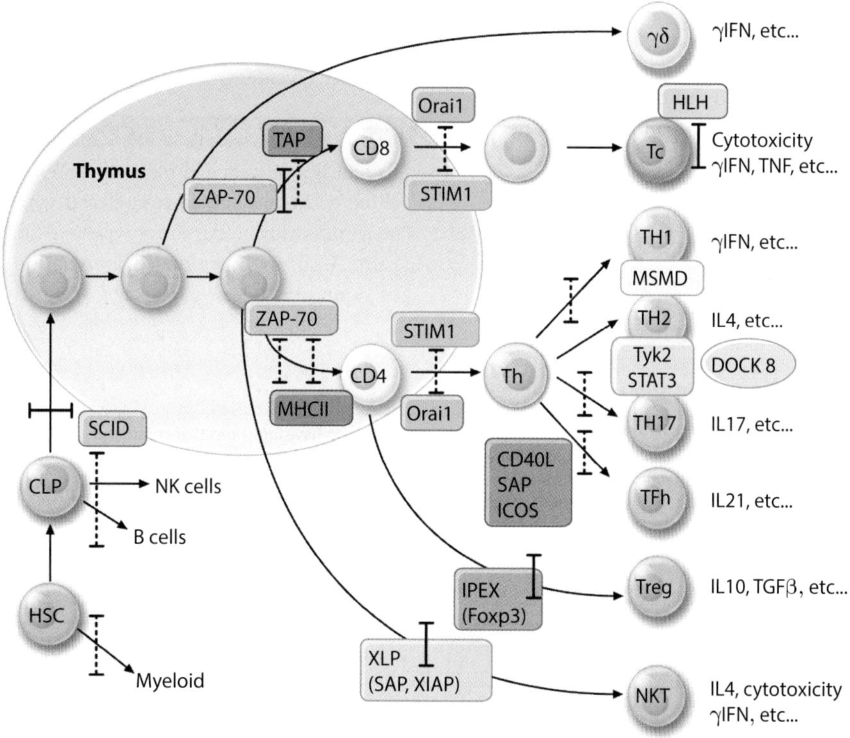

FIGURE 48-1 T cell differentiation, effector pathways, and related primary immunodeficiencies (PIDs). Hematopoietic stem cells (HSCs) differentiate into common lymphoid progenitors (CLPs), which, in turn, give rise to the T cell precursors that migrate to the thymus. The development of CD4+ and CD8+ T cells is shown. Known T cell effector pathways are indicated, that is, γδ cells, cytotoxic T cells (Tc), TH1, TH2, TH17, TFh (follicular helper) CD4 effector T cells, regulatory T cells (Treg), and natural killer T cells (NKTs); abbreviations for PIDs are contained in boxes. Vertical bars indicate a complete deficiency; broken bars a partial deficiency. SCID, severe combined immunodeficiency; ZAP 70, zeta-associated protein deficiency, MHCII, major histocompatibility complex class II deficiency; TAP, TAP1 and 2 deficiencies; Orai1, Stim1 deficiencies; HLH, hematopoietic lymphohistiocytosis; MSMD, Mendelian susceptibility to mycobacterial disease; Tyk2, DOCK8, autosomal recessive form of hyper-IgE syndrome; STAT3, autosomal dominant form of hyper-IgE syndrome; CD40L, ICOS, SAP deficiencies; IPEX, immunodysregulation polyendocrinopathy enteropathy X-linked syndrome; XLP, X-linked proliferative syndromes. (From Longo DL, Fauci AS, Kasper DL, Hauser SL, JamesonJL, Loscalzo J, eds. *Harrison's Principles of Internal Medicine*. 18th ed. New York, NY: McGraw-Hill; 2012.)

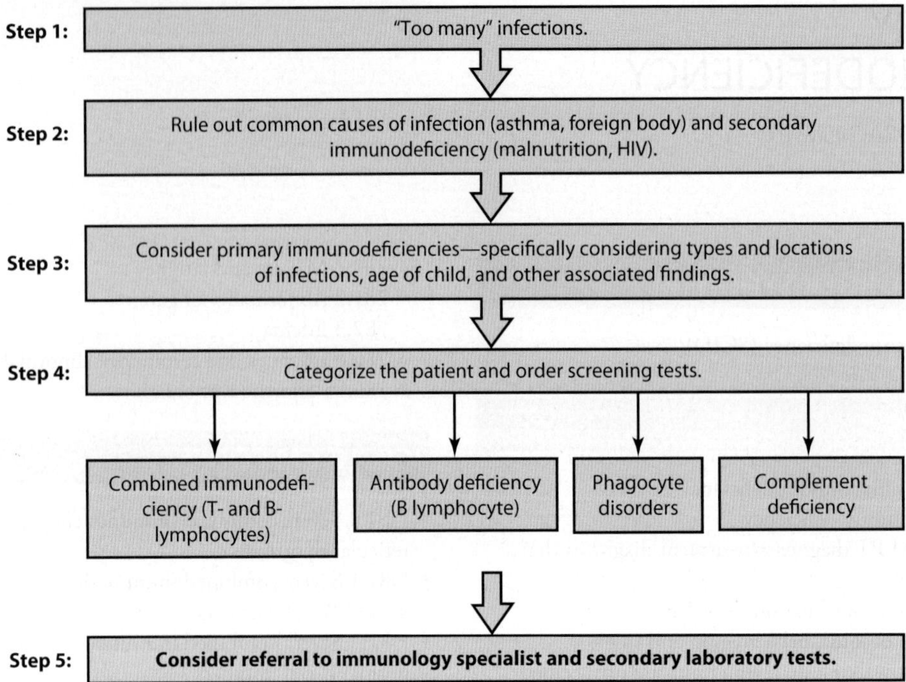

FIGURE 48-2 General approach to primary immunodeficiencies. (From Hay WM, et al. *Current Diagnosis & Treatment: Pediatrics*, 21st ed. New York, NY: McGraw-Hill. www.accessmedicine.com. Copyright © The McGraw-Hill Companies, Inc. All rights reserved.)

PREFERRED PRACTICE PATTERNS[1]

- Note: The APTA *Guide to Physical Therapist Practice* includes practice patterns for neuromuscular and musculoskeletal systems; as primary immunodeficiency is medical in nature, the practice patterns addressed are those for associated disorders that may occur and impair aerobic capacity.
- 4D: Impaired Joint Mobility, Motor Function, Muscle Performance, and Range of Motion Associated with Connective Tissue Dysfunction
- 4E: Impaired Joint Mobility, Motor Function, Muscle Performance, and Range of Motion Associated with Localized Inflammation
- 6B: Impaired Aerobic Capacity/Endurance Associated with Deconditioning
- 7B: Impaired Integumentary Integrity Secondary to Superficial Skin Involvement

PATIENT PRESENTATION

Patient is a 38-year-old male who presents to the physical therapy clinic without a physician's referral with a primary complaint of generalized lower-extremity weakness and bilateral knee and hip pain, 4/10, with prolonged ambulation and cycling. The onset of symptoms began a year ago around the same time he had a

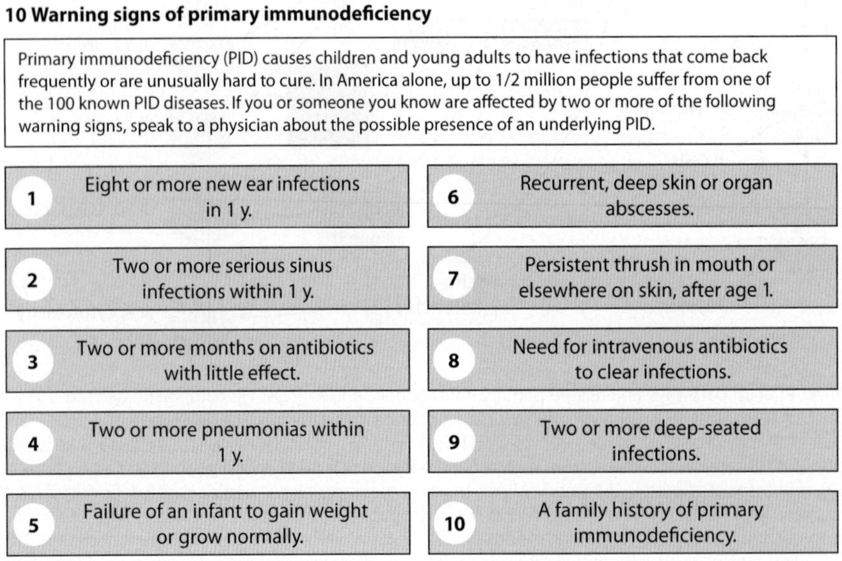

10 Warning signs of primary immunodeficiency

Primary immunodeficiency (PID) causes children and young adults to have infections that come back frequently or are unusually hard to cure. In America alone, up to 1/2 million people suffer from one of the 100 known PID diseases. If you or someone you know are affected by two or more of the following warning signs, speak to a physician about the possible presence of an underlying PID.

1. Eight or more new ear infections in 1 y.
2. Two or more serious sinus infections within 1 y.
3. Two or more months on antibiotics with little effect.
4. Two or more pneumonias within 1 y.
5. Failure of an infant to gain weight or grow normally.
6. Recurrent, deep skin or organ abscesses.
7. Persistent thrush in mouth or elsewhere on skin, after age 1.
8. Need for intravenous antibiotics to clear infections.
9. Two or more deep-seated infections.
10. A family history of primary immunodeficiency.

FIGURE 48-3 Warning signs of primary immunodeficiency. (Data from the Jeffrey Modell Foundation.)

respiratory infection. The respiratory infection has been chronic and treated with multiple courses of antibiotics. Rest alleviates the symptoms mildly. Patient states he walked 2 miles last night for exercise and feels "feverish" this morning. Patient is also an avid cyclist and has not been able to train at previous level of intensity the last few months due to fatigue, joint pain, and shortness of breath. Patient would like to get stronger and get back to previous level of activity. Patient's vitals: BP 130/64 mm Hg; Pulse rate 86 bpm; SPO_2% of 98%, RR 21 per minute. Patient's skin feels moist and warm to touch.

KEY FEATURES

Description

- Failure of the body to provide defense against bacterial or viral invasion as there is no or insufficient production of antibodies
- There are 70 to 100 types in approximately six categories
  - Primary immunodeficiency disorders
  - Congenital immunodeficiency diseases
- B-cell (antibody) deficiencies
- T-cell deficiencies
- Combination B- and T-cell deficiencies
- Defective phagocytes
- Complement deficiencies
- Unknown (idiopathic)
- SCID (bubble boy disease) is considered the most severe form of the disease
  - Chronic infections
  - Frequent infections
  - Multiple body-system involvement
  - Onset often vague with misdiagnosis of underlying disease

Essentials of Diagnosis

- Must be made by a physician and confirmed by medical diagnostic testing
- Warning signs of primary immunodeficiency
  - Eight or more new ear infections within 1 year
  - Two or more serious sinus infections within 1 year
  - Two or more months on antibiotics with little effect
  - Two or more pneumonias within 1 year
  - Failure of an infant to gain weight or grow normally
  - Recurrent, deep skin or organ abscesses
  - Persistent thrush in mouth or elsewhere on skin, after age 1
  - Need for intravenous antibiotics to clear infections
  - Two or more deep-seated infections such as sepsis, meningitis, or cellulitis
  - A family history of primary immune deficiency
- Frequent/recurrent Infections
- Blood infections
- Inflammation of internal organs: Liver, spleen, pancreas
- Autoimmune disorders
- Blood disorders
- Digestive problems
- Delayed growth and development
- Genetic factors
- Abscessed wounds
- Ineffective use of antibiotics

General Considerations

- May result in secondary problems such as aerobic capacity and muscle endurance impairment, sarcopenia, weakness/impaired muscle performance, musculoskeletal problems, neuromuscular problems, weight loss indicating the need for PT intervention depending on severity.
- Once thought to be rare, now recognized on a spectrum of severity.
- Because immune disorders frequently refer pain or are causative of pain in various body areas, individuals may be referred to PT inappropriately or appropriately.
  - Possible inappropriate referral when referred to the lower back, upper back, or chest.
- History of heartburn or indigestion may be indicative of GI or cardiac problems, primary immune deficiency, or associated autoimmune disorders.

Demographics

- Can affect individuals of all ages
- More common in boys
- Some indication of genetic familial tendency
- Serious forms are apparent at birth, about 400/year
- Between 25,000 and 50,000 in the United States

CLINICAL FINDINGS

SIGNS AND SYMPTOMS

- The signs and symptoms indicated here may be characteristic of multiple immune systemic disorders, often confounding medical diagnosis.
- It is not the purview of a PT to medically diagnose an immune pathology but rather to recognize the possibilities in the differential diagnosis process, especially when the findings are not consistent with conditions commonly treated.
  - Musculoskeletal
  - Neuromuscular
  - Integumentary
  - Cardiopulmonary
  - Functional and mobility dysfunction secondary to medical pathology
- Susceptibility to bacterial infections and viral infections, which become chronic and difficult to cure
  - Pneumonia
  - Meningitis
  - Osteomyelitis
  - Cellulitis
  - Chronic sinusitis
  - Chronic bronchitis
  - Chronic ear infections
  - Blood poisoning
  - Abscesses
  - Pneumocystis
  - Toxoplasmosis
- Delayed growth
- Autoimmune disorders
  - Lupus
  - Rheumatoid arthritis
  - Diabetes, type 1
- Blood disorders
- Loss of appetite
- Intestinal/abdominal cramping
- Skin abscesses
- Wound abscesses
- Joint pain, frequently bilaterally and simultaneously
- Muscle pain
- Vomiting
- Diarrhea
- Nausea
- Dehydration
- Inflammation and infection of internal organs
  - Liver
  - Pancreas
  - Spleen
- If there are associated autoimmune disorders or infections
  - Anemia
  - Anxiety
  - Atherosclerosis
  - Depression

- Difficulty concentrating
- Edema in extremities
- Fatigue
- Headaches
- High blood pressure
- Kidney dysfunction/disease, nephritis
- Low-grade fever
- Morning stiffness
- Numbness in extremities
- Pericarditis (left side chest pain) with referral to neck, back, shoulders, arms
- Pleurisy
- Psychosis
- Raynaud phenomenon
- Seizures
- Swollen glands, lymph nodes
- Vasculitis
- Weakness in extremities
- Weight loss

Functional Implications

- Activity-limiting fatigue
- Anxiety and depression
- Avoidance of others who are sick
- Blood clots in women
- Can be indicative of serious medical conditions
- Cardiac disease
- Changes in lifestyle, secondary to pain and fatigue, limiting physical activity
- Decreased exercise tolerance
- Dehydration with loss of appetite
- Diffuse pain
- Eating disorders if GI system affected
- Frequent hand washing
- Impotence in males secondary to medication side effects
- Inability to ambulate secondary to joint deformity and/or pain
- Inability to concentrate
- Inability to take live vaccines
- Inappropriate self-medication
- Increased risk of pregnancy resulting in child with primary immune disease if both parents have the gene or another child has the disease
- Isolation to prevent infection
- Joint deformity
- Joint pain
- Limitations in activity secondary to cardiac pathology
- Limitations in ADLs or IADLs
- Management of cholesterol
- Need to stop smoking
- Psychological and concentration challenges
- Respiratory disease
- Sarcopenia resulting in weakness, muscle-mass loss, inability to ambulate or perform self-care, and aerobic capacity limitation secondary to inactivity
- Severe symptoms may be disabling, resulting in the inability to leave home
- Shortness of breath
- Sleep disturbances, sleeplessness
- Water retention, decreased urination, or other changes in urination
- Wearing a face mask in public for protection

Possible Contributing Causes

- Environmental factors such as chemicals, toxins
- Heredity
- Immune deficiencies
- Infection such as HIV
- Infectious (bacterial or viral) diseases
- Relationship of various pathogens to infection in primary immunodeficiency disorders
- Side effects of drugs, such as disease-modifying antirheumatic drugs (DMARDS), chemotherapy
- Systemic immunological condition, inflammatory: Autoimmune disease
- Vaccinations containing live virus
- Viral or bacterial infections

Differential Diagnosis

- Autoimmune/inflammatory diseases that affect the upper and lower GI tracts
- Barrett esophagus
- Celiac disease
- Chronic fatigue syndrome
- Crohn disease
- Endocrine disorders
- Esophageal cancer
- Fibromyalgia
- Gastroparesis
- Gastroenteritis
- Glomerulonephritis
- HIV
- Inflammation of the spleen
- Inflammatory bowel disease
- Irritable bowel syndrome
- Lupus
- Non-malignant tumors in the abdomen or organs
- Organ dysfunction as a result of cancer or malignancy
- Pancreatitis
- Post–weight-loss surgery complications: Bariatric surgeries for weight loss
- Referred pain from heart, spine, hip
- Rheumatoid arthritis
- Scleroderma
  - Side effects of gastric bypass, lap bands, and sleeves, although considered safe and medically indicated, may cause reflux, malabsorption, and other conditions
- Sjögren syndrome
- Stomach disorders
- Stomach ulcers
- Vasculitis

MEANS OF CONFIRMATION OR DIAGNOSIS

Laboratory Tests

- Blood tests/lab tests: Complete blood count (CBC), chemistry panel (kidney function, liver, electrolytes, blood sugar, cholesterol, triglycerides)
  - Erythrocyte sedimentation rate (ESR)
  - Antinuclear antibody (ANA)
  - Antiphospholipid antibodies (APLs)
  - Anti-Sm
  - Anti-dsDNA
  - Anti-Ro (SSA) and anti-La (SSB)
  - C-reactive protein (CRP)
  - Hemoglobin and hematocrit (H & H)
- Glomerular filtration rate and proteinuria for kidney function
- Protein/creatinine ratio for kidney function, protein loss

- Urinalysis for kidney disease
- Liver function studies

Imaging

- Radiography
  - Upper GI series
  - Lower GI series
- CT scans
- MRIs

Diagnostic Procedures

- Endoscopy
- Acid: Measurement
- Genetic testing
- Skin tests
- Prenatal amniocentesis
- Observation
  - Pallor
  - Sickly looking

FINDINGS AND INTERPRETATION

- H & H for signs of bleeding, anemia, pathogens, immune status, vitamin deficiencies, check white blood cell count for infection

TREATMENT

- Face masks to prevent infection
- Stem cell transplantation
- Protective clothing
- Appropriate therapies to manage functional and movement problems
- Avoidance of estrogen therapy
  - Estrogen may be causative or contributory
- Kidney dialysis if kidneys fail
- Dietary modifications if kidney disease present
- Bone marrow transplant

Medication

- NSAIDs
- Antimalarials (hydroxychloroquine) for concomitant diseases
- Corticosteroids
- Immunosuppressants (azathioprine, belimumab, cyclophosphamide, mycophenolate mofetil or methotrexate for concomitant diseases
- Gamma interferon
- Immunoglobulin therapy
- Anticoagulants including aspirin for blood clots
- Cardiac medications as indicated
- Antihypertensive as indicated
- Cholesterol-lowering medications
- Growth factor therapy
- If GI symptoms present
  - Acid blockers
    - Proton pump inhibitors: Available over the counter and prescription for GI symptoms
  - Acid reducers
    - H-2 receptors: Available over the counter and prescription
  - Prokinetic agents
    - Facilitate stomach emptying and valve tightening between stomach and esophagus
- Antibiotics specific to infection
- Bone marrow transplants
- Cytokines

REFERRALS/ADMITTANCE

- If a patient is referred for PT and the causative problem is not considered appropriate for PT, refer to the appropriate physician.
- If an emergency is identified, refer to an ER.

IMPAIRMENTS

- Impairments for which PT is indicated
  - Muscle weakness
  - Joint pain
  - Diffuse soft tissue pain
  - Soft tissue and/or joint contracture
  - Soft tissue and/or joint deformity with biomechanical malalignment
  - Muscle atrophy
  - Gait abnormality/difficulty walking
  - Contractures of soft tissue, fascia, muscle; joint limitations
  - Shortness of breath
  - Inability to perform self-care
  - Limited aerobic endurance
  - Functional decline, decrease in functional abilities
  - Coordination deficits
  - Balance dysfunction
  - Postural abnormalities
  - Developmental delay

TESTS AND MEASURES

- History
- Palpation
- Vital signs
- Muscle performance testing
- ROM measurements
- Joint integrity and mobility
- Edema measurements
- Peripheral nerve integrity
- Gait
- Balance
- Locomotion
- Motor function
- Orthotic, protective, and supportive device
- Pain
- Posture
- Reflex integrity
- Self-care and home management
- Sensory integrity
- Ventilation and respiration
- Work/community and leisure integration including ADLs
- Integumentary
- As primary immunodeficiency causes inflammation in multiple organ systems, the following tests and measures are included.
- Palpation
  - Liver: In supine, with left hand under trunk parallel to 11th and 12th rib, lift upward; right hand lateral to rectus and press in and up: +/= reproduction of symptoms with deep breath indicates liver involvement

- Ascites: With the fingers, percuss outward from center, if sound is dull, ascites may be present.
- Spleen: it is not recommended for PT to palpate an enlarged spleen (only palpable if enlarged) because of the potential of rupture.
- Gallbladder (Murphy sign): Place fingers right of rectus abdominus below rib cage: +/= sudden pain and muscle tensing with deep breath.
- Kidneys: In supine, place one hand under client between ribs and iliac crest and other hand on abdomen below ribs pointing in opposite direction: +/− tenderness or reproduction of symptoms.
- Bladder not usually palpable unless it is distended and rises above pubic bone.
  - In supine, place hand above pubis and press down: +/= tenderness, reproduction of pain, or ability to feel the bladder.

- Observation
  - Pink or purplish striae may be indicative of Cushing syndrome, and dilated veins may indicate hepatic pathology or inferior vena cava obstruction, not diverticulitis.
  - Contour: Roundedness, concavity/hollowness, asymmetry, distension, pregnancy signs.
  - Cullen sign: Bluish discoloring around umbilicus which may be a sign of retroperitoneal bleeding.
  - Bluish discoloration in lower abdomen: Grey Turner sign, which is a sign of hemorrhagic pancreatitis.
  - Pulsing in the area of the navel may be abdominal aortic aneurysm.
  - Left lower quadrant pain.
  - Palpable abdominal tenderness: On left or generalized.
  - Psoas sign: Provide resistance over patient's right knee as they flex the hip; pain is indicative of appendicitis or possible inflammation of the abdomen.
  - Obturator sign: Internal rotation of right lower extremity (RLE) and flexion may be indicative of appendicitis or pelvic inflammation.
  - Rovsing sign: Pain on the right side of abdomen when pressure is put on the left may be indicative of appendicitis.

INTERVENTION

- PT intervention is consistent with the movement-related problems that occur as a result of the effects of the condition or secondary problems.
- Gait training
- Therapeutic exercise: All relevant categories, energy conservation, aerobic-capacity related
- Therapeutic activities for bed-mobility training, transfer-, and transitional-movement training
- Neuromuscular re-education
- Self-care management training including use of adaptive equipment/home-modification assessment
- Physical agents for management of pain and inflammation
  - Heat, cold
  - Electrical stimulation
  - Laser
  - Soft tissue mobilization

FUNCTIONAL GOALS

- Patient will be able to
  - Demonstrate reduction in pain from ___ to ___ in (body part) in order to ___ (state function) or use sleep (e.g., in order to facilitate continuous sleep up to ___ hours to enable alertness during waking hours required for work).
  - Increase muscle performance in ___ (body part; specify muscle group or functional activity) from ___ to ___ in order to ___ (state function).
  - Achieve adequate functional aerobic capacity, and the ability to talk during activity in order to achieve functional gait and activity tolerance for work, play, school, self-care; ADLs and IADLs.
  - Have functional gait in the home and community (with or without a device, allowing for work, play, self-care; ADLs, and IADLs, up to ___ feet based on patient's need and prior functional level.
  - Achieve 600 m or greater in a 6-minute walk test for initiation of safe functional gait in the community.
  - Perform active verbalization with increasing taxonomy for safety during gait, including negotiation of even and uneven surfaces, opening and closing doors, transferring in and out of a car.
  - Perform activities requiring abdominals with appropriate muscle splinting/guarding to prevent retraction of stoma, if patient has a colostomy or ileostomy.
  - Tolerate 30 minutes of continuous moderate exercise three times a week in ___ weeks, and five times a week in ___ weeks, depending on the severity of the disease.

PROGNOSIS

- As this pathology is primarily medical in nature, the physician establishes the medical prognosis.
- Chronic diseases may go unnoticed for years or be so severe as to cause poor prognosis secondary to acquired infections.
- Shown to decrease lifespan; with appropriate medical management, individuals should be able to lead an active lifestyle.
- If the individual contracts one of the associated immune disorders such as lupus or rheumatism, the prognosis would be consistent with immune deficiency compounded by other diseases.
- For the PT prognosis, establish goals that the patient can achieve based on their overall condition.
- Unless the medical condition is unstable or the goals unrealistic, the prognosis from a PT perspective should be good.
  - "Good" refers only to the realistic functional goals established.

PATIENT RESOURCES

- Drugs & Medications. WebMD. http://www.webmd.com. Accessed July 3, 2013.
- Immune Deficiency Foundation. http://primaryimmune.org. Accessed July 3, 2013.
- Primary Immunodeficiency Association. http://www2.kenes.com/ukpin2011/GeneralInformation/Pages/PrimaryImmunodeficiencyAssociation.aspx. Accessed July 3, 2013.

REFERENCE

1. APTA. *Guide to Physical Therapy Practice*. Alexandria, VA: American Physical Therapy Association; 2003. http://guidetoptpractice.apta.org. Accessed July 4, 2013.

ADDITIONAL REFERENCES

- Chapel HM. Primary immune deficiencies—improving our understanding of their role in immunological disease. *Clin Exp Immunol*. 2005;139(1):11–12. doi: 10.1111/j.1365–2249.2005.02655.x.

- Chandrasoma P, Taylor CR. Deficiencies of the host response. In: Chandrasoma P, Taylor CR, eds. *Concise Pathology*. 3rd ed. New York, NY: McGraw-Hill; 1998. http://www.accessphysiotherapy.com/content/183828. Accessed July 4, 2013.
- Cunningham-Rundles C. Immune deficiency: office evaluation and treatment. *Allergy Asthma Proc*. 2003;24(6):409–415.
- Dutton M. Fundamentals and core concepts. In: Dutton M, ed. *McGraw-Hill's NPTE (National Physical Therapy Examination)*. 2nd ed. New York, NY: McGraw-Hill; 2012. http://www.accessphysiotherapy.com/content/5396365. Accessed April 4, 2013.
- Goodman CC, Fuller KS. *Pathology: Implications for the Physical Therapist*. 3rd ed. Philadelphia, PA: Saunders Elsevier; 2009.
- Goodman CC, Snyder TK. *Differential Diagnosis for Physical Therapists: Screening for Referral*. 4th ed. St. Louis, MO: Saunders Elsevier; 2007.
- Hauk PJ, Johnston RB, Liu AH. Immunodeficiency. In: Hay WW, Levin MJ, Sondheimer JM, Deterding RR, eds. *CURRENT Diagnosis & Treatment: Pediatrics*. 20th ed. New York, NY: McGraw-Hill; 2011. http://www.accessphysiotherapy.com/content/6587666. Accessed July 4, 2013.
- Kishiyama JL. Disorders of the immune system. In: McPhee SJ, Hammer GD, eds. *Pathophysiology of Disease*. 6th ed. New York, NY: McGraw-Hill; 2010. http://www.accessphysiotherapy.com/content/5366878. Accessed July 4, 2013.

49 LUPUS ERYTHEMATOSUS, SYSTEMIC

Debra F. Stern, DPT, DBA, MSM, PT
Eric Shamus, PhD, DPT, PT, CSCS

CONDITION/DISORDER SYNONYM

- Lupus erythematosus

ICD-9-CM CODES

- 695.4 Lupus erythematosus
- PT diagnoses/treatment diagnoses that may be associated with immune disorders affecting movement
  - 315.4 Developmental coordination disorder
  - 718.07 Articular cartilage disorder, ankle and foot
  - 718.03 Articular cartilage disorder, forearm
  - 718.04 Articular cartilage disorder, hand
  - 718.45 Contracture of joint, pelvic region and thigh
  - 719.39 Palindromic rheumatism involving multiple sites
  - 719.4 Pain in joint
  - 719.70 Difficulty in walking involving joint site unspecified
  - 728.2 Muscular wasting and disuse atrophy, not elsewhere classified
  - 729.9 Other and unspecified disorders of soft tissue
  - 729.1 Myalgia and myositis, unspecified
  - 729.9 Other disorders of soft tissue
  - 736.9 Acquired deformity of limb site unspecified
  - 780.7 Malaise and fatigue
  - 781.2 Abnormality of gait
  - 782.3 Edema
  - 786.0 Dyspnea and respiratory abnormalities
  - 786.05 Shortness of breath

ICD-10-CM CODES

- L93.0 Discoid lupus erythematosus
- L93.2 Other local lupus erythematosus

PREFERRED PRACTICE PATTERNS[1]

- 4D: Impaired Joint Mobility, Motor Function, Muscle Performance, and Range of Motion Associated with Connective Tissues Dysfunction
- 4E: Impaired Joint Mobility, Motor Function, Muscle Performance, and Range of Motion Associated with Localized Inflammation
- 7B: Impaired Integumentary Integrity Associated with Superficial Skin Involvement

PATIENT PRESENTATION

A 28-year-old Asian female is referred to physical therapy 6 months postpartum with her first child. Since the baby's birth, she has been suffering from what she describes as severe fatigue with muscle weakness and pain in her legs and hands, making it difficult to take care of her baby. She also has some mild back pain. She is upset because her husband thinks she is just depressed. Her history reveals that during her last trimester she complained of a rash on her face that the obstetrician told her was a "rash of pregnancy" and not anything to worry about. A mild rash is evident on her cheeks at the time of her initial PT evaluation. Throughout the initial examination she is drinking water because her mouth is dry and she is also complaining of dry eyes.

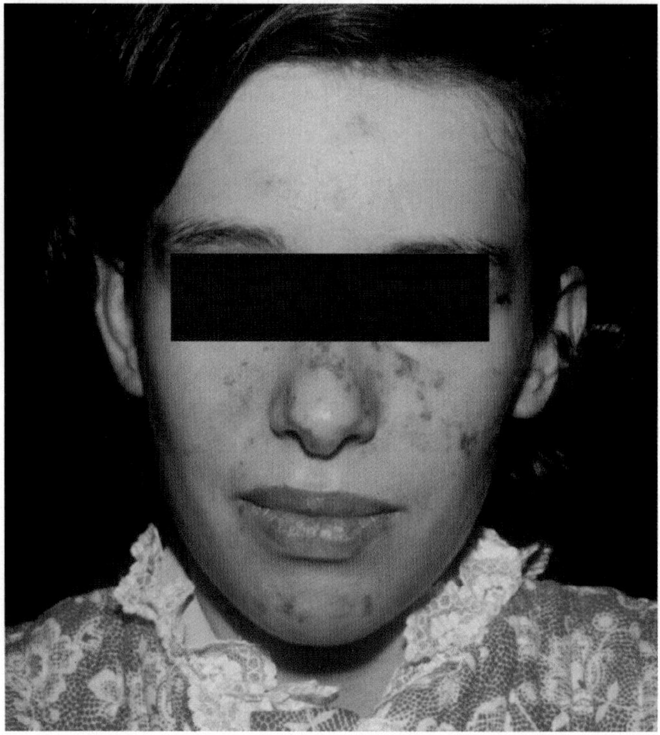

FIGURE 49-1 Systemic lupus erythematosus: butterfly rash associated with pericardial, myocardial, and endocardial disease. (From Fuster V, Walsh RA, Harrington RA. *Hurst's The Heart,* 13th ed. www.accessmedicine.com. Copyright © The McGraw-Hill Companies, Inc. All rights reserved.)

KEY FEATURES

Description

- A long term autoimmune disease that attacks the body's tissues and organ systems as if they were foreign substances.
- Affects skin, joints, kidneys, brain, and other organs.
- Although systemic lupus erythematosus (SLE) is a most common form, there are others: Discoid or cutaneous lupus, drug-induced systemic lupus, neonatal lupus, and subacute cutaneous lupus.
- Onset often vague with misdiagnosis.

Essentials of Diagnosis

- Must be made by a physician and confirmed by medical diagnostic testing

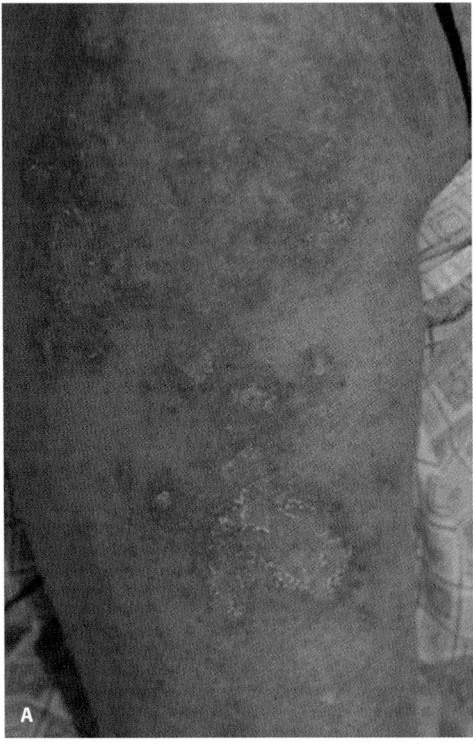
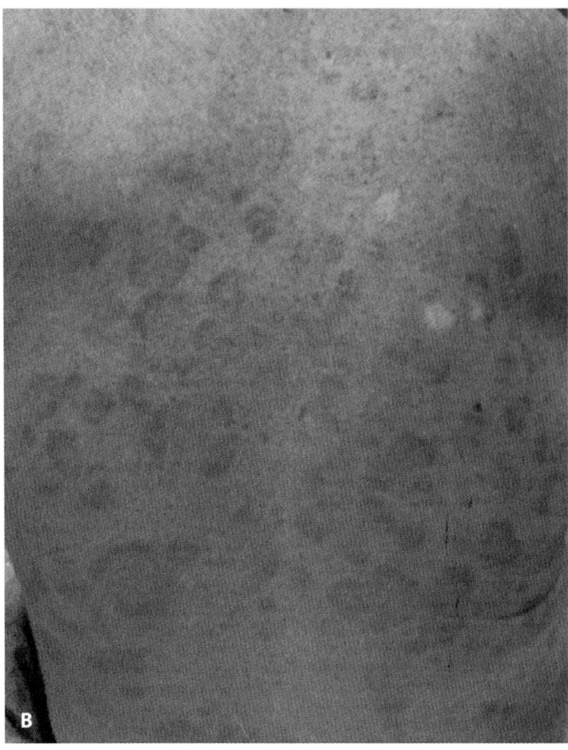

FIGURE 49-2 Subacute cutaneous lupus (SCLE). There are two main clinical variants: psoriasiform, scaly erythematous plaques (**A**) and erythematous, annular plaques (**B**). (From McKean SC, Ross JJ, Dressler DD, Brotman DJ, Ginsberg JS. *Principles and Practice of Hospital Medicine*. www.accessmedicine.com. Copyright © The McGraw-Hill Companies, Inc. All rights reserved.)

- According to the American College of Rheumatology (ACR)[2] 4 of 11 of the following must be present:
  - Malar rash: A rash over the cheeks and nose, often in the shape of a butterfly
  - Discoid rash: A rash that appears as red, raised, disk-shaped patches
  - Photosensitivity: A reaction to sun or light that causes a skin rash to appear or get worse
  - Oral ulcers: Sores appearing in the mouth
  - Arthritis: Joint pain and swelling of two or more joints in which the bones around the joints do not become destroyed
  - Serositis: Inflammation of the lining around the lungs (pleuritis) or inflammation of the lining around the heart that causes chest pain, which is worse with deep breathing (pericarditis)
  - Kidney disorder: Persistent protein or cellular casts in the urine
  - Neurological disorder: Seizures or psychosis
  - Blood disorder: Anemia (low red blood cell count), leukopenia (low white blood cell count), lymphopenia (low level of specific white blood cells), or thrombocytopenia (low platelet count)
  - Immunologic disorder: Abnormal anti-double-stranded DNA or anti-Sm, positive antiphospholipid antibodies
  - Abnormal antinuclear antibody (ANA)

General Considerations

- Diagnosis for more occult problems may take time and require intensive medical diagnostic testing.
- May result in secondary problems
  - Aerobic capacity and muscle-endurance impairment.
  - Sarcopenia.
  - Weakness/impaired muscle performance
  - Musculoskeletal problems
  - Neuromuscular problems
  - Weight loss indicating the need for physical therapy
- Because lupus and other immune disorders frequently refer pain or are causative of pain in various body areas, individuals may be referred to PT inappropriately or appropriately; inappropriate referral may be such as when referred to the lower back or upper back or chest.
- History of heartburn or indigestion may be indicative of GI or cardiac problems.

Demographics

- Females more likely than males: 9 out of 10 cases are women of childbearing age
- More common in African Americans
- Can affect individuals of all ages
- Some indication of genetic familial tendency

CLINICAL FINDINGS

SIGNS AND SYMPTOMS

- The signs and symptoms indicated here may be characteristic of multiple immune systemic disorders, which often confound medical diagnosis.
- It is not the purview of a PT to medically diagnose an immune pathology but rather to recognize the possibility in the differential diagnosis process, especially when the findings are not consistent with conditions commonly treated such as
  - Musculoskeletal
  - Neuromuscular

- Integumentary
- Cardiopulmonary
- Functional and mobility dysfunction secondary to medical pathology
- Anemia
- Anxiety
- Atherosclerosis
- Blood clots in women
- Dehydration with loss of appetite
- Depression
- Difficulty concentrating
- Edema in extremities
- Episodic hair loss with regrowth
- Fatigue
- Headaches
- High blood pressure
- Joint pain, frequently bilaterally and simultaneously
- Kidney dysfunction or disease, nephritis
- Low-grade fever
- Morning stiffness
- Multiple body system involvement
- Muscle pain
- Numbness in extremities
- Pericarditis (left-side chest pain) with referral to neck, back, shoulders, arms
- Pleurisy
- Psychosis
- Raynaud phenomenon
- Seizures
- Sensitivity to light, photosensitivity
- Skin rashes, often characteristic butterfly rash on face
- Skin sore, flakiness on extremities and ears
- Swollen glands; lymph nodes
- Vasculitis
- Weakness in extremities
- Weight loss

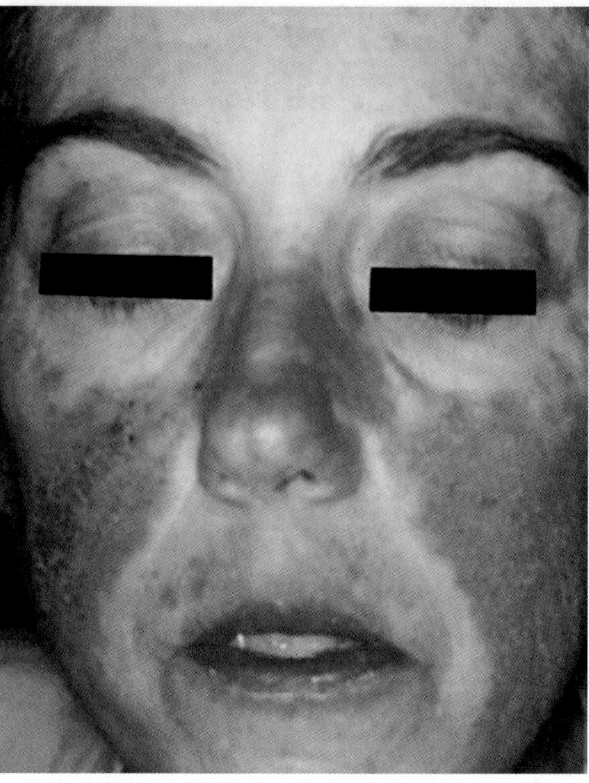

FIGURE 49-3 Acute cutaneous lupus erythematosus (ACLE) typically manifests as the characteristic malar "butterfly" rash. (Reproduced with permission from Wolff K, Johnson RA, Suurmond D. *Fitzpatrick's Color Atlas & Synopsis of Clinical Dermatology*. 5th ed. New York, NY: McGraw-Hill; 2005: Fig. 156-3.)

Functional Implications

- Severe symptoms may be disabling, resulting in the inability to leave home
- Inability to concentrate
- Inability to ambulate secondary to joint deformity and or pain
- Activity-limiting fatigue
- Sleep disturbances, sleeplessness
- Sarcopenia resulting in weakness, muscle-mass loss, inability to ambulate or perform self-care, as well as aerobic capacity limitation secondary to inactivity
- Decreased exercise tolerance
- Changes in lifestyle secondary to pain and fatigue limiting physical activity
- Limitations in activity secondary to cardiac pathology
- Limitations in ADLs or IADLs
- Psychological challenges
- Increased chance of a miscarriage
- Impotence in males secondary to medication side effects

Possible Contributing Causes

- Unknown, but may be attributable to the following:
  - Ultraviolet (UV) light
  - Drugs that cause sensitivity to the sun such as sulfa drugs and tetracycline drugs
  - Effects of medications such as penicillin or related antibiotic drugs
  - Viral infections or bacterial infections
  - Physical stress
  - Emotional stress
  - Vaccinations containing live virus
  - Pregnancy
  - Heredity
  - Environmental factors such as chemicals and toxins
  - Immune deficiencies
  - Infectious bacterial or viral diseases
  - Stress and anxiety
  - Systemic immunological condition: Inflammatory, autoimmune disease
  - Postsurgical scarring/adhesions
  - Pregnancy
  - Smoking
  - Side effects from medication/drugs

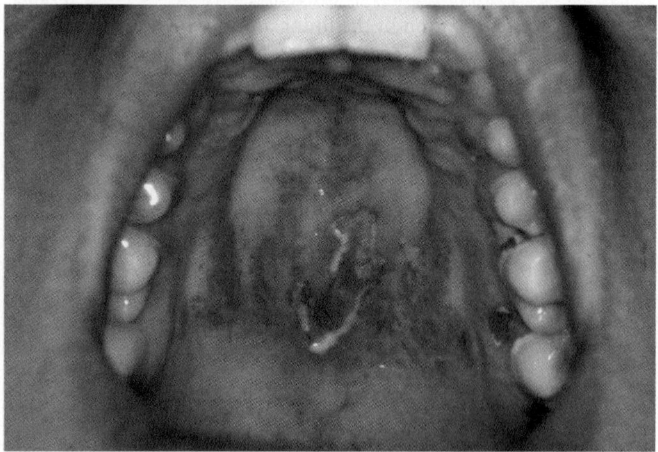

FIGURE 49-4 Lupus erythematosus (LE): hard palate erythematous eroded plaques were associated with chronic cutaneous LE. (From Wolff K, Johnson RA. *Fitzpatrick's Color Atlas and Synopsis of Clinical Dermatology*. 6th ed. www.accessmedicine.com. Copyright © The McGraw-Hill Companies, Inc. All rights reserved.)

Differential Diagnosis

- Fibromyalgia
- Scleroderma
- Glomerulonephritis
- Chronic fatigue syndrome
- Sjögren syndrome
- Vasculitis
- Rheumatoid arthritis
- Organ dysfunction as a result of cancer or malignancy
- Non-malignant tumors in the abdomen or organs
- Endocrine disorders
- Autoimmune/inflammatory diseases that affect the upper and lower GI tracts
- Irritable bowel syndrome
- Crohn disease
- Barrett esophagus
- Gastroparesis
- Stomach ulcers
- Esophageal cancer
- Inflammatory bowel disease
- Celiac disease
- Gastroenteritis
- Stomach disorders
- Referred pain from heart, spine, hip
- Post–weight-loss surgery complications
  - Bariatric surgeries for weight loss
  - Side effects of gastric bypass, lap bands, and sleeves, although considered safe and medically indicated, may cause reflux, malabsorption, and other conditions

MEANS OF CONFIRMATION OR DIAGNOSIS

Laboratory Tests

- Blood tests/lab tests: Complete blood count (CBC), chemistry panel (kidney function, liver, electrolytes, blood sugar, cholesterol, triglycerides)
- Erythrocyte sedimentation rate (ESR)
- Antinuclear antibody (ANA)
- Antiphospholipid antibodies (APLs)
- Anti-Sm
- Anti-dsDNA
- Anti-Ro/SSA and anti-La/SSB
- C-reactive protein (CRP)
- Hemoglobin and hematocrit
- Glomerular filtration rate and proteinuria for kidney function
- Protein/creatinine ratio for kidney function: Protein loss
- Urinalysis for kidney disease

Imaging

- Radiography
  - Upper GI series
  - Lower GI series
- CT scans
- MRIs

Diagnostic Procedures

- Endoscopy
- Acid: Measurement
- Esophageal motility

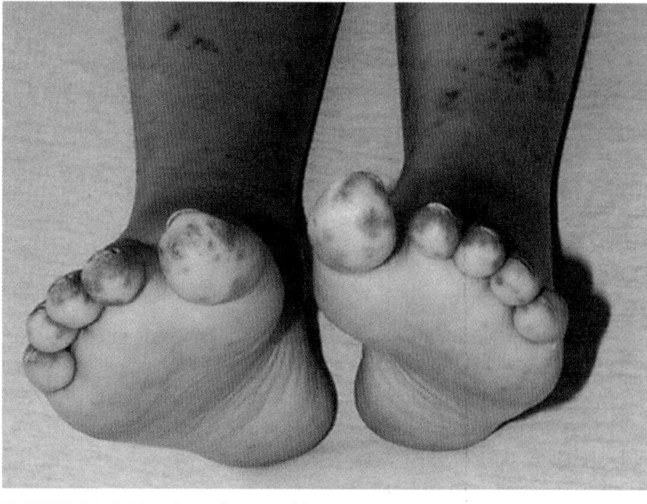

FIGURE 49-5 Vasculitis of toes and legs in a patient with systemic lupus erythematosus. (From Goldsmith LA, Katz S, Gilchrest B, Paller A, Leffell D, Wolff K. *Fitzpatrick's Dermatology in General Medicine*, 8th ed. www.accessmedicine.com.)

FINDINGS AND INTERPRETATION

- Hemoglobin and hematocrit for signs of bleeding, anemia, pathogens, immune status, and vitamin deficiencies, check white blood cell count for infection

TREATMENT

Medication

- Avoidance of estrogen therapy, as estrogen may be causative or contributory
- NSAIDs
- Antimalarials: Hydroxychloroquine (plaquenil)
- Corticosteroids
- Immunosuppressants (azathioprine, belimumab, cyclophosphamide, mycophenolate mofetil, or methotrexate)
- Anticoagulants including aspirin for blood clots
- Cardiac medications as indicated
- Antihypertensive as indicated
- Cholesterol-lowering medications
- If GI symptoms present
  - Acid blockers
    - Proton pump inhibitors: Available over the counter and prescription for GI symptoms
  - Acid reducers
    - H-2 receptors: Available over the counter and prescription
  - Prokinetic agents
    - Facilitate stomach emptying and valve tightening between stomach and esophagus

MEDICAL PROCEDURES

- Surgical management
  - Not generally for lupus, but problems with organ systems may necessitate surgical intervention
- Other
  - Sunscreen to minimize effects of UV
  - Protective clothing
  - Kidney dialysis if kidneys fail
  - Dietary modifications if kidney disease present

REFERRALS/ADMITTANCE

- If a patient is referred for PT and the causative problem is not considered to be appropriate for PT, make referral to the appropriate physician.
- If an emergency is identified, refer to an ER.

IMPAIRMENTS

- Balance dysfunction
- Contractures of soft tissue: Fascia, muscle
- Coordination deficits
- Diffused soft tissue pain
- Functional decline: Decrease in functional abilities
- Gait abnormality/difficulty walking
- Inability to perform self-care
- Joint limitations
- Joint pain
- Limited aerobic endurance
- Muscle atrophy
- Muscle weakness
- Postural abnormalities
- Shortness of breath
- Soft tissue and/or joint contracture/deformity with biomechanical malalignment

TESTS AND MEASURES

- History
- Palpation
- Vital signs
- Muscle performance testing
- Range of motion measurements
- Joint integrity and mobility
- Edema measurements
- Peripheral nerve integrity
- Gait
- Balance
- Locomotion
- Motor function
- Orthotic: Protective and supportive device
- Pain
- Posture
- Reflex integrity
- Self-care and home management
- Sensory integrity
- Ventilation and respiration
- Work/community and leisure integration including ADLs
- Integumentary
- Because lupus affects multiple systems, the tests and measures here are included
- Observation
  - Pink or purplish striae may be indicative of Cushing syndrome, dilated veins may indicate hepatic pathology or inferior vena cava obstruction, not diverticulitis.
  - Abdomen contour
    - Roundedness
    - Concavity/hollowness
    - Asymmetry
    - Distension
    - Pregnancy signs
  - Cullen sign: Bluish discoloring around umbilicus, which may be a sign of retroperitoneal bleeding.
  - Bluish discoloration in lower abdomen: Grey Turner sign, which is a sign of hemorrhagic pancreatitis.
  - Pulsing in the area of the navel may be abdominal aortic aneurysm.
  - Left lower quadrant pain.
  - Palpable abdominal tenderness on left or generalized.
  - Psoas sign: Provide resistance over patient's right knee as they flex the hip; pain is indicative of appendicitis or possible inflammation of the abdomen.
  - Obturator sign: Internal rotation of right lower extremity and flexion may be indicative of appendicitis or pelvic inflammation.
  - Rovsing sign: Pain on the right side of abdomen when pressure is put on the left may be indicative of appendicitis.
- Palpation
  - Liver: In supine, with left hand under trunk parallel to 11th and 12th rib, lift upward; right hand lateral to rectus and press in and up: +/= reproduction of symptoms with deep breath indicates liver involvement.
  - Ascites: With the fingers, percuss outward from center, if sound is dull, ascites may be present.
  - Spleen: It is not recommended for PT to palpate an enlarged spleen (only palpable if enlarged) because of the potential of rupture.
  - Gallbladder (Murphy's): Place fingers right of rectus abdominus below rib cage: +/= sudden pain and muscle tensing with deep breath.
  - Kidneys: In supine, place one hand under client between ribs and iliac crest, and other hand on abdomen below ribs and pointing in opposite direction: +/− tenderness or reproduction of symptoms.
  - Bladder: Not usually palpable unless it is distended and rises above pubic bone; in supine, place hand above pubis and press down: +/= tenderness, reproduction of pain, or ability to feel the bladder.

INTERVENTION

- PT intervention is consistent with the movement-related problems that occur as a result of the effects of
  - Gait training
  - Therapeutic exercise: All relevant categories, energy conservation, aerobic capacity-related
  - Therapeutic activities for bed-mobility training, transfer-, and transitional-movement training
  - Neuromuscular re-education
  - Wheelchair management
  - Self-care management training including the use of adaptive equipment/home modification assessment
  - Physical agents for management of pain and inflammation
    - Heat, cold
    - Electrical stimulation
    - Laser
    - Soft tissue mobilization
  - Orthotic instruction/management; check out for same
  - Interprofessional
    - Lifestyle modification
    - Smoking cessation
    - Weight management

- Dietary counseling
- Psychological intervention
- Pastoral counseling
- Occupational therapy
- Speech-language pathology

FUNCTIONAL GOALS

- Patient will be able to
  - Demonstrate reduction in pain from __ to __ in (body part) in order to __ (state function) or use sleep (e.g., in order to facilitate continuous __, sleep up to __ hours to enable alertness during waking hours required for work).
  - Increase muscle performance in __ (body part; specify muscle group or functional activity) from __ to __ in order to __ (state function).
  - Achieve adequate functional aerobic capacity, and the ability to talk during activity in order to achieve functional gait and activity tolerance for work, play, school, self-care; ADLs and IADLs.
  - Have functional gait in the home and community (with or without a device), allowing for work, play, self-care; ADLs and IADLs, up to __ feet based on patient need and prior functional level.
  - Achieve 600 m or greater in a 6-minute walk test for initiation of safe functional gait in the community.
  - Perform active verbalization with increasing taxonomy for safety during gait, including negotiation of even and uneven surfaces, opening and closing doors, transferring in and out of a car.
  - Perform activities requiring abdominals with appropriate muscle if patient has a colostomy or ileostomy splinting/guarding to prevent retraction of stoma.
  - Tolerate 30 minutes of continuous moderate exercise three times a week in __ weeks, and five times a week in __ weeks, depending on the severity of the disease.

PROGNOSIS

- As this pathology is primarily medical in nature, the physician establishes the medical prognosis.
- It is a chronic disease but with appropriate medical management, individuals should be able to lead an active lifestyle.
- For the PT prognosis, establish goals that the patient can achieve based on their overall condition.
- Unless the medical condition is unstable or the goals unrealistic, the prognosis from a PT perspective should be good.
  - "Good" refers only to the realistic functional goals established.

PATIENT RESOURCES

- Lupus Foundation of America. www.lupus.org. Accessed July 5, 2013.
- Systemic Lupus Erythematosus. NIH, National Institute of Arthritis and Musculoskeletal and Skin Diseases. http://www.niams.nih.gov/health_info/Lupus/default.asp. Accessed July 5, 2013.

REFERENCES

1. APTA. *Guide to Physical Therapy Practice.* Alexandria, VA: American Physical Therapy Association; 2003. http://guidetoptpractice.apta.org. Accessed July 1, 2013.
2. American College of Rheumatology. The 1982 Revised Criteria for Classification of Systemic Lupus Erythematosus. http://www.rheumatology.org/practice/clinical/classification/SLE/sle.asp. Accessed July 1, 2013.

ADDITIONAL REFERENCES

- Choi ST, Kang JI, Park IH, et al. Subscale analysis of quality of life in patients with systemic lupus erythematosus: association with depression, fatigue, disease activity and damage. *Clin Exp Rheumatol.* 2012;30(5):665–672.
- Goodman CC, Fuller KS. *Pathology: Implications for the Physical Therapist.* 3rd ed. Philadelphia, PA: Saunders Elsevier; 2009.
- Goodman CC, Snyder TK. *Differential Diagnosis for Physical Therapists: Screening for Referral.* 4th ed. St. Louis, MO: Saunders Elsevier; 2007.
- Hahn BH, Tsao BP. Pathogenesis of systemic lupus erythematosus. In: Firestein GS, Budd RC, Harris ED Jr, et al., eds. *Kelley's Textbook of Rheumatology.* 8th ed. Philadelphia, PA: Saunders Elsevier; 2008.
- Kosinski M, Gajria K, Fernandes A, Cella D. Qualitative validation of the FACIT-Fatigue scale in systemic lupus erythematosus. *Lupus.* 2013;22(5):422–430.
- McOmber MA, Shulman RJ. Pediatric functional gastrointestinal disorders. *Nutr Clin Pract.* 2008;23(3):268–274.
- Ruiz-Irastorza G, Ramos-Casals M, Brito-Zeron P, Khamashta MA. Clinical efficacy and side effects of antimalarials in systemic lupus erythematosus: a systematic review. *Ann Rheum Dis.* 2010;69(1):20–28. doi:10.1136/ard.2008.101766.
- Suleiman S, Johnston DE. The abdominal wall: an overlooked source of pain. *Am Fam Physician.* 2001;64(3):431–438.

50 SCLERODERMA

Debra F. Stern, DPT, DBA, MSM, PT
Eric Shamus, PhD, DPT, PT, CSCS

CONDITION/DISORDER SYNONYMS

- CREST syndrome
- Localized scleroderma
- Systemic sclerosis

ICD-9-CM CODES

- 701.0 Circumscribed scleroderma
- 710.1 Systemic sclerosis
- Associated physical therapy diagnoses
  - 315.4 Developmental coordination disorder
  - 718.03 Articular cartilage disorder, forearm
  - 718.04 Articular cartilage disorder, hand
  - 718.07 Articular cartilage disorder, ankle and foot
  - 718.45 Contracture of joint, pelvic region and thigh
  - 719.39 Palindromic rheumatism involving multiple sites
  - 719.4 Pain in joint
  - 719.70 Difficulty in walking
  - 728.2 Muscular wasting and disuse atrophy
  - 728.89 Other disorders of muscle, ligament, and fascia
  - 729.1 Myalgia and myositis, unspecified
  - 729.9 Other disorders of soft tissue
  - 736.9 Acquired deformity of limb
  - 780.7 Malaise and fatigue
  - 781.2 Abnormality of gait
  - 782.3 Edema
  - 786.0 Dyspnea and respiratory abnormalities
  - 786.05 Shortness of breath

ICD-10-CM CODES

- L94.0 Localized scleroderma [morphea]
- L94.3 Sclerodactyly
- M34.0 Progressive systemic sclerosis
- M34.1 CR(E)ST syndrome
- M34.9 Systemic sclerosis, unspecified

PREFERRED PRACTICE PATTERNS

- 4D: Impaired Joint Mobility, Motor Function, Muscle Performance, and Range of Motion Associated with Connective Tissues Dysfunction[1]
- 4E: Impaired Joint Mobility, Motor Function, Muscle Performance, and Range of Motion Associated with Localized Inflammation[2]
- 7B: Impaired Integumentary Integrity Associated with Superficial Skin Involvement[3]

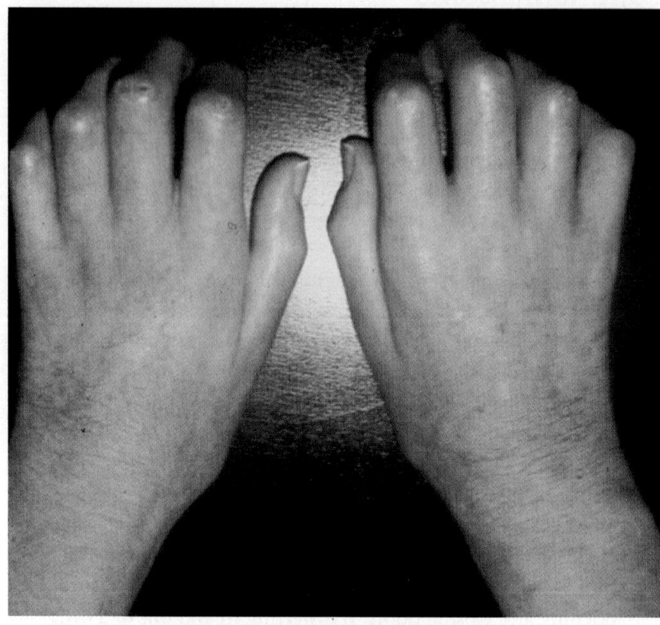

FIGURE 50-1 Scleroderma: claw-like hand deformity and shiny, tight skin. It can be linked with myocardial fibrosis. (From Fuster V, Walsh RA, Harrington RA. *Hurst's The Heart.* 13th ed. www.accessmedicine.com. Copyright © The McGraw-Hill Companies, Inc. All rights reserved.)

- 7E: Impaired Integumentary Integrity Associated With Skin Involvement Extending Into Fascia, Muscle, or Bone, and Scar Formation[4]

PATIENT PRESENTATION

A 40-year-old female who is a CrossFit competitor, is referred to OP PT with low back pain and generalized stiffness. While you are conducting the initial interview, you notice that her hands are getting mottled and her fingers red. She constantly rubs her fingers and periodically scratches her forearms and face. She has had some recent weight loss without dieting, and is happy about it, but not that her legs look skinnier. Upon questioning, she does describe that she is eating less because of intermittent heartburn not necessarily relieved with antacids. Observation reveals some red spots on her face, which she states have appeared over the past year or so.

KEY FEATURES

Description

- Autoimmune skin disorder
- Chronic, commonly progressive connective tissue disease considered an autoimmune rheumatic disease
- Skin hardening
- Intense fibrosis
- Finger sensitivity to cold
- Decreased sweating
- Multiple body system involvement
- Onset often vague, misdiagnoses common

Essentials of Diagnosis

- Etiology unknown
- Systemic scleroderma
  - Prolonged history of Raynaud phenomenon before presenting with swollen fingers, heartburn, shortness of breath
- Localized scleroderma
  - Morphea: Oval-shaped skin patches with purplish borders that may fade over time
  - Linear scleroderma: Bands of hardened skin on extremities or forehead, usually on one side of the body

General Considerations

- May result in secondary problems indicating need for PT intervention depending on severity: Aerobic capacity and muscle endurance impairment, sarcopenia, weakness, musculoskeletal problems, neuromuscular problems, weight loss.
- Because scleroderma frequently refers or causes pain in various body areas, individuals may be inappropriately referred to PT, such as when referred to low back, upper back, chest.
- History of heartburn or indigestion may be related to scleroderma or may indicate GI or cardiac problem.
- Individuals with scleroderma have twice the incidence of breast and bronchoalveolar cancer than the rest of the population.

Demographics

- Females-to-male ratio: 7:1
- Systemic scleroderma more common in adults; localized scleroderma most common in children
- Between 2 and 20 cases per million people
- Can affect individuals of any age: Most frequent onset between 25 and 55 years of age, average onset in 40s
- Decreased incidence after age 60
- Some indication of genetic familial tendency
- More common in Caucasians
- More severe in African and Native Americans

FIGURE 50-2 Barium esophagogram of a patient with scleroderma and stricture. Note the markedly dilated esophagus and retained food material. (Reproduced with permission from Waters PF, DeMeester TR. Foregut motor disorders and their surgical management. *Med Clin North Am.* 1981;65:1253. Copyright Elsevier.)

CLINICAL FINDINGS

SIGNS AND SYMPTOMS

- Alveolitis
- Anemia
- Anxiety, depression
- Arrhythmias
- Atherosclerosis
- Bloating
- Chest pain
- Coughing
- CREST Syndrome
  - Calcium deposits in body tissues
  - Raynaud phenomenon
  - Esophageal reflux (heartburn)
  - Sclerodactyly or thick skin on fingers
  - Telangiectasias: Enlarged blood vessels, appear as red spots on face and other areas
- Decreased sweating
- Diarrhea, constipation
- Difficulty swallowing
- Dry mouth or eyes (characteristic of Sjogren's, may be present with scleroderma)
- Dry skin
- Edema in fingers, hands, especially in morning
- Entrapment neuropathies
- Fatigue
- Gastroesophageal reflux disease (GERD)
- Hair loss in areas with thickened skin or other skin changes
- Headache
- High blood pressure
- Intestinal paresis
- Itchiness
- Joint or muscle pain
- Kidney dysfunction
- Malabsorption
- Mouth ulcers
- Nausea
- Numbness in extremities
- Pericardial effusion
- Pulmonary fibrosis
- Raynaud phenomenon
- Restricted movement, especially in digits, secondary to skin changes
- Shiny appearance of skin
- Shortness of breath
- Skin changes: Change in color or thickening (sclerodactyly) usually on fingers, hands, face, mouth
- Sores or ulcerations on fingers
- Stiffness
- Tendon rubs
- Vasculitis
- Vomiting
- Weakness in extremities
- Weight loss

Functional Implications

- Anxiety, depression, psychological changes
- Cardiac or respiratory disease
- Decreased exercise tolerance
- Dehydration, loss of appetite
- Diffuse pain
- Eating disorder if GI system effected

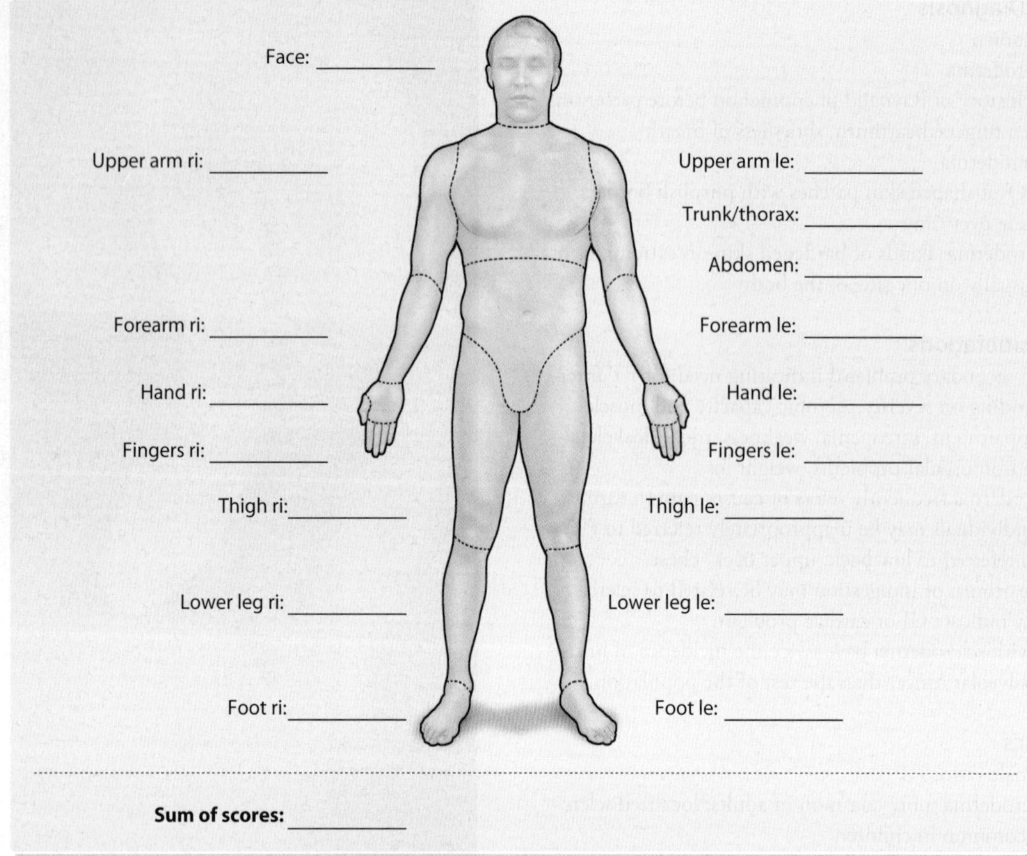

FIGURE 50-3 Modified Rodnan skin score (mRSS). Skin hardening will be evaluated with the modified mRSS that is usually performed by assessing the skin thickness at 17 different areas. The skin sclerosis is categorized by palpation to grade 1, corresponding to mild; 2, moderate; and 3, corresponding to severe, ri = right, le = left. (From Goldsmith LA, Katz S, Gilchrest B, Paller A, Leffell D, Wolff K. *Fitzpatrick's Dermatology in General Medicine*. 8th ed. www.accessmedicine.com. Copyright © The McGraw-Hill Companies, Inc. All rights reserved.)

- Erectile dysfunction
- Inability to ambulate secondary to joint deformity, weakness, pain
- Inability to concentrate
- Inappropriate self-medication
- Joint deformity
- Joint pain
- Lifestyle changes secondary to pain and fatigue
- Limited activity secondary to cardiac pathology
- Limited range of motion (ROM), ADLs, IADLs
- May indicate serious medical conditions in multiple organ systems
- Medication side effects (cardiac)
- Need to stop smoking
- Sarcopenia resulting in weakness, muscle-mass loss, inability to ambulate or perform self-care, limited aerobic capacity secondary to inactivity
- Severe symptoms may cause inability to leave home
- Shortness of breath
- Sleep disturbances, inability to lay flat secondary to reflux
- Vaginal dryness, pain associated with sex
- Water retention, decreased urination or other changes in urination

Possible Contributing Causes

- Unknown etiology
- May be attributable to the following
  - Overproduction of collagen
  - Physical or emotional stress, anxiety
  - Heredity
  - Environmental factors (chemicals, toxins)
  - Exposure to toxic substances, such as mercury
  - Immune deficiencies
  - Systemic immunological condition (inflammatory autoimmune disease)
  - Medication side effects
  - Possible association with pregnancy

Differential Diagnosis

- Autoimmune/inflammatory diseases affecting upper and lower GI tracts
- Barrett esophagus
- Celiac disease
- Chronic fatigue syndrome
- Crohn disease
- Endocrine disorder
- Esophageal cancer
- Fibromyalgia
- Gastroparesis
- Gastroenteritis
- Glomerulonephritis
- Inflammatory bowel disease
- Irritable bowel syndrome
- Lupus erythematosus
- Non-malignant tumor in abdomen or organs

- Organ dysfunction from cancer or malignancy
- Referred pain from heart, spine, hip
- Rheumatoid arthritis
- Sjögren syndrome
- Stomach disorder
- Stomach ulcers
- Vasculitis

MEANS OF CONFIRMATION OR DIAGNOSIS

Laboratory Tests

- Blood tests, complete blood count (CBC)
- Chemistry panel (kidney function, liver, electrolytes, blood sugar, cholesterol, triglycerides)
  - Erythrocyte sedimentation rate (ESR)
  - Antinuclear antibody (ANA)
  - Antiphospholipid antibodies (APLs)
  - Anti-Sm
  - Anti-dsDNA
  - Anti-Ro(SSA) and anti-La(SSB)
  - C-reactive protein (CRP)

Imaging

- Radiography
  - Upper GI series
  - Lower GI series
- CT
- MRI

Diagnostic Procedures

- Acid measurement
- ECG
- Endoscopy
- Esophageal motility
- Skin assessment: 17 points for integrity
- Skin biopsy

FINDINGS AND INTERPRETATION

- Arrhythmias

TREATMENT

Medication

- NSAIDs[5]
  - Anti-inflammatories
  - Antifibrotics
- Corticosteroids
- Immunosuppressants: Azathioprine, belimumab, cyclophosphamide, mycophenolate mofetil or methotrexate
- Anticoagulants, including aspirin for blood clots
- Cardiac medications as indicated (i.e., ACE inhibitors)
- Antihypertensives as indicated
- Vasodilators
- Topical nitroglycerin
- Cholesterol-lowering medications
- If GI symptoms present
  - Acid blockers
    - Proton pump inhibitors: OTC and prescription for GI symptoms
  - Acid reducers
    - H2 receptors: OTC and prescription

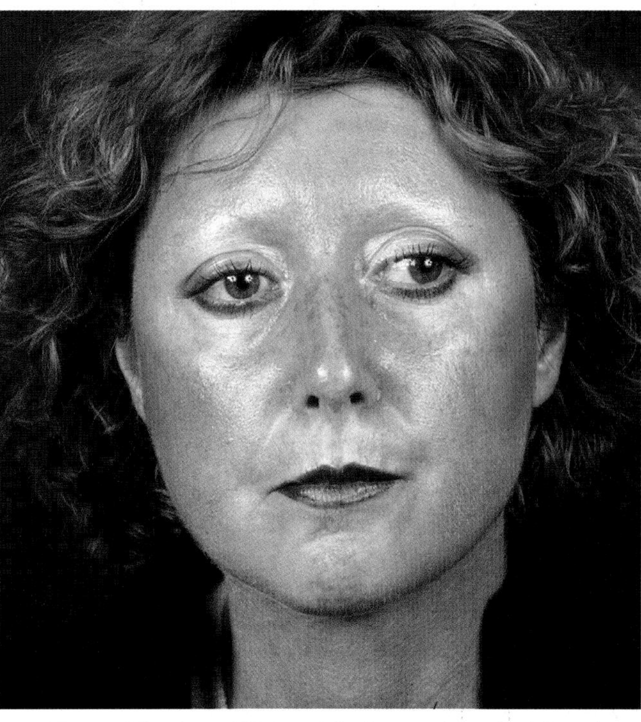

FIGURE 50-4 Scleroderma (dSSc) Mask-like facies with stretched, shiny skin and loss of normal facial lines giving a younger appearance than actual age; the hair is dyed. Thinning of the lips and perioral sclerosis result in a small mouth. Sclerosis (whitish, glistening areas) and multiple telangiectases (not visible at this magnification) are also present. (From Wolff K, Johnson RA. *Fitzpatrick's Color Atlas and Synopsis of Clinical Dermatology*. 6th ed. www.accessmedicine.com. Copyright © The McGraw-Hill Companies, Inc. All rights reserved.)

  - Prokinetic agents
    - Facilitate stomach emptying, valve tightening between stomach and esophagus

MEDICAL PROCEDURES

- Protective clothing
- Surgery
  - Amputation
  - Kidney transplant
  - Lung transplant
- Dietary modifications if kidney disease present
- Psoralen photochemotherapy (PUVA)
- Topical photodynamic therapy

REFERRALS/ADMITTANCE

- If causative problem is not considered appropriate for PT intervention, refer to appropriate physician.
- If emergency identified, refer to ER.

IMPAIRMENTS

- Muscle weakness
- Joint pain
- Diffuse soft tissue pain
- Soft tissue, skin, and or joint contracture
- Soft tissue and or joint deformity with biomechanical malalignment
- Muscle atrophy

- Gait abnormality/difficulty walking
- Contractures of soft tissue; skin, fascia, muscle; joint limitations
- Shortness of breath
- Inability to perform self-care
- Limited aerobic endurance
- Functional decline; decrease in functional abilities
- Coordination deficits
- Balance dysfunction
- Postural abnormalities

TESTS AND MEASURES

- Medical history
- Palpation
- Vital signs
- Muscle performance
- ROM
- Joint integrity, mobility
- Edema measurements
- Peripheral nerve integrity
- Gait, balance, locomotion, motor function
- Orthotic, protective and supportive device
- Pain
- Posture
- Reflex integrity
- Self-care and home management
- Sensory integrity
- Ventilation and respiration
- Work/community and leisure integration, including ADLs
- Integumentary
- As scleroderma affects multiple systems, the following tests and measures are included.
- Palpation
  - Liver: In supine, with left hand under trunk parallel to 11th and 12th ribs, lift upward; right hand lateral to rectus, press in and up: +/= reproduction of symptoms with deep breath, indicates liver involvement.
  - Ascites: Percuss outward from center with fingers; if sound is dull, ascites may be present.
  - Spleen: Not recommended for PT to palpate enlarged spleen secondary to ease of rupture (only palpable if enlarged).
  - Gallbladder (Murphy's): Place fingers right of rectus abdominus below rib cage: +/= sudden pain and muscle tensing with deep breath.
  - Kidneys: In supine, place one hand under client between ribs and iliac crest, other hand on abdomen below ribs and ribs pointing in opposite direction: +/− tenderness or reproduction of symptoms.
  - Bladder: Not usually palpable unless distended and raised above pubic bone; in supine, place hand above pubis and press down: +/= tenderness, reproduction of pain, ability to feel the bladder: __+.
- Skin observation

INTERVENTION

- Physical therapy intervention is consistent with movement-related problems occurring from the effects of scleroderma.
- Gait training
- Therapeutic exercise: All relevant categories, energy conservation, aerobic capacity related, stretching
- Therapeutic activities for bed mobility, transfer and transitional movement
- Neuromuscular re-education
- Self-care management, including use of adaptive equipment or home modification
- Physical agents for management of pain, inflammation, edema
  - Heat
  - Electrical stimulation
  - Laser
  - Soft tissue mobilization
- Orthotic instruction
- Prosthetic instruction in presence of amputation
- Biofeedback to facilitate vasodilatation in fingers

FUNCTIONAL GOALS

- Patient will be able to
  - Demonstrate reduction in pain from ___ to ___in (body part) in order to ________ (state function) or use sleep; in order to facilitate continuous sleep up to ______ hours to enable alertness during waking hours.
  - Reduce edema from _____ to or by ____ in (body part) in order to (state function, such as ability to wear shoes or protect skin on feet).
  - Demonstrate volitional vasodilatation in fingers to avoid vasoconstriction and minimize/eliminate response to cold and finger ulcerations.
  - Increase muscle performance in (body part; specify muscle group or functional activity) from ____ to ____ in order to (state function).
  - Achieve functional aerobic capacity, ability to talk during activity so as to achieve functional gait and activity tolerance for ADLs/IADLs.
  - Achieve 600 m or greater in a 6-minute walk test for initiation of safe, functional gait in the community.
  - Perform active verbalization with increasing taxonomy for safety during gait, including negotiation of even and uneven surfaces, opening and closing doors, transferring in and out of car.
  - Tolerate 30 minutes of continuous, moderate exercise three times per week in ______ weeks, and five times per week in ____________ weeks, depending on disease severity.

PROGNOSIS

- Highly variable, chronic disease.
- Stabilization or remission sometimes possible.
- May result in severe systemic problems or death.
- Patients should be able to lead an active lifestyle with appropriate medical management.
- Physician establishes the medical prognosis, as pathology is primarily medical in nature.
- For PT prognosis, goals should be established that the patient can achieve based on overall condition.
- Prognosis from a PT perspective should be good, unless medical condition is unstable or goals unrealistic.

PATIENT RESOURCE

- Scleroderma Foundation. http://www.scleroderma.org/site/PageServer. Accessed June 11, 2013.

REFERENCES

1. The American Physical Therapy Association. Pattern 4D: impaired joint mobility, motor function, muscle performance, and range of motion associated with connective tissue dysfunction. *Interactive Guide to Physical Therapist Practice.* 2003. doi: 10.2522/ptguide.3.1_4. http://guidetoptpractice.apta.org/content/1/SEC11.extract. Accessed May 5, 2014.
2. The American Physical Therapy Association. Pattern 4E: impaired joint mobility, motor function, muscle performance, and range of motion associated with localized inflammation. *Interactive Guide to Physical Therapist Practice.* 2003. doi: 10.2522/ptguide.3.1_5. http://guidetoptpractice.apta.org/content/1/SEC12.extract. Accessed May 5, 2014.
3. The American Physical Therapy Association. Pattern 7B: impaired integumentary integrity associated with superficial skin involvement. *Interactive Guide to Physical Therapist Practice.* 2003. doi: 10.2522/ptguide.3.4_2. http://guidetoptpractice.apta.org/content/1/SEC36.extract. Accessed May 5, 2014.
4. The American Physical Therapy Association. Pattern 7E: impaired integumentary integrity associated with skin involvement extending into fascia, muscle, or bone and scar formation. *Interactive Guide to Physical Therapist Practice.* 2003. doi: 10.2522/ptguide.3.4_5. http://guidetoptpractice.apta.org/content/1/SEC39.extract. Accessed May 5, 2014.
5. Panus PC, Jobst EE, Masters SB, Katzung B, Tinsley SL, Trevor AJ. *Pharmacology for the Physical Therapist.* New York, NY: McGraw-Hill; 2009. http://www.accessphysiotherapy.com/resource/615. Accessed June 10, 2013.

ADDITIONAL REFERENCES

- Bulpitt KJ, Clements PJ, Lachenbruch PA, et al. Early undifferentiated connective tissue disease: III. Outcome and prognostic indicators in early scleroderma (systemic sclerosis). *Ann Intern Med.* 1993;118(8):602–609.
- Dutton M. Integumentary physical therapy. In: Dutton M, ed. *McGraw-Hill's NPTE (National Physical Therapy Examination).* 2nd ed. New York, NY: McGraw-Hill; 2012. http://www.accessphysiotherapy.com/content/5403118. Accessed June 10, 2013.
- Dutton M. Differential diagnosis. In: Dutton M, ed. *Dutton's Orthopaedic Examination, Evaluation, and Intervention.* 2nd ed. New York, NY: McGraw-Hill; 2008. http://www.accessphysiotherapy.com/content/5547841. Accessed June 10, 2013.
- Goodman CC, Fuller KS. *Pathology: Implications for the Physical Therapist.* 3rd ed. Philadelphia, PA: Saunders Elsevier; 2009.
- Goodman CC, Snyder TK. *Differential Diagnosis for Physical Therapists: Screening for Referral.* 4th ed. St. Louis, MO: Saunders Elsevier; 2007.
- Lambe M, Björnådal L, Neregård P, Nyren O, Cooper GS. Childbearing and the risk of scleroderma: a population based study in Sweden. *Am J Epidemiol.* 2004;159(2):162–166.
- Minai OA, Dweik RA, Arroliga AC. Manifestations of scleroderma pulmonary disease. *Clin Chest Med.* 1998;19(4):713–731.
- Mills JC, Stappenbeck TS, Bunnett N. Gastrointestinal disease. In: McPhee SJ, Hammer GD, eds. *Pathophysiology of Disease: An Introduction to Clinical Medicine.* 6th ed. New York, NY: McGraw-Hill; 2010. http://www.accessphysiotherapy.com/content/5369615. Accessed June 11, 2013.
- Prakash UB. Respiratory complications in mixed connective tissue disease. *Clin Chest Med.* 1998;19(4):733–746.

51 SJÖGREN SYNDROME

Debra F. Stern, DPT, DBA, MSM, PT
Eric Shamus, PhD, DPT, PT, CSCS

CONDITION/DISORDER SYNONYMS

- Primary Sjögren's (dry eyes and mouths only)
- Secondary Sjögren's (associated with other immune disorders)

ICD-9-CM CODES

- 710.2 Sicca syndrome
- PT diagnoses/treatment diagnoses that may be associated with immune disorders affecting movement
  - 315.4 Developmental coordination disorder
  - 718.03 Articular cartilage disorder, forearm
  - 718.04 Articular cartilage disorder, hand
  - 718.07 Articular cartilage disorder, ankle and foot
  - 718.45 Contracture of joint, pelvic region and thigh
  - 719.39 Palindromic rheumatism involving multiple sites
  - 719.4 Pain in joint
  - 728.2 Muscular wasting and disuse atrophy, not elsewhere classified
  - 728.89 Other disorders of muscle, ligament, and fascia
  - 729.1 Myalgia and myositis, unspecified
  - 729.9 Other and unspecified disorders of soft tissue
  - 729.9 Other disorders of soft tissue
  - 736.9 Acquired deformity of limb site unspecified
  - 780.7 Malaise and fatigue
  - 781.2 Abnormality of gait
  - 782.3 Edema
  - 786.0 Dyspnea and respiratory abnormalities
  - 786.05 Shortness of breath

ICD-10-CM CODES

- M35.00 Sicca syndrome, unspecified
- M35.01 Sicca syndrome with keratoconjunctivitis

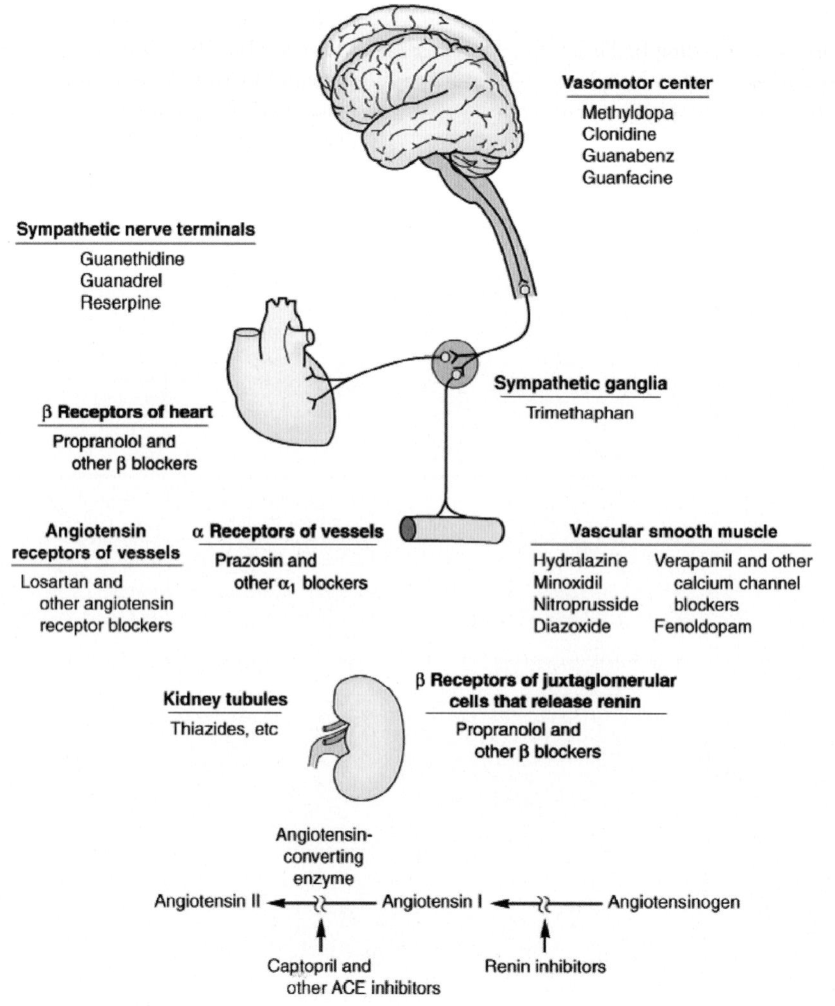

FIGURE 51-1 Sites of blood pressure control and actions of the major classes of antihypertensive drugs. (From Panus PC, Katzung B, Jobst E, Tinsley S, Masters S, Trevor A. *Pharmacology for the Physical Therapist*. New York, NY: McGraw-Hill; 2009.)

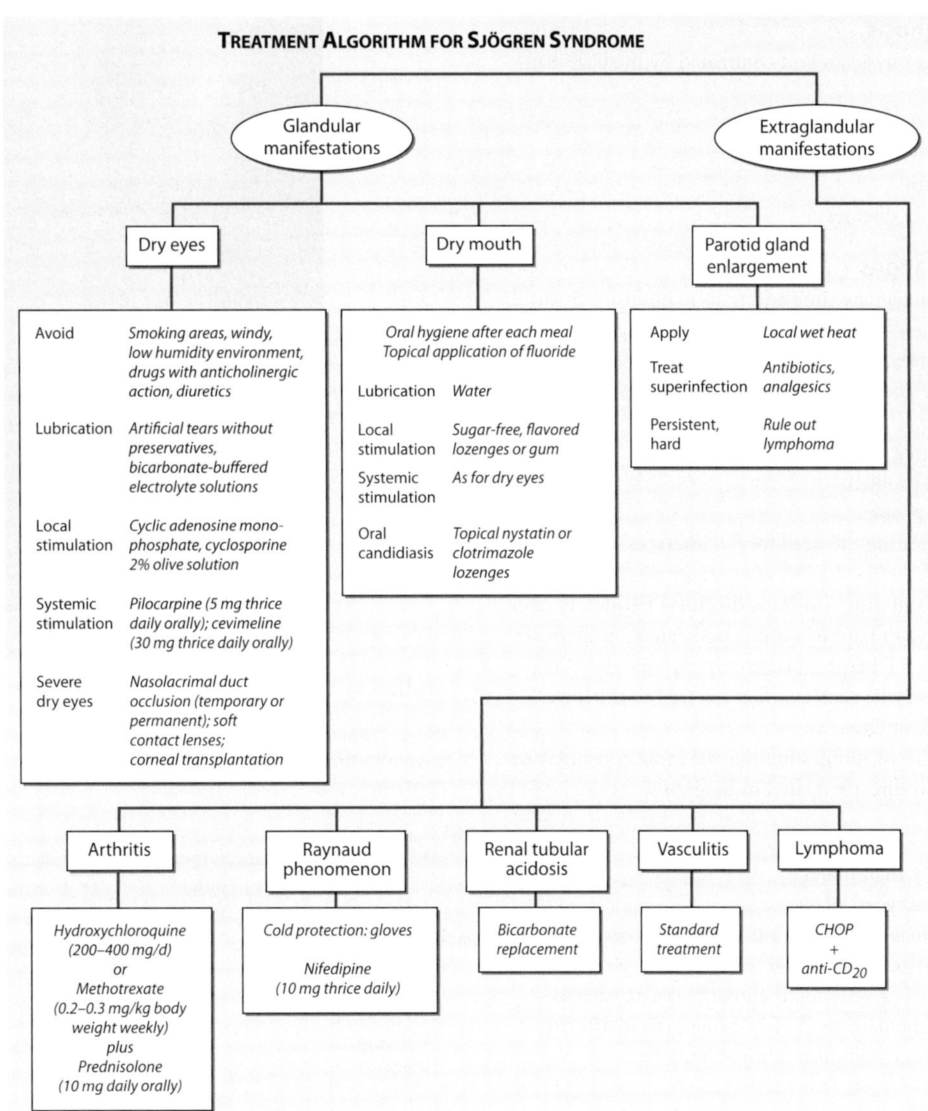

FIGURE 51-2 Treatment algorithm for Sjögren syndrome. (From Longo DL, Fauci AS, Kasper DL, Hauser SL, Jameson JL, Loscalzo J, eds. *Harrison's Principles of Internal Medicine*. 18th ed. New York, NY: McGraw-Hill; 2012.)

PREFERRED PRACTICE PATTERNS[1]

- 4D: Impaired Joint Mobility, Motor Function, Muscle Performance, and Range of Motion Associated with Connective Tissues Dysfunction
- 4E: Impaired Joint Mobility, Motor Function, Muscle Performance, and Range of Motion Associated with Localized Inflammation
- 7B: Impaired Integumentary Integrity Associated with Superficial Skin Involvement

PATIENT PRESENTATION

A 40-year-old female is referred to PT with onset of pain in both hands and wrists. Her pain started 2 weeks before when she was preparing food for a large house party and doing a lot of "chopping and slicing" with a large chef's knife. Her family history includes a mother with rheumatoid arthritis (RA) and father with OA. She describes "self diagnosed" wrist tendinitis in the past for which she used wrist splints for short periods of time and took NSAIDs until the pain resolved. The tendinitis was episodic and often followed the hours at the computer (she is a full-time receptionist). She recently had pink eye that has resolved with medication. She also related that she complained to her dentist several years ago that her mouth was always dry and he recommended hard, sugar free sucking candies as well as staying well hydrated. X-rays of her hands taken 1 week prior were negative. At this time she is taking NSAIDs, but they are not helping so her physician referred her to PT.

KEY FEATURES

Description

- Condition in which healthy tissue is mistaken by the body as foreign substances
- Affects the exocrine glands
- Limits production of body secretions
- Multiple body system involvement
- Onset often vague with misdiagnosis

Essentials of Diagnosis

- Must be made by a physician and confirmed by medical diagnostic testing
- History
- Presence of markers
- Dry eyes and mouth
- Elimination of other diseases

General Considerations

- Specific diagnosis may take time and require intensive medical diagnostic testing
- May result in secondary problems such as
  - Aerobic capacity and muscle endurance impairment
  - Sarcopenia
  - Weakness/impaired muscle performance
  - Musculoskeletal problems
  - Neuromuscular problems
  - Weight loss, indicating the need for PT intervention depending on severity
- Because Sjögren's and other immune disorders frequently refer pain or are causative of pain in various body areas, individuals may get referred to PT inappropriately or appropriately; inappropriate referral may be such as when referred to the lower back or upper back or chest
- History of heartburn or indigestion may be indicative of GI or cardiac problems or directly related to Sjögren's

Demographics

- Females more likely than males
- Adults older than 40 years of age
- Can affect individuals of all ages, but is rare in children
- Some indication of genetic familial tendency
- More likely if there is a systemic rheumatic disease such as systemic lupus erythematosus (SLE) or rheumatoid arthritis
- Estimated one to four million in United States

CLINICAL FINDINGS

SIGNS AND SYMPTOMS[2]

- The signs and symptoms indicated below may be characteristic of multiple immune systemic disorders, often confounding medical diagnosis.
- It is not the purview of a PT to medically diagnose an immune pathology but rather to recognize the possibility in the differential diagnosis process, especially when the findings are not consistent with conditions commonly treated; musculoskeletal, neuromuscular, integumentary, cardiopulmonary, or functional and with mobility dysfunction secondary to medical pathology.

- Anger
- Anxiety
- Arrhythmias
- Cancer of lymph nodes in small percentage
- Cavities
- Chest pain
- Coughing
- Cracked, sore tongue
- Decreased sweating
- Depression
- Diarrhea or constipation
- Difficulty concentrating
- Difficulty speaking
- Difficulty swallowing
- Difficulty with digestion
- Diffuse pain
- Diminished taste
- Dry eyes characteristic of Sjögren's and may be present with scleroderma

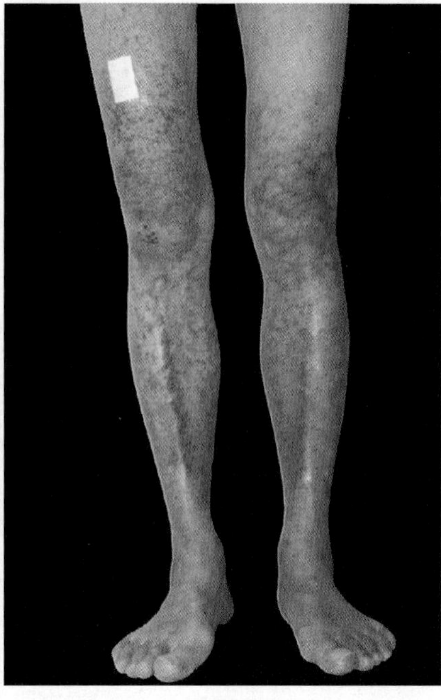

FIGURE 51-3 Cutaneous vasculitis in primary Sjögren syndrome. Biopsy showed leukocytoclastic vasculitis. (From Goldsmith LA, Katz SI, Gilchrest BA, Paller A, Leffell DJ, Wolff K. *Fitzpatrick's Dermatology in General Medicine*. 8th ed. www.accessmedicine.com. Copyright © The McGraw-Hill Companies, Inc. All rights reserved.)

- Dry mouth (characteristic of Sjögren's and may be present with scleroderma)
- Dry skin
- Dry throat
- Esophagitis
- Fatigue
- Fear
- Gastroparesis
- Gastric/intestinal paresis
- Gastroesophageal reflux disease (GERD)
- Headache
- High blood pressure
- Interstitial lung disease
- Itchiness

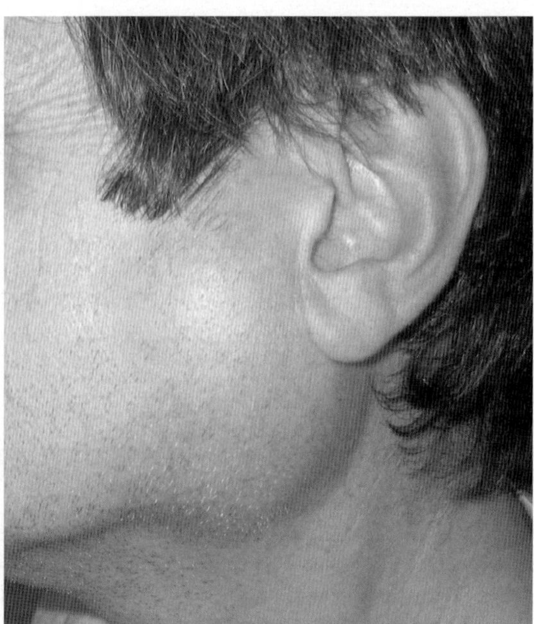

FIGURE 51-4 Parotid enlargement. (From Imboden J, Hellmann DB, Stone JH. *Current Rheumatology Diagnosis & Treatment*. 2nd ed. www.accessmedicine.com. Copyright © The McGraw-Hill Companies, Inc. All rights reserved.)

- Joint deformity
- Joint pain/arthritis
- Joint swelling/inflammation
- Kidney dysfunction or disease, nephritis
- Liver dysfunction, cirrhosis
- Lung disease, inflammation
- Malabsorption with GI dysfunction
- May be cardiac problems in newborns of mothers with Sjögren's
- Memory loss
- Mouth ulcers
- Muscle pain
- Nausea
- Nosebleeds
- Numbness in extremities, neuropathy
- Pancreatitis
- Respiratory disease
- Shortness of breath
- Side effects of medications used to treat organ or circulatory dysfunction associated with Sjögren's
- Sinusitis
- Skin rashes
- Stiffness
- Swollen glands, salivary
- Thyroid dysfunction
- Vasculitis
- Vision problems such as light sensitivity, blurriness, corneal ulcers
- Vomiting
- Weakness in extremities
- Weight loss
- Yeast infections, especially in mouth

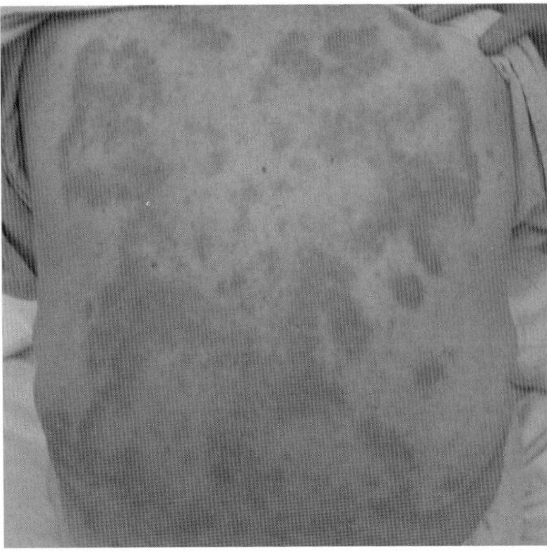

FIGURE 51-5 Polycyclic, photosensitive cutaneous lesions in a 67-year-old woman with primary SS and anti-Ro/SS-A antibodies. (From Goldsmith LA, Katz SI, Gilchrest BA, Paller A, Leffell DJ, Wolff K. *Fitzpatrick's Dermatology in General Medicine*. 8th ed. www.accessmedicine.com. Copyright © The McGraw-Hill Companies, Inc. All rights reserved.)

Functional Implications

- Severe symptoms may be disabling, resulting in the inability to leave home
- Vaginal dryness and pain associated with sex because of inability to find comfortable position
- Inability to concentrate
- Sensitivity to light
- Inability to ambulate secondary to joint deformity, weakness, and/or pain
- Activity-limiting fatigue
- ROM limitations
- Sleep disturbances and sleeplessness
- Dehydration with loss of appetite or trouble swallowing
- Eating disorders, inability or difficulty swallowing
- Sarcopenia resulting in weakness, muscle-mass loss, inability to ambulate or perform self-care as well as aerobic capacity limitation secondary to inactivity
- Decreased exercise tolerance
- Changes in lifestyle secondary to pain and fatigue, limiting physical activity
- Limitations in activity secondary to kidney, thyroid, liver, or lung pathology
- Inappropriate self-medication
- Limitations in ADLs or IADLs
- Psychological challenges

Possible Contributing Causes

- Unknown, but may be attributable to
  - Decreased levels of estrogen, menopause
  - Environmental factors such as chemicals and toxins
  - Exposure to toxic substances such as mercury
  - Heredity
  - Immune deficiencies
  - Lymphocytes that do not die, apoptosis
  - Side effects from medication/drugs
  - Smoking
  - Stress and anxiety
  - Systemic immunological condition, inflammatory: Autoimmune disease
  - Viral infections

Differential Diagnosis

- Fibromyalgia
- SLE
- Glomerulonephritis
- Chronic fatigue syndrome
- Vasculitis
- Scleroderma
- RA
- Organ dysfunction as the result of cancer or malignancy
- Non-malignant tumors in the abdomen or organs
- Endocrine disorders
- Autoimmune/inflammatory diseases that affect the upper and lower GI tracts
- Irritable bowel syndrome
- Crohn disease
- Barrett esophagus
- Gastroparesis
- Stomach ulcers
- Esophageal cancer
- Inflammatory bowel disease
- Celiac disease
- Gastroenteritis
- Stomach disorders
- Referred pain from heart, spine, hip
- Post–weight-loss surgery complications: Bariatric surgeries for weight loss; side effects of gastric bypass, lap bands, and sleeves, although considered safe and medically indicated, may cause reflux, malabsorption, inability to eat and other conditions

MEANS OF CONFIRMATION OR DIAGNOSIS

Laboratory Tests

- Blood tests/lab tests: Complete blood count (CBC), chemistry panel (kidney function, liver, electrolytes, blood sugar, cholesterol, triglycerides)
- Presence of antibodies common in Sjögren syndrome
  - Rheumatoid factor; ~60% in Sjögren's
  - Anti-Ro/SSA and anti-La/SSB (may also be present in SLE); Sjögren markers
- Erythrocyte sedimentation rate (ESR)
- Antinuclear antibody (ANA)
- C-reactive protein (CRP)
- Levels of different types of blood cells
- Immunoglobulins (Ig)
- Glomerular filtration rate and proteinuria for kidney function
- Protein/creatinine ratio
- Urinalysis

Imaging

- Radiography
  - Upper GI series
  - Sialogram, injectable dye to determine saliva production
  - Salivary scintigraphy for salivary function
  - Chest X-ray
- CT scans
- MRIs

Diagnostic Procedures

- Eyes: Schirmer test for dryness, slit lamp for cornea, rose bengal and lissamine green for dry spots
- Biopsies
- Spit test

FINDINGS AND INTERPRETATION

- Ig
  - To determine hemoglobin and hematocrit for signs of bleeding, anemia, pathogens, immune status, and vitamin deficiencies, check white blood cell count for infection
- Glomerular filtration rate and proteinuria for kidney function
- Protein/creatinine ratio for kidney function; protein loss

TREATMENT

Medication

- Pharmacologic management
  - Drugs to increase saliva production such as pilocarpine (Salagen) and cevimeline (Evoxac)
  - Drugs to facilitate tear production such as cyclosporine ophthalmic emulsion (Restasis)
  - Hydroxypropyl cellulose ophthalmic inserts such as Lacrisert
  - Eye drops: Over the counter or prescription
  - Artificial saliva
  - Disease-modifying antirheumatic drugs (DMARDs)
  - Drugs that suppress the immune system, such as methotrexate or cyclosporine, may also be prescribed
  - Antimalarials (plaquenil, also used with SLE)
  - NSAIDs
  - Anti-inflammatory agents
  - Corticosteroids
  - Antifungals
  - Immunosuppressants (azathioprine, belimumab, cyclophosphamide, mycophenolate mofetil, or methotrexate)
  - Anticoagulants, including aspirin for blood clots
  - Cardiac medications as indicated
  - Antihypertensives as indicated
    - Vasodilators
    - Topical nitroglycerin
    - Cholesterol-lowering medications
  - If GI symptoms present
    - Acid blockers; proton-pump inhibitors: Available over the counter and prescription for GI symptoms
    - Acid reducers; H-2 receptors: Available over the counter and prescription
    - Prokinetic agents; facilitate stomach emptying and valve tightening between stomach and esophagus

MEDICAL PROCEDURES

- Surgical management
  - Surgical sealing of tear ducts
  - Problems with organ systems may necessitate surgical intervention including amputation or organ transplantation

REFERRALS/ADMITTANCE

- If a patient is referred for PT and the causative problem is not considered appropriate for PT, refer to the appropriate physician.
- If an emergency is identified, refer to an ER.

IMPAIRMENTS

- Balance dysfunction
- Contractures of soft tissue such as skin, fascia, and muscle; joint limitations
- Coordination deficits
- Diffuse soft tissue pain
- Functional decline, decrease in functional abilities
- Gait abnormality/difficulty walking
- Inability to perform self-care
- Joint pain
- Joint swelling
- Limited aerobic endurance
- Muscle atrophy
- Muscle weakness
- Postural abnormalities
- Shortness of breath
- Soft tissue and or joint deformity with biomechanical malalignment
- Soft tissue, skin, and or joint contracture

TESTS AND MEASURES

- Balance
- Edema measurements
- Gait
- History
- Integumentary
- Joint integrity and mobility
- Locomotion
- Motor function
- Muscle performance testing
- Orthotic: Protective and supportive device(s)

- Pain
- Peripheral nerve integrity
- Posture
- Reflex integrity
- ROM measurements
- Self-care and home management
- Sensory integrity
- Ventilation and respiration
- Vital signs
- Work/community and leisure integration including ADL
- As Sjögren's affects multiple systems, the tests and following measures are included.
- Observation
  - Pink or purplish striae may be indicative of Cushing syndrome, and dilated veins may indicate hepatic pathology or inferior vena cava obstruction, not diverticulitis.
  - Abdomen contour: Roundedness, concavity/hollowness, asymmetry, distension, and pregnancy signs.
  - Cullen sign: Bluish discoloring around the umbilicus, which may be a sign of retroperitoneal bleeding.
  - Bluish discoloration in lower abdomen: Grey Turner sign, which is a sign of hemorrhagic pancreatitis.
  - Pulsing in the area of the navel may be abdominal aortic aneurysm.
  - Left lower quadrant pain.
  - Palpable abdominal tenderness on left or generalized.
  - Psoas sign: Provides resistance over patient's right knee as they flex the hip; pain is indicative of appendicitis or possible inflammation of the abdomen.
  - Obturator sign: Internal rotation of right lower extremity (RLE) and flexion may be indicative of appendicitis or pelvic inflammation.
  - Rovsing sign: Pain on the right side of abdomen when pressure is put on the left may be indicative of appendicitis.
- Palpation
  - Liver: In supine, with left hand under trunk parallel to 11th and 12th rib, lift upward; right hand lateral to rectus and press in and up: +/= reproduction of symptoms with deep breath, indicates liver involvement.
  - Ascites: With the fingers, percuss outward from center, if sound is dull, ascites may be present.
  - Spleen: It is not recommended for PT to palpate an enlarged spleen (only palpable if enlarged) because of the potential of rupture.
  - Gallbladder (Murphy's): Place fingers to the right of rectus abdominus below rib cage: +/= sudden pain and muscle tensing with deep breath.
  - Kidneys: In supine, place one hand under client between ribs and iliac crest, and other hand on abdomen below ribs and pointing in opposite direction: +/− tenderness or reproduction of symptoms.
  - Bladder: Not usually palpable unless it is distended and rises above pubic bone; in supine, place hand above pubis and press down: +/= tenderness, reproduction of pain, or ability to feel the bladder.

INTERVENTION

- PT intervention is consistent with the movement-related problems that occur as a result of the dysfunctions.
- If there is a stoma from a colostomy or ileostomy, activities should be avoided if they cause retraction.
- Gait training
- Therapeutic exercise in all relevant categories: Energy conservation, aerobic-capacity related, and stretching
- Therapeutic activities for bed-mobility training, transfer-, and transitional-movement training
- Neuromuscular re-education
- Wheelchair management
- Self-care management training including use of adaptive equipment/home-modification assessment
- Physical agents for management of pain, inflammation, and edema
  - Heat
  - Electrical stimulation
  - Laser
  - Soft tissue mobilization
- Orthotic instruction/management
- Prosthetic instruction/management in the presence of amputation
- Biofeedback to facilitate vasodilatation in fingers
- Interprofessional
  - Lifestyle modification
  - Smoking cessation
  - Weight management
  - Dietary counseling
  - Psychological intervention
  - Pastoral counseling
  - Occupational therapy
  - Speech-language pathology
- Other appropriate therapies to manage functional and movement problems
  - Frequently sipping liquids
  - Sucking on candies that facilitate saliva production to lubricate mouth
  - Chewing gum
  - Dietary modifications if kidney disease present
  - Increasing humidity
  - Wearing goggles outside to prevent dry eye
  - Frequent fluid intake

FUNCTIONAL GOALS

- Patient will be able to
  - Demonstrate reduction in pain from ___ to ___ in (body part) in order to ___ (state function) or use sleep (e.g., in order to facilitate continuous sleep up to ___ hours to enable alertness during waking hours required for work).
  - Reduce edema from ___ to or by ___ in (body part) in order to ___ (state function such as ability to wear shoes or protect skin on feet).
  - Increase muscle performance in ___ (body part, specify muscle group or functional activity) from ___ to ___ in order to ___ (state function).
  - Achieve adequate functional aerobic capacity and the ability to talk during activity in order to achieve functional gait and activity tolerance for work, play, school, self-care; ADLs and IADLs.
  - Functional gait in the home and community (with or without a device), allowing for work, play, self-care, ADLs and IADLs, up to ___ feet based on patient need and prior functional level.
  - Achieve 600 m or greater in a 6-minute walk test for initiation of safe functional gait in the community.

- Perform active verbalization with increasing taxonomy for safety during gait, including negotiation of even and uneven surfaces, opening and closing doors, and transferring in and out of a car.
- Perform activities requiring abdominals with appropriate muscle splinting/guarding to prevent retraction of stoma, if patient has a colostomy or ileostomy.
- Tolerate 30 minutes of continuous moderate exercise three times a week in ___ weeks, and five times a week in ___ weeks, depending on the severity of the disease.

PROGNOSIS

- As this pathology is primarily medical in nature, the physician establishes the medical prognosis.
- It is a highly variable chronic disease; however, most individuals with appropriate medical management should be able to lead an active lifestyle.
- For the PT prognosis, goals should be established that the patient can achieve based on the overall condition.
- Unless the medical condition is unstable or the goals unrealistic, the prognosis from a PT perspective should be good.
  - "Good" refers to the realistic functional goals established.

PATIENT RESOURCES

- Sjögren's Syndrome Foundation. http://www.sjogrens.org./ Accessed July 10, 2013.

REFERENCES

1. APTA. *Guide to Physical Therapy Practice*. Alexandria, VA: American Physical Therapy Association; 2003. http://guidetoptpractice.apta.org. Accessed July 10, 2013.
2. Locke GR III. EGJ and GER Disease. In: Giuli R, Galmiche JP, Jamieson GG, Scarpignato C, eds. *The Esopagogastric Junction*. Paris: John Libbey Eurotext; 1998. https://www.hon.ch/OESO/books/Vol_5_Eso_Junction/Articles/art126.html. Accessed July 10, 2013.

ADDITIONAL REFERENCES

- Goodman CC, Fuller KS. *Pathology: Implications for the Physical Therapist*. 3rd ed. Philadelphia, PA: Saunders Elsevier; 2009.
- Goodman CC, Snyder TK. *Differential Diagnosis for Physical Therapists: Screening for Referral*. 4th ed. St. Louis, MO: Saunders Elsevier; 2007.
- Malandraki GA, Kaufman A, Hind J, et al. The effects of lingual intervention in a patient with inclusion body myositis and Sjögren's syndrome: a longitudinal case study. *Arch Phys Med Rehabil*. 2012;93(8):1469–1475. doi: 10.1016/j.apmr.2012.02.010.
- McOmber MA, Shulman RJ. Pediatric functional gastrointestinal disorders. *Nutr Clin Pract*. 2008;23(3):268–274.
- Mills JC, Stappenbeck TS, Bunnett N. Gastrointestinal disease. In: McPhee SJ, Hammer GD, eds. *Pathophysiology of Disease: An Introduction to Clinical Medicine*. 6th ed. New York, NY: McGraw-Hill; 2010. http://www.accessphysiotherapy.com/content/5369615. Accessed January 10, 2013.
- Ozgocmen S, Gur A. Treatment of central nervous system involvement associated with primary Sjögren's syndrome. *Curr Pharm Des*. 2008;14(13):1270–1273.
- Panus PC, Jobst EE, Masters SB, Katzung B, Tinsley SL, Trevor AJ. Drugs affecting the respiratory system. In: Panus PC, Jobst EE, Masters SB, Katzung B, Tinsley SL, Trevor AJ, eds. *Pharmacology for the Physical Therapist*. New York, NY: McGraw-Hill; 2009. http://www.accessphysiotherapy.com/content/6095983. Accessed July 10, 2013.
- Suleiman S, Johnston DE. The abdominal wall: an overlooked source of pain. *Am Fam Physician*. 2001;64(3);431–438.
- Ulcerative Colitis. National Digestive Diseases Information Clearinghouse (NDDIC). U.S. Department of Health and Human Services. *NIH Publication No. 12-1597*. October 2011. http://digestive.niddk.nih.gov/ddiseases/pubs/colitis/. Accessed July 10, 2013.
- Wang KK, Sampliner RE. Updated guidelines 2008 for the diagnosis, surveillance and therapy of Barrett's esophagus. *Am J Gastroenterol*. 2008;103(3):788–797. doi:10.1111/j.1572-0241.2008.01835.x.

SECTION I INFECTIOUS DISORDERS

52 OSTEOMYELITIS

Eric Shamus, PhD, DPT, PT, CSCS
Shallen (McClain) Flory, DPT

CONDITION/DISORDER SYNONYMS

- Bone infection
- Pyogenic osteomyelitis

ICD-9-CM CODES

- 730 Osteomyelitis periostitis and other infections involving bone
- 730.0 Acute osteomyelitis

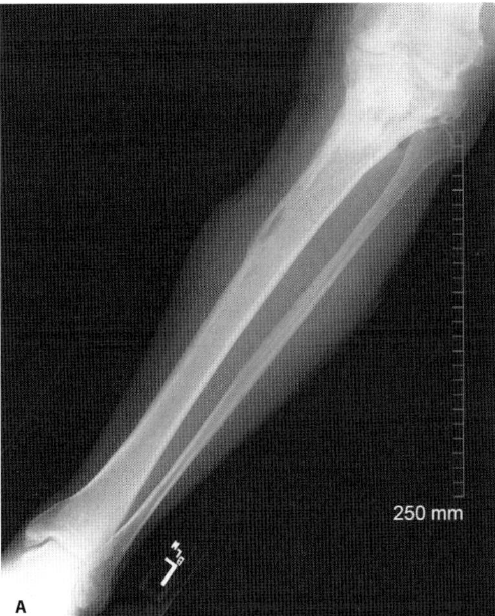

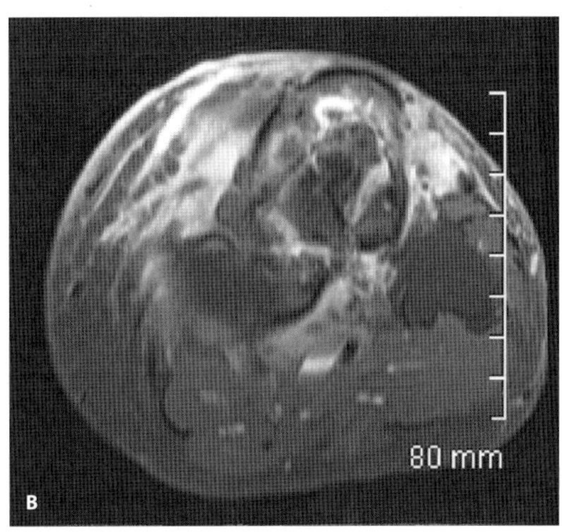

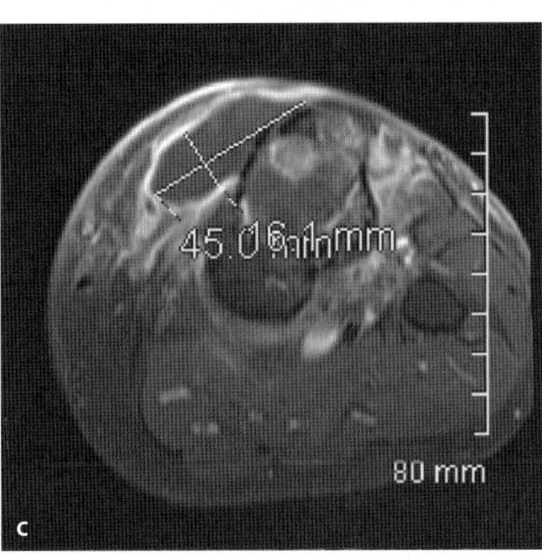

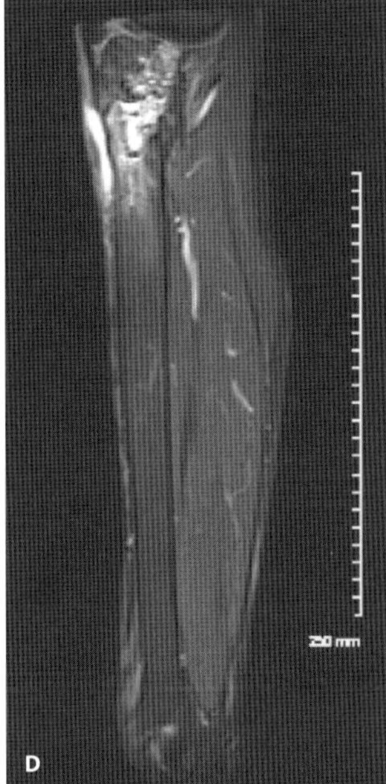

FIGURE 52-1 **A.** Standard radiology image indicates infection with sclerosis of the proximal tibia and periosteal elevation and obvious bone destruction with an apparent cavity and the suggestion of a sequestrum in the proximal medial tibia. **B** and **C.** Magnetic resonance images more clearly visualize the bone and soft tissue anatomy, confirming an extensive infection with destruction within the proximal tibia that has extended into the surrounding soft tissues and the joint as well as a ring of calcification most consistent with an abscess. **D.** A longitudinal MRI shows the extent of longitudinal bone destruction and soft tissue involvement with contrast enhancement that suggests viable marrow from the middle to the distal tibial shaft. (From Longo DL, Fauci AS, Kasper DL, Hauser SL, Jameson JL, Loscalzo J, eds. *Harrison's Principles of Internal Medicine*. 18th ed. New York, NY: McGraw-Hill; 2012.)

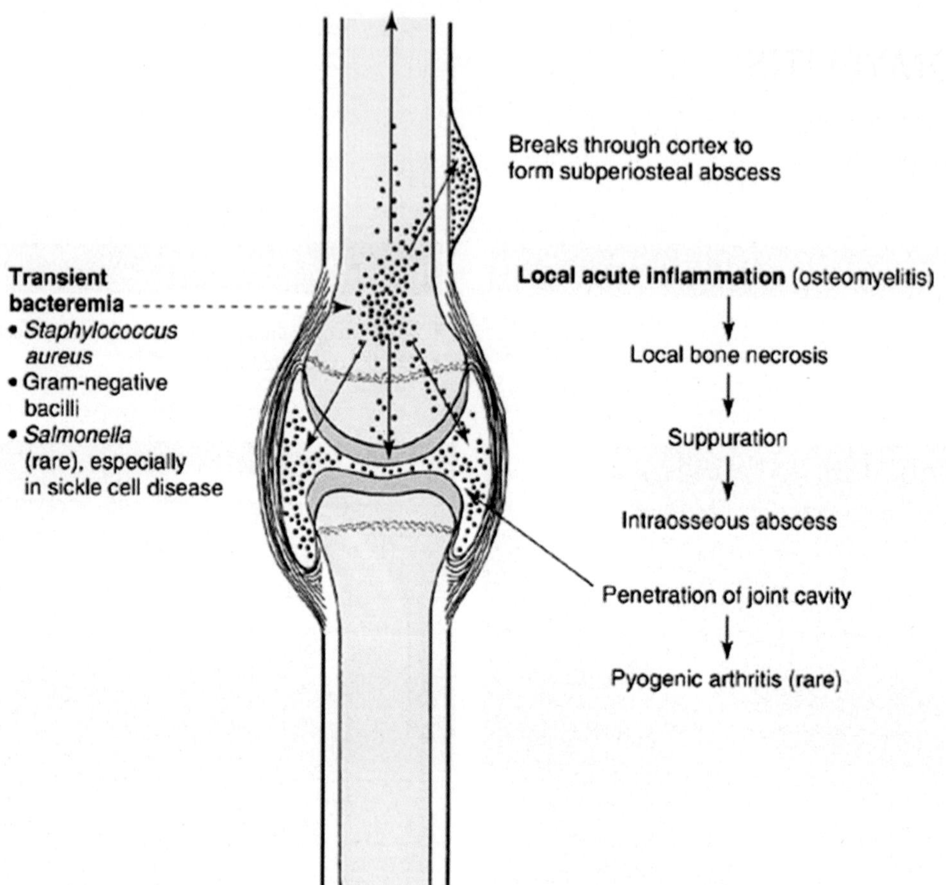

FIGURE 52-2 Acute osteomyelitis. The primary site of infection is usually in the metaphysial region, from which the infection may spread to involve the cortex and form a subperiosteal abscess; may spread into the medullary cavity; or, rarely, may spread into the adjacent joint space. (From Chandrasoma P, Taylor CR. *Concise Pathology*. 3rd ed. www.accessmedicine.com. Copyright © The McGraw-Hill Companies, Inc. All rights reserved.)

- 730.00 Acute osteomyelitis, site unspecified
- 730.01 Acute osteomyelitis, shoulder region
- 730.02 Acute osteomyelitis, upper arm
- 730.03 Acute osteomyelitis, forearm
- 730.04 Acute osteomyelitis, hand
- 730.05 Acute osteomyelitis, pelvic region and thigh
- 730.06 Acute osteomyelitis, lower leg
- 730.07 Acute osteomyelitis, ankle and foot
- 730.08 Acute osteomyelitis, other specified sites
- 730.09 Acute osteomyelitis, multiple sites
- 730.1 Chronic osteomyelitis
- 730.10 Chronic osteomyelitis, site unspecified
- 730.11 Chronic osteomyelitis, shoulder region
- 730.12 Chronic osteomyelitis, upper arm
- 730.13 Chronic osteomyelitis, forearm
- 730.14 Chronic osteomyelitis, hand
- 730.15 Chronic osteomyelitis, pelvic region and thigh
- 730.16 Chronic osteomyelitis, lower leg
- 730.17 Chronic osteomyelitis, ankle and foot
- 730.18 Chronic osteomyelitis, other specified sites
- 730.19 Chronic osteomyelitis, multiple sites
- 730.2 Unspecified osteomyelitis
- 730.20 Unspecified osteomyelitis, site unspecified
- 730.21 Unspecified osteomyelitis, shoulder region
- 730.22 Unspecified osteomyelitis, upper arm
- 730.23 Unspecified osteomyelitis, forearm
- 730.24 Unspecified osteomyelitis, hand
- 730.25 Unspecified osteomyelitis, pelvic region and thigh
- 730.26 Unspecified osteomyelitis, lower leg
- 730.27 Unspecified osteomyelitis, ankle and foot
- 730.28 Unspecified osteomyelitis, other specified sites
- 730.29 Unspecified osteomyelitis, multiple sites
- 730.3 Periostitis without mention of osteomyelitis
- 730.30 Periostitis, without mention of osteomyelitis, site unspecified
- 730.31 Periostitis, without mention of osteomyelitis, shoulder region
- 730.32 Periostitis, without mention of osteomyelitis, upper arm
- 730.33 Periostitis, without mention of osteomyelitis, forearm
- 730.34 Periostitis, without mention of osteomyelitis, hand
- 730.35 Periostitis, without mention of osteomyelitis, pelvic region and thigh
- 730.36 Periostitis, without mention of osteomyelitis, lower leg
- 730.37 Periostitis, without mention of osteomyelitis, ankle and foot

The Cierney and Mader Staging System.

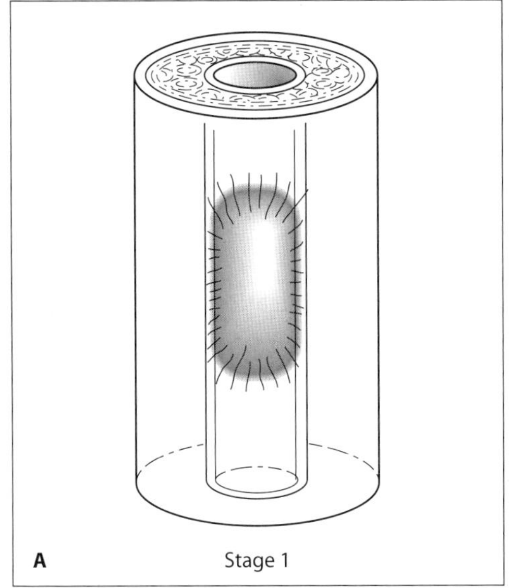

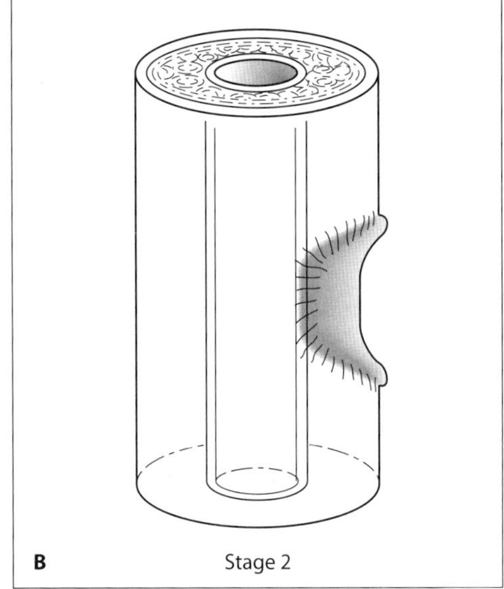

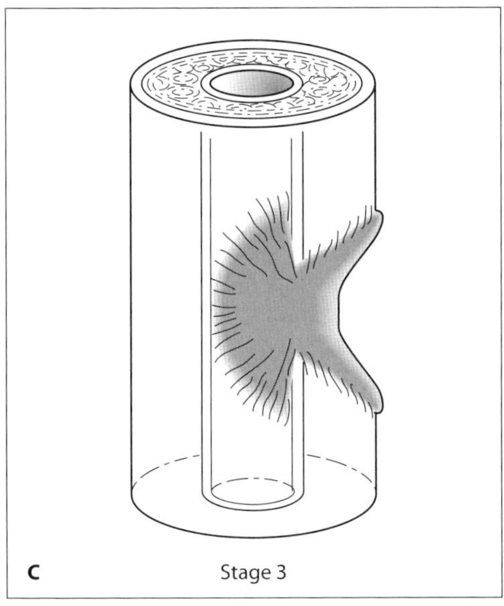

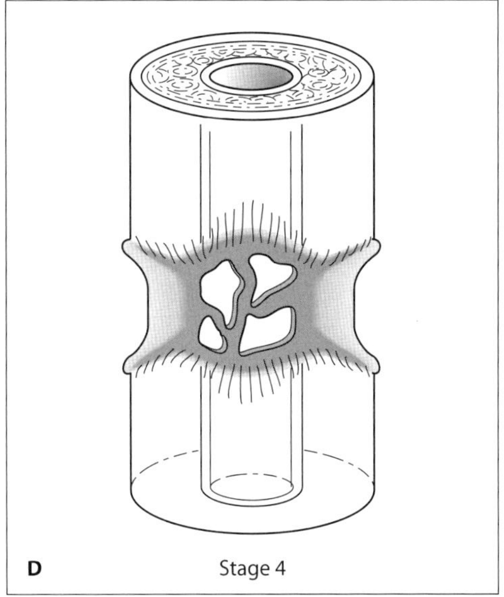

FIGURE 52-3 The Cierny and Mader staging system for osteomyelitis is classified by the anatomic extent of the infection and by the physiologic status of the host rather than by chronicity or etiology. The four stages are characterized by the pattern of bony involvement of the infection in order of increasing complexity: stage 1—medullary only, stage 2—superficial cortex only, stage 3—localized medullary and cortical, and stage 4—diffuse medullary and cortical. (From Skinner HB. *Current Diagnosis & Treatment in Orthopedics*. 4th ed. www.accessmedicine.com. Copyright © The McGraw-Hill Companies, Inc. All rights reserved.)

- 730.38 Periostitis, without mention of osteomyelitis, other specified sites
- 730.39 Periostitis, without mention of osteomyelitis, multiple sites

ICD-10-CM CODES

- M46.20 Osteomyelitis of vertebra, site unspecified
- M86.10 Other acute osteomyelitis, unspecified site
- M86.119 Other acute osteomyelitis, unspecified shoulder
- M86.129 Other acute osteomyelitis, unspecified humerus
- M86.139 Other acute osteomyelitis, unspecified radius and ulna
- M86.149 Other acute osteomyelitis, unspecified hand
- M86.159 Other acute osteomyelitis, unspecified femur
- M86.169 Other acute osteomyelitis, unspecified tibia and fibula
- M86.179 Other acute osteomyelitis, unspecified ankle and foot
- M86.18 Other acute osteomyelitis, other site
- M86.19 Other acute osteomyelitis, multiple sites
- M86.20 Subacute osteomyelitis, unspecified site
- M86.219 Subacute osteomyelitis, unspecified shoulder
- M86.229 Subacute osteomyelitis, unspecified humerus
- M86.239 Subacute osteomyelitis, unspecified radius and ulna
- M86.249 Subacute osteomyelitis, unspecified hand
- M86.259 Subacute osteomyelitis, unspecified femur
- M86.269 Subacute osteomyelitis, unspecified tibia and fibula
- M86.279 Subacute osteomyelitis, unspecified ankle and foot
- M86.28 Subacute osteomyelitis, other site
- M86.29 Subacute osteomyelitis, multiple sites
- M86.60 Other chronic osteomyelitis, unspecified site
- M86.619 Other chronic osteomyelitis, unspecified shoulder

- M86.629 Other chronic osteomyelitis, unspecified humerus
- M86.639 Other chronic osteomyelitis, unspecified radius and ulna
- M86.642 Other chronic osteomyelitis, left hand
- M86.659 Other chronic osteomyelitis, unspecified thigh
- M86.669 Other chronic osteomyelitis, unspecified tibia and fibula
- M86.679 Other chronic osteomyelitis, unspecified ankle and foot
- M86.68 Other chronic osteomyelitis, other site
- M86.69 Other chronic osteomyelitis, multiple sites
- M86.9 Osteomyelitis, unspecified

PREFERRED PRACTICE PATTERNS[1]

- 4C: Impaired Muscle Performance
- 4F: Impaired Joint Mobility, Motor Function, Muscle Performance, ROM, and Reflex Integrity Association with Spinal Disorders

PATIENT PRESENTATION

A 33-year-old male presents with complaints of low back pain with insidious onset and duration of 5 weeks. He reports that he has pain while trying to sleep, particularly in his hips. The patient describes the pain as a deep ache that may be coming from his bones. He reports that he has chills and has had a running fever. He also reports pain 7/10 in his feet at the end of the day. He later reports that he had a skin infection approximately 2 months ago that was treated and cleared with topical antibiotics.

He is referred to physical therapy by his primary care physician. The physician ordered blood cultures, a complete blood count (CBC), and an X-ray. The results of the lab tests are not in yet, but the X-ray shows necrosis in the right ankle with soft tissue swelling. The physical therapy evaluation shows generalized muscle weakness in the lower extremities as well as localized swelling and redness in the right ankle. The patient has normal reflexes and dermatome response.

KEY FEATURES

Description

- Bone infection by bacteria (*Staphylococcus aureus*) or fungi
- Can spread to the bone through a skin ulcer or skin infection
- Can be spread throughout the body by the bloodstream
- Can begin after surgery

Essentials of Diagnosis

- Cultured bone biopsy
- High fever
- Tenderness
- Bone pain
- Local swelling and redness
- Pyogenic osteomyelitis caused by bacterial infection

General Considerations

- Widespread bone infection
- Can occur after dental work
- Higher incidence once spleen is removed
- Can cause the need for amputation
- Can be caused by *Mycobacterium kansasii* and *Mycobacterium fortuitum*

Demographics

- Can occur across the lifespan
- In children: In the long bones
- In adults: In the spine, feet

CLINICAL FINDINGS

SIGNS AND SYMPTOMS

- Pain with movement
- Bone pain at night
- Abscess
- Soft tissue swelling
- Muscle weakness
- Fever
- Malaise
- Chills
- Low back pain
- Swelling in the lower legs
- Bone pain (common in the hips)

Functional Implications

- Causes disability for aging and elderly women and men
- Necrosis of the bone
- Removal of prosthesis or metal implant

Possible Contributing Causes

- Compromised immune system
- Diabetes
- Poor blood supply
- Poor dietary habits or eating disorders
- Sickle cell disease
- Spleen removal
- Surgery
- Trauma

Differential Diagnoses

- Cushing syndrome or glucocorticoid administration
- Excessive vitamin D/A
- History of drug abuse or misuse (alcohol, tobacco)
- Hyperparathyroidism
- Hyperthyroidism
- Leukemia
- Multiple myeloma, lymphoma, or metastatic cancer
- Osteogenesis imperfecta
- Paget disease
- Pathologic fracture from neoplasm
- Trauma
- Tuberculosis

MEANS OF CONFIRMATION OR DIAGNOSIS

Laboratory Tests

- Blood cultures
- C-reactive protein (CRP)
- CBC
- Erythrocyte sedimentation rate (ESR)

Imaging

- X-ray
- Computer assisted tomography (CT)
- Diagnostic ultrasound
- Spinal and pelvic x-rays may demonstrate demineralization, vertebral compression
- Posterior, anterior, and lateral x-rays of affected areas of spine are utilized to identify location and severity of fracture(s)
- MRI of the area of possible infection
- Single-energy x-ray absorptiometry (SXA); quantitative computed tomography (QCT); radiographic absorptiometry (RA)

Diagnostic Procedures

- Needle aspiration

FINDINGS AND INTERPRETATION

- ESR
- Necrosis on X-ray

TREATMENT

Medication

- Oral and IV antibiotics

MEDICAL PROCEDURES

- Surgical removal of metal appliance
- Removal of infection
- Removal of bone and followed bone graft

REFERRALS/ADMITTANCE

- To endocrinologist
- To general practitioner
- To geriatrician
- To orthopedist for joint assessment
- To rheumatologist
- To pharmacist for bone supplements
- To occupational therapist for ADL training
- To registered dietitian for nutrition education

IMPAIRMENTS

- Physical impairment
  - Chronic or recurrent pain or discomfort
  - Incomplete use of arms or fingers
  - Incomplete use of feet or legs
  - Disfigurement or deformity
  - Disability with reduced use of the limb
- Activity limitations
  - Self-care
  - Mobility
  - Physical transport
  - ADLs
  - Socialization and social activities
  - Work loss or employment restrictions
- Quality of life (QoL) and health-related quality of life (HQoL)
- Environment and adjustments
  - Assistive devices
  - Home and occupational modifications
  - Family assistance

TESTS AND MEASURES

- Fall risk assessments: FRAS® score (10-year risk assessment)

INTERVENTION

- Therapeutic exercise
- Progressive weight-bearing exercises, for example, aquatic therapy
- Patient education and lifestyle changes
- Transcutaneous electric nerve stimulation (TENS)
- Manual therapy/joint mobilization with precaution of bone density
- Soft tissue massage
- Orthotics to decrease flexion forces and reduce pain or dysfunction

FUNCTIONAL GOALS

- Adequate control of pain/infection
- Prevention of disability
- Improve strength, flexibility, posture, and balance
- Decrease in risks for falls

PROGNOSIS

- If poor blood supply, outcome less positive with possible need for amputation
- Depends on type of infection
- Depends on general health
- Depends on location and duration of infection

PATIENT RESOURCE

- Osteomyelitis. MedlinePlus, US National Library of Medicine, NIH National Institutes of Health. http://www.nlm.nih.gov/medlineplus/ency/article/000437.htm. Accessed July 7, 2013.

REFERENCE

1. APTA Guide to PT Practice. http://guidetoptpractice.apta.org/search?fulltext=osteoporosis&submit=yes&x=0&y=0. Accessed July 7, 2013.

ADDITIONAL REFERENCES

- Chandrasoma P, Taylor CR. Infections of bone. In: Chandrasoma P, Taylor CR, eds. *Concise Pathology*. 3rd ed. New York, NY: McGraw-Hill; 2011. http://www.accessphysiotherapy.com/content/193548. Accessed July 7, 2013.
- Chandrasoma P, Taylor CR. Metabolic bone disease. In: Chandrasoma P, Taylor CR, eds. *Concise Pathology*. 3rd ed. New York, NY: McGraw-Hill; 2011. http://www.accessphysiotherapy.com/content/193568. Accessed July 7, 2013.
- Dutton M. Metabolic disease. In: Dutton M, ed. *Orthopaedic Examination, Evaluation, and Intervention*. 2nd ed. New York, NY: McGraw-Hill; 2008. http://www.accessphysiotherapy.com/content/5546939. Accessed July 7, 2013.
- Dutton M. Pathology of bone. In: Dutton M, ed. *McGraw-Hill's NPTE (National Physical Therapy Examination)*. 2nd ed. New York, NY: McGraw-Hill; 2012. http://www.accessphysiotherapy.com/content/5396057. Accessed July 7, 2013.
- Hay WW, Levin MJ, Sondheimer JM, Deterding RR. General considerations. In: Hay WW, Levin MJ, Sondheimer JM, Deterding RR, eds. *CURRENT Diagnosis & Treatment: Pediatrics*. 20th ed. New York, NY: McGraw-Hill; 2011. http://www.accessphysiotherapy.com/content/6591503. Accessed July 7, 2013.
- McPhee SJ, Hammer GD. Pathophysiology of selected disorders of calcium metabolism. In: McPhee SJ, Hammer GD, eds. *Pathophysiology of Disease: An Introduction to Clinical Medicine*. 6th ed. New York, NY: McGraw-Hill; 2010. http://www.accessphysiotherapy.com/content/5370820. Accessed July 7, 2013.
- Osteoporosis Handout on Health (*NIH Publication No. 11-5158*). NIH Osteoporosis and Related Bone Diseases Resource Center. 2011; Bethesda, MD. http://www.niams.nih.gov/Health_Info/Bone/Osteoporosis/osteoporosis_hoh.asp. Accessed July 7, 2013.
- Rahman N, Bhatia K. Impairments and disability associated with arthritis and osteoporosis. Arthritis Series No .4. Cat. No. PHE 90. Canberra: Australian Institute of Health and Welfare (AIHW); 2007. http://www.aihw.gov.au/publication-detail/?id=6442468025. Accessed July 7, 2013.

53 PRION DISEASES

Eric Shamus, PhD, DPT, PT, CSCS
Mollie Venglar, DSc, MSPT, NCS

CONDITION/DISORDER SYNONYMS

- Creutzfeldt–Jakob disease (CJD)
- Fatal familial insomnia
- Gerstmann– Sträussler –Scheinker syndrome
- Kuru
- Transmissible spongiform encephalopathies (TSEs)
- Variant Creutzfeldt–Jakob disease (vCJD)

ICD-9-CM CODES

- 046.0 Kuru
- 046.1 Jakob–Creutzfeldt disease
- 046.11 Variant Creutzfeldt–Jakob disease
- 046.19 Other and unspecified Creutzfeldt–Jakob disease
- 046.2 Subacute sclerosing panencephalitis
- 046.3 Progressive multifocal leukoencephalopathy
- 046.7 Other specified prion diseases of central nervous system
- 046.71 Gerstmann–Sträussler–Scheinker syndrome
- 046.72 Fatal familial insomnia
- 046.79 Other and unspecified prion disease of central nervous system
- 046.8 Other specified slow virus infection of central nervous system
- 046.9 Unspecified slow virus infection of central nervous system

ICD-10-CM CODES

- A81.00 Creutzfeldt–Jakob disease, unspecified
- A81.01 Variant Creutzfeldt–Jakob disease
- A81.09 Other Creutzfeldt–Jakob disease
- A81.1 Subacute sclerosing panencephalitis
- A81.2 Progressive multifocal leukoencephalopathy
- A81.81 Kuru
- A81.82 Gerstmann–Sträussler–Scheinker syndrome
- A81.83 Fatal familial insomnia
- A81.89 Other atypical virus infections of central nervous system
- A81.9 Atypical virus infection of central nervous system, unspecified

PREFERRED PRACTICE PATTERNS[1]

- 5A: Primary Prevention/Risk Reduction for Loss of Balance and Falling
- 5C: Impaired Motor Function and Sensory Integrity Associated with Nonprogressive Disorders of the Central Nervous System—congenital origin or acquired in infancy or childhood
- 5D: Impaired Motor Function and Sensory Integrity Associated with Nonprogressive Disorders of the Central Nervous System—acquired in adolescence or adulthood
- 5I: Impaired Arousal, Range of Motion and Motor Control Associated with Coma, Near Coma, or Vegetative State

PATIENT PRESENTATION

A 52-year-old man was admitted to the hospital following a fall that resulted in a fractured right ankle. The ankle fractured was surgically repaired. The family reports that the patient had become increasingly unstable while walking; he struggles to get out of his favorite chair at home, and needs help with getting dressed. He is also very confused and seems to struggle with remembering things from one moment to the next. These concerns started approximately 3 weeks ago. Before that time, he was completely independent and worked successfully at a job that required him to think and act quickly.

Physical therapy was ordered in the hospital to address ambulation, non-weight bearing on the right lower extremity.

KEY FEATURES

Description

- Progressive neurodegenerative disorders
- Abnormal pathogenic agent

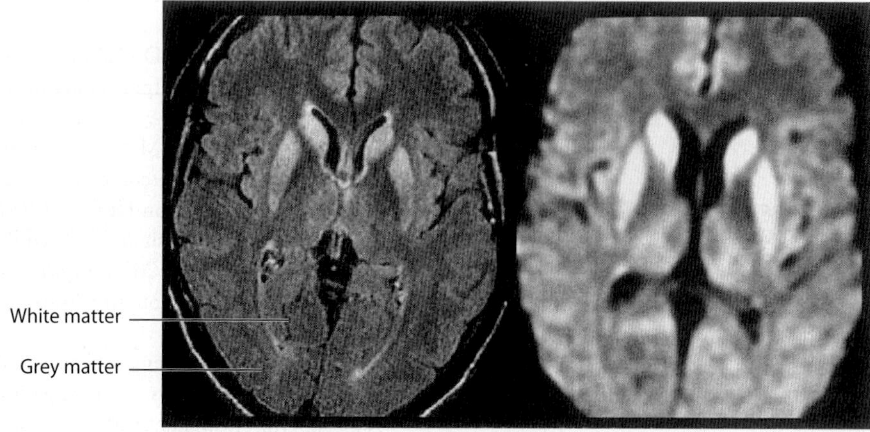

FIGURE 53-1 Appearance of brain with spongiform encephalopathy. (*Left*) Normal brain. (*Right*) Brain infected with a prion. Note the spongelike appearance. (Reproduced with permission from Nester EW, Anderson DG, Roberts CE Jr, Nester MT. *Microbiology: A Human Perspective*. 6th ed. New York, NY: McGraw-Hill; 2008.)

- Leads to brain damage
- Affects the central nervous system
- Rapidly progressive and fatal
- Human prion diseases
  - Kuru
  - Fatal familial insomnia
  - CJD
  - vCJD
  - Gerstmann–Sträussler–Scheinker syndrome
- Animal prion diseases
  - Bovine spongiform encephalopathy (BSE)
  - Chronic wasting disease (CWD)
  - Scrapie
  - Transmissible mink encephalopathy
  - Feline spongiform encephalopathy
  - Ungulate spongiform encephalopathy
- Three classifications
  - Sporadic
  - Familial
  - Acquired

Essentials of Diagnosis

- Presence of microscopic vacuolization of the brain tissue, spongy

General Considerations

- Can affect both humans and animals
- Currently no cure, fatal
- Long incubation periods

Demographics

- Familial type is genetic: Defect in the prion protein gene

CLINICAL FINDINGS

SIGNS AND SYMPTOMS

- Dementia
- Convulsions
- Ataxia
- Behavior or personality changes
- Neuronal loss
- Loss of inflammatory response

Functional Implications

- Inability to perform ADLs independently
- Inability to perform functional mobility independently
- Inability to perform cognitive tasks appropriate to age and educational level
- Inability to execute fine and gross motor tasks independently

Possible Contributing Causes

- Increased risk
  - Immunosuppressed
  - Perinatal to early childhood period
- Prior meningitis

Differential Diagnosis

- Stroke
- Subdural empyema
- Cerebral abscess

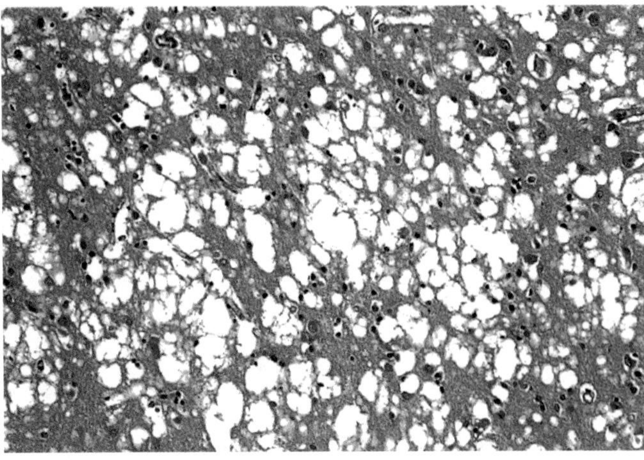

FIGURE 53-2 Spongiform changes. (Reproduced with permission from Connor DH, Chandler FW, Schwartz DQA, Manz HJ, Lack EE, eds. *Pathology of Infectious Diseases*. vol 1. Stamford, CT: Appleton & Lange; 1997.)

- Cerebral venous thrombosis
- Septic embolism
- Meningitis

MEANS OF CONFIRMATION OR DIAGNOSIS

Laboratory Tests

- Cerebral spinal fluid testing
- Immunohistochemical analysis of brain tissue
- Electroencephalogram (EEG)

Imaging

- CT scan for detailed imaging
- MRI

FINDINGS AND INTERPRETATION

- Pulvinar sign on MRI
- Periodic sharp waves on EEG

REFERRALS/ADMITTANCE

- Emergency room if encephalitis is suspected
- Neurologist both during infection and for follow-up
- Social work and case management

IMPAIRMENTS

- Aerobic capacity
- Arousal
- Attention
- Bed mobility
- Behavior
- Cognition
- Cranial nerve integrity
- Deep tendon reflexes
- Endurance
- Fine motor control
- Gait
- Home management
- Muscle strength
- Muscle tone
- Postural control

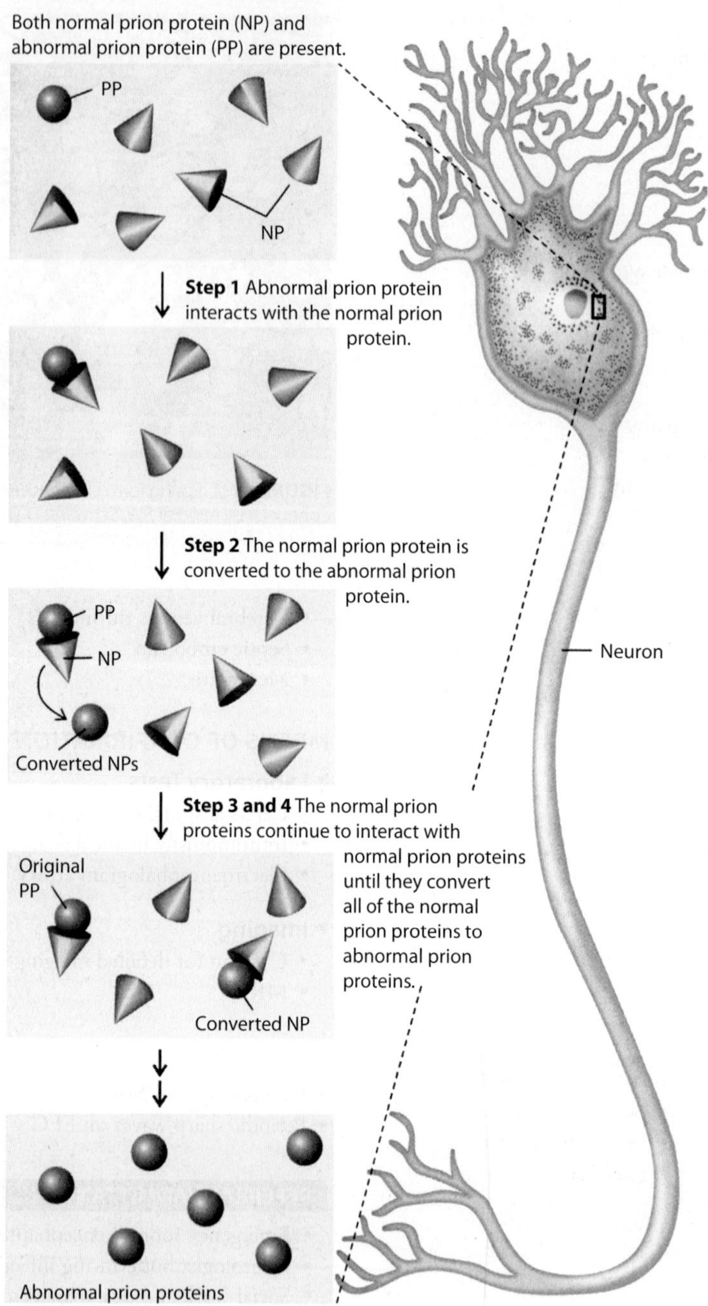
Both normal prion protein (NP) and abnormal prion protein (PP) are present.
PP
NP
Step 1 Abnormal prion protein interacts with the normal prion protein.
Step 2 The normal prion protein is converted to the abnormal prion protein.
PP
NP
Converted NPs
Step 3 and 4 The normal prion proteins continue to interact with normal prion proteins until they convert all of the normal prion proteins to abnormal prion proteins.
Original PP
Converted NP
Abnormal prion proteins
Neuron

FIGURE 53-3 Proposed mechanism of how prions are converted to abnormal proteins. The normal and abnormal prion proteins differ in their tertiary structures. (Reproduced with permission from Nester EW, Anderson DG, Roberts CE Jr, Nester MT. *Microbiology: A Human Perspective*. 6th ed. New York, NY: McGraw-Hill; 2008.)

- Range of motion (ROM)
- Respiratory control
- Self-care
- Sensation
- Sitting and standing balance
- Transfers

TESTS AND MEASURES

- Test of level of consciousness: Glasgow Coma Scale
- Cognition: Mini-mental state examination (MMSE), executive function tests, memory, comprehension
- Pain: Subjective report, Visual Analog Scale (VAS) or verbal report
- Strength and muscle endurance
- Coordination
- Muscle tone
- Joint ROM
- Cranial nerve testing
- Sensation
- Postural alignment
- Balance (timed up and go [TUG], multi-directional reach test [MDRT], Tinetti, BBS)
- Gait (TUG, Tinetti, 10-m walk test, dynamic gait index [DGI])
- Respiratory function (spirometer, oxygen saturation, auscultation)
- Functional mobility: (Functional Independence Measure [FIM^{TM}])

INTERVENTION

- Interventions are based on the extent and location of central nervous system damage
- If in coma
  - Instruct others in positioning and joint ROM
  - Coma stimulation activities
- Once cleared for more active treatment
  - Functional mobility: Bed mobility, transfers, gait
  - Balance and coordination activities: Postural control, balance strategies, speed/reaction time, multi-tasking
  - Flexibility and stretching
  - Strength and resistance training
  - Pulmonary and cardiovascular re-conditioning
  - Problem-solving and motor planning skills
- Note: Patients will fatigue quickly; consider options such as proprioceptive neuromuscular facilitation to address multiple movement plains simultaneously, thus reducing sets/reps and controlling fatigue.

FUNCTIONAL GOALS

- Goals for people recovering from an infectious disease of the brain are specific to the identified impairments; these are general goals and would need to be made more specific for each patient.
- Short-term goals
  - The patient will perform transfers to and from level surfaces with minimal physical assistance and minimal verbal cues for sequencing.
  - The patient will ambulate on level tile surfaces with appropriate assistive device and moderate assistance for balance and sequencing.
  - The patient will consistently perform a two-step motor task without verbal or visual cuing.
- Long-term goals
  - The patient will maintain postural control independently while ambulating on community surfaces for greater than 15 minutes.
  - The patient will ambulate distances greater than 1000 feet without physical assistance, with occasional verbal cues for safety.
  - The patient will complete a multi-step task (greater than three steps) successfully without verbal, visual, or physical cuing.

PROGNOSIS

- No known cure.
- Rapidly progressive.
- Fatal.
- Life expectancy with CJD is 4 to 5 months.

PATIENT RESOURCES

- National Prion Disease Pathology Surveillance Center. (From the Division of Neuropathology, Case Western Reserve University. National CJD surveillance system established in collaboration with CDC.) http://www.cjdsurveillance.com Accessed July 5, 2013.
- Prion Diseases. CDC, Centers for Disease Control and Prevention. http://www.cdc.gov/ncidod/dvrd/prions. Accessed July 5, 2013.

REFERENCE

1. APTA. *Guide to Physical Therapy Practice*. http://guidetoptpractice.apta.org. Accessed July 5, 2013.

ADDITIONAL REFERENCES

- Chandrasoma P, Taylor CR, eds. *Concise Pathology*. 3rd ed. New York, NY: McGraw-Hill; 2011. http://www.accessphysiotherapy.com/resource/7. Accessed July 5, 2013.
- Dewane JA, Porter RE. Inflammatory and infectious disorders of the brain. In: Umphred DA, ed. *Neurological Rehabilitation*. 5th ed. St. Louis, MO: Mosby Elsevier; 2006:661–663.
- Dutton M. *Orthopaedic Examination, Evaluation, and Intervention*. 2nd ed. New York, NY: McGraw-Hill; 2008. http://www.accessphysiotherapy.com/content/5548968. Accessed July 5, 2013.
- Dutton M. *McGraw-Hill's NPTE (National Physical Therapy Examination)*.2nd ed. New York, NY: McGraw-Hill; 2012. http://www.accessphysiotherapy.com/resource/611. Accessed July 5, 2013.
- Geriatric Examination Toolkit. University of Missouri. http://web.missouri.edu/~proste/tool/. Accessed July 5, 2013.
- Malone TR, Hazle C, Grey ML, eds. *Imaging in Rehabilitation*. New York, NY: McGraw-Hill; 2008. http://www.accessphysiotherapy.com/resource/613. Accessed July 5, 2013.
- Panus PC, Jobst EE, Masters SB, Katzung B, Tinsley SL, Trevor AJ, eds. *Pharmacology for the Physical Therapist*. New York, NY: McGraw-Hill; 2009. http://www.accessphysiotherapy.com/resource/615. Accessed July 5, 2013.
- Ropper AH, Samuels MA. *Adams and Victor's Principles of Neurology*. 9th ed. New York, NY: McGraw-Hill; 2009:716–723.
- Shamus E, Stern DF. *Effective Documentation for Physical Therapy Professionals*. 2nd ed. New York, NY: McGraw-Hill; 2011. http://www.accessphysiotherapy.com/content/55665155. Accessed July 5, 2013.
- Tinetti Balance and Gait Evaluation. http://www.bhps.org.uk/falls/documents/TinettiBalanceAssessment.pdf. Accessed May 5, 2014.
- TraumaticBrainInjury.com. http://www.traumaticbraininjury.com/symptoms-of-tbi/glasgow-coma-scale Accessed July 5, 2013.

54 RHEUMATIC FEVER

Shari Rone-Adams, DBA, MHSA, PT

CONDITION/DISORDER SYNONYM

- Acute rheumatic fever

ICD-9-CM CODES

- 390 Rheumatic fever without mention of heart involvement
- 391 Rheumatic fever with heart involvement
- 392 Rheumatic chorea

ICD-10-CM CODES

- I00 Rheumatic fever without heart involvement
- I01.0 Acute rheumatic pericarditis
- I01.1 Acute rheumatic endocarditis
- I01.2 Acute rheumatic myocarditis
- I01.8 Other acute rheumatic heart disease
- I01.9 Acute rheumatic heart disease, unspecified
- I02.0 Rheumatic chorea with heart involvement
- I02.9 Rheumatic chorea without heart involvement

PREFERRED PRACTICE PATTERNS[1]

- 4C: Impaired Muscle Performance
- 4D: Impaired Joint Mobility, Motor Function, Muscle Performance, and Range of Motion Associated with Connective Tissue Dysfunction
- 6D: Impaired Aerobic Capacity/Endurance Associated with Cardiovascular Pump Dysfunction or Failure
- 6E: Impaired Ventilation and Respiration/Gas Exchange Associated with Ventilatory Pump Dysfunction or Failure

PATIENT PRESENTATION

A 9-year-old female presents with joint pain and swelling. Three days ago the left knee was the most painful but on the day the left knee is better, but increased pain and swelling is present in the right ankle. The right ankle is swollen, tender and very warm to the touch. Mother reports a low-grade fever over the past week. The client reports that she has been very tired and was unable to participate in PE as they were running laps and she was short of breath. She also reports shortness of breath when lying down at night.

KEY FEATURES

Description

- Autoimmune inflammatory disease that can develop as a sequela of streptococcal infection, group A
- Characterized by inflammatory lesions of the joints, heart, blood vessels, subcutaneous tissue, and central nervous system
- Form of endocarditis

Essentials of Diagnosis

- Rheumatic fever has variable manifestations; therefore, no specific diagnostic test exists for diagnosis
- Usually occurs approximately 20 days after strep throat or scarlet fever
- Diagnosis is based on the Jones criteria; major and minor criteria used to confirm diagnosis
- Diagnosed if individual meets two major criteria or one major and one minor criteria with previous strep infection
  - Major criteria
    - Carditis
    - Polyarthritis
    - Sydenham chorea (SC)
    - Erythema marginatum
    - Subcutaneous nodules
  - Minor criteria
    - Polyarthralgia
    - Previous rheumatic fever or rheumatic heart disease
    - Fever
    - Elevated erythrocyte sedimentation rate (ESR) or C-reactive protein (CRP) levels
    - Prolonged PR interval
- Evidence of preceding group A streptococcal infection: Positive throat culture or rapid antigen test result
- Elevated or rising streptococcal antibody titer

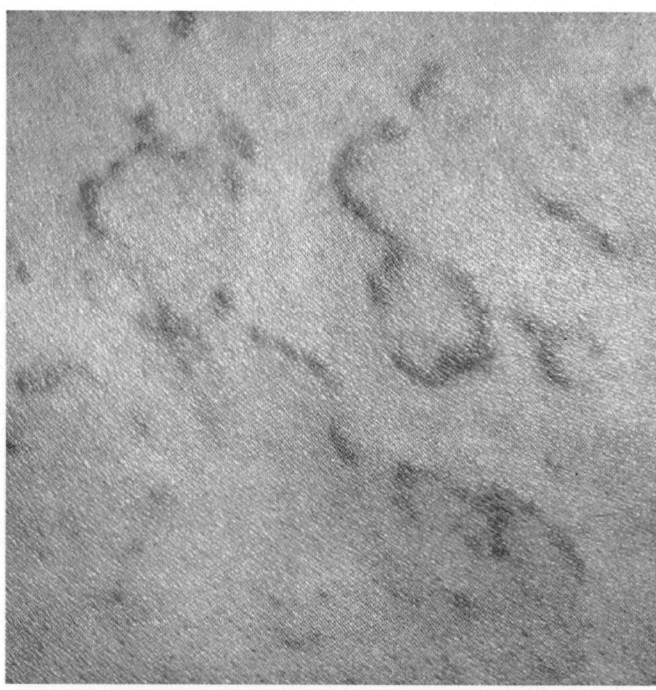

FIGURE 54-1 Erythema marginatum of rheumatic fever. Enlarging and shifting transient annular and polycyclic lesions. (From Goldsmith LA, Katz SI, Gilchrest BA, Paller A, Leffell DJ, Wolff K. *Fitzpatrick's Dermatology in General Medicine*. 8th ed. www.accessmedicine.com. Copyright © The McGraw-Hill Companies, Inc. All rights reserved.)

General Considerations

- The most significant complication is rheumatic heart disease, which usually occurs after repeated bouts of acute illness.
  - It can present as valvular stenosis, most commonly involving the mitral valve.
  - These patients are prone to infective endocarditis and stroke.
- Chorea can present months after the inciting infection.
- Some physicians monitor ESR and restart activity when it normalizes.

Demographics

- Rheumatic fever is predominantly a disease of developing countries and is concentrated in areas of deprivation and crowding.
- The risk of developing rheumatic fever after an episode of streptococcal pharyngitis has been estimated at 0.3% to 3%.
- Overall incidence in the United States is less than 1 per 100,000.
- It is most common in 5- to 15-year-old children.
- A genetic predisposition to rheumatic fever does exist.
- The disease does not have a major racial or gender predisposition.

CLINICAL FINDINGS

SIGNS AND SYMPTOMS

- Signs and symptoms result from inflammation in the heart, joints, skin, or central nervous system
- Sore throat: 35% to 60% of patients with rheumatic fever recall having upper respiratory symptoms in the preceding several weeks
- Swollen and painful joints, particularly knees, ankles, elbows, and wrists
- Erythema marginatum: Flat or raised red lattice-like rash found on trunk and proximal extremities
- Subcutaneous nodules over bony surfaces
- SC: Characterized by emotional lability, personality change, muscular weakness, and uncoordinated, involuntary, purposeless movements
- Abdominal pain
- Fever
- Muscle aches
- Nose bleeds
- Skin nodules
- Skin rash
- Joint pain and swelling
- Carditis
- Clinical manifestations of valvular heart disease
- Arthralgia
- Malaise
- Epistaxis
- Heart failure

Functional Implications

- Fatigue
- Muscle aches and weakness
- Chorea resulting in muscular weakness, and uncoordinated, involuntary, purposeless movements
- Swollen and painful joints limiting functional mobility
- Inability to perform ADLs and IADLs independently
- Inability to perform functional mobility independently
- Impaired aerobic capacity

Possible Contributing Causes

- Bed rest during initial illness and decreased activity level leading to a decline in functional status
- Cardiac involvement
  - Pancarditis
  - Congestive heart failure (CHF)
  - Heart blocks
  - Pericardial effusion
  - Value replacement
  - Rheumatic heart disease
- SC
- Polyarthritis

Differential Diagnosis

- Gonococcal arthritis
- Juvenile rheumatoid arthritis
- Lyme disease
- Mixed connective tissue disease

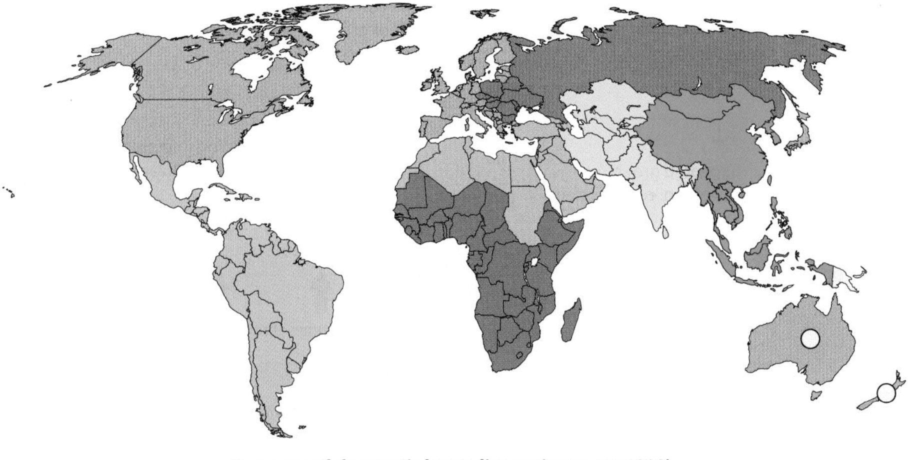

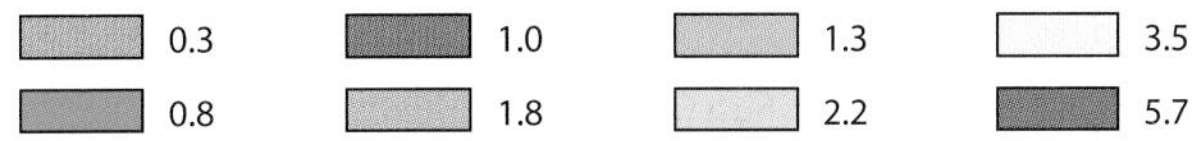

FIGURE 54-2 Prevalence of rheumatic heart disease in children 5–14 years old. The circles within Australia and New Zealand represent indigenous populations (and also Pacific Islanders in New Zealand). (From Carapetis JR, Steer AC, Mulholland EK, Weber M. The global burden of group A streptococcal diseases. *Lancet Infect Dis*. 2005;5:685–694, with permission.)

- Reactive arthritis
- Rheumatoid arthritis
- Septic arthritis
- Sickle cell anemia
- Systemic lupus erythematosus

MEANS OF CONFIRMATION OR DIAGNOSIS

Laboratory Tests

- No single laboratory test can confirm the diagnosis of rheumatic fever.
- Evidence of preceding group A streptococcal infection is an important part of the diagnosis.
- Throat culture remains the criterion standard for confirmation of group A streptococcal infection.
- Antibody titer tests are also used and include antistreptolysin O (ASO) test, anti-DNase B test, and the anti-streptococcal-hyaluronidase test.
- Blood cultures are obtained to help rule out infective endocarditis, bacteremia, and disseminated gonococcal infection.
- Electrocardiography

Imaging

- Chest X-ray
- Echocardiography

FINDINGS AND INTERPRETATION

- Chest X-ray for diagnosis of cardiomegaly and CHF in patients with carditis
- Electrocardiography is used to diagnosis a prolongation of the PR interval
- Echocardiography for diagnosis of valvular regurgitant lesions

TREATMENT

Medication

- Anti-inflammatory agents
- Steroids
- Intravenous immunoglobulin
- Penicillin prophylaxis: Low doses of antibiotics over the long term to prevent strep throat from returning

REFERRALS/ADMITTANCE

- Cardiologist
- Infectious disease specialist
- Neurologist or psychiatrist for diagnosis and management of chorea
- Occupational therapy for ADL
- Rheumatologist
- Social work and case management

IMPAIRMENTS

- Aerobic capacity
- Bed mobility
- Endurance
- Gait
- Home management
- Joint pain
- Joint ROM
- Muscle strength
- Self-care
- Transfers

TESTS AND MEASURES

- Aerobic capacity (assessment of performance during established exercise protocols (e.g., using treadmill, ergometer, 6-minute walk test, 3-minute step test)
- Autonomic responses to positional changes
- Physiologic responses during functional mobility
- Analysis of thoracoabdominal movements and breathing patterns
  - At rest, during activity, and during exercise
- Ability to clear airway
- Capillary refill time
- Classification of edema through volume and girth measurements

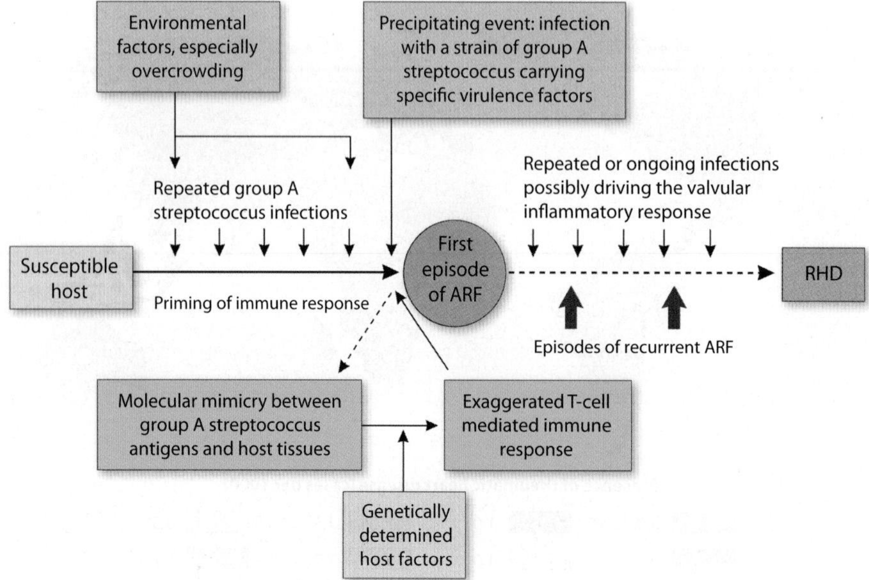

FIGURE 54-3 Pathogenetic pathway for acute rheumatic fever and rheumatic heart disease. (From Carapetis JR, McDonald M, Wilson NJ. Acute rheumatic fever. *Lancet*. 2005;366:155–168. Copyright 2005, with permission from Elsevier.)

- Cough and sputum assessment
- Perceived exertion and dyspnea
- Standard vital signs (e.g., blood pressure, heart rate, respiratory rate) at rest and during and after activity
- Chest wall mobility, expansion, and excursion
- Ventilatory muscle strength, power, and endurance
- Auscultation of the heart and lungs
- Pulse oximetry
- Pulmonary function
- Soft tissue swelling, inflammation, or restriction
- Joint hypermobility and hypomobility
- Strength and muscle endurance
- Joint ROM
- Pain
- Sensation
- Postural alignment
- Balance
- Gait
- Functional mobility

INTERVENTION

- Individuals may require PT due to prolonged bed rest or cardiac involvement including value replacement, polyarthritis
- Aerobic endurance activities
- Breathing exercises and ventilatory muscle training
- Assistive cough techniques
- Techniques to maximize ventilation (e.g., maximum inspiratory hold, staircase breathing, manual hyperinflation)
- Pulmonary and cardiovascular re-conditioning
  - Active aerobic exercises
- Joint protection
- Postural awareness
- Functional mobility: Bed mobility, transfers, gait
- Flexibility and stretching
- Strength and resistance training
- Cryotherapy (e.g., cold pack, ice massage)
- Superficial thermal modalities
- Aquatic exercises
- Endurance training
- ADL and IADL training
- Orthotic: Protective and supportive devices
- Patients with rheumatic fever are typically advised to rest (bed rest) through the acute illness and then to gradually increase activity.
  - This is particularly important for patients with carditis.

FUNCTIONAL GOALS

- PT goals would be consistent with the cardiovascular and movement-related problems that occur secondary to the condition
- Goals related to the condition could include the following:
  - Increase aerobic capacity
  - Improve ability to perform physical tasks related to self-care, home management, community, work, and leisure
  - Improve physiologic response to increased oxygen demand
  - Increased strength, power, and endurance
  - Decrease symptoms associated with increased oxygen demand
  - Improve joint integrity and mobility
  - Improve airway clearance
  - Improve exercise tolerance
  - Improve ventilation, respiration and circulation
  - Improve ability to perform functional mobility (bed mobility, transfers, gait)
  - Increase ability to perform physical tasks related to self-care and home
  - Decrease joint pain
  - Improve joint integrity and mobility
  - Reduce secondary impairment
  - Reduce soft tissue swelling, inflammation, and restriction
  - Increase tolerance to positions and activities

PROGNOSIS

- Rheumatic fever is likely to come back in people who do not take low-dose antibiotics continually, for 3 to 5 years after the first episode of the disease.
- Prognosis is directly related to the severity of cardiac involvement.
- Approximately 60% of patients with carditis improve over a 10-year period.
  - Prognosis is worse in those with severe carditis and most develop rheumatic heart disease.

PATIENT RESOURCE

- What about my child and Rheumatic fever? American Heart Association. http://www.heart.org/idc/groups/heart-public/@wcm/@hcm/documents/downloadable/ucm_300321.pdf. Accessed June 1, 2013.

REFERENCE

1. APTA. *Guide to Physical Therapy Practice*. Atlanta, GA: American Physical Therapy Association; 2003. http://guidetoptpractice.apta.org. Accessed June 1, 2013.

ADDITIONAL REFERENCES

- Armstrong C. Practice guidelines: AHA guidelines on prevention of rheumatic fever and diagnosis and treatment of acute streptococcal pharyngitis. *Am Fam Physician*. 2010;81(3):346–359.
- Bisno AL, Stevens DL. Streptococcus pyogenes. In: Mandell GL, Bennett JE, Dolin R, eds. *Mandell, Douglas, and Bennett's Principles and Practice of Infectious Diseases*. 7th ed. Philadelphia, PA: Elsevier Churchill Livingstone; 2009.
- Cilliers AM. Rheumatic fever and its management. *BMJ*. 2006;333(7579):1153–1156. doi: 10.1136/bmj.39031.420637.BE.
- DeTurk WE, Cahalin LP, eds. *Cardiovascular and Pulmonary Physical Therapy: An Evidence-Based Approach*. 2nd ed. New York, NY: McGraw-Hill; 2011. http://www.accessphysiotherapy.com/resource/652. Accessed June 1, 2013.
- Dutton M. Cardiovascular Physical Therapy. In: Dutton M, ed. *McGraw-Hill's NPTE (National Physical Therapy Examination)*.2nd ed. New York, NY: McGraw-Hill; 2012. http://www.accessphysiotherapy.com/content/5401746. Accessed June 1, 2013.
- Hay WW, Levin MJ, Sondheimer JM, Deterding RR, eds. *CURRENT Diagnosis & Treatment: Pediatrics*. 20th ed. New York, NY: McGraw-Hill; 2011. http://www.accessphysiotherapy.com/resource/14. Accessed June 1, 2013.
- Watts RL, Standaertt DG, Obeso JA, eds. *Movement Disorders*. 3rd ed. New York, NY: McGraw-Hill; 2012. http://www.accessphysiotherapy.com/resource/721. Accessed June 1, 2013.

SECTION J INTEGUMENTARY DISORDERS

55 DERMATITIS

Shari Rone-Adams, DBA, MHSA, PT

COMMON/DISORDER SYNONYMS

- Contact dermatitis
- Seborrheic dermatitis
- Atopic dermatitis (AD)

ICD-9-CM CODES

- 692.0 Contact dermatitis and other eczema due to detergents
- 692.1 Contact dermatitis and other eczema due to oils and greases
- 692.2 Contact dermatitis and other eczema due to solvents
- 692.3 Contact dermatitis and other eczema due to drugs and medicines in contact with skin
- 692.4 Contact dermatitis and other eczema due to other chemical products
- 692.5 Contact dermatitis and other eczema due to food in contact with skin
- 692.6 Contact dermatitis and other eczema due to plants [except food]
- 692.7 Contact dermatitis and other eczema due to solar radiation
- 692.8 Contact dermatitis and other eczema due to other specified agents
- 692.84 Contact dermatitis and other eczema due to animal (cat) (dog) dander
- 692.89 Contact dermatitis and other eczema due to other specified agents
- 692.9 Contact dermatitis and other eczema, unspecified cause

ICD-10-CM CODE

- L20–L30 Dermatitis and eczema

PREFERRED PRACTICE PATTERN[1]

- 7B: Impaired Integumentary Integrity Associated with Superficial Skin Involvement[2]

PATIENT PRESENTATION

A 32-year-old female presents with a pink scaly rash on her antecubital fossae, bilaterally. The rash is moderately erythematous and localized. There are excoriated areas indicating scratching due to itching. She reports the rash started on the weekend when she was pulling weeds in the back yard. She did use an over-the-counter hydrocortisone cream that provided some relief from the itching.

KEY FEATURES

Description

- Dermatitis is an inflammation of the skin.
- Dermatitis is a common condition that usually is not life threatening or contagious.
- It embraces a range of ailments that in most cases are characterized by red, itchy skin.
- Common types of dermatitis include
  - Contact dermatitis: Inflammation that occurs when substances touching the skin cause irritation or an allergic reaction.
  - AD or eczema: Chronic, relapsing, and inflammatory condition that results in itchy, inflamed, irritated skin.
    - These diseases often have an inherited tendency to develop alongside other allergic conditions such as asthma and hay fever.
  - Seborrheic dermatitis: Common skin disorder occurring in areas rich in sebaceous glands such as the scalp, ears, eyebrows, and chest, causing scaly, itchy red skin, and stubborn dandruff.

Essentials of Diagnosis

- Diagnosis is generally based on medical history and examination of the skin.
- Contact dermatitis: Diagnosis is based on medical history, the appearance of the skin, and a history of exposure to irritants or allergens.
- Seborrheic dermatitis: Diagnosis is based on history, appearance of the skin, physical, and skin biopsy.
- AD (eczema): Diagnosis is based on history and appearance of the skin.
- Skin lesion biopsies or skin cultures may be used to rule out other causes.

General Considerations

- Individuals in certain outdoor and manufacturing occupations are at higher risk for exposure to allergens and irritants that may cause dermatitis.
- Treatment is similar for most types of skin irritation and inflammation.
- Individuals often have an inherited tendency to develop other allergic conditions such as asthma and hay fever.

Demographics

- Dermatitis occurs in about 3% to 5% of the general population and affects all races as well as males and females equally.
- Contact dermatitis accounts for 90% of occupational skin disorders.

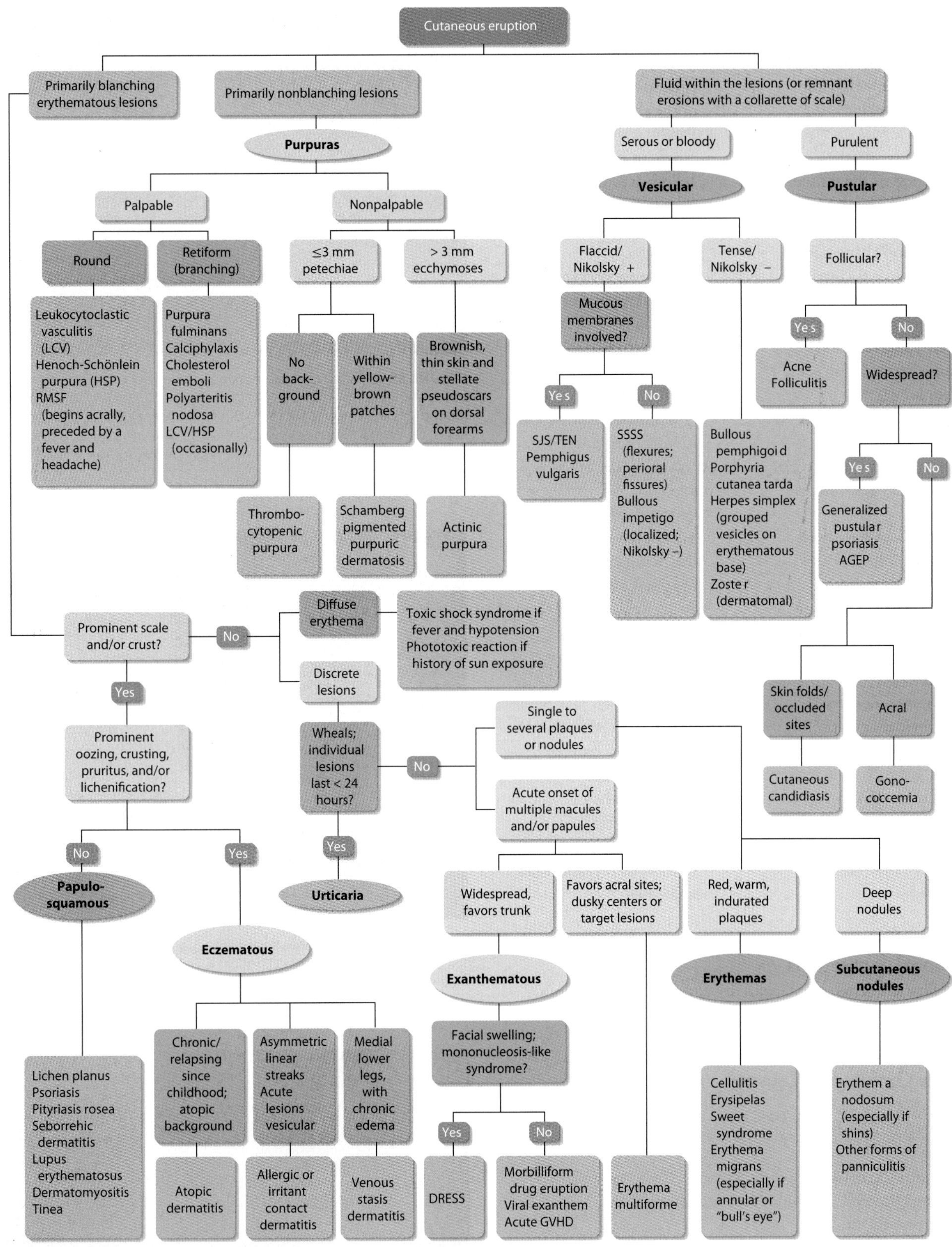

FIGURE 55-1 Diagnostic approach: inflammatory dermatoses ("rashes"). AGEP, acute generalized exanthematous pustulosis; DRESS, drug rash with eosinophilia and systemic symptoms; GVHD, graft-versus-host disease; RMSF, Rocky Mountain spotted fever; SJS, Stevens-Johnson syndrome; SSSS, staphylococcal scalded skin syndrome; TEN, toxic epidermal necrolysis. (From Henderson MC, Tierney LM, Smetana GW. *The Patient History: An Evidence-Based Approach to Differential Diagnosis.* www.accessmedicine.com.)

CLINICAL FINDINGS

SIGNS AND SYMPTOMS

- Redness or inflammation
- Localized swelling
- Itching
- Skin lesions or rash
- Tenderness of the skin in the exposed area
- Warmth of the exposed area
- Scarring and changes in skin color
- Contact dermatitis
  - Certain flowers, herbs, fruits, and vegetables can cause dermatitis in some people
  - Itching, which may be severe
  - Dry, cracked, red patches, which may resemble a burn
  - Blisters, draining fluid, and crusting in severe reactions
  - Skin rash limited to an exposed area, for example, directly under a watch-band
  - Pain or tenderness
- Seborrheic dermatitis
  - Greasy, yellowish, or reddish scaling on the scalp and other hairy areas
  - Often causes dandruff
  - Called cradle cap in infants, may be aggravated by stress
  - Inflammation (redness) of the skin
  - Patchy scaling or thick crusts on the scalp
  - Yellow or white flakes (dandruff) on the scalp, hair, eyebrows, beard, or mustache
  - Red, greasy skin covered with flaky white or yellow scales on other areas of the body, including chest, arm-pits, the area where the thigh meets the abdomen (groin) or the male scrotum
  - Itching or soreness
- AD (commonly called eczema)
  - Chronic, relapsing, and inflammatory condition that results in itchy, inflamed, irritated skin
  - Scaly, itchy skin that may swell or blister
  - Red to brownish-gray colored patches
  - Itching, which may be severe, especially at night
  - Small, raised bumps, which may leak fluid and crust over when scratched
  - Thickened, cracked, or scaly skin
  - Raw, sensitive skin from scratching

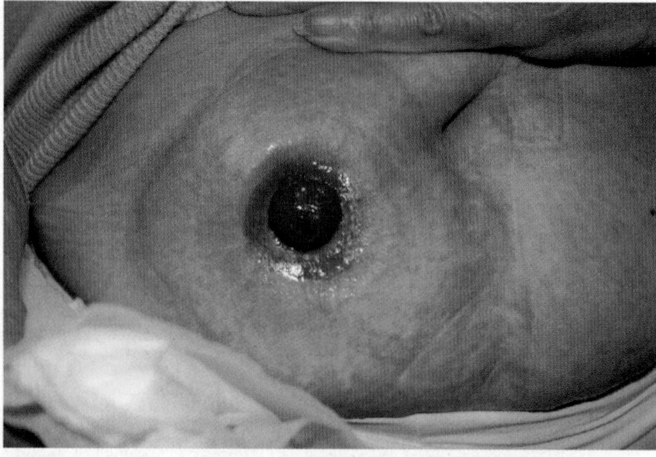

FIGURE 55-2 Irritant contact dermatitis circumferentially around an ileostomy because the bag aperture was cut too big thereby allowing soiling of the skin around this short stoma. (From Goldsmith LA, Katz SI, Gilchrest BA, Paller A, Leffell DJ, Wolff K. *Fitzpatrick's Dermatology in General Medicine*. 8th ed. www.accessmedicine.com. Copyright © The McGraw-Hill Companies, Inc. All rights reserved.)

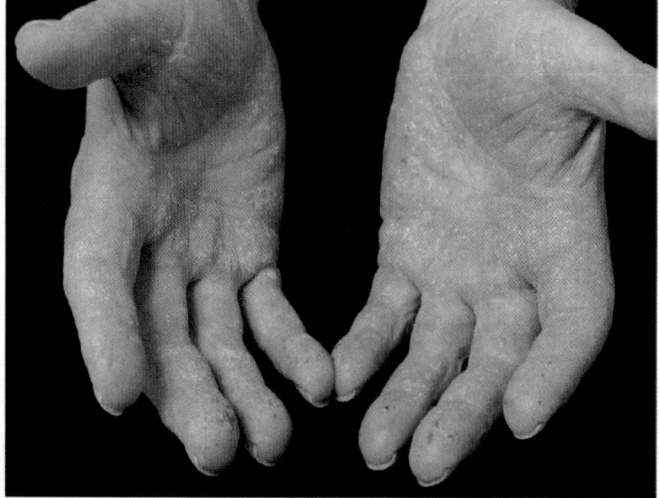

FIGURE 55-3 Irritant contact dermatitis in a welder. (From Goldsmith LA, Katz SI, Gilchrest BA, Paller A, Leffell DJ, Wolff K. *Fitzpatrick's Dermatology in General Medicine*. 8th ed. www.accessmedicine.com. Copyright © The McGraw-Hill Companies, Inc. All rights reserved.)

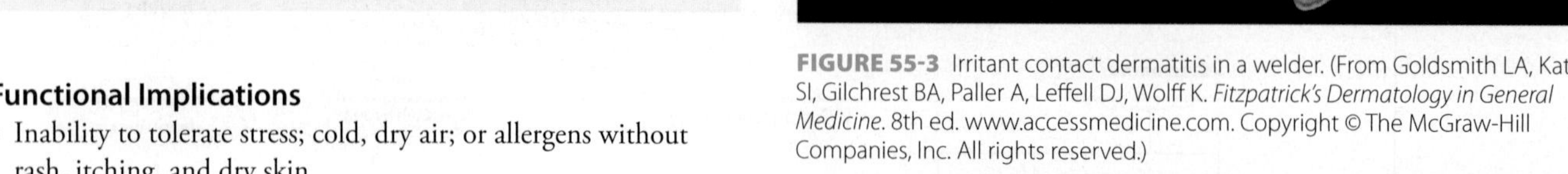

▶ Functional Implications

- Inability to tolerate stress; cold, dry air; or allergens without rash, itching, and dry skin
- Limitation of the use of some modalities

▶ Possible Contributing Causes

- Skin lesions
- Circulation impairment
- Edema
- The following make symptoms worse:
  - Allergies to pollen, mold, dust mites, or animals
  - Colds or the flu
  - Diet
  - Contact with rough materials
  - Dry skin
  - Exposure to environmental irritants
  - Exposure to water
  - Feeling too hot or too cold
  - Fragrances or dyes added to skin lotions or soaps
  - Stress

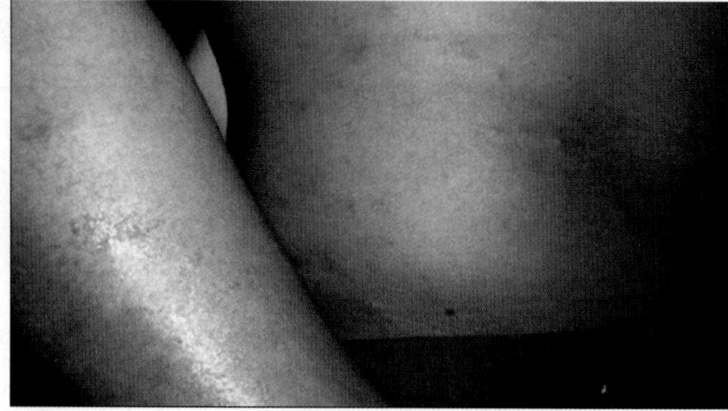

FIGURE 55-4 Irritant pustular dermatitis from nickel salts. (From Goldsmith LA, Katz SI, Gilchrest BA, Paller A, Leffell DJ, Wolff K. *Fitzpatrick's Dermatology in General Medicine*. 8th ed. www.accessmedicine.com. Copyright © The McGraw-Hill Companies, Inc. All rights reserved.)

- Contact dermatitis: Results from either repeated contact with irritants or contact with allergy-producing substances such as poison ivy, poison oak, flowers, herbs, fruits, and vegetables

Differential Diagnosis

- Dermatophytid
- Fungal infection
- Impetigo
- Pompholyx
- Psoriasis
- Scabies

MEANS OF CONFIRMATION OR DIAGNOSIS

Laboratory Tests

- Scraping of the lesion and examination under the microscope
- Skin biopsy
- Skin patch tests
- Immunological testing
- Elevated total immunoglobulin (IgE) denotes an underlying allergy

FINDINGS AND INTERPRETATION

- Skin biopsy (when eczema does not respond to treatment)
- Skin patch tests: May be used to isolate the allergens causing the skin reaction

TREATMENT

Medication

- Corticosteroid creams or ointments[3]
- Calcineurin inhibitors (Tacrolimus and Pimecrolimus)[3]
- Coal tar[3]
- Antihistamines and steroids
- Oral or injected corticosteroids[3]
- Immunomodulators
- Antibiotics
- Tricyclic antidepressants
- Wet dressings and soothing anti-itch (antipruritic) or drying lotions may be recommended to reduce other symptoms
- Other treatments
  - Phototherapy
  - Wrap therapy, emollient oils during bathing, and wrapping affected areas after bathing

REFERRALS/ADMITTANCE

- Allergist/immunologist
- Dermatologist

IMPAIRMENTS

- Skin integrity
- Circulation
- Pain
- Sensation
- Gait
- Joint ROM
- Muscle strength
- Functional mobility
- Self-care
- Home management

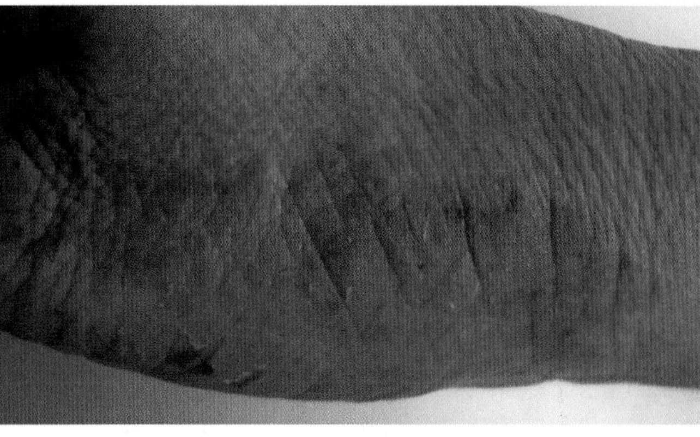

FIGURE 55-5 Contact Dermatitis. This lesion on the side of the thumb resulted from latex allergy in a nurse. The skin is erythematous, itchy, thickened, and fissured (lichenoid) due to scratching. (From LeBlond RF, DeGowin RL, Brown DD. *DeGowin's Diagnostic Examination*. 9th ed. www.accessmedicine.com. Copyright © The McGraw-Hill Companies, Inc. All rights reserved.)

TESTS AND MEASURES

- Integumentary integrity tests
  - Pigmentation
  - Shape and size of skin involvement
  - Presence of rash, fungi, blistering, ecchymosis, hair growth, signs of infection
  - Skin temperature
  - Tissue mobility, turgor, texture
- Circulation tests
  - Capillary refill, palpation of pulses
- Volume and girth measurement for edema and effusion
- Pain: Subjective report, visual analog pain (VAS) scale, or verbal report
- Gait
- Sensation
- Joint ROM
- Strength
- Functional mobility

INTERVENTION

- Not typically treated by PT, but PT should be able to recognize the condition and check the skin before and after application of modalities
- Depending on the extent of condition and secondary impairments, the following may apply
  - Dressings (e.g., wound coverings)
  - Topical agents (e.g., ointments, moisturizers, creams, cleansers, sealants)
  - Athermal modalities (e.g., pulsed ultrasound, pulsed electromagnetic fields)
  - Hydrotherapy
  - Phototherapy (e.g., ultraviolet)
  - Compression therapies (e.g., vasopneumatic compression devices, compression bandaging, compression garments)
  - Orthotic: Protective and supportive devices
  - Electrical muscle stimulation
  - Transcutaneous electrical nerve stimulation (TENS)
  - Functional training
  - ADL/IADL training

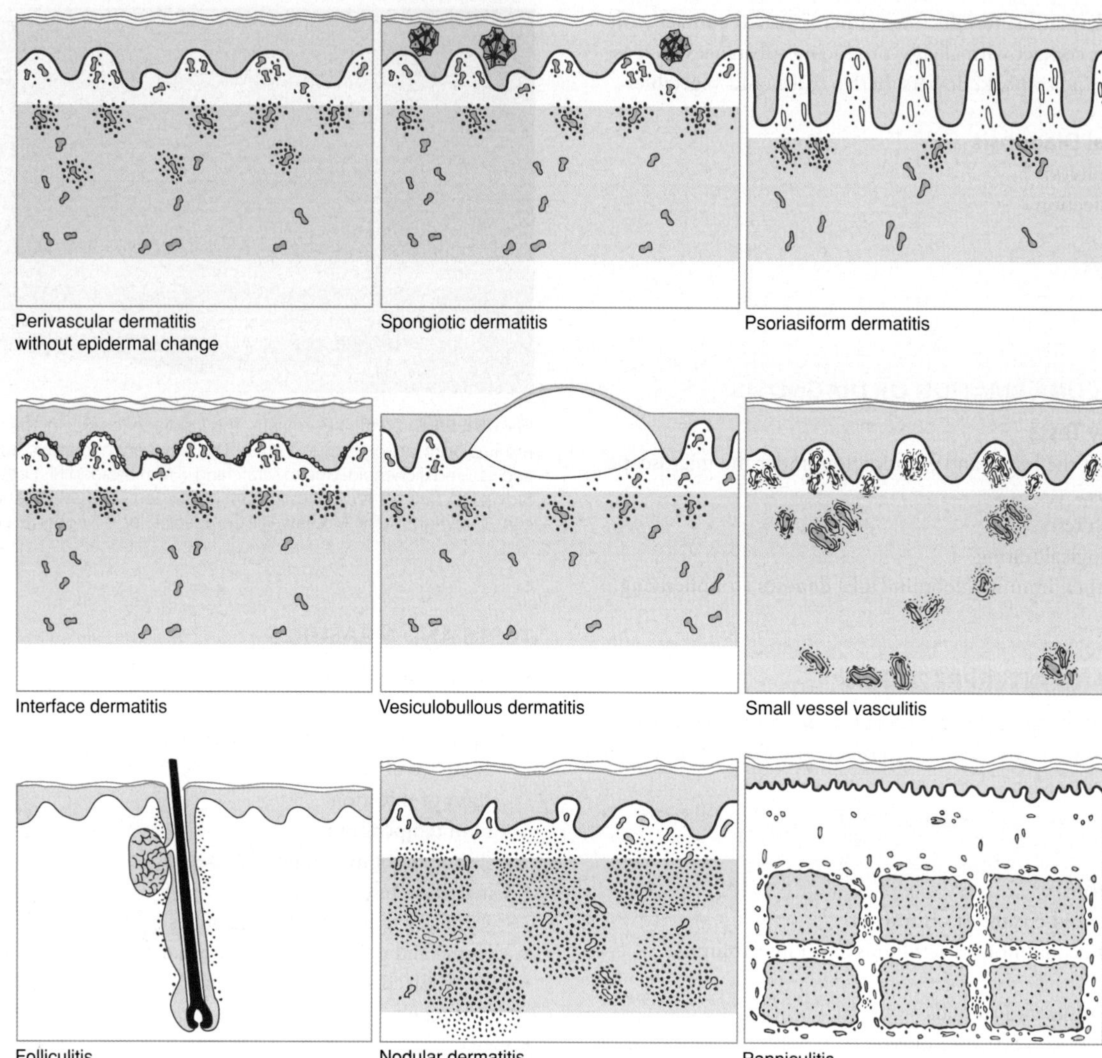

FIGURE 55-6 Nine patterns of inflammatory skin disease. (From McPhee SJ, Hammer GD. *Pathophysiology of Disease: An Introduction to Clinical Medicine.* 6th ed. New York, NY: McGraw-Hill. http://www.accessmedicine.com. Copyright © The McGraw-Hill Companies, Inc. All rights reserved.)

FUNCTIONAL GOALS

- PT goals would be consistent with the movement-related problems that occur secondary to the condition.
- Goals related to the condition could include the following:
  - Ability to perform physical tasks is increased.
  - Awareness and use of community resources are improved.
  - Risk of recurrence of condition is reduced.
  - Risk of secondary impairments is reduced.
  - Self-management of symptoms is improved.
  - Pain is decreased.
  - Sense of well-being is improved.
  - Soft tissue swelling, inflammation, or restriction is reduced.
  - Tolerance to positions and activities is increased.
  - Ability to recognize and initiate treatment of a recurrence is improved through increased self-management of symptoms.
  - Deformities are prevented.
  - Wound and soft tissue healing is enhanced.
  - Complications of soft tissue and circulatory disorders are decreased.

PROGNOSIS

- Generalized hypersensitivity reaction (anaphylaxis and angioedema) in hypersensitive individuals is potentially fatal and can occur upon exposure to an allergen.
- Contact dermatitis usually clears up without complications within 2 or 3 weeks but may return if the substance or material that caused it cannot be identified or avoided.
- Seborrheic dermatitis and AD are chronic conditions that are likely to recur after treatment.

PATIENT RESOURCES

- American Contact Dermatitis Society. www.contactderm.org. Accessed June 1, 2013.
- British Contact Dermatitis Society. www.bcds.org.uk. Accessed June 1, 2013.
- National Eczema Association. www.nationaleczema.org. Accessed June 1, 2013.

REFERENCES

1. APTA. *Guide to Physical Therapy Practice*. Atlanta, GA: American Physical Therapy Association; 2003. http://guidetoptpractice.apta.org. Accessed June 1, 2013.
2. The American Physical Therapy Association. Pattern 7B: impaired integumentary integrity associated with superficial skin involvement. *Interactive Guide to Physical Therapist Practice*. 2003. doi: 10.2522/ptguide.3.4_2. http://guidetoptpractice.apta.org/content/1/SEC36.extract?sid=4f656fd4-2c4a-4749-9738-3f247f01b18c. Accessed May 6, 2014.
3. Hay WW, Levin MJ, Sondheimer JM, Deterding RR. Treatment. In: Hay WW, Levin MJ, Sondheimer JM, Deterding RR, eds. *CURRENT Diagnosis & Treatment: Pediatrics*. 20th ed. New York, NY: McGraw-Hill; 2011. http://www.accessphysiotherapy.com/content/6589527. Accessed June 1, 2013.

ADDITIONAL REFERENCES

- Cork MJ, Danby SG, Vasilopoulos Y, et al. Epidermal barrier dysfunction in atopic dermatitis. *J Invest Dermatol.* 2009;129(8):1892–1908. doi:10.1038/jid.2009.133.
- Dutton M. Integumentary physical therapy. In: Dutton M, ed. *McGraw-Hill's NPTE (National Physical Therapy Examination).* 2nd ed. New York, NY: McGraw-Hill; 2012. http://www.accessphysiotherapy.com/content/5403045. Accessed June 1, 2013.
- Morelli JG, Burch JM. Skin. In: Hay WW, Levin MJ, Sondheimer JM, Deterding RR, eds. *CURRENT Diagnosis & Treatment: Pediatrics*. 20th ed. New York, NY: McGraw-Hill; 2011. http://www.accessphysiotherapy.com/content/6580310. Accessed June 1, 2013.
- McCalmont TH. Diseases of the skin. In: McPhee SJ, Hammer GD, eds. *Pathophysiology of Disease: An Introduction to Clinical Medicine*. 6th ed. New York, NY: McGraw-Hill; 2010. http://www.accessphysiotherapy.com/content/5368775. Accessed June 1, 2013.
- Nicol NH, Boguniewicz M. Successful strategies in atopic dermatitis management. *Dermatol Nurs*. 2008;(Suppl):3–18.
- Peters J. Managing Eczema. *Nurs Times*. 2011;107(47):22, 24–6.

56 ECZEMA

Shari Rone-Adams, DBA, MHSA, PT

CONDITION/DISORDER SYNONYMS

- Atopic dermatitis (AD)
- Atopic eczema
- Infantile eczema
- Nummular eczema

ICD-9-CM CODES

- 692.0 Contact dermatitis and other eczema due to detergents
- 692.1 Contact dermatitis and other eczema due to oils and greases
- 692.2 Contact dermatitis and other eczema due to solvents
- 692.3 Contact dermatitis and other eczema due to drugs and medicines in contact with skin
- 692.4 Contact dermatitis and other eczema due to other chemical products
- 692.5 Contact dermatitis and other eczema due to food in contact with skin
- 692.6 Contact dermatitis and other eczema due to plants [except food]
- 692.7 Contact dermatitis and other eczema due to solar radiation
- 692.8 Contact dermatitis and other eczema due to other specified agents
- 692.84 Contact dermatitis and other eczema due to animal (cat) (dog) dander
- 692.89 Contact dermatitis and other eczema due to other specified agents
- 692.9 Contact dermatitis and other eczema, unspecified cause

ICD-10-CM CODE

- L20–L30 Dermatitis and eczema

PREFERRED PRACTICE PATTERN[1]

- 7B: Impaired Integumentary Integrity Secondary to Superficial Skin Involvement[2]

PATIENT PRESENTATION

A 15-year-old female presents with a dry, rough, red rash on her arms, legs, and trunk. The rash is itchy and inflamed. The itchiness is intense and she often scratches till it bleeds. During times of stress, the rash spreads to her face and neck. The rash has gotten worse over time. As a baby, she had small patches on her arm which have now spread to her legs and trunk. The patient states that when it is testing time at school the skin condition becomes worse.

KEY FEATURES

Description

- Eczema is a common group of skin conditions
- Form of dermatitis

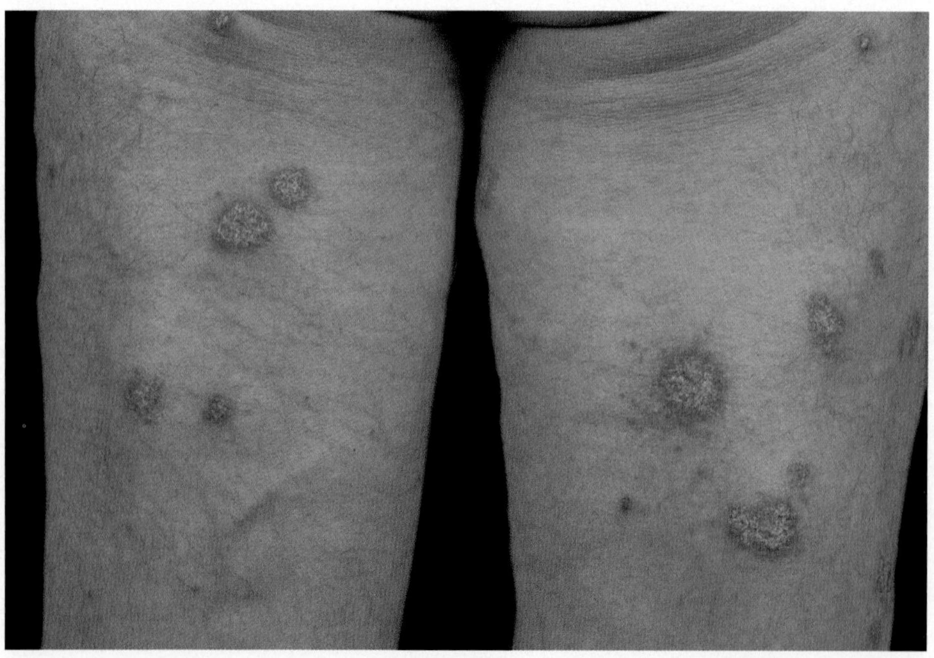

FIGURE 56-1 Nummular eczema. Pruritic, round, nummular (coin-shaped) plaques with erythema, scales, and crusts on the posterior legs. (From Wolff K, Johnson RA, Saavedra AP. *Fitzpatrick's Color Atlas and Synopsis of Clinical Dermatology*, 7th ed. http://www.accessmedicine.com. Copyright © The McGraw-Hill Companies, Inc. All rights reserved.)

- A chronic, relapsing, and inflammatory skin condition
- Results in itchy, inflamed, irritated skin
- Often has an inherited tendency to develop other allergic conditions such as asthma and hay fever

Essentials of Diagnosis

- There are no laboratory tests used to diagnose eczema
- Clinical features of the disease are used for diagnosis, including the itchiness and the biology and spread (appearance) of the lesions
- Ruling out other skin diseases like contact dermatitis and seborrheic dermatitis is used to confirm the diagnosis
- Skin lesion biopsies or skin cultures may be used to rule out other causes

General Considerations

- There are three stages of the disease: Infantile, childhood, and adult
  - Often with latent phases in between
  - At each stage, the condition may be diagnosed as acute, subacute, or chronic
- Intrinsic
  - Nonallergic with xerosis and occurrence at a younger age
- Extrinsic
  - Generally associated with a medical history (personal or hereditary) of respiratory allergy

Demographics

- Eczema is the most common skin problem for which people seek medical treatment
- Affects about 10% of the U.S. population

CLINICAL FINDINGS

SIGNS AND SYMPTOMS

- Itching, which may be severe, especially at night
- Small, raised bumps, which may leak fluid and crust over when scratched
- Rash, most common on face, back of knees, wrists, hands, and feet
- Thickened, cracked, or scaly skin
- Change in skin pigmentation making affected area lighter or darker
- Red to brownish-gray colored patches
- Areas with loss of hair and skin color changes

Functional Implications

- Inability to tolerate stress; cold, dry air; allergens without rash, itching, and dry skin
- Limitation of the use of some modalities

Possible Contributing Causes

- Skin lesions
- Celiac disease
- Gluten sensitivity
- Circulation impairment
- Pain
- Edema
- The following can make symptoms worse
  - Allergies to pollen, mold, dust mites, or animals
  - Colds or the flu
  - Diet
  - Contact with rough materials
  - Dry skin
  - Exposure to environmental irritants
  - Exposure to water
  - Feeling too hot or too cold

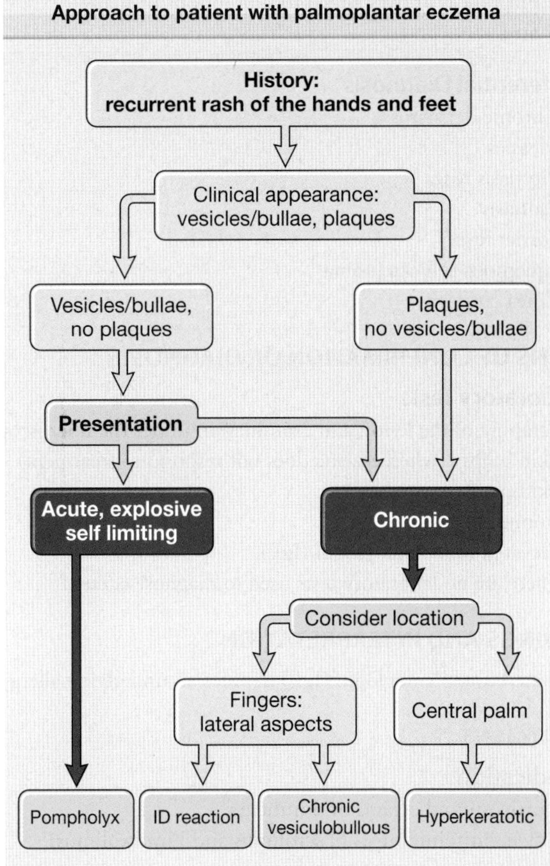

FIGURE 56-2 Approach to the patient with vesicular palmoplantar eczema. (From Goldsmith LA, et al. *Fitzpatrick's Dermatology in General Medicine*, 8th ed. www.accessmedicine.com. Copyright © The McGraw-Hill Companies, Inc. All rights reserved.)

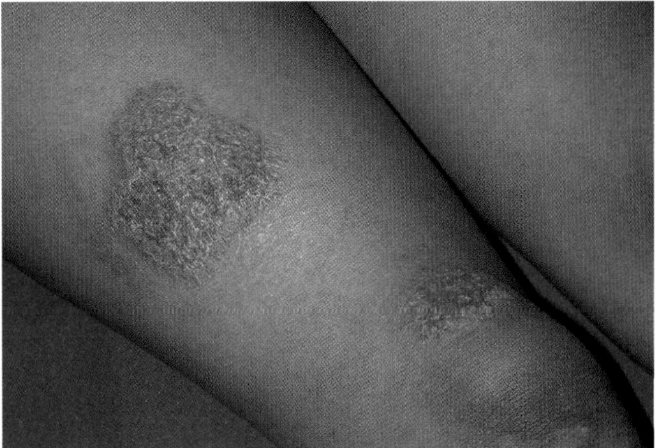

FIGURE 56-3 Nummular dermatitis. (From Stern SDC, Cifu AS, Aitkorn D. *Symptom to Diagnosis: An Evidence-Based Guide*, 2nd ed. www.accessmedicine.com. Copyright © The McGraw-Hill Companies, Inc. All rights reserved.)

- Fragrances or dyes added to skin lotions or soaps
- Stress

▶ Differential Diagnosis

- Chronic dermatoses
- Measles
- Pityriasis rosea
- Psoriasis
- Scarlet fever
- Squamous cell carcinoma
- Tinea corporis

MEANS OF CONFIRMATION OR DIAGNOSIS

▶ Laboratory Tests

- Scraping of the lesion and examination under the microscope
- Skin biopsy (when eczema does not respond to treatment)
- Skin patch tests
- Immunological testing
- Elevated total hemoglobin (IgE)
- There are no laboratory tests used to diagnose eczema

FINDINGS AND INTERPRETATION

- Elevated total hemoglobin (IgE) denotes an underlying allergy

TREATMENT

▶ Medication

- Corticosteroid creams or ointments[3]
- Calcineurin inhibitors (Tacrolimus and Pimecrolimus)[3]
- Coal tar[3]
- Antihistamines and steroids
- Oral or injected corticosteroids[3]
- Immunomodulators
- Antibiotics
- Tricyclic antidepressants
- Other treatments
  - Phototherapy
  - Wrap therapy
    - Emollient oils during bathing and wrapping affected areas after bathing

REFERRALS/ADMITTANCE

- Allergist/immunologist
- Dietician
- Dermatologist

IMPAIRMENTS

- Skin integrity
- Circulation
- Pain
- Sensation
- Joint ROM
- Muscle strength
- Functional mobility
- Self-care
- Home management

TESTS AND MEASURES

- Integumentary integrity
  - Pigmentation

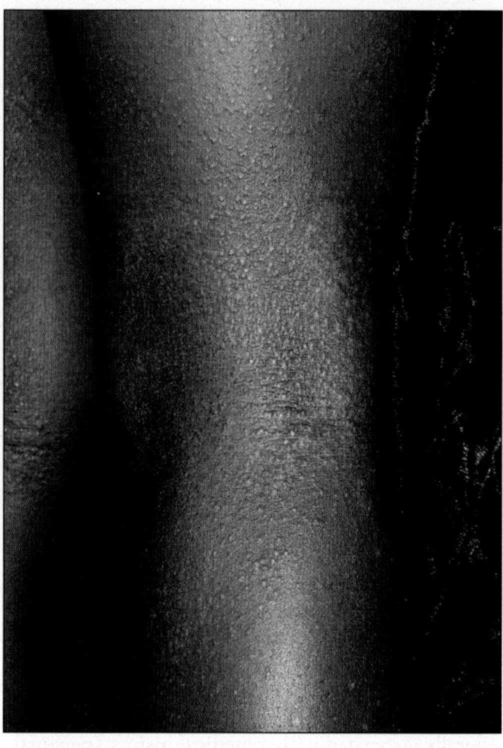

FIGURE 56-4 Atopic dermatitis in Black child: follicular. Pruritic follicular papules on the posterior leg. Follicular eczema is a reaction pattern that occurs more commonly in African and Asian children. (From Wolff K, Johnson RA. *Fitzpatrick's Color Atlas & Synopsis of Clinical Dermatology*. 6th ed. New York, NY:McGraw-Hill; 2009.)

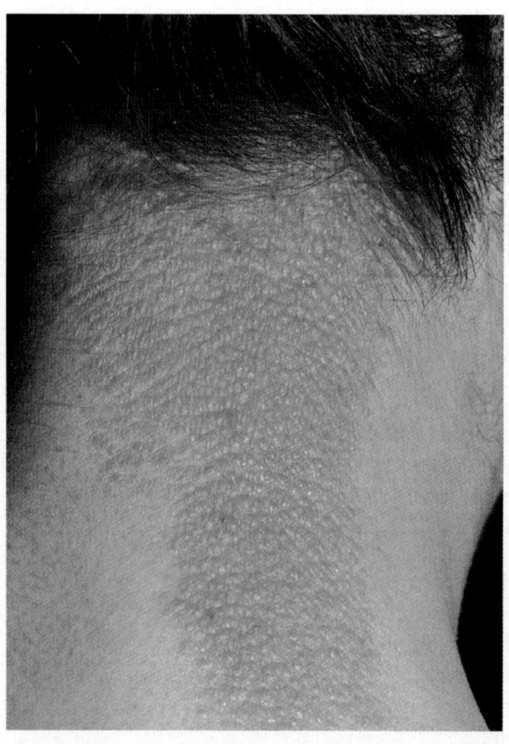

FIGURE 56-5 Lichen simplex chronicus. Confluent, popular, follicular eczema, creating a plaque of lichen simplex chronicus of the posterior neck and occipital scalp. Condition had been present for many years as a result of chronic rubbing of the area. (From Wolff K, Johnson RA. *Fitzpatrick's Color Atlas & Synopsis of Clinical Dermatology*. 6th ed. New York, NY:McGraw-Hill; 2009.)

- Shape and size of skin involvement
- Presence of rash, fungi, blistering, ecchymosis, hair growth, signs of infection
- Skin temperature
- Tissue mobility: Turgor, texture

- Circulation
  - Capillary refill, palpation of pulses
- Volume and girth measurement for edema and effusion
- Pain: Subjective report, visual analog pain (VAS) scale, or verbal report
- Sensation
- Joint ROM
- Strength and muscle endurance
- Functional mobility
- Orthotic: Protective and supportive devices

INTERVENTION

- Not typically treated by PT, but PT should be able to recognize the condition and check the skin before and after application of modalities
- Depending on the extent of the condition and secondary impairments, the following may apply:
  - Dressings (e.g., wound coverings)
  - Topical agents (e.g., ointments, moisturizers, creams, cleansers, sealants)
  - Athermal modalities (e.g., pulsed ultrasound, pulsed electromagnetic fields)
  - Hydrotherapy
  - Phototherapy (e.g., ultraviolet)
  - Compression therapies (e.g., vasopneumatic compression devices, compression bandaging, compression garments)
  - Orthotic: Protective and supportive devices
  - Electrical muscle stimulation
  - Transcutaneous electrical nerve stimulation (TENS)
  - Functional training
  - ADL/IADL training

FUNCTIONAL GOALS

- PT goals would be consistent with the movement-related problems that occur secondary to the condition.
- Goals related to the condition could include the following:
  - Ability to perform physical tasks is increased.
  - Awareness and use of community resources are improved.
  - Risk of recurrence of the condition is reduced.
  - Risk of secondary impairments is reduced.
  - Self-management of symptoms is improved.
  - Pain is decreased.
  - Soft tissue swelling, inflammation, or restriction is reduced.
  - Tolerance to positions and activities is increased.
  - Ability to recognize and initiate treatment of a recurrence is improved through increased self-management of symptoms.
  - Deformities are prevented..
  - Wound and soft tissue healing is enhanced.
  - Complications of soft tissue and circulatory disorders are decreased.

PROGNOSIS

- Chronic condition, but is controllable with treatment.
- With childhood onset, it often resolves in the teens.
- In adults, it is often long term and reoccurring.
- Flare-ups are most likely in the winter when there is dry, cold air.

PATIENT RESOURCES

- Atopic Dermatitis. National Institute of Arthritis and Musculoskeletal and Skin Diseases. http://www.niams.nih.gov/Health_Info/Atopic_Dermatitis/default.asp. Accessed August 8, 2014.
- Eczema Society of Canada. http://www.eczemahelp.ca. Accessed June 2, 2013.
- National Eczema Association. http://www.eczema.org. Accessed June 2, 2013.

REFERENCES

1. APTA. *Guide to Physical Therapy Practice*. Atlanta, GA: American Physical Therapy Association; 2003. http://guidetoptpractice.apta.org. Accessed June 2, 2013.
2. The American Physical Therapy Association. Pattern 7B: impaired integumentary integrity associated with superficial skin involvement. *Interactive Guide to Physical Therapist Practice*. 2003. doi: 10.2522/ptguide.3.4_2. http://guidetoptpractice.apta.org/content/1/SEC36.extract?sid=4f656fd4-2c4a-4749-9738-3f247f01b18c. Accessed May 6, 2014.
3. Hay WW, Levin MJ, Sondheimer JM, Deterding RR. Treatment. In: Hay WW, Levin MJ, Sondheimer JM, Deterding RR, eds. *CURRENT Diagnosis & Treatment: Pediatrics*. 20th ed. New York, NY: McGraw-Hill; 2011. http://www.accessphysiotherapy.com/content/6589527. Accessed June 2, 2013.

ADDITIONAL REFERENCES

- Cork MJ, Danby SG, Vasilopoulos Y, et al. Epidermal barrier dysfunction in atopic dermatitis. *J Invest Dermatol.* 2009;129(8):1892–1908. doi:10.1038/jid.2009.133.
- Dutton M. Integumentary physical therapy. In: Dutton M, ed. *McGraw-Hill's NPTE (National Physical Therapy Examination)*.2nd ed. New York, NY: McGraw-Hill; 2012. http://www.accessphysiotherapy.com/content/5403045. Accessed June 2, 2013.
- Morelli JG, Burch JM. Skin. In: Hay WW, Levin MJ, Sondheimer JM, Deterding RR, eds. *CURRENT Diagnosis & Treatment: Pediatrics*. 20th ed. New York, NY: McGraw-Hill; 2011. http://www.accessphysiotherapy.com/content/6580310. Accessed June 2, 2013.
- McCalmont TH. Diseases of the skin. In: McPhee SJ, Hammer GD, eds. *Pathophysiology of Disease*. 6th ed. New York, NY: McGraw-Hill; 2010. http://www.accessphysiotherapy.com/content/5368775. Accessed June 2, 2013.
- Nicol NH, Boguniewicz M. Successful strategies in atopic dermatitis management. *Dermatol Nurs*. 2008;(Suppl);3–18.

57 SKIN INFECTIONS, STREPTOCOCCAL

Shari Rone-Adams, DBA, MHSA, PT

CONDITION/DISORDER SYNONYMS

- Superficial pyoderma
- Streptococcal impetigo
- Impetigo contagiosa

ICD-9-CM CODE

- 041.01 *Streptococcus* infection in conditions classified elsewhere and of unspecified site, *Streptococcus*, group A

ICD-10-CM CODE

- B95.0 *Streptococcus*, group A, as the cause of diseases classified elsewhere

PREFERRED PRACTICE PATTERN[1]

- 7B*:* Impaired Integumentary Integrity Secondary to Superficial Skin Involvement

PATIENT PRESENTATION

A 62-year-old male presents with swelling, pain, and discoloration of the right foot. His wife reports that he stepped on a sharp object on the floor 3 days ago. He now has fever, diarrhea, and is showing some confusion. The patient has no complaints of pain. He has a history of type II diabetes. Because of the possible associated and unidentifiable fever and confusion the patient was referred to a walk in medical clinic.

KEY FEATURES

Description

- *Streptococcus* pyogenes (group A *Streptococcus*) is responsible for infections in the skin
- Group A infections
  - Cellulitis and erysipelas
  - Impetigo
  - Scarlet fever
  - Severe strep infections
- Highly infectious skin rash, spreads rapidly
- It occurs most often in tropical climates or during the summer months in nontropical climates
- With this infection, the patient is usually afebrile and has no pain
- Lesions are most often on the face and extremities and may become a mild but chronic illness if untreated
- Most common in children, particularly those in unhealthy living conditions
- In adults, it may follow other skin disorders or a recent upper respiratory infection, such as a cold or other virus
- Preceding a streptococcal respiratory infection

Essentials of Diagnosis

- Diagnosis is usually made by considering medical history and signs and symptoms, including the distinctive sores.
- A culture may be used to confirm the diagnosis or to rule out another cause.

General Considerations

- Highly contagious and can be spread through close contact or sharing items.
- Scratching can spread the sores to other parts of the body.

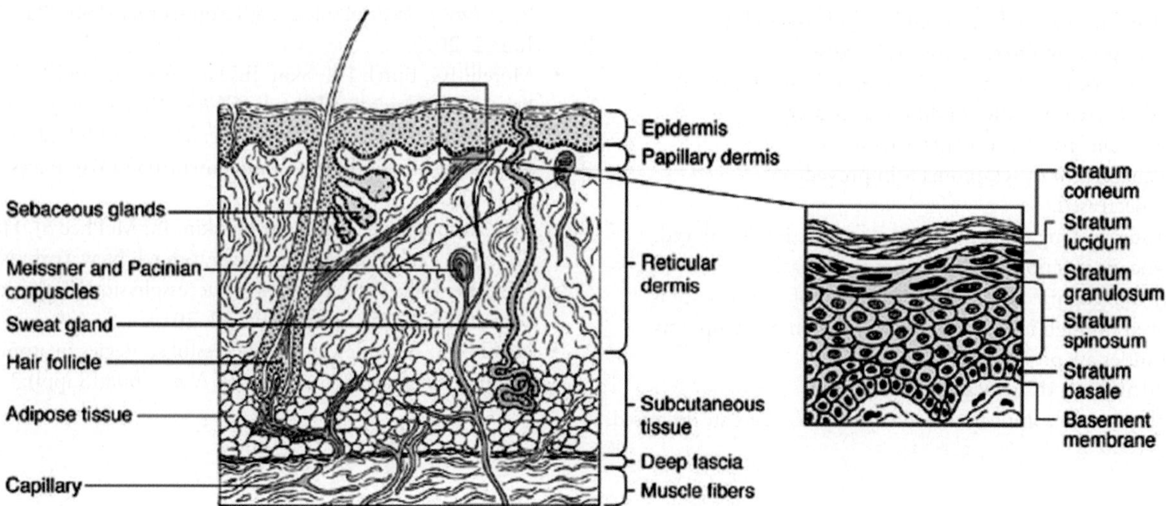

FIGURE 57-1 Structure of the skin. (From Chandrasoma P, Taylor CR. *Concise Pathology*. 3rd ed. www.accessmedicine.com. Copyright © The McGraw-Hill Companies, Inc. All rights reserved.)

- It can be difficult to distinguish clinically between skin infection caused by streptococci and other bacteria such as *Staphylococcus*

Demographics

- Highest prevalence in children 2 to 5 years of age
- Can be seen in adults, but is more prevalent in children

CLINICAL FINDINGS

SIGNS AND SYMPTOMS

- Impetigo
- Erysipelas
- Rash
- Blisters filled with pus
- Fever
- Malaise
- Vomiting: Childhood type
- Itching blister
- Erythematous denuded areas
- Honey-colored crusts
- Localized area of redness
- Purulent vesicles covered with a thick, confluent, honey-colored fluid
- Swollen lymph nodes near the infection
- Lesions most often on face, lips, arms, and legs

Functional Implications

- Very contagious, limiting contact and social status

Possible Contributing Causes

- Skin lesions
- Circulation impairment
- Pain
- Edema
- Contact with someone with the skin infection

Differential Diagnosis

- Erysipelas
- Follicular mucinosis
- Folliculitis
- Herpetic impetigo
- Insect bites
- Lymphadenitis
- Lymphadenopathy
- Pemphigus foliaceus
- Pemphigus vulgaris
- Pseudomonas folliculitis
- *Staphylococcus aureus* infection
- Tinea

MEANS OF CONFIRMATION OR DIAGNOSIS

Laboratory Tests

- Culture of the skin or lesion
- Blood cultures: Leukocytosis tests

FINDINGS AND INTERPRETATION

- Streptozyme screening test to detect antibodies
- Antistreptolysin O titer (ASO), increased levels are seen

TREATMENT

Medication

- Parental antibiotics
  - Penicillin
  - Cefazolin

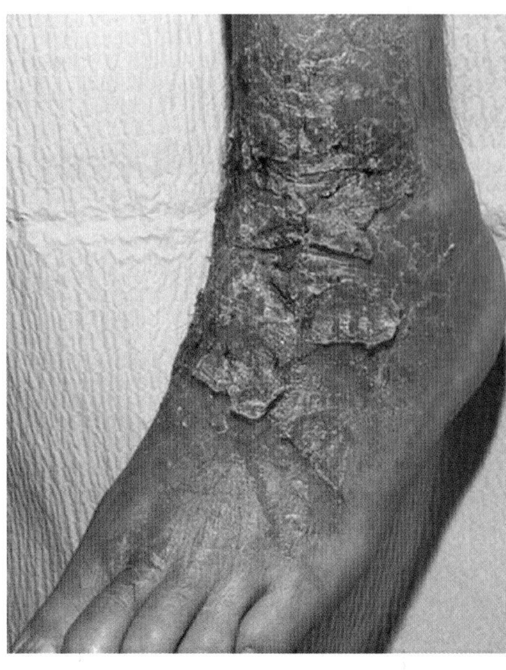

FIGURE 57-2 Infectious eczematoid dermatitis frequently follows contact dermatitis that is untreated and in an area where there is constant rubbing. In this case, the patient was a logger working in an area with poor access to medical attention. (From Goldsmith LA Katz SI, Gilchrest BA, Paller A, Leffell DJ, Wolff K. *Fitzpatrick's Dermatology in General Medicine*. 8th ed. www.accessmedicine.com. Copyright © The McGraw-Hill Companies, Inc. All rights reserved.)

REFERRALS/ADMITTANCE

- Allergist/immunologist
- Dermatologist

IMPAIRMENTS

- Skin integrity
- Circulation

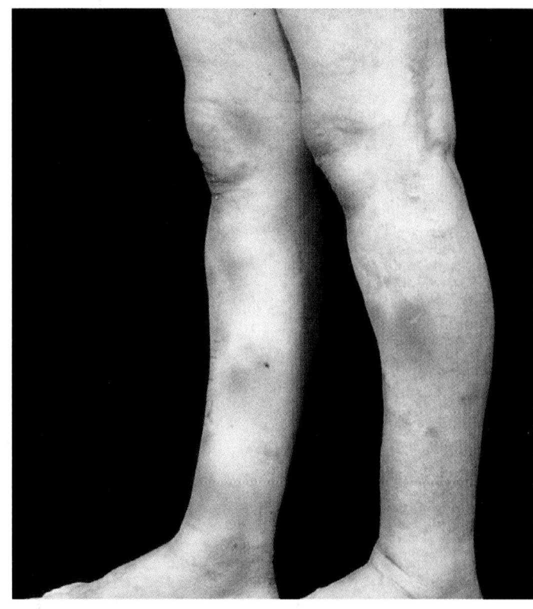

FIGURE 57-3 Erythema nodosum. Erythematous nodules located mainly on the anterior of the legs. (From Goldsmith LA, et al. *Fitzpatrick's Dermatology in General Medicine*, 8th ed. www.accessmedicine.com. Copyright © The McGraw-Hill Companies, Inc. All rights reserved.)

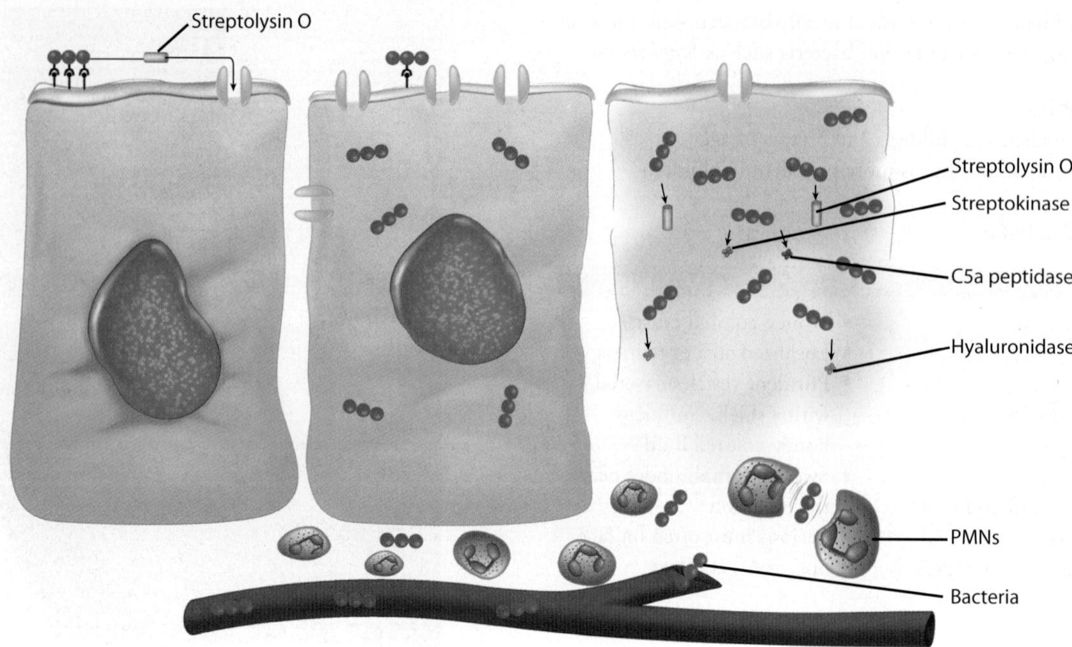

FIGURE 57-4 Group A streptococcal disease, cellular view. The cellular events are similar to *Staphylococcus aureus*. Streptolysin O is a pore-forming toxin (like α-toxin), and there are many extracellular products. A difference is that although *S aureus* tends to be localized, group A streptococci (GAS) tend to spread diffusely, as shown in the cell on the right. This may be due to hyaluronidase (spreading factor) or resistance to phagocytosis. Below the cells, factor H binding is mediating GAS escaping the polymorphonuclear neutrophils (PMNs). (From Ryan KJ, Ray CG. *Sherris Medical Microbiology*. 5th ed. www.accessmedicine.com.)

- Pain
- Sensation
- Joint ROM
- Muscle strength
- Functional mobility
- Self-care
- Home management

TESTS AND MEASURES

- Integumentary integrity
  - Pigmentation
  - Shape and size of skin involvement
  - Presence of rash, fungi, blistering, ecchymosis, hair growth, signs of infection
  - Skin temperature
  - Tissue mobility: Turgor, texture
- Circulation
  - Capillary refill, palpation of pulses
- Volume and girth measurement for edema and effusion
- Pain: Subjective report, Visual Analog Scale (VAS) or verbal report
- Sensation
- Joint ROM
- Strength and muscle endurance
- Functional mobility
- Orthotic: Protective and supportive devices

INTERVENTION

- Not typically treated by PT, but PT should be able to recognize the condition and understand that the condition is highly contagious.
- Precautions should be taken to prevent the spread of the disease to healthcare professionals and other patients.
- Depending on the extent of the condition and secondary impairments, the following may apply:
  - Dressings (e.g., wound coverings)
  - Topical agents (e.g., ointments, moisturizers, creams, cleansers, sealants)
  - Athermal modalities (e.g., pulsed ultrasound, pulsed electromagnetic fields)
  - Hydrotherapy
  - Phototherapy (e.g., ultraviolet)
  - Compression therapies (e.g., vasopneumatic compression devices, compression bandaging, compression garments
  - Orthotic: Protective and supportive devices
  - Electrical muscle stimulation
  - Transcutaneous electrical nerve stimulation (TENS)
  - Functional training
  - ADL/IADL training

FUNCTIONAL GOALS

- PT goals would be consistent with the movement-related problems that occur secondary to the condition.
- Goals related to the condition could include the following:
  - Ability to perform physical tasks is increased.
  - Awareness and use of community resources are improved.
  - Risk of recurrence of the condition is reduced.
  - Risk of secondary impairments is reduced.
  - Self-management of symptoms is improved.
  - Sense of well-being is improved.
  - Soft tissue swelling, inflammation, or restriction is reduced.
  - Tolerance to positions and activities is increased.
  - Ability to recognize and initiate treatment of a recurrence is improved through increased self-management of symptoms.

- Wound and soft tissue healing is enhanced
- Complications of soft tissue and circulatory disorders are decreased.
- Pain is decreased.

PROGNOSIS

- With treatment, usually heals within 2 to 3 weeks.
- Lesions usually resolve after 7 to 10 days.
- Cellulitis, lymphangitis, and suppurative lymphadenitis occur in about 10% of patients.

PATIENT RESOURCE

- Streptococcal Infections. MedlinePlus. US National Library of Medicine, NIH National Institutes of Health, 2013. http://www.nlm.nih.gov/medlineplus/streptococcalinfections.html. Accessed June 5, 2013.

REFERENCE

1. APTA. *Guide to Physical Therapy Practice*. Atlanta, GA: American Physical Therapy Association; 2003. http://guidetoptpractice.apta.org. Accessed June 5, 2013.

ADDITIONAL REFERENCES

- Chandrasoma P, Taylor CR. Diseases of the skin. In: Chandrasoma P, Taylor CR, eds. *Concise Pathology*. 3rd ed. New York, NY: McGraw-Hill; 2011. http://www.accessphysiotherapy.com/content/192507. Accessed June 5, 2013.
- Denegar CR, Prentice WE. Managing pain with therapeutic modalities. In: Prentice WE, Quillen WS, Underwood F, eds. *Therapeutic Modalities in Rehabilitation*. 4th ed. New York, NY: McGraw-Hill; 2011. http://www.accessphysiotherapy.com/content/8135782. Accessed June 5, 2013.
- Dutton M, ed. *McGraw-Hill's NPTE (National Physical Therapy Examination)*.2nd ed. New York, NY: McGraw-Hill; 2012. http://www.accessphysiotherapy.com/resource/611. Accessed June 5, 2013.
- Hay WW, Levin MJ, Sondheimer JM, Deterding RR, eds. *CURRENT Diagnosis & Treatment: Pediatrics*. 20th ed. New York, NY: McGraw-Hill; 2011. http://www.accessphysiotherapy.com/resource/14. Accessed June 5, 2013.
- Panus PC, Jobst EE, Masters SB, Katzung B, Tinsley SL, Trevor AJ. Antibacterial agents. In: Panus PC, Jobst EE, Masters SB, Katzung B, Tinsley SL, Trevor AJ, eds. *Pharmacology for the Physical Therapist*. New York, NY: McGraw-Hill; 2009. http://www.accessphysiotherapy.com/content/6093975. Accessed June 5, 2013.
- Pattern 7B: impaired integumentary integrity associated with superficial skin involvement. In: *Guide to Physical Therapist Practice 2003*. 2nd ed. Alexandria, VA: American Physical Therapy Association; 2003. doi: 10.2522/ptguide.3.4_2
- Skin Infections, Streptococcal. *Quick Answers to Medical Diagnosis and Therapy*. New York, NY: McGraw-Hill;2011. http://www.accessmedicine.com/content.aspx?aid=3271991. Accessed June 5, 2013.

SECTION K METABOLIC DISORDERS

58 GAUCHER DISEASE

Eric Shamus, PhD, DPT, PT, CSCS
Amber Yampolsky, MPT, ATP

CONDITION/DISORDER SYNONYMS

- Glucocerebrosidase deficiency
- Glucosylceramidase

ICD-9-CM CODE

- 272.7 Lipidoses

ICD-10-CM CODE

- E75.22 Gaucher disease

PREFERRED PRACTICE PATTERNS[1]

- 4A: Primary Prevention/Risk Reduction for Skeletal Demineralization
- 4C: Impaired Muscle Performance
- 4F: Impaired Joint Mobility, Motor Function, Muscle Performance, Rom, and Reflex Integrity Association with Spinal Disorders
- 4G: Impaired Joint Mobility, Muscle Performance, and Rom Associated with Fracture

PATIENT PRESENTATION

A 36-year-old female recently had a fall resulting in a fracture of her right radius/ulna. She was walking and became tired and had pain in her knees causing her to fall. Her X-ray revealed generalized osteoporosis. Abdominal CT was positive for an enlarged liver and spleen. Laboratory CBC showed anemia. She reports that she has had generalized pain in her legs for about 2 years and that she bruises easily. She works as a cashier and has had difficulty tolerating her shifts due to the need for prolonged standing. Her PMH is positive for asthma. Upon examination patient was found to have decreased hamstring length with popliteal angle = 50 degrees bilaterally, decreased hip strength = 4/5 for abduction and extension, decreased hamstring strength = 3+/5. No tenderness to palpation and no edema but she complained of generalized pain in BLE's 4/10 on Visual Analogue Scale. The pain is intermittently present at rest but fairly consistent with activity.

KEY FEATURES

Description

- Lysosomal storage disorder (LSD)[2]
- Called a storage disease
- Lipid cells are stored in the liver and spleen causing enlargement
- Genetic disorder where there is a lack of enzyme glucocerebrosidase[2]
- Bruising, fatigue, and liver/spleen enlargement

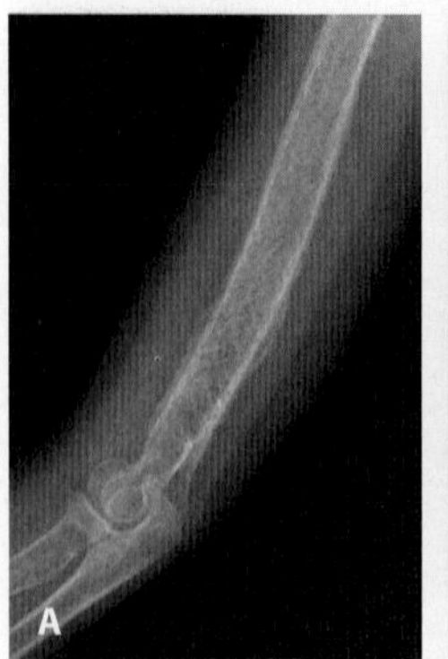

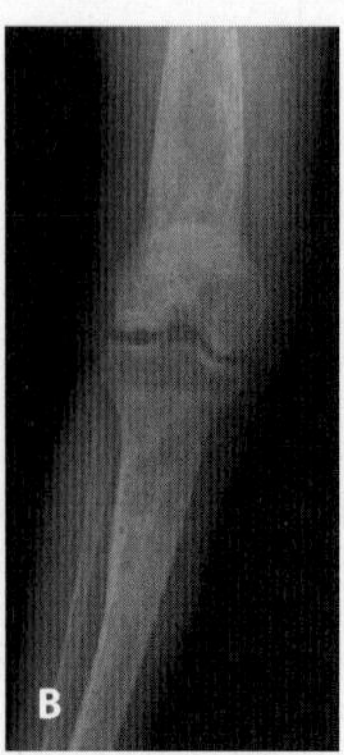

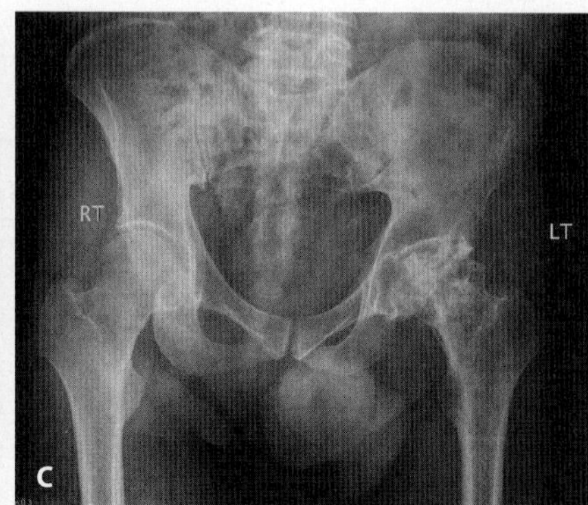

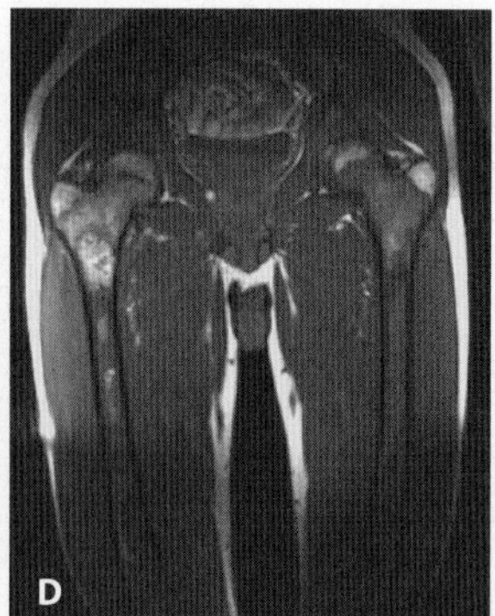

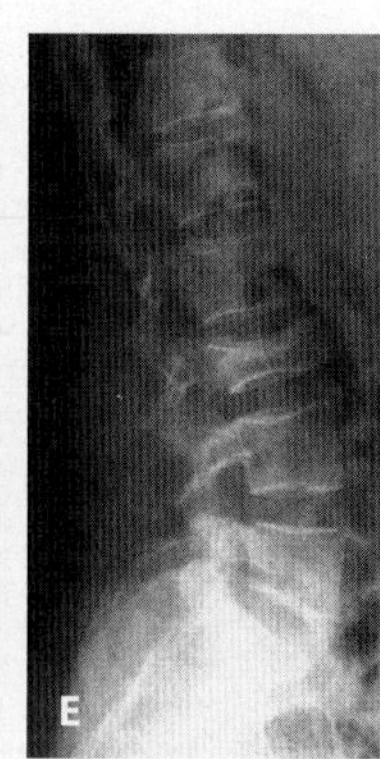

FIGURE 58-1 Gaucher-related skeletal involvement including (**A**) humerus with chevron or herring-bone pattern; (**B**) Erlenmeyer flask deformity of the proximal femur; (**C**) plain radiograph of osteonecrosis of the left hip; (**D**) MRI of pelvis and thighs performed 2 weeks after bone crisis of the right thigh. Bone edema is seen in the upper part of the femur at the level of lesser trochanter. Chronic marrow signal changes are seen in both femurs; (**E**) vertebral collapse. (From Kaushansky K, Lichtman MA, Beutler E, Kipps T, Prchal J, Seligsohn U. *Williams Hematology*. 8th ed. McGraw-Hill. Courtesy of Dr. Ehud Lebel, Shaare Zedek Medical Center, Jerusalem, Israel.)

Essentials of Diagnosis

- Juvenile form: There may be increased swelling at birth
- Three subtypes: Types 1, 2, and 3
  - Type 1: Most common
  - Type 2: Neurologic involvement in babies; fatal
  - Type 3a and 3b: Neurologic; liver, spleen, lung involvement
- Can be tested through blood or saliva

General Considerations

- Autosomal recessive disease
- Genetic mutation from both parents
- Type 2: Acute
- Type 3: Chronic

Demographics

- Type 1: Individuals of Jewish (Ashkenazi) heritage are at higher risk
  - An individual can be a carrier and not know it
  - Individuals from eastern and central Europe are at higher risk
- Type 2: Infants, any ethnic group
- Type 3: 20 to 40 years of age, northern Swedish decent

CLINICAL FINDINGS

SIGNS AND SYMPTOMS

- Fractures
- Bone pain
- Newborn skin changes
- Fatigue
- Anemia
- Nosebleeds
- Enlarged liver
- Enlarged spleen
- Increased clotting time
- Osteoporosis
- Bruise easily
- Lung disease
- Seizures
- Swelling at birth
- Heart valve problems

Functional Implications

- Fatigue with activity
- Cognitive impairment
- Joint pain that limits activity
- Hearing loss
- Increased clotting time

Possible Contributing Causes

- Genetic disorder
- Family history

Differential Diagnosis

- Trauma
- Pathologic fracture from neoplasm
- Osteogenesis imperfecta
- Inadequate mineralization of existing bone matrix (osteoid) or poor bone quality
- Osteoporosis
  - Juvenile osteoporosis occurs in children or young adults of both genders with normal gonadal function
    - Onset typically occurs around 8 to 14 years of age, and hallmarks include rapid onset of bone pain and/or fracture secondary to trauma
  - Type 1 (postmenopausal osteoporosis) typically occurs in women 50 to 65 years of age and is characterized by accelerated bone loss (trabecular bone)
  - Type 2 (age-associated or senile osteoporosis) presents in women and men older than 70 years of age as a result of bone loss associated with the aging process; fractures occur in both cortical and trabecular bones
- Infections (such as tuberculosis)
- Fibrous dysplasia
- Peripheral neuropathy
- Repetitive stress fractures
- Multiple myeloma, lymphoma, or metastatic cancer
- Leukemia
- Renal osteodystrophy
- Hormone deficiency (estrogen in women; androgen in men)
- Cushing syndrome or glucocorticoid administration
- Hyperthyroidism
- Hyperparathyroidism
- History of drug abuse or misuse (i.e., alcohol, tobacco, or excessive vitamin D or A)

MEANS OF CONFIRMATION OR DIAGNOSIS

Laboratory Tests

- Blood test for enzyme activity, glucocerebrosidase[2]

Imaging

- Spinal and pelvic radiographs, X-ray
- CT
- Bone scan or radiography
- Diagnostic ultrasound (mobile community-based screening)

Diagnostic Procedures

- Genetic testing
- Bone marrow test
- Biopsy spleen

FINDINGS AND INTERPRETATION

- Anemia
- Pulmonary hypertension

TREATMENT

Medication

- Enzyme replacement
  - Enzyme infusion for type 1
  - Enzyme infusion does not cross blood–brain barrier for types 2 and 3
- Stimulation of bone formation
  - Bisphosphonates
  - Vitamin D, phosphorus, and calcium supplements

REFERRALS/ADMITTANCE

- Endocrinologists
- Family physicians or general practitioners
- Geriatricians
- Orthopedists for joint assessment
- Genetic counselor
- Pharmacists for bone supplements
- Occupational therapists for ADL training
- Registered dietitians for nutrition

IMPAIRMENTS

- Physical impairment
  - Chronic or recurrent pain or discomfort
  - Hearing impairment
  - Heart failure
  - Fatigue
- Activity limitations
  - Self-care
  - Mobility
  - ADLs
  - Work loss or employment restrictions

TESTS AND MEASURES

- Vertebral fracture assessment (VFA)
- Fall risk assessments: World Health Organization fracture risk assessment tool (FRAX); 10-year risk assessment
- Quality of life (QoL) and health-related quality of life (HQoL)

INTERVENTION

- Therapeutic exercise
- Progressive weight-bearing exercises (ie., aquatic therapy)
- Patient education and lifestyle changes
- Transcutaneous electric nerve stimulation (TENS)
- Manual therapy/joint mobilization with precaution of bone density
- Soft tissue massage

FUNCTIONAL GOALS

- Prevention of future fractures
- Adequate control of pain
- Improve strength, flexibility, posture, and balance
- Decreases risks for falls

PROGNOSIS

- Type 1: Normal life expectancy
- Type 2: Life expectancy to 3 years old
- Type 3: Life expectancy to 30s and 40s

PATIENT RESOURCES

- Children's Gaucher Research Fund. http://www.childrensgaucher.org. Accessed May 6, 2014.
- National Gaucher Foundation. http://www.gaucherdisease.org. Accessed May 6, 2014.

REFERENCES

1. APTA. *Guide to Physical Therapy Practice*. American Physical Therapy Association. http://guidetoptpractice.apta.org. Accessed April 20, 2013.
2. Thomas JA, Van Hove JL. Inborn errors of metabolism. In: Hay WW, Levin MJ, Sondheimer JM, Deterding RR, eds. *CURRENT Diagnosis & Treatment: Pediatrics*. 20th ed. New York, NY: McGraw-Hill; 2011:Chapter 34. http://www.accessphysiotherapy.com/content/6588542. Accessed April 20, 2013.

ADDITIONAL REFERENCES

- Biegstraaten M, van Schaik IN, Aerts JM, Hollak CE. "Non-neuronopathic" Gaucher disease reconsidered. Prevalence of neurological manifestations in a Dutch cohort of type I Gaucher disease patients and a systematic review of the literature. *J Inherit Metab Dis*. 2008;31:337–349.
- Chandrasoma P, Taylor CR. Diseases of bones. In: Chandrasoma P, Taylor CR, eds. *Concise Pathology*. 3rd ed. New York, NY: McGraw-Hill; 1998. http://www.accessphysiotherapy.com/content/193568. Accessed April 20, 2013.
- Charrow J. Enzyme replacement therapy for Gaucher disease. *Expert Opin Biol Ther*. 2009;9:121–131.
- Dutton M. Cardiovascular physical therapy. In: Dutton M, ed. *McGraw-Hill's NPTE (National Physical Therapy Examination)*. 2nd ed. New York, NY: McGraw-Hill; 2012. http://www.accessphysiotherapy.com/content/5401859. Accessed April 20, 2013.
- Dutton M. Differential diagnosis. In: Dutton M, ed. *Dutton's Orthopaedic Examination, Evaluation, and Intervention*. 2nd ed. New York, NY: McGraw-Hill; 2008. http://www.accessphysiotherapy.com/content/5546939. Accessed April 20, 2013.
- Prentice WE. Therapeutic massage. In: Prentice WE, Quillen WS, Underwood F, eds. *Therapeutic Modalities in Rehabilitation*. 4th ed. New York, NY: McGraw-Hill; 2011. http://www.accessphysiotherapy.com/content/8140761. Accessed April 20, 2013.
- Zimran A, Gelbart T, Westwood B, Grabowski GA, Beutler E. High frequency of the Gaucher disease mutation at nucleotide 1226 among Ashkenazi Jews. *Am J Hum Genet*. 1991;49(4):855–859.

SECTION L NEPHROLOGICAL DISORDERS

59 PYELONEPHRITIS, ACUTE

Debra F. Stern, DPT, DBA, MSM, PT
Eric Shamus, PhD, DPT, PT, CSCS

CONDITION/DISORDER SYNONYM

- Kidney Infection

ICD-9-CM CODE

- 590.9 Infection of kidney, unspecified
- Associated physical therapy diagnoses
  - 315.4 Developmental coordination disorder (clumsiness, dyspraxia and/or specific motor development disorder)
  - 718.45 Contracture of joint, pelvic region and thigh
  - 719.70 Difficulty in walking
  - 728.2 Muscular wasting and disuse atrophy
  - 728.89 Other disorders of muscle, ligament, and fascia
  - 729.9 Other disorders of soft tissue
  - 780.7 Malaise and fatigue
  - 781.2 Abnormality of gait
  - 782.3 Edema
  - 786.0 Dyspnea and respiratory abnormalities
  - 786.05 Shortness of breath

ICD-10-CM CODE

- N15.9 Renal tubulo-interstitial disease, unspecified

PREFERRED PRACTICE PATTERN[1]

As of July, 2014, the APTA Guide to Physical Therapist Practice does not include practice patterns for organ system pathology; therefore, the associated or secondary musculoskeletal,

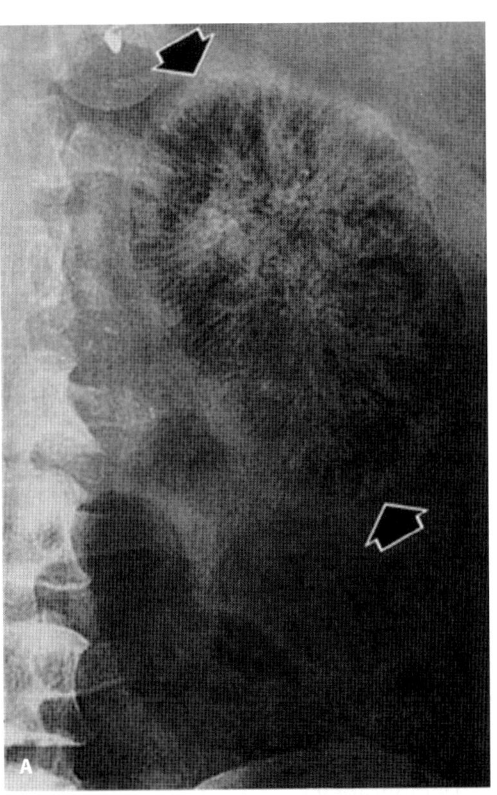
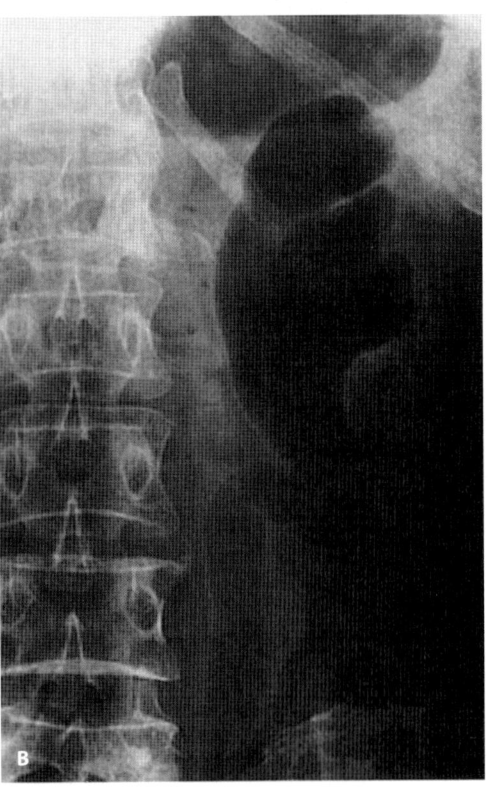

FIGURE 59-1 Plain films of the abdomen with abnormal radiolucencies. (**A**) Emphysematous pyelonephritis. Interstitial striated pattern of radiolucent gas throughout the entire left kidney. Similar changes were present in the right kidney. 58-year-old diabetic man with pyuria and septic shock. (**B**) Gas pyelogram. No interstitial gas, but gas fills dilated left kidney calices, pelvis, and ureter. 50-year-old diabetic woman with sepsis and left upper urinary tract infection caused by gas-forming microorganisms. (From Tanagho EA, McAninch JW. *Smith's General Urology*. 17th ed. www.accessmedicine.com.)

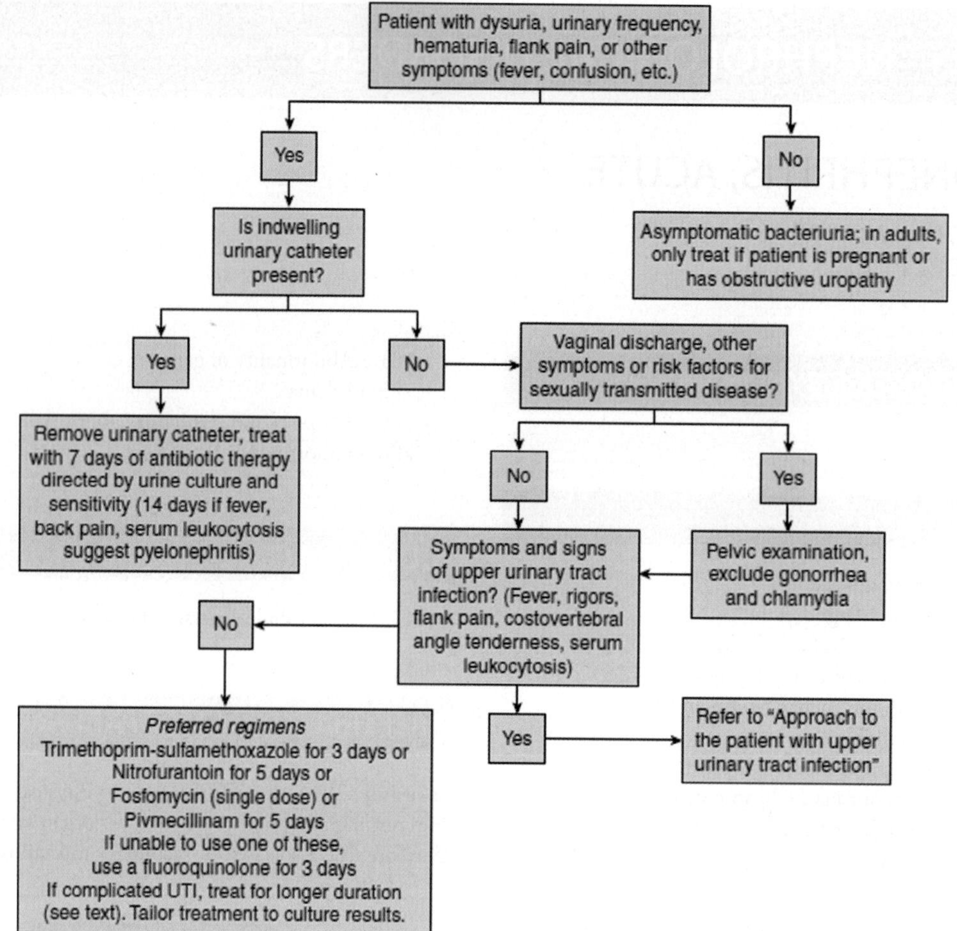

FIGURE 59-2 Approach to the patient with urine culture, urine dipstick, or urine microscopy suggestive of urinary tract infection (UTI). (From McKean S, Ross JJ, Dressler DD, Brotman DJ, Ginsberg JS. *Principles and Practice of Hospital Medicine*. www.accessmedicine.com. Copyright © The McGraw-Hill Companies, Inc. All rights reserved.)

cardiovascular/pulmonary, or potential neuromuscular patterns would be indicated.

PATIENT PRESENTATION

Patient is a 38-year-old female that presents with low back and groin pain. She states it has been bothering her for 2 days. The patient has a fever of 100.4°F. The patient also states she has had a urinary tract infection (UTI) that has not gone away. The low back and groin pain are not reproducible. She has negative slump and SLR test. She does have lumbar spasms. The patient was referred to her family physician. The patient was sent to the hospital 2 days later with increased fever and decreased kidney functioning.

KEY FEATURES

Description

- Bacteria build up in the kidneys
- Usually begins in the bladder and works up to the kidneys
- Kidney and renal pelvis infection
- Severe pain, with or without attempts at urination, in adult males and females; no pain at all, especially in the elderly and children
- Pain in the low back with possible tenderness to palpation of the kidneys.

Essential of Diagnosis

- May be indicative of serious medical conditions
- May mimic colon cancer or tumors, irritable bowel, colitis or, in females, gynecological problems such as endometriosis, uterine fibroids, or ectopic pregnancies
- Recognize the possibility of UG pathology in the differential diagnosis process, especially when findings are not consistent with conditions commonly treated (i.e., musculoskeletal, neuromuscular, integumentary, cardiopulmonary)

General Considerations

- When urine sits too long in the bladder, it is prone to infection.
- Diagnosis for more occult problems may take time and require intensive medical diagnostic testing.
- Possible referred pain to back, pelvic region, or rectal area (in men).
- Symptoms are frequently referred to the back and abdominal areas, so it may be common to have patients inappropriately referred to PT.

Demographics

- Females more susceptible than males to cystitis secondary to the anatomical proximity of the urethra to the anus and the bladder
- Females more susceptible than males to urethritis because of anatomical proximity of the urethra to the vagina; urethritis can

also be caused by sexually transmitted diseases (e.g., herpes, gonorrhea, chlamydia)

- Approximately 50% of all women will have a UTI in their lifetimes
- Children are at greater risk, with approximately 3% annually having a UTI

CLINICAL FINDINGS

SIGNS AND SYMPTOMS[2,3]

- Urethra (urethritis)
  - Burning with urination
  - Difficulty urinating
- Bladder (cystitis)
  - Pelvic pressure
  - Lower abdomen discomfort
  - Frequent, painful urination
  - Blood in urine
- Kidneys (acute pyelonephritis)
  - Urinary urgency
  - Dysuria
  - Nocturia
  - Hematuria
  - Upper back and side (flank) pain
  - Fatigue
  - High fever
  - Shaking and chills
  - Nausea
  - Vomiting
  - Painful urination
  - Malodorous urine
  - Change in color of urine
  - Positive cultures
- Possible secondary problems may, depending on severity, indicate the need for physical therapy intervention
  - Impairment of aerobic capacity and muscle endurance
  - Sarcopenia
  - Weakness or impaired muscle performance
  - Musculoskeletal problems
  - Neuromuscular problems
  - Weight loss or weight gain

Functional Implications

- Severe symptoms, such as urgent need to urinate, may be disabling and result in the inability to leave home
- Pain
- Dehydration secondary to fear of drinking
- Emesis, loss of appetite, and inability to drink or eat secondary to nausea or inability to swallow
- Sarcopenia resulting in weakness, loss of muscle mass, inability to ambulate or perform self-care
- Aerobic capacity limitation secondary to inactivity
- Need for catheters: External, indwelling, or intermittent
  - May present a problem with stoma retraction associated with abdominal contraction
- Decreased exercise tolerance
- Changes in lifestyle limit physical activity
- Eating disorders/anorexia
- Fatigue
- Inappropriate self-medication
- Anxiety and depression
- Limitations in ADLs or IADLs
- Infection
- Requires dietary changes to reduce irritants (e.g., caffeine, coffee, alcohol, citrus)
- Urinary retention

Possible Contributing Causes

- Antibiotics
- Birth control, especially insertion of a diaphragm and use of spermicides
- Blockages in urinary tract (i.e., kidney stones, enlarged prostate, benign mass)
- Catheter use, especially indwelling
- Cystoscopy
- Diabetes
- Environmental irritants
- *Escherichia coli* (*E. coli*)
- Gender (females are more susceptible)
- Immunological compromise
- Infection (bacterial or viral, including food poisoning)
- Kidney dialysis
- Low estrogen
- Menopause
- Poor UG hygiene
- Pregnancy

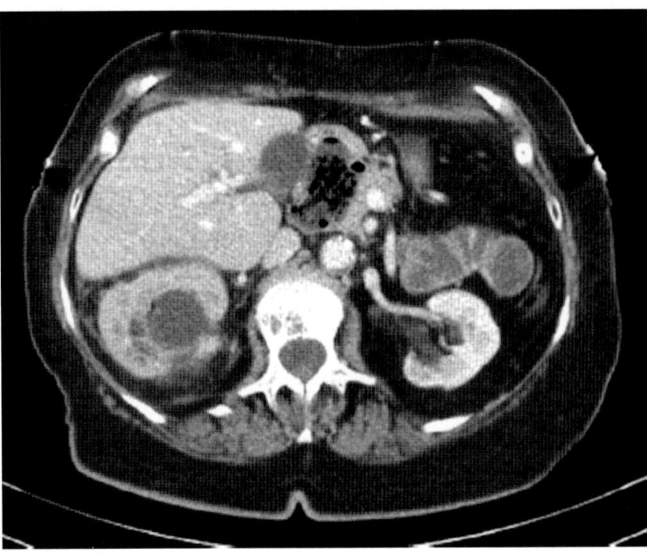

FIGURE 59-3 Computed tomography scan of the abdomen showing pyelonephritis in a patient with a urinary tract obstruction from a stone at the ureteropelvic junction. The right kidney is significantly enlarged, with hydronephrosis and perinephric fat stranding. (From McKean S, Ross JJ, Dressler DD, Brotman DJ, Ginsberg JS. *Principles and Practice of Hospital Medicine*. www.accessmedicine.com. Copyright © The McGraw-Hill Companies, Inc. All rights reserved.)

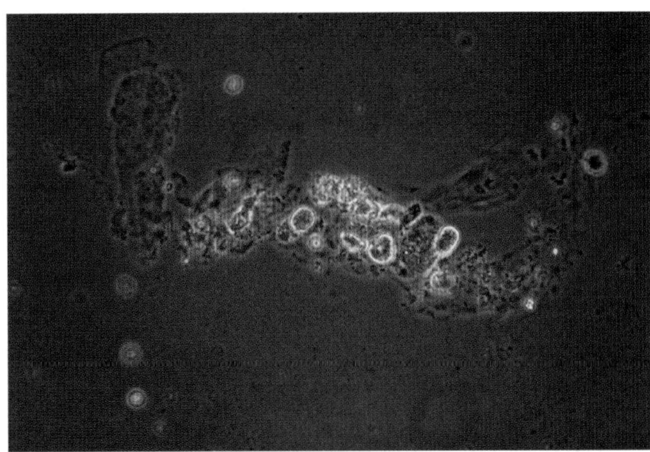

FIGURE 59-4 White blood cell casts seen in pyelonephritis. These can be differentiated from a clump of WBCs by their cylindrical shape and the presence of a hyaline matrix. (From Longo DL, Fauci AS, Kasper DL, Hauser SL, Jameson JL, Loscalzo J, eds. Harrison's Principles of Internal Medicine. 18th ed. New York, NY:McGraw-Hill; 2012.)

- Sexual activity; new sex partner or multiple partners
- *Staphylococcus saprophyticus*
- Stress and anxiety
- Urinary tract abnormalities
- Urologic surgery

Differential Diagnosis

- Cystitis of bladder
- Urethritis
- Organ dysfunction resulting from cancer or malignancy
- Non-malignant tumors in the abdomen or organs
- Endocrine disorders
- Gynecologic problems in females
  - Endometriosis
  - Menses
  - Ectopic pregnancies
  - Ovarian cysts
  - Fibroids
  - Menopause
- Autoimmune diseases that affect the upper and lower gastrointestinal (GI) tracts
- Crohn disease
- Irritable bowel syndrome
- Appendicitis
- Peritonitis
- Prostatitis
- Benign prostatic hypertrophy
- Pelvic inflammatory disease
- Gastroenteritis
- Perforated ulcers in GI system
- Kidney pathology
- Infections in the abdomen
- Bowel disorders
  - Constipation or diarrhea
  - Inflammation of the abdominal or organ linings
  - Obstructions
  - Torsions
- Referred pain from heart, spine, or hip
- Post–bariatric-surgery complications

MEANS OF CONFIRMATION OR DIAGNOSIS

Laboratory Tests

- Urine culture/urinalysis
- Blood tests for hemoglobin and hematocrit for signs of bleeding, anemia, pathogens, immune status, vitamin deficiencies, and white blood cell count

Imaging

- Ultrasound
- Intravenous urinary pyelogram using dye
- CT
- Bladder scan
- MRI

Diagnostic Procedures

- Patient history and clinical examination
  - History of urination
- Cystoscopy
- Urodynamic testing
- Manual palpation for tenderness

FINDINGS AND INTERPRETATION

- Most common bacteria
  - *E. Coli*
  - *Proteus Pseudomonas*
  - *Staphylococcus aureus*
  - *Streptococcus Faecalis*
- Pyuria (>5 WBCs/high-power field)[3]
- Uric nitrate by dipstick, most children (70%) have negative nitrite tests

TREATMENT

Medication

- Intravenous doripenem
- Antibiotics specific to causative bacteria[2]
  - Sulfamethoxazole/trimethoprim
  - Amoxicillin, Nitrofurantoin, Ampicillin
  - Ciprofloxacin, Levofloxacin
  - For sexually active females prone to UTI, instruct to take antibiotic following sexual intercourse
- Vaginal estrogen if estrogen levels low
- Pain medication

MEDICAL PROCEDURES

- Hospitalization with IV antibiotics if severe
- If catheterized, frequent changing of catheter, frequent emptying, bladder training to wean off of catheter if possible
- Instructions for self-testing of urine if infections are frequent
- Recommend heating pads to abdomen for pain management

REFERRAL/ADMITTANCE

- If an emergency is identified, refer to ER.
- If a patient is referred for PT and the causative problem is not considered to be appropriate for PT, referral to the appropriate physician must be made.
- If appropriate for PT, referral or treatment for UG pathology is usually performed by PT specialists in women's or men's health.

IMPAIRMENTS

- Muscle weakness in the pelvic floor
- Muscle atrophy
- Gait abnormality or difficulty walking
- Contractures of soft tissue (i.e., fascia, muscle)
- Muscle impairment in the pelvic floor
- Inability to perform self-care

TESTS AND MEASURES

- Observation
  - Scars may indicate adhesions or abdominal surgeries that may be causative of diverticula.
  - Striae, pink or purplish may be indicative of Cushing syndrome.
  - Dilated veins may indicate hepatic pathology or inferior vena cava obstruction, not diverticulitis.
  - Contour: Roundedness, concavity/hollowness, asymmetry, distension, pregnancy signs.
  - Cullen sign: Bluish discoloration around the umbilicus, which may be a sign of retroperitoneal bleeding.
  - Grey Turner sign: Bluish discoloration in lower abdomen, which is a sign of hemorrhagic pancreatitis.

- Bulging in groin or other areas of abdomen especially apparent with contraction of musculature in area may be hernia.
- Pulsing in the area of the navel may be abdominal aortic aneurysm
- Left lower quadrant pain, often following a meal.
- Palpable abdominal tenderness on left/right or generalized.
- Psoas sign: Provides resistance over patient's right knee as they flex the hip; pain would be indicative of appendicitis or possible inflammation of the abdomen.
- Obturator sign: Internal rotation of RLE and flexion may be indicative of appendicitis or pelvic inflammation.
- Rovsing sign: Pain on the right side of abdomen when pressure is put on the left may be indicative of appendicitis.

- Palpation
  - Kidneys: In supine, place one hand under client between ribs and iliac crest; other hand on abdomen below ribs, and ribs pointing in opposite direction: +/– tenderness or reproduction of symptoms.
  - Bladder: Not usually palpable unless it is distended and rises above pubic bone; in supine, place hand above pubis and press down.
    - +/= tenderness, reproduction of pain, or ability to feel the bladder: __+ ___–.
  - Appendix (McBurney's): Apply vertical pressure halfway between right ASIS and umbilicus.
  - Liver: In supine, with left hand under trunk parallel to 11th and 12th rib, lift upward; right hand lateral to rectus and press in and up.
    - +/= reproduction of symptoms with deep breath.
  - Ascites: With the fingers, percuss outward from center; if sound is dull, ascites may be present.
  - Spleen: Not recommended for PT to palpate an enlarged spleen (only palpable if enlarged) because of the potential.
  - Gallbladder (Murphy's): Place fingers to the right of rectus abdominus below rib cage.
    - +/= sudden pain and muscle tensing with deep breath.

INTERVENTION

- Physical therapy intervention is indicated for movement-related problems that occur secondary to UG infection and include
  - Gait training
  - Therapeutic exercise: All relevant categories, energy conservation
    - If there is a stoma from a colostomy or ileostomy, PT must be aware that activities should be avoided if they cause retraction
  - Therapeutic activities for bed-mobility training, transfer- and transitional-movement training, and pelvic floor retraining
  - Self-care management training
    - If a male has an external catheter, ensure it is secure to prevent accidental loss.
    - For indwelling catheters, ensure they are not pulled out and that drainage clamps are locked.
    - Determine if a leg bag or tube and "hanging bag" are in use.
    - Bag should be below waist/bladder level at all times and should not touch the floor.
    - If full, bag should be emptied to prevent backflow.
  - Neuromuscular re-education
  - Electrical stimulation
  - Interprofessional
    - Lifestyle modification
    - Hydration
    - Smoking cessation
    - Weight management
    - Dietary counseling
    - Psychological intervention

FUNCTIONAL GOALS

- The patient will be able to
  - Achieve adequate functional aerobic capacity and ability to talk during activity in order to achieve functional gait and activity tolerance for work, play, school, self-care; ADLs and IADLs.
  - Perform with functional, independent gait in the home and community (with or without a device), allowing for work, play, self-care; ADLs and IADLs, up to __________ feet based on patient's need and prior functional level.
  - Achieve 600 m or greater in a 6-minute walk test for initiation of safe functional gait in the community.
  - Perform active verbalization with increasing taxonomy for safety during gait, including negotiation of even and uneven surfaces, opening and closing doors, transferring in and out of a car.
  - Perform activities requiring abdominals with appropriate muscle splinting or guarding to prevent retraction of stoma, if patient has a colostomy or ileostomy.
  - Tolerate 30 minutes of continuous moderate exercise three times a week in ______ weeks, and five times a week in____________ weeks) depending on the severity of the disease.

PROGNOSIS

- As this pathology is primarily medical in nature, it is the physician who establishes the medical prognosis.
- If treated promptly and effectively with antibiotics, UTIs should resolve.
- If left untreated, acute, and or chronic kidney infections can result in permanent kidney damage.
- For females with a history of approximately three UTIs, it is likely that they will recur over time.
- For the physical therapy prognosis, established goals should be achievable based on the patient's overall condition.
- Unless the medical condition is unstable or the goals unrealistic, the prognosis from a physical therapy perspective should be good.
  - "Good" refers only to the realistic functional goals established.
  - This includes UG problems managed by PTs specifically.

PATIENT RESOURCES

- The Official Foundation of the American Urological Association. http://www.urologyhealth.org. Accessed June 5, 2013.
- Urology Care Foundation. The Official Foundation of the American Urological Association. http://www.urologyhealth.org. Accessed June 5, 2013.
- Urinary Tract Infections in Children. National Kidney & Urologic Diseases Information Clearinghouse (NKUDIC), National Institutes of Health. http://kidney.niddk.nih.gov/kudiseases/pubs/utichildren. Accessed June 5, 2013.
- Urinary Tract Infection in Children—Symptoms. WebMD. http://children.webmd.com/tc/urinary-tract-infections-in-children-symptoms. Accessed June 5, 2013.

REFERENCES

1. APTA. *Guide to Physical Therapy Practice*. Atlanta, GA: American Physical Therapy Association; 2003. http://guidetoptpractice.apta.org. Accessed June 5, 2013.
2. Urinary tract infection(UTI). Mayo Clinic. http://www.mayoclinic.com/health/urinary-tract-infection/DS00286. Accessed June 5, 2013.
3. Lum GM. Kidney & urinary tract. In: Hay WW, Levin MJ, Sondheimer JM, Deterding RR, eds. *CURRENT Diagnosis & Treatment: Pediatrics*. 20th ed. New York, NY: McGraw-Hill; 2011:Chapter 22. http://www.accessphysiotherapy.com/content/6584756. Accessed June 14, 2013.

ADDITIONAL REFERENCES

- Dutton M. Pathology, gynecology, and psychology. In: Dutton M, ed. *McGraw-Hill's NPTE (National Physical Therapy Examination)*.2nd ed. New York, NY: McGraw-Hill; 2012. http://www.accessphysiotherapy.com/content/5402339. Accessed June 5, 2013.
- Dutton M. Differential diagnosis. In: Dutton M, ed. *Orthopaedic Examination, Evaluation, and Intervention*. 2nd ed. New York, NY: McGraw-Hill; 2008. http://www.accessphysiotherapy.com/content/5547094. Accessed January 5, 2013.
- Grover ML, Bracamonte JD, Kanodia AK, et al. Assessing adherence to evidence-based guidelines for the diagnosis and management of uncomplicated urinary tract infection. *Mayo Clin Proc.* 2007;82(2):181–185.
- Hickerson AD, Carson CC. The treatment of urinary tract infections and use of ciprofloxacin extended release. *Expert Opin Investig Drugs.* 2006;15(5):519–532.
- ICD9DATA. http://www.icd9data.com. Accessed June 5, 2013.
- ICD10DATA. http://www.icd10data.com. Accessed June 5, 2013.
- NIH National Kidney & Urolgic Diseases Information Clearinghouse (NKUDIC). *Urinary Tract Infections in Children.* http://kidney.niddk.nih.gov/kudiseases/pubs/utichildren/. Accessed June 5, 2013.
- Ochoa Sangrador C, Malaga Guerrero S; Panel de Expertos de la Conferencia de Consenso; Grupo Investigador de la Conferencia de Consenso. Recommendations of the consensus conference "diagnostic and therapeutic management of urinary tract infection in childhood." *An Pediatr (Barc).* 2007;67(5):517–525.
- van Pinxteren B, van Vliet SM, Wiersma TJ, Goudswaard AN; Nederlands Huisartsen Genootschap. Summary of the practice guidline 'Urinary-tract infections' (second revision) from the Dutch College of General Practitioners. *Ned Tijdschr Geneeskd.* 2006;150(13):718–722.

60 URETHRITIS

Debra F. Stern, DPT, DBA, MSM, PT
Eric Shamus, PhD, DPT, PT, CSCS
Wendy Song, DO

CONDITION/DISORDER SYNONYM

- Nongonococcal urethritis

ICD-9-CM CODES

- 590.9 Infection of kidney, unspecified
- Associated ICD-9-CM PT diagnoses/treatment diagnosis that may be directly related to urogenital (UG) disorders or consequences from bed rest, surgery, or inactivity or directly related to UG disorders specifically
  - 315.4 Developmental coordination disorder
  - 718.45 Contracture of joint, pelvic region and thigh
  - 719.70 Difficulty in walking
  - 728.2 Muscular wasting and disuse atrophy
  - 728.89 Other disorders of muscle, ligament, and fascia
  - 729.9 Other and unspecified disorders of soft tissue
  - 780.7 Malaise and fatigue
  - 781.2 Abnormality of gait
  - 782.3 Edema
  - 786.0 Dyspnea and respiratory abnormalities
  - 786.05 Shortness of breath

ICD-10-CM CODE

- N15.9 Renal tubulo-interstitial disease, unspecified

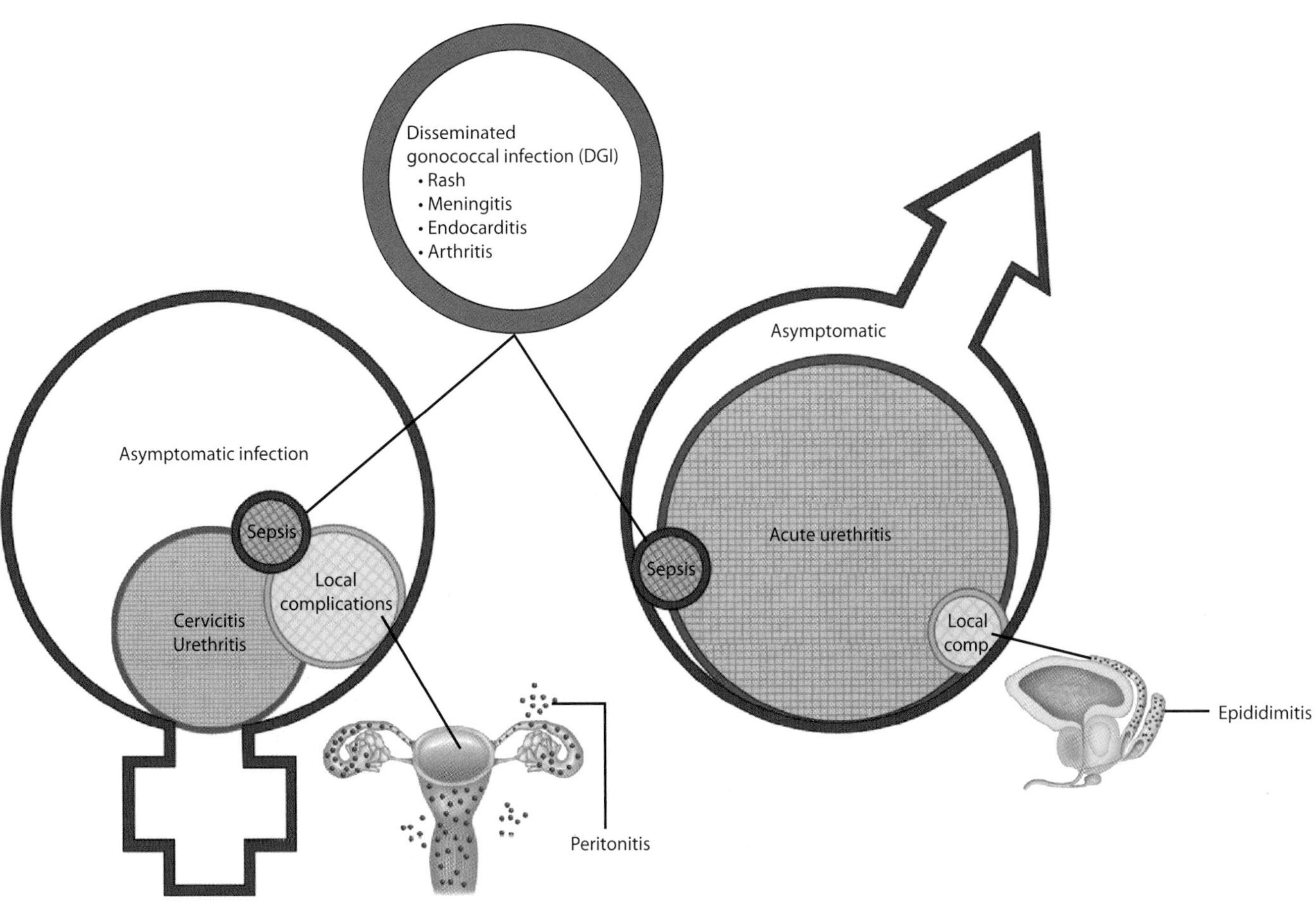

FIGURE 60-1 Gonorrhea in men and women. The majority of cases in women are asymptomatic. Local extension up the fallopian tubes causes salpingitis. The majority of men have acute urethritis, and only a small percentage have local extension the epididymitis. A very small part of either spectrum results in bacteremia and disseminated gonococcal infection. (From Ryan KJ, Ray CG. *Sherris Medical Microbiology*. 5th ed. www.accessmedicine.com. Copyright © The McGraw-Hill Companies, Inc. All rights reserved.)

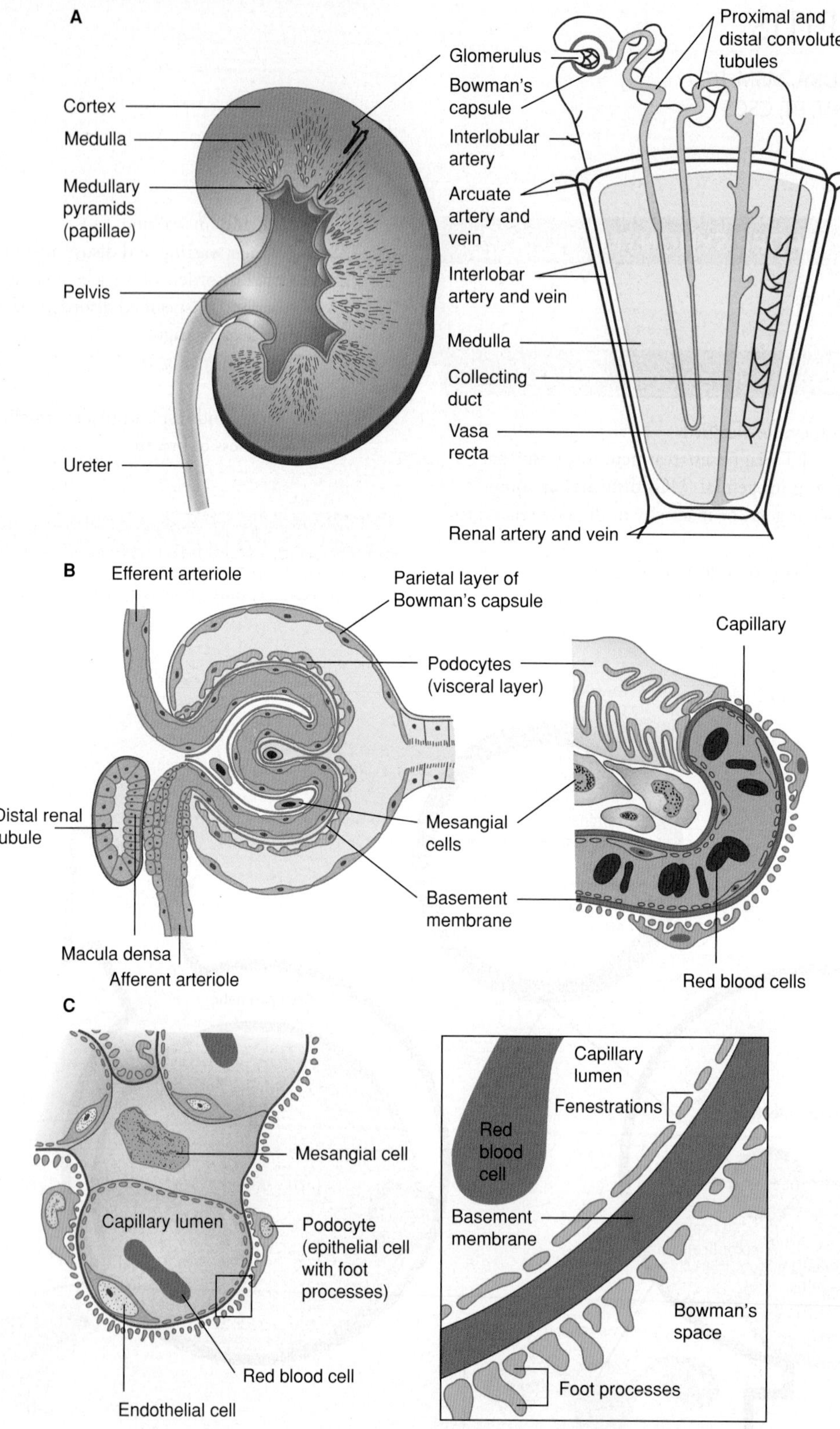

FIGURE 60-2 Structures of the kidney. **A.** Landmarks of the normal kidney. **B.** Glomerulus and glomerular capillary. **C.** Detailed structure of the glomerulus and the glomerular filtration membrane composed of endothelial cell, basement membrane, and podocyte. Note that for clarity the distal tubule is separated from the glomerulus in **A;** however, its true anatomic relationship, which is essential for physiologic function, is illustrated in **B.** (Redrawn with permission from Chandrasoma P, Taylor CE. *Concise Pathology*. 3rd ed. Originally published by Appleton & Lange. Copyright © 1998 by the McGraw-Hill Companies, Inc.)

PREFERRED PRACTICE PATTERN

- As of June, 2014, the APTA *Guide to Physical Therapist Practice* does not include practice patterns for organ system pathology; therefore, the associated or secondary musculoskeletal, cardiovascular/pulmonary, or potential neuromuscular patterns would be indicated.

PATIENT PRESENTATION

A 45-year-old male presents to the clinic with groin and low back pain. After questioning he is having increased urinary urgency, burning, and pain in his penis during urination for 5 days. He also noticed a small amount of penile discharge. He denies sexual intercourse in the past 2 years. Vitals are: Temperature: 98.9; Pulse: 76; Respiration: 18; Blood pressure: 126/83; and SpO_2% of 99%. Physical exam reveals a scant amount of clear penile discharge and inflammation of the urethral meatus. The patient was referred to the urologist.

KEY FEATURES

Description

- Swelling and Inflammation of the urethra
- Males and females frequently asymptomatic[1]
- Females present with symptoms of urinary tract infection: Burning with urination
- Males present with a clear or purulent discharge[1]
- If spread to kidneys, symptoms more severe and pain is located in the low back with possible tenderness to palpation of the kidneys

Essentials of Diagnosis

- Difficulty urinating
- Painful urination
- Malodorous urine
- Pelvic pain in women
- Change in color of urine
- Positive cultures

General Considerations

- Most infections of the urethra are sexually transmitted.
- Most common bacterial causes in males[1]
  - *Neisseria gonorrhoeae*
  - *Chlamydia trachomatis*
  - Coliforms in males practicing insertive anal intercourse
- May refer pain to back, pelvic region
- May result in secondary problems such as
  - Reiter syndrome
  - Epididymitis or prostatitis
  - Aerobic capacity and muscle-endurance impairment
  - Sarcopenia
  - Weakness/impaired muscle performance
  - Neuromuscular problems
  - Weight loss or weight gain indicating the need for PT intervention depending on severity
- May mimic colon cancer or tumors, irritable bowel, colitis, or gynecological problems in females such as endometriosis, uterine fibroids, or ectopic pregnancies.
- There are specific UG pathologies that may be appropriate for PT, but PT usually does not have a role specifically in the treatment.

Demographics

- Women more susceptible to cystitis, secondary to the anatomical proximity of the urethra to the anus and the urethra to the bladder
- Frequently associated with sexual intercourse
- *Escherichia coli* is the common bacterial cause
- Women more susceptible to urethritis because of anatomical proximity of urethra to vagina and can be caused by sexually transmitted diseases such as herpes, gonorrhea, and chlamydia

CLINICAL FINDINGS

SIGNS AND SYMPTOMS

- Symptoms are frequently referred to the back and abdominal area; it may be more common than previously identified for patients to be inappropriately referred to PT.
- Urethra (urethritis): Main symptoms
  - Severe pain with or without attempts at urination in males and females, or no pain at all, especially in the elderly and children
  - Burning with urination
  - Discharge from the penis
  - Blood in the urine or semen
- Bladder (cystitis): Main symptoms
  - Pelvic pressure
  - Lower abdomen discomfort
  - Frequent, painful urination
  - Blood in urine
- Kidneys (acute pyelonephritis): Main symptoms
  - Upper back and side (flank) pain
  - High fever
  - Shaking and chills
  - Nausea
  - Vomiting

Functional Implications

- Severe symptoms such as immediacy of need to urinate may be disabling, resulting in the inability to leave home
- Pain
- Dehydration secondary to fear of drinking, emesis, loss of appetite, inability to drink or eat secondary to nausea, or inability to swallow
  - Medically, should be drinking copious amounts of water
- Sarcopenia resulting in weakness, muscle-mass loss, inability to ambulate or perform self-care, as well as aerobic capacity limitation secondary to inactivity
- Need for catheters, external or indwelling or intermittent
  - Presence of the same may present a problem with stoma retraction associated with abdominal contraction
- Decreased exercise tolerance
- Changes in lifestyle limiting physical activity
- Eating disorders/anorexia
- Fatigue
- Inappropriate self-medication
- Anxiety and depression
- Can be indicative of serious medical conditions
- Limitations in ADLs or IADLs
- Infection, systemic
- Need for dietary changes, reducing irritants such as caffeine, coffee, alcohol, and citrus
- Urinary retention
- Need to drink fluids to flush urinary system

Possible Contributing Causes

- Injury
- Sensitivity to spermicidal or contraceptive chemicals
- Poor UG hygiene

- Sexually transmitted diseases[2]
  - Gonorrhea
  - Nongonococcal urethritis
- Birth control such as insertion of a diaphragm and use of spermicides
- Urinary tract abnormalities
- Blockages in urinary tract such as kidney stones in males/females; enlarged prostate
- Immunological compromise
- Catheter use, especially indwelling
- Infection, bacterial or viral, including food poisoning
- Kidney dialysis

Differential Diagnosis

- Cystitis of bladder
- Acute pyelonephritis
- Organ dysfunction as a result of cancer or malignancy
- Non-malignant tumors in the abdomen or organs
- Endocrine disorders
- Gynecologic problems in females such as
  - Endometriosis
  - Menses
  - Ectopic pregnancies
  - Ovarian cysts
  - Fibroids
  - Menopause
- Autoimmune diseases that affect the upper and lower GI tracts
- Crohn disease
- Irritable bowel syndrome
- Appendicitis
- Peritonitis
- Prostatitis
- Benign prostatic hypertrophy
- Pelvic inflammatory disease
- Gastroenteritis
- Perforated ulcers anywhere in GI system
- Kidney pathology
- Infections in the abdomen
- Bowel disorders including
  - Constipation or diarrhea
  - Inflammation of the lining of the of the abdomen or organs
  - Obstructions
  - Torsions
- Referred pain from heart, spine, hip
- Post–weight-loss surgery complications

MEANS OF CONFIRMATION OR DIAGNOSIS

Laboratory Tests

- Blood tests/lab tests
- Urine culture/urinalysis
- Hemoglobin and hematocrit for signs of bleeding, anemia, pathogens, immune status, and vitamin deficiencies; check white blood cell count for infection

Imaging

- Ultrasound
- Intravenous urinary pyelogram using dye
- CT scans
- Bladder scans
- MRIs

Diagnostic Procedures

- Cystoscopy
- Urodynamic testing
- Manual palpation for tenderness
- History of urination

FINDINGS AND INTERPRETATION

- Positive leukocyte esterase test on first-void urine
- Microscopic examination of first-void urine: More than 10 WBCs per high-power test[1]
- Gram strain of urethral secretions: More than 5 WBCs per high-power test[1]

TREATMENT

Medications

- Antibiotics specific to causative bacteria
  - Sulfamethoxazole/trimethoprim (such as Bactrim and Septra)
  - Amoxicillin (such as Larotid and Moxatag)
  - Nitrofurantoin (such as Furadantin and Macrodantin)
  - Ampicillin
  - Ciprofloxacin (Cipro)
  - Levofloxacin (Levaquin)
  - For sexually active females prone to UTI, there may be instruction to take antibiotics following sexual intercourse
- Pain medication
- Hospitalization with IV antibiotics if severe
- Vaginal estrogen if levels low

MEDICAL PROCEDURES

- If catheterized, frequent changing of catheter, frequent emptying, and bladder training to wean off catheter if possible
- Instructions for self-testing of urine if infections frequent
- Recommendations for heating pads to abdomen for pain management

REFERRALS/ADMITTANCE

- If a patient is referred for PT and the causative problem is not considered appropriate for PT, make referral to the appropriate physician.
- If appropriate for PT, referral or treatment for UG pathology is usually performed by PT specialists in women's and men's health.
- If an emergency is identified, referral to an ER may be necessary.

IMPAIRMENTS

- Muscle weakness, pelvic floor
- Muscle atrophy
- Gait abnormality/difficulty walking
- Contractures of soft tissue, fascia, muscle
- Pelvic floor muscle impairment
- Inability to perform self-care

TESTS AND MEASURES

- Observation
  - Scars may indicate adhesions of abdominal surgeries that may be causative of diverticula.

- Pink or purplish striae may be indicative of Cushing syndrome; dilated veins may indicate hepatic pathology or inferior vena cava obstruction, not diverticulitis.
- Abdominal contour: Roundedness, concavity/hollowness, asymmetry, distension, pregnancy signs.
- Cullen sign: Bluish discoloring around the umbilicus, which may be a sign of retroperitoneal bleeding.
- Bluish discoloration in lower abdomen: Grey Turner sign, which is a sign of hemorrhagic pancreatitis.
- Bulging in groin or other areas of abdomen especially apparent with contraction of musculature in area, may be hernia.
- Pulsing in the area of the navel may be abdominal aortic aneurysm.
- Left lower quadrant pain, often following a meal.
- Palpable abdominal tenderness on left/right or generalized.
- Psoas sign: Provides resistance over patient's right knee as they flex the hip; pain would be indicative of appendicitis or possible inflammation of the abdomen.
- Obturator sign: Internal rotation of right lower extremity (RLE) and flexion may be indicative of appendicitis or pelvic inflammation.
- Rovsing sign: Pain on the right side of abdomen when pressure is put on the left may be indicative of appendicitis.

- Palpation
  - Kidneys: In supine, place one hand under client between ribs and iliac crest and other hand on abdomen below ribs and pointing in opposite direction: +/– tenderness or reproduction of symptoms.
  - Bladder : Not usually palpable unless distended and rises above pubic bone; in supine, place hand above pubis and press down: +/= tenderness, reproduction of pain, or ability to feel the bladder:__ + __ –.
  - Appendix (McBurney's): Apply vertical pressure halfway between right anterior superior iliac spine (ASIS) and umbilicus.
  - Liver: In supine, with left hand under trunk parallel to 11th and 12th rib, lift upward; right hand lateral to rectus and press in and up: +/= reproduction of symptoms with deep breath.
  - Ascites: With the fingers, percuss outward from center, if sound is dull, ascites may be present.
  - Spleen: It is not recommended for PT to palpate an enlarged spleen (only palpable if enlarged) because of the potential of rupture.
  - Gallbladder (Murphy's): Place fingers to the right of rectus abdominus below rib cage: +/= sudden pain and muscle tensing with deep breath.

INTERVENTION

- PT intervention is consistent with movement-related problems that occur secondary to the UG problem and include.
  - Gait training
  - Therapeutic exercise: All relevant categories, energy conservation
    - If there is a stoma from a colostomy or ileostomy, PT must be aware that activities are avoided if they cause retraction.
  - Therapeutic activities for bed-mobility training, transfer- and transitional-movement training, pelvic floor retraining.
  - Self-care management training
    - If a male has an external catheter, ensure it is secure to prevent accidental loss.
    - With indwelling catheters, ensure they are not pulled out and that drainage clamps are locked.
    - Determine if a leg bag or tube and hanging bag is in use.
    - Bag should be below waist/bladder level at all times and should not touch the floor.
    - If full, bag should be emptied to prevent backflow.
  - Neuromuscular re-education
  - Electrical stimulation
  - Interprofessional
    - Lifestyle modification
    - Smoking cessation
    - Weight management
    - Dietary counseling
    - Psychological intervention

FUNCTIONAL GOALS

- Patient will be able to
  - Achieve adequate functional aerobic capacity and ability to talk during activity in order to achieve functional gait and activity tolerance for work, play, school, self-care; ADLs, and IADLs.
  - Achieve functional independent gait in the home and community (with or without a device), allowing for work, play, self-care; ADLs, and IADLs, up to ___ feet based on patient's need and prior functional level.
  - Achieve 600 m or greater in a 6-minute walk test for initiation of safe functional gait in the community.
  - Perform active verbalization with increasing taxonomy for safety during gait, including negotiation of even and uneven surfaces, opening and closing doors, and transferring in and out of a car.
  - Perform activities requiring abdominals with appropriate muscle splinting/guarding to prevent retraction of stoma, if patient has a colostomy or ileostomy.
  - Tolerate 30 minutes of continuous moderate exercise three times a week in ___ weeks, and five times a week in ___ weeks, depending on the severity of the disease.

PROGNOSIS

- As this pathology is primarily medical in nature, the physician establishes the medical prognosis.
- If treated promptly and effectively with antibiotics, UTIs should resolve.
- If left untreated, acute, and/or chronic, kidney infections can result in permanent kidney damage.
- Once a female has a history of approximately three UTIs, it is likely that they will recur over time.
- For the PT prognosis, establish goals that the patient can achieve based on the overall condition.
- Unless the medical condition is unstable or the goals unrealistic, the prognosis from a PT perspective should be good.
  - This includes UG problems managed by PTs specifically.
    - "Good" refers only to the realistic functional goals established.

PATIENT RESOURCES

- Urology Care Foundation. The Official Foundation of the American Urological Association. http://www.urologyhealth.org. Accessed July 14, 2013.
- Urinary Tract Infection (UTI). Mayo Clinic. http://www.mayoclinic.com/health/urinary-tract-infection/DS00286. Accessed July 14, 2013.

REFERENCES

1. Hay WW, Levin MJ, Sondheimer JM, Deterding RR. The spectrum of signs & symptoms of sexually transmitted infections. In: Hay WW, Levin MJ, Sondheimer JM, Deterding RR, eds. *CURRENT Diagnosis & Treatment: Pediatrics*. 20th ed. New York, NY: McGraw-Hill; 2011. http://www.accessphysiotherapy.com/content/6592382. Accessed July 14, 2013.
2. Chandrasoma P, Taylor CR. Sexually transmitted infections. In: Chandrasoma P, Taylor CR, eds. *Concise Pathology*. 3rd ed. New York, NY: McGraw-Hill; 2011:Chapter 54. http://www.accessphysiotherapy.com/content/191565. Accessed July 14, 2013.

ADDITIONAL REFERENCES

- Bradshaw CS, Tabrizi SN, Read TR, et al. Etiologies of non-gonococcal urethritis: bacteria, viruses, and the association with orogenital exposure. *J Infect Dis*. 2006;193(3):336–345.
- Brill JR. Diagnosis and treatment of urethritis in men. *Am Fam Physician*. 2010;81(7):873–878.
- Gaydos C, Maldeis NE, Hardick A, Hardick J, Quinn TC. *Mycoplasma genitalium* compared to *Chlamydia*, gonorrhoea and *Trichomonas* as an aetiological agent of urethritis in men attending STD clinics. *Sex Transm Infect*. 2009;85(6):438–440. doi: 10.1136/sti.2008.035477.
- He W, Chen M, Zu X, Li Y, Ning K, Qi L. Chronic prostatitis presenting with dysfunctional voiding and effects of pelvic floor biofeedback treatment. *BJU Int*. 2010;195(7):975–977. doi: 10.1111/j.1464-410X.2009.08850.x.
- McCormack WM. Urethritis. In: Mandell GL, Bennett JE, Dolin R, eds. *Principles and Practice of Infectious Diseases*. 7th ed. Philadelphia, PA: Elsevier Churchill Livingstone; 2009:Chapter 106.
- Urinary Tract Infections in Children. National Kidney and Urologic Diseases Information Clearinghouse (NKUDIC). National Institutes of Health. http://kidney.niddk.nih.gov/kudiseases/pubs/utichildren./ Accessed July 14, 2013.

61 URINARY TRACT INFECTION

Debra F. Stern, DPT, DBA, MSM, PT
Eric Shamus, PhD, DPT, PT, CSCS

CONDITION/DISORDER SYNONYM

- Urinary tract infection (UTI)

ICD-9-CM CODES

- 590.9 Infection of kidney, unspecified
- Associated ICD-9-CM PT diagnoses/treatment diagnosis that may be directly related to urogenital (UG) disorders or consequences from bed rest, surgery, or inactivity or directly related to UG disorders specifically
  - 315.4 Developmental coordination disorder
  - 718.45 Contracture of joint, pelvic region and thigh
  - 719.70 Difficulty in walking
  - 728.2 Muscular wasting and disuse atrophy
  - 728.89 Other disorders of muscle, ligament, and fascia
  - 729.9 Other and unspecified disorders of soft tissue
  - 780.7 Malaise and fatigue
  - 781.2 Abnormality of gait
  - 782.3 Edema
  - 786.0 Dyspnea and respiratory abnormalities
  - 786.05 Shortness of breath

ICD-10-CM CODE

- N15.9 Renal tubulo-interstitial disease, unspecified

PREFERRED PRACTICE PATTERN

- As of June, 2014, the APTA *Guide to Physical Therapist Practice* does not include practice patterns for organ system pathology; therefore, the associated or secondary musculoskeletal, cardiovascular/pulmonary, or potential neuromuscular patterns would be indicated.[1]

PATIENT PRESENTATION

A 29-year-old woman complains of a 2-day history of dysuria, urgency, and urinary frequency. She denies the use of medications and has no significant past medical history. On examination, her blood pressure (BP) is 100/70 mm Hg, heart rate (HR) 90 beats per minute, and temperature 98°F (36.6°C). The thyroid is normal on palpation. The heart and lung examinations are normal. She does not have back tenderness. The abdomen is nontender and without masses. The pelvic examination reveals normal female genitalia. There is no adnexal tenderness or masses.[2]

KEY FEATURES

Description

- Can occur in any component of the urinary system: Upper UTIs (kidneys and ureters) and lower UTIs (urethra and bladder)
- Sudden onset of confusion in elderly without fever
- Severe pain with or without attempts at urination in males and females or no pain at all, especially in the elderly and children
- Changes in color, volume (decrease), and odor of urine
- Most common in bladder and urethra
  - Cystitis
  - Urethritis
- If spread to kidneys, symptoms more severe, and pain is located in the lower back with possible tenderness to palpation of the kidneys

Essentials of Diagnosis

- Difficulty urinating
- Painful urination
- Malodorous urine
- Pelvic pain in women
- Rectal pain in men
- Change in color of urine
- Positive cultures

General Considerations

- Diagnosis for more occult problems may take time and require intensive medical diagnostic testing
- May refer pain to back, pelvic region, or rectal area (men)
- May result in secondary problems such as
  - Aerobic capacity and muscle-endurance impairment

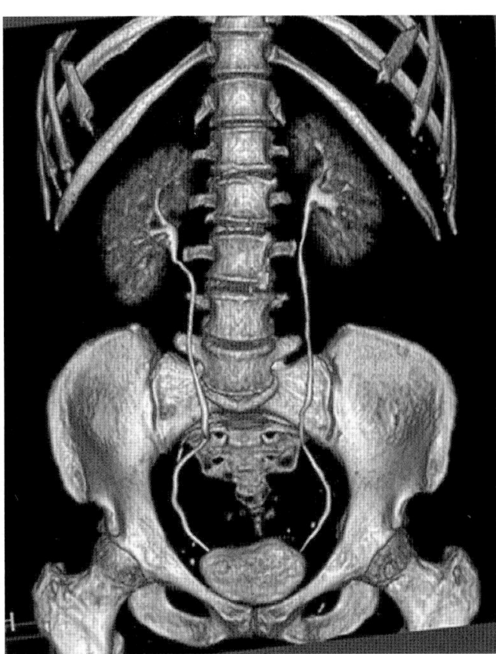

FIGURE 61-1 3-D reconstruction. Three-dimensional postprocessed volume-rendered image of the urinary tract beautifully demonstrates the kidneys, ureters, and bladder. (From Chen MYM, Pope TL, Ott DJ. *Basic Radiology*. 2nd ed. www.accessmedicine.com.)

  - Sarcopenia
  - Weakness/impaired muscle performance
  - Musculoskeletal problems
  - Neuromuscular problems
- May mimic colon cancer or tumors, irritable bowel, colitis, or gynecological problems in females such as endometriosis, uterine fibroids, or ectopic pregnancies
- May or may not be associated with fever

▶ Demographics

- More common in women than men in general
- Women more susceptible to cystitis, secondary to the anatomical proximity of the urethra to the anus and the urethra to the bladder
- Frequently associated with sexual intercourse
- Women more susceptible to urethritis because of anatomical proximity of urethra to vagina, and can be caused by sexually transmitted diseases such as herpes, gonorrhea, and chlamydia
- About half of all women will have a UTI in their lifetime
- Children are at greater risk, 8% of girls and 2% of boys will acquire UTIs in childhood[3]

CLINICAL FINDINGS

SIGNS AND SYMPTOMS

- It is not the purview of a PT to medically diagnose a UG pathology but rather to recognize the possibility in the differential diagnosis process, especially when the findings are not consistent with conditions commonly treated: Musculoskeletal, neuromuscular, integumentary, and cardiopulmonary.
- As the symptoms are frequently referred to the back and abdominal area, it may be more common than previously identified for patients to be inappropriately referred to PT.[4,5]
- There are specific UG pathologies that may be appropriate for PT, but PT usually does not have a role specifically in the treatment of UTIs.
- Dysfunctional voiding
- Urethra (urethritis): Main symptoms
  - Burning with urination
  - Blood in the urine or semen
  - Discharge from the penis
- Bladder (cystitis): Main symptoms
  - Pelvic pressure
  - Lower abdomen discomfort
  - Frequent, painful urination
  - Blood in urine
- Kidneys (acute pyelonephritis): Main symptoms
  - Upper back and side (flank) pain
  - High fever
  - Shaking and chills
  - Nausea
  - Vomiting
- Abdominal or stomach pain or cramping
- Abdominal (stomach or intestinal) pain after ingesting food or liquid
- Nausea
- Emesis
- Changes in clarity of urine: Cloudy, sediment
- Change in color of urine: Brown or pink, indicating blood
- Urge to urinate, may or may not produce urine or have difficulty initiating
- Pain or burning associated with urination or defecation
- Urine has strong odor
- Changes in urinary habits
- Bloated or swollen abdomen, abdominal distention
- Unexplained weight loss
- Fever
- Fistulas
- General abdominal/pelvic pain in women more than men
- Rectal pain in males
- Middle and lower abdominal pain in children
- Abdominal muscle spasm, guarding
- In older adults, sudden changes in mental status

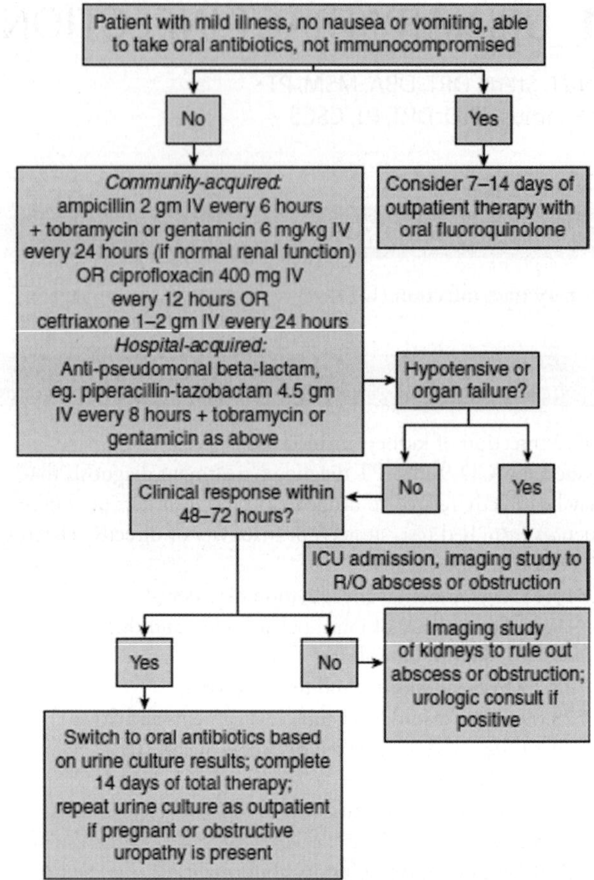

FIGURE 61-2 Approach to the patient with upper UTI (ICU, intensive care unit; R/O, rule out). (From McKean S, Ross J, Dressler DD, Brotman DJ, Ginsberg JS. *Principles and Practice of Hospital Medicine*. www.accessmedicine.com. Copyright © The McGraw-Hill Companies, Inc. All rights reserved.)

▶ Functional Implications

- Severe symptoms such as immediacy of need to urinate may be disabling, resulting in the inability to leave home
- Pain
- Dehydration secondary to fear of drinking, emesis, loss of appetite, inability to drink or eat secondary to nausea, or inability to swallow
  - Medically, should be drinking copious amounts of water
- Sarcopenia resulting in weakness, muscle-mass loss, inability to ambulate or perform self-care as well as aerobic capacity limitation secondary to inactivity
- Need for catheters, external or indwelling or intermittent
  - Presence of same may present a problem with stoma retraction associated with abdominal contraction
- Decreased exercise tolerance
- Changes in lifestyle limiting physical activity
- Eating disorders/anorexia
- Fatigue

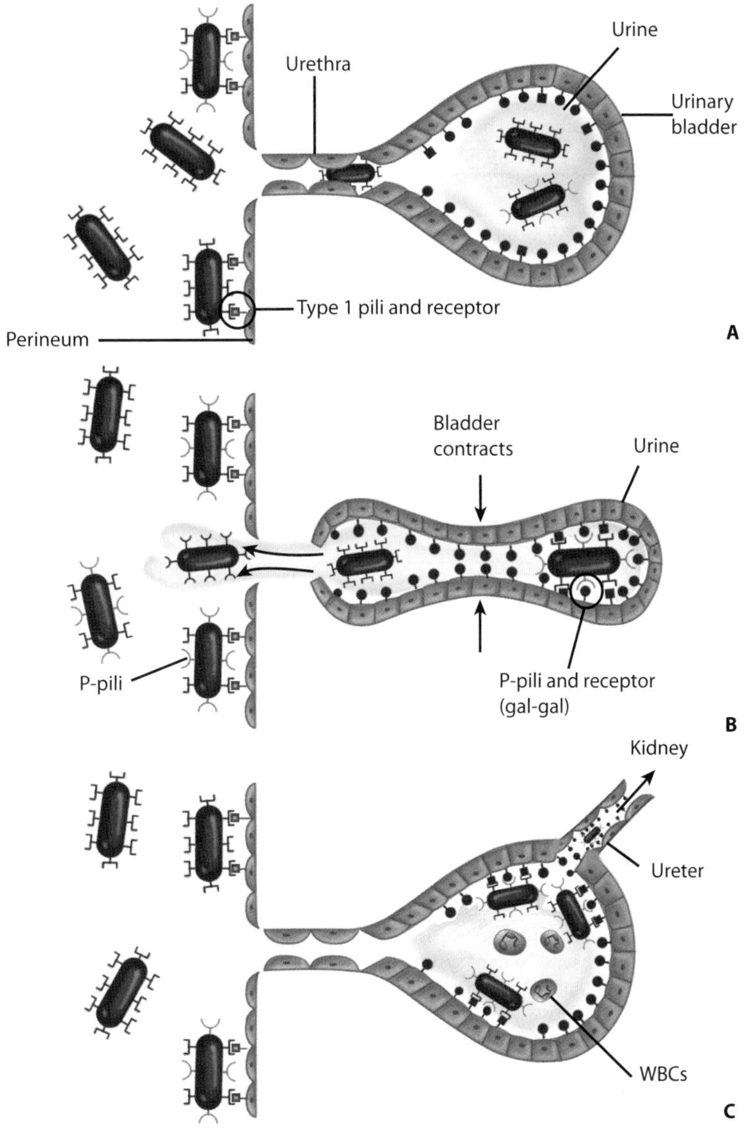

FIGURE 61-3 Urinary tract infection due to *Escherichia coli*. The urinary bladder, perineal mucosa, and short female urethra are shown. *E. coli* from the nearby rectal flora have colonized the perineum, utilizing binding by type 1 (common) pili. *E. coli* with P pili are also present but are of no use at this site. **A.** A few *E. coli* have gained access to the bladder owing to mechanical disruptions such as sexual intercourse or instrumentation (catheters). Note that receptors for the P pili not present on the perineal mucosa are found on the surface of bladder mucosal cells. **B.** During voiding, the bladder has expelled the *E. coli*, which have only type 1 pili. The P pili-containing bacteria remain behind due to the strong binding to the P (Gal-Gal) receptor. **C.** The remaining *E. coli* have multiplied and are causing a urinary tract infection (cystitis) with inflammation and hemorrhage. In some cases, the bacteria ascend the ureter to cause pyelonephritis. WBCs, white blood cells. (From Ryan KJ, Ray CG. *Sherris Medical Microbiology*. 5th ed. www.accessmedicine.com. Copyright © The McGraw-Hill Companies, Inc. All rights reserved.)

- Inappropriate self-medication
- Anxiety and depression
- Can be indicative of serious medical conditions
- Limitations in ADLs or IADLs
- Infection, systemic
- Need for dietary changes, reducing irritants such as caffeine, coffee, alcohol, and citrus
- Urinary retention
- Need to drink fluids to flush urinary system

Possible Contributing Causes

- Female
- Stress and anxiety
- Poor UG hygiene
- Sexual activity
- Birth control such as insertion of a diaphragm and use of spermicides
- Urinary tract abnormalities
- Blockages in urinary tract such as kidney stones in males/females; enlarged prostate
- Menopause
- Lack of estrogen
- Immunological compromise
- Catheter use, especially indwelling
- Environmental irritant
- Infection, bacterial or viral including food poisoning
- *Escherichia coli* is the common bacterial cause
- Kidney dialysis

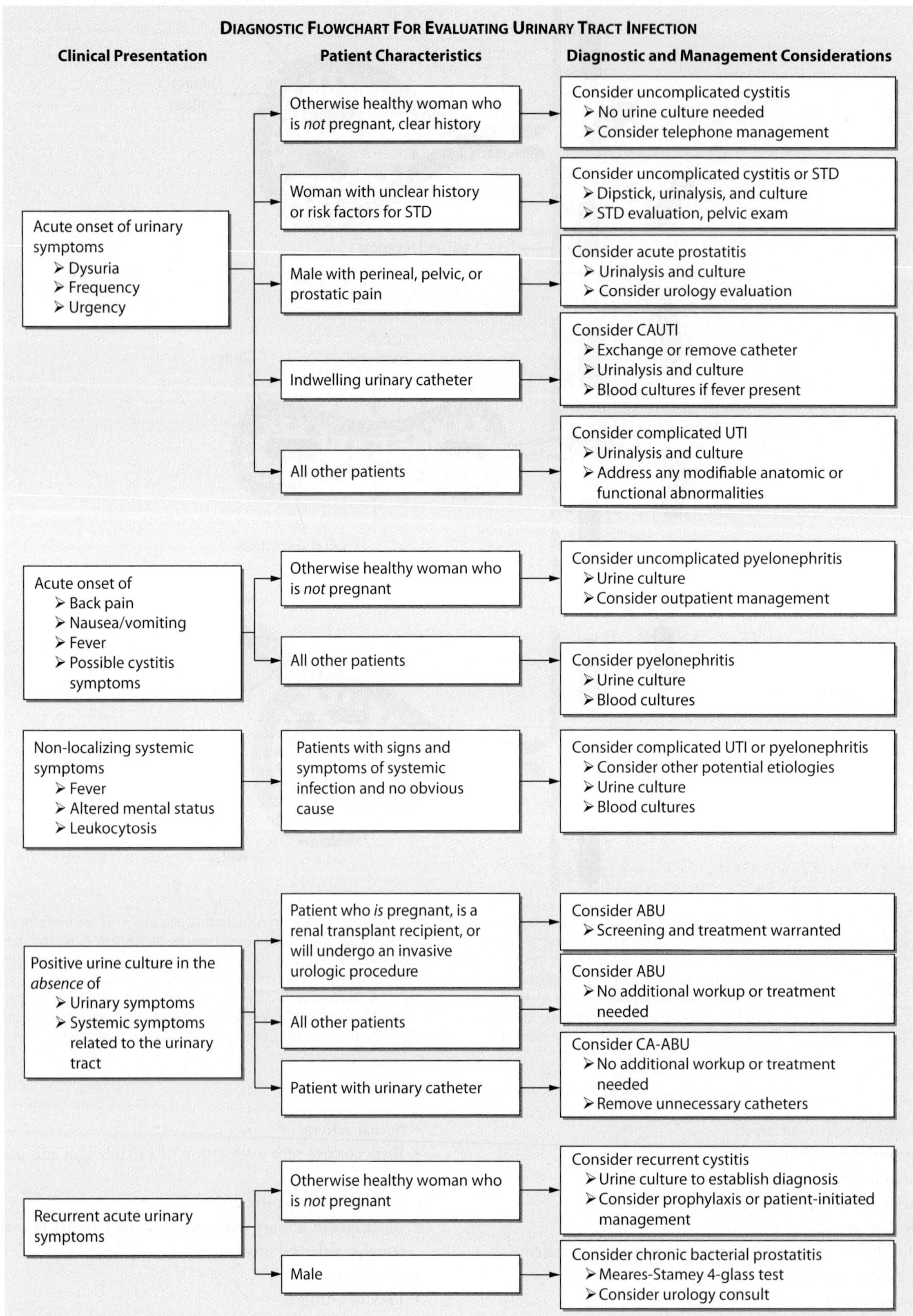

FIGURE 61-4 Diagnostic approach to urinary tract infection. STD, sexually transmitted disease; CAUTI, catheter-associated UTI; ABU, asymptomatic bacteriuria; CA-ABU, catheter-associated ABU. (From Longo DL, Fauci AS, Kasper DL, Hauser SL, Jameson JL, Loscalzo J, eds. *Harrison's Principles of Internal Medicine*. 18th ed. New York, NY: McGraw-Hill; 2012.)

Differential Diagnosis

- Organ dysfunction as a result of cancer or malignancy
- Non-malignant tumors in the abdomen or organs
- Endocrine disorders
- Gynecologic problems in females such as
  - Endometriosis
  - Menses
  - Ectopic pregnancies
  - Ovarian cysts
  - Fibroids
  - Menopause
- Autoimmune diseases that affect the upper and lower GI tracts
- Crohn disease
- Irritable bowel syndrome
- Appendicitis
- Peritonitis
- Prostatitis
- Benign prostatic hypertrophy
- Pelvic inflammatory disease
- Gastroenteritis
- Perforated ulcers anywhere in GI system
- Kidney pathology
- Infections in the abdomen
- Bowel disorders including
  - Constipation or diarrhea
  - Inflammation of the lining of the of the abdomen or organs
  - Obstructions
  - Torsions
- Referred pain from heart, spine, hip
  - Post–weight-loss surgery complications

MEANS OF CONFIRMATION OR DIAGNOSIS

Laboratory Tests

- Blood test, CBC/lab tests
- Urine culture/urinalysis
- Hemoglobin and hematocrit for signs of bleeding, anemia, pathogens, immune status, and vitamin deficiencies; check white blood cell count for infection

Imaging

- Radiographic[3]
- Ultrasound
- Intravenous urinary pyelogram using dye
- CT scans
- Bladder scans
- MRIs

Diagnostic Procedures

- Cystoscopy
- Urodynamic testing
- Manual palpation for tenderness
- History of urination

FINDINGS AND INTERPRETATION

- Pyuria (>5 WBCs/high-power field)[3]
- Uric nitrate by dipstick, most children (70%) have negative nitrite tests[2]

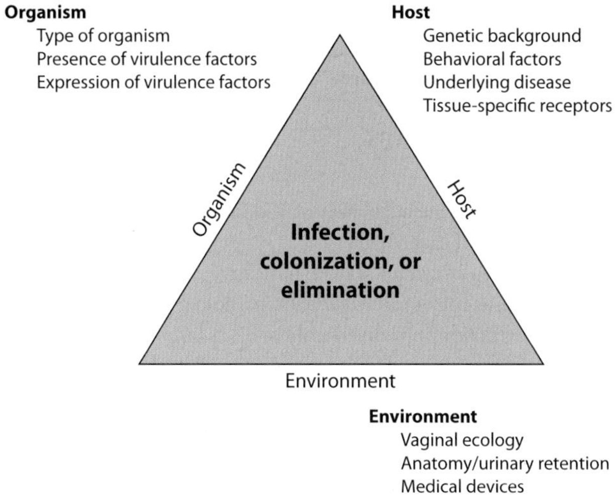

FIGURE 61-5 Pathogenesis of urinary tract infection. The relationship between specific host, pathogen, and environmental factors determines the clinical outcome. (From Longo DL, Fauci AS, Kasper DL, Hauser SL, Jameson JL, Loscalzo J, eds. *Harrison's Principles of Internal Medicine*. 18th ed. New York, NY:McGraw-Hill; 2012.)

TREATMENT

Medication

- Antibiotics specific to causative bacteria
  - Sulfamethoxazole/trimethoprim (such as Bactrim and Septra)
  - Amoxicillin (such as Larotid and Moxatag)
  - Nitrofurantoin (such as Furadantin and Macrodantin)
  - Ampicillin
  - Ciprofloxacin (Cipro)
  - Levofloxacin (Levaquin)
  - For sexually active females prone to UTI, there may be instruction to take antibiotics following sexual intercourse
- Pain medication
- Vaginal estrogen if levels low

MEDICAL PROCEDURES

- If catheterized, frequent changing of catheter, frequent emptying, and bladder training to wean off catheter if possible
- Instructions of self-testing of urine if infections frequent
- Recommendations for heating pads to abdomen for pain management
- Hospitalization with IV antibiotics if severe

REFERRALS/ADMITTANCE

- If a patient is referred for PT and the causative problem is not considered appropriate for PT, make referral to the appropriate physician.
- If appropriate for PT, referral or treatment for UG pathology is usually performed by PT specialists in women's and men's health.
- If an emergency is identified, referral to an ER may be necessary.

IMPAIRMENTS

- Muscle weakness, pelvic floor
- Muscle atrophy
- Gait abnormality/difficulty walking

- Contractures of soft tissue; fascia, muscle
- Pelvic floor muscle impairment
- Inability to perform self-care

TESTS AND MEASURES

- Observation
  - Scars may indicate adhesions of abdominal surgeries that may be causative of diverticula.
  - Pink or purplish striae may be indicative of Cushing syndrome; dilated veins may indicate hepatic pathology or inferior vena cava obstruction, not diverticulitis.
  - Abdominal contour: Roundedness, concavity/hollowness, asymmetry, distension, pregnancy signs.
  - Cullen sign: Bluish discoloring around the umbilicus, which may be a sign of retroperitoneal bleeding.
  - Bluish discoloration in lower abdomen, Grey Turner sign, which is a sign of hemorrhagic pancreatitis.
  - Bulging in groin or other areas of abdomen especially apparent with contraction of musculature in area, may be hernia.
  - Pulsing in the area of the navel may be abdominal aortic aneurysm.
  - Left lower quadrant pain, often following a meal.
  - Palpable abdominal tenderness on left/right or generalized.
  - Psoas sign: Provides resistance over patient's right knee as they flex the hip; pain would be indicative of appendicitis or possible inflammation of the abdomen.
  - Obturator sign: Internal rotation of right lower extremity (RLE) and flexion may be indicative of appendicitis or pelvic inflammation.
  - Rovsing sign: Pain on the right side of abdomen when pressure is put on the left may be indicative of appendicitis.
- Palpation
  - Kidneys: In supine, place one hand under client between ribs and iliac crest and other hand on abdomen below ribs and pointing in opposite direction: +/– tenderness or reproduction of symptoms.
  - Bladder: Not usually palpable unless distended and rises above pubic bone; in supine, place hand above pubis and press down: +/= tenderness, reproduction of pain, or ability to feel the bladder: __ + __ –.
  - Appendix (McBurney's): Apply vertical pressure halfway between right anterior superior iliac spine (ASIS) and umbilicus.
  - Liver: In supine, with left hand under trunk parallel to 11th and 12th rib, lift upward; right hand lateral to rectus and press in and up: +/= reproduction of symptoms with deep breath.
  - Ascites: With the fingers, percuss outward from center, if sound is dull, ascites may be present.
  - Spleen: It is not recommended for PT to palpate an enlarged spleen (only palpable if enlarged) because of the potential of rupture.
  - Gallbladder (Murphy's): Place fingers to the right of rectus abdominus below rib cage: +/= sudden pain and muscle tensing with deep breath.

INTERVENTION

- PT intervention is consistent with movement-related problems that occur secondary to the UG problem and include
  - Gait training
  - Therapeutic exercise: All relevant categories, energy conservation
    - If there is a stoma from a colostomy or ileostomy, PT must be aware that activities are avoided if they cause retraction.
  - Therapeutic activities for bed-mobility training, transfer- and transitional-movement training, pelvic floor retraining
  - Self-care management training
    - If a male has an external catheter, ensure it is secure to prevent accidental loss.
    - With indwelling catheters, ensure they are not pulled out and that drainage clamps are locked.
    - Determine if a leg bag or tube and hanging bag is in use.
    - Bag should be below waist/bladder level at all times and should not touch the floor.
    - If full, bag should be emptied to prevent backflow.
  - Neuromuscular re-education
  - Electrical stimulation
  - Biofeedback
  - Interprofessional
    - Lifestyle modification
    - Smoking cessation
    - Weight management
    - Dietary counseling
    - Psychological intervention

FUNCTIONAL GOALS

- Patient will be able to
  - Achieve adequate functional aerobic capacity and ability to talk during activity, in order to achieve functional gait and activity tolerance for work, play, school, self-care; ADLs, and IADLs.
  - Achieve functional independent gait in the home and community (with or without a device), allowing for work, play, self-care; ADLs and IADLs, up to ___ feet based on patient's need and prior functional level.
  - Achieve 600 m or greater in a 6-minute walk test for initiation of safe functional gait in the community.
  - Perform active verbalization with increasing taxonomy for safety during gait, including negotiation of even and uneven surfaces, opening and closing doors, and transferring in and out of a car.
  - Perform activities requiring abdominals with appropriate muscle splinting/guarding to prevent retraction of stoma, if patient has a colostomy or ileostomy.
  - Tolerate 30 minutes of continuous moderate exercise three times a week in ___ weeks, and five times a week in ___ weeks, depending on the severity of the disease.

PROGNOSIS

- As this pathology is primarily medical in nature, the physician establishes the medical prognosis.
- If treated promptly and effectively with antibiotics, UTIs should resolve.
- If left untreated, acute, and/or chronic, kidney infections can result in permanent kidney damage.
- Once a female has a history of approximately three UTIs, it is likely that they will recur over time.
- For the PT prognosis, establish goals that the patient can achieve based on their overall condition.
- Unless the medical condition is unstable or the goals unrealistic, the prognosis from a PT perspective should be good.
  - This includes UG problems managed by PTs specifically
  - "Good" refers only to the realistic functional goals established.

PATIENT RESOURCES

- Urology Care Foundation, The Official Foundation of the American Urological Association. http://www.urologyhealth.org. Accessed July 14, 2013.
- Urinary Tract Infections in Children. National Kidney and Urologic Diseases Information Clearinghouse (NKUDIC). http://kidney.niddk.nih.gov/kudiseases/pubs/utichildren. Accessed July 14, 2013.
- Urinary Tract Infections in Children—Symptoms. WebMD. http://children.webmd.com/tc/urinary-tract-infections-in-children-symptoms. Accessed July 14, 2013.
- Urinary Tract Infection (UTI). Mayo Clinic. http://www.mayoclinic.com/health/urinary-tract-infection/DS00286. Accessed July 14, 2013.

REFERENCES

1. APTA. *Guide to Physical Therapy Practice*. Alexandria, VA: American Physical Therapy Association; 2003. http://guidetoptpractice.apta.org. Accessed July 14, 2013.
2. Toy EC. Urinary tract infection, Case 115. *LANGE Case Files*. www.accessmedicine.com. Accessed May 6, 2014.
3. Lum GM. Kidney & urinary tract. In: Hay WW, Levin MJ, Sondheimer JM, Deterding RR, eds. *CURRENT Diagnosis & Treatment: Pediatrics*. 20th ed. New York, NY: McGraw-Hill; 2011:Chapter 22. http://www.accessphysiotherapy.com/content/6584756. Accessed July 14, 2013.
4. Dutton M. Genitourinary. In: Dutton M, ed. *McGraw-Hill's NPTE (National Physical Therapy Examination)*. 2nd ed. New York, NY: McGraw-Hill; 2012. http://www.accessphysiotherapy.com/content/56509801. Accessed July 14, 2013.
5. Dutton M. Renal origin. In: Dutton M, ed. *Dutton's Orthopaedic Examination, Evaluation, and Intervention*. 3rd ed. New York, NY: McGraw-Hill; 2012. http://www.accessphysiotherapy.com/content/56525908. Accessed July 14, 2013.

ADDITIONAL REFERENCES

- DeMuri GP, Wald ER. Imaging and antimicrobial prophylaxis following the diagnosis of urinary tract infection in children. *Pediatr Infect Dis J*. 2008;27(6):553–554. doi: 10.1097/INF.0b013e31817a739c.
- He W, Chen M, Zu X, Li Y, Ning K, Qi L. Chronic prostatitis presenting with dysfunctional voiding and effects of pelvic floor biofeedback treatment. *BJU Int*. 2010;195(7):975–977. doi: 10.1111/j.1464-410X.2009.08850.x.
- Williams G, Craig JC. Prevention of recurrent urinary tract infection in children. *Curr Opin Infect Dis*. 2009;22(1):72–76. doi: 10.1097/QCO.0b013e328320a885.

SECTION M ONCOLOGICAL DISORDERS

62 BREAST CANCER

Eric Shamus, PhD, DPT, PT, CSCS
Adrian Taylor, DPT
Elizabeth E. Demarse, DPT, MTC
Stephanie N. Wright, MOT, OTR/L

ICD-9-CM CODES

- 198.81 Secondary malignant neoplasm of breast
- 233 Carcinoma in situ of breast and genitourinary system
- 233.0 Carcinoma in situ of breast

ICD-10-CM CODES

- C79.81 Secondary malignant neoplasm of breast
- D05.90 Unspecified type of carcinoma in situ of unspecified breast

PREFERRED PRACTICE PATTERNS

- 4E: Impaired Joint Mobility, Motor Function, Muscle Performance, and Range of Motion Associated with Localized Inflammation[1]
- 6B: Impaired Aerobic Capacity/Endurance Associated with Deconditioning[2]
- 6H: Impaired Circulation and Anthropometric Dimensions Associated with Lymphatic System Disorders[3]

PATIENT PRESENTATION

A 60-year-old woman is noted to have a 2-cm mass in the left breast. The patient's physician recommends that a core needle biopsy be performed. Tissue analysis by the pathologist under the microscope reveals intraductal carcinoma. The patient is advised by the surgeon to have surgery to remove the primary breast mass in addition to some lymph nodes. The patient undergoes wide excision of the breast mass and lymph node removal.[4] Patient comes to physical therapy for scar and lymphedema management.

KEY FEATURES

Description

- Cancer originating in the tissue of the Breast
  - Ductal or lobular
  - Invasive or noninvasive (in situ)

Essentials of Diagnosis

- Mammography
- MRI
- Ultrasound

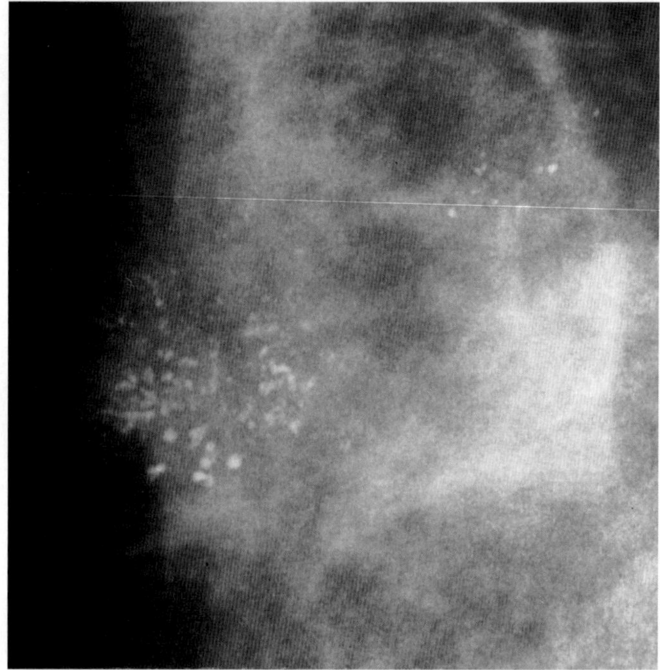

FIGURE 62-1 Magnification view of microcalcifications seen on a screening mammogram of a patient. Note the pleomorphism of the microcalcifications. The size varies from very fine to coarse, and shapes are bizarre. This appearance is typical of comedocarcinoma. (From Chen MYM, Pope TL, Ott DJ. *Basic Radiology*. 2nd ed. www.accessmedicine.com. Copyright © The McGraw-Hill Companies, Inc. All rights reserved.)

- Biomarkers
- Axillary sentinel lymph node biopsy
- PET/CT to determine spread
- Biopsy of tumor
  - Needle or core/open

General Considerations

- Not always associated with pain
- Lumps in breast or axilla
- Change in breast/nipple shape or color
- Nipple discharge

Demographics

- Accounts for one-third of all cancers diagnosed in American women
- Women 100 times more likely to be diagnosed than men
- Increased risk with age

Definitive diagnosis

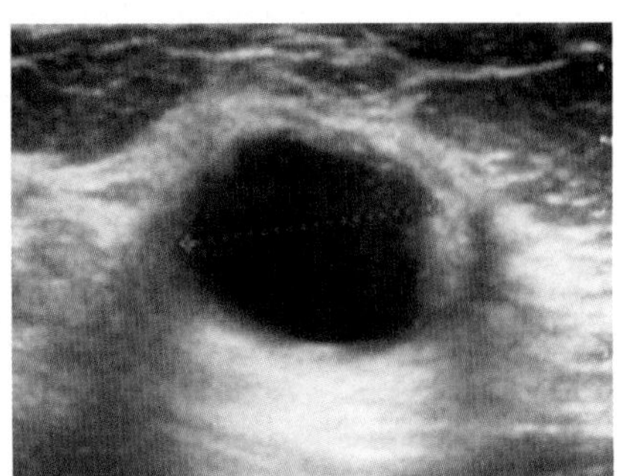
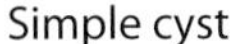
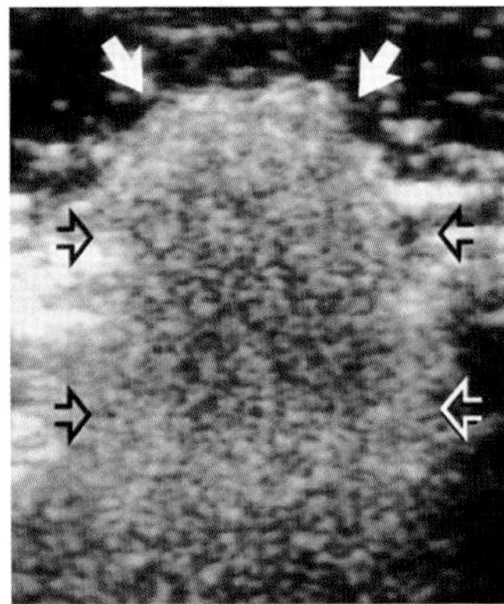
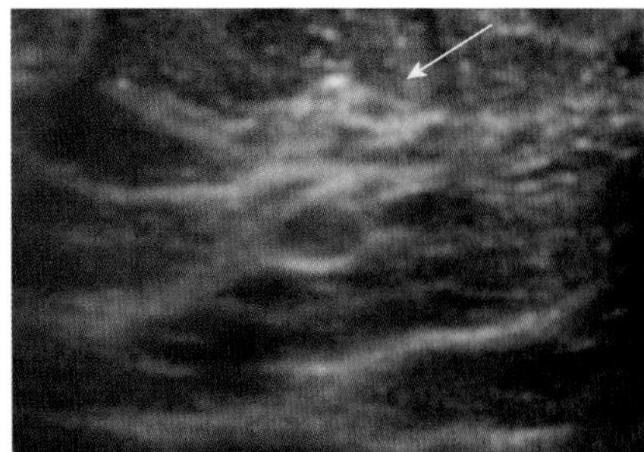

Simple cyst   Silicone   Fibroglandular ridge

Requires needle biopsy

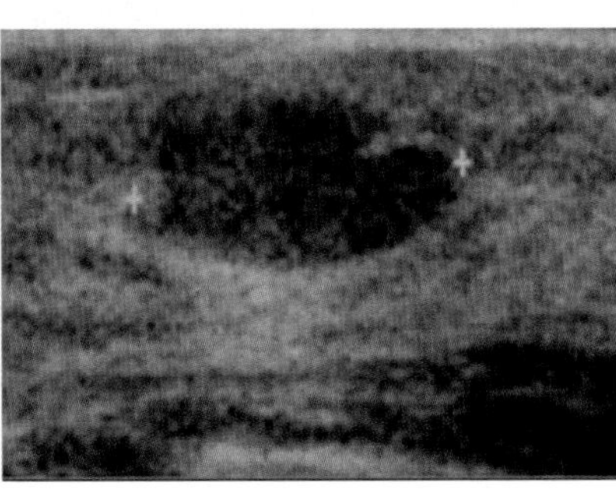
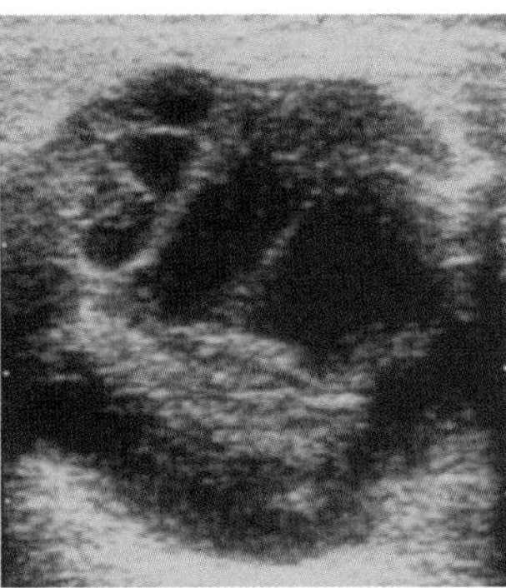
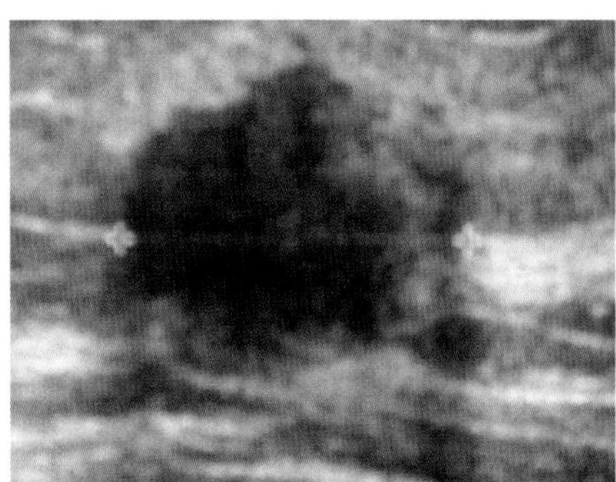

Solid - benign   Complex cyst   Suspicious

FIGURE 62-2 Sonographic appearance of palpable breast masses. (From Hoffman BL, Schorge.j, Schaffer j, Halvorson l, Bradshaw k, Cunningham F. *Williams Gynecology*. 2nd ed. www.accessmedicine.com. Copyright © The McGraw-Hill Companies, Inc. All rights reserved.)

CLINICAL FINDINGS

SIGNS AND SYMPTOMS

- Lumps, hard knots, or thickening in any part of the breast
- Swelling, warmth, redness, darkening
- Change in size or shape of breast
- Dimpling or puckering of the skin
- Itchy, scaly sore or rash on the nipple
- New pain in one spot that does not go away
- Pulling in of nipple or other area of breast
- Chest, breast, axillary, or shoulder pain of unknown etiology
- Nipple discharge

Functional Implications

- Decreased ROM
- Impaired posture
- Pain with mobility
- Endurance deficits
- Self-care or ADL deficits

Possible Contributing Causes

- Female sex
- Hormone replacement therapy
- Weight gain and obesity
- Older age
- Personal or family history; heredity
- Race/ethnicity
- Excessive alcohol consumption
- BRCA-1 gene
- Childbirth
- Radiation
- Age of menarche

Differential Diagnosis

- Fibroadenomas
- Lipomas
- Mammary dysplasia (fibrocystic breast disease)

MEANS OF CONFIRMATION OR DIAGNOSIS

Laboratory Test

- Blood test

Imaging

- Digital mammography
- MRI
- PET
- Ultrasound

Diagnostic Procedures

- Biopsy
  - Needle
  - Lymph node
  - Open

- Staging
  - Stages 0 through IV

FINDINGS AND INTERPRETATION

- Hormone receptor test
  - Estrogen receptor
  - Progesterone receptor
- HER2/neu test
  - FISH test
  - SPoT-Light HER2 CISH test
  - Inform HER2 Dual ISH test

TREATMENT

Medication

- Tamoxifen
- Chemotherapy
  - Side effects include
    - Nausea
    - Vomiting
    - Diarrhea
    - Alopecia
    - Mouth sores
    - Conjunctivitis
    - Ulcers
    - Leukopenia
    - Anemia
    - Thrombocytopenia
    - Headaches
    - Dizziness
    - Menstrual irregularities
    - Infertility
    - Peripheral neuropathies
- Hormonal therapy

MEDICAL PROCEDURES

- Radiation
  - Side effects
    - Pain
    - Lesions
    - Fatigue
    - Secondary neoplasm
    - Integumentary compromise (burns)
    - Radiation fibrosis
- Mastectomy
  - Bilateral or single
  - Radical
  - Skin sparing
  - Modified radical
- Axillary lymph node dissection
- Sentinel lymph node dissection
- Reconstruction
  - Tissue expander (TE) placement
  - Latissimus dorsi (Lat) flap
  - Transverse rectus abdominus muscle (TRAM) flap
  - Deep inferior epigastric perforator (DIEP) flap

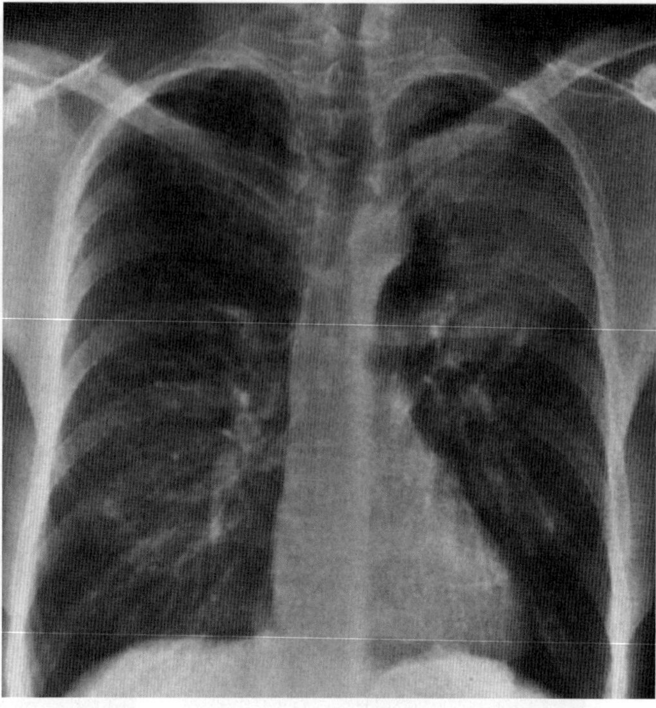

FIGURE 62-3 PA view of the chest. A large mass in the left upper lobe represents primary lung carcinoma. (From Chen MYM, Pope TL, Ott DJ. *Basic Radiology*. 2nd ed. www.accessmedicine.com. Copyright © The McGraw-Hill Companies, Inc. All rights reserved.)

REFERRALS/ADMITTANCE

- To oncologist, radiologist, or neurologist for medical treatment
- To plastic surgeon for reconstruction/cosmetic procedure
- To physician for treatment of lymphedema
- To respiratory therapist if respiratory symptoms involved

IMPAIRMENTS

- Pulmonary and circulatory complications
- Lymphedema
- Restricted mobility/ROM of upper extremity
- Postural/structural misalignment
- Weakness
- Impaired functional use of the upper extremity
- Fatigue, impaired endurance
- Soft tissue integrity (scar, fibrosis)
- Pain

TEST AND MEASURES

- Disabilities of the arm, shoulder, and hand (DASH) score to assess physical function
- Karnofsky Performance Status Scale (KPS)
- Aerobic endurance
- Functional strength, manual muscle testing (MMT)
- Upper-extremity ROM
- Posture
- Structural (shoulder complex, cervical, thoracic)

- Sensory integrity
- Community and work integration
- Integumentary integrity
- Pain
- Lymphedema (see lymphedema diagnosis)

INTERVENTION

- Postsurgical breathing exercises
- Pain management
- Strengthening exercises
- Posture and body-mechanics education
- Aerobic conditioning
- ROM exercises
- Scar/fibrotic tissue management
- ADL training
- Lymphedema management (see lymphedema diagnosis)
- Precautions with reconstruction
  - TRAM or DIEP: Trunk flexion 45 degrees
  - TE placed: No repetitive movement

FUNCTIONAL GOALS

- Patient will be able to
  - Perform self-care tasks independently (particularly washing body or hair, grooming, toileting).
  - Carry one load of groceries weighing <5 lb without significant dyspnea or increased lymphedema as measured by patient report of 3 or lower on Borg Dyspnea Scale.
  - Reach for objects above shoulder- or head level using appropriate shoulder mechanics without verbal cue.

PATIENT RESOURCES

- Breast Cancer. American Cancer Society. http://www.cancer.org/cancer/breastcancer/detailedguide/breast-cancer-breast-cancer-types. Accessed April 2, 2013.
- National Cancer Institute at the National Institutes of Health. Lymphedema. http://www.cancer.gov/cancertopics/pdq/supportivecare/lymphedema/healthprofessional/page1. Accessed April 2, 2013.
- National Lymphedema Network. Lymphedema risk reduction practices. Position Statement of the National Lymphedema Network. www.lymphnet.org. Accessed April 2, 2013.
- National Lymphedema Network. What is lymphedema? http://www.lymphnet.org/lymphedemaFAQs/overview.htm. Accessed April 2, 2013.
- Multiple Myeloma. MDGuidelines. http://www.mdguidelines.com/multiple-myeloma/differential-diagnosis. Accessed April 2, 2013.

REFERENCES

1. The American Physical Therapy Association. Pattern 4E: impaired joint mobility, motor function, muscle performance, and range of motion associated with localized inflammation. *Interactive Guide to Physical Therapist Practice*. 2003. doi: 10.2522/ptguide.3.1_5. http://guidetoptpractice.apta.org/content/1/SEC12.extract?sid=a85bc719-efdb-4ada-bfa2-fad1333a3620. Accessed May 6, 2014.
2. The American Physical Therapy Association. Pattern 6B: impaired aerobic capacity/endurance associated with deconditioning. *Interactive Guide to Physical Therapist Practice*. 2003. doi: 10.2522/ptguide.3.3_2. http://guidetoptpractice.apta.org/content/1/SEC28.extract?sid=4da3cb00-dbc7-4a83-bf51-ab4f93c35cfc. Accessed May 6, 2014.
3. The American Physical Therapy Association. Pattern 6H: impaired circulation and anthropometric dimensions associated with lymphatic system disorders. *Interactive Guide to Physical Therapist Practice*. 2003. doi: 10.2522/ptguide.3.3_8. http://guidetoptpractice.apta.org/content/1/SEC34.extract?sid=06452a17-58d4-4c18-a6f6-676a7f40405c. Accessed May 6, 2014.
4. Troy EC. Breast Cancer. Lange Case Files Series. http://www.accessmedicine.com/caseHome.aspx?lange=0#AC4. Accessed April 2, 2013.

ADDITIONAL REFERENCES

- Dutton M. *Pathology. McGraw-Hill's NPTE (National Physical Therapy Examination)*.2nd ed. New York, NY: McGraw-Hill; 2012. http://www.accessphysiotherapy.com/content/5402112. Accessed April 2, 2013.
- ICD9DATA. http://www.icd9data.com. Accessed March 16, 2013.
- ICD10DATA. http://www.icd10data.com. Accessed March 16, 2013.
- McPhee SJ, Hammer GD. *Epithelial Neoplasia. Pathophysiology of Disease*. 6th ed. New York, NY: McGraw-Hill; 2010. http://www.accessphysiotherapy.com/content/5367250. Accessed January 31, 2013.
- Panus PC, Jobst EE, Masters SB, Katzung B, Tinsley SL, Trevor AJ. *Cancer Chemotherapy. Pharmacology for the Physical Therapist*. New York, NY: McGraw-Hill; 2009:Chapter 31. http://www.accessphysiotherapy.com/content/6095262. Accessed April 2, 2013.
- Rossy KM, Scheinfeld NS, et al. *Dermatologic Manifestations of Lymphedema Differential Diagnoses*. Emedicine Medscape. http://emedicine.medscape.com/article/1087313-differential. Online August 2, 2011. Accessed April 2, 2013.

63 COLORECTAL CANCER

Debra F. Stern, DPT, DBA, MSM, PT
Eric Shamus, PhD, DPT, PT, CSCS
Elizabeth E. Demarse, DPT, MTC

ICD-9-CM CODES

- 153.9 Malignant neoplasm of colon, unspecified site
- Associated physical therapy diagnoses
  - 315.4 Coordination disorder (clumsiness, dyspraxia and/or specific motor development disorder)
  - 718.45 Contracture of joint, pelvic region and thigh
  - 719.70 Difficulty in walking
  - 728.2 Muscular wasting and disuse atrophy
  - 728.89 Disorders of muscle, ligament and fascia
  - 729.9 Other disorders of soft tissue
  - 780.7 Malaise and fatigue
  - 781.2 Abnormality of gait: Ataxic, paralytic, spastic, staggering
  - 782.3 Edema
  - 786.0 Dyspnea and respiratory abnormalities
  - 786.05 Shortness of breath

ICD-10-CM CODE

- C18.9 Malignant neoplasm of colon, unspecified

PREFERRED PRACTICE PATTERN

As of July, 2014, the APTA Guide to Physical Therapist Practice does not include practice patterns for organ system pathology.

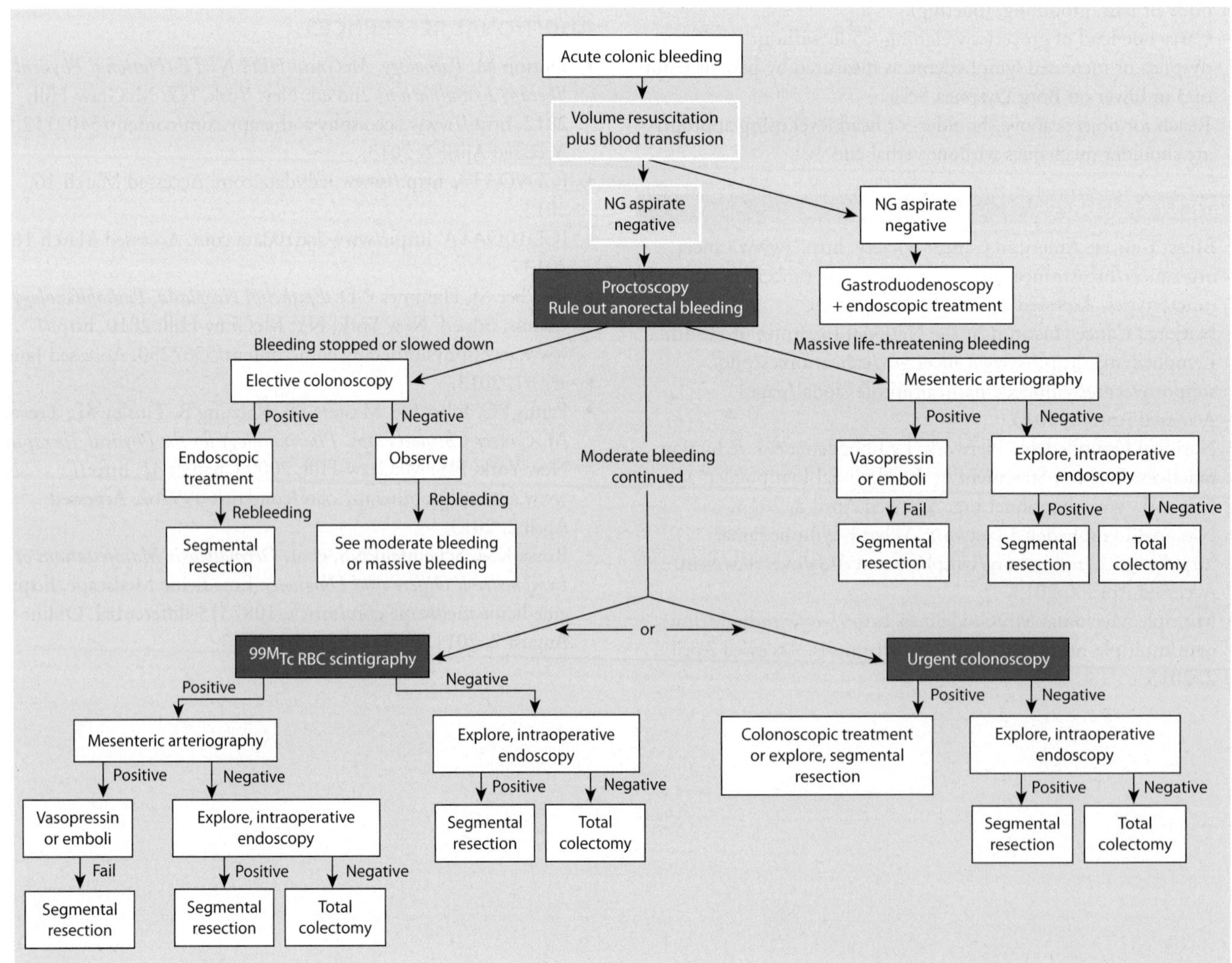

FIGURE 63-1 Algorithm for treatment of colorectal hemorrhage. NG = nasogastric; ^{99m}Tc = technetium-99; RBC = red blood cell. (Reproduced with permission from Gordon PH, Nivatvongs S, eds. *Principles and Practice of Surgery for the Colon, Rectum, and Anus*. 2nd ed. New York, NY: Marcel Dekker, Inc.; 1999: p. 1279.)

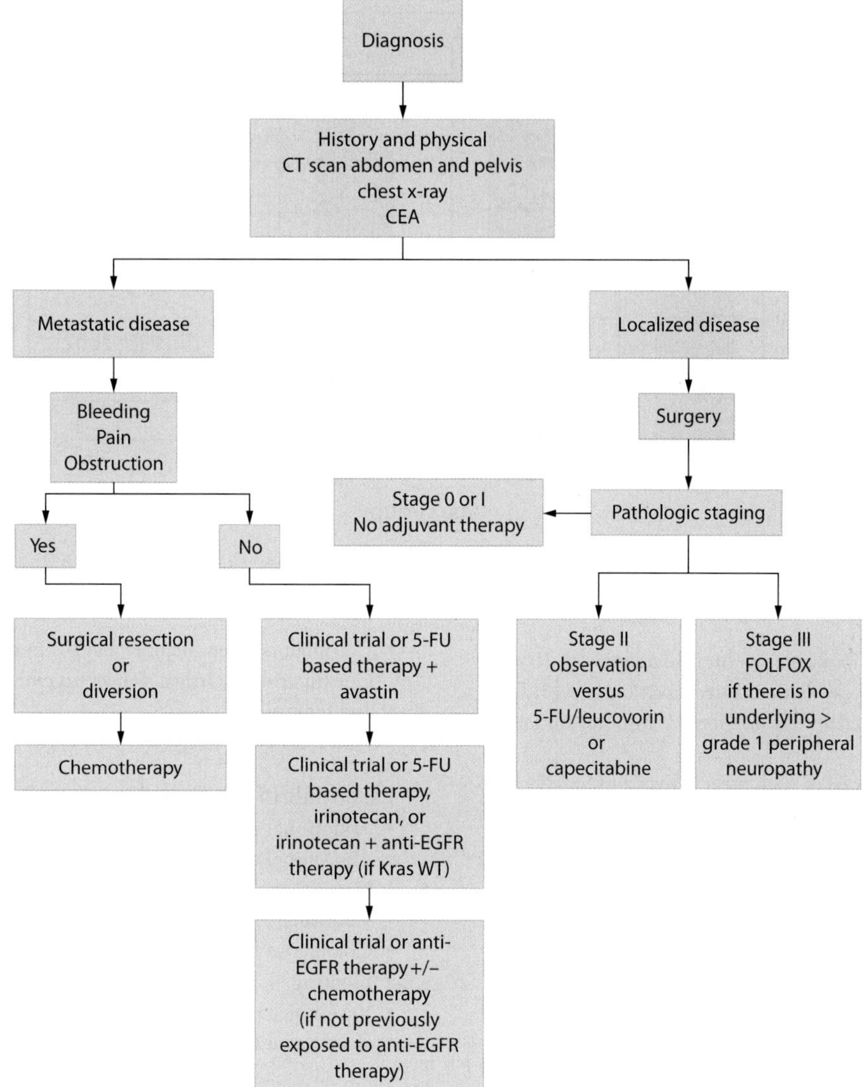

FIGURE 63-2 Diagnostic and therapeutic algorithm for colon cancer. (From Kantarjian HM, Wolff RA, Koller CA. *The MD Anderson Manual of Medical Oncology*. 2nd ed. www.accessmedicine.com. Copyright © The McGraw-Hill Companies, Inc. All rights reserved.)

Therefore, the associated or secondary musculoskeletal, cardiovascular/pulmonary, or potential neuromuscular patterns would be indicated.

PATIENT PRESENTATION

A 34-year-old female presents to PT with complaints of general weakness, 2 weeks after being discharged from a 40-day admission to the hospital. She was previously employed as a CAN nurse, but has not worked in the past year since her diagnosis. She went into respiratory failure after her surgery (colon tumor resection, hemidiaphragm hernia repair, and hysterectomy with bilateral salpingo-oophorectomy). She was intubated and still has her feeding tube in, although, she is not using it currently. She expects to get it removed in the next few weeks. She lives in a two-level home with her family. She has difficulty getting up the stairs and has to use both arms to pull herself up them. She is independent with ADLs; however, uses supervision assist during showering for safety. She also uses hand held assist when getting into the shower as it is a step-over tub/shower. She is experiencing daily vomiting, usually in the mornings and constipation from the pain medicines. She has a lot of pain and numbness in her whole body with sleeping at night; however, she feels that the right side of her body is worse than the left. It also feels weaker than the left side. In addition, she has low back pain that started during her hospital admission.

Structural assessment includes: flat lumbar spine with patient maintaining a forward bent torso during standing, walking, and sitting. She is able to lay flat only for a short period of time (<5 min) because of pain and nausea. She has a well-healed esophageal and abdominal incision, and a clean and covered G-tube. No other structural abnormalities noted. She appears with good muscular tone throughout (except low back) despite complaints of weakness.

Her strength is WNL except for hip extension which is 4/5 on the left and 3+/5 on the right, and ankle PF 4/5 bilateral. She has decreased lumbar paraspinal recruitment observed with prone ipsilateral hip extension. She is not able to maintain terminal knee extension with a unilateral heel raise and clears the heels aproximately ½ inch. Patient is also unable to maintain an appropriate erect sitting posture for more than 30 seconds.

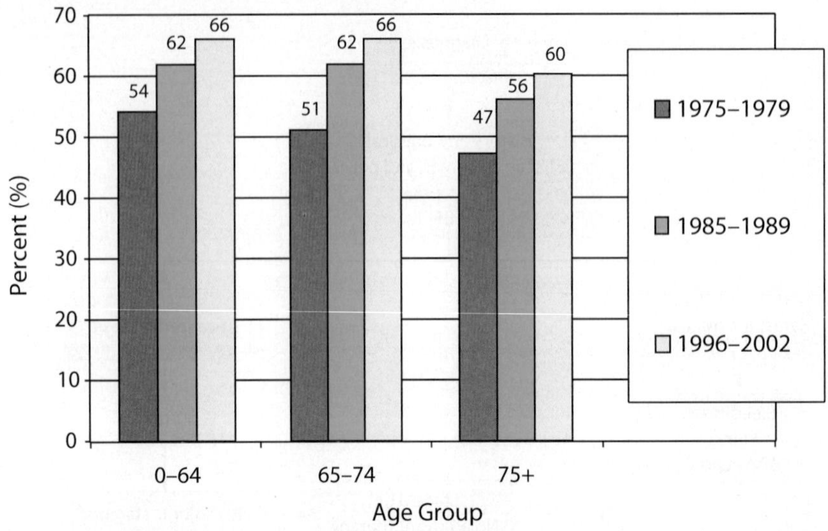

FIGURE 63-3 All-stage 5-year survival by age group for colon and rectal cancer. (From Halter JB, Ouslander JG, Tinetti M, Studenski S, High K, Asthana S. *Hazzard's Geriatric Medicine and Gerontology*. 6th ed. www.accessmedicine.com. Copyright © The McGraw-Hill Companies, Inc. All rights reserved.)

She has decreased cardiovascular endurance tested with 10 minutes on recumbent elliptical. Patient rated exertion as #15, hard, on Borg Scale of Perceived Exertion, after 10 minutes on level 1 using UE and LE.

PMH: Stage IV colorectal ca with mets to liver and lung, chemo

PSH: Liver metastasectomy, right hepatectomy, Bartholin gland excision, sigmoid resection

KEY FEATURES

Description

- Malignancy of the colon
- May metastasize and result in death if untreated, curable if caught in early stages
- Complaints often include changes in bowel habits: Constipation, diarrhea, bowel urgency, incontinence, and cramping
- Pain frequently referred to low back

Essentials of Diagnosis

- Abdominal pain (constant or intermittent)
- Abdominal tenderness
- Nausea
- Vomiting
- Changes in bowel habits: Diarrhea, constipation
- Bloating
- Rectal bleeding possible
- Rectal/anal irritation

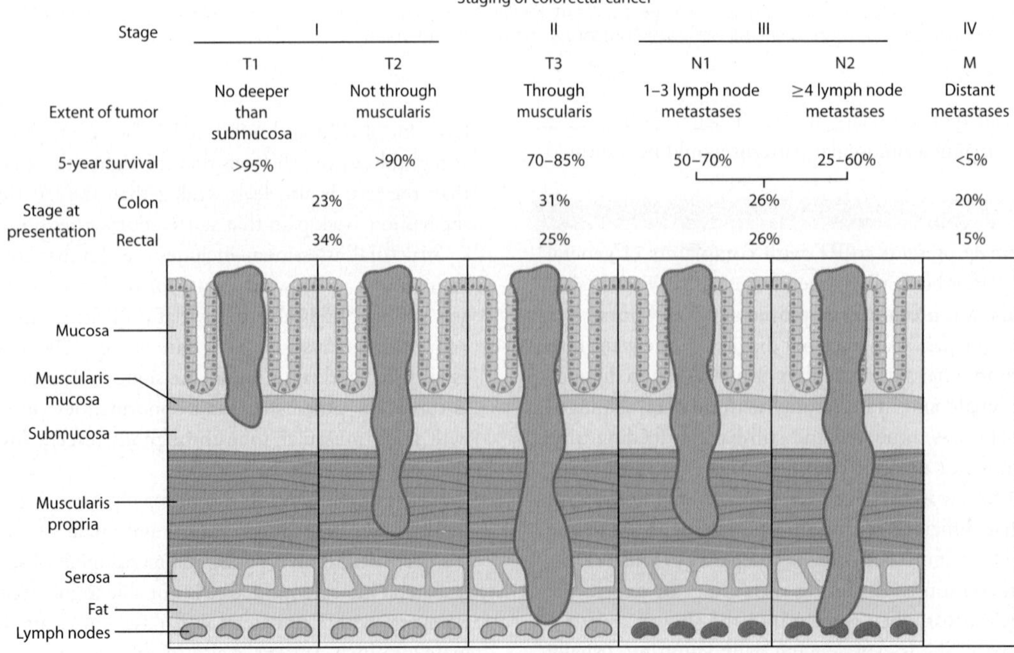

FIGURE 63-4 Staging and prognosis for patients with colorectal cancer. (From Longo DL, Fauci AS, Kasper DL, Hauser SL, Jameson JL, Loscalzo J, eds. *Harrison's Principles of Internal Medicine*. 18th ed. New York, NY:McGraw-Hill; 2012.)

- Acute drop in blood pressure may cause decreased blood flow to intestines
- Inability to swallow
- Lack of appetite
- Unexplained weight loss
- Abdominal pain upon ingesting food
- Joint pain possible
- Dark stool or bright red blood in stool
- Malaise, fatigue

General Considerations

- While PT may not manage GI disorders specifically, clients may receive care for secondary problems: Weakness, gait abnormalities, limited aerobic endurance, musculoskeletal problems, neuromuscular problems, weight loss, or weight gain
- Symptoms may include chronic or episodic diarrhea, incontinence or urgency of bowel movements, blood in stool
  - May be symptomatic of inflammatory disease, precancerous condition, cancer
- Diagnosis for occult problems may take time and require intensive diagnostic testing
- GI disorders frequently refer pain to other body areas; individuals may be inappropriately referred to PT
- May be related to stress, constipation
- More serious problems include autoimmune conditions like Crohn's
- Acute pain indicative of appendicitis
- GI complaints in females may indicate cancer/tumors in reproductive organs, or gynecological problems: Endometriosis, uterine fibroids, ectopic pregnancies
- May indicate inguinal or umbilical hernia
- History of heartburn/indigestion may indicate GI or cardiac problems

Demographics

- GI disorders occur throughout the lifespan (birth through geriatric)
- More common in people aged 50 years or older
- Increased risk with older age
- More common if history of polyps or personal history of cancer
- Overall incidence of colon and rectal cancer 45.5 per 100,000[1]
- Caucasians 44.3 per 100,000
- African Americans 53.1 per 100,00
- Asians 34.9 per 100,000
- American Indians 31.1 per 100,000

CLINICAL FINDINGS

SIGNS AND SYMPTOMS

- Symptoms may be characteristic of multiple GI disorders, confounding medical diagnosis.
- PT should recognize the possibility of GI pathology in differential diagnosis, especially when findings are not consistent with conditions commonly treated.
- Pain
  - Abdominal/stomach pain, cramping (constant or intermittent, severe)
  - Pain upon ingesting food or liquid
    - May be cardiac in nature
  - Lower abdominal pain
- Bowel changes
  - Diarrhea (acute, chronic)

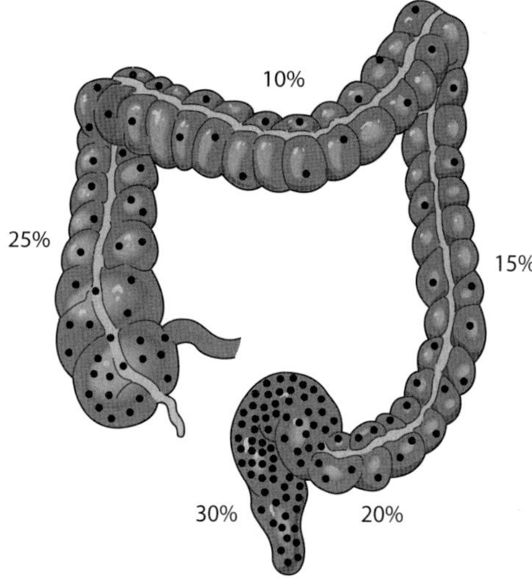

FIGURE 63-5 Distribution of cancer of the colon and rectum. (From Doherty GM. *Current Diagnosis & Treatment: Surgery*. 13th ed. www.accessmedicine.com. Copyright © The McGraw-Hill Companies, Inc. All rights reserved.)

  - Constipation (acute, chronic)
  - Blood in stool, dark or fresh bleeding
  - Rectal bleeding
  - Change in stool odor or color
  - Feeling of having to move bowels constantly
  - Mucous in the stool or just mucous discharge
  - Rectal bleeding
  - Narrowing of stool
- Abdominal distention
- Abdominal muscle spasm, guarding
- Unexplained weight loss
- Loss of appetite, cachexia
- Fatigue
- Anemia
- Flatulence
- Nausea
- Emesis
- Complaints of "feeling full" regardless of having ingested food
- Symptoms may be vague

Functional Implications

- Severe symptoms associated with immediacy of defecation may be disabling, causing inability to leave home.
- Chronic constipation may cause severe pain and result in fecal material backing up through the esophagus, require manual extraction, surgery, and/or bowel retraining.
- Dehydration secondary to diarrhea, emesis, appetite loss, nausea, inability to swallow
- Eating disorder/anorexia secondary to fear of pain upon ingesting food
- Anemia
- Sarcopenia resulting in weakness, decreased muscle mass, inability to ambulate or perform self-care, limited aerobic capacity secondary to inactivity
- Need for temporary or permanent colostomies/ileostomies (usually with intestinal problems vs. upper GI)
  - May present problem with stoma retraction associated with abdominal contraction
- Decreased exercise tolerance
- Limited physical activity
- Reluctance to leave home
- Fatigue

- Psychological challenges: Anxiety, depression
- Limitations in ADLs, or IADLs.

Possible Contributing Causes
- High-fat, low-fiber diet
- Diabetes
- Inflammatory bowel disease (IBD), Crohn disease, ulcerative colitis
- Stress, anxiety
- Inflammatory cause, autoimmune disease
- Chemical
- Environmental irritants
- Obesity
- Lack of exercise
- Heredity
- Cancer: Esophageal, colon, liver, bile duct, pancreatic, metastatic, anal/rectal
- Smoking

Differential Diagnosis
- Abdominal infections
- Appendicitis
- Autoimmune diseases affecting upper and lower GI tracts
- Bladder or urinary tract infection, kidney pathology
- Bowel disorder
  - Constipation or diarrhea
  - Inflammation of abdominal lining, organ obstruction
  - Torsion
- Celiac disease, gluten intolerance
- Colitis (ulcerative, non-ulcerative)
- Crohn disease
- Endocrine disorder
- Gastroenteritis
- Gynecologic problems in females
  - Endometriosis
  - Menses
  - Ectopic pregnancies
  - Ovarian cysts
  - Fibroids
- IBD
- Irritable bowel syndrome (IBS)
- Non-malignant tumor in abdomen or organs
- Organ dysfunction from cancer or malignancy
  - Colon cancer
  - Ovarian cancer
- Pelvic inflammatory disease
- Perforated ulcer in GI system
- Post–weight-loss (bariatric) surgery complications
  - Side effects may mimic diverticulitis or cause a flare-up
- Referred pain from heart, spine, hip
- Rheumatoid arthritis

MEANS OF CONFIRMATION OR DIAGNOSIS

Laboratory Tests
- Fecal occult blood test/stool sample
- Blood test
- Hemoglobin and Hematocrit (H & H)

Imaging
- Abdominal scans
- Radiography
- Barium enemas
- CT

Diagnostic procedures
- Biopsy
- Colonoscopy
- Digital rectal examination
- Endorectal ultrasound
- Manual palpation for tenderness
- Medical history
- Sigmoidoscopy

FINDINGS AND INTERPRETATION
- H & H for signs of bleeding, anemia, pathogens, immune status, vitamin deficiencies, white blood cell count

TREATMENT

Medication
- Chemotherapy[2]
- Biologics; monoclonal antibody[2]

MEDICAL PROCEDURES
- Radiation
  - Internal
  - External
  - Intraoperative
- Bowel diversion surgery
  - Bowel resection
  - Bowel resection with colostomy or ileostomy
  - Ileoanal reservoir surgery
  - Continent ileostomy
- Removal of tumors/growths
- Nasogastric tube
- Feeding tube
- Total/peripheral parenteral nutrition (TPN/PPN)
- IV for hydration

REFERRALS/ADMITTANCE
- If causative problem is not considered appropriate for PT intervention, refer to appropriate physician
- Refer to ER if emergency identified
- Dietary counseling
- Psychological intervention
- Pastoral counseling
- Surgical management
- Occupational therapist

IMPAIRMENTS
- Muscle weakness
- Muscle atrophy
- Gait abnormality/difficulty walking
- Contractures of soft tissue (fascia, muscle); joint limitations
- Shortness of breath
- Potential rectal muscle impairment
- Inability to perform self-care
- Limited aerobic endurance
- Functional decline
- Postsurgical abdominal pain
- Radiation burns and resulting open areas, scars, adhesions

TESTS AND MEASURES

- Palpation
  - Appendix (McBurney's): Apply vertical pressure halfway between right ASIS and umbilicus: −/+ may indicate appendicitis.
  - Liver: In supine, with left hand under trunk parallel to 11th and 12th ribs, lift upward; right hand lateral to rectus, press in and up: +/= reproduction of symptoms with deep breath, indicates liver involvement.
  - Ascites: Percuss outward from center with fingers; if sound is dull, ascites may be present.
  - Spleen: Not recommended for PT to palpate enlarged spleen (only palpable if enlarged).
  - Gallbladder (Murphy's): Place fingers to the right of rectus abdominus below rib cage: +/= sudden pain and muscle tensing with deep breath.
  - Kidneys: In supine, place one hand under client between ribs and iliac crest, other hand on abdomen below ribs and ribs pointing in opposite direction: +/− tenderness or reproduction of symptoms.
  - Bladder: Not usually palpable unless distended and raised above pubic bone; in supine, place hand above pubis and press down: +/= tenderness, reproduction of pain, ability to feel the bladder: __+ ___−.
- Observation
  - Scars may indicate adhesions or abdominal surgeries causative of diverticula.
  - Pink or purplish striae may be indicative of Cushing syndrome.
  - Dilated veins may indicate hepatic pathology or inferior vena cava obstruction, not diverticulitis.
  - Contour: Roundness, concavity, asymmetry, distension, pregnancy signs.
  - Cullen sign: Bluish discoloring around the umbilicus may be a sign of retroperitoneal bleeding.
  - Bluish discoloration in lower abdomen: Grey Turner sign, signals hemorrhagic pancreatitis.
  - Bulging in groin and abdomen especially apparent with contraction of musculature in area may be hernia.
  - Pulsing in navel area may be abdominal aortic aneurysm.
  - Left lower quadrant pain, often following a meal.
  - Palpable abdominal tenderness: On left side or generalized.
  - Psoas sign: Provides resistance over patient's right knee as they flex the hip; pain indicates appendicitis, possible inflammation of abdomen.
  - Obturator sign: Internal rotation and flexion of right lower extremity may indicate appendicitis, pelvic inflammation.
  - Roving sign: Pain on the right side of abdomen when pressure applied to the left may indicate appendicitis.

INTERVENTION

- PT intervention is consistent with movement-related problems secondary to GI disorder; include
  - Gait training
  - Therapeutic exercise: All relevant categories, energy conservation
    - If stoma from colostomy or ileostomy, avoid activities that cause retraction.
  - Therapeutic activities for bed-mobility training, transfer- and transitional-movement training
  - Wheelchair management
  - Neuromuscular re-education
  - Self-care training
  - Electrical stimulation to rectus/anus in cases of incontinence or muscle control/coordination with reversal of bowel diversion surgery
  - Manual therapy
  - Massage
  - Interprofessional
    - Lifestyle modification
    - Smoking cessation
    - Weight management
    - Pharmacologic management

FUNCTIONAL GOALS

- Patient will be able to
  - Achieve functional aerobic capacity, ability to talk during activity so as to achieve functional gait and activity tolerance for ADLs/IADLs.
  - Achieve 600 m or greater in a 6-minute walk test for initiation of safe, functional gait in the community.
  - Perform active verbalization with increasing taxonomy for safety during gait, including negotiation of even and uneven surfaces, opening and closing doors, transferring in and out of car.
  - Perform activities requiring abdominals with appropriate muscle splinting/guarding to prevent retraction of stoma, if patient has colostomy or ileostomy.
  - Tolerate 30 minutes of continuous, moderate exercise three times a week in ______ weeks, and five times a week in ____________ weeks, depending on the severity of the disease.

PROGNOSIS

- Physician establishes the medical prognosis, as pathology is primarily medical in nature.
- Colorectal cancer is curable if caught early; depending on the stage of disease, could result in death.
- For PT prognosis, goals should be established that the patient can achieve based on their overall condition.
- Prognosis from a PT perspective should be good, unless medical condition is unstable or goals unrealistic.

PATIENT RESOURCES

- Colonrectal Cancer. American Cancer Society. http://www.cancer.org/cancer/colonandrectumcancer/index. Accessed February 6, 2013.
- Genetics and Colorectal Cancer. American Society of Colon and Rectal Surgeons. http://www.fascrs.org/patients/treatments_and_screenings/genetics_and_colorectal_cancer. Accessed February 9, 2013.
- Ulcerative Colitis. National Digestive Diseases Information Clearinghouse (NDDIC). US Department of Health and Human Services. *NIH Publication No. 12-1597.* October 2011. http://digestive.niddk.nih.gov/ddiseases/pubs/colitis/. Accessed February 9, 2013.

REFERENCES

1. Centers for Disease Control and Prevention. United States Cancer Statistics Top 10 Cancers. National Program for Cancer Registries. http://apps.nccd.cdc.gov/uscs/toptencancers.aspx#Footnotes. Accessed February 9, 2013.

2. Panus PC, Jobst EE, Masters SB, Katzung B, Tinsley SL, Trevor AJ. *Pharmacology for the Physical Therapist.* New York, NY: McGraw-Hill; 2009. http://www.accessphysiotherapy.com/resource/615. Accessed February 9, 2013.

ADDITIONAL REFERENCES

- Goodman CC, Fuller KS. *Pathology: Implications for the Physical Therapist.* 3rd ed. Philadelphia, PA: Saunders Elsevier; 2009.
- Goodman CC, Snyder TK. *Differential Diagnosis for Physical Therapists: Screening for Referral.* 4th ed. St. Louis, MO: Saunders Elsevier; 2007.
- ICD9DATA. http://www.icd9data.com. Accessed February 9, 2013.
- ICD10DATA. http://www.icd10data.com. Accessed February 9, 2013.
- McOmber M, Shulman RJ. Pediatric functional gastrointestinal disorders. *Nutr Clin Prac.* 2008;23:268–274.
- McPhee SJ, Hammer GD. Pathophysiology of disorders of the esophagus. In: McPhee SJ, Hammer GD, eds. *Pathophysiology of Disease.* 6th ed. New York, NY: McGraw-Hill; 2010. http://www.accessphysiotherapy.com/content/5369615. Accessed February 9, 2013.
- Suleiman S, Johnston DE. The abdominal wall: an overlooked source of pain. *Am Fam Physician.* 2001;64(3);431–439.
- Wang KK, Sampliner RE. Updated guidelines 2008 for the diagnosis, surveillance and therapy of Barrett's esophagus. *Am J Gastroenterol.* 2008;103(3):788–797.

64 OVARIAN CANCER

Stephanie N. Wright, MOT, OTR/L
Elizabeth E. Demarse, DPT, MTC
Eric Shamus, PhD, DPT, PT, CSCS
Adrian Taylor, DPT

CONDITION/DISORDER SYNONYMS

- Extraovarian primary peritoneal carcinoma (EOPPC)
- Germ cell tumor (in egg cells)

ICD-9-CM CODES

- 183 Malignant neoplasm of ovary and other uterine adnexa[1]
- 183.0 Malignant neoplasm of ovary[1]
- 198.6 Secondary malignant neoplasm of ovary[2]

ICD-10-CM CODES

- C56.9 Malignant neoplasm of unspecified ovary
- C79.60 Secondary malignant neoplasm of unspecified ovary

PREFERRED PRACTICE PATTERNS

- 4C: Impaired Muscle Performance
- 6B: Impaired Aerobic Capacity/Endurance Associated With Deconditioning

PATIENT PRESENTATION

A 55-year-old female presents with left LE pain 12 weeks s/p pelvic tumor debulking with end-block appendectomy, omentectomy, proctectomy, lower anterior resection of bowels with primary coloproctostomy and hyperthermic intraperitoneal chemotherapy, and G and J tube placement. Prior to her surgery she worked full-time as an interior decorator. She jogged and walked her dog on a regular basis for exercise. Since her surgery she has progressed from walking with a walker to a cane, and now does not need an assistive device for walking. She states that she walks slower than her normal pace and has a slight limp. Yesterday she was able to navigate a flight of stairs for the first time since her surgery (patient lives in a 2-level home). She has recently stopped wearing the knee brace because it was not allowing her to bend her knee. She received a few weeks of outpatient PT initially after her surgery. They did strengthening and balance exercises, endurance activities, electrical stimulation (for pain) and massage. She feels these helped somewhat; however, she has been newly diagnosed with left femoral nerve neurapraxia secondary to nerve compression during surgery. She is now recommended for neuromuscular re-education and would like to get back to her active lifestyle.

Past medical history (PMH) and past surgical history (PSH): Total abdominal hysterectomy-bilateral salpingo-oophorectomy (TAH-BSO), loop colostomy, rhinoplasty. The patient has visible atrophy of left (L) proximal LE musculature. Left hip MMT 3+/5 (extension 4/5), knee flexion and extension 5/5, and all ankle 5/5. Passive ROM of left LE all within normal limits (WNL). Active ROM hip flexion 95 degrees, extension (sidelying) 10 degrees, ABD 30 degrees, IR 45 degrees, ER 30 degrees. Patient notes minor pain with hip ABD and knee flexion. She is unable to perform supine active straight leg raise unassisted. Maintains single leg stance (SLS) for 30 seconds on right and left LE.

Thomas Test: Pain provoking, lacking approximately 20 degrees hip extension on left

Bilateral IT band tightness with tenderness to palpation only on left.

She reports current left LE pain to be 3/10, with increase to 6/10 with walking. She is currently taking pain medications on a regular basis and uses Lidoderm patches at night.

Sensation: Numbness in left anteromedial leg and WNL in foot. Distal reflexes WNL.

Gait deviations: Antalgic gait, decreased step length on left, lacking left terminal knee extension (TKE) on heel strike and left full hip extension on toe off, decreased speed, and Trendelenburg sign.

KEY FEATURES

Description

- Either EOPPC or germ cell tumor (in egg cells)
- Second-most common female urogenital cancer
- EOPCC is the most lethal of ovarian cancers
- Epithelial tumors make up for 90% of the cases

Essentials of Diagnosis

- Diagnosis is difficult and most women present with metastasis at time of diagnosis.
- Most primary malignant ovarian neoplasms are either carcinomas (serous, mucinous, or endometrioid adenocarcinomas) or malignant germ cell tumors.[1]
- Metastatic malignant neoplasms to the ovary include carcinomas, lymphomas, and melanomas.[1]
- This may be from a primary ovarian cancer involving the opposite ovary, or from a cancer at a distant site.[2]

General Considerations

- Most symptoms are common with noncancer diagnoses, and therefore are overlooked (e.g., abdominal/pelvic pain)

Demographics

- Occurs in women
- Incidence peaks in women during their fifth and sixth decade of life
- White and Hawaiian women have the highest incidence of ovarian cancer in the United States

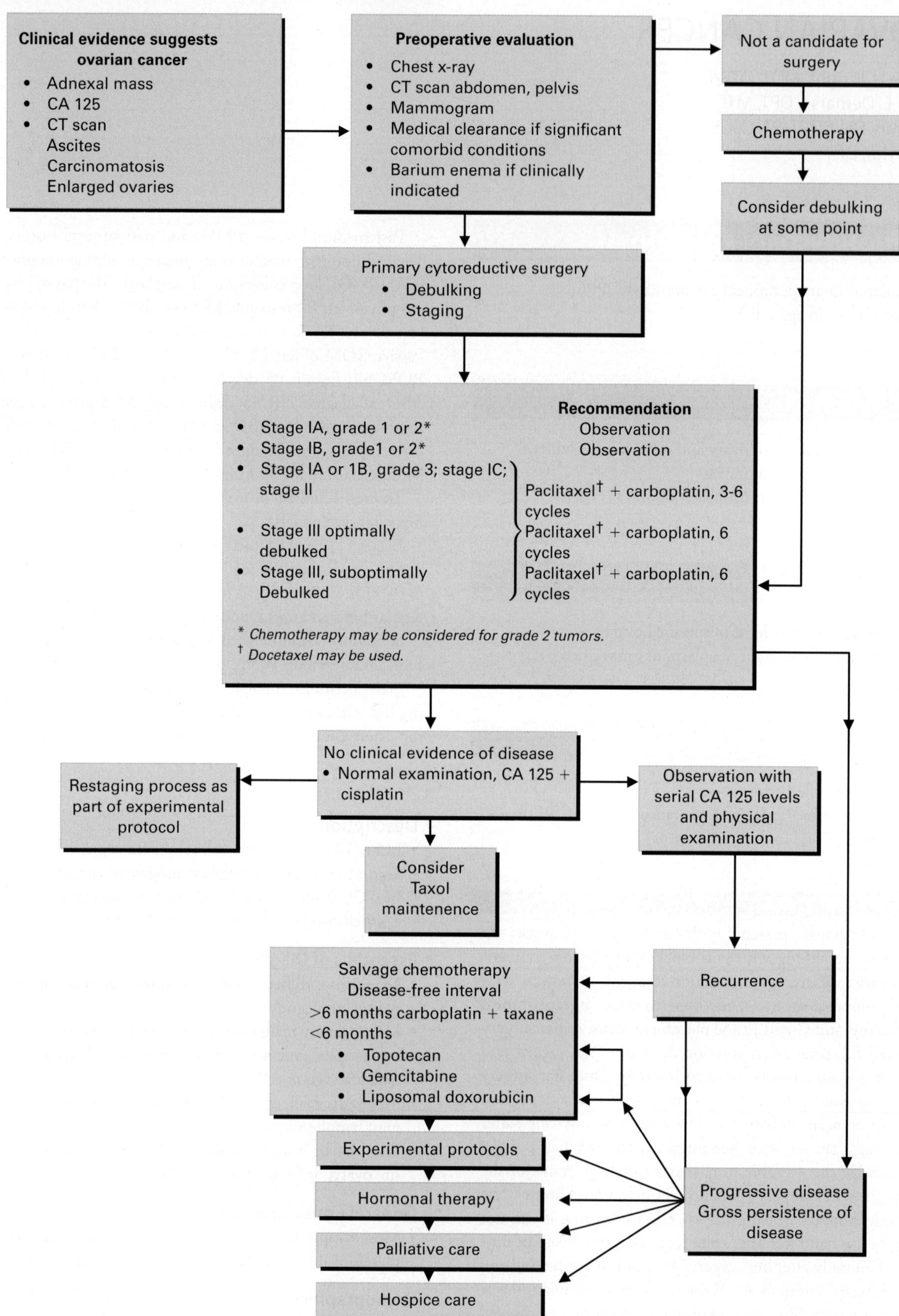

FIGURE 64-1 Summary of treatment of ovarian cancer. (From Kantarjian HM, Wolff RA, Koller CA. *The MD Anderson Manual of Medical Oncology*. 2nd ed. www.accessmedicine.com. Copyright © The McGraw-Hill Companies, Inc. All rights reserved.)

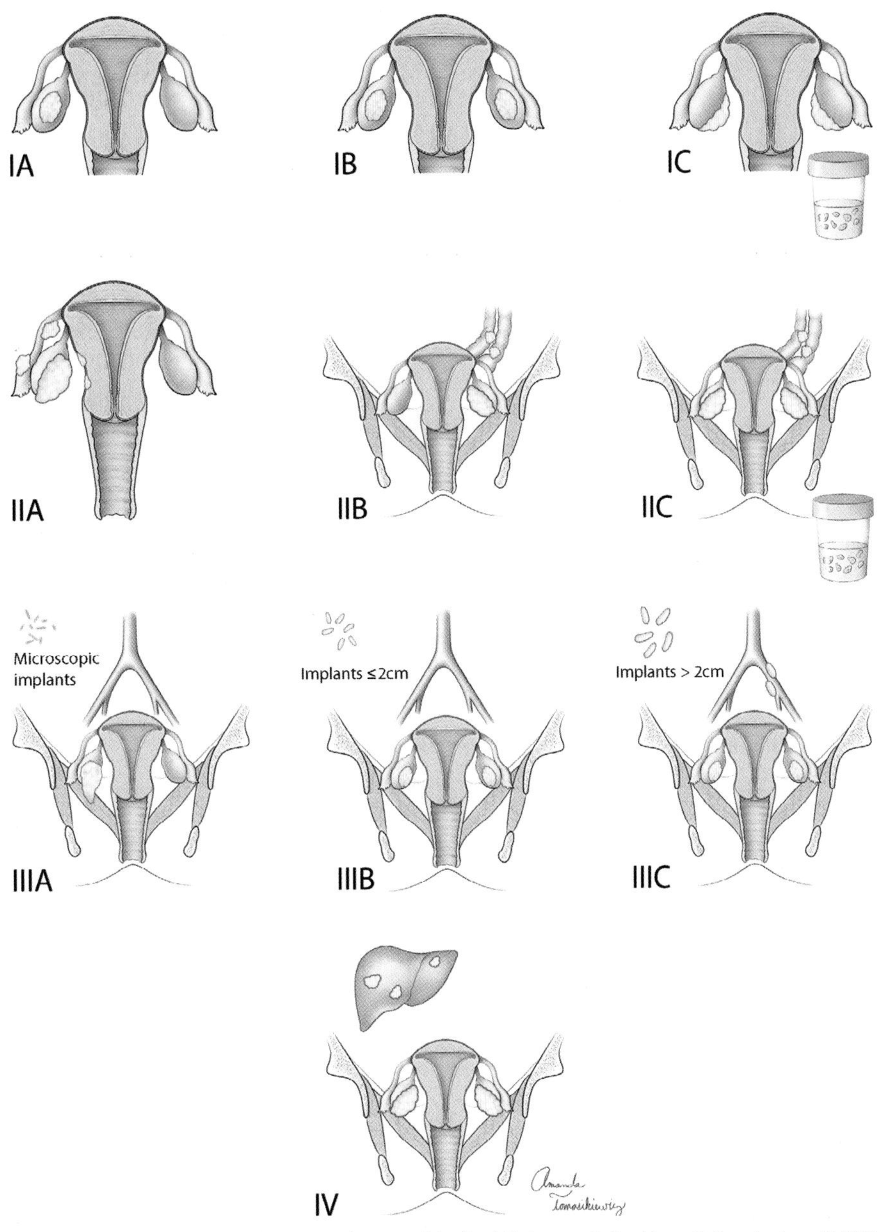

FIGURE 64-2 FIGO staging for ovarian cancer. (From Hoffman BL, Schorge J, Schaffer J, Halvorson L, Bradshaw K, Cunningham F. *Williams Gynecology*. 2nd ed. www.accessmedicine.com. Copyright © The McGraw-Hill Companies, Inc. All rights reserved.)

CLINICAL FINDINGS

SIGNS AND SYMPTOMS

- Typically asymptomatic or vague symptoms
  - Abdominal bloating
  - Flatulence
  - Fatigue and malaise
  - Gastritis
  - General abdominal discomfort
  - Antalgic gait
  - Postural abnormality
  - Abdominal/back pain
- Less common symptoms
  - Abnormal vaginal bleeding
  - Leg pain
  - Pelvic mass
  - Low back pain
  - Local pelvic pain (occurs late in the disease)
- Symptoms associated with metastasis
  - Unexplained weight loss
  - Weakness
  - Pleurisy
  - Ascites
  - Cachexia
- Paraneoplastic cerebellar degeneration (PCD): Primarily affects women with gynecologic cancers
  - Ataxic gait
  - Truncal and appendicular ataxia
  - Nystagmus
  - Speech impairment (dysarthria)
- Radiation side effects
  - Fatigue
  - Secondary neoplasm
  - Integumentary compromise (burns)
  - Radiation fibrosis
- Chemotherapy side effects
  - Alopecia
  - Anemia
  - Conjunctivitis
  - Diarrhea
  - Dizziness
  - Headaches
  - Infertility
  - Leukopenia
  - Menstrual irregularities
  - Mouth sores
  - Nausea
  - Peripheral neuropathies
  - Thrombocytopenia
  - Ulcers
  - Vomiting

Functional Implications

- Antalgic gait
- Decreased endurance
- Pain with mobility (guarded pelvic/hip movements)
- Postural abnormality
- Postural muscle imbalance
- Self-care/ADL deficits

Possible Contributing Causes

- Etiology unknown
- Risk factors include
  - Hormonal factors
  - Environmental factors
  - Genetic factors
    - Family history of ovarian or breast cancer
    - First-degree relative with ovarian cancer or who has the BRCA1 mutation has a 45% lifetime chance of developing ovarian cancer
  - Nulliparous women

Differential Diagnoses

- Adnexal tumors
- Anovulation
- Appendicitis (acute); appendiceal tumors
- Ascites
- Bladder distention/urinary retention
- Borderline ovarian cancer
- Bowel adhesions
- Cervicitis
- Colon cancer
- Colon cancer (adenocarcinoma)
- Colonic obstruction
- Ectopic pregnancy
- Embryologic remnants
- Endometriosis
- Fecal impaction
- Gastric cancer (Gastric adenocarcinoma)
- Hydrosalpinx/pyosalpinx
- Irritable bowel syndrome (IBS)
- Low-lying cecum
- Malignant gastric tumors
- Metastatic gastrointestinal carcinoma
- Ovarian cysts; torsion
- Pancreatic cancer
- Pelvic inflammatory disease (PID); pelvic abscess
- Peritoneal cancer; cysts
- Rectal cancer
- Retroperitoneal mass
- Urinary tract obstruction
- Uterine cancer; fibroids; anomalies

MEANS OF CONFIRMATION OR DIAGNOSIS

Laboratory Tests

- Alpha-fetoprotein (AFP)
- CA-125 test
- Human chorionic gonadotropin (HCG)
- Kidney and liver function
- Lactate dehydrogenase (LDH)
- White blood count

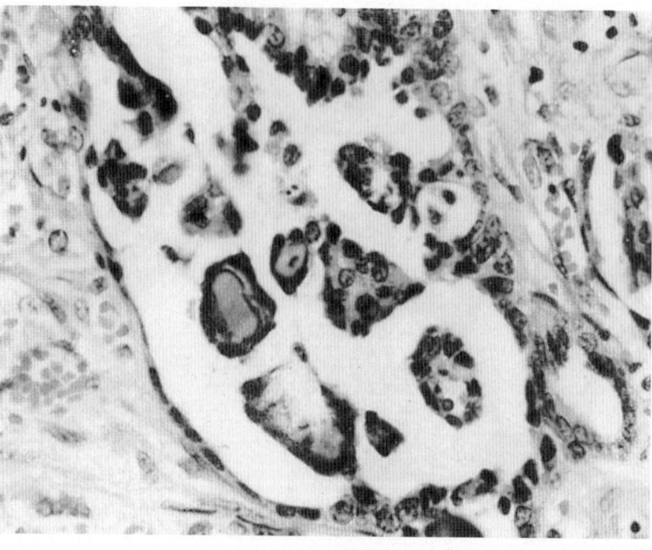

FIGURE 64-3 Papillary lesion with incorporated talc granules. (From DeCherney AH, Nathan L. *Current Diagnosis & Treatment Obstetrics & Gynecology*. 10th ed. www.accessmedicine.com. Copyright © The McGraw-Hill Companies, Inc. All rights reserved.)

Imaging

- Barium enema X-ray
- Bone scan
- Chest X-ray: Metastasis
- CT scans
- MRI
- Positron emission tomography (PET) scan
- Ultrasound

Diagnostic Procedures

- Biopsy
- Exploratory laparotomy
- Laparoscopy

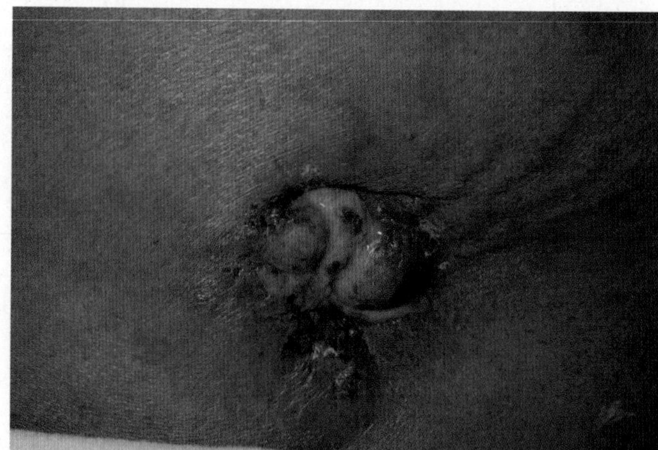

FIGURE 64-4 Sister Mary Joseph Node. This 63-year-old woman presents with abdominal swelling and ascites. She was diagnosed with ovarian cancer. Axial CT scan of the abdomen at the level of the umbilicus demonstrates ascitic fluid and the umbilical nodularity (*arrows*). (From Knoop KJ, Stack LB, Storrow AB, Thurman RJ. *The Atlas of Emergency Medicine*. 3rd ed. www.accessmedicine.com. Copyright © The McGraw-Hill Companies, Inc. All rights reserved. Photo contributor: R. Jason Thurman, MD.)

FINDINGS AND INTERPRETATION

- Chest X-ray: Metastasis

TREATMENT

Medication

- Chemotherapy
  - Intraperitoneal (IP)
  - Intravenous (IV)
- Radiation
  - External beam
  - Brachytherapy

MEDICAL PROCEDURES

- Cytoreductive surgery
  - Total abdominal hysterectomy (TAH)
  - Bilateral salpingo-oophorectomy (BSO)
  - Omentectomy
  - Lymphadenectomy

REFERRALS/ADMITTANCE

- To oncologist
- To gynecologist

IMPAIRMENTS

- Balance
- Endurance
- Impaired circulation and anthropometric dimensions related to lymphatic system disorders
- Impaired gait
- Impaired muscle performance (pelvic floor/core)
- Impaired posture
- Impaired ROM (hip, lumbar, sacral)
- Internal organ/connective tissue fibrosis (external beam radiation)
- Self-care/ADL

TESTS AND MEASURES

- Aerobic capacity
- Balance
- Circumferential and volumetric measurements of involved extremities
- Functional strength
- Gait
- Karnofsky Performance Status Scale (KPS)
- Mobility/Transfers
- Pain
- Posture
- ROM; Thomas test
- Self-care/ADL
- Skin integrity

INTERVENTION

- ADL training
- Aerobic conditioning
- Balance training
- Gait training
- Manual lymphatic drainage, if warranted
- ROM exercises
- Strengthening exercises

FUNCTIONAL GOALS

For postsurgical intervention without surgery, PT usually involved mostly with pelvic dysfunction and bladder control

- The patient will
  - Control urination flow, that is, start/stop.
  - Carry in one load of groceries (<15 lb) without significant pelvic or back pain.
  - Pick object up from ground without loss of balance.

PROGNOSIS

- Dependent on stage at detection
- 75% survival at 1 year post-diagnosis
- 50% survival at 5 years post-diagnosis

PATIENT RESOURCE

- *Ovarian cancer*. American Cancer Society website. http://www.cancer.org/Cancer/OvarianCancer/DetailedGuide/ovarian-cancer-diagnosis. Accessed June 12, 2013.

REFERENCES

1. Malignant neoplasm of ovary and other uterine adnexa 183-. ICD-9Data.com. http://www.icd9data.com. Accessed June 12, 2013.
2. Secondary malignant neoplasm of other specified sites 198-. ICD-9Data.com. http://www.icd9data.com. Accessed June 12, 2013.

ADDITIONAL REFERENCES

- Chandrasoma P, Taylor CR. The ovaries. In: Chandrasoma P, Taylor CR, eds. *Concise Pathology*. 3rd ed. New York, NY: McGraw-Hill; 2011. http://www.accessphysiotherapy.com/content/191173. Accessed June 12, 2013.
- Hay WW, Levin MJ, Sondheimer JM, Deterding RR. Gonads (ovaries & testes). In: Hay WW, Levin MJ, Sondheimer JM, Deterding RR, eds. *CURRENT Diagnosis & Treatment: Pediatrics*. 20th ed. New York, NY: McGraw-Hill; 2011. http://www.accessphysiotherapy.com/content/6588186. Accessed June 12, 2013.
- Lee AH, Su D, Pasalich M, Wong YL, Binns CW. Habitual physical activity reduces risk of ovarian cancer: A case-control study in southern China. *Prev Med*. 2012. doi:pii: S0091-7435(12)00586-5. 10.1016/j.ypmed.2012.11.009.
- Liang W, Lee AH, Binns CW, Zhou Q, Huang R, Hu D. Habitual physical activity reduces the risk of ischemic stroke: a case-control study in southern china. *Cerebrovasc Dis*. 2009;28(5):454–459. doi: 10.1159/000235990.
- Purcell KJ, Taylor RN. Disorders of the female reproductive tract. In: McPhee SJ, Hammer GD, eds. *Pathophysiology of Disease: An Introduction to Clinical Medicine*. 6th ed. New York, NY: McGraw-Hill; 2010. http://www.accessphysiotherapy.com/content/5372181. Accessed June 12, 2013.

65 PROSTATE CANCER

Elizabeth E. Demarse, DPT, MTC
Eric Shamus, PhD, DPT, PT, CSCS
Stephanie N. Wright, MOT, OTR/L
Adrian Taylor, DPT

ICD-9-CM CODES[1]

- 185 Malignant neoplasm of prostate
- 233.4 Carcinoma in situ of prostate

ICD-10-CM CODES[2]

- C61 Malignant neoplasm of prostate
- D07.5 Carcinoma in situ of prostate

PREFERRED PRACTICE PATTERNS[3]

- 4C: Impaired Muscle Performance
- 6B: Impaired Aerobic Capacity/Endurance Associated With Deconditioning

PATIENT PRESENTATION

A 73-year-old male presents with intermittent urinary leakage that is worse with activity. He is retired but stays active in his home doing repairs and renovations. He uses a Kotex sized protective pad which he changes once a day. He gets up an average of 2×/night for urination and does not need pad protection with sleep. He complains that Viagra does not help as much with his erection as it did when he first started taking it. He avoids acidic drinks and drinks water throughout the day. He is pending C-pap for his recently diagnosed sleep apnea. He denies any signs or symptoms of infection and has no bowel issues. PMH includes prostate cancer, external beam radiation (XRT) to prostate, erectile dysfunction (uses penile pump and Viagra), urinary leakage s/p XRT, O/A, dyslipidemia, pneumonia, sleep apnea.

Flow cytometry with WNL for fluid retention. Sensation/neurological: patient is able to sense leakage (can have pudendal nerve damage secondary to XRT). MMT: is able to maintain pelvic floor contraction (verbal cue—to engage muscles as if attempting to stop urine flow or draw the testicles inward).First trial: 25 seconds, second: 38 seconds, third: 55 seconds. Quick flicks (engaging and releasing using aforementioned cueing) in 10 seconds. First trial: 3×, second: 3×, third: 5×.

KEY FEATURES

Description

- Cancer begins in prostate gland
- Wraps around the urethra
- 98% of prostatic tumors are adenocarcinomas[1]
- Aggressive and slow-growing forms

Essentials of Diagnosis

- Prostate-specific antigen (PSA) screens
- Needle biopsy

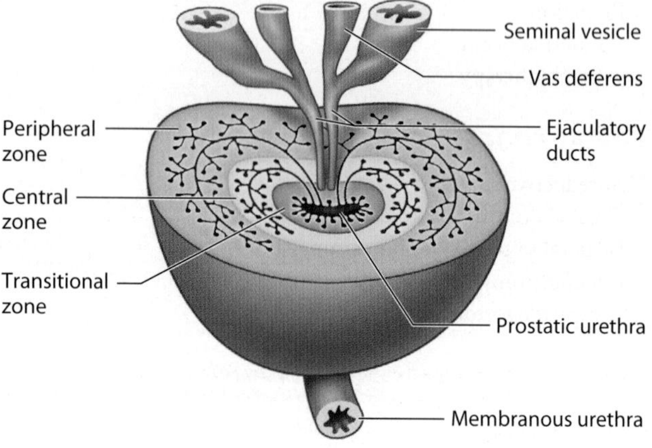

FIGURE 65-1 Organization of the prostate gland. (From Mescher AL. *Junqueira's Basic Histology: Text and Atlas*. 12th ed. www.accessmedicine.com. Copyright © The McGraw-Hill Companies, Inc. All rights reserved.)

- Gleason grade to assess risk of cancer spreading
  - The Gleason scale assigns cancer cells a score from 1 to 10, by combining the two most common patterns of cells to give a total score (i.e., 3 + 4 = grade 7). These scores are broken down into three main levels.
    - **Gleason score of 4 or less** = Low-grade (well differentiated)
    - **Gleason score between 4 and 7** = Intermediate grade (moderately differentiated)
    - **Gleason score between 8 and 10** = High-grade (poorly differentiated)
- ABCD stages of prostate cancer
  - Stage A: Cancer found when not suspected or due to a high PSA level
  - Stage B: Cancer found due to abnormal digital rectal examination and is held in the prostate
  - Stage C: Cancer that has spread to the tissues outside of the prostate
  - Stage D: Cancer that has spread to the lymph nodes or bone

General Considerations

- Prostate wraps around the urethra causing urination issues
- Enlarged prostate does not increase risk of cancer
- Vegetarians have a lower rate of prostate cancer

Demographics

- Most frequently diagnosed visceral malignancy in American men
- Increased risk for
  - African American men
  - Brother or father with prostate cancer
  - Men older than 60 years of age
- Second-most common cause of male death from cancer

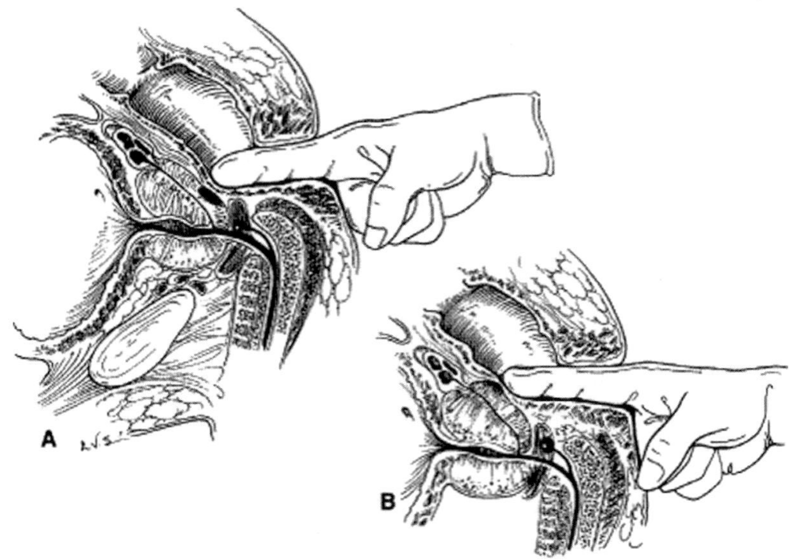

FIGURE 65-2 Differential diagnosis of prostatic nodules. **A.** Cancerous nodules are not raised; there is an abrupt change in consistency at its edges. **B.** Inflammatory area is raised above the surface of the gland; induration decreases gradually at its periphery. (From Tanagho EA, McAninch JW. *Smith's General Urology*. 17th ed. www.accessmedicine.com. Copyright © The McGraw-Hill Companies, Inc. All rights reserved.)

CLINICAL FINDINGS

SIGNS AND SYMPTOMS

- May be asymptomatic until late stages
- Need to urinate frequently, especially at night
- Difficulty urinating, slow start
- Decreased force in the stream of urine
- Leakage of urine after urination
- Blood in urine
- Blood in semen
- Painful ejaculation
- Swelling in legs
- Pain or stiffness in the lower back, hips, or upper thighs
- Sciatica
- Bone pain (if cancer has spread)
- Chemotherapy side effects
  - Alopecia
  - Anemia
  - Conjunctivitis
  - Diarrhea
  - Dizziness
  - Headaches
  - Infertility
  - Leukopenia
  - Mouth sores
  - Nausea
  - Peripheral neuropathies
  - Thrombocytopenia
  - Ulcers
  - Vomiting
- Radiation side effects
  - Fatigue
  - Secondary neoplasm
  - Integumentary compromise (burns)
  - Radiation fibrosis

Functional Implications

- Incontinence
- Sexual dysfunction

Possible Contributing Causes

- Alcohol abuse
- Androgens
- Exposure to Agent Orange
- Exposure to cadmium
- Familial history
- Genetics
- High animal fat diets
- Xenotropic murine leukemia virus-related virus (XMRV)

Differential Diagnoses

- Benign prostatic hyperplasia (BPH)
- Calculi
- Lumbar spine radiculopathy
- Prostatic cysts
- Prostatic tuberculosis
- Prostatitis
- Sacral dysfunction
- Urinary tract infection (UTI)

MEANS OF CONFIRMATION OR DIAGNOSIS

Laboratory test

- PSA Screen
- Reverse transcription-polymerase chain reaction (RT-PCR)

Imaging

- Transrectal and prostate ultrasounds
- X-rays
- MRI
- To determine if cancer has spread
  - Bone scan
  - Positron emission tomography (PET) scan
  - CT scan

Diagnostic Procedures

- Bladder scope
- Cystoscopy
- Digital rectal exam
- Transperineal biopsy
- Transrectal US-guided biopsy

FINDINGS AND INTERPRETATION

- Abnormal rectal examination; hard irregular surface
- Gleason Grading System
  - Grades tumors on a 1 to 5 scale based on normalcy of tissue
  - Higher the score, the more likely the spread of cancer

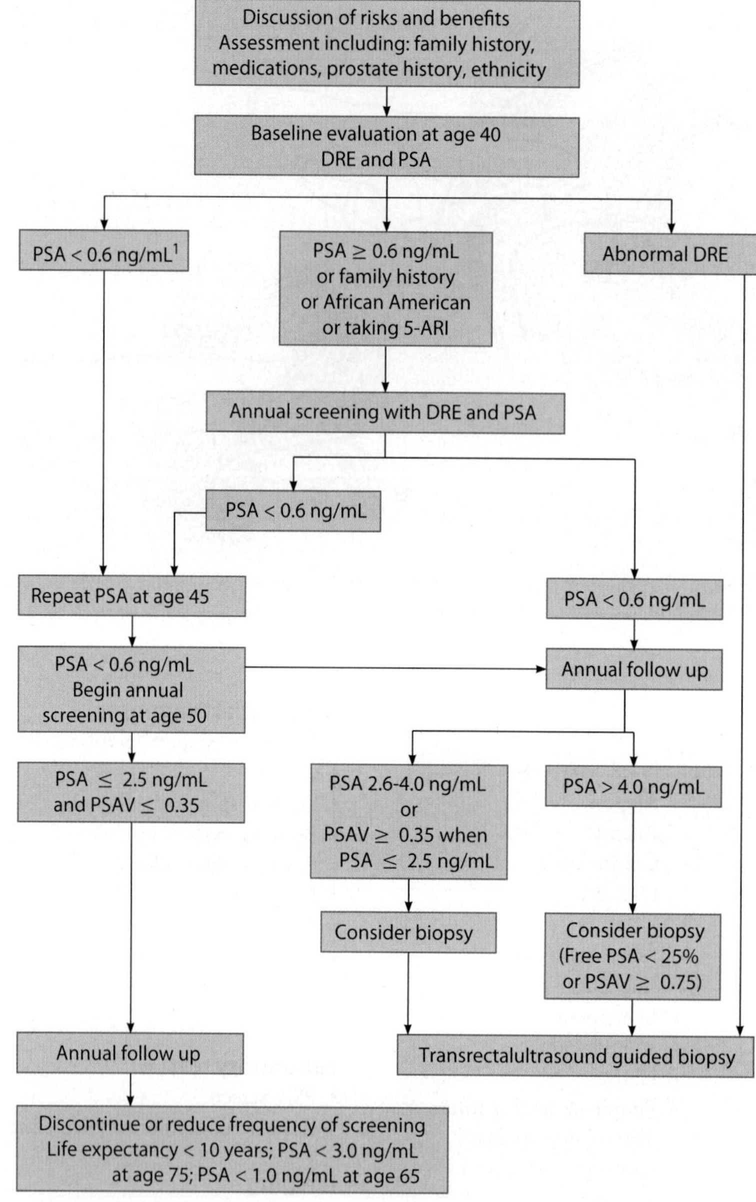

FIGURE 65-3 An algorithm for prostate cancer early detection. DRE, digital rectal examination; 5-ARI, 5α-reductase inhibitor; PSAV, PSA velocity (ng/mL/yr) calculated on at least three consecutive values over at least an 18- to 24-month period. (Based on NCCN guidelines, data from the *Baltimore Longitudinal Study on Aging*, and *Prostate Cancer Prevention Trial*.)

TREATMENT

Medication

- Radiation (external beam or prostate brachytherapy)
- Hormonal therapy
  - Androgen deprivation therapy
  - Estrogen replacement therapy
  - Reduction of testosterone
- Chemotherapy
  - Docetaxel
  - Cytotoxic agents: Satraplatin and ixabepilone
- Immunotherapy
  - For control of metastatic prostate cancer
- Post-treatment vaccine
  - Provenge

MEDICAL PROCEDURES

- Radical prostatectomy

REFERRALS/ADMITTANCE

- To oncologist for cancer assessment
- To urologist for other possible dysfunctions
- To occupational therapist (OT) for postsurgical for ADL training
- To a radiologist for imaging
- To the Prostate Cancer Foundation for support and information

IMPAIRMENTS

- Urinary incontinence
- Lumbosacral plexopathy
- Lymphedema

- Sexual dysfunction
- Decreased bone marrow density (BMD)/osteoporosis
- Fatigue
- Muscle performance
- Balance
- Posture

TESTS AND MEASURES

- Functional strength
- Karnofsky Performance Status Scale (KPS)
- Circumferential and volumetric measurements of involved extremities
- Aerobic capacity
- Pelvic floor
- Sensory integrity
- Balance
- Posture

INTERVENTION

- Pelvic floor exercises
- Lymphedema prevention/education
- Manual lymphatic drainage
- Lower abdominal core exercises
- Therapeutic exercise
- Ambulation
- ADL/functional-activity training

FUNCTIONAL GOALS

For postsurgical intervention without surgery, PT usually involved mostly with pelvic dysfunction and bladder control

- The patient will be able to
  - Control urination flow, that is, start/stop.
  - Not have any incidents of leakage.
  - Maintain an erection for ____
  - Carry in one load of groceries (<15 lb) without significant pelvic or back pain.

PROGNOSIS

- Variable based on
  - Extent of tumor
    - Gleason Grading System results
    - Speed of growth and location of tumor
    - Time from onset to medical intervention
    - Age and overall health of patient

ADDITIONAL INFORMATION

- For additional information, please see Presenting Problem 3. In: *Basic & Clinical Biostatistics*. 4th ed. Textbook on www.Access-Physiotherapy.com

PATIENT RESOURCE

- Prostate Cancer Foundation (PCF). www.pcf.org. Accessed June 2, 2013.

REFERENCES

1. ICD-9-CM. http://www.icd9data.com. Accessed June 1, 2013.
2. ICD-10-CM. http://www.icd10data.com. Accessed June 1, 2013.
3. APTA Guide to Physical Therapist Practice. http://guidetoptpractice.apta.org. Accessed June 1, 2013.

ADDITIONAL REFERENCES

- Dawson B, Trapp RG. Presenting problems. In: Dawson B, Trapp RG, eds. *Basic & Clinical Biostatistics*. 4th ed. New York, NY: McGraw-Hill; 2004. http://www.accessphysiotherapy.com/content/2048209. Accessed June 1, 2013.
- Dutton M. Causes of pelvic pain. In: Dutton M, ed. *Dutton's Orthopaedic Examination, Evaluation, and Intervention*. 3rd ed. New York, NY: McGraw-Hill; 2012. http://www.accessphysiotherapy.com/content/5547528. Accessed June 2, 2013.

66 LYMPHEDEMA, POSTMASTECTOMY

Eric Shamus, PhD, DPT, PT, CSCS
Elizabeth E. Demarse, DPT, MTC
Stephanie N. Wright, MOT, OTR/L
Adrian Taylor, DPT

ICD-9-CM CODES

- 457.0 Postmastectomy lymphedema syndrome
- 457.1 Other lymphedema

ICD-10-CM CODES

- I89.0 Lymphedema, not elsewhere classified
- I97.2 Postmastectomy lymphedema syndrome

PREFERRED PRACTICE PATTERNS

- 4E: Impaired Joint Mobility, Motor Function, Muscle Performance, and Range of Motion Associated with Localized Inflammation[1]
- 6H: Impaired Circulation and Anthropometric Dimensions Associated with Lymphatic System Disorders[2]

PATIENT PRESENTATION

Patient is a 52-year-old female diagnosed with right invasive breast cancer 2 years ago with a right modified radical mastectomy and axillary node dissection. Patient deferred reconstruction due to the need for chemotherapy and radiation to right axilla and chest wall. She reports healing well from surgery and completed radiation and chemotherapy with limited side effects and only mild radiation fibrosis.

Patient reports going on a canoe trip with her family and soon after, noticing her rings and bracelets becoming tight and some edema in her knuckles and hand that subsided with elevation. In the next week, the edema became worse, did not subside and she began to notice tingling and mild numbness in her fingertips that worsened in the evening and also when she first woke up in the morning. An ultrasound was negative for DVT in right upper extremity.

Patient now presents with limitations in available AROM in elbow flexion, wrist extension and flexion and finger flexion. Full AROM measured in shoulder flexion and abduction. Grip is 10 lb less than nondominant left hand and lateral pinch strength also is 5 lb below left. Patient has limited muscle endurance in right shoulder due to weight of her arm and has begun using left arm for many tasks. There is a shiny appearance to the skin over the hand and forearm and pitting is noted. Stemmer's sign is positive as well as a 15% greater limb volume noted with arm-volume measurement than unaffected left arm.

KEY FEATURES

Description

- Occurs when lymph system is damaged or blocked and buildup of lymph fluid occurs in soft tissues, causing swelling
- Obstruction of lymphatic vessels or lymph nodes
- Increased water and protein in the interstitial space[3]
- Lymphedema can occur as a result of surgery, chemotherapy, or radiation causing interruption of the lymphatic system
- Postmastectomy, axillary, or sentinel lymph node dissection affects upper extremities
- Considered secondary lymphedema

Essentials of Diagnosis

- Detailed medical history (e.g., surgical procedures, chemotherapy, radiation)
- Presence of nonpitting edema
- MRI or CT
- Circumferential upper-extremity measurement

General Considerations

- Commonly occurs following breast cancer surgery
- Axillary or sentinel node dissections and radiation therapy increase risk of occurrence

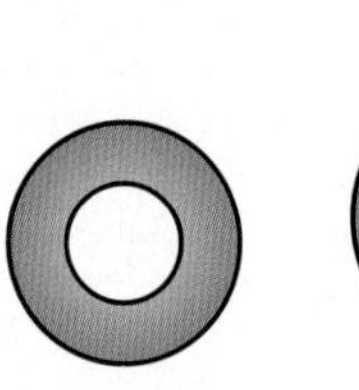

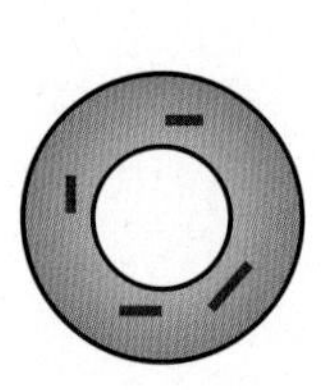

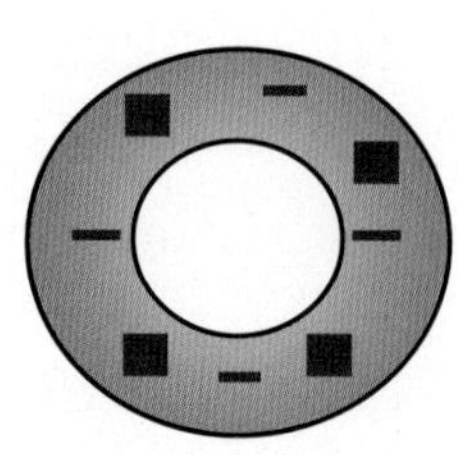

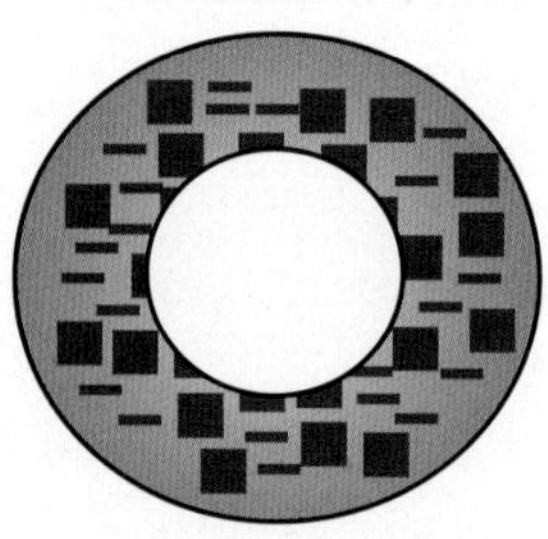

FIGURE 66-1 Stages of lymphedema. Edema mainly located above the fascia. Increased interstitial protein concentration marked by dashes; fibrosis marked by squares. (From DeTurk WE, Cahalin LP. *Cardiovascular and Pulmonary Physical Therapy: An Evidence-Based Approach*. 2nd ed. http://www.accessphysiotherapy.com. Copyright © The McGraw-Hill Companies, Inc. All rights reserved.)

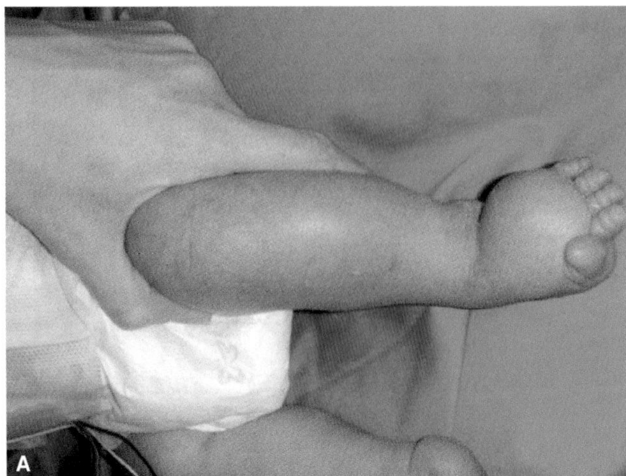

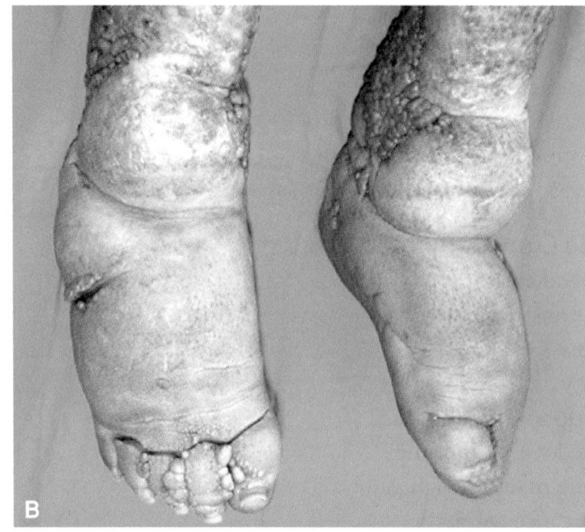

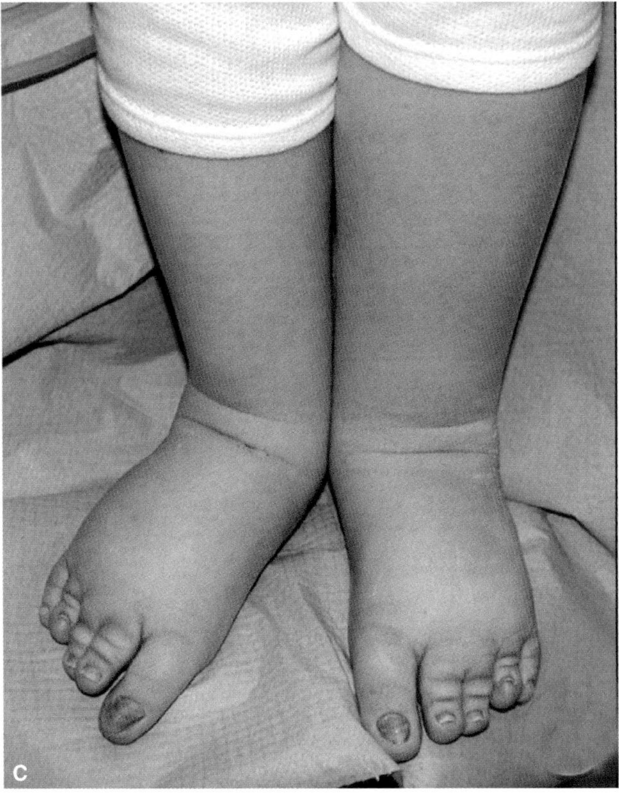

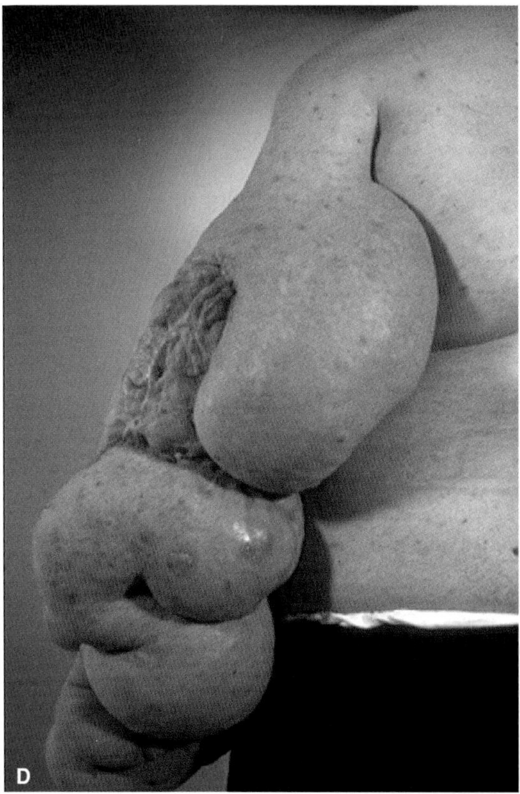

FIGURE 66-2 Various types of congenital primary lymphedema characterized by lymphedema of lower limb, below the knees (**A**), with papillomatosis (**B**), and with upslanting toenails (**C**), that can evolve into elephantiasis (**D**). (From Goldsmith LA, Katz SI, Gilchrest BA, Paller A, Leffell DJ, Wolff K. *Fitzpatrick's Dermatology in General Medicine.* 8th ed. www.accessmedicine.com. Copyright © The McGraw-Hill Companies, Inc. All rights reserved.)

- Classification for lymphedema[3]
- Mild: Less than 3 cm difference between the affected and unaffected limb[3]
- Moderate: Between 3 and 5 cm difference between the unaffected and affected limb[3]
- Severe: 5+ cm difference between the unaffected and affected limb
- Graded 1 (least severe) to 4 (most severe)[3]
- Pitting only present in stages 1 and 2[3]

Demographics

- Parallels those of breast cancer

CLINICAL FINDINGS

SIGNS AND SYMPTOMS

- Pitting/nonpitting lymphedema of extremity
  - Pitting only present in stages 1 and 2[3]
- Skin feeling tight or shiny
- Decreased flexibility/ROM in the hand or wrist
- Difficulty fitting into clothing in one specific area
- Ring, wristwatch, bracelet tightness
- Usually unilateral
- Asymmetrical appearance
- Localized presentation
- Warmth, tenderness
- Redness

▶ Functional Implications
- Stiffness, limited ROM
- Sensory disturbances
- Decreased resistance to infection
- Susceptibility to skin breakdown
- Decreased self-care, ADLs

▶ Possible Contributing Causes
- Lymphadenectomy
- Limb constriction
- Overuse
- Obesity
- Radiation fibrosis
- Delayed wound healing
- Scarring of left or right subclavian lymphatic ducts
- Breast cancer surgery
- Diagnostic dissection
- Mastectomy
- Radiation

▶ Differential Diagnosis
- Edema[3]
- Cellulitis
- Dermatologic manifestations of cardiac or renal disease
- Erysipelas
- Filariasis
- Lymphangioma
- Thrombophlebitis
- Venous insufficiency

MEANS OF CONFIRMATION OR DIAGNOSIS

▶ Imaging
- Indirect lymphangiography
- Direct lymphography
- Fluorescent microlymphography
- MRI
- Lymphoscintigram

▶ Diagnostic Procedures
- Doppler study
- Surgical history (axillary lymph node dissection [ALND], modified radical mastectomy)
- Visual inspection
- Circumferential measurements

FINDINGS AND INTERPRETATION
- Common clinical findings include
- Increased circumferential limb girth
- Postural changes
- Neuromuscular deficits
- Integumentary complications (atrophic skin changes)
- Edema
- Decreased ROM
- Decreased strength
- Pain (axillary cording postmastectomy with lymph node dissection)

TREATMENT

▶ Medication
- Diuretics (limited success)
- Benzopyrenes

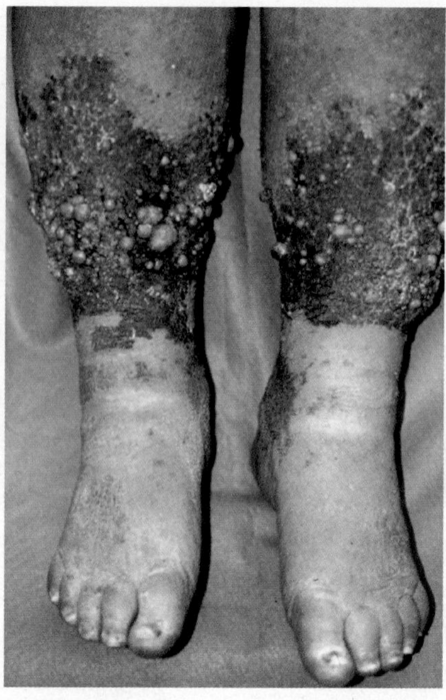

FIGURE 66-3 Verrucous skin changes in chronic lymphedema. (From Goldsmith LA, Katz SI, Gilchrest BA, Paller A, Leffell DJ, Wolff K. *Fitzpatrick's Dermatology in General Medicine.* 8th ed. www.accessmedicine.com.)

MEDICAL PROCEDURES
- Surgical (limited success)
    - Liposuction
    - Removal of abnormal lymphatic tissue

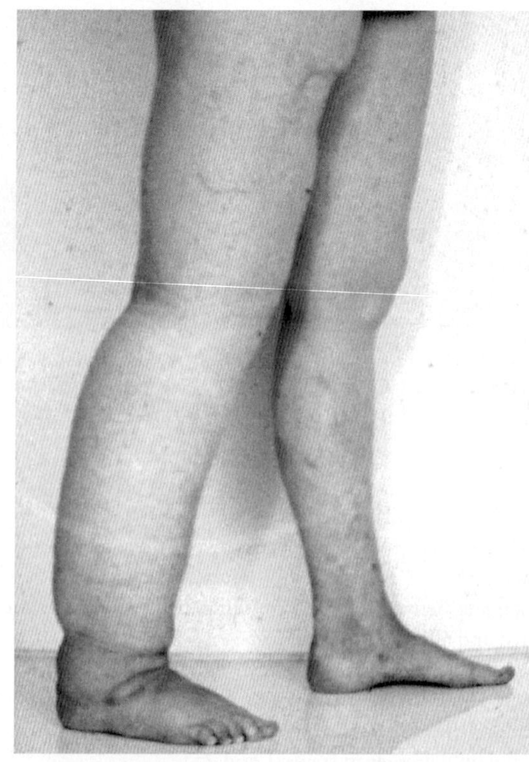

FIGURE 66-4 Acquired lymphedema. Edema is centered at the ankle and involves the foot and toes. (From Doherty GM. *Current Diagnosis & Treatment: Surgery.* 13th ed. www.accessmedicine.com.)

- Venous graft
- Amputation

REFERRAL/ADMITTANCE

- Lymphedema specialist

IMPAIRMENTS

- Discomfort in affected upper extremity
- Weakness
- Neuropathy
- Decreased ROM
- Impaired skin healing
- Impaired functional use of affected upper extremity
- Pain

TESTS AND MEASURES

- Aerobic capacity
- Ankle brachial index (ABI or ABPI)
- Circumferential and volumetric measurements of involved upper extremity
- Integumentary integrity
- Joint integrity and mobility
- Muscle performance and strength
- Pain
- Posture
- Range of motion
- Self-care/ADL abilities
- Sensory integrity
- Stemmer's sign

INTERVENTION

- Lymphedema therapy, manual lymph drainage
- Short-stretch compression bandages
- Multi-layered bandaging
- Retrograde massage
- Low-level laser
- Exercise
  - Avoid excessive activities that may cause fluid buildup.
  - Begin with lower-extremity exercises.
  - Monitor during and after activity for limb swelling.
  - Follow postsurgical weight lifting precautions.
- Compression therapy.
- Compression garments (sleeve), especially for flying
- Initial stage may improve with elevation
- Mechanical pump
- Electrotherapeutic modalities
- Skin care
  - Keep skin clean and dry
  - Wear gloves for skin protection
  - Sunblock, insect repellant

FUNCTIONAL GOALS

- Patient will be able to
  - Perform manual lymphatic drainage (MLD) and proper skin care in order to prevent progression of lymphedema and maintain functional use of upper extremity.
  - Perform daily activities without increased upper-extremity swelling

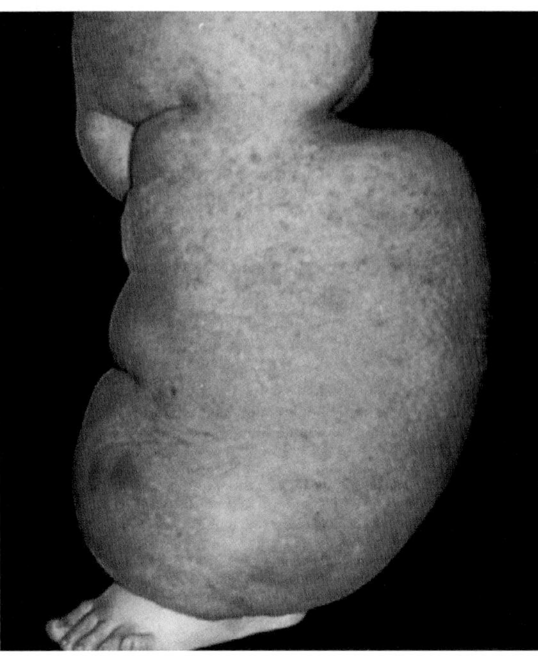

FIGURE 66-5 Lymphedema of the left leg in a 47-year-old fireman. The extreme swelling began at birth and was painless. Note the lack of stasis pigmentation or ulceration. The patient functioned normally at work and wanted no treatment. (From Goldsmith LA, Katz SI, Gilchrest BA, Paller A, Leffell DJ, Wolff K. *Fitzpatrick's Dermatology in General Medicine.* 8th ed. www.accessmedicine.com. Copyright © The McGraw-Hill Companies, Inc. All rights reserved.)

PROGNOSIS

- Chronic, requires lifelong management.
- A comprehensive intervention can significantly reduce lymphedema during treatment and after with ongoing home-exercise program.
- Dependent on complications and compliance with intervention.

ADDITIONAL INFORMATION

- See case study in Chapter 22. *Cardiovascular and Pulmonary Physical Therapy: An Evidence-Based Approach.* 2nd ed. http://www.accessphysiotherapy.com/content/6887974. Accessed July 5, 2013.

PATIENT RESOURCES

- National Cancer Institute at the National Institutes of Health. Lymphedema. http://www.cancer.gov/cancertopics/pdq/supportivecare/lymphedema/healthprofessional/page1. Accessed July 5, 2013.
- National Lymphedema Network. What is lymphedema? http://www.lymphnet.org/lymphedemaFAQs/overview.htm. Accessed July 5, 2013.
- Rossy KM, Scheinfeld NS, et al. Lymphedema differential diagnoses. Medscape. http://emedicine.medscape.com/article/1087313-differential. Accessed July 5, 2013.

REFERENCES

1. The American Physical Therapy Association. Pattern 4E: impaired joint mobility, motor function, muscle performance, and range of motion associated with localized inflammation. *Interactive Guide to Physical Therapist Practice.* 2003. doi: 10.2522/ptguide.3.1_5. http://guidetoptpractice.apta.org/content/1/SEC12.

extract?sid=b3838417-fbe3-4d63-9090-5ce260a287a3. Accessed May 6, 2014.

2. The American Physical Therapy Association. Pattern 6H: impaired circulation and anthropometric dimensions associated with lymphatic system disorders. *Interactive Guide to Physical Therapist Practice.* 2003. doi: 10.2522/ptguide.3.3_8. http://guidetoptpractice.apta.org/content/1/SEC34.extract?sid=06452a17-58d4-4c18-a6f6-676a7f40405c. Accessed May 6, 2014.
3. Leaird KD. Physical therapy associated with lymphatic system disorders. In: DeTurk WE, Cahalin LP, eds. *Cardiovascular and Pulmonary Physical Therapy: An Evidence-Based Approach.* 2nd ed. New York, NY: McGraw-Hill: 2011. http://www.accessphysiotherapy.com/abstract/6887974-6887974. Accessed July 5, 2013.

ADDITIONAL REFERENCES

- American Cancer Society. *Ovarian Cancer.* http://www.cancer.org/Cancer/OvarianCancer/DetailedGuide/ovarian-cancer-diagnosis. Accessed July 5, 2013.
- Dutton M. *McGraw-Hill's NPTE (National Physical Therapy Examination).* 2nd ed. New York, NY: McGraw-Hill; 2012. http://www.accessphysiotherapy.com/resource/611. Accessed July 5, 2013.
- MDGuidelines. *Multiple Myeloma.* http://www.mdguidelines.com/multiple-myeloma/differential-diagnosis. Accessed July 5, 2013.
- Panus PC, Jobst EE, Masters SB, Katzung B, Tinsley SL, Trevor AJ, eds. *Pharmacology for the Physical Therapist.* New York, NY: McGraw-Hill; 2009. http://www.accessphysiotherapy.com/resource/615. Accessed July 5, 2013.
- Ridner SH, Poage-Hooper E, Kanar C, Doersam JK, Bond SM, Dietrich MS. A pilot randomized trial evaluating low-level laser therapy as an alternative treatment to manual lymphatic drainage for breast cancer-related lymphedema. *Oncol Nurs Forum.* 2013;40(4):383–393. doi: 10.1188/13.ONF.383-393.

67 MULTIPLE MYELOMA

Eric Shamus, PhD, DPT, PT, CSCS
Elizabeth E. Demarse, DPT, MTC
Stephanie N. Wright, MOT, OTR/L
Adrian Taylor, DPT

CONDITION/DISORDER SYNONYMS

- Plasma cell myeloma
- Kahler's disease

ICD-9-CM CODES

- 140-239 Neoplasms
- 200-209 Malignant neoplasm of lymphatic and hematopoietic tissue
- 203 Multiple myeloma and immunoproliferative neoplasms
- 203.0 Multiple myeloma
- 203.00 Multiple myeloma without remission
- 203.01 Multiple myeloma in remission
- 203.02 Multiple myeloma, in relapse

ICD-10-CM CODES

- C90.00 Multiple myeloma not having achieved remission
- C90.01 Multiple myeloma in remission
- C90.02 Multiple myeloma in relapse

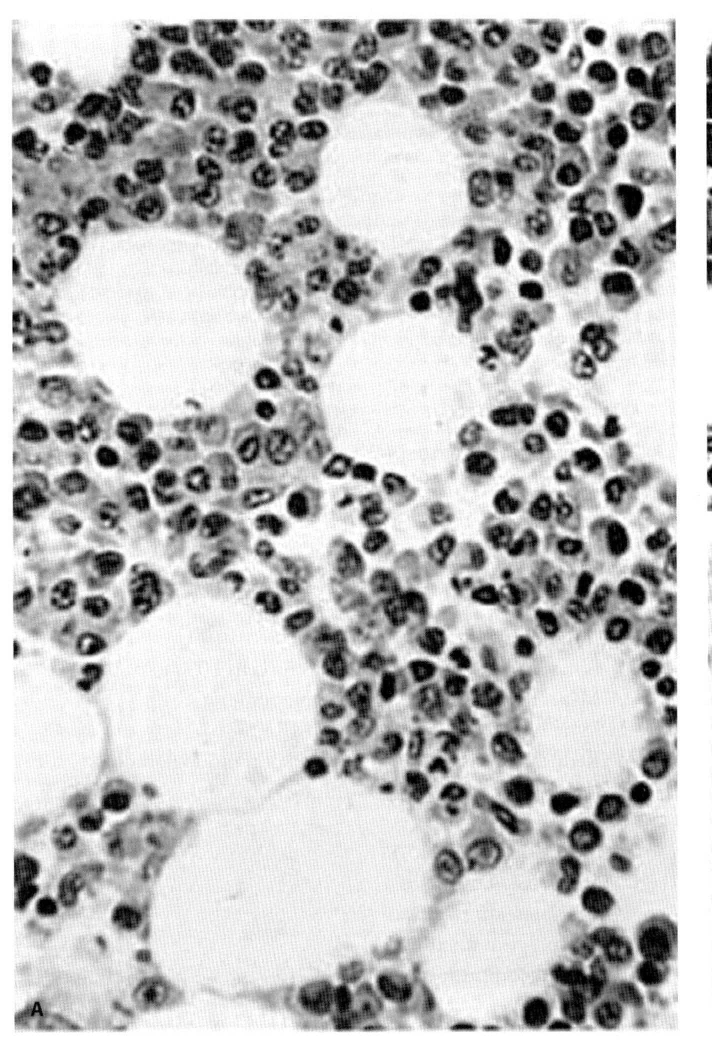

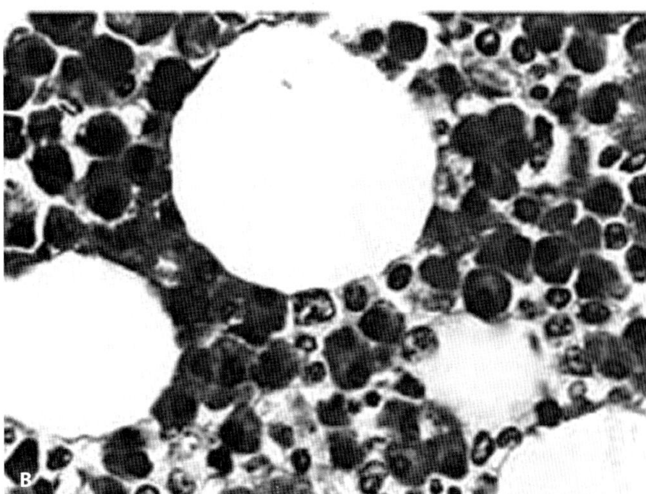

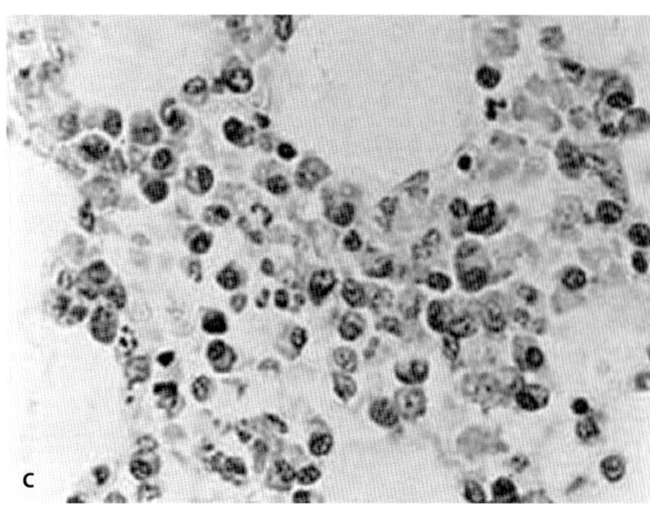

FIGURE 67-1 Section of a needle biopsy of bone marrow from a patient with marrow involvement by multiple myeloma. **A.** Numerous plasma cells have replaced most of the marrow; a few fat cells remain. **B** and **C.** Same case after staining for immunoglobulin light chains by the immunoperoxidase technique. In **B**, staining with anti-kappa reveals a positive reaction (*black*) in the plasma cells, whereas in **C**, staining with anti-lambda shows no reactivity. This demonstrates the monoclonal nature of this neoplasm. An IgA-kappa monoclonal spike was detected in serum. (From Chandrasoma P, Taylor CR. *Concise Pathology*. 3rd ed. www.accessmedicine.com. Copyright © The McGraw-Hill Companies, Inc. All rights reserved.)

PREFERRED PRACTICE PATTERNS[1]

- 4E: Impaired Joint Mobility, Motor Function, Muscle Performance, and Range of Motion Associated with Localized Inflammation
- 6B: Impaired Aerobic Capacity/Endurance Associated with Deconditioning
- 6H: Impaired Circulation and Anthropometric Dimensions Associated with Lymphatic System Disorders

PATIENT PRESENTATION

A 62-year-old female that is retired, complains of a recent onset of left-sided back pain that radiates from her left lower scapula area down the left side of her back and into her left leg. The pain began about 5 weeks ago after she was hospitalized for pneumonia. She was admitted for 3 weeks. She did not receive her monthly chemotherapy treatment during this time. The pain is worse when she does activities that require her to use her arms. She describes it as aching pain in the middle back and she feels weak and stiff in the lower left side of her back and left thigh. She lives alone, however, has a caregiver who assists as need. She is able to perform her self-care independently; however, she is not able to vacuum, sweep, or mop, as these activities increase her pain.

The patient has a moderately kyphotic posture with a flattened lumbar curve. The thoracic and lumbar paraspinals are tight with greater tightness in the right thoracic paraspinals. Strength is WNL in bilateral UE except for left scapular muscle weakness. She has LE weakness in left hip muscles (abduction and extension), as well as bilateral ankle plantar flexion (PF). She is unable to perform unilateral heel raise on right or left. She complains of increased pain with UE and LE testing. The pain complaint was greater with UE testing, particularly shoulder MMT. She presents with postural muscle weakness with the inability to maintain an appropriate erect sitting posture for more than 15 seconds secondary to increased back pain and feeling fatigued. She is neurologically intact with patellar reflex; however, has severe bilateral foot neuropathy (chemotherapy-induced peripheral neuropathy) affecting distal reflexes. She is able to transfer independent from sitting to supine and to sidelying on both sides, however, complains of increased pain during transfer from supine to sidelying in both directions. Patient transfers sit–stand requiring bilateral UE and moves slowly with transfer. She walks with a cane in left hand and has used this since her discharge from the hospital. Gait is appropriate and non-antalgic. The patient was diagnosed with T7-9 compression fractures secondary to disease.

KEY FEATURES

Description

- Multiple small tumors in the bone marrow
- Overgrowth of plasma cells in bone marrow
- Plasma decreases
- RBCs/WBCs/platelets decrease
- Primary malignant neoplasm of plasma cells arising in the bone marrow
- Most common form of plasma cell dyscrasia[2]
- Initial weakening of the bones and bone marrow of the vertebrae, ribs, skull, pelvis, and femur
- Progression causes damage to the kidneys, leads to recurrent infections, and can affect the nervous system

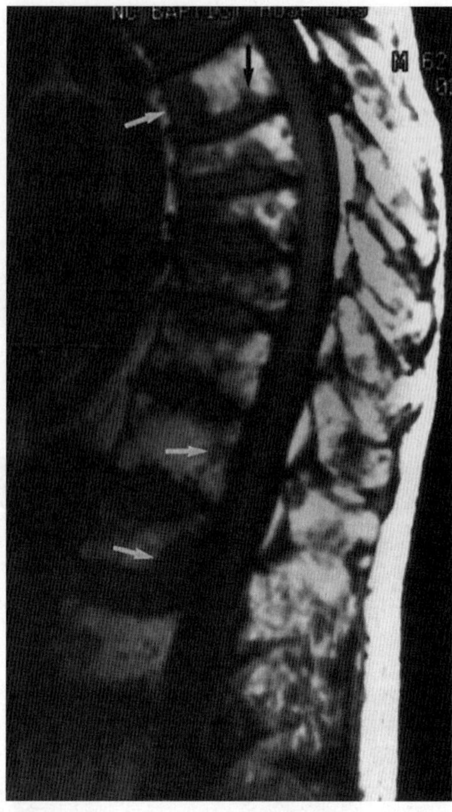

FIGURE 67-2 Sagittal T1-weighted MR image of the thoracic spine shows multiple small hypointense foci of myeloma (*arrows*) replacing normal bone marrow. Compression fractures are also seen, indicated by loss of height of several upper thoracic vertebral bodies. The spinal cord is intact, but spread of tumor or retropulsion of fractured bone could result in cord compression. Note that metastatic tumor other than myeloma could have an identical appearance. (From Chen MYM, Pope TL, Ott DJ. *Basic Radiology*. 2nd ed. www.accessmedicine.com. Copyright © The McGraw-Hill Companies, Inc. All rights reserved.)

Essentials of Diagnosis

- Major criteria
  - Plasmacytoma by biopsy of tissue
  - Bone marrow shows clonal plasma cells >30%
  - High M-protein (IgG >3.5 g/dL, IgA >2.0 g/dL)
  - Bence Jones Proteinuria >1.0 g/24 h
- Minor criteria
  - Bone marrow shows clonal plasma cells 10% to 30%
  - M-protein less than that for major criteria
  - Lytic bone lesions on x-ray or MRI
  - Reduced levels of non-monoclonal immunoglobulins (IgM <50 mg/dL, IgA <100 mg/dL, or IgG <600 mg/dL)

General Considerations

- Spine/pelvis/femur/ribs
  - Compression fractures
  - Pathological fractures
  - Neural compromise

Demographics

- Median age of diagnosis is 68 years for men, 70 years for women
- More common in men
- African American men are affected twice as often as White men

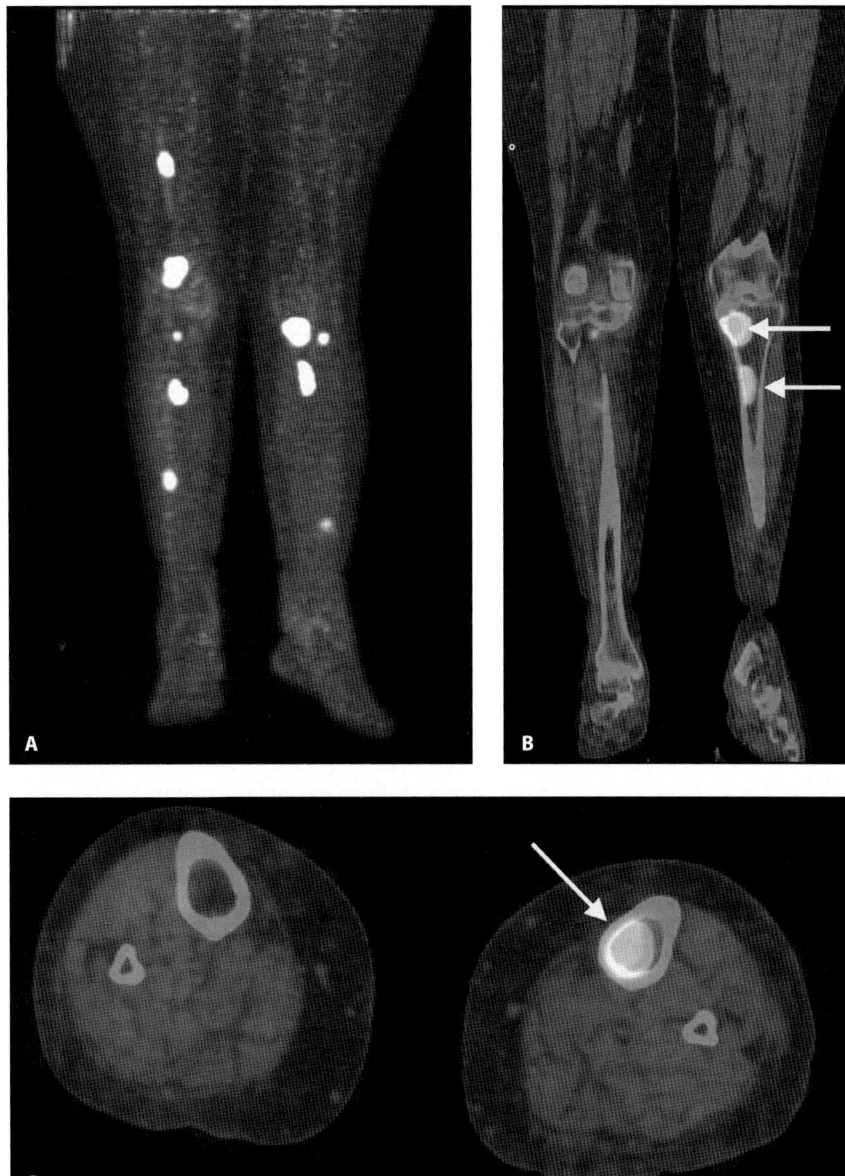

FIGURE 67-3 **A.** Maximum intensity projection (MIP) image from a PET-CT. The bright white spots scattered in the bones of the lower extremities bilaterally represent areas of actively growing myeloma. **B.** Coronal section of fused PET-CT. The two lesions in the left tibia (*arrows*) represent the lesions that are causing cortical destruction. A color image of this same section is located on the cover of the book. **C.** Axial section of fused PET-CT at the level of the more distal of the two left tibial lesions confirms the location of the lesion inside the medullary cavity of the proximal left tibia (*arrow*). (From Chen MYM, Pope TL, Ott DJ. *Basic Radiology*. 2nd ed. www.accessmedicine.com. Copyright © The McGraw-Hill Companies, Inc. All rights reserved.)

CLINICAL FINDINGS

SIGNS AND SYMPTOMS

- Clinicopathologic correlates[2]
- Unexplained back pain
- Anemia due to accelerated red cell destruction, nutritional factors, and replacement of marrow[2]
- Fractures due to bone marrow involvement
- Infection due to decreased ability to produce specific antibody[2]
- Bone pain[2]
- Nerve root compression if in the spine bones
- Fatigue
- Arthritis[2]
- Neuropathy[2]
- Bone loss
  - Pathological fractures
- Renal disease[2]
- Hyperviscosity
- Frequent urination
- Muscular weakness
- Bruises easily
- Weight loss
- Radiation side effects
  - Fatigue
  - Secondary neoplasm
  - Integumentary compromise (burns)
  - Radiation fibrosis
- Chemotherapy side effects
  - Nausea
  - Vomiting
  - Diarrhea
  - Alopecia
  - Mouth sores
  - Conjunctivitis
  - Ulcers
  - Leukopenia
  - Anemia
  - Thrombocytopenia
  - Headaches
  - Dizziness
  - Menstrual irregularities
  - Infertility
  - Peripheral neuropathies

Functional Implications
- Pain with mobility
- Risk for pathological fractures
- Decreased independence
- Impaired performance with ADLs
- Decreased participation in work and leisure
- Infection risk
- Endurance
- Impaired gait

Possible Contributing Causes
- No precise etiology
- Possibly genetic
- Environmental
- Radiation
- Infection
- Chronic inflammation
- Possible due to exposure to Agent Orange

Differential Diagnosis
- Bone neoplasms
- Chronic lymphocytic leukemia (plasma cell leukemia)
- Metastatic cancer (carcinoma)
- Monoclonal gammopathy of undetermined significance (MGUS)
- Non-Hodgkin lymphoma
- Other protein disorders such as macroglobulinemia
- Primary amyloidosis

MEANS OF CONFIRMATION OR DIAGNOSIS

Laboratory Tests
- Complete blood count (CBC), plus differential and platelet counts
- Serum calcium and albumin levels
- Beta-2 microglobulin levels
- Blood urea nitrogen (BUN) and serum creatinine levels to measure kidney function
- C-reactive protein test
- Lactate dehydrogenase levels

Imaging
- X-rays
- Positron emission tomography (PET) scan

Diagnostic Procedures
- Bone marrow biopsy
- Needle biopsy of bone marrow

FINDINGS AND INTERPRETATIONS
- Structural abnormality particularly with compression fractures in spine
- Multiple lytic lesions in ribs, skull, long bones on x-ray
- Bone lysis
- Decreased or no lumbar lordosis with severe kyphosis

TREATMENT

Medication
- Immunotherapy
- Chemotherapy
- Immunosuppression
- Interferon alpha therapy
- Radiation (Treat symptoms: Pain, lesions)
- Bisphosphonate therapy

MEDICAL PROCEDURES
- Bone marrow transplantation
- Stem cell transplant
- Transplantation
- Allogeneic (consider graft-versus-host disease [GVHD] and steroid myopathy)
- Autogeneic
- Adjunctive therapy
- Prophylactic fixation of pending fractures
- Decompression of the spinal cord when indicated
- Treatment of pathologic fractures

REFERRALS/ADMITTANCE
- To hospital for acute exacerbation of symptoms
- To occupational therapist for functional activities of daily-living training
- To oncologist, hematologist, neurologist, orthopedic surgeon

IMPAIRMENTS
- Bone loss and osteoporosis
- Posture: Skeletal deformity
- Bone pain
- Mobility compromised
- Fall risk
- Peripheral nerve integrity
- Aerobic endurance
- Difficulty performing self-care/ADLs
- Fatigue
- Skeletal muscle wasting

TESTS AND MEASURES
- Karnofsky Performance Status Scale (KPS)
- Aerobic capacity
- Mobility/transfers assessment
- Balance tests
- Gait tests
- Functional strength test
- ROM

INTERVENTION
- Aerobic conditioning
- Resistance training
- Gait training
- Weight bearing
  - >50% (cortical metastatic involvement), nonweight bearing with crutches or walking; touch down permitted
  - 25% to 50%, partial weight bearing; avoid twisting or stretching
  - 0% to 25%, full weight bearing; avoid lifting or straining
  - Use guidelines with caution: Consider age, general health, overall level of fitness, and level of pain
- Balance training
- Posture training

FUNCTIONAL GOALS

- The patient will be able to
  - Don/doff shoes and socks independently using appropriate body mechanics.
  - Perform 10-minute standing activity rating exertion as <#13 on Borg Scale of Perceived Exertion.

PROGNOSIS

- Variable based on severity, treatment, and complications
- Recovery period of 45 to 60 months with bone marrow transplant
- 35% to 40% survival rate at 5 years

PATIENT RESOURCE

- Multiple Myeloma. MDGuidelines.com. http://www.mdguidelines.com/multiple-myeloma/differential-diagnosis. Accessed June 2, 2013.

REFERENCES

1. APTA. *Guide to Physical Therapy Practice*. Atlanta, GA: American Physical Therapy Association; 2003. http://guidetoptpractice.apta.org. Accessed June 2, 2013.
2. Chandrasoma P, Taylor CR. Plasma cell neoplasms. In: Chandrasoma P, Taylor CR, eds. *Concise Pathology*. 3rd ed. New York, NY: McGraw-Hill; 2011. http://www.accessphysiotherapy.com/content/194083. Accessed June 2, 2013.

ADDITIONAL REFERENCES

- Dutton M. Differential diagnosis. In: Dutton M, ed. *Dutton's Orthopaedic Examination, Evaluation, and Intervention.* 2nd ed. New York, NY: McGraw-Hill; 2008. http://www.accessphysiotherapy.com/content/5546925. Accessed June 2, 2013.
- McDonald RJ, Trout AT, Gray LA, Dispenzieri A, Thielen KR, Kallmes DF. Vertebroplasty in multiple myeloma: outcomes in a large patient series. *The American Journal of Neuroradiology.* 2008;29(4):642–648.
- Simon RR, Sherman SC. Primary bone tumors. In: Simon RR, Sherman SC, eds. *Emergency Orthopedics*. 6th ed. New York, NY: McGraw-Hill; 2011. http://www.accessphysiotherapy.com/content/7702663. Accessed June 2, 2013.

68 SKIN CANCER (MELANOMA)

Shari Rone-Adams, DBA, MHSA, PT

CONDITION/DISORDER SYNONYMS

- Cutaneous melanoma
- Malignancy of melanocytes
- Malignant melanoma
- Melanoma

ICD-9-CM CODES

- 172 Malignant melanoma of skin
- 172.0 Malignant melanoma of skin of lip
- 172.1 Malignant melanoma of skin of eyelid, including canthus
- 172.2 Malignant melanoma of skin of ear and external auditory canal
- 172.3 Malignant melanoma of skin of other and unspecified parts of face
- 172.4 Malignant melanoma of skin of scalp and neck
- 172.5 Malignant melanoma of skin of trunk, except scrotum
- 172.6 Malignant melanoma of skin of upper limb, including shoulder
- 172.7 Malignant melanoma of skin of lower limb, including hip
- 172.8 Malignant melanoma of other specified sites of skin
- 172.9 Melanoma of skin, site unspecified

ICD-10-CM CODES

- C43.0 Malignant melanoma of lip
- C43.10 Malignant melanoma of unspecified eyelid, including canthus
- C43.20 Malignant melanoma of unspecified ear and external auricular canal
- C43.30 Malignant melanoma of unspecified part of face
- C43.31 Malignant melanoma of nose
- C43.39 Malignant melanoma of other parts of face
- C43.4 Malignant melanoma of scalp and neck
- C43.59 Malignant melanoma of other part of trunk
- C43.60 Malignant melanoma of unspecified upper limb, including shoulder
- C43.70 Malignant melanoma of unspecified lower limb, including hip
- C43.8 Malignant melanoma of overlapping sites of skin
- C43.9 Malignant melanoma of skin, unspecified
- D03.0 Melanoma in situ of lip
- D03.10 Melanoma in situ of unspecified eyelid, including canthus
- D03.11 Melanoma in situ of right eyelid, including canthus
- D03.12 Melanoma in situ of left eyelid, including canthus
- D03.20 Melanoma in situ of unspecified ear and external auricular canal
- D03.21 Melanoma in situ of right ear and external auricular canal

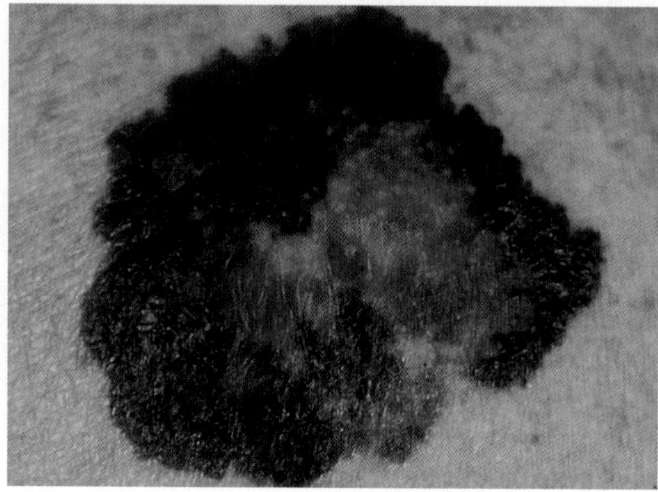

FIGURE 68-1 Superficial spreading melanoma. This is the most common type of melanoma. Such lesions usually demonstrate asymmetry, border irregularity, color variegation (black, blue, brown, pink, and white), a diameter >6 mm, and a history of change (e.g., an increase in size or development of associated symptoms such as pruritus or pain.) (From Longo DL, Fauci AS, Kasper DL, Hauser SL, Jameson JL, Loscalzo J, eds. *Harrison's Principles of Internal Medicine.* 18th ed. New York, NY: McGraw-Hill; 2012.)

- D03.22 Melanoma in situ of left ear and external auricular canal
- D03.30 Melanoma in situ of unspecified part of face
- D03.39 Melanoma in situ of other parts of face
- D03.4 Melanoma in situ of scalp and neck
- D03.51 Melanoma in situ of anal skin
- D03.52 Melanoma in situ of breast (skin) (soft tissue)
- D03.59 Melanoma in situ of other part of trunk
- D03.60 Melanoma in situ of unspecified upper limb, including shoulder
- D03.61 Melanoma in situ of right upper limb, including shoulder
- D03.62 Melanoma in situ of left upper limb, including shoulder
- D03.70 Melanoma in situ of unspecified lower limb, including hip
- D03.71 Melanoma in situ of right lower limb, including hip
- D03.72 Melanoma in situ of left lower limb, including hip
- D03.8 Melanoma in situ of other sites
- D03.9 Melanoma in situ, unspecified

PREFERRED PRACTICE PATTERNS

- 7B: Impaired Integumentary Integrity Secondary to Superficial Skin Involvement[1]
- 7C: Impaired Integumentary Integrity Secondary to Partial-Thickness Skin Involvement and Scar Formation[2]
- 7D: Impaired Integumentary Integrity Secondary to Full-Thickness Skin Involvement and Scar Formation[3]
- 7E: Impaired Integumentary Integrity Secondary to Skin Involvement Extending into Fascia, Muscle, or Bone[4]

PATIENT PRESENTATION

A 56-year-old male construction worker presents with right shoulder bursitis. Upon skin inspection, the patient had a black mole on his right upper arm. He reports that it has been there for a few years and has changed shape, size, and color over the past year. Previously it was a flat brownish color and was round. Presently, it presents as a black, raised area, with irregular boarders. As a construction worker, the area is regularly exposed to the sun and he reports he does not use sunblock. The patient received physical therapy treatment for his shoulder. Upon discussion with his orthopedists, the patient was referred to a dermatologist.

KEY FEATURES

Description

- Melanoma is a cancer that develops in melanocytes (pigment cells present in the skin)
- Majority of melanomas are in the skin; other sites include eyes, mucosa, gastrointestinal tract, genitourinary tract, leptomeninges
- Least common form of skin cancer but most aggressive, metastasizing to other body areas
- Risk factors include blond or red hair, light-colored skin, blue eyes, and freckles

Essentials of Diagnosis

- Clark staging of melanomas
  - Level I: All tumor cells above basement membrane (in situ)
  - Level II: Tumor extends into papillary dermis
  - Level III: Tumor extends to interface between papillary and reticular dermis
  - Level IV: Tumor extends between bundles of collagen of reticular dermis (extends into reticular dermis)
  - Level V: Tumor invasion of subcutaneous tissue

General Considerations

- Sun exposure increases risk of melanoma
- Five different forms (histologic types) of melanoma
  - Superficial spreading melanomas (70% of melanomas)
  - Nodular melanomas
  - Lentigo maligna melanomas
  - Acral lentiginous melanomas
  - Mucosal lentiginous melanomas

Demographics

- Approximately 50,000 new cases diagnosed in United States annually
- Approximately 10% of patients with melanoma have a family history
- Previous history of melanoma increases risk of developing a second melanoma
- Annual incidence has increased dramatically over the past few decades, as have deaths from melanoma
- Ten times more common in Caucasians than in African Americans
- Men have a higher rate of melanoma than women in the United States
- Tends to run in families

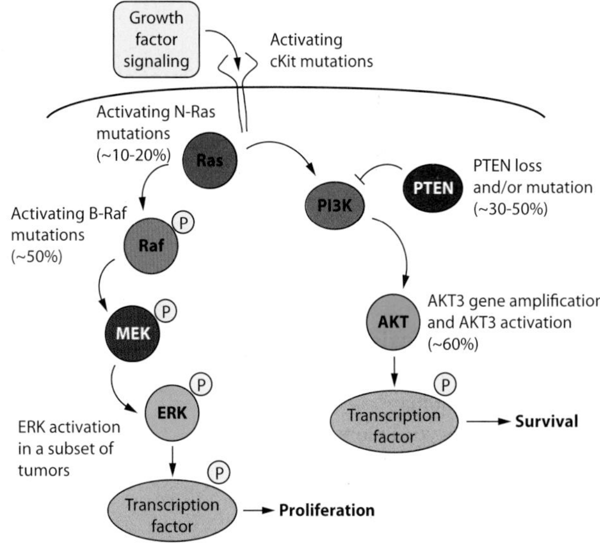

FIGURE 68-2 Major pathways involved in melanoma. The MAP kinase and AKT pathways, which promote proliferation and inhibit apoptosis, respectively, are subject to mutations in melanoma. ERK, extracellular signal-regulated kinase; MEK, methylethylketone; PTEN, pentaerythritol tetranitrate. (From Longo DL, Fauci AS, Kasper DL, Hauser SL, Jameson JL, Loscalzo J, eds. *Harrison's Principles of Internal Medicine*. 18th ed. New York, NY: McGraw-Hill; 2012.)

CLINICAL FINDINGS

SIGNS AND SYMPTOMS

- Any change in size, shape, color of a mole, or other skin growth
- Pneumonic ABCDE
  - Asymmetry
  - Border irregularity
  - Color variegation
  - Diameter
  - Evolving
- Moles with the following characteristics
  - Flat, brown, black
  - Uneven edges
  - Irregular or asymmetrical shape
  - Usually 6 mm (0.25 in) or larger in diameter
  - Crusty, oozing, bleeding
  - Itching
  - Swelling
  - Painful sensitivity
- Sore that does not heal
- Bleeding
- Pigmented lesion
- Melanocytic lesions[5]

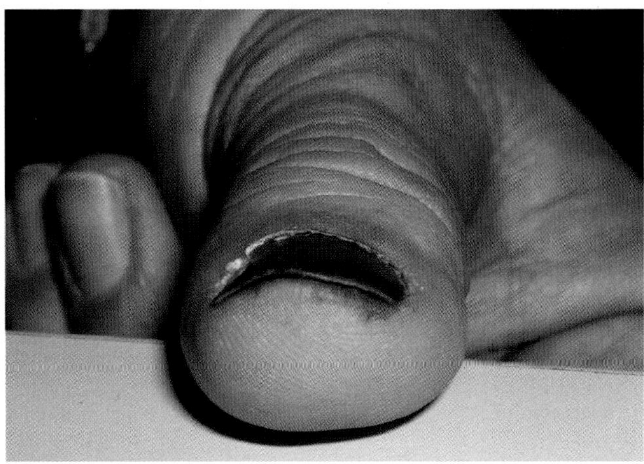

FIGURE 68-3 Nail melanoma: note Hutchinson's sign of the hyponychium. (From Goldsmith LA, Katz SI, Gilchrest BA, Paller A, Leffell DJ, Wolff K. *Fitzpatrick's Dermatology in General Medicine*. 8th ed. www.accessmedicine.com. Copyright © The McGraw-Hill Companies, Inc. All rights reserved.)

Functional Implications

- Limited use of some modalities
- Systemic illness possible depending on the stage of melanoma and presence of metastatic disease

Possible Contributing Causes

- Edema
- Skin lesions
- Sun exposure
- Tanning beds

Differential Diagnosis

- Atypical fibroxanthoma
- Basal cell carcinoma
- Benign melanocytic lesions
- Blue nevus
- Dysplastic nevus
- Epithelioid (Spitz) tumor
- Halo nevus
- Histiocytoid hemangioma
- Lentigo maligna melanoma
- Metastasis of other tumors to skin
- Mycosis fungoides
- Pigmented actinic keratosis
- Pigmented spindle cell tumor
- Sebaceous carcinoma
- Squamous cell carcinoma

MEANS OF CONFIRMATION OR DIAGNOSIS

Laboratory Tests

- Skin biopsy
- Epiluminescence microscopy (dermatoscopy)
- Elevated alkaline phosphatase level
- Elevated liver function test
- Elevated lactate dehydrogenase (LDH)

Imaging

- Chest X-ray[6]
- MRI[7]
- Bone scan[7]
- Ultrasonography to diagnose lymph node involvement[7]
- PET/CT to look for other sites of metastasis[8]

FINDINGS AND INTERPRETATION

- Elevated alkaline phosphatase level may signal metastatic disease
- Elevated liver function test may represent metastatic disease to the liver
- Elevated LDH may indicate metastases to lung or liver

TREATMENT

Medications

- Carmustine[9]
- Cisplatin[10]
- Dacarbazine[9]
- Interferon[10]
- Interleukin-2[9]
- Ipilimumab[9]
- Peginterferon alfa-2b[10]
- Tamoxifen[10]
- Vemurafenib[9]
- Vinblastine[10]

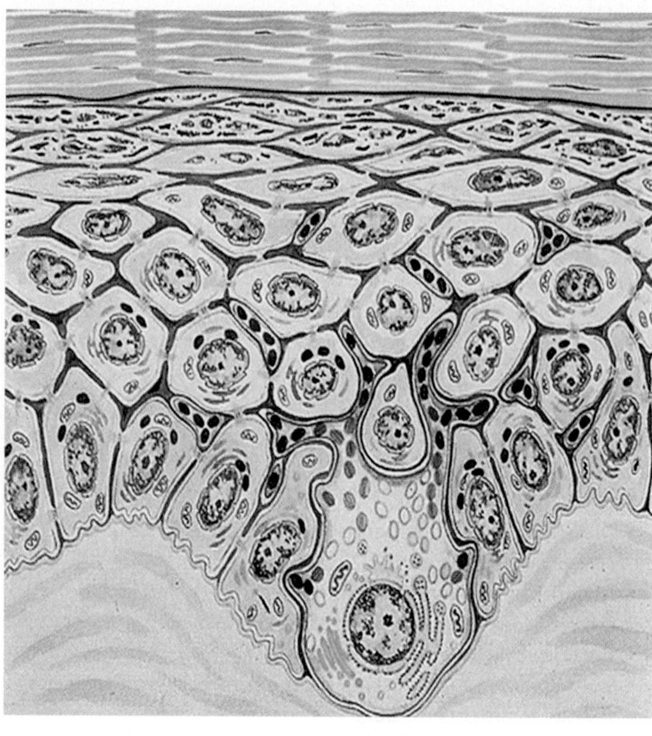

FIGURE 68-4 Following malignant transformation, invasive melanoma cells replicate, penetrate surrounding epidermal layers, and migrate to more distant tissues. (From Brunicardi FC, Andersen C, Billiar T, et al. *Schwartz's Principles of Surgery*. 9th ed. www.accessmedicine.com. Copyright © The McGraw-Hill Companies, Inc. All rights reserved.)

MEDICAL PROCEDURES

- Surgical removal of tumor and nearby lymph glands if necessary
- If spread to other parts of the body
  - Immunotherapy[11]
  - Chemotherapy[10]
  - Radiation

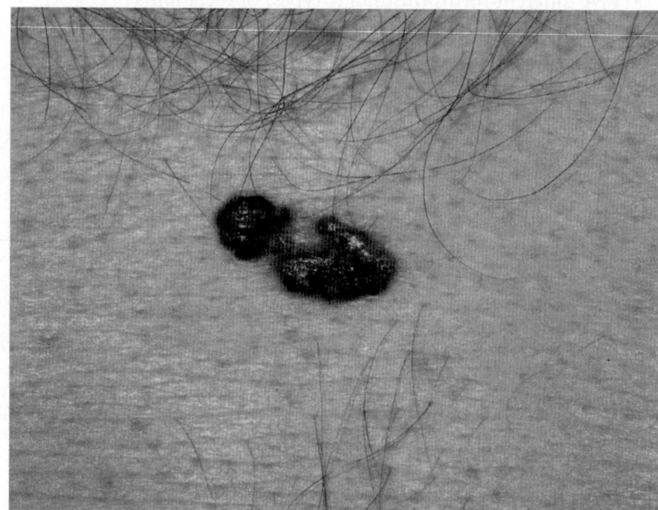

FIGURE 68-5 Superficial spreading melanoma. Breslow depth 1.1 mm. (From Halter JB, Ouslander J, Tinetti M, Studenski S, High K, Asthana S. *Hazzard's Geriatric Medicine and Gerontology*. 6th ed. www.accessmedicine.com. Copyright © The McGraw-Hill Companies, Inc. All rights reserved.)

REFERRALS/ADMITTANCE

- To dermatologist for diagnosis
- To oncologist for treatment

IMPAIRMENTS

- Circulation
- Functional mobility
- Gait
- Home management
- Joint ROM
- Muscle strength
- Pain
- Self-care
- Sensation
- Skin integrity

TESTS AND MEASURES

- Integumentary integrity and observation
    - Pigmentation
    - Shape and size of skin involvement
    - Presence of edema, effusion, open areas, signs of infection
    - Skin temperature
    - Tissue mobility: Tugor, texture
    - Wound characteristics
- Circulation
- Volume and girth measurement for edema and effusion
- Pain: Subjective report, Visual Analogue Scale (VAS), verbal report[12]
- Gait and balance
- Sensation
- Joint ROM
- Strength and muscle endurance
- Functional mobility
- Orthotic: Protective and supportive devices

INTERVENTION

- Not typically treated by PT, but PT should recognize the condition and check skin before and after application of modalities.
- PT should refer patient appropriately if melanoma suspected.
- Depending on the extent of the condition and secondary impairments, the following interventions may apply
    - Dressings (wound coverings)
    - Topical agents (ointments, moisturizers, creams, cleansers, sealants)
    - Compression therapies (vasopneumatic compression devices, compression bandaging, compression garments)
    - Orthotic: Protective and supportive devices
    - Electrical muscle stimulation
    - Transcutaneous electrical nerve stimulation (TENS)[13]
    - Functional training
    - ADL and IADL training

FUNCTIONAL GOALS

- Physical therapy goals should be consistent with secondary movement-related problems, including
    - Ability to perform physical tasks
    - Awareness and use of community resources
    - Reduced risk of recurrence or secondary impairments
    - Self-management of symptoms

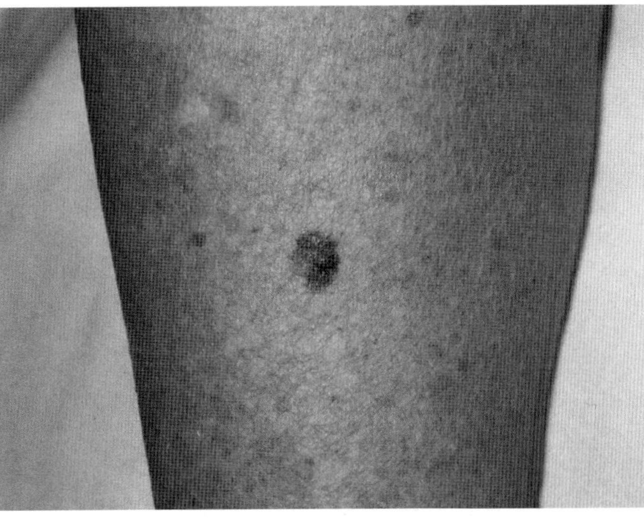

FIGURE 68-6 Early superficial spreading melanoma. Note the asymmetry and irregular border. (From Halter, JB Ouslander J, Tinetti M, Studenski S, High K, Asthana S. *Hazzard's Geriatric Medicine and Gerontology.* 6th ed. www.accessmedicine.com. Copyright © The McGraw-Hill Companies, Inc. All rights reserved.)

    - Decreased pain
    - Improved sense of well-being
    - Reduced swelling, inflammation, restriction of soft tissue
    - Increased tolerance for positions and activities
    - Ability to recognize recurrence and initiate treatment
    - Enhanced wound and soft tissue healing

PROGNOSIS

- Thin melanomas (less than 1 mm in diameter) have excellent cure rates.
- Caught early, most melanomas can be cured with relatively minor surgery.
- The thicker a melanoma, the less optimistic the prognosis.
- See method of estimating the prognosis of malignant melanoma.[5]

PATIENT RESOURCE

- Melanoma. Skin Cancer Foundation. http://www.skincancer.org/skin-cancer-information/melanoma. Accessed July 2, 2013.

REFERENCES

1. The American Physical Therapy Association. Pattern 7B: impaired integumentary integrity associated with superficial skin involvement. *Interactive Guide to Physical Therapist Practice* 2003. doi: 10.2522/ptguide.3.4_2. http://guidetoptpractice.apta.org/content/1/SEC36.extract?sid=f85321a8-7cc4-406c-b73c-e8fa0c26de11. Accessed May 6, 2014.
2. The American Physical Therapy Association. Pattern 7C: impaired integumentary integrity associated with partial-thickness skin involvement and scar formation. *Interactive Guide to Physical Therapist Practice* 2003. doi: 10.2522/ptguide.3.4_3. http://guidetoptpractice.apta.org/content/1/SEC37.extract?sid=4f92d3c0-b83f-4ae5-864f-15a4d1f04448. Accessed May 6, 2014.
3. The American Physical Therapy Association. Pattern 7D: impaired integumentary integrity associated with full-thickness skin involvement and scar formation. *Interactive Guide to*

Physical Therapist Practice 2003. doi: 10.2522/ptguide.3.4_4. http://guidetoptpractice.apta.org/content/1/SEC38.extract?sid=4092b3c3-a0a9-4a05-9f9c-d98c1f8b59c6. Accessed May 6, 2014.

4. The American Physical Therapy Association. Pattern 7E: impaired integumentary integrity associated with skin involvement extending into fascia, muscle, or bone and scar formation. *Interactive Guide to Physical Therapist Practice*. 2003.doi: 10.2522/ptguide.3.4_5. http://guidetoptpractice.apta.org/content/1/SEC39.extract?sid=187e3020-f30e-4afc-a20d-82a3a3a1e763. Accessed May 6, 2014.
5. Chandrasoma P, Taylor CR. Blood: II. Hemolytic anemias; polycythemia. In: Chandrasoma P, Taylor CR, eds. *Concise Pathology*. 3rd ed. Stamford, CT: Appleton & Lang; 1998. http://www.accessphysiotherapy.com/content/187050. Accessed July 2, 2013.
6. Miyamoto SD, Sondheimer HM, Fagan TE, Collins KK. Cardiovascular diseases. In: Hay W, Levin MJ, Sondheimer JM, Deterding RR, eds. *CURRENT Diagnosis & Treatment: Pediatrics*. 20th ed. New York, NY: McGraw-Hill; 2011. http://www.accessphysiotherapy.com/abstract/6583154#6583208. Accessed July 2, 2013.
7. Dutton M. *Orthopaedic Examination, Evaluation, and Intervention*. 3rd ed. New York, NY: McGraw-Hill; 2008. http://www.accessphysiotherapy.com/resource/612. Accessed July 2, 2013.
8. Waxman SG. *Clinical Neuroanatomy*. 26th ed. New York, NY: McGraw-Hill; 2010. http://www.accessphysiotherapy.com/resource/22. Accessed July 2, 2013.
9. American Physical Therapy Association. Drug Monographs. McGraw-Hill. http://www.accessphysiotherapy.com/drugs. Accessed July 2, 2013.
10. Panus PC, Jobst EE, Masters SB, Katzung B, Tinsley SL, Trevor AJ. *Pharmacology for the Physical Therapist*. New York, NY: McGraw-Hill; 2009. http://www.accessphysiotherapy.com/resource/615. Accessed July 2, 2013.
11. Covar RA, Fleischer DM, Boguniewicz M. Allergic disorders. In: Hay WW, Levin MJ, Sondheimer JM, Deterding RR, eds. *CURRENT Diagnosis & Treatment: Pediatrics*. 20th ed. New York, NY: McGraw-Hill; 2011. http://www.accessphysiotherapy.com/abstract/6589468#6589505. Accessed July 2, 2013.
12. Denegar CR, Prentice WE. Managing pain with therapeutic modalities. In: Prentice WE, Quillen WS, Underwood F, eds. *Therapeutic Modalities in Rehabilitation*. 4th ed. New York, NY: McGraw-Hill; 2011. http://www.accessphysiotherapy.com/abstract/8135800#8135806. Accessed July 2, 2013.
13. Hooker DN, Prentice WE. Basic principles of electricity and electrical stimulating currents. In: Prentice WE, Quillen WS, Underwood F, eds. *Therapeutic Modalities in Rehabilitation*. 4th ed. New York, NY: McGraw-Hill; 2011. http://www.accessphysiotherapy.com/content/8136367#8136367. Accessed July 2, 2013.

ADDITIONAL REFERENCES

- Dutton M. Integumentary physical therapy. In: Dutton M, ed. *McGraw-Hill's NPTE (National Physical Therapy Examination)*. 2nd ed. New York, NY: McGraw-Hill; 2012. http://www.accessphysiotherapy.com/content/5403146. Accessed July 2, 2013.
- Morelli JG, Burch JM. Skin. In: Hay WW, Levin MJ, Sondheimer JM, Deterding RR, eds. *CURRENT Diagnosis & Treatment: Pediatrics*. 20th ed. New York, NY: McGraw-Hill; 2011. http://www.accessphysiotherapy.com/content/6580229. Accessed July 2, 2013.

69 TUMOR, BONE

Eric Shamus, PhD, DPT, PT, CSCS
Stephanie N. Wright, MOT, OTR/L

CONDITION/DISORDER SYNONYMS

- Chondrosarcoma
- Ewing (or Ewing's) sarcoma
- Osteosarcoma

ICD-9-CM CODES

- 170 Malignant neoplasm of bone and articular cartilage
- 170.0 Malignant neoplasm of bones of skull and face except mandible
- 170.1 Malignant neoplasm of mandible
- 170.2 Malignant neoplasm of vertebral column excluding sacrum and coccyx
- 170.3 Malignant neoplasm of ribs sternum and clavicle
- 170.4 Malignant neoplasm of scapula and long bones of upper limb
- 170.5 Malignant neoplasm of short bones of upper limb
- 170.6 Malignant neoplasm of pelvic bones sacrum and coccyx
- 170.7 Malignant neoplasm of long bones of lower limb
- 170.8 Malignant neoplasm of short bones of lower limb
- 170.9 Malignant neoplasm of bone and articular cartilage site unspecified

ICD-10-CM CODES

- C40.00 Malignant neoplasm of scapula and long bones of unspecified upper limb
- C40.10 Malignant neoplasm of short bones of unspecified upper limb
- C40.20 Malignant neoplasm of long bones of unspecified lower limb
- C40.30 Malignant neoplasm of short bones of unspecified lower limb
- C41.0 Malignant neoplasm of bones of skull and face
- C41.1 Malignant neoplasm of mandible
- C41.2 Malignant neoplasm of vertebral column
- C41.3 Malignant neoplasm of ribs, sternum and clavicle
- C41.4 Malignant neoplasm of pelvic bones, sacrum and coccyx
- C41.9 Malignant neoplasm of bone and articular cartilage, unspecified

PREFERRED PRACTICE PATTERNS

- 4E: Impaired Joint Mobility, Motor Function, Muscle Performance, and Range of Motion Associated With Localized Inflammation[1]
- 6B: Impaired Aerobic Capacity/Endurance Associated With Deconditioning[2]

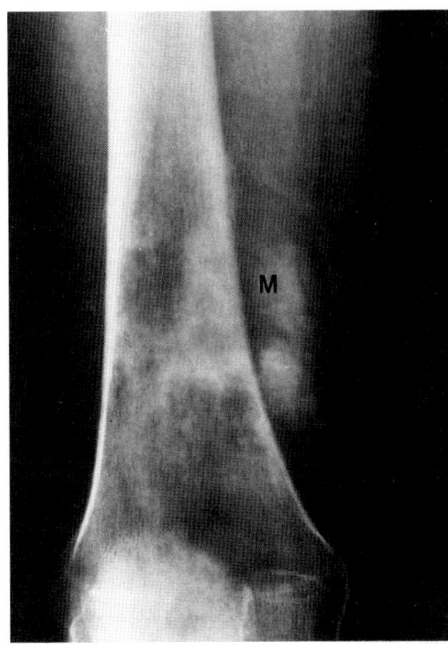

FIGURE 69-1 AP view of the distal femur. Many of the radiographic features of this osteosarcoma mark it as a malignant tumor. The abnormal area of mottled lucent and sclerotic tumor in the metaphysis fades gradually into the shadows of surrounding normal bone. It is difficult to see where the tumor begins and ends; there is a large soft tissue mass adjacent to the bone (M). The periosteum has been unable to maintain a shell of mineralized new bone around this mass. The sclerotic areas within the bone and the mineralized portions of the soft tissue mass both have a relatively amorphous, smudged appearance that is seen with calcified osteoid matrix. (From Chen MYM, Pope TL, Ott DJ. *Basic Radiology*. 2nd ed. www.accessmedicine.com. Copyright © The McGraw-Hill Companies, Inc. All rights reserved.)

PATIENT PRESENTATION

A 21-year-old female began noticing severe low back pain after working out at her local gym. After a week of back rest, the pain continued and she made an appointment with her primary care physician who provided anti-inflammatory medications and continued back rest. The patient reports the symptoms continued and she began to notice additional pain and a lump on her right scapula.

After a PET scan, CT and MRI she was diagnosed with Ewing sarcoma and has received five rounds of chemotherapy, radiation to right scapula, left distal humerus and currently to lumbar vertebrae L2 and L3. She reports she will be having an autologous stem cell transplant in 3 months.

Her shoulder flexion and external rotation is limited by pain and weakness (4/5) in right shoulder. Biceps and triceps strength is also limited at 3+/5 in left arm, pain when resistance applied and is limiting her ability to dress and bathe herself. The pain is present in her left arm when attempting to lift heavy items or pushing self to standing. Opening heavy doors, trying to wash her own hair and putting on a seat belt aggravates the pain in her right shoulder. Her back is painful and aches after walking or standing for more than 10 minutes, but is relieved with sitting or lying in a recliner. She reports having difficulty lying flat at night.

KEY FEATURES

Description

- Considered either osteoclastic or osteoblastic
- Abnormal growth of cells within the bone
- Can be either benign or malignant (cancerous)
- Often spreads to bone from cancerous tumors in other areas
  - Breast
  - Kidney
  - Lung
  - Prostate
  - Thyroid

Essentials of Diagnosis

- Some benign tumors have no symptoms until fracture
- Malignant tumors
  - Bone pain at site, worse at night
  - Fracture from simple trauma or no trauma at all
  - Mass or swelling at the site of tumor
  - Fracture through cortical bone

General Considerations

- Gradual onset of signs and symptoms
- Distal femur accounts for more than 40% of cases, with proximal tibia, proximal humerus, and mid and proximal femur following in frequency[3]
- Clinical correlation[4]

Demographics

- Sixth most common malignancy in childhood[3]
- Third most common malignancy among adolescents[3]
- Occurs at an earlier age in girls than boys, corresponding to growth spurt[3]
- Ewing sarcoma most common in toddlers and young Caucasian males

CLINICAL FINDINGS

SIGNS AND SYMPTOMS

- Bone pain: Constant, not dependent on position or activity
- Fractures
- Swelling, localized
- Fever[3]
- Weight loss[3]
- Presence of mass
- Spontaneous pain from nerve-root irritation
- Motor weakness
- Muscle wasting
- Lower or upper motor neuron changes
- Sensory changes
- Hydrocephalus
- Papilledema
- Elevated intracranial pressure
- Chemotherapy; side effects include
  - Nausea
  - Vomiting
  - Diarrhea
  - Alopecia
  - Mouth sores
  - Conjunctivitis
  - Ulcers
  - Leukopenia
  - Anemia
  - Thrombocytopenia
  - Headaches
  - Dizziness
  - Menstrual irregularities
  - Infertility
  - Peripheral neuropathies

Functional Implications

- Loss of independence with ADLs, self-care, and locomotion in home and community environments

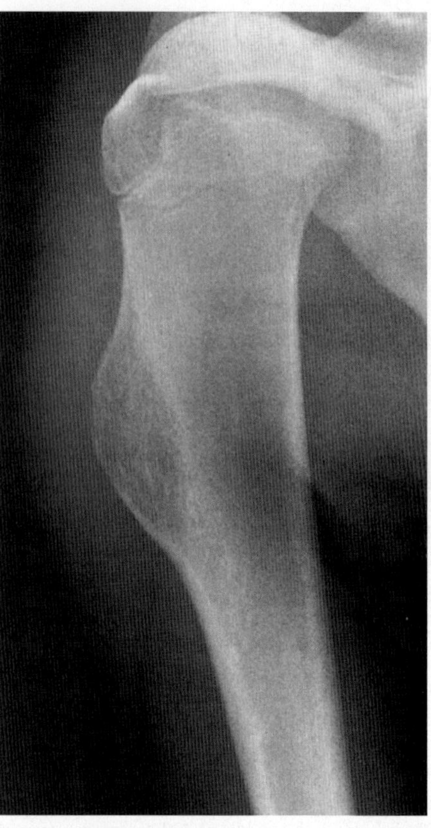

FIGURE 69-2 AP view of the proximal humerus. There is a sessile osteochondroma on the lateral aspect of this child's humerus. (From Chen MYM, Pope TL, Ott DJ. *Basic Radiology*. 2nd ed. www.accessmedicine.com. Copyright © The McGraw-Hill Companies, Inc. All rights reserved.)

- Altered sensation predisposing patient to injury
- Lost or altered ability to work and participate in leisure activity

Possible Contributing Causes

- Cause usually unknown
- Genetic mutation
- Trauma for detection

Differential Diagnosis

- Degenerative or protruding disc
- Fracture
- Gall bladder, kidney, or stomach/intestinal disease
- Leukemia
- Lymphoma
- Muscle strain
- Myeloma
- Spondylitis
- Stenosis

MEANS OF CONFIRMATION OR DIAGNOSIS

Laboratory Tests

- Complete blood count (CBC)
- Urinalysis
- Erythrocyte sedimentation rate (ESR)
- Serum calcium
- Phosphorus
- Alkaline phosphatase
- Serum protein electrophoresis
- Lactic dehydrogenase

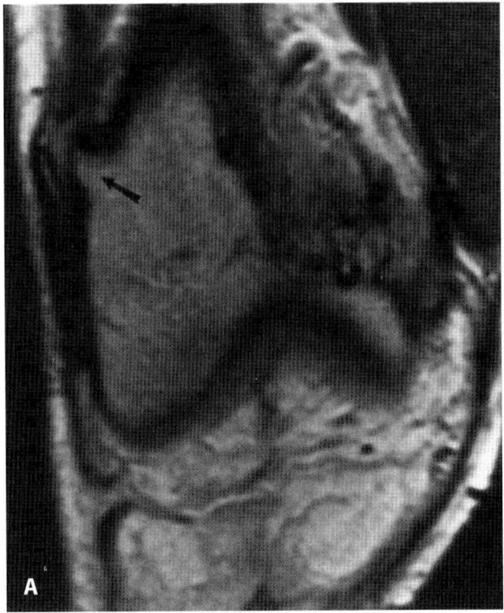

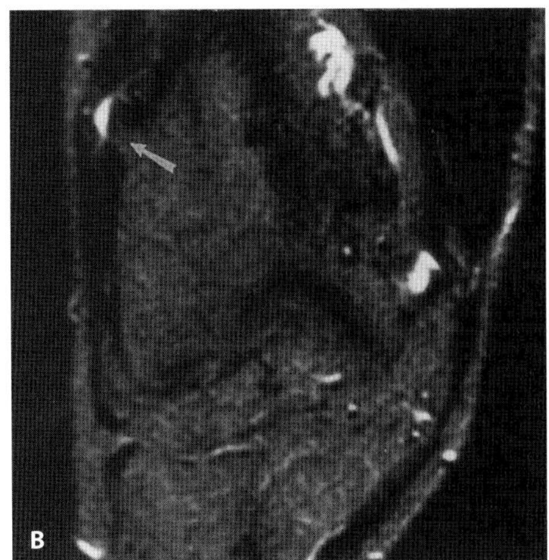

FIGURE 69-3 (**A, B**) Proton-density (**A**) and T2-weighted (**B**) coronal MR images of the knee. A very tiny osteochondroma arises from the lateral metaphysis of the distal femur (*arrow*). Notice that the signal intensity (*shade of gray*) inside this diminutive tumor is the same as that of the adjoining marrow space. The bright area over the osteochondroma in Figure 70-3B represents a small, fluid-filled bursa. This patient complained of a snapping sensation which most likely was due to movement of the iliotibial band back and forth over the osteochondroma. (From Chen MYM, Pope TL, Ott DJ. *Basic Radiology*. 2nd ed. www.accessmedicine.com. Copyright © The McGraw-Hill Companies, Inc. All rights reserved.)

Imaging

- Radiographs
- Radionuclide bone scan (scintigraphy)
- CT scan with contrast[3]
- MRI, more sensitive in defining the extent of the primary tumor[3]
- Angiography
- Ultrasonography

Diagnostic Procedures

- Biopsy

FINDINGS AND INTERPRETATION

- ESR
  - Elevated in Ewing sarcoma
- Serum calcium
  - Elevated in metastatic bone disease

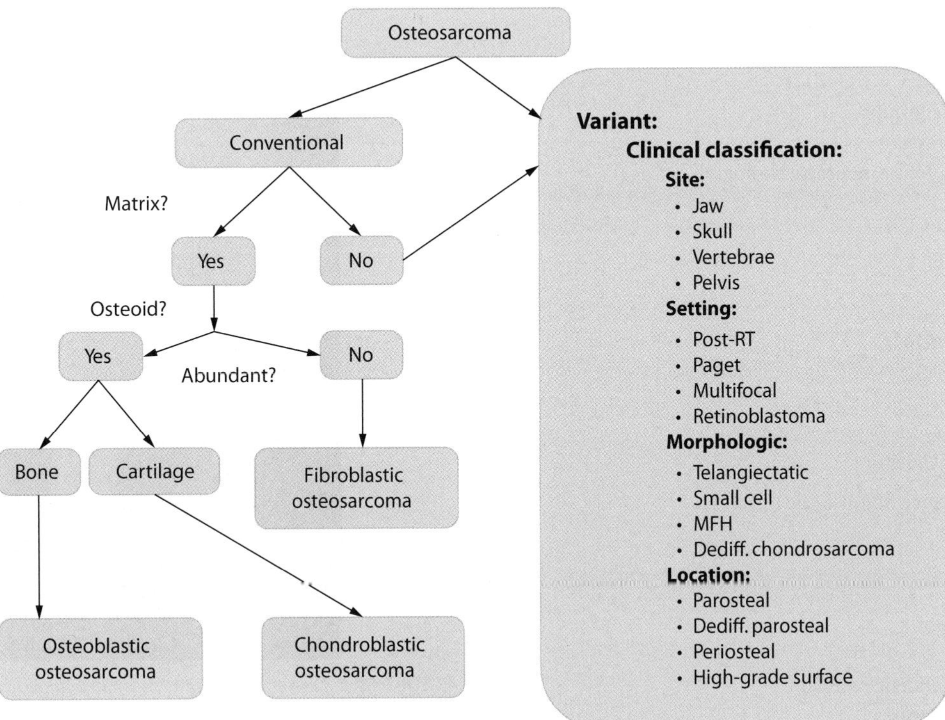

FIGURE 69-4 Flowchart of osteosarcoma: pathologic diagnosis rationale. (From Kantarjian HM, Wolff RA, Koller CA. *The MD Anderson Manual of Medical Oncology*. 2nd ed. www.accessmedicine.com. Copyright © The McGraw-Hill Companies, Inc. All rights reserved.)

- Phosphorus
  - Decreased with "brown tumors" associated with hyperthyroidism
- Alkaline phosphatase
  - Elevated in osteosarcoma and Paget disease
- Serum protein electrophoresis
  - Abnormal in metastatic bone disease
- Lactic dehydrogenase
  - Elevated with osteosarcoma
- Radiographs

TREATMENT

▶ Medication

- Hormonal therapy
- Chemotherapy[3]
  - Doxorubicin
  - Cisplatin
  - Methotrexate
  - Ifosfamide

MEDICAL PROCEDURES

- Tumor resection
  - Marginal excision
  - Wide excision
- Limb salvage
- Stem cell transplantation
- Biologic therapy
- Radiation: Osteosarcomas are highly radioresistant; limited treatment role at this time[3]

REFERRALS/ADMITTANCE

- Neurologist
- Oncologist, neurooncologist
- Spinal cord support group
- Custom durable medical equipment (DME) provider
- Recreational therapy
- Challenged athlete groups
- Occupational therapist
- Counselor, psychologist, neuropsychologist

IMPAIRMENTS

- Posture
- Gait[5]
- Range of motion (ROM)
- Balance
- Aerobic endurance

TESTS AND MEASURES

- Karnofsky Performance Status Scale (KPS)
- Functional strength
- Posture
- Sensory integrity
- Functional Measures
  - Barthel index
  - Functional independence measure
- Gait and balance measures
  - Tinetti
  - Motor assessment scale

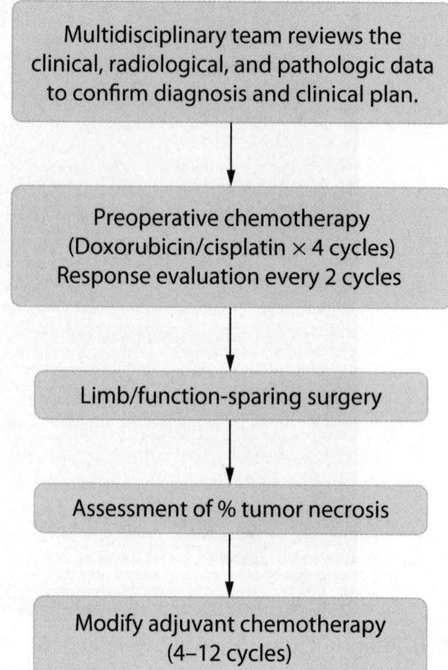

FIGURE 69-5 Treatment approach for patients with osteosarcoma/malignant fibrous histiocytoma/dedifferentiated chondrosarcoma. (From Kantarjian HM, Wolff RA, Koller CA. *The MD Anderson Manual of Medical Oncology*. 2nd ed. www.accessmedicine.com. Copyright © The McGraw-Hill Companies, Inc. All rights reserved.)

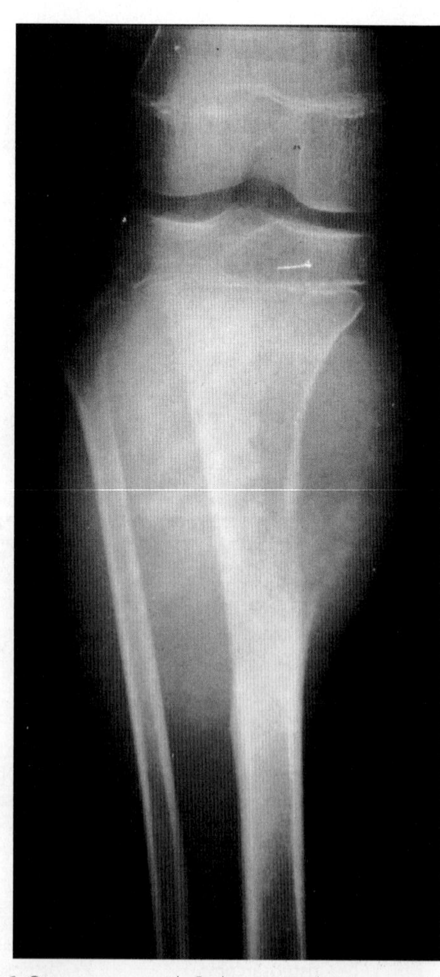

FIGURE 69-6 Osteosarcoma with Codman triangle, a new area of subperiosteal bone formed when a tumor raises the periosteum away from the bone. (From Doherty GM. *Current Diagnosis & Treatment: Surgery*. 13th ed.; www.accessmedicine.com. Copyright © The McGraw-Hill Companies, Inc. All rights reserved.)

    - Gait assessment rating scale
    - Rancho Los Amigo Observational Gait Analysis
    - 6-minute walk test
- Multi-directional reach test
- Active and passive ROM; flexibility
- Pain scale

INTERVENTION

- Pain management
- Strengthening exercises
- Aerobic conditioning
- ROM exercises
- Scar management

FUNCTIONAL GOALS

- Due to the variability of location and extent of the tumor, goals will need to be very specific to the patient. These goals are very general and relate to general functional mobility.
- Short-term goals
    - The patient will be able to
        - Perform wheelchair to/from bed transfer via sit (lateral) pivot with minimal assist and moderate verbal cues for sequencing in order to increase safe functional mobility on returning home.
        - Transition sit to and from stand from a 90-degree hip angle with and contact guard assist consistently to increase safe functional mobility.
        - Ambulate more than 50 feet with minimal assistance and appropriate assistive device to improve mobility in preparation to return home.
        - Tolerate 8 minutes of continuous exercise without exceeding a Borg perceived exertion rating of greater than 12 to improve cardiovascular endurance and increase tolerance for daily activity.
- Long-term goals
    - The patient will be able to
        - Improve Berg Balance Scale score to greater than or equal to 50/56 to demonstrate a decreased fall risk during functional activities.
        - Ambulate on a variety of indoor/outdoor surfaces with distant supervision and assistive device as needed to maximize safe and functional ambulation and return to appropriate premorbid activities.
        - The patient will tolerate 15 minutes of continuous activity without exceeding a Borg perceived exertion rating of greater than 12.
        - Patient will carry one load of groceries weighing <15 lb without significant dyspnea, as measured by patient report of 3 or lower on Borg Dyspnea Scale.

PROGNOSIS

- Varies, on the basis of the extent of tumor, speed of growth, location, and time from onset to medical intervention.

PATIENT RESOURCE

- Osteosarcoma. American Cancer Society. http://www.cancer.org/cancer/osteosarcoma/index. Accessed July 14, 2013.

REFERENCES

1. The American Physical Therapy Association. Pattern 4E: impaired joint mobility, motor function, muscle performance, and range of motion associated with localized inflammation. *Interactive Guide to Physical Therapist Practice.* 2003. doi: 10.2522/ptguide.3.1_5. http://guidetoptpractice.apta.org/content/1/SEC12.extract?sid=f5461de3-99ce-4f0a-9b25-18549885b18e. Accessed May 6, 2014.
2. The American Physical Therapy Association. Pattern 6B: impaired aerobic capacity/endurance associated with deconditioning. *Interactive Guide to Physical Therapist Practice.* 2003. doi: 10.2522/ptguide.3.3_2. http://guidetoptpractice.apta.org/content/1/SEC28.extract?sid=b615195c-10f9-432c-b2f1-70ce116681c1. Accessed May 6, 2014.
3. Hay WW, Levin MJ, Sondheimer JM, Deterding RR. Major pediatric neoplastic diseases. In: Hay WW, Levin MJ, Sondheimer JM, Deterding RR, eds. *CURRENT Diagnosis & Treatment: Pediatrics.* 20th ed. New York, NY: McGraw-Hill; 2011. http://www.accessphysiotherapy.com/content/6587229. Accessed July 14, 2013.
4. Waxman SG. *Clinical Neuroanatomy.* New York, NY: McGraw-Hill; 2010. http://www.accessphysiotherapy.com/resource/22. Accessed July 14, 2013.
5. Shamus E, Stern DF. *Effective Documentation for Physical Therapy Professionals.* 2nd ed. New York, NY: McGraw-Hill; 2011. http://www.accessphysiotherapy.com/resource/696. Accessed July 14, 2013.

ADDITIONAL REFERENCES

- Bernstein M, Kovar H, Paulussen M, et al. Ewing's sarcoma family of tumors: current management. *Oncologist.* 2006;11:503–519.
- Dutton M. Pediatric physical therapy. In: Dutton M, ed. *McGraw-Hill's NPTE (National Physical Therapy Examination).* 2nd ed. New York, NY: McGraw-Hill; 2012. http://www.accessphysiotherapy.com/content/5404760. Accessed July 14, 2013.
- Grimer RJ. Surgical options for children with osteosarcoma. *Lancet Oncol.* 2005;6(2):85–92.
- Heare T, Hensley MA, Dell'Orfano S. Bone tumors: osteosarcoma and Ewing's sarcoma. *Curr Opin Pediatr.* 2009;21(3):365–372.
- ICD9DATA. http://www.icd9data.com. Accessed June 16, 2013.
- ICD10DATA. http://www.icd10data.com. Accessed June 16, 2013.
- Malone TR, Hazle C, Grey ML. Imaging of the pelvis and hip. In: Malone TR, Hazle C, Grey ML, eds. *Imaging in Rehabilitation.* New York, NY: McGraw-Hill; 2008. http://www.accessphysiotherapy.com/content/5941062. Accessed July 14, 2013.
- Maloney K, Foreman NK, Giller RH, et al. Neoplastic disease. In: Hay WW, Levin MJ, Sondheimer JM, Deterding RR, eds. *CURRENT Diagnosis & Treatment: Pediatrics.* 20th ed. New York, NY: McGraw-Hill; 2011. http://www.accessphysiotherapy.com/content/6587229. Accessed July 14, 2013.

SECTION N RESPIRATORY DISORDERS

70 ASTHMA

Angela S. Garcia, PharmD, MPH, CPh
Eric Shamus, PhD, DPT, PT, CSCS

CONDITION/DISORDER SYNONYMS

- Extrinsic asthma
- Intrinsic asthma
- Exercise-induced asthma
- Asthmatic bronchitis
- Bronchial asthma
- Bronchial hyperresponsiveness
- Chronic lung disease

ICD-9-CM CODES

- 493.00 Extrinsic asthma, unspecified
- 493.01 Extrinsic asthma with status asthmaticus
- 493.02 Extrinsic asthma with (acute) exacerbation
- 493.10 Intrinsic asthma, unspecified
- 493.11 Intrinsic asthma with status asthmaticus
- 493.12 Intrinsic asthma with (acute) exacerbation
- 493.20 Chronic obstructive asthma, unspecified
- 493.21 Chronic obstructive asthma with status asthmaticus
- 493.22 Chronic obstructive asthma with (acute) exacerbation
- 493.81 Exercise induced bronchospasm
- 493.82 Cough variant asthma
- 493.90 Asthma unspecified type, unspecified
- 493.91 Asthma unspecified type with status asthmaticus
- 493.92 Asthma, unspecified type, with (acute) exacerbation
- 780.7 Malaise and fatigue
- 786.0 Dyspnea and respiratory abnormalities
- 786.05 Shortness of breath

ICD-10-CM CODES

- J44.9 Chronic obstructive pulmonary disease, unspecified
- J44.0 Chronic obstructive pulmonary disease with acute lower respiratory infection
- J44.1 Chronic obstructive pulmonary disease with (acute) exacerbation
- J45.20 Mild intermittent asthma, uncomplicated
- J45.22 Mild intermittent asthma with status asthmaticus
- J45.21 Mild intermittent asthma with (acute) exacerbation
- J45.901 Unspecified asthma with (acute) exacerbation
- J45.902 Unspecified asthma with status asthmaticus
- J45.909 Unspecified asthma, uncomplicated
- J45.990 Exercise induced bronchospasm
- J45.991 Cough variant asthma
- J45.998 Other asthma

PREFERRED PRACTICE PATTERNS

- 6A: Primary Prevention/Risk Reduction for Cardiovascular/Pulmonary Disorders[1]
- 6B: Impaired Aerobic Capacity/Endurance Associated with Deconditioning[2]
- 6C: Impaired Ventilation, Respiration/Gas Exchange, and Aerobic Capacity/Endurance Associated with Airway Clearance Dysfunction[3]
- 6F: Impaired Ventilation and Respiration/Gas Exchange Associated with Respiratory Failure[4]

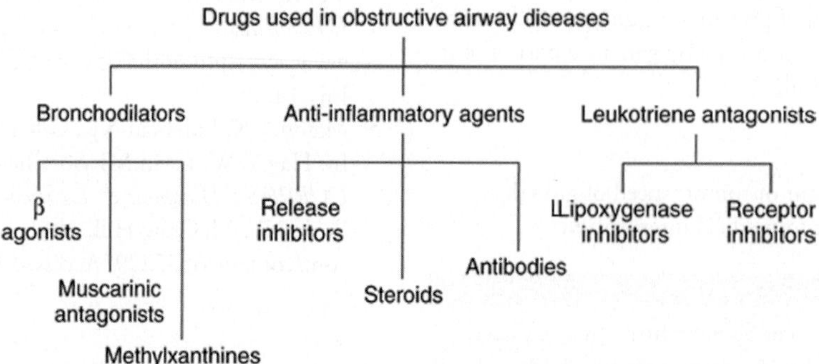

FIGURE 70-1 Drug classes useful in obstructive airway disorders include bronchodilators (smooth muscle relaxants) and anti-inflammatory drugs. Bronchodilators include beta$_2$-selective agonists, muscarinic antagonists, and methylxanthines. Anti-inflammatory drugs include mast cell release inhibitors, corticosteroids, and an anti-IgE antibody. Leukotriene antagonists have both bronchodilator and anti-inflammatory mechanisms of action. (From Panus PC, Katzung BG, Jobst EE, Tinsley S, Masters SB, Trevor AJ. *Pharmacology for the Physical Therapist*. New York, NY: McGraw-Hill; 2009.)

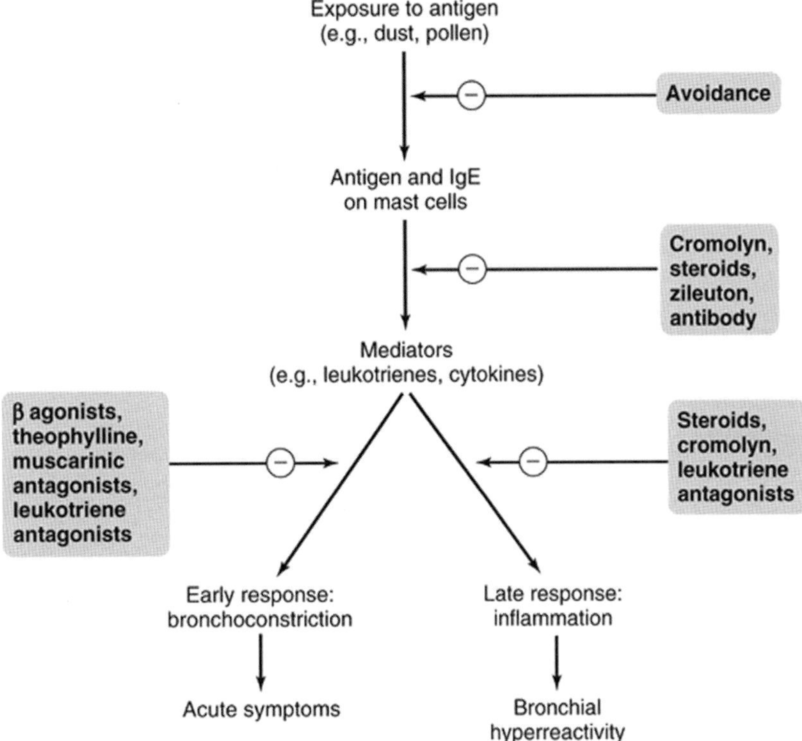

FIGURE 70-2 Summary of treatment strategies in asthma. (Reproduced with permission from Cockcroft DW. The bronchial late response in the pathogenesis of asthma and its modulation by therapy. *Ann Allergy*. 1985;55:857.)

PATIENT PRESENTATION

A 37-year-old nonsmoking man complains of a 3-month history of a nonproductive cough that is worse at night and with exercise. He does not have fevers or other symptoms to suggest infection. He is normotensive, and his lungs are clear to auscultation bilaterally, except for an occasional expiratory wheeze on forced expiration. A chest radiograph is read as normal.[5]

KEY FEATURES

Description

- Form of bronchial disorder associated with airway obstruction, marked by recurrent attacks of paroxysmal dyspnea, with wheezing due to spasmodic contraction of the bronchi.[6–8]
- Chronic respiratory disease manifested as difficulty breathing due to the narrowing of bronchial passageways.
- Chronic lung disease that inflames and narrows the airways leading to recurrent periods of wheezing, chest tightness, shortness of breath, and cough.
- Coughing often occurs at night or early in the morning, but may go unnoticed during the day or be considered an allergic response to an inhaled (airborne or environmental) trigger.
- Affects people of all ages, but most often starts during childhood.
- More than 22 million people are known to have asthma in the United States; nearly 6 million are children.[6]
- People with asthma have inflamed airways, which may become sensitive and tend to react strongly to certain inhaled substances.
- When airways react, the muscles around them tighten, narrowing the lumen wall leading to less air-flow into the lungs; swelling of the lumen may result in narrowing, leading to further restriction and triggering a cascade of cells to thicken mucus or increase mucus production.
- Symptoms may be mild and self-resolve or require minimal treatment with prescription medication; some symptoms are persistent and require ongoing prescription medication for control.
- Symptom recognition is important, to prevent long-term damage.

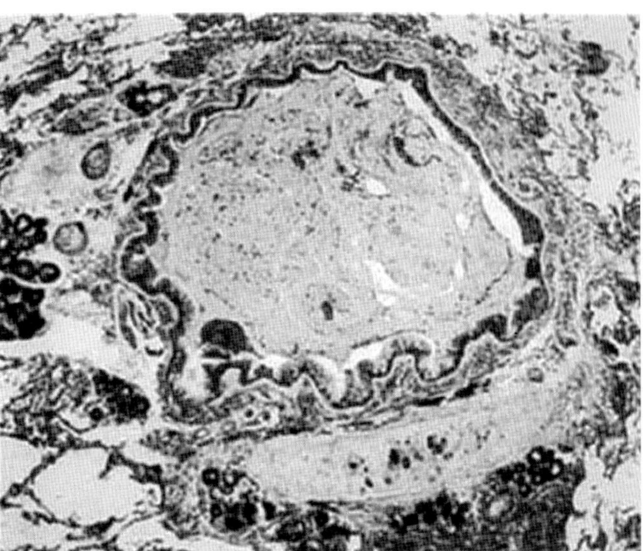

FIGURE 70-3 Bronchial asthma, showing a small bronchus filled with a plug of viscid mucus and inflammatory cells. (From Chandrasoma P, Taylor CR. *Concise Pathology*. 3rd ed. www.accessmedicine.com. Copyright © The McGraw-Hill Companies, Inc. All rights reserved.)

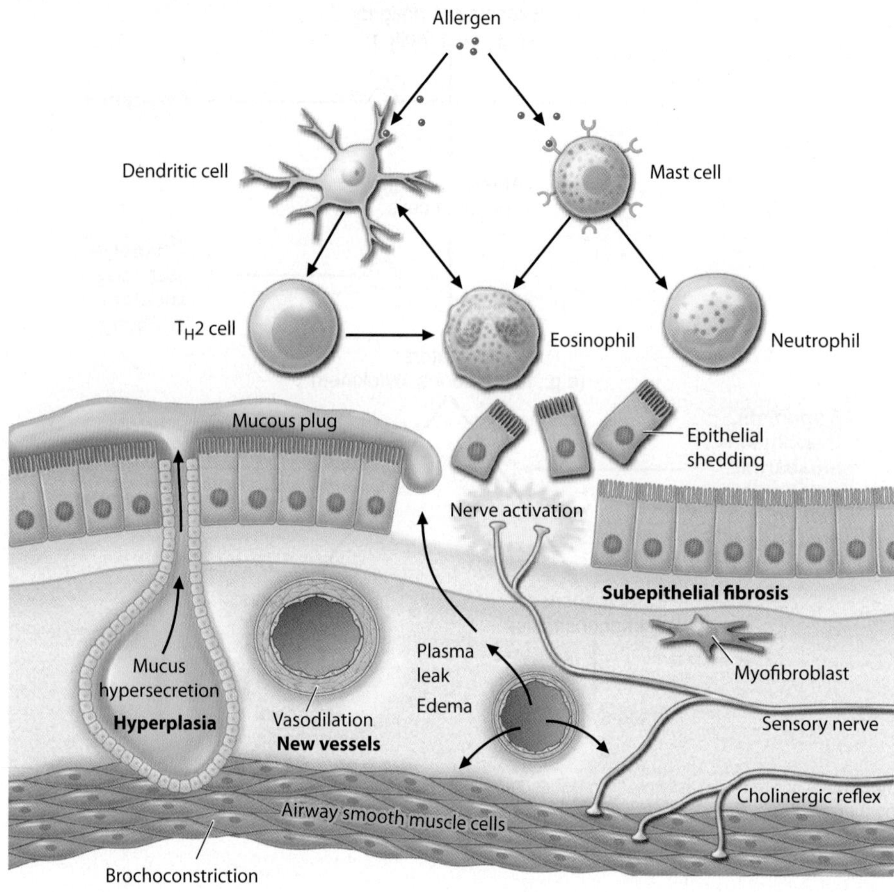

FIGURE 70-4 The pathophysiology of asthma is complex with participation of several interacting inflammatory cells, which result in acute and chronic inflammatory effects on the airway. (From Longo DL, Fauci AS, Kasper DL, Hauser SL, Jameson JL, Loscalzo J, eds. *Harrison's Principles of Internal Medicine*. 18th ed. New York, NY:McGraw-Hill; 2012.)

- Children often have difficulties expressing symptoms of an attack, so adults must be aware of a child's presentation so that treatment can be initiated to prevent a severe attack, which may require emergency care or be fatal
- Comorbidities may exacerbate the symptoms or make management more difficult (sleep apnea, reflux disease, upper respiratory infections, psychological stress, etc.)
- Common allergens include dust mites, cockroaches, animal dander, seasonal pollens; reducing exposure to these may reduce clinical symptoms or exacerbations of asthma

Essentials of Diagnosis

- Guidelines[6–8]
  - EPR-3 (Expert Panel Report 3rd revision)
  - National Institutes of Health
- Previous life-threatening asthma attack
- Episodic or chronic symptoms of airflow obstruction
- Medical history indicative of hallmark symptoms or worsening condition over time
- Prolonged expiration and diffuse wheezes on physical examination
- Reversibility of airflow obstruction, either spontaneously or following bronchodilator therapy
- Limitation of airflow on pulmonary function testing or positive bronchoprovocation challenge

General Considerations

- Assessing asthma control, classifying severity of exacerbations, and responsiveness to pharmacotherapy are critical to initiating treatment and successful management of the disease[7,9]
- Classifying severity of asthma exacerbations involves
  - Mild, moderate, or severe with a subset of life-threatening
  - Symptoms and signs are reflective of worsening dyspnea, changes in initial peak expiratory flow (compared to predicted or personal best)
  - Response to short-acting beta-agonist treatment before the emergency department (at home or in transit)

Demographics

- Minorities have increased risk for incidence and prevalence
- Among children, more common in boys than girls; among adults, more common in women

CLINICAL FINDINGS

SIGNS AND SYMPTOMS

- Hallmark signs (not required to be present): Coughing; which may be worse at night, wheezing, chest tightness, shortness of breath[6–8]
- These symptoms may be a temporary response or secondary to some exposure, but do not equate with having asthma.

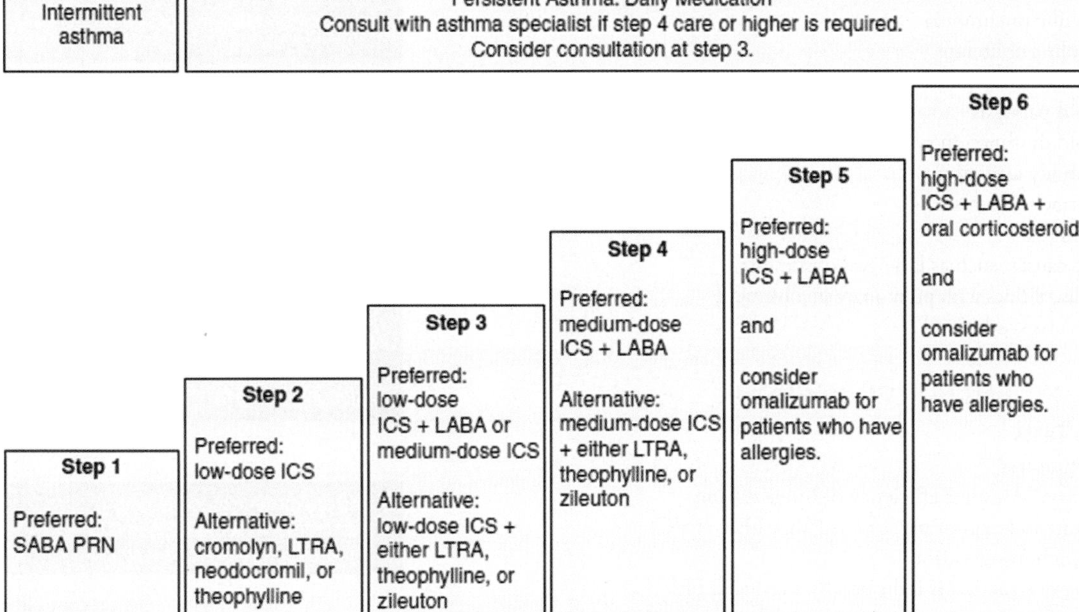

FIGURE 70-5 Stepwise approach for managing asthma in adults and youths 12 years of age or older.
Alphabetical order is used when more than one treatment option is listed within either preferred or alternative therapy.
Notes:
- *The stepwise approach is meant to assist, not replace, the clinical decision-making required to meet individual patient needs.*
- *If alternative treatment is used and response is inadequate, discontinue it, and use the preferred treatment before stepping up.*
- *Zileuton is a less desirable alternative due to limited studies as adjunctive therapy and the need to monitor liver function. Theophylline requires monitoring of serum concentration levels.*
- *In step 6, before oral corticosteroids are introduced, a trial of high-dose ICS + LABA + either LTRA, theophylline, or zileuton may be considered, although this approach has not been studied in clinical trials.*
- *Clinicians who administer immunotherapy or omalizumab should be prepared and equipped to identify and treat anaphylaxis that may occur.*

ICS, inhaled corticosteroid; LABA, long-acting inhaled beta$_2$-agonist; LTRA, leukotriene receptor antagonist; SABA, inhaled short acting beta$_2$-agonist. (From the Guidelines for the Diagnosis and Management of Asthma of the National Asthma Education and Prevention Program (NAEPP) Expert Panel Report 3, 2007.)

Functional Implications

- Type, frequency, and severity of asthma symptoms may vary over time between absent or unnoticeable to severe with life-threatening exacerbations[6–8]

Possible Contributing Causes

- Use of medications known to increase risk for bronchospasm[6–8]
- Certain comorbid diseases
- Inherited tendency toward allergies (atopy) is the strongest identifiable predisposing factor for development of asthma; not all people with asthma have allergies
- Parents who have asthma
- Certain respiratory infections during childhood
- Contact with some airborne allergens, exposure to some viral infections in infancy or early childhood when the immune system is developing
- Contact with certain chemicals or irritants (industrial or environmental exposures)
- Eczema

Differential Diagnosis

- Lower airway disorders[7]
  - Chronic obstructive pulmonary disease (COPD)
  - Bronchiectasis
  - Allergic bronchopulmonary mycosis

- Cystic fibrosis
- Eosinophilic pneumonia
- Bronchiolitis obliterans
- Upper airway disorders[7]
  - Vocal fold paralysis
  - Vocal fold dysfunction syndrome
  - Foreign body aspiration
  - Laryngotracheal masses
  - Airway edema
- Psychiatric causes, such as laryngeal dyskinesia
- Systemic vasculitides with pulmonary involvement (Churg–Strauss syndrome)

MEANS OF CONFIRMATION OR DIAGNOSIS

Laboratory Tests

- Lung function test[6–8]
  - Spirometry: Measures efficiency of lungs during inspiration and expiration (FEV_1, FVC, FEV_1/FVC) with bronchoprovocation
    - Airflow obstruction is indicated by a reduced FEV_1/FVC ratio
  - Body plethysmography
- Significant reversibility of airflow obstruction is indicated by increased FEV_1 and FVC after inhalation of bronchodilator therapy[6–8]
- Arterial blood gas and pH[6–8]
- Peak expiratory flow[6–8]

Imaging

- Chest radiograph[6–8]
- EKG[6–8]

Diagnostics Procedures

- Medical history and physical examination
- Allergy testing
- Usually done in children aged 5 years or older

FINDINGS AND INTERPRETATION

- Mortality rates increase with recurrent, uncontrolled exacerbations and exposure to triggers
- Reversibility of airway obstruction decreases with repeated exacerbations or uncontrolled inflammation and may develop into irreversible obstructive lung diseases

TREATMENT

Medication

- Goals of pharmacotherapy are to reduce airway constriction or bronchospasm and prevent recurrent inflammation that may lead to irreversible lung damage if not properly controlled[6–8]
- Rescue medication: Acute symptoms (bronchoconstriction)[6–8]
  - Inhaled short-acting beta-agonist
  - Inhaled anticholinergics
  - Systemic corticosteroids (oral or IV)
- Controller medication: Chronic symptoms (inflammation)[6,8]
  - Inhaled corticosteroids
  - Inhaled long-acting beta-agonist

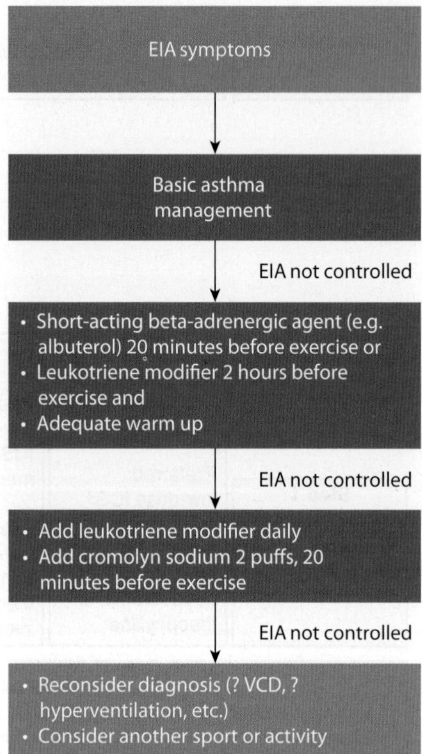

FIGURE 70-6 Flow diagram for the treatment of exercise-induced asthma. (From Patel DR, Greydanus DE, Baker RJ. *Pediatric Practice: Sports Medicine*. www.accesspediatrics.com Copyright © The McGraw-Hill Companies, Inc. All rights reserved.)

  - Leukotriene modifiers
  - Long-acting bronchodilators (mediator inhibitors)
  - Recombinant antibody
- Antihistamines[6,8]

MEDICAL PROCEDURES

- Immunizations highly recommended (influenza, pneumococcal)[6,8]
- Trigger recognition and avoidance are critical to avoiding or preventing exacerbations[6,8]
- Rehabilitative therapy[6,8]
  - Breathing technique and stress management may decrease risk of exacerbation or improve lung function

REFERRALS/ADMITTANCE

- To pulmonologist
- To allergist
- To respiratory therapist
- To pharmacist

IMPAIRMENTS

- Physical impairment
  - Lung function
  - Normal activity or exercise tolerance
  - Sleep
  - Memory

- Prophylaxis during surgery may be necessary to avoid respiratory complications
- Pregnancy complications and oxygen flow to the baby (potential issues of low-birth-weight babies)
- Activity limitations
  - Self-care
- Quality of life (QoL) and health-related quality of life (HQoL)
  - May be diminished with uncontrolled asthma for the patient and family
- Environment and adjustments
  - Indoor air quality
  - Environmental pollutants

TESTS AND MEASURES

- Spirometry
- X-ray
- Peak flow meter

INTERVENTION

- Patient education and lifestyle changes
- Chest physical therapy
- Manual therapy to loosen congestion in the lungs
- Exercise (aerobic, strength, flexibility, posture, breathing)
- Airway clearance
- Pursed-lip breathing
- Coughing techniques
- Pulmonary rehabilitation (PR)[9]
  - Improves exercise capacity
- Inspiratory muscle training (IMT)

FUNCTIONAL GOALS

- Patient will be able to
  - Ambulate over 600 m in a 6-minute walk test.
  - Score above 80% of their predicted FEV_1 score.
  - Tolerate 1 hour of moderate exercise three times a week.
  - Achieve symptom and exacerbation prevention.
  - Increase respiratory level to normal pulmonary function.
  - Achieve optimized activity levels.

PROGNOSIS

- Very good.
- Asthma cannot be cured but can be successfully managed; asthma exacerbations can occur at any time, even without the presence of symptoms.
- National Heart, Lung, and Blood Institute (NHLBI) maintains ongoing research aimed at prevention and treatment of heart, lung, and blood diseases, has led to advances in medical knowledge and management of chronic lung diseases such as asthma.[6,8]

PATIENT RESOURCES

- American Asthma Foundation. http://www.americanasthmafoundation.org. Accessed June 17, 2013.
- Asthma and Allergy Foundation of America. http://www.aafa.org. Accessed June 17, 2013.
- National Heart and Lung Institute, National Institute of Health. What is asthma? http://www.nhlbi.nih.gov/health/health-topics/topics/asthma/. Accessed June 17, 2013.
- World Asthma Foundation. http://worldasthmafoundation.org/. Accessed June 17, 2013.

REFERENCES

1. The American Physical Therapy Association. Pattern 6A: primary prevention/risk reduction for cardiovascular/pulmonary disorders. *Interactive Guide to Physical Therapist Practice.* 2003. doi: 10.2522/ptguide.3.3_1. http://guidetoptpractice.apta.org/content/1/SEC27.extract?sid=bdee9b9c-7de0-412b-bb5c-daade0f852e2. Accessed May 6, 2014.
2. The American Physical Therapy Association. Pattern 6B: impaired aerobic capacity/endurance associated with deconditioning. *Interactive Guide to Physical Therapist Practice.* 2003. doi: 10.2522/ptguide.3.3_2. http://guidetoptpractice.apta.org/content/1/SEC28.extract?sid=86db7488-0373-439e-a256-4f779b081866. Accessed May 6, 2014.
3. The American Physical Therapy Association. Pattern 6C: impaired ventilation, respiration/gas exchange, and aerobic capacity/endurance associated with airway clearance dysfunction. *Interactive Guide to Physical Therapist Practice.* 2003. doi: 10.2522/ptguide.3.3_3. http://guidetoptpractice.apta.org/content/1/SEC29.extract?sid=ede5cb60-c2b9-4da5-8446-fc9fa4616c0d. Accessed May 6, 2014.
4. The American Physical Therapy Association. Pattern 6F: impaired ventilation and respiration/gas exchange associated with respiratory failure. *Interactive Guide to Physical Therapist Practice.* 2003. doi: 10.2522/ptguide.3.3_6. http://guidetoptpractice.apta.org/content/1/SEC32.extract?sid=6ebaffc7-f596-4c8c-a286-342e52371352. Accessed May 6, 2014.
5. McPhee Sj, Hammer GD. Case 81. In: McPhee Sj, Hammer GD, eds. *Pathophysiology of Disease: An Introduction to Clinical Medicine.* 6th ed. New York, NY: McGraw-Hill; 2010. http://www.accessphysiotherapy.com/resource/17. Accessed June 17, 2013.
6. National Heart and Lung Institute, National Institute of Health. What is asthma? http://www.nhlbi.nih.gov/health/health-topics/topics/asthma/. Accessed June 17, 2013.
7. AccessMedicine. Asthma. Quick Answers to Medical Diagnosis and Therapy. http://www.accessmedicine.com/quickam.aspx. Accessed January 5, 2013.
8. National Asthma Education and Prevention Program. Expert Panel Report 3: Guidelines for the Diagnosis and Management of Asthma. *National Institutes of Health Pub.* No. 08-4051. Bethesda, MD; 2007. http://www.nhlbi.nih.gov/guidelines/asthma/asthgdln.htm. Accessed June 17, 2013.
9. Certo CM, DeTurk WE, Cahalin LP. History of cardiopulmonary rehabilitation. In: DeTurk WE, Cahalin LP, eds. *Cardiovascular and Pulmonary Physical Therapy.* 2nd ed. New York, NY; McGraw-Hill: 2011. http://www.accessphysiotherapy.com/abstract/6870102#6870104. Accessed June 17, 2013.

ADDITIONAL REFERENCES

- Goodman CC, Fuller KS. *Pathology Implications for the Physical Therapist.* 3rd ed. St. Louis, MO: Saunders; 2009.

- Goodman CC, Snyder TK. *Differential Diagnosis for Physical Therapists: Screening for Referral.* 4th ed. St. Louis, MO: Saunders; 2007.
- ICD9Data.com. http://www.icd9data.com. Accessed June 17, 2013.
- ICD10Data.com. http://www.icd10data.com. Accessed June 17, 2013.
- Panus PC, Jobst EE, Masters SB, Katzung B, Tinsley SL, Trevor AJ. Drugs affecting the respiratory system. In: Panus PC, Jobst EE, Masters SB, Katzung B, Tinsley SL, Trevor AJ, eds. *Pharmacology for the Physical Therapist.* New York, NY: McGraw-Hill; 2009. http://www.accessphysiotherapy.com/content/6095983. Accessed June 17, 2013.
- Wells Cl. Pulmonary pathology. In: DeTurk WE, Cahalin LP, eds. *Cardiovascular and Pulmonary Physical Therapy: An Evidence-Based Approach.* 2nd ed. New York, NY: McGraw-Hill; 2011. http://www.accessphysiotherapy.com/content/6873405#6873405. Accessed June 17, 2013.
- Williams SG, Schmidt DK, Redd SC, et al. National Asthma Education and Prevention Program. Key clinical activities for quality asthma care. Recommendations of the National Asthma Education and Prevention Program. *MMWR Recomm Rep.* 2003; 52(RR-6):1–8.

71 BRONCHITIS

Eric Shamus, PhD, DPT, PT, CSCS
Marangela Obispo, MSPT, GCS

CONDITION/DISORDER SYNONYMS

- Acute bronchitis
- Inflammation-bronchi

ICD-9-CM CODES

- 466 Acute bronchitis and bronchiolitis
- 490 Bronchitis not specified as acute or chronic
- 491 Chronic bronchitis
- Associated physical therapy diagnosis
  - 780.7 Malaise and fatigue
  - 786.0 Dyspnea and respiratory abnormalities
  - 786.05 Shortness of breath

ICD-10-CM CODES

- J20.9 Acute bronchitis, unspecified
- J41.0 Simple chronic bronchitis

PREFERRED PRACTICE PATTERNS

- 6C: Impaired Ventilation, Respiration/Gas Exchange, and Aerobic Capacity/Endurance Associated With Airway Clearance Dysfunction[1]
- 6F: Impaired Ventilation and Respiration/Gas Exchange Associated With Respiratory Failure[2]

PATIENT PRESENTATION

A 39-year-old female arrives to the clinic with a diagnosis of back pain. She reports difficulty performing her job duties as a waitress in a casino due to symptoms of pain and tiredness. She has been a second-hand smoker for the past 3 years due to her job setting. Patient revealed that she had a mild fever 3 days ago which went away after taking acetaminophen—which she continues to take due to frequent headaches. She also reports onset of a cold approximately 1 week ago with current symptoms of sore throat, productive cough, and chest pain after coughing. She reports presence of sputum when coughing which turned from clear to yellowish in the last 2 days. Upon examination patient presents with normal vital signs with an O_2 saturation of 94% at rest, normal ROM of all extremities and lumbar spine, and normal strength of all extremities. Functional mobility was normal with increased time required mainly due to fatigue. Her breathing sounds were abnormal with wheezing present after coughing. Blood tests, chest x-ray, and sputum culture were normal.

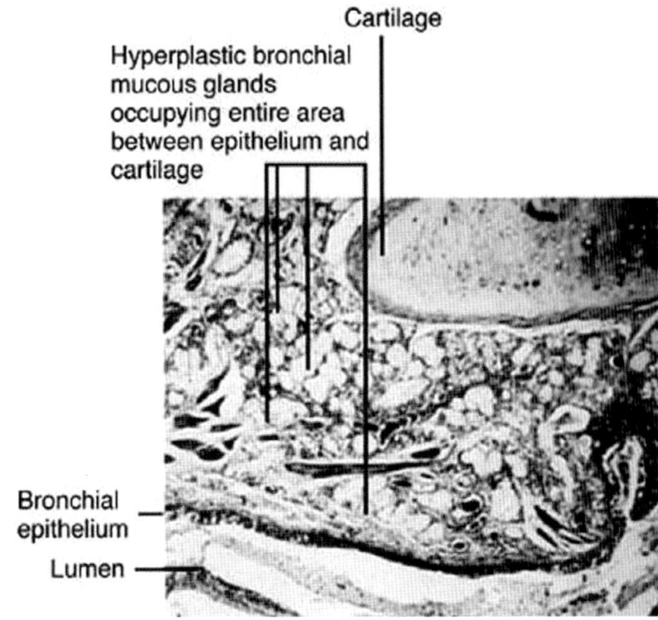

FIGURE 71-1 Chronic bronchitis, showing marked hyperplasia of the bronchial mucous glands. In this case, the glands occupy almost the entire area between the surface epithelium and cartilage, giving a Reid index of almost 1. (From Chandrasoma P, Taylor CR. *Concise Pathology*. 3rd ed. www.accessmedicine.com. Copyright © The McGraw-Hill Companies, Inc. All rights reserved.)

KEY FEATURES

Description

- Inflammation of the air passageways in the lungs
- Categorized as chronic obstructive pulmonary disease (COPD)
- Acute or chronic

Essentials of Diagnosis

- Can be acute or chronic
- Diagnosis based on clinical manifestation
- Acute bronchitis usually after a common cold (viral respiratory infection)
- May get secondary bacterial infection

General Considerations

- Influenza is a systemic illness involving the respiratory tract
- Antibiotics have limited or no role in the treatment of a virus
- Can develop into pneumonia

Demographics

- Infants and young children
- Elderly with weak immune system

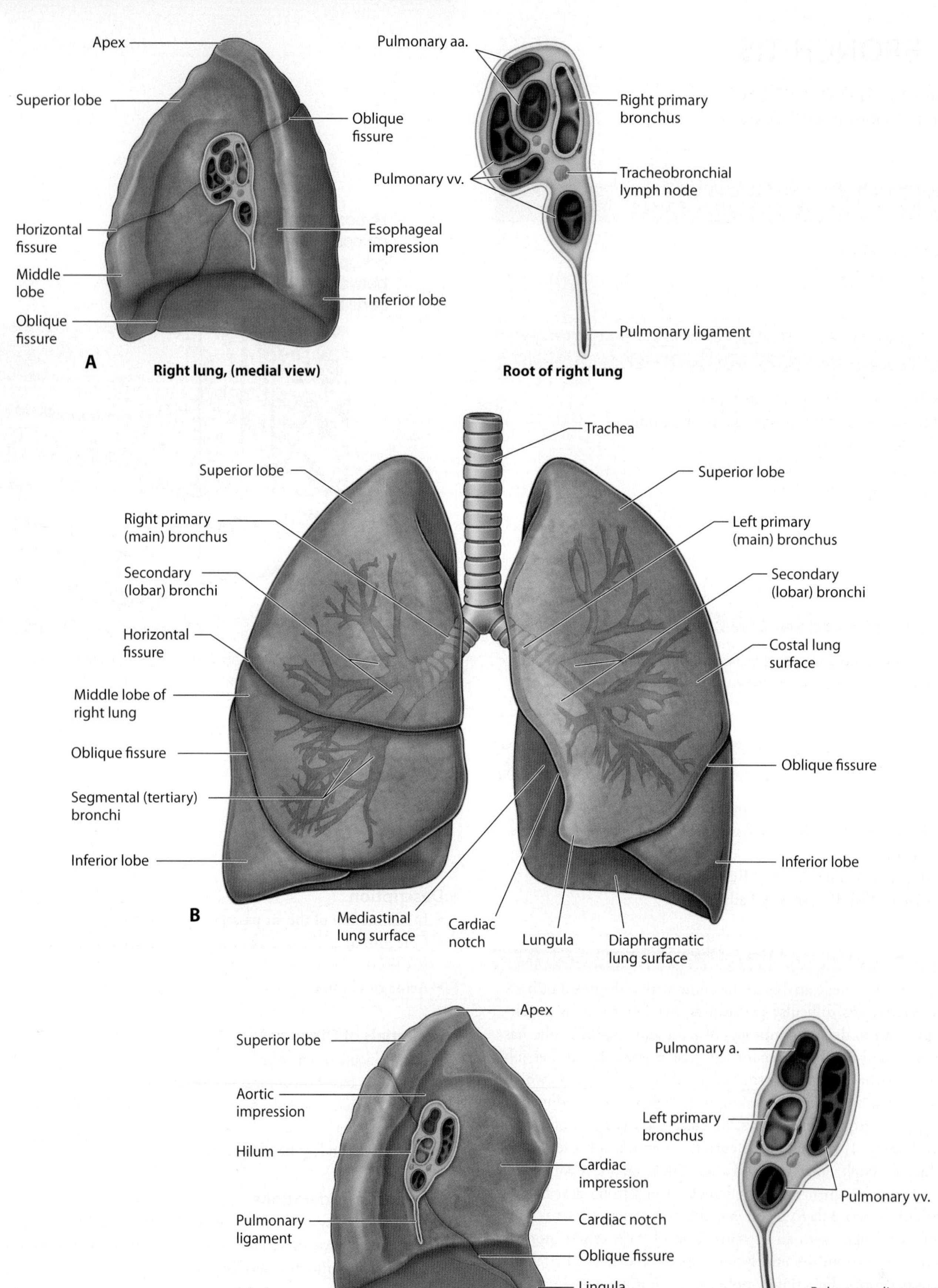

FIGURE 71-2 **A.** Right lung in medial view. **B.** Bronchial tree and lungs. **C.** Left lung in medial view. (From Morton DA, Foreman KB, Albertine KH. *The Big Picture: Gross Anatomy*. www.accessmedicine.com. Copyright © The McGraw-Hill Companies, Inc. All rights reserved.)

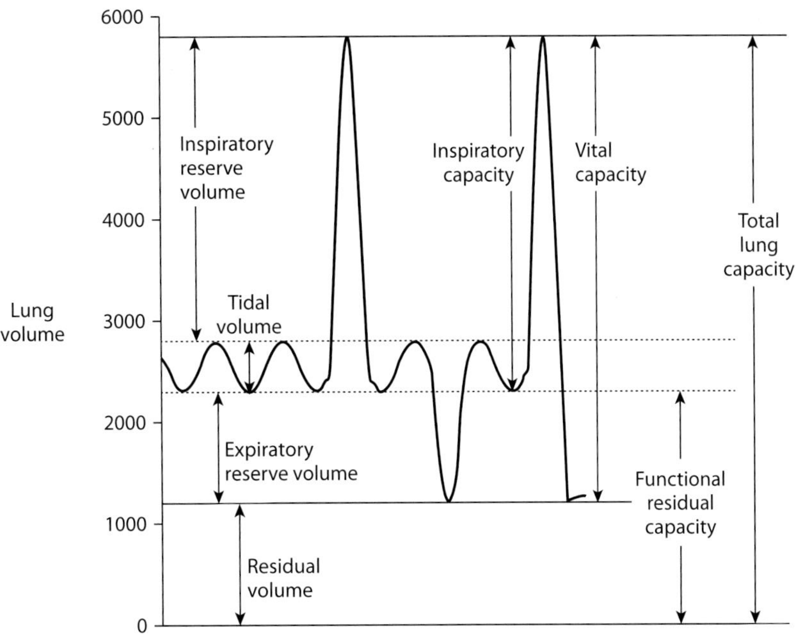

FIGURE 71-3 Pulmonary spirometry. Lung volumes in milliliters are depicted. (From Toy EC, Weisbrodt N, Dubinsky W, O'Neil R, Walters E, Harms K. *Case Files: Physiology*. 2nd ed. www.accessmedicine.com. Copyright © The McGraw-Hill Companies, Inc. All rights reserved.)

CLINICAL FINDINGS

SIGNS AND SYMPTOMS

- Low-grade fever
- Runny nose
- Malaise
- Pleurisy
- Sore throat
- Cough with productive mucus
- Edema
- Chest tightness
- Rales sounds
- Ankle, feet, leg swelling
- Wheezing
- Shoulder raised to allow increased air flow to lungs
- Shortness of breath
- Tensed muscles from dyspnea

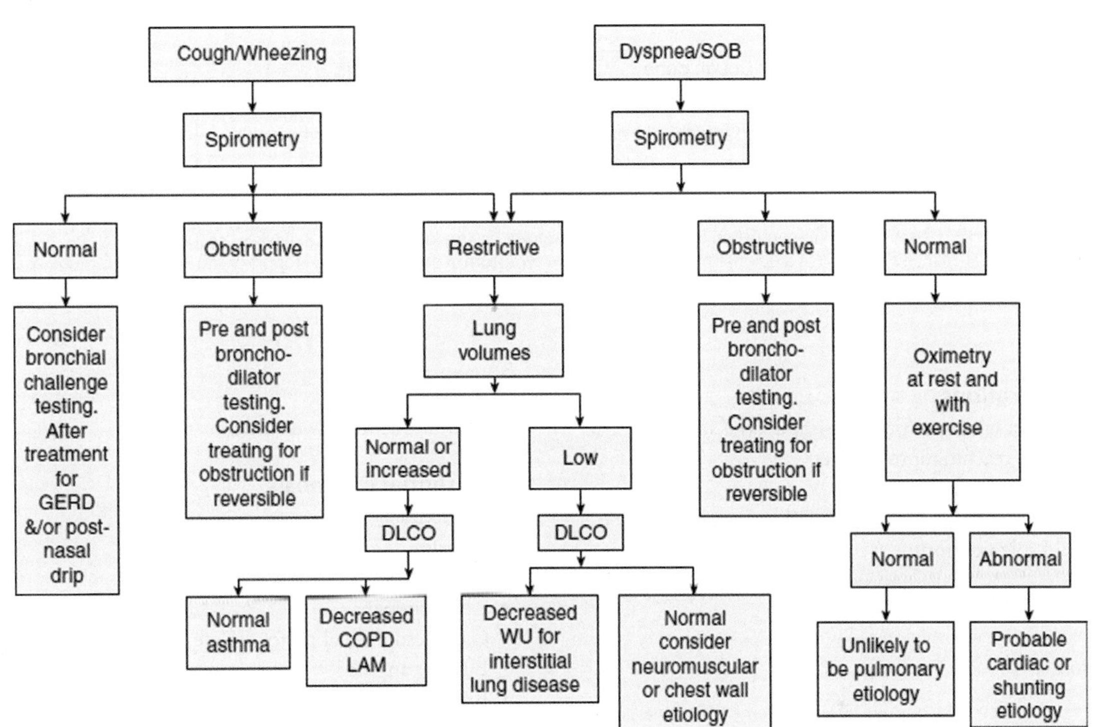

FIGURE 71-4 Assessment of symptoms. (From McKean S, Ross JJ, Dressler DD, Brotman DJ, Ginsberg JS. *Principles and Practice of Hospital Medicine*. www.accessmedicine.com. Copyright © The McGraw-Hill Companies, Inc. All rights reserved.)

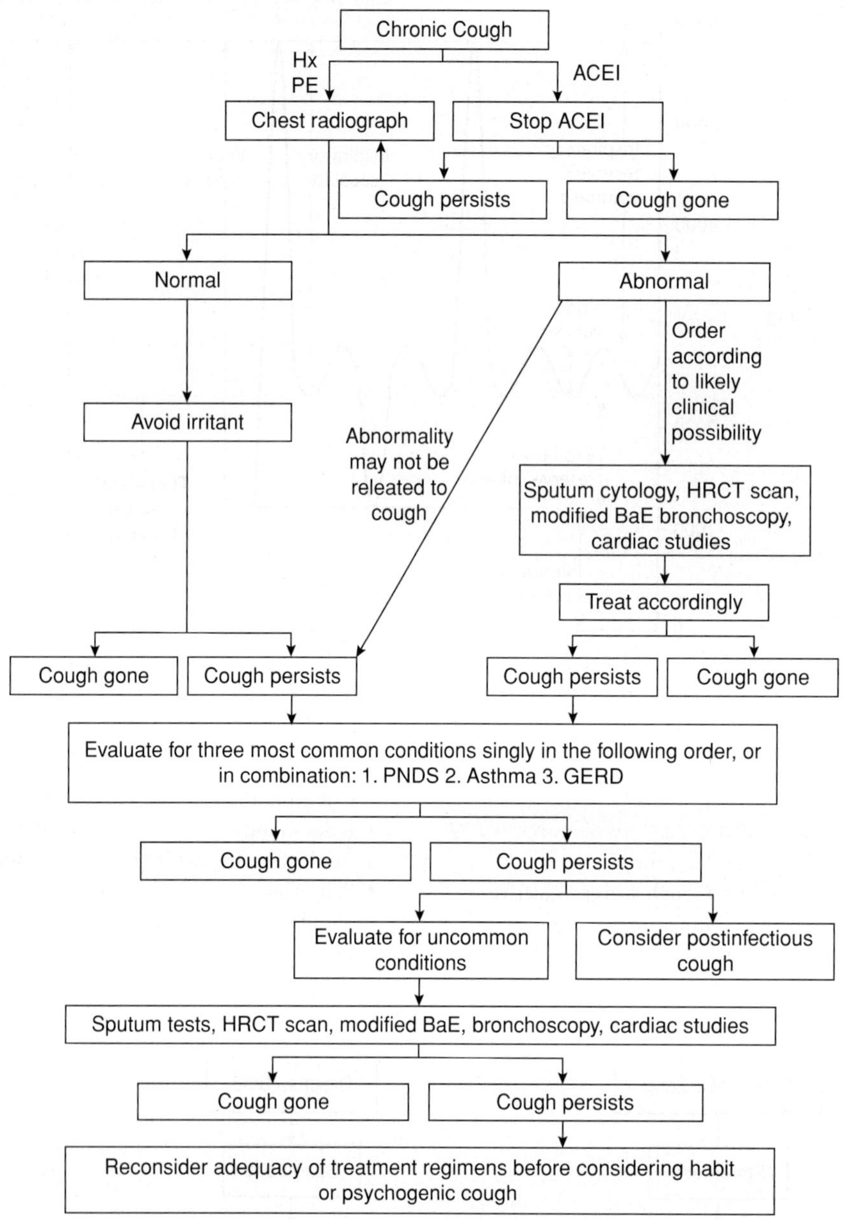

FIGURE 71-5 Algorithm for diagnosis and treatment of chronic cough. ACEI, angiotensin-converting enzyme inhibitor; BaE, barium esophagography; GERD, gastroesophageal reflux disease; HRCT, high-resolution computed tomography; Hx, history; PE, physical examination; PNDS, postnasal drip syndrome. (Data from Irwin RS, Boulet L-P, Cloutier MM, et al. Managing cough as a defense mechanism and as a symptom: a consensus panel report of the American College of Chest Physicians. *Chest*. 1998;114(suppl):133S–181S.)

Functional Implications

- Disabling dyspnea when performing simple tasks involving arm elevation, such as reaching into cabinet
- Decreased exercise tolerance
- Patients with mononucleosis should avoid contact sports for 6 weeks to avoid splenic rupture

Possible Contributing Causes

- Smoking
- Air pollution
- Allergies
- Occupations with poor air quality
- Long-term exposure to lung irritants
- Environmental irritants
- Periodontal disease
- Immunodeficiency disorders

Differential Diagnosis

- Influenza
- Measles
- Asthma
- Chickenpox
- Gastroesophageal reflux disease
- Ludwig angina
- Bronchiectasis
- Adult cystic fibrosis
- Kawasaki disease
- Pneumonia

- Goiter
- Upper respiratory tract infection
- Asthma (reversible)
- Central airway obstruction
- Lung tumor
- Tuberculosis

MEANS OF CONFIRMATION OR DIAGNOSIS

Laboratory Tests

- Viral culture
- Nasopharyngeal swab for influenza

Imaging

- Chest radiograph[3]
- CT for sinuses

Diagnostic Procedures

- Lung function tests
- Pulse oximetry
- Abnormal lung sounds

FINDINGS AND INTERPRETATION

- Mucus that is yellow-green in color likely indicates bacterial infection
- Acute sinusitis on CT will show complete opacification and air–fluid level[1]

REFERRALS/ADMITTANCE

- For imaging, x-ray
- For medication, anti-inflammatory agents, bronchodilators, expectorants, antihistamines, or vaccines
- For surgical consult if deviated septum
- For ENT consult
- For pulmonologist consult

IMPAIRMENTS

- Exercise limitation
- Shortness of breath
- Limited endurance capacity

INTERVENTION

- Fluid intake
- Smoking cessation
- Manual sinus drainage
- Coughing techniques
- Manual lobe drainage
- Pulmonary rehabilitation (PR)[4]
  - Enhances patient's sense of well-being
  - Improves exercise capacity
- Inspiratory muscle training (IMT)
- Once controlled: Exercise (aerobic, strength, flexibility, posture, breathing) to regain prior level of function

FUNCTIONAL GOALS

- Patient will have improved oxygenation, achieved by
  - Reduced airway edema secondary to inflammation and bronchospasm
  - Elimination of bronchial secretions
  - Prevention/treatment of respiratory infection
  - Increased exercise tolerance
  - Avoiding irritants/allergens
  - Relief/treatment of anxiety or depression
  - Improved muscle oxidative capacity
- Patient will be able to ambulate over 600 m in a 6-minute walk test
- Patient will score above 80% of their predicted forced expiratory volume in one second (FEV1) score.
- Patient will tolerate 1 hour of moderate exercise three times a week

PROGNOSIS

- Very good with rest and medication
- Symptoms usually disappear in 7 to 10 days
- Immunocompromised individuals are at high risk of complications
- Caution should be taken to prevent development of pneumonia

PATIENT RESOURCE

- Mossad SB. Upper Respiratory Tract Infections. Cleveland Clinic Center for Continuing Education. http://www.clevelandclinicmeded.com/medicalpubs/diseasemanagement/infectious-disease/upper-respiratory-tract-infection/. Accessed January 2, 2013.

REFERENCES

1. The American Physical Therapy Association. Pattern 6C: impaired ventilation, respiration/gas exchange, and aerobic capacity/endurance associated with airway clearance dysfunction. *Interactive Guide to Physical Therapist Practice.* 2003. doi: 10.2522/ptguide.3.3_3. Accessed March 1, 2013.
2. The American Physical Therapy Association. Pattern 6F: impaired ventilation and respiration/gas exchange associated with respiratory failure. *Interactive Guide to Physical Therapist Practice.* 2003. doi: 10.2522/ptguide.3.3_6. http://guidetoptpractice.apta.org/content/1/SEC32.extract?sid=6ebaffc7-f596-4c8c-a286-342e52371352. Accessed May 6, 2014.
3. Wells Cl.. Pulmonary pathology. In: DeTurk WE, Cahalin LP, eds. *Cardiovascular and Pulmonary Physical Therapy: An evidence based Approach.* 2nd ed. New York, NY: McGraw-Hill; 2011:Chapter 7. http://www.accessphysiotherapy.com/content/6873405#6873405. Accessed March 13, 2013.
4. Certo CM, DeTurk WE, Cahalin LP. History of cardiopulmonary rehabilitation. In: DeTurk WE, Cahalin LP, eds. *Cardiovascular and Pulmonary Physical Therapy: An evidence based Approach.* 2nd ed. New York, NY: McGraw-Hill; 2011:Chapter 1. http://www.accessphysiotherapy.com/abstract/6870102#6870104. Accessed March 13, 2013.

ADDITIONAL REFERENCES

- Aagaard E, Gonzales R. Management of acute bronchitis in healthy adults. *Infect Dis Clin North Am.* 2004;18(4):919–937.
- Aliverti A, Quaranta M, Chakrabarti B, Albuquerque A, Calverley P. Paradoxical movement of the lower ribcage at rest and during exercise in COPD patients. *Eur Respir J.* 2009;33(1):49-60.
- Arroll B, Kenealy T. Antibiotics for the common cold and acute purulent rhinitis. *Cochrane Database Syst Rev.* 2005;(3):CD000247.

- Bateman ED, Feldman C, O'Brien J, Plit M, Joubert JR. Guideline for the management of chronic obstructive pulmonary disease (COPD): 2004 revision. *S Afr Med J.* 2004;94(7):559–587.
- Batra PS. Radiologic imaging in rhinosinusitis. *Cleve Clin J Med.* 2004;71(11):886–888.
- Goodman CC, Fuller KS. *Pathology Implications for the Physical Therapist.* 3rd ed. St. Louis, MO: Saunders Elsevier; 2009.
- Goodman CC, Snyder TE. *Differential Diagnosis for Physical Therapists Screening for Referral.* 4th ed. St. Louis, MO: Saunders Elsevier; 2007.
- Gwaltney JM. Acute bronchitis. In: Mandell GL, Bennett JE, Dolin R, eds. *Principles and Practice of Infectious Diseases.* 6th ed. Philadelphia, PA: Elsevier Churchill Livingstone; 2005.
- Hirschman JV. Antibiotics for common respiratory tract infections in adults. *Arch Intern Med.* 2002;162(3):256–264.
- ICD9DATA. http://www.icd9data.com. Accessed March 13, 2013.
- ICD10DATA. http://www.icd10data.com. Accessed March 13, 2013.
- Panus PC, Jobst EE, Masters SB, Katzung B, Tinsley SL, Trevor AJ. Drugs affecting the respiratory system. In: Panus PC, Jobst EE, Masters SB, Katzung B, Tinsley SL, Trevor AJ, eds. *Pharmacology for the Physical Therapist.* New York, NY: McGraw-Hill; 2009:Chapter 35. http://www.accessphysiotherapy.com/content/6095983. Accessed March 13, 2013.

72 CHRONIC OBSTRUCTIVE PULMONARY DISEASE

Eric Shamus, PhD, DPT, PT, CSCS
Marangela Obispo, MSPT, GCS
Christopher S. Ellis, DPT

CONDITION/DISORDER SYNONYMS

- Nonseptic obstructive airway disease
- Septic obstructive airway disease

ICD-9-CM CODES

- 490 Bronchitis, not specified as acute or chronic
- 491 Chronic bronchitis
- 492 Emphysema
- 493 Asthma
- 494 Bronchiectasis
- 495 Extrinsic allergic alveolitis
- 496 Chronic airway obstruction, not elsewhere classified
- Associated physical therapy diagnoses
  - 780.7 Malaise and fatigue
  - 786.0 Dyspnea and respiratory abnormalities
  - 786.05 Shortness of breath

ICD-10-CM CODES

- F17 Nicotine dependence
- J44 Other chronic obstructive pulmonary disease
- J41 Chronic simple and mucopurulent chronic bronchitis
- J42 Unspecified chronic bronchitis
- J43 Emphysema
- J45 Asthma
- J47 Bronchiectasis
- Z57.31 Occupational exposure to environmental tobacco smoke
- Z72.0 Tobacco use
- Z77.22 Exposure to environmental tobacco smoke
- Z87.891 Personal history of nicotine dependence

PREFERRED PRACTICE PATTERNS

- 6C: Impaired Ventilation, Respiration/Gas Exchange, and Aerobic Capacity/Endurance Associated with Airway Clearance Dysfunction[1]
- 6F: Impaired Ventilation and Respiration/Gas Exchange Associated with Respiratory Failure[2]

PATIENT PRESENTATION

A 60-year-old man presents to your office with a prescription of functional decline. The patient complains of frequent coughing and shortness of breath (SOB). He is well known to you because of multiple office visits in the past few years for similar reasons. He has a chronic "smoker's cough," but reports that in the past 2 days his cough has increased, his sputum has changed from white to green in color, and he has had to increase the frequency with which he uses his Albuterol inhaler. He denies having a fever, chest pain, peripheral edema, or other symptoms. His medical history is significant for hypertension, peripheral vascular disease, and two hospitalizations for pneumonia in the past 5 years. He has a 60-pack-year history of smoking and continues to smoke two packs of cigarettes a day. Patient reports decreased ability to walk inside his home and difficulty with all ADLs due to fatigue and SOB. He denies having any assistive device at home and denies use of supplemental O_2.

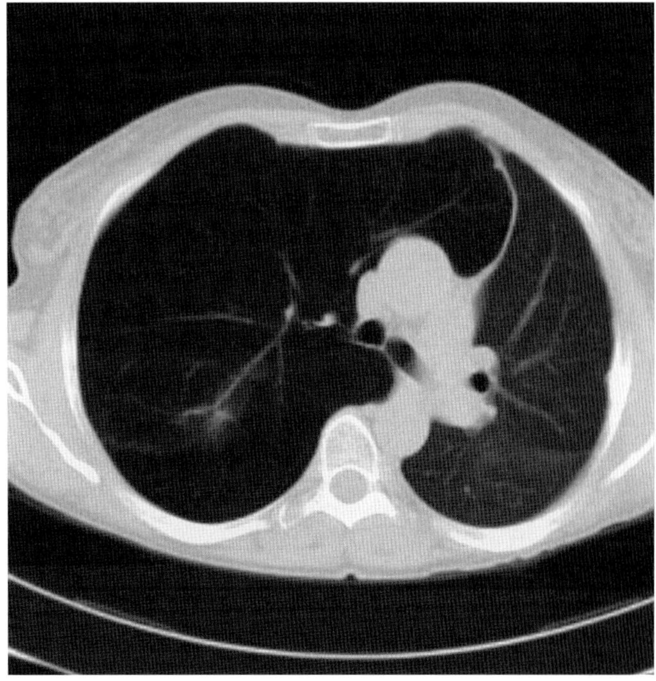

FIGURE 72-1 Chest CT scan of a patient with COPD who underwent a left single-lung transplant. Note the reduced parenchymal markings in the right lung (*left side of figure*) as compared to the left lung, representing emphysematous destruction of the lung, and mediastinal shift to the left, indicative of hyperinflation. (From Longo DL, Fauci AS, Kasper DL, Hauser SL, Jameson JL, Loscalzo J. *Harrison's Principles of Internal Medicine.* 18th ed. New York, NY: McGraw-Hill; 2012.)

On examination, patient appears with barrel chest. He is in moderate respiratory distress. His temperature is 98.4°F, his blood pressure is 152/95 mm Hg, his pulse is 98 beats/min, his respiratory rate is 24 breaths/min, and he has an oxygen saturation of 91% on room air at rest. His lung examination is significant for diffuse expiratory wheezing, use of accessory muscles of respiration and a prolonged expiratory phase of respiration. There are no

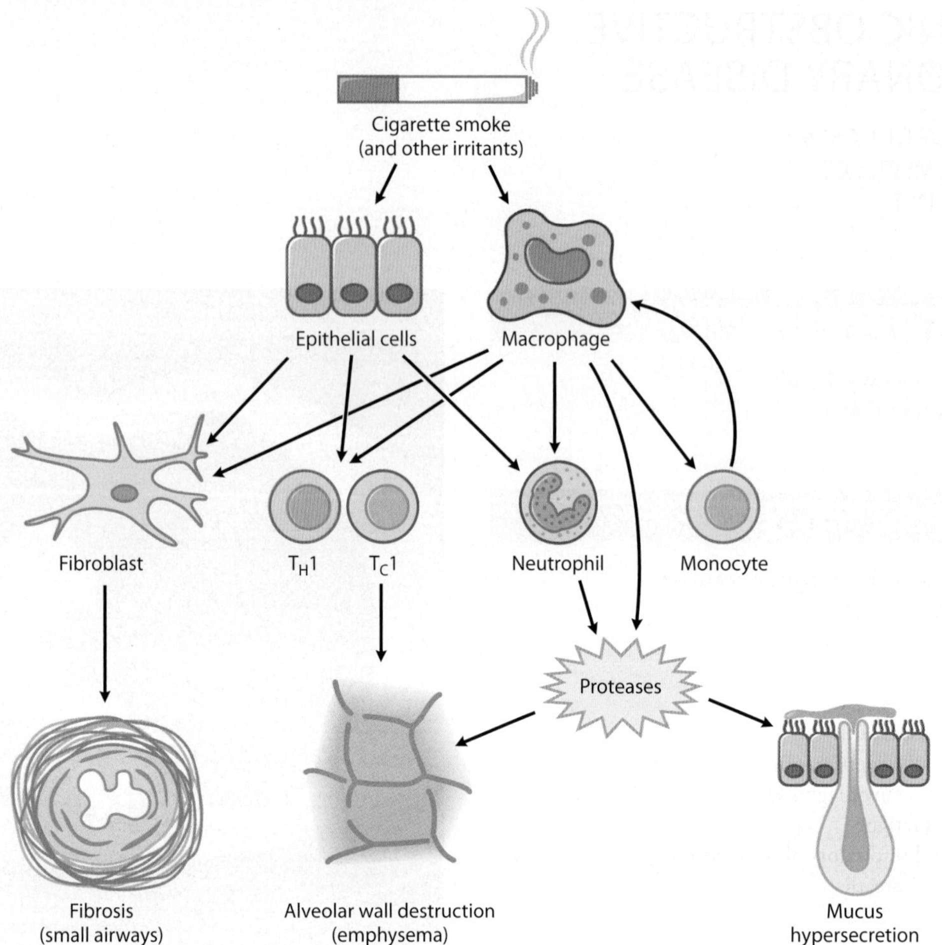

FIGURE 72-2 *Cellular mechanisms in* chronic obstructive pulmonary disease. Cigarette smoke and other irritants activate epithelial cells and macrophages in the lung to release mediators that attract circulating inflammatory cells, including monocytes (which differentiate to macrophages within the lung), neutrophils, and T lymphocytes (T_H1 and T_C1 cells). Fibrogenic factors released from epithelial cells and macrophages lead to fibrosis of small airways. Release of proteases results in alveolar wall destruction (emphysema) and mucus hypersecretion (chronic bronchitis). (From Brunton LL, Chabner BA, Knollmann BC. *Goodman & Gilman's The Pharmacological Basis of Therapeutics*. 12th ed. www.accessmedicine.com. Copyright © The McGraw-Hill Companies, Inc. All rights reserved.)

signs of cyanosis. Patient presents with impaired strength in bilateral LEs. Endurance is impaired and by demonstrated a decreased 2MWT with increased, tachycardia, tachypnea, and decreased O_2 saturation after performance requiring 5 min to recover. Patient presents with increased labor of breathing after minimal activity. Patient requires increased time for bed mobility, transfers, and gait with multiple rest breaks. A chest X-ray shows an increased anteroposterior (AP) diameter and flattened diaphragms, but otherwise he has clear lung fields.[3]

KEY FEATURES

Description

- A cluster of chronic lung diseases that cause air to be trapped in lungs and hyperinflation
- Afflicted individuals usually have both emphysema and chronic bronchitis
- Chronic airflow limitation (CAL), narrowing of airways (not fully reversible)
- Disorders
  - Chronic bronchitis: Inflammation of airway with increased mucus production
  - Obstructive bronchiolitis
  - Emphysema: Damaged air sacs and small tubes of the lungs
  - Chronic obstructive lung disease (COLD)
  - Chronic obstructive airway disease (COAD)
  - CAL
  - Chronic obstructive respiratory disease (CORD)
- Subdivided into septic and nonseptic[4]
  - Nonseptic
    - Cough is productive
    - Breathing sounds: Rales, wheezing
  - Septic
    - Cough can be variable
    - Breathing sounds decreased

Essentials of Diagnosis

- Most individuals have lost 50% lung function when diagnosed
- Diagnostic guidelines
  - GOLD (the Global Initiative for COLD)
  - Guidelines from American Thoracic Society and European Respiratory Society
- Diagnosis
  - Physical examination
  - Air-flow limitation on pulmonary function test (spirometer)

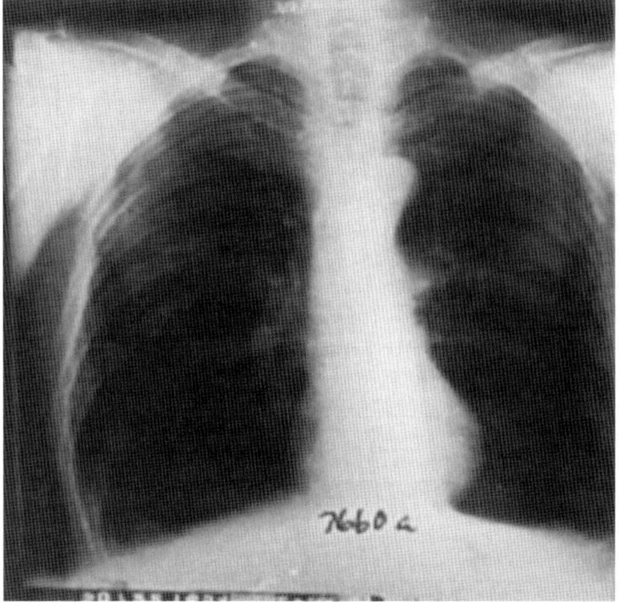

A

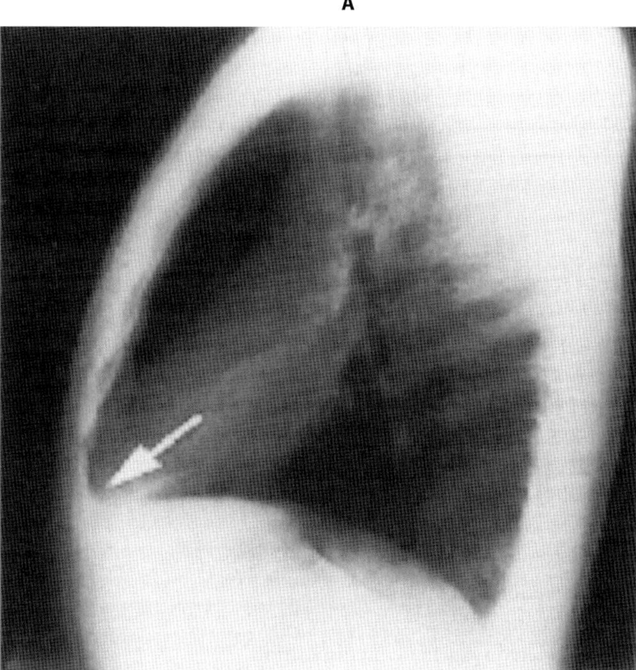

Normal

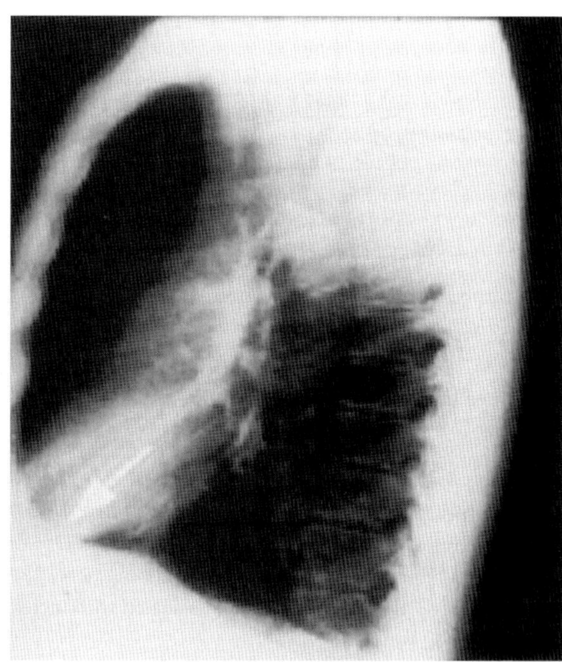

Hyperinflation

B

FIGURE 72-3 Chest radiograph of a patient with COPD. It shows flattened diaphragm and lung markings are reduced with hyperinflation. Heart is teardrop-shaped. (From Halter JB, Ouslander J, Tinetti M, Studenski S, High K, Asthana S. *Hazzard's Geriatric Medicine and Gerontology*. 6th ed. www.accessmedicine.com.)

   - Spirometer measures compared to predicted values for age, height, body weight, gender
   - Expressed as function expiratory volume (FEV)
  - Chronic cough
  - Hypoxemia
  - Hypercapnia

General Considerations

- Mortality rates increase with repeated exposure to irritant or causative factors
- Most cases include cigarette smoking
  - Acute exacerbations often caused by lung infection, exposure to air pollution, smoke, cold air temperature, dust, chemical smells
- Adults with asthma are 12 times more likely to develop chronic obstructive pulmonary disease (COPD) than adults without asthma
- Must monitor oxygen levels in patients with COPD; can become apneic
- Loss of airflow usually due to
  - Lost elasticity in airways and air sacs

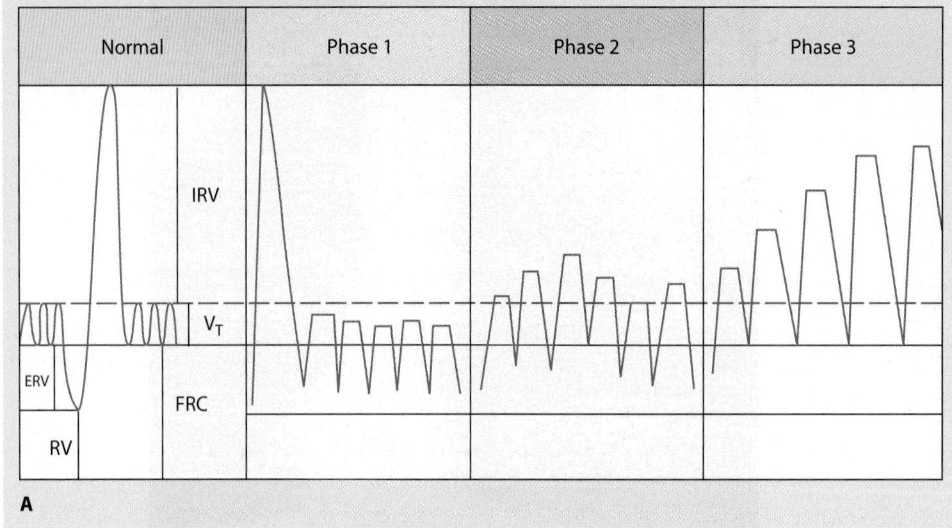

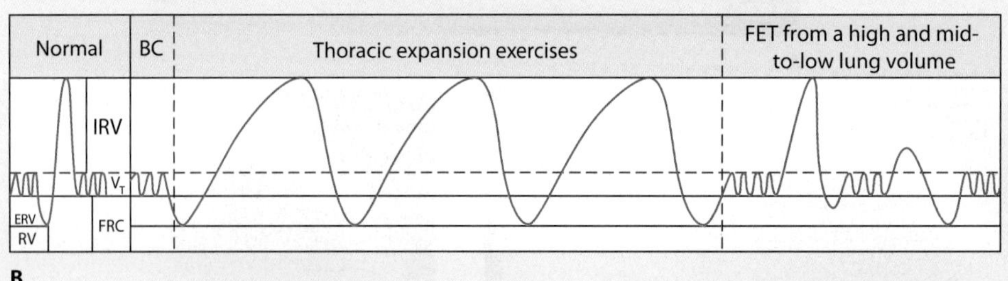

FIGURE 72-4 Autogenic drainage (AD) (**A**) versus active cycle of breathing (ACB) (**B**), both from spirograms of normal individuals. AD: phase 1, peripheral loosening of mucus; phase 2, collection of mucus in large airways; phase 3, transport of mucus to the mouth. ACB: BC, breathing control; FET, forced expiration technique. (Republished with permission of Lippincott Williams & Wilkins, from Savci S, Ince DI, Arikan H. A comparison of autogenic drainage and the active cycle of breathing in patients with chronic obstructive pulmonary disorders. *J Cardiopulm Rehabil.* 2000;20(1); permission conveyed through Copyright Clearance Center, Inc.)

- Increased mucus production
- Damage to air sac
- Inflammation, thickening of airway walls

Demographics

- Most commonly presents at age 55 to 60 years
- More common in men than women in middle age
- Increasing prevalence among women (associated with increased smoking among women)

CLINICAL FINDINGS

SIGNS AND SYMPTOMS

- Chest tightness[4]
- Wheezing
- Dyspnea
- Cough
- Shoulder raised to allow increased airflow to lungs
- SOB
- Tensed muscles from dyspnea
- Depression
- Paradoxical inspiration
- Digital clubbing
- Barrel chest deformity[4]

Functional Implications

- Disabling dyspnea when performing simple tasks (i.e., arm elevation to reach into cabinets)
- Decreased exercise tolerance

Possible Contributing Causes

- Smoking
- Air pollution
- Long-term exposure to lung irritants
- Environmental irritants
- Sinusitis
- Periodontal disease
- Aging process
- Heredity, genetic predisposition
- Deficiency of alpha-1 protease inhibitor

Differential Diagnosis

- Bronchiectasis
- Adult cystic fibrosis (CF)
- Asthma (reversible)
- Central airway obstruction
- Lung tumor
- Tuberculosis

MEANS OF CONFIRMATION OR DIAGNOSIS

Laboratory Tests

- Blood gas measurements
- Blood pH (indicating hypoxemia or hypercapnia)

Imaging

- Chest radiograph[4]
- High-resolution CT

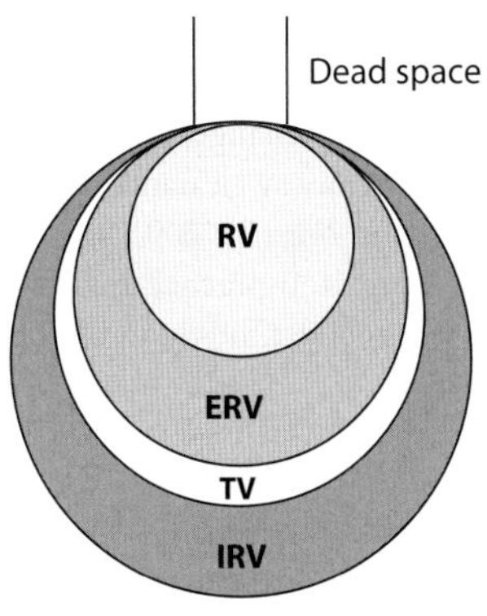

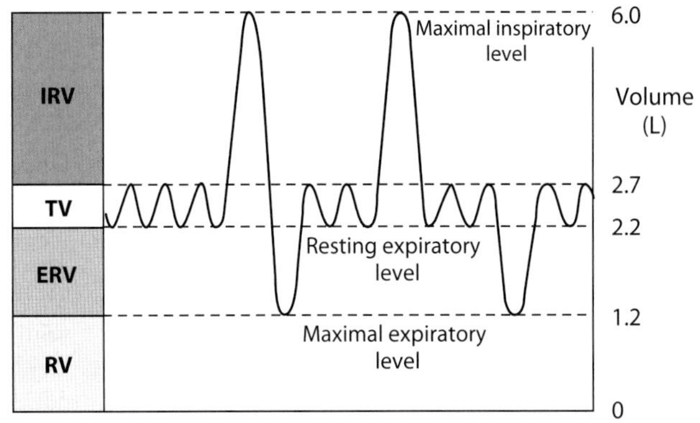

IRV = Inspiratory reserve volume
ERV = Expiratory reserve volume
TV = Tidal volume
RV = Residual volume

		Volume (L)		
		Men	Women	
Vital capacity	IRV	3.3	1.9	Inspiratory capacity
	TV	0.5	0.5	
	ERV	1.0	0.7	Functional residual capacity
	RV	1.2	1.1	
Total lung capacity		6.0	4.2	

Respiratory minute volume (rest): 6 L/min
Alveolar ventilation (rest): 4.2 L/min
Maximal voluntary ventilation (BTPS): 125–170 L/min

Timed vital capacity: 83% of total in 1 s; 97% in 3 s
Work of quiet breathing: 0.5 kg-m/min
Maximal work of breathing: 10 kg-m/breath

FIGURE 72-5 Lung volumes and some measurements related to the mechanics of breathing. The diagram at the upper right represents the excursions of a spirometer plotted against time. (Reproduced, with permission, from Ganong WF. *Review of Medical Physiology*. New York, NY: McGraw-Hill; 2005:652.)

- Ventilation/perfusion lung scan
- X-ray: Usually shows hyperinflation and lowered diaphragm

Diagnostic Procedures

- Seattle Obstructive Lung Disease Questionnaire (SOLQ)
- Lung or pulmonary function tests
  - Body plethysmography
  - Peak expiratory flow
  - Nitrogen washout

FINDINGS AND INTERPRETATION

- FEV_1/forced vital capacity (FVC) ratio <70% confirms presence of airflow obstruction
- FEV_1 usually reduced, used to measure severity
- Spirometry should be performed before and after taking a bronchodilator
  - Improvement in $FEV_1 \geq 12\%$ indicates reversibility; is concordant with asthma, not COPD
- FVC decreased
- D_{LCO} and T_{LCO} decreased
- Residual volume (RV) decreased

REFERRALS/ADMITTANCE

- Hospital for imaging, X-ray
- Physician for medication: Anti-inflammatories, bronchodilators, expectorants, antihistamines, vaccine
- Surgeon for surgical consult
- Pulmonologist for oxygen treatment

IMPAIRMENTS

- Exercise limitation
- SOB
- Impaired proximal upper-limb strength
- Limited endurance capacity
- Depression

TESTS AND MEASURES

- Spirometry
- Ribcage expansion
- FVC

INTERVENTION

- Smoking cessation
- Exercise (aerobic, strength, flexibility, posture, breathing)
- Airway clearance
- Pursed-lip breathing
- Coughing techniques
- Pharmacologic management[5]
  - Bronchodilator
    - B2-adrenergic agonists
    - Leukotriene antagonists
    - Anticholinergics (antagonize bronchial secretions)
    - Methylxanthines
  - Anti-inflammatories
    - Inhaled corticosteroids
    - Oral corticosteroids

    - Antibiotics
    - Mast cell stabilizers
  - Mucolytic expectorants
  - Antihistamines
  - Pneumococcal vaccine
  - Annual prophylactic influenza vaccination
- Long-term oxygen treatment (LTOT)
- Oxygen therapy
- Lung transplant
- Lung-volume reduction surgery (LVRS) alternative to lung transplant
- Pulmonary rehabilitation (PR)[6]
  - Enhances patient's sense of well-being
  - Improves exercise capacity
- Inspiratory muscle training (IMT)

FUNCTIONAL GOALS

- Patient will have
  - Improved oxygenation, decreased carbon dioxide retention, achieved by
    - Reducing airway edema secondary to inflammation and bronchospasm
    - Facilitating elimination of bronchial secretions
    - Preventing/treating respiratory infection
    - Increased exercise tolerance
    - Controlling complications
    - Avoiding irritants/allergens
    - Treating anxiety, depression
    - Improved muscle oxidative capacity
- Patient will be able to ambulate over 600 m in a 6-minute walk test.
- Patient will score above 80% of predicted FEV_1.
- Patient will tolerate 1 hour of moderate exercise three times per week.

PROGNOSIS

- Poor: Condition is chronic, progressive, and debilitating
- Survival rates
  - 80% at 1 year
  - 50% at 5 years
  - 35% at 10 years
- No known cure to reverse damage

PATIENT RESOURCES

- COPD Alliance. http://www.copd.org. Accessed June 12, 2013.
- COPD Foundation. http://www.copdfoundation.org. Accessed June 12, 2013.

REFERENCES

1. The American Physical Therapy Association. Pattern 6C: impaired ventilation, respiration/gas exchange, and aerobic capacity/endurance associated with airway clearance dysfunction. *Interactive Guide to Physical Therapist Practice*. 2003. doi: 10.2522/ptguide.3.3_3. http://guidetoptpractice.apta.org/content/1/SEC29.extract?sid=ede5cb60-c2b9-4da5-8446-fc9fa4616c0d. Accessed May 6, 2014.
2. The American Physical Therapy Association. Pattern 6F: impaired ventilation and respiration/gas exchange associated with respiratory failure. *Interactive Guide to Physical Therapist Practice*. 2003. doi: 10.2522/ptguide.3.3_6. http://guidetoptpractice.apta.org/content/1/SEC32.extract?sid=6ebaffc7-f596-4c8c-a286-342e52371352. Accessed May 6, 2014.
3. Toy EC. Dyspnea (COPD), Case 61. LANGE Case Files. http://www.accessmedicine.com/caseContent.aspx?aid=510023002&tabid=1. Accessed May 12, 2013.
4. Wells Cl. Pulmonary pathology. In: DeTurk WE, Cahalin LP, eds. *Cardiovascular and Pulmonary Physical Therapy: An Evidence-Based Approach*. 2nd ed. New York, NY: McGraw-Hill; 2011. http://www.accessphysiotherapy.com/content/6873405#6873405. Accessed May 12, 2013.
5. Panus PC, Jobst EE, Masters SB, Katzung B, Tinsley SL, Trevor AJ. Drugs affecting the respiratory system. In: Panus PC, Jobst EE, Masters SB, Katzung B, Tinsley SL, Trevor AJ, eds. *Pharmacology for the Physical Therapist*. New York, NY: McGraw-Hill; 2009. http://www.accessphysiotherapy.com/content/6095983. Accessed May 12, 2013.
6. Certo CM, DeTurk WE, Cahalin LP. History of cardiopulmonary rehabilitation. In: DeTurk WE, Cahalin LP, eds. *Cardiovascular and Pulmonary Physical Therapy*. 2nd ed. New York, NY; McGraw-Hill: 2011. http://www.accessphysiotherapy.com/abstract/6870102#6870104. Accessed May 12, 2013.

ADDITIONAL REFERENCES

- Aliverti A, Quaranta M, Chakrabarti B, Albuquerque AL, Calverley PM. Paradoxical movement of the lower ribcage at rest and during exercise in COPD patients. *Eur Respir J*. 2009;33(1):49–60.
- Bateman ED, Feldman C, O'Brien J, Plit M, Joubert JR. Guideline for the management of chronic obstructive pulmonary disease (COPD): 2004 revision. *S Afr Med J*. 2004;94(7 Pt 2):559–575.
- Goodman CC, Fuller KS. *Pathology Implications for the Physical Therapist*. 3rd ed. St. Louis, MO: Saunders; 2009.
- Goodman CC, Snyder TK. *Differential Diagnosis for Physical Therapists: Screening for Referral*. 4th ed. St. Louis, MO: Saunders; 2007.

73 CYSTIC FIBROSIS

Eric Shamus, PhD, DPT, PT, CSCS
Amber Yampolsky, MPT, ATP

CONDITION/DISORDER SYNONYMS

- Mucoviscidosis
- Cystic fibrosis (CF)

ICD-9-CM CODES

- 277.0 Cystic fibrosis
- Associated physical therapy diagnoses
  - 780.7 Malaise and fatigue
  - 786.0 Dyspnea and respiratory abnormalities
  - 786.05 Shortness of breath

ICD-10-CM CODES

- E84 Cystic fibrosis
- E84.9 Cystic fibrosis, unspecified

PREFERRED PRACTICE PATTERNS

- 6C: Impaired Ventilation, Respiration/Gas Exchange, and Aerobic Capacity/Endurance Associated with Airway Clearance Dysfunction[1]
- 6F: Impaired Ventilation and Respiration/Gas Exchange Associated with Respiratory Failure[2]

PATIENT PRESENTATION

A 14-year-old male presents with CF diagnosed via sweat chloride test at 1-month old. He is complaining of increased sputum production and decreased activity/exercise tolerance with difficulty in walking the necessary distances around school without having shortness of breath. Therefore, he has recently been placed on homebound schooling. He likes school and misses being with his friends. When he is not having an exacerbation, he reports increased coughing with moderately intense activity/exercise and that he participates in a walking program 3×/wk for 20 minutes. He performs airway clearance using vest treatment (high-frequency chest wall oscillation) 2 times/day for 30 minutes at variable frequency. He has an acapella PEP device but does not use it much. He does nebulizer treatments with Pulmozyme and bronchodilators 2 times/day. He has had progressively increasing frequency of hospitalizations over the past 2 years for CF exacerbation and pneumonia. His past medical history includes: positive cultures for pseudomonas and burkholderia cepacia, as well as g-tube placement. Pulmonary function testing shows an FEV1 of 85%. Physical examination reveals moderate clubbing of his nail beds, flattened thoracic spine with elevated and forward rounded shoulders. He is thin. He is able to complete a 6-minute walk test for a distance of 1800 ft, with O_2 saturation, 90% (96% at rest), increased HR from 100 at rest to 120, and report of dyspnea on the modified Borg scale, 3, perceived rating of exertion on the modified Borg scale, 2.

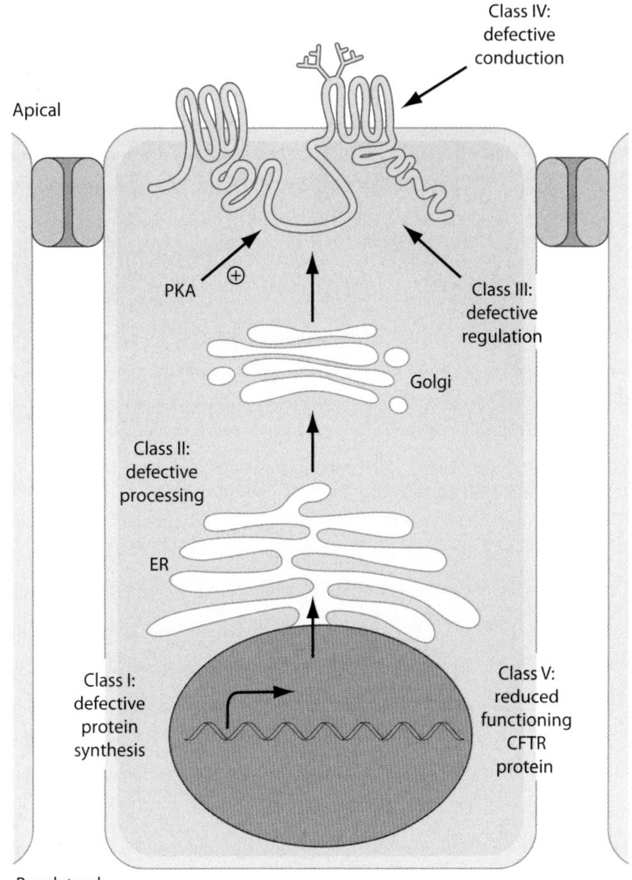

FIGURE 73-1 Schema describing classes of genetic mutations in CFTR gene and effects on CFTR protein/function. Note the ΔF_{508} mutation is a class II mutation and, like class I mutations, would be predicted to produce no mature CFTR protein in the apical membrane. CFTR, cystic fibrosis transmembrane conductance regulator. (From Longo DL, Fauci AS, Kasper DL, Hauser SL, Jameson JL, Loscalzo J. *Harrison's Principles of Internal Medicine*. 18th ed. New York, NY: McGraw-Hill; 2012.)

KEY FEATURES

Description

- Genetic disease
- Mucus buildup, blocks airways
- Mutation on chromosome pair 7

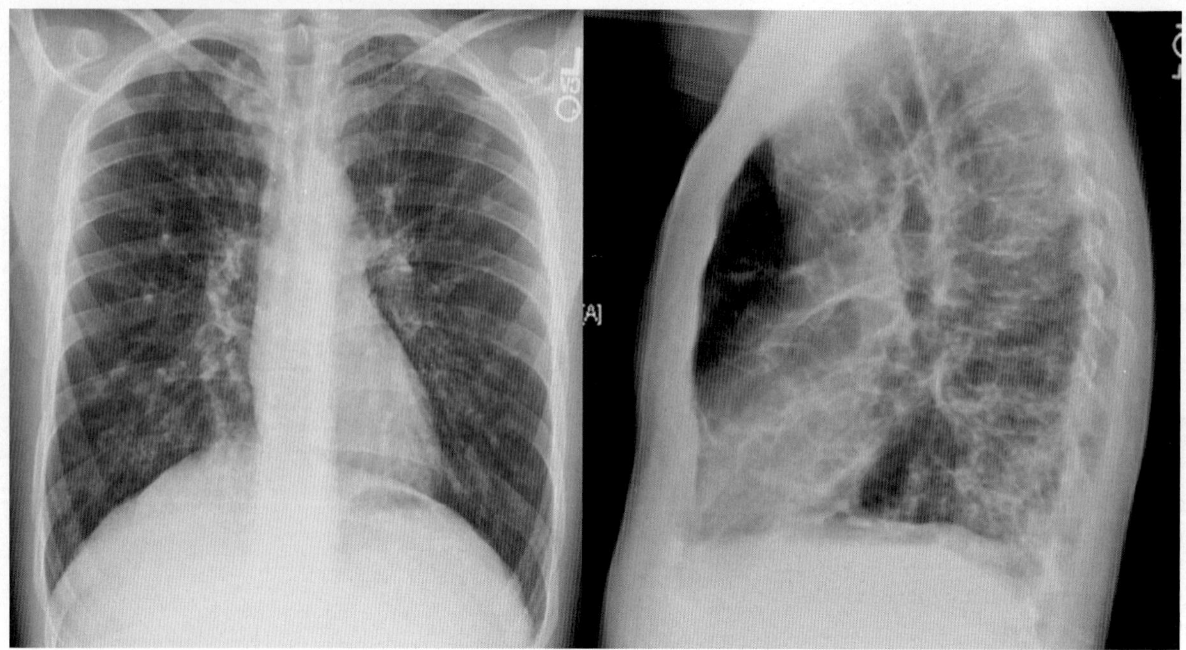

FIGURE 73-2 Cystic fibrosis with bronchiectasis, apical disease. (From Longo DL, Fauci AS, Kasper DL, Hauser SL, Jameson JL, Loscalzo J. *Harrison's Principles of Internal Medicine*. 18th ed. New York, NY: McGraw-Hill; 2012.)

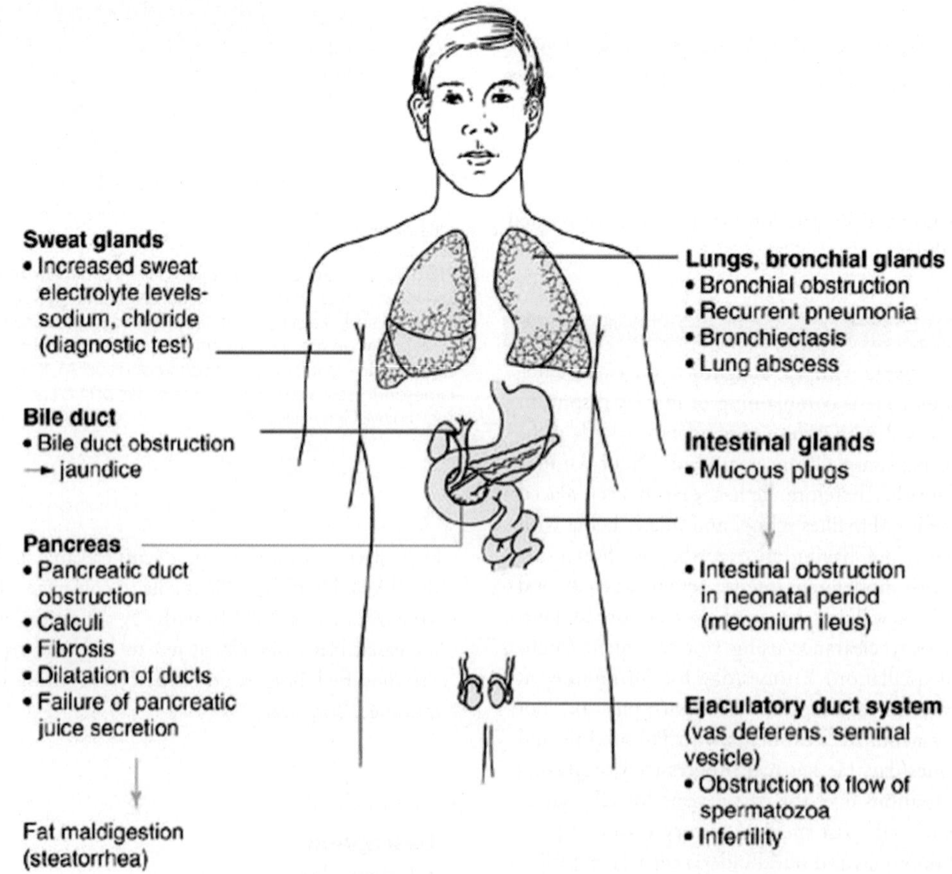

FIGURE 73-3 Clinical features of cystic fibrosis. Many of the features of this disease are caused by obstruction of exocrine ducts due to the increased viscosity of secretions. (From Chandrasoma P, Taylor CR. *Concise Pathology*. 3rd ed. www.accessmedicine.com.)

Essentials of Diagnosis

- Productive cough
- Early diagnosis critical
- Autosomal recessive heritability
- Thick, sticky mucus
- Salty sweat

General Considerations

- Exocrine glands affected
- Bacteria can grow in the built-up mucus
- Mucus blocks pancreatic digestive enzymes from small intestines
  - Intestines cannot absorb fats, proteins, vitamins
  - Malnutrition
- Affects lungs, pancreas, liver, intestines, sinuses

Demographics

- Usually diagnosed in newborns
- Children of Caucasian descent most commonly affected
- Individuals can live to middle age with medical care

CLINICAL FINDINGS

SIGNS AND SYMPTOMS

- Baby's skin tastes salty
- Mucus in the lungs
- Dehydration
- Chest tightness, limited ribcage mobility
- Fatigue
- Malnutrition
- Constipation
- Clubbing of finger tips
- Wheezing
- Sinusitis
- Chronic cough
- Shoulder raised to allow increased air-flow to lungs
- Shortness of breath
- Tensed muscles from dyspnea
- Anxiety
- Postural abnormality
- Depression

Functional Implications

- Disabling dyspnea when performing simple tasks
- Decreased exercise tolerance
- Malnutrition causes fatigue

Possible Contributing Causes

- Genetic: Inherited gene from both parents
- Each parent must be a carrier of the gene; parents might not be aware that they are a carrier
- Children have 25% chance of inheriting CF if both parents are carriers

Differential Diagnosis

- Bronchiectasis
- Fungal or parasitic infection
- Lung abscess
- Cat scratch fever
- Sarcoidosis
- Hodgkin lymphoma
- Asthma
- Central airway obstruction
- Lung cancer

MEANS OF CONFIRMATION OR DIAGNOSIS

Laboratory Tests

- Prenatal screening
- Genetic test

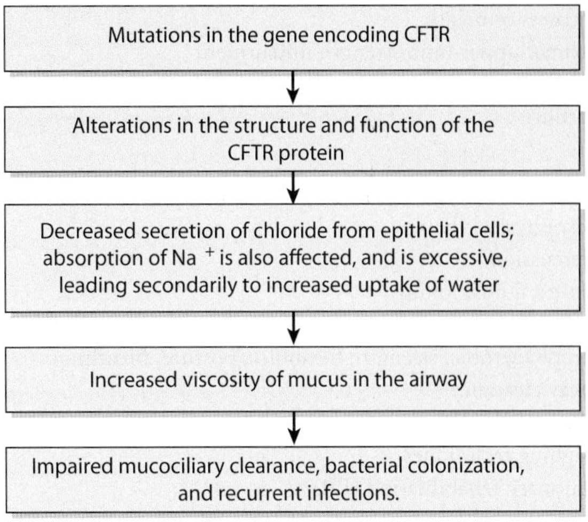

Mutations in the gene encoding CFTR
↓
Alterations in the structure and function of the CFTR protein
↓
Decreased secretion of chloride from epithelial cells; absorption of Na^+ is also affected, and is excessive, leading secondarily to increased uptake of water
↓
Increased viscosity of mucus in the airway
↓
Impaired mucociliary clearance, bacterial colonization, and recurrent infections.

FIGURE 73-4 Summary of possible mechanisms involved in cells in the airways of individuals with cystic fibrosis (OMIM 219700) who have pulmonary pathology. In individuals of Caucasian origin, 70% of the mutations occur at one locus, resulting in deletion of ΔF508 from the CTR protein. However, over 1000 mutations have been identified in the *CFTR* gene. Basically, the CFTR protein acts normally as a cAMP-regulated transporter involved in secretion of Cl^-, but in addition normally inhibits absorption of Na^+ by a Na^+ channel. The viscosity of the mucus in the pancreatic ductules is also increased, leading to their obstruction. The details of how abnormalities of CFTR affect ion transport in the pancreas are somewhat different than in the lung. (From Murray RK, Bender D, Botham KM, Kennelly PJ, Rodwell V, Weil PA. *Harper's Illustrated Biochemistry*. 29th ed. www.accessmedicine.com. Copyright © The McGraw-Hill Companies, Inc. All rights reserved.)

- Sputum culture
- Blood test
- Sweat chloride test

Imaging

- Chest radiograph[3]
- Chest CT, high resolution
- Ventilation/perfusion lung scan

Diagnostic Procedures

- Lung function or pulmonary function tests
  - Spirometry
  - Body plethysmography
  - Peak expiratory flow

FINDINGS AND INTERPRETATION

- May show osteoporosis on x-ray

TREATMENT

Medication

- For lung infection, antibiotics
- Pancreatic enzyme

REFERRALS/ADMITTANCE

- To hospital for imaging, X-ray
- To physician for medication
- To pulmonologist for medical assessment
- To respiratory therapist for disease management

IMPAIRMENTS

- Exercise limitation
- Excess loss of salts/electrolytes from sweating

- Shortness of breath
- Proximal upper-limb strength impairment
- Limited endurance capacity
- Infertility

INTERVENTION

- Chest physical therapy
  - Percussion
  - Postural positioning
- Manual therapy to loosen ribcage, diaphragm, thoracic spine
- Exercise (aerobic, strength, flexibility, posture, breathing)
- Airway clearance
- Pursed-lip breathing
- Coughing techniques
- Pulmonary rehabilitation (PR)[4]
  - Improves exercise capacity
- Inspiratory muscle training (IMT)

FUNCTIONAL GOALS

- Patient will be able to
  - Ambulate over 600 m in a 6-minute walk test.
  - Score above 80% of their predicted FEV_1 score.
  - Tolerate 1 hour of moderate exercise three times per week.

PROGNOSIS

- Infection can overload the system.
- No cure.

PATIENT RESOURCE

- Cystic Fibrosis Foundation. www.cff.org. Accessed May 6, 2013.

REFERENCES

1. The American Physical Therapy Association. Pattern 6C: impaired ventilation, respiration/gas exchange, and aerobic capacity/ endurance associated with airway clearance dysfunction. *Interactive Guide to Physical Therapist Practice*. 2003. doi: 10.2522/ ptguide.3.3_3. http://guidetoptpractice.apta.org/content/1/ SEC29.extract?sid=ede5cb60-c2b9-4da5-8446-fc9fa4616c0d. Accessed May 6, 2014.
2. The American Physical Therapy Association. Pattern 6F: impaired ventilation and respiration/gas exchange associated with respiratory failure. *Interactive Guide to Physical Therapist Practice 2003.* doi: 10.2522/ptguide.3.3_6. http://guidetoptpractice.apta.org/ content/1/SEC32.extract?sid=6ebaffc7-f596-4c8c-a286-342e52371352. Accessed May 6, 2014.
3. Wells Cl.. Pulmonary pathology. In: DeTurk WE, Cahalin LP, eds. *Cardiovascular and Pulmonary Physical Therapy: An evidence base d Approach*. 2nd ed. New York, NY: McGraw-Hill; 2011:Chapter 7. http://www.accessphysiotherapy.com/ content/6873405#6873405 Accessed May 19, 2013.
4. Certo CM, DeTurk WE, Cahalin LP. History of cardiopulmonary rehabilitation. In: DeTurk WE, Cahalin LP, eds. *Cardiovascular and Pulmonary Physical Therapy*. New York, NY; McGraw-Hill: 2011:Chapter 1. http://www.accessphysiotherapy.com/ abstract/6870102#6870104. Accessed May 24, 2013.

ADDITIONAL REFERENCES

- Fitzgerald DW, Sterling TR, Haas DW. Mycobacterium tuberculosis. In: Mandell GL, Bennett JE, Dolan R, eds. *Mandell, Douglas, and Bennett's Principles and Practice of Infectious Diseases*. 7th ed. Orlando, FL: Saunders Elsevier; 2009:Chapter 250.
- Golden MP, Vikram HR. Extrapulmonary tuberculosis: an overview. *American Family Physician*. 2005;72(9):1761--1768.
- Goodman CC, Fuller KS. *Pathology Implications for the Physical Therapist*. 3rd ed. St. Louis, MO: Saunders Elsevier; 2009.
- Goodman CC, Snyder TE. *Differential Diagnosis for Physical Therapists Screening for Referral*. 4th ed. St. Louis, MO: Saunders Elsevier; 2007.
- Hay WW, Levin MJ, Sondheimer JM, Deterding RR. Bacterial infections. In: Hay WW, Levin MJ, Sondheimer JM, Deterding RR, eds. *CURRENT Diagnosis & Treatment: Pediatrics*. 20th ed. New York, NY: McGraw-Hill; 2011. http://www.accessphysiotherapy.com/content/6590639. Accessed May 14, 2013.
- ICD9DATA. http://www.icd9data.com. Accessed May 16, 2013.
- ICD10DATA. http://www.icd10data.com. Accessed May 19, 2013.
- Iseman MD. Tuberculosis. In: Goldman L, Ausiello D, eds. *Cecil Medicine*. 23rd ed. Philadelphia, PA: Saunders Elsevier; 2007: Chapter 345.
- Konstantinos A. Testing for tuberculosis. *Australian Prescriber*. 2010;33(1):12–18. http://www.australianprescriber.com/ magazine/33/1/12/18. Accessed May 19, 2013.
- Panus PC, Jobst EE, Masters SB, Katzung B, Tinsley SL, Trevor AJ. Drugs affecting the respiratory system. In: Panus PC, Jobst EE, Masters SB, Katzung B, Tinsley SL, Trevor AJ, eds. *Pharmacology for the Physical Therapist*. New York, NY: McGraw-Hill; 2009:Chapter 35. http://www.accessphysiotherapy.com/content/ 6095983. Accessed May 19, 2013.
- Pulmonary Tuberculosis. PubMed Health, US National Library of Medicine. http://www.ncbi.nlm.nih.gov/pubmedhealth/ PMH0001141. Accessed May 26, 2013.

74 PNEUMONIA

Eric Shamus, PhD, DPT, PT, CSCS
Jennifer Shamus, PhD, DPT, COMT, CSCS

CONDITION/DISORDER SYNONYMS

- Acute interstitial pneumonia
- Bronchial pneumonia
- Lobar pneumonia
- Lung inflammation
- Pneumonitis

ICD-9-CM CODES

- 480 Viral pneumonia
- 481 Pneumococcal pneumonia [streptococcus pneumoniae pneumonia
- 482 Other bacterial pneumonia
- 483 Pneumonia due to other specified organism
- 484 Pneumonia in infectious diseases classified elsewhere
- 485 Bronchopneumonia, organism unspecified
- 486 Pneumonia, organism unspecified
- Associated physical therapy diagnoses/treatment diagnosis
  - 780.7 Malaise and fatigue
  - 786.0 Dyspnea and respiratory abnormalities
  - 786.05 Shortness of breath

ICD-10-CM CODES

- J12.0 Adenoviral pneumonia
- J12.1 Respiratory syncytial virus pneumonia
- J12.2 Parainfluenza virus pneumonia
- J12.81 Pneumonia due to SARS-associated coronavirus
- J12.89 Other viral pneumonia
- J12.9 Viral pneumonia, unspecified
- J13 Pneumonia due to Streptococcus pneumoniae
- J15.0 Pneumonia due to Klebsiella pneumoniae
- J18.1 Lobar pneumonia, unspecified organism

PREFERRED PRACTICE PATTERNS[1]

- 6C: Impaired Ventilation, Respiration/Gas Exchange, and Aerobic Capacity/Endurance Associated with Airway Clearance Dysfunction
- 6F: Impaired Ventilation and Respiration/Gas Exchange Associated with Respiratory Failure

PATIENT PRESENTATION

A 61-year-old woman presents to the emergency room complaining of cough for 2 weeks. The cough is productive of green sputum and is associated with sweating, shaking chills, and fever up to 102°F (38.8°C). She was exposed to her grandchildren who were

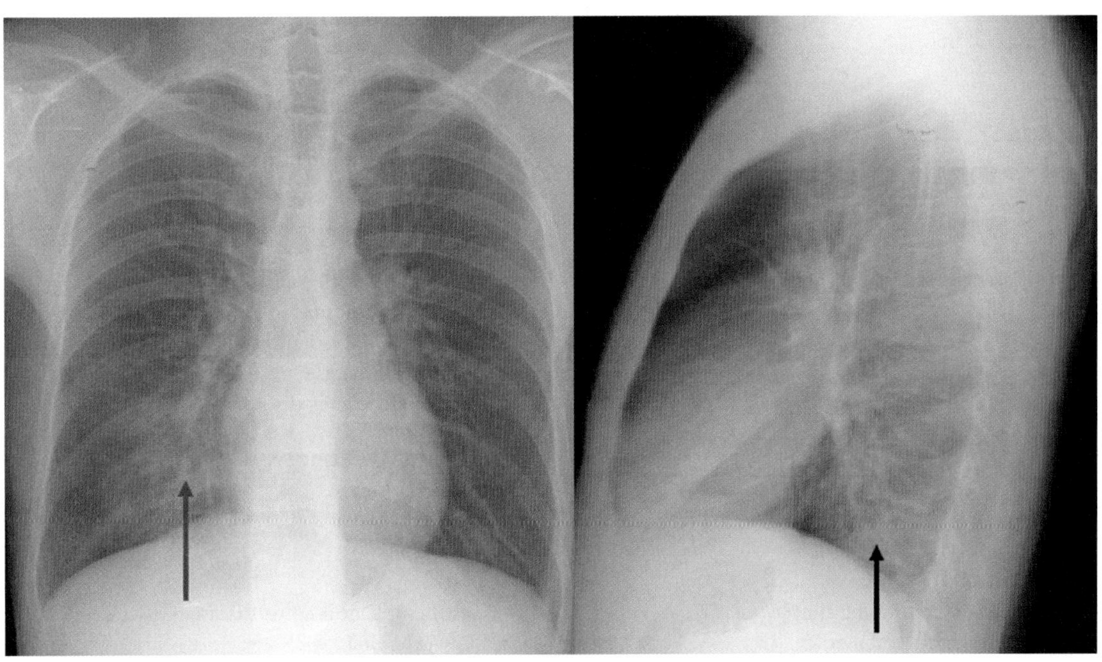

FIGURE 74-1 Right lower lobe pneumonia—subtle opacity on PA film (*red arrow*), while the lateral film illustrates the "spine sign" (*black arrow*) where the lower spine does not become more lucent. (From Longo DL, Fauci AS, Kasper DL, Hauser SL, Jameson JL, Loscalzo J, eds. *Harrison's Principles of Internal Medicine*. 18th ed. New York, NY: McGraw-Hill; 2012.)

told that they had upper respiratory infections 2 weeks ago but now are fine. Her past medical history is significant for diabetes for 10 years, which is under good control using oral hypoglycemics. She denies tobacco, alcohol, or drug use. On examination, she looks ill and in distress, with continuous coughing and chills. Her blood pressure is 100/80 mm Hg, her pulse is 110 beats/min, her temperature is 101°F (38.3°C), her respirations are 24 breaths/min, and her oxygen saturation is 97% on room air. Examination of the head and neck is unremarkable. Her lungs have rhonchi and decreased breath sounds, with dullness to percussion in bilateral bases. Her heart is tachycardic but regular. Her extremities are without signs of cyanosis or edema. The remainder of her examination is normal. A complete blood count (CBC) shows a high white blood cell (WBC) count of 17,000 cells/mm^3, with a differential of 85% neutrophils and 20% lymphocytes. Her blood sugar is 120 mg/dL.[2]

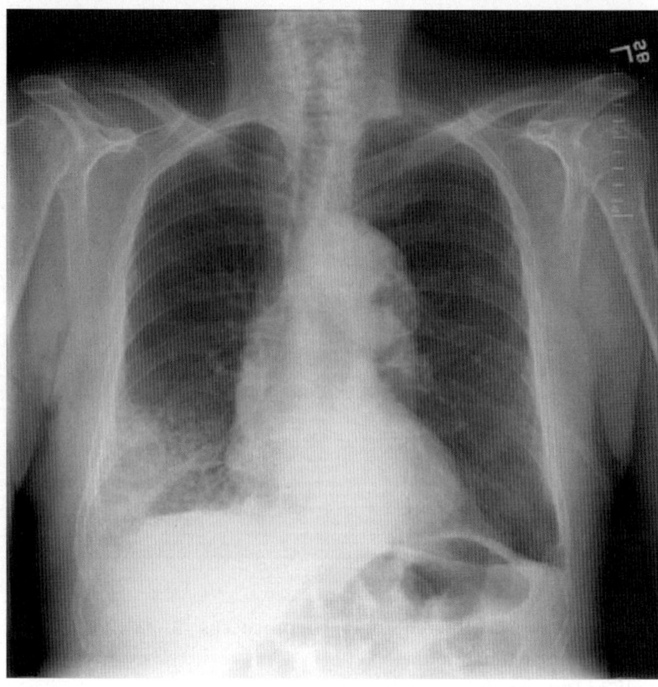

FIGURE 74-2 Pneumococcal lobar pneumonia. A 78-year-old man with chronic lung disease had subjective fever, right-sided pleuritic chest pain, and greatly increased shortness of breath for 2 days. He was afebrile, and his WBC count was 10,600 with 40% band forms. Blood cultures were positive for Streptococcus pneumoniae. A sputum submitted for culture more than 24 hours after antibiotics were begun yielded no pneumococci. (From McKean S, Ross JJ, Dressler DD, Brotman DJ, Ginsberg JS. *Principles and Practice of Hospital Medicine*. www.accessmedicine.com. Copyright © The McGraw-Hill Companies, Inc. All rights reserved.)

KEY FEATURES

Description

- Inflammation of the lungs (specifically the alveoli)
- Infection can be bacterial, viral, fungal, or parasitic
- Pneumonitis is lung inflammation
- Pneumonia is pneumonitis with pulmonary consolidation

Essentials of Diagnosis

- Can develop from bronchitis, which is usually after a common cold (viral respiratory infection)
- Case with mild symptoms is called walking pneumonia

General Considerations

- Influenza is a systemic illness involving the respiratory tract
- Antibiotics have limited to no role in the treatment of a virus
- If caused by bacteria, antibiotics will be prescribed
- Can develop secondary bacterial infection
- Pneumonia can be life threatening

Demographics

- Infants and young children
- Elderly or frail

CLINICAL FINDINGS

SIGNS AND SYMPTOMS[3]

- Diarrhea
- Increased heart beat
- Low-grade fever
- Runny nose
- Malaise
- Pleurisy
- Sore throat
- Cough with productive mucus
- Edema
- Chest tightness
- Rales (crackling sounds in lungs)
- Swelling of ankles, feet, legs
- Wheezing
- Raising shoulders allows increased lung air flow
- Shortness of breath
- Tensed muscles from dyspnea

Functional Implications

- Disabling dyspnea when performing simple tasks
  - Arm elevation to reach into cabinet
  - Decreased exercise tolerance
  - Patients with mononucleosis should avoid contact sports for 6 weeks to avoid splenic rupture
  - Respiratory dysfunction limiting one's ability to function at work

Possible Contributing Causes

- Flu virus
- Respiratory syncytial virus
- Rhinovirus
- Herpes simplex virus
- Severe acute respiratory syndrome (SARS)
- Smoking
- Air pollution
- Allergies
- Occupations with poor air quality
- Long-term exposure to lung irritants
- Environmental irritants
- Periodontal disease
- Immunodeficiency disorders

Differential Diagnosis

- Influenza
- Measles
- Asthma
- Chickenpox
- Gastroesophageal reflux disease (GERD)
- Ludwig angina
- Bronchiectasis
- Adult cystic fibrosis (CF)
- Kawasaki disease (KD)

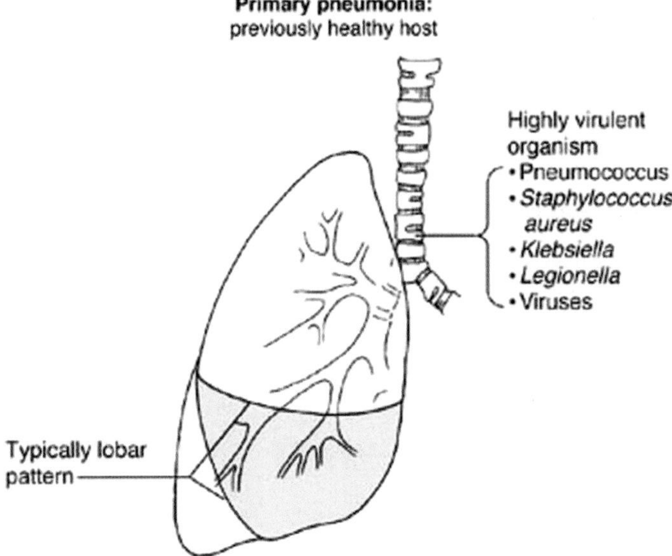

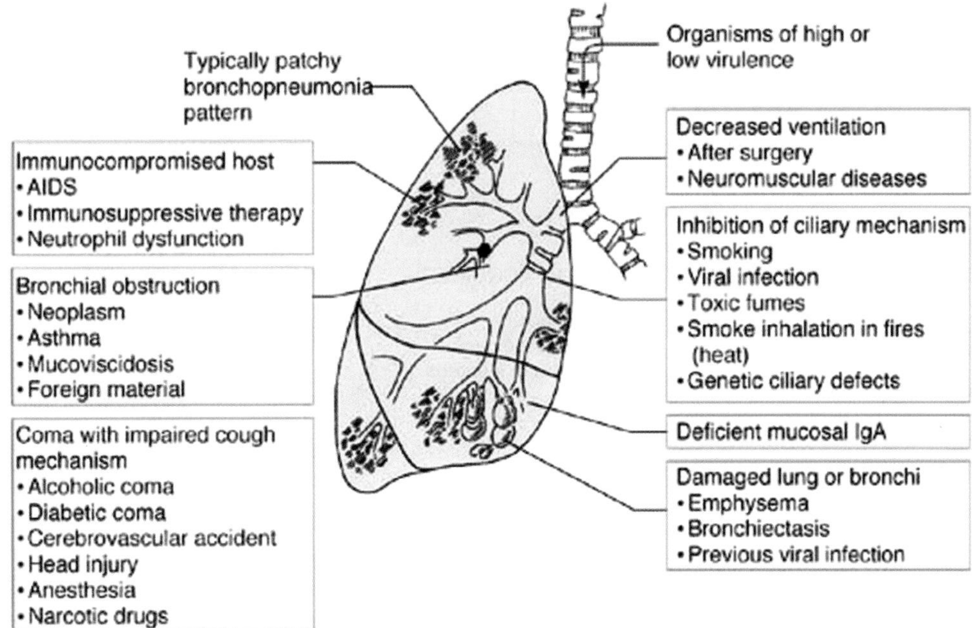

FIGURE 74-3 Primary versus secondary pneumonia. Note that predisposing diseases (*in boxes*) are important in the pathogenesis of secondary pneumonia. (From Chandrasoma P, Taylor CR. *Concise Pathology*. 3rd ed. www.accessmedicine.com. Copyright © The McGraw-Hill Companies, Inc. All rights reserved.)

- Bronchitis
- Goiter
- Upper respiratory tract infection
- Asthma (reversible)
- Central airway obstruction
- Lung tumor
- Tuberculosis

MEANS OF CONFIRMATION OR DIAGNOSIS

Laboratory Tests

- Viral culture
- Blood test
- Nasopharyngeal swab for influenza

Imaging

- Chest X-ray
- CT scan of sinuses

Diagnostic Procedures

- Pulse oximetry for monitoring oxygenation
- Abnormal lung sounds

FINDINGS AND INTERPRETATION

- Lack of air space on chest X-ray
- Mucus that is yellow-green likely has a bacterial infection.
- Acute sinusitis on CT will show complete opacification and air–fluid level.[3]

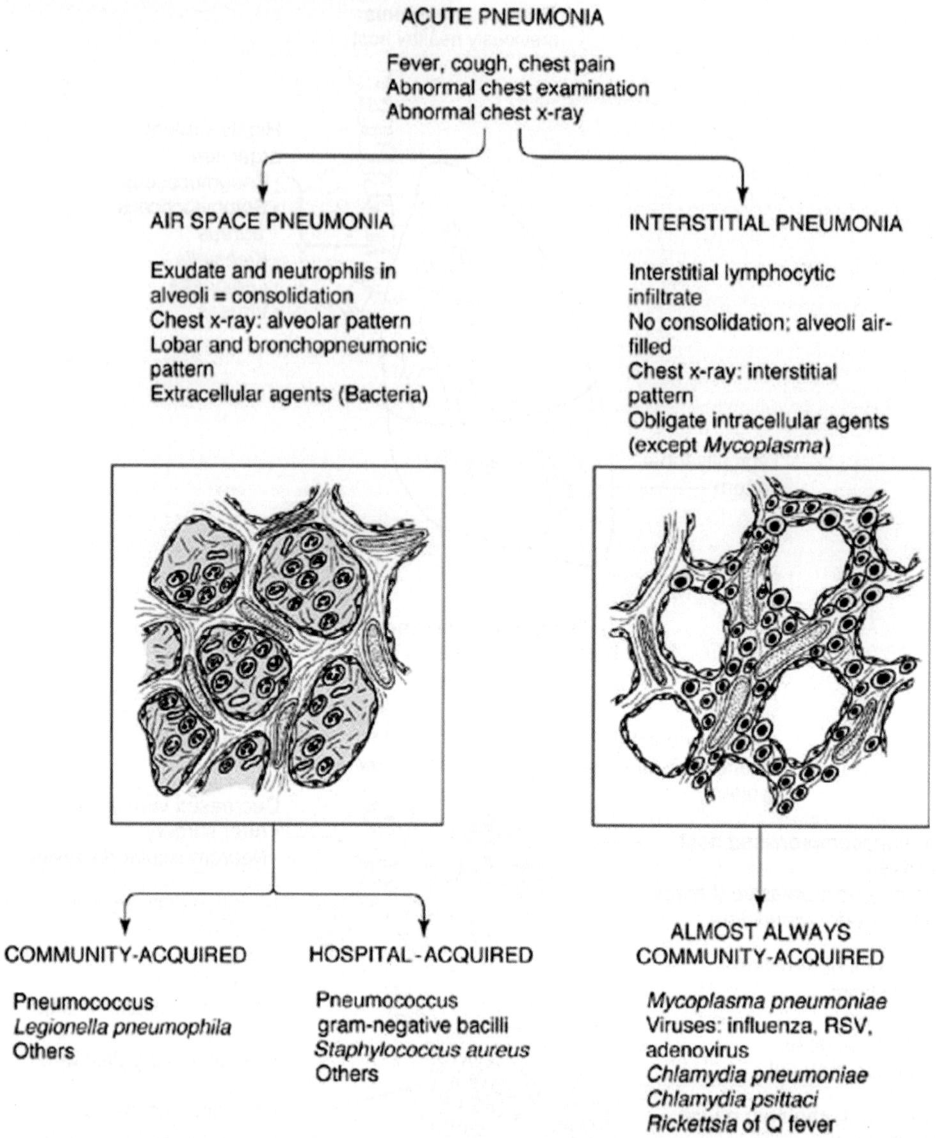

ACUTE PNEUMONIA

Fever, cough, chest pain
Abnormal chest examination
Abnormal chest x-ray

AIR SPACE PNEUMONIA

Exudate and neutrophils in alveoli = consolidation
Chest x-ray: alveolar pattern
Lobar and bronchopneumonic pattern
Extracellular agents (Bacteria)

INTERSTITIAL PNEUMONIA

Interstitial lymphocytic infiltrate
No consolidation; alveoli air-filled
Chest x-ray: interstitial pattern
Obligate intracellular agents (except *Mycoplasma*)

COMMUNITY-ACQUIRED

Pneumococcus
Legionella pneumophila
Others

HOSPITAL-ACQUIRED

Pneumococcus
gram-negative bacilli
Staphylococcus aureus
Others

ALMOST ALWAYS COMMUNITY-ACQUIRED

Mycoplasma pneumoniae
Viruses: influenza, RSV, adenovirus
Chlamydia pneumoniae
Chlamydia psittaci
Rickettsia of Q fever

FIGURE 74-4 Classification of acute pneumonias based on the pattern of lung involvement and etiology. (From Chandrasoma P, Taylor CR. *Concise Pathology*. 3rd ed. www.accessmedicine.com.)

TREATMENT

▸ Medication

- Anti-inflammatory agents
- Bronchodilators
- Expectorants
- Antihistamines
- Vaccines

MEDICAL PROCEDURES

- Lung function tests

REFERRALS/ADMITTANCE

- To hospital ER if in severe respiratory distress
- To radiologist for imaging; chest X-ray, CT scan of sinuses
- To surgeon for deviated septum consult
- To ear, nose, and throat (ENT) specialist
- To pulmonologist

IMPAIRMENTS

- Exercise limitation
- Shortness of breath
- Limited endurance capacity

TESTS AND MEASURES

- Lung sounds
- Vital capacity: Spirometry

INTERVENTION

- Fluid intake
- Smoking cessation
- Manual sinus drainage
- Coughing techniques
- Manual lobe drainage once infection is gone
- Pulmonary rehabilitation (PR)
  - Enhances the patient's sense of well-being
  - Improves exercise capacity

- Inspiratory muscle training (IMT)
- Exercise to return to prior level of function (once infection under control)
  - Aerobic
  - Strength
  - Flexibility
  - Postural
  - Breathing

FUNCTIONAL GOALS

- Improve oxygenation by
  - Reducing airway edema secondary to inflammation and bronchospasm
  - Facilitating elimination of bronchial secretions
  - Preventing/treating respiratory infection
  - Increasing exercise tolerance
  - Avoiding irritants/allergens
  - Relieving anxiety; treating depression
  - Improving muscle oxidative capacity
- Patient will be able to
  - Ambulate over 600 m in a 6-minute walk test.
  - Score above 80% of their predicted FEV_1 score.
  - Tolerate 1 hour of moderate exercise three times a week.

PROGNOSIS

- Symptoms usually go away in 7 to 21 days.
- Individuals that are immunocompromised are at high risk of complications.
- Can be life threatening.

PATIENT RESOURCES

- Pneumonia, American Lung Association. http://www.lung.org/lung-disease/pneumonia. Accessed July 2, 2103.
- Pneumonia, Canadian Lung Association. http://www.lung.ca/diseases-maladies/a-z/pneumonia-pneumonie/bacterial-bacterienne_e.php. Accessed July 2, 2103.

REFERENCES

1. APTA. *Guide to Physical Therapy Practice*. Atlanta: American Physical Therapy Association; 2003. http://guidetoptpractice.apta.org. Accessed July 2, 2013.
2. Toy EC. Pneumonia, Case 64. LANGE Case Files. http://www.accessmedicine.com/casecontent.aspx?aid=510023118&tabid=1. Accessed July 4, 2013.
3. Mossad SB. Upper respiratory tract infections. Cleveland Clinic, Center for Continuing Education. http://www.clevelandclinicmeded.com/medicalpubs/diseasemanagement/infectious-disease/upper-respiratory-tract-infection. Accessed July 2, 2013.

ADDITIONAL REFERENCES

- Aagaard E, Gonzales R. Management of acute bronchitis in healthy adults. *Infect Dis Clin N Am*. 2004;18(4):919–937.
- Aliverti A, Quaranta M, Chakrabarti B, Albuquerque AL, Calverley PM. Paradoxical movement of the lower ribcage at rest and during exercise in COPD patients. *Eur Respir J*. 2009;33(1):49–60. doi: 10.1183/09031936.00141607.
- Arroll B, Kenealy T. Antibiotics for the common cold and acute purulent rhinitis. *Cochrane Database Syst Rev*. 2005;(3):CD000247.
- Batra PS. Radiologic imaging in rhinosinusitis. *Cleve Clin J Med*. 2004;71(11):886–888.
- Bateman ED, Feldman C, O'Brien J, Plit M, Joubert JR; COPD Guideline Working Group of the South African Thoracic Society. Guideline for the management of chronic obstructive pulmonary disease (COPD): 2004 revision. *S Afr Med J*. 2004;94(7 Pt 2):559–575.
- Goodman CC, Fuller KS. *Pathology: Implications for the Physical Therapist*. 3rd ed. Philadelphia, PA: Saunders Elsevier; 2009.
- Goodman CC, Snyder TK. *Differential Diagnosis for Physical Therapists: Screening for Referral*. 4th ed. St. Louis, MO: Saunders Elsevier; 2007.
- Gwaltney JM. Acute bronchitis. In: Mandell GL, Bennett JE, Dolin R, eds. *Principles and Practice of Infectious Diseases*. 6th ed. Philadelphia, PA: Elsevier Churchill Livingstone; 2005.
- Hirschmann JV. Antibiotics for common respiratory tract infections in adults. *Arch Intern Med*. 2002;162(3):256–264.
- Panus PC, Jobst EE, Masters SB, Katzung B, Tinsley SL, Trevor AJ. Drugs affecting the respiratory system. In: Panus PC, Jobst EE, Masters SB, Katzung B, Tinsley SL, Trevor AJ, eds. *Pharmacology for the Physical Therapist*. New York, NY: McGraw-Hill; 2009. http://www.accessphysiotherapy.com/content/6095983. Accessed July 4, 2013.
- Wells Cl. Pulmonary pathology. In: DeTurk WE, Cahalin LP, eds. *Cardiovascular and Pulmonary Physical Therapy: An Evidence-Based Approach*. 2nd ed. New York, NY: McGraw-Hill; 2011. http://www.accessphysiotherapy.com/content/6873405#6873405. Accessed July 4, 2013.

75 PNEUMOTHORAX

Eric Shamus, PhD, DPT, PT, CSCS
Lindsey (Davis) Hornecke, DPT

CONDITION/DISORDER SYNONYMS

- Collapsed lung
- Pneumothoraces (plural form of disorder)
- Spontaneous pneumothorax
- Tension pneumothorax
- Traumatic pneumothorax

ICD-9-CM CODES

- 512.0 Pneumothorax and air leak
- 860 Traumatic pneumothorax and hemothorax
- Associated physical therapy diagnoses
  - 780.7 Malaise and fatigue
  - 786.0 Dyspnea and respiratory abnormalities
  - 786.05 Shortness of breath

ICD-10-CM CODES

- J93.0 Spontaneous tension pneumothorax
- J93.11 Primary spontaneous pneumothorax
- J93.12 Secondary spontaneous pneumothorax
- J93.81 Chronic pneumothorax
- J93.82 Other air leak
- J93.83 Other pneumothorax
- J93.9 Pneumothorax, unspecified
- J95.811 Postprocedural pneumothorax
- J95.812 Postprocedural air leak
- S21.309A Unspecified open wound of unspecified front wall of thorax with penetration into thoracic cavity, initial encounter
- S27.0XXA Traumatic pneumothorax, initial encounter
- S27.1XXA Traumatic hemothorax, initial encounter
- S27.2XXA Traumatic hemopneumothorax, initial encounter

PREFERRED PRACTICE PATTERNS[1]

- 6A: Primary Prevention/Risk Reduction for Cardiovascular/Pulmonary Disorders
- 6B Impaired Aerobic Capacity/Endurance Associated with Deconditioning
- 6C: Impaired Ventilation, Respiration/Gas Exchange, and Aerobic Capacity/Endurance Associated with Airway Clearance Dysfunction
- 6F: Impaired Ventilation and Respiration/Gas Exchange Associated with Respiratory Failure

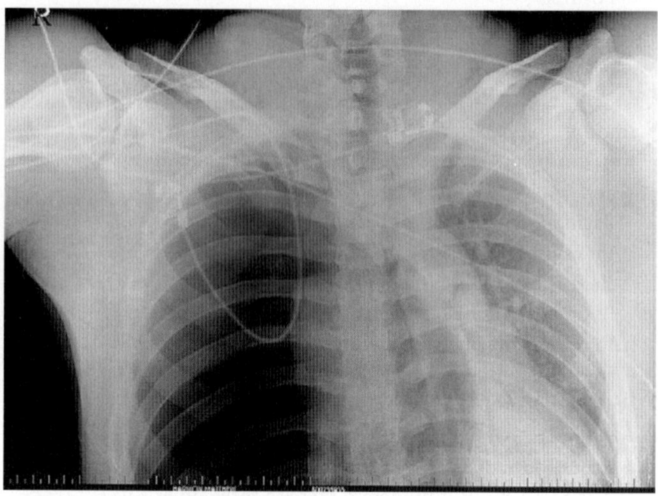

FIGURE 75-1 Tension pneumothorax with collapse of right lung field and deviation of heart and trachea. (From Patel DR, Greydanus DE, Baker RJ. *Pediatric Practice: Sports Medicine.* www.accesspediatrics. Copyright © The McGraw-Hill Companies, Inc. All rights reserved.)

PATIENT PRESENTATION

A 68-year-old male presents with complaints of shortness of breath and chest pain. His chest pain is worse while coughing and deep breathing. His symptoms began after a motor vehicle accident 8 weeks ago. Chest x-ray revealed two broken ribs, which most likely occurred when the air bag deployed. He has chronic obstructive pulmonary disease (COPD) and a history of cigarette smoking, which he has quit 3 months ago.

After his ribs have healed, his primary care physician refers him to physical therapy. The physician tested his pulmonary function

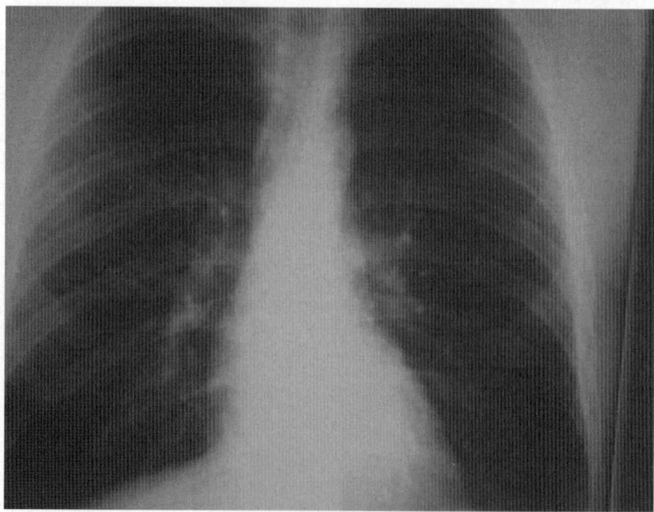

FIGURE 75-2 Pneumothorax involving 40% of lung field. (From Patel DR, Greydanus DE, Baker RJ. *Pediatric Practice: Sports Medicine.* www.accesspediatrics. Copyright © The McGraw-Hill Companies, Inc. All rights reserved.)

and noted he has decreased vital capacity and total lung capacity and increased residual volume. Physical therapy examination reveals postural abnormalities of rounded shoulders, forward head, and increased thoracic kyphosis. His scalene musculature is shortened and rope like on palpation. The PT also notices he mostly uses his accessory muscles for normal breathing. He ambulated 450 m on a 6-minute walk test.

KEY FEATURES

Description

- Collapsed lung occurs from air in the region around the lung
- Pressure on the lung prevents expansion of the lung with inhalation
- Chest pain with breathing

Essentials of Diagnosis

- Spontaneous pneumothorax (PTX) can occur with no etiology
- Focal area of absent breath sounds[2,3]
- Iatrogenic PTX[4]
  - From a complication, from a diagnostic, or treatment procedure
- Tension PTX[4]
  - Air enters the pleural space but cannot escape
  - Can be a traumatic or a severe spontaneous event
- Primary PTX
  - Unknown cause
- Secondary PTX
  - Known cause

General Considerations

- Can be caused by
  - Rib fracture
  - Gunshot wound
  - Penetration trauma into the lung
- Can be life threatening
- May need a chest tube

Demographics

- More common in tall and thin individuals
- Familial
- Spontaneously in newborns and in older children
- Males (16–24) with high-risk trauma activities[3]

CLINICAL FINDINGS

SIGNS AND SYMPTOMS

- Sudden shortness of breath[2]
- Focal area of absent breath sounds[2]
- Chest pain; worsens with deep breath or cough
- Cyanosis
- Fatigue
- Increased heart rate
- Decreased oxygenation throughout the body
- Nasal flaring
- Hypotension (low blood pressure)
- Chest tightness
- Raising shoulders allows increased lung air flow
- Tensed muscles from dyspnea

Functional Implications

- If spontaneous PTX, patient prohibited from air travel until completely healed
- Disabling dyspnea when performing simple tasks
  - Arm elevation to reach into cabinet

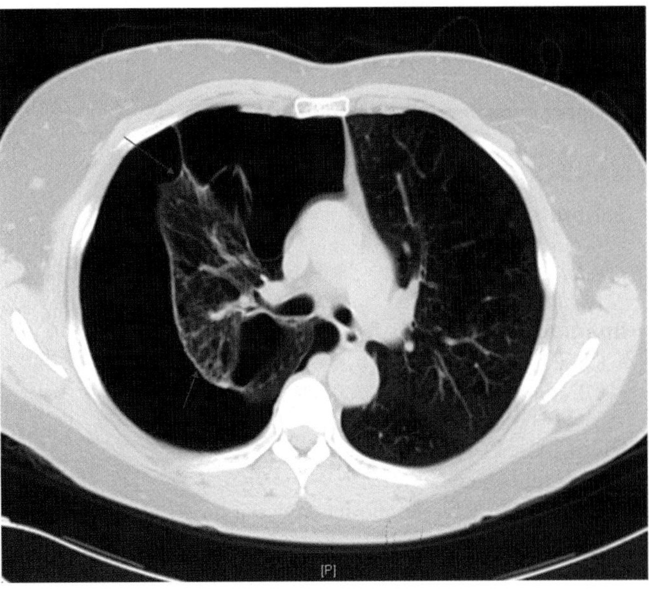

FIGURE 75-3 CT scan of large right-sided pneumothorax. Note significant collapse of right lung with adhesion to anterior chest wall. Pleural reflection highlighted with *red arrows*. The patient has severe underlying emphysema. (From Longo DL, Fauci AS, Kasper DL, Hauser SL, Jameson JL, Loscalzo J, eds. *Harrison's Principles of Internal Medicine*. 18th ed. New York, NY: McGraw-Hill; 2012.)

  - Decreased exercise tolerance
  - Inability to function at work secondary to respiratory problems

Possible Contributing Causes

- Acute complication of tracheostomy[2]
- Asthma
- COPD
- Congenital malformation
- Cystic fibrosis (CF)
- Familial
- Gunshot to lungs
- Having had a previous PTX
- Loud music
- Lung rupture (small region)
- Measles
- Puncture wound to lungs
- Rib fracture
- Smoking
- Tuberculosis
- Whooping cough

Differential Diagnoses

- Asthma
- Bronchiectasis
- Bronchitis
- Central airway obstruction
- Chickenpox
- Congenital lobar emphysema
- CF
- Diaphragmatic hernia
- Gastroesophageal reflux disease (GERD)
- Goiter
- Influenza
- Kawasaki disease (KD)
- Ludwig angina

- Lung cysts/tumor
- Measles
- Tuberculosis
- Upper respiratory tract infection

MEANS OF CONFIRMATION OR DIAGNOSIS

Laboratory Tests

- Arterial blood gases
- Blood test

Imaging

- Chest x-ray
- CT scan

Diagnostic Procedures

- Lung function tests
- Pulse oximetry for monitoring oxygenation
- Lung sounds
- Percussion of the chest/lungs

FINDINGS AND INTERPRETATION

- Increased free air in the pleural space
- Focal area of absent lung sounds
- Shift of the trachea away from the area with absent breath sounds[2]

TREATMENT

Medication

- Oxygen to wash out blood nitrogen[2]

MEDICAL PROCEDURES

- Needle aspiration
- Lung function tests

REFERRALS/ADMITTANCE

- To hospital ER for shortness of breath or chest pain
- To radiologist for imaging; chest x-ray
- To surgeon for chest tube consult
- To pulmonologist

IMPAIRMENTS

- Exercise limitation
- Shortness of breath
- Oxygen deprivation
- Hypotension
- Limited endurance capacity

TESTS AND MEASURES

- Lung sounds
- Vital capacity: Spirometry
- O_2 saturation

INTERVENTION

- Oxygen
- Fluid intake
- Smoking cessation
- Rest
- Once scarring has occurred
  - Pulmonary rehabilitation (PR)
    - Improves exercise capacity
  - Inspiratory muscle training (IMT)
  - Ribcage and thoracic mobility
  - Exercise to return to prior level of function
    - Aerobic
    - Strength
    - Flexibility
    - Postural
    - Breathing

FUNCTIONAL GOALS

- Improve oxygenation by
  - Reducing airway edema secondary to inflammation and bronchospasm
  - Facilitating elimination of bronchial secretions
  - Preventing/treating respiratory infection
  - Increasing exercise tolerance
  - Avoiding irritants/allergens
  - Relieving anxiety; treating depression
  - Improving muscle oxidative capacity
- Patient will be able to
  - Ambulate over 600 m in a 6-minute walk test.
  - Score above 80% of their predicted FEV1 score.
  - Tolerate 1 hour of moderate exercise three times a week.

PROGNOSIS

- Prognosis is related to the size.[4]
  - PTX has a 15% mortality rate.
  - 32% recurrence rate within the first 2 years.
- Small PTX may go away on its own.
- Large PTX may need a chest tube.
- Can be life threatening.
- Once a person has had a PTX, there is a high probability of having another one.

PATIENT RESOURCE

- Pneumothorax. www.pneumothorax.org. Accessed July 4, 2013.

REFERENCES

1. APTA. *Guide to Physical Therapy Practice*. Atlanta: American Physical Therapy Association; 2003. http://guidetoptpractice.apta.org. Accessed July 2, 2013.
2. Hay WW, Levin MJ, Sondheimer JM, Deterding RR. Disorders of the pleura & pleural cavity. In: Hay WW, Levin MJ, Sondheimer JM, Deterding RR, eds. *CURRENT Diagnosis & Treatment: Pediatrics*. 20th ed. New York, NY: McGraw-Hill; 2011. http://www.accessphysiotherapy.com/content/6582681. Accessed July 4, 2013.
3. Patel DR, Greydanus DE, Baker RJ. Chest trauma. In: Patel DR, Greydanus DE, Baker RJ, eds. *Pediatric Practice: Sports Medicine*. New York, NY: McGraw-Hill; 2009. http://www.accessphysiotherapy.com/content/6982825. Accessed July 4, 2013.
4. DeTurk WE, Cahalin LP. Pleural diseases and disorders. In: DeTurk WE, Cahalin LP, eds. *Cardiovascular and Pulmonary Physical Therapy: An Evidence-Based Approach*. 2nd ed. New York, NY: McGraw-Hill; 2011. http://www.accessphysiotherapy.com/content/6873810. Accessed July 4, 2013.

ADDITIONAL REFERENCES

- Aagaard E, Gonzales R. Management of acute bronchitis in healthy adults. *Infect Dis Clin N Am.* 2004;18:919–937.
- Aliverti A, Quaranta M, Chakrabarti B, Albuquerque AL, Calverley PM. Paradoxical movement of the lower ribcage at rest and during exercise in COPD patients. *Eur Respir J.* 2009;33(1):49–60.
- Arroll B, Kenealy T. Antibiotics for the common cold and acute purulent rhinitis. *Cochrane Database Syst Rev.* 2005;(3): CD000247.
- Bateman ED, Feldman C, O'Brien J, Plit M, Joubert JR. Guideline for the management of chronic obstructive pulmonary disease (COPD): 2004 revision. *S Afr Med J.* 2004; 94(7):559–575.
- Batra PS. Radiologic imaging in rhinosinusitis. *Cleve Clin J Med.* 2004;71:886–888.
- Baumann MH, et al. Management of spontaneous pneumothorax: an American College of Chest Physicians Delphi Consensus Statement. ACCP Pneumothorax Consensus Group. *Chest.* 2001;119:590.
- Damore DT, Dayan PS. Medical causes of pneumomediastinum in children. *Clin Pediatr.* 2001;40:87.
- Goodman CC, Fuller KS. *Pathology: Implications for the Physical Therapist.* 3rd ed. Philadelphia, PA: Saunders Elsevier; 2009.
- Goodman CC, Snyder TK. *Differential Diagnosis for Physical Therapists: Screening for Referral.* 4th ed. St. Louis, MO: Saunders Elsevier; 2007.
- Gwaltney JM. Acute bronchitis. In: Mandell GL, Bennett JE, Dolin R, eds. *Principles and Practice of Infectious Diseases.* 6th ed. Philadelphia, PA: Elsevier Churchill Livingstone; 2005.
- Hirschmann JV. Antibiotics for common respiratory tract infections in adults. *Arch Intern Med.* 2002;162:256–264.
- Light RW, Lee GY. Pneumothorax, chylothorax, hemothorax, and fibrothorax. In: Mason RJ, Murray JF, Broaddus VC, Nadel JA, eds. *Textbook of Respiratory Medicine.* 4th ed. Philadelphia, PA: Saunders Elsevier; 2005.
- Mossad SB. Upper respiratory tract infections. Cleveland Clinic Center for Continuing Education. http://www.clevelandclinic-meded.com/medicalpubs/diseasemanagement/infectious-disease/upper-respiratory-tract-infection. Accessed July 2, 2013.
- Noppen M, De Keukeleire T. Pneumothorax. *Respiration.* 2008; 76(2):121–127.
- Panitch HB, Papastamelos C, Schidlow DV. Abnormalities of the pleural space. In: Taussig LM, Landau LI eds. *Pediatric Respiratory Medicine.* Mosby; 1999.
- Panus PC, Jobst EE, Masters SB, Katzung B, Tinsley SL, Trevor AJ. *Pharmacology for the Physical Therapist.* New York, NY: McGraw-Hill; 2009. http://www.accessphysiotherapy.com/content/6095983. Accessed July 4, 2013.
- Wells Cl. Pulmonary pathology. In: DeTurk WE, Cahalin LP, eds. *Cardiovascular and Pulmonary Physical Therapy: An Evidence-Based Approach.* 2nd ed. New York, NY: McGraw-Hill; 2011. http://www.accessphysiotherapy.com/content/6873405#6873405. Accessed July 4, 2013.

76 PULMONARY EDEMA

Eric Shamus, PhD, DPT, PT, CSCS
Greg W. Hartley, DPT, PT, GCS, CEEAA

CONDITION/DISORDER SYNONYM

- Oedema

ICD-9-CM CODES

- 514 Pulmonary congestion and hypostasis
- 518.4 Acute edema of lung, unspecified
- PT diagnoses/treatment diagnoses that may be associated with respiratory disorders
  - 780.7 Malaise and fatigue
  - 786.0 Dyspnea and respiratory abnormalities
  - 786.05 Shortness of breath

ICD-10-CM CODES

- J81.0 Acute pulmonary edema
- J81.1 Chronic pulmonary edema

PREFERRED PRACTICE PATTERNS[1]

- 6A: Primary Prevention/Risk Reduction for Cardiovascular/Pulmonary Disorders
- 6B Impaired Aerobic Capacity/Endurance Associated with Deconditioning
- 6C: Impaired Ventilation, Respiration/Gas Exchange, and Aerobic Capacity/Endurance Associated with Airway Clearance Dysfunction
- 6F: Impaired Ventilation and Respiration/Gas Exchange Associated with Respiratory Failure

PATIENT PRESENTATION

A 77-year-old male in a telemetry unit of an acute care facility for exacerbation of congestive heart failure (CHF) presents to the physical therapist during the second day of treatment with a sudden (new) onset of shortness of breath (respiration rate, 24; PO_2 84% while on 2 L of O_2 via nasal canula), crackles without wheezing heard upon auscultation, elevated blood pressure (177/109), anxiety, profuse diaphoresis, frothy pink sputum, and edema in both feet. The patient's current relevant medications include furosemide as a diuretic, and enalapril for an angiotensin-converting enzyme (ACE) inhibitor. He is in some distress and is unable to respond to questions reliably or without further anxiety. The physical therapist notified the nurse and the physician who obtained the following STAT test results: a standard chest radiograph revealed fluid in the alveolar walls and upper lobe diversion; an echocardiogram confirmed impaired left ventricular function; a complete blood count (CBC) with differential revealed a mildly elevated white count (10,800 cells/μL/mm^3); the blood urea nitrogen (BUN) was 30 mg/dL; creatinine was 1.5 mg/dL; B-type natriuretic peptide (BNP) was 600 pg/mL; and arterial blood gases revealed elevated carbon dioxide and low oxygen concentration.

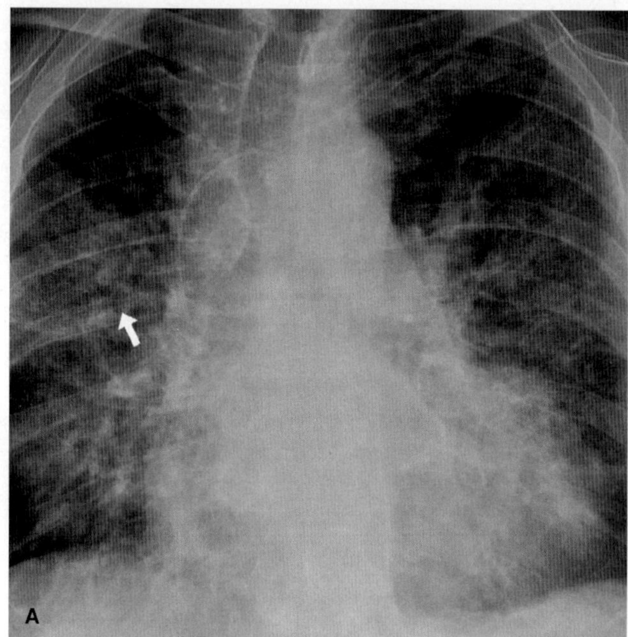

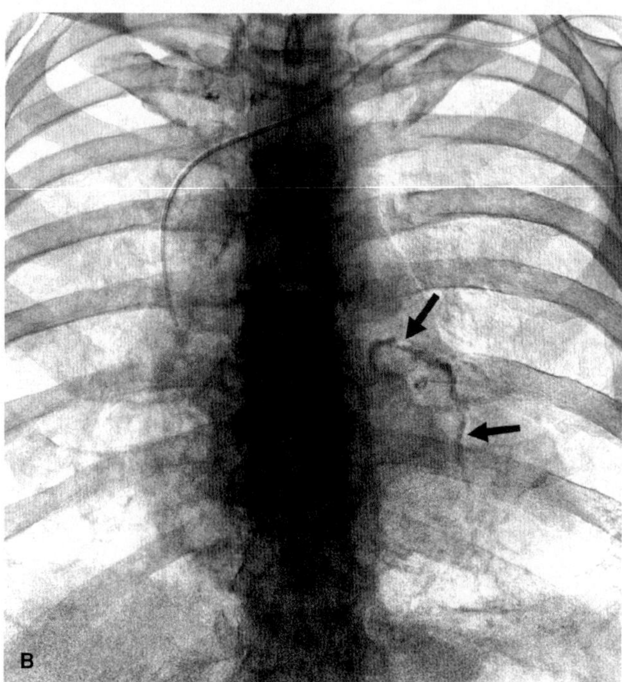

FIGURE 76-1 Radiographs of a 67-year-old man with dyspnea. **A.** Standard radiography demonstrates cardiomegaly and pulmonary edema (*arrow*). **B.** Dual-energy subtraction radiograph demonstrates extensive calcification within the left anterior descending artery (LAD) (*arrows*). (*continued*)

KEY FEATURES

Description

- Fluid accumulation in the air sacs/spaces and parenchyma of the lungs
- Respiratory failure
- Impaired gas exchange
- Peripheral edema
- Shortness of breath/difficulty breathing

Essentials of Diagnosis

- Sudden onset shortness of breath (dyspnea)
- Cyanosis
- Circulatory dysfunction
- Coughing up blood
- Pleural effusion

General Considerations

- Injury to the lung parenchyma
- Cardiac arrest secondary to lack of oxygen

Demographics

- Elderly, usually associated with heart failure, are most affected

CLINICAL FINDINGS

SIGNS AND SYMPTOMS

- Anxiety
- Crackles
- Cyanosis
- Diaphoresis
- Difficulty breathing
- Dyspnea
- Excessive sweating
- Fatigue
- Increased heart rate/tachycardia
- Pale skin
- Peripheral edema
- Pink sputum
- Rales
- Rhonchi
- Third heart sound
- Wheezing

Functional Implications

- Decreased exercise tolerance
- Exercising at high altitude can worsen edema
- Inability to speak secondary to shortness of breath
- Disabling dyspnea when performing simple tasks (i.e., arm elevation to reach into cabinet)

Possible Contributing Causes

- Acute myocardial infarction, heart attack
- Cardiogenic verse noncardiogenic
- CHF
- Electrocution
- Exercising at high altitude
- Head trauma
- Increased intracerebral pressure
- Ischemia
- Kidney failure
- Mitral stenosis
- Opiod/heroin use
- Seizures
- Sepsis
- Transfusion
- Valvular regurgitation

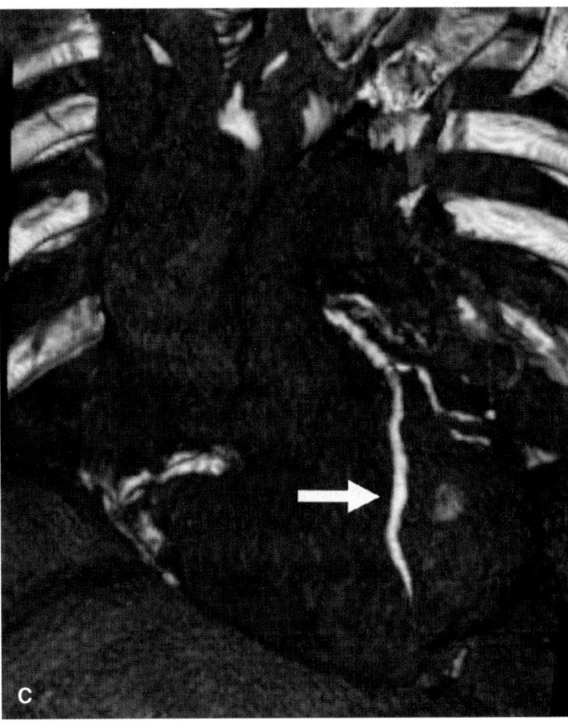

FIGURE 76-1 *(Continued)* **C.** Three-dimensional computed tomography reconstruction of the chest confirms extensive calcifications in the LAD territory (*arrow*). (From Fuster V, Walsh RA, Harrington RA. *Hurst's The Heart*. 13th ed. www.accessmedicine.com. Copyright © The McGraw-Hill Companies, Inc. All rights reserved.)

Differential Diagnosis

- CHF
- Influenza
- Cystic fibrosis
- Asthma
- Gastroesophageal reflux disease
- Bronchiectasis
- Kawasaki disease
- Bronchitis

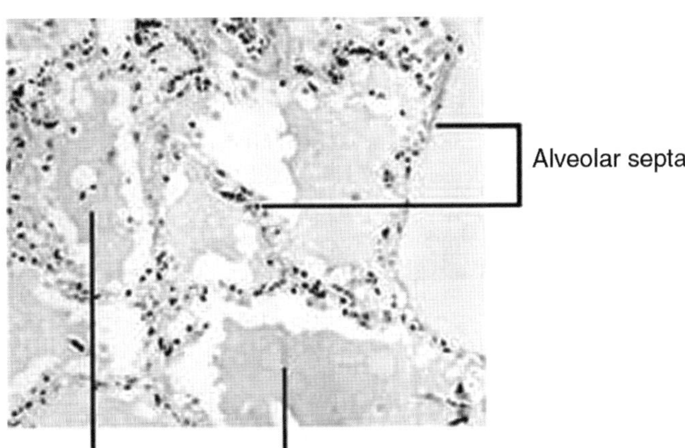

FIGURE 76-2 Pulmonary edema, characterized by the presence of fluid in the alveoli. The fluid has a frothy appearance resulting from admixture with air. (From Chandrasoma P, Taylor CR. *Concise Pathology*. 3rd ed. www.accessmedicine. com. Copyright © The McGraw-Hill Companies, Inc. All rights reserved.)

- Upper respiratory tract infection
- Central airway obstruction
- Lung tumor
- Tuberculosis

MEANS OF CONFIRMATION OR DIAGNOSIS

▶ Laboratory Tests

- Blood test for electrolytes
- Arterial blood gases
- Lung function tests
- Pulse oximetry
- Auscultation
- Percussion of the chest/lungs

▶ Imaging

- Pulmonary capillary wedge pressure
- Pulmonary angiography
- Chest radiograph
- CT
- Lung ventilation/perfusion scan
- Echocardiogram

FINDINGS AND INTERPRETATION

- Chest X-ray demonstrates interstitial and alveolar edema
- Crackle sound with auscultation

TREATMENT

▶ Medication

- Diuretic
- Morphine

REFERRALS/ADMITTANCE

- For imaging, X-ray
- To pulmonologist, for respiratory assessment

IMPAIRMENTS

- Exercise limitation
- Shortness of breath
- Oxygen deprivation
- Limited endurance capacity

TEST AND MEASURES

- 6-minute walk test for mild or nonsymptomatic cases
- BORG Rating of Perceived Exertion (RPE)
- Monitor vital signs to include lung auscultations
- Short-Form 36 Health Survey (SF-36)
- New York Heart Association Functional Classification scale

INTERVENTION

- Oxygen
- Rest
- Fluid intake
- Smoking cessation
- Pulmonary rehabilitation (PR) to improve exercise capacity
- Inspiratory muscle training (IMT)
- Exercise (aerobic, strength, flexibility, posture, breathing) to return to prior level of function

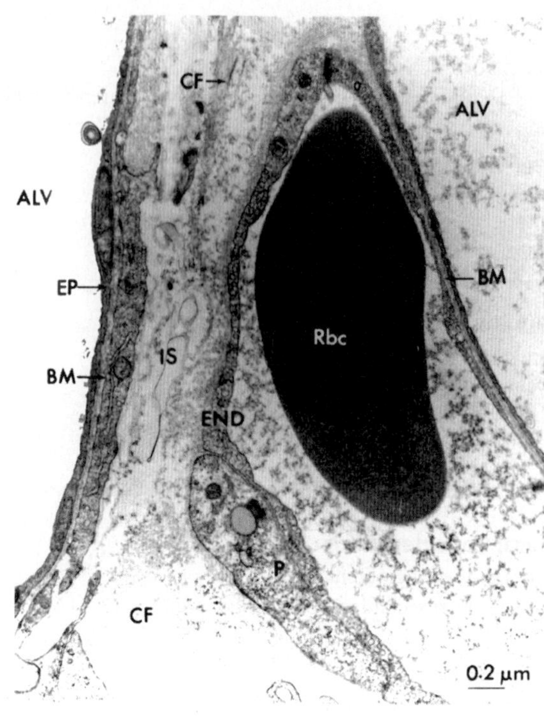

FIGURE 76-3 Interstitial pulmonary edema. Electron micrograph showing the alveolar septum and a pulmonary capillary in cross section. On the right, the basement membrane of the alveolar epithelium and the capillary endothelium are fused. This barrier is, therefore, thin (0.2 μm), which optimizes gas exchange and inhibits accumulation of edema fluid. On the other side, the interstitial space contains connective tissue that is in continuity with the loose connective tissue of the perivascular and peribronchial interstitium. Edema fluid first accumulates in this pericapillary space. The continuity of the interstitial spaces provides a pathway for movement of edema fluid centrally away from areas of gas exchange. ALV, alveolus; EP, epithelial cell; BM, basement membrane; IS, interstitial space; Rbc, red blood cell; CF, pericapillary fluid; END, endothelial cell. (Reproduced with permission from Fishman AP. Pulmonary edema. *Circulation*. 1972;46:390.)

FUNCTIONAL GOALS

- Improve oxygenation
- Patient will be able to
  - Ambulate over 600 m in a 6-minute walk test.

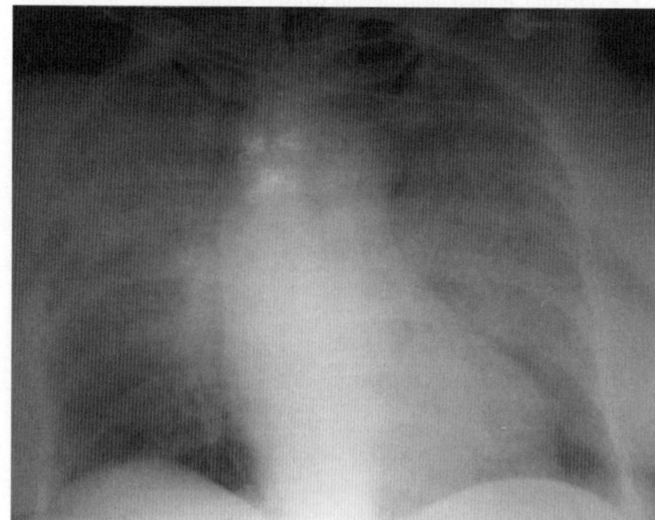

FIGURE 76-4 The radiographic appearance of severe pulmonary edema. (From Stone CK, Humphries RL. *Current Diagnosis & Treatment: Emergency Medicine*. 7th ed. www.accessmedicine.com. Copyright © The McGraw-Hill Companies, Inc. All rights reserved.)

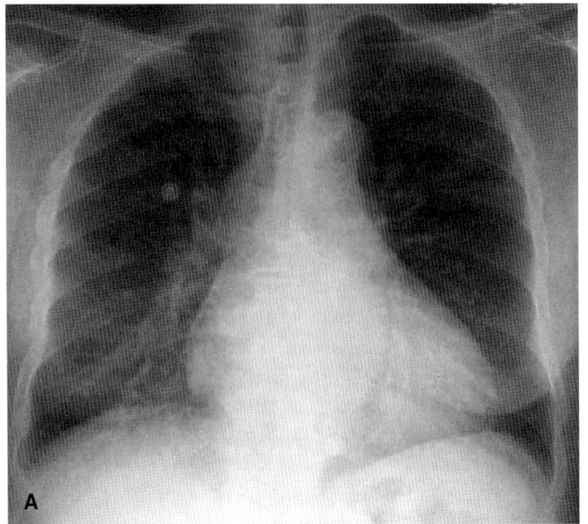

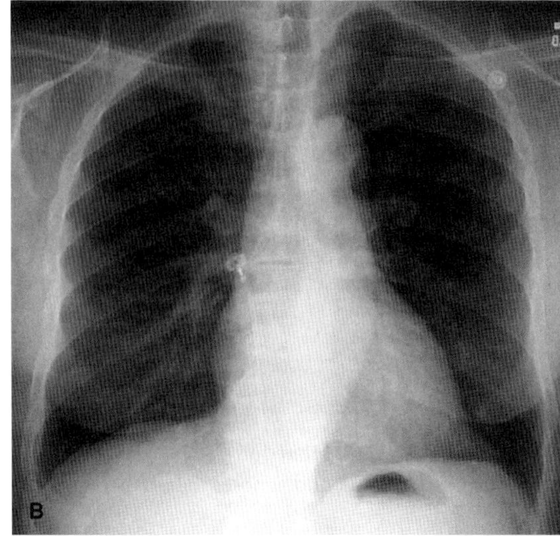

FIGURE 76-5 **A.** 55-year-old woman with an acute shortness of breath. **B.** Chest radiograph of the same patient obtained 1 month earlier. (From Chen MYM, Pope TL, Ott DJ. *Basic Radiology*. 2nd ed. www.accessmedicine.com. Copyright © The McGraw-Hill Companies, Inc. All rights reserved.)

- Score more than 80% of predicted FEV_1 score.
- Tolerate 1 hour of moderate exercise three times a week.

PROGNOSIS

- Depends on the amount of fluid in the lung.
- Can be life threatening, lead to respiratory failure.

PATIENT RESOURCE

- Who is at Risk for Pulmonary Embolism? National Heart Lung and Blood Institute, National Institutes of Health. http://www.nhlbi.nih.gov/health/health-topics/topics/pe/atrisk.html. Accessed July 3, 2013.

REFERENCE

1. APTA. *Guide to Physical Therapy Practice*. Atlanta: American Physical Therapy Association; 2003. http://guidetoptpractice.apta.org. Accessed July 3, 2013.

ADDITIONAL REFERENCES

- Aagaard E, Gonzales R. Management of acute bronchitis in healthy adults. *Infect Dis Clin North Am*. 2004;18(4):919–937. http://dx.doi.org/10.1016/j.idc.2004.07.001. Accessed May 9, 2014.
- Aliverti A, Quaranta M, Chakrabarti B, Albuquerque AL, Calverley PM.. Paradoxical movement of the lower ribcage at rest and during exercise in COPD patients. *Eur Respir J*. 2009;33(1):49–60. doi: 10.1183/09031936.00141607.
- Arroll B, Kenealy T. Antibiotics for the common cold and acute purulent rhinitis. *Cochrane Database Syst Rev*. 2005;(3):CD000247. doi: 10.1002/14651858.CD000247.
- Bateman ED, Feldman C, O'Brien J, Plit M, Joubert JR. Guideline for the management of chronic obstructive pulmonary disease (COPD): 2004 Revision. *S Afr Med J*. 2004;94(7 Pt 2):559–575.
- Batra PS. Radiologic imaging in rhinosinusitis. *Cleve Clin J Med*. 2004;71(11):886–888. doi:10.3949/ccjm.71.11.886.
- Goodman CC, Fuller KS. *Pathology: Implications for the Physical Therapist*. 3rd ed. Philadelphia, PA: Saunders Elsevier; 2009.
- Goodman CC, Snyder TK. *Differential Diagnosis for Physical Therapists: Screening for Referral*. 4th ed. St. Louis, MO: Saunders Elsevier; 2007.
- Gwaltney JM. Acute bronchitis. In: Mandell GL, Bennett JE, Dolin R, eds. *Principles and Practice of Infectious Diseases*. 6th ed. Philadelphia, PA: Elsevier Churchill Livingstone; 2005.
- Hirschmann JV. Antibiotics for common respiratory tract infections in adults. *Arch Intern Med*. 2002;162(3):256–264.
- ICD9Data.com. http://www.icd9data.com. Accessed July 3, 2013.
- ICD10Data.com. http://www.icd10data.com. Accessed July 3, 2013.
- Light RW, Lee GY. Pneumothorax, chylothorax, hemothorax, and fibrothorax. In: Mason RJ, Murray JF, Broaddus VC, Nadel JA, eds. *Textbook of Respiratory Medicine*. 4th ed. Philadelphia, PA: Saunders Elsevier; 2005.
- Mossad SB. Upper Respiratory Tract Infections. Cleveland Clinic Center for Continuing Education. http://www.clevelandclinicmeded.com/medicalpubs/diseasemanagement/infectious-disease/upper-respiratory-tract-infection. Accessed July 3, 2013.
- Noppen M, De Keukeleire T. Pneumothorax. *Respiration*. 2008;76(2):121–127. doi: 10.1159/000135932.
- O'Leary R, McKinlay J. Neurogenic pulmonary oedema. *Continuing Education in Anaesthesia, Critical Care & Pain*. 2011;11(3):87–92. doi:10.1093/bjaceaccp/mkr006. http://ceaccp.oxfordjournals.org/content/11/3/87.extract. Accessed May 9, 2014.
- Panus PC, Jobst EE, Masters SB, Katzung B, Tinsley SL, Trevor AJ. Drugs affecting the respiratory system. In: Panus PC, Jobst EE, Masters SB, Katzung B, Tinsley SL, Trevor AJ, eds. *Pharmacology for the Physical Therapist*. New York, NY: McGraw-Hill; 2009:Chapter 35. http://www.accessphysiotherapy.com/content/6095983. Accessed July 3, 2013.
- Wells Cl. Pulmonary pathology. In: DeTurk WE, Cahalin LP, eds. *Cardiovascular and Pulmonary Physical Therapy: An Evidence-Based Approach*. 2nd ed. New York, NY: McGraw-Hill; 2011. http://www.accessphysiotherapy.com/content/6873405#6873405. Accessed July 3, 2013.
- Wells PS, Hirsh J, Anderson DR, et al. Accuracy of clinical assessment of deep-vein thrombosis. *Lancet*. 1995;345(8961):1326–1330.

77 PULMONARY EMBOLISM

Eric Shamus, PhD, DPT, PT, CSCS
Jennifer Shamus, PhD, DPT, COMT, CSCS

CONDITION/DISORDER SYNONYM

- Venous thromboembolism (VTE)

ICD-9-CM CODES

- 415.1 Pulmonary embolism and infarction
- Associated PT diagnoses/treatment diagnoses that may be associated with respiratory disorders
  - 780.7 Malaise and fatigue
  - 786.0 Dyspnea and respiratory abnormalities
  - 786.05 Shortness of breath

ICD-10-CM CODE

- I26 Pulmonary embolism

PREFERRED PRACTICE PATTERNS[1]

- 6A: Primary Prevention/Risk Reduction for Cardiovascular/Pulmonary Disorders
- 6B Impaired Aerobic Capacity/Endurance Associated with Deconditioning
- 6C: Impaired Ventilation, Respiration/Gas Exchange, and Aerobic Capacity/Endurance Associated with Airway Clearance Dysfunction
- 6F: Impaired Ventilation and Respiration/Gas Exchange Associated with Respiratory Failure

PATIENT PRESENTATION

A 34-year-old man presents to the emergency department complaining of shortness of breath and chest pain that he describes as right sided and increased with deep breathing. He states it started suddenly when he woke up and started moving. He denies fever, chills, nausea, vomiting, or cough. He has a recent history of multiple gunshot wounds resulting in ongoing pain in his upper back and T-10 paraplegia. One week ago, he was discharged from the hospital to a rehabilitation facility. He is currently taking acetaminophen/hydrocodone and ibuprofen for his pain, which has increased with his physical therapy and occupational therapy. He is also taking hydrochlorothiazide and captopril for hypertension and fluoxetine for depression. He recently quit smoking tobacco since he was hospitalized and denies any alcohol or illicit drug use. On physical examination, he is an otherwise fit young man who

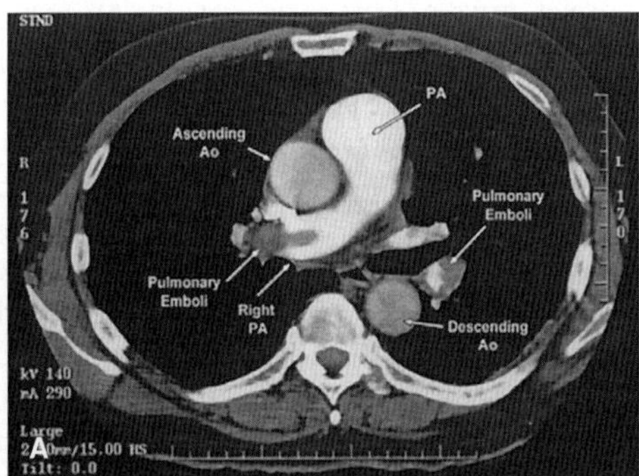

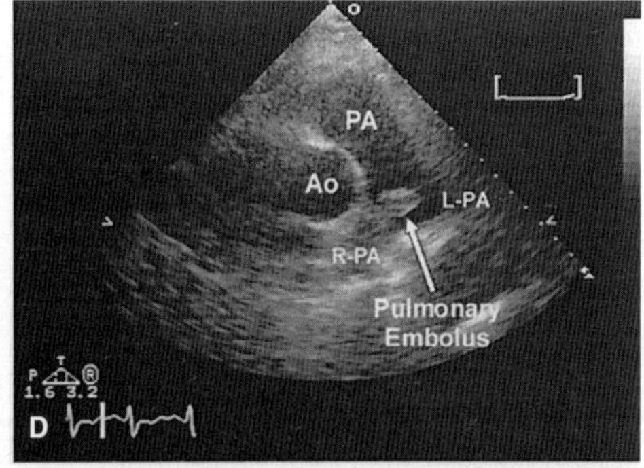

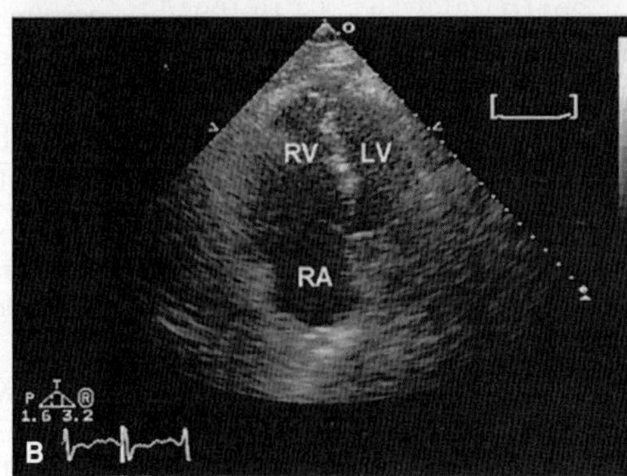

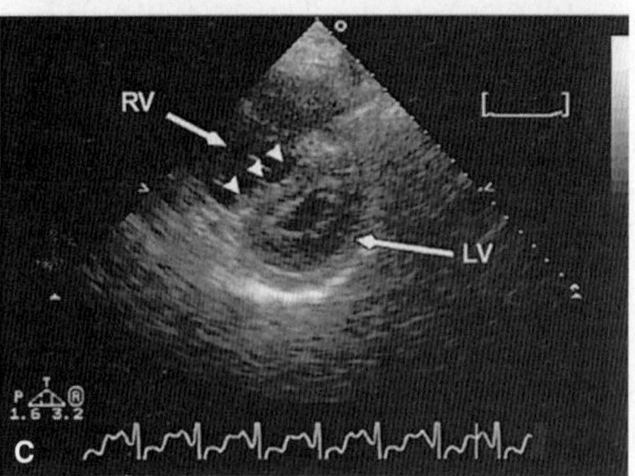

FIGURE 77-1 Chest computed tomography and echocardiographic findings in a 55-year-old man with submassive **pulmonary embolism**. **A.** Chest computed tomography scan demonstrating multiple segmental emboli, including a central embolus in main pulmonary artery and extending into right pulmonary artery (R-PA). **B.** Transthoracic apical four-chamber view with severe right ventricular (RV) dilatation. **C.** Transthoracic parasternal short-axis view showing flattening of interventricular septum ("D-shaped" left ventricle [LV], *arrowheads*). **D.** Transthoracic short-axis view demonstrating the central clot in the main and R-PAs. Ao, aorta; L-PA, left pulmonary artery; PA, pulmonary artery; RA, right atrium; R-PA, right pulmonary artery. (From Garg RK, Bednarz J, Spencer KT, Lang RM. Acute pulmonary embolism. *Circulation.* 2000;102:2441, with permission.)

appears slightly short of breath and uncomfortable. His heart rate is 101 beats per minute, his blood pressure is 110/78 mm Hg, and his respiratory rate is 26 breaths per minute. His pulse oximetry is 96% on 2 L of O_2 by nasal canula. His lungs are clear to auscultation. There is mild swelling of his left calf. He has no sensation in his lower extremities. Laboratory studies reveal a white blood cell count (WBC) of 10,000/mm^3. Hemoglobin, hematocrit, electrolytes, and renal function are all within normal limits. A 12-lead electrocardiogram (ECG) reveals a sinus rhythm at a rate of 103 beats per minute. His chest radiograph reveals minimal bibasilar atelectasis but no evidence of infiltrates or effusions.[2]

KEY FEATURES

Description

- Blockage of the artery of the lung
- Thrombus (blood clot), commonly from deep veins in the legs
- Chest pain with breathing
- Embolism can be fat or air
- Increased pressure in the right ventricle of the heart

Essentials of Diagnosis

- Sudden onset shortness of breath (dyspnea)
- Cyanosis
- Circulatory dysfunction
- Pleural effusion

General Considerations

- Can be life threatening; sudden death can occur
- Can damage part of the lung
- Organ damage secondary to reduced oxygen levels

Demographics

- For every 10 years older than 60 years old, the risk of pulmonary embolism (PE) doubles[3]
- Pregnancy increases risk
- Obesity increases risk

CLINICAL FINDINGS

SIGNS AND SYMPTOMS

- Calf pain
- Chest pain
- Chest tightness
- Coughing
- Cyanosis
- Decreased oxygenation throughout the body
- Fatigue
- Increased heart rate
- Increased respiratory rate
- Light-headedness
- Pain worse with deep breath or cough
- Palpitations
- Pulmonary component of the second heart sound
- Shortness of breath
- Shoulder raised to allow increased lung air flow
- Sudden death
- Sweating
- Swelling in one leg
- Tensed muscles from dyspnea

Functional Implications

- Bleeding problems from blood-thinner medication
  - Caution with massage and cross-friction techniques secondary to bruising and bleeding
  - Increased with bleeding and bruising with minimal activities

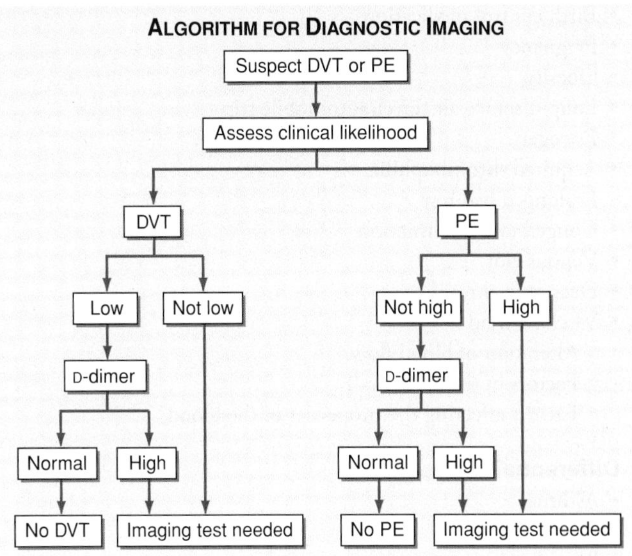

FIGURE 77-2 How to decide whether diagnostic imaging is needed. (From Longo DL, Fauci AS, Kasper DL, Hauser SL, Jameson JL, Loscalzo J, eds. *Harrison's Principles of Internal Medicine.* 18th ed. New York, NY: McGraw-Hill; 2012.)

- Disabling dyspnea when performing simple tasks (i.e., arm elevation to reach into cabinet)
- Decreased exercise tolerance

Possible Contributing Causes

- Recent surgery
- Fractures
- High blood pressure
- Air bubble or tumor breaks loose
- Cancer
- Female hormone therapy

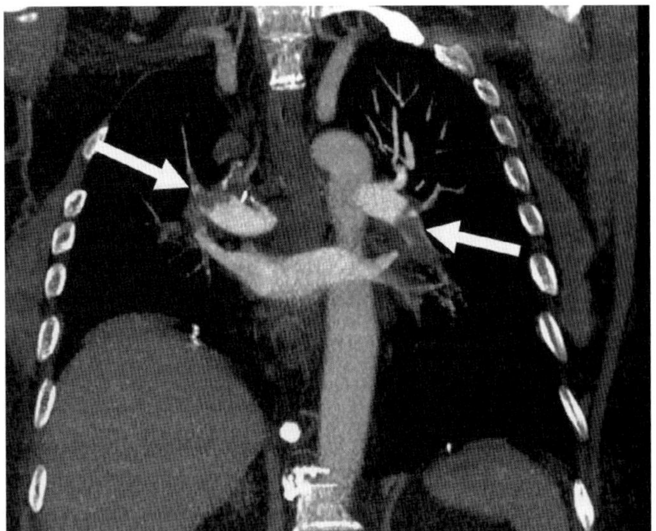

FIGURE 77-3 Large bilateral proximal PE on a coronal chest CT image in a 54-year-old man with lung cancer and brain metastases. He had developed sudden onset of chest heaviness and shortness of breath while at home. There are filling defects in the main and segmental pulmonary arteries bilaterally (*white arrows*). Only the left upper lobe segmental artery is free of thrombus. (From Longo DL, Fauci AS, Kasper DL, Hauser SL, Jameson JL, Loscalzo J, eds. *Harrison's Principles of Internal Medicine.* 18th ed. New York, NY: McGraw-Hill; 2012.)

- Birth control medication
- Pregnancy
- Obesity
- Long-distance air travel/automobile trip
- Estrogen
- Acquired thrombophilia
- Prolonged bed rest
- Congenital malformation
- Venous clot
- Deep vein thrombosis
- Virchow triad
  - Alteration of blood flow
  - Factors in the vessel wall
  - Factors affecting the properties of the blood

Differential Diagnosis

- Asthma
- Bronchiectasis
- Bronchitis
- Central airway obstruction
- Congestive heart failure
- Cystic fibrosis
- Gastroesophageal reflux disease
- Goiter
- Influenza
- Kawasaki disease
- Ludwig angina
- Lung tumor
- Tuberculosis
- Upper respiratory tract infection

MEANS OF CONFIRMATION OR DIAGNOSIS

Laboratory Tests

- Blood test, clotting status
- Arterial blood gases
- Lung function tests
- Pulse oximetry
- Wells score
- Geneva rule
- Percussion of the chest/lungs

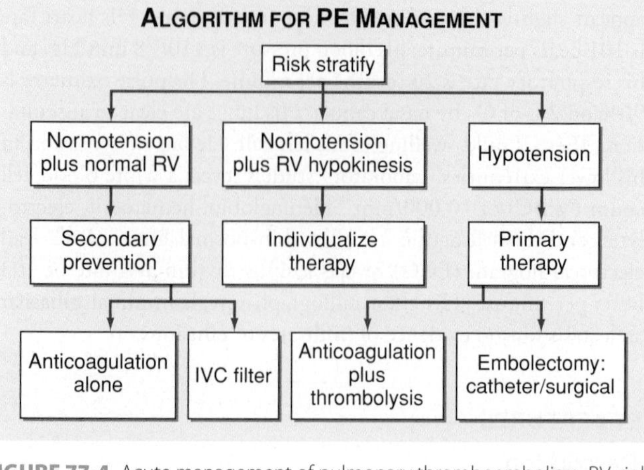

FIGURE 77-4 Acute management of pulmonary thromboembolism. RV, right ventricular; IVC, inferior vena cava. (From Longo DL, Fauci AS, Kasper DL, Hauser SL, Jameson JL, Loscalzo J, eds. *Harrison's Principles of Internal Medicine.* 18th ed. New York, NY: McGraw-Hill; 2012.)

Imaging

- Pulmonary angiography
- Chest radiograph
- CT
- Lung ventilation/perfusion scan
- Echocardiogram
- Ultrasound legs for blood clots

FINDINGS AND INTERPRETATION

- Normal D-dimer level can exclude thrombotic PE
- McConnell sign on electrocardiogram

TREATMENT

Medication

- Anticoagulants
- Thrombolysis drugs

MEDICAL PROCEDURES

- Embolism must be eliminated

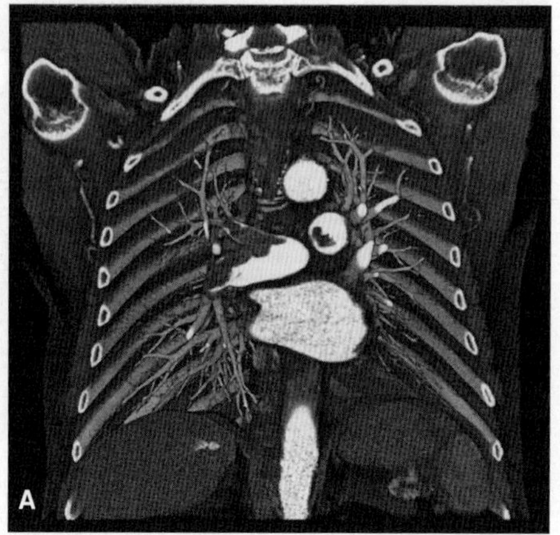

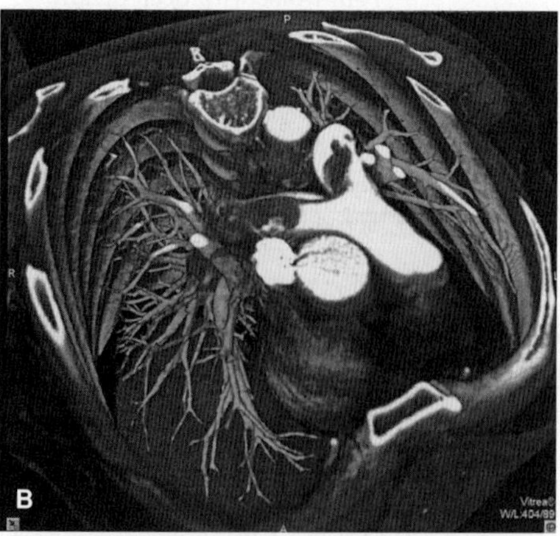

FIGURE 77-5 Contrast-enhanced 16-slice computed tomography scan in a 72-year-old man with extensive, acute central pulmonary embolism showing a "saddle embolus" (*arrows*) extending into both central pulmonary arteries. Colored volume-rendering technique seen from an anterocranial (**A**) and anterior (**B**) perspective allows intuitive visualization of location and extent of embolism. (From Fuster V, Walsh RA, Harrington RA. *Hurst's The Heart.* 13th ed. www.accessmedicine.com. Copyright ©The McGraw-Hill Companies, Inc. All rights reserved.)

REFERRALS/ADMITTANCE

- For imaging, X-ray
- Surgical consult/hospital for pulmonary thrombectomy, vena cava filter
- Pulmonologist for respiratory assessment

IMPAIRMENTS

- Exercise limitation
- Shortness of breath
- Oxygen deprivation
- Limited endurance capacity

TEST AND MEASURES

- 6-minute walk test for mild or nonsymptomatic cases
- BORG Rating of Perceived Exertion (RPE)
- Monitor vital signs to include lung auscultations
- Short-Form 36 Health Survey (SF-36)
- New York Heart Association Functional Classification scale

INTERVENTION

- Oxygen
- Rest
- Fluid intake
- Smoking cessation
- Pulmonary rehabilitation (PR) once clot is eliminated
  - Improves exercise capacity
  - Inspiratory muscle training (IMT)
- Exercise (aerobic, strength, flexibility, posture, breathing) to return to prior level of functioning

FUNCTIONAL GOALS

- Improve oxygenation
- Patient will be able to
  - Ambulate more than 600 m in a 6-minute walk test.
  - Score more than 80% of predicted FEV_1 score.
  - Tolerate 1 hour of moderate exercise three times a week.

PROGNOSIS

- Immediate diagnosis and treatment can be life-saving.
- Geneva prediction rule.
- Depends on the amount of the lung affected.
- Can be life threatening.

PATIENT RESOURCE

- Acute Pulmonary Embolism. European Society of Cardiology. http://www.escardio.org/guidelines-surveys/esc-guidelines/Pages/acute-pulmonary-embolism.aspx. Accessed July 3, 2013.

REFERENCES

1. APTA. *Guide to Physical Therapy Practice*. Atlanta: American Physical Therapy Association; 2003. http://guidetoptpractice.apta.org. Accessed July 3, 2013.
2. Toy EC. Pulmonary embolism, Case 55. *LANGE Case Files*. http://www.accessmedicine.com/casecontent.aspx?aid=8651625&tabid=1. Accessed July 4, 2013.
3. Who is at Risk for Pulmonary Embolism? National Heart Lung and Blood Institute, National Institutes of Health. http://www.nhlbi.nih.gov/health/health-topics/topics/pe/atrisk.html. Accessed July 3, 2013.

ADDITIONAL REFERENCES

- Aagaard E, Gonzales R. Management of acute bronchitis in healthy adults. *Infect Dis Clin North Am*. 2004;18(4):919–937. http://dx.doi.org/10.1016/j.idc.2004.07.001. Accessed May 9, 2014.
- Aliverti A, Quaranta M, Chakrabarti B, Albuquerque AL, Calverley P. Paradoxical movement of the lower ribcage at rest and during exercise in COPD patients. *Eur Respir J*. 2009;33(1):49–60. doi: 10.1183/09031936.00141607.
- Arroll B, Kenealy T. Antibiotics for the common cold and acute purulent rhinitis. *Cochrane Database Syst Rev*. 2005;(3):CD000247. doi: 10.1002/14651858.CD000247.pub2.
- Wells CL. Pulmonary pathology. In: DeTurk WE, Cahalin LP, eds. *Cardiovascular and Pulmonary Physical Therapy: An Evidence-Based Approach*. 2nd ed. New York, NY: McGraw-Hill; 2011. http://www.accessphysiotherapy.com/content/6873405#6873405 Accessed July 3, 2013.
- Goodman CC, Fuller KS. *Pathology: Implications for the Physical Therapist*. 3rd ed. Philadelphia, PA: Saunders Elsevier; 2009.
- Goodman CC, Snyder TK. *Differential Diagnosis for Physical Therapists: Screening for Referral*. 4th ed. St. Louis, MO: Saunders Elsevier; 2007.
- Gwaltney JM. Acute bronchitis. In: Mandell GL, Bennett JE, Dolin R, eds. *Principles and Practice of Infectious Diseases*. 6th ed. Philadelphia, PA: Elsevier Churchill Livingstone; 2005.
- Hirschmann JV. Antibiotics for common respiratory tract infections in adults. *Arch Intern Med*. 2002;162(3):256–264.
- Light RW, Lee GY. Pneumothorax, chylothorax, hemothorax, and fibrothorax. In: Mason RJ, Murray JF, Broaddus VC, Nadel JA, eds. *Textbook of Respiratory Medicine*. 4th ed. Philadelphia, PA: Saunders Elsevier; 2005.
- Mossas SB. Upper Respiratory Tract Infections. Cleveland Clinic Center for Continuing Education. http://www.clevelandclinicmeded.com/medicalpubs/diseasemanagement/infectious-disease/upper-respiratory-tract-infection. Accessed July 2, 2013.
- Noppen M, De Keukeleire T. Pneumothorax. *Respiration*. 2008;76(2):121–127. doi: 10.1159/000135932.
- Panus PC, Jobst EE, Masters SB, Katzung B, Tinsley SL, Trevor AJ. Drugs affecting the respiratory system. In: Panus PC, Jobst EE, Masters SB, Katzung B, Tinsley SL, Trevor AJ, eds. *Pharmacology for the Physical Therapist*. New York, NY: McGraw-Hill; 2009. http://www.accessphysiotherapy.com/content/6095983. Accessed July 3, 2013.
- Wells PS, Hirsh J, Anderson DR, et al. Accuracy of clinical assessment of deep-vein thrombosis. *Lancet*. 1995;345(8961):1326–1330.

78 UPPER RESPIRATORY TRACT INFECTION

Eric Shamus, PhD, DPT, PT, CSCS
Jennifer Shamus, PhD, DPT, COMT, CSCS

CONDITION/DISORDER SYNONYMS

- Epiglottitis
- Laryngitis
- Laryngotracheitis
- Nasopharyngitis
- Pharyngitis
- Rhinitis
- Rhinosinusitis
- Sinusitis
- Tracheitis

ICD-9-CM CODES

- 465.9 Acute upper respiratory infections of unspecified site
- PT diagnoses/treatment diagnoses that may be associated with respiratory disorders
    - 780.7 Malaise and fatigue
    - 786.0 Dyspnea and respiratory abnormalities
    - 786.05 Shortness of breath

ICD-10-CM CODE

- J06.9 Acute upper respiratory infection, unspecified

PREFERRED PRACTICE PATTERNS[1]

- 6C: Impaired Ventilation, Respiration/Gas Exchange, and Aerobic Capacity/Endurance Associated with Airway Clearance Dysfunction
- 6F: Impaired Ventilation and Respiration/Gas Exchange Associated with Respiratory Failure

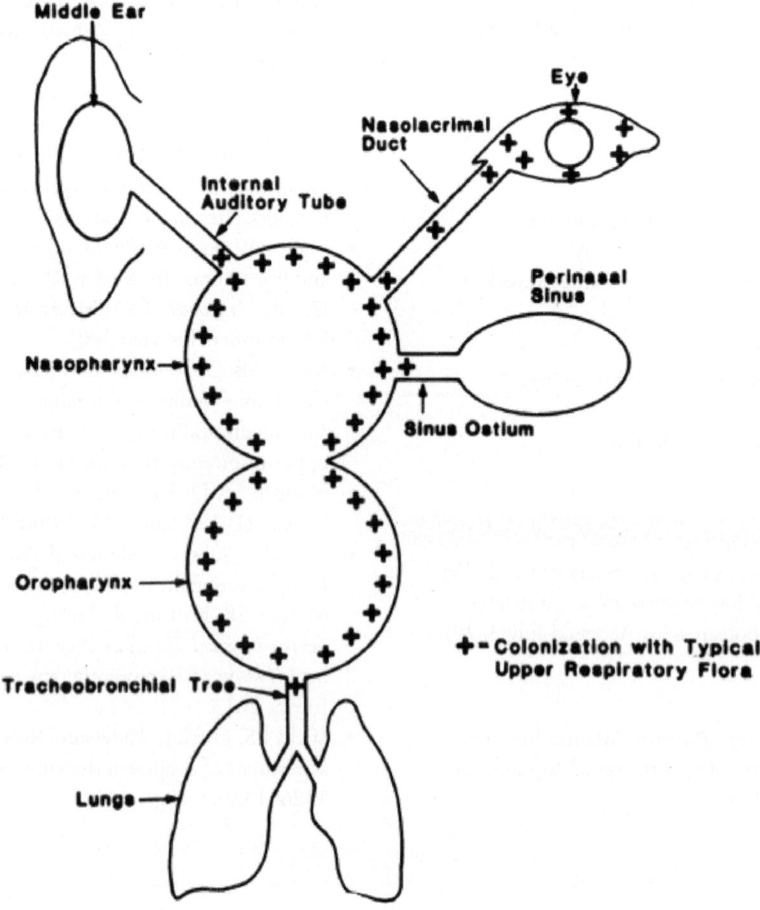

FIGURE 78-1 Diagram of the anatomic relations of head and neck structures and distribution of the indigenous flora. (Reproduced with permission from Todd JK. Bacteriology and clinical relevance of nasopharyngeal and oropharyngeal cultures. *Pediatr Infect Dis.* 1984;3:159.)

PATIENT PRESENTATION

A 10-year-old girl is brought to her pediatrician's office complaining of headache for the past 2 weeks. Her mother had taken the girl to an optometrist, and her vision was normal. The patient states that she has been in good health and that she received a cat as a birthday present 1 month previously. On examination, she has a normal temperature, the tympanic membranes appear normal, and her throat is clear. There is some tenderness of the right cheek and over the right orbit.[2]

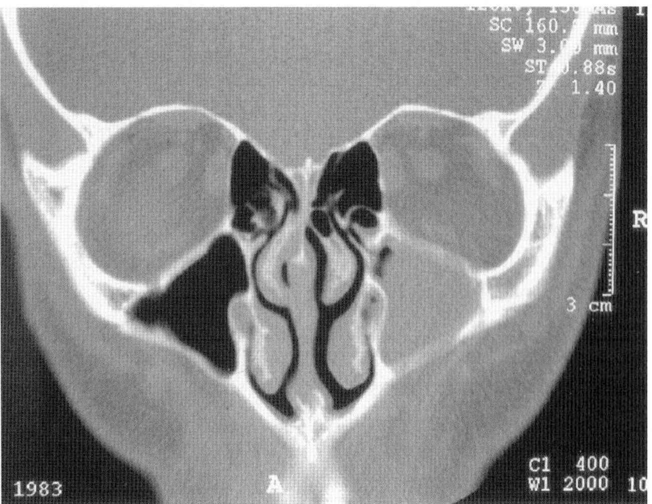

FIGURE 78-2 Acute sinusitis with opacification of the maxillary sinus. (Reproduced with permission from Brunicardi FC, Andersen D, Billiar T, et al. *Schwartz's Principles of Surgery.* 8th ed. New York, NY: McGraw-Hill; 2004.)

KEY FEATURES

Description

- Nonspecific term for acute infections in the nose, paranasal, sinuses, pharynx, larynx, trachea, and bronchi
- Viruses are the main cause

Essentials of Diagnosis

- Diagnosis is based upon clinical manifestation[3]
- Sinusitis and acute bronchitis usually occur after a common cold

General Considerations

- Influenza is a systemic illness involving the respiratory tract that is separate from upper respiratory tract infections (URI or UTI)
- Spread by aerosol, droplet, hand-to-hand contact
- Antibiotics have no-to-limited role in the treatment of the common cold or URI[3]

Demographics

- Across the lifespan

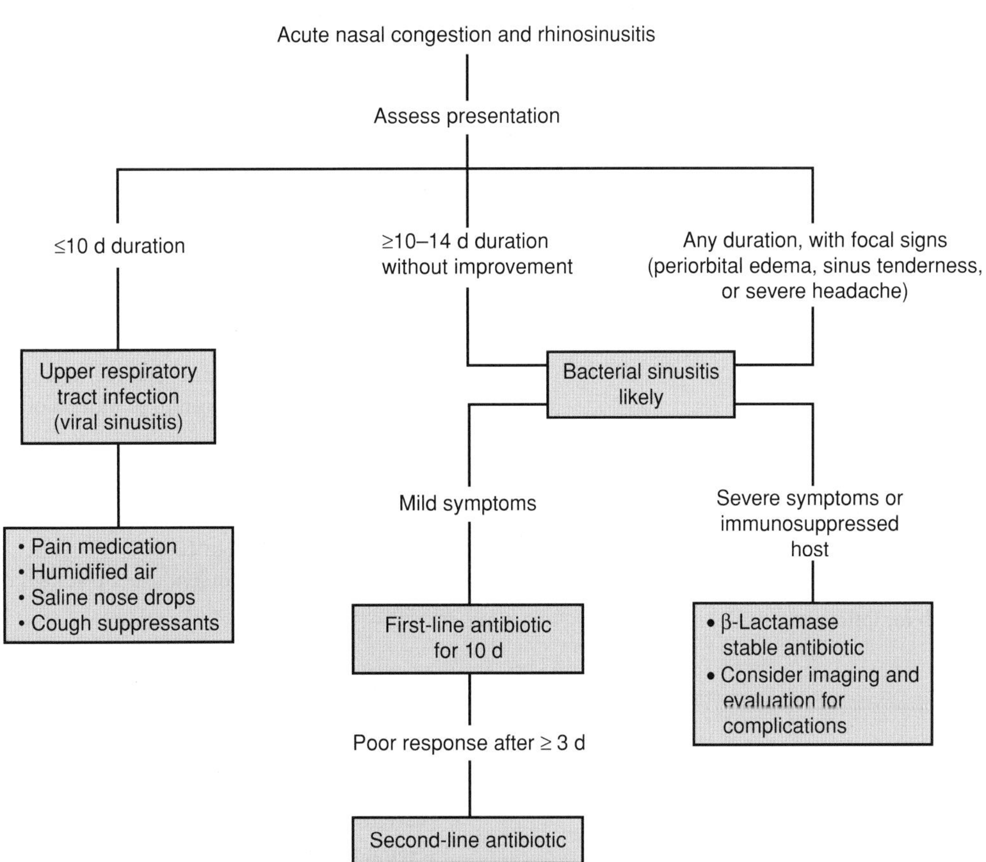

FIGURE 78-3 Algorithm for acute nasal congestion and rhinosinusitis. (From Hay WM et al. *Current Diagnosis & Treatment: Pediatrics.* 21st ed. www.accessmedicine.com. Copyright © The McGraw-Hill Companies, Inc. All rights reserved.)

CLINICAL FINDINGS

SIGNS AND SYMPTOMS[4]

- Chest tightness
- Cough
- Edema
- Fever
- Headache
- Local swelling
- Nasal congestion
- Shortness of breath
- Shoulder raised to allow increased lung air flow
- Sneezing
- Sore throat
- Tensed muscles from dyspnea
- Wheezing

Functional Implications

- Disabling dyspnea when performing simple tasks such as
  - Arm elevation to reach into cabinet
  - Decreased exercise tolerance
- Patients with mononucleosis should avoid contact sports for 6 weeks as fear of splenic rupture.

Possible Contributing Causes

- Air pollution
- Cocaine use
- Deviated septum
- Environmental irritants
- Immunodeficiency disorders
- Long-term exposure to lung irritants
- Periodontal disease
- Smoking

Differential Diagnosis

- Adult cystic fibrosis
- Asthma/Asthma (reversible)
- Bronchiectasis
- Bronchitis
- Central airway obstruction
- Chickenpox
- Gastroesophageal reflux disease
- Goiter
- Influenza
- Kawasaki disease
- Ludwig angina
- Lung tumor
- Measles
- Pneumonia
- Tuberculosis

MEANS OF CONFIRMATION OR DIAGNOSIS

Laboratory Tests

- Viral culture
- Nasopharyngeal swab for influenza

Imaging

- Chest radiograph
- CT for sinuses

FINDINGS AND INTERPRETATION

- Acute sinusitis on CT will show complete opacification and air–fluid level[1]

REFERRALS/ADMITTANCE

- For imaging, X-ray
- Medication: Anti-inflammatory agents, bronchodilators, expectorants, antihistamines, or vaccines
- Surgical consult, deviated septum
- Ear, nose, and throat (ENT) physician
- Pulmonologist

IMPAIRMENTS

- Exercise limitation
- Shortness of breath
- Limited endurance capacity

INTERVENTION

- Increased fluid intake
- Smoking cessation
- Manual sinus drainage
- Coughing techniques
- Pulmonary rehabilitation (PR)
  - Enhances the patient's sense of well-being
  - Improves exercise capacity
- Inspiratory muscle training (IMT)

FUNCTIONAL GOALS

- Improve oxygenation
  - Achieved by
    - Reducing airway edema secondary to inflammation and bronchospasm
    - Facilitating elimination of bronchial secretions
    - Preventing/treating respiratory infection
    - Increase exercise tolerance
    - Avoid irritants/allergens
    - Relieve anxiety/treat depression
    - Improve muscle oxidative capacity
- Patient will be able to
  - Ambulate more than 600 m in a 6-minute walk test.
  - Score more than 80% of their predicted FEV1 score.
  - Tolerate 1 hour of moderate exercise three times a week.
- Once under control, exercise (aerobic, strength, flexibility, posture, breathing) to return to prior level of function.

PROGNOSIS

- Very good with rest and medication.
- Most URIs resolve in 3 to 10 days.[4]
- Immunocompromised individuals are at high risks of complications.

PATIENT RESOURCE

- Acute Respiratory Tract Infection Guideline Summaries. AMA, American Medical Association. http://www.ama-assn.org//ama/pub/physician-resources/medical-science/infectious-diseases/topics-interest/other-infectious-diseases/acute-respiratory-tract.page. Accessed July 5, 2013.

REFERENCES

1. APTA. *Guide to Physical Therapist Practice*. 2nd ed. Alexandria, VA: American Physical Therapy Association; 2001. Revised 2003.
2. Toy EC. Sinusitis, Case 30. LANGE Case Files. http://www.accessmedicine.com/casecontent.aspx?aid=8650631&tabid=1. Accessed July 3, 2013.
3. Hirschmann JV. Antibiotics for common respiratory tract infections in adults. *Arch Intern Med.* 2002;162(3):256–264.
4. Mossad SB. Upper Respiratory Tract Infections. Cleveland Clinic, Center for Continuing Education. http://www.clevelandclinicmeded.com/medicalpubs/diseasemanagement/infectious-disease/upper-respiratory-tract-infection./ Accessed July 5, 2013.

ADDITIONAL REFERENCES

- Aagaard E, Gonzales R. Management of acute bronchitis in healthy adults. *Infect Dis Clin North Am.* 2004;18(4):919–937.
- Aliverti A, Quaranta M, Chakrabarti B, Albuquerque AL, Calverley PM. Paradoxical movement of the lower ribcage at rest and during exercise in COPD patients. *Eur Respir J.* 2009;33 (1):49–60. doi: 10.1183/09031936.00141607.
- Arroll B, Kenealy T. Antibiotics for the common cold and acute purulent rhinitis. *Cochrane Database Syst Rev.* 2005;(3): CD000247.
- Bateman ED, Feldman C, O'Brien J, Plit M, Joubert JR; COPD Guideline Working Group of the South African Thoracic Society. Guideline for the management of chronic obstructive pulmonary disease (COPD): 2004 revision. *S Afr Med J.* 2004;94(7 Pt 2):559–575.
- Batra PS. Radiologic imaging in rhinosinusitis. *Cleve Clin J Med.* 2004;71(11):886–888.
- Goodman CC, Fuller KS. *Pathology: Implications for the Physical Therapist.* 3rd ed. Philadelphia, PA: Saunders Elsevier; 2009.
- Goodman CC, Snyder TK. *Differential Diagnosis for Physical Therapists: Screening for Referral.* 4th ed. St. Louis, MO: Saunders Elsevier; 2007.
- Panus PC, Jobst EE, Masters SB, Katzung B, Tinsley SL, Trevor AJ. Drugs affecting the respiratory system. In: Panus PC, Jobst EE, Masters SB, Katzung B, Tinsley SL, Trevor AJ, eds. *Pharmacology for the Physical Therapist.* New York, NY: McGraw-Hill; 2009. http://www.accessphysiotherapy.com/content/6095983. Accessed July 5, 2013.
- Schuetz P, Briel M, Christ-Crain M, et al. Procalcitonin to guide initiation and duration of antibiotic treatment in acute respiratory infections: an individual patient data meta-analysis. *Clin Infect Dis.* 2012;55(5):651–662.
- Wells CL. Pulmonary pathology. In: DeTurk WE, Cahalin LP, eds. *Cardiovascular and Pulmonary Physical Therapy: An Evidence-Based Approach.* 2nd ed. New York, NY: McGraw-Hill; 2011. http://www.accessphysiotherapy.com/content/6873405#6873405 Accessed July 5, 2013.

79 TUBERCULOSIS, PULMONARY

Eric Shamus, PhD, DPT, PT, CSCS
Jennifer Shamus, PhD, DPT, COMT, CSCS

CONDITION/DISORDER SYNONYM

- Tuberculosis, pulmonary

ICD-9-CM CODES

- 011 Pulmonary tuberculosis
- 011.0 Tuberculosis of lung infiltrative
- 011.00 Tuberculosis of lung, infiltrative, unspecified
- 011.01 Tuberculosis of lung, infiltrative, bacteriological or histological examination not done
- 011.02 Tuberculosis of lung, infiltrative, bacteriological or histological examination unknown (at present)
- 011.03 Tuberculosis of lung, infiltrative, tubercle bacilli found (in sputum) by microscopy
- 011.04 Tuberculosis of lung, infiltrative, tubercle bacilli not found (in sputum) by microscopy but found by bacterial culture
- 011.05 Tuberculosis of lung, infiltrative, tubercle bacilli not found by bacteriological examination, but tuberculosis confirmed histologically
- 011.06 Tuberculosis of lung, infiltrative, tubercle bacilli not found bacteriological or histological examination, but tuberculosis confirmed by other methods (inoculation of animals)
- 011.1 Tuberculosis of lung nodular
- 011.10 Tuberculosis of lung, nodular, unspecified examination
- 011.11 Tuberculosis of lung, nodular, bacteriological or histological examination not done
- 011.12 Tuberculosis of lung, nodular, bacteriological or histological examination unknown (at present)
- 011.13 Tuberculosis of lung, nodular, tubercle bacilli found (in sputum) by microscopy
- 011.14 Tuberculosis of lung, nodular, tubercle bacilli not found (in sputum) by microscopy, but found by bacterial culture
- 011.15 Tuberculosis of lung, nodular, tubercle bacilli not found by bacteriological examination, but tuberculosis confirmed histologically
- 011.16 Tuberculosis of lung, nodular, tubercle bacilli not found by bacteriological or histological examination, but tuberculosis confirmed by other methods (inoculation of animals)
- 011.2 Tuberculosis of lung with cavitation
- 011.20 Tuberculosis of lung with cavitation, unspecified
- 011.21 Tuberculosis of lung with cavitation, bacteriological or histological examination not done
- 011.22 Tuberculosis of lung with cavitation, bacteriological or histological examination unknown (at present)
- 011.23 Tuberculosis of lung with cavitation, tubercle bacilli found (in sputum) by microscopy
- 011.24 Tuberculosis of lung with cavitation, tubercle bacilli not found (in sputum) by microscopy, but found by bacterial culture
- 011.25 Tuberculosis of lung with cavitation, tubercle bacilli not found by bacteriological examination, but tuberculosis confirmed histologically

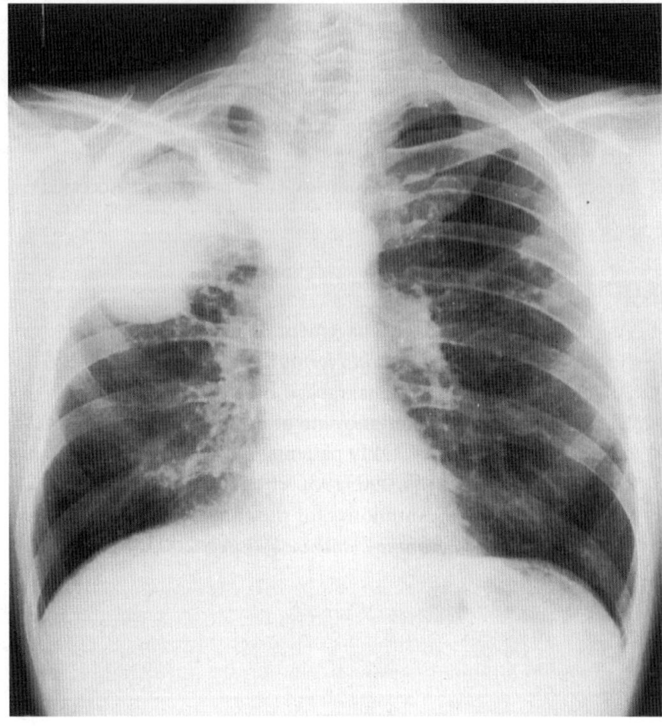

FIGURE 79-1 Cavitary tuberculosis of the right upper lobe. (From Tintinalli JE, Stapczynski J, Ma OJ, Cline D, Cydulka R, Meckler G. *Tintinalli's Emergency Medicine: A Comprehensive Study Guide.* 7th ed. www.accessmedicine.com. © The McGraw-Hill Companies, Inc. All rights reserved.)

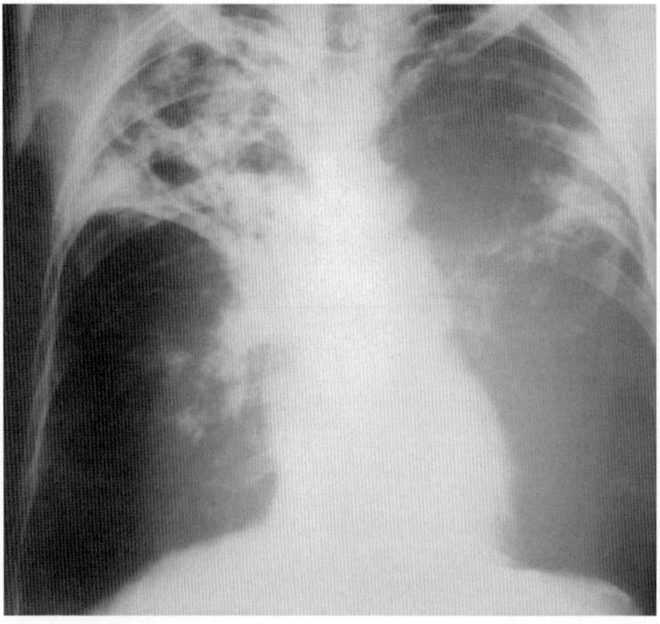

FIGURE 79-2 Advanced bilateral pulmonary tuberculosis. (Public Health Image Library, CDC.)

- 011.26 Tuberculosis of lung with cavitation, tubercle bacilli not found by bacteriological or histological examination, but tuberculosis confirmed by other methods (inoculation of animals)
- 011.3 Tuberculosis of bronchus
- 011.30 Tuberculosis of bronchus, unspecified
- 011.31 Tuberculosis of bronchus, bacteriological or histological examination not done
- 011.32 Tuberculosis of bronchus, bacteriological or histological examination results unknown (at present)
- 011.33 Tuberculosis of bronchus, tubercle bacilli found (in sputum) by microscopy
- 011.34 Tuberculosis of bronchus, tubercle bacilli not found (in sputum) by microscopy, but found in bacterial culture
- 011.35 Tuberculosis of bronchus, tubercle bacilli not found by bacteriological examination, but tuberculosis confirmed histologically
- 011.36 Tuberculosis of bronchus, tubercle bacilli not found by bacteriological or histological examination, but tuberculosis confirmed by other methods (inoculation of animals)
- 011.4 Tuberculous fibrosis of lung
- 011.40 Tuberculous fibrosis of lung, unspecified
- 011.41 Tuberculous fibrosis of lung, bacteriological or histological examination not done
- 011.42 Tuberculous fibrosis of lung, bacteriological or histological examination unknown (at present)
- 011.43 Tuberculous fibrosis of lung, tubercle bacilli found (in sputum) by microscopy
- 011.44 Tuberculous fibrosis of lung, tubercle bacilli not found (in sputum) by microscopy, but found by bacterial culture
- 011.45 Tuberculous fibrosis of lung, tubercle bacilli not found by bacteriological examination, but tuberculosis confirmed histologically
- 011.46 Tuberculous fibrosis of lung, tubercle bacilli not found by bacteriological or histological examination, but tuberculosis confirmed by other methods (inoculation of animals)
- 011.5 Tuberculous bronchiectasis
- 011.50 Tuberculous bronchiectasis, unspecified
- 011.51 Tuberculous bronchiectasis, bacteriological or histological examination not done
- 011.52 Tuberculous bronchiectasis, bacteriological or histological examination unknown (at present)
- 011.53 Tuberculous bronchiectasis, tubercle bacilli found (in sputum) by microscopy
- 011.54 Tuberculous bronchiectasis, tubercle bacilli not found (in sputum) by microscopy, but found by bacterial culture
- 011.55 Tuberculous bronchiectasis, tubercle bacilli not found by bacteriological examination, but tuberculosis confirmed histologically
- 011.56 Tuberculous bronchiectasis, tubercle bacilli not found by bacteriological or histological examination, but tuberculosis confirmed by other methods (inoculation of animals)
- 011.6 Tuberculous pneumonia (any form)
- 011.60 Tuberculous pneumonia (any form), unspecified
- 011.61 Tuberculous pneumonia (any form), bacteriological or histological examination not done
- 011.62 Tuberculous pneumonia (any form), bacteriological or histological examination unknown (at present)
- 011.63 Tuberculous pneumonia (any form), tubercle bacilli found (in sputum) by microscopy
- 011.64 Tuberculous pneumonia (any form), tubercle bacilli not found (in sputum) by microscopy, but found by bacterial culture

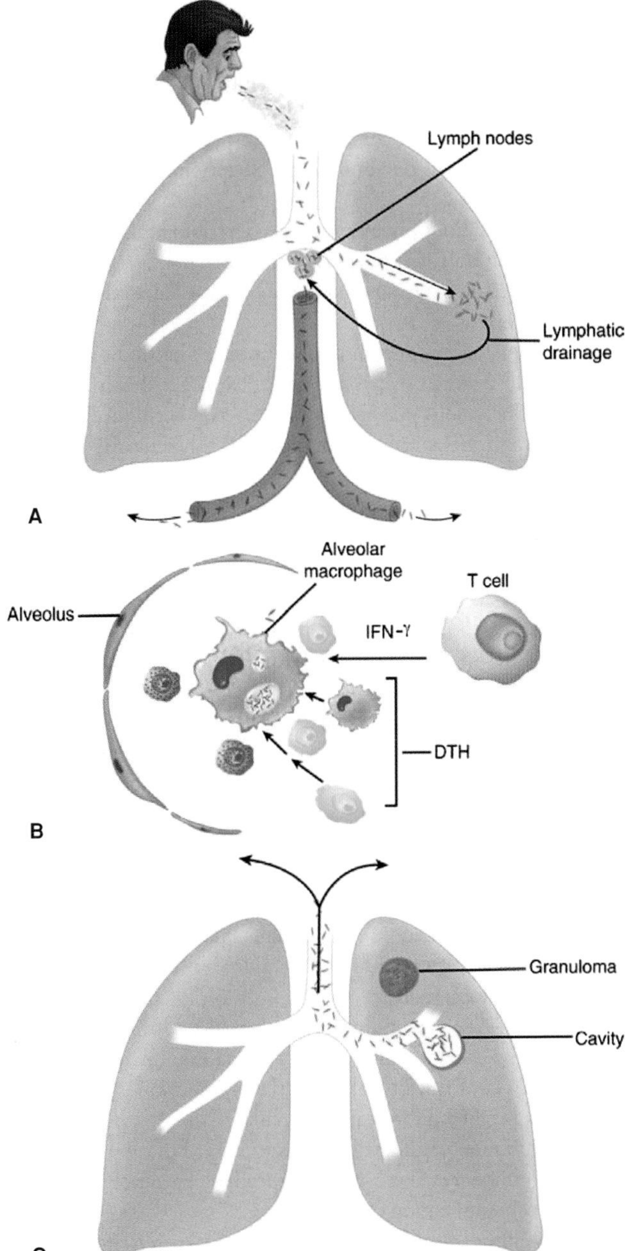

FIGURE 79-3 Tuberculosis. **A.** Primary tuberculosis. *Mucobacterium tuberculosis* is inhaled in droplet nuclei from an active case of tuberculosis. Initial multiplication is in the alveoli with spread through lymphatic drainage to the hilar lymph nodes. After further lymphatic drainage to the bloodstream, the organisms are spread throughout the body. **B.** Alveolar macrophage. The two-front battle being carried out between **A** and **C** is shown. Ingested bacteria multiply in the nonactivated macrophage. (1) T_H1 cellular immune responses attempt to activate the macrophage by secreting cytokines (interferon gamma [IFN-γ]). If successful, the disease is arrested. (2) Inflammatory elements of delayed-type hypersensitivity (DTH) are attracted and cause destruction. If activation is not successful, disease and injury continue. **C.** Reactivation tuberculosis. Reactivation typically starts in the upper lobes of the lung with granuloma formation. DTH-mediated destruction can form a cavity, which allows the organisms to be coughed up to infect another person. (From Ryan KJ, Ray CG. *Sherris Medical Microbiology.* 5th ed. New York, NY: McGraw-Hill; 2010.)

- 011.65 Tuberculous pneumonia (any form), tubercle bacilli not found by bacteriological examination, but tuberculosis confirmed histologically
- 011.66 Tuberculous pneumonia (any form), tubercle bacilli not found by bacteriological or histological examination, but tuberculosis confirmed by other methods (inoculation of animals)
- 011.7 Tuberculous pneumothorax
- 011.70 Tuberculous pneumothorax, unspecified
- 011.71 Tuberculous pneumothorax, bacteriological or histological examination not done
- 011.72 Tuberculous pneumothorax, bacteriological or histological examination results unknown (at present)
- 011.73 Tuberculous pneumothorax, tubercle bacilli found (in sputum) by microscopy
- 011.74 Tuberculous pneumothorax, tubercle bacilli not found (in sputum) by microscopy, but found by bacterial culture
- 011.75 Tuberculous pneumothorax, tubercle bacilli not found by bacteriological examination, but tuberculosis confirmed histologically
- 011.76 Tuberculous pneumothorax, tubercle bacilli not found by bacteriological or histological examination, but tuberculosis confirmed by other methods (inoculation of animals)
- 011.8 Other specified pulmonary tuberculosis
- 011.80 Other specified pulmonary tuberculosis, unspecified
- 011.81 Other specified pulmonary tuberculosis, bacteriological or histological examination not done
- 011.82 Other specified pulmonary tuberculosis, bacteriological or histological examination unknown (at present)
- 011.83 Other specified pulmonary tuberculosis, tubercle bacilli found (in sputum) by microscopy
- 011.84 Other specified pulmonary tuberculosis, tubercle bacilli not found (in sputum) by microscopy, but found by bacterial culture
- 011.85 Other specified pulmonary tuberculosis, tubercle bacilli not found by bacteriological examination, but tuberculosis confirmed histologically
- 011.86 Other specified pulmonary tuberculosis, tubercle bacilli not found by bacteriological or histological examination, but tuberculosis confirmed by other methods (inoculation of animals)
- 011.9 Unspecified pulmonary tuberculosis
- 011.90 Pulmonary tuberculosis, unspecified
- 011.91 Pulmonary tuberculosis, unspecified, bacteriological or histological examination not done
- 011.92 Pulmonary tuberculosis, unspecified, bacteriological or histological examination unknown (at present)
- 011.93 Pulmonary tuberculosis, unspecified, tubercle bacilli found (in sputum) by microscopy
- 011.94 Pulmonary tuberculosis, unspecified, tubercle bacilli not found (in sputum) by microscopy, but found by bacterial culture
- 011.95 Pulmonary tuberculosis, unspecified, tubercle bacilli not found by bacteriological examination, but tuberculosis confirmed histologically
- 011.96 Pulmonary tuberculosis, unspecified, tubercle bacilli not found by bacteriological or histological examination, but tuberculosis confirmed by other methods (inoculation of animals)
- Associated ICD-9-CM PT diagnoses/treatment diagnosis that may be directly related to respiratory disorders
  - 786.05 Shortness of breath
  - 780.7 Malaise and fatigue
  - 786.0 Dyspnea and respiratory abnormalities

ICD-10-CM CODES

- A15.0 Tuberculosis of lung
- A15.5 Tuberculosis of larynx, trachea and bronchus

PREFERRED PRACTICE PATTERNS[1]

- 6C: Impaired Ventilation, Respiration/Gas Exchange, and Aerobic Capacity/Endurance Associated with Airway Clearance Dysfunction
- 6F: Impaired Ventilation and Respiration/Gas Exchange Associated with Respiratory Failure

PATIENT PRESENTATION

A 62-year-old man is brought to the clinic for a 3-month history of unintentional weight loss (12 lb). His appetite has diminished, but he reports no vomiting or diarrhea. He does report some depressive symptoms since the death of his wife a year ago, at which time he moved from Hong Kong to the United States to live with his daughter. He denies a smoking history. He complains of a 3-month history of productive cough with greenish sputum. He has not felt feverish. He takes no medications regularly. On examination, his temperature is 100.4°F and respiratory rate 16 breaths per minute. His neck has a normal thyroid gland and no cervical or supraclavicular lymphadenopathy. His chest has few scattered rales in the left mid-lung fields and a faint expiratory wheeze on the right. His heart rhythm is regular with no gallops or murmurs. His abdominal examination is benign, his rectal examination shows no masses, and his stool is negative for occult blood.[2]

KEY FEATURES

Description

- Contagious only from people with active tuberculosis, pulmonary (TB)
- Bacterial infection in the lungs
- Bacteria mycobacterium tuberculosis
- Glandular: Chronic cervical adenitis
- Miliary: X-ray, snowstorm (millet seed) appearance
- Meningitis: Fever, vomiting, headache, convulsions
- Extrapulmonary tuberculosis
  - Spread to lymph system
  - Spread to pleura
  - Spread to bones
  - Usually in young children and immunosuppressed

Essentials of Diagnosis

- Positive skin test means positive exposure
- X-ray
- Most infections are asymptomatic
- Chest pain
- Productive cost
- Chronic scarring in the lungs

General Considerations

- Transmitted by respiratory air droplets from coughing or sneezing
- If untreated, can cause permanent lung damage
- Can spread to other parts of the body

- Latent TB is asymptomatic and noncontagious
- If infected, takes almost a month to be contagious
- Bacillus Calmette–Guérin vaccine for children (will have false-positive skin test)

Demographics

- Most common with patients who are immunosuppressive
- Countries with poor nutrition and poor water quality
- Prisoners

CLINICAL FINDINGS

SIGNS AND SYMPTOMS

- Chest tightness
- Chronic cough
- Clubbing of fingers
- Crackles
- Enlarged lymph nodes
- Fatigue
- Fever
- Loss of appetite
- Night sweats
- Shortness of breath
- Shoulder raised to allow increased lung air flow
- Tensed muscles from dyspnea
- Weight loss
- Wheezing

Functional Implications

- Disabling dyspnea when performing simple tasks such as arm elevation to reach into cabinets
- Decreased exercise tolerance

Possible Contributing Causes

- In contact with individuals with TB
- Poor nutrition
- Weak immune system, AIDS
- Diabetes
- Chemotherapy
- Smoking
- Alcoholism
- Corticosteroids

Differential Diagnosis

- Actinomycosis
- Aspergillosis
- Blastomycosis
- Bronchiectasis
- Cat scratch fever
- Central airway obstruction
- Fungal or parasitic infection
- Hodgkin lymphoma
- Lung abscess
- Lung cancer
- Pericarditis
- Sarcoidosis
- Squamous cell carcinoma
- Syphilis
- Syringoma

MEANS OF CONFIRMATION OR DIAGNOSIS

Laboratory Tests

- Tuberculin skin test (Mantoux test)
  - Interpretation of tuberculin skin test reaction
- Biopsy
- Bronchoscopy
- Sputum culture
- Thoracentesis
- Amplified mycobacterium tuberculosis direct (MTD) test
- Interferon gamma release assay (IGRA)
- Blood gas measurements
- Blood test
- Seattle Obstructive Lung Disease Questionnaire (SOLQ)
- Lung function tests or pulmonary function tests
  - Spirometry
  - Body plethysmography
  - Peak expiratory flow

Imaging

- Chest radiograph
- Chest CT scan
- High-resolution CT
- Ventilation/perfusion lung scan

FINDINGS AND INTERPRETATION

- Scarring on the lungs
- Often false positive with skin test, follow-up X-ray needed

TREATMENT

Medication[3]

- Antibiotics
- Isoniazid
- Rifampin
- Pyrazinamide
- Ethambutol

REFERRALS/ADMITTANCE

- Imaging, X-ray
- Medication
- Pulmonologist

IMPAIRMENTS

- Exercise limitation
- Shortness of breath
- Proximal upper-limb strength impairment
- Limited endurance capacity

INTERVENTION

- Smoking cessation
- Exercise (aerobic, strength, flexibility, posture, breathing)
- Airway clearance
- Pursed-lip breathing
- Coughing techniques
- Pulmonary rehabilitation (PR)
  - Enhances the patient's sense of well-being
  - Improves exercise capacity
  - Decreases the need for hospitalization
  - Lowers overall health costs
- Inspiratory muscle training (IMT)

FUNCTIONAL GOALS

- Patient will be able to
  - Ambulate more than 600 m in a 6-minute walk test.
  - Score higher than 80% of their predicted FEV1 score.
  - Tolerate 1 hour of moderate exercise three times a week.

PROGNOSIS

- Infection can be dormant.
- Excellent for recovery if bacteria are sensitive.

PATIENT RESOURCES

- Tuberculosis, American Lung Association. http://www.lung.org/lung-disease/tuberculosis. Accessed July 11, 2013.
- Tuberculosis. South Carolina Tuberculosis Association. http://sctuberculosis.org. Accessed May 9, 2014.

REFERENCES

1. APTA. *Guide to Physical Therapy Practice*. Alexandria, VA: American Physical Therapy Association; 2003. http://guidetoptpractice.apta.org. Accessed July 11, 2013.
2. Toy EC. Tuberculosis (pulmonary), cavity lung lesions, Case 80. http://www.accessmedicine.com/casecontent.aspx?aid=510023809&tabid=1. Accessed July 11, 2013.
3. Pulmonary Tuberculosis. A.D.A.M. Encyclopedia. PubMed Health. http://www.ncbi.nlm.nih.gov/pubmedhealth/PMH0001141/. Accessed July 11, 2013.

ADDITIONAL REFERENCES

- DeTurk WE, Cahalin LP, eds. *Cardiovascular and Pulmonary Physical Therapy: An Evidence-Based Approach.* 2nd ed. New York, NY: McGraw-Hill; 2011. http://www.accessphysiotherapy.com/resource/652. Accessed July 11, 2013.
- Fitzgerald DW, Sterling TR, Haas DW. Mycobacterium tuberculosis. In: Mandell GL, Bennett JE, Dolan R, eds. *Mandell, Douglas, and Bennett's Principles and Practice of Infectious Diseases.* 7th ed. Orlando, FL: Saunders Elsevier; 2009:Chapter 250.
- Golden MP, Vikram HR. Extrapulmonary tuberculosis: an overview. *Am Fam Physician.* 2005;72(9):1761–1768.
- Goodman CC, Fuller KS. *Pathology: Implications for the Physical Therapist.* 3rd ed. Philadelphia, PA: Saunders Elsevier; 2009.
- Goodman CC, Snyder TK. *Differential Diagnosis for Physical Therapists: Screening for Referral.* 4th ed. St. Louis, MO: Saunders Elsevier; 2007.
- Iseman MD. Tuberculosis. In: Goldman L, Ausiello D, eds. *Cecil Medicine.* 23rd ed. Philadelphia, PA: Saunders Elsevier; 2007: Chapter 345.
- Konstantinos A. Testing for tuberculosis. *Australian Prescriber.* 2010;33(1):12–18. http://www.australianprescriber.com/magazine/33/1/12/18/. Accessed July 11, 2013
- Ogle JW, Anderson MS. Infections: bacterial & spirochetal. In: Hay WW, Levin MJ, Sondheimer JM, Deterding RR, eds. *CURRENT Diagnosis & Treatment: Pediatrics.* 20th ed. New York, NY: McGraw-Hill; 2011. http://www.accessphysiotherapy.com/content/6590639. Accessed July 11, 2013.
- Panus PC, Jobst EE, Masters SB, Katzung B, Tinsley SL, Trevor AJ. Drugs affecting the respiratory system. In: Panus PC, Jobst EE, Masters SB, Katzung B, Tinsley SL, Trevor AJ, eds. *Pharmacology for the Physical Therapist.* New York, NY: McGraw-Hill; 2009. http://www.accessphysiotherapy.com/content/6095983. Accessed July 11, 2013.

PART 3

NEUROLOGICAL DISORDERS

80 BRAIN ABSCESS

Mollie Venglar, DSc, MSPT, NCS

CONDITION/DISORDER SYNONYM

- Cerebral abscess

ICD-9-CM CODE

- 324.0 Intracranial abscess

ICD-10-CM CODES

- G06.0 Intracranial abscess and granuloma
- G06.2 Extradural and subdural abscess, unspecified

PREFERRED PRACTICE PATTERNS

- 5C: Impaired Motor Function and Sensory Integrity Associated with Nonprogressive Disorders of the Central Nervous System—congenital origin or acquired in infancy or childhood[1]
- 5D: Impaired Motor Function and Sensory Integrity Associated with Nonprogressive Disorders of the Central Nervous System—acquired in adolescence or adulthood[2]

PATIENT PRESENTATION

A 37-year-old female was brought to the emergency department (ED) when her roommate was unable to arouse her in the morning. The roommate reported that for several days the woman had increasing difficulties with maintaining conversations and managing her normal

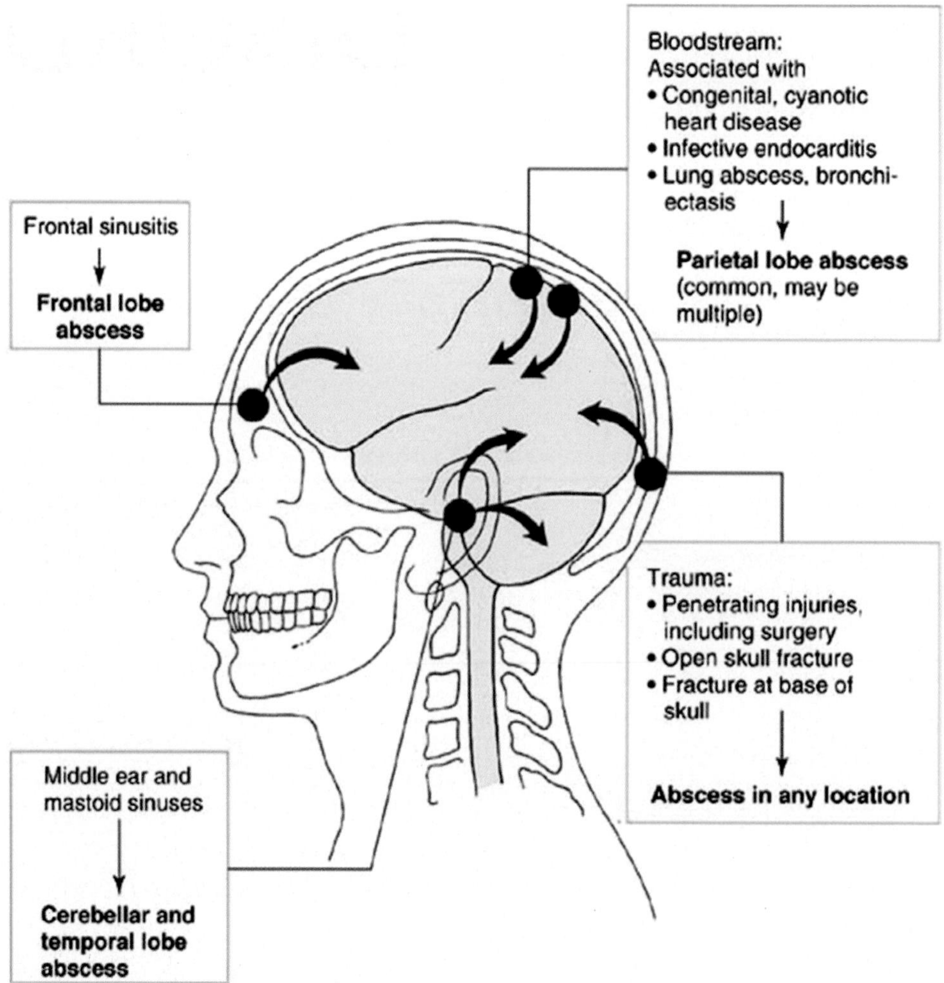

FIGURE 80-1 Cerebral abscess—common sites and routes of infection. (From Chandrasoma P, Taylor CR. *Concise Pathology*. 3rd ed. http://www.accessmedicine.com. Copyright © The McGraw-Hill Companies, Inc. All rights reserved.)

schedule. For several months she had complained of tooth and jaw pain but had not been to the dentist. In the ED, she continued to be unconscious and her respirations were inadequate to maintain life. She was placed on a ventilator. Brain imaging revealed an abscess in the area of the inferior aspect of left frontal lobe and anterior left temporal lobe.

KEY FEATURES

Description

- Confined area of infection within the cranium
- Cerebral abscess: Common sites of infection[3]

Essentials of Diagnosis

- Greater than 90% of brain abscesses due to external causes: Compound fracture of skull, bullet wound, surgical complication involving brain or cranium
- May be secondary to infectious process elsewhere in the body including
  - Paranasal sinus (rhinogenic): Usually leads to abscess in frontal and temporal lobes
  - Middle ear (otogenic): Usually leads to abscess in anterolateral cerebellum, middle and inferior temporal lobe
  - Pulmonary infection
  - Bacterial endocarditis
- Rupture of abscess can advance to irreversible coma

General Considerations

- Approximately 50% are metastatic
- Approximately 20% cannot be traced to the site of origin

Demographics

- All ages and genders, who experience one of the contributing causes, are at risk for developing a brain abscess.
- 60% of children who develop a brain abscess have congenital heart disease.

CLINICAL FINDINGS

SIGNS AND SYMPTOMS

- Headache
- Drowsiness
- Confusion
- Focal or generalized seizure
- Focal motor, sensory, or speech disturbance
- Fever (inconsistent)
- Leukocytosis (inconsistent)
- Increased intracranial pressure (later in the course of illness)
- Papilledema (later in the course of illness)

Functional Implications

- Loss of independence with all aspects of mobility, ADLs, self-care
- Impaired ability to interact with others effectively
- Difficulty with cognitive processing, particularly executive function

Possible Contributing Causes

- Bacterial endocarditis
- Pulmonary infection
- Sinus infection
- Middle-ear infection
- Congenital heart disease
- Infected pelvic organs

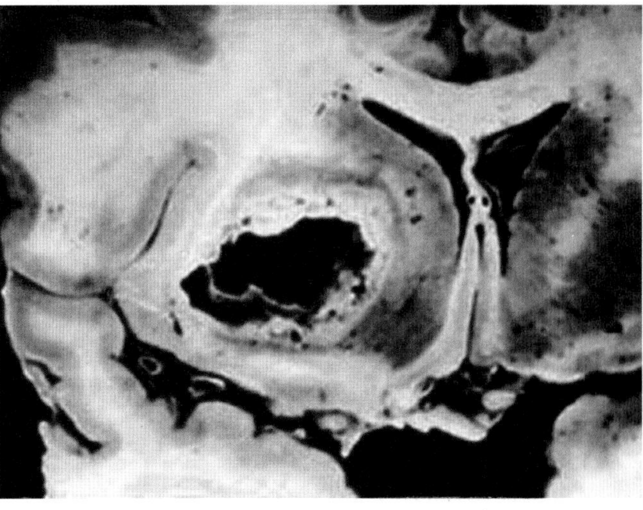

FIGURE 80-2 Cerebral abscess, showing a cavity in the region of the basal ganglia lined by inflammatory exudate. The cavity was filled with pus that drained when the brain was cut. (From Chandrasoma P, Taylor CR. *Concise Pathology*. 3rd ed. http://www.accessmedicine.com. Copyright © The McGraw-Hill Companies, Inc. All rights reserved.)

- Infected tonsils
- Abscessed teeth
- Osteomyelitis
- Pulmonary arteriovenous malformation
- Surgical trauma
- Cranial injury

Differential Diagnosis

- Brain tumor
- Stroke
- Subdural empyema

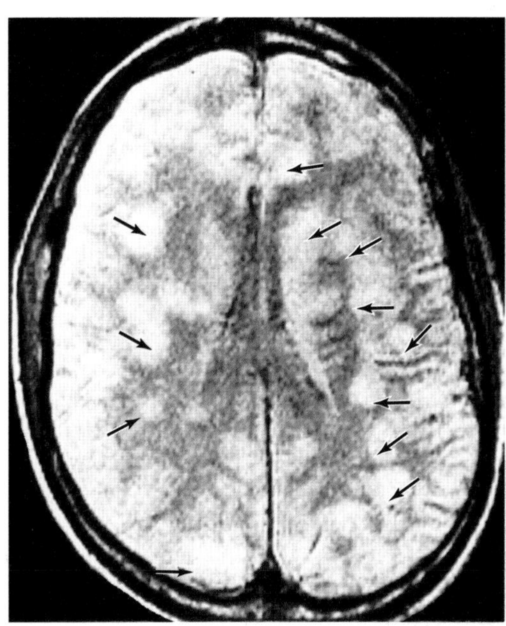

FIGURE 80-3 Magnetic resonance image of a horizontal section through the lateral ventricles in a patient with AIDS. Notice the multiple high-intensity regions throughout both hemispheres, representing cerebral abscesses (*arrows*). (From Waxman SG. *Clinical Neuroanatomy*. 26th ed. http://www.accessmedicine.com. Copyright © The McGraw-Hill Companies, Inc. All rights reserved.)

MEANS OF CONFIRMATION OR DIAGNOSIS

Laboratory Tests

- Sedimentation rate
- Cerebrospinal fluid (CSF) pressure
- Mild-to-moderate pleocytosis
- Complete blood count (CBC)

Imaging

- CT with contrast[4]
- MRI[4]

FINDINGS AND INTERPRETATION

- Blood protein moderately elevated
- Elevated sedimentation rate
- Moderately increased CSF pressure

TREATMENT

Medication

- Antibiotics, usually intravenous, for several weeks
- Intravenous mannitol or dexamethasone to prevent cerebellar herniation and temporal-lobe damage

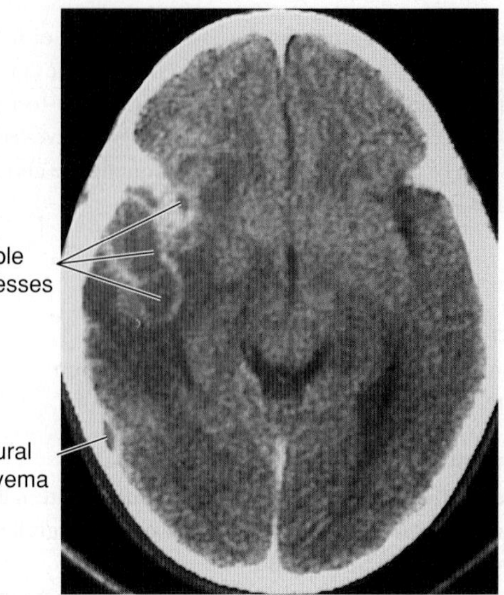

FIGURE 80-4 Computed tomography image of a horizontal section through the temporal lobes, showing an epidural lesion and multiple rounded confluent masses in the right lobe. (From Waxman SG. *Clinical Neuroanatomy*. 26th ed. http://www.accessmedicine.com. Copyright © The McGraw-Hill Companies, Inc. All rights reserved.)

REFERRALS/ADMITTANCE

- To emergency room physician if emergency identified
- To neurologist or neurosurgeon for diagnosis and treatment of infection
- To neuropsychologist for cognitive testing after resolution of the active infection
- To physiatrist for specific rehabilitation if residual neurologic deficit requires rehabilitation
- To occupational therapist for ADL, cognitive, and fine-motor task retraining
- To speech/language pathologist for speech, cognition, and swallowing impairments
- To respiratory therapist as needed (depending on respiratory impact of the brain injury)
- To case management or social work for coordination of care

IMPAIRMENTS

- Arousal
- Attention
- Behavior
- Cognition
- Cranial nerve integrity
- Peripheral nerve integrity: Possibly from a comorbid diagnosis
- Gait
- Wheelchair mobility
- Balance
  - Static sit
  - Dynamic sit
  - Static stand
  - Dynamic stand
  - Moving base of support
- Muscle strength
- Muscle recruitment
- Coordination
- Posture and postural control
- Range of motion (ROM)
- Reflexes
  - Deep-tendon reflexes
  - Babinski
  - Clonus
- Muscle tone: Anticipate hypertonicity or spasticity
- Sensation
- Motor planning
- Bed mobility
- Transfers
- Neglect: Evident in cases of primary damage to one side of the brain
- Endurance
- Aerobic capacity
- Self-care
- Home management
- Fine-motor skills
- Respiratory compromise

TESTS AND MEASURES

- Glasgow Outcome Scale[5]
- Glasgow Coma Scale[6]
- Ranchos Los Amigos Scale[6]
- Modified Ashworth Scale[7]
- Functional measures
  - Barthel Index[8]
  - Functional Independence Measure[9]
- Gait and balance measures
  - Tinetti[10]
  - Motor Assessment Scale[11]
  - Gait Assessment Rating Scale[12]
  - Rancho Los Amigo Observational Gait Analysis[13]
  - 6-minute walk test[14]
  - Multi-directional reach test[15]
  - HiMAT (if appropriate based on patient's Berg Balance Scale and Dynamic Gait Index scores)[16]

- Cognitive testing
- Sensory testing: May be limited by cognition or consciousness
- Strength: Include speed of force production and ability to change force production
- Active and passive ROM, flexibility
- Bed mobility
- Transfers
- Cranial nerves: Particularly vision
- Vestibular assessment

INTERVENTION

- ROM, stretching, positioning
- Tone management
- Orientation to vertical position
- Strengthening
- Balance training
- Gait training (if appropriate and with appropriate bracing and assistive devices)
- Transfer training
- Bed-mobility training
- Wheelchair-mobility training (curbs, ramps, varied surfaces, negotiating obstacles)
- Cardiovascular and pulmonary endurance

FUNCTIONAL GOALS

- Due to the variability of abscess location and resulting neurologic deficits, goals should be specific to the patient. The following goals relate to general functional mobility.
- Short-term goals
  - Patient will be able to
    - Transfer between wheelchair and bed via sit (lateral) pivot with minimal assistance and moderate verbal cues for sequencing in order to increase safe functional mobility on return home.
    - Transition consistently between sit and stand from a 90-degree hip angle and contact guard assistance in order to increase safe functional mobility.
    - Ambulate >50 ft with minimal assistance and appropriate assistive device to improve mobility in preparation for return home.
    - Tolerate 10 minutes of continuous exercise without significant change in vital signs to improve cardiovascular endurance and increase tolerance for daily activity.
- Long-term goals
  - The patient will be able to
    - Achieve ≥1500 ft on 6-minute walk test with supervision and appropriate assistive device indoors over level surfaces to increase efficient functional mobility and endurance for daily activities.
    - Perform static tandem standing without upper-extremity support for 30 seconds with supervision to improve standing balance and postural control.
    - Achieve a Berg Balance Scale score to ≥53 out of 56 to demonstrate decreased fall risk during functional activities.
    - Ambulate on a variety of indoor and outdoor surfaces with distant supervision and assistive device as needed to maximize safe and functional ambulation and return to appropriate premorbid activities.

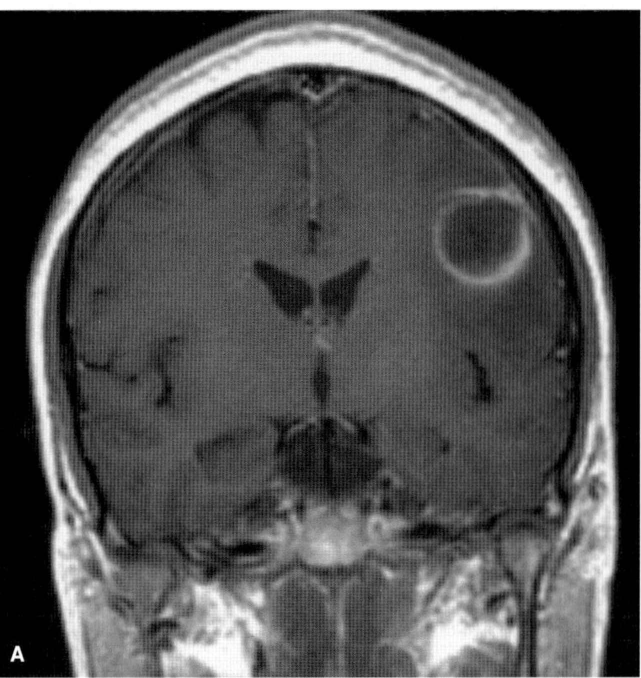

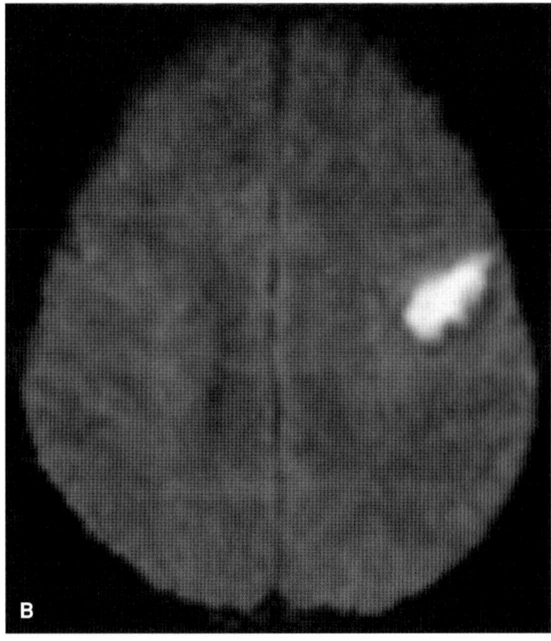

FIGURE 80-5 Cerebral abscess in a patient with fever and a right hemiparesis. **A.** Coronal postcontrast T1-weighted image demonstrates a ring enhancing mass in the left frontal lobe. **B.** Axial diffusion-weighted image demonstrates restricted diffusion (high signal intensity) within the lesion, which in this setting is highly suggestive of cerebral abscess. (From Longo DL, Fauci AS, Kasper DL, Hauser SL, Jameson JL, Loscalzo J, eds. *Harrison's Principles of Internal Medicine.* 18th ed. http://www.accessmedicine.com. Copyright © The McGraw-Hill Companies, Inc. All rights reserved.)

PROGNOSIS

- More than 50% of patients who are comatose before initiation of treatment will die.
- Cases identified and treated early have a 5% to 10% mortality rate.
- Approximately 30% of patients will have residual neurologic deficit.

ADDITIONAL INFORMATION

- For additional information, please see Case 12 in Chapter 10 of *Clinical Neuroanatomy* on AccessPhysiotherapy.com.[4]

PATIENT RESOURCE

- Practice Guidelines. American Academy of Neurology. http://www.aan.com/news/?event=read&article_id=9580. Accessed January 24, 2013.

REFERENCES

1. The American Physical Therapy Association. Pattern 5C: impaired motor function and sensory integrity associated with nonprogressive disorders of the central nervous system - congenital origin or acquired in infancy or childhood. *Interactive Guide to Physical Therapist Practice*. 2003. doi: 10.2522/ptguide.3.2_3. Accessed February 22, 2013.
2. The American Physical Therapy Association. Pattern 5D: impaired motor function and sensory integrity associated with nonprogressive disorders of the central nervous system - acquired in adolescence or adulthood. *Interactive Guide to Physical Therapist Practice*. 2003. doi: 10.2522/ptguide.3.2_4. Accessed February 22, 2013.
3. Chandrasoma P, Taylor CR. *Concise Pathology*. 3rd ed. Stamford, CT: Appleton & Lang; 1998. http://www.accessphysiotherapy.com/content/187050. Accessed February 22, 2013.
4. Waxman SG. *Clinical Neuroanatomy*. New York, NY: McGraw-Hill; 2010. http://www.accessphysiotherapy.com/resource/22. Accessed February 22, 2013.
5. Introduction to the Extended Glasgow Outcome Scale. The Center for Outcome Measurement in Brain Injury. http://tbims.org/combi/gose/index.html. Accessed February 22, 2013.
6. Wilson PE, Clayton GH. Rehabilitation medicine. In: Hay W, Levin MJ, Sondheimer JM, Detering RR, eds. *CURRENT Diagnosis & Treatment: Pediatrics*. New York, NY: McGraw-Hill; 2011:Chapter 26. http://www.accessphysiotherapy.com/abstract/6586373#6586380. Accessed February 22, 2013.
7. Levine P. Testing spasticity: The Modified Ashworth Scale. *Advance for Physical Therapy and Rehab Medicine*. http://physical-therapy.advanceweb.com/Article/Testing-Spasticity-The-Modified-Ashworth-Scale.aspx. Accessed February 22, 2013.
8. Barthel Index (BI). *StrokEngine Assess*. http://www.strokecenter.org/wp-content/uploads/2011/08/barthel.pdf. Accessed May 9, 2014.
9. Functional Independence Measure (FIM). *StrokEngine Assess*. http://strokengine.ca/assess/PDF/FIMappendixD.pdf. Accessed May 9, 2014.
10. Tinetti Balance and Gait Evaluation. http://www.bhps.org.uk/falls/documents/TinettiBalanceAssessment.pdf. Accessed May 9, 2014.
11. Carr JH, Shepherd RB, Nordholm L, Lynne D. Investigation of a new motor assessment scale for stroke patients. *Phys Ther*. 1985;65:175–180.
12. Components of the Gait Assessment Rating Score (GARS). http://ojaischoolofmassage.com/documents/Previewof_GAITASSESSMENTRATINGSCALE_.pdf. Accessed May 9, 2014.
13. Oregon Health and Science University. Observational gait analysis. http://moon.ouhsc.edu/dthompso/gait/knmatics/oga.htm. Accessed February 22, 2013.
14. Six-minute Walk Test (6MWT). http://strokengine.ca/assess/module_6mwt_intro-en.html. Accessed May 9, 2014.
15. Temple University Gait Study Center. Multidirectional Reach Test. http://podiatry.temple.edu/gaitlab/facilities/mdrt.html. Accessed February 22, 2013.
16. Introduction to the High Level Mobility Assessment Tool. The Center for Outcome Measurement in Brain Injury. http://tbims.org/combi/himat/index.html. Accessed January 6, 2013.

ADDITIONAL REFERENCES

- Hay WW, Levin MJ, Sondheimer JM, Deterding RR. Infections & inflammatory disorders of the central nervous system. In: Hay WW, Levin MJ, Sondheimer JM, Deterding RR, eds. *CURRENT Diagnosis & Treatment: Pediatrics*. 20th ed. New York, NY: McGraw-Hill; 2011. http://www.accessphysiotherapy.com/content/6585600. Accessed January 24, 2013.
- ICD9DATA. http://www.icd9data.com. Accessed January 24, 2013.
- ICD10DATA. http://www.icd10data.com. Accessed January 24, 2013.
- Ropper AL, Samuels MA. *Adams and Victor's Principles of Neurology*. 9th ed. New York, NY: McGraw-Hill; 2009:683–686.

81 ALZHEIMER'S DISEASE

Mollie Venglar, DSc, MSPT, NCS

CONDITION/DISORDER SYNONYM

- Alzheimer's dementia

ICD-9-CM CODE

- 331.0 Alzheimer's disease

ICD-10-CM CODE

- G30.9 Alzheimer's disease, unspecified

PREFERRED PRACTICE PATTERN

- 5E: Impaired Motor Function and Sensory Integrity Associated with Progressive Disorders of the Central Nervous System[1]

PATIENT PRESENTATION

Physical therapy has been requested for a 78-year-old woman with Alzheimer's disease. She is presently calm, she speaks only when spoken to, she moves only when asked to move. On questioning she is unable to accurately report the day of the week, the month, or the year. She states she is in a medical building but cannot be more specific. Her husband reports that she seems to walk around the house fairly well, but when he takes her to public places such as their church, a restaurant, or a grocery store, she seems to struggle with her balance while walking and she gets somewhat agitated and very confused. He is unable to adequately calm her until they return home and she returns to sitting in her favorite chair. Upper and lower quarter screens reveal slightly decreased strength bilaterally but no loss of range or motion.

KEY FEATURES

Description

- A degenerative neurologic disorder characterized by progressive dementia
- Results in inability to care for oneself or interact in the environment

Essentials of Diagnosis

- Insidious onset
- Gradual development of forgetfulness that degenerates into other failures of cerebral function
- Concise pathology that accounts for 50% of all dementia cases[2]

General Considerations

- Definitive diagnosis is made upon autopsy
- Imaging in late stages of the disease reveals hippocampal and frontal lobe atrophy[3]

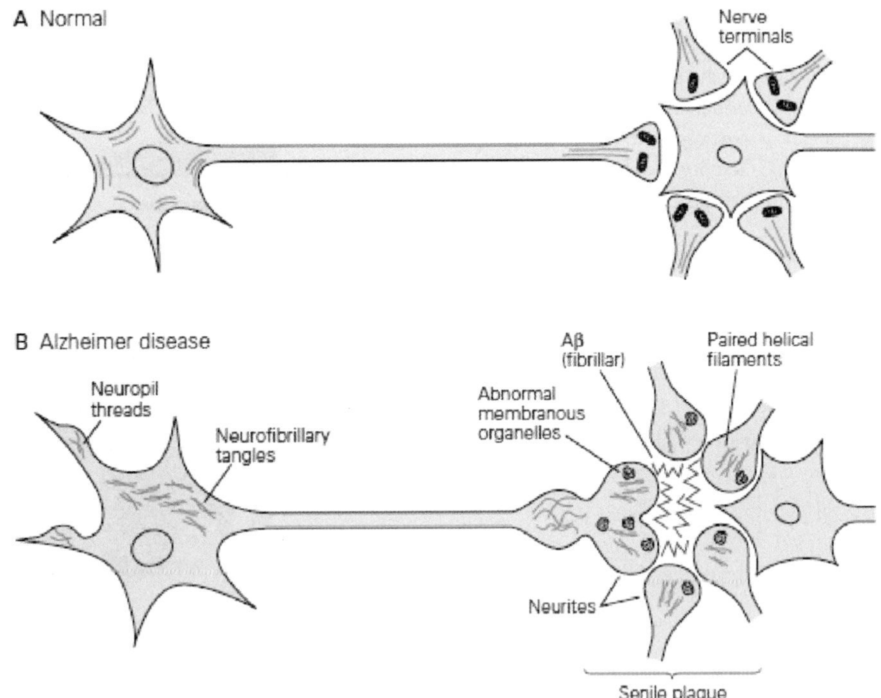

FIGURE 81-1 Comparison of a normal neuron and one with abnormalities associated with Alzheimer's disease. The cytopathologic hallmarks are intracellular neurofibrillary tangles and extracellular senile plaques that have a core of β-amyloid peptides surrounded by altered nerve fibers and reactive glial cells. (From Kandel ER, Schwartz JH, Jessell TM, Siegelbaum SA, Hudspeth AJ, eds. *Principles of Neural Science.* 4th ed. McGraw-Hill; 2000.)

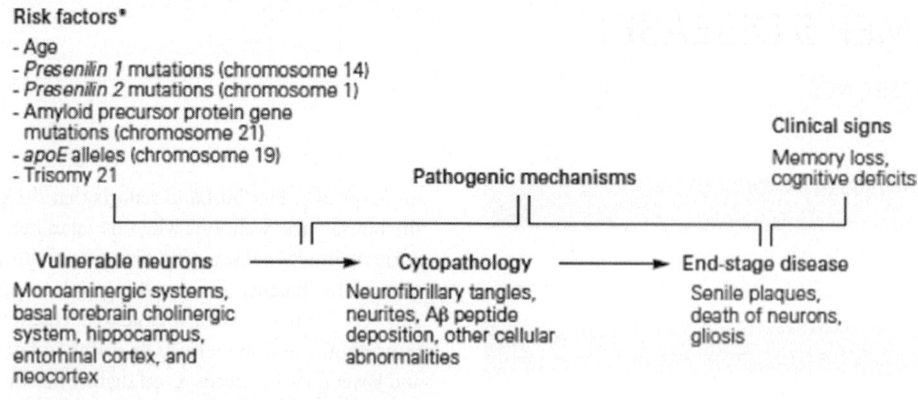

FIGURE 81-2 Relationships of risk factors, pathogenic processes, and clinical signs to cellular abnormalities in the brain during's Alzheimer disease. (From Kandel ER, Schwartz JH, Jessell TM, Siegelbaum SA, Hudspeth AJ eds. *Principles of Neural Science.* 4th ed. McGraw-Hill; 2000.)

- Early in the disease process, all other possible causes of dementia are ruled out to diagnose Alzheimer's disease

Demographics

- Onset primarily occurs at age 60 years and older
- Women three times more likely than men
- Weak genetic link; most commonly idiopathic

CLINICAL FINDINGS

SIGNS AND SYMPTOMS

- Loss of cognitive function, most commonly in the following sequence
  - Abstract thinking
  - Judgment and problem-solving
  - Language for communication
  - Personality changes
- Eventually the person loses ability to perform self-care or ADLs
- Although the ability to perform automatic movements is maintained, the understanding of purpose behind the activities is lost
- As the person loses this understanding, he/she may participate in less physical activity, resulting in disuse atrophy

Functional Implications

- Loss of
  - Interaction in the environment
  - Memory and goal-directed behavior
  - Independence with ADLs
  - Strength and mobility

Possible Contributing Causes

- Unknown, primarily idiopathic

Differential Diagnosis

- Age-related dementia
- Dementia of AIDS
- Hydrocephalus
- Lewy-body disease

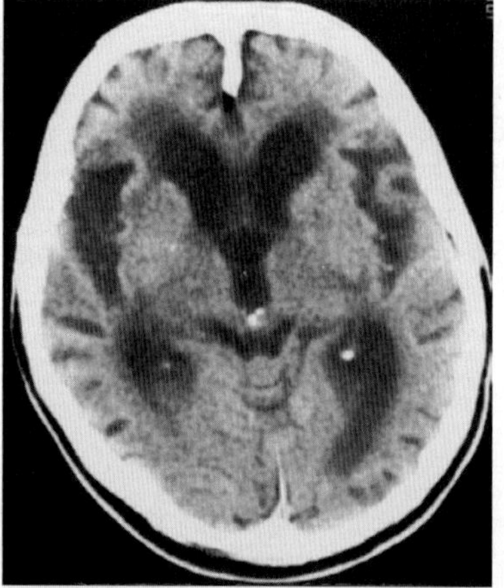

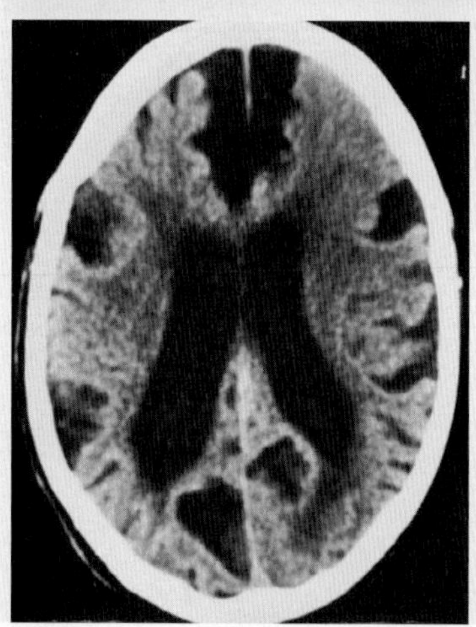

FIGURE 81-3 **Top:** Alzheimer's disease. Axial CT section demonstrating severe generalized cerebral cortical atrophy and moderately severe ventricular enlargement. **Bottom:** Pick disease. Pronounced selective atrophy of the frontal and temporal lobes. (Reproduced by permission from Lee SH, Rao KCVG, Zimmerman RA. *Cranial MRI and CT.* New York, NY: McGraw-Hill; 1992.)

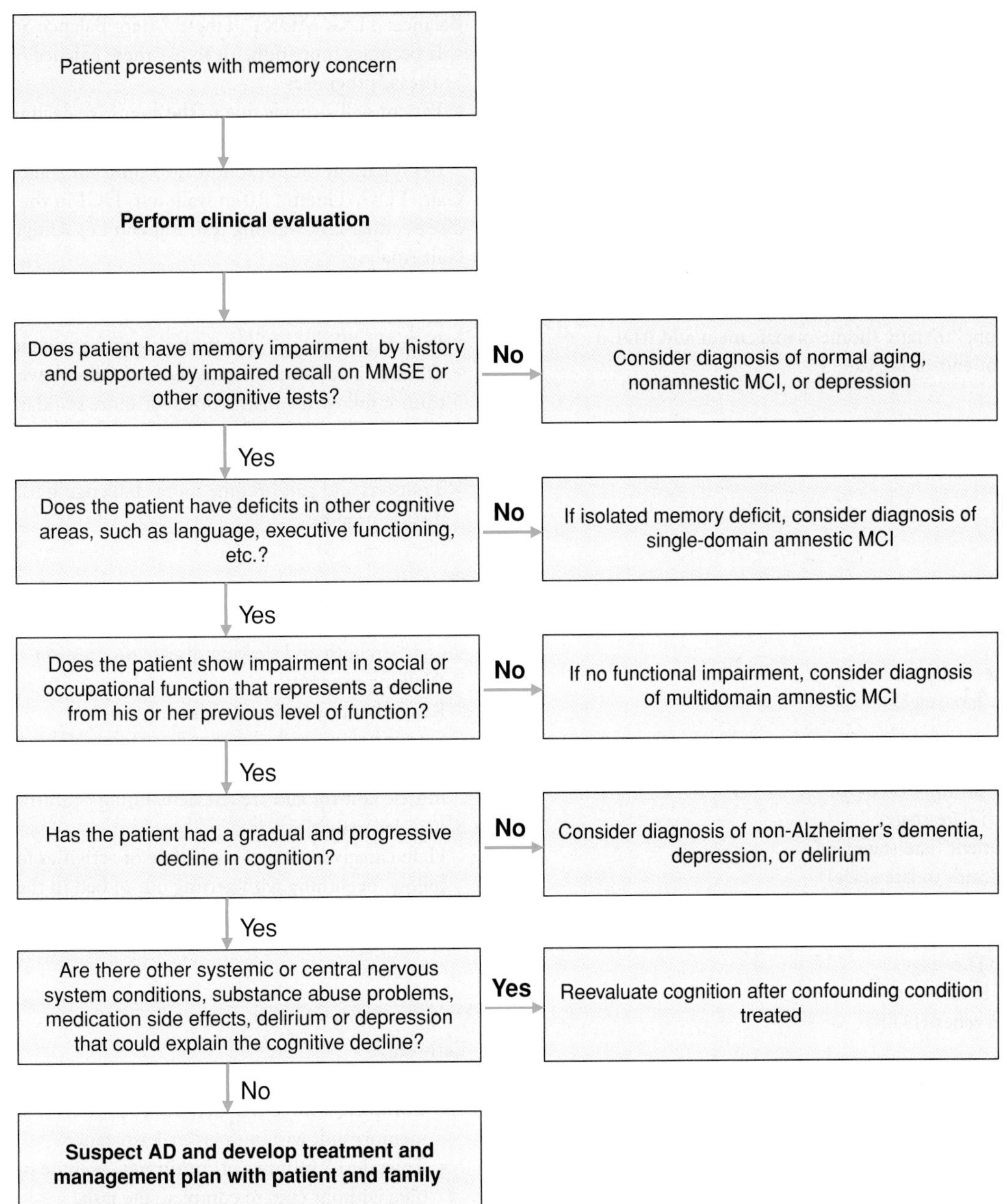

FIGURE 81-4 Algorithm for the clinical diagnosis of Alzheimer's disease. (From Halter JB, Ouslander JG, Tinetti ME, et al. *Hazzard's Geriatric Medicine and Gerontology*. 6th ed. http://www.accessmedicine.com. Copyright © The McGraw-Hill Companies, Inc. All rights reserved.)

- Metabolic disorders
- Nutritional deficiencies
- Paraneoplastic limbic encephalitis
- Pseudodementia of depression
- Stroke (multi-infarct dementia)
- Subdural hematoma
- Supranuclear palsy
- Tumor

MEANS OF CONFIRMATION OR DIAGNOSIS

Laboratory Tests

- CSF for protein analysis
- Neuropsychologic testing

Imaging

- CT of the brain[4]
- MRI of the brain[5]
- SPECT for hypoperfusion in the parietal and temporal regions
- PET scan for abnormal brain proteins[5]

Diagnostic Procedures

- EEG for brain function

FINDINGS AND INTERPRETATION

- In advanced stages of Alzheimer disease, MRI will show frontal lobe atrophy.
- In early stages, EEG may show resting alpha frequency declines.

- Most imaging and tests are designed to rule out other causes of the apparent dementia.

TREATMENT

Medication

- Aricept

REFERRALS/ADMITTANCE

- To neurologist for imaging, disease management, medication
- To social worker for family support and coordination of care
- For occupational therapy (home management and ADLs)
- To hospice for end-of-life care

IMPAIRMENTS

- Arousal
- Attention
- Behavior
- Cognition
- Gait training (late-stage)[6]
- Wheelchair (w/c) mobility (late-stage)[6]
- Balance[5]
  - Static sit (late-stage)
  - Dynamic sit (late-stage)
  - Static stand
  - Dynamic stand
  - Moving base of support (BOS)
- Muscle strength (late-stage)
- Muscle recruitment (late-stage)
- Coordination (mid- to late-stage)
- Postural control
- Posture
- ROM (mid- to late-stage)
- Reflexes (mid- to late-stage)
  - Deep tendon reflex (DTR)
  - Babinski
  - Clonus
- Motor planning (mid- to late-stage)
- Bed mobility (mid- to late-stage)
- Transfers (mid- to late-stage)
- Endurance (late-stage)
- Aerobic capacity (late-stage)
- Self-care (mid-stage)
- Home management (mid-stage)
- Respiratory compromise (late-stage)

TESTS AND MEASURES

- Cognition: Mini-Mental State Examination (MMSE), executive function tests, memory, comprehension, speed of processing, attention and concentration[7]
- Barthel Index
- Strength: May have to report functional strength if the patient is unable to follow directions for a manual muscle test (MMT)
- Active and passive range of motion
- Reflexes
- Coordination: Gross and fine motor
- Flexibility: Specific muscle length as well as spinal flexibility during functional activities
- Postural alignment
- Balance: TUG, MDRT, Tinetti,[8] Berg Balance Scale
  - It becomes more difficult to use these balance measures as disease progresses
  - Patient will struggle due to the cognitive decline
  - Observe balance strategies and fall-risk during functional activities if patient cannot follow directions for standardized measures
- Gait: TUG, Tinetti,[8] 10-m walk test, DGI in the early stage of the disease, dual-task walking test, Rancho Los Amigo Observational Gait Analysis[9]
  - It becomes more difficult to use these gait measures as disease progresses
  - Patient will struggle due to the cognitive decline
  - Observe gait pattern, strategies, and fall-risk when the patient cannot follow the instructions for more standardized measures
- Integumentary: More of a concern in late-stage
- Functional mobility: Basic bed mobility
  - Transfers and gait become more challenging for the patient as disease progresses

INTERVENTION

- Movement has shown effectiveness in maintaining functional muscle strength and slowing disease progression
  - Walking program
  - Recumbent or stationary bike
  - Strengthening with therabands or free weights initially, seated weight machines later (weight machines require less internal muscle control and are less demanding cognitively)
- Scheduled activities
  - Help caregivers design a schedule of activities for the patient to follow, beginning with getting out of bed in the morning
  - Repetitive sequence of daily events decrease cognitive demand and reduce anxiety and frustration for both patient and caregiver

FUNCTIONAL GOALS

- Early-stage
  - Patient will
    - Complete a three-step activity 100% accurately with use of a memory aid, without personal assistance.
    - Tolerate 15 minutes of continuous exercise on a recumbent bike without cues to complete the task.
- Mid-stage
  - Patient will
    - Complete a one-step activity 100% accurately with the use of a memory aid, without personal assistance.
    - Ambulate 200 ft with contact guard assistance in a controlled indoor environment without cues to complete the activity.
- Late-stage
  - Caregiver will
    - Demonstrate appropriate safety and body mechanics during all bed mobility and transfer activities with the patient in the home.
    - Demonstrate appropriate guarding and assistance for ambulating short distances with patient in the home.

PROGNOSIS

- Poor; the disease is progressive and degenerative.
- Death is usually the result of respiratory or cardiovascular causes and inanition.

PATIENT RESOURCE

- Alzheimers. Alzheimer's Association. http://www.alz.org/research/overview.asp. Accessed January 21, 2013.

REFERENCES

1. The American Physical Therapy Association. Pattern 5E: impaired motor function and sensory integrity associated with progressive disorders of the central nervous system [abstract]. *Guide to Physical Therapy Practice*. 2003. http://guidetoptpractice.apta.org/content/1/SEC22.extract?sid=319647e3-433c-4720-84ac-edd5ded1eb4b. Accessed February 22, 2013.
2. Chandrasoma P, Taylor CR. *Concise Pathology*. 3rd ed. New York, NY: McGraw-Hill; 1998. http://www.accessphysiotherapy.com/abstract/193218. Accessed February 22, 2013.
3. Anatomy and Physiology Revealed. Accessphysiotherapy. http://www.accessphysiotherapy.com/APR. Accessed February 22, 2013.
4. Waxman SG. *Clinical Neuroanatomy*. New York, NY: McGraw-Hill; 2010. http://www.accessphysiotherapy.com/resource/22. Accessed February 22, 2013.
5. Dutton M. *Orthopaedic Examination, Evaluation, and Intervention*. New York, NY: McGraw-Hill; 2008. http://www.accessphysiotherapy.com/resource/612. Accessed February 22, 2013.
6. Shamus E, Stern D. *Effective Documentation for Physical Therapy Professionals*. 2nd ed. New York, NY: McGraw-Hill; 2011. http://www.accessphysiotherapy.com/resource/696. Accessed February 22, 2013.
7. Dutton M. *McGraw-Hill's NPTE (National Physical Therapy Examination)*. 2nd ed. New York, NY: McGraw-Hill; 2012. http://www.accessphysiotherapy.com/content/5399379. Accessed February 22, 2013.
8. Tinetti Balance and Gait Evaluation. http://www.bhps.org.uk/falls/documents/TinettiBalanceAssessment.pdf. Accessed January 19, 2013.
9. The University of Oklahoma Health Sciences Center. Observational gait analysis. http://moon.ouhsc.edu/dthompso/gait/knmatics/oga.htm. Accessed February 22, 2013.

ADDITIONAL REFERENCES

- ICD9DATA. http://www.icd9data.com. Accessed January 21, 2013.
- ICD10DATA. http://www.icd10data.com. Accessed January 21, 2013.
- Malone TR, Hazle C, Grey ML. Imaging of the brain. In: Malone TR, Hazle C, Grey ML, eds. *Imaging in Rehabilitation*. New York, NY: McGraw-Hill; 2008. http://www.accessphysiotherapy.com/content/5940348#5940348. Accessed February 6, 2013.
- Ropper AL, Samuels MA. *Adams and Victor's Principles of Neurology*. 9th ed. New York, NY: McGraw-Hill; 2009:1014–1023.
- Schulte OJ, Stephens J, Ann J. Brain function, aging and dementia. In: Umphred DA, ed. *Neurological Rehabilitation*. 5th ed. St. Louis, MO: Mosby Elsevier. 2007: 904, 910, 917–923.

82 AMYOTROPHIC LATERAL SCLEROSIS

Mollie Venglar, DSc, MSPT, NCS

CONDITION/DISORDER SYNONYMS

- Lou Gehrig disease
- Amyotrophic lateral sclerosis (ALS)
- Motor neuron disease

ICD-9-CM CODE

- 728.2 Muscular wasting and disuse atrophy not elsewhere classified

ICD-10-CM CODE

- M62.50 Muscle wasting and atrophy, not elsewhere classified, unspecified site

PREFERRED PRACTICE PATTERN

- 5E: Impaired Motor Function and Sensory Integrity Associated with Progressive Disorders of the Central Nervous System[1]

PATIENT PRESENTATION

In home health, the physical therapist sees a 51-year-old man who is transitioning from moderate to severe ALS. Following examination the physical therapist determines that he is no longer capable of safe ambulation; he tolerates sitting upright but only with

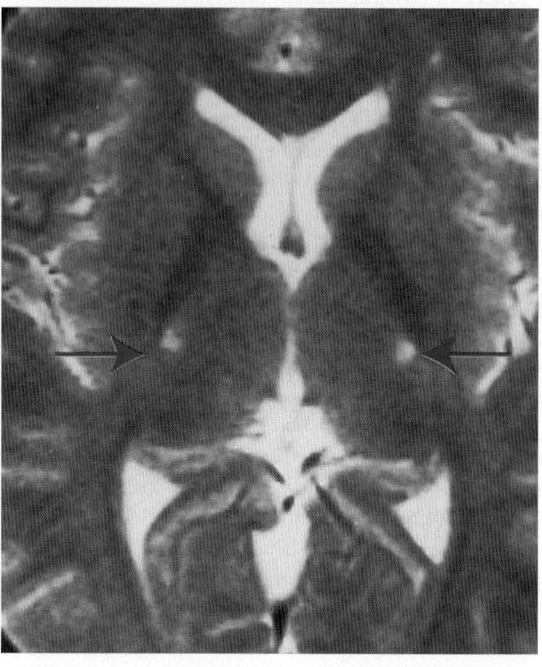

FIGURE 82-1 Amyotrophic lateral sclerosis. Axial T2-weighted MRI scan through the lateral ventricles of the brain reveals abnormal high signal intensity within the corticospinal tracts (*red arrows*). This MRI feature represents an increase in water content in myelin tracts undergoing Wallerian degeneration secondary to cortical motor neuronal loss. This finding is commonly present in ALS, but can also be seen in AIDS-related encephalopathy, infarction, or other disease processes that produce corticospinal neuronal loss in a symmetric fashion. (From Longo DL, Fauci AS, Kasper DL, Hauser SL, Jameson JL, Loscalzo J, eds. *Harrison's Principles of Internal Medicine*. 18th ed. http://www.accessmedicine.com. Copyright © The McGraw-Hill Companies, Inc. All rights reserved.)

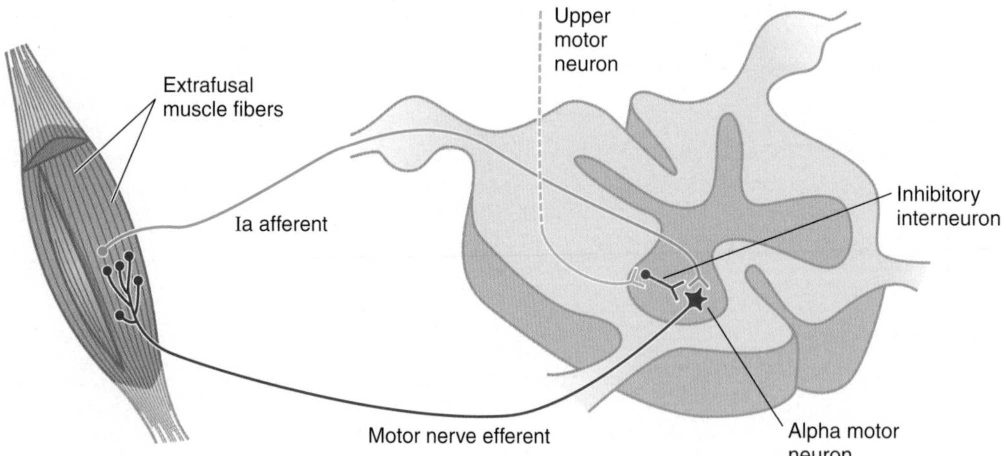

FIGURE 82-2 Monosynaptic muscle stretch reflex with descending control via inhibitory interneurons. Primary Ia afferents (*green*) from muscle spindles, activated when the muscle is stretched rapidly, synapse directly on motor neurons (*blue*) going to the stretched muscle, causing it to contract and resist the movement. Pyramidal upper motor neurons (*aqua*) from the cerebral cortex suppress spinal reflexes and the lower motor neurons indirectly by activating the spinal cord inhibitory interneuron pools (*red*). When the pyramidal influences are removed, the reflexes are released from inhibition and become more active, leading to hyperreflexia and spasticity. Baclofen acts to restore the lost inhibition by stimulating postsynaptic GABA receptors. Tizanidine acts presynaptically to stimulate GABA release from spinal cord inhibitory interneuron. (From Brunton LL, Chabner BA, Knollmann BC. *Goodman & Gilman's The Pharmacological Basis of Therapeutics*. 12th ed. http://www.accessmedicine.com. Copyright © The McGraw-Hill Companies, Inc. All rights reserved.)

full support. He reports he is having increased difficulty with his coughing and his chest feels heavy. His care giver is getting increasingly concerned about his skin and would like advice on how to manage him better. Presently he is able to communicate verbally, but the activity is fatiguing and his oxygen saturation drops to 83% during conversation. On muscle testing he demonstrates gross strength of 2+/5 in bilateral upper extremities and 3/5 in bilateral lower extremities. Sensation is intact.

KEY FEATURES

Description

- Quickly progressive, degenerative motor disorder caused by the loss of nerve cells in the anterior horn of the spinal cord and motor nuclei of the brain stem[2]
- Loss of muscle strength and coordination

Essentials of Diagnosis

- Rapid, progressive loss of motor function not attributable to internal or external injury
- Diagnosis made by evidence of motor loss in multiple parts of the body, speed of degeneration, and ruling out other progressive neurologic disorders

General Considerations

- Onset may be either in the extremities or in the bulbar region initially; eventually all patients experience degeneration in both areas
- Diagnosis requires evidence of denervation in at least three motor regions
- Usually does not affect the senses

Demographics

- Male-to-female ratio 2:1[3]
- Most patients aged above 45 years, but can be much younger[3]
- 10% familial (tend to have onset at younger age)[3]

CLINICAL FINDINGS

SIGNS AND SYMPTOMS

- Both upper motor neuron and lower motor neuron signs and symptoms
- Limb onset ALS
  - One side will be involved initially; spread to both sides within months
  - Patients usually report unexplained tripping while walking, or difficulty managing buttons and small objects
  - Muscle fasciculation evident
  - Spasticity remains mild
- Bulbar onset ALS
  - Difficulty with speech production, voice changes, hoarseness
  - Difficulty with swallowing, gagging, choking easily
  - Difficulty with saliva management, drooling
- Sensation is spared, may experience transient paresthesias due to position or nerve compression
- Bowel and bladder control usually maintained
- Respiratory compromise evident with both bulbar and limb onset

Functional Implications

- Loss of independence in mobility, self-care, eating, breathing
- Dependence on others and on technology for survival

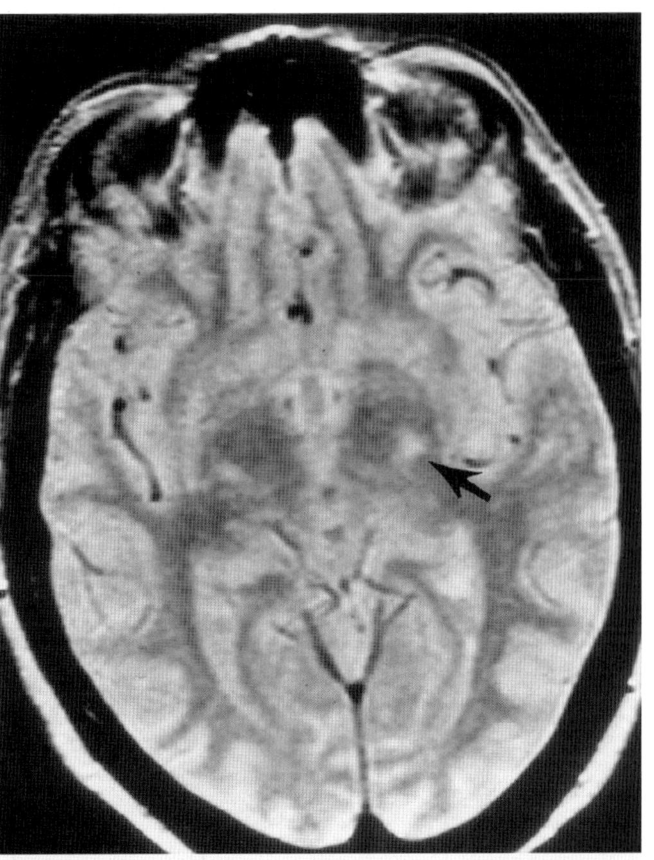

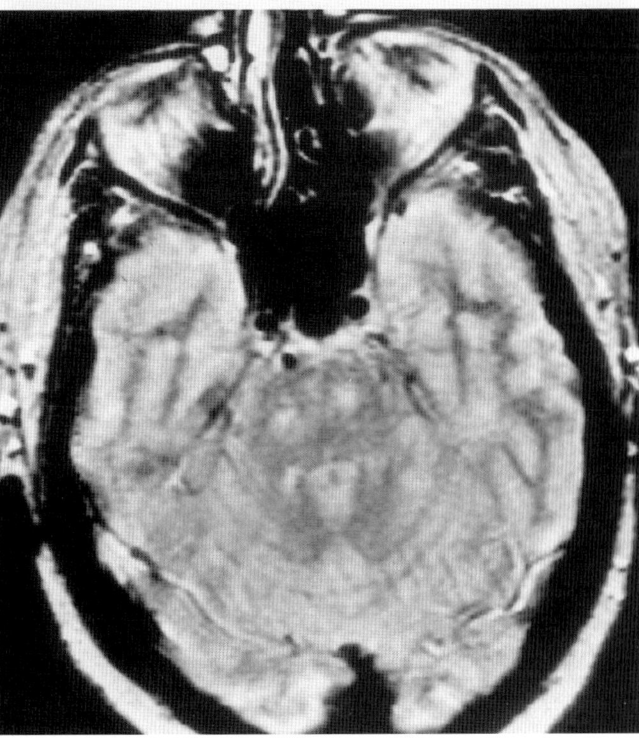

FIGURE 82-3 T2-weighted MRI showing signal changes that reflect Wallerian change in the corticospinal tracts at the level of the internal capsule (*top, black arrow*) and the pons (*bottom*) in a case of ALS. (From Ropper AH, Samuels MA. *Adams & Victor's Principles of Neurology*. 9th ed. http://www.accessmedicine.com. Copyright © The McGraw-Hill Companies, Inc. All rights reserved.)

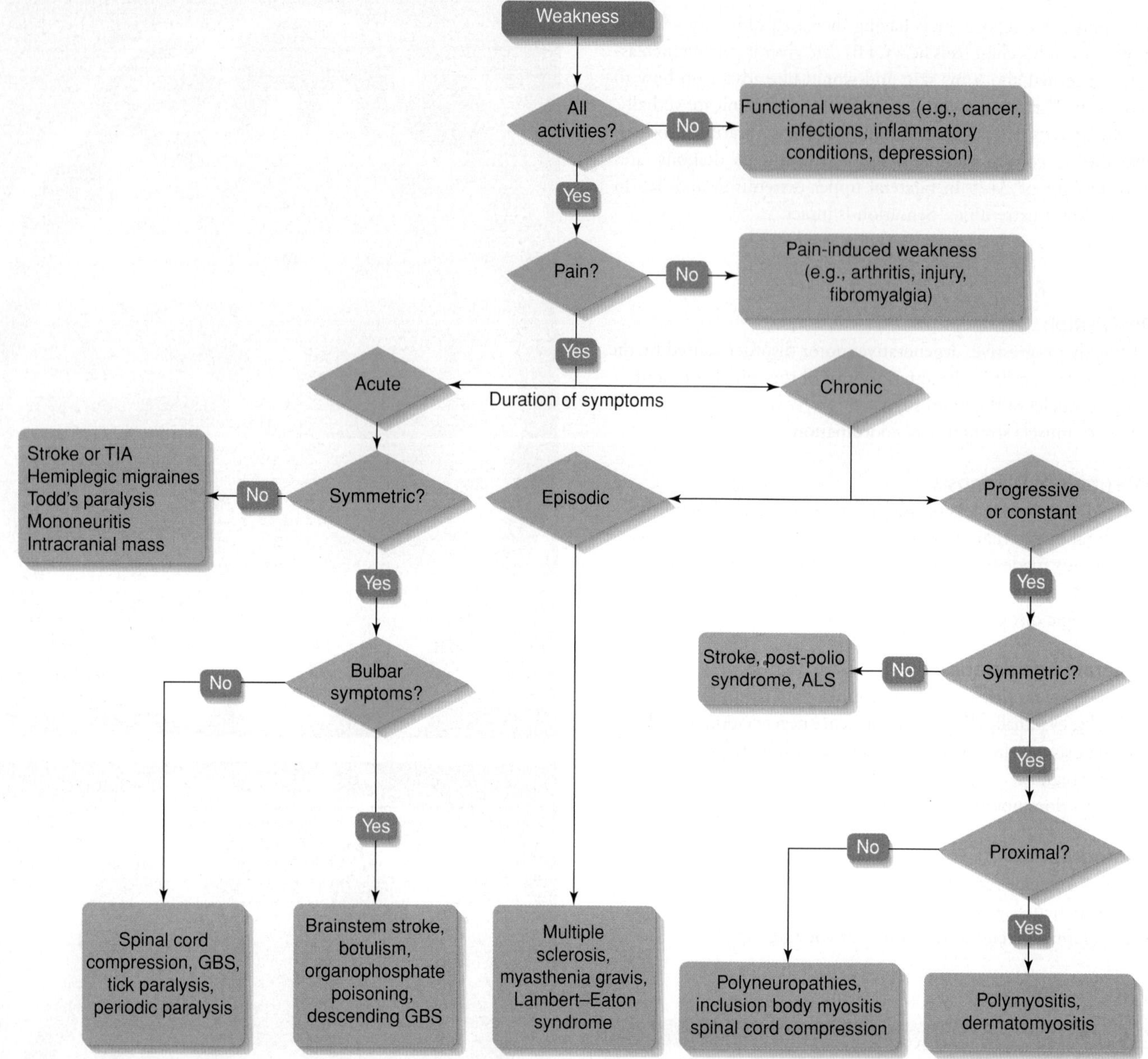

FIGURE 82-4 Diagnostic algorithm: Muscle weakness. ALS, amyotrophic lateral sclerosis; DM, dermatomyositis; GBS, Guillain–Barré syndrome; TIA, transient ischemic attack. (From Henderson MC, Tierney LM, Smetana GW. *The Patient History: An Evidence-Based Approach to* Differential Diagnosis. http://www.accessmedicine.com.)

Possible Contributing Causes

- Primarily idiopathic
- Family member who has a hereditary form

Differential Diagnosis

- Progressive spinal muscular atrophy
- Progressive bulbar palsy
- Primary lateral sclerosis
- Parkinson disease
- Muscular dystrophy
- Multiple sclerosis
- Cervical spondylosis
- Inflammatory myopathy
- Myasthenia gravis
- Inclusion body myositis

MEANS OF CONFIRMATION OR DIAGNOSIS

Laboratory Tests

- Serum creatine kinase may be moderately elevated
- Muscle biopsy
- Genetic test for family history of ALS
- Blood tests to rule out other conditions

Imaging

- MRI

Diagnostic Procedures

- Electromyography (EMG): Widespread fasciculation and fibrillation
- Motor nerve conduction velocity test (NCV) if positive demonstrates slight slowing with focal motor conduction block

- Swallowing study
- Breathing test for lung involvement

FINDINGS AND INTERPRETATIONS

- MRI may show slight atrophy of the motor cortices and Wallerian degeneration of the motor tracts

TREATMENT

Medication

- Medicine: Riluzole (bulbar onset), baclofen or tizanidine for spasticity

REFERRALS/ADMITTANCE

- Neurologist for confirmation of diagnosis and initiation of disease management
  - Feeding tube referral when needed
  - Hospice referral when needed
- ALS Association for support
- Respiratory therapy for progressive respiratory management

IMPAIRMENTS

- Cranial nerve integrity
- Peripheral nerve integrity
- Gait impairment or loss
- Wheelchair mobility
- Sitting balance
- Standing balance
- Weakness
- Poor muscle recruitment
- Poor or lost coordination
- Postural control and posture deficits
- Active range of motion (AROM) loss, eventually passive ROM loss
- Change in deep tendon reflexes
- Muscle tone changes (could be either flaccid or spastic)
- Bed-mobility impairment
- Difficulty with transfers
- Declining endurance
- Reduced aerobic capacity
- Self-care decline
- Home-management decline
- Loss of fine motor control
- Limited respiratory function

TESTS AND MEASURES

- Cognition: Mini-mental State Examination (MMSE), executive function tests, memory, comprehension
- Pain: Subjective report, Visual Analog Scale (VAS), or verbal report
- Strength and muscle endurance
- Coordination
- Muscle tone
- Joint ROM
- Cranial nerve integrity
- Sensation (only needed if patient reports sensory symptoms or if sensory compromise is suspected; loss of sensation is not a common impairment in this diagnosis)
- Postural alignment

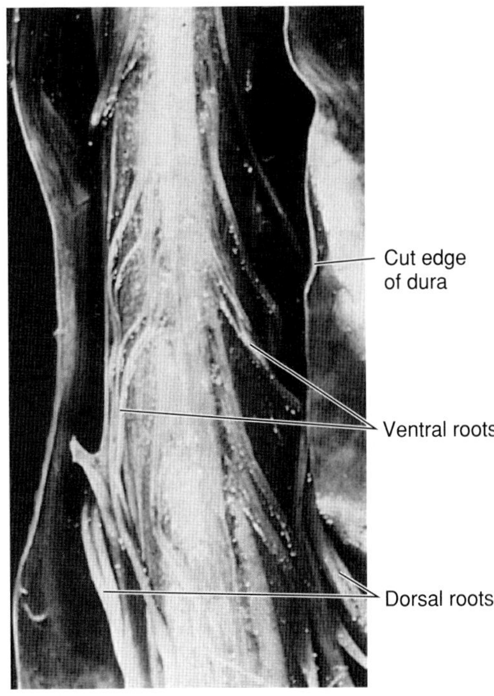

FIGURE 82-5 Ventral view of the spinal cord (with the dura opened) of a patient with motor neuron disease (amyotrophic lateral sclerosis). Notice the reduction in size of the ventral roots (resulting from the degeneration of the axons of motor neurons) compared with the normal dorsal roots. (From Waxman SG. *Clinical Neuroanatomy*. 26th ed. http://www.accessmedicine.com. Copyright © The McGraw-Hill Companies, Inc. All rights reserved.)

- Balance (TUG, MDRT, Tinetti, BBS)
- Gait (TUG, Tinetti, 10-m walk test, DGI in the early stage of the disease)
- Respiratory function (spirometer, oxygen saturation, breathing pattern, auscultation)
- Integumentary: More of a concern in the mid and late stages
- Functional mobility: FIM™
- Fatigue: Fatigue Severity Scale
- Disease-specific measure: ALS Functional Rating Scale

INTERVENTION

- Aggressive strengthening is contraindicated. Avoid fatiguing the person as a whole, or individual muscles.
- Fatigue
  - Energy conservation
  - Coordinate breathing with activity
  - Adaptive equipment to reduce fatigue
- Functional mobility
  - Adaptive equipment as needed (hospital bed, four-wheeled walker, wheelchair)
  - LE bracing as needed
  - Caregiver training on patient handling/guarding for ambulation, transfers, and bed mobility
- Balance and postural control
  - Balance reaction in sitting and standing with and without a moving base of support
    - If the muscle is already denervated, it will not produce a balance reaction.
      - Example: If the person has lost dorsiflexion function, they will not gain an ankle strategy regardless of the amount of practice.

- Example: If the person has lost shoulder function, they will not gain a protective response regardless of the amount of practice.
  - Assistive device as needed (walker, bracing)
- Exercise
  - If MMT is 3/5 or greater, moderate intensity is acceptable.
  - If MMT is less than 3/5, low intensity should be used.
    - Overwork damage will occur faster in the weakened or denervated muscle.
  - Use functional activities for strengthening whenever possible.
  - Aquatic exercise is beneficial.
  - Aerobic exercise is helpful but moderated by respiratory status and fatigue.
  - Self or caregiver assisted mild stretching to maintain ROM in all appendicular joints as well as cervical spine.
- Respiratory
  - Postural drainage as tolerated. (This is not appropriate in late-stage ALS.)
  - Active cough techniques as tolerated.
  - Encourage use of suction, cough-assist, and ventilation during therapy.
- Pain
  - Adaptive equipment to prevent pain from joint malalignment or skin breakdown (e.g., supportive back/seat in wheelchair, neck brace, arm trough or lap tray on wheelchair, bracing or taping to decrease shoulder subluxation).

FUNCTIONAL GOALS

- Early-stage
  - Patient will
    - Ambulate with four-wheeled rolling walker independently over community surfaces for 3 minutes while maintaining oxygen saturation above 92%.
    - Demonstrate accurate stepping strategy with minimal challenge to standing balance while using an assistive device in 75% of trials.
- Mid-stage
  - Patient will
    - Transfer between wheelchair and bed via sit pivot transfer with minimal assistance from caregiver in 50% of trials.
    - Accurately navigate home environment in power-controlled wheelchair without assistance from caregiver.
    - Perform transition between sit and supine on bed with no greater than moderate assistance from caregiver.
- Late-stage
  - Patient will
    - Self-direct transfer between bed and wheelchair with at least 85% accuracy.
    - Self-direct wheelchair positioning to prevent pressure/pain and optimize ability to access controls with 100% accuracy.

PROGNOSIS

- Average lifespan after diagnosis is 4 years.[4]
- Death usually from respiratory failure or pulmonary infection.[4]

ADDITIONAL INFORMATION

- For additional information, please see spinal cord case (part of *Clinical Neuroanatomy*) on AccessPhysiotherapy.com

PATIENT RESOURCE

- ALS Association. http://www.alsa.org. Accessed August 8, 2014.

REFERENCES

1. The American Physical Therapy Association. Pattern 5E: impaired motor function and sensory integrity associated with progressive disorders of the central nervous system. *Interactive Guide to Physical Therapist Practice*. 2003. doi: 10.2522/ptguide.3.2_5. http://guidetoptpractice.apta.org/content/1/SEC22.extract?sid=23e64db7-53b2-4adc-bd47-08b58118ccd2. Accessed May 14, 2014.
2. Anatomy & Physiology Revealed. AccessPhysiotherapy. Accessphysiotherapy.com. Accessed February 22, 2013.
3. Bello-Haas VD. Amyotrophic lateral sclerosis. In: O'Sullivan SB, Schmitz TJ, eds. *Physical Rehabilitation*. 5th ed. Philadelphia, PA: FA Davis; 2007:819–852.
4. Lomen-Hoerth C, Messing RO. Pathophysiology of selected neurologic disorders. In: McPhee SJ, Hammer GD, eds. *Pathophysiology of Disease*.6th ed. New York, NY: McGraw-Hill; 2010. http://www.accessphysiotherapy.com/content/5368605#5368605. Accessed February 22, 2013.

ADDITIONAL REFERENCES

- Denegar CR, Prentice WE. Managing pain with therapeutic modalities. In: Prentice WE, Quillen WS, Underwood F, eds. *Therapeutic Modalities in Rehabilitation*. 4th ed. New York, NY: McGraw-Hill; 2011:Chapter 4. http://www.accessphysiotherapy.com/abstract/8135087#8135091. Accessed February 22, 2013.
- Dutton M. *McGraw-Hill's NPTE (National Physical Therapy Examination)*. 2nd ed. New York, NY: McGraw-Hill; 2012. http://www.accessphysiotherapy.com/content/5400153#5400153. Accessed February 22, 2013.
- Dutton M. *Orthopaedic Examination, Evaluation, and Intervention*. New York, NY: McGraw-Hill; 2008. http://www.accessphysiotherapy.com/resource/612. Accessed February 22, 2013.
- ICD10DATA. http://www.icd10data.com. Accessed January 21, 2013.
- ICD9DATA. http://www.icd9data.com. Accessed January 21, 2013.
- Panus PC, Jobst EE, Masters SB, Katzung B, Tinsley SL, Trevor AJ. *Pharmacology for the Physical Therapist*. New York, NY: McGraw-Hill; 2009. http://www.accessphysiotherapy.com/resource/615. Accessed February 22, 2013.
- Ropper AL, Samuels MA. *Adams and Victor's Principles of Neurology*. 9th ed. New York, NY: McGraw-Hill; 2009:1058–1065.
- Waxman SG. *Clinical Neuroanatomy*. New York, NY: McGraw-Hill; 2010. http://www.accessphysiotherapy.com/resource/22. Accessed February 22, 2013.

83 CEREBELLAR STROKE

Mollie Venglar, DSc, MSPT, NCS

CONDITION/DISORDER SYNONYM

- Cerebellar hemorrhage

ICD-9-CM CODE

- 431 Intracerebral hemorrhage

ICD-10-CM CODE

- I61.4 Nontraumatic intracerebral hemorrhage in cerebellum

PREFERRED PRACTICE PATTERN

- 5D: Impaired Motor Function and Sensory Integrity Associated with Nonprogressive Disorders of the Central Nervous System—acquired in adolescence or adulthood[1]

PATIENT PRESENTATION

A 42-year-old woman experiences surgical evacuation of a hemorrhage in the midline of her cerebellum. Intracranial pressures appear to be controlled and she is now allowed to participate in therapies. She reports nausea with most upright, unsupported activities. She struggles to maintain proper trunk alignment and control during static sitting at the side of the hospital bed and relies on her upper extremities to help her stay upright. She has no difficulty with cognitive tests but is easily distracted by the sensations of vertigo and nausea. On attempts to ambulate, she lists to the left and requires maximum assistance to keep her trunk in midline. She does not demonstrate any visual field cuts. She does not tolerate testing for dynamic visual acuity, vestibulo-ocular reflex (VOR), or head thrust due to nausea.

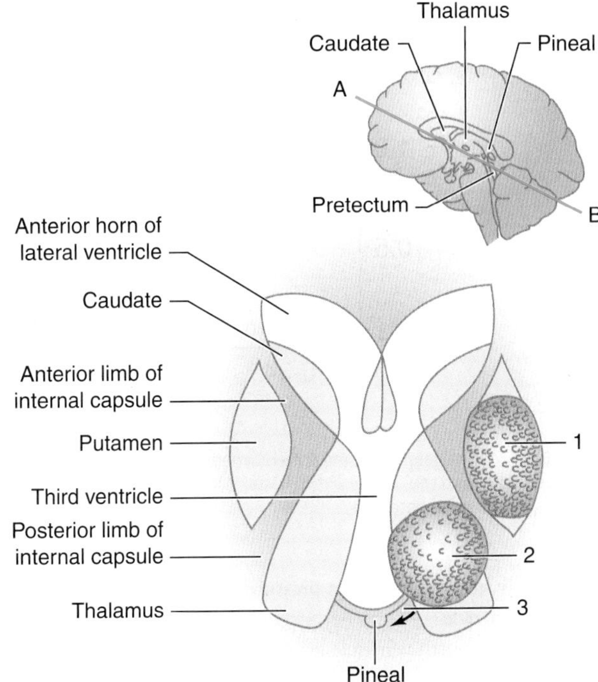

FIGURE 83-1 Anatomic relationships in deep cerebral hemorrhage. **Top:** Plane of section. **Bottom:** Putaminal (1) and thalamic (2) hemorrhages can compress or transect the adjacent posterior limb of the internal capsule. Thalamic hemorrhages can also extend into the ventricles or compress the hypothalamus or midbrain upgaze center (3). (From Greenberg DA, Aminoff MJ, Simon RP. *Clinical Neurology*. 8th ed. http://www.accessmedicine.com. Copyright © The McGraw-Hill Companies, Inc. All rights reserved.)

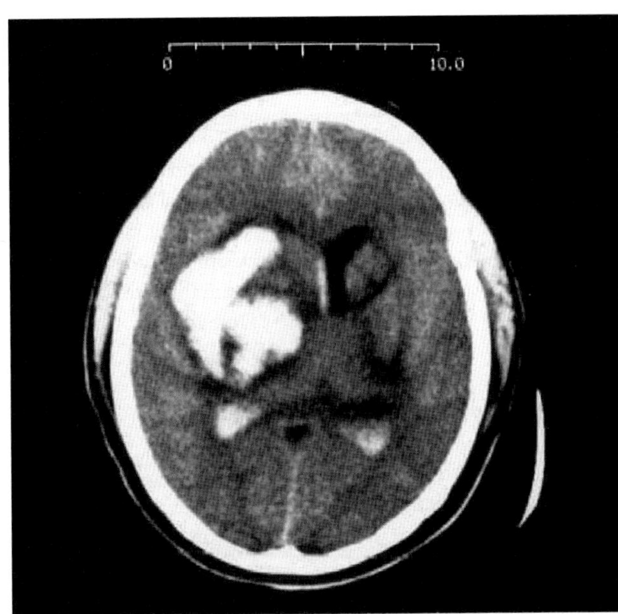

FIGURE 83-2 Large intracerebral hemorrhage caused by hypertensive stroke in a nulliparous woman whose blood pressure was recorded at 270/140 mm Hg. (From Cunningham FG, Leveno K, Bloom S, Hauth J, Rouse D, Spong C. *Williams Obstetrics*. 23rd ed. http://www.accessmedicine.com. Copyright © The McGraw-Hill Companies, Inc. All rights reserved.)

KEY FEATURES

Description

- Stroke, usually due to hemorrhage, affecting the hemispheres, vermis, or flocculonodular lobe of the cerebellum

Essentials of Diagnosis

- Most prominent feature of acute cerebellar stroke is repeated vomiting.
- Patient will experience occipital headache, vertigo, difficulty remaining upright, walking.
- Most cases show mild unilateral facial weakness and decreased corneal reflex.
- May exhibit dysarthria or dysphagia.

General Considerations

- Can be life threatening depending on the size of hematoma

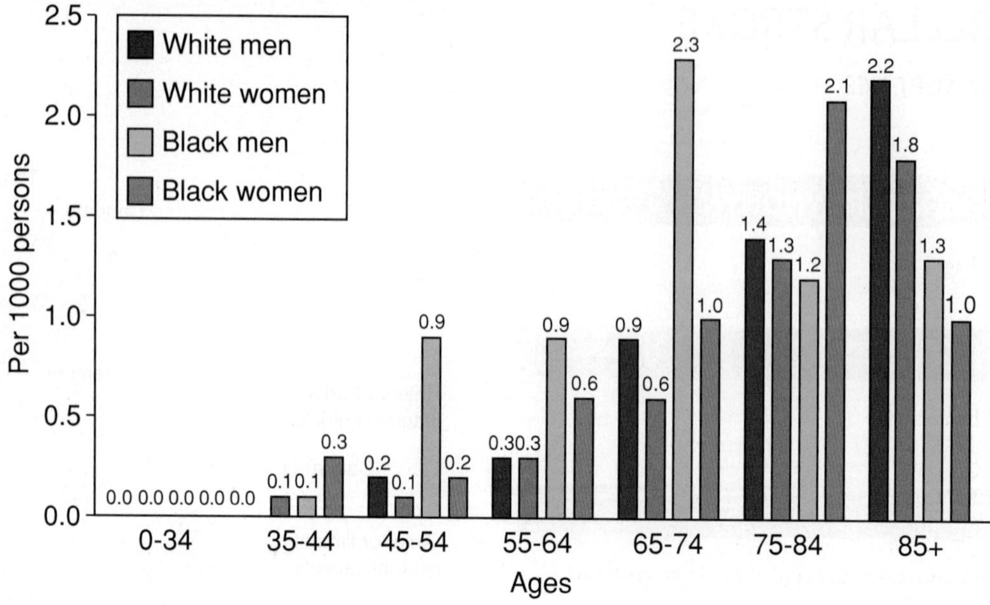

FIGURE 83-3 Annual rate of first intracerebral hemorrhage by age, sex, and race in the Greater Cincinnati/Northern Kentucky Stroke Study (GNKSS; 1993–1994). Unpublished data from the GNKSS. (From Fuster V, Walsh RA, Harrington RA. *Hurst's The Heart*. 13th ed. http://www.accessmedicine.com. Copyright © The McGraw-Hill Companies, Inc. All rights reserved.)

- Generally hematoma causes pressure in area of the fourth ventricle
  - Blocking fourth ventricle leads to hydrocephalus
  - Increased pressure in area of the fourth ventricle causes damage to the brain stem
  - Patient's status can quickly deteriorate to coma as pressure builds
  - Cerebellar stroke due to hemorrhage considered medical emergency

▶ Demographics

- Can occur in any age group, either gender

CLINICAL FINDINGS

SIGNS AND SYMPTOMS

- Asthenia
- Asynergia
- Dysarthria
- Dysdiadochokinesia
- Dysmetria
- Dysphagia[2]
- Dyssynergia
- Gait ataxia
- Hypotonia[3]
- Limb ataxia
- Mild facial weakness
- Nystagmus[4]
- Occipital headache
- Postural instability
- Titubation
- Tremor[4]
- Vertigo[5]
- Vomiting

▶ Functional Implications

- Loss of independence with all aspects of mobility, ADLs, self-care
- Safety concerns for any activity requiring upright control
- Impaired ability to interact effectively with immediate and community environments

▶ Possible Contributing Causes

- Hypertension (HTN)
- Arteriovenous malformation (AVM)
- Hyperlipidemia
- Obesity[6]
- Smoking
- Sedentary lifestyle
- Peripheral vascular disease
- Birth trauma

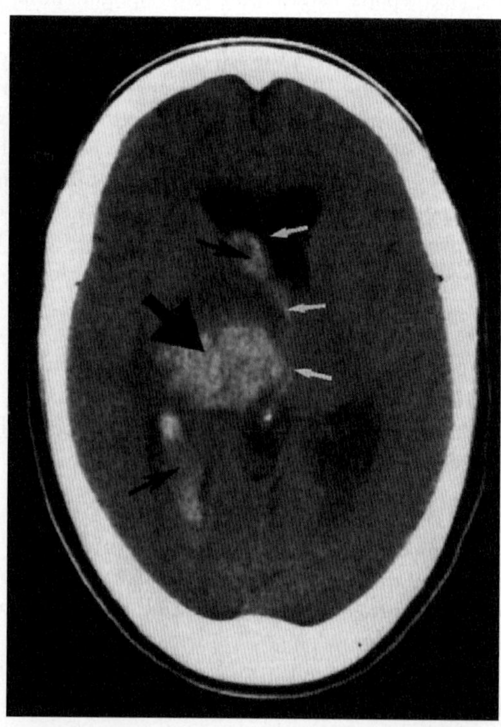

FIGURE 83-4 Hemorrhagic stroke seen on CT. The CT image demonstrates bleeding in the right basal ganglia (*large black arrow*) into the ventricles (*small black arrows*) with midline shift (*white arrows*). (From Chen MYM, Pope TL Jr., Ott DJ. *Basic Radiology*. New York, NY: McGraw-Hill; 2004:p. 337.)

Differential Diagnosis

- Cerebellar ataxia
- Cerebellar degeneration
- Hydrocephalus
- Transient ischemic attack (TIA)

MEANS OF CONFIRMATION OR DIAGNOSIS

Imaging

- CT[7]

Diagnostic Procedures

- Neurovascular tests
  - Neck flexion for meningeal irritation
  - Palpation of arteries
  - Auscultation of heart and blood vessels
  - Ophthalmic pressures

FINDINGS AND INTERPRETATION

- CT:[7] Accurate for cerebellar hemorrhage; to determine need for surgical evacuation

TREATMENT

Medications

- Mannitol at initial identification of hydrocephalus

REFERRALS/ADMITTANCE

- To emergency room to assessment and management of medical emergency
- To neurosurgeon for surgical evacuation of cerebellar hematoma
- To physiatrist for specific rehabilitation; physiatrist will manage medications, symptoms, future needs if not managed by neurologist
- To occupational therapist for ADL, fine motor task retraining
- To speech/language pathologist for speech and swallowing impairments
- To support groups for patients and caregivers
- To case management or social work for coordination of care

IMPAIRMENTS

- Arousal
- Cranial nerve integrity
- Peripheral nerve integrity
- Gait[8]
- Wheelchair mobility
- Balance
  - Static sit
  - Dynamic sit
  - Static stand
  - Dynamic stand
  - Moving base of support
- Muscle strength (appearance of weakness may be an issue of low tone)
- Muscle recruitment
- Coordination
- Postural control
- Posture
- Reflexes
  - Deep tendon
  - Babinski
  - Clonus
- Muscle tone
- Motor planning
- Bed mobility
- Transfers
- Endurance
- Aerobic capacity (usually related to being sedentary in the hospital)
- Self-care
- Home management
- Fine motor coordination

TESTS AND MEASURES

- Bed mobility
- Transfers
- Sitting balance: Static and dynamic
- Standing balance: Static and dynamic[9]
  - Eyes open and eyes closed
  - Narrow versus wide base of support
  - Sternal nudge
- Postural control
- Gait[9]
  - Backward
  - Tandem
  - Variable speed
  - Sudden stops
  - Sideways
  - Turns
  - Walk on toes/heels
  - Stepping over objects
  - Standardized measures: Dynamic Gait Index, Timed Up and Go
- Muscle tone
- Muscle strength
- Coordination
  - Adiadochokinesis (Dysdiadochokinesia)[7]
  - Heel-shin slide
  - Toe/heel
  - Tap
  - Dysmetria testing (finger-to-nose, finger-to-finger)
- Vestibular testing
  - Vestibulo–ocular (VOR) reflex testing
  - Optokinetics

INTERVENTION

- Head control
- Trunk and core control
- Posture and postural control, balance training
- Bed-mobility training
- Transfer training
- Wheelchair-mobility training
- Gait training
- Frenkel exercises[10]
- Proprioceptive neuromuscular facilitation: stability techniques
- Vestibular retraining as needed
- Interactive metronome

FUNCTIONAL GOALS

- Goals based on presentation and prognosis; following are general goals to be considered.
- Patient will be able to
  - Demonstrate accurate vestibulo–ocular reflex at a pace of 50 beats per minute in order to scan environment in the community.
  - Accurately and independently transition supine-to-sit in 10 seconds without loss of balance to improve general independence.
  - Maintain static standing balance with feet together, without upper-extremity support, for 30 seconds (or other age-appropriate target) to demonstrate improved postural control.
  - Ambulate on variety of surfaces with supervision for >250 ft with assistive device as needed in preparation for return to community.
  - Demonstrate appropriate balance control while walking with sudden 180-degree turns on level surfaces to demonstrate improved dynamic postural control.

PROGNOSIS

- High risk for hydrocephalus with cerebellar hemorrhage or hematoma; compression of brain stem causes highest risk for rapid deterioration.
- Cerebellar hemorrhage or hematoma responds better than most hemorrhages to surgical evacuation if found quickly enough.
- Few patients survive after onset of coma.
- 5228 deaths were reported in the United States under the ICD-10 Code I61.4 from 1999 to 2007.

PATIENT RESOURCE

- Stroke. National Stroke Association. http://www.stroke.org/site/PageNavigator/HOME. Accessed February 22, 2013.

REFERENCES

1. The American Physical Therapy Association. Pattern 5D: impaired motor function and sensory integrity associated with nonprogressive disorders of the central nervous system - acquired in adolescence or adulthood. *Interactive Guide to Physical Therapist Practice*. 2003. doi: 10.2522/ptguide.3.2_4. http://guidetoptpractice.apta.org/content/1/SEC21.extract. Accessed May 14, 2014.
2. Chandrasoma P, Taylor CR. *Concise Pathology*. 3rd ed. Stamford, CT: Appleton & Lang; 1998. http://www.accessphysiotherapy.com/content/187050. Accessed February 22, 2013.
3. Dutton M. *McGraw Hill's NPTE (National Physical Therapy Examination)*.2nd ed. New York, NY: McGraw-Hill; 2012. http://www.accessphysiotherapy.com/resource/611. Accessed February 22, 2013.
4. Bernard TJ, Knupp K, Yang ML, Arndt D, Levinson P, Moe PG. Neurologic & muscular disorders. In: Hay W, Levin MJ, Sondheimer JM, Detering RR, eds. *CURRENT Diagnosis & Treatment: Pediatrics*. New York, NY: McGraw-Hill; 2011:Chapter 23. http://www.accessphysiotherapy.com/abstract/6585385#6585406. Accessed February 22, 2013.
5. Dutton M. *Orthopaedic Examination, Evaluation, and Intervention*. New York, NY: McGraw-Hill; 2008. http://www.accessphysiotherapy.com/resource/612. Accessed February 22, 2013.
6. Gostic CL, Blatt DM. Physical therapy associated with obesity. In: DeTurk WE, Cahalin LP, eds. *Cardiovascular and Pulmonary Physical Therapy*. New York, NY; McGraw-Hill: 2011:Chapter 16. http://www.accessphysiotherapy.com/abstract/6880859. Accessed February 22, 2013.
7. Waxman SG. *Clinical Neuroanatomy*. New York, NY: McGraw-Hill; 2010. http://www.accessphysiotherapy.com/resource/22. Accessed February 22, 2013.
8. Shamus E, Feingold Stern D. *Effective Documentation for Physical Therapy Professionals*. 2nd ed. New York, NY: McGraw-Hill; 2011. http://www.accessphysiotherapy.com/resource/696. Accessed February 22, 2013.
9. University of Missouri. Geriatric Examination Tool Kit. http://web.missouri.edu/~proste/tool. Accessed February 22, 2013.
10. Dutton M. *Dutton's Orthopedic Survival Guide: Managing Common Conditions*. New York, NY: McGraw-Hill; 2011. http://www.accessphysiotherapy.com/resource/685. Accessed February 22, 2013.

ADDITIONAL REFERENCES

- ICD9DATA. http://www.icd9data.com. Accessed February 22, 2013.
- ICD10DATA. http://www.icd10data.com. Accessed February 22, 2013.
- Melnick ME. Clients with cerebellar dysfunction. In: Umphred DA, ed. *Neurological Rehabilitation*. 5th ed. St. Louis, MO: Mosby Elsevier; 2007:845–850.
- Ropper AL, Samuels MA. *Adams and Victor's Principles of Neurology*. 9th ed. New York, NY: McGraw-Hill; 2009:805–806.
- Schmitz TJ. Examination of coordination. In: O'Sullivan SB, Schmitz TJ, eds. *Physical Rehabilitation*. 5th ed. Philadelphia, PA: FA Davis; 2007:198–199, 201, 212–218.

84 CEREBROVASCULAR ACCIDENT

Mollie Venglar, DSc, MSPT, NCS
Megan Samantha Rosga, DPT, MSPT, NCS

CONDITION/DISORDER SYNONYMS

- Cerebral vascular accident
- Stroke

ICD-9-CM CODES[1]

- 430 Subarachnoid hemorrhage
- 431 Intracerebral hemorrhage
- 432 Other and unspecified intracranial hemorrhage
- 433 Occlusion and stenosis of precerebral arteries
- 434 Occlusion of cerebral arteries
- 434.0 Cerebral thrombosis
- 434.00 Cerebral thrombosis without cerebral infarction
- 434.01 Cerebral thrombosis with cerebral infarction
- 434.1 Cerebral embolism
- 434.10 Cerebral embolism without cerebral infarction
- 434.11 Cerebral embolism with cerebral infarction
- 434.9 Cerebral artery occlusion unspecified
- 434.90 Cerebral artery occlusion unspecified without cerebral infarction
- 434.91 Cerebral artery occlusion unspecified with cerebral infarction
- 435 Transient cerebral ischemia
- 436 Acute but ill-defined cerebrovascular disease
- 437 Other and ill-defined cerebrovascular disease
- 438 Late effects of cerebrovascular disease

ICD-10-CM CODES[2]

- I63.30 Cerebral infarction due to thrombosis of unspecified cerebral artery
- I63.40 Cerebral infarction due to embolism of unspecified cerebral artery
- I63.50 Cerebral infarction due to unspecified occlusion or stenosis of unspecified cerebral artery
- I66.09 Occlusion and stenosis of unspecified middle cerebral artery
- I66.19 Occlusion and stenosis of unspecified anterior cerebral artery
- I66.29 Occlusion and stenosis of unspecified posterior cerebral artery
- I66.9 Occlusion and stenosis of unspecified cerebral artery

PREFERRED PRACTICE PATTERN

5D: Impaired Motor Function and Sensory Integrity Associated with Nonprogressive Disorders of the Central Nervous System—acquired in adolescence or adulthood[3]

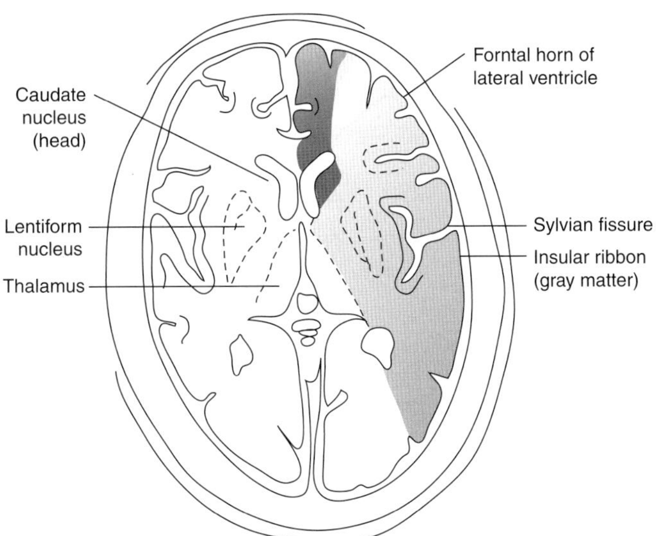

FIGURE 84-1 Brain is supplied by anterior cerebral artery (*darker gray* region anterior-medial), middle cerebral artery (*lighter gray* region comprising the majority of the cerebral cortex), and posterior cerebral artery (*unshaded* portion posterior). (Modified with permission from Schwartz DT. *Emergency Radiology: Case Studies*. New York, NY: McGraw-Hill; 2008:505.)

PATIENT PRESENTATION

A 59-year-old man with a history of hypertension (HTN) presents to the emergency department (ED) with right-sided paralysis and aphasia. The patient's wife states he was in his normal state of health until 1 hour ago, when she heard a thud in the bathroom and walked in to find him collapsed on the floor. She immediately called emergency medical services, which transported the patient to the ED. En route, his finger-stick blood sugar was 108 mg/dL. On arrival in the ED, the patient is placed on monitors and an IV is established. His temperature is 36.8°C (98.2°F), blood pressure is 169/93 mm Hg, heart rate 86 beats per minute, and respiratory rate is 20 breaths per minute. The patient has a noticeable left-gaze preference and is verbally unresponsive, although he will follow simple commands such as raising his left thumb. He has a normal neurological examination on the left, but on the right has a facial droop, no motor activity, decreased deep tendon reflexes (DTRs), and no sensation to light-touch.[4]

KEY FEATURES

Description

- Results in sudden, specific neurological deficit based on location and extent of ischemia or hemorrhage.
- May occur over seconds, minutes, hours, or few days.
- Symptoms include sensory dysfunction, aphasia, dysarthria, dysphagia, visual field defects, cognitive impairment, and most commonly hemiplegia.

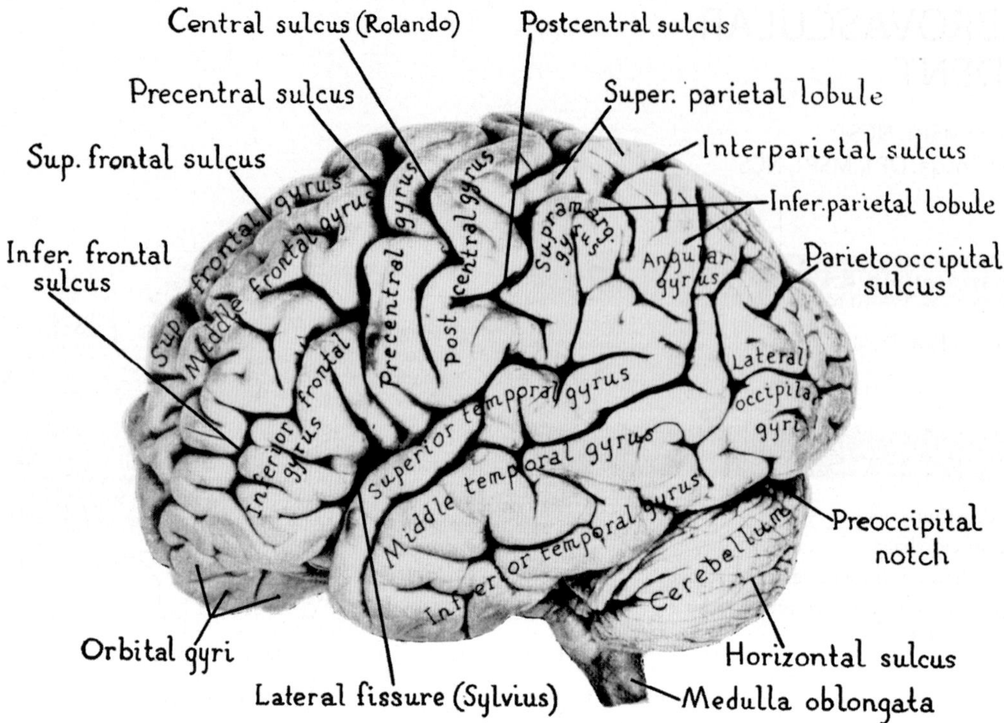

FIGURE 84-2 Photograph of the lateral surface of the human brain. (Reproduced by permission from Carpenter MB, Sutin J. *Human Neuroanatomy*. 8th ed. Baltimore, MD: Williams & Wilkins; 1982.)

▶ Essentials of Diagnosis

- Brain damage may result in the following changes or dysfunction
  - Motor loss
  - Sensory loss
  - Visual impairment
  - Autonomic dysfunction
  - Perceptual changes
  - Cognitive, personality, behavioral changes
  - Changes in consciousness

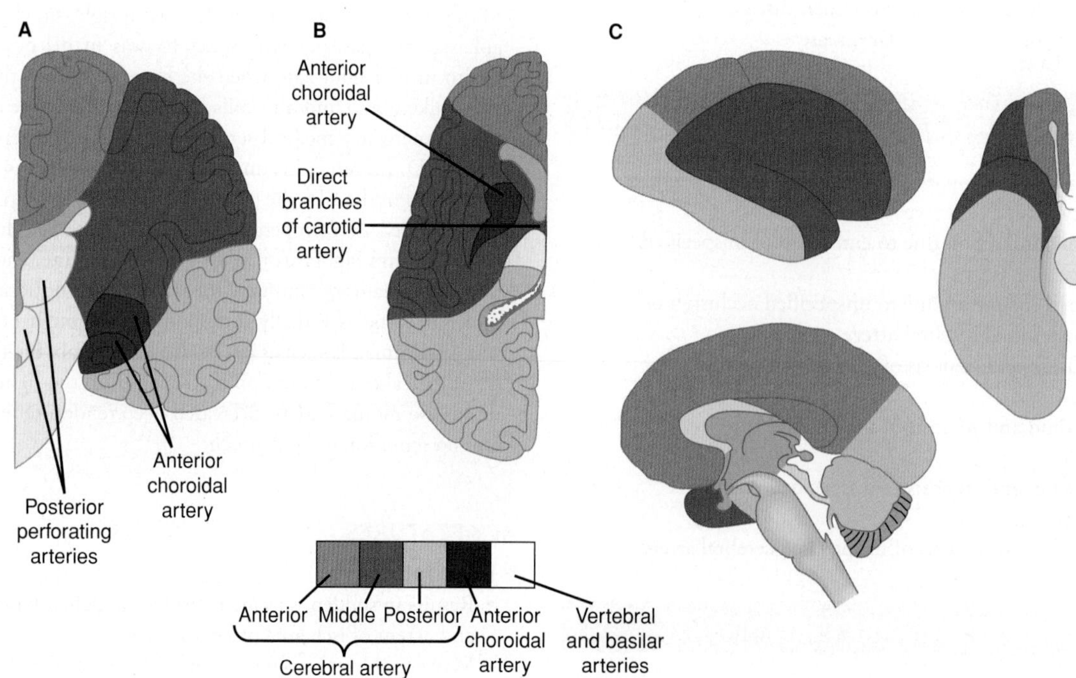

FIGURE 84-3 Vascular territories of the major cerebral arteries. **A.** Coronal section through the cerebrum. **B.** Horizontal section through the cerebrum. **C.** Vascular supply to the cerebral cortex. (Redrawn with permission from Chusid JG. *Correlative Neuroanatomy and Functional Neurology*. 19th ed. Originally published by Appleton & Lange. Copyright © 1985 by the McGraw-Hill Companies, Inc.)

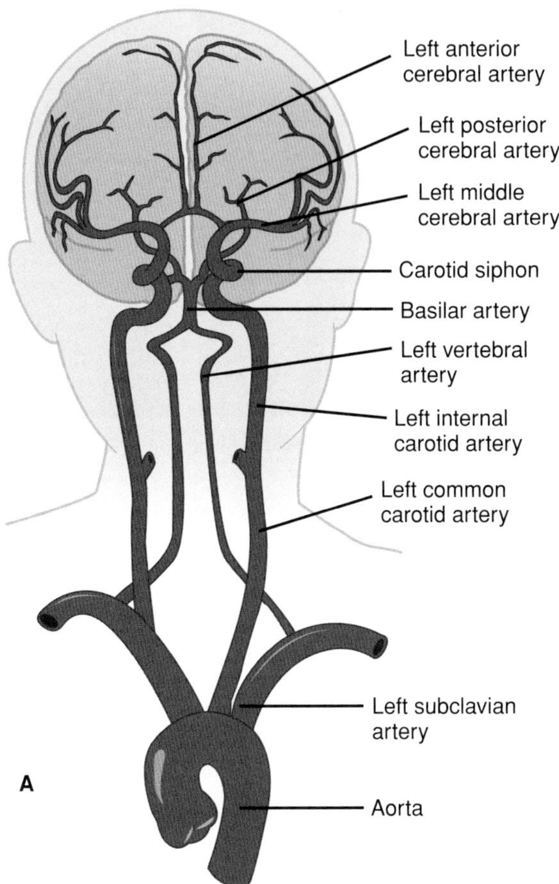

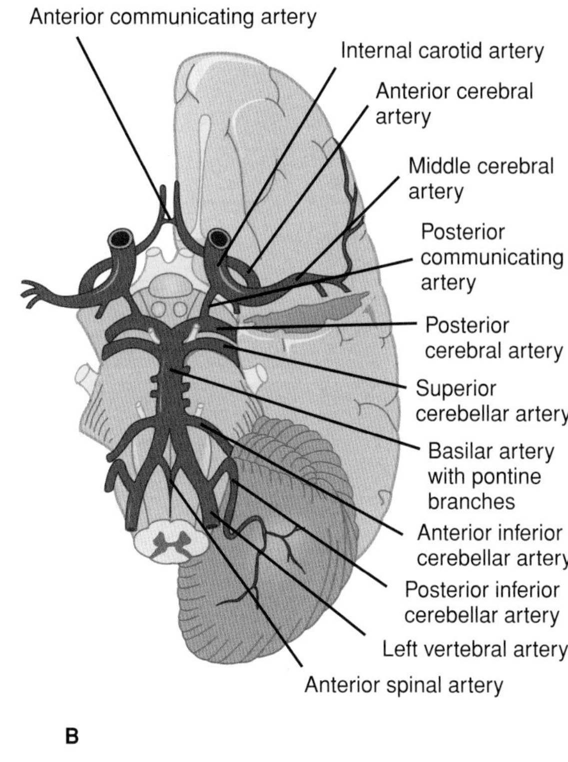

FIGURE 84-4 Major cerebral arteries. **A.** Anterior view. **B.** Inferior view showing the circle of Willis and principal arteries of the brainstem. (Redrawn with permission from Waxman SG. *Neuroanatomy with Clinical Correlations.* 25th ed. McGraw-Hill; 2003.)

  - Communication difficulties
  - Eating, swallowing, bowel and bladder changes

General Considerations

- Two major classification groups
  - Ischemic (2 types)
    - Thrombotic: Atherosclerotic plaques and HTN produce cerebrovascular accident (CVA) due to plaques that form at the branching and curves of arteries[5]
    - Embolic: An embolus that causes CVA can travel from the heart, internal carotid artery thrombosis, or atheromatous plaque of the carotid sinus; branches of middle cerebral artery (MCA) most commonly affected[5]
  - Hemorrhagic: HTN, ruptured saccular aneurysm, or arteriovenous malformation (AVM) can cause a bleed in the brain[5]

Demographics

- Largest single cause of neurological disability.
- Approximately four million Americans suffer physical impairments and disability from stroke.
- Two thirds of all strokes occur in individuals aged 65 years or older Risk of stroke doubles every 10 years after age 55.
- Greater incidence in men than women; twice as likely in African Americans versus Caucasians.
- Cerebral infarction (thrombosis or embolism) is most common form (70% of all strokes), followed by hemorrhages (20%) and unspecified cause (10%).

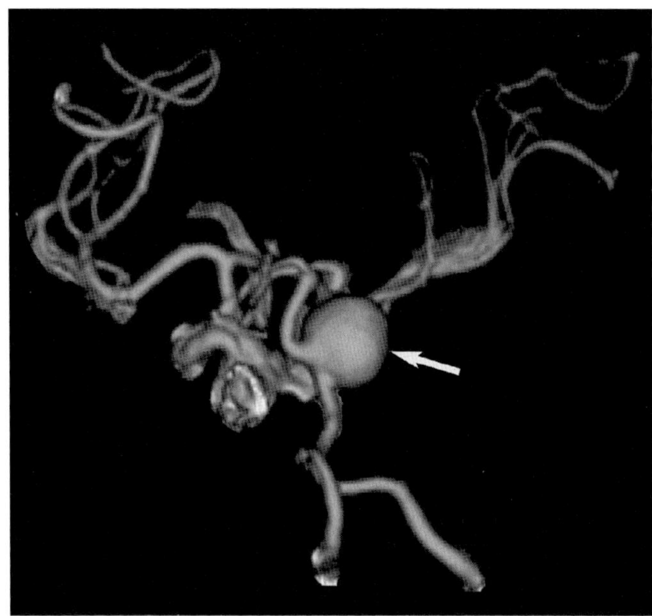

FIGURE 84-5 3D reformatted image from CT angiography of brain shows a 16-mm aneurysm (*arrow*) arising from the left lateral aspect of the mid basilar artery. (From Chen MYM, Pope TL, Ott DJ. *Basic Radiology.* 2nd ed. http://www.accessmedicine.com.)

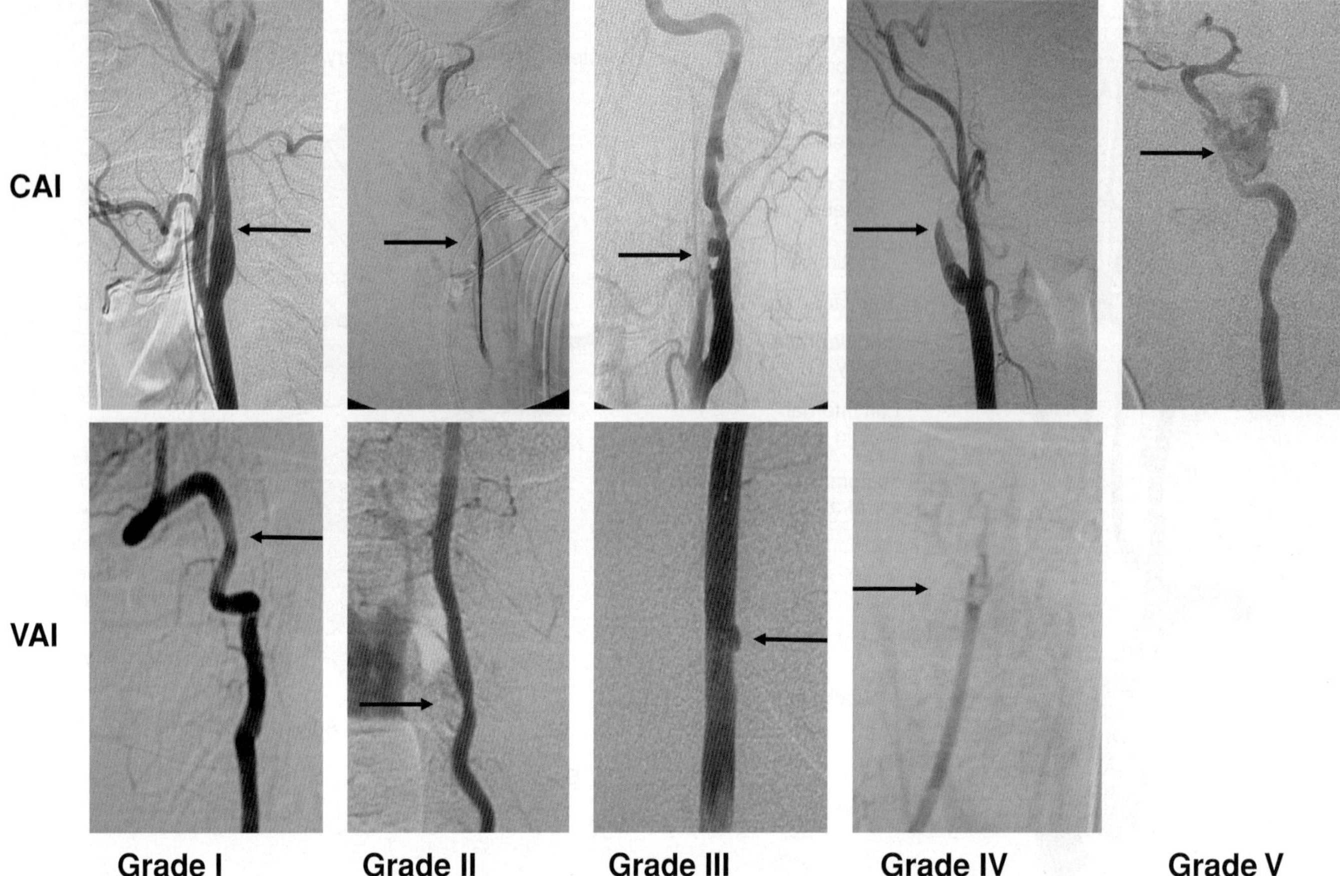

FIGURE 84-6 The Denver grading scale for blunt cerebrovascular injuries. Grade I: irregularity of the vessel wall, dissection/intramural hematoma with <25% luminal stenosis. Grade II: visualized intraluminal thrombus or raised intimal flap, or dissection/intramural hematoma with 25% or more luminal narrowing. Grade III: pseudoaneurysm. Grade IV: vessel occlusion. Grade V: vessel transection. CAI, carotid artery injury; VAI,vertebral artery injury. (From Brunicardi FC, Andersen D, Billiar T, et al., eds. *Schwartz's Principles of Surgery*. 9th ed. http://www.accessmedicine.com. Copyright © The McGraw-Hill Companies, Inc. All rights reserved.)

CLINICAL FINDINGS

SIGNS AND SYMPTOMS

- Dependent on part(s) of the brain affected by CVA and amount of tissue damage from obstruction or hemorrhage[5]
- Common sequelae treated by PT include
  - Behavioral changes
  - Cognitive changes
  - Motor and motor-planning deficits
  - Sensory deficits
  - Spasticity or hypertonicity

Functional Implications

- Loss of independence with all aspects of mobility, ADLs, self-care
- Loss of ability to interact with others effectively
- Difficulty with cognitive processing, particularly executive function

Possible Contributing Causes

- HTN
- AVM
- Hyperlipidemia
- Cardiovascular disease, coronary artery disease, atrial fibrillation
- Obesity
- Smoking
- Sedentary lifestyle
- Pulmonary insufficiency
- Peripheral vascular disease
- Diabetes
- Previous stroke or transient ischemic attack (TIA)
- Patent foramen ovale
- Fibromuscular dysplasia

Differential Diagnosis

- Hydrocephalus
- Hypertensive encephalopathy[5]
- Meningitis
- TIA[5]

MEANS OF CONFIRMATION OR DIAGNOSIS

Laboratory Tests

- Urinalysis to detect infection, renal failure, hyperglycemia, dehydration
- Blood analysis: Complete blood count, platelet count, prothrombin time, erythrocyte sedimentation rate
- Lipid profile
- Thyroid function

Imaging

- CT most often used with contrast to enhance density of intravascular blood; inaccurate during acute phase of ischemic stroke, but often used to rule out other brain lesions (tumor, abscess); accurate for hemorrhagic stroke[6]

- MRI more sensitive than CT for acute ischemic stroke (within 2–6 hours)[7]
- PET scan: Images regional blood flow and localized cerebral metabolism; helps identify areas where ischemia may be reversible[4]
- Transcranial and carotid doppler: Non-invasive, helps identify areas of decreased blood flow
- Cerebral angiography: Invasive, primarily used when surgery indicated in cases of stenosis, aneurysm, AVM

Diagnostic Procedures

- Timing profile: Look for pattern and speed of onset, and initial neurologic symptoms
  - Abrupt onset with rapid coma suggests cerebral hemorrhage
  - Variable and uneven onset typical of cerebral ischemia from thrombosis
- Vital signs
- Neurovascular tests
  - Neck flexion for meningeal irritation
  - Palpation of arteries
  - Auscultation of heart and blood vessels
  - Ophthalmic pressures
- Full cardiac evaluation including radiographs, electrocardiogram
- Echocardiography
- Lumbar puncture to diagnose subarachnoid hemorrhage, focal neurologic deficit, and nuchal rigidity present

TREATMENT

Medication

- Antihypertensive[8]
- Antidepressive[8]
- Gabapentin for intractable neurogenic pain or seizure[8]
- Antiseizure medications[8]
- Spasmolytics (oral, intrathecal, intramuscular) for spasticity management[8]
- Thrombolytics (in ischemic stroke only)[8]
- Antiplatelet (in ischemic stroke only)[8]
- Anticoagulants (in ischemic stroke only)[8]

REFERRALS/ADMITTANCE

- To ER physician in emergency
- To neurologist or neurosurgeon as needed (based on location/severity of injury, management of medications, management of future needs)
- To neuropsychologist for cognitive testing
- To physiatrist for management of medications, symptoms, future needs
- To occupational therapist for ADL training, cognitive retraining, fine motor tasks
- To speech/language pathologist for speech, cognition, swallowing impairments
- To respiratory therapist as needed (depending on respiratory impact of the brain injury)
- To support groups for patients, family, caregivers
- To case management or social work for coordination-of-care assistance

IMPAIRMENTS

- Arousal
- Attention
- Behavior
- Cognition
- Cranial nerve integrity
- Peripheral nerve integrity: Possibly from a comorbid diagnosis
- Gait
- Wheelchair mobility[9]
- Balance
  - Static sit
  - Dynamic sit
  - Static stand
  - Dynamic stand
  - Moving BOS
- Muscle strength
- Muscle recruitment
- Coordination
- Postural control
- Posture
- ROM
- Reflexes
  - DTR
  - Babinski
  - Clonus
- Muscle tone (common synergy patterns after stroke)[10]
- Sensation
- Motor planning
- Bed mobility
- Transfers
- Neglect or inattention to single side of body
- Endurance
- Aerobic capacity
- Self-care
- Home management
- Fine motor
- Respiratory compromise
- Neurogenic pain

TESTS AND MEASURES

- NIH Stroke Scale[10]
- Glasgow Coma Scale
- Modified Ashworth Scale
- Functional measures
  - Barthel Index
  - Functional Independence Measure[9]
- Gait and balance measures[11]
  - Tinetti Performance Oriented Mobility Assessment
  - Berg Balance Scale (BBS)
  - Motor Assessment Scale
  - Gait Assessment Rating Scale
  - Rancho Los Amigo Observational Gait Analysis
  - 6-minute walk test
  - Timed up and Go (TUG)
  - 10-m walk test
  - Romberg
  - Dynamic Gait Index (DGI)
  - Functional Gait Assessment (FGA)
  - Multi-directional reach test
  - Physical performance test
  - HiMAT (if appropriate for patients who have requisite scores on BBS and DGI)

- Cognitive testing
- Sensory testing: May be limited by cognition, consciousness, aphasias
- Strength: Include speed of force production and ability to change force production
- Active and passive ROM, flexibility, muscle length
- Bed mobility
- Transfers
- Cranial nerves, particularly vision[10]
- Vestibular assessment
- Cardiovascular assessment (include Borg scale)
- Pulmonary assessment
- Detailed study of outcome measures completed by the Neurology Section of the American Physical Therapy Association StrokEDGE Task Force; a compendium of outcome tools is provided on the Neurology Section website

INTERVENTION

- ROM/stretching/positioning
- Tone management
- Strengthening (including biofeedback, functional electrical stimulation)[12]
- Balance training[13]
- Gait training (appropriate bracing and assistive devices), body-weight supported treadmill training[14]
- Transfer training
- Orthotics management
- Bed-mobility training
- Wheelchair-mobility training
- Cardiovascular and pulmonary endurance[15]
- Specific approaches:[10] NDT, motor learning and motor control (including constraint-induced movement therapy,[16] forced use), proprioceptive neuromuscular facilitation
- Postural retraining, shoulder subluxation management

FUNCTIONAL GOALS

- Short-term goals
  - Patient will
    - Perform wheelchair transfer to/from bed via sit (lateral) pivot to the right and left with appropriate lower-extremity bracing, minimal assist, moderate verbal cues for sequencing to increase safe functional mobility on return home.
    - Transition consistently between sit and stand from 90-degree hip angle with contact-guard assist to increase safe functional mobility.
    - Ambulate greater than 50 ft with minimal assistance, appropriate assistive device, lower-extremity bracing to improve mobility on return home.
    - Tolerate 10 minutes of continuous exercise on Nustep machine at low resistance without significant change in vital signs or Borg Scale report to improve cardiovascular endurance and increase tolerance for ADLs.
- Long-term goals
  - Patient will
    - Increase 6-minute walk test to ≥1500 ft indoors, over level surfaces, with supervision and assistive device to increase efficient functional mobility and endurance for ADLs.
    - Perform static tandem standing without upper-extremity support for 30 seconds with supervision for improved standing balance and postural control.
    - Improve score on Berg Balance Scale score to ≥53 out of 56 to demonstrate decreased fall-risk during functional activities.
    - Ambulate on a variety of indoor/outdoor surfaces with distant supervision, assistive device as needed to maximize safe and functional ambulation, and return to appropriate premorbid activities.

PROGNOSIS

- Brunnström stages of recovery.[10]
- Fugl–Meyer stages of recovery.[10]
- 70% regain independence in ADLs within 1 year of onset.
- 82% relearn to walk within 1 year of onset.
- 30% to 60% will not regain arm function on the hemiplegic side; failure to recover grip-strength within first month after onset is correlated with no recovery of arm function at 3 months without continued intervention.
- Research shows functional recovery may continue for months or years with appropriate intervention (function-induced recovery).
- Patients with smaller lacunar infarcts show better motor recovery than patients with larger hemispheric damage.
- No significant difference between type of stroke (ischemic vs. hemorrhagic) or location of stroke (hemisphere vs. brainstem) with regard to potential for motor recovery.

PATIENT RESOURCES

- National Stroke Association. www.stroke.org. Accessed February 21, 2013.
- American Stroke Association. www.strokeassociation.org. Accessed February 21, 2013.

REFERENCES

1. ICD9DATA. http://www.icd9data.com. Accessed February 3, 2013.
2. ICD10DATA. http://www.icd10data.com. Accessed February 3, 2013.
3. The American Physical Therapy Association. Pattern 5D: impaired motor function and sensory integrity associated with nonprogressive disorders of the central nervous system - acquired in adolescence or adulthood. *Interactive Guide to Physical Therapist Practice.* 2003. doi: 10.2522/ptguide.3.2_4. http://guidetoptpractice.apta.org/content/1/SEC21.extract. Accessed May 14, 2014.
4. Toy CE. Stroke, Case 54. LANGE Case Files. http://www.accessmedicine.com/casecontent.aspx?aid=8651576&tabid=1. Accessed February 21, 2013.
5. Chandrasoma P, Taylor CR. *Concise Pathology.* 3rd ed. Stamford, CT: Appleton & Lang; 1998. http://www.accessphysiotherapy.com/content/187050. Accessed February 21, 2013.
6. Waxman SG. *Clinical Neuroanatomy.* New York, NY: McGraw-Hill; 2010. http://www.accessphysiotherapy.com/resource/22. Accessed February 21, 2013.
7. Dutton M. *Orthopaedic Examination, Evaluation, and Intervention.* New York, NY: McGraw-Hill; 2008. http://www.accessphysiotherapy.com/resource/612. Accessed February 21, 2013.
8. Panus PC, Jobst EE, Masters SB, Katzung B, Tinsley SL, Trevor AJ. *Pharmacology for the Physical Therapist.* New York, NY: McGraw-Hill; 2009. http://www.accessphysiotherapy.com/resource/615. Accessed February 21, 2013.
9. Shamus E, Feingold Stern D. *Effective Documentation for Physical Therapy Professionals.* 2nd ed.New York, NY: McGraw-Hill; 2011.

http://www.accessphysiotherapy.com/resource/696. Accessed February 21, 2013.
10. Dutton M. *McGraw Hill's NPTE (National Physical Therapy Examination)*.2nd ed. New York, NY: McGraw-Hill; 2012. http://www.accessphysiotherapy.com/resource/611. Accessed February 21, 2013.
11. University of Missouri. Geriatric examination tool kit. http://web.missouri.edu/~proste/tool. Accessed February 21, 2013.
12. Canadian Stroke Network. Strength training – lower extremity. StrokEngine. http://strokengine.ca/intervention/index.php?page=topic&id=50. Accessed February 21, 2013.
13. Canadian Stroke Network. Balance training. StrokEngine. http://strokengine.ca/intervention/index.php?page=topic&id=30. Accessed February 21, 2013.
14. Canadian Stroke Network. Body Weight Supported Treadmill Training. StrokEngine. http://strokengine.ca/intervention/index.php?page=topic&id=33. Accessed February 21, 2013.
15. Sisto SA. Cardiopulmonary concerns in the patient with neurological deficits: an evidence-based approach. In: DeTurk WE, Cahalin LP, eds. *Cardiovascular and Pulmonary Physical Therapy.* New York, NY; McGraw-Hill: 2011:Chapter 14. http://www.accessphysiotherapy.com/abstract/6879516#6879520. Accessed February 21, 2013.
16. Canadian Stroke Network. Constraint-induced movement therapy – upper extremity. http://strokengine.ca/intervention/index.php?page=topic&id=52. Accessed February 21, 2013.

ADDITIONAL REFERENCES

- Neurology Section of the American Physical Therapy Association. StrokEDGE Documents. *Neurology Section Outcome Measures Recommendations.* http://www.neuropt.org/go/healthcare-professionals/neurology-section-outcome-measures-recommendations/stroke. Accessed February 21, 2013.
- O'Sullivan SB. Stroke. In: O'Sullivan SB, Schmitz TJ, eds. *Physical Rehabilitation*. 5th ed. Philadelphia, PA: FA Davis; 2007:705–776.
- Ryerson SD. Hemiplegia. In: Umphred DA, ed. *Neurological Rehabilitation*. 5th ed. St. Louis, MO: Mosby Elsevier; 2007: 857–896.

85 CONCUSSION

Ben Greenberg, PhD
Stephen A. Russo, PhD
Brady L. Tripp, PhD, ATC

CONDITION/DISORDER SYNONYMS

- Mild traumatic brain injury (mTBI)
- Post-concussion syndrome (PCS)
- Second impact syndrome
- Sport-related concussion

ICD-9-CM CODES

- 850 Concussion
- 850.0 With no loss of consciousness
- 850.11 With brief loss of consciousness (less than 30 minutes)
- 850.12 With brief loss of consciousness (31 to 59 minutes)
- 850.2 With moderate loss of consciousness (1 to 24 hours)
- 850.3 With prolonged loss of consciousness and return to pre-existing consciousness level (24 hours + with full recovery)
- 850.4 With prolonged loss of consciousness, without return to pre-existing consciousness level
- 850.5 Loss of consciousness of unspecified duration
- 850.9 Concussion unspecified

ICD-10-CM CODES

- S06.0 Concussion
- S06.0X0A Without loss of consciousness, initial encounter
- S06.0X0D Without loss of consciousness, subsequent encounter
- S06.0X0S Without loss of consciousness, sequela
- S06.0X1 Concussion with loss of consciousness of 30 minutes or less
- S06.0X2 Concussion with loss of consciousness of 31 minutes to 59 minutes
- S06.0X3 Concussion with loss of consciousness of 1 hour to 5 hours 59 minutes
- S06.0X4 Concussion with loss of consciousness of 6 hours to 24 hours, initial encounter
- S06.0X5 Concussion with loss of consciousness greater than 24 hours with return to pre existing conscious level
- S06.0X6 Concussion with loss of consciousness greater than 24 hours without return to pre-existing conscious level with patient surviving
- S06.0X7 Concussion with loss of consciousness of any duration with death due to brain injury prior to regaining consciousness
- S06.0X8 Concussion with loss of consciousness of any duration with death due to other cause prior to regaining consciousness
- S06.0X9 Concussion with loss of consciousness of unspecified duration

PREFERRED PRACTICE PATTERNS

- 5C: Impaired Motor Function and Sensory Integrity Associated with Nonprogressive Disorders of the Central Nervous System—congenital origin or acquired in infancy or childhood[1]

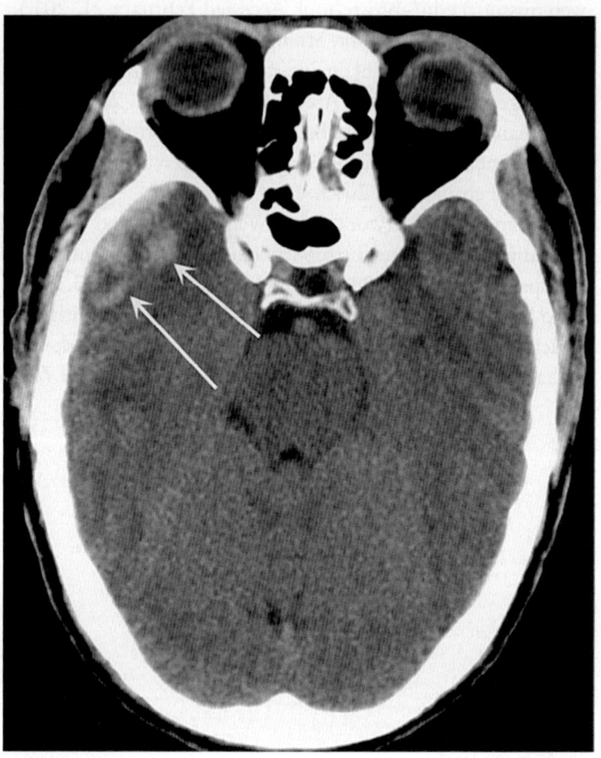

FIGURE 85-1 Traumatic cerebral contusion. Noncontrast CT scan demonstrating a hyperdense hemorrhagic region in the anterior temporal lobe. (From Longo DL, Fauci AS, Kasper DL, Hauser SL, Jameson JL, Loscalzo J, eds. *Harrison's Principles of Internal Medicine*. 18th ed. New York, NY: McGraw-Hill; 2012.)

- 5D: Impaired Motor Function and Sensory Integrity Associated with Nonprogressive Disorders of the Central Nervous System—acquired in adolescence or adulthood[2]
- 5I: Impaired Arousal, Range of Motion, and Motor Control Associated with Coma, Near Coma, or Vegetative State[3]

PATIENT PRESENTATION

A 15-year-old, male, high-school football player presents with headache, photosensitivity, balance problems, and dizziness that began approximate 5 days ago. He also reported experiencing persistent fatigue, "fogginess," and mental sluggishness that has been present during the same period. He has a personal and family history of migraine headaches, but believes that he suffered an injury 6 days ago when he tried to tackle the starting running back for the varsity football team during the first day of summer practice.

The patient described the collision with the running back as him "putting [his] helmet in my chest" and then recalled that he was subsequently hit in the frontal area of the head by the running back's helmet as he was falling to the ground. He denied any loss of consciousness or amnesia because of the hit, but noted that he felt "dazed" for approximately 2 minutes after the collision. He did not report the hit or any of his symptoms to athletic trainer who was attending to the team during practice and finished the remaining 45 minutes of practice and conditioning drills.

The patient reported that he felt "tired" after practice and slept an estimated 9.5 hours (9:00 PM to 6:30 AM) that night. The next day, he began experiencing a "migraine" headache in school, which was accompanied by his other symptoms. He also noted that his headache discomfort (i.e., 7 out of 10 on a 10-point scale), prompted a visit to a local emergency department (ED) 2 days after the collision at football practice. He underwent a chest X-ray and computerized tomography (CT) of the brain during this ED visit, both of which were negative. He was "given a shot" for his migraine pain and ultimately released from the ED. Three days after the collision, the patient began taking daily naps after school, lasting approximately 2 to 3 hours, without a change in his normal sleep cycle. He also noted experiencing an increase in photosensitivity, lethargy, and dizziness when watching TV or working on the computer. He complained of a persistent, constant bilateral headache at a 4/10 level and described the pain as "sharp," "pounding," and "throbbing." He also reported an increase in his symptoms throughout the day at school, typically beginning in fourth period. He presented to the clinic wearing sunglasses secondary to his photophobia, but the physical examination completed during his office visit is essentially normal.

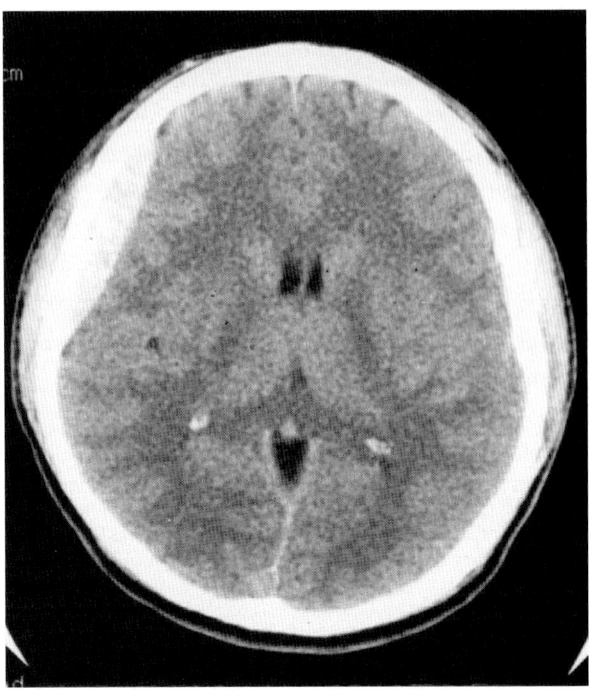

FIGURE 85-2 Acute epidural hematoma. Unenhanced CT scan showing a typical lens-shaped frontal epidural clot. (From Ropper AH, Samuels MA. *Adams and Victor's Principles of Neurology*. 9th ed. New York, NY: McGraw-Hill; 2009.)

KEY FEATURES

Description

- Complex pathophysiological process affecting the brain, induced by traumatic biomechanical force[4]
- May be caused by direct blow to the head, face, neck, elsewhere on the body with impulsive force transmitted to the head
- May occur from linear deceleration injury or rotational injury[5]
  - Seventeen times more likely to occur with linear acceleration >100 g
  - Fourteen times more likely to occur with rotational acceleration >5000 rad/s
- "Simple" versus "Complex" concussions[6,7]
  - Simple: Symptoms resolve in 7 to 10 days, neurocognitive testing, no intervention beyond limiting play, physical and cognitive rest until symptoms resolve
  - Complex: Symptoms persist more than 10 days or loss of consciousness for more than 1 minute; neuropsychological testing and multidisciplinary approach recommended for individuals with history of head injuries
  - Complex concussions 18 times more likely than simple concussions to have impaired composite scores on neurocognitive testing for 3 out of 4 on visual memory, reaction time, processing speed, or symptom scores
- Second impact syndrome: Life-threatening condition, may be triggered by very minor impact while individual still suffering symptoms of initial concussion[8]

Essentials of Diagnosis

- More prevalent and severe in children/adolescents[9,10]
- Short-term impairment of neurological functioning that resolves spontaneously over time
- In athletic populations, concussed patients frequently minimize or deny symptoms in effort to resume practice and competition[11]
- Most accurate diagnosis from clinical examination and neurocognitive evaluation[12]
- Baseline neurocognitive testing is helpful to determine neurocognitive deficits post-injury[4,13]

General Considerations

- Most common form of mTBI
- Neurometabolic cascade following concussions: Dynamic changes in cerebral blood flow, glutamate, glucose, potassium, calcium; may persist from minutes to days[14]
- Functional deficits positively associated with physical and cognitive exertion levels, with impairment persisting in those who attempt to "fight through" signs and symptoms of concussion[15]
- Repeated injury (particularly more than three concussions) may result in increased symptom severity, protracted recovery, reduced threshold to concussive injuries, increased risk of depression, cognitive impairment later in life[16–20]

Demographics

- Estimated 1.6 to 3.8 million sport-related concussions per year[20]
- 30% to 80% of mTBIs cause concussion symptoms; severity of injury not always related to persistence of symptoms[21]
- 50% to 60% of soccer and football players sustain concussions[22]
- Developmental differences in response to concussion[9,10]
  - The younger the individual and longer the duration of post-concussion symptoms, greater the risk of second impact syndrome
  - Younger individuals demonstrate slower recovery and greater decrease from baseline in neurocognitive measures post-concussion
- Approximately one out of four adolescents injured during sports fail to report concussion (66% of whom do not think it serious enough)[12]

TABLE 85-1 Signs and Symptoms Associated with Minor Traumatic Brain Injury

Cognitive Symptoms	Physical Signs and Symptoms	Behavioral Changes
Attention difficulties	Headaches	Irritability
Concentration problems	Dizziness	Depression
Amnesia and perseveration	Insomnia	Anxiety
Short-term and long-term memory problems	Fatigue	Sleep disturbances
	Uneven gait	Emotional lability
Orientation problems	Nausea, vomiting	Loss of initiative
Altered processing speed	Blurred vision	Loneliness and helplessness
Altered reaction time	Seizures	Problems related to job, relationship, home, or school management
Calculation difficulties and problems with executive function		

Note: At 3 after injury, <30% are symptomatic; at 1 yr, 15% are symptomatic.
Source: From Tintinalli JE, Stapczynski J, Ma OJ, Cline D, Cydulka R, Meckler G. *Tintinalli's Emergency Medicine: A Comprehensive Study Guide*. 7th ed. www.accessmedicine.com.

- Those who sustain one concussion during sports are three times more likely to sustain another concussion within the same sport season[23]
- Those who sustain more than three concussions are eight times more likely to have cognitive deficits with future concussions[19]

CLINICAL FINDINGS

SIGNS AND SYMPTOMS

- Loss of consciousness only occurs in 8% to 19% of concussion cases[24]
- Post-traumatic amnesia, dizziness, mental "fogginess" may be more salient than loss of consciousness in determining injury severity and potential persistence of concussion symptoms
  - Amnesia 10 times more predictive of neurocognitive deficits than loss of consciousness[24,25]
- Symptoms persisting 5 to 15 minutes (compared with <5 minutes) result in significantly more frequent symptom reporting and decreased neurocognitive functioning for up to 1 week post-injury[13]
- Four aspects of post-concussion symptoms[26]
  - Somatic symptoms
    - Visual problems
    - Dizziness
    - Balance difficulty
    - Headache
    - Photosensitivity
    - Phonosensitivity
    - Nausea
  - Emotionality
    - Emotional liability
    - Nervousness
    - Sadness
    - Irritability
  - Cognitive symptoms
    - Attention problems
    - Memory dysfunction
    - Fogginess
    - Fatigue
    - Cognitive slowing
  - Sleep disturbance
    - Difficulty falling asleep
    - Sleeping more or less than usual
- Most common symptoms in adolescent athletes[13]
  - Headache (71% of cases)
  - Feeling "slowed down" (58%)
  - Difficulty concentrating (57%)
  - Dizziness (55%)
- Second impact syndrome may result in intracranial pressure, causing[8,27]
  - Vasomotor paralysis
  - Edema
  - Herniation
  - Coma
  - Ocular involvement
  - Respiratory failure
  - Death
  - More rapid occurrence of symptoms than with epidural hematoma

Functional Implications

- Poor task performance in school or work due to cognitive symptoms
- Possible re-emergence of symptoms with increased physical or cognitive exertion[15]
- Interpersonal conflict due to emotionality
- Inability to resume sports activity before complete resolution of the condition, despite pressure to resume practice or competition

TABLE 85-2 Return-to-Activity Program

Sports Related	Non-Sports Related
No activity (rest until symptom-free)	No activity (rest until symptom-free)
Light aerobic exercise	Light aerobic exercise
Sport-specific training (noncontact)	Moderate aerobic exercise
Noncontact drills	Return to normal activities
Full-contact drills	
Game play	

Note: Patient must remain asymptomatic for 24 h between each step. Development of symptoms at any level requires return to the previous symptom-free level.
Source: From Tintinalli JE, Stapczynski J, Ma OJ, Cline D, Cydulka R, Meckler G. *Tintinalli's Emergency Medicine: A Comprehensive Study Guide*. 7th ed. www.accessmedicine.com.

TABLE 85-3 Clinical and Radiographic Characteristics of the Main Traumatic Brain Lesions

	Epidural Hematoma	Acute Subdural Hematoma	Chronic Subdural Hematoma	Contusion/Parenchymal Hemorrhage	Intraventricular Hematoma	Subarachnoid Hemorrhage	Subdural Hygroma	Diffuse Axonal Injury
Causative factor	Laceration of middle cerebral artery or dural sinus	Tearing of bridging pial veins and arteries	Trauma (may be absent or minimal) Risk factors: coagulopathy and severe brain atrophy	Shearing of parenchymal vessels. Risk factors: coagulopathy and amyloid vasculopathy	Shearing of parenchymal vessels; rule out vascular defects	Exclude underlying aneurysmal rupture	Arachnoid tear, following meningitis	Deceleration or rotational forces
Typical location	Lateral cerebral convexities	Lateral cerebral convexities	Lateral cerebral convexities, may be bilateral	Inferior frontal and temporal lobes	Lateral and third ventricles blood filled	Basilar cisterns	Lateral cerebral convexities	Deep white matter, corpus callosum, dorsolateral pons
Evolution	Hours	Many hours	Days to weeks	Expand over 12–48 h	Rapid	Minutes to hours	Days to weeks	From time of injury
Clinical profile	Classically, lucid interval then coma, but more variable; pupillary dilatation with contralateral then bilateral limb weakness; slowly evolving stupor then coma	Drowsiness, coma; pupillary dilatation with contralateral then bilateral limb weakness; progressive stupor then coma	Headache, progressive alteration in mental status ± focal neurologic signs	Stupor → coma, dilated pupil, progressive hemiplegia, spasticity	Progressive signs of hydrocephalus	Headache, meningismus, delayed manifestations, vasospasm	Mimics chronic subdural hematoma	Coma, posturing, normal intracranial pressure
Age at risk	Children, young adults	Any	Elderly	Any	Any	Any	Infants, children, adults	Any
Radiologic features	Acute bulging epidural clot bounded by cranial sutures; lenticular in shape	Acute blood rimming broad region of cerebral convexity	Hyper- or isodense, unilateral or bilateral	Multiple, confluent regions of edema intermixed with focal, acute blood	Focal, acute blood within ventricles; may layer with gravity	Acute blood lining cortex in subarachnoid space	Focal, CSF density, fluid collection	CT may be normal; MRI shows evolving small deep contusions
Surgical intervention	Urgent evacuation	Urgent evacuation if large enough to cause symptoms	Evacuation in some circumstances	Evacuate if large	Shunting	May cause secondary vasospasm or late hydrocephalus	Aspiration of fluid	None

Source: From Ropper AH, Samuels MA. *Adams and Victor's Principles of Neurology*. 9th ed. New York, NY: McGraw-Hill; 2009.

Possible Contributing Causes

- Use of mouth guard does not reduce occurrence of neurocognitive symptoms or deficits.[28]
- Personal or family history of migraine increases recovery time.[29]
- Learning disabilities, attention deficit disorders are also possible risk factors for protracted recovery.[21]
- Repeated concussions reduce threshold for sustaining additional injuries.[16]

Differential Diagnosis

- Skull fracture
- Cervical spine injury
- Cerebral laceration and contusion
- Subarachnoid, subdural, and extradural hemorrhage
- Chronic traumatic encephalopathy (dementia pugilistica)

MEANS OF CONFIRMATION OR DIAGNOSIS

Imaging

- CT and MRI typically grossly normal
- Functional magnetic resonance image (fMRI) to detect brain abnormalities
- For post-concussion symptoms that persist or worsen, a focal neurological deficit, Glasgow Coma Scale (GCS) score <15, or seizures
  - CT or MRI recommended to rule out other conditions[21]
- PET/SPECT do not differentiate severity of symptoms

Diagnostic Procedures

- Mental status evaluation of orientation, concentration, amnesia recommended immediately after injury[30,31]
- Neurocognitive testing improves accurate diagnosis rate from 65% (based on symptom reporting alone) to 93%[12]
- GCS
- McCrea, et al. Sideline Evaluation[28,32]
- Sport Concussion Assessment Tool (SCAT 3) (Child SCAT 3)
- Immediate Post-Concussion Assessment and Cognitive Test (ImPACT)
- Romberg testing
- Balance Error Scoring System (BESS)
- GCS to assess patients in a coma

FINDINGS AND INTERPRETATION

- Report of post-concussion symptoms
- Reduced performance on neurocognitive testing compared to baseline

REFERRALS/ADMITTANCE

- To hospital for imaging if symptoms persist/worsen or focal neurological deficit

IMPAIRMENTS

- Impaired processing and memory possible following concussion: Importance of written treatment recommendations and inclusion of parent/guardian when treating more severe cases

INTERVENTION

- Cognitive rest
- Restrict activity level while symptomatic or persisting neurocognitive deficits
- Graduated return to play protocol, stepwise process and the patient should be asymptomatic at each level for 24 hours before moving to the next level[33]
  - No activity
  - Light aerobic exercise
  - Sport specific exercise
  - Noncontact training drills
  - Full-contact practice
  - Return to play
- More conservative return to activity with children/adolescents due to increased risk of second impact syndrome at younger age
- No recommended medications
  - NSAIDs may mask symptom patterns, dangerous with too early return
  - Avoid narcotics to avoid confusion between medication side effects and symptoms of concussion[22]
  - Medical management of persistent post-concussion symptoms with SSRIs, beta-blockers, calcium-channel blockers, or neurostimulant medications are not presently FDA-approved[34]
- For second impact syndrome
  - Immediate treatment: Rapid intubation, hyperventilation, intravenous administration of osmotic diuretic (e.g., 20% mannitol)[27]
  - Foley catheterization necessary for osmotic diuresis

FUNCTIONAL GOALS

- Patient will
  - Be symptom-free at rest.
  - Be symptom-free with cognitive/physical exertion.
- Have normal neurocognitive data defined as matching baseline neurocognitive scores or obtaining normative scores consistent with pre-injury level of functioning.[3,7,20,35]

PROGNOSIS

- Days 1 to 10 post-injury: Symptoms most severe, highest risk of second impact syndrome.[21]
- Day 30 post-injury: Symptoms improved, often subclinical (neurocognitive tests should match baseline).[21]
- Days 30 to 90 post-injury: Majority of individuals recover.[21]
- Actual rate of PCS between 1% to 5% of all mTBI patients.[21]
  - Previous reports of PCS rates between 10% to 15% determined to be severely inflated.[21]
- Psychological factors, social influences, and pre-injury level of functioning appear to be involved in persistent cases of PCS.
- Prognosis for second impact syndrome poor unless immediate intervention initiated.[27]
- Surgical intervention ineffective.

PATIENT RESOURCES

- Centers for Disease Control and Prevention. *Heads up: Concussion in youth sports.* http://www.cdc.gov/concussioninyouthsports. Accessed June 12, 2013.
- Concussions. American Association of Neurological Surgeons. http://www.aans.org/Patient%20Information/Conditions%20and%20Treatments/Concussion.aspx. Accessed June 12, 2013.
- Facts about sports concussions. American Headache Society. http://www.aans.org/Patient%20Information/Conditions%20and%20Treatments/Concussion.aspx. Accessed June 12, 2013.

REFERENCES

1. The American Physical Therapy Association. Pattern 5C: impaired motor function and sensory integrity associated with nonprogressive disorders of the central nervous system - congenital origin or acquired in infancy or childhood. *Interactive Guide to Physical Therapist Practice*. 2003. doi: 10.2522/ptguide.3.2_3. http://guidetoptpractice.apta.org/content/1/SEC20.extract. Accessed May 14, 2014.
2. The American Physical Therapy Association. Pattern 5D: impaired motor function and sensory integrity associated with nonprogressive disorders of the central nervous system - acquired in adolescence or adulthood. *Interactive Guide to Physical Therapist Practice*. 2003. doi: 10.2522/ptguide.3.2_4. http://guidetoptpractice.apta.org/content/1/SEC21.extract. Accessed May 14, 2014.
3. The American Physical Therapy Association. Pattern 5I: impaired arousal, range of motion, and motor control associated with coma, near coma, or vegetative state. *Interactive Guide to Physical Therapist Practice*. 2003. doi: 10.2522/ptguide.3.2_9. http://guidetoptpractice.apta.org/content/1/SEC26.extract. Accessed May 14, 2014.
4. Aubry M, Cantu R, Dvorak J, et al. Summary and agreement statement of the First International Conference on Concussion in Sport, Vienna 2001. Recommendations for the improvement of safety and health of athletes who may suffer concussive injuries. *Br J Sports Med.* 2002;36(1):6–10.
5. Guskiewicz K. Emotional and cognitive problems in football players. In: Raw V, chair, ed. *Long Term Outcomes of Football Injuries*. Continuing medical education plenary session conducted at the John Hopkins Medicine Traumatic Brain Injury in Professional Football: An Evidence Based Perspective. Washington, DC. June, 2010.
6. Iverson G. Predicting slow recovery from sport-related concussion: The new simple-complex distinction. *Clin J Sport Med.* 2007;17(1):31–37.
7. McCrory P, Johnston K, Meeuwisse W, et al. Summary and agreement statement of the 2nd International Conference on Concussion in Sport, Prague 2004. *Clin J Sport Med.* 2005; 15(2):196–204.
8. Saunders RL, Harbaugh RE. The second impact in catastrophic contact-sports head trauma. *JAMA*. 1984;252(4):538–539.
9. Field M, Collins MW, Lovell MR, Maroon J. Does age play a role in recovery from sports-related concussion? A comparison of high school and collegiate athletes. *J Pediatr*. 2003:142(5); 546–553.
10. Lovell MR, Collins MW, et al. Recovery from mild concussion in high school athletes. *J Neurosurg.* 2003;98(2): 296–301.
11. McCrea M, Hammeke T, Olsen G, Leo P, Guskiewicz K. Unreported concussion in high school football players: Implications for prevention. *Clin J Sport Med.* 2004;14(1):13–17.
12. Van Kampen DA, Lovell MR, Pardini JE, Collins MW, Fu FH. The "value added" of neurocognitive testing after sports-related concussion. *Am J Sports Med.* 2006;34(10):1630–1635.
13. Lovell MR, Collins MW, Iverson GL, Johnston KM, Bradley JP. Grade 1 or "Ding" concussions in high school athletes. *Am J Sports Med.* 2004;32(1):47–54.
14. Giza CC, Hovda DA. The neurometabolic cascade of concussion. *J Athl Train.* 2003;36(3):228–235.
15. Majerske CW, Mihalik JP, Ren D, et al. Concussion in sports: postconcussive activity levels, symptoms, and neurocognitive performance. *J Athl Train.* 2008;43(3):265–274.
16. Guskiewicz KM, Weaver NL, Padua DA, Garrett WE Jr. Epidemiology of concussion in collegiate and high school football players. *Am J Sports Med.* 2000;28(5):643–650.
17. Guskiewicz KM, Marshall SW, Bailes J, et al. Association between recurrent concussion and late-life cognitive impairment in retired professional football players. *Neurosurgery*. 2005;57(4): 719–726.
18. Guskiewicz KM, Marshall SW, Bailes J, et al. Recurrent concussion and risk of depression in retired professional football players. *Med Sci Sport Exerc.* 2007;39(6):903–909.
19. Iverson GL, Gaetz M, Lovell MR, Collins MW. Cumulative effects of concussion in amateur athletes. *Brain Inj.* 2004;18(5): 433–443.
20. McCrory P, Meeuwisse W, Johnston K, et al. Consensus statement on concussion in sport 3rd International Conference on Concussion in Sport held in Zurich, November 2008. *Clin J Sport Med.* 2009;19(3):185–200.
21. McCrae MA. *Mild Traumatic Brain Injury and Postconcussion Syndrome*. New York, NY: Oxford University Press; 2008.
22. Delaney JS, Lacroix VJ, Leclerc S, Johnston KM. Concussions among university football and soccer players. *Clin J Sport Med.* 2002;12(6):331–338.
23. Guskiewicz KM, McCrea M, Marshall SW, et al. Cumulative effects associated with recurrent concussion in collegiate football players: The NCAA study. *JAMA*. 2003;290(19):2549–2555.
24. Collins MW, Iverson GL, Lovell MR, McKeag DB, Norwig J, Maroon J. On-field predictors of neuropsychological and symptom deficit following sports-related concussion. *Clin J Sport Med.* 2003;13(4):222–229.
25. Cantu R. Posttraumatic retrograde and anterograde amnesia: pathophysiology and implications in grading and safe return to play. *J Athl Train.* 2001;36(3):244–248.
26. Pardini J, Stump J, Lovell MR, Collins MW, Moritz K, Fu F. The Post Concussion Symptom Scale (PCSS): a factor analysis [abstract]. *Br J Sports Med.* 2004;38:661–662.
27. Cantu RC. Second impact syndrome. *Clin Sports Med.* 1998; 17(1):37–44.
28. Mihalik JP, McCaffery MA, Rivera EM, et al. Effectiveness of mouthguards in reducing neurocognitive defecits following sports-related cerebral concussion. *Dent Traumatol.* 2007; 23(1):14–20.
29. Mihalik JP, Stump JE, Collins MW, Lovell MR, Field M, Maroon JC. Posttraumatic migraine characteristics in athletes following sports-related concussion. *J Neurosurg.* 2005;102(5): 850–855.
30. McCrea M, Kelly JP, Randolph C, et al. Standardized assessment of concussion (SAC): on-site mental status evaluation of the athlete. *J Head Trauma Rehabil.* 1998;13(2):27–35.
31. McCrea M, Kelly JP, Randolph C, Cisler R, Berger L. Immediate neurocognitive effects of concussion. *Neurosurgery*. 2002;50(5): 1032–1040.
32. McCrea M, Kelly JP, Kluge J, Ackley B, Randolph C. Standardized assessment of concussion in football players. *Neurology*. 1997;48(3):586–588.
33. McCrory P, Meeuwisse W, Aubry M, et al. Consensus statement on Concussion in Sport - The 4th International Conference on Concussion in Sport held in Zurich, November 2012. *Br J*

Sports Med. 2013;47(5):250–258. doi: 10.1136/bjsports-2013-092313.

34. Reddy CC, Lombard LA. A treatment paradigm for sports concussion. *Brain Injury / professional.* 2007;4(4):24–25.
35. Centers for Disease Control and Prevention. *Heads up: Concussion in youth sports.* http://www.cdc.gov/concussion/HeadsUp/youth.html. Accessed September 6, 2014.

ADDITIONAL REFERENCES

- Bernard TJ, Knupp K, Yang ML, Arndt D, Levinson P, Moe PG. Neurologic & muscular disorders. In: Hay W, Levin MJ, Sondheimer JM, Detering RR, eds. *CURRENT Diagnosis & Treatment: Pediatrics.* New York, NY: McGraw-Hill; 2011:Chapter 23. http://www.accessphysiotherapy.com/abstract/6585385#6585406. Accessed June 12, 2013.
- ICD9DATA. http://www.icd9data.com. Accessed June 12, 2013.
- ICD10DATA. http://www.icd10data.com. Accessed June 12, 2013.
- Pitto A, Chen JK, Johnston KM. Contributions of functional magnetic resonance imaging (fMRI) to sport concussion evaluation. *NeuroRehabilitation.* 2007;22(3):217–227.
- Waxman SG. *Clinical Neuroanatomy.* New York, NY: McGraw-Hill; 2010. http://www.accessphysiotherapy.com/resource/22. Accessed June 12, 2013.
- Wilson PE, Clayton GH. Rehabilitation medicine. In: Hay W, Levin MJ, Sondheimer JM, Detering RR, eds. *CURRENT Diagnosis & Treatment: Pediatrics.* New York, NY: McGraw-Hill; 2011:Chapter 26. http://www.accessphysiotherapy.com/abstract/6586373#6586380. Accessed June 12, 2013.

86 ENCEPHALITIS

Mollie Venglar, DSc, MSPT, NCS

CONDITION/DISORDER SYNONYMS

- Meningoencephalitis
- Acute disseminated encephalomyelitis

ICD-9-CM CODE

- 323.9 Unspecified cause of encephalitis, myelitis, and encephalomyelitis

ICD-10-CM CODE

- G04.90 Encephalitis and encephalomyelitis, unspecified

PREFERRED PRACTICE PATTERNS

- 5A: Primary Prevention/Risk Reduction for Loss of Balance and Falling[1]
- 5C: Impaired Motor Function and Sensory Integrity Associated with Nonprogressive Disorders of the Central Nervous System—congenital origin or acquired in infancy or childhood[2]
- 5D: Impaired Motor Function and Sensory Integrity Associated with Nonprogressive Disorders of the Central Nervous System—acquired in adolescence or adulthood[3]
- 5I: Impaired Arousal, Range of Motion and Motor Control Associated with Coma, Near Coma, or Vegetative State[4]

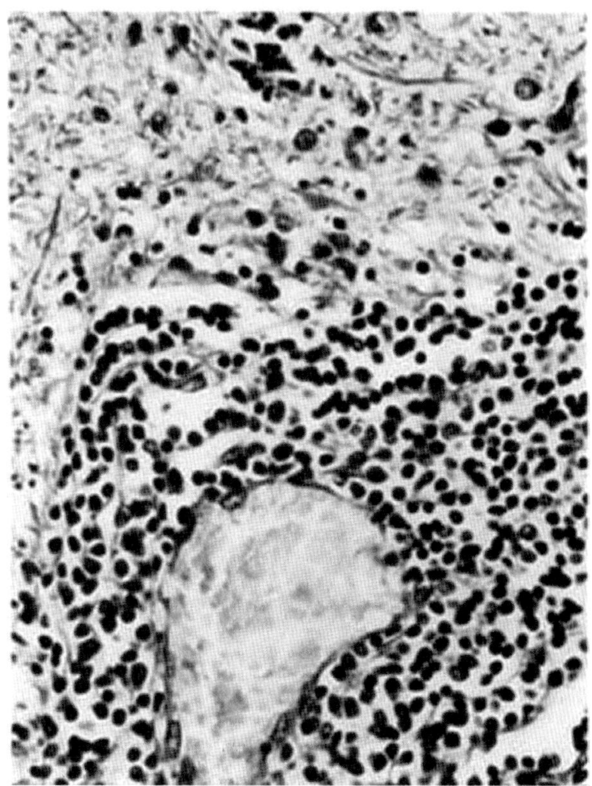

FIGURE 86-1 Viral encephalitis, showing perivascular lymphocytic cuffing. (From Chandrasoma P, Taylor CR. *Concise Pathology*. 3rd ed. http://www.accessmedicine.com. Copyright © The McGraw-Hill Companies, Inc. All rights reserved.)

PATIENT PRESENTATION

Three weeks after a regimen of cyclosporine to treat his psoriasis, a 42-year-old man developed a fever, headache, and nausea that were unresponsive to medication or position change. Within a few days he struggled with balance and gait ataxia and became progressively more disoriented. By the end of the week he was comatose, with Glasgow Coma Scale score of 5. Magnetic resonance imaging (MRI) reveals mediotemporal lobe necrosis. The patient is placed on intravenous acyclovir.

KEY FEATURES

Description

- Infection of the brain parenchyma
- Most commonly results in infection of the entire brain, but some viruses attack specific nervous system structures

Essentials of Diagnosis

- May occur with meningitis; some overlap of signs and symptoms
- Two primary forms: Viral and bacterial
- Postinfectious encephalitis: Autoimmune reaction to systemic viral infection
- Causative factor must be identified to initiate appropriate medical treatment prior to physical therapy involvement
- Common forms include
  - Herpes simplex encephalitis (most common cause of sporadic encephalitis in adults)
  - Arboviral encephalitis (most common epidemic forms): West Nile virus, Eastern and Western equine encephalitis, and rabies

General Considerations

- Rapid differential diagnosis of encephalitis versus meningitis should be made due to similarities of initial symptoms and response to medication.
- Severity may progress over a period of 1 week; PT should monitor for changing neurologic signs and symptoms, refer accordingly.

Demographics

- Approximately 20,000 cases of acute viral encephalitis are reported annually in the United States.
- Death occurs in 5% to 20%.
- All ages and genders are susceptible; some forms are more common in specific geographic locations.

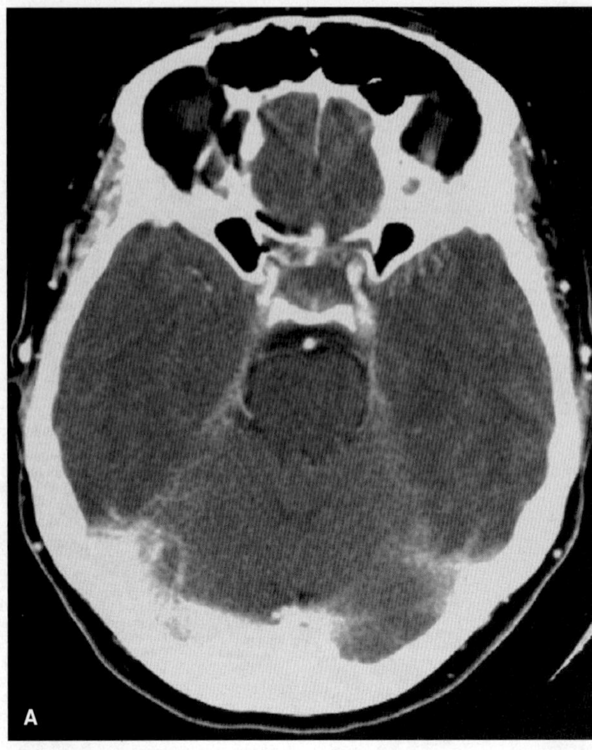

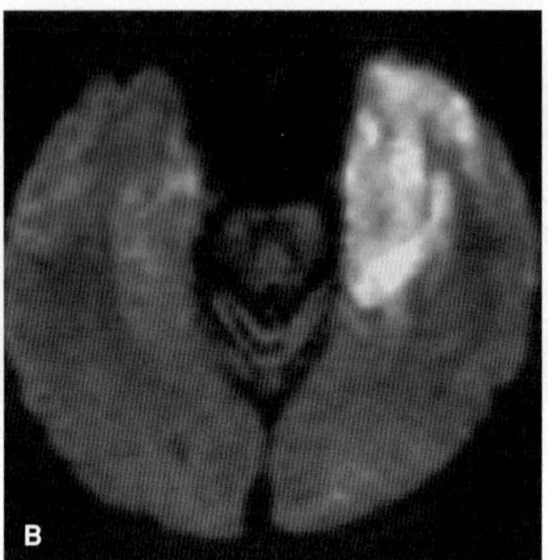

FIGURE 86-2 CT (**A**) and diffusion-weighted MRI (**B**) scans of the brain of a patient with left-temporal-lobe HSV encephalitis. (From Longo DL, Fauci AS, Kasper DL, et al., eds. *Harrison's Principles of Internal Medicine*. 18th ed. http://www.accessmedicine.com. Copyright © The McGraw-Hill Companies, Inc. All rights reserved.)

CLINICAL FINDINGS

SIGNS AND SYMPTOMS

- Fever
- Headache
- Nuchal rigidity
- Vomiting
- General malaise
- Coma
- Cranial nerve palsy
- Hemiplegia
- Involuntary movements
- Ataxia

Functional Implications

- Inability to perform activities of daily living (ADLs) independently
- Loss of independent functional mobility
- Inability to perform age and education appropriate cognitive tasks
- Inability to execute fine and gross motor tasks independently

Possible Contributing Causes

- Increased risk
  - Immunosuppressed
  - Perinatal to early childhood period
- Prior meningitis

Differential Diagnosis

- Stroke
- Subdural empyema
- Cerebral abscess
- Cerebral venous thrombosis
- Septic embolism
- Meningitis

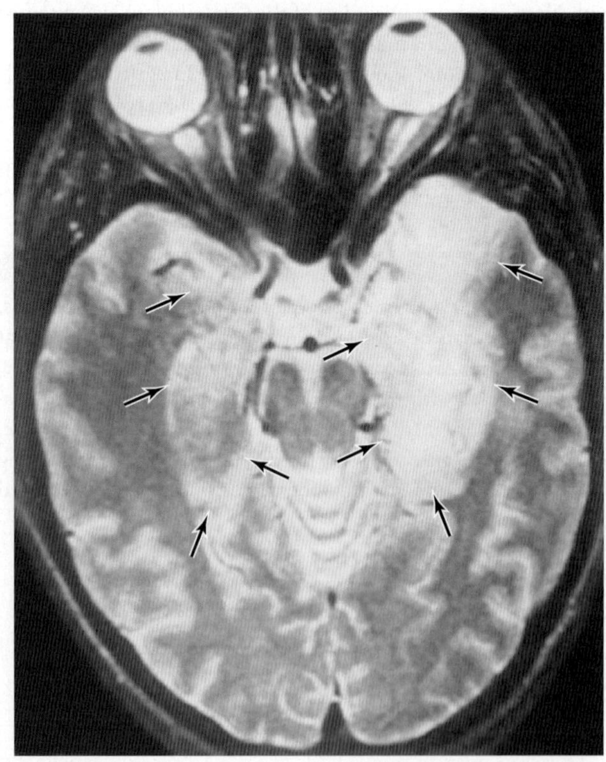

FIGURE 86-3 Magnetic resonance image of horizontal section through the head at the level of the temporal lobe. The large lesion in the left temporal lobe and a smaller one on the right side are indicated by arrowheads. Computed tomography scans confirmed the presence of multiple small hemorrhagic lesions in both temporal lobes. (From Waxman SG. *Clinical Neuroanatomy*, 26th ed. http://www.accessmedicine.com. Copyright © The McGraw-Hill Companies, Inc. All rights reserved.)

MEANS OF CONFIRMATION OR DIAGNOSIS

Laboratory Tests

- Cerebral spinal fluid testing
- Intracranial pressure

▶ Imaging

- CT scan for detailed imaging[5]
- MRI with gadolinium enhancement[5]

FINDINGS AND INTERPRETATION

- MRI may reveal (e.g., mediotemporal) lobe necrosis

TREATMENT

▶ Medications

- Antiviral agents[6]
- Corticosteroids if cerebral edema present[6]

REFERRALS/ADMITTANCE

- To ER if encephalitis is suspected
- To neurologist during infection and for follow-up
- To physician for respiratory therapy if source of infection is pulmonary in origin
- To occupational therapist for ADL- and cognitive-retraining
- To social worker for case management

IMPAIRMENTS

- Arousal
- Attention
- Behavior
- Cognition
- Cranial nerve integrity
- Gait[7]
- Sitting and standing balance
- Muscle strength
- Postural control
- Range of motion
- Deep tendon reflexes
- Muscle tone
- Sensation
- Bed mobility
- Transfers
- Endurance
- Aerobic capacity
- Self-care
- Home management
- Fine motor control
- Respiratory control

TESTS AND MEASURES

- Test level of consciousness: Glasgow coma scale[8]
- Cognition[9]: Mini-Mental State Examination (MMSE), executive function tests, memory, comprehension[10]
- Pain: Subjective report, visual analog scale (VAS), verbal report
- Strength and muscle endurance
- Coordination
- Muscle tone
- Joint range-of-motion (ROM)
- Cranial nerve testing[10]
- Sensation
- Postural alignment
- Balance (TUG, MDRT, Tinetti,[11] BBS)[9]
- Gait (TUG, Tinetti,[11] 10-m walk test, DGI)[9]
- Respiratory function (spirometer, oxygen saturation, auscultation)
- Functional mobility: Functional Independence Measure (FIM™)[7]

TABLE 86-1 Causes of Viral Encephalitis

Diffuse encephalitis
Epidemic (arbovirus) encephalitis
Eastern equine encephalitis
Western equine encephalitis
Venezuelan equine encephalitis
St. Louis encephalitis
California encephalitis
Japanese B encephalitis
Sporadic encephalitis
Herpes simplex encephalitis
Enterovirus encephalitis
Measles encephalitis
Varicella (chickenpox) encephalitis
Encephalitis in the immunocompromised patient
Herpes simplex encephalitis
Progressive multifocal leukoencephalopathy (PML)
Cytomegalovirus
HIV (AIDS) encephalitis
Specific types of encephalitis
Poliomyelitis
Rabies
Subacute sclerosing panencephalitis (SSPE)
Prion (slow virus) infections

Source: From Chandrasoma P, Taylor CR. *Concise Pathology*. 3rd ed. www.accessmedicine.com.

INTERVENTION

- Interventions based on extent and location of central nervous system damage
- If in coma
  - Instruct caregivers in positioning and joint ROM
  - Coma stimulation activities
- Once cleared for more active treatment
  - Functional mobility: Bed mobility, transfers, gait
  - Balance and coordination activities: Postural control, balance strategies, speed/reaction time, multitasking[7]
  - Flexibility and stretching
  - Strength and resistance training
  - Pulmonary and cardiovascular reconditioning
  - Problem solving and motor planning skills
- Note: Patients will fatigue quickly; consider options such as proprioceptive neuromuscular facilitation to address multiple movement planes simultaneously, reducing sets/reps, and controlling fatigue.

FUNCTIONAL GOALS

- Goals for people recovering from infectious disease of the brain are specific to impairments identified; general goals should be made more specific for each patient.
- Short-term goals
  - Patient will
    - Perform transfers to and from level surfaces with minimal physical assistance or verbal cues for sequencing.

- Ambulate on level tile surfaces with appropriate assistive device and moderate assistance for balance and sequencing.
- Consistently perform a two-step motor task without verbal or visual cues.
- Long-term goals
  - Patient will
    - Maintain postural control independently while ambulating on community surfaces for longer than 15 minutes
    - Ambulate distances >1000 feet without physical assistance, occasional verbal cues for safety.
    - Complete a multistep task (>3 steps) successfully without verbal, visual, or physical cues.

PROGNOSIS

- Death rate is high.
- Likelihood of persistent neurologic deficits depends partly on the infecting agent.
  - Patients with mumps meningoencephalitis have excellent prognosis.
  - Approximately 55% of patients with herpes simplex encephalitis have some neurologic sequelae.
- Speed of medical intervention at onset relates directly to prognosis for recovery.

PATIENT RESOURCE

- Encephalitis Society. http://www.encephalitis.info. Accessed February 22, 2013.

REFERENCES

1. The American Physical Therapy Association. Pattern 5A: Primary prevention/risk reduction for loss of balance and falling. *Interactive Guide to Physical Therapist Practice*. 2003. DOI: 10.2522/ptguide.3.2_1. http://guidetoptpractice.apta.org/content/1/SEC18.extract. Accessed May 14, 2014.
2. The American Physical Therapy Association. Pattern 5C: Impaired motor function and sensory integrity associated with nonprogressive disorders of the central nervous system—congenital origin or acquired in infancy or childhood. *Interactive Guide to Physical Therapist Practice*. 2003. DOI: 10.2522/ptguide.3.2_3. http://guidetoptpractice.apta.org/content/1/SEC20.extract. Accessed May 14, 2014.
3. The American Physical Therapy Association. Pattern 5D: Impaired motor function and sensory integrity associated with nonprogressive disorders of the central nervous system - acquired in adolescence or adulthood. *Interactive Guide to Physical Therapist Practice*. 2003. DOI: 10.2522/ptguide.3.2_4. http://guidetoptpractice.apta.org/content/1/SEC21.extract. Accessed May 14, 2014.
4. The American Physical Therapy Association. Pattern 5I: Impaired arousal, range of motion, and motor control associated with coma, near coma, or vegetative state. *Interactive Guide to Physical Therapist Practice* 2003. DOI: 10.2522/ptguide.3.2_9. Accessed February 22, 2013.
5. Malone TR, Hazle C, Grey ML. *Imaging in Rehabilitation*. New York, NY: McGraw-Hill; 2008. http://www.accessphysiotherapy.com/resource/613. Accessed February 22, 2013.
6. Panus PC, Jobst EE, Masters SB, Katzung B, Tinsley SL, Trevor AJ. *Pharmacology for the Physical Therapist*. New York, NY: McGraw-Hill; 2009. http://www.accessphysiotherapy.com/resource/615. Accessed February 22, 2013.
7. Shamus E, Feingold Stern D. *Effective Documentation for Physical Therapy Professionals, 2e*. New York, NY: McGraw-Hill; 2011. http://www.accessphysiotherapy.com/resource/696. Accessed February 22, 2013.
8. Glasgow Coma Scale. *TraumaticBrainInjury.com*. http://www.traumaticbraininjury.com/content/symptoms/glasgowcomascale.html. Accessed February 22, 2013.
9. The University of Missouri. *Geriatric Examination Toolkit*. http://web.missouri.edu/~proste/tool/cog/index.htm. Accessed February 22, 2013.
10. Dutton M. *McGraw Hill's NPTE (National Physical Therapy Examination), 2e*. New York, NY: McGraw-Hill; 2012. http://www.accessphysiotherapy.com/resource/611. Accessed February 22, 2013.
11. *Tinetti Balance and Gait Evaluation*. http://www.bhps.org.uk/falls/documents/TinettiBalanceAssessment.pdf. Accessed February 22, 2013.

ADDITIONAL REFERENCES

- Chandrasoma P, Taylor CR. *Concise Pathology*. 3rd ed. New York, NY: McGraw-Hill; 2011. http://www.accessphysiotherapy.com/content/193000. Accessed February 22, 2013.
- Dewane JA, Porter RE. Inflammatory and infectious disorders of the brain. In: Umphred DA, ed. *Neurological Rehabilitation*. 5th ed. St. Louis, MO: Mosby Elsevier; 2007: 661–663.
- ICD9DATA web site. http://www.icd9data.com. Accessed January 21, 2013.
- ICD10DATA web site. http://www.icd10data.com. Accessed January 21, 2013.
- Ropper AL, Samuels MA. *Adams and Victor's Principles of Neurology*. 9th ed. New York, NY: McGraw-Hill; 2009:716–723.

87 EPILEPSY

Mollie Venglar, DSc, MSPT, NCS

ICD-9-CM CODE

- 345.9 Epilepsy

ICD-10-CM CODE

- G40.909 Epilepsy, epileptic, epilepsia (attack) (cerebral) (convulsion) (fit) (seizure)

PREFERRED PRACTICE PATTERNS

- 5A: Primary Prevention/Risk Reduction for Loss of Balance and Falling[1]
- 5C: Impaired Motor Function and Sensory Integrity Associated with Nonprogressive Disorders of the Central Nervous System—congenital origin or acquired in infancy or childhood[2]
- 5D: Impaired Motor Function and Sensory Integrity Associated with Nonprogressive Disorders of the Central Nervous System—acquired in adolescence or adulthood[3]

PATIENT PRESENTATION

A physical therapist is evaluating a 15-year-old boy with a history of epilepsy since the age of 12. The boy suffered a medial collateral ligament tear during the last epileptic seizure 2 weeks ago. During the interview, the boy states that he has heard exercise will help him not have epileptic episodes. The physical therapist explains the interaction between exercise and epilepsy and proceeds to develop a plan of care to address the knee instability and exercise tolerance.

KEY FEATURES

Description

- Chronic disorder of various causes characterized by recurrent seizures
- Seizures result from sudden and excessive electrical discharge of large groups of neurons.

Essentials of Diagnosis

- Diagnosis requires that the individual experience seizures, but not all seizures are indicative of epilepsy.
- Epilepsy can be caused by any major category of serious disease or human disorder.
- Approximately 1% of cases result from genetic disease
- People with idiopathic or primary epilepsies share the following features:
  - Variable family history
  - Generalized spike-wave abnormality on electroencephalogram (EEG)
  - Onset in childhood or adolescence
- Development of epilepsy in an individual who suffers brain injury is influenced by family history and premorbid and postmorbid EEG abnormalities.

General Considerations

- Third most common serious neurologic disease in the elderly, following stroke and dementia.
- Depression commonly occurs in people with epilepsy.
  - Suggested that the hippocampus, implicated in both mood disorders and seizures, is likely link between depression and epilepsy.
- Events that may trigger seizure in people with epilepsy include
  - Stress
  - Poor nutrition
  - Missed medication
  - Skipping meals
  - Flickering lights
  - Illness
  - Fever and allergies
  - Lack of sleep
  - Strong emotions
  - Heat and humidity
- Fear of seizure may cause self-restriction of activities resulting in deconditioning, reduced balance strategy, loss of muscle strength, and endurance.

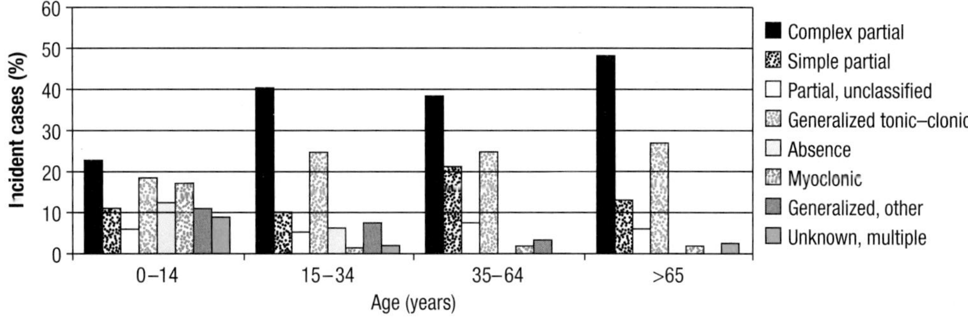

FIGURE 87-1 Distribution of the main types of epilepsy by age. Apparent is the overrepresentation of absence and myoclonic seizures in childhood and of complex partial seizures in older individuals. (Adapted from Hauser WA, Annegers JF: Epidemiology of epilepsy. In: Laidlaw JP, Richens A, Chadwick D, eds. Textbook of Epilepsy, 4th ed. New York, NY: Churchill Livingstone; 1992: 23–45 and Engel J Jr, Pedley TA. Epilepsy: *A Comprehensive Textbook*. Philadelphia, PA: Davis, 1998.)

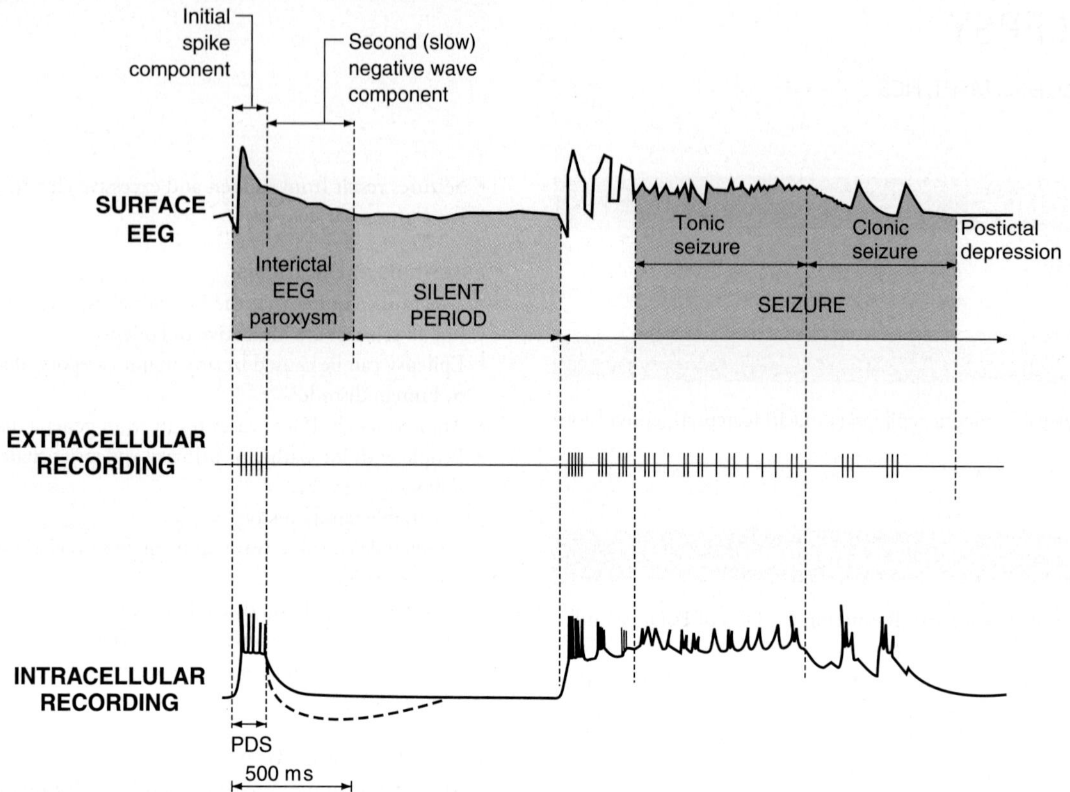

FIGURE 87-2 Relations among cortical EEG, extracellular, and intracellular recordings in a seizure focus induced by local application of a convulsant agent to the mammalian cortex. The extracellular recording was made through a high-pass filter. Note the high-frequency firing of the neuron evident in both extracellular and intracellular recording during the paroxysmal depolarization shift (PDS). (Modified with permission from Ayala GF, Dichter M, Gumnit RJ, et al. Genesis of epileptic interictal spikes. New knowledge of cortical feedback systems suggests a neurophysiological explanation of brief paroxysms. *Brain Res.* 1973;52:1–17. Copyright © Elsevier.)

Demographics

- Affects approximately 45 million people worldwide
- Highest incidence in young children and elderly populations; 75% of cases have onset before age 20 years
- Men affected slightly more than women

CLINICAL FINDINGS

SIGNS AND SYMPTOMS

- Many people with epilepsy have no outward signs or symptoms except during seizure.
- Most signs and symptoms related to medication use, such as
  - Ataxia
  - Nystagmus
  - Dizziness
  - Confusion
  - Slurred speech
  - Nausea
  - Vomiting
  - Fatigue
  - Lethargy

Functional Implications

- Injury from fall at onset of seizures or collision with objects during the seizure
- Asphyxia, if seizure occurs while eating, drinking, and swimming
- Deconditioning resulting in poor activity tolerance and increased fall risk

Possible Contributing Causes

- Stroke
- Intracranial mass
- Traumatic brain injury
- Subdural hematoma
- Pneumonia
- Hypoxia
- Alcohol abuse
- Brain abscess
- High doses of caffeine can trigger seizure in people with epilepsy.

Differential Diagnosis

- Transient ischemic attack
- Hypoglycemia
- Other seizure disorder
- Syncope
- Transient cerebral anoxia
- Recurrent cardiac arrhythmia
- Nonspecific dizziness or episodic vertigo

MEANS OF CONFIRMATION OR DIAGNOSIS

Imaging

- EEG
- MRI to rule out other pathologies causing epilepsy or seizure[4]

REFERRALS/ADMITTANCE

- To EMS or ER if patient develops status epilepticus
- To neurologist for pharmacologic control of seizure
  - Important aspect of epilepsy management
  - Common antiseizure medications include[5]

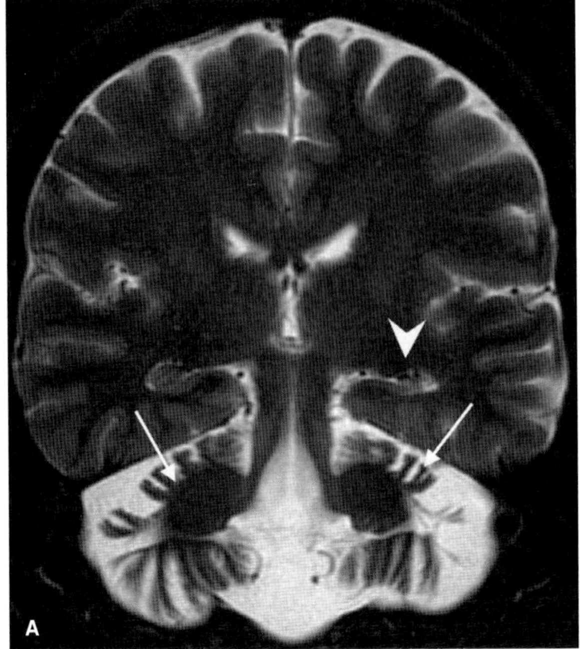

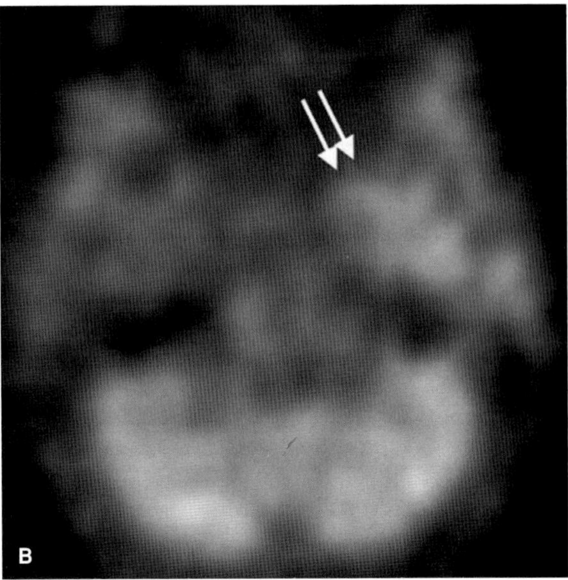

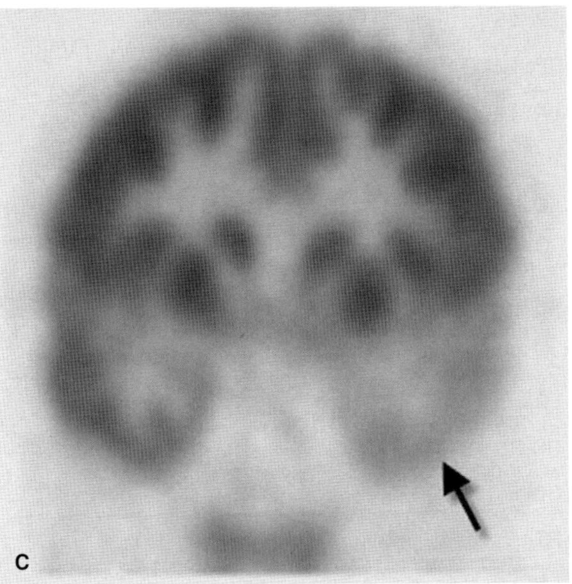

FIGURE 87-3 Coronal fast multiplanar inversion recovery (FMPIR) MRI (**A**), axial ictal SPECT (**B**), and coronal interictal PET images (**C**) in a 34-year-old woman with a long-standing history of medical refractory epilepsy who presents with increasing seizure frequency. (From Chen MYM, Pope TL, Ott DJ. *Basic Radiology.* 2nd ed. http://www.accessmedicine.com.)

- Gabapentin (Neurontin)
- Lamotrigine (Lamictal)
- Topiramate (Topamax)
- Tiagabine (Gabitril)
- Levetiracetam (Keppra)
- Divalproex sodium (Depakote)
- Sodium valproate (Valproate)
- Benzodiazepines
- Carbamazepine
- Ethosuximide
- Phenobarbital
- Primidone
- Phenytoin
- Vigabatrin

- To neurosurgeon if drug therapy inadequate or levels become toxic, one of the following may be recommended
  - Lobectomy
  - Cortical resection
  - Corpus callosum sectioning
  - Vagal nerve stimulation
- To neuropsychologist
- To dietician: Ketogenic diet often recommended
- To support group

IMPAIRMENTS

- Decreased cardiovascular function
- Decreased cardiovascular endurance
- Decreased muscle endurance
- Decreased muscle strength
- Impaired balance reactions

TESTS AND MEASURES

- Vital-sign monitoring
- Balance testing (avoid altered-vision testing, may trigger seizure in some patients)[6]
- Gait[7]
- Muscle strength
- Muscle endurance
- Cardiovascular endurance

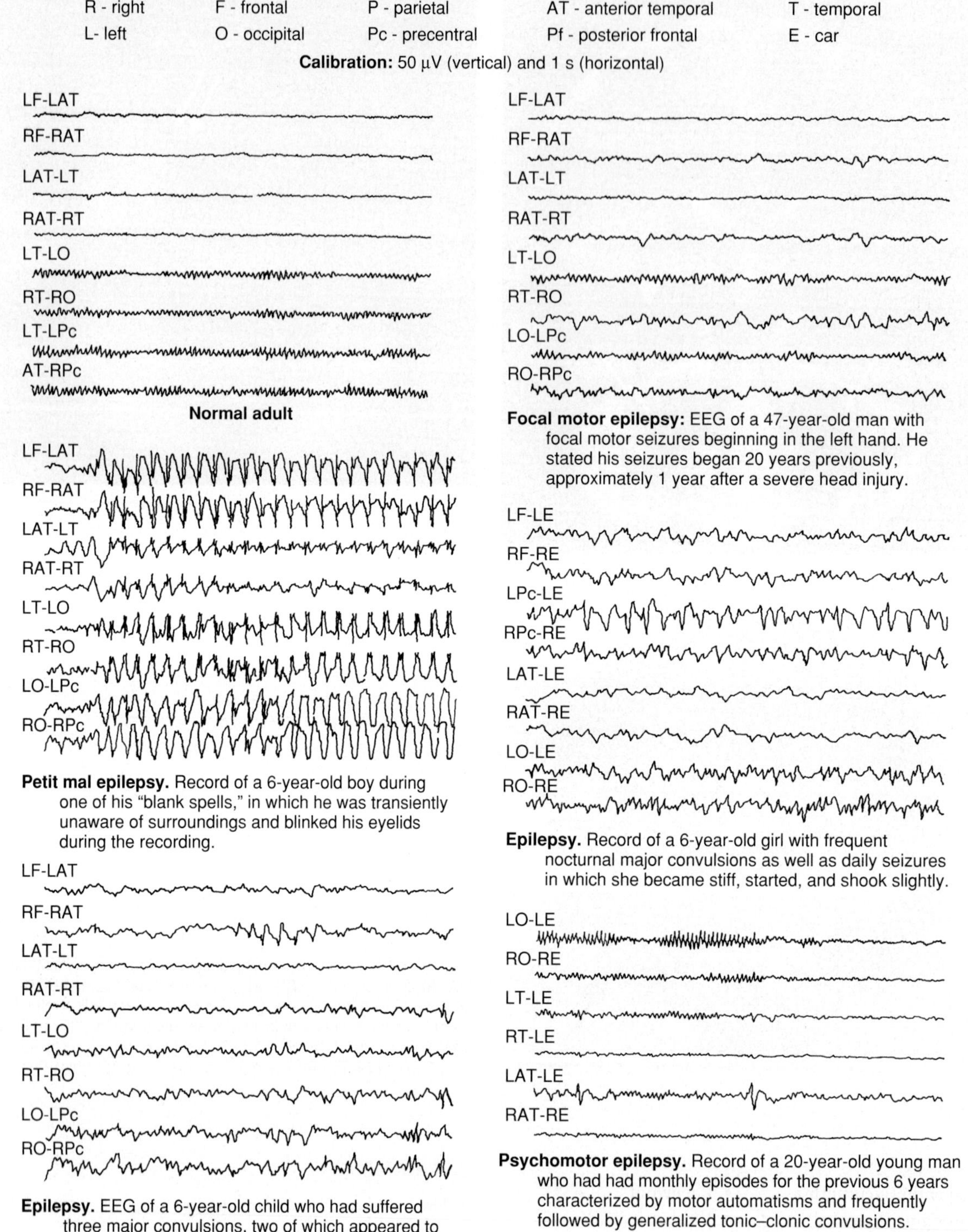

FIGURE 87-4 Representative electroencephalograms. (From Waxman SG. *Clinical Neuroanatomy.* 26th ed. http://www.accessmedicine.com. Copyright © The McGraw-Hill Companies, Inc. All rights reserved.)

INTERVENTION

- Assessment of home, school, work environments for seizure triggers, and recommended modifications
- General cardiovascular and muscular reconditioning
- Encourage group activities, such as recreational sport
- Integrate hydration with exercise as dehydration often leads to seizure
- Provide safety training to compensate for medication side effects

FUNCTIONAL GOALS

- Patient will be able to
  - Tolerate 20 minutes of continuous activity on an exercise bike at 60% maximum heart rate without adverse event.
  - Walk through grocery store while pushing the grocery cart for 30 minutes without excess fatigue or adverse event.
  - Consistently demonstrate appropriate balance reactions without assistance while walking on outdoor surfaces for 1000 feet.

PROGNOSIS

- Increased mortality rate compared to general population.
- Death from asphyxia may occur if an individual experiences seizure while eating or drinking and airway remains blocked in postictal phase.
- Attempted suicide more common in people with epilepsy compared to general population.
- In people with epilepsy of unknown cause diagnosed before 10 years of age, 75% remission rate (defined as 5 years without seizure) is possible.

PATIENT RESOURCES

- Epilepsy Association. http://epilepsyassociation.com. Accessed February 22, 2013.
- Epilepsy Foundation. http://www.epilepsyfoundation.org. Accessed February 22, 2013.
- American Epilepsy Society. http://www.aesnet.org. Accessed February 22, 2013.

REFERENCES

1. The American Physical Therapy Association. Pattern 5A: primary prevention/risk reduction for loss of balance and falling. *Interactive Guide to Physical Therapist Practice*. 2003. DOI: 10.2522/ptguide.3.2_1. http://guidetoptpractice.apta.org/content/1/SEC18.extract. Accessed May 14, 2014.
2. The American Physical Therapy Association. Pattern 5C: impaired motor function and sensory integrity associated with nonprogressive disorders of the central nervous system—congenital origin or acquired in infancy or childhood. *Interactive Guide to Physical Therapist Practice*. 2003. DOI: 10.2522/ptguide.3.2_3. http://guidetoptpractice.apta.org/content/1/SEC20.extract. Accessed May 14, 2014.
3. The American Physical Therapy Association. Pattern 5D: impaired motor function and sensory integrity associated with nonprogressive disorders of the central nervous system—acquired in adolescence or adulthood. *Interactive Guide to Physical Therapist Practice*. 2003. DOI: 10.2522/ptguide.3.2_4. http://guidetoptpractice.apta.org/content/1/SEC21.extract. Accessed May 14, 2014.
4. Malone TR, Hazle C, Grey ML. *Imaging in Rehabilitation*. New York, NY: McGraw-Hill; 2008. http://guidetoptpractice.apta.org/content/1/SEC26.extract. Accessed May 14, 2014.
5. Panus PC, Jobst EE, Masters SB, Katzung B, Tinsley SL, Trevor AJ. *Pharmacology for the Physical Therapist*. New York, NY: McGraw-Hill; 2009. http://www.accessphysiotherapy.com/resource/615. Accessed February 22, 2013.
6. The University of Missouri. Geriatric Examination Tool Kit. http://web.missouri.edu/~proste/tool/. Accessed February 22, 2013.
7. Shamus E, Stern D. *Effective Documentation for Physical Therapy Professionals, 2e*. New York, NY: McGraw-Hill; 2011. http://www.accessphysiotherapy.com/resource/696. Accessed February 22, 2013.

ADDITIONAL REFERENCES

- Burke-Doe A, Runion HI, Smith TJ. Impact of drug therapy on patients receiving neurological rehabilitation. In: Umphred DA, ed. *Neurological Rehabilitation*. 5th ed. St. Louis, MO: Mosby Elsevier; 2007:1122–1123.
- Fuller KS. Epilepsy. In: Goodman CC, Fuller KS, eds. *Pathology: Implications for the Physical Therapist*. 3rd ed. St. Louis, MO: Saunders Elsevier; 2009: 1532–1546.
- ICD9DATA web site. http://www.icd9data.com. Accessed February 22, 2013.
- ICD10DATA web site. http://www.icd10data.com. Accessed February 22, 2013.

88 GUILLAIN–BARRÉ SYNDROME

Mollie Venglar, DSc, MSPT, NCS

CONDITION/DISORDER SYNONYMS

- Landry—Guillain–Barré–Strohl syndrome
- Acute inflammatory demyelinating polyneuropathy
- Acute demyelinating polyneuritis

ICD-9-CM CODE

- 357.0 Acute infective polyneuritis

ICD-10-CM CODE

- G61.0 Guillain–Barré syndrome

PREFERRED PRACTICE PATTERN

- 5G: Impaired motor function and sensory integrity associated with acute or chronic polyneuropathies[1]

PATIENT PRESENTATION

A 25-year-old woman is brought into the emergency department (ED) after sinking to the ground during a volleyball match. Her teammate notes that she had been stumbling and was starting to have more difficulty with her serve for the past week. On arrival, she can no longer raise her legs and labors to adjust herself in bed. She has also begun to complain of shortness of breath. She denies fever but states that 3 weeks ago the entire team suffered from abdominal cramps and diarrhea after a championship cookout. The patient denies previous health problems. Her temperature is 36.6°C (98°F); heart rate, 50 beats/min; respiration rate, 26 breaths/min; and blood pressure, 90/60 mmHg. She can only keep her arms up against gravity for 5 seconds, and her hands are limp. She has slight movement of her legs with decreased sensation of pain and fine touch in her lower legs. Her reflexes are absent. She has no skin lesions. Her heart and lung examinations are unremarkable except for bradycardia and poor inspiratory effort. MRI of the brain and spine is normal.[2]

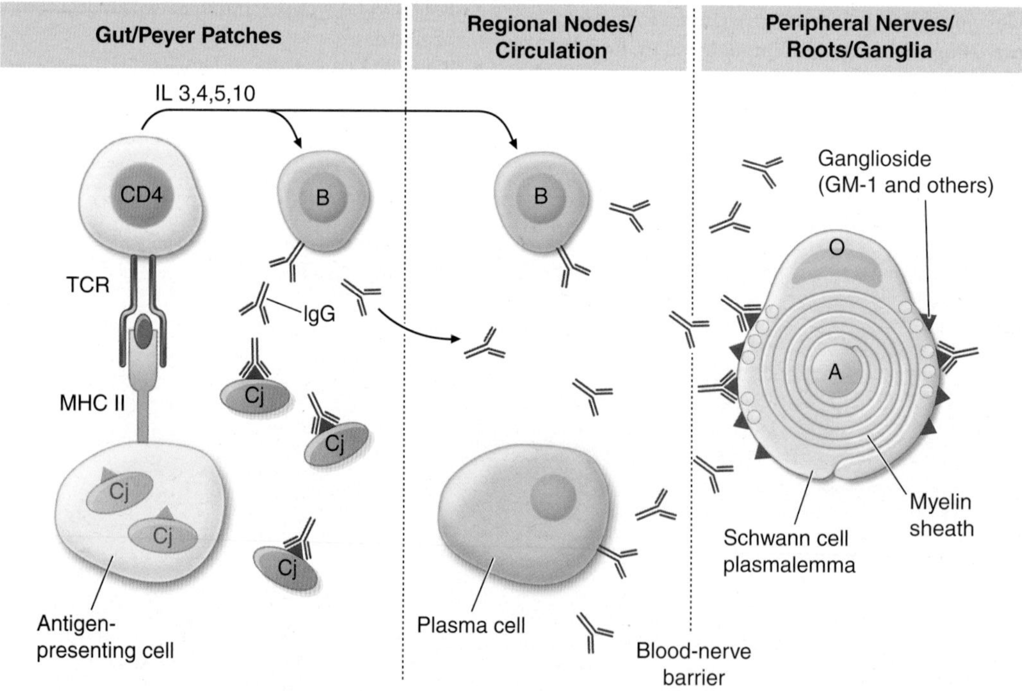

FIGURE 88-1 Postulated immunopathogenesis of GBS associated with *Campylobacter jejuni* infection. B cells recognize glycoconjugates on *C. jejuni* (Cj) (triangles) that cross-react with ganglioside present on Schwann cell surface and subjacent peripheral nerve myelin. Some B cells, activated via a T cell–independent mechanism, secrete primarily IgM (not shown). Other B cells (upper left side) are activated via a partially T cell–dependent route and secrete primarily IgG; T cell help is provided by CD4 cells activated locally by fragments of Cj proteins that are presented on the surface of antigen-presenting cells (APCs). A critical event in the development of GBS is the escape of activated B cells from Peyer patches into regional lymph nodes. Activated T cells probably also function to assist in opening of the blood-nerve barrier, facilitating penetration of pathogenic autoantibodies. The earliest changes in myelin (right) consist of edema between myelin lamellae and vesicular disruption (shown as circular blebs) of the outermost myelin layers. These effects are associated with activation of the C5b–C9 membrane attack complex and probably mediated by calcium entry; it is possible that the macrophage cytokine tumor necrosis factor (TNF) also participates in myelin damage. B, B cell; MHC II, class II major histocompatibility complex molecule; TCR, T cell receptor; A, axon; O, oligodendrocyte. (From Longo DL et al., eds. *Harrison's Principles of Internal Medicine.* 18th ed. http://www.accessmedicine.com. Copyright © McGraw-Hill Education. All rights reserved.)

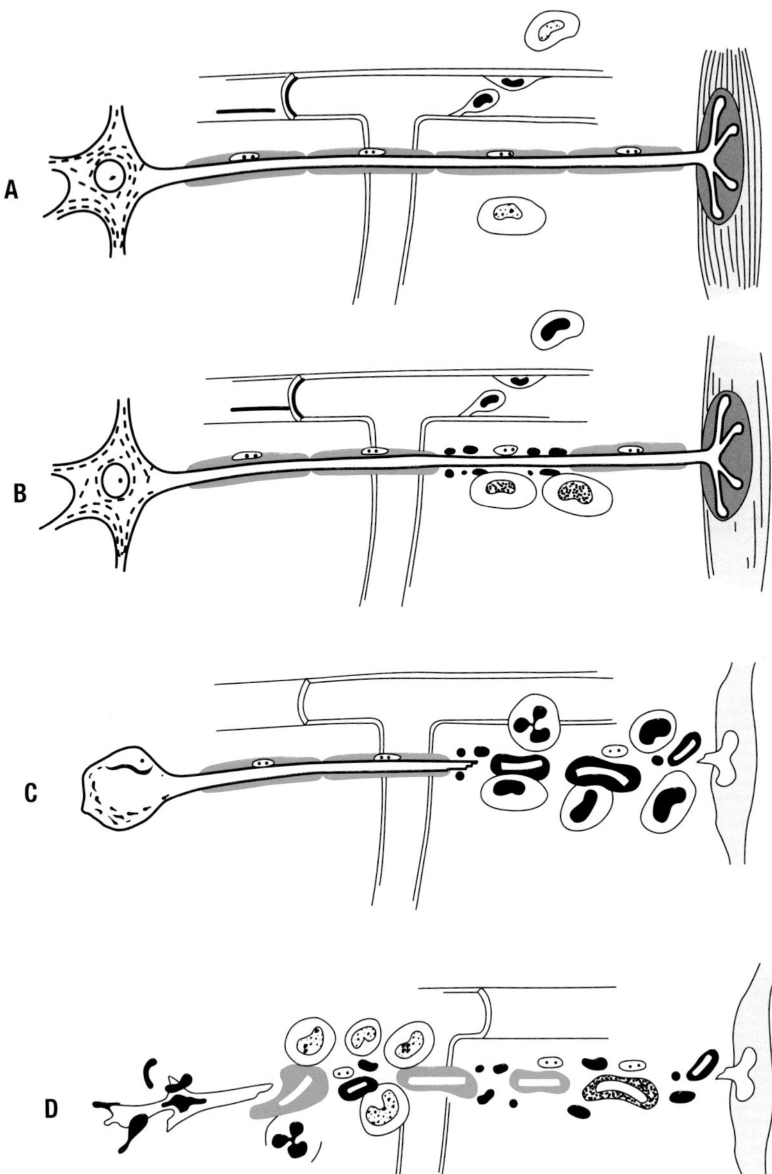

FIGURE 88-2 Diagram of probable cellular events in acute inflammatory polyneuropathy (Guillain–Barré syndrome). **A.** Lymphocytes attach to the walls of endoneurial vessels and migrate through the vessel wall, enlarging and transforming as they do so. At this stage no nerve damage has occurred. **B.** More lymphocytes have migrated into the surrounding tissue. The first effect on the nerve is breakdown of myelin, the axon being spared (segmental demyelination). This change appears to be mediated by the mononuclear exudate, but the mechanism is uncertain. **C.** The lesion is more intense, polymorphonuclear leukocytes are present as well as lymphocytes. There is interruption of the axon in addition to myelin sheath damage; as a result, the muscle undergoes denervation atrophy, and the nerve cell body shows central chromatolysis. If the axonal damage is distal, the nerve cell body will survive, and regeneration and clinical recovery are likely. If, as in **D**, axonal interruption has occurred proximally because of a particularly intense root or proximal nerve lesion, the nerve cell body may die and undergo dissolution. In this situation, there is no regeneration, only the possibility of collateral reinnervation of muscle from surviving motor fibers. (From Asbury AK, Arnason BGW, Adams RD. *The inflammatory lesion in acute idiopathic polyneuritis.* Medicine [Baltimore]. 1969;48:173.)

KEY FEATURES

Description

- Demyelination of the peripheral nervous system, resulting in quickly progressing paralysis beginning distally, potentially ending full quadriplegic presentation with respiratory failure[3–5]

Essentials of Diagnosis

- Most common bacteria identified with Guillain–Barré syndrome (GBS) is *Campylobacter jejuni*;[6] other common infections include cytomegalovirus and Epstein–Barr virus
- Sixty percent of cases have preceding upper respiratory illness or vaccination 1 to 3 weeks prior to onset.

General Considerations

- Two forms of GBS are common, though several other variants exist.
  - Nonaxonal form
    - Peripheral nerves undergo demyelination, but no damage to axons
    - High likelihood of regaining full function with appropriate medical and therapeutic intervention
  - Axonal form
- Axon of the peripheral nerve is damaged, does not remyelinate
  - Function through that nerve is lost, patient will likely have permanent functional loss of associated muscle

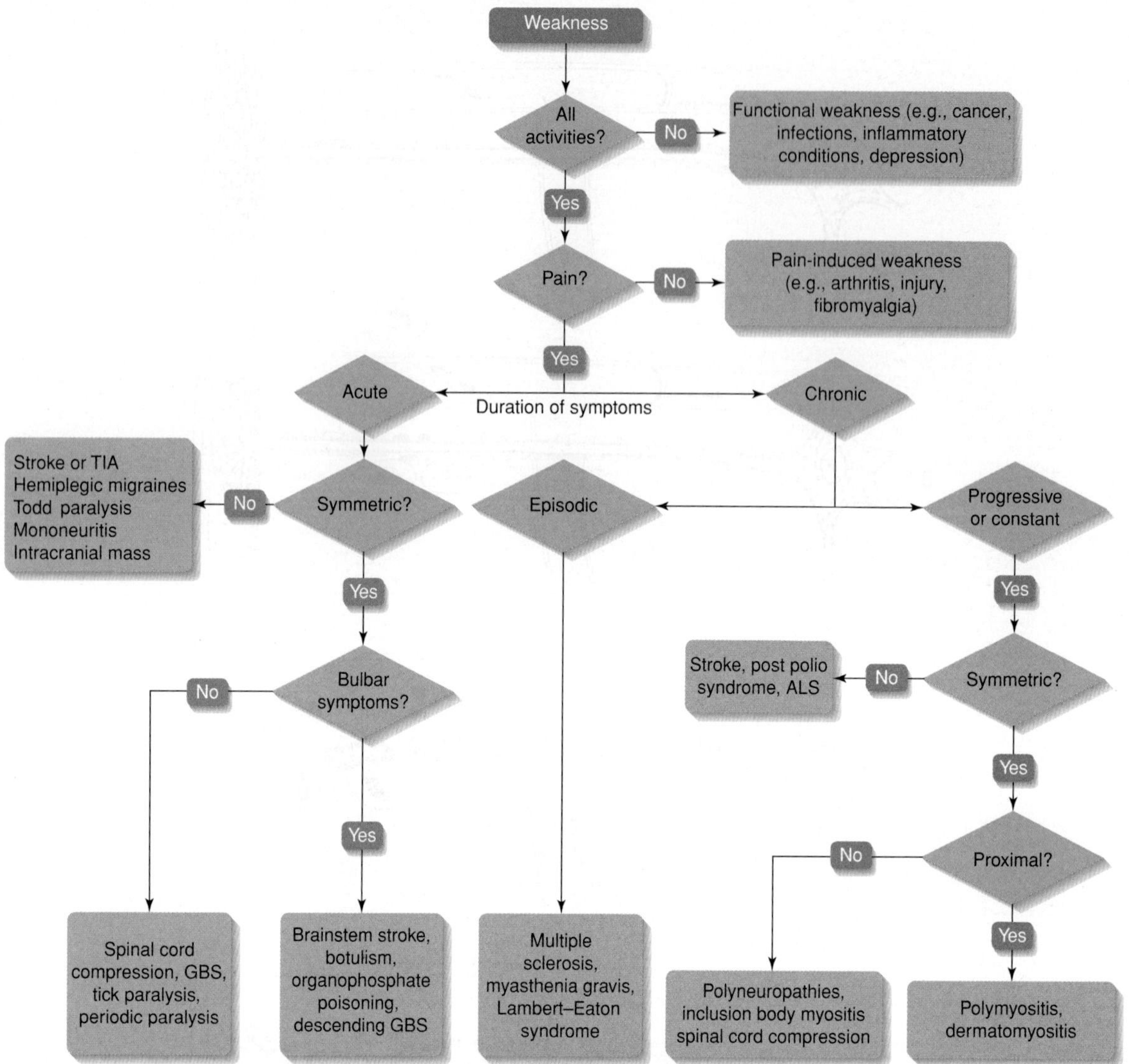

FIGURE 88-3 Diagnostic algorithm: Muscle weakness. ALS, amyotrophic lateral sclerosis; DM, dermatomyositis; GBS, Guillain–Barré syndrome; TIA, transient ischemic attack. (From Henderson MC, Tierney LM, Smetana GW. The Patient History: *An Evidence-Based Approach to Differential Diagnosis.* http://www.accessmedicine.com.)

TABLE 88-1 Subtypes of Guillain–Barré Syndrome (GBS)

Subtype	Features	Electrodiagnosis	Pathology
Acute inflammatory demyelinating polyneuropathy (AIDP)	Adults affected more than children; 90% of cases in the Western world; recovery rapid; anti-GM1 antibodies (<50%)	Demyelinating	First attack on Schwann cell surface; widespread myelin damage, macrophage activation, and lymphocytic infiltration; variable secondary axonal damage
Acute motor axonal neuropathy (AMAN)	Children and young adults; prevalent in China and Mexico; may be seasonal; recovery rapid; anti-GD1a antibodies	Axonal	First attack at motor nodes of Ranvier; macrophage activation, few lymphocytes, frequent periaxonal macrophages; extent of axonal damage highly variable
Acute motor sensory axonal neuropathy (AMSAN)	Mostly adults; uncommon; recovery slow, often incomplete; closely related to AMAN	Axonal	Same as AMAN, but also affects sensory nerves and roots; axonal damage usually severe
M. Fisher syndrome (MFS)	Adults and children; uncommon; ophthalmoplegia, ataxia, and areflexia; anti-GQ1b antibodies (90%)	Demyelinating	Few cases examined; resembles AIDP

Source: From Longo DL, Fauci AS, Kasper DL, et al., eds. *Harrison's Principles of Internal Medicine.* 18th ed. http://www.accessmedicine.com.

- Rapid progression from onset to potential respiratory failure; should be identified and treated very quickly.
- Most patients show gradual return of strength beginning 2 to 4 weeks after the point at which progression of the disease stops ("nadir").
- Approximately 50% of patients experience dysfunction of the autonomic nervous system, including
  - Low cardiac output
  - Cardiac dysrhythmias
  - Marked fluctuation in blood pressure
  - Poor venous return
  - Bowel and bladder retention

Demographics

- Males and females of all ages susceptible
- Approximately 4 in 100,000 people afflicted each year

CLINICAL FINDINGS

SIGNS AND SYMPTOMS

- Progressive weakness in distal to proximal direction resulting in quadriplegia
  - Decreased muscle strength, recruitment, endurance
  - Decreased active range of motion (AROM)
  - Decreased sensation in stocking/glove pattern
- Loss of deep tendon reflexes, initially at the calcaneal (Achilles) tendon
- Deep muscle aching
- Respiratory failure

Functional Implications

- Bed mobility, transfers, gait, basic and complex activities of daily living (ADLs)
- Decreased independence with all self-care
- Decreased ability to interact with environment physically, verbally, sometimes visually (if cranial nerves controlling vision are affected)

Possible Contributing Causes

- Definitive cause is unknown.
- *Campylobacter jejuni* is the most common bacterium associated with GBS.[6]
- Pre-morbid respiratory illness (severe cold or flu) is also a common contributing cause.

Differential Diagnosis

- Spinal cord compression (myelopathy)
- Miller–Fisher syndrome (GBS variant)
- Chronic inflammatory demyelinating polyradiculoneuropathy
- Acute spinal cord disease
- Myasthenia gravis
- Sarcoidosis
- Upper motor neuron (UMN) disorder
- Tick paralysis
- Poliomyelitis
- Polyarteritis nodosa
- Polyneuropathy of critical illness
- Transverse myelitis
- Cervical stenosis
- Spinal tumor
- Diabetic neuropathy

TABLE 88-2 Variants of Guillain-Barré Syndrome

Regional
Fisher syndrome of ophthalmoplegia, ataxia, and areflexia
Cervical-brachial-pharyngeal, often with ptosis
Oculopharyngeal weakness
Predominant paraparesis
Bilateral facial or abducens weakness with distal paresthesias
Ophthalmoplegia with GQ_1b autoantibodies
Functional
Generalized ataxia without dysarthria or nystagmus
Pure sensory
Pure motor
Pandysautonomia
Axonal (AMAN)

Source: From Ropper AH, Samuels MA. *Adams & Victor's Principles of Neurology.* *9th* ed. http://www.accessmedicine.com.

MEANS OF CONFIRMATION OR DIAGNOSIS

Laboratory Tests

- Test of cerebral spinal fluid (CSF)

Imaging

- MRI with contrast

Diagnostic Procedures

- Electrodiagnostics

FINDINGS AND INTERPRETATION

- Test of CSF: Positive if protein levels elevated.
- MRI with contrast will show gadolinium enhancement of cauda equina roots.[7]
- Electrodiagnostics: Abnormalities of nerve conduction occur early in disease process; reduction in amplitude of action potential in muscle.

REFERRALS/ADMITTANCE

- To ER if early signs and symptoms are noted
- To ICU: Necessary to appropriately manage disease until patient reaches nadir[8]
  - Respiratory therapy to manage ventilation decline
  - After nadir is reached, other therapies may begin to intervene
  - Plasmapheresis or intravenous immunoglobulin (IVIg)
- To occupational therapist for ADLs, self-care, fine-motor training
- To social worker for case management and coordination of care.

IMPAIRMENTS

- Cranial nerve integrity
- Peripheral nerve integrity
- Gait[9]
- Wheelchair mobility[9]
- Balance
  - Static sit
  - Dynamic sit

- Static stand
- Dynamic stand
- Moving base of support
- Muscle strength
- Muscle recruitment
- Coordination
- Posture, postural control
- ROM
- Deep tendon reflexes
- Muscle tone
- Sensation
- Bed mobility
- Transfers
- Endurance
- Aerobic capacity
- Self-care
- Home management
- Fine motor
- Respiratory compromise

TESTS AND MEASURES

- Manual muscle testing: Identify patterns of weakness, fasciculations[7]
- Muscle tone
- Active and passive ROM
- Sensory integrity[7]
- Cranial nerve examination[10]
- Vital signs: Resting and active[11]
- Respiratory capacity
- Functional assessment: Functional Independence Measure (FIM™)
  - Gait (observational gait analysis, 10-m walk test)
  - Wheelchair mobility[9]
  - Transfers
  - Bed mobility
  - ADLs
  - Sitting and standing balance (balance reactions, protective responses)

INTERVENTION

- Except for positioning and passive ROM, physical therapy should not be initiated until patient reaches nadir and disease is stabilized.
- Fatigue and muscle overuse may lead to further damage; should be avoided, especially in early stage of recovery.
- Graduated functional exercise program
  - Early stage: Passive ROM, moving to active-assisted, supported-sitting tolerance, assisted bed mobility.
  - Middle stage: Antigravity ROM, specific and function-resistive exercises beginning with patient's own limb/body weight, sitting balance, standing tolerance.
  - Late stage: Functional exercises working on muscle control and endurance, standing balance, balance reactions, progressive aerobic activity while monitoring for fatigue.
- Proprioceptive neuromuscular facilitation for mobility and stability within graduated exercise program.[10]
- Adaptive equipment as needed: Wheelchair with cushion, orthotics, gait devices, eating utensils.
- Energy conservation, patient self-awareness of fatigue.

FUNCTIONAL GOALS

- In hospital (after nadir)
  - Patient will
    - Tolerate sitting at the edge of bed for 3 minutes with moderate to maximal assistance and no evidence of orthostatic hypotension.
    - Maintain head control with minimal assistance for 2 minutes while seated in a wheelchair.
- In-patient rehabilitation or skilled nursing facility
  - Patient will
    - Consistently transition from supine to sit with minimal assistance and fewer than two verbal cues for safety.
    - Demonstrate independent unsupported sitting at an edge of a mat for 3 minutes during upper-extremity activity. without loss of balance
- Out-patient therapy
  - Patient will
    - Ambulate >150 feet with a wheeled walker on level surfaces with supervision and no loss of balance.
    - Transfer between all surfaces via lateral pivot transfer with supervision for safety.

PROGNOSIS

- Eighty percent of GBS cases will regain ambulation within 6 months of onset.
- Three to five percent pass away from cardiac, respiratory, or other systemic organ failure.
- Poor prognosis associated with severity of muscle weakness, need for respiratory support, cranial nerve involvement, older age at onset, length of time to nadir, recent cytomegalovirus infection.

PATIENT RESOURCES

- Guillain–Barré Syndrome/Chromic Inflammatory Demyelinating Polyneuropathy. http://www.gbs-cidp.org. Accessed February 6, 2013.
- Guillain–Barré Syndrome Support Group. http://www.gbs.org.uk. Accessed February 6, 2013.

REFERENCES

1. The American Physical Therapy Association. Pattern 5G: impaired motor function and sensory integrity associated with acute or chronic polyneuropathies. *Interactive Guide to Physical Therapist Practice*. 2003. DOI: 10.2522/ptguide.3.2_7. http://guidetoptpractice.apta.org/content/1/SEC24.extract. Accessed May 14, 2014.
2. Waxman SG. *Clinical Neuroanatomy*. New York, NY: McGraw-Hill; 2010. http://www.accessphysiotherapy.com/resource/22. Accessed February 22, 2013.
3. American Physical Therapy Association. *Anatomy and Physiology Revealed*. New York, NY: McGraw-Hill; 2007. http://anatomy.mcgraw-hill.com/apt.html?login=1318852389155&system=Nervous§ion=Dissection&topic=Peripheral%20nerves&topicAbbr=Pne&view=Brachial%20plexus&viewAbbr=Brp. Accessed February 22, 2013.
4. Longo DL, Fauci AS, Kasper DL, Hauser SL, Jameson L, Loscalzo J, eds. *Harrison's Principles of Internal Medicine, 18e*. New York, NY: McGraw-Hill; 2012. http://accessmedicine.com/content.aspx?aID=9148788&searchStr=guillain-barre+syndrome# 9148788. Accessed February 22, 2013.

5. Ogle JW, Anderson MS. Chapter 40. Infections: bacterial & spirochetal. In: Hay WW, Levin MJ, Sondheimer JM, Deterding RR, eds. *CURRENT Diagnosis & Treatment: Pediatrics*. 20th ed. New York, NY: McGraw-Hill; 2011. http://www.accessphysiotherapy.com/abstract/6591272#6591272. Accessed February 22, 2013.
6. Dutton M. *Orthopaedic Examination, Evaluation, and Intervention*. New York, NY: McGraw-Hill; 2008. http://www.accessphysiotherapy.com/resource/612. Accessed February 22, 2013.
7. Hall JB, Schmidt GA, Wood LDH, eds. *Principles of Critical Care, 3e*. New York, NY: McGraw-Hill; 2005. http://accessmedicine.com/content.aspx?aID=2293039&searchStr=guillain-barre+syndrome#2293039. Accessed February 22, 2013.
8. Shamus E, Feingold Stern D. *Effective Documentation for Physical Therapy Professionals, 2e*. New York, NY: McGraw-Hill; 2011. http://www.accessphysiotherapy.com/resource/696. Accessed February 22, 2013.
9. Dutton M. *Dutton's Orthopedic Survival Guide: Managing Common Conditions*. New York, NY: McGraw-Hill; 2011. http://www.accessphysiotherapy.com/resource/685. Accessed February 22, 2013.
10. Dutton M. *McGraw Hill's NPTE (National Physical Therapy Examination), 2e*. New York, NY: McGraw-Hill; 2012. http://www.accessphysiotherapy.com/resource/611. Accessed February 22, 2013.

ADDITIONAL REFERENCES

- Hallum A. Neuromuscular diseases. In: Umphred DA, ed *Neurological Rehabilitation*. 5th ed. St. Louis, MO: Mosby Elsevier. 2007: 498–508.
- ICD9DATA web site. http://www.icd9data.com. Accessed February 22, 2013.
- ICD10DATA web site. http://www.icd10data.com. Accessed February 22, 2013.
- Ropper AL, Samuels MA. *Adams and Victor's Principles of Neurology*. 9th ed. New York, NY: McGraw-Hill; 2009: 1261–1270.

89 HUNTINGTON DISEASE

Mollie Venglar, DSc, MSPT, NCS

CONDITION/DISORDER SYNONYMS

- Huntington chorea
- Huntington's disease (HD)

ICD-9-CM CODE

- 333.4 Huntington chorea

ICD-10-CM CODE

- G10 Huntington disease (HD)

PREFERRED PRACTICE PATTERN

- 5E: Impaired Motor Function and Sensory Integrity Associated with Progressive Disorders of the Central Nervous System[1]

PATIENT PRESENTATION

A 40-year-old man presents to the psychiatry emergency room for inappropriate behavior and confusion. He works as a janitor and has had reasonably good work attendance. His coworkers say that he has appeared "fidgety" for several years. They specifically mention jerky movements that seem to affect his entire body more recently. His mother is alive and well, although his father died at age 28 in an auto accident. On examination, he is alert but easily distracted. His speech is fluent but is noted to be tangential. He has trouble with spelling the word "world" backwards and counting in serial sevens, but recalls three objects at 3 minutes. When he walks, there is a lot of distal hand movement, and his balance is precarious, although he can stand with both feet together for several seconds. His deep tendon reflexes are increased bilaterally, and there is bilateral ankle clonus. A urine drug screen is negative.[2]

KEY FEATURES

Description

- Degeneration of nerve cells in the brain
- Hereditary disorder
- Children of people with Huntington disease have 50% chance of inheriting the gene

Essentials of Diagnosis

- Genetic dysfunction on fourth chromosome
- Autosomal dominant inheritance
- Characterized by choreoathetosis and dementia

General Considerations

- Family history and genetic testing to confirm diagnosis

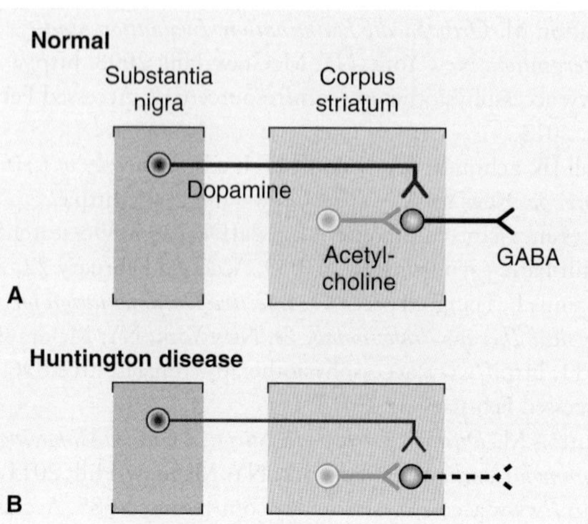

FIGURE 89-1 Schematic representation of the sequence of neurons involved in Huntington disease. **A.** Dopaminergic neurons (red) originating in the substantia nigra normally inhibit the GABAergic output from the striatum (caudate and putamen), whereas cholinergic neurons (green) exert an excitatory effect. **B.** In Huntington disease, GABAergic neurons (black) are preferentially lost, resulting in reduced inhibitory output from the striatum. (From Aminoff MJ. Pharmacologic management of parkinsonism and other movement disorders. In: Katzung BG, Masters SB, Trevor AJ, eds. *Basic and Clinical Pharmacology.* 12th ed. New York, NY: McGraw-Hill; 2012.)

Demographics

- Adult onset generally in fourth or fifth decade of life
- Early onset, not common but may occur in adolescence
- Most common in people who are Caucasian of European ancestry

CLINICAL FINDINGS

SIGNS AND SYMPTOMS

- Slight but evident alteration in character initially, followed by issues of self-control, eventually leading to failure of all cognitive functions
- Difficulty with attention and concentration, poor mental flexibility
- Movement abnormalities begin in the hands and face, initial slowing of movement and loss of coordination, progressing to chorea, then athetosis
- Degree and continuous nature of movement cause most patients to experience extreme weight loss and malnutrition
- Behavioral changes
- Irritability
- Rigidity
- Tremors
- Paranoia
- Dementia
- Unsteady gait
- Abnormal reflexes
- Memory loss

Functional Implications

- Loss of ability to interact in society and eventually with family members
- Loss of ability to care for self mentally, emotionally, physically
- Loss of functional mobility and associated cognitive processes

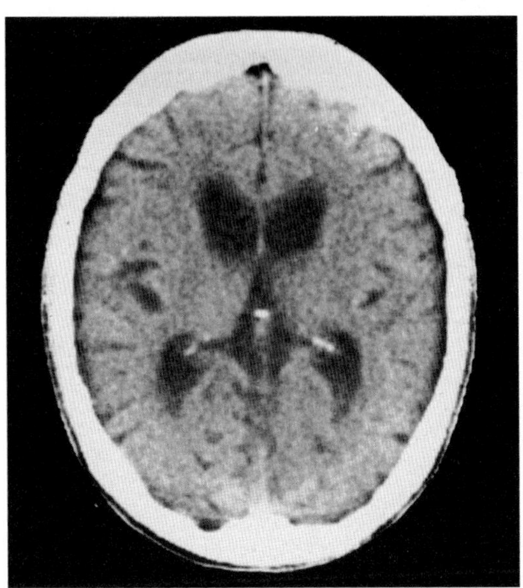
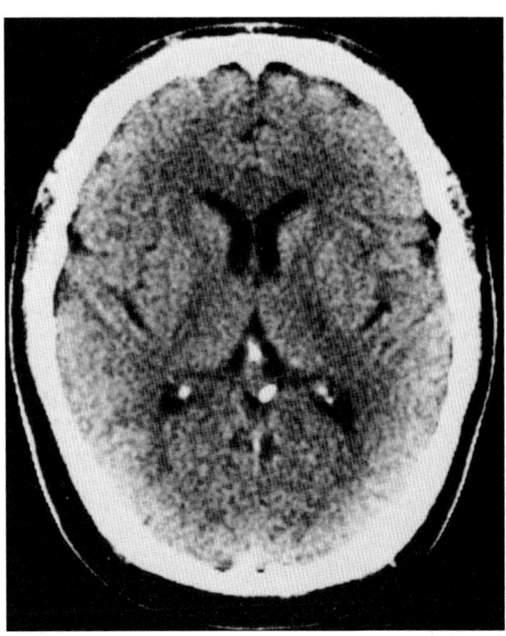

FIGURE 89-2 CT brain in Huntington dementia. (Reproduced, with permission, from Ropper AH, Brown RH. *Adams and Victor's Principles of Neurology*. 8th ed. New York, NY: McGraw-Hill, 2005: 912.)

- Difficulty swallowing
- Limited ambulation
- Poor communication, speech impairments

Possible Contributing Causes

- Genetic disorder; no other known contributing causes

Differential Diagnosis

- Alzheimer disease
- Cerebral infection
- Hyperglycemia
- Lupus
- Parkinsondisease
- Stroke
- Sydenham chorea
- Tardive dyskinesia
- Thyrotoxicosis

MEANS OF CONFIRMATION OR DIAGNOSIS

Laboratory Tests

- DNA/genetic testing

Imaging

- Head CT[3]

FINDINGS AND INTERPRETATION

- Head CT may show loss of brain tissue[3]

TREATMENT

Medication

- Fluoxetine
- Carbamazepine
- Antipsychotic agents

REFERRALS/ADMITTANCE

- To neurologist for imaging, disease management
- To support groups for psychological support
  - Huntington Disease Society of America
- To hospice for end-of-life care
- To geneticist for genetic counseling

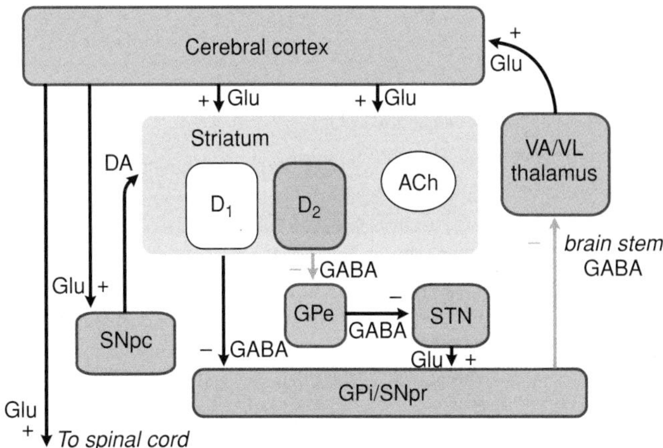

FIGURE 89-3 The basal ganglia in Huntington disease. HD is characterized by loss of neurons from the striatum. The neurons that project from the striatum to the GPe and form the indirect pathway are affected earlier in the course of the disease than those which project to the GPi. This leads to a loss of inhibition of the GPe. The increased activity in this structure, in turn, inhibits the STN, SNpr, and GPi, resulting in a loss of inhibition to the VA/VL thalamus and increased thalamocortical excitatory drive. Structures in purple have reduced activity in HD, whereas structures in purple have increased activity. Light blue line indicates primary pathways of reduced activity. (From Bunton LL, Chabner BA, Knollmann BC. *Goodman & Gilman's The Pharmacological Basis of Therapeutics*. 12th ed. http://www.accessmedicine.com. Copyright © The McGraw-Hill Companies, Inc. All rights reserved.)

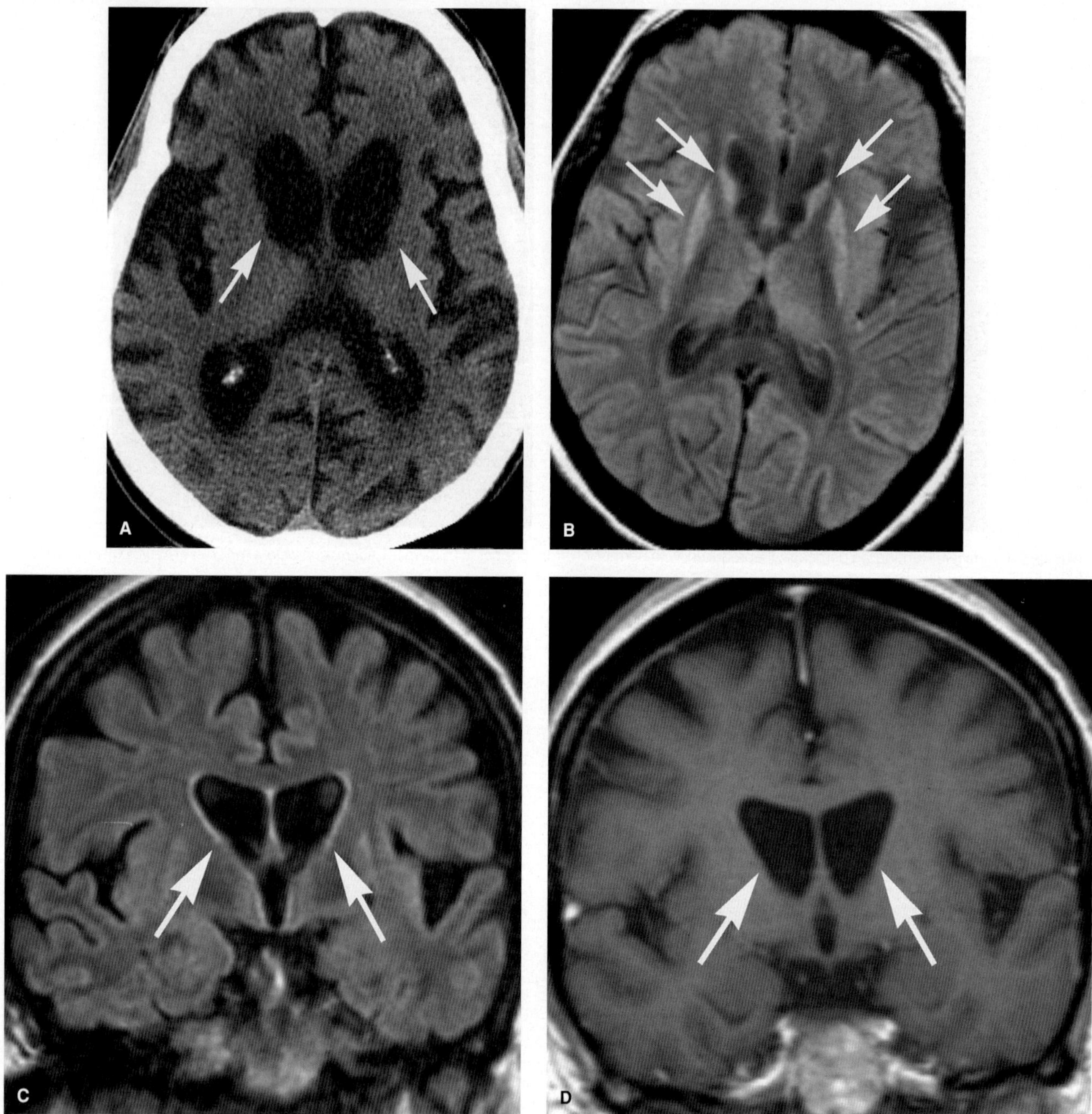

FIGURE 89-4 Axial noncontrast CT (**A**) demonstrates symmetric bilateral severe atrophy involving the caudate nuclei, putamen, and globus pallidi bilaterally with consequent enlargement of the frontal horns of the lateral ventricles (***arrows***). There is also diffuse prominence of the sulci indicating generalized cortical atrophy. Axial (**B**) and coronal (**C**) FLAIR images demonstrate bilateral symmetric abnormal high signal in the caudate and putamen. Coronal T1-weighted image (**D**) demonstrates enlarged frontal horns with abnormal configuration. Also note diffusely decreased marrow signal, which could represent anemia or myeloproliferative disease. (From Longo DL, et al., eds. *Harrison's Principles of Internal Medicine.* 18th ed. http://www.accessmedicine.com.)

IMPAIRMENTS

- Arousal
- Attention
- Behavior
- Cognition
- Gait[3]
- Wheelchair mobility[4]
- Balance
  - Static sit
  - Dynamic sit
  - Static stand
  - Dynamic stand
  - Moving base of support (BOS)
- Muscle strength
- Muscle recruitment
- Coordination
- Postural control (due to choreoathetosis)
- Posture (later stages)
- Range of motion (ROM)
- Reflexes

- Deep tendon reflexes (DTR)
- Babinski
- Clonus
- Muscle tone
- Motor planning
- Bed mobility
- Transfers
- Endurance
- Aerobic capacity
- Self-care
- Home management
- Fine motor
- Respiratory compromise

TESTS AND MEASURES

- Cognition: Mini-Mental State Examination (MMSE),[5] executive function tests, memory, comprehension, speed of processing, attention, and concentration
- Strength and muscle endurance
- Coordination: Gross and fine motor
- Muscle tone: Look for fluctuations between normal and high tones; tone changes with patient's level of anxiety, frustration
- Joint ROM: passive and active; note end-feel, any contractures, particularly later stages of disease
- Flexibility: specific muscle length, spinal flexibility during functional activities
- Cranial nerve integrity, especially related to swallowing
- Sensation, especially deep and combined cortical sensations
- Postural alignment
  - Balance (TUG, multi-directional reach test (MDRT),[6] Tinetti,[7] BBS)
  - As disease progresses, it becomes more difficult to use balance measures; patient will struggle due to the cognitive decline and extraneous movements
- Gait (TUG, Tinetti, 10-m walk test, DGI in early stage of disease, dual-task walking test)
  - As disease progresses, it becomes more difficult to use gait measures; patient will struggle due to the cognitive decline and extraneous movements
- Respiratory function: May be difficult for patient to understand more involved measures of respiratory function; monitor breath rate and patterns
- Integumentary: Greater concern in middle and late stages
- Functional mobility: Bed mobility, transfers, gait become more challenging as disease progresses
- United Huntington Disease Rating Scale: Examines cognitive and motor function specific to Huntington disease

INTERVENTION

- Increase aerobic capacity and endurance
  - Passive and active stretching of accessory muscles
  - Spirometry if patient can understand testing procedure[8]
  - Aerobic training
- Balance and coordination: Keep as functional and automatic as possible
  - Balance strategies
  - Speed/reaction-time training with small amplitude, controlled movements
  - Multitasking
- Gait
  - With or without assistive device
  - Direction changes and turning
  - Auditory cues (rhythmic metronome) for assistance as cognition declines
- Postural activities: Focus on coactivation of the trunk; proprioceptive neuromuscular facilitation (PNF) techniques[9]
- Flexibility and stretching
- Strength and resistance training

FUNCTIONAL GOALS

- Early stage
  - Patient or caregiver will report less than two episodes of falling in the home within 1 month of starting physical therapy.
  - Patient will demonstrate aerobic endurance appropriate to age range on recumbent stationary bike.
- Middle stage
  - Patient will
    - Perform car transfers with moderate physical assistance and maximal verbal cues from caregiver.
    - Ambulate >150 feet with one handheld and consistent cadence without significant increase in respiratory rate.
- Late stage
  - Caregiver will
    - Demonstrate consistent and safe transfers between bed and wheelchair to allow patient greater interaction with environment.
    - Demonstrate knowledge and physical ability to monitor pressure sores, prevent patient skin breakdown.

PROGNOSIS

- Poor: Disease is progressive and degenerative.
- Decline to vegetative state within 10 to 20 years of symptom onset for most patients.[10]

PATIENT RESOURCE

- Huntington's Disease Society of America. http://www.hdsa.org/. Accessed June 30, 2013.

REFERENCES

1. The American Physical Therapy Association. Pattern 5E: Impaired motor function and sensory integrity associated with progressive disorders of the central nervous system. *Interactive Guide to Physical Therapist Practice*. 2003. DOI: 10.2522/ptguide.3.2_5. http://guidetoptpractice.apta.org/content/1/SEC22.extract. Accessed May 14, 2014.
2. Toy EC. Huntington Disease, Case 91. LANGE Case Files. www.accessmedicine.com. Accessed May 14, 2014.
3. Waxman SG. *Clinical Neuroanatomy*. New York, NY: McGraw-Hill; 2010. http://www.accessphysiotherapy.com/resource/22. Accessed June 30, 2013.
4. Shamus E, Feingold Stern D. *Effective Documentation for Physical Therapy Professionals, 2e*. New York, NY: McGraw-Hill; 2011. http://www.accessphysiotherapy.com/resource/696. Accessed June 30, 2013.
5. Dutton M. *McGraw Hill's NPTE (National Physical Therapy Examination), 2e*. New York, NY: McGraw-Hill; 2012. http://www.accessphysiotherapy.com/resource/611. Accessed June 30, 2013.

6. Temple University Gait Study Center. Multi-direction reach test. http://podiatry.temple.edu/research/gait-study-center/techniques-and-methods/multi-directional-reach-test. Accessed May 14, 2014.
7. Tinetti Balance and Gait Evaluation. http://www.bhps.org.uk/falls/documents/TinettiBalanceAssessment.pdf. Accessed June 30, 2013.
8. Federico MJ, Kerby GS, Detering RR, et al. Chapter 19. Respiratory tract & mediastinum. In: Hay W, Levin MJ, Sondheimer JM, Detering RR, eds. *CURRENT Diagnosis & Treatment: Pediatrics*. New York, NY: McGraw-Hill; 2011. http://accessphysiotherapy.mhmedical.com/content.aspx?bookid=497§ionid=40851686. Accessed May 14, 2014.
9. Dutton M. *Dutton's Orthopedic Survival Guide: Managing Common Conditions*. New York, NY: McGraw-Hill; 2011. http://www.accessphysiotherapy.com/resource/685. Accessed June 30, 2013.
10. Chandrasoma P, Taylor CR. Degenerative diseases. In: Chandrasoma P, Taylor CR, eds. *Concise Pathology*. 3rd ed. Stamford, CT: Appleton & Lang; 1998. http://www.accessphysiotherapy.com/content/193234#193234. Accessed June 30, 2013.

ADDITIONAL REFERENCES

- Standaert DG, Roberson ED. Treatment of central nervous system degenerative disorders. In: Brunton LL, Chabner BA, Knollmann BC, eds. *Goodman & Gilman's The Pharmacological Basis of Therapeutics, 12e*. New York, NY: McGraw-Hill; 2011. http://accesspharmacy.com/Content.aspx?searchStr=huntington's+disease&aid=16665971. Accessed June 30, 2013.
- ICD9DATA web site. http://www.icd9data.com. Accessed June 30, 2013.
- ICD10DATA web site. http://www.icd10data.com. Accessed June 30, 2013.
- Gövert F, Schneider SA. Huntington's disease and Huntington's disease-like syndromes: an overview. *Curr Opin Neurol.* 2013;26(4):420–427. DOI: 10.1097/WCO.0b013e3283632d90.
- Melnick ME. Metabolic, hereditary, and genetic disorders in adults with basal ganglia movement disorders. In: Umphred DA, ed. *Neurological Rehabilitation*. 5th ed. St. Louis, MO: Mosby Elsevier. 2007: 793–799.
- Ropper AL, Samuels MA. *Adams and Victor's Principles of Neurology*. 9th ed. New York, NY: McGraw-Hill; 2009: 1027–1031. http://www.accessphysiotherapy.com/content/6092290. Accessed June 30, 2013.
- Ropper AH, Samuels MA. Degenerative diseases of the nervous system. In: *Adams and Victor's Principles of Neurology, 9e*. New York, NY: McGraw-Hill; 2009. http://accessmedicine.com/content.aspx?aID=3639135&searchStr=huntington's+disease. Accessed June 30, 2013.

90 HYDROCEPHALUS

Mollie Venglar, DSc, MSPT, NCS

CONDITION/DISORDER SYNONYM

- Raised/increased intracranial pressure

ICD-9-CM CODE

- 331.4 Hydrocephalus

ICD-10-CM CODE

- G91.9 Hydrocephalus (acquired) (external) (internal) (malignant) (recurrent)

PREFERRED PRACTICE PATTERNS

- 5C: Impaired Motor Function and Sensory Integrity Associated with Nonprogressive Disorders of the Central Nervous System—congenital origin or acquired in infancy or childhood[1]
- 5D: Impaired Motor Function and Sensory Integrity Associated with Nonprogressive Disorders of the Central Nervous System—acquired in adolescence or adulthood[2]
- 5E: Impaired Motor Function and Sensory Integrity Associated with Progressive Disorders of the Central Nervous System[3]

PATIENT PRESENTATION

On a recent visit to her father's house a woman noted that her 73-year-old father seemed to move slower than he recalled from previous visits. Her father seemed to struggle to follow involved conversations and he got frustrated with "losing" objects around the house. Her father had bruising on his left elbow and forearm but would only say that he lost his balance "a little". In his past medical history, the man had suffered a mild stroke 4 years ago with subsequent hydrocephalus. At that time, he had a ventriculoperitoneal shunt placed. He had no physical or cognitive sequelae from the stroke after the first year. The woman took her father to his neurologist. Testing revealed that the shunt had malfunctioned and his intracranial pressure (ICP) exceeded 25 mm Hg.

KEY FEATURES

Description

- ICP beyond what cranium and vertebral column can accommodate
- Reduced cerebrospinal fluid (CSF) production, decreased cerebral blood volume

Essentials of Diagnosis

- Two types of hydrocephalus
  - Noncommunicating
  - Communicating

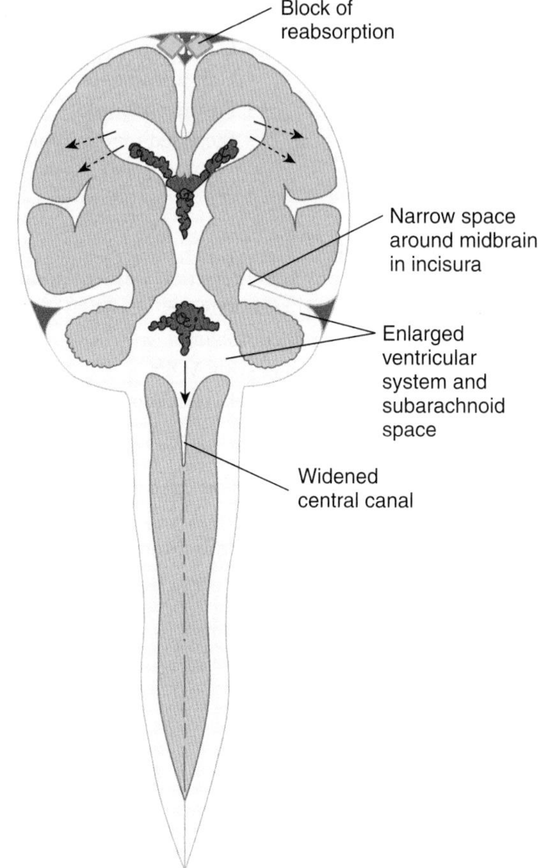

FIGURE 90-1 Schematic illustration of the effect of obstruction of reabsorption of CSF causing communicating hydrocephalus. *Arrows* indicate transependymal flow. Another possible site of obstruction is at the narrow space around the midbrain in the incisura. (From Waxman SG. *Clinical Neuroanatomy*. 26th ed. http://www.accessmedicine.com. Copyright © The McGraw-Hill Companies, Inc. All rights reserved.)

- Change in ICP for a given change in intracranial volume is called intracranial compliance.
- Normal compliance curve begins steep rise at approximately 25 mm Hg.
- If brain, blood, CSF volumes continue to increase, accommodative mechanisms fail and ICP rises exponentially.
- Diagnosis made via monitoring intracranial pressure
  - Above 25 mm Hg considered hydrocephalus

General Considerations

- Numerical difference between ICP and mean blood pressure in cerebral vessels is the cerebral perfusion pressure.
  - A widespread reduction in cerebral perfusion occurs as ICP approaches the mean systemic blood pressure, resulting in ischemia and brain death.
  - Reduced cerebral perfusion pressure can result in cerebral infarction.
- Normal ICP range between 2 to 5 mm Hg

Demographics
- Hydrocephalus can occur in any age group

CLINICAL FINDINGS

SIGNS AND SYMPTOMS
- Headache
- Neck pain
- Nausea
- Vomiting
- Drowsiness
- Ocular palsy
- Papilledema
- Confusion
- Gait disturbance
- Positive Babinski
- Increased tone in limbs

Functional Implications
- Decreased cognitive or physical interaction with environment
- Poor safety with gait and balance activities
- Decline in judgment or problem solving
- Decline or loss of independence with ADLs
- Inability to participate school, work, recreational activities

Possible Contributing Causes
- Cerebral or extracerebral mass (tumor, edema, abscess)
- Generalized brain swelling
- Increased venous pressure (venous sinus thrombosis, heart failure)
- Choroid plexus tumor
- Meningitis
- Ventricle obstruction
- Chiari malformation[4]
- Arteriovenous malformation
- Myelomeningocele

Differential Diagnosis
- Brain tumor
- Chiari malformation
- Cerebrovascular accident
- Parkinson disease

MEANS OF CONFIRMATION OR DIAGNOSIS

Imaging
- CT for detailed imaging of brain[5]

Diagnostic Procedures
- ICP monitoring
- Lumbar puncture with progressive fluid reduction

REFERRALS/ADMITTANCE
- To ER physician if acute onset
- To neurologist for monitoring
- To neurosurgeon for shunt placement if patient is a candidate
- Other services as needed based on impairments (occupational therapy, speech therapy, neuropsychologist)

IMPAIRMENTS
- Attention
- Bed mobility
- Cognition
- Cranial nerve integrity
- Endurance

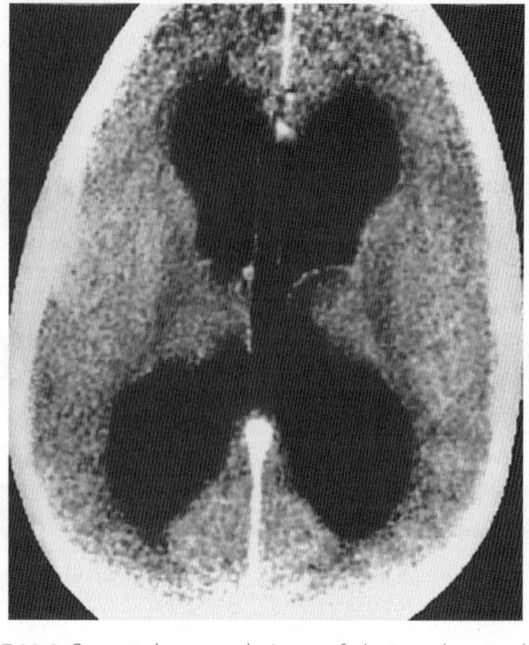

FIGURE 90-2 Computed tomography image of a horizontal section through the head of a 7-year-old child with noncommunicating hydrocephalus owing to the obstruction of the outflow foramens by a medulloblastoma. (From Waxman SG. *Clinical Neuroanatomy*. 26th ed. http://www.accessmedicine.com. Copyright © The McGraw-Hill Companies, Inc. All rights reserved.)

- Fine motor control
- Gait
- Home management
- Motor planning
- Muscle strength, coordination
- Muscle tone
- Postural control
- Self-care
- Sensation
- Sitting and standing balance (static and dynamic)
- Transfers

TESTS AND MEASURES
- Glasgow Coma Scale
- Modified Ashworth Scale
- Functional Independence Measure[6]

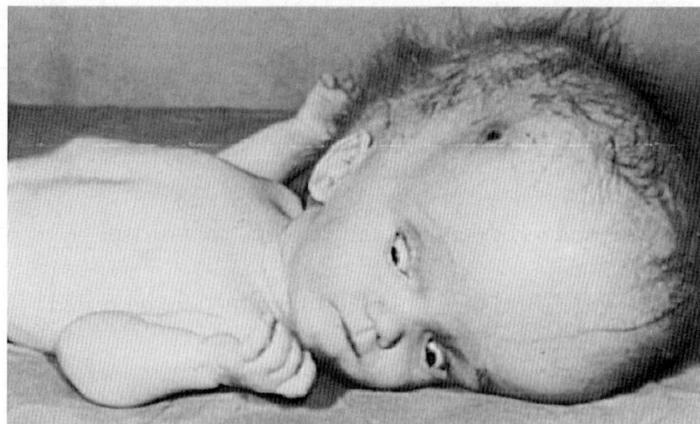

FIGURE 90-3 Hydrocephalus in a 14-month-old infant. (From Waxman SG. *Clinical Neuroanatomy*. 26th ed. http://www.accessmedicine.com. Copyright © The McGraw-Hill Companies, Inc. All rights reserved.)

- Gait and balance measures[7]
  - Tinetti performance-oriented mobility assessment[8]
  - Berg Balance Scale (BBS)
  - 6-minute walk test
  - Timed Up and Go (TUG)
  - Dynamic Gait Index (DGI)
  - Functional Gait Assessment (FGA)
  - Multi-directional reach test
  - Physical performance test
  - High-level mobility assessment tool (HiMAT) if appropriate for patients with appropriate scores on BBS and DGI
- Cognitive testing
- Sensory testing: May be limited by cognition, consciousness, aphasias
- Strength: Includes speed of force production and ability to change force production
- Active and passive ROM, flexibility, muscle length
- Bed mobility
- Transfers
- Cranial nerves: Particularly vision

INTERVENTION

- ROM, stretching, positioning
- Tone management
- Strengthening (including biofeedback, functional electrical stimulation)
- Balance training
- Gait training (appropriate bracing and assistive devices)
- Transfer training
- Orthotics management
- Bed-mobility training
- Wheelchair-mobility training
- Cardiovascular and pulmonary endurance
- Postural retraining

FUNCTIONAL GOALS

- Goals dependent on individual's age, degree of damage from elevated ICP. Following goals aimed at adult with mild-to-moderate impairment:
  - Patient will
    - Have 10% improved Dynamic Gait Index score to show improved balance safety during functional activities.
    - Be able to walk >500 ft with supervision, without assistive device on outdoor surfaces.
    - Perform a four-step task with no more than one verbal cue to show improved memory and learning.

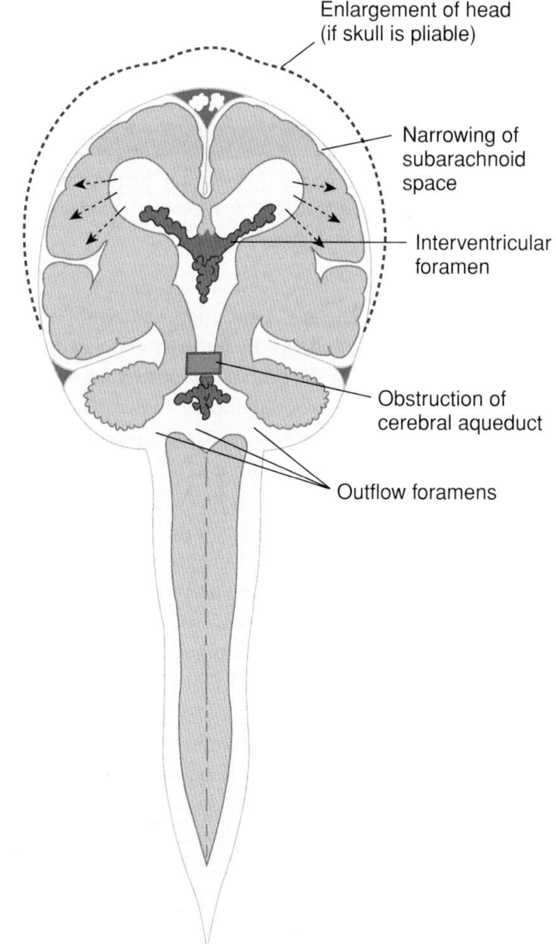

FIGURE 90-4 Schematic illustration of the effects of obstruction of the cerebral aqueduct causing noncommunicating hydrocephalus. *Arrows* indicate transependymal flow. Other possible sites of obstruction are the interventricular foramen and the outflow foramens of the fourth ventricle. (From Waxman SG. *Clinical Neuroanatomy*. 26th ed. http://www.accessmedicine.com. Copyright © The McGraw-Hill Companies, Inc. All rights reserved.)

    - Perform independent path-finding within healthcare facility with supervision and assistance to show improved problem-solving and functional mobility.

PROGNOSIS

- Use of the ventroperitoneal shunt improves likelihood of ICP control; however, the shunt may become obstructed or displaced, any change in the patient's presentation should be addressed immediately.

TABLE 90-1 Hydrocephalus

Type	Cause	Effect
Noncommunicating (obstructive)	Obstruction of interventricular foramen	Enlargement of lateral ventricle
	Obstruction of cerebral aqueduct	Enlargement of lateral and third ventricles
	Obstruction of outflow foramens of fourth ventricle	Enlargement of all ventricles
Communicating	Obstruction of perimesencephalic cistern (occlusion of incisura tentorii)	Enlargement of all ventricles; widening of posterior fossa cisterns
	Obstruction of subarachnoid CSF flow over the cerebral convexities	Enlargement of all ventricles, widening of all basal cisterns

Source: From Waxman SG: *Clinical Neuroanatomy*. 26th ed. http://www.accessmedicine.com. Copyright © The McGraw-Hill Companies, Inc. All rights reserved.

- Uncontrolled ICP will result in death.
- Poorly controlled ICP will result in brain damage, degree of which depends on the extent and duration of elevated ICP.

PATIENT RESOURCE

- Hydrocephalus. Hydrocephalus Association. http://www.hydroassoc.org. Accessed June 15, 2013.

REFERENCES

1. The American Physical Therapy Association. Pattern 5C: impaired motor function and sensory integrity associated with nonprogressive disorders of the central nervous system - congenital origin or acquired in infancy or childhood. *Interactive Guide to Physical Therapist Practice.* 2003. doi: 10.2522/ptguide.3.2_3. http://guidetoptpractice.apta.org/content/1/SEC20.extract?sid=f364ed2a-f329-410e-aca6-3b959af5ba40. Accessed May 15, 2014.
2. The American Physical Therapy Association. Pattern 5D: impaired motor function and sensory integrity associated with nonprogressive disorders of the central nervous system - acquired in adolescence or adulthood. *Interactive Guide to Physical Therapist Practice.* 2003. doi: 10.2522/ptguide.3.2_4. http://guidetoptpractice.apta.org/content/1/SEC21.extract?sid=37e24d1e-1855-428d-8c69-67ddb5a343c4. Accessed May 15, 2014.
3. The American Physical Therapy Association. Pattern 5E: impaired motor function and sensory integrity associated with progressive disorders of the central nervous system. *Interactive Guide to Physical Therapist Practice.* 2003. doi: 10.2522/ptguide.3.2_5. http://guidetoptpractice.apta.org/content/1/SEC22.extract?sid=c24e223f-732e-42eb-b48a-3159d816e6a2. Accessed May 15, 2014.
4. Bernard TJ, Knupp K, Yang ML, Arndt D, Levinson P, Moe PG. Neurologic & muscular disorders. In: Hay W, Levin MJ, Sondheimer JM, Detering RR, eds. *CURRENT Diagnosis & Treatment: Pediatrics.* New York, NY: McGraw-Hill; 2011: Chapter 23. http://www.accessphysiotherapy.com/abstract/6585385#6585406. Accessed June 22, 2013.
5. Malone TR, Hazle C, Grey ML. *Imaging in Rehabilitation.* New York: McGraw-Hill; 2008. http://www.accessphysiotherapy.com/resource/613. Accessed June 22, 2013.
6. Shamus E, Stern DF. *Effective Documentation for Physical Therapy Professionals.* 2nd ed.New York, NY: McGraw-Hill; 2011. http://www.accessphysiotherapy.com/resource/696. Accessed June 22, 2013.
7. University of Missouri. *Geriatric Examination Tool Kit.* http://web.missouri.edu/~proste/tool/. Accessed June 22, 2013.
8. Tinetti Balance and Gait Evaluation. http://accessphysiotherapy.mhmedical.com/book.aspx?bookID=441. Accessed May 14, 2014.

ADDITIONAL REFERENCES

- Barkovich AJ, Kuzniecky RI, Jackson GD, Guerrini R, Dobyns WB. A developmental and genetic classification for malformations of cortical development. *Neurology.* 2005;65(12):1873–1887.
- Doherty D, Shurtleff DB. Pediatric perspective on prenatal counseling for myelomeningocele. *Birth Defects Res A Clin Mol Teratol.* 2006;76(9):645–653.
- ICD9DATA. http://www.icd9data.com. Accessed June 22, 2013.
- ICD10DATA. http://www.icd10data.com. Accessed June 22, 2013.
- Kotrikova B, Krempien R, Freier K, MuHling J. Diagnostic imaging in the management of craniosynostoses. *Eur Radiol.* 2007;17(8):1968–1978.
- Patel DR, Greydanus DE, Baker RJ. Meningomyelocele. In: Patel DR, Greydanus DE, Baker RJ, eds. *Pediatric Practice: Sports Medicine.* New York, NY: McGraw-Hill; 2009. http://www.accessphysiotherapy.com/content/6982280. Accessed June 15, 2013.
- Paul LK, Brown WS, Adolphs R, et al. Agenesis of the corpus callosum: Genetic, developmental and functional aspects of connectivity. *Nat Rev Neurosci.* 2007;8(4):287–299.
- Ropper AL, Samuels MA. Adams *and Victor's Principles of Neurology.* 9th ed. New York, NY: McGraw-Hill; 2009.
- Vertinsky AT, Barnes PD. Macrocephaly, increased intracranial pressure, and hydrocephalus in the infant and young child. *Top Magn Reson Imaging.* 2007;18(1):31–51.

91 MENINGITIS

Mollie Venglar, DSc, MSPT, NCS

CONDITION/DISORDER SYNONYMS

- Leptomeningitis
- Bacterial meningitis
- Cryptococcal meningitis
- Haemophilus meningitis

ICD-9-CM CODES[1]

- 320 Bacterial meningitis
- 320.0 Haemophilus meningitis
- 320.1 Pneumococcal meningitis
- 320.2 Streptococcal meningitis
- 320.3 Staphylococcal meningitis
- 320.7 Meningitis in other bacterial diseases classified elsewhere
- 320.89 Meningitis due to other specified bacteria
- 321 Meningitis due to other organisms
- 321.0 Cryptococcal meningitis

ICD-10-CM CODES[2]

- B45.1 Cerebral cryptococcosis
- G00.0 Haemophilus meningitis
- G00.1 Pneumococcal meningitis
- G00.2 Streptococcal meningitis
- G00.3 Staphylococcal meningitis
- G00.8 Other bacterial meningitis
- G00.9 Bacterial meningitis, unspecified
- G01 Meningitis in other bacterial diseases classified elsewhere

PREFERRED PRACTICE PATTERNS[3]

- 5A: Primary Prevention/Risk Reduction for Loss of Balance and Falling
- 5C: Impaired Motor Function and Sensory Integrity Associated With Nonprogressive Disorders of the Central Nervous System—congenital origin or acquired in infancy or childhood
- 5D: Impaired Motor Function and Sensory Integrity Associated With Nonprogressive Disorders of the Central Nervous System—acquired in adolescence or adulthood
- 5I: Impaired Arousal, Range of Motion and Motor Control Associated With Coma, Near Coma, or Vegetative State

PATIENT PRESENTATION

A 27-year-old woman is seen in the in-patient rehabilitation center for physical rehabilitation following meningitis. The woman suffered heart and lung failure and generalized convulsions before responding to the medications provided in the ICU. Presently, the woman presents with poor postural control and reduced muscle tone in her trunk and extremities. She tolerates very little time in a fully upright position. Her cognition is impaired and her attention to task is limited to approximately 10 seconds.

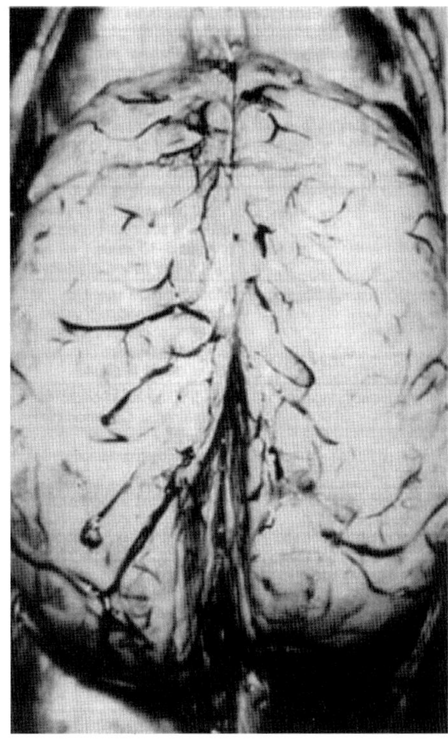

FIGURE 91-1 Pyogenic meningitis, showing obliteration of the gyri of the brain surface by the purulent exudate. (From Chandrasoma P, Taylor CR. *Concise Pathology*. 3rd ed. http://www.accessmedicine.com. Copyright © The McGraw-Hill Companies, Inc. All rights reserved.)

KEY FEATURES

Description

- Infection of the meninges of the brain and spinal cord caused by a microorganism
- Severity and extent of the infection causes a wide range of neurologic signs and symptoms, generally nonfocal in nature

Essentials of Diagnosis

- Headache and neck stiffness are common with all infections of the central nervous system.
- No physical test distinguishes a bacterial from a viral infection; must rely on body fluid cultures.
- If a central nervous system infection is suspected, the therapist should seek information regarding a potential source of infection or a condition that predisposed the patient to infection.

General Considerations

- Haemophilus meningitis is caused by the *haemophilus influenzae* bacteria.
  - The most common form of meningitis.
  - Acquired following an upper respiratory infection.

- Bacterial meningitis is caused by a wide range of bacteria.
  - Onset of symptoms is very rapid and considered a medical emergency.
- Cryptococcal meningitis is caused by the fungus *Cryptococcus neoformans.*
  - Found in soil around the world.
  - Onset is slower than bacterial meningitis.

Demographics

- Commonly nosocomial or iatrogenic
- Most common worldwide forms of meningitis include: Pneumococcal, influenza, and meningococcal
- Other bacteria cause meningitis, but may be less common in some parts of the world than others
- Approximately 3/100,000 in the United States; 500/100,000 in Africa

CLINICAL FINDINGS

SIGNS AND SYMPTOMS

- Headache, stiff neck
- Change in mental status (confusion, delirium)
- Fever or hypothermia
- Malaise
- Impaired heart, lung, liver, kidney function
- Seizure, generalized convulsions
- Sensory deficit/change
- Motor deficit/change
- With increased intracranial pressure, papilledema may develop
- With prolonged infection, cranial nerves may become effected

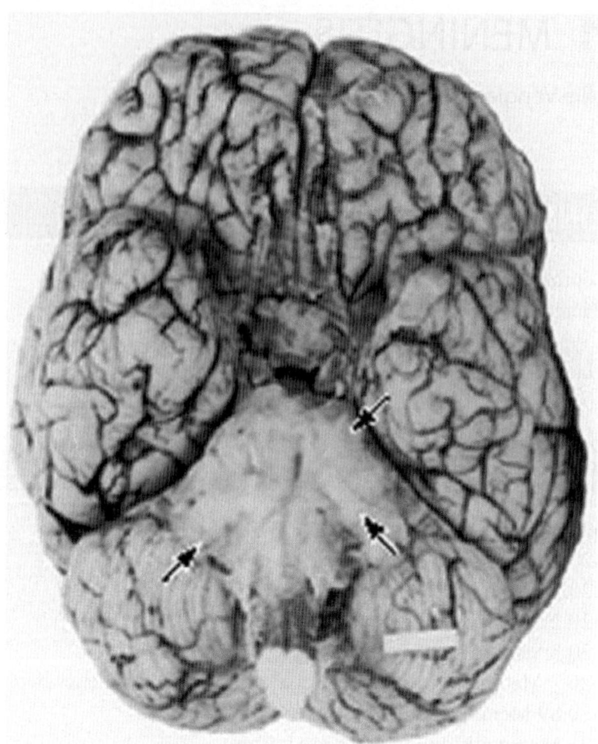

FIGURE 91-2 Autopsy specimen in a patient with tuberculous meningitis, with prominent basilar exudate (*arrows*). (Reproduced with permission from Waxman SG. *Clinical Neuroanatomy*. 26th ed. New York, NY: McGraw-Hill; 2010:Fig. 25-17.)

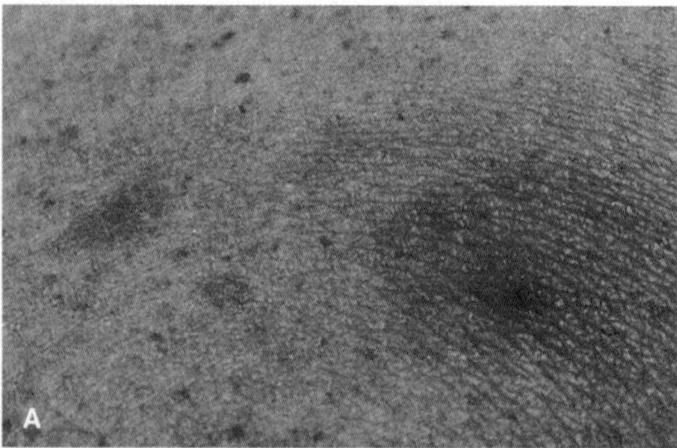

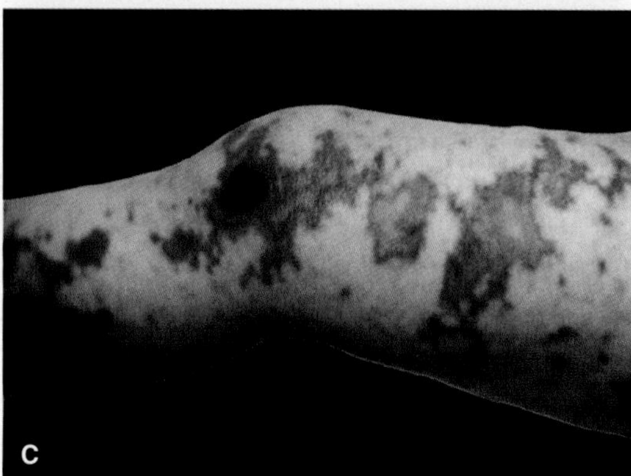

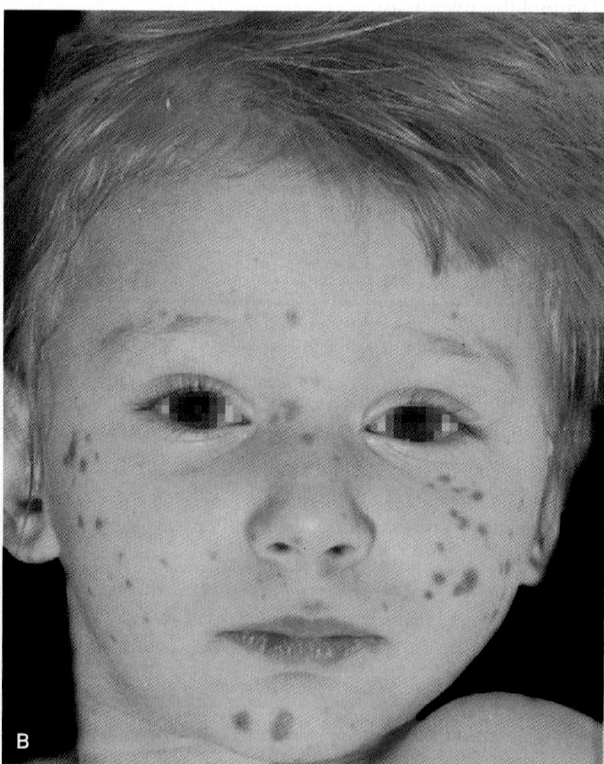

FIGURE 91-3 *Neisseria meningitidis* infection. Acute meningococcemia. **A.** Transient macular and papular lesions on the upper chest. **B.** Discrete pink-to-purple macules and papules, as well as purpura, on the face of a young child. These lesions represent early diffuse intravascular coagulation (DIC). **C.** Map-like gray-to-black areas of cutaneous infarction are seen in this child with DIC. (From Goldsmith LA, Katz SI, Gilchrest BA, Paller A, Leffell DJ, Wolff K eds. *Fitzpatrick's Dermatology in General Medicine*. 8th ed. http://www.accessmedicine.com. Copyright © The McGraw-Hill Companies, Inc. All rights reserved.)

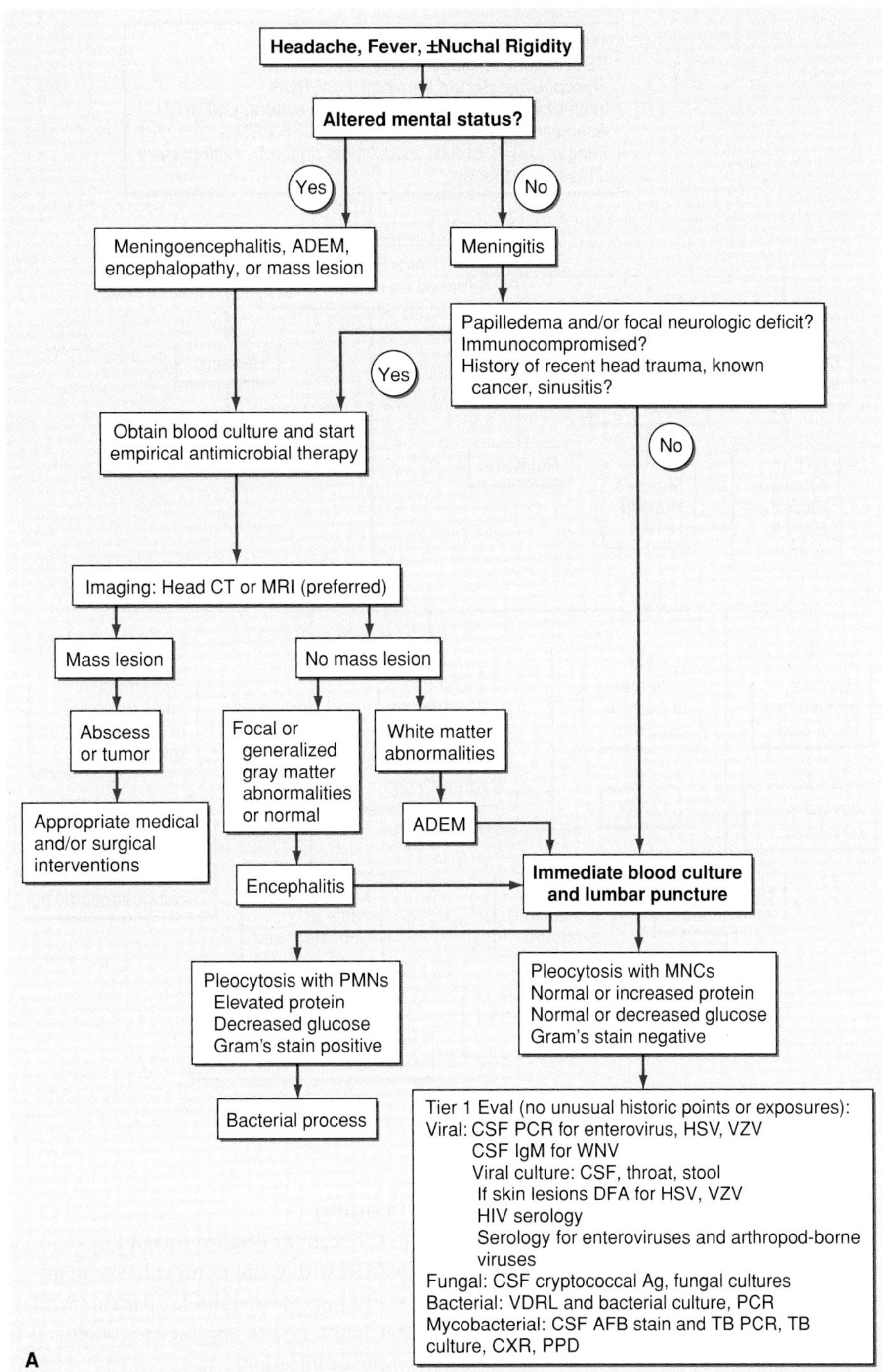

FIGURE 91-4 The management of patients with suspected CNS infection. ADEM, acute disseminated encephalomyelitis; AFB, acid-fast bacillus; Ag, antigen; CSF, cerebrospinal fluid; CT, computed tomography; CTFV, Colorado tick fever virus; CXR, chest x-ray; DFA, direct fluorescent antibody; EBV, Epstein–Barr virus; HHV, human herpesvirus; HSV, herpes simplex virus; LCMV, lymphocytic choriomeningitis virus; MNCs, mononuclear cells; MRI, magnetic resonance imaging; PCR, polymerase chain reaction; PMNs, polymorphonuclear leukocytes; PPD, purified protein derivative; TB, tuberculosis; VDRL, Venereal Disease Research Laboratory; VZV, varicella-zoster virus; WNV, West Nile virus. (From Longo DL, Fauci AS, Kasper DL, Hauser SL, Jameson JL, Loscalzo J, eds. *Harrison's Principles of Internal Medicine.* 18th ed. http://www.accessmedicine.com. Copyright © The McGraw-Hill Companies, Inc. All rights reserved.) *(continued)*

Functional Implications

- Loss of mobility temporarily with permanent loss possible
- Loss of hearing/vestibular function in some cases
- Temporary loss of coordination, fine and gross motor skills; permanent loss possible.
- Loss of independence with activities of daily living
- Reduced cognitive function, particularly executive functions

Possible Contributing Causes

- Severe sinus infection
- Cranial or spinal surgery
- Shunt placement
- Open head injury
- Diseases of the middle ear and paranasal sinuses
- Dural tears from remote trauma

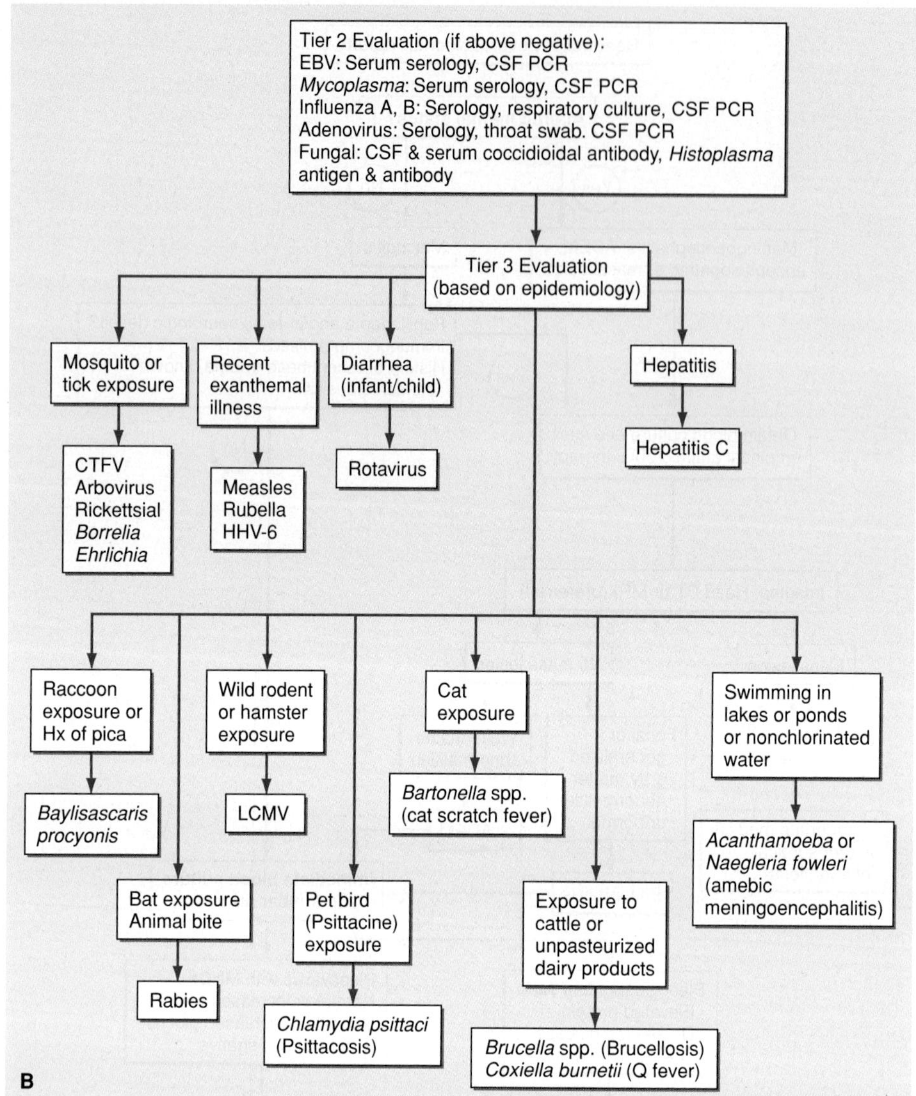

FIGURE 91-4 *(Continued)*

- Ruptured brain abscess
- Congenital anomaly
- Diabetes

Differential Diagnoses

- Extrapyramidal rigidity
- Hydrocephalus
- Alcoholic intoxication or withdrawal
- Hepatic encephalopathy
- Subarachnoid hemorrhage
- Meningoencephalitis
- Epstein–Barr virus
- Behçet's disease

MEANS OF CONFIRMATION OR DIAGNOSIS

Laboratory Tests

- Complete blood count, general chemistry panel, and culture to determine the microorganism involved and the extent of the infection
  - Lumbar puncture to test cerebral spinal fluid

Imaging

- CT scan for detailed imaging
- MRI with gadolinium enhancement
- EEG may be helpful for patients with seizure due to infection
- Chest x-rays to disclose area of abscess that may be the original site of infection

FINDINGS AND INTERPRETATION

- Lumbar puncture to test cerebral spinal fluid for presence of red and white blood cells, protein concentration, glucose, and microorganisms.
  - Presence of high polymorphonuclear leukocytes, high protein, low glucose suggests bacterial infection.
  - Presence of predominant lymphocytes, high protein, low glucose suggests infection with mycobacteria, fungi, uncommon bacteria, and viruses, such as herpes simplex, mumps, arbovirus
  - Presence of high lymphocytes, normal protein, normal glucose suggests viral infection.
  - Spinal fluid concentrations of various central nervous system infections.

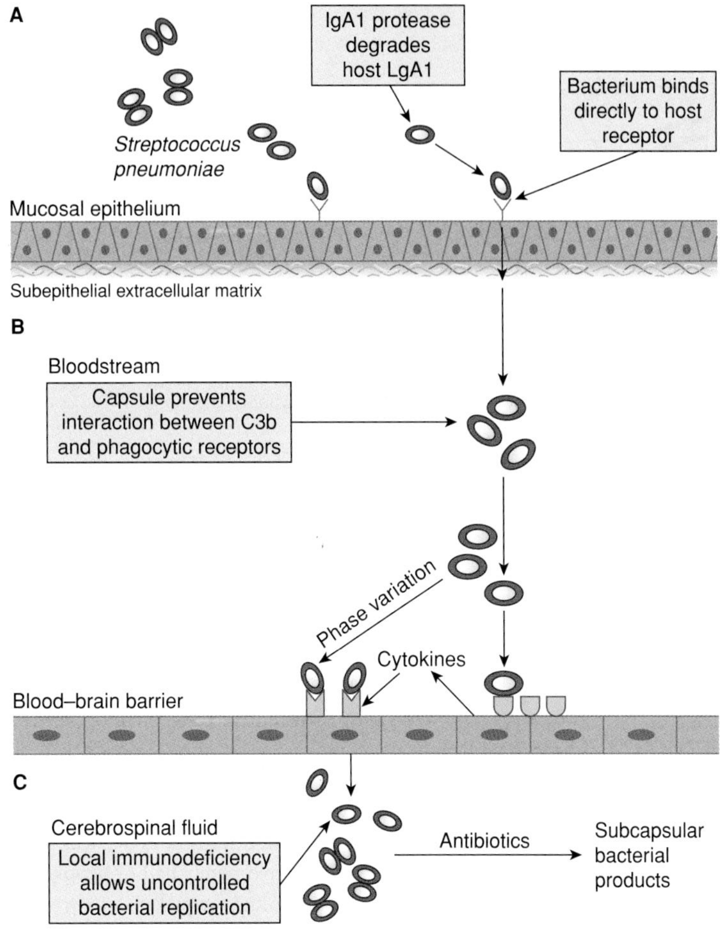

FIGURE 91-5 Pathogenic steps leading to pneumococcal meningitis. The pneumococcus adheres to and colonizes the nasopharynx. IgA1 protease protects the pneumococcus from host antibody (**A**). Once in the bloodstream, the bacterial capsule helps the pneumococcus to evade opsonization (**B**). The pneumococcus accesses the cerebrospinal fluid through receptors on the endothelial surface of the blood-brain barrier (**C**). (Redrawn with permission from Koedel U, Scheld WM, Pfister HW. Pathogenesis and pathophysiology of pneumococcal meningitis. *Lancet Infect Dis.* 2002;2:731.)

TREATMENT

Medications

- Broad-spectrum antibiotics until microorganism is identified, then specific antibiotic
- Third- and fourth-generation cephalosporins
- Corticosteroids

REFERRALS/ADMITTANCE

- To hospital emergency department if meningitis is suspected
- To OT for ADL and cognitive retraining
- To respiratory therapy if source of infection is pulmonary in origin
- To neurologist both during infection and for follow-up
- To otolaryngologist for middle- and inner-ear testing
- To social worker and case management team for multiple resources

IMPAIRMENTS

- Aerobic capacity
- Arousal
- Attention
- Bed mobility
- Behavior
- Cognition
- Cranial nerve integrity
- Deep tendon reflexes
- Endurance
- Fine motor control
- Gait
- Hearing Loss
- Home management
- Muscle strength
- Muscle tone
- Postural control
- Range of motion (ROM)
- Respiratory control
- Self-care
- Sensation
- Sitting and standing balance
- Transfers

TESTS AND MEASURES

- Kernig sign: Inability to extend the knees when hips flexed
- Brudzinski sign: Flexion of hip and knee in response to flexion of the neck
- Cognition: Mini-Mental State Examination (MMSE), executive function tests, memory, comprehension
- Pain: Subjective report, Visual Analog Scale (VAS), or verbal report

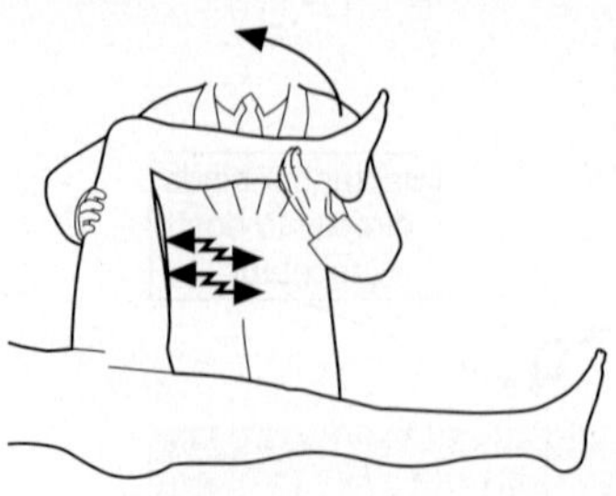

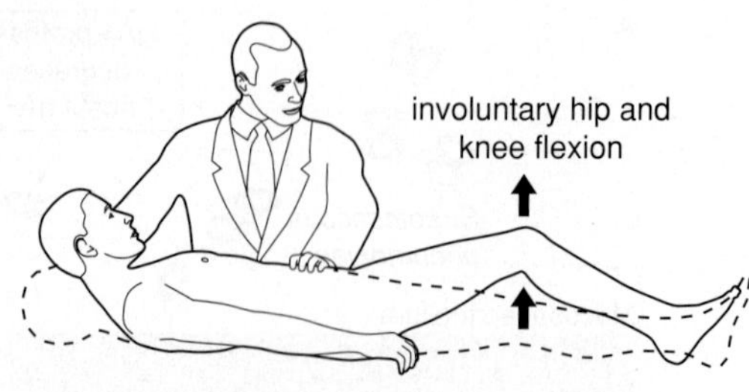

FIGURE 91-6 Two signs of meningeal irritation. **A.** Kernig sign: With the patient supine, flex the hip and knee, each to about 90 degrees. With the hip immobile, attempt to extend the knee. In meningeal irritation, this attempt is resisted and causes pain in the hamstring muscles. **B.** Brudzinski sign: Place the patient supine and hold the thorax down on the bed. Attempt to flex the neck. With meningeal irritation this causes involuntary flexion of the hips. (From LeBlond RF, DeGowin RL, Brown DD. *DeGowin's Diagnostic Examination*. 9th ed. http://www.accessmedicine.com. Copyright © The McGraw-Hill Companies, Inc. All rights reserved.)

- Strength and muscle endurance
- Coordination
- Muscle tone
- Joint ROM
- Cranial nerve integrity: Specific tests of vestibular function if deficits are evident
- Sensation
- Postural alignment
- Balance: Timed Up and Go test (TUG), Mutidirectional Reach Test (MDRT), Tinetti Balance and Gait Evaluation, Berg Balance Scale (BBS)
- Gait: TUG, Tinetti, 10-m walk test, Dynamic Gait Index (DGI)
- Respiratory function (spirometer, oxygen saturation, auscultation)
- Functional mobility (Functional Independence Measure [FIM^{tm}])

INTERVENTION

- Should be based on the extent and location of central nervous system damage resulting from the infection.
- Patients with active infection should be cautiously treated by a physical therapist due to high risk of developing communicating hydrocephalus and/or ischemic stroke early in the disease.
- Once cleared for more active treatment, interventions can include
  - Functional mobility: Bed mobility, transfers, gait
  - Balance and coordination activities: Postural control, balance strategies, speed/reaction time, multi tasking
  - Flexibility and stretching
  - Strength and resistance training
  - Pulmonary and cardiovascular reconditioning
  - Problem-solving and motor-planning skills

FUNCTIONAL GOALS

Note: Goals for people recovering from an infectious disease of the brain are specific to the identified impairments. These are general goals and would need to be made more specific for each patient.

- Short-term goals
  - Patient will be able to
    - Perform transfers to and from level surfaces with minimal physical assistance and minimal verbal cues for sequencing.
    - Ambulate on level tile surfaces with appropriate assistive device and moderate assistance for balance and sequencing.
    - Consistently perform a two-step motor task without verbal or visual cueing.
- Long-term goals
  - Patient will be able to
- Maintain postural control independently while ambulating on community surfaces for >15 minutes.
- Ambulate distances greater than 1000 ft without physical assistance, with occasional verbal cues for safety.
- Complete a multi step task (greater than three steps) successfully without verbal, visual, or physical cueing.

PROGNOSIS

- Left untreated, meningitis is usually fatal.
- Highest death rates occur in children and the elderly.
- Approximately half of people who survive have serious neurologic sequelae.
- Persistent neurologic deficit is a predictor of later seizure activity.
- Use of certain antibiotics commonly results in ototoxicity; hearing loss may be a result of the meningitis or the medication.

PATIENT RESOURCES

- Kernig's sign of meningitis. In: Medline Plus. http://www.nlm.nih.gov/medlineplus/ency/imagepages/19077.htm. Accessed July 5, 2013.
- Meningitis. In: Medline Plus. http://www.nlm.nih.gov/medlineplus/ency/article/000680.htm. Accessed July 5, 2013.
- Meningitis-cryptococcal. In: Medline Plus. http://www.nlm.nih.gov/medlineplus/ency/article/000642.htm. Accessed July 5, 2013.

REFERENCES

1. APTA Guide to Physical Therapist Practice. http://guidetoptpractice.apta.org/. Accessed July 5, 2013.
2. ICD-9-CM. http://www.icd9data.com. Accessed July 5, 2013.
3. ICD-10-CM. http://www.icd10data.com. Accessed July 5, 2013.

ADDITIONAL REFERENCES

- Brudzinski's sign of meningitis. In: Medline Plus. http://www.nlm.nih.gov/medlineplus/ency/imagepages/19069.htm. Accessed July 5, 2013.
- Dewane JA, Porter RE. Inflammatory and infectious disorders of the brain. In: Umphred DA, ed. *Neurological Rehabilitation*. 5th ed. St. Louis, MO: Mosby Elsevier. 2007:659–661.
- Dutton M. Causes of head, face, and temporomandibular joint symptoms. In: Dutton M, ed. *Orthopaedic Examination,*

Evaluation, and Intervention. 2nd ed. New York, NY: McGraw-Hill; 2008. http://www.accessphysiotherapy.com/content/5547000. Accessed July 5, 2013.

- Geriatric Examination Tool Kit. University of Missouri School of Health Professions Department of Physical Therapy. http://web.missouri.edu/~proste/tool. Accessed July 5, 2013.
- Hay WW, Levin MJ, Sondheimer JM, Deterding RR. Lumbar puncture. In: Hay WW, Levin MJ, Sondheimer JM, Deterding RR, eds. *CURRENT Diagnosis & Treatment: Pediatrics*. 20th ed. New York, NY: McGraw-Hill; 2011. http://www.accessphysiotherapy.com/content/6585067. Accessed July 5, 2013.
- Hay WW, Levin MJ, Sondheimer JM, Deterding RR. Neurologic and muscular disorders. In: Hay WW, Levin MJ, Sondheimer JM, Deterding RR, eds. *CURRENT Diagnosis & Treatment: Pediatrics*. 20th ed. New York, NY: McGraw-Hill; 2011. http://www.accessphysiotherapy.com/content/6585048. Accessed July 5, 2013.
- Panus PC, Jobst EE, Masters SB, Katzung B, Tinsley SL, Trevor AJ. Corticosteroids and corticosteroid antagonists. In: Panus PC, Jobst EE, Masters SB, Katzung B, Tinsley SL, Trevor AJ, eds. *Pharmacology for the Physical Therapist*. New York, NY: McGraw-Hill; 2009. http://www.accessphysiotherapy.com/content/6093458. Accessed July 5, 2013.
- Panus PC, Jobst EE, Masters SB, Katzung B, Tinsley SL, Trevor AJ. Inhibitors of bacterial cell wall synthesis. In: Panus PC, Jobst EE, Masters SB, Katzung B, Tinsley SL, Trevor AJ, eds. *Pharmacology for the Physical Therapist*. New York, NY: McGraw-Hill; 2009. http://www.accessphysiotherapy.com/content/6093998. Accessed July 5, 2013.
- Ropper AL, Samuels MA. *Adams and Victor's Principles of Neurology*. 9th ed. New York, NY: McGraw-Hill; 2009:667–678.

92 BACTERIAL MENINGITIS

Mollie Venglar, DSc, MSPT, NCS

CONDITION/DISORDER SYNONYMS

- Meningitis
- Haemophilus meningitis

ICD-9-CM CODES

- 320 Bacterial meningitis
- 320.0 Haemophilus meningitis
- 320.1 Pneumococcal meningitis
- 320.2 Streptococcal meningitis
- 320.3 Staphylococcal meningitis
- 320.7 Meningitis in other bacterial diseases classified elsewhere
- 320.89 Meningitis due to other specified bacteria
- 321.0 Cryptococcal meningitis

ICD-10-CM CODES

- A48.8 Meningitis in other bacterial diseases classified elsewhere
- G00.8 Meningitis due to other specified bacteria
- G00.9 Bacterial meningitis

PREFERRED PRACTICE PATTERNS[1]

- 5A: Primary Prevention/Risk Reduction for Loss of Balance and Falling
- 5C: Impaired Motor Function and Sensory Integrity Associated with Nonprogressive Disorders of the Central Nervous System—congenital origin or acquired in infancy or childhood
- 5D: Impaired Motor Function and Sensory Integrity Associated with Nonprogressive Disorders of the Central Nervous System—acquired in adolescence or adulthood

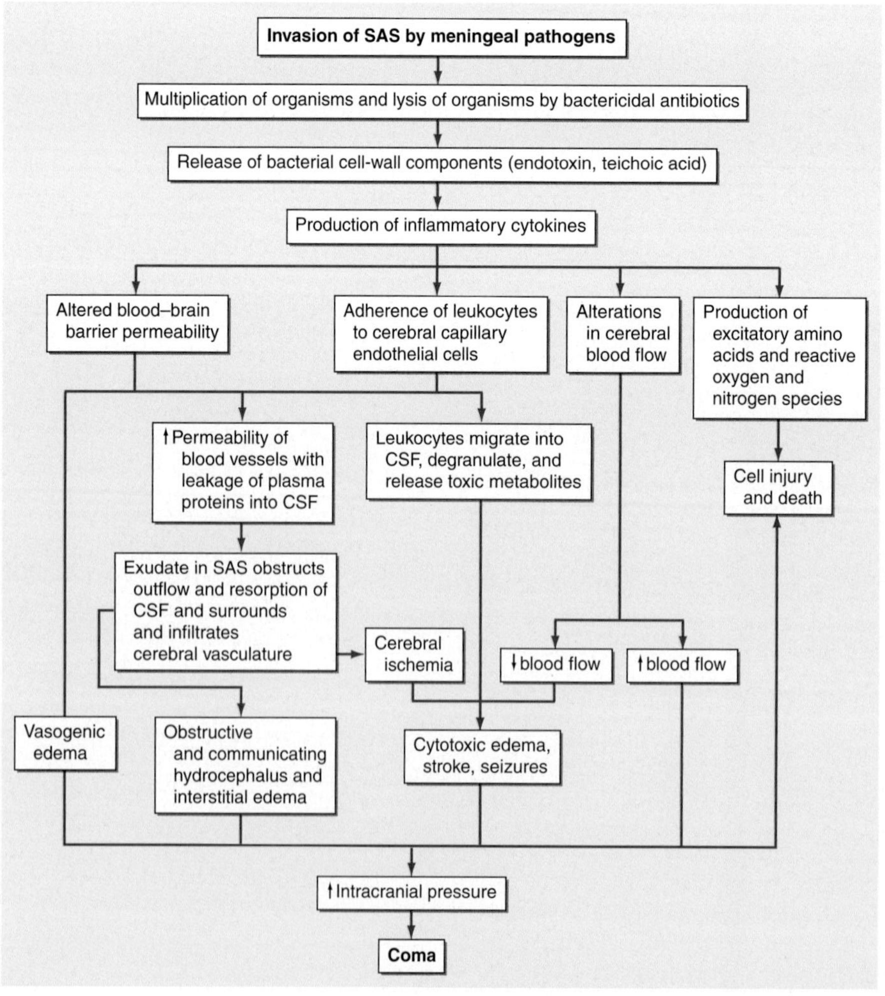

FIGURE 92-1 The pathophysiology of the neurologic complications of bacterial meningitis. CSF, cerebrospinal fluid; SAS, subarachnoid space. (From Longo DL, Fauci AS, Kasper DL, Hauser SL, Jameson JL, Loscalzo J, eds. *Harrison's Principles of Internal Medicine*. 18th ed. http://www.accessmedicine.com.)

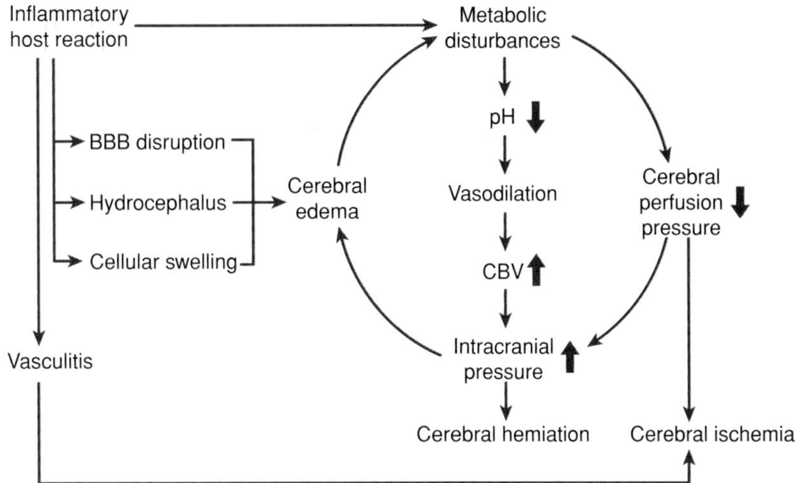

FIGURE 92-2 Pathophysiological alterations leading to neuronal injury during bacterial meningitis. BBB, blood–brain barrier; CBV, cerebral blood volume. (Redrawn with permission from Koedel U, Scheld WM, Pfister HW. Pathogenesis and pathophysiology of pneumococcal meningitis. *Lancet Infect Dis*. 2002;2:731.)

- 5I: Impaired Arousal, Range of Motion and Motor Control Associated with Coma, Near Coma, or Vegetative State

PATIENT PRESENTATION

An otherwise healthy 19-year-old man is brought to the emergency department (ED) by his roommate who states that he has "not been acting right" for the past 24 hours. As per the roommate, the patient had complained of a headache and fever for 2 days prior to arrival, and has been progressively somnolent and confused since then. His roommate states that the patient is a college student who does not use any illegal drugs and occasionally drinks alcohol. The patient has a fever of 38.5°C (101°F), a heart rate of 120 beats per minute, blood pressure of 114/69, and respiratory rate of 20 breaths per minute. His oxygen saturation is 98% on room air. The head and neck examination are significant for dry mucous membranes and nuchal rigidity. His skin is noted to be warm and without any rash. In the ED, he has a Glasgow Coma Score (GCS) of 10 (eyes open to voice [3], patient moans to painful stimuli [2], and localizes painful stimuli [5]). The motor examination is symmetric, and the patient appears to be sensate in all extremities. His reflexes are 2+ bilaterally throughout the upper and lower extremities with a negative Babinski. Blood work reveals a leukocytosis of 24,000/mm but is otherwise unremarkable. A computed tomography (CT) scan is completed which shows no mass, shift, bleed, or edema.[2]

KEY FEATURES

Description

- Infection of the meninges of the brain and spinal cord caused by a spread of bacteria
- Severity and extent causes a wide range of neurologic signs and symptoms, generally nonfocal in nature

Essentials of Diagnosis

- Bacterial meningitis is rare.
- Infection can result due to the following:
  - Head injury
  - Severe local infection
  - Ear infection (otitis media)
  - Nasal sinuses infection
- Onset of symptoms is very rapid and considered a medical emergency.
- Commonly nosocomial or iatrogenic.
- No physical test distinguishes a bacterial from a viral infection; must rely on body fluid cultures.
- If a central nervous system infection is suspected, the therapist should seek information regarding a potential source of infection or a condition that predisposed the patient to infection.

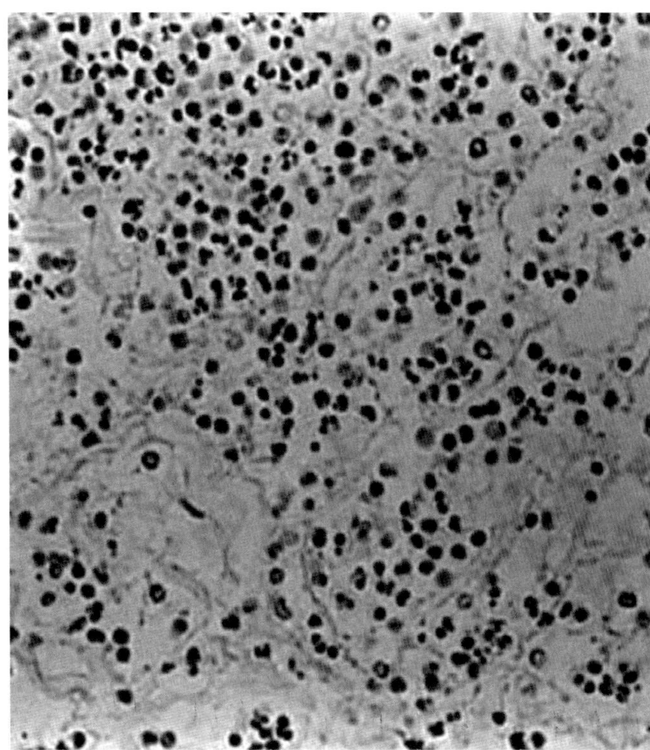

FIGURE 92-3 Acute bacterial meningitis, showing the acute inflammatory exudate on the meningeal surface. The exudate is characterized by large numbers of neutrophils. (From Chandrasoma P, Taylor CR. *Concise Pathology*. 3rd ed. http://www.accessmedicine.com. Copyright © The McGraw-Hill Companies, Inc. All rights reserved.)

▶ General Considerations

- Bacterial meningitis is caused by a wide range of bacteria.
  - Most common forms of meningitis include pneumococcal, influenza, and meningococcal worldwide; other bacteria cause meningitis but may be less common in some parts of the world.
  - Haemophilus meningitis is caused by the *Haemophilus influenzae* bacteria (Hib)
    - Most common form of meningitis
    - Acquired most likely following an upper respiratory infection
    - Rare; mostly limited to secondary to vaccine

▶ Demographics

- Approximately 3/100,000 in the United States; 500/100,000 in Africa[3]

CLINICAL FINDINGS

SIGNS AND SYMPTOMS

- Flu-like symptoms
- Headache
- Stiff neck
- Skin rash
- Change in mental status (confusion, delirium)
- Fever or hypothermia
- Malaise
- Impaired heart, lung, liver, kidney function
- Seizure, generalized convulsions
- Sensory deficit/change
- Motor deficit/change
- With increased intracranial pressure, papilledema may develop
- With prolonged infection, cranial nerves may become effected

▶ Functional Implications

- Loss of mobility temporarily with permanent loss possible
- Loss of hearing/vestibular function in some cases
- Loss of coordination (fine and gross motor) temporarily with permanent loss possible
- Loss of independence with activities of daily living
- Reduced cognitive function, particularly executive functions

▶ Possible Contributing Causes

- Severe sinus infection
- Cranial or spinal surgery
- Shunt placement
- Open head injury
- Diseases of the middle ear and paranasal sinuses
- Dural tears from remote trauma
- Ruptured brain abscess
- Congenital anomaly
- Diabetes

▶ Differential Diagnosis

- Alcoholic intoxication or withdrawal
- Behcet disease
- Epstein–Barr virus
- Extrapyramidal rigidity
- Hepatic encephalopathy
- Hydrocephalus
- Meningoencephalitis
- Subarachnoid hemorrhage

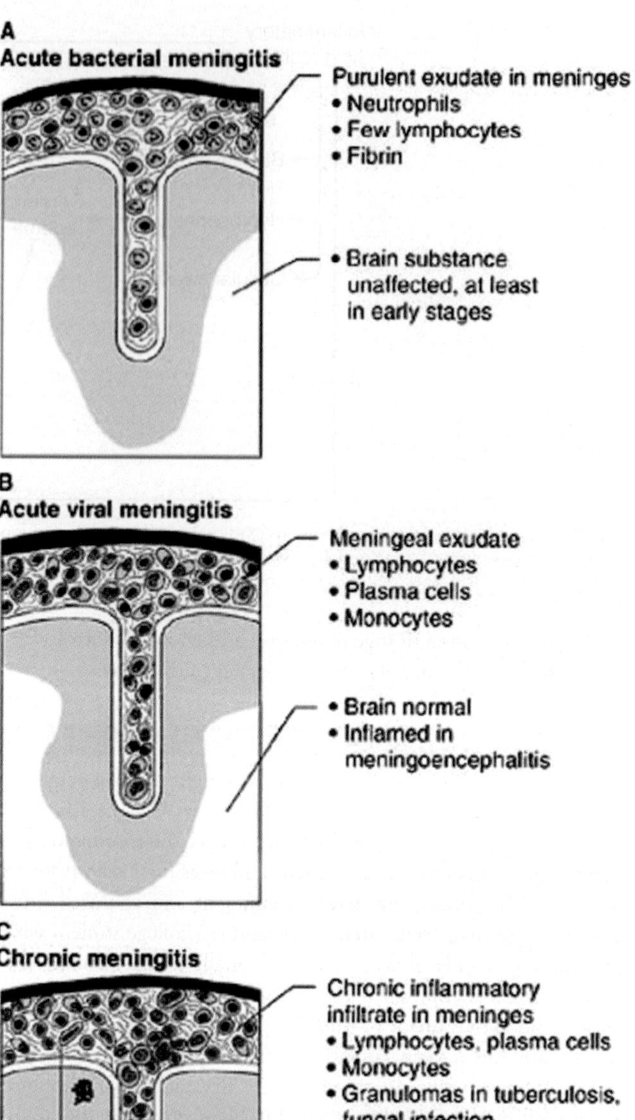

FIGURE 92-4 Contrasting histologic features in different types of meningitis. (From Chandrasoma P, Taylor CR. *Concise Pathology*. 3rd ed. http://www.accessmedicine.com.)

MEANS OF CONFIRMATION OR DIAGNOSIS

▶ Laboratory Tests

- Lab tests for complete blood count, general chemistry panel, and culture are used to determine the microorganism involved and the extent of the infection.

▶ Imaging

- CT scan for detailed imaging
- MRI with gadolinium enhancement
- Electroencephalography (EEG) may be helpful for patients with seizure due to infection

TABLE 92-1 Pathogenetic Sequence of Bacterial Neurotropism

Neurotropic Stage	Host Defense	Strategy of Pathogen
1. Colonization or mucosal invasion	Secretory IgA Ciliary activity Mucosal epithelium	IgA protease secretion Ciliostasis Adhesive pili
2. Intravascular survival	Complement	Evasion of alternative pathway by polysaccharide capsule
3. Crossing of blood–brain barrier	Cerebral endothelium	Adhesive pili
4. Survival within CSF	Poor opsonic activity	Bacterial replication

Source: Reproduced with permission from Quagliarello V, Scheld WM. Bacterial meningitis: pathogenesis, pathophysiology, and progress. *N Engl J Med.* 1992;327:864.

- Chest X-rays to disclose area of abscess that may be the original site of infection

Diagnostic Procedures

- Lumbar puncture to test the cerebral spinal fluid for presence of red and white blood cells, protein concentration, glucose, and microorganisms
  - High polymorphonuclear leukocytes, high protein, low glucose suggests bacterial infection
  - Predominant lymphocytes, high protein, low glucose suggests infection with mycobacteria, fungi, uncommon bacteria, and viruses such as herpes simplex, mumps, arbovirus
    - High lymphocytes, normal protein, normal glucose suggests viral infection

TREATMENT

Medications

- Broad-spectrum antibiotics until microorganism is identified, then specific antibiotic
- Third- and fourth-generation cephalosporins
- Corticosteroids

REFERRALS/ADMITTANCE

- To ER if meningitis is suspected
- To neurologist both during infection and for follow-up
- To otolaryngologist for middle and inner ear testing
- To respiratory therapy if source of infection is pulmonary in origin
- To occupational therapy for ADL and cognitive retraining
- To social work and case management

IMPAIRMENTS

- Aerobic capacity
- Arousal
- Attention
- Bed mobility
- Behavior
- Cognition
- Cranial nerve integrity
- Deep tendon reflexes
- Endurance
- Fine motor control
- Gait
- Home management
- Muscle strength
- Muscle tone
- Postural control
- Range of motion
- Respiratory control
- Self-care
- Sensation
- Sitting and standing balance
- Transfers

TESTS AND MEASURES

- Kernig sign: Inability to extend the knees when the hips are flexed
- Brudzinski sign: Flexion of hip and knee in response to flexion of the neck
- Cognition: Mini-Mental State Examination (MMSE), executive function tests, memory, comprehension

TABLE 92-2 Common Causes of Bacterial Meningitis in the United States by Host Age

	Age			
Pathogen	**<3 Months**	**3 Months–18 Years**	**18–50 Years**	**>50 Years**
Group B streptococci	X			
E coli	X			
Listeria monocytogenes	X			X
N. meningitidis		X	X	X
S. pneumoniae		X	X	X
Aerobic gram-negative bacilli	X			X

Source: McPhee SJ, Hammer GD. *Pathophysiology of Disease: An Introduction to Clinical Medicine.* 6th ed. http://www.accessmedicine.com.

- Pain: Subjective report, VAS or verbal report
- Strength and muscle endurance
- Coordination
- Muscle tone
- Joint ROM
- Cranial nerve integrity: Specific tests of vestibular function if deficits are evident
- Sensation
- Postural alignment
- Balance (TUG, MDRT, Tinetti, BBS)
- Gait (TUG, Tinetti, 10-m walk test, DGI)
- Respiratory function (spirometer, oxygen saturation, auscultation)
- Functional mobility (Functional Independence Measure [FIM™])

INTERVENTION

- Interventions are based on the extent and location of central nervous system damage resulting from the infection.
- Patients with active infection should be cautiously treated by a physical therapist due to high risk of developing communicating hydrocephalus and/or ischemic stroke early in the disease.
- Once cleared for more active treatment
  - Functional mobility: Bed mobility, transfers, gait
  - Balance and coordination activities: Postural control, balance strategies, speed/reaction time, multi tasking
  - Flexibility and stretching
  - Strength and resistance training
  - Pulmonary and cardiovascular reconditioning
  - Problem-solving and motor planning skills

FUNCTIONAL GOALS

Note: Goals for people recovering from an infectious disease of the brain are specific to the identified impairments; these are general goals and would need to be made more specific for each patient.

- Short-term goals
  - Patient will
    - Perform transfers to and from level surfaces with minimal physical assistance and minimal verbal cues for sequencing.
    - Ambulate on level tile surfaces with appropriate assistive device and moderate assistance for balance and sequencing.
    - Consistently perform a 2-step motor task without verbal or visual cuing.
- Long-term goals
  - Patient will
    - Maintain postural control independently while ambulating on community surfaces for greater than 15 minutes.
    - Ambulate distances >1000 ft without physical assistance, with occasional verbal cues for safety.
    - Complete a multistep task (>3 steps) successfully without verbal, visual, or physical cuing.

PROGNOSIS

- Untreated, meningitis is usually fatal.
- Greatest percentages of death are in children and the elderly.
- Approximately half of people who survive have serious neurologic sequelae.
- Persistent neurologic deficit is a predictor of later seizure activity.
- Use of certain antibiotics commonly results in ototoxicity; hearing loss may be a result of the meningitis or the medication.

PATIENT RESOURCES

- Kernig's sign of meningitis. MedlinePlus. http://www.nlm.nih.gov/medlineplus/ency/imagepages/19077.htm. Accessed July 5, 2013.
- Meningitis. MedlinePlus. http://www.nlm.nih.gov/medlineplus/ency/article/000680.htm. Accessed July 5, 2013.
- National Meningitis Association. http://www.nmaus.org. Accessed July 5, 2013.

REFERENCES

1. The American Physical Therapy Association. *Interactive Guide to Physical Therapist Practice*. Alexandria, VA: The American Physical Therapy Association; 2003. http://guidetoptpractice.apta.org/. Accessed July 5, 2013.
2. Toy EC. Bacterial Meningitis, Case 57. *LANGE Case Files*. http://www.accessmedicine.com/casecontent.aspx?aid=8651699&tabid=1. Accessed July 5, 2013.
3. Weisfelt M, van de Beek D, Spanjaard L, Reitsma JB, de Gans J. Community-acquired bacterial meningitis in older people. *J Am Geriatr Soc*. 2006;54(10):1500–1507.

ADDITIONAL REFERENCES

- Bernard TJ, Knupp K, Yang ML, Arndt D, Levisohn P, Moe PG. Neurologic & muscular disorders. In: Hay WW, Levin MJ, Sondheimer JM, Deterding RR, eds. *CURRENT Diagnosis & Treatment: Pediatrics*. 20th ed. New York, NY: McGraw-Hill; 2011. http://www.accessphysiotherapy.com/content/6585048. Accessed July 5, 2013.
- Brudzinski's sign of meningitis. MedlinePlus. http://www.nlm.nih.gov/medlineplus/ency/imagepages/19069.htm. Accessed July 5, 2013.
- Dewane JA, Porter RE. Inflammatory and infectious disorders of the brain. In: Umphred DA, ed. *Neurological Rehabilitation*. 5th ed. St. Louis, MO: Mosby Elsevier. 2007:659–661.
- Dutton M. Differential diagnosis. In: Dutton M, ed. *Orthopaedic Examination, Evaluation, and Intervention*. 2nd ed. New York, NY: McGraw-Hill; 2008. http://www.accessphysiotherapy.com/content/5547000. Accessed July 5, 2013.
- Geriatric Examination Tool Kit. University of Missouri School of Health Professions Department of Physical Therapy. http://web.missouri.edu/~proste/tool. Accessed July 5, 2013.
- McPhee SJ, Hammer GD. Pathophysiology of selected infectious disease syndromes. In: McPhee SJ, Hammer GD, eds. *Pathophysiology of Disease*. 6th ed. New York, NY: McGraw-Hill; 2010. http://www.accessphysiotherapy.com/content/5367060. Accessed July 5, 2013.
- Meningitis—Cryptococcal. MedlinePlus. http://www.nlm.nih.gov/medlineplus/ency/article/000642.htm. Accessed July 5, 2013.
- Panus PC, Jobst EE, Masters SB, Katzung B, Tinsley SL, Trevor AJ. Antibacterial agents. In: Panus PC, Jobst EE, Masters SB, Katzung B, Tinsley SL, Trevor AJ, eds. *Pharmacology for the Physical Therapist*. New York, NY: McGraw-Hill; 2009. http://www.accessphysiotherapy.com/content/6093998. Accessed July 5, 2013.
- Panus PC, Jobst EE, Masters SB, Katzung B, Tinsley SL, Trevor AJ. Corticosteroids and corticosteroid antagonists. In: Panus PC, Jobst EE, Masters SB, Katzung B, Tinsley SL, Trevor AJ, eds. *Pharmacology for the Physical Therapist*. New York, NY: McGraw-Hill; 2009. http://www.accessphysiotherapy.com/content/6093458. Accessed July 5, 2013.
- Ropper AH, Samuels MA. *Adams and Victor's Principles of Neurology*. 9th ed. New York, NY: McGraw-Hill; 2009:667–678.

93 CRYPTOCOCCAL MENINGITIS

Mollie Venglar, DSc, MSPT, NCS
Eric Shamus, PhD, DPT, PT, CSCS

CONDITION/DISORDER SYNONYM

- Meningitis

ICD-9-CM CODE

- 321.0 Cryptococcal meningitis

ICD-10-CM CODE

- B45.1 Cerebral cryptococcosis

PREFERRED PRACTICE PATTERNS[1]

- 5A: Primary Prevention/Risk reduction for Loss of Balance and Falling
- 5C: Impaired Motor Function and Sensory Integrity Associated with Nonprogressive Disorders of the Central Nervous System—Congenital Origin or Acquired in Infancy or Childhood
- 5D: Impaired Motor Function and Sensory Integrity Associated with Nonprogressive Disorders of the Central Nervous System—Acquired in Adolescence or Adulthood
- 5I: Impaired Arousal, Range of Motion, and Motor Control Associated with Coma, Near Coma, or Vegetative State

PATIENT PRESENTATION

After returning from a mission trip to promote farming in rural areas of Africa, a 28-year-old man noted increasing stiffness in his neck and headaches that responded poorly to acetaminophen and rest. He had little appetite and felt feverish after a couple of days. His friends noticed he seemed to be progressively more confused and took him to the doctor. Meningitis was suspected so the man was sent to the emergency department of the local hospital. Lumbar puncture revealed normal glucose and protein levels but elevated lymphocytes in the cerebrospinal fluid.

KEY FEATURES

Description

- Fungal infection of the meninges of the brain and spinal cord.
- Fungus *Cryptococcus neoformans* is found in the soil.

Essentials of Diagnosis

- Severity and extent of the infection causes a wide range of neurologic signs and symptoms, generally nonfocal in nature.
- Different from bacterial meningitis as symptoms emerge over a few days.
- No physical test distinguishes a bacterial from a viral infection; must rely on body fluid cultures.

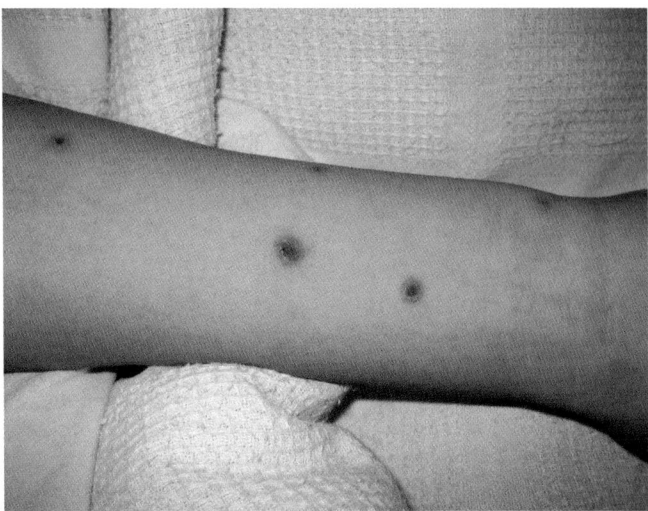

FIGURE 93-1 India ink preparation. *Cryptococcus neoformans* seen as encapsulated yeast on India ink preparation of the CSF from an HIV patient with cryptococcal meningitis. (From Knoop KJ, Stack LB, Storrow AB, Thurman RJ. *The Atlas of Emergency Medicine.* 3rd ed. Photo contributor: Seth W. Wright, *MD.* http://www.accessmedicine.com. Copyright © The McGraw-Hill Companies, Inc. All rights reserved.)

- Commonly nosocomial or iatrogenic.
- If a central nervous system infection is suspected, the therapist should seek information regarding a potential source of infection or a condition that predisposed the patient to infection.

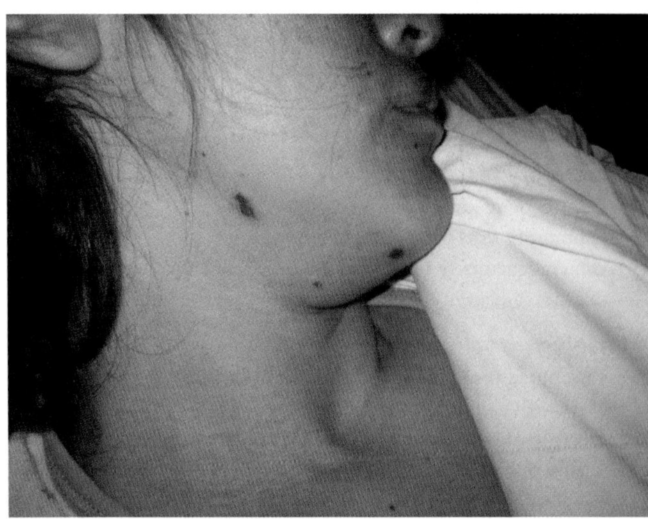

FIGURE 93-2 Cryptococcal infection. This patient had extensive cutaneous involvement with disseminated cryptococcal infection. (From Knoop KJ, Stack LB, Storrow AB, Thurman RJ. *The Atlas of Emergency Medicine.* 3rd ed. Photo contributors: Seth W. Wright, MD, and Universidad Peruana Cayetano Heredia, Lima, Peru. http://www.accessmedicine.com. Copyright © The McGraw-Hill Companies, Inc. All rights reserved.)

▶ **General Considerations**

- If a central nervous system infection is suspected, the therapist should seek information regarding a potential source of infection or a condition that predisposed the patient to infection.

▶ **Demographics**

- Individuals with weak immune systems

CLINICAL FINDINGS

SIGNS AND SYMPTOMS

- Symptoms emerge over a few days
- Fever or hypothermia
- Hallucinations
- Nausea
- Sensitivity to light
- Headache, stiff neck
- Change in mental status (confusion, delirium)
- Increased heart rate
- Malaise

▶ **Functional Implications**

- Loss of mobility temporarily with permanent loss possible
- Loss of hearing/vestibular function in some cases
- Temporary loss of coordination (fine and gross motor) with permanent loss possible
- Loss of independence with activities of daily living
- Reduced cognitive function, particularly executive functions

▶ **Possible Contributing Causes**

- Contact with fungus *C. neoformans* in the soil
- Severe sinus infection
- Cranial or spinal surgery
- Shunt placement
- Open head injury

▶ **Differential Diagnosis**

- Extrapyramidal rigidity
- Hydrocephalus
- Alcohol intoxication or withdrawal
- Hepatic encephalopathy
- Subarachnoid hemorrhage
- Meningoencephalitis
- Epstein–Barr virus
- Behçet disease

MEANS OF CONFIRMATION OR DIAGNOSIS

▶ **Laboratory Tests**

- Cryptococcal antigen in the CSF or blood
- Laboratory tests for complete blood count
- General chemistry panel and culture are used to determine the microorganism involved and the extent of the infection

▶ **Imaging**

- Computed tomography (CT) scan for detailed imaging
- MRI with gadolinium enhancement
- Electroencephalogram (EEG) may be helpful for patients with seizure due to infection
- Chest radiographs to disclose area of abscess that may be the original site of infection

▶ **Diagnostic Procedures**

- Lumbar puncture to test the cerebral spinal fluid for presence of red and white blood cells, protein concentration, glucose, and microorganisms

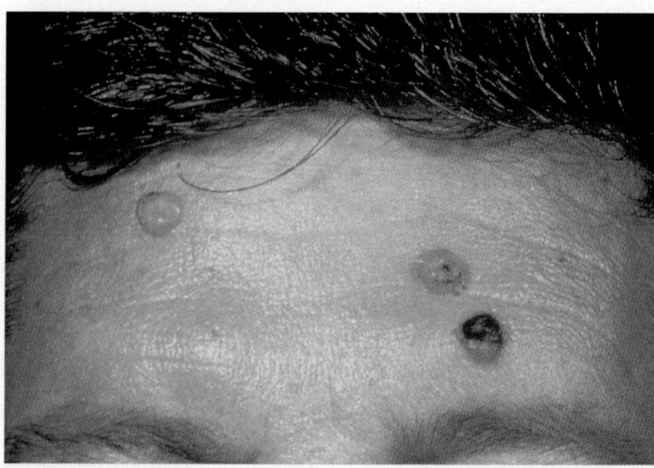

FIGURE 93-3 Cryptococcal infection. Cutaneous cryptococcal lesions are often clinically difficult to distinguish from other cutaneous eruptions. (From Knoop KJ, Stack LB, Storrow AB, Thurman RJ. *The Atlas of Emergency Medicine.* 3rd ed. Photo contributors: Seth W. Wright, MD, and Universidad Peruana Cayetano Heredia, Lima, Peru. http://www.accessmedicine.com. Copyright © The McGraw-Hill Companies, Inc. All rights reserved.)

  - High polymorphonuclear leukocytes, high protein, and low glucose suggest bacterial infection
  - Predominant lymphocytes, high protein, low glucose suggests infection with mycobacteria, fungi, uncommon bacteria, and viruses such as herpes simplex, mumps, arbovirus
  - High lymphocytes, normal protein, and normal glucose suggest viral infection

TREATMENT

▶ **Medication**

- Antifungal medication
- Intravenous therapy with amphotericin B
- Fluconazole
- Corticosteroids

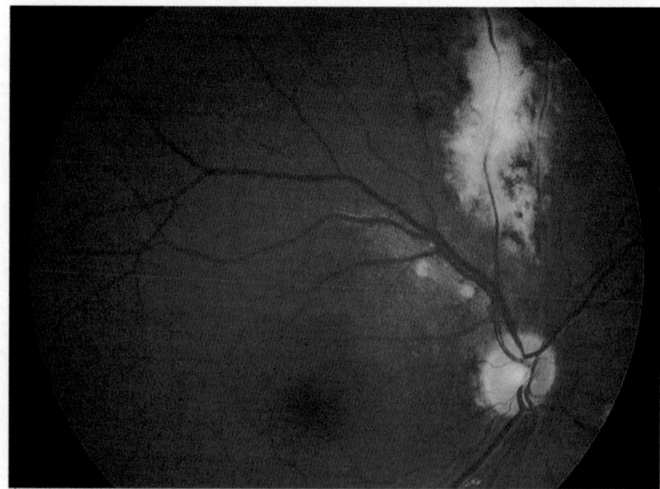

FIGURE 93-4 Cryptococcal infection. Cryptococcal skin lesions in disseminated form. Note that the umbilicated centers give a similar appearance to that of molluscum contagiosum. (From Knoop KJ, Stack LB, Storrow AB, Thurman RJ. *The Atlas of Emergency Medicine.* 3rd ed. Photo contributor: Briana Hill, MD. http://www.accessmedicine.com. Copyright © The McGraw-Hill Companies, Inc. All rights reserved.)

REFERRALS/ADMITTANCE

- To ER room if meningitis suspected
- To neurologist both during infection and for follow-up
- To otolaryngologist for middle and inner ear testing
- To respiratory therapy if source of infection is pulmonary in origin
- To occupational therapy for ADL and cognitive retraining
- To social work and case management

IMPAIRMENTS

- Arousal
- Attention
- Behavior
- Cognition
- Cranial nerve integrity
- Gait
- Sitting and standing balance
- Muscle strength
- Postural control
- Range of motion
- Deep tendon reflexes
- Muscle tone
- Sensation
- Bed mobility
- Transfers
- Endurance
- Aerobic capacity
- Self-care
- Home management
- Fine motor control
- Respiratory control

TESTS AND MEASURES

- Kernig sign: Inability to extend the knees when the hips are flexed
- Brudzinski sign: Flexion of the hip and knee in response to flexion of the neck
- Cognition: Mini-Mental State Examination (MMSE), executive function tests, memory, comprehension
- Pain: Subjective report, VAS, or verbal report
- Strength and muscle endurance
- Coordination
- Muscle tone
- Joint ROM
- Cranial nerve integrity: Specific tests of vestibular function if deficits are evident
- Sensation
- Postural alignment
- Balance (TUG, MDRT, Tinetti, BBS)
- Gait (TUG, Tinetti, 10-m walk test, DGI)
- Respiratory function (spirometer, oxygen saturation, auscultation)
- Functional mobility (Functional Independence Measure [FIM^{TM}])

INTERVENTION

- Interventions based on the extent and location of central nervous system damage resulting from the infection
- Patients with active infection to be cautiously treated by a physical therapist due to high risk of the disease being spread person to person though respiratory droplets
- Once cleared for more active treatment

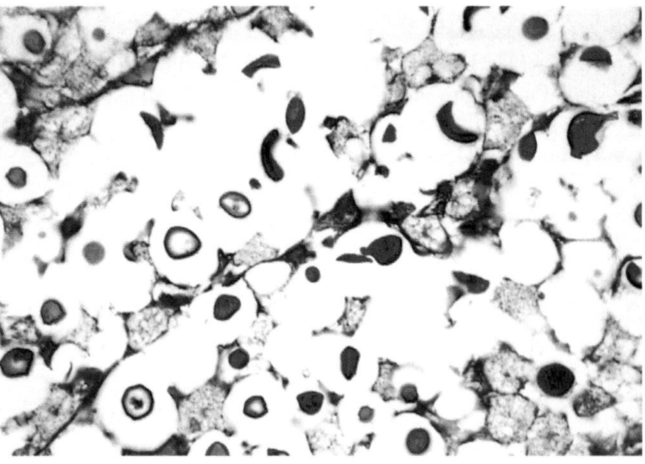

FIGURE 93-5 Cryptococcal meningitis. The *C. neoformans* cells are stained red by the PAS (periodic acid-Schiff) stain. The capsule is not stained, but is creating the halo around the organisms. Note the lack of inflammatory cells. (Reproduced with permission from Connor DH, Chandler FW, Schwartz DQA, Manz HJ, Lack EE, eds. *Pathology of Infectious Diseases,* vol. 1. Stamford, CT: Appleton & Lange; 1997.)

  - Functional gait
  - Balance and coordination activities: Postural control, balance strategies, speed/reaction time, multitasking
  - Flexibility and stretching
  - Strength and resistance training
  - Pulmonary and cardiovascular reconditioning
  - Problem-solving and motor-planning skills

FUNCTIONAL GOALS

Note: Goals for people recovering from an infectious disease of the brain are specific to the identified impairment. These are general goals and would need to be made more specific for each patient.

- Short-term goals
  - Patient will
    - Perform transfers to and from level surfaces with minimal physical assistance and minimal verbal cues for sequencing.
    - Ambulate on level tile surfaces with appropriate assistive device(s) and moderate assistance for balance and sequencing.
    - Consistently perform a two-step motor task without verbal or visual cuing.
- Long-term goals
  - Patient will
    - Maintain postural control independently while ambulating on community surfaces for >15 minutes.
    - Ambulate distances >1000 feet without physical assistance, with occasional verbal cues for safety.
    - Complete a multistep task (>3 steps) successfully without verbal, visual, or physical cuing.

PROGNOSIS

- Untreated meningitis is usually fatal.
- Greatest percentages of death are in children and the elderly.
- Approximately half of people who survive have serious neurologic sequelae.
- Persistent neurologic deficit is a predictor of later seizure activity.
- Use of certain antibiotics commonly results in ototoxicity; hearing loss may be a result of the meningitis or the medication.

PATIENT RESOURCES

- MedlinePlus. U.S. National Library of Medicine, NIH. Kernig's sign of meningitis. http://www.nlm.nih.gov/medlineplus/ency/imagepages/19077.htm. Accessed July 5, 2013.
- MedlinePlus. U.S. National Library of Medicine, NIH. Meningitis—Cryptococcal. http://www.nlm.nih.gov/medlineplus/ency/article/000642.htm. Accessed July 5, 2013.
- MedlinePlus. U.S. National Library of Medicine, NIH. Meningitis. http://www.nlm.nih.gov/medlineplus/ency/article/000680.htm. Accessed July 5, 2013.

REFERENCE

1. The American Physical Therapy Association. *Interactive Guide to Physical Therapist Practice*. Alexandria, VA: The American Physical Therapy Association; 2003. http://guidetoptpractice.apta.org/. Accessed July 5, 2013.

ADDITIONAL REFERENCES

- Bernard TJ, Knupp K, Yang ML, Arndt D, Levisohn P, Moe PG. Neurologic & muscular disorders. In: Hay WW, Levin MJ, Sondheimer JM, Deterding RR, eds. *Current Diagnosis & Treatment: Pediatrics*. 20th ed. New York, NY: McGraw-Hill; 2011. http://www.accessphysiotherapy.com/content/6585048. Accessed July 5, 2013.
- Brudzinski's sign of meningitis. MedlinePlus. http://www.nlm.nih.gov/medlineplus/ency/imagepages/19069.htm. Accessed July 5, 2013.
- Dewane JA, Porter RE. Inflammatory and infectious disorders of the brain. In: Umphred DA, ed. *Neurological Rehabilitation*. 5th ed. St. Louis, MO: Mosby Elsevier; 2007:659–661.
- Dutton M. Differential diagnosis. In: Dutton M, ed. *Dutton's Orthopaedic Examination, Evaluation, and Intervention*. 2nd ed. New York, NY: McGraw-Hill; 2008. http://www.accessphysiotherapy.com/content/5547000. Accessed July 5, 2013.
- Geriatric Examination Tool Kit. University of Missouri School of Health Professions Department of Physical Therapy. http://web.missouri.edu/~proste/tool./ Accessed July 5, 2013.
- Kauffman CA. Cryptococcosis. In: Goldman L, Ausiello D, eds. *Cecil Medicine*. 23rd ed. Philadelphia, PA: Saunders Elsevier; 2007: Chapter 357.
- Panus PC, Jobst EE, Masters SB, Katzung B, Tinsley SL, Trevor AJ. Antibacterial agents. In: Panus PC, Jobst EE, Masters SB, Katzung B, Tinsley SL, Trevor AJ, eds. *Pharmacology for the Physical Therapist*. New York, NY: McGraw-Hill; 2009. http://www.accessphysiotherapy.com/content/6093998. Accessed July 5, 2013.
- Panus PC, Jobst EE, Masters SB, Katzung B, Tinsley SL, Trevor AJ. Corticosteroids and corticosteroid antagonists. In: Panus PC, Jobst EE, Masters SB, Katzung B, Tinsley SL, Trevor AJ, eds. *Pharmacology for the Physical Therapist*. New York, NY: McGraw-Hill; 2009. http://www.accessphysiotherapy.com/content/6093458. Accessed July 5, 2013.
- Ropper AH, Samuels MA. *Adams and Victor's Principles of Neurology*. 9th ed. New York, NY: McGraw-Hill; 2009:667–678.

94 HEMOPHILUS MENINGITIS

Mollie Venglar, DSc, MSPT, NCS
Eric Shamus, PhD, DPT, PT, CSCS

CONDITION/DISORDER SYNONYMS

- Meningitis
- Bacterial meningitis
- Haemophilus meningitis (HIB)

ICD-9-CM CODE

- 320.0 Haemophilus meningitis

ICD-10-CM CODES

- A48.8 Other specified bacterial diseases
- G00.8 Other bacterial meningitis
- G00.9 Bacterial meningitis, unspecified

PREFERRED PRACTICE PATTERNS[1]

- 5A: Primary Prevention/Risk Reduction for Loss of Balance and Falling
- 5C: Impaired Motor Function and Sensory Integrity Associated With Nonprogressive Disorders of the Central Nervous System—congenital origin or acquired in infancy or childhood
- 5D: Impaired Motor Function and Sensory Integrity Associated With Nonprogressive Disorders of the Central Nervous System—acquired in adolescence or adulthood
- 5I: Impaired Arousal, Range of Motion and Motor Control Associated With Coma, Near Coma, or Vegetative State

PATIENT PRESENTATION

An "as-needed" (PRN) physical therapist called in sick to work with reports of flu-like symptoms, particularly sinus congestion, and increasing stiffness in her neck. She also noticed a skin rash and unusual sensations in her hands and feet, and she felt clumsy. She treated patients at the acute care hospital a couple of weeks ago and, because she had not had a flu shot yet, wore a mask while working with most of the patients. She reported to employee health and was sent immediately to the emergency department with suspicion of meningitis. Cerebrospinal fluid testing revealed high leukocyte count, high protein volume, and low glucose.

KEY FEATURES

Description

- A type of bacterial meningitis found in the nose and throat
- Infection of the meninges of the brain and spinal cord caused by a spread of bacteria
- Caused by the *haemophilus influenza* bacteria (Hib)
  - Most common form of meningitis
  - Acquired following an upper respiratory infection

Essentials of Diagnosis

- Bacteria contracted by exhaled droplets from an infected adult or child or by the following:
  - Head injury
  - Severe local infection
  - Ear infection (otitis media)
  - Nasal sinus infection

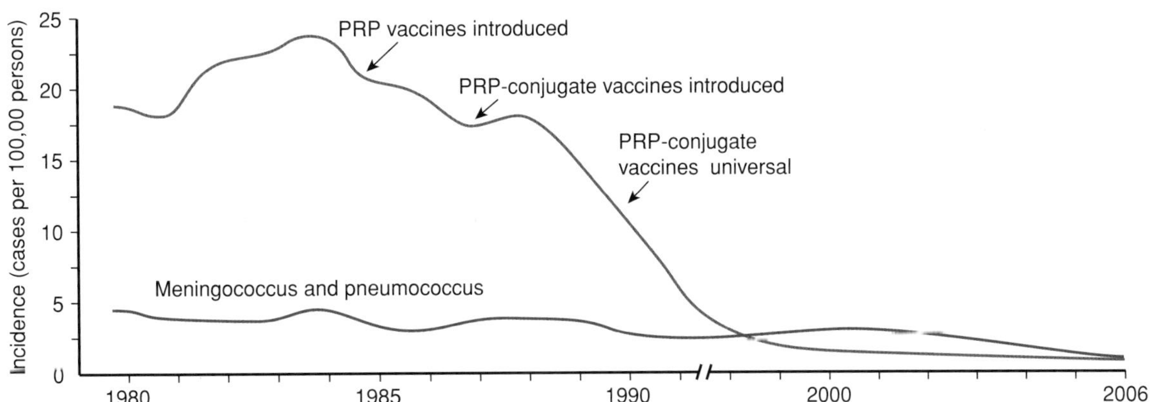

FIGURE 94-1 The decline in *Haemophilus influenzae* type b (Hib) meningitis in association with the introduction of new vaccines is shown. Note also the steady state of the other major causes of childhood meningitis. They did not increase to "fill in the gap" nor did *H. influenzae* invasive disease caused by other serotypes. (From Ryan KJ, Ray CG. *Sherris Medical Microbiology*. 5th ed. http://www.accessmedicine.com. Copyright © The McGraw-Hill Companies, Inc. All rights reserved.)

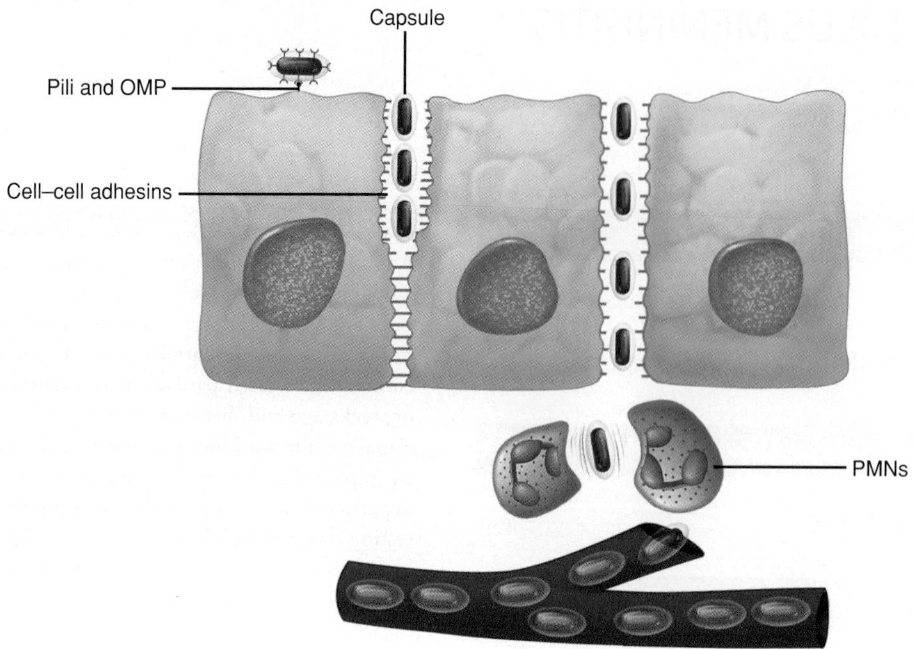

FIGURE 94-2 *Haemophilus influenzae* disease, cellular view. Organisms attach to epithelial cells using pili and outer membrane proteins (OMP). Invasion takes place between cells by disruption of cell–cell adhesion molecules. In the submucosa, the capsule allows the bacteria to evade phagocytosis and enter the bloodstream. PMNs, polymorphonuclear neutrophils. (From Ryan KJ, Ray CG. *Sherris Medical Microbiology*. 5th ed. http://www.accessmedicine.com. Copyright © The McGraw-Hill Companies, Inc. All rights reserved.)

- Hib can enter the bloodstream and cause infection in the meninges or lungs.
- No physical test distinguishes a bacterial from a viral infection; must rely on body fluid cultures.
- If a central nervous system infection is suspected, the therapist should seek information regarding a potential source of infection or a condition that predisposed the patient to infection.

General Considerations

- Generally, bacterial meningitis is rare; secondary to vaccine
- Individual may not know they have the bacteria

Demographics

- Usually seen in children under 5 years old

CLINICAL FINDINGS

SIGNS AND SYMPTOMS

- Severity and extent causes a wide range of neurologic signs and symptoms, generally nonfocal in nature
- Flu-like symptoms
- Pneumonia
- Swollen throat, difficulty breathing
- Headache
- Stiff neck
- Skin rash
- Change in mental status (confusion, delirium)
- Fever or hypothermia
- Malaise
- Impaired heart, lung, liver, kidney function
- Seizure, generalized convulsions
- Sensory deficit/change
- Motor deficit/change
- With increased intracranial pressure, papilledema may develop
- With prolonged infection, cranial nerves may become affected

Functional Implications

- Loss of mobility temporarily with permanent loss possible
- Loss of hearing/vestibular function in some cases
- Loss of coordination, fine and gross motor temporarily with permanent loss possible
- Loss of independence with activities of daily living
- Reduced cognitive function, particularly executive functions

Possible Contributing Causes

- Bone marrow transplant
- Cranial or spinal surgery
- Dural tears from remote trauma
- HIV/AIDS, immunosuppressive
- Open head injury
- Removal of spleen
- Ruptured brain abscess
- Severe sinus infection
- Shunt placement
- Sickle cell disease

Differential Diagnosis

- Alcohol intoxication or withdrawal
- Behçet disease
- Epstein–Barr virus (EBV)
- Extrapyramidal rigidity
- Hepatic encephalopathy
- Hydrocephalus
- Meningoencephalitis
- Subarachnoid hemorrhage

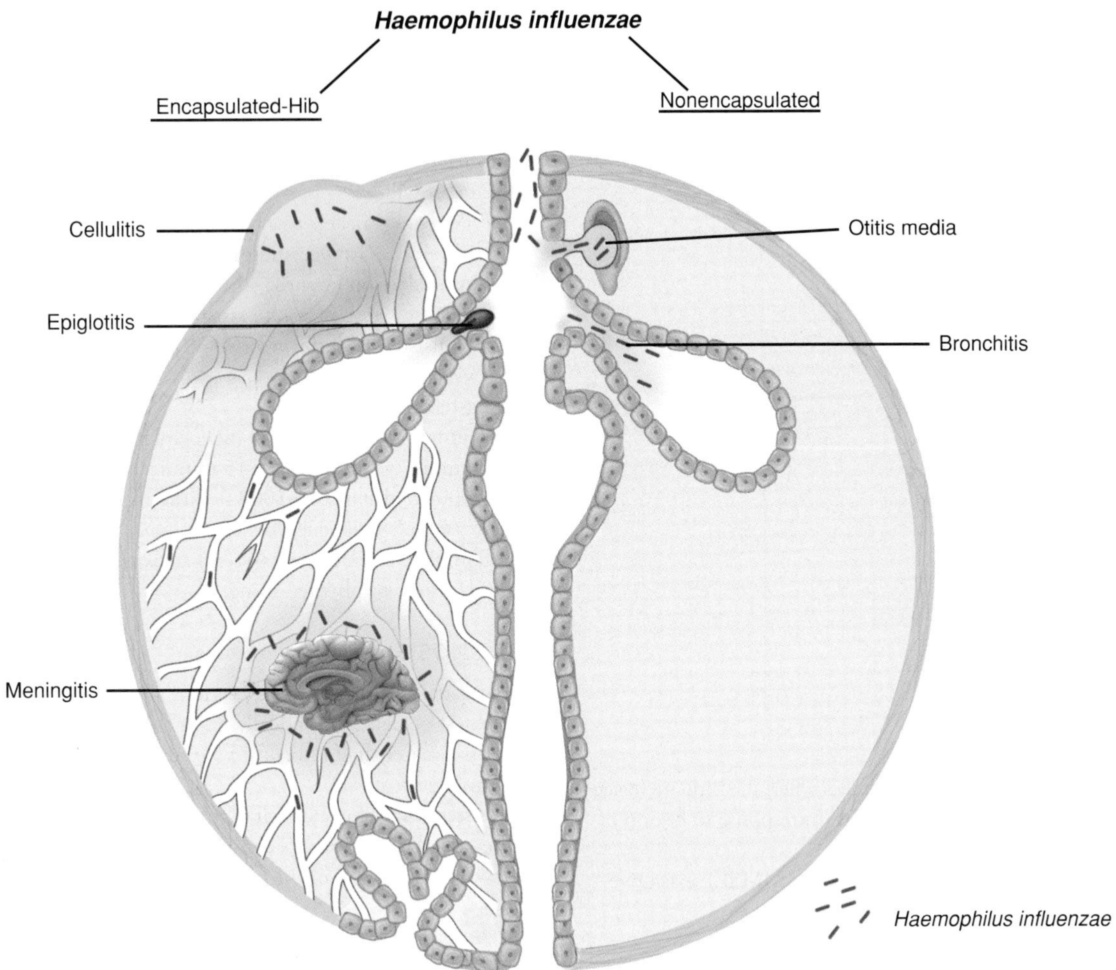

FIGURE 94-3 Haemophilus disease overview. *(Left)* Invasive disease is caused by encapsulated strains, mostly type b (Hib). From a nasopharyngeal colonization site, the organisms invade locally to produce cellulitis or epiglottitis. Invasion of the blood occurs in all Hib forms and most frequently leads to meningitis. *(Right)* Localized disease is produced when nonencapsulated strains from the nasopharynx are trapped in the middle ear paranasal sinuses or compromised bronchi. (From Ryan KJ, Ray CG. *Sherris Medical Microbiology*. 5th ed. http://www.accessmedicine.com. Copyright © The McGraw-Hill Companies, Inc. All rights reserved.)

MEANS OF CONFIRMATION OR DIAGNOSIS

Laboratory Tests

- Lab tests for complete blood count, general chemistry panel, and culture are used to determine the microorganism involved and the extent of the infection

Imaging

- Computed tomography (CT) scan for detailed imaging
- MRI with gadolinium enhancement
- Electroencephalogram (EEG) may be helpful for patients with seizure due to infection
- Chest radiographs to disclose area of abscess that may be the original site of infection

Diagnostic Procedures

- Lumbar puncture to test the cerebral spinal fluid for presence of red and white blood cells, protein concentration, glucose, and microorganisms

FINDINGS AND INTERPRETATION

- Lumbar puncture to test the cerebral spinal fluid
  - High polymorphonuclear leukocytes, high protein, and low glucose suggests bacterial infection
  - Predominant lymphocytes, high protein, low glucose suggests infection with mycobacteria, fungi, uncommon bacteria, and viruses such as herpes simplex, mumps, and arbovirus.
  - High lymphocytes, normal protein, and normal glucose suggests viral infection.

TREATMENT

Medications

- Antibiotics
- Third and fourth generation cephalosporins
- Corticosteroids

REFERRALS/ADMITTANCE

- To emergency room if meningitis is suspected
- To neurologist both during infection and for follow-up
- To otolaryngologist for middle and inner ear testing
- To respiratory therapy if source of infection is pulmonary in origin
- To occupational therapy for ADL and cognitive retraining
- To social work and case management

IMPAIRMENTS

- Aerobic capacity
- Arousal
- Attention
- Bed mobility
- Behavior
- Cognition
- Cranial nerve integrity
- Deep tendon reflexes
- Endurance
- Fine motor control
- Gait
- Home management
- Muscle strength
- Muscle tone
- Postural control
- Range of motion
- Respiratory control
- Self-care
- Sensation
- Sitting and standing balance
- Transfers

TESTS AND MEASURES

- Kernig sign: Inability to extend the knees when the hips are flexed
- Brudzinski sign: Flexion of hip and knee in response to flexion of the neck
- Cognition: Mini-Mental State Examination (MMSE), executive function tests, memory, comprehension
- Pain: Subjective report, VAS or verbal report
- Strength and muscle endurance
- Coordination
- Muscle tone
- Joint ROM
- Cranial nerve integrity: Specific tests of vestibular function if deficits are evident
- Sensation
- Postural alignment
- Balance (TUG, MDRT, Tinetti, BBS)
- Gait (TUG, Tinetti, 10-m walk test, DGI)
- Respiratory function (spirometer, oxygen saturation, auscultation)
- Functional mobility (Functional Independence Measure (FIM™)

INTERVENTION

- Interventions are based on the extent and location of central nervous system damage resulting from the infection.
- Patients with active infection should be cautiously treated by a physical therapist due to high risk of developing communicating hydrocephalus and/or ischemic stroke early in the disease.
- Once cleared for more active treatment
  - Functional mobility: Bed mobility, transfers, gait
  - Balance and coordination activities: Postural control, balance strategies, speed/reaction time, multi tasking
  - Flexibility and stretching
  - Strength and resistance training
  - Pulmonary and cardiovascular reconditioning
  - Problem-solving and motor planning skills

FUNCTIONAL GOALS

Note: Goals for people recovering from an infectious disease of the brain are specific to the identified impairments; these are general goals and would need to be made more specific for each patient.

- Short-term goals
  - Patient will
    - Perform transfers to and from level surfaces with minimal physical assistance and minimal verbal cues for sequencing.
    - Ambulate on level tile surfaces with appropriate assistive device(s) and moderate assistance for balance and sequencing.
    - Consistently perform a two-step motor task without verbal or visual cuing.
- Long-term goals
  - Maintain postural control independently while ambulating on community surfaces for >15 minutes.
  - Ambulate distances >1000 ft without physical assistance, with occasional verbal cues for safety.
  - Complete a multi step task (>3 steps) successfully without verbal, visual, or physical cuing.

PROGNOSIS

- Untreated, meningitis is very serious and usually fatal.
- Greatest percentages of death are in children and the elderly.
- Approximately half of people who survive have serious neurologic sequelae.
- Persistent neurologic deficit is a predictor of later seizure activity.
- Use of certain antibiotics commonly results in ototoxicity; hearing loss may be a result of the meningitis or the medication.

PATIENT RESOURCES

- Kernig's sign of meningitis. MedlinePlus. U.S. National Library of Medicine, NIH. http://www.nlm.nih.gov/medlineplus/ency/imagepages/19077.htm. Accessed July 6, 2013.
- Meningitis-Cryptococcal. MedlinePlus. U.S. National Library of Medicine, NIH. http://www.nlm.nih.gov/medlineplus/ency/article/000642.htm. Accessed July 6, 2013.
- Meningitis. MedlinePlus. U.S. National Library of Medicine, NIH. Medline Plus. http://www.nlm.nih.gov/medlineplus/ency/article/000680.htm. Accessed July 6, 2013.

REFERENCE

1. The American Physical Therapy Association. *Interactive Guide to Physical Therapist Practice*. Alexandria, VA: The American Physical Therapy Association; 2003. http://guidetoptpractice.apta.org/. Accessed July 6, 2013.

ADDITIONAL REFERENCES

- Bernard TJ, Knupp K, Yang ML, Arndt D, Levisohn P, Moe PG. Neurologic & muscular disorders. In: Hay WW, Levin MJ, Sondheimer JM, Deterding RR, eds. *CURRENT Diagnosis & Treatment: Pediatrics*. 20th ed. New York, NY: McGraw-Hill; 2011. http://www.accessphysiotherapy.com/content/6585048. Accessed July 6, 2013.
- Brudzinski's sign of meningitis. MedlinePlus. http://www.nlm.nih.gov/medlineplus/ency/imagepages/19069.htm. Accessed July 6, 2013.

- Dewane JA, Porter RE. Inflammatory and infectious disorders of the brain. In: Umphred DA, ed. *Neurological Rehabilitation*. 5th ed. St. Louis, MO: Mosby Elsevier; 2007:659–661.
- Dutton M. Differential diagnosis. In: Dutton M, ed. *Dutton's Orthopaedic Examination, Evaluation, and Intervention*. 2nd ed. New York, NY: McGraw-Hill; 2008. http://www.accessphysiotherapy.com/content/5547000. Accessed July 6, 2013.
- Geriatric Examination Tool Kit. University of Missouri School of Health Professions Department of Physical Therapy. http://web.missouri.edu/~proste/tool. Accessed July 6, 2013.
- Hay WW, Levin MJ, Sondheimer JM, Deterding RR. Neurologic & muscular disorders. In: Hay WW, Levin MJ, Sondheimer JM, Deterding RR, eds. *CURRENT Diagnosis & Treatment: Pediatrics*. 20th ed. New York, NY: McGraw-Hill; 2011. http://www.accessphysiotherapy.com/content/6585067. Accessed July 6, 2013.
- Panus PC, Jobst EE, Masters SB, Katzung B, Tinsley SL, Trevor AJ. Antibacterial agents. In: Panus PC, Jobst EE, Masters SB, Katzung B, Tinsley SL, Trevor AJ, eds. *Pharmacology for the Physical Therapist*. New York, NY: McGraw-Hill; 2009. http://www.accessphysiotherapy.com/content/6093998. Accessed July 6, 2013.
- Panus PC, Jobst EE, Masters SB, Katzung B, Tinsley SL, Trevor AJ. Corticosteroids and corticosteroid antagonists. In: Panus PC, Jobst EE, Masters SB, Katzung B, Tinsley SL, Trevor AJ, eds. *Pharmacology for the Physical Therapist*. New York, NY: McGraw-Hill; 2009. http://www.accessphysiotherapy.com/content/6093458. Accessed July 6, 2013.
- Ropper AL, Samuels MA. *Adams and Victor's Principles of Neurology*. 9th ed. New York, NY: McGraw-Hill; 2009.

95 MULTIPLE SCLEROSIS

Eric Shamus, PhD, DPT, PT, CSCS
Mollie Venglar, DSc, MSPT, NCS
Annie Burke-Doe, PhD, MPT, PT

CONDITION/DISORDER SYNONYM

- Disseminated sclerosis

ICD-9-CM CODE

- 340 Multiple sclerosis

ICD-10-CM CODE

- G35 Multiple sclerosis

PREFERRED PRACTICE PATTERNS

- 4C: Impaired Muscle Performance
- 5E: Impaired Motor Function and Sensory Integrity Associated with Progressive Disorders of the Central Nervous System
- 6B: Impaired Aerobic Capacity/Endurance Associated with Deconditioning
- 6C: Impaired Ventilation, Respiration/Gas Exchange, and Aerobic Capacity/Endurance Associated with Airway Clearance Dysfunction
- 6E: Impaired Ventilation and Respiration/Gas Exchange Associated with Ventilatory Pump Dysfunction or Failure

PATIENT PRESENTATION

A 24-year-old graduate student was studying late at night for an examination when he realized that his left arm and left leg were numb. He dismissed the complaint, recalling that 6 or 7 months ago he had similar symptoms. He rose from his desk and noticed that he had poor balance. His vision was blurred, and remembered that he had some blurred vision approximately 1 to 2 years earlier, but that this resolved. He had not seen a physician for any of these previous symptoms. He went to bed and decided that he would seek medical consultation the next day.[1]

KEY FEATURES

Description

- Chronic disease
- Progressive disorder characterized by demyelination (or demyelinating plaques) in the central nervous system attacking the brain, spinal cord, and optic nerves
- The disease process causes areas of inflammation, lesions, in random and unpredictable areas of the central nervous system. The inflammation leads to irreversible axonal damage and scarring that interferes with nerve impulse.

Essentials of Diagnosis

- Etiology is unknown[2]
- Episodic neurologic symptoms
- Usually under 55 years of age at onset.[3]
- Single pathologic lesion cannot explain clinical findings.
- Multiple foci is best visualized by MRI.

General Considerations

- Diagnosis of clinically definite disease can be made when there is dissemination of symptoms in time and space.
  - Time: Any new lesion in the central nervous systems in a follow-up MRI
  - Space: One or more lesions identified in two distinct locations in the central nervous system
- The diagnosis is probable in patients with multifocal white matter disease, but only one clinical attack.
- Four categories of the disease
  - Relapsing/Remitting: Clearly defined relapses, or episodes of loss of function, followed by relative recovery
  - Primary progressive: Continuous decline in function, not interrupted by plateaus or periods of faster decline/relapse
  - Secondary progressive: Begins as relapsing/remitting, and later becomes slow progressive decline without periods of remittance
  - Progressive relapsing: Continuous decline with periods of faster decline/relapse, time between relapses shows progressive decline

Demographics

- 90% of people with multiple sclerosis (MS) are diagnosed between the ages of 16 and 60 years; more common in women (2.5:1)
- Much more common in persons of western European lineage who live in temperate zones
- No population with a high risk for MS exists between latitudes 40° N and 40° S[3]
- Genetic susceptibility to the disease possible, based on twin studies, familial cases, and an association with specific human leukocyte antigen (HLA) antigens (HLA-DR2)

CLINICAL FINDINGS

SIGNS AND SYMPTOMS

- Symptoms may develop quickly (within hours) or over days/weeks
- Most common initial symptoms
  - Fatigue
  - Incoordination
  - Speech disturbances
  - Motor weakness
  - Paresthesia
  - Difficulty with walking
  - Vision difficulties (most commonly diplopia)
  - Tremor
  - Bowel and/or bladder dysfunction
- Less common initial presentations
  - Hemiplegia
  - Trigeminal neuralgia
  - Facial palsy
- Other signs and symptoms as the disease progresses
  - Spasticity and reflex spasm
  - Contractures

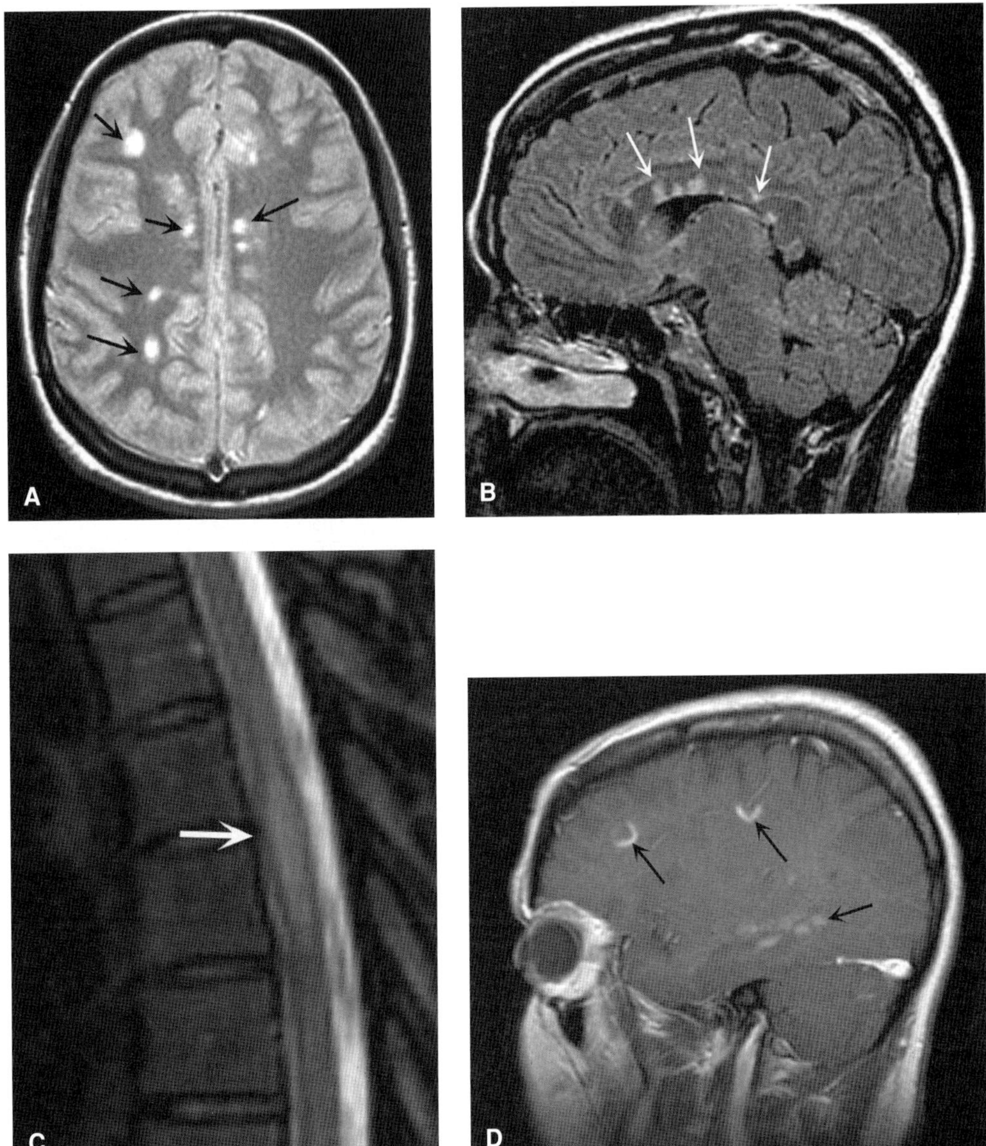

FIGURE 95-1 MRI findings in MS. **A.** Axial first-echo image from T2-weighted sequence demonstrates multiple bright signal abnormalities in white matter, typical for MS. **B.** Sagittal T2-weighted FLAIR (fluid attenuated inversion recovery) image in which the high signal of CSF has been suppressed. CSF appears dark, while areas of brain edema or demyelination appear high in signal as shown here in the corpus callosum (*arrows*). Lesions in the anterior corpus callosum are frequent in MS and rare in vascular disease. **C.** Sagittal T2-weighted fast spin echo image of the thoracic spine demonstrates a fusiform high-signal-intensity lesion in the midthoracic spinal cord. **D.** Sagittal T1-weighted image obtained after the intravenous administration of gadolinium DTPA reveals focal areas of blood–brain barrier disruption, identified as high-signal-intensity regions (*arrows*). (From Longo DL, Fauci AS, Kasper DL, Hauser SL, Jameson JL, Loscalzo J, eds. *Harrison's Principles of Internal Medicine*. 18th ed. http://www.accessmedicine.com. Copyright © The McGraw-Hill Companies, Inc. All rights reserved.)

- Cerebellar and bulbar symptoms
- Sensory symptoms
  - Numbness
  - Musculoskeletal pain
  - Paresthesia
  - Dysesthesia
  - Distortion of superficial sensation
- Visual symptoms
  - Decreased acuity
  - Scotoma
  - Ocular pain
- Sexual symptoms
  - Impotence
  - Decreased genital sensation
  - Decreased genital lubrication
- Emotional and cognitive symptoms
  - Depression
  - Lability
  - Disorders of judgment
  - Agnosia
  - Memory disturbance
  - Poor conceptual thinking
  - Limited attention
  - Dysphasia
- About 50% of people will have cognitive deficits, 10% to 20% have significant deficits. The following are most commonly affected:
  - Short-term memory
  - Conceptual reasoning
  - Problem solving
  - Verbal fluency

Functional Implications

- Excessive fatigue must be avoided.
- Depending on the area of the central nervous system demyelination, the person may struggle with functional loss in the range

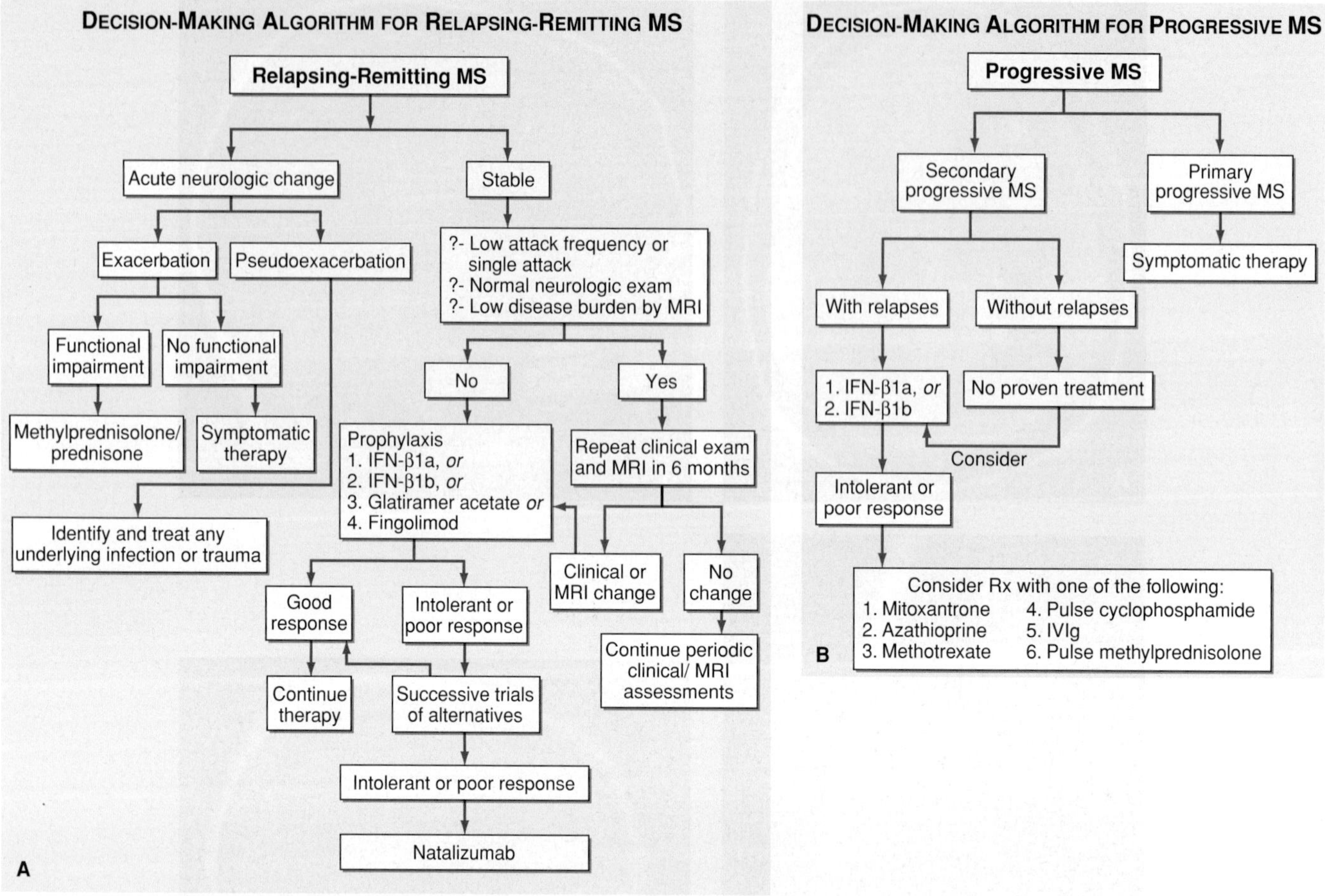

DECISION-MAKING ALGORITHM FOR RELAPSING-REMITTING MS

- Relapsing-Remitting MS
  - Acute neurologic change
    - Exacerbation
      - Functional impairment → Methylprednisolone/ prednisone
      - No functional impairment → Symptomatic therapy
    - Pseudoexacerbation → Identify and treat any underlying infection or trauma
  - Stable → ?- Low attack frequency or single attack; ?- Normal neurologic exam; ?- Low disease burden by MRI
    - No → Prophylaxis: 1. IFN-β1a, *or* 2. IFN-β1b, *or* 3. Glatiramer acetate *or* 4. Fingolimod
      - Good response → Continue therapy
      - Intolerant or poor response → Successive trials of alternatives (→ Good response) → Intolerant or poor response → Natalizumab
    - Yes → Repeat clinical exam and MRI in 6 months
      - Clinical or MRI change → Prophylaxis
      - No change → Continue periodic clinical/ MRI assessments

A

DECISION-MAKING ALGORITHM FOR PROGRESSIVE MS

- Progressive MS
  - Secondary progressive MS
    - With relapses → 1. IFN-β1a, *or* 2. IFN-β1b → Intolerant or poor response → Consider Rx with one of the following: 1. Mitoxantrone 2. Azathioprine 3. Methotrexate 4. Pulse cyclophosphamide 5. IVIg 6. Pulse methylprednisolone
    - Without relapses → No proven treatment (Consider → 1. IFN-β1a, *or* 2. IFN-β1b)
  - Primary progressive MS → Symptomatic therapy

B

FIGURE 95-2 Therapeutic decision-making for MS. (From Longo DL, Fauci AS, Kasper DL, Hauser SL, Jameson JL, Loscalzo J, eds. *Harrison's Principles of Internal Medicine.* 18th ed. http://www.accessmedicine.com.)

of minor aspects of function, such as raising one arm over head to all aspects of function where the person experiences total paralysis.

- The progressive forms of MS result in declining function over time causing the person to become technology- and assistant-dependent for all aspects of mobility, activities of daily living (basic to complex), communication, and socialization.

Possible Contributing Causes

- Region of birth
- Genetic susceptibility
- Viral attack of the myelin resulting in an autoimmune response to the damaged myelin

Differential Diagnoses

- Acute disseminated encephalomyelitis
- Antiphospholipid antibody syndrome
- Behçet disease
- Cavernous angiomas of the brainstem
- Embolic infarcts
- Foramen magnum lesion (Arnold–Chiari malformation)
- Guillain–Barré syndrome
- HIV-associated myelopathy
- Human T-cell lymphotropic virus type I-associated myelopathy
- Lupus erythematosus

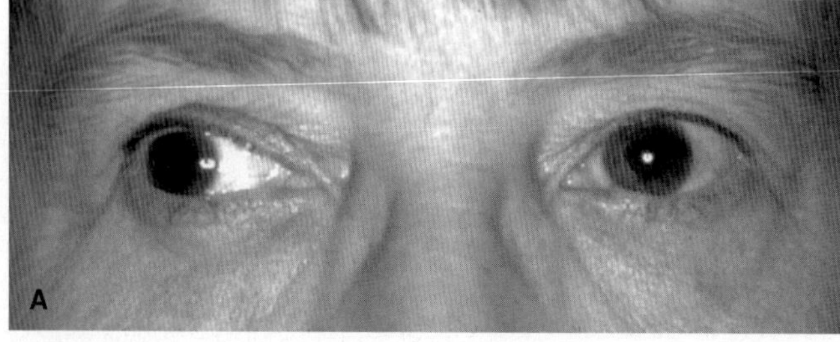

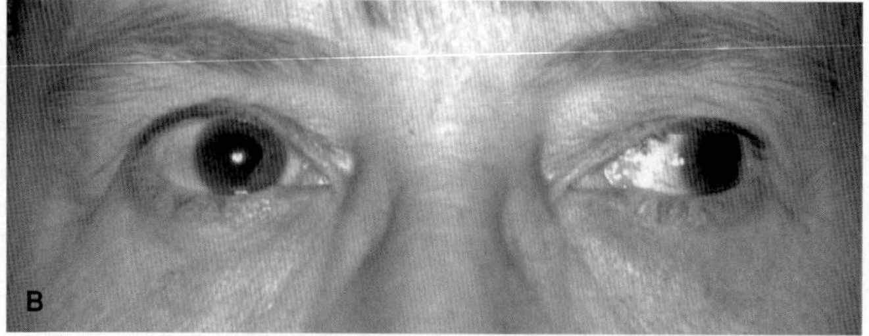

FIGURE 95-3 Bilateral internuclear ophthalmoplegia due to multiple sclerosis. (Reproduced with permission from Riordan-Eva P, Witcher JP. *General Ophthalmology.* 17th ed. New York, NY: McGraw-Hill. Copyright © 2008 by The McGraw-Hill Companies, Inc.)

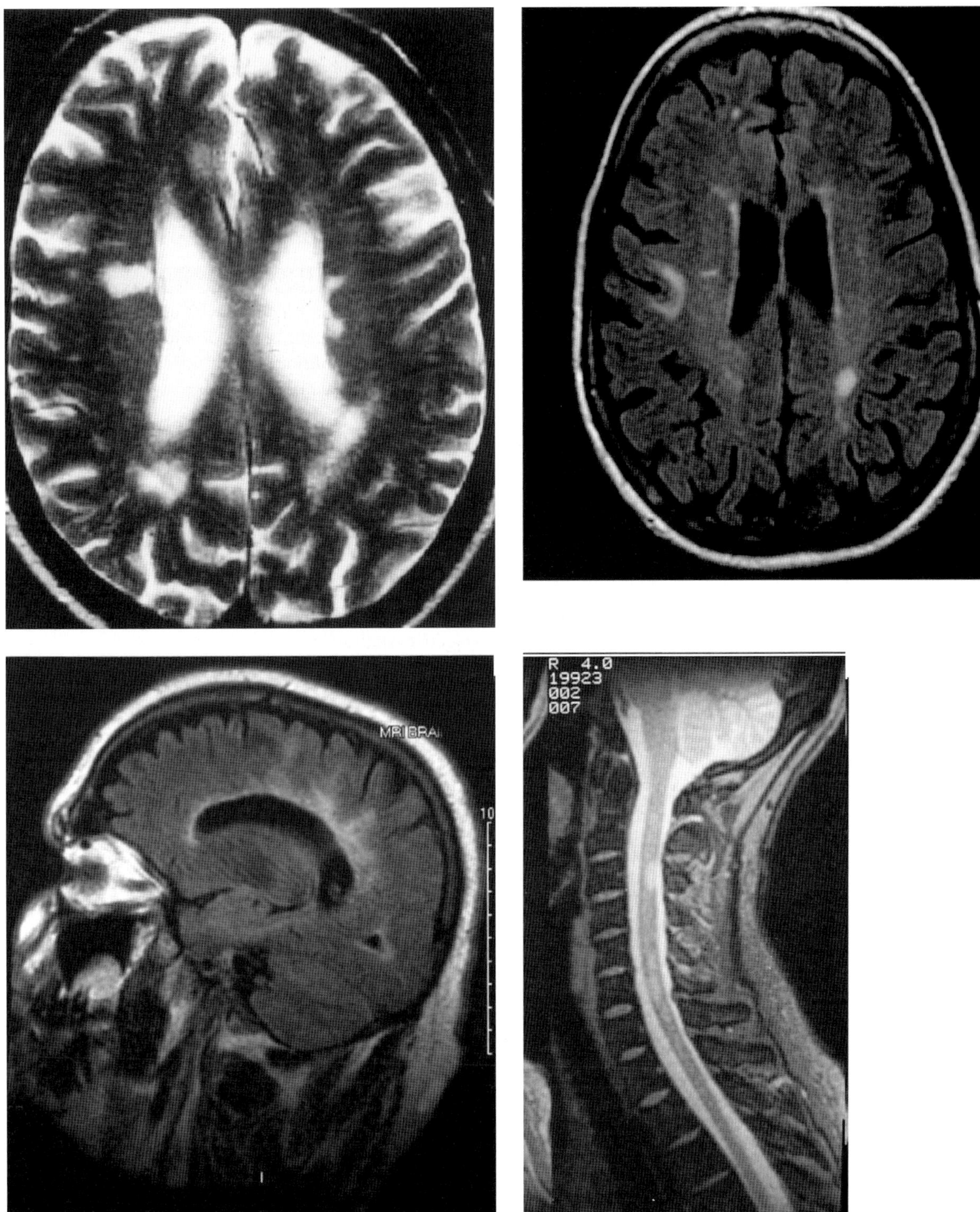

FIGURE 95-4 Multiple sclerosis. T2-weighted and fluid-attenuated inversion recovery (FLAIR) sequence MRIs demonstrating multiple plaques in the periventricular white matter (*upper left*), emanating radially from the corpus callosum ("Dawson fingers"; *lower left*), a "C-like"–shaped lesion in the right subcortical white matter that is created by interruption of the lesion by the adjacent cortex (*upper right*), and cervical spinal cord (*lower right*). The radial orientation and periventricular location of cerebral lesions are typical of the disease. (From Ropper AH, Samuels MA. *Adams & Victor's Principles of Neurology*. 9th ed. http://www.accessmedicine.com. Copyright © The McGraw-Hill Companies, Inc. All rights reserved.)

- Lyme disease
- Neurosyphilis
- Optic neuritis
- Progressive multifocal leukoencephalopathy
- Spinal cord tumor
- Subacute combined degeneration of the spinal cord (B_{12} deficiency)
- Syringomyelia
- Transverse myelitis
- Vasculitis

MEANS OF CONFIRMATION OR DIAGNOSIS

Laboratory Tests

- A definitive diagnosis can never be based solely on the laboratory findings
- Cerebrospinal fluid (CSF) testing is not routine to diagnose MS
- Elevated IgG and discrete bands of IgG (oligoclonal bands), which are not specific, having been found in a variety of inflammatory neurologic disorders and occasionally in patients with vascular or neoplastic disorders of the nervous system

Imaging

- MRI with gadolinium shows both new and active lesions; inaccurate for older lesions.
- Visual evoked potentials, brain stem auditory evoked potentials, somatosensory evoked potentials to measure nerve condition.
- May be necessary in patients presenting with myelopathy alone and in whom there is no clinical or laboratory evidence of more widespread disease to exclude a congenital or acquired surgically treatable lesion.
- The foramen magnum region must be visualized to exclude the possibility of Arnold–Chiari malformation, in which part of the cerebellum and the lower brainstem are displaced into the cervical canal, producing mixed pyramidal and cerebellar deficits in the limbs.

FINDINGS AND INTERPRETATION

- Many people with MS have elevated levels of gamma globulin.
- Approximately 25% of people with MS have white cells present in the CSF.

TREATMENT

Medications

- Disease-modifying agents
  - Avonex: For treatment of all relapsing forms and single clinical episodes confirmed by MRI
  - Betaseron: For treatment of all relapsing forms
  - Copaxone: For treatment of relapsing/remitting
  - Rebif: For treatment of all relapsing forms
  - Novantrone: For treatment of worsening relapsing/remitting and for progressive relapsing or secondary progressive
  - Tysabri: Monotherapy for relapsing forms, recommended for patients who had poor response or poor tolerance for other medications
- Corticosteroids (such as methylprednisolone) for acute relapses to limit the effect of the inflammatory process
- Symptomatic therapy
  - Spasticity
    - Baclofen (oral and intrathecal), tizanidine, dantrolene sodium
    - Diazepam: Most frequently used for night spasms
    - Flexeril: For back spasms
    - Botulinum toxin or phenol blocks for individual muscle spasticity.
  - Fatigue
    - Amantadine hydrochloride and modafinil commonly prescribed, but not FDA-approved specifically for MS-related fatigue.
  - Neurogenic bladder
    - Propantheline bromide, imipramine, oxybutynin to reduce bladder spasm
    - Bethanechol, phenoxybenzamine to reduce urinary retention
  - Pain
    - Gabapentin for dysesthetic pain

MEDICAL PROCEDURES

- Severing peripheral nerves to address specific intractable nerve pain
- Tendon lengthening for contractures

REFERRALS/ADMITTANCE

- All patients, but especially those with progressive disease despite standard therapy, should be referred
- To hospital for admission when
  - Patients requiring plasma exchange
  - During severe relapses
  - Patient unable to manage at home
- To occupational therapist: Manage fine motor dysfunction, retraining of ADLs, job retraining, if applicable
- To respiratory therapist: For patients with bulbar symptoms
- To speech/language pathologist: For patients with dysarthria and dysphagia
- To neurologist: Manage medications and progression of disease
- To psychologist: To help manage depression and cognitive symptoms

IMPAIRMENTS

- Aerobic compactly limitation
- Weakness
- Spasticity
- Incoordination, tremor, impaired balance
- Pain
- Visual impairment
- Fatigue
- Memory, cognitive impairment
- Ambulation, transfer
- ADLs
- Community skills
- Bowel and bladder dysfunction
- Sexual dysfunction
- Dysarthria
- Dysphasia
- Adjustment motivation
- Medical complications
  - Decubitus ulcer
  - Contracture
  - Nutrition
  - Respiratory problems
- Vocation
- Family adjustment
- Avocation
- Homemaking

TESTS AND MEASURES

- Ashworth and modified Ashworth spasticity scale
- Balance testing (Berg Balance Scale, Multi-directional reach test [MDRT], Tinetti Balance and Gait Evaluation, Dynamic Gait Index, etc.)

- Barthel Index
- Bed mobility and transfers
- Borg Rating of Perceived Exertion (RPE) to help patient monitor fatigue
- Box and Block Test of manual dexterity
- Canadian Occupational Performance Measure
- Cranial nerve testing
- Deep tendon reflex, Babinski
- Functional mobility (Functional Independence Measure [FIM™])
- Gait (Timed Up and Go, Tinetti, Dynamic Gait Index, 6-minute walk test)
- Health Status Questionnaire
- Joint ROM and muscle length testing
- Kurtzke Expanded Disability Status Scale (EDSS)
- Kurtzke Functional System Scores (FSS)
- Manual muscle testing
- Minimal Assessment of Cognitive Function in MS (MACFIMS)
- Modified Fatigue Impact Scale (MFIS)
- Multiple Sclerosis Quality of Life Inventory (MSQLI)
- Sensory testing
- The Dallas Pain Questionnaire

INTERVENTION

- Fatigue
  - Energy conservation techniques
  - Adaptive equipment and assistive technology
  - Planned exercise and rest activities
  - Adaptation of work environment
  - Exercise for general strength, cardiovascular and overall conditioning
  - Cooling may be beneficial in reducing fatigue, especially during exercise
- Weakness
  - Active assistive exercise
  - Active exercise
  - Progressive resistive exercise with caution for fatigue
  - Compensatory strengthening
  - Bracing as needed (ankle foot orthosis, hand/wrist splinting, etc.)
- Spasticity
  - Stretching
  - Cold
  - Inhibitory relaxation techniques
    - Joint approximation
    - Slow rolling from supine to side
    - Slow rocking
    - Slow stroking of the paravertebrals
    - Pressure on muscle tendons
  - Reflex-inhibiting movement patterns and positioning
  - Functional and weight-bearing exercise in various positions may normalize tone
- Balance and coordination
  - Sequence in functional activities
  - Balance from wide to narrow base
  - Static to dynamic activities
  - Low to high center of gravity
  - Strengthening in fixation
  - Visual cues
  - Biofeedback
  - Adaptive equipment in ADLs
    - Cuff weights for tremor
    - Weighted canes
- Sensory dysfunction
  - Sensory integration activities
  - Compensation for loss of sensation
  - Visual compensation to overcome/manage dysesthesias
- Dysarthria and dysphagia: Refer to speech therapy
- Ambulation and mobility
- Cognitive dysfunction
- General conditioning and fitness
- Activities of daily living
- Employment
- Psychosocial issues

FUNCTIONAL GOALS

Note: Due to the varying nature of the disease and the stage of progression, goals should be made specific to the patient's needs while accounting for fatigue.

- Patient will be able to
  - Demonstrate physical independence with bed mobility with the use of assistive devices as needed to control fatigue.
  - Demonstrate independent ambulation on a variety of surfaces for short community distances with assistive devices as needed to control fatigue.
  - Tolerate 15 minutes of continuous exercise on a stationary bike three times a week without evidence of excessive fatigue.

PROGNOSIS

- Relapses occur without warning.
- There is no means of preventing progression of the disorder; appropriately managing fatigue will help to manage symptoms.
- About half of all patients are without significant disability even 10 years after onset of symptoms.
- More favorable outcomes are linked to female gender, onset before age 35, monoregional versus polyregional attack, and relapsing/remitting form of MS.
- Less favorable outcomes are linked to male gender, brain stem symptoms (dysarthria, nystagmus, tremor, ataxia), high frequency of attacks (progressive relapsing form), and poor recovery after attacks (secondary progressive form).

PATIENT RESOURCES

- MSAA: The Multiple Sclerosis Association of America. http://www.mymsaa.org. Accessed June 21, 2013.
- National Multiple Sclerosis Society. http://www.nationalmssociety.org/index.aspx. Accessed June 21, 2013.

REFERENCES

1. Toy EC. Multiple Sclerosis, Case 96. *LANGE Case Files.* http://www.accessmedicine.com. Accessed May 15, 2014.
2. Multiple sclerosis. http://www.icd9data.com/2011/Volume1/320-389/340-349/340/default.htm. Accessed June 21, 2013.
3. World Health Organization. Version 2007. http://apps.who.int/classifications/apps/icd/icd10online/?gg35.htm+g35. Accessed June 21, 2013.

ADDITIONAL REFERENCES

- APTA Guide to Physical Therapist Practice. http://guidetoptpractice.apta.org. Accessed June 21, 2013.
- Fox EJ. Management of worsening multiple sclerosis with mitoxantrone: a review. *Clin Ther*. 2006;28(4):461–474.
- Frankel DI. Multiple sclerosis. In: Umphred DA, ed. *Neurological Rehabilitation*. 5th ed. St. Louis, MO: Mosby Elsevier; 2007: 709–731.
- ICD-9-CM. http://www.icd9data.com. Accessed June 21, 2013.
- ICD-10-CM. http://www.icd10data.com. Accessed June 21, 2013.
- Panus PC, Jobst EE, Masters SB, Katzung B, Tinsley SL, Trevor AJ. Skeletal muscle relaxants. In: Panus PC, Jobst EE, Masters SB, Katzung B, Tinsley SL, Trevor AJ, eds. *Pharmacology for the Physical Therapist*. New York, NY: McGraw-Hill; 2009. http://www.accessphysiotherapy.com/content/6095608. Accessed June 21, 2013.
- Ropper AL, Samuels MA. *Adams and Victor's Principles of Neurology*. 9th ed. New York, NY: McGraw-Hill; 2009:874–896.
- Waxman SG. Signaling in the nervous system. In: Waxman SG, ed. *Clinical Neuroanatomy*. 26th ed. New York, NY: McGraw-Hill; 2010. http://www.accessphysiotherapy.com/content/5271216. Accessed June 21, 2013.

96 PARAPLEGIA

Mollie Venglar, DSc, MSPT, NCS
Megan Samantha Rosga, DPT, MSPT, NCS

ICD-9-CM CODE

- 344.1 Paraplegia

ICD-10-CM CODE

- G82.20 Paraplegia, unspecified

PREFERRED PRACTICE PATTERN

- 5H: Impaired Motor Function, Peripheral Nerve Integrity, and Sensory Integrity Associated with Nonprogressive Disorders of the Spinal Cord

PATIENT PRESENTATION

An 18-year-old male was injured on a motorbike he had received for his birthday. His friends dared the young man to jump the pond on the family property. In mid-jump he lost his hold on the bike, the bike fell into the pond, and he continued through the air. He landed on his back and was knocked unconscious. In the emergency department, radiographs revealed a complete dislocation of T4 on T5 with fractures of the bodies of T3, 4, 5 as well as the pedicles of T4 and laminae of T3, 5. Patient underwent surgical fixation with Harrington rods and was placed in a thoraco-lumbar stabilizing orthosis (TLSO). Prior to his injury he participated in high school football and basketball, he worked in the family business, and was planning to enter college in the fall. His past medical history was unremarkable. His injury is assessed as a T4, ASIA A (American Spinal Injury Association).

KEY FEATURES

Description

- Complete paralysis of the trunk and bilateral lower extremities
- Result of damage to the spinal cord in the thoracic, lumbar, sacral spine, or cauda equina

Essentials of Diagnosis[1]

- Complete neurological examination
  - Muscle strength testing of the upper extremity (UE), lower extremity (LE), core musculature
  - Reflexes, deep tendon reflexes (DTRs)
  - Sensation
  - Coordination
  - Proprioception
- Diagnosis is made by level of injury, severity of injury, and use of the ASIA assessment.
- Complete loss of sensory and motor function due to damage in the thoracic or lumbar spine.
- Paraparesis is the partial loss of sensory or motor function due to damage in the thoracic or lumbar spine
- Commonly the result of trauma, but can also occur due to infarction or hemorrhage
- Spinal cord ends at or near the first lumbar vertebra (L1); damage at or above this level will produce upper motor neuron (UMN) signs and symptoms
- Damage below L1 will produce lower motor neuron (LMN) signs and symptoms

General Considerations

- Damage to the spinal cord results in potential complications to many body systems
- Be aware of wide range of complications to be safe and effective with patient care

Demographics

- Men four times as likely as women
- Most common cause is motor vehicle accident (MVA)
- Second most common cause is falls

CLINICAL FINDINGS

SIGNS AND SYMPTOMS

- UMN signs present if the injury is above the conus medullaris
- LMN signs present if the injury is in the conus medullaris or cauda equina
- Complete injury is defined as no motor or sensory function spared in the lowest sacral segments
- Incomplete injury is defined as partial or full function spared in the lowest sacral segments
- Altered or lost trunk control and balance
- Autonomic dysfunction if the injury is above the T6
- Orthostatic hypotension
- Loss of bone density
- Decreased ventilatory capability for paraplegics with damage in the mid- to upper-thoracic region
- Altered or lost ambulation/locomotion
- Altered or lost bed mobility
- Altered or lost transfer ability
- Altered or lost muscle strength
- Altered or lost sensations
- Altered DTRs
- Altered or lost bowel and bladder function
- Altered or lost autonomic control
- Altered blood pressure
- Spasticity
- Altered thermoregulation
- Changes in muscle tone
- Edema of legs, ankles, feet
  - Typically symmetrical and pitting in nature

Functional Implications

- Bladder and bowel dysfunction
- Decreased endurance and energy efficiency
- Dysesthesias
- Gait abnormalities

ASIA AMERICAN SPINAL INJURY ASSOCIATION

INTERNATIONAL STANDARDS FOR NEUROLOGICAL CLASSIFICATION OF SPINAL CORD INJURY (ISNCSCI)

ISCOS INTERNATIONAL SPINAL CORD SOCIETY

Patient Name________ Date/Time of Exam________

Examiner Name________ Signature________

RIGHT

	MOTOR KEY MUSCLES		SENSORY KEY SENSORY POINTS Light Touch (LTR)	Pin Prick (PPR)
		C2		
		C3		
		C4		
UER (Upper Extremity Right)	Elbow flexors C5			
	Wrist extensors C6			
	Elbow extensors C7			
	Finger flexors C8			
	Finger abductors (little finger) T1			
		T2		
		T3		
		T4		
		T5		
		T6		
		T7		
		T8		
		T9		
		T10		
		T11		
		T12		
		L1		
LER (Lower Extremity Right)	Hip flexors L2			
	Knee extensors L3			
	Ankle dorsiflexors L4			
	Long toe extensors L5			
	Ankle plantar flexors S1			
		S2		
		S3		
		S4-5		
RIGHT TOTALS (MAXIMUM)	(50)		(56)	(56)

Comments (Non-key Muscle? Reason for NT? Pain?):

(VAC) Voluntary anal contraction (Yes/No)

LEFT

SENSORY KEY SENSORY POINTS Light Touch (LTL)	Pin Prick (PPL)		MOTOR KEY MUSCLES	
		C2		
		C3		
		C4		
			C5 Elbow flexors	UEL (Upper Extremity Left)
			C6 Wrist extensors	
			C7 Elbow extensors	
			C8 Finger flexors	
			T1 Finger abductors (little finger)	
		T2		
		T3		
		T4		
		T5		
		T6		
		T7		
		T8		
		T9		
		T10		
		T11		
		T12		
		L1		
			L2 Hip flexors	LEL (Lower Extremity Left)
			L3 Knee extensors	
			L4 Ankle dorsiflexors	
			L5 Long toe extensors	
			S1 Ankle plantar flexors	
		S2		
		S3		
		S4-5		
(56)	(56)		(50)	LEFT TOTALS (MAXIMUM)

(DAP) Deep anal pressure (Yes/No)

MOTOR (SCORING ON REVERSE SIDE)

0 = total paralysis
1 = palpable or visible contraction
2 = active movement, gravity eliminated
3 = active movement, against gravity
4 = active movement, against some resistance
5 = active movement, against full resistance
5* = normal corrected for pain/disuse
NT = not testable

SENSORY (SCORING ON REVERSE SIDE)

0 = absent
1= altered
2 = normal
NT = not testable

C2 C3 C4 T2 T3 T4 T5 T6 T7 T8 T9 T10 T11 T12 L1 C5 C6 T1 L2 L3 L4 L5 S1 S2 S3 S4-5 C7 C8

Palm

Dorsum

• Key Sensory Points

MOTOR SUBSCORES

UER ___ + UEL ___ = UEMS TOTAL ___
MAX (25) (25) (50)

LER ___ + LEL ___ = LEMS TOTAL ___
MAX (25) (25) (50)

SENSORY SUBSCORES

LTR ___ + LTL ___ = LT TOTAL ___
MAX (56) (56) (112)

PPR ___ + PPL ___ = PP TOTAL ___
MAX (56) (56) (112)

NEUROLOGICAL LEVELS
Steps 1-5 for classification as on reverse

	R	L
1. SENSORY		
2. MOTOR		

3. NEUROLOGICAL LEVEL OF INJURY (NLI)

4. COMPLETE OR INCOMPLETE?
Incomplete = Any sensory or motor function in S4-5

5. ASIA IMPAIRMENT SCALE (AIS)

(In complete injuries only)
ZONE OF PARTIAL PRESERVATION
Most caudal level with any innervation

	R	L
SENSORY		
MOTOR		

A

REV 02/13

Muscle Function Grading

0 = total paralysis

1 = palpable or visible contraction

2 = active movement, full range of motion (ROM) with gravity eliminated

3 = active movement full ROM against gravity

4 = active movement full ROM against gravity and moderate resistance in a muscle specific position.

5 = (normal) active movement, full ROM against gravity and full resistance in a functional muscle position expected from an otherwise unimpaired person.

5* = (normal) active movement, full ROM against gravity and sufficient resistance to be considered normal if identified inhibiting factors (i.e. pain, disuse) were not present.

NT = not testable (i.e. due to immobilization, severe pain such that the patient cannot be graded, amputation of limb, or contracture of > 50% of the normal range of motion).

Sensory Grading

0 = Absent

1 = Altered, either decreased/impaired sensation or hypersensitivity

2 = Normal

NT = Not testable

Non Key Muscle Functions (optional)

May be used to assign a motor level to differentiate AIS B vs. C

Movement	Root level
Shoulder: Flexion, extension, abduction, adduction, internal and external rotation **Elbow:** Supination	C5
Elbow: Pronation **Wrist:** Flexion	C6
Finger: Flexion at proximal joint, extension. **Thumb:** Flexion, extension and abduction in plane of thumb	C7
Finger: Flexion at MCP joint **Thumb:** Opposition, adduction and abduction perpendicular to palm	C8
Finger: Abduction of the index finger	T1
Hip: Adduction	L2
Hip: External rotation	L3
Hip: Extension, abduction, internal rotation **Knee:** Flexion **Ankle:** Inversion and eversion **Toe:** MP and IP extension	L4
Hallux and Toe: DIP and PIP flexion and abduction	L5
Hallux: Adduction	S1

B

ASIA Impairment Scale (AIS)

A = Complete. No sensory or motor function is preserved in the sacral segments S4-5.

B = Sensory Incomplete. Sensory but not motor function is preserved below the neurological level and includes the sacral segments S4-5 (light touch or pin prick at S4-5 or deep anal pressure) AND no motor function is preserved more than three levels below the motor level on either side of the body.

C = Motor Incomplete. Motor function is preserved below the neurological level**, and more than half of key muscle functions below the neurological level of injury (NLI) have a muscle grade less than 3 (Grades 0-2).

D = Motor Incomplete. Motor function is preserved below the neurological level**, and <u>at least half</u> (half or more) of key muscle functions below the NLI have a muscle grade ≥ 3.

E = Normal. If sensation and motor function as tested with the ISNCSCI are graded as normal in all segments, and the patient had prior deficits, then the AIS grade is E. Someone without an initial SCI does not receive an AIS grade.

** For an individual to receive a grade of C or D, i.e. motor incomplete status, they must have either (1) voluntary anal sphincter contraction or (2) sacral sensory sparing <u>with</u> sparing of motor funtion more than three levels below the motor level for that side of the body. The International Standards at this time allows even non-key muscle function more than 3 levels below the motor level to be used in determining motor incomplete status (AIS B versus C).

NOTE: When assessing the extent of motor sparing below the level for distingusihing between AIS B and C, the ***motor level*** on each side is used; whereas to differentiate between AIS C and D (based on proportion of key muscle functions with strength grade 3 or greater) the ***neurological level of injury*** is used.

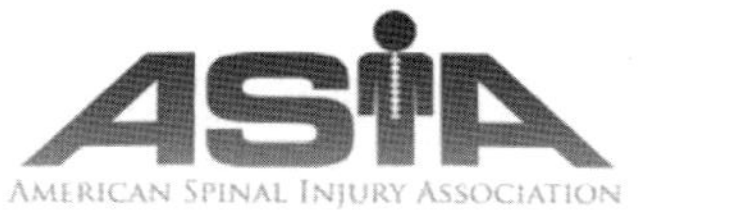

INTERNATIONAL STANDARDS FOR NEUROLOGICAL CLASSIFICATION OF SPINAL CORD INJURY

ISCoS
INTERNATIONAL SPINAL CORD SOCIETY

Steps in Classification

The following order is recommended for determining the classification of individuals with SCI.

1. Determine sensory levels for right and left sides.
The sensory level is the most caudal, intact dermatome for both pin prick and light touch sensation.

2. Determine motor levels for right and left sides.
Defined by the lowest key muscle function that has a grade of at least 3 (on supine testing), providing the key muscle functions represented by segments above that level are judged to be intact (graded as a 5).
Note: in regions where there is no myotome to test, the motor level is presumed to be the same as the sensory level, if testable motor function above that level is also normal.

3. Determine the neurological level of injury (NLI)
This refers to the most caudal segment of the cord with intact sensation and antigravity (3 or more) muscle function strength, provided that there is normal (intact) sensory and motor function rostrally respectively.
The NLI is the most cephalad of the sensory and motor levels determined in steps 1 and 2.

4. Determine whether the injury is Complete or Incomplete.
(i.e. absence or presence of sacral sparing)
*If voluntary anal contraction = **No** AND all S4-5 sensory scores = **0** AND deep anal pressure = **No,** then injury is **Complete.***
*Otherwise, injury is **Incomplete.***

5. Determine ASIA Impairment Scale (AIS) Grade:

Is injury <u>Complete</u>? **If YES, AIS=A** and can record ZPP (lowest dermatome or myotome on each side with some preservation)

NO

Is injury Motor <u>Complete</u>? **If YES, AIS=B**

NO (No=voluntary anal contraction OR motor function more than three levels below the motor level on a given side, if the patient has sensory incomplete classification)

Are <u>at least</u> half (half or more) of the key muscles below the <u>neurological</u> level of injury graded 3 or better?

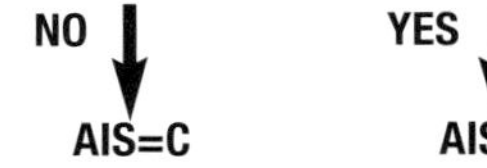

NO → **AIS=C**

YES → **AIS=D**

If sensation and motor function is normal in all segments, AIS=E
Note: AIS E is used in follow-up testing when an individual with a documented SCI has recovered normal function. If at initial testing no deficits are found, the individual is neurologically intact; the ASIA Impairment Scale does not apply.

FIGURE 96-1 The American Spinal Injury Association system for categorizing spinal cord injury patients according to level and degree of neurologic deficit. (From the American Spinal Injury Association. *International Standards for Neurological Classification of Spinal Cord Injury*, revised 2013; Atlanta, GA. Reprinted 2013. Reprinted with permission.)

- Impaired balance
- Impaired bed mobility
- Impaired coordination
- Impaired muscular strength
- Impaired transfers
- Increased risk of contracture
- Increased risk of deep vein thrombosis
- Increased risk of heterotopic ossification
- Increased risk of urinary tract infection (the first sign is often a change in tone or spasticity)
- Neuropathic pain
- Osteoporosis
- Postural/orthostatic hypotension
- Pressure sores
- Renal calculi
- Sexual dysfunction
- UE and shoulder pain/over use

Possible Contributing Causes

- Traumatic[2]
  - Most frequent cause in adults
  - MVAs 45.6%
  - Falls 19.6%
  - Acts of violence, including gun shots 17.8%
  - Recreational sports 10.7%
  - Other 6.3%
- Nontraumatic/pathological influence[1]
  - 30% of all spinal cord injuries
  - Vascular malfunctions (arteriovenous malformation [AVM]), thrombosis, embolus, or hemorrhage
  - Vertebral subluxations due to rheumatoid arthritis (RA) or degenerative joint disease (DJD)
  - Infections: Syphilis, transverse myelitis
  - Spinal neoplasms
  - Syringomyelia
  - Abscesses of the spinal cord
  - Neurological diseases: Multiple sclerosis (MS), amyotrophic lateral sclerosis (ALS; also known as Lou Gehrig disease)

Differential Diagnoses

- Spinal shock
- Traumatic brain injury
- Spinal cord concussion
- Hysterical paralysis
- Caisson disease (decompression sickness)

MEANS OF CONFIRMATION OR DIAGNOSIS

Imaging

- MRI
- Computed tomography (CT) scan for detailed imaging
- X-ray for spinal vertebra damage

Diagnostic Procedures

- Reflex testing
- Manual muscle testing
- EMG testing

FINDINGS AND INTERPRETATION

- Anterior cord injury
  - Flexion injury results in greatest damage to the anterior spinal cord

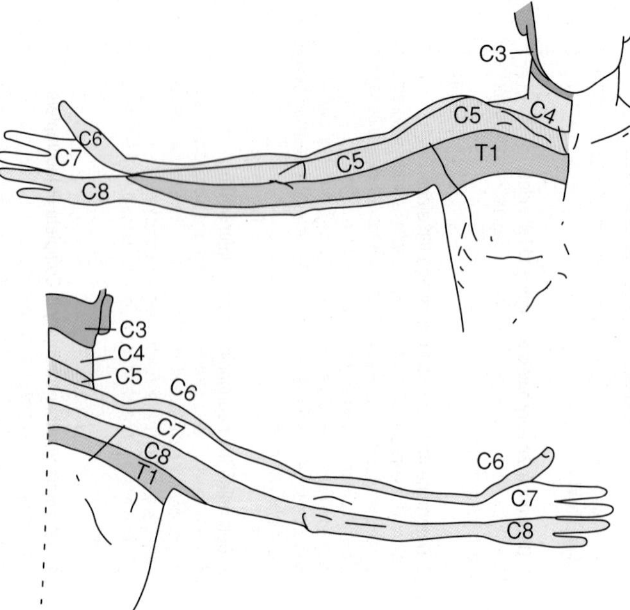

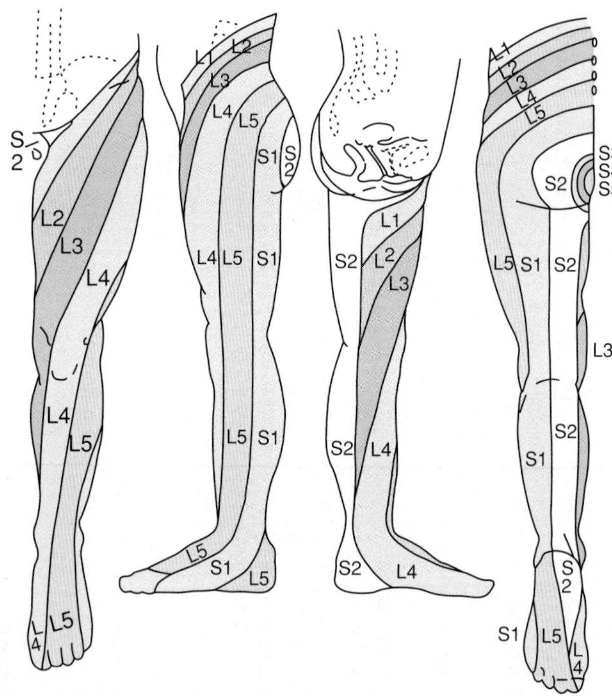

FIGURE 96-2 Dermatomes of the upper and lower extremities, outlined by the pattern of sensory loss following lesions of single nerve roots. (From JJ Keegan, FD Garrett. *Anat Rec*. 1948;102:409–437.)

  - Producing loss of motor function below the level of the injury, but sparing of some sensory function
- Posterior cord injury
  - Hyperextension injury results in greatest damage to the posterior spinal cord
  - Producing profound loss of sensation, but some sparing of motor function below the level of the injury
- Damage to the cauda equina or the conus medullaris of the spinal cord
  - Results in LMN signs and symptoms

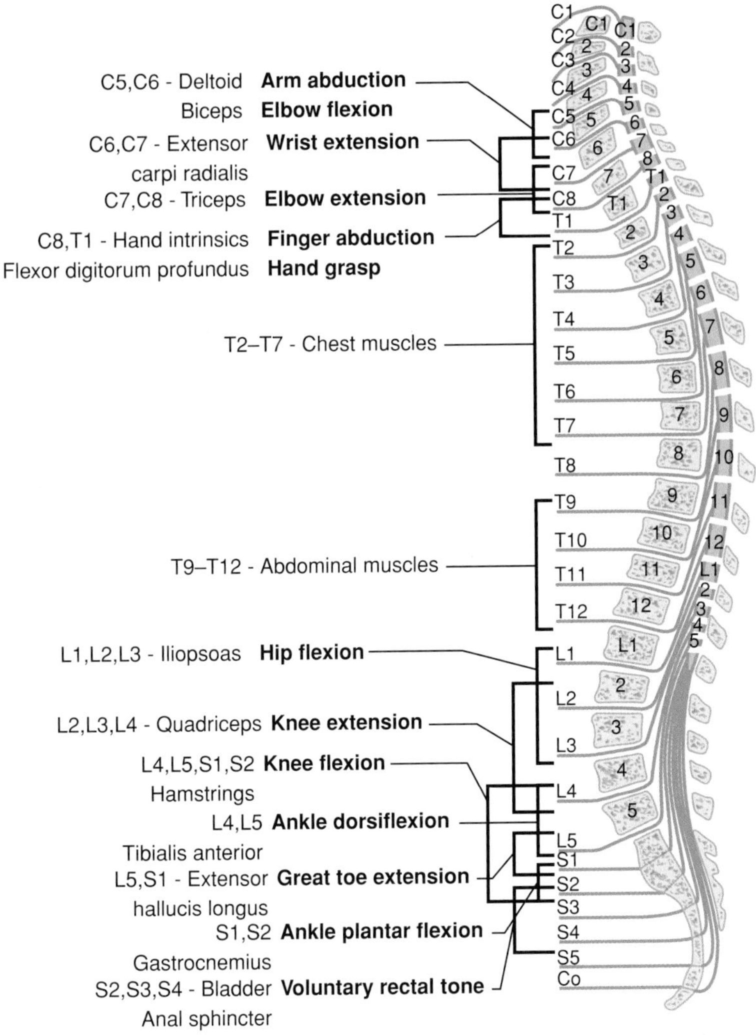

FIGURE 96-3 Spinal cord level. The spinal cord level of injury can be delineated by physical examination, including a detailed neurologic examination. (From Tintinalli JE, Stapczynski J, Ma OJ, Cline D, Cydulka R, Meckler G. *Tintinalli's Emergency Medicine: A Comprehensive Study Guide*. 7th ed. http://www.accessmedicine.com.

REFERRALS/ADMITTANCE

- To trauma center (ER) at time of injury
  - Proper relocation of patient with avoiding active and passive movement
  - Proper medical stabilization of patient
  - Vertebral realignment/early immobilization of fractures
- To neurologist if the injury is chronic, but patient is losing more sensation or motor function
- To spinal cord support group
- To custom durable medical equipment provider
- To recreational therapy
- To challenged athlete groups
- To OT, as needed
- To vocational rehabilitation for job site modification or job retraining
- To counselor or psychologist

IMPAIRMENTS

- Peripheral nerve integrity
- Gait
- Wheelchair (w/c) mobility
- Transfers
- Balance
  - Static sit
  - Dynamic sit
  - Static stand
  - Dynamic stand
  - Moving base of support (BOS)
- Muscle strength
- Muscle recruitment
- Coordination
- Postural control
- Posture
- ROM
- Reflexes
  - DTRs
  - Babinski
  - Clonus
- Muscle tone
- Sensation
- Bed mobility

TABLE 96-1 Cardiopulmonary Risk Factors Following an SCI

Impaired respiratory mechanics	• Paralysis/weakness of respiratory/trunk muscles. • Abnormal tone: spasms, spasticity, flaccidity. May limit potential inspiratory/expiratory efforts. • Posture: thoracic kyphosis, shoulder protraction with internal rotation. May limit chest expansion. • Decreased ROM of spine, rib cage, shoulders or pelvis, caused by spinal fixation devices, spasticity, immobility, etc. • Decreased cough effectiveness caused by weakness, poor posture, etc. • Poor breath support for speech. • Presence of a tracheostomy tube or cervical fixation devices such as a Halo or Somi brace. • Pain: limiting motion or force.
Sleep dysfunction	• Impaired respiratory mechanics. May result in retention of CO_2 at night. • Potentially fatal if not detected and attended to.
Autonomic dysfunction and cardiovascular dysfunction	• Autonomic dysreflexia: potentially severe cardiopulmonary responses. Can be fatal. • Inability to regulate body temperature. • Inability to regulate sweating. • Orthostatic hypotension. • Significant bradycardia. • Risk for development of deep vein thrombosis (DVT) and potential for pulmonary embolus (PE).
Increased risk of infections	• Ongoing risk for urinary tract infections: foley catheter, dehydration, inadequate or infrequent voiding, etc. • Ongoing risk for respiratory infections: dehydration, secretion retention, hypoventilation, etc. • Ongoing risk for septicemia: unhealed or infected skin injuries/bed sores, loss of sensation (possibly not aware of injury), etc.
Heterotopic bone formation	• Limitations in ROM which could limit chest movements and inspiratory efforts.
Decubiti (bed sores)	• Skin breakdown which could limit postural changes and secretion mobilization. • Invites infections.
Poor nutrition/hydration	• Swallowing dysfunction (secondary to tracheostomy tube, cervical fixation device, trauma to vocal folds, etc.). • Gastrointestinal bleeds/ulcers, irregularities, etc. • Inadequate caloric intake: reduce energy level. • Inadequate liquid intake: dehydration.
Other inherent risks	• Age: older patients carry higher respiratory risks. • Obesity. • Other medical history concurrent with SCI. • Other past medical/social history. • Previous lifestyle.

Source: DeTurk WE, Cahalin LP. *Cardiovascular and Pulmonary Physical Therapy*. 2nd ed.

- Transfers
- Endurance
- Aerobic capacity
- Self care
- Home management
- Respiratory compromise

TESTS AND MEASURES

- ASIA
  - Motor
  - Sensation
  - ASIA neurologic level
  - Complete versus incomplete
- Functional mobility (Functional Independence Measure [FIM™])
  - Bed mobility
  - W/c mobility
  - Transfers
  - Gait
    - Timed Up and Go Test (TUG)
    - 10-meter walk test
    - Functional gait assessment (FGA)
    - Walking index for spinal cord injury (WISCI)
- Sitting and standing (for people with incomplete injuries or damage in the lower lumbar and sacral levels)
  - Balance tests
    - Sit-and-reach test
    - Tinetti Gait and Balance Evaluation
    - Berg Balance Scale (BBS)
  - Cardiovascular and pulmonary endurance (6-minute walk test, if appropriate; UE ergometer test)
- Muscle endurance
- Skin assessment
- Active and passive ROM, muscle length
- Posture in sitting (w/c and edge of mat, supported/unsupported) and standing if applicable
- Pain scale (1–10)

INTERVENTION

- ROM/stretching/positioning
- Orientation to vertical position
- Strengthening
- Balance training
- Gait training (if appropriate and with appropriate bracing and assistive devices)
- Transfer training
- Bed-mobility training
- W/c-mobility training (curbs, ramps, various surfaces, negotiating obstacles, wheelies, floor recovery)
- Cardiovascular and pulmonary endurance

FUNCTIONAL GOALS

- Spinal cord injury to T1-6 levels (intercostals and trunk above the waist)
    - Patient will
        - Transfer between the w/c and the edge of mat via lateral pivot transfer with contact guard assist for safety to maximize safety and independence with functional mobility.
        - Propel ultra-light weight manual w/c >500 feet indoors over level surfaces, while negotiating obstacles with close supervision and minimal verbal cues for technique to maximize safe functional independence and mobility.
- Spinal cord injury to the T7-L1 levels (abdominal muscles)
    - Patient will
        - Safe and independent with all aspects of bed mobility.
        - Propel an ultra-light weight manual w/c on community surfaces >1500 feet with supervision for safety to increase safe and efficient functional independence.
- Spinal cord injury to the L2-S2 levels
    - Patient will
        - Assessed and fitted for proper LE bracing for a trial of gait training in parallel bars with appropriate assist.
        - Independent with transfers to and from all surfaces via lateral pivot transfer to maximize safe functional independence.

PROGNOSIS

- Good for becoming functional with some/all activities for patients who obtain appropriate services and participate in maintaining the health of their body systems.
- Variable for recovery of prior function based on degree, location, severity of injury. Patients at ASIA A and B are less likely to recover prior function than those at ASIA C and D.

PATIENT RESOURCE

- Canadian Paraplegic Association. http://www.cpa-ab.org. Accessed July 7, 2013.

REFERENCES

1. Kirshblum SC, Biering-Sorensen F, Betz R, Burns S, Donovan W, et al. International Standards for Neurological Classification of Spinal Cord Injury: Cases with Classification Challenges. *The Journal of Spinal Cord Medicine.* 2014;37(2):120–127.
2. Fulk GD, Schmitz TJ, Behrman AL. Traumatic spinal cord injury. In: O'Sullivan SB, Schmitz TJ, eds. *Physical Rehabilitation.* 5th ed. Philadelphia, PA: F.A. Davis Company; 2007:937–991.

ADDITIONAL REFERENCES

- Kirshblum SC, Biering-Sorensen F, Betz R, Burns S, Donovan W, et al. International Standards for Neurological Classification of Spinal Cord Injury: Cases with Classification Challenges. *The Journal of Spinal Cord Medicine.* 2014;37(2):120–127.
- Raskob GE, Hull RD, Pineo GF. Venous thrombosis. In: Lichtman MA, Kipps TJ, Seligsohn U, Kaushansky K, Prchal JT, eds. *Williams Hematology.* 8th ed. New York, NY: McGraw-Hill; 2011. http://www.accessmedicine.com/content.aspx?aID=6241628. Accessed July 7, 2013.
- Ropper AL, Samuels MA. *Adams and Victor's Principles of Neurology.* 9th ed. New York, NY: McGraw-Hill; 2009:1181–1188.

97 PARKINSON'S DISEASE

Mollie Venglar, DSc, MSPT, NCS

CONDITION/DISORDER SYNONYM

- Paralysis agitans

ICD-9-CM CODE

- 332.0 Paralysis agitans

ICD-10-CM CODE

- G20 Parkinsonism (idiopathic) (primary)

PREFERRED PRACTICE PATTERN

- 5E: Impaired Motor Function and Sensory Integrity Associated with Progressive Disorders of the Central Nervous System[1]

PATIENT PRESENTATION

A 75-year-old male with a 7-year history of Parkinson's disease (PD) was admitted to the hospital following a fall. He did not suffer any fractures, but reports pain in his back when he exerts himself. He has been admitted to in-patient rehabilitation for mobility retraining. He has a festinating gait pattern with poor disassociation in his trunk and no arm swing. He demonstrates bilateral upper-extremity (UE) tremors that increase in amplitude when he is under physical, mental, or emotional stress. He struggles both to initiate a movement and to control the movement once it is initiated. His wife reports that he walks better when he holds on to her arm and they walk together, but that walking seems more effortful for him over the past several months.[2]

KEY FEATURES

Description

- Progressive degenerative disorder of the central nervous system
- Death of dopamine-producing cells in the substantia nigra
- Named after English MD, James Parkinson
- Parkinsonian syndromes (4 types)
- Primary or idiopathic, no known cause
- Secondary or acquired
- Hereditary parkinsonism
- Parkinson plus syndrome or multiple system degeneration

Essentials of Diagnosis

- Core features include a tetrad of hypo- or bradykinesia, resting tremor, postural instability, and rigidity
- Some people have a rigidity-dominant presentation; others have a dyskinesia-dominant presentation (predominantly those with onset at a young age)
- Pathophysiology

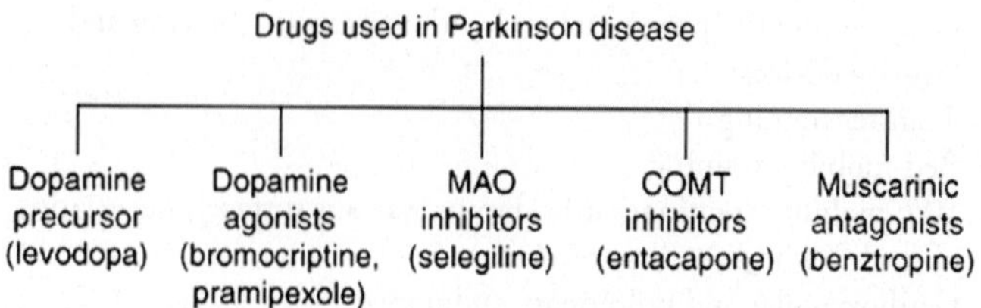

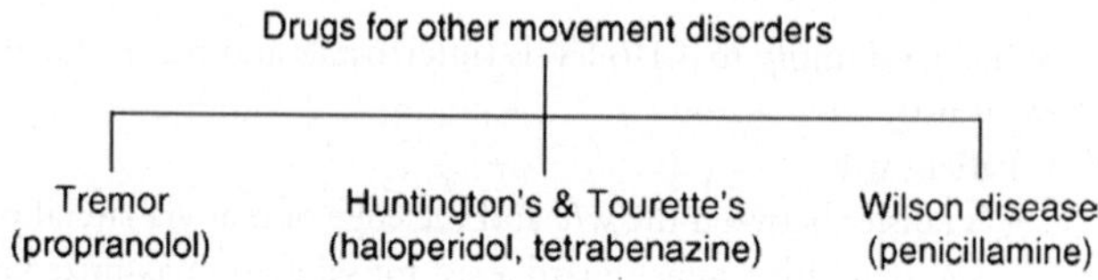

FIGURE 97-1 Classification of drugs used in the treatment of Parkinson's disease. (From Panus PT, Katzung B, Jobst E, Tinsley S, Masters S, Trevor A. *Pharmacology for the Physical Therapist*. New York, NY: McGraw-Hill; 2009: p. 228.)

General Considerations

- Positive diagnosis of PD is made with a successful levodopa (l-dopa) trial

Demographics

- Onset generally between 45 to 70 years of age
- More common in men
- Impacts all ethnic groups and socioeconomic classes
- Most cases are idiopathic; genetic variants exist, but are rare

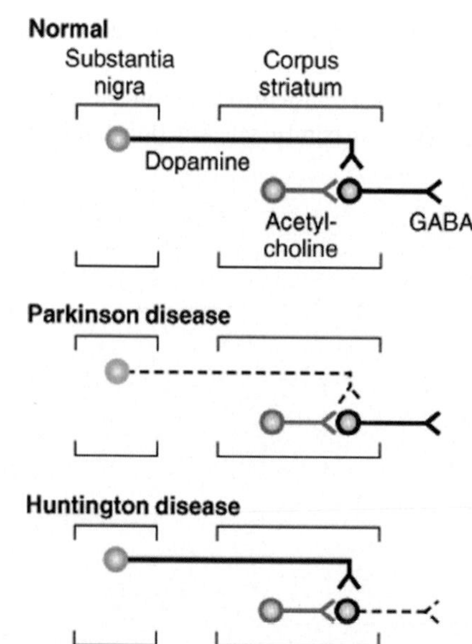

FIGURE 97-2 Schematic representation of the sequences of neurons involved in Parkinson's disease and Huntington's chorea. **Top.** Dopaminergic neurons (light gray) originating in the substantia nigra normally inhibit the GABAergic output from the striatum, whereas cholinergic neurons (gray) exert an excitatory effect. **Middle.** Neurons in Parkinson's disease. The dopaminergic neuron (dashed, light gray) is lost with a relative increase in cholinergic activity. **Bottom.** Neurons in Huntington's disease. The cholinergic neurons may be lost (gray), but even more GABAergic neurons (dashed black) degenerate. (From Panus PT, Katzung B, Jobst E, Tinsley S, Masters S, Trevor A. *Pharmacology for the Physical Therapist*. New York, NY: McGraw-Hill; 2009:p. 229.)

CLINICAL FINDINGS

SIGNS AND SYMPTOMS

- Tremor: Usually asymmetrical
- Gait disturbance, usually described as "festinating"
- Postural instability
- Stooped posture
- Stiffness/rigidity: Begins on one side
- Slowness of movement
- Dizziness
- Freezing of movement
- Bradykinesia or hypokinesia
- Muscle ache
- Loss of dexterity
- Mask-like facial expression
- Micrographia (small, cramped handwriting)
- Depression
- Neuropsychiatric problems
- Speech disturbance: Decreased volume and pitch, as well as motoric loss
- Dementia in the later stages of the disease
- Loss of smell
- Constipation

Functional Implications

- Progressive loss of
  - Balance reactions
  - Ambulation ability and safety
  - Respiratory capacity to support activity
  - Interaction with home and community environments

Possible Contributing Causes

- Unknown
- Drug-induced parkinsonism (DIP)

Differential Diagnoses

- Hemiparkinson-hemiatrophy syndrome
- Progressive supranuclear palsy (PSP)
- Basal ganglia tumors
- Vascular pathology
- Multiple system atrophy (MSA)
- Lewy body disease
- Corticobasal ganglionic degeneration (CBGD)
- Encephalitis
- Pseudobulbar palsy
- Binswanger disease
- Normal-pressure hydrocephalus (NPH)
- Multiple sclerosis (MS)

MEANS OF CONFIRMATION OR DIAGNOSIS

Laboratory Tests

- Blood test to help rule out other disorders

Imaging

- Positron emission tomography (PET) scan
- Magnetic resonance imaging (MRI) and computed tomography (CT) usually normal

Diagnostic Procedures

- Confirmation is made by a positive response to l-dopa trial in a patient with the tetrad of symptoms brady- or hypokinesia, resting tremor, postural changes and instability, cogwheel rigidity.

FINDINGS AND INTERPRETATION

- PET scan would demonstrate decreased activity in the basal ganglia.

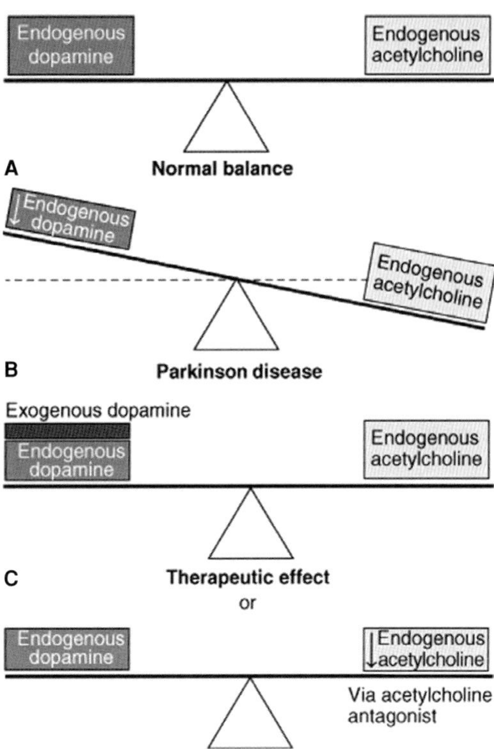

FIGURE 97-3 Schematic representation of the imbalance of neurotransmitters. **A.** Normal balance of acetylcholine and dopamine in the CNS. **B.** In Parkinson's disease, a decrease in dopamine results in an imbalance and tips the scale toward acetylcholine. **C.** Drug therapy in Parkinson's disease is aimed at correcting the imbalance between acetylcholine and dopamine. This can be accomplished by either (1) increasing the supply of dopamine or (2) blocking or lowering acetylcholine levels to restore normal balance. (From Panus PT, Katzung B, Jobst E, Tinsley S, Masters S, Trevor A. *Pharmacology for the Physical Therapist*. New York, NY: McGraw-Hill; 2009:p. 229.)

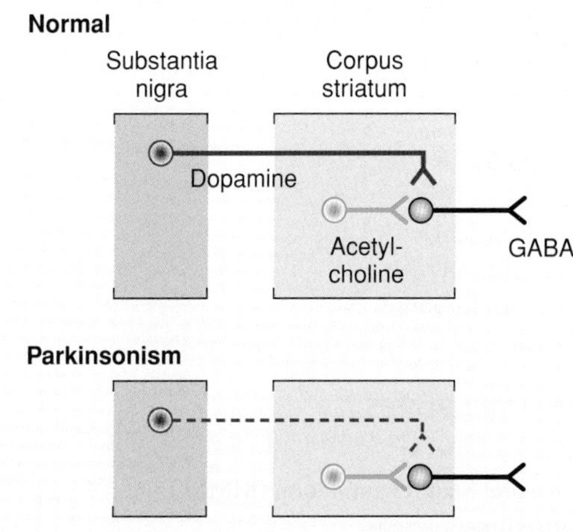

FIGURE 97-4 Schematic representation of the sequence of neurons involved in parkinsonism. **Top:** Dopaminergic neurons (*red*) originating in the substantia nigra normally inhibit the GABAergic output from the striatum (caudate and putamen), whereas cholinergic neurons (*green*) exert an excitatory effect. **Bottom:** In parkinsonism, there is a selective loss of dopaminergic neurons (*dashed, red*). This leads to increased inhibitory output from the striatum. (From Aminoff MJ. Pharmacologic management of parkinsonism and other movement disorders. In: Katzung BG, Masters SB, Trevor AJ, eds. *Basic and Clinical Pharmacology*. 12th ed. New York, NY: McGraw-Hill; 2012.)

TREATMENT

▸ Medications

- Sinemet
- Ropinirole
- Symmetrel
- Cogentin
- Entacapone
- Rasagiline
- Selegiline

REFERRALS/ADMITTANCE

- To neurologist for imaging; disease management
- To neurosurgeon for deep brain stimulation
- To the National Parkinson Foundation for support

IMPAIRMENTS

- Attention
- Cognition
- Gait training
- Wheelchair (w/c) mobility
- Balance
  - Static sit
  - Dynamic sit
  - Static stand
  - Dynamic stand
  - Moving base of support (BOS)
- Muscle strength
- Muscle recruitment and control
- Coordination (fine and gross motor skills)
- Posture and postural control
- ROM
- Reflexes
  - Deep tendon reflexes (DTRs)
  - Babinski
  - Clonus
- Muscle tone
- Motor planning
- Bed mobility
- Transfers
- Endurance
- Aerobic capacity
- Self-care
- Home management
- Fine motor control
- Respiratory compromise
- Loss of smell

TESTS AND MEASURES

- Cognition
  - Mini-Mental State Examination (MMSE)
  - Executive function tests
    - Memory
    - Comprehension
    - Speed of processing
    - Attention and concentration
- Strength and muscle endurance
- Coordination: Gross and fine motor skills
- Muscle tone: Look for rigidity (cogwheel is the most common in PD) and tremors

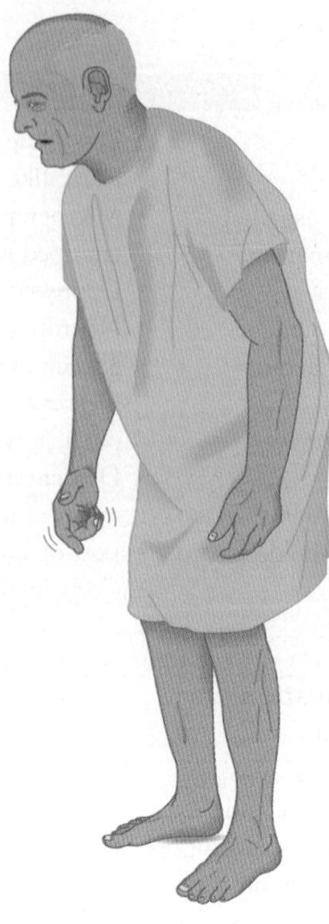

FIGURE 97-5 Typical flexed posture of a patient with parkinsonism. (From Greenberg DA, Aminoff MJ, Simon RP. *Clinical Neurology*. 8th ed. http://www.accessmedicine.com. Copyright © The McGraw-Hill Companies, Inc. All rights reserved.)

- Joint ROM: Passive and active (note end feel and any contractures from the rigidity)
- Flexibility: Specific muscle length, as well as spinal flexibility during functional activities
- Cranial nerve integrity (especially related to vision and swallowing)
- Sensation (especially deep and combined cortical sensations)
- Postural alignment (note if appears fixed or still flexible)
- Balance
  - Timed Up and Go Test (TUG)
  - Multi-directional reach test (MDRT)
  - Tinetti Performance Oriented Mobility Assessment (POMA)
  - Berg Balance Scale (BBS)
  - Retropulsion test
  - Clinical test of sensory organization and balance (CTSIB)
- Gait
  - TUG
  - Tinetti gait and balance evaluation
  - 10-meter walk test
  - Dynamic Gait Index (DGI) in the early stage of the disease
  - Walking dual-task assessment
- Respiratory function
  - Spirometry
  - Oxygen saturation
  - Breathing pattern
  - Auscultation
- Integumentary: More of a concern in the mid- and late stages
- Functional mobility: Functional Independence Measure (FIM™)
- Disease-specific measures
  - Unified Parkinson's Disease Rating Scale (UPDRS)
  - Parkinson's Disease Rating Scale-39

- Hoehn and Yahr scale (HY)[1]
- Schwab and England Activities of Daily Living Scale (ADL)

INTERVENTION

- Increase aerobic capacity and endurance
  - Passive and active stretching of accessory muscles
  - Spirometry
  - Aerobic training
- Balance and coordination activities (agility, if appropriate)
  - Balance strategies
  - Speed/reaction time training
  - Multi tasking
- Gait training
  - With/without assistive device
  - Change of direction/turning
  - Visual cues if needed to prevent/release freezing
  - Treadmill on decline
- Body mechanics training
- Postural awareness and control
- Flexibility/stretching
- Relaxation
- Proprioceptive neuromuscular facilitation (PNF) techniques
- Strength/resistance training
- Aquatic exercise

FUNCTIONAL GOALS

- For patients that fit into the HY[2] ratings of 1 to 1.5
  - Patient will
    - Tolerate a 30-minute aerobic exercise program, three times a week, with age-appropriate heart rate and VO_2 maximum measurements to maintain cardiorespiratory function.
    - Demonstrate age-appropriate bilateral joint ROM and muscle length in both UE and lower extremities (LE) to maintain current physical abilities/activities.
- For patients that fit into the HY[2] ratings of 2 to 2.5
  - Patient will
    - Ambulate with normal arm swing bilaterally >50% of the time when they are in a visually stimulating environment to decrease the frequency of "freezing" events.
    - Demonstrate normal and consistent ankle, hip, and stepping strategies to maintain balance on a variety of surfaces and in a variety of environments without loss of balance.
- For patients that fit into the HY[2] rating of 3.0
    - Effectively use visual or auditory cues to decrease episodes of freezing by >50% in the home and community environments.
    - Demonstrate the ability to turn 180 degrees in >5 steps and without loss of balance.
- For patients that fit into the HY[2] rating of 4.0
  - Patient will
    - Demonstrate safe and appropriate use of the U-Step walker in the home and community environment with less than two verbal cues for every 250 ft of ambulation.
    - Demonstrate the ability to get in and out of bed with minimally physical assistance and short, precise, verbal commands from caregiver.
- For patients that fit into the HY[2] rating of 5.0
  - Caregiver will
    - Demonstrate consistent and safe transfers of patient between the bed and the w/c to allow patient greater interaction with the environment.
    - Demonstrate knowledge of and physical ability to monitor for pressure sores to prevent patient skin breakdown.

PROGNOSIS

- Poor ultimately; the disease is progressively degenerative.
- Therapy can help plateau the disease temporarily, improve quality of life, and maintain function for as long as possible.
- Average length of time from onset of the disease to w/c bound is 7.5 years.

ADDITIONAL INFORMATION

- For additional information, please see Case Study #17 in Chapter 13 (Control of Movement) of the *Clinical Neuroanatomy*. 26th ed. Textbook on www.AccessPhysiotherapy.com

PATIENT RESOURCE

- National Parkinson Foundation. 1-800-4PD-INFO (1-800-473-4636) http://www.parkinson.org/. Accessed July 14, 2013.

REFERENCES

1. APTA Guide to PT Practice. http://guidetoptpractice.apta.org/content/1/SEC22.extract?sid=617be7ac-5357-4271-914a-04c15040f7fb. Accessed July 14, 2013.
2. O'Sullivan SB. Parkinson's disease. In: O'Sullivan SB, Schmitz TJ, eds. *Physical Rehabilitation*. 5th ed. Philadelphia, PA: F.A. Davis Company; 2007:853–893.

ADDITIONAL REFERENCES

- Malone TR, Hazle C, Grey ML. Imaging of the brain. In: Malone TR, Hazle C, Grey ML, eds. *Imaging in Rehabilitation*. New York, NY: McGraw-Hill; 2008. http://www.accessphysiotherapy.com/content/5940267. Accessed July 14, 2013.
- Panus PC, Jobst EE, Masters SB, Katzung B, Tinsley SL, Trevor AJ. Pharmacologic management of Parkinson's disease and other movement disorders. In: Panus PC, Jobst EE, Masters SB, Katzung B, Tinsley SL, Trevor AJ, eds. *Pharmacology for the Physical Therapist*. New York, NY: McGraw-Hill; 2009. http://www.accessphysiotherapy.com/content/6092281. Accessed July 14, 2013.
- Ropper AL, Samuels MA. *Adams and Victor's Principles of Neurology*. 9th ed. New York, NY: McGraw-Hill: 2009;1033–1045.
- Waxman SG. Control of movement. In: Waxman SG, ed. *Clinical Neuroanatomy*. 26th ed. New York, NY: McGraw-Hill; 2010. http://www.accessphysiotherapy.com/content/5274060. Accessed July 14, 2013.

98 POLYNEUROPATHY, CHEMOTHERAPY INDUCED

Mollie Venglar, DSc, MSPT, NCS

CONDITION/DISORDER SYNONYMS

- Antineoplastic neuropathy
- Drug-induced neuropathy or neuronopathy

ICD-9-CM CODE[1]

- 357.6 Polyneuropathy due to drugs

ICD-10-CM CODE[2]

- G62.0 Drug-induced polyneuropathy

PREFERRED PRACTICE PATTERN

- 5G Impaired Motor Function and Sensory Integrity Associated with Acute or Chronic Polyneuropathies[3]

PATIENT PRESENTATION

A 69-year-old man reports increasing difficulty working in his woodshop. He was successfully treated for non-Hodgkin lymphoma with radiation and chemotherapy. All treatments ended 3 weeks ago. He noticed numbness in his hands and feet and felt clumsy shortly after starting his chemotherapy, but was told it would likely go away later. Yesterday, he felt like going for a walk but found he struggled with what used to be an easy distance. He regularly catches his toes on the carpet at home and on the grass in the yard when he is walking. His wife passed away 2 years ago and he is concerned about being able to live on his own. Other medical history includes osteoarthritis in his right knee, impingement in the left shoulder, and hyperlipidemia which is controlled by 20 mg Lipitor daily.

KEY FEATURES

Description

- Damage to nerve cells of the peripheral nervous system
- Numbness, tingling in the hands and feet
- Peripheral neuropathy
- Patients may experience painful peripheral neuropathy
- Predominantly sensory polyneuropathy beginning several weeks after the completion of antineoplastic drug therapy

Essentials of Diagnosis

- Change in symptoms can be sudden or appear slowly.
- Severity of polyneuropathy is dose- and time-dependent.

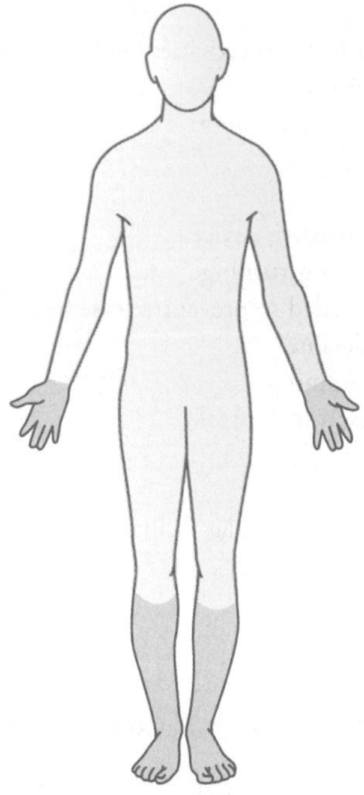

FIGURE 98-1 Distribution of sensory and lower-motor-neuron deficits in a patient with peripheral polyneuropathy. Notice the "stocking-and-glove" pattern of sensory loss. (From Waxman SG. *Clinical Neuroanatomy*. 26th ed. http://www.accessmedicine.com. Copyright © The McGraw-Hill Companies, Inc. All rights reserved.)

- Concentration of platinum in the peripheral nervous system is correlated to degree of pathologic changes; greatest concentrations generally found in the dorsal root ganglia, but can become concentrated in dorsal columns of the spinal cord.

General Considerations

- Most common medications involved are
  - Cisplatin
  - Carboplatin
  - Paclitaxel
  - Docetaxel
  - Vincristine
  - Vinblastine
  - Vinorelbine
  - Thalidomide
- Many are also ototoxic, cause autonomic dysfunction, or lead to seizures.
- Chemotherapy-related fatigue is common, will impact assessment and treatment of those with chemotherapy-induced polyneuropathy.

Demographics

- Adults more commonly affected than children

CLINICAL FINDINGS

SIGNS AND SYMPTOMS

- Altered gait pattern
- Constipation
- Impaired balance
- Impaired vestibular function
- Loss of sensation to light touch
- Loss or impairment of deep-tendon reflexes
- Loss or impairment of vibration and proprioception
- Numbness of hand, feet, mouth area
- Pain, burning, stabbing
- Tingling

Functional Implications

- Difficulty with fine motor tasks (e.g., writing, grooming, cooking, feeding, bathing) due to loss of sensation
- Fall risk with mobility on uneven/unpredictable surfaces
- Injury risk with items of unknown sharpness or temperature
- Difficulty with gross motor tasks (e.g., transfers, gait, stair climbing, dressing) due to loss of sensation
- Balance problems due to loss of sensation or ototoxicity

Possible Contributing Causes

- Chemotherapy to treat cancers may cause polyneuropathy, depending on duration of chemotherapy treatment
- Diabetes
- Alcoholism
- Malnutrition

Differential Diagnosis

- Diabetes mellitus
- Guillain–Barré syndrome
- HIV-related neuropathy
- Peripheral vascular disease
- Polyarteritis nodosa
- Tabes dorsalis

MEANS OF CONFIRMATION OR DIAGNOSIS

Diagnostic Procedures

- Nerve conduction velocity (NCV) testing

FINDINGS AND INTERPRETATION

- Most of the drugs used cause axonal damage with secondary demyelination; may be partially reversible after the drug is discontinued.

REFERRALS/ADMITTANCE

- To oncologist if chemotherapy-related
- To occupational therapist for assistance with fine motor activities and activities of daily living (ADLs)

IMPAIRMENTS

- Peripheral nerve integrity
- Gait training
- Balance
  - Static standing
  - Dynamic standing
  - Moving base-of-support standing
- Range of motion (ROM)
- Endurance
- Aerobic capacity
- Self-care
- Home management

TESTS AND MEASURES

- Sensory testing
- Cranial nerve testing
- Reflex testing
- Muscle tone
- Manual muscle test
- Active and passive ROM testing, muscle-length testing
- Functional assessment (assist, device, environment)
  - Bed mobility
  - Transitions
  - Sitting balance
  - Standing balance
  - Transfers
  - Gait
  - Stairs
- Pain assessment
- Postural assessment
- Cardiovascular endurance

INTERVENTION

- Massage to increase circulation
- Lotion and creams for skin care
- Fatigue management
- Hydration
- Mobility: Walking or wheelchair mobility
  - Include devices, bracing, shoe selection
    - Balance strategies
    - Compensatory strategies for lost sensory feedback
- Pain management
- Cardiovascular exercise while monitoring fatigue (submaximum)
- Bracing as needed for comfort or joint support

FUNCTIONAL GOALS

- Patient will
  - Demonstrate accurate and consistent grasping and finger control.
  - Tolerate 15 minutes of submaximal aerobic exercise without reporting excessive fatigue.
  - Demonstrate ability to walk independently on all community surfaces without loss of balance and with appropriate assistive device as needed.

PROGNOSIS

- Polyneuropathy due to demyelination may improve, though studies report mixed outcomes.
- Most chemotherapy-induced polyneuropathies are permanent, require individual to compensate for the deficit.

PATIENT RESOURCES

- Managing Chemotherapy Side Effects. Chemocare.com. http://www.chemocare.com/managing/numbness__tingling.asp. Accessed July 7, 2013.
- National Cancer Institute. Chemotherapy induced Peripheral neuropathy. *NCI Cancer Bulletin*. 2010;7(4). http://www.cancer.gov/aboutnci/ncicancerbulletin/archive/2010/022310/page6. Accessed July 7, 2013.

REFERENCES

1. ICD9DATA. http://www.icd9data.com. Accessed July 7, 2013.
2. ICD10DATA. http://www.icd10data.com. Accessed July 7, 2013.
3. The American Physical Therapy Association. Pattern 5G Impaired motor function and sensory integrity associated with acute or chronic polyneuropathies. *Interactive Guide to Physical Therapist Practice*. 2003. doi: 10.2522/ptguide.3.2_7. Accessed July 7, 2013.

ADDITIONAL REFERENCES

- Pachman DR, Barton DL, Watsin JC, Loprinzi CL. Chemotherapy-Induced Peripheral Neuropathy: Prevention and Treatment. *Clinical Pharmacology & Therapeutics*. 2011;90(3):377–387.
- Ropper AL, Samuels MA. *Adams and Victor's Principles of Neurology*. 9th ed. New York, NY: McGraw-Hill; 2009: 1171–1173, 1275-7.

99 POSTPOLIO SYNDROME

Mollie Venglar, DSc, MSPT, NCS

CONDITION/DISORDER SYNONYMS

- Late effects of polio
- Postpolio sequelae

ICD-9-CM CODES

- 138 Late effects of acute poliomyelitis
- 344 Other paralytic syndromes
- 357.4 Polyneuropathy in other diseases classified elsewhere

ICD-10-CM CODES[1]

- G14 Postpolio syndrome
- G63 Polyneuropathy in diseases classified elsewhere

PREFERRED PRACTICE PATTERNS

- 4A: Primary Prevention/Risk Reduction for Skeletal Demineralization
- 5H: Impaired Motor Function, Peripheral Nerve Integrity, and Sensory Integrity Associated with Nonprogressive Disorders of the Spinal Cord
- 5G: Impaired Motor Function and Sensory Integrity Associated with Acute or Chronic Polyneuropathies
- 6B Impaired Aerobic Capacity/Endurance Associated with Deconditioning
- 6E: Impaired Ventilation and Respiration/Gas Exchange Associated with Ventilatory Pump Dysfunction or Failure
- 7A: Primary Prevention/Risk Reduction for Integumentary Disorders
- 7B: Impaired Integumentary Integrity Associated with Superficial Skin Involvement
- 7C: Impaired Integumentary Integrity Associated with Partial-Thickness Skin Involvement and Scar Formation

PATIENT PRESENTATION

Diagnosed with polio 32 years ago, the client reports to physical therapy with left foot and ankle pain. She states that her left leg was primarily impacted by the disease, and she wore braces for about 3 years after the polio subsided. She does not participate in organized sports, but goes for twice daily walks with her dog, each ½ to ¾ miles. She notes that it is taking longer and longer to complete the walk. She has developed a flat foot on the left with little ability to achieve push-off during gait. After approximately 3 minutes of walking, she develops an audible foot slap on the left. Ankle strategies are delayed in both ankles during balance testing, though much slower on the left. She is able to maintain single-leg stance on the left leg for 3 to 4 seconds on a solid surface, but unable to maintain at all on a compliant surface. She is able to maintain single-leg stance on the right leg for 10 seconds on a solid surface, and 4 seconds on a compliant surface.

KEY FEATURES

Description

- Onset of polio symptoms in people who suffered the effects of the poliovirus in the past

Essentials of Diagnosis

- The poliovirus was eradicated in the United States by 1994 due to the introduction of nationally required polio vaccines in 1955 and 1960.

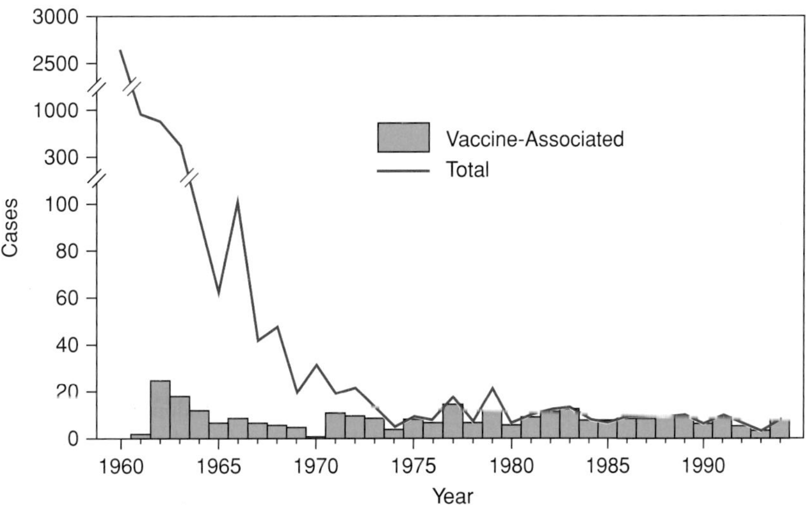

FIGURE 99-1 Total number of reported paralytic poliomyelitis cases (excluding imported cases) and number of reported vaccine-associated cases–United States, 1960–1994. (Reproduced from Paralytic poliomyelitis–United States, 1980–1994. MMWR Morb Mortal Wkly Rep 1997;46:79.)

- Following are the two types of acute poliovirus infection:
  - Paralytic
  - Nonparalytic
- The poliovirus attacks the motor neurons by destroying anterior horn cells. In the recovery process, anterior horn cells that survived the virus attempted to reinnervate muscle cells by extensive sprouting of any undamaged motor neurons.
- In postpolio syndrome (PPS), the motor neurons with the extensive sprouting appear to be degenerating and the associated muscle cells are losing innervation.
- Following are several hypotheses discussed for the onset of PPS:
  - The degree of loss of anterior horn cells with the initial virus is the primary factor.
  - Age-related changes on the already limited motor neuron pool cause the "late-effect" symptoms.
  - Overuse and fatigue of the already weakened muscles are factors in the development of new-muscle weakness.
  - Neurons that recovered from the initial attack were not physiologically normal, thus susceptible to premature aging and failure.
  - The dormant poliovirus was reactivated by an unknown mechanism.

▸ General Considerations

- Predictive factors for the onset of PPS are
  - Time since initial polio
  - Degree of weakness during the acute polio
  - Muscle pain during exercise
  - Joint pain
  - Recent weight gain
- For most of the people who suffered from polio in the past, the diagnosis of PPS can be devastating.
- Often patients will not identify deficits for several years after onset.
- Symptoms appear after a long period of neurological and functional stability after recovery from the acute poliovirus infection.
- Symptoms will appear in muscles that were not noticeably impacted from the initial poliovirus attack.

▸ Demographics

- Estimates of the number of people with the original poliovirus are uncertain so the number of people with PPS is also uncertain.
- The time from polio to PPS onset is on average 35 years, but reportedly ranges from 10 to 80 years.

CLINICAL FINDINGS

SIGNS AND SYMPTOMS

- Breathing problems
- Cold intolerance
- Fasciculations
- General fatigue[2]
- Hypoventilations
- Muscle and joint pain
- Muscle atrophy
- Muscle cramps
- New muscle weakness
- Sleep disorders
- Swallowing difficulties

▸ Functional Implications

- Symptoms tend to occur as a group, thus impacting all aspects of living, including
  - ADLs
  - Mobility
  - Home management
  - Self-care
  - Work
  - Leisure activities
  - Family commitments

▸ Possible Contributing Causes

- People who previously had either paralytic or nonparalytic polio are susceptible to PPS.
- Often a fall, injury, major illness, or surgery will precipitate the onset.

▸ Differential Diagnoses

- Amyotrophic lateral sclerosis (ALS)
- Hypothyroid myopathy
- Multiple sclerosis (MS)
- Myasthenia gravis
- Spinal cord injury or tumor
- Spinal muscular atrophy (SMA)

MEANS OF CONFIRMATION OR DIAGNOSIS

▸ Imaging

- Electromyography (EMG)

FINDINGS AND INTERPRETATION

- EMG will show neuropathic changes.

REFERRALS/ADMITTANCE

- To neurologist who specializes in PPS
- To multidisciplinary team that specializes in PPS
  - Occupational therapist
  - Respiratory therapist
  - Social worker or neuropsychologist
  - Therapeutic recreation specialist
  - Vocational rehabilitation
  - Orthotist
  - Adaptive technology specialist/practitioner
- To PPS support group

IMPAIRMENTS

- Peripheral nerve integrity
- Gait training
- Wheelchair (w/c) mobility
- Balance
  - Static standing
  - Dynamic standing
  - Moving base of support (BOS) standing
- Muscle strength
- Muscle recruitment
- Coordination
- Posture and postural control
- ROM
- Reflexes (deep tendon reflexes [DTRs] are reduced or absent)
- Muscle tone (muscles become flaccid and atrophied)
- Bed mobility
- Transfers
- Endurance declines for individual muscles, as well as the whole body
- Aerobic capacity

- Self-care
- Home management
- Fine motor control declines in people who have upper-extremity involvement
- Respiratory compromise

TESTS AND MEASURES

- Manual muscle testing (MMT)
- Active and passive ROM testing
- Muscle length testing
- Sensory testing
- Reflex testing
- Muscle tone testing
- Functional assessment (assist, device, environment)
  - Bed mobility
  - Transitions
  - Sitting balance
  - Standing balance
  - Transfers
  - Wheelchair (w/c) mobility
  - Gait
  - Stairs
- Fatigue impact questioning
- Pain assessment
- Postural assessment and endurance to maintain upright posture
- Respiratory assessment
- Cardiovascular endurance

INTERVENTION

- Lifestyle modification
- Postural correction
- Energy conservation
- Modified strengthening and conditioning
- Mobility: Walking and/or w/c mobility
  - Using devices, bracing, etc.
- Balance strategies
- As needed for home and work activities
- Pain management
- Aerobic exercise[2], endurance for functional activities
- Decreasing fatigue/effort during functional activities like transfers, bathing, home management
- Respiratory care
- Diet modifications: Controlling weight gain

FUNCTIONAL GOALS

- The patient will
  - Demonstrate effective energy management in daily life by report of no greater than one episode of excessive fatigue in the past week.
  - Demonstrate decreased fatigue during walking with prescribed adaptive equipment by increasing distance during a 5-minute walk by 50%.
  - Tolerate submaximal aerobic training for 20 minutes three times a week to help maintain general health and fitness.

PROGNOSIS

- Unknown, but impacted by the lifestyle changes necessary to manage fatigue.

PATIENT RESOURCES

- Polio Survivors Association. http://www.polioassociation.org. Accessed July 2, 2013.
- Poliomyelitis. World Health Organization. http://www.who.int/mediacentre/factsheets/fs114/en. Accessed July 2, 2013.

REFERENCES

1. ICD10DATA.com. http://www.icd10data.com/ICD10CM/Codes/G00-G99/G10-G14/G14-/G14. Accessed July 2, 2013.
2. Oncu J, Durmaz B, Karapolat H. Short-term effects of aerobic exercise on functional capacity, fatigue, and quality of life in patients with post-polio syndrome. *Clin Rehabil.* 2009;23(2):155–163. doi: 10.1177/0269215508098893.

ADDITIONAL REFERENCES

- Brooks GF, Carroll KC, Butel JS, Morse SA, Mietzneron TA. Picornaviruses (enterovirus & rhinovirus groups). In: Brooks GF, Carroll KC, Butel JS, Morse SA, Mietzneron TA, eds. *Jawetz, Melnick, & Adelberg's Medical Microbiology.* 25th ed. New York, NY: McGraw-Hill; 2010:Chapter 36. http://accessmedicine.mhmedical.com/content.aspx?bookid=504§ionid=40999958. Accessed May 15, 2014.
- Keenan MA, Mehta S. Rehabilitation. In: Skinner HB, ed. *CURRENT Diagnosis & Treatment in Orthopedics.* 4th ed. New York, NY: McGraw-Hill; 2006:Chapter 13. http://www.accessmedicine.com/content.aspx?aID=2316716. Accessed July 2, 2013.
- Quiben MU. The challenges of the late effects of polio: postpolio syndrome. In: Umphred DA, ed. *Neurological Rehabilitation.* 5th ed. St. Louis, MO: Mosby Elsevier; 2007: 940–958.

100 PRIMARY LATERAL SCLEROSIS

Mollie Venglar, DSc, MSPT, NCS

CONDITION/DISORDER SYNONYM

- Motor neuron disease

ICD-9-CM CODE

- 335.24 Primary lateral sclerosis

ICD-10-CM CODE

- G12.2 Motor neuron disease

PREFERRED PRACTICE PATTERN

- 5E: Impaired Motor Function and Sensory Integrity Associated with Progressive Disorders of the Central Nervous System

PATIENT PRESENTATION

A 49-year-old man reports to physical therapy stating that he has had an increase in the number of falls he experiences weekly. He was diagnosed with primary lateral sclerosis (PLS) 2 years ago, works as a handyman at a small island resort, is married and has two teenage children. He walks without an assistive device. On testing, his lower extremities test grossly 3/5 to 3+/5 with an increase in tone on fast, passive motion testing. His dynamic gait index (DGI) score is 19/24 with the greatest difficulty when changing gait speed, stepping over obstacles, and going up/down steps. He was out of breath following administration of the DGI and his oxygen saturation dropped from 98% to 92%. During static balance testing, he was able to maintain standing with his feet together for 8 seconds with his eyes open and 7 seconds with his eyes closed. He maintained single-leg stance on each leg for 4 seconds with his eyes open.

KEY FEATURES

Description

- Motor neuron disease
- Degenerative neurologic disorder of the upper motor neurons in the brain and spinal cord
- First described by Dr Jean-Martin Charcot
- Progressive weakness in the voluntary muscles
- Nerve cells degenerate causing weakness

Essentials of Diagnosis[1]

- Progression of symptoms over 3 years without evidence of lower motor neuron dysfunction
- Disease is progressive, but may persist for decades
- Evidence of loss of function in the lower extremities (LEs) first, then progressing to the muscles of speech and swallowing, and then loss in the upper extremities (UEs)

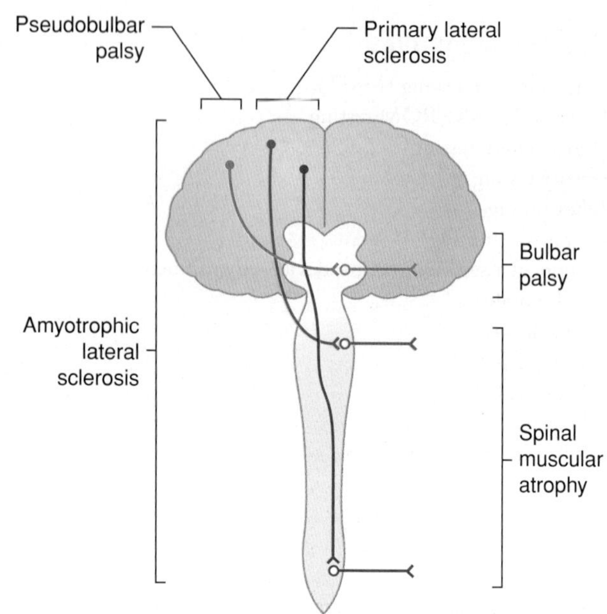

FIGURE 100-1 Adult-onset motor neuron disease syndromes. Upper motor neurons are shown with filled circles and lower motor neurons with open circles for cell bodies. Cerebral cortex is indicated with *dark*, brainstem *white*, and spinal cord *light shading*. (From Greenberg DA, Aminoff MJ, Simon RP. *Clinical Neurology*. 8th ed. http://www.accessmedicine.com. Copyright © The McGraw-Hill Companies, Inc. All rights reserved.)

General Considerations

- Spontaneous onset for adults.
- Breathing may be affected in the later stages of the disease.
- Juvenile primary lateral sclerosis (JPLS) is linked to a mutation in the ALS2 gene.

Demographics

- Onset 40 to 60 years old; mean of 50 years old
- JPLS

CLINICAL FINDINGS

SIGNS AND SYMPTOMS

- Antalgic gait
- Dysarthria
- Drooling, weakness of bulbar muscles
- LE onset with spastic paraparesis
- Later develop symptoms in the UEs and oropharyngeal muscles
- Entirely upper motor neuron signs and symptoms
- Sensation is spared
- Hyperactive reflexes
- Babinski sign
- Painful muscle spasms
- Speech problems

Functional Implications

- Declining independence with bed mobility, transfers, ambulation
- Declining balance in sitting and standing
- Declining respiratory support for all daily and recreational activities
- Increasing need for advanced adaptive equipment

Possible Contributing Causes

- Sporadic, no known familial link for adults
- Juvenile form linked to gene mutation: ALS2

Differential Diagnoses

- Amyotrophic lateral sclerosis (ALS)
- Cerebral palsy (CP)
- Familial spastic paraplegia
- Henoch–Schönlein purpura (HSP)
- Meningioma
- Multiple sclerosis (MS)
- Spondylosis
- Tropical spastic paraparesis (TSP)

MEANS OF CONFIRMATION OR DIAGNOSIS

Laboratory Tests

- Blood tests to help rule out other diagnoses

Imaging

- MRI

Diagnostic Procedures

- Electromyography (EMG)

FINDINGS AND INTERPRETATION

- EMG will show neuropathic changes.
- MRI may show slight atrophy of the motor cortices and Wallerian degeneration of the motor tracts.

TREATMENT

Medication

- Benzodiazepines or dantrolene sodium for spasticity

REFERRALS/ADMITTANCE

- To neurologist for confirmation of diagnosis and disease management
- To respiratory therapist for breathing support and devices
- To occupational therapist for ADL, UE splinting, and adaptive equipment
- To ALS Association for support and services
- To speech therapy for individuals with speech and facial muscle involvement

IMPAIRMENTS

- Gait
- Wheelchair (w/c) mobility
- Depression
- Balance
  - Static sit
  - Dynamic sit
  - Static stand
  - Dynamic stand
  - Moving base of support (BOS)
- Muscle strength
- Muscle recruitment
- Coordination
- Postural control (as disease progresses)

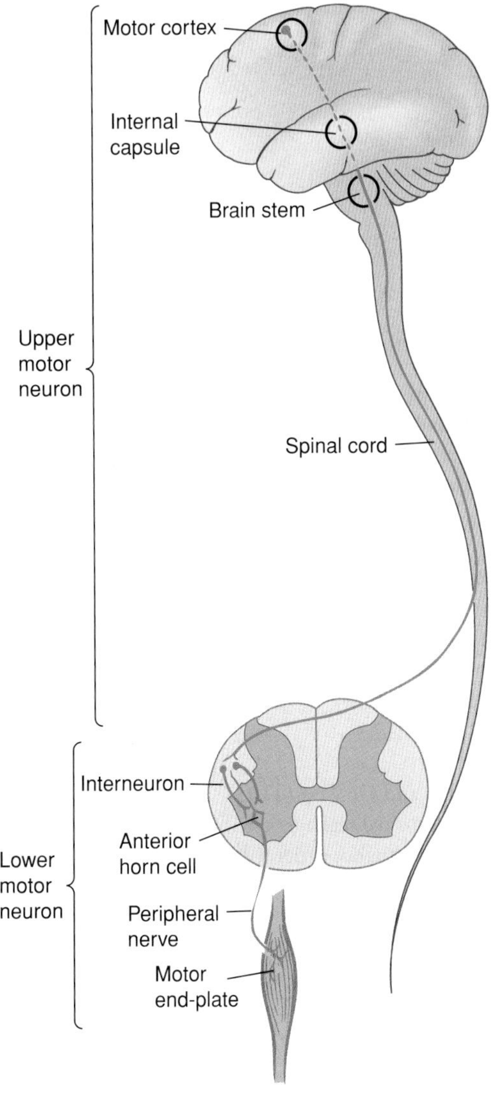

FIGURE 100-2 Motor pathways divided into upper- and lower motor neuron regions. (From Waxman SG. *Clinical Neuroanatomy*. 26th ed. http://www.accessmedicine.com. Copyright © The McGraw-Hill Companies, Inc. All rights reserved.)

- Posture (as disease progresses)
- ROM
- Reflexes
  - Deep tendon reflexes (DTRs)
  - Babinski
  - Clonus

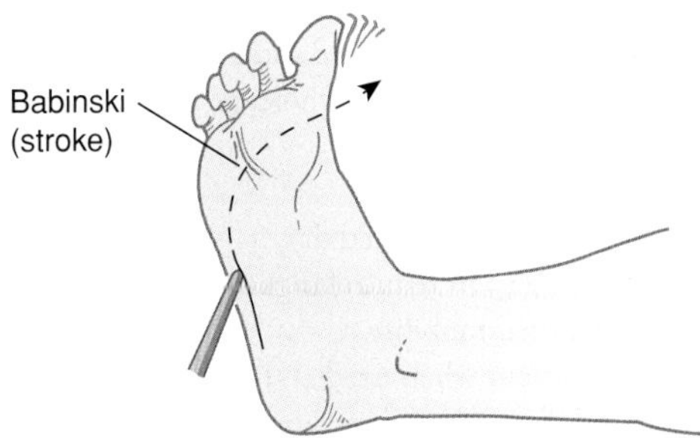

FIGURE 100-3 Testing for extensor plantar reflexes. (From Waxman SG. *Clinical Neuroanatomy*. 26th ed. http://www.accessmedicine.com. Copyright © The McGraw-Hill Companies, Inc. All rights reserved.)

- Muscle tone
- Bed mobility
- Transfers
- Self care
- Home management
- Fine motor skills

TESTS AND MEASURES

- Cognition
  - Mini-Mental State Examination (MMSE)
  - Executive function tests (memory, comprehension)
- Pain
  - Subjective report
  - Visual Analog Scale (VAS)
  - Verbal report
- Strength and muscle endurance
- Coordination: Gross and fine motor skills
- Muscle tone
- Joint ROM: Passive and active
- Cranial nerve examination
- Sensation (only needed if patient reports sensory symptoms or if sensory compromise is suspected; loss of sensation is not a common impairment)
- Postural alignment
- Balance
  - Timed Up and Go Test (TUG)
  - Multi-directional reach test (MDRT)
  - Tinetti Performance Oriented Mobility Assessment (POMA)
  - Berg Balance Scale (BBS)
- Gait
  - TUG
  - Tinetti gait and balance evaluation
  - 10-m walk test
  - DGI in the early stage of the disease
- Respiratory function
  - Spirometry
  - Oxygen saturation
  - Breathing pattern
  - Auscultation
- Integumentary: More of a concern in the mid- and late stages
- Functional mobility: Functional Independence Measure (FIM™)
- Fatigue: Fatigue Severity Scale (FSS)
- Disease-specific measure: ALS Functional Rating Scale is frequently used due to the similarities between ALS and PLS

INTERVENTION

- No known treatments to stop or reverse progression of the disease
- Aggressive strengthening contraindicated
- Must not fatigue the person as a whole, or individual muscles
- Addressing fatigue
  - Energy conservation
  - Coordinate breathing with activity
  - Adaptive equipment to reduce fatigue
- Addressing functional mobility
  - Adaptive equipment when needed (hospital bed, four-wheeled walker, w/c). Often the progression of weakness and the degree of spasticity will make the need for power mobility evident before the individual loses all ability to walk.
  - LE bracing when needed
  - Caregiver training on patient handling/guarding for ambulation, transfers, and bed mobility
- Addressing balance and postural control
  - Balance strategies in sitting and standing with and without a moving base of support
    - Balance reactions training is possible early on in the disease, but will need to be compensated for later. Degree of spasticity will limit success with balance reaction training.
  - Assistive device, as needed (walker, bracing)
- Addressing exercise
  - If manual muscle test (MMT) is 3/5 or greater, moderate intensity is acceptable
  - If MMT is less than 3/5, low intensity should be used.
    - Overwork damage will occur faster in the weakened or denervated muscle.
  - Use functional activities for strengthening whenever possible.
  - Aquatic exercise is beneficial.
  - Aerobic exercise is helpful, but moderated by respiratory status and fatigue.
  - Mild-to-moderate stretching by patient or caregiver to maintain ROM in all appendicular joints, as well as cervical spine
- Addressing respiratory issues
  - Postural drainage as tolerated (in late-stage ALS, this is not appropriate)
  - Active cough techniques, as tolerated
  - Encourage use of suction, cough-assist, and ventilation during therapy
- Addressing pain
  - Adaptive equipment to prevent pain from joint malalignment or skin breakdown
    - Supportive back/seat in w/c
    - Neck brace
    - Arm trough or lap tray on w/c
    - Bracing or taping to decrease shoulder subluxation

TABLE 100-1 Lower- versus Upper Motor Neuron Lesions

Variable	Lower Motor Neuron Lesion	Upper Motor Neuron Lesion
Weakness	Flaccid paralysis	Spastic paralysis
Deep tendon reflexes	Decreased or absent	Increased
Babinski reflex	Absent	Present
Atrophy	May be marked	Absent or resulting from disuse
Fasciculations and fibrillations	May be present	Absent

Source: Waxman SG. *Clinical Neuroanatomy.* 26th ed. http://www.accessmedicine.com.

FUNCTIONAL GOALS

- Early stage
  - The patient will
    - Ambulate with a four-wheeled rolling walker in both home and community environments for up to 8 minutes prior to requiring a rest break.
    - Demonstrate performance of >19/28 on the Tinetti POMA, as a measure of moderate risk of falls.

- Middle stage
  - The patient will
    - Navigate home and community obstacle in their power w/c with minimal verbal cues for safety.
    - Perform a lateral pivot transfer between the w/c and the bed with moderate assistance from a caregiver.
- Late stage
  - The caregiver will demonstrate appropriate body mechanics to safely manage patient between bed and w/c without external verbal cues.

PROGNOSIS

- Poor; the disease is progressively degenerative.
- Death most commonly the result of significant respiratory impairment.
- Prognosis is related to the care received and the willingness of the patient and caregiver to pursue respiratory support.

PATIENT RESOURCES

- ALS Association Website. http://www.alsa.org/?gclid=CMilyrHmoasCFQtb7Aod10azpA. Accessed July 6, 2013.
- Primary lateral sclerosis. NINDS Primary Lateral Sclerosis Information. National Institue of Neurological Disorders and Stroke. http://www.ninds.nih.gov/disorders/primary_lateral_sclerosis/primary_lateral_sclerosis.htm. Accessed August 8, 2014.

REFERENCE

1. Brown RH. Amyotrophic lateral sclerosis and other motor neuron diseases. In: Longo DL, Fauci AS, Kasper DL, Hauser SL, Jameson JL, Loscalzo J, eds. *Harrison's Principles of Internal Medicine*. 18th ed. New York, NY: McGraw-Hill; 2011. http://www.accessmedicine.com/content.aspx?aID=9146812. Accessed July 6, 2013.

ADDITIONAL REFERENCES

- Dutton M. Guillain–Barré syndrome. In: Dutton M, ed. *McGraw-Hill's NPTE (National Physical Therapy Examination)*. 2nd ed. New York, NY: McGraw-Hill; 2012. http://www.accessphysiotherapy.com/content/5400147. Accessed July 6, 2013.
- Hibbs RE, Zambon AC. Agents acting at the neuromuscular junction and autonomic ganglia. In: Brunton LL, Chabner BA, Knollmann BC, eds. *Goodman & Gilman's The Pharmacological Basis of Therapeutics*. 12th ed. New York, NY: McGraw-Hill; 2010. http://www.accesspharmacy.com/content.aspx?aID=16661089. Accessed July 6, 2013.
- Ropper AL, Samuels MA. *Adams and Victor's Principles of Neurology*. 9th ed. New York, NY: McGraw-Hill; 2009:1061, 1064.

101 TETRA/QUADRIPLEGIA

Mollie Venglar, DSc, MSPT, NCS
Megan Samantha Rosga, DPT, MSPT, NCS

CONDITION/DISORDER SYNONYMS

- Tetraplegia
- Quadriplegia

ICD-9-CM-CODE[1]

- 344.0 Quadriplegia unspecified

ICD-10-CM CODE[2]

- G82.50 Quadriplegia unspecified

PREFERRED PRACTICE PATTERN

- 5H: Impaired Motor Function, Peripheral Nerve Integrity, and Sensory Integrity Associated with Nonprogressive Disorders of the Spinal Cord

PATIENT PRESENTATION

A 20-year-old man was transferred to the in-patient rehabilitation unit one week after a shallow water accident in which he hit a sandbar while surfing. He sustained a fracture in the cervical region. He has intact perianal sensation and all sensations intact to C7. His cervical fracture was stabilized via anterior approach with an iliac crest bone graft and screws. He wears a sternal-occipital-mandibular immobilizer (SOMI), abdominal binder, and compression stockings. He presents to in-patient rehabilitation in a reclined wheelchair due to orthostatic hypotension and lack of trunk control. His injury is assessed as a C7 incomplete, ASIA B (American Spinal Injury Association). Past medical history is unremarkable except for childhood illnesses/injuries.

KEY FEATURES

Description

- Loss of motor and/or sensory function due to damage in the cervical spinal cord

Essentials of Diagnosis

- Diagnosis is made by level of injury, severity of injury, and use of the ASIA assessment.
- Quadriplegia is complete loss of sensory and motor function due to damage in cervical spine.
- Quadriparesis is the partial loss of sensory or motor function due to damage in the cervical spine.
- Quadriplegia is most commonly the result of trauma but can also occur due to infarction, hemorrhage, spinal stenosis.

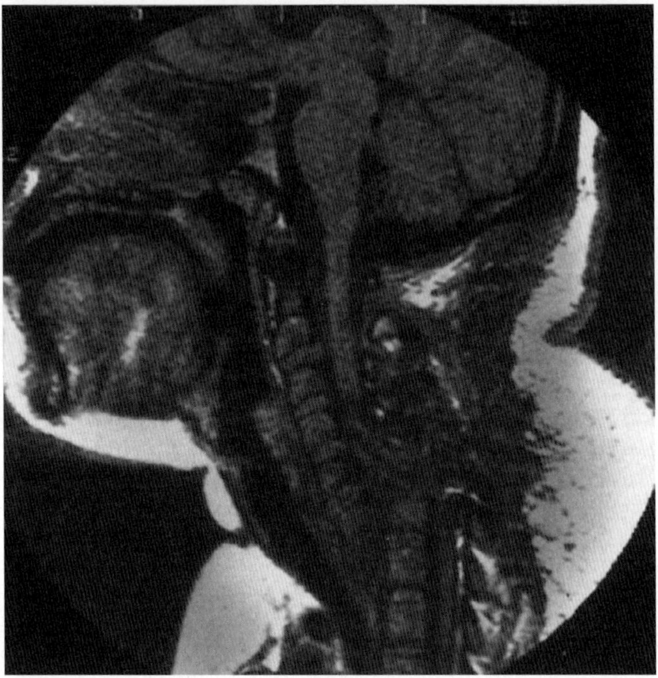

FIGURE 101-1 A 21-year-old quadriplegic woman who had a motor vehicle accident 4 weeks ago. (From Chen MYM, Pope TL, Ott DJ. *Basic Radiology*. 2nd ed. http://www.accessmedicine.com. Copyright © The McGraw-Hill Companies, Inc. All rights reserved.)

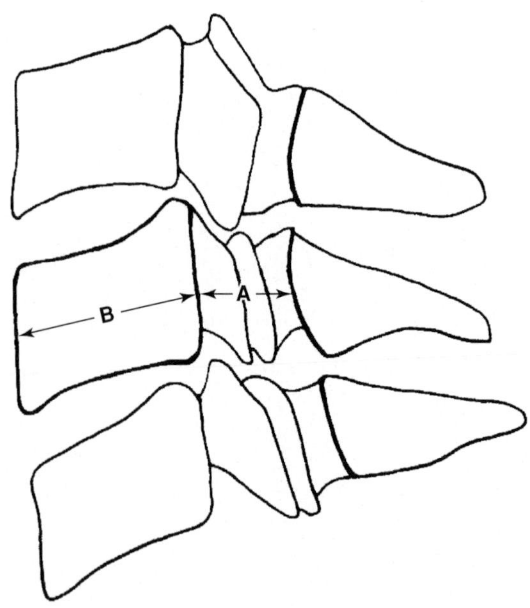

FIGURE 101-2 The ratio of the spinal canal to the vertebral body is the distance from the midpoint of the posterior aspect of the vertebral body to the nearest point on the corresponding spinolaminar line (**A**) divided by the anteroposterior width of the vertebral body (**B**). (Reproduced with permission from Torg JS, Pavlov H, Genuaria SE. Neuropraxia of the cervical spinal cord with transient quadriplegia. *J Bone Joint Surg Am.* 1986;68:1354.)

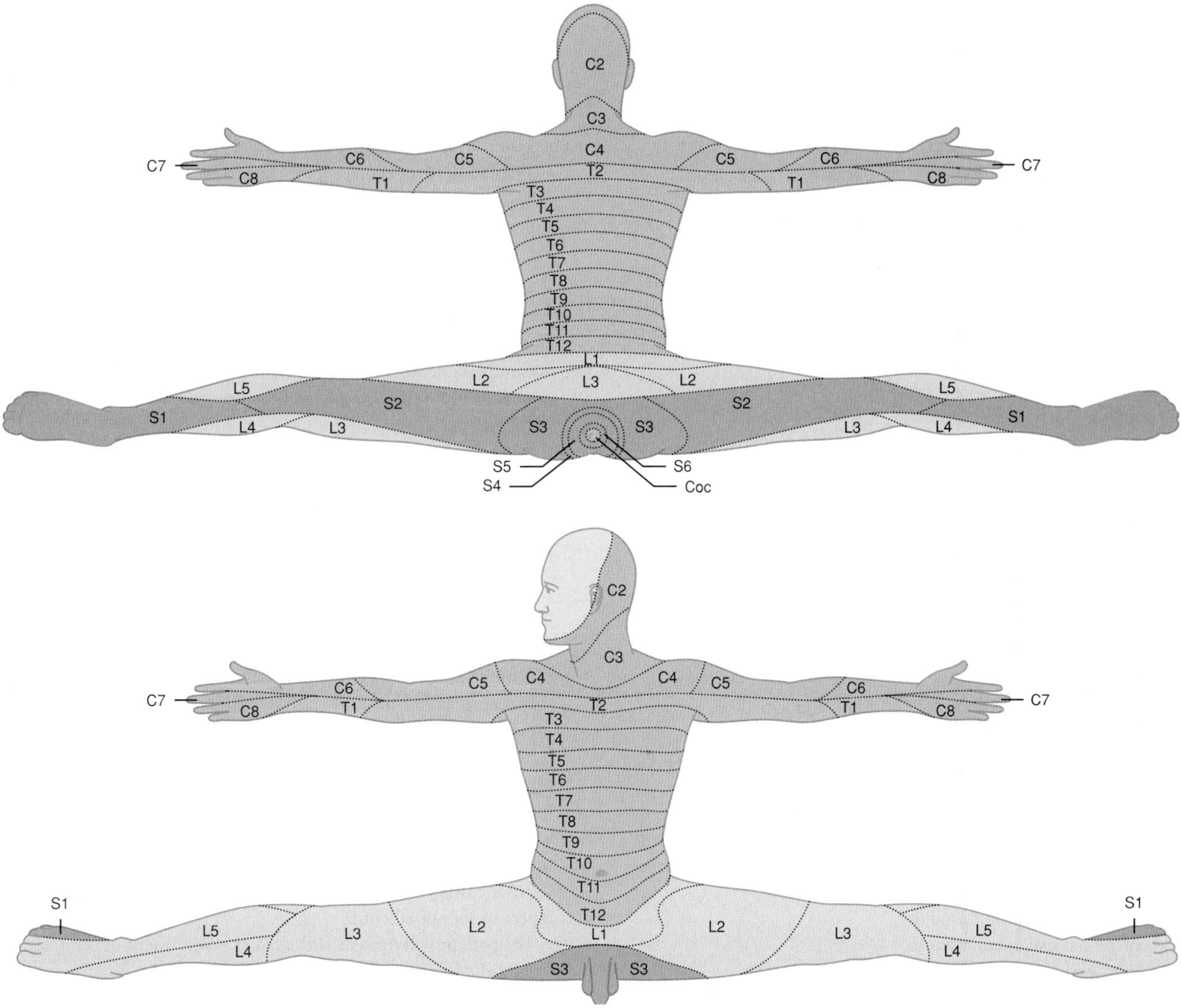

FIGURE 101-3 Dermatomes for sensory examination. (From Tintinalli JE, Stapczynski J, Ma OJ, Cline D, Cydulka R, Meckler G. *Tintinalli's Emergency Medicine: A Comprehensive Study Guide*. 7th ed. http://www.accessmedicine.com. Copyright © The McGraw-Hill Companies, Inc. All rights reserved.)

General Considerations

- Damage to the cervical spinal cord results in complications to many body systems.
  - The individual will likely experience most of the following:
    - Loss of motor and/or sensory function
    - Neurogenic bowel and bladder
    - Autonomic dysfunction
    - Orthostatic hypotension
    - Loss of bone density
    - Decreased ventilatory capability
    - Cardiac deconditioning
- Working with this population requires the PT to be aware of this wide range of complications to be safe and effective with patient care.

Demographics

- Men four times as likely as women[1]
- Most common cause is motor vehicle accident (MVA), second is falls[3]

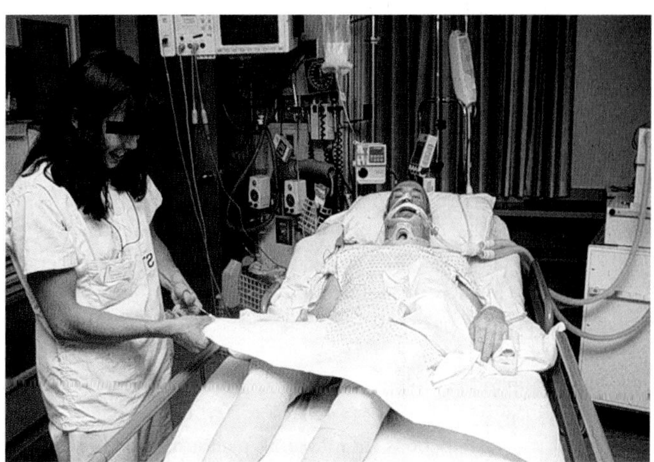

FIGURE 101-4 Abdominal binder. (From DeTurk WE, Cahalin LP. *Cardiovascular and Pulmonary Physical Therapy: An Evidence-Based Approach*. 2nd ed. http://www.accessphysiotherapy.com. Copyright © The McGraw-Hill Companies, Inc. All rights reserved.)

CLINICAL FINDINGS

SIGNS AND SYMPTOMS

- Upper motor neuron signs present
- Complete injury is defined as no motor or sensory function spared in the lowest sacral segments; incomplete injury is defined as partial or full function spared in the lowest sacral segments.
- Altered or lost trunk control and balance
- Altered or lost head/neck control
- Altered or lost ambulation/locomotion
- Altered or lost bed mobility
- Altered or lost transfer ability
- Altered or lost muscle strength
- Altered or lost sensations
- Altered deep tendon reflexes (DTRs)
- Altered or lost bowel and bladder function
- Altered or lost autonomic control
- Altered blood pressure
- Spasticity
- Altered thermoregulation

Functional Implications

- Bladder and bowel dysfunction
- Decreased endurance and energy efficiency
- Dysesthesias
- Gait abnormalities
- Impaired bed mobility
- Impaired coordination
- Impaired movement of upper extremity (UE)/lower extremity (LE), trunk, head, and neck
- Impaired muscular strength
- Impaired sitting balance
- Impaired transfers
- Impaired upright tolerance
- Impaired wheelchair mobility
- Increased risk of contracture
- Increased risk of deep vein thrombosis
- Increased risk of heterotopic ossification
- Increased risk of pressure sores
- Neuropathic pain
- Osteoporosis and renal calculi
- Postural/orthostatic hypotension
- Respiratory impairment
- Sexual dysfunction

Possible Contributing Causes

- Traumatic
  - Most frequent cause in adults
  - MVA, 45.6%[3]
  - Fall, 19.6%[3]
  - Acts of violence, including gun shots, 17.8%[3]
  - Recreational sports, 10.7%[3]
  - Other, 6.3%[3]
- Nontraumatic/pathological influence: 30% of all spinal cord injuries (SCIs)
  - Vascular malfunctions (arteriovenous malformation, thrombosis, embolus, or hemorrhage)
  - Vertebral subluxations due to rheumatoid arthritis or degenerative joint disease
  - Infections: Syphilis, transverse myelitis
  - Spinal neoplasms
  - Syringomyelia
  - Abscesses of the spinal cord

Differential Diagnosis

- Spinal shock
- Traumatic brain injury
- Spinal cord concussion
- Hysterical paralysis
- Decompression sickness

MEANS OF CONFIRMATION OR DIAGNOSIS

- Tests
  - Complete neurological examination
  - Muscle strength testing (UE, LE, core, and head/neck)
  - DTRs
  - Sensation, coordination, proprioception

Imaging

- MRI
- CT scan for detailed imaging
- Radiograph for spinal vertebra damage

FINDINGS AND INTERPRETATION

- Flexion injury results in greatest damage to the anterior spinal cord (anterior cord Injury), producing loss of motor function below the level of the injury but sparing of some sensory function.
- Hyperextension injury results in greatest damage to the posterior spinal cord (posterior cord injury), producing profound loss of sensation but some sparing of motor function below the level of the injury.
- Central cord syndrome results from damage to the more central aspect of the spinal cord.
  - The patient will present with greater involvement of the UEs than the LEs.
- Brown–Séquard syndrome results from damage to one side of the spinal cord (hemi-section).
  - Due to the locations of crossing of the long tracts of the spinal cord, motor will be lost on the side of the lesion but spared on the opposite side.
  - Cutaneous sensations (temperature, pain) will be maintained on the side of the lesion and lost on the opposite side.

REFERRALS/ADMITTANCE

- To trauma center, emergency room (ER) at time of injury
  - Proper relocation of patient avoiding active and passive movement
  - Proper medical stabilization of patient
  - Vertebral realignment/early immobilization of fractures
- To neurologist if the injury is chronic but patient is losing more sensation or motor function
- To spinal cord support group
- To custom durable medical equipment provider
- To recreational therapy
- To challenged athlete groups
- To occupational therapy as needed
- To vocational rehabilitation for job site modification or job retraining
- To counselor or psychologist

IMPAIRMENTS

- Peripheral nerve integrity
- Gait
- Wheelchair mobility
- Balance
  - Static sit
  - Dynamic sit
  - Static stand
  - Dynamic stand
  - Moving base of support (BOS)
- Muscle strength
- Muscle recruitment
- Coordination
- Proprioception
- Postural control
- Posture
- ROM
- Reflexes
  - DTRs
  - Babinski
  - Clonus
- Muscle tone
- Sensation
- Bed mobility
- Transfers
- Endurance
- Aerobic capacity
- Self-care
- Home management
- Fine motor
- Respiratory compromise

TESTS AND MEASURES

- ASIA Assessment
  - Motor
  - Sensation
  - ASIA neurologic level
  - Complete versus incomplete
- Functional independence measure (FIM™)
  - Wheelchair mobility
  - Bed mobility
  - Transfers
  - Gait if appropriate (Timed Up and Go, 10-m walk test, Functional Gait Assessment, Walking Index for Spinal Cord Injury, Dynamic Gait Index)
- Sitting and standing (for people with incomplete injuries or damage in the lower lumbar and sacral levels)
  - Balance tests (sitting reach test, Tinetti, Berg Balance Scale)
  - Cardiovascular and pulmonary endurance (6-minute walk test if appropriate, UE ergometer test)
- Muscle endurance
- Skin assessment
- Active and passive ROM, muscle length
- Posture in sitting (wheelchair and edge of mat, supported, unsupported) and standing if applicable)
- Pain

INTERVENTION

- Balance training (sitting, standing if appropriate)
- Bed-mobility training
- Cardiovascular endurance
- Family training/education
- Gait training (if appropriate and with appropriate bracing and assistive devices)
- Orientation to vertical position
- ROM/stretching/positioning
- Strengthening of intact musculature
- Transfer training
- Wheelchair-mobility training (curbs, ramps, various surfaces, negotiating obstacles, wheelies, and floor recovery)

FUNCTIONAL GOALS

- Level of injury as well as the degree of completeness directly impacts potential functioning.
- C3-4
  - Patient will
    - Self-direct wheelchair to/from bed transfer via mechanical lift with minimal verbal cues for safety and technique to improve safe functional mobility and decrease caregiver burden.
    - Perform 5/10 cervical head rotations right and left with close supervision for potential trial of head array wheelchair for increased functional independence.
- C5-6
  - Patient will
    - Perform rolling in bed with use of loop ladder and supervision assistance for improved independence with bed mobility.
    - Tolerate standing frame at 70% of standing position for 10 minutes with stable vital signs to promote weight-bearing activities through LEs.
- C7-8
  - Patient will
    - Propel an ultra-light-weight manual wheelchair over community surfaces with supervision assistance to improve safe and efficient functional independence.
    - Transfer between wheelchair and bed via lateral pivot transfer with supervision assistance to improve independence at home.

PROGNOSIS

- Good for becoming functional with some activities for patients who obtain appropriate services and participate in maintaining the health of their body systems.
- Variable for recovery of prior function based on degree, location, and severity of injury.
- Patients at ASIA scale A and B are less likely to recover prior function than those at ASIA C and D.

ADDITIONAL INFORMATION

- See Case Study: Patient with C5 Tetraplegia on AccessPhysiotherapy.com for more information.

PATIENT RESOURCES

- American Association of People with Disabilities. http://www.aapd.com/. Accessed July 2, 2013.
- Paraquad, Paraplegic Quadripelgic Association. Independent living institute. http://www.independentliving.org/donet/407_paraquad_paraplegic_quadriplegic_association.html. Accessed July 2, 2013.

REFERENCES

1. ICD9Data.com. www.icd9data.com. Accessed May 21, 2014.
2. ICD10Data.com. http://www.icd10data.com/ICD10CM/Codes. Accessed July 2, 2013.
3. Fulk GD, Schmitz TJ, Behrman AL. Traumatic spinal cord injury. In: O'Sullivan SB, Schmitz TJ, eds. *Physical Rehabilitation*. 5th ed. Philadelphia, PA: F.A. Davis Company; 2007:937–991.

ADDITIONAL REFERENCES

- Ciesla ND, Kuramoto JD. Physical therapy associated with respiratory failure. In: DeTurk WE, Cahalin LP, eds. *Cardiovascular and Pulmonary Physical Therapy, Second Edition: An Evidence-Based Approach*. 2nd ed. New York, NY: McGraw-Hill; 2010:Chapter 19. http://www.accessphysiotherapy.com/abstract/6885040#6885040. Accessed July 2, 2013.
- Dutton M. Intervention principles. In: Dutton M, ed. *Orthopaedic Examination, Evaluation, and Intervention*. 2nd ed. New York, NY: McGraw-Hill; 2008:Chapter 10. http://www.accessphysiotherapy.com/content/5548968. Accessed July 2, 2013.
- Dutton M, Dutton M. Therapeutic exercise. In: Dutton M, Dutton M, eds. *Dutton's Orthopedic Survival Guide: Managing Common Conditions*. New York, NY: McGraw-Hill; 2011:Chapter 4. http://www.accessphysiotherapy.com/content/8651381. Accessed July 2, 2013.
- Halter J, Ouslander J, Tinetti M, Studenski S, High K, Asthana S, eds. *Hazzard's Geriatric Medicine and Gerontology*. 6th ed. New York, NY; 2009.
- Lichtman MA, Kipps TJ, Seligsohn U, Kaushansky K, Prchal JT. *Williams Hematology*. 8th ed. New York, NY: McGraw-Hill; 2010.
- Malone TR, Hazle C, Grey ML. The ankle and foot. In: Malone TR, Hazle C, Grey ML, eds. *Imaging in Rehabilitation*. New York, NY: McGraw-Hill; 2008:Chapter 10. http://www.accessphysiotherapy.com/content/5940084. Accessed July 2, 2013.
- Pattern 5H: impaired motor function, peripheral nerve integrity, and sensory integrity associated with nonprogressive disorders of the spinal cord. In: *Guide to Physical Therapist Practice*. 2nd ed. Alexandria, VA: American Physical Therapy Association; 2001. Revised 2003.
- Ropper AL, Samuels MA. *Adams and Victor's Principles of Neurology*. 9th ed. New York, NY: McGraw-Hill; 2009:1181–1188. http://accessmedicine.mhmedical.com/book.aspx?bookID=690. Accessed May 21, 2014.
- Shamus E, Stern DF, eds. *Effective Documentation for Physical Therapy Professionals*. 2nd ed. New York, NY: McGraw-Hill; 2011. http://www.accessphysiotherapy.com/resource/696. Accessed July 2, 2013.
- Six-minute Walk Test (6MWT). StrokEngine. http://strokengine.ca/assess/module_6mwt_intro-en.html. Accessed May 21, 2014.
- Tinetti Balance and Gait Evaluation. http://www.bhps.org.uk/falls/documents/TinettiBalanceAssessment.pdf. Accessed July 2, 2013.

102 SYRINGOMYELIA

Mollie Venglar, DSc, MSPT, NCS

CONDITION/DISORDER SYNONYMS

- Spinal cord cavitation
- Syringomyelia type III
- Syrinx

ICD-9-CM CODE[1]

- 336.0 Syringomyelia and syringobulbia

ICD-10-CM CODE[2]

- G95.0 Syringomyelia and syringobulbia

PREFERRED PRACTICE PATTERN[3]

- 5H: Impaired Motor Function, Peripheral Nerve Integrity, and Sensory Integrity Associated with Nonprogressive Disorders of the Spinal Cord

PATIENT PRESENTATION

A 21-year-old male with a 2-year history of C7 quadriplegia reports to his neurologist with report of loss of tenodesis grip and triceps strength bilaterally. Although he is still able to perform his daily functions it is taking longer to do so, and his ability to complete his transfers is becoming more impaired. He denies any injuries or traumas to his spine since the accident that caused the C7 quadriplegia. He has no fever, headache, or nausea. He demonstrates normal cognition. He has not been exposed to any illnesses or viruses, of which he is aware, for several months. MRI reveals a fluid-filled syrinx in the spinal cord at the level of C5.

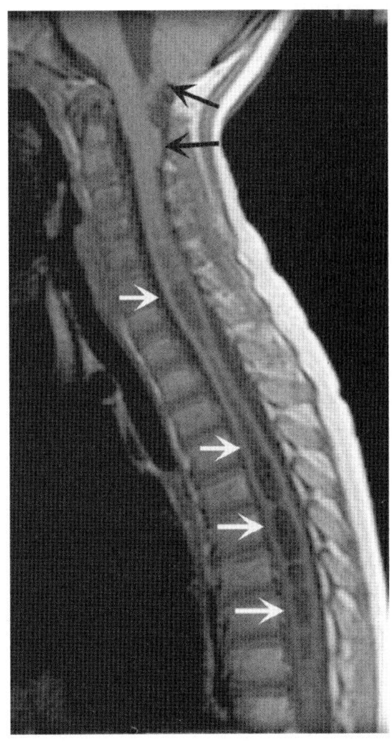

FIGURE 102-1 MRI of syringomyelia associated with a Chiari malformation. Sagittal T1-weighted image through the cervical and upper thoracic spine demonstrates descent of the cerebellar tonsils and vermis below the level of the foramen magnum (*black arrows*). Within the substance of the cervical and thoracic spinal cord, a CSF collection dilates the central canal (*white arrows*). (From Longo DL, Fauci AS, Kasper DL, Hauser SL, Jameson JL, Loscalzo J, eds. *Harrison's Principles of Internal Medicine*. 18th ed. http://www.accessmedicine.com. Copyright © The McGraw-Hill Companies, Inc. All rights reserved.)

KEY FEATURES

Description

- Damage to the spinal cord is caused due to the formation of a fluid-filled cavity within the spinal cord.[4]
- The fluid forms a cavity called a syrinx that can elongate over time, destroying the interior of the spinal cord.

Essentials of Diagnosis

- Four types of syringomyelia
  - Types I, II, IV are developmental
  - Type III is acquired and associated with one of the following
    - Spinal cord tumor
    - Traumatic myelopathy
    - Spinal arachnoiditis and pachymeningitis
    - Secondary myelomalacia from cord compression, infarction, or hematomyelia

General Considerations

- Type III syrinx is suspected when a person with a previously stable presentation experiences changes in sensorimotor function after a spinal cord injury that extends above the level of the original injury.

Demographics

- Occurs more often in people with tetra/quadriplegia than in those with paraplegia

CLINICAL FINDINGS

SIGNS AND SYMPTOMS

- Bowel and bladder dysfunction
- Hot and cold sensory loss
- Headaches
- Pain
- Paralysis
- Scoliosis
- Spreading sensory loss
- Spreading motor loss
- Spasticity or involuntary muscle contraction

Functional Implications

- Progressive loss of function until the problem is treated.
- Loss of functional mobility and independence with ADLs.

▶ Possible Contributing Causes

- Arachnoiditis
- Previous spinal cord trauma is a risk factor
- Congenital spinal malformations
- Meningitis
- Tethered spinal cord
- Trauma
- Tumor

▶ Differential Diagnosis

- Amyloid polyneuropathy
- Arachnoiditis
- Fabry disease
- Meningitis
- Spondylitis
- Stenosis
- Tangier disease

MEANS OF CONFIRMATION OR DIAGNOSIS

▶ Laboratory Tests

- Spinal tap via lumbar puncture

▶ Imaging

- MRI
- CT scan for detailed imaging

FINDINGS AND INTERPRETATION

- Fluid-filled cavity within the spinal cord[4]

REFERRALS/ADMITTANCE

- To neurologist
- To neurosurgeon to repair syrinx, restore normal cerebral spinal fluid flow, and relieve pressure on spinal cord
- To neuro-oncologist
- To occupational therapist
- To counselor, psychologist, neuropsychologist

IMPAIRMENTS

- Peripheral nerve integrity
- Gait
- Wheelchair mobility
- Balance
  - Static sit
  - Dynamic sit
  - Static stand
  - Dynamic stand
  - Moving outside the base of support (BOS)
- Muscle strength
- Muscle recruitment
- Coordination
- Postural control
- Posture
- ROM
- Reflexes
  - Deep tendon reflex (DTR)
  - Babinski
  - Clonus
- Muscle tone

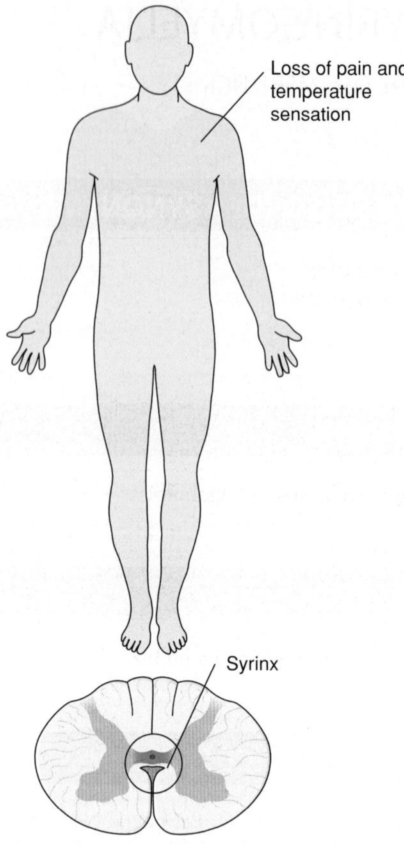

FIGURE 102-2 Syringomyelia (the presence of a cavity in the spinal cord due to breakdown of gliomatous new formations, presenting clinically with pain and paresthesias followed by muscular atrophy of the hands) involving the cervicothoracic portion of the cord. (Reproduced with permission from Waxman SG, deGroot J. *Clinical Neuroanatomy*. 22nd ed. Originally published by Appleton & Lange. Copyright © 1995 by The McGraw-Hill Companies, Inc.)

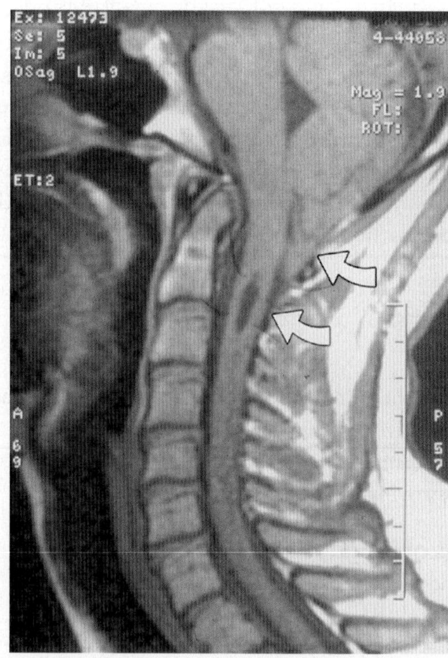

FIGURE 102-3 Chiari-type malformation and developmental syringomyelia. T1-weighted MRI of the low-lying cerebellar tonsils below the foramen magnum and behind the upper cervical cord (*upper arrow*) and the syrinx cavity in the upper cord (*lower arrow*). (From Ropper AH, Samuels MA. *Adams & Victor's Principles of Neurology*. 9th ed. http://www.accessmedicine.com. Copyright © The McGraw-Hill Companies, Inc. All rights reserved.)

- Sensation
- Bed mobility
- Transfers
- Endurance
- Aerobic capacity
- Self-care
- Home management
- Fine motor
- Respiratory compromise

TESTS AND MEASURES

- American Spinal Injury Association (ASIA) assessment
  - Motor
  - Sensation
  - ASIA classification neurologic level
  - Complete versus incomplete
  - Functional mobility
    - Functional independence measure (FIM™)
  - Wheelchair mobility
  - Transfers
  - Gait (Timed Up and Go, 10-meter walk test, Functional Gait Assessment, Walking Index for Spinal Cord Injury)
- Sitting and standing (for people with incomplete injuries or damage in the lower lumbar and sacral levels)
- Balance tests (sitting reach test, Tinetti, Berg Balance Scale)
  - Cardiovascular and pulmonary endurance (6-minute walk test) if appropriate, upper extremity (UE) ergometer test)
- Muscle endurance
- Skin assessment
- Active and passive ROM, muscle length
- Posture sitting (wheelchair and edge of mat, supported/unsupported) and standing if applicable
- Pain

INTERVENTION

- Balance retraining
- Bed-mobility retraining
- Cardiovascular and pulmonary endurance
- Gait retraining (if appropriate and with appropriate bracing and assistive devices)
- Orientation to vertical position if needed: Assessing orthostatic hypotension during treatment
- ROM/stretching/positioning
- Strengthening
- Transfer retraining
- Wheelchair-mobility retraining (curbs, ramps, various surfaces, negotiating obstacles, wheelies, floor recovery)

FUNCTIONAL GOALS

Note: Goals for syringomyelia depend on the level of the lesion and will result in similar functional expectations as those of the varying spinal levels indicated in the paraplegia and quad/tetraplegia sections.

- T1–T6
  - Patient will
    - Transfer between wheelchair and edge of mat via lateral pivot transfer with contact guard assistance to maximize safety and independence with functional mobility.

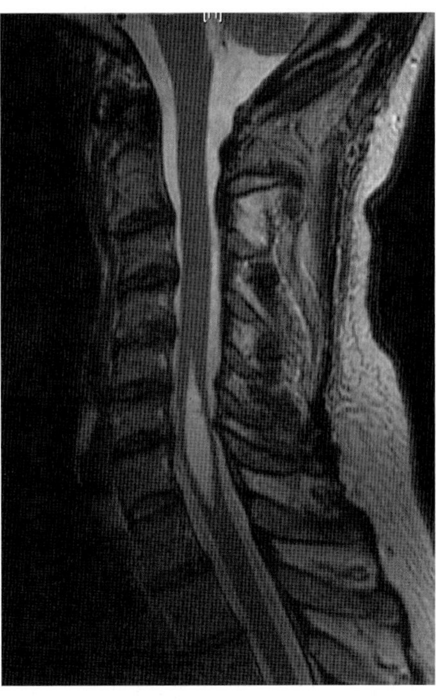

FIGURE 102-4 A developmental syringomyelia without Chiari malformation. The cord is greatly expanded but there were only signs of spinothalamic sensory loss over the arms. (From Ropper AH, Samuels MA. *Adams & Victor's Principles of Neurology*. 9th ed. http://www.accessmedicine.com.)

    - Propel ultra-light-weight manual wheelchair >500 ft indoors over level surfaces while negotiating obstacles with close supervision and minimal verbal cues for technique to maximize safe functional independence and mobility.

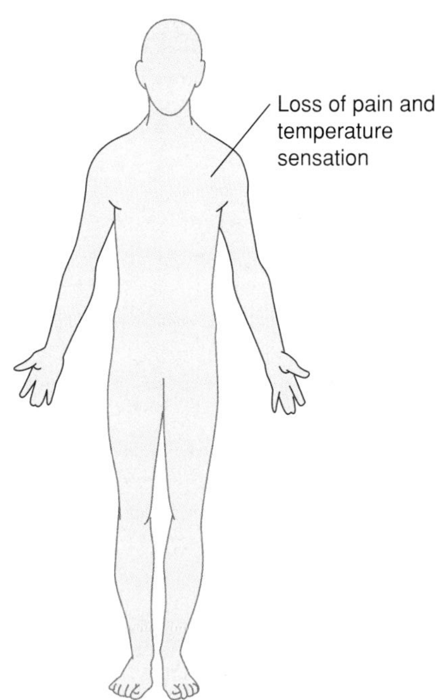

FIGURE 102-5 Syringomyelia involving the cervicothoracic portion of the spinal cord. (From Waxman SG. *Clinical Neuroanatomy*. 26th ed. http://www.accessmedicine.com.)

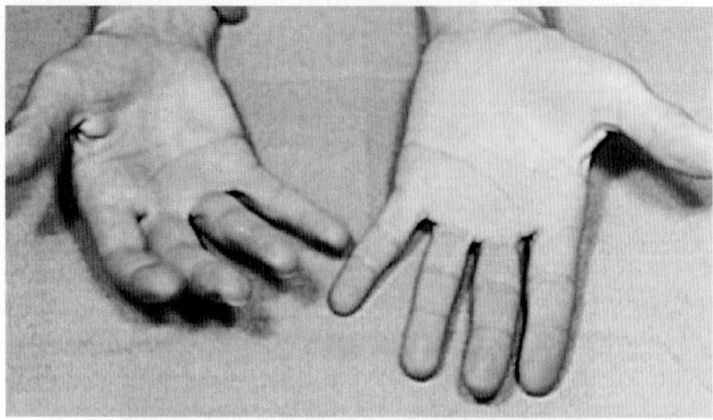

FIGURE 102-6 Wasting of the small muscles of the hands in a woman with syringomyelia. (From Waxman SG. *Clinical Neuroanatomy*. 26th ed. http://www.accessmedicine.com. Copyright © The McGraw-Hill Companies, Inc. All rights reserved.)

- T7–L1
  - Patient will
    - Be safe and independent with all aspects of bed mobility.
    - Propel an ultra-light-weight manual wheelchair on community surfaces >1500 ft with supervision for safety to increase safe and efficient functional independence.
- L2–S2
  - Patient will be
    - Assessed and fitted for proper LE bracing for a trial of gait training in parallel bars with appropriate assistance.
    - Independent with transfers to and from all surfaces via lateral pivot transfer to maximize safe functional independence.

PROGNOSIS

- Variable, based on length of time and resulting necrosis caused by the syringomyelia,

PATIENT RESOURCE

- Syringomyelia. American Syringomyelia & Chiari Alliance Project. http://www.asap.org/index.php/disorders/syringomyelia. Accessed July 10, 2013.

REFERENCES

1. ICD9Data.com. http://www.icd9data.com. Accessed July 10, 2013.
2. ICD10Data.com. http://www.icd10data.com/ICD10CM/Codes. Accessed July 10, 2013.
3. Pattern 5H. Impaired motor function, peripheral nerve integrity, and sensory integrity associated with nonprogressive disorders of the spinal cord. In: *Guide to Physical Therapist Practice*. 2nd ed. Alexandria, VA: American Physical Therapy Association; 2001. Revised 2003.
4. Syringomyelia. A.D.A.M Medical Encyclopedia. Pubmed Health. http://www.ncbi.nlm.nih.gov/pubmedhealth/PMH0002373/ Accessed July 10, 2013.

ADDITIONAL REFERENCES

- Dutton M. Intervention principles. In: Dutton M, ed. *Orthopaedic Examination, Evaluation, and Intervention*. 2nd ed. New York, NY: McGraw-Hill; 2008:Chapter 10. http://www.accessphysiotherapy.com/content/5548968. Accessed July 10, 2013.
- Dutton M, Dutton M. Therapeutic exercise. In: Dutton M, Dutton M, eds. *Dutton's Orthopedic Survival Guide: Managing Common Conditions*. New York, NY: McGraw-Hill; 2011:Chapter 4. http://www.accessphysiotherapy.com/content/8651381. Accessed July 10, 2013.
- Malone TR, Hazle C, Grey ML, eds. *Imaging in Rehabilitation*. New York, NY: McGraw-Hill; 2008. http://www.accessphysiotherapy.com/resource/613. Accessed July 10, 2013.
- Ropper A, Samuels MA. *Adams and Victor's Principles of Neurology*. 9th ed. New York, NY: McGraw-Hill; 2009:1222–1226.
- Shamus E, Stern DF, eds. *Effective Documentation for Physical Therapy Professionals*. 2nd ed. New York, NY: McGraw-Hill; 2011. http://www.accessphysiotherapy.com/resource/696. Accessed July 10, 2013.
- Six-Minute Walk Test (6MWT). StrokEngine. http://strokengine.ca/assess/module_6mwt_intro-en.html. Accessed May 21, 2014.
- Tinetti Balance and Gait Evaluation. http://www.bhps.org.uk/falls/documents/TinettiBalanceAssessment.pdf. Accessed July 10, 2013.

103 TRAUMATIC BRAIN INJURY

Megan Samantha Rosga, DPT, MSPT, NCS
Mollie Venglar, DSc, MSPT, NCS

CONDITION/DISORDER SYNONYM

- Brain contusion

ICD-9-CM CODES

- 854 Intracranial injury of other and unspecified nature
- 854.0 Intracranial injury of other and unspecified nature without mention of open intracranial wound
- 854.00 Intracranial injury of other and unspecified nature without open intracranial wound with state of consciousness unspecified
- 854.01 Intracranial injury of other and unspecified nature without open intracranial wound with no loss of consciousness
- 854.02 Intracranial injury of other and unspecified nature without open intracranial wound with brief (less than 1 hour) loss of consciousness
- 854.03 Intracranial injury of other and unspecified nature without open intracranial wound with moderate (1 to 24 hours) loss of consciousness
- 854.04 Intracranial injury of other and unspecified nature without open intracranial wound with prolonged (more than 24 hours) loss of consciousness and return to pre-existing conscious level
- 854.05 Intracranial injury of other and unspecified nature without open intracranial wound with prolonged (more than 24 hours) loss of consciousness without return to pre-existing conscious level
- 854.06 Intracranial injury of other and unspecified nature without open intracranial wound with loss of consciousness of unspecified duration
- 854.09 Intracranial injury of other and unspecified nature without open intracranial wound with concussion unspecified
- 854.1 Intracranial injury of other and unspecified nature with open intracranial wound
- 854.10 Intracranial injury of other and unspecified nature with open intracranial wound with state of consciousness unspecified
- 854.11 Intracranial injury of other and unspecified nature with open intracranial wound with no loss of consciousness
- 854.12 Intracranial injury of other and unspecified nature with open intracranial wound with brief (less than 1 hour) loss of consciousness
- 854.13 Intracranial injury of other and unspecified nature with open intracranial wound with moderate (1 to 24 hours) loss of consciousness
- 854.14 Intracranial injury of other and unspecified nature with open intracranial wound with prolonged (more than 24 hours) loss of consciousness and return to pre-existing conscious level
- 854.15 Intracranial injury of other and unspecified nature with open intracranial wound with prolonged (more than 24 hours) loss of consciousness without return to pre-existing conscious level

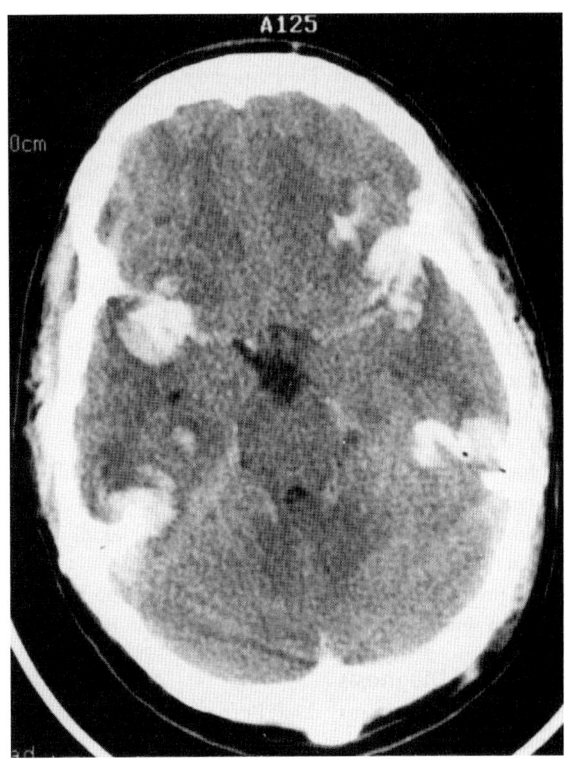

FIGURE 103-1 CT scan without contrast infusion showing areas of hemorrhagic contusion adjacent to bony prominences. There is also slight subarachnoid blood along the tentorium and in the insular cisterns, both typical of traumatic bleeding. (From Ropper AH, Samuels MA. 9th ed. http://www.accessmedicine.com. Copyright © The McGraw-Hill Companies, Inc. All rights reserved.)

- 854.16 Intracranial injury of other and unspecified nature with open intracranial wound with loss of consciousness of unspecified duration
- 854.19 Intracranial injury of other and unspecified nature with open intracranial wound with concussion unspecified

ICD-10-CM CODES

- S06.2X Diffuse traumatic brain injury
- S06.3 Focal traumatic brain injury
- S06 Intracranial Injury

PREFERRED PRACTICE PATTERNS

- 5C: Impaired Motor Function and Sensory Integrity Associated with Nonprogressive Disorders of the Central Nervous System—congenital origin or acquired in infancy or childhood
- 5D: Impaired Motor Function and Sensory Integrity Associated with Nonprogressive Disorders of the Central Nervous System—acquired in adolescence or adulthood

PATIENT PRESENTATION

A 47-year-old male was driving when involved in a single vehicle rollover, while unbelted and intoxicated. He was thrown from his vehicle and found in a ditch. Glasgow Coma Scale (GCS) was initially 3. He required intubation and ventilation. He remained comatose for 31 days. Once he was medically stable, he was transferred to an inpatient rehabilitation institute for individuals with brain injury. Presently he is highly confused and agitated when he is out of his bed. He frequently tries to get up from his wheelchair without staff and has had numerous falls since arriving at institute. He has full movement and good strength in bilateral upper extremities. On the Modified Ashworth Scale he tests at a level 2 or 3 for his lower extremities depending on his degree of agitation.

KEY FEATURES

Description

- Defined as external trauma to the skull that results in damage to one or more parts of the brain
- May or may not include fracture of the skull
  - Open head injury (penetrating): Fracture of the skull with brain injury
  - Closed head injury (blunt, non-penetrating): Skull remains intact, but brain injury is evident
- Initial presentation will range from comatose to ambulatory and verbal depending on the extent and location of damage

Essentials of Diagnosis

- Damage to the brain may result in changes or dysfunction to any body functions including:
  - Motor loss
  - Sensory loss
  - Autonomic dysfunction
  - Perceptual changes
  - Cognitive, personality, and behavioral changes
  - Changes in consciousness
  - Communication difficulties
  - Eating, swallowing, bowel and bladder changes

General Considerations

- Delayed effects of the trauma are common
- Full extent of the injury is not known at the time of injury
- Intracranial swelling must be addressed/controlled before the full extent of the damage can be identified
- Seizures are common
- Swelling will cause secondary damage to parts of the brain that were not impacted by the initial trauma
- Physical activity is contraindicated until the full effects of the brain injury are known and the patient has stable intracranial pressures

Demographics

- Approximately 500,000 people are admitted to the hospital each year in America due to cerebral trauma[1]; 75,000 to 90,000 die from the cerebral trauma and many others remain permanently disabled.
- Most commonly injured are between the ages of 15 and 24 years.[1]
- Men are twice as likely as women to suffer a brain injury.[1]

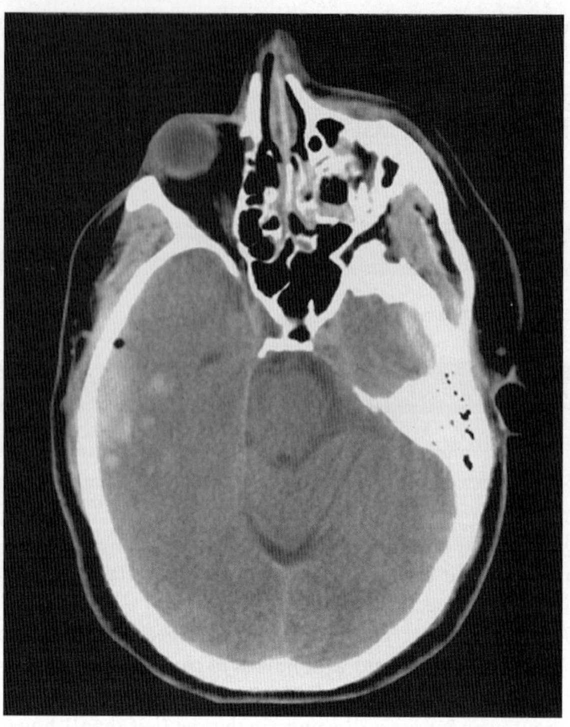

FIGURE 103-2 Temporal Lobe Contusion**.** A temporal lobe contusion is seen on the right. The quadrigeminal cistern is partially effaced suggesting early herniation. (From Knoop KJ, Stack L, Storrow A, Thurman RJ. *The Atlas of Emergency Medicine*. 3rd ed. http://www.accessmedicine.com. Copyright © The McGraw-Hill Companies, Inc. All rights reserved. Photo contributor: Lawrence B. Stack, MD.)

- Leading cause of brain injury in the young adult is motor vehicle crash.[1]
- Leading cause of brain injury in people over the age of 65 is falls.[1]

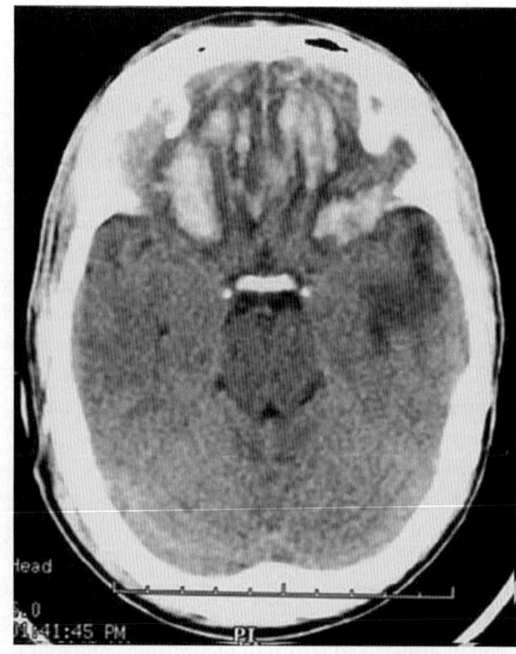

FIGURE 103-3 Severe bilateral contusions in the basal aspect of the frontal lobes, caused by the brain moving over the rough, irregular skull base during sudden cranial acceleration. (From Brunicardi FC, Andersen D, Billiar T, et al., eds. *Schwartz's Principles of Surgery*. 9th ed. http://www.accessmedicine.com. Copyright © The McGraw-Hill Companies, Inc. All rights reserved.)

CLINICAL FINDINGS

SIGNS AND SYMPTOMS

- Signs and symptoms are dependent on the part(s) of the brain that are injured and the extent of the injury.
- Common sequela treated by a PT include:
  - Behavioral changes
  - Cognitive function changes
  - Motor and motor planning deficits
  - Sensory deficits
  - Spasticity or hypertonicity

Functional Implications

- Loss of independence with all aspects of mobility, ADLs, self-care
- Loss of ability to interact with others effectively
- Difficulty with cognitive processing, particularly executive function

Possible Contributing Causes

- Automobile accident
- Falls
- Physical assault
- PA previous brain injury
- Risk-taking behaviors
- Sports

Differential Diagnosis

- The mechanism of injury indicates the diagnosis.

MEANS OF CONFIRMATION OR DIAGNOSIS

Laboratory Tests

- Intracranial pressure
- Oxygen saturation
- Hemoglobin
- Electrolyte and acid-base levels

Imaging

- CT
- MRI
- Radiographs

FINDINGS AND INTERPRETATION

- Cerebral hypoxia and/or ischemia
- Cerebral hemorrhages
- Electrolyte imbalances
- Infections from open wounds/open head injury

TREATMENT

Medications

- Antibiotics for nosocomial or opportunistic infections
- Baclofen pump
- Blood pressure management
- Carbamazepine or propranolol to treat aggression and agitation
- Corticosteroids
- Dantrolene sodium for general spasticity; botulinum toxin type A for specific muscle spasticity
- Gabapentin for intractable neurogenic pain
- Hyperosmolar therapy
- Oral baclofen for increased tone
- Valproic acid for seizure control

REFERRALS/ADMITTANCE

- To emergency room physician
- To neurologist or neurosurgeon as needed, based on location and severity of injury, management of medications, and management of future needs
- To neuropsychologist for cognitive testing
- To physiatrist for specific rehabilitation physician care. If not managed by a neurologist, the physiatrist will manage medications, symptoms, future needs, etc.
- To occupational therapist for ADLs, cognitive retraining, fine motor tasks
- To speech/language pathologist for speech, cognition, and swallowing impairments
- To respiratory therapist as needed (depending on the respiratory impact of the brain injury)
- To support groups for patients and family/caregivers
- To case management or social work for assistance with coordination of care

IMPAIRMENTS

- Arousal
- Attention
- Behavior
- Cognition
- Cranial nerve integrity
- Peripheral nerve integrity: Possibly from a comorbid diagnosis
- Gait
- Wheelchair mobility
- Balance
  - Static sit
  - Dynamic sit
  - Static stand
  - Dynamic stand
  - Moving base of support
- Muscle strength
- Muscle recruitment
- Coordination
- Postural control
- Posture
- ROM
- Reflexes
  - Deep tendon reflexes
  - Babinski
  - Clonus
- Muscle tone: Anticipate hypertonicity or spasticity
- Sensation
- Motor planning
- Bed mobility
- Transfers
- Neglect: Evident in cases of primary damage to one side of the brain
- Endurance
- Aerobic capacity
- Self-care
- Home management
- Fine motor
- Respiratory compromise

TESTS AND MEASURES

- Glasgow Outcome Scale
- Glasgow Coma Scale
- Rancho Los Amigos Scale
- Modified Ashworth scale
- Functional measures
  - Barthel Index
  - Functional independence measure
- Gait and balance measures
  - Berg Balance Scale (BBS)
  - Tinetti
  - Dynamic Gait Index (DGI)
  - Motor assessment scale
  - Gait assessment rating scale
  - Rancho Los Amigo Observational Gait Analysis
  - 6-minute walk test
  - Multi-directional reach test
  - HiMAT if appropriate for patients who have appropriate scores on Berg Balance Scale (BBS) and Dynamic Gait Index (DGI)
- Cognitive testing and cognitive behavioral level via Rancho Los Amigos
- Sensory testing may be limited by cognition or consciousness
- Strength: Includes speed of force production and ability to change force production
- Active and passive ROM, flexibility
- Bed mobility
- Transfers
- Cranial nerves, particularly vision
- Vestibular assessment

INTERVENTION

- ROM/stretching/positioning
- Tone management
- Orientation to vertical position
- Strengthening
- Balance training
- Gait training (if appropriate and with appropriate bracing and assistive devices)
- Transfer training
- Bed-mobility training
- Wheelchair-mobility training (curbs, ramps, various surfaces, negotiating obstacles)
- Cardiovascular and pulmonary endurance

FUNCTIONAL GOALS

Note: Goals are based on the cognitive behavioral levels identified in the Rancho Los Amigos Cognitive Scale. These will have to be modified on the basis of the likely comorbidities acquired concurrently with the brain injury.

- Rancho levels 1 and 2
  - Patient will demonstrate a response to tactile or verbal stimulation 80% of the time to show improving brain function.
  - Patient's caregiver will demonstrate appropriate bed and wheelchair positioning to prevent skin breakdown.
- Rancho level 3
  - Patient will
    - Tolerate tilt table at 75% of upright position for 10 minutes with vital signs stable to increase tolerance and orientation to vertical position.
    - Tolerate sitting at the edge of the mat with minimal physical support and maximal verbal cues to attend to the task for 3 minutes without loss of balance.
- Rancho level 4
  - Patient will
    - Demonstrate escalation less than 25% of treatment time during PT treatment in a closed environment.
    - Demonstrate escalation less than 75% of treatment time during PT treatment in an open environment.
- Rancho level 5
  - Patient will ambulate 250 ft with minimal assistance for balance indoors over level surfaces in a nondistracting environment to increase safe functional independence and mobility.
- Rancho level 6
  - Patient will ambulate indoors over level surfaces while negotiating obstacles for 500 ft with contact guard assistance for safety and moderate verbal cues for path-finding and attention to task in order to increase safe functional independence and mobility.
- Rancho level 7
  - Patient will perform floor recovery with supervision and upper extremity (UE) support on stable surface to increase safe functional independence.
- Rancho level 8
  - Patient will ambulate >500 ft indoors/outdoors over level and unlevel surfaces in a distracting environment with distant supervision and occasional cues for attention to task in order to increase safe and efficient functional mobility and independence.
- Rancho level 9
  - Patient will
    - Be completely independent with bilateral rolling, supine to/from sit, and scooting to ensure safe functional independence.
- Rancho level 10
  - Patient will
    - Increase BBS score ≥6 points to increase safe functional independence, increase balance, and decrease fall risk.
    - Tolerate assessment of HiMAT balance assessment to determine additional deficits in functional mobility to promote safe return to appropriate premorbid activities.

PROGNOSIS

- The following have been indicated to impact prognosis:
  - Age: Those older than 40 years tend to have a worse prognosis compared to people younger than 40.
  - Rehabilitation: Early rehabilitation (shorter time between brain injury and start of rehabilitation) has been shown to produce better outcomes.
  - Size of lesion: Some evidence supports that people suffering from smaller lesions will have better outcomes.
  - Type of lesion: Most patients with corpus callosum and dorsolateral brainstem lesions will not recover from a persistent vegetative state.
- Several factors contribute to the severity of an injury and the ability to access health care. Speed at which an individual receives emergency care following the head trauma will also impact prognosis.

PATIENT RESOURCE

- American Trauma Society. www.amtrauma.org. Accessed July 2, 2013.

REFERENCE

1. American Trauma Society. www.amtrauma.org. Accessed July 2, 2013.

ADDITIONAL REFERENCES

- Barthel Index. StrokEngine. http://www.strokecenter.org/wp-content/uploads/2011/08/barthel.pdf. Accessed May 9, 2014.
- Biros MH, Heegaard WE. Head injury. In: Marx JA, ed. *Rosen's Emergency Medicine: Concepts and Clinical Practice*. 7th ed. Philadelphia, PA: Mosby Elsevier; 2009:Chapter 38.
- Components of the Gait Assessment Rating Score (GARS). University of missouri. http://ojaischoolofmassage.com/documents/GARS.pdf. Accessed May 20, 2014.
- Dutton M, ed. *Orthopaedic Examination, Evaluation, and Intervention*. 2nd ed. New York, NY: McGraw-Hill; 2008. http://www.accessphysiotherapy.com/resource/612. Accessed July 2, 2013.
- Functional Independence Measure (FIM). StrokEngine. http://strokengine.ca/assess/PDF/FIMappendixD.pdf. Accessed May 9, 2014.
- Hay WW, Levin MJ, Sondheimer JM, Deterding RR. Rehabilitation medicine. In: Hay WW, Levin MJ, Sondheimer JM, Deterding RR, eds. *CURRENT Diagnosis & Treatment: Pediatrics*. 20th ed. New York, NY: McGraw-Hill; 2011:Chapter 26. http://www.accessphysiotherapy.com/content/6586370. Accessed July 2, 2013.
- ICD9Data.com. http://www.icd9data.com. Accessed July 2, 2013.
- ICD10Data.com. http://www.icd10data.com/ICD10CM/Codes. Accessed July 2, 2013.
- Introduction to the Extended Glasgow Outcome Scale. The Center for Outcome Measurement in Brain Injury. http://tbims.org/combi/gose/index.html. Accessed July 2, 2013.
- Introduction to the High Level Mobility Assessment Tool. The Center for Outcome Measurement in Brain Injury. http://tbims.org/combi/himat/index.html. Accessed July 2, 2013.
- Leveque JC, Hoff JT. Neurosurgery. In: Greenfield LJ, Mulholland MW, Oldham KT, Zelenock GB, Lillemoe KD, eds. *Greenfield's Surgery: Scientific Principles and Practice*. 4th ed. Philadelphia, PA: Lippincott Williams & Wilkins; 2005:Chapter 114.
- Malone TR, Hazle C, Grey ML. Imaging of the brain. In: Malone TR, Hazle C, Grey ML, eds. *Imaging in Rehabilitation*. New York, NY: McGraw-Hill; 2008:Chapter 2. http://www.accessphysiotherapy.com/content/5940267. Accessed July 2, 2013.
- Panus PC, Jobst EE, Masters SB, Katzung B, Tinsley SL, Trevor AJ, eds. *Pharmacology for the Physical Therapist*. New York, NY: McGraw-Hill; 2009. http://www.accessphysiotherapy.com/resource/615. Accessed July 2, 2013.
- Motor Assessment Scale (MAS). StrokEngine. http://strokengine.ca/assess/module_mas_indepth-en.html. Accessed May 20, 2014.
- Multidirectional Reach Test. Temple University. Gait Study Center. Temple University. http://podiatry.temple.edu/research/gait-study-center/techniques-and-methods/multi-directional-reach-test. Accessed May 14, 2014.
- Observational Gait Analysis. University of Oklahoma Health Sciences Center. http://moon.ouhsc.edu/dthompso/gait/knmatics/oga.htm. Accessed July 2, 2013.
- Pattern 5D. Impaired motor function and sensory integrity associated with nonprogressive disorders of the central nervous system - acquired in adolescence or adulthood. In: *Guide to Physical Therapist Practice*. 2nd ed. Alexandria, VA: American Physical Therapy Association; 2001. Revised 2003.
- Rancho Los Amigos Cognitive Scale Revised. Northeast Center for Special Care. http://www.northeastcenter.com/rancho_los_amigos_revised.htm. Accessed July 2, 2013.
- Ropper A, Samuels MA. *Adams and Victor's Principles of Neurology*. 9th ed. New York, NY: McGraw-Hill; 2009:846–873.
- Shamus E, Stern DF, eds. *Effective Documentation for Physical Therapy Professionals*. 2nd ed. New York, NY: McGraw-Hill; 2011. http://www.accessphysiotherapy.com/resource/696. Accessed July 2, 2013.
- Six-minute Walk Test (6MWT). StrokEngine. http://strokengine.ca/assess/module_6mwt_intro-en.html. Accessed May 21, 2014.
- Testing Spasticity. The Modified Ashworth Scale. Advance for Physical Therapy & Rehab Medicine. http://physical-therapy.advanceweb.com/Article/Testing-Spasticity-The-Modified-Ashworth-Scale.aspx. Accessed July 2, 2013.
- Tinetti Balance and Gait Evaluation. http://www.bhps.org.uk/falls/documents/TinettiBalanceAssessment.pdf. Accessed July, 2013.
- Waxman SG. Imaging of the brain. In: Waxman SG, ed. *Clinical Neuroanatomy*. 26th ed. New York, NY: McGraw-Hill; 2010: Chapter 22. http://www.accessphysiotherapy.com/content/5275385. Accessed July 2, 2013.
- Winkler PA. Traumatic brain injury. In: Umphred DA, ed. *Neurological Rehabilitation*. 5th ed. St. Louis, MO: Mosby Elsevier. 2007:532–566.

104 TUMOR, BRAIN

Mollie Venglar, DSc, MSPT, NCS

ICD-9-CM CODES

- 191.7 Malignant neoplasm of brain stem
- 191.8 Malignant neoplasm of other parts of brain
- 191.9 Malignant neoplasm of brain unspecified site
- 198.3 Secondary malignant neoplasm of brain and spinal cord
- 225.0 Benign neoplasm of brain
- 237.5 Neoplasm of uncertain behavior of brain and spinal cord
- 239.6 Neoplasm of unspecified nature of brain
- V10.85 Personal history of malignant neoplasm of brain
- V12.41 Personal history of benign neoplasm of the brain

ICD-10-CM CODES

- C71.7 Malignant neoplasm of brain stem
- C71.8 Malignant neoplasm of overlapping sites of brain
- C71.9 Malignant neoplasm of brain, unspecified
- C79.31 Secondary malignant neoplasm of brain
- D33.0 Benign neoplasm of brain, supratentorial
- D33.1 Benign neoplasm of brain, infratentorial
- D33.2 Benign neoplasm of brain, unspecified
- D43.0 Neoplasm of uncertain behavior of brain, supratentorial
- D43.2 Neoplasm of uncertain behavior of brain, unspecified
- D43.1 Neoplasm of uncertain behavior of brain, infratentorial
- D49.6 Neoplasm of unspecified behavior of brain
- H47.631 Disorders of visual cortex in (due to) neoplasm, right side of brain
- H47.632 Disorders of visual cortex in (due to) neoplasm, left side of brain
- Z85.841 Personal history of malignant neoplasm of brain
- Z86.011 Personal history of benign neoplasm of the brain

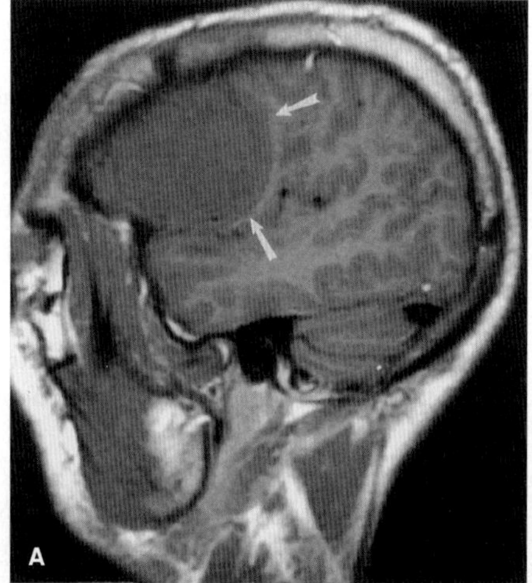

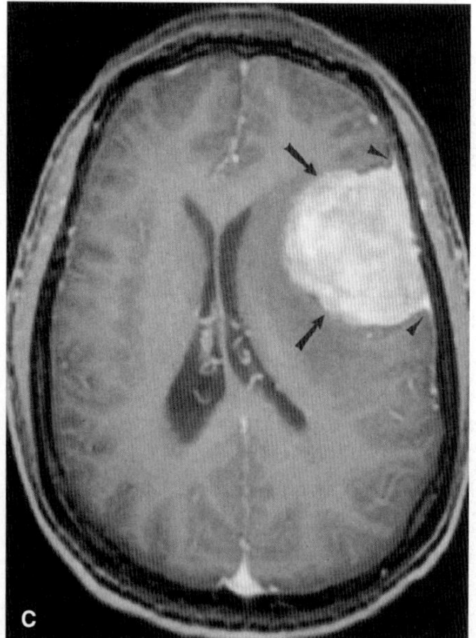

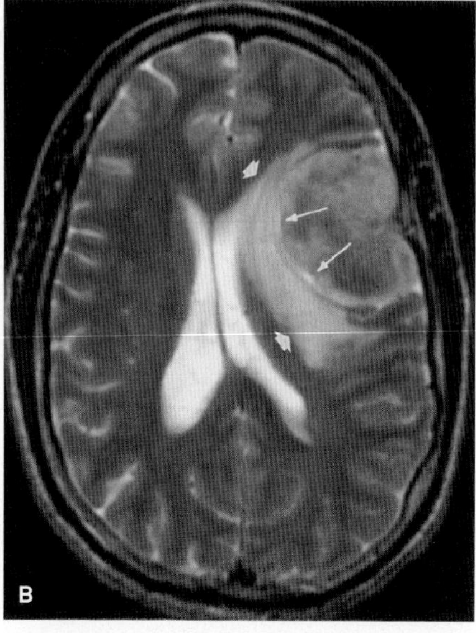

FIGURE 104-1 Noncontrast sagittal T1-weighted (**A**) and axial T2-weighted (**B**) images, as well as postcontrast axial T1-weighted image (**C**) in a 33-year-old Hispanic man who presents with a syncopal episode and involuntary tremors. (From Chen MYM, Pope TL, Ott DJ. *Basic Radiology*. 2nd ed. http://www.accessmedicine.com. Copyright © The McGraw-Hill Companies, Inc. All rights reserved.)

TABLE 104-1 Pediatric Brain Tumors

Classification	Type	Description
Infratentorial	Astrocytomas	Neoplasms in which the predominant cell type is derived from an astrocyte. Regional effects of astrocytomas include compression, invasion, and destruction of brain parenchyma, arterial and venous hypoxia, competition for nutrients, release of metabolic end products (e.g., free radicals, altered electrolytes, neurotransmitters), release and recruitment of cellular mediators (e.g., cytokines) that disrupt normal parenchymal function. The type of neurological symptoms that result from astrocytoma development depends foremost on the site and extent of tumor growth in the CNS. Astrocytomas of the spinal cord or brainstem are less common and present with motor/sensory or cranial nerve deficits referable to the tumor's location. The etiology of diffuse astrocytomas has been the subject of analytic epidemiological studies that have yielded associations with various disorders and exposures.
	Ependymomas	Found in the infratentorial region about 65% of the time, and represent 10% of all childhood brain tumors. These tumors arise from ependymal cells in the ventricles and spinal column. Initial signs and symptoms relate to increased intracranial pressure in posterior fossa ependymomas.
	Medulloblastoma	Infiltrate the floor or lateral wall of the fourth ventricle and extend into the cavity. These are fast growing tumors and they may spread throughout the CNS via cerebrospinal fluid.
Supratentorial	Craniopharyngioma	Benign tumors located near the pituitary gland. Cause problems from compression rather than invasion of tissues. Progression of the tumor is related to symptoms of increasing intracranial pressure, visual complaints, and endocrine disturbances.
	Optic tract glioma	Generally slow growing astrocytomas. Visual disturbances are the predominant clinical symptom.
	Pineal	Symptoms are often related to increased intracranial pressure and include headache.

Source: Data from Kerkering GA. Brain injuries: traumatic brain injuries, near drowning, and brain tumors. In: Campbell SK, Vander Linden DW, Palisano RJ, eds. *Physical Therapy for Children.* 3rd ed. St. Louis, MO: Saunders. 2006:709–734.

PREFERRED PRACTICE PATTERNS

- 5C: Impaired Motor Function and Sensory Integrity Associated with Nonprogressive Disorders of the Central Nervous System—congenital origin or acquired in infancy or childhood
- 5D: Impaired Motor Function and Sensory Integrity Associated with Nonprogressive Disorders of the Central Nervous System—acquired in adolescence or adulthood
- 5E: Impaired Motor Function and Sensory Integrity Associated with Progressive Disorders of the Central Nervous System
- 6B: Impaired Aerobic Capacity/Endurance Associated with Deconditioning[1]

PATIENT PRESENTATION

A 13-year-old girl suffered a mild concussion during physical education class at school. The school nurse noted that the girl's pupillary reflexes were absent so she was sent to the local emergency department. She was very drowsy and dizzy and required help to sit upright without falling over. She was unable to walk safely as her accuracy of stepping was impaired and she could not maintain

TABLE 104-2 Common Impairments, Activity Limitations, and Participation Restrictions in Children with Brain Injuries

Impairments	Activity limitations	Participation Restrictions
Abnormal muscle tone	Decreased age-appropriate mobility	Dependent mobility
Postural asymmetry	Delayed gross motor skills	Dependent self-help skills
Decreased muscle strength	Poor school performances	Social isolation
Loss of range of motion	Decreased attention to environment	Limited play with peers
Ataxia		
Poor balance		
Behavior state changes		
Poor motor planning		
Poor visual perceptual skills		
Impaired cognition		

Source: Reproduced with permission from Kerkering GA. Brain injuries: traumatic brain injuries, near drowning, and brain tumors. In: Campbell SK, Vander Linden DW, Palisano RJ, eds. *Physical Therapy for Children.* 3rd ed. St. Louis, MO: Saunders. 2006:709–734.

an upright posture in her trunk. MRI revealed a 4 cm tumor in the midline of the cerebellum. The doctors postulate that the concussion caused just enough increase in intracranial pressure for the effects of the tumor to be identified.

KEY FEATURES

Description

- Neoplasm in the brain tissue of either primary or secondary origin
- Brain tumor types according to age and site

Essentials of Diagnosis

- Classic triad[2]
  - Morning headache
  - Vomiting
  - Papilledema
- Breast, lung, melanoma, and renal cell cancers are most likely to metastasize to brain tissue.
- Tumor can occur in any part of the brain, symptoms help identify location of tumor prior to diagnostic imaging.
- Confirmation is commonly by stereotactic biopsy or craniotomy.

General Considerations

- Secondary metastatic deposits are more common in adults than in children
- Frequency and location of pediatric brain tumors
  - Posterior fossa most common frequency and location in pediatric brain tumors[2]
- AIDS, neurofibromatosis, and systemic cancers predispose the patient to development of a tumor in the nervous system
- Growth rates and invasiveness vary
  - Glioblastomas are highly malignant and invasive
  - Meningiomas are benign and slowly progressive

Demographics

- Approximately 20,000 people die annually in the United States from a malignant glioma.
- Approximately 130,000 people who die with cancer have evidence of metastases to the brain.
- In children, primary brain tumors constitute the most common solid tumor and represent 25% to 30% of childhood neoplasms.[2]
- Medulloblastomas, spongioblastomas, optic nerve gliomas, and pinealomas occur most frequently before age 20.
- Meningiomas and glioblastomas occur more frequently after age 50.
- Glioblastomas occur slightly more frequently in men.
- Almost all gliomas occur sporadically.

CLINICAL FINDINGS

SIGNS AND SYMPTOMS

- Classic triad[2]
  - Morning headache
  - Vomiting
  - Papilledema
- Drowsiness
- Confusion, altered mental functions
- Increased intracranial pressure
- Increased head circumference[2]
- Focal or generalized seizure[2]
- Personality change[2]
- Blurred vision/Diplopia
- Focal or regional motor, sensory, or speech disturbance
- Dizziness
- Decreased coordination/Unsteadiness[2]
- Ataxia[2]
- Hemiplegia[2]
- Hyperreflexia

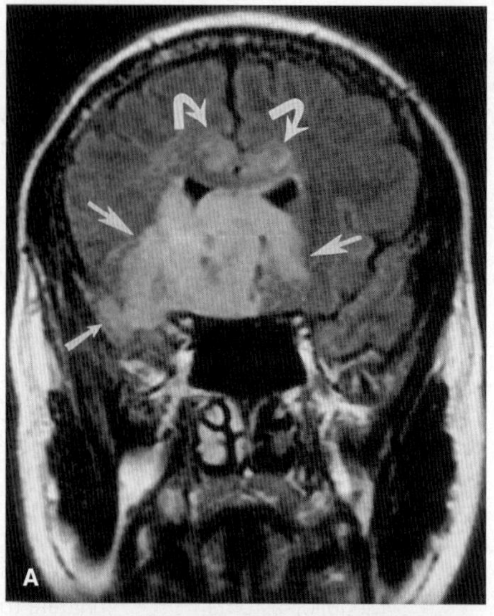

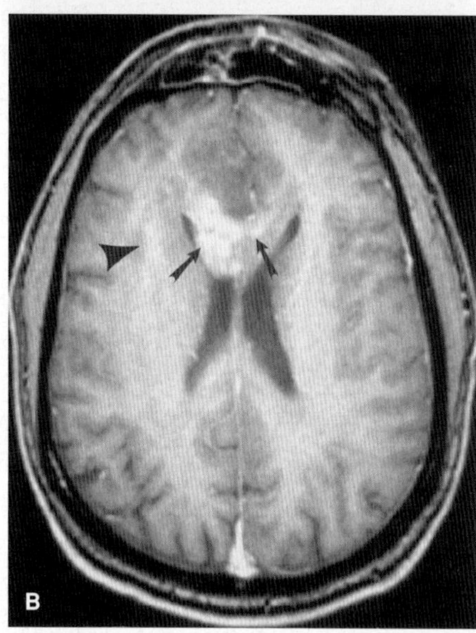

FIGURE 104-2 Initial coronal T2 FLAIR-weighted (**A**) and axial contrast-enhanced T1-weighted (**B**) images in a 48-year-old woman who presents with a history of headaches and seizures. (From Chen MYM, Pope TL, Ott DJ. *Basic Radiology*. 2nd ed. http://www.accessmedicine.com. Copyright © The McGraw-Hill Companies, Inc. All rights reserved.)

Functional Implications

- Loss of independence with all aspects of mobility, ADLs, and self-care
- Loss of ability to interact with others effectively
- Difficulty with all aspects of cognitive processing

Possible Contributing Causes

- AIDS
- Breast cancer
- Epstein–Barr virus
- Hereditary predisposition
- Human papilloma virus

- Human T-lymphotropic virus
- Lung cancer
- Lymphoma
- Melanoma
- Neurofibromatosis
- Renal cancer

Differential Diagnosis

- Brain abscess
- Hydrocephalus
- Normal pressure hydrocephalus
- Stroke
- Subdural empyema
- Subdural hematoma

MEANS OF CONFIRMATION OR DIAGNOSIS

Laboratory Tests

- Stereotactic biopsy
- Complete blood count (CBC)
- Craniotomy for highly suspicious lesion with intent to remove as much as possible during diagnosis

Imaging

- CT scan with contrast
- MRI

FINDINGS AND INTERPRETATION

- MRI can reveal tumors (i.e., in the midline of the cerebellum)

TREATMENT

Medication

- High-potency glucocorticoids to address brain edema related to the neoplasm
  - Methylprednisolone
  - Dexamethasone
- Anti-epileptic medications for patients with seizures or to pre-empt convulsions
- Phenytoin during radiation
- Chemotherapy
  - Side effects
    - Nausea
    - Vomiting
    - Diarrhea
    - Alopecia
    - Mouth sores
    - Conjunctivitis
    - Ulcers
    - Leukopenia
    - Anemia
    - Thrombocytopenia
    - Headaches
    - Dizziness
    - Menstrual irregularities
    - Infertility
    - Peripheral neuropathies
- Radiation, general or stereotactic
  - Side effects
    - Fatigue
    - Secondary neoplasm
    - Integumentary compromise (burns)

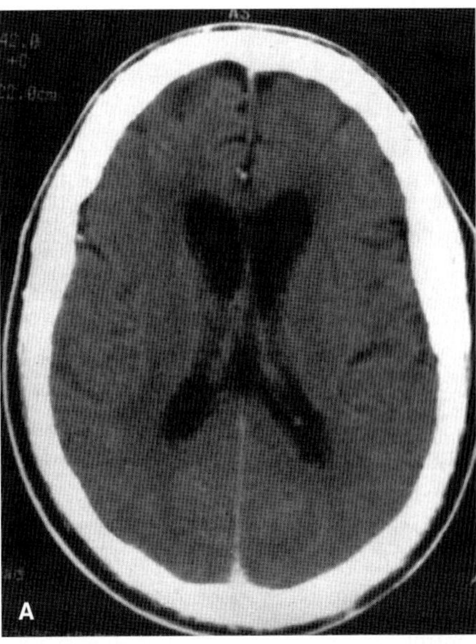

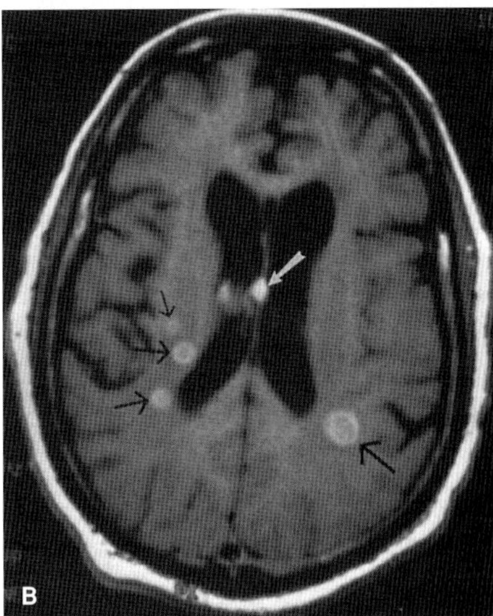

FIGURE 104-3 A contrast-enhanced axial CT scan (**A**) and a gadolinium-enhanced axial T1-weighted MR image (**B**) in a 58-year-old man who presents with a history of lung cancer and mental status changes. (From Chen MYM, Pope TL, Ott DJ. *Basic Radiology*. 2nd ed. http://www.accessmedicine.com. Copyright © The McGraw-Hill Companies, Inc. All rights reserved.)

REFERRALS/ADMITTANCE

- To emergency room physician
- To multidisciplinary team[2]
  - Neurosurgeon
  - Neuro-oncology
  - Endocrinologist
  - Neuropsychologist for cognitive testing after resolution of tumor
  - Physiatrist for specific rehabilitation physician care if residual neurologic deficit requires rehabilitation
  - Occupational therapist for ADLs, cognitive retraining, fine motor tasks
  - Speech/language pathologist for speech, cognition, and swallowing impairments
  - Case management or social work for assistance with coordination of care

IMPAIRMENTS

- Arousal
- Attention
- Behavior
- Cognition
- Cranial nerve integrity
- Peripheral nerve integrity, possibly from a comorbid diagnosis
- Gait
- Wheelchair mobility
- Balance
  - Static sit
  - Dynamic sit
  - Static stand
  - Dynamic stand
  - Moving base of support
- Muscle strength
- Muscle recruitment
- Coordination
- Postural control
- Posture
- ROM
- Reflexes
  - Deep tendon reflexes
  - Babinski
  - Clonus
- Muscle tone, anticipate hypertonicity or spasticity
- Sensation
- Motor planning
- Bed mobility
- Transfers
- Neglect, evident in cases of primary damage to one side of the brain
- Endurance
- Aerobic capacity

TABLE 104-3 Frequency of Major Types of Intracranial Tumors

Types of Tumors[a]		Frequency of Occurrence
Gliomas		50%
Glioblastoma multiforme	50%	
Astrocytoma	20%	
Ependymoma	10%	
Medulloblastoma	10%	
Oligodendroglioma	5%	
Mixed	5%	
Meningiomas		20%
Nerve sheath tumors		10%
Metastatic tumors		10%
Congenital tumors		5%
Miscellaneous tumors		5%

[a]Exclusive of pituitary tumors.

Source: Reproduced with permission from Way LW, ed. *Current Surgical Diagnosis & Treatment.* 10th ed. Appleton & Lange, 1994.

- Self-care
- Home management
- Fine motor
- Respiratory compromise

TESTS AND MEASURES

- Functional Measures
  - Barthel Index
  - Functional Independence Measure
- Gait and balance measures
  - Tinetti
  - Motor Assessment Scale

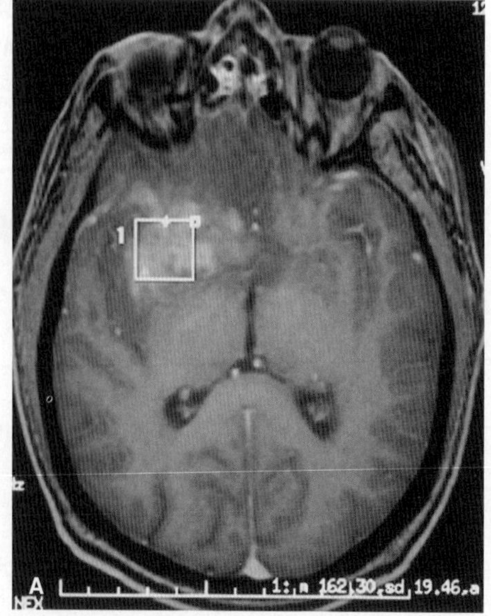

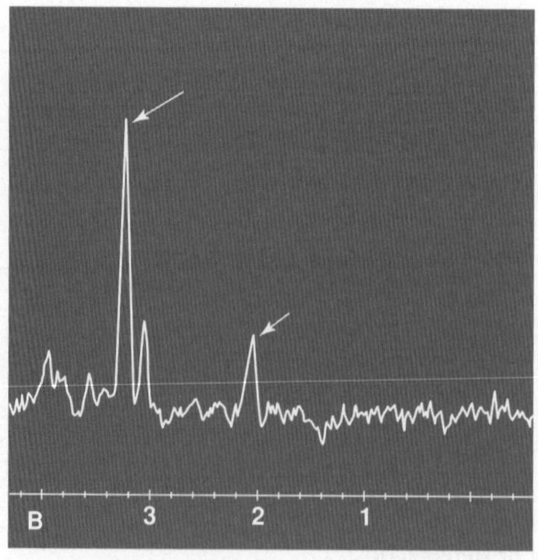

FIGURE 104-4 The same patient as in Figure 104-2. (**A**) At a more inferior level, the patchy, heterogeneous enhancement of this mass within the right inferior frontal/temporal regions is better appreciated. A region-of-interest or volume element (i.e., voxel) was centered within the enhancing tumor volume, and an MR spectrum was obtained. (**B**) MR spectrum. The NAA peak is abnormally decreased (*short arrow* at 2.0), and the choline signal is elevated (*long arrow* at 3.2), supporting the diagnosis of a malignant brain tumor. (From Chen MYM, Pope TL, Ott DJ. *Basic Radiology.* 2nd ed. http://www.accessmedicine.com. Copyright © The McGraw-Hill Companies, Inc. All rights reserved.)

- Gait assessment rating scale
- Rancho Los Amigo Observational Gait Analysis
- 6-minute walk test
- Multi-directional reach test
- Cognitive testing
- Sensory testing may be limited by cognition or consciousness
- Strength, includes speed of force production and ability to change force production
- Active and passive ROM, flexibility
- Bed mobility
- Transfers
- Cranial nerves, particularly vision
- Vestibular assessment
- Fatigue impact

INTERVENTION

- Fatigue management
- ROM/stretching/positioning
- Orientation to vertical position
- Strengthening
- Balance training
- Gait training (if appropriate and with appropriate bracing and assistive devices)
- Transfer training
- Bed-mobility training
- Wheelchair-mobility training (curbs, ramps, various surfaces, negotiating obstacles)
- Cardiovascular and pulmonary endurance

FUNCTIONAL GOALS

Note: Due to the variability of location and extent of the tumor, goals will need to be very specific to the patient. These goals are very general and relate to general functional mobility.

- Short-term goals
  - Patient will:
    - Perform wheelchair to/from bed transfer via sit (lateral) pivot with minimal assist and moderate verbal cues for sequencing to increase safe functional mobility on return home.
    - Transition to sit to stand with a 90-degree hip angle and progress from contact guard assist independence to increase safe functional mobility.
    - Ambulate >50 ft with minimal assistance and appropriate assistive device to improve mobility in preparation to return home.
    - Tolerate 8 minutes of continuous exercise without exceeding a Borg perceived exertion rating of >12 to improve cardiovascular endurance and increase tolerance for daily activity.
- Long-term goals
  - The patient will:
    - Improve Berg Balance Scale score to greater than or equal to 50/56 to demonstrate a decreased fall risk during functional activities.
    - Ambulate on a variety of indoor/outdoor surfaces with distant supervision and assistive device as needed to maximize safe and functional ambulation and return to appropriate premorbid activities.
    - Tolerate 15 minutes of continuous activity without exceeding a Borg perceived exertion rating of >12.

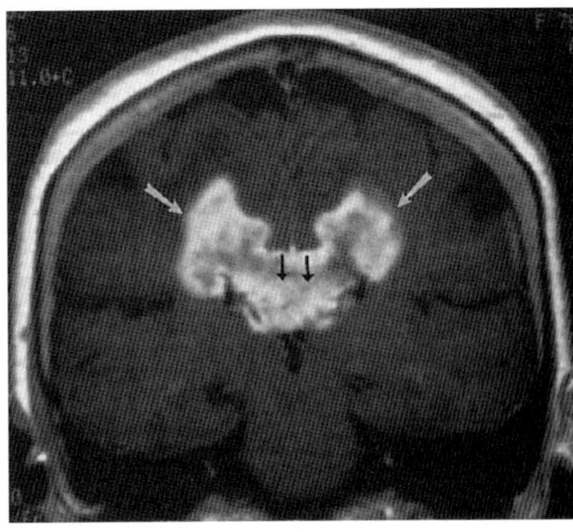

FIGURE 104-5 A 76-year-old woman presents with a 6-month history of progressive gait ataxia and frequent falling. Coronal contrast-enhanced T1-weighted MR image of a glioblastoma multiforme is shown. An enhancing mass (*white arrows*) extends through the corpus callosum (*black arrows*) into both hemispheres. (From Chen MYM, Pope TL, Ott DJ. *Basic Radiology*. 2nd ed. http://www.accessmedicine.com. Copyright © The McGraw-Hill Companies, Inc. All rights reserved.)

    - Carry one load of groceries weighing <15 lb without significant dyspnea, as measured by patient report of ≤3 on Borg Dyspnea Scale.

PROGNOSIS

- Children have a better prognosis than do adults.[2]
- For children with medulloblastoma, more favorable in cases older than 4 years of age.
- Brain glioblastomas have a poor prognosis for treatment and high mortality rate.
- Untreated malignant brain tumors result in death within 9 to 18 months.

PATIENT RESOURCE

- National Brain Tumor Society. http://www.braintumor.org/patients-family-friends. Accessed July 14, 2013.

REFERENCES

1. The American Physical Therapy Association. Pattern 6B: impaired aerobic capacity/endurance associated with deconditioning. *Interactive Guide to Physical Therapist Practice*. 2003. doi: 10.2522/ptguide.3.3_2. http://guidetoptpractice.apta.org/content/1/SEC28.extract. Accessed May 21, 2014.
2. Hay WW, Levin MJ, Sondheimer JM, Deterding RR. Major pediatric neoplastic diseases. In: Hay WW, Levin MJ, Sondheimer JM, Deterding RR, eds. *CURRENT Diagnosis & Treatment: Pediatrics*. 20th ed. New York, NY: McGraw-Hill; 2011. http://www.accessphysiotherapy.com/content/6587229. Accessed July 14, 2013.

ADDITIONAL REFERENCES

- Barthel Index. StrokEngine. http://www.medicine.mcgill.ca/strokengine-assess/module_bi_intro-en.html. Accessed July 14, 2013.

- Chandrasoma P, Taylor CR. Infections of the brain parenchyma. In: Chandrasoma P, Taylor CR, eds. *Concise Pathology*. 3rd ed. New York, NY: McGraw-Hill; 2011. http://www.accessphysiotherapy.com/content/193000. Accessed July 14, 2013.
- Components of the Gait Assessment Rating Score (GARS). University of Missouri. http://web.missouri.edu/~proste/tool/GARS.pdf. Accessed July 14, 2013.
- Functional Independence Measure (FIM). StrokEngine. http://www.medicine.mcgill.ca/strokengine-assess/module_fim_intro-en.html. Accessed July 14, 2013.
- Hay WW, Levin MJ, Sondheimer JM, Deterding RR. Infections & inflammatory disorders of the central nervous system. In: Hay WW, Levin MJ, Sondheimer JM, Deterding RR, eds. *CURRENT Diagnosis & Treatment: Pediatrics*. 20th ed. New York: McGraw-Hill; 2011. http://www.accessphysiotherapy.com/content/6585600. Accessed July 14, 2013.
- ICD9Data.com. http://www.icd9data.com. Accessed July 14, 2013.
- ICD10Data.com. http://www.icd10data.com/ICD10CM/Codes. Accessed July 14, 2013.
- Introduction to the Extended Glasgow Outcome Scale. The center for outcome measurement in brain injury. http://tbims.org/combi/gose/index.html. Accessed July 14, 2013.
- Introduction to the High Level Mobility Assessment Tool. The center for outcome measurement in brain injury. http://tbims.org/combi/himat/index.html. Accessed July 14, 2013.
- Motor Assessment Scale (MAS). StrokEngine. http://www.medicine.mcgill.ca/strokengine-assess/module_mas_intro-en.html. Accessed July 14, 2013.
- Multidirectional Reach Test. Temple University. Gait Study Center. Temple University. http://podiatry.temple.edu/gaitlab/facilities/mdrt.html. Accessed July 14, 2013.
- Rancho Los Amigos Cognitive Scale Revised. Northeast Center for Special Care. http://www.northeastcenter.com/rancho_los_amigos_revised.htm. Accessed July 14, 2013.
- Ropper AL, Samuels MA. *Adams and Victor's Principles of Neurology*. 9th ed. New York, NY: McGraw-Hill. 2009:683–686.
- Six-minute Walk Test (6MWT). StrokEngine. http://www.medicine.mcgill.ca/strokengine-assess/module_6mwt_intro-en.html. Accessed July 14, 2013.
- Tinetti Balance and Gait Evaluation. http://www.ohsu.edu/sgimhartford/toolbox/TinettiBalanceAndGaitEvaluation.pdf. Accessed July 14, 2013.
- Tinetti Balance and Gait Evaluation. http://www.bhps.org.uk/falls/documents/TinettiBalanceAssessment.pdf Accessed July 14, 2013.
- Waxman SG, ed. *Clinical Neuroanatomy*. 26th ed. New York, NY: McGraw-Hill; 2010. http://www.accessphysiotherapy.com/resource/22. Accessed July 14, 2013.

105 TUMOR, SPINAL

Mollie Venglar, DSc, MSPT, NCS
Adrian Taylor, DPT

CONDITION/DISORDER SYNONYMS

- Intraspinal tumor
- Spinal cord neoplasm
- Spinal cord space-occupying lesion

ICD-9-CM CODES

- 237.5 Neoplasm of uncertain behavior of brain and spinal cord
- 238.0 Neoplasm of uncertain behavior of bone and articular cartilage

ICD-10-CM CODES

- C72.0 Malignant neoplasm of spinal cord
- D33.4 for benign neoplasm of spinal cord
- D43.4 Neoplasm of uncertain behavior of spinal cord
- D48.0 Neoplasm of uncertain behavior of bone and articular cartilage

PREFERRED PRACTICE PATTERNS[1]

- 5H: Impaired Motor Function, Peripheral Nerve Integrity, and Sensory Integrity Associated with Nonprogressive Disorders of the Spinal Cord
- 6B: Impaired Aerobic Capacity/Endurance Associated with Deconditioning

PATIENT PRESENTATION

During an MRI to determine the extent of a disc lesion, the radiologist discovered a spinal tumor at the level of L3 in a 60-year-old patient. The patient had reported symptoms of "pins and needles" on the anterior and medial thigh, and progressive difficulty ascending and descending steps for the past 4 months to his primary care physician. The physician ordered an MRI assuming the radicular symptoms were related to a disc lesion in the lumbar spine. The patient was referred to a neurooncologist for further work up. The spinal tumor was determined to be extramedullary.

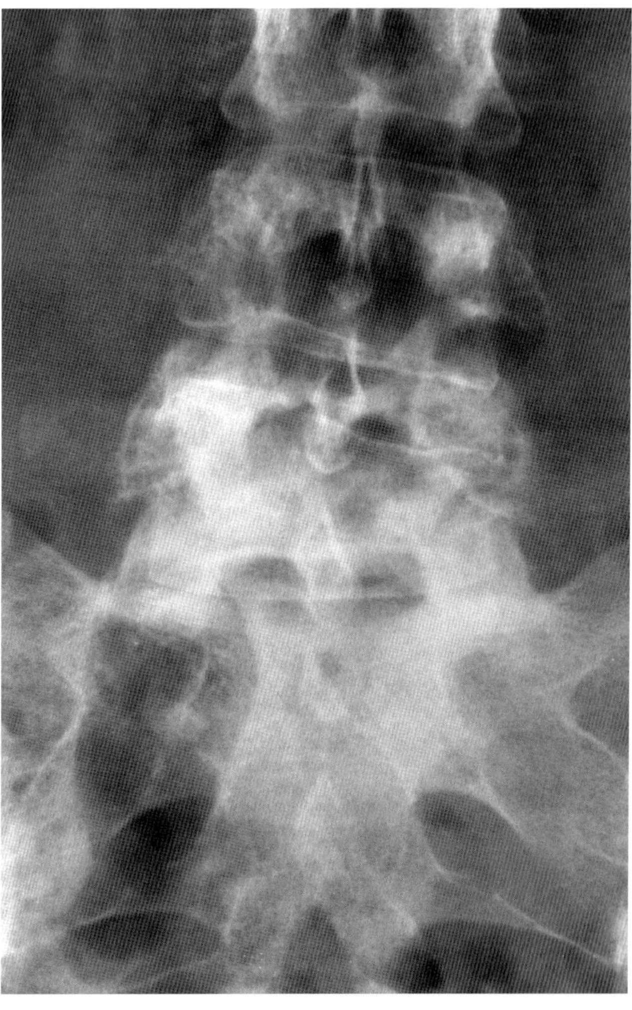

FIGURE 105-1 Radiograph of the spine of a 45-year-old woman whose cancer had metastasized from the breast. (From Skinner HB. *Current Diagnosis & Treatment in Orthopedics*. 4th ed. http://www.accessmedicine.com. Copyright © The McGraw-Hill Companies, Inc. All rights reserved.)

KEY FEATURES

Description

- Cell growth in or around the spinal cord
- Spinal tumors account for approximately 15% of primary CNS tumors

Essentials of Diagnosis

- Primary spinal tumors are ones that start in spinal tissue
- Secondary spinal tumors are spread from other sites (metastasis)

General Considerations

- Spinal tumors are divided into two groups:
  - Intramedullary (those that arise within the spinal cord tissue)
  - Extramedullary (those that arise within the spinal column but outside of the spinal cord, in the meninges)
- Most common primary extramedullary tumors are neurofibromas and meningiomas.
- Physical presentation is the result of the location and extent of the tumor (see paraplegia and tetra/quadriplegia).
- Onset of signs/symptoms is gradual.
- Clinical correlation.

Demographics

- Equal male and female incidence; can impact any age

CLINICAL FINDINGS

SIGNS AND SYMPTOMS

- Atrophy
- Back pain: Usually worse with lying down or made worse by an extended time in a recumbent position
- Brown–Séquard syndrome-like symptoms
- Gait disturbances
- Hydrocephalus
- Hyperreflexia
- Hyporeflexia
- Increased intracranial pressure
- Loss or alternation of bowel and bladder function
- Loss or alteration of motor function
- Loss or alteration of sensation
- Pain to palpation over the involved spinal segment in 50% of patients
- Papilledema
- Paralysis
- Radicular pain
- Sexual dysfunction
- Spasticity
- Sphincter disturbances
- Stiffness of the back muscles
- Syringomyelia-like symptoms
- Urinary frequency
- Urinary urgency
- Vascular changes: Cold sensation upper or lower extremity
- Tumors can affect
  - Spinal cord cells
  - Nerve root compression
  - Circulatory system
  - Bone strength

Functional Implications[2]

- Loss of independence with ADLs and self-care
- Loss of independence with locomotion in home and community environments
- Altered sensation predisposing patient to injury
- Loss of (or altered) ability to work and participate in leisure activity

Possible Contributing Causes

- Unknown cause for primary spinal tumors.
- Spine and spinal cord are common metastatic sites for other forms of cancer including breast, bone, lung, lymphoma.

Differential Diagnosis[3]

- Blood clot of the retroperitoneal space
- Degenerative or protruding disc
- Disease of the gall bladder
- Disease of the kidney
- Disease of the pleura
- Disease of the stomach or intestine
- Leukemia
- Lymphoma
- Muscle strain
- Myeloma
- Spondylitis
- Stenosis

MEANS OF CONFIRMATION OR DIAGNOSIS

Laboratory Tests

- Complete blood count (CBC)
- Urinalysis
- Erythrocyte sedimentation rate (ESR)
  - Elevated in Ewing sarcoma

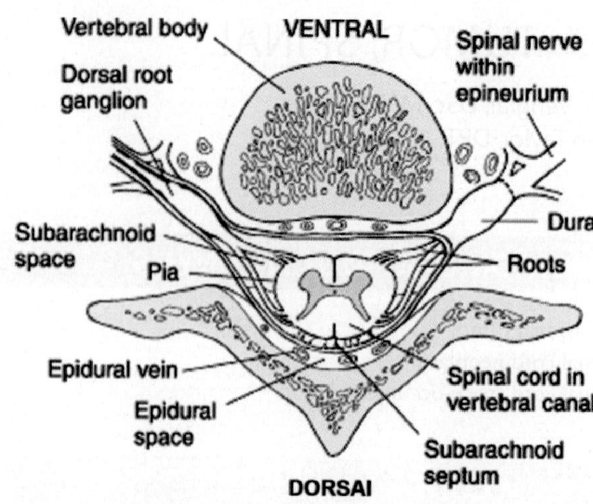

FIGURE 105-2 Exit of the spinal nerves. (Adapted with permission from Waxman SG. *Correlative Neuroanatomy*. 24th ed. McGraw-Hill; 2000.)

- Serum calcium
  - Elevated in metastatic bone disease
- Phosphorus
  - Decreased with brown tumors associated with hyperthyroidism
- Alkaline phosphatase
  - Elevated in osteosarcoma and Paget disease
- Serum protein electrophoresis
  - Abnormal in metastatic bone disease
- Lactic dehydrogenase
  - Elevated with osteosarcoma

Imaging

- MRI of the spine
- Spinal CT scan
- Radiographs, X-ray
- Radionuclide bone scan (scintigraphy)
- Angiography
- Ultrasonography
- Cerebrospinal fluid (CSF) examination
- Cytology (cell studies)

FINDINGS AND INTERPRETATION

- Sensorimotor spinal tract syndrome is due to compression of the spinal cord tracts and produces an asymmetrical spastic weakness, altered or loss of sensory function, and spastic bladder with weak voluntary control.
- Radicular-spinal cord syndrome is a combination of cord compression and radicular pain.
- The pain is worsened by events that increase intrathoracic pressure.
- Intramedullary syringomyelic syndrome produces a segmental or dissociated sensory loss, amyotrophy, early incontinence, and late corticospinal weakness.

TREATMENT

Medication

- Hormonal therapy
- Chemotherapy

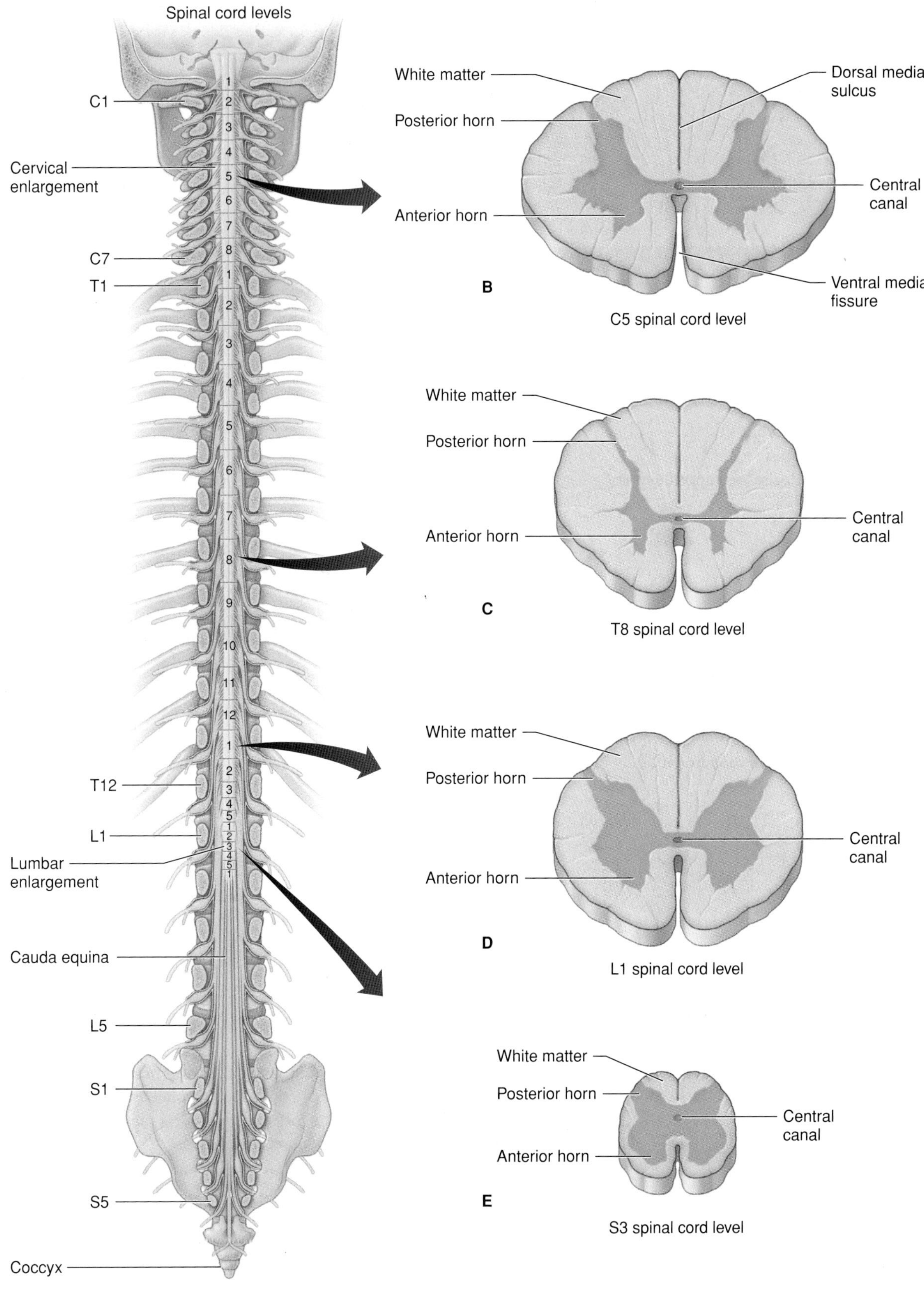

FIGURE 105-3 (**A**) Posterior view of the coronal section of the vertebral canal. Compare and contrast the spinal cord, spinal nerve, and vertebral levels. (**B–E**) C5, T8, L1, and S3 cross-sections of the spinal cord, respectively. Compare and contrast gray and white matter at the various levels. (From Morton DA, Foreman KB, Albertine KH. *The Big Picture: Gross Anatomy*. http://www.accessmedicine.com. Copyright © The McGraw-Hill Companies, Inc. All rights reserved.)

MEDICAL PROCEDURES

- Tumor resection
  - Marginal excision
  - Wide excision
- Limb salvage
- Radiation
- Radiation therapy
- Stem cell transplantation
- Biologic therapy

REFERRALS/ADMITTANCE

- To neurologist
- To oncologist
- To neurooncologist
- To spinal cord support group
- To custom durable medical equipment (DME) provider
- To recreational therapy
- To challenged athlete groups
- To occupational therapist
- To counselor, psychologist, neuropsychologist

IMPAIRMENTS

- Peripheral nerve integrity
- Gait
- Wheelchair mobility
- Balance
  - Static sit
  - Dynamic sit
  - Static stand
  - Dynamic stand
  - Moving outside the base of support (BOS)
- Muscle strength
- Muscle recruitment
- Coordination
- Postural control
- Posture
- ROM
- Reflexes
  - Deep tendon reflexes (DTR)
  - Babinski
  - Clonus
- Muscle tone
- Sensation
- Bed mobility
- Transfers
- Endurance
- Aerobic capacity
- Self-care
- Home management
- Fine motor
- Respiratory compromise
- Autonomic compromise

TEST AND MEASURES

- Aerobic endurance
- Community and work integration
- Functional strength
- Gait analysis

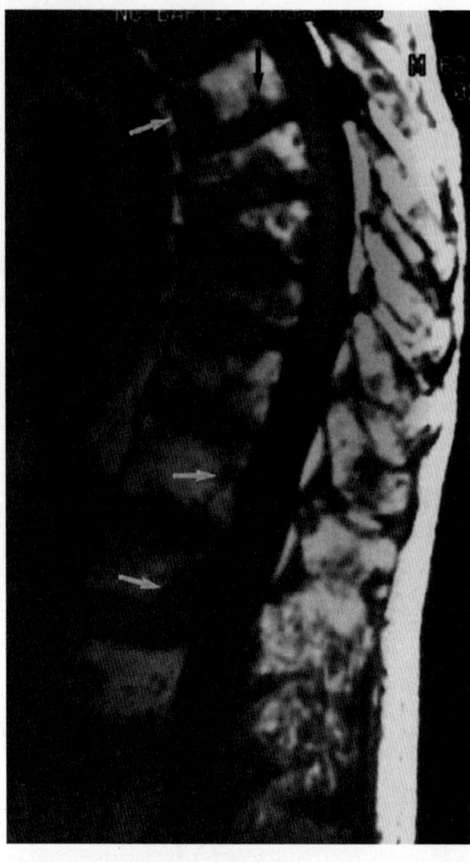

FIGURE 105-4 Sagittal T1-weighted MR image of the thoracic spine shows multiple small hypointense foci of myeloma (*arrows*) replacing normal bone marrow. Compression fractures are also seen, indicated by loss of height of several upper thoracic vertebral bodies. The spinal cord is intact, but spread of tumor or retropulsion of fractured bone could result in cord compression. Note that metastatic tumor other than myeloma could have an identical appearance. (From Chen MYM, Pope TL, Ott DJ. *Basic Radiology*. 2nd ed. http://www.accessmedicine.com. Copyright © The McGraw-Hill Companies, Inc. All rights reserved.)

- Integumentary integrity
- Karnofsky performance scale (KPS)
- Lower-extremity range of motion (ROM)
- Pain scale
- Posture analysis
- Sensory integrity

INTERVENTION

- Bed-mobility training including leg management and use of assistive devices (loop ladder, bed rail, etc.)
- Transfer training: Bed, wheelchair, toilet, shower bench, car, furniture in the home, etc.
- Wheelchair mobility/management training
- Gait training: Depending on the location and severity of the tumor
- Sitting balance
- Scar management
- Standing balance, if appropriate
- Strengthening for any muscles still innervated
- Active and passive ROM of all joints
- Skin inspection training, pressure relief training
- Respiratory intervention: To produce adequate secretion clearance/cough, maintain adequate vital capacity to support functional activities and leisure activities

FUNCTIONAL GOALS

Note: Please refer to goals for spinal cord injury (SCI) quadriplegia and paraplegia for information based on the level of the spinal cord lesion.

- Patient will be able to
  - Transfer between the bed and wheelchair using a slide board with contact guard assistance for balance and no more than two verbal cues for safety.
  - Transition between supine and long-sitting in bed with supervision assistance to facilitate dressing activities.
  - Verbally identify all areas of their body at risk for skin breakdown, without cueing, to direct a caregiver in appropriate skin inspection.
  - Carry in one load of groceries (<15 lb) without significant dyspnea, measured by patient report of 3 or less on Borg Dyspnea Scale.

PROGNOSIS

- Variable, based on extent of tumor, speed of growth, location, and time from onset to medical intervention.

PATIENT RESOURCES

- A Brief Overview. National Lymphedema Network. http://www.lymphnet.org/lymphedemaFAQs/overview.htm. Accessed July 14, 2013.
- Lymphedema (PDQ®). National Cancer Institute at the National Institutes of Health. http://www.cancer.gov/cancertopics/pdq/supportivecare/lymphedema/healthprofessional/page1. Accessed July 14, 2013.
- Sama AA. Spinal tumors. Medscape Reference. http://emedicine.medscape.com/article/1267223-overview#aw2aab6b3. Accessed July 14, 2013.
- Seiter K. Multiple myeloma treatment & management. Medscape Reference. http://emedicine.medscape.com/article/204369-treatment#aw2aab6b6b8aa. Accessed July 14, 2013.

REFERENCES

1. *Guide to Physical Therapist Practice*. 2nd ed. Alexandria, VA: American Physical Therapy Association; 2001. Revised 2003.
2. Aminoff MJ, Greenberg DA, Simon RP. Motor deficits. In: Aminoff MJ, Greenberg DA, Simon RP, eds. *Clinical Neurology*. 7th ed. New York, NY: McGraw-Hill; 2011: Chapter 5. http://www.accessmedicine.com/content.aspx?aID=5147390. Accessed July 14, 2013.
3. Goodman CC, Snyder TEK. *Differential Diagnosis for Physical Therapists, Screening for Referral*. 4th ed. St. Louis, MO: Saunders Elsevier; 2007:570.

ADDITIONAL REFERENCES

- Dutton M. Intervention principles. In: Dutton M, ed. *Orthopaedic Examination, Evaluation, and Intervention*. 2nd ed. New York, NY: McGraw-Hill; 2008:Chapter 10. http://www.accessphysiotherapy.com/content/5548968. Accessed July 14, 2013.
- Hu SS, Tribus CB, Tay BK, Bhatia NN. Disorders, diseases, & injuries of the spine. In: Skinner HB, ed. *CURRENT Diagnosis & Treatment in Orthopedics*. 4th ed. New York, NY: McGraw-Hill; 2011:Chapter 5. http://www.accessmedicine.com/content.aspx?aID=2319334. Accessed July 14, 2013.
- ICD9Data.com. http://www.icd9data.com. Accessed July 14, 2013.
- ICD10Data.com. http://www.icd10data.com/ICD10CM/Codes. Accessed July 14, 2013.
- Malone TR, Hazle C, Grey ML. Imaging of the cervical spine and temporomandibular joint. In: Malone TR, Hazle C, Grey ML, eds. *Imaging in Rehabilitation*. New York, NY: McGraw-Hill;2008:Chapter 3. http://www.accessphysiotherapy.com/content/5940352. Accessed July 14, 2013.
- Multiple Myeloma. MD Guidelines. http://www.mdguidelines.com/multiple-myeloma/differential-diagnosis. Accessed July 14, 2013.
- Ropper AL, Samuels MA. *Adams and Victor's Principles of Neurology*. 9th ed. New York, NY: McGraw-Hill; 2009:1216–1221.
- Rossy KM. Dermatologic manifestations of lymphedema differential diagnoses. Medscape Reference. http://emedicine.medscape.com/article/1087313-differential. Accessed July 14, 2013.
- Shamus E, Stern DF, eds. *Effective Documentation for Physical Therapy Professionals*. 2nd ed. New York, NY: McGraw-Hill; 2011. http://www.accessphysiotherapy.com/resource/696. Accessed July 14, 2013.
- Waxman SG. The vertebral column and other structures surrounding the spinal cord. In: Waxman SG, ed *Clinical Neuroanatomy*. 26th ed. New York, NY: McGraw-Hill; 2010:Chapter 6. http://www.accessphysiotherapy.com/content/5272198. Accessed July 14, 2013.

PART 4

ORTHOPAEDIC DISORDERS

SECTION A HEAD AND JAW DISORDERS

106 HEADACHES

Eric Shamus, PhD, DPT, PT, CSCS
Jennifer Shamus, PhD, DPT, COMT, CSCS

CONDITION/DISORDER SYNONYMS

- Cephalgia
- Vascular headache
- Muscular tension/myogenic headache
- Cervicogenic headache
- Traction/inflammatory headaches

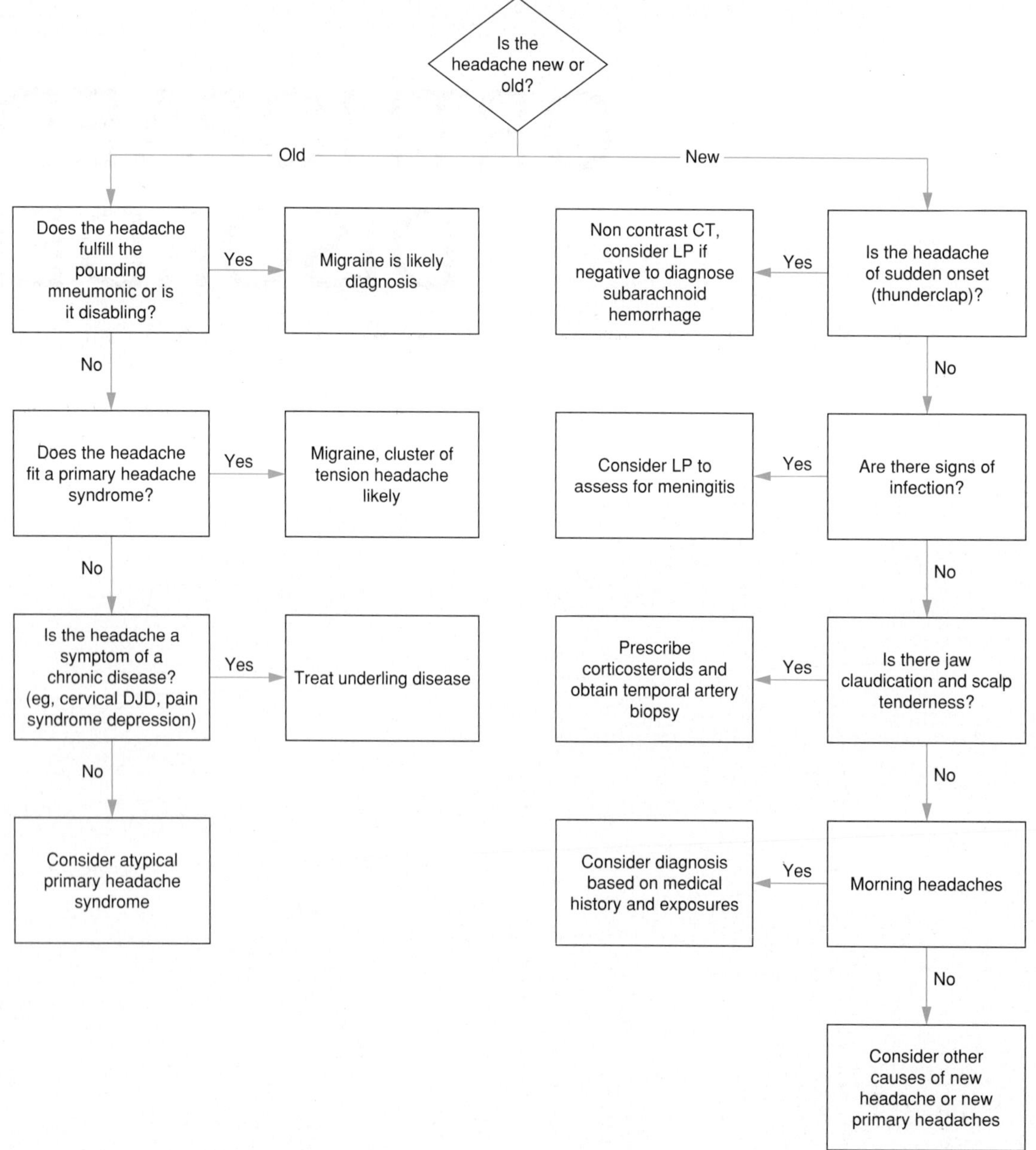

FIGURE 106-1 Diagnostic approach: headache. DJD, degenerative joint disease; LP, lumbar puncture; SAH, subarachnoid hemorrhage. (From Stern SDC, Cifu AS, Altkorn D. *Symptom to Diagnosis: An Evidence-Based Guide*. 2nd ed. http://www.accessmedicine.com. Copyright © The McGraw-Hill Companies, Inc. All rights reserved.)

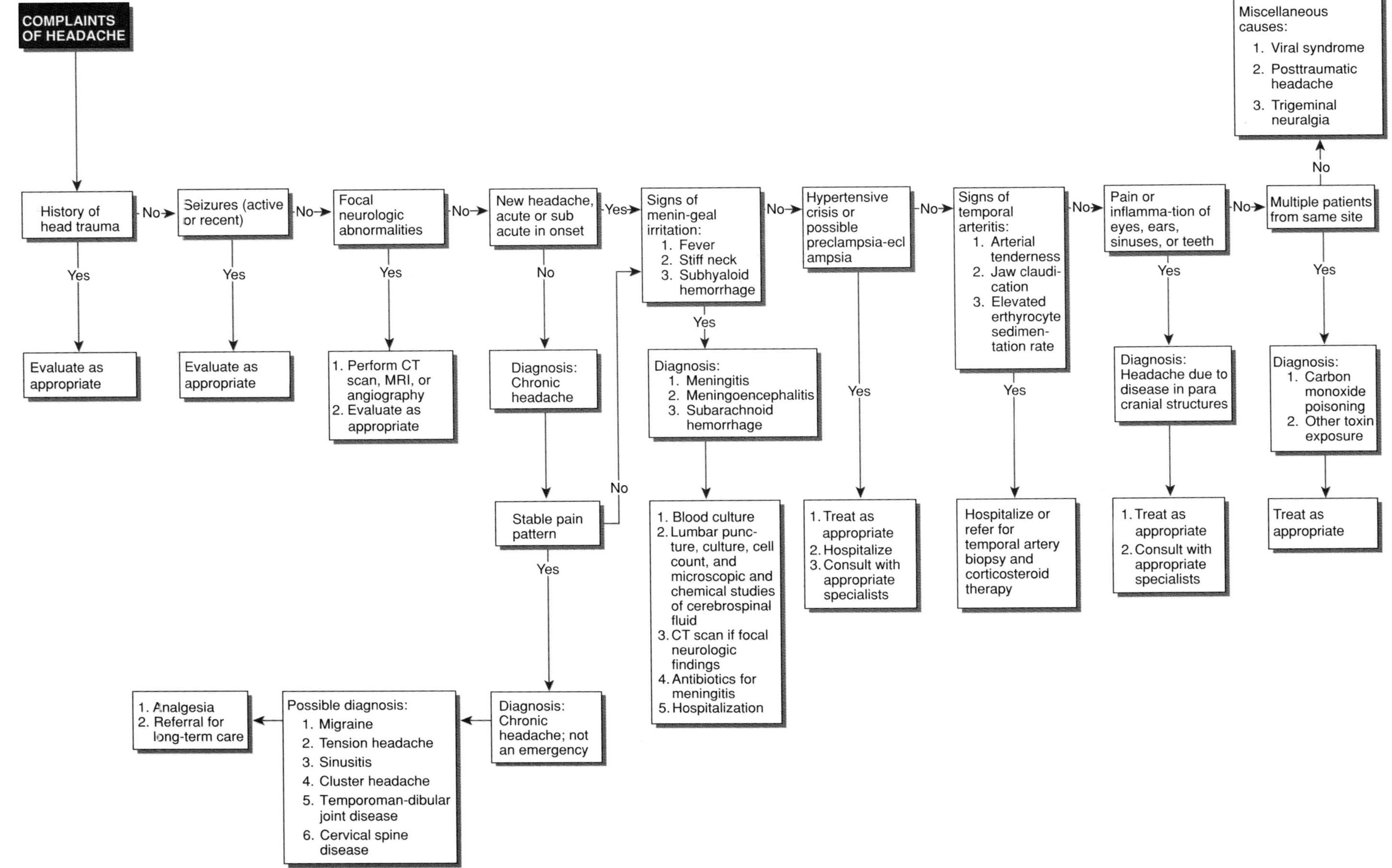

FIGURE 106-2 Management of complaints of headache. (From Stone CK, Humphries RL. *Current Diagnosis & Treatment: Emergency Medicine.* 7th ed. http://www.accessmedicine.com.)

ICD-9-CM CODES

- 307.81 Tension headache
- 339 Other headache syndromes
- 339.0 Cluster headaches and other trigeminal autonomic cephalgias
- 339.1 Tension type headache
- 339.2 Post-traumatic headache
- 339.3 Drug induced headache, not elsewhere classified
- 339.4 Complicated headache syndromes
- 339.8 Other specified headache syndromes

ICD-10-CM CODES

- G43 Migraine
- G44 Cluster headache and other trigeminal autonomic cephalgias
- G44.009 Cluster headache syndrome, unspecified, not intractable
- G44.209 Tension-type headache, unspecified, not intractable
- G44.309 Post-traumatic headache, unspecified, not intractable
- G44.41 Drug-induced headache, not elsewhere classified, intractable
- G44.51 Hemicrania continua
- G44.80 Other primary headaches
- G44.81 Hypnic headache
- G44.82 Headache associated with sexual activity
- G44.88 Headache attributed to head and or neck trauma

PREFERRED PRACTICE PATTERN

- 4E: Impaired Joint Mobility, Motor Function, Muscle Performance, and ROM Associated with Localized Inflammation[1]

PATIENT PRESENTATION

A 17-year-old female is complaining of headaches. She states she is not sure why she gets headaches. She has gone to the doctor for a workup and is scheduled for a brain CT examination. She reports to physical therapy because she has headaches that are interfering with her functional activities. She started taking a log of her headaches and has not noted any pattern with food or with her menstrual cycle.

KEY FEATURES

Description

- Pain in the head or neck region
- International Classification of Headache Disorders-II (ICDH-II), 2004
  - 13 headache classification groups
- National Institute of Health (NIH) has five classifications of headaches
  - Vascular headache
  - Muscular tension/myogenic headache
  - Cervicogenic headache
  - Traction headaches
  - Inflammatory headaches

Essentials of Diagnosis

- ICDH-II classifications
  - First four are primary headaches: Migraines, tension headaches, cluster headaches, trigeminal headaches

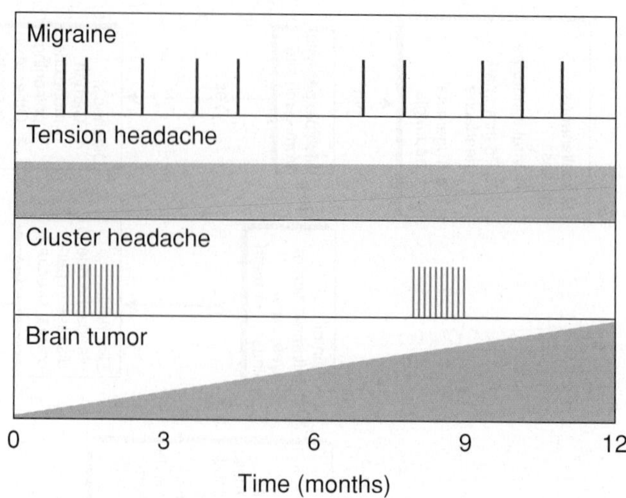

FIGURE 106-3 Temporal patterns of headache. Migraine headache is episodic and may occur at varying intervals. Tension headache may be present every day. Cluster headache occurs in bouts separated by symptom-free periods. Headache caused by brain tumor often increases in severity with time. (From Greenberg DA, Aminoff MJ, Simon RP. *Clinical Neurology*. 8th ed. http://www.accessmedicine.com. Copyright © The McGraw-Hill Companies, Inc. All rights reserved.)

- Headaches caused by cough, exertion, sexual activity, and stabbing are primary headaches
- Groups 5 through 12 are secondary headaches, based upon their etiology: Whiplash injury, intracranial headaches, neck injury, vascular disorders
- NIH: Vascular headache
  - Migraine[2]
  - Cluster headaches[2]
- NIH: Muscular tension/myogenic headache
  - Tension headache
- NIH: Cervicogenic headache
  - Disorder of the cervical spine
- NIH: Traction headaches
  - Can be caused by stroke
- NIH: Inflammatory headaches
  - Can be caused by sinus infection with inflammation
  - Increased intracranial pressure

General Considerations

- Headaches can be harmless, disabling, or life threatening.
- Headaches may indicate more severe pathology in the head/brain region.
- Vision and sinus problems can cause headaches.

Demographics

- Cluster headaches more common in men than in women[2]
- Migraine headaches more common in women[2]

CLINICAL FINDINGS

SIGNS AND SYMPTOMS

- Differential features of headaches in children[3]
- Migraine[2]
  - Pulsating pain
  - Nausea
  - Sensitivity to light or sound
  - One or both sides of the head
  - Aggravated with routine activity
- Cluster headaches[2]
  - Severe headaches
  - Short-lasting

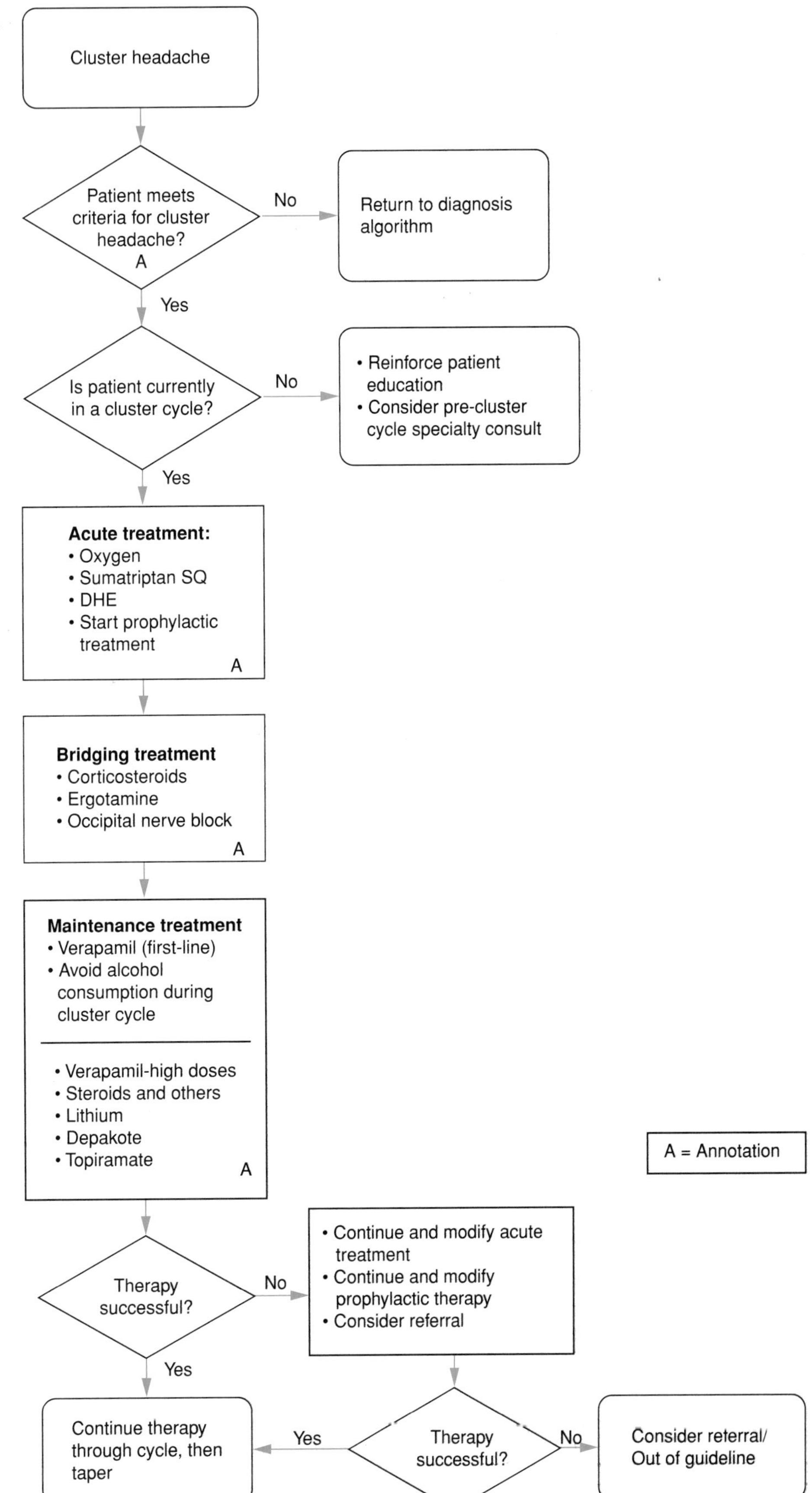

FIGURE 106-4 Cluster headache algorithm. (From Esherick JS, Clark DS, Slater ED. *Current Practice Guidelines in Primary Care 2012*. http://www.accessmedicine.com.)

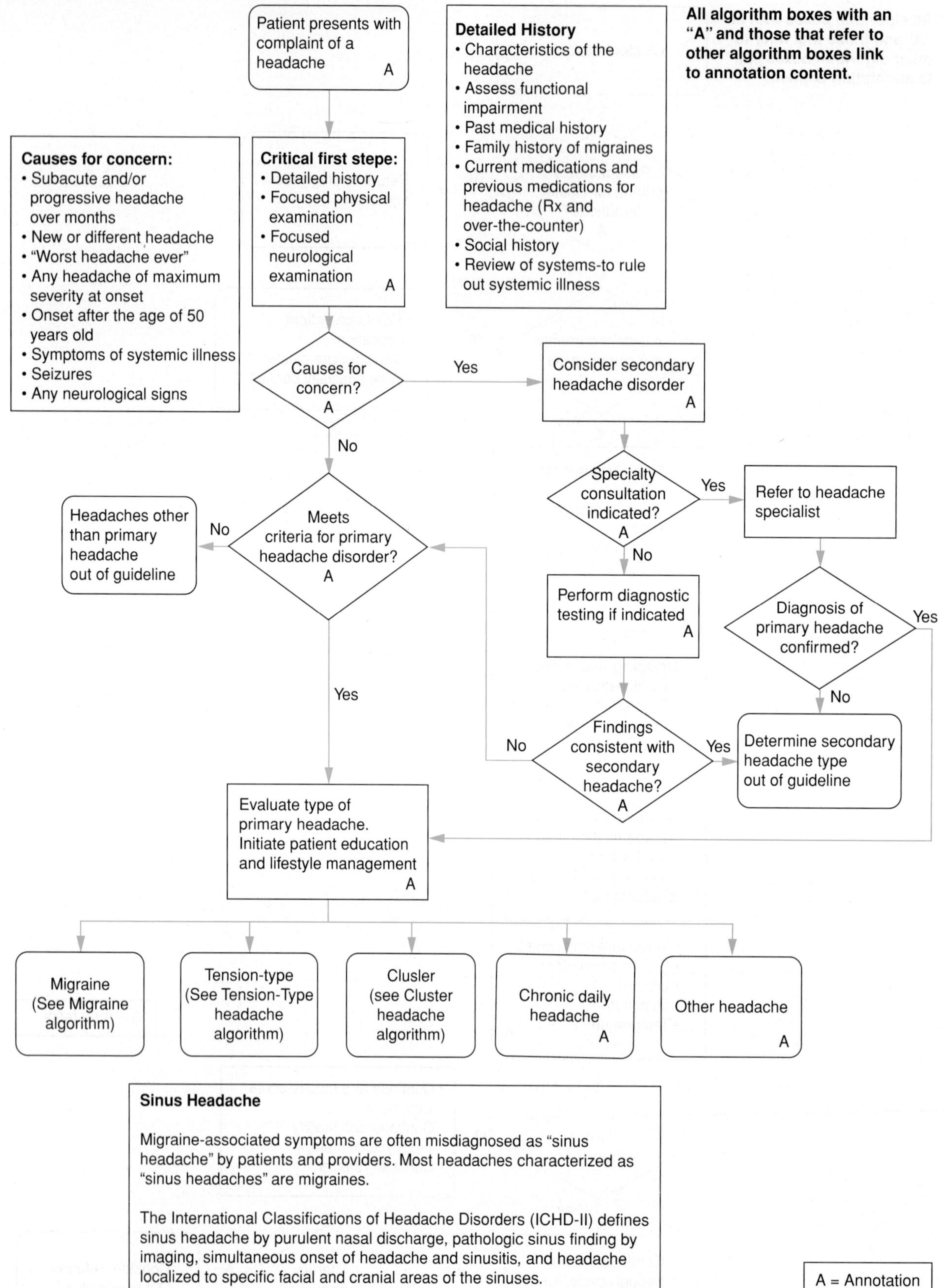

FIGURE 106-5 Headache diagnosis algorithm. (From Esherick JS, Clark DS, Slater ED. *Current Practice Guidelines in Primary Care 2012*. http://www.accessmedicine.com.)

- Symptoms around the eye
- Toxic headaches
  - Fever
- Muscular tension/myogenic headache[2]
  - Squeezing or tightening on head
  - Mild-to-moderate pain
  - Still able to perform routine activity
- Cervicogenic headache
  - Stiff neck
  - Limited mobility
  - One-sided
  - Pain radiating into arm

Functional Implications

- Difficulty maintaining sitting posture secondary to neck pain
- Inability to sleep
- Weakness with upper-extremity lifting
- Inability to drive or work secondary to light or sound sensitivity
- Difficulty with neck movements (driving) secondary to pain

Possible Contributing Causes

- Forward-head, rounded-shoulders posture due to tight pectoralis, weak periscapular, deep neck-flexor muscles
- Prolonged position of cervical side bending toward impaired nerve or prolonged extension
- Facet hypertrophy
- Trauma
- Light
- Sounds
- Hydration
- Nutritional deficiency
- Vascular insufficiency
- Muscular tightness
- Stress

Differential Diagnosis

- Tumor
- Glaucoma
- Sinusitis
- Myofascial pain syndrome
- Rhomboid or trapezius spasms
- Degenerative disk disease
- Lyme disease
- Temporomandibular joint dysfunction
- Arnold–Chiari malformation

MEANS OF CONFIRMATION OR DIAGNOSIS

Imaging

- MRI[2]
- X-ray/Plain-film radiograph[4]
- CT[4]

FINDINGS AND INTERPRETATION

- MRI helps visualize the head/brain region in diagnosis.[2]
- X-ray/Plain-film radiograph is helpful if osteophyte located in intervertebral foramen of cervical spine.[4]

REFERRALS/ADMITTANCE

- To hospital for imaging
- To nutritionist for dietary counseling
- To optometrist for eye examination
- To neurologist for imaging

IMPAIRMENTS

- Restricted mobility of the upper-/mid-thoracic spine and subcranial spine
- Hypermobile mid-cervical spine
- Tight pectoralis major and minor
- Noted weakness of longus colli and longus capitis
- Noted weakness of periscapular muscles

TESTS AND MEASURES

- Cervical spine AROM
- Physical examination cluster to rule in cervical radiculopathy[3]
  - Spurling test[2]
  - Rotation limited to ipsilateral side
  - Upper limb nerve tension test[2]
  - Diminished brachioradialis reflex

INTERVENTION

- Rest
- Hydration
- Joint manipulation to the thoracic and upper-cervical spine
  - Suboccipital release
  - Myofascial release
- Cervical distraction and traction to relieve nerve compression
- Cranio cervical flexion exercises
- Address pain
  - Electrical stimulation
  - Heat/ice
- Address hypertonicity
  - Soft tissue massage
  - Heat
- Address muscle weakness
  - Deep neck-flexor training
  - Strengthening of lower/middle trapezius, rhomboids, rotator cuff, serratus anterior, latissimus dorsi

FUNCTIONAL GOALS

- Patient will be able to
  - Sit with neutral cervical and thoracic spine posture for >30 minutes with 0/10 pain rating.
  - Sit at work station and perform computer work for 45 minutes with 0/10 pain rating.
  - Rotate cervical spine 70 degrees to talk on the telephone with 0/10 pain rating in neck and arm.

PROGNOSIS

- Fair to very good, depending on etiology of headaches.

PATIENT RESOURCE

- American Headache Society. http://www.americanheadachesociety.org/ Accessed July 6, 2013.

REFERENCES

1. The American Physical Therapy Association. Pattern 4E: impaired joint mobility, motor function, muscle performance, and range of motion associated with localized inflammation. *Interactive Guide to Physical Therapist Practice*. 2003. doi: 10.2522/ptguide.3.1_5. Accessed July 1, 2013.

2. Dutton M. Differential diagnosis within specific regions. In: Dutton M, ed. *Orthopaedic Examination, Evaluation, and Intervention.* 2nd ed. New York, NY: McGraw-Hill; 2008. http://www.accessphysiotherapy.com/content/5546998. Accessed July 2, 2013.
3. Bernard TJ, Knupp K, Yang ML, Arndt D, Levinson P, Moe PG. Neurologic & muscular disorders. In: Hay WW, Levin MJ, Sondheimer JM, Deterding RR, eds. *CURRENT Diagnosis & Treatment: Pediatrics.* 20th ed. New York, NY: McGraw-Hill; 2011:Chapter 23. http://www.accessphysiotherapy.com/content/6585098. Accessed July 6, 2013.
4. Malone TR, Hazle C, Grey ML. *Imaging in Rehabilitation.* New York, NY: McGraw-Hill; 2008. http://www.accessphysiotherapy.com/resource/613. Accessed July 6, 2013.

ADDITIONAL REFERENCES

- Chaibi A, Russell MB. Manual therapies for cervicogenic headache: a systematic review. *J Headache Pain.* 2012;13(5):351–359. doi: 10.1007/s10194-012-0436-7. Epub 2012 Mar 30.
- Dutton M. Systems review. In: Dutton M, ed. *Dutton's Orthopedic Survival Guide: Managing Common Conditions.* New York, NY: McGraw-Hill; 2011. http://www.accessphysiotherapy.com/content/8656096. Accessed July 5, 2013.
- Huang Q, Li W, Li N, et al. Elevated blood pressure and analgesic overuse in chronic daily headache: an outpatient clinic-based study from China. *J Headache Pain.* 2013;14(1):51. doi: 10.1186/1129-2377-14-51.
- ICD9DATA web site. http://www.icd9data.com. Accessed July 6, 2013.
- ICD10DATA web site. http://www.icd10data.com. Accessed July 1, 2013.

107 HEADACHE, CERVICOGENIC

Eric Shamus, PhD, DPT, PT, CSCS
Mollie Venglar, Dsc, MSPT, NCS

CONDITION/DISORDER SYNONYMS

- Cephalgia
- Headache

ICD-9-CM CODES

- 307.81 Tension headache
- 339 Other headache syndromes

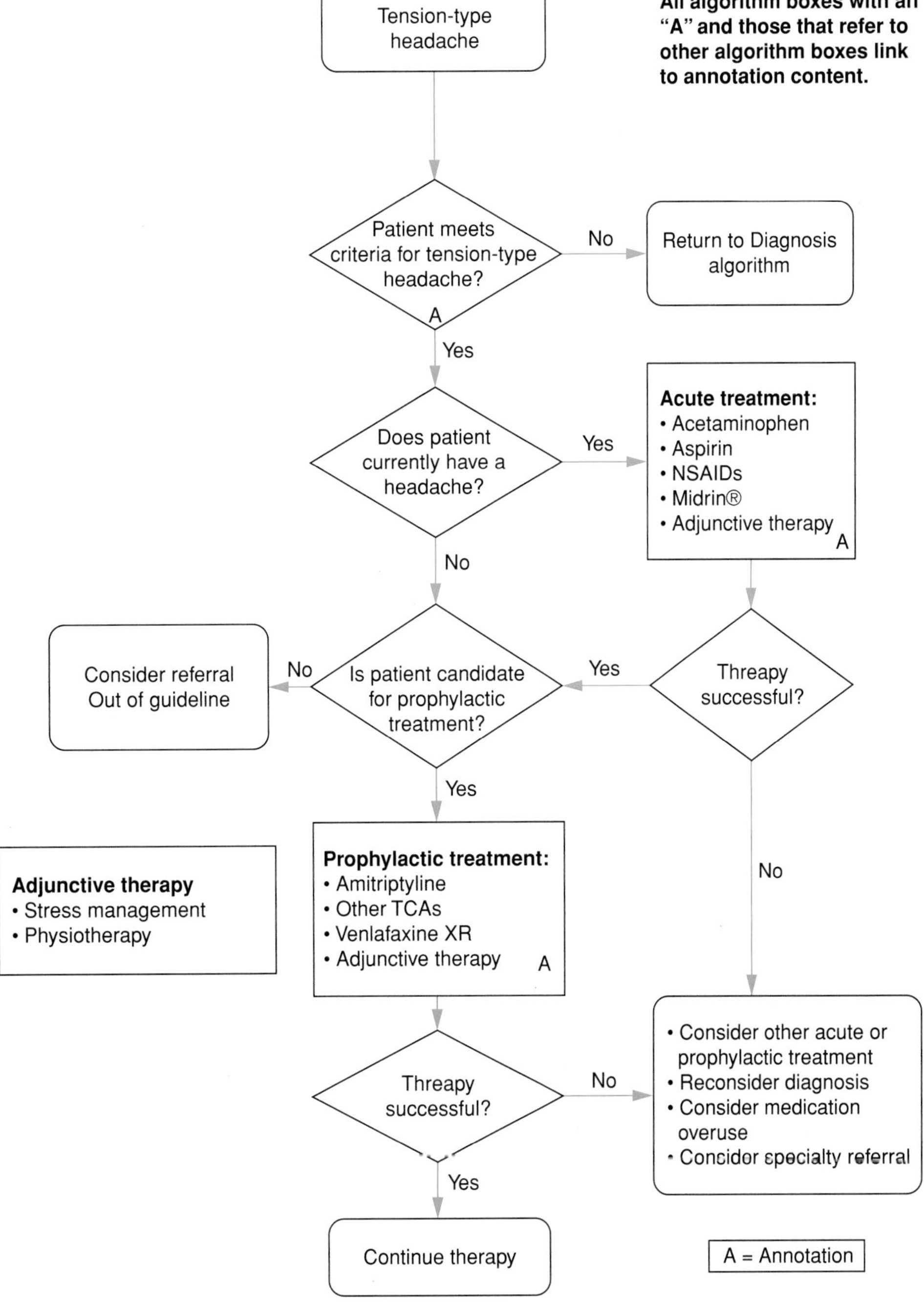

FIGURE 107-1 Tension-type headache algorithm. (From Esherick JS, Clark DS, Slater ED. *Current Practice Guidelines in Primary Care*. 2013. http://www.accessmedicine.com. Copyright © The McGraw-Hill Companies, Inc. All rights reserved.)

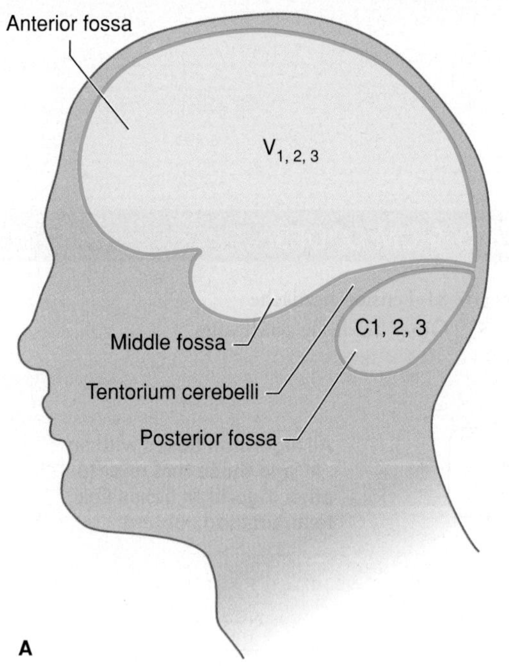

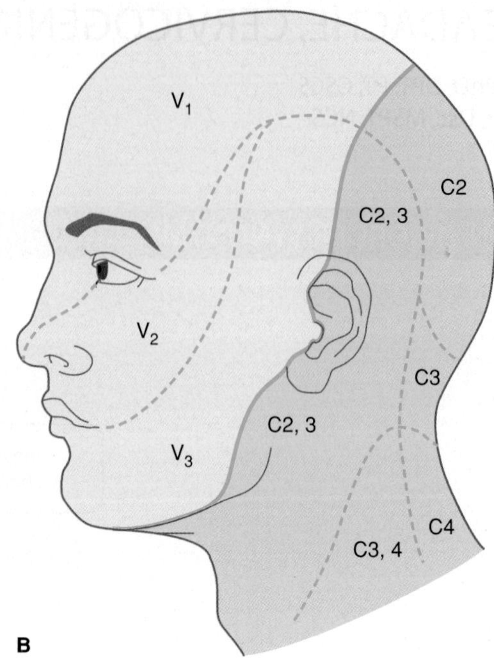

FIGURE 107-2 Innervation of pain-sensitive intracranial compartments (**A**) and corresponding extracranial sites of pain radiation (**B**). The trigeminal (V) nerve, especially its ophthalmic (V1) division, innervates the anterior and middle cranial fossae; lesions in these areas can produce frontal headache. The upper-cervical nerve roots (especially C2) innervate the posterior fossa; lesions here can cause occipital headache. (From Greenberg DA, Aminoff MJ, Simon RP. *Clinical Neurology*. 8th ed**.** http://www.accessmedicine.com. Copyright © The McGraw-Hill Companies, Inc. All rights reserved.)

- 339.1 Tension type headache
- 339.2 Post-traumatic headache
- 339.8 Other specified headache syndromes

ICD-10-CM CODES

- G44.209 Tension-type headache, unspecified, not intractable
- G44.309 Post-traumatic headache, unspecified, not intractable
- G44.88 Headache attributed to head and or neck trauma

PREFERRED PRACTICE PATTERN

- 4E: Impaired Joint Mobility, Motor Function, Muscle Performance, and ROM Associated with Localized Inflammation[1]

PATIENT PRESENTATION

A 17-year-old female is studying long nights for college entrance examinations. She is not involved in any other activities, but rather spends all of her spare time on the computer reading or studying. She reports to physical therapy because she has a headache that won't subside and she can no longer turn her head fully to the right. It has become painful even to sit at her computer or to sit through class. Now the pain is interfering with her sleep, which is causing even more anxiety about her upcoming examinations. On initial observation when the client arrives, the physical therapist notes that she has a forward head and rounded shoulders. She turns her whole body to look at the physical therapist when speaking. She is having spasms in her upper traps and scalene muscles.

KEY FEATURES

Description

- Pain in the head or neck region
- Dysfunction in the cervical spine
  - Suboccipital
  - C1 to C3 vertebral region

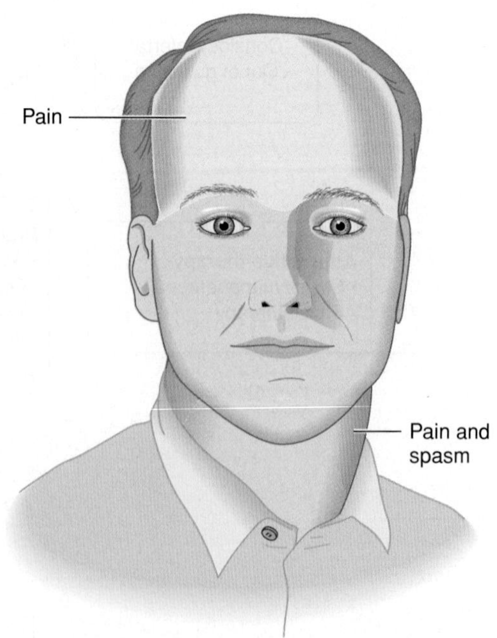

FIGURE 107-3 Distribution of symptoms and signs in tension headache. (From Greenberg DA, Aminoff MJ, Simon RP. *Clinical Neurology*. 8th ed. http://www.accessmedicine.com. Copyright © The McGraw-Hill Companies, Inc. All rights reserved.)

- One of five National Institute of Health (NIH) headache classifications
  - Cervicogenic headache

Essentials of Diagnosis

- International classification of headache disorders, 2nd ed. (ICHD-II) criteria
  - Secondary headaches are based on etiology
    - May be caused by whiplash injury, intracranial headaches, neck injury, vascular disorders
- NIH definition for cervicogenic headache
  - Disorder of the cervical spine

General Considerations

- Headaches can be harmless or disabling.
- May be a sign of more severe pathology in head or brain region.
- Sinuses and vision problems can cause headaches.

Demographics

- Cervical spine injury can affect any age group

CLINICAL FINDINGS

SIGNS AND SYMPTOMS

- Differential features of headaches in children[2]
- Muscular tension/myogenic headache[3]
  - Squeezing or tightening on head
  - Mild-to-moderate pain
  - Okay with routine activity
- Cervicogenic headache
  - Stiff neck
  - Limited mobility
  - One-sided
  - Pain may radiate to the arm

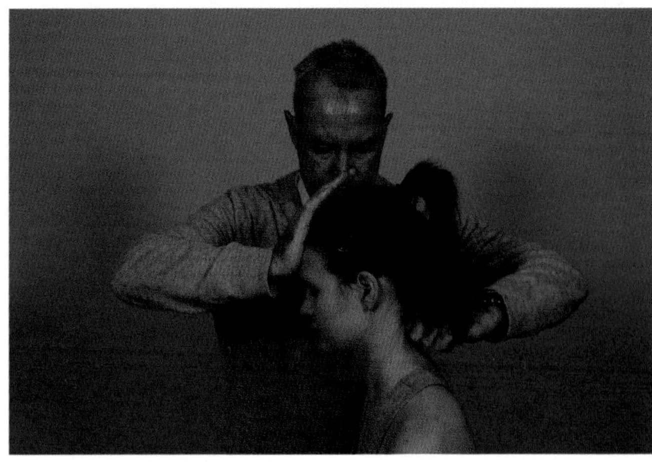

FIGURE 107-4 Modified Sharp–Purser test. (From Dutton M. *Dutton's Orthopaedic Examination, Evaluation, and Intervention*. 3rd ed. http://www.accessphysiotherapy.com. Copyright © The McGraw-Hill Companies, Inc. All rights reserved.)

- Degenerative disk disease
- Lyme disease
- Temporomandibular joint dysfunction
- Arnold–Chiari malformation
- Trigeminal nucleus central sensitization
- Migraine headaches[3]
  - Pulsating pain
  - Nausea
  - Sensitivity to light
  - Sensitivity to sound
  - One or both sides of the head
  - Aggravated with routine activity
- Cluster headaches[3]
  - Severe headaches
  - Short-lasting
  - Symptoms around the eye
- Toxic headaches
  - Fever

Functional Implications

- Difficulty maintaining sitting postures secondary to neck pain
- Inability to sleep
- Weakness with upper-extremity lifting
- Inability to drive or work secondary to intolerance for light or sound
- Difficulty with neck movements (driving) secondary to pain

Possible Contributing Causes

- Forward-head, rounded-shoulders posture due to tight pectoralis, weak periscapular, and deep neck-flexor muscles
- Prolonged position of cervical side bending toward impaired nerve or prolonged extension
- Facet hypertrophy
- Trauma
- Hydration
- Nutrition deficiency
- Muscular tightness
- Stress

Differential Diagnosis

- Tumor
- Glaucoma
- Sinusitis
- Myofascial pain syndrome
- Rhomboid/trapezius spams

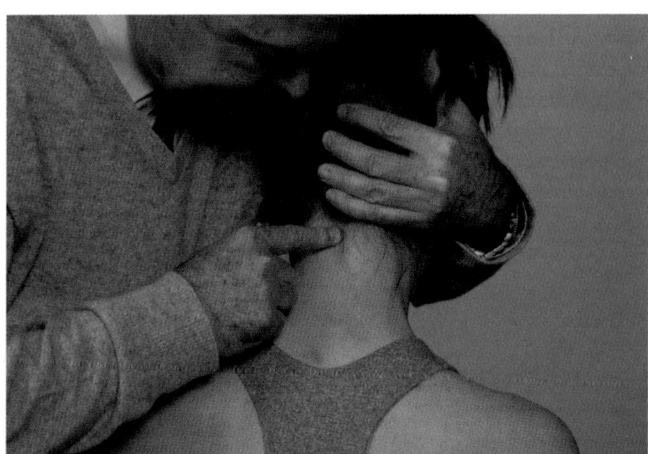

FIGURE 107-5 Confirmatory test for alar ligament in sitting. (From Dutton M. *Dutton's Orthopaedic Examination, Evaluation, and Intervention*. 3rd ed. http://www.accessphysiotherapy.com. Copyright © The McGraw-Hill Companies, Inc. All rights reserved.)

MEANS OF CONFIRMATION

▶ **Imaging**
- MRI[3]
- X-ray/Plain-film radiograph[4]
- CT[4]

FINDINGS AND INTERPRETATION

- MRI helps to visualize the head/brain region in diagnosis.[3]
- X-ray/Plain-film radiograph helpful if osteophyte located in intervertebral foramen of cervical spine.[4]

REFERRALS/ADMITTANCE

- To hospital for imaging
- To nutritionist for dietary/nutritional counseling, evaluate for nutritional deficiency
- To optometrist for eye examination
- To neurologist for imaging

IMPAIRMENTS

- Restricted mobility of the upper-/mid-thoracic spine and subcranial spine
- Hypermobile mid-cervical spine
- Tight pectoralis major and minor
- Noted weakness of longus colli and longus capitis
- Noted weakness of periscapular muscles

TESTS AND MEASURES

- Physical examination cluster to rule in cervical radiculopathy[2]
  - Spurling test[3]
  - Rotation limited to ipsilateral side
  - Upper limb nerve tension test[3]
  - Diminished brachioradialis reflex
- Cervical spine AROM
- Sharp-Purser: Atlantoaxial instability
- Cervical passive intervertebral motion testing
- Sub-cranial translation instability testing
- Passive physiological intervertebral mobility testing (PPIVM)
- Upper-extremity screening examination
- Neck Disability Index (NDI)
- Postural examination
- Muscle length testing, including upper trapezius, levator scapulae, pectoral muscles
- Upper limb nerve tension test
- Deep neck-flexor endurance test
- Upper-extremity neurological screen (dermatome, myotome, reflexes)

INTERVENTION

- Rest
- Hydration
- Joint manipulation to the thoracic and upper-cervical spine
  - Suboccipital release
  - Myofascial release
- Cervical distraction and traction to relieve nerve compression
- Cranio Cervical flexion exercises
- Address pain
  - Electrical stimulation
  - Heat/Ice
- Address hypertonicity
  - Soft tissue massage
  - Ice to decrease inflammatory process
- Address muscle weakness
  - Deep neck-flexor training
    - Pressure cuff training: Start at 20 mm Hg and doing 10 times 10 seconds before progressing to 22 mm Hg
  - Strengthening of lower/middle trapezius, rhomboids, rotator cuff
  - Serratus anterior, latissimus dorsi

FUNCTIONAL GOALS

- Patient will be able to
  - Sit with a neutral cervical and thoracic spine posture for more than 30 minutes with 0 out of 10 pain rating.
  - Sit at work station and perform computer work for 45 minutes with 0 out of 10 pain rating.
  - Rotate cervical spine 70 degrees so as to talk on the telephone with 0 out of 10 pain rating in the neck/arm.

PROGNOSIS

- Fair to very good, depending on severity of cervical spine injury.

PATIENT RESOURCE

- American Headache Society. http://www.americanheadachesociety.org/. Accessed July 6, 2013.

REFERENCES

1. The American Physical Therapy Association. Pattern 4E: impaired joint mobility, motor function, muscle performance, and range of motion associated with localized inflammation. *Interactive Guide to Physical Therapist Practice*. 2003. doi: 10.2522/ptguide.3.1_5. http://guidetoptpractice.apta.org/content/1/SEC12.extract. Accessed May 20, 2014.
2. Bernard TJ, Knupp K, Yang ML, Arndt D, Levisohn P, Moe PG. Disorders affecting the nervous system in infants & children. In: Hay WW, Levin MJ, Sondheimer JM, Deterding RR, eds. *CURRENT Diagnosis & Treatment: Pediatrics*. 20th ed. New York, NY: McGraw-Hill; 2011. http://www.accessphysiotherapy.com/content/6585098. Accessed July 6, 2013.
3. Dutton M. *Orthopaedic Examination, Evaluation, and Intervention*. 2nd ed. New York, NY: McGraw-Hill; 2008. http://www.accessphysiotherapy.com/content/5546998. Accessed July 6, 2013.
4. Malone TR, Hazle C, Grey ML. *Imaging in Rehabilitation*. New York, NY: McGraw-Hill; 2008. http://www.accessphysiotherapy.com/resource/613. Accessed July 7, 2013.

ADDITIONAL REFERENCES

- Dutton M. *Dutton's Orthopedic Survival Guide: Managing Common Conditions*. New York, NY: McGraw-Hill; 2011. http://www.accessphysiotherapy.com/content/8656096. Accessed July 6, 2013.
- ICD9DATA web site. http://www.icd9data.com. Accessed July 6, 2013.
- ICD10DATA web site. http://www.icd10data.com. Accessed July 1, 2013.
- Youssef EF, Shanb AS. Mobilization versus massage therapy in the treatment of cervicogenic headache: a clinical study. *J Back Musculoskelet Rehabil.* 2013;26(1):17–24. doi: 10.3233/BMR-2012-0344.

108 HEADACHE, MYOGENIC

Eric Shamus, PhD, DPT, PT, CSCS
Jennifer Shamus, PhD, DPT, COMT, CSCS
Mollie Venglar, Dsc, MSPT, NCS

CONDITION/DISORDER SYNONYMS

- Cephalgia
- Headache
- Tension headache

ICD-9-CM CODES[1]

- 307.81 Tension headache
- 339 Other headache syndromes
- 339.1 Tension-type headache

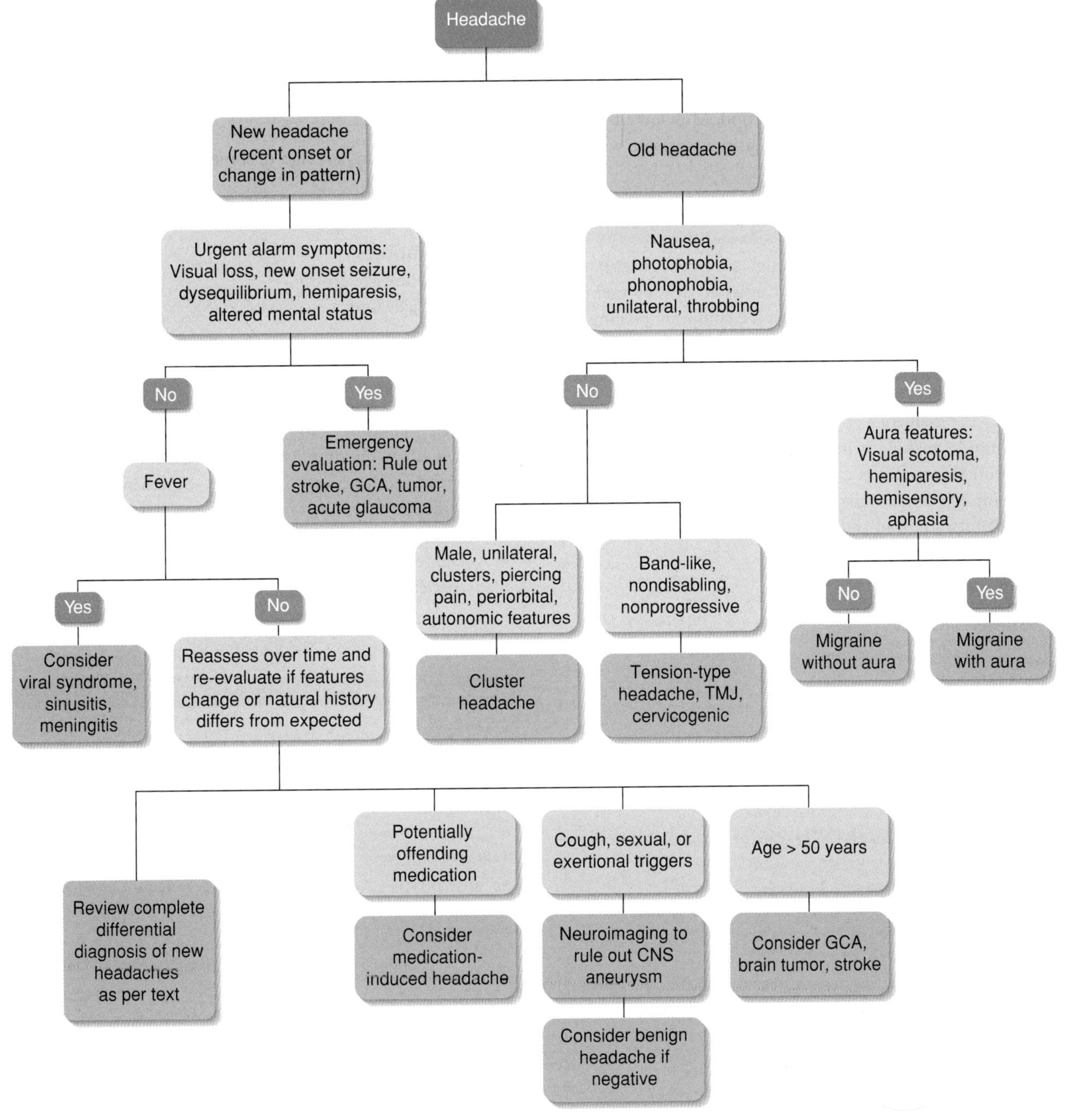

FIGURE 108-1 Algorithm for headache. CNS, central nervous system; GCA, giant cell arteritis; TMJ, temporomandibular joint. (From Henderson MC, Tierney LM, Smetana GW. *The Patient History: An Evidence-Based Approach to Differential Diagnosis*. http://www.accessmedicine.com. Copyright © The McGraw-Hill Companies, Inc. All rights reserved.)

- 339.2 Post-traumatic headache
- 339.8 Other specified headache syndromes

ICD-10-CM CODES[2]

- G44.209 Tension-type headache, unspecified, not intractable
- G44.309 Post-traumatic headache, unspecified, not intractable
- G44.81 Hypnic headache
- G44.82 Headache associated with sexual activity
- G44.83 Primary cough headache
- G44.84 Primary exertional headache
- G44.85 Primary stabbing headache
- G44.89 Other headache syndrome

PREFERRED PRACTICE PATTERN[3]

- 4E: Impaired Joint Mobility, Motor Function, Muscle Performance, and ROM Associated with Localized Inflammation
- 4F: Impaired Joint Mobility, Motor Function, Muscle Performance, Range of Motion, and Reflex Integrity Associated with Spinal Disorders

PATIENT PRESENTATION

A 17-year-old female is studying long nights for college entrance examinations. She is not involved in any other activities presently, but rather spends all of her spare time on the computer reading or studying. After about 2 hours of studying she notices a tight feeling at the base of her skull and a dull headache pain. Over the next 30 to 45 minutes the pain intensifies and she has to lie down to get any relief. The frequency of these headaches has increased over the past 2 months making it increasingly more difficult to study for her examinations. This is causing her a great deal of anxiety. During the interview with this client, the physical therapist notes that she has a forward head and rounded shoulders.

KEY FEATURES

Description

- Pain in the head or neck region
- Muscular in origin
- Squeezing feeling in the head
- Referred pattern depending on Travell trigger points
- International Classification of Headache Disorders-2 (ICDH-2), 2004
  - 13 headache groups
- National Institute of Health (NIH) one of five classifications of headaches
  - Muscular tension/myogenic headache

Essentials of Diagnosis

- ICDH-2
  - Migraines, tension headaches, cluster headaches and trigeminal headaches are classified as the four primary headaches
- NIH
  - Muscular tension/myogenic headache
  - Tension headache

General Considerations

- Headaches can be harmless or disabling.

TABLE 108-1 Classification of TTH and Migraine

	Migraine Without Aura	Tension-Type Headache
Duration	1–72 h[a]	30 min to 7 d
Quality	Throbbing/pounding	Pressure tight band
Severity	Moderate to severe	Mild to moderate
Location	Unilateral/bilateral[a]	Bilateral
Physical activity	Worsens headache	No effect
Associated factors		
a. Nausea+/− vomiting	a or b	Not present
b. Photo + phonophobia		One feature but not both

[a]Modified for children based on the IHCD-II classification criteria.

Source: Hay WW, Levin MJ, Deterding RR, Abzug MJ. *Current Diagnosis & Treatment: Pediatrics*. 21st ed. New York, NY: McGraw-Hill; 2012.

- Headaches can be a sign of something more severe in the head/brain region.
- Vision and sinus problems can cause headaches.

Demographics

- Can be any age group
- Individuals under excess stress

CLINICAL FINDINGS

SIGNS AND SYMPTOMS

- Differential features of headaches in children
  - Muscle contraction
  - Diffuse
  - Time course
  - Depression
  - Anxiety
- Muscular tension/myogenic headache
  - Squeezing or tightening on head
  - Mild-to-moderate pain
  - Okay with routine activity

TABLE 108-2 Differential Diagnosis of Headaches

Primary Causes	Secondary Causes	
• Migraine without aura • Migraine with aura • Childhood pediatric syndromes • Tension-type headache • Trigeminal autonomic cephalgias	• Trauma • Hypertension • Arterial dissection • Medication overuse headache • Idiopathic intracranial hypertension • Intracranial hypotension • Chiari malformation • Seizure • Mass/Neoplasm • Sleep apnea	• Substance withdrawal • Infection • Sinusitis • Hypoxia • Hypercapnia • Mitochondrial disorders • Thyroid dysfunction • Anemia • Asthenopia (eye strain) • Temporomandibular joint dysfunction • Substance use

Source: Hay WW, Levin MJ, Deterding RR, Abzug MJ. *Current Diagnosis & Treatment: Pediatrics*. 21st ed. New York, NY: McGraw-Hill; 2012.

TABLE 108-3 Summary of Published Studies Investigating Manual Therapy Treatment for Upper Cervical Dysfunction and Headache

Author	Sample Size	Intervention Group	Control Group	Outcome Measured	Number of Visits and Duration of Care
Boline et al.[a]	150	Manipulation	Medication	Headache frequency and intensity. Number of medications. SF-36 score	12 visits 6 wk
Howe et al.[b]	52	Manipulation ± Injection + Medication	Medication only	Cervical range of motion. Neck, scapular, arm, and hand pain. Neck stiffness. Headache intensity	1 visit only
Jensen et al.[c]	19	Mobilization Muscle energy	Cold packs	Frequency of medications. Pain intensity, dizziness, visual, and hearing	6 visits 12 wk
Nilsson[d]	39	Manipulation	Laser friction massage	Headache duration and intensity. The number of nonsteroidal anti-inflammatory drugs	6 visits 3 wk
Nilsson et al.[e]	39	Manipulation	Laser friction massage	Cervical passive range of motion	6 visits 3 wk
Osterbauer et al.[f]	20	Manipulation electrical ± stimulation ± Medication	No treatment (10 nonimpaired)	Pain intensity. Cervical range of motion. Kinesthesia	2–3 visits per wk 6 wk
Parker et al.[g]	85	Manipulation by chiropractor Manipulation by physical therapist	Mobilization by a physical therapist	Migraine frequency, intensity, and duration. Disability	Up to 16 visits 8 wk
Rogers[h]	20	Manipulation	Stretching	Pain. Kinesthesia	6 visits
Schoensee et al.[156,i]	10	Mobilization	None	Headache frequency, duration, and intensity	3–4 wk 9–12 visits 3–4 wk
Vernon[j]	33	Manipulation	None	Headache frequency, duration, and intensity	9 visits Unspecified
Whittingham et al.[k]	26	Manipulation at C1 and C2	None	Headache frequency, duration, and intensity	4 visits 2 wk
Yeomans[l]	58	Manipulation	None	Cervical intersegmental range of motion	3 visits per wk 2–6 wk

[a]Data from Boline PD, Kassak K, Bronfort G, Nelson C, Anderson AV. Spinal manipulation vs. amitriptyline for the treatment of chronic tension-type headaches: a randomized clinical trial. *J Manip Physiol Ther.* 1995;18:148–154.
[b]Data from Howe DH, Newcombe RG, Wade MT. Manipulation of the cervical spine—a pilot study. *J R Coll Gen Pract.* 1983;33:574–579.
[c]Data from Jensen OK, Nielsen FF, Vosmar L. An open study comparing manual therapy with the use of cold packs in the treatment of post-traumatic headache. *Cephalgia.* 1990;10:241–250.
[d]Data from Nilsson N. A randomized controlled trial of the effect of spinal manipulation in the treatment of cervicogenic headache. *J Manip Physiol Ther.* 1995;18:435–440.
[e]Data from Nilsson N, Christensen HW, Hartvigsen J. Lasting changes in passive range motion after spinal manipulation: a randomized, blind, controlled trial. *J Manip Physiol Ther.* 1996;19:165–168.
[f]Data from Osterbauer PJ, Derickson KL, Peles JD, DeBoer KF, Fuhr AW, Winters JM. Three-dimensional head kinematics and clinical outcome of patients with neck injury treated with spinal manipulative therapy: a pilot study. *J Manip Physiol Ther.* 1992;15:501–511.
[g]Data from Parker GB, Tupling H, Pryor DS. A controlled trial of cervical manipulation of migraine. *Aust N Z J Med.* 1978;8:589–593.
[h]Data from Rogers RG. The effects of spinal manipulation on cervical kinesthesia in patients with chronic neck pain: a pilot study. *J Manip Physiol Ther.* 1997;20:80–85.
[i]Data from Schoensee SK, Jensen G, Nicholson G, Gossman M, Katholi C. The effect of mobilization on cervical headaches. *J Orthop Sports Phys Ther.*1995; 21:184–196.
[j]Data from Vernon H. Chiropractic manipulative therapy in the treatment of headaches: a retrospective and prospective study. *J Manip Physiol Ther.* 1982;5:109–112.
[k]Data from Whittingham W, Ellis WB, Molyneux TP. The effect of manipulation (toggle recoil technique) for headaches with upper cervical joint dysfunction: a pilot study. *J Manip Physiol Ther.* 1994;17:369–375.
[l]Data from Yeomans SG. The assessment of cervical intersegmental mobility before and after spinal manipulative therapy. *J Manip Physiol Ther.* 1992;15:106–114. With permission from Molina P. Upper cervical dysfunction and cervicogenic headache. In: Wilmarth MA, ed. *Evidence-Based Practice for the Upper and Lower Quarter. Orthopaedic Physical Therapy Home Study Course 13.2.1.* La Crosse, WI: Orthopaedic Section, APTA, Inc, 2003:1–44.
Source: Dutton M: *Dutton's Orthopaedic Examination, Evaluation, and Intervention.* 3rd ed. New York, NY: McGraw-Hill; 2012.

Functional Implications

- Difficulty maintaining sustained sitting postures secondary to neck pain
- Inability to sleep
- Weakness with upper-extremity lifting
- Inability to drive or work secondary to the inability to tolerate light or sound
- Difficulty with neck movements secondary to pain; driving

Possible Contributing Causes

- Forward head rounded shoulders posture due to tight pectoralis, weak periscapular, and deep neck-flexor muscles
- Prolonged position of cervical side bending toward impaired nerve or prolonged extension
- Facet hypertrophy
- Trauma
- Hydration
- Nutritional deficiency
- Vascular insufficiency
- Muscular tightness
- Stress

Differential Diagnoses

- Tumor
- Glaucoma
- Sinusitis
- Myofascial pain syndrome
- Rhomboid/Trapezius spasms
- Degenerative disk disease
- Lyme disease
- Temporomandibular joint dysfunction
- Arnold–Chiari malformation
- Migraine
  - Pulsating pain on one or both sides of the head
  - Nausea
  - Sensitivities to light and sound
  - Aggravated with routine activity
- Cluster headaches
  - Severe headaches
  - Short-lasting
  - Symptoms around the eye
- Toxic headaches
  - Fever
- Cervicogenic headache
  - Stiff neck
  - Limited mobility
  - One-sided
  - Can radiate into arm

MEANS OF CONFIRMATION OF DIAGNOSIS

Imaging

- MRI to visualize the head/brain region
- X-ray/Plain-film radiograph helpful if osteophyte located in intervertebral foramen in cervical spine
- CT scan

FINDINGS AND INTERPRETATION

- Laboratory tests are negative.
- Brain MRI is negative.
- Increase EMG signal of the upper trapezius and scalenes.

REFERRALS/ADMITTANCE

- To hospital for imaging of the brain and sinuses
- To nutritionist for diet and food allergies that maybe contributing
- To optometrist for an eye examination
- To neurologist for nerve conduction test (EMG)

IMPAIRMENTS

- Restricted mobility of the upper-/mid-thoracic spine and subcranial spine
- Hypermobile mid-cervical spine
- Tight pectoralis major and minor
- Weakness noted of longus colli and longus capitis
- Weakness noted of periscapular muscles

TESTS AND MEASURES

- Physical examination cluster to rule in cervical radiculopathy[4]
  - Spurling test
  - Rotation limited to ipsilateral side
  - Upper limb neural tension test
  - Diminished brachioradialis reflex

INTERVENTION

- Rest
- Hydration
- Joint manipulation to the thoracic and upper-cervical spine
  - Suboccipital release
  - Myofascial release
- Cervical distraction and traction to relieve nerve compression
- Craniocervical flexion exercises
- Addressing pain
  - Electrical stimulation
  - Heat/Ice
- Addressing hypertonicity
  - Soft tissue massage
  - Heat
- Addressing muscle weakness
  - Deep neck-flexor training
  - Strengthening of lower/middle trapezius, rhomboids, rotator cuff
  - Serratus anterior, latissimus dorsi

FUNCTIONAL GOALS

- Patient will be able to
  - Sit with a neutral cervical and thoracic spine posture for more than 30 minutes with 0/10 pain.
  - Sit at workstation and perform computer work for 45 minutes with 0/10 pain.
  - Rotate cervical spine 70 degrees with 0/10 neck/arm pain to communicate on the telephone.

PROGNOSIS

- Fair to very good depending upon etiology of headaches.
- Once tension and posture improves, headaches should go away.

PATIENT RESOURCE

- American Headache Society. http://www.americanheadachesociety.org. Accessed July 6, 2013.

REFERENCES

1. ICD-9-CM. http://www.icd9data.com. Accessed July 1, 2013.
2. ICD-10-CM. http://www.icd10data.com. Accessed July 1, 2013.
3. APTA Guide to Physical Therapist Practice. http://guidetoptpractice.apta.org. Accessed July 1, 2013.
4. Hay WW, Levin MJ, Sondheimer JM, Deterding RR. Disorders affecting the nervous system in infants and children. In: Hay WW, Levin MJ, Sondheimer JM, Deterding RR, eds. *CURRENT Diagnosis & Treatment: Pediatrics*. 20th ed. New York, NY: McGraw-Hill; 2011. http://www.accessphysiotherapy.com/content/6585098. Accessed July 6, 2013.

ADDITIONAL REFERENCES

- Dutton M. Differential diagnosis within specific regions. In: Dutton M, ed. *Orthopaedic Examination, Evaluation, and Intervention*. 2nd ed. New York, NY: McGraw-Hill; 2008. http://www.accessphysiotherapy.com/content/5546998. Accessed July 6, 2013.
- Dutton M. Pattern 4F: impaired joint mobility, motor function, muscle performance, and range of motion, or reflex integrity, secondary to spinal disorders. In: Dutton M, ed. *Orthopaedic Examination, Evaluation, and Intervention*. 2nd ed. New York, NY: McGraw-Hill; 2008. http://www.accessphysiotherapy.com/content/55590375. Accessed July 6, 2013.
- Dutton M. Systems review. In: Dutton M, ed. *Dutton's Orthopedic Survival Guide: Managing Common Conditions*. New York, NY: McGraw-Hill; 2011. http://www.accessphysiotherapy.com/content/8656096. Accessed July 22, 2013.
- Sun-Edelstein C, Mauskop A. Complementary and alternative approaches to the treatment of tension-type headache. *Curr Pain Headache Rep*. 2012;16(6):539–544. doi: 10.1007/s11916-012-0295-6.

109 VASCULAR HEADACHES

Eric Shamus, PhD, DPT, PT, CSCS
Jennifer Shamus, PhD, DPT, COMT, CSCS
Mollie Venglar Dsc, MSPT, NCS

CONDITION/DISORDER SYNONYMS

- Cephalgia
- Headache

ICD-9-CM CODES

- 307.81 Tension headache
- 339 Other headache syndromes
- 339.0 Cluster headaches and other trigeminal autonomic cephalgias
- 339.1 Tension type headache
- 339.2 Post-traumatic headache
- 339.3 Drug induced headache, not elsewhere classified
- 339.4 Complicated headache syndromes
- 339.8 Other specified headache syndromes

ICD-10-CM CODES

- G43 Migraine
- G44 Other headache syndromes
- G44.009 Cluster headache syndrome, unspecified, not intractable

PREFERRED PRACTICE PATTERN

- 4E: Impaired Joint Mobility, Motor Function, Muscle Performance, and Range of Motion Associated with Localized Inflammation

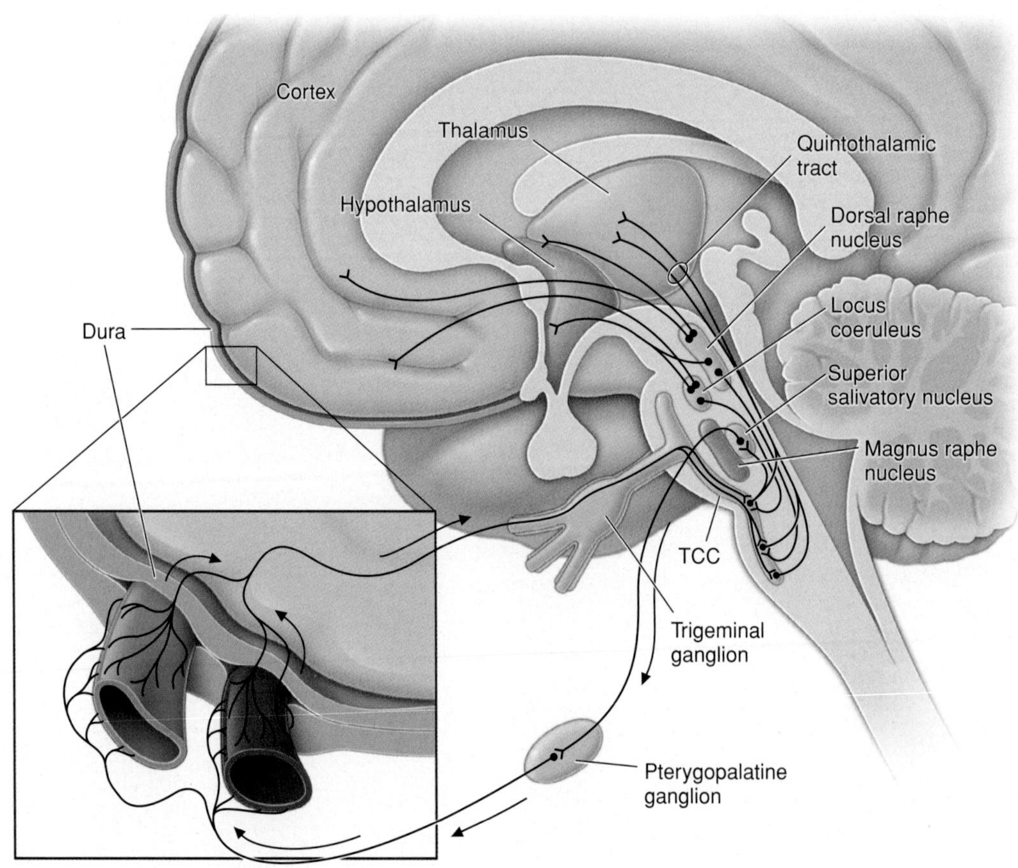

FIGURE 109-1 Brain stem pathways that modulate sensory input. The key pathway for pain in migraine is the trigeminovascular input from the meningeal vessels, which passes through the trigeminal ganglion and synapses on second-order neurons in the trigeminocervical complex (TCC). These neurons in turn project in the quintothalamic tract and, after decussating in the brain stem, synapse on neurons in the thalamus. Important modulation of the trigeminovascular nociceptive input comes from the dorsal raphe nucleus, locus coeruleus, and nucleus raphe magnus. (From Longo DL, Fauci AS, Kasper DL, Hauser SL, Jameson JL, Loscalzo J, eds. *Harrison's Principles of Internal Medicine*. 18th ed. http://www.accessmedicine.com. Copyright © The McGraw-Hill Companies, Inc. All rights reserved.)

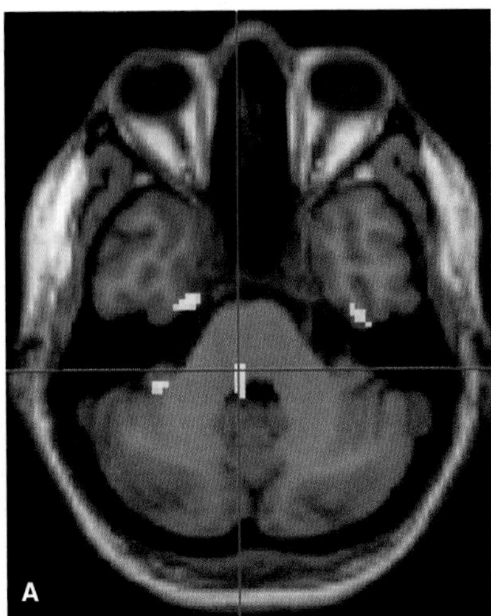

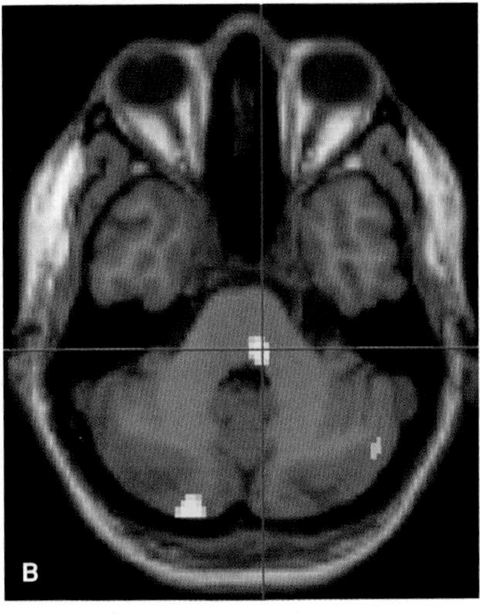

FIGURE 109-2 Positron emission tomography (PET) activation in migraine. In spontaneous attacks of episodic migraine there is activation of the region of the dorsolateral pons; an identical pattern is found in chronic migraine (*not shown*). This area, which includes the noradrenergic locus coeruleus, is fundamental to the expression of migraine. Moreover, lateralization of changes in this region of the brain stem correlates with lateralization of the head pain in hemicranial migraine; the scans shown in panels **A** and **B** are of patients with acute migraine headache on the right and left side, respectively. (From Afridi SK, et al. *Brain.* 2005;128:932.)

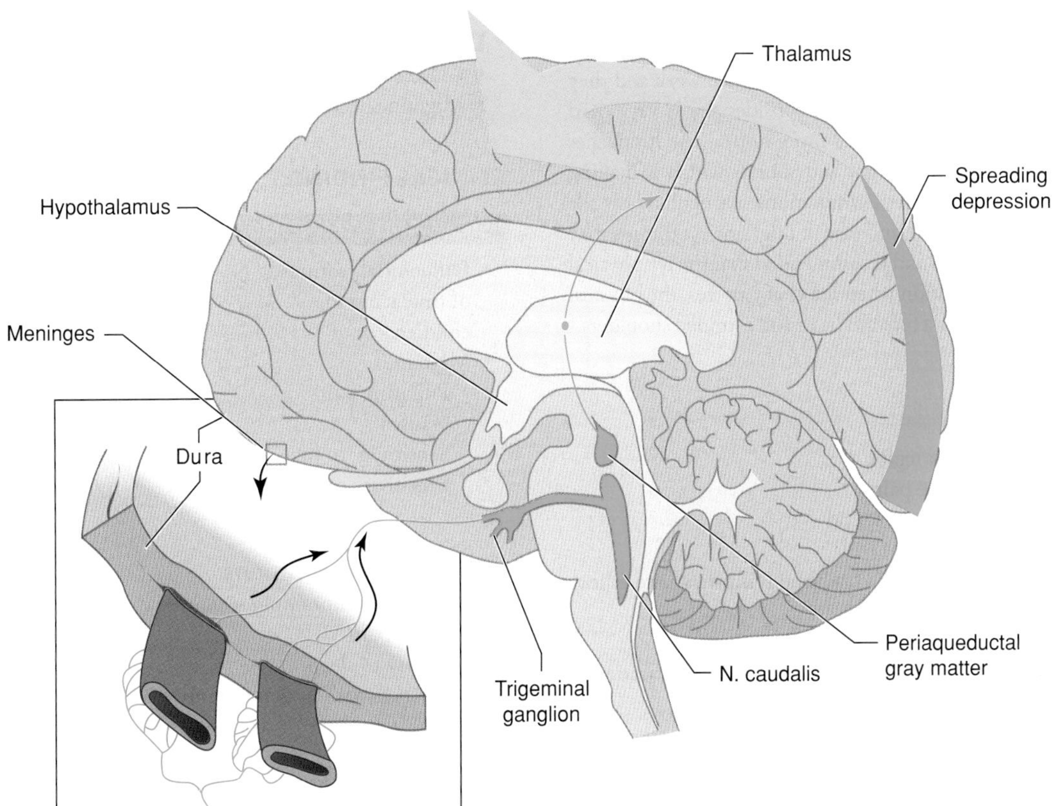

FIGURE 109-3 Central and peripheral nervous system sites proposed to be involved in migraine pathogenesis. During the aura phase, a reduction in cortical blood flow spreads anteriorly from the occipital cortex (*large arrow*), which is thought to be due to spreading depression. During the headache phase, sterile inflammation in the meninges may activate trigeminal (V) nerve sensory fibers that project to the nucleus caudalis, periaqueductal gray, sensory thalamic nuclei, and primary somatosensory cortex (*small arrows*). Alternatively, this central sensory pathway may convey normal afferent signals that are interpreted as noxious. (From Greenberg DA, Amnioff MJ, Simon RP. *Clinical Neurology*. 8th ed. http://www.accessmedicine.com. Copyright © The McGraw-Hill Companies, Inc. All rights reserved.)

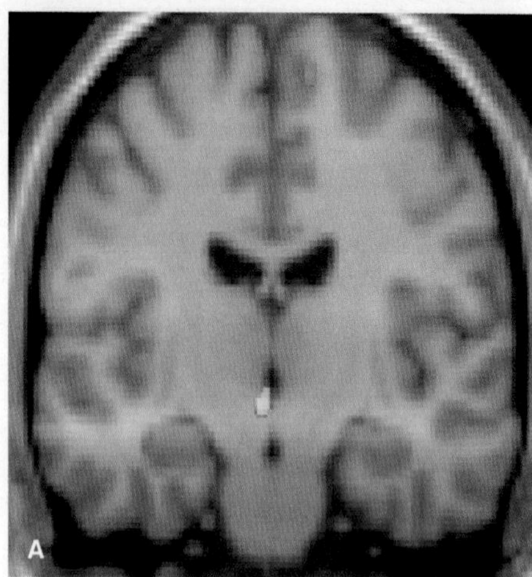

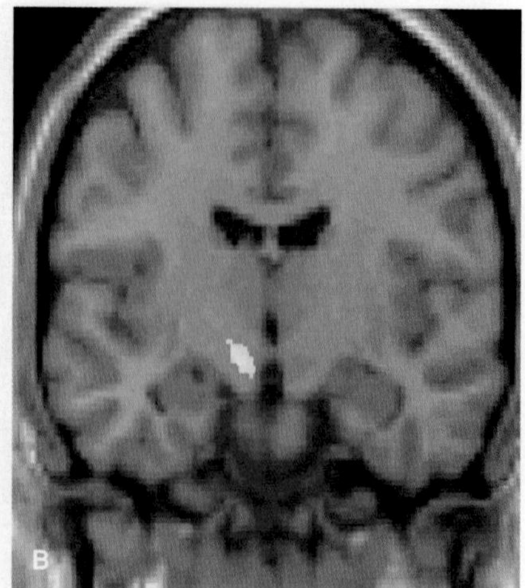

FIGURE 109-4 Posterior hypothalamic gray matter activation on positron emission tomography (PET) in a patient with acute cluster headache (**A**). (From A May et al: *Lancet.* 1998;352:275.) High-resolution T1 weighted MRI obtained using voxel-based morphometry demonstrates increased gray matter activity, lateralized to the side of pain in a patient with cluster headache (**B**). (From A May et al. *Nat Med.* 1999;5:836.)

PATIENT PRESENTATION

A 17-year-old female is studying long nights for college entrance examinations. She is not involved in any other activities presently, but rather spends all of her spare time on the computer reading or studying. She reports to physical therapy because she has had increasing frequency of migraine headaches. She started having headaches in sixth grade but they were generally only a few times each year. Now she has them a couple of times each week and they last about 6 hours. Once the headache subsides she is very tired and has difficulty focusing for several more hours. The headaches are accompanied by sensitivity light and sounds which is making it very difficult to study for her examinations, particularly on the computer. Her doctor feels the increase in migraine symptoms may be partly due to her posture and recommended that she try physical therapy. On initial observation when the client arrives, the physical therapist notes that she has a forward head and rounded shoulders.[1]

KEY FEATURES

Description

- Pain in the head or neck region
- Severe episodes of intense pain
- Hypersensitivity to light and sound
- Many triggers
- International Classification of Headache Disorders, 2nd edition (ICDH-II)
  - 13 headache groups
- National Institute of Health (NIH): one of five classifications of headaches
  - Vascular headache

Essentials of Diagnosis

- ICDH-II:
  - First four are primary headaches
  - Migraines, tension headaches, cluster headaches, and trigeminal headaches are primary
- NIH: Vascular headache
  - Migraine
  - Cluster headaches

General Considerations

- Headaches can be harmless, disabling, or life threatening.
- Headaches can be a sign of something more severe in the head/brain region.
- Vision problems and sinuses can cause headaches.

Demographics

- Cluster headaches are more common in men.
- Migraine headaches are more common in women.

CLINICAL FINDINGS

SIGNS AND SYMPTOMS

- Differential features of headaches in children
- Migraine
  - Pulsating pain
  - Nausea
  - Sensitivity to light
  - Sensitivity to sound
  - One or both sides of the head
  - Aggravated with routine activity
- Cluster headaches
  - Severe headaches
  - Short-lasting
  - Symptoms around the eye

Functional Implications

- Difficulty maintaining sustained sitting postures secondary to neck pain
- Inability to sleep
- Weakness with upper-extremity (UE) lifting
- Inability to drive or work secondary to the inability to tolerate light or sound

Possible Contributing Causes

- Forward-head, rounded-shoulders posture due to tight pectoralis, weak periscapular, and deep neck-flexor muscles
- Prolonged position of cervical side bending toward impaired nerve or prolonged extension
- Facet hypertrophy
- Trauma

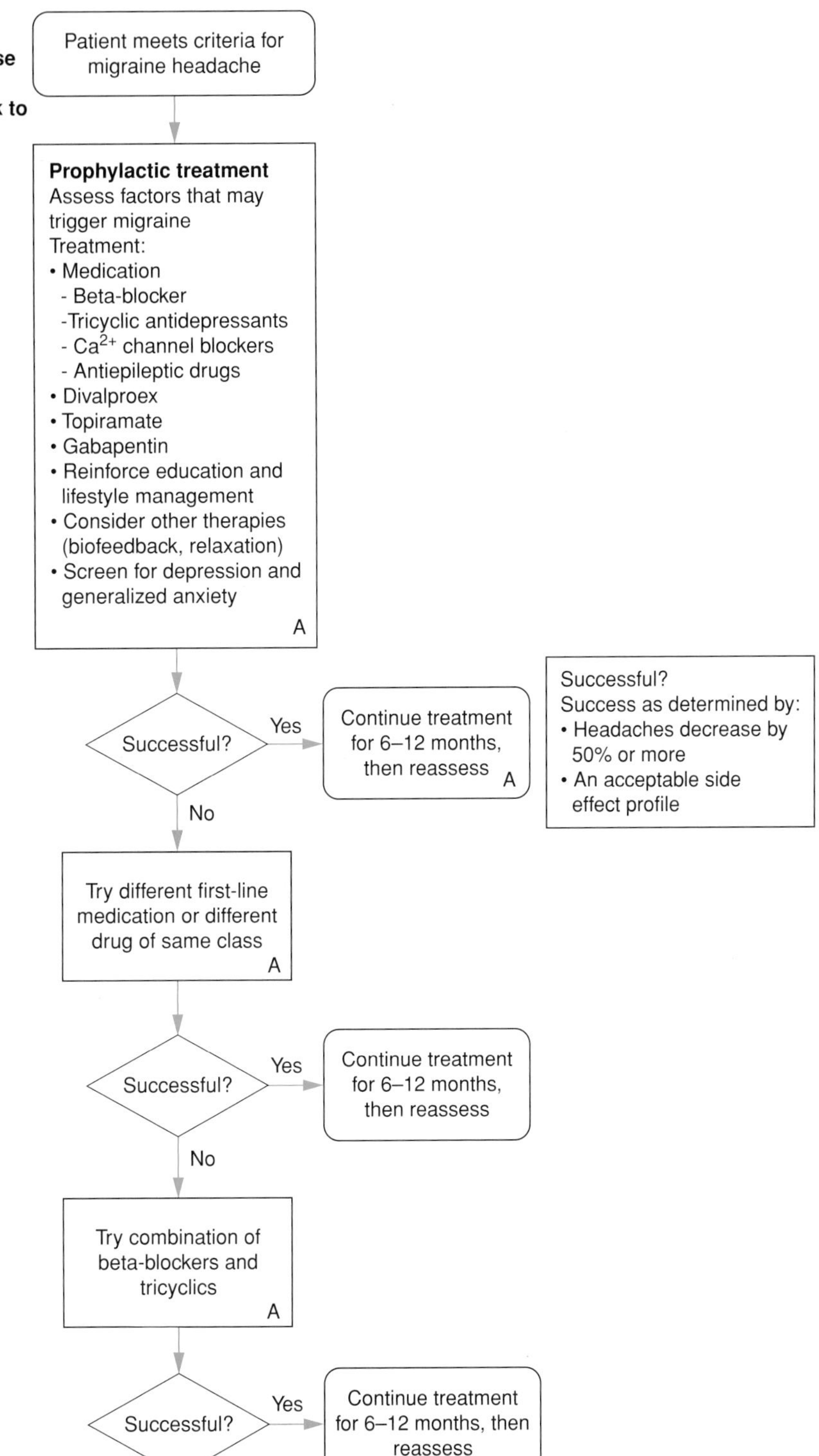

FIGURE 109-5 Migraine prophylactic treatment algorithm. (From Esherick JS, Clark DS, Slater ED. *Current Practice Guidelines in Primary Care 2012*. http://www.accessmedicine.com. Copyright © The McGraw-Hill Companies, Inc. All rights reserved.)

- Light
- Sounds
- Hydration
- Nutrition deficiency
- Vascular insufficiency
- Muscular tightness
- Stress

Differential Diagnosis

- Tumor
- Glaucoma
- Sinusitis
- Myofascial pain syndrome
- Rhomboid/Trapezius spams
- Degenerative disk disease

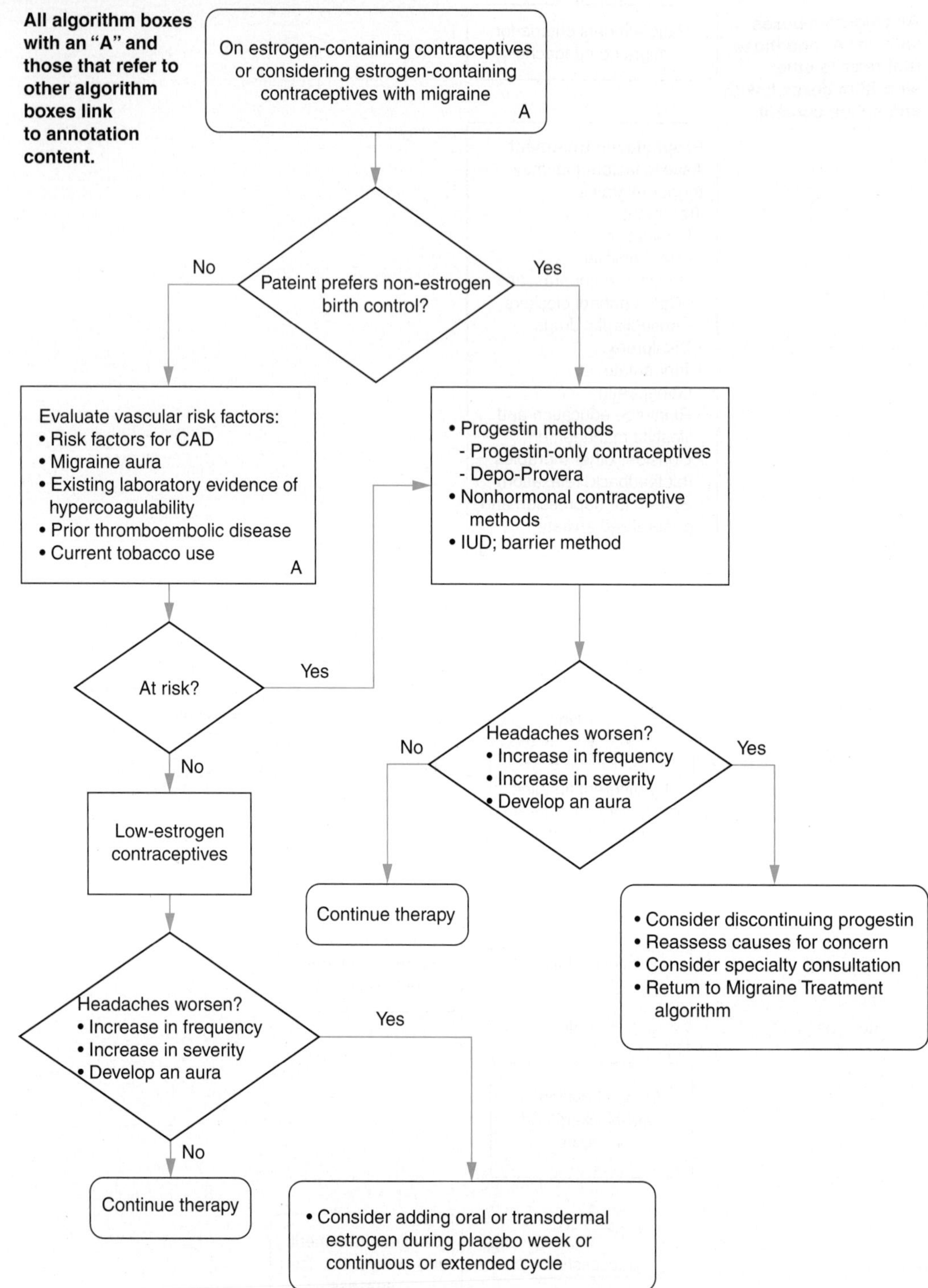

FIGURE 109-6 On estrogen-containing contraceptives or considering estrogen-containing contraceptives with migraine algorithm. (From Esherick JS, Clark DS, Slater ED. *Current Practice Guidelines in Primary Care 2012*. http://www.accessmedicine.com. Copyright © The McGraw-Hill Companies, Inc. All rights reserved.)

- Lyme disease
- Temporomandibular joint dysfunction
- Arnold–Chiari malformation
- Toxic headaches
  - Fever
- Muscular tension/myogenic headache
  - Squeezing or tightening on head
  - Mild-to-moderate pain
  - Okay with routine activity
- Cervicogenic headache
  - Stiff neck
  - Limited mobility
  - One-sided
  - Can radiate into arm

MEANS OF CONFIRMATION OR DIAGNOSIS

▶ **Imaging**
- MRI helpful in diagnosis to visualize the head/brain region
- X-ray/Plain-film radiograph helpful if osteophyte located in intervertebral foramen in cervical spine
- Doppler blood flow test
- CT

FINDINGS AND INTERPRETATION

- Laboratory tests are negative
- Brain MRI is negative
- EMG signal of the upper trapezius and scalenes

REFERRALS/ADMITTANCE

- To imaging
- To nutritionist
- To optometrist for an eye examinations
- To neurologist
  - Imaging

IMPAIRMENTS

- Vision
- Hearing
- Restricted mobility of the upper-/mid-thoracic spine and subcranial spine
- Hypermobile mid-cervical spine
- Tight pectoralis major and minor
- Weakness noted of longus colli and longus capitis
- Weakness noted of periscapular muscles

TESTS AND MEASURES

- Physical examination cluster to rule in cervical radiculopathy[2]
  - Spurling test
  - Rotation limited to ipsilateral side
  - Upper limb nerve tension test
  - Diminished brachioradialis reflex

INTERVENTION

- Rest
- Hydration
- Joint manipulation to the thoracic and upper-cervical spine
  - Suboccipital release
  - Myofascial release
- Cervical distraction and traction to relieve nerve compression
- Cranio cervical flexion exercises
- Addressing pain
  - Electrical stimulation
  - Heat/Ice
- Addressing hypertonicity
  - Soft tissue massage
  - Heat
- Addressing muscle weakness
  - Deep neck-flexor training
  - Strengthening of lower/middle trapezius, rhomboids, rotator cuff, serratus anterior, latissimus dorsi

FUNCTIONAL GOALS

- Patient will be able to
  - Sit with a neutral cervical and thoracic spine posture for more than 30 minutes with 0/10 pain.
  - Sit at work station and perform computer work for 45 minutes with 0/10 pain.
  - Rotate cervical spine 70 degrees with 0/10 neck/arm pain to communicate on the telephone.

PROGNOSIS

- Fair to very good dependent on etiology.

PATIENT RESOURCES

- American Headache Society. http://www.americanheadachesociety.org/ Accessed July 6, 2013.
- M.A.G.N.U.M. The National Migraine Association. http://www.migraines.org./ Accessed July 6, 2013.

REFERENCES

1. Toy EC. Migraine Headache, Case 94. LANGE Case Files. http://www.accessmedicine.com/casecontent.aspx?aid=510024251&tabid=1. Accessed July 6, 2013.
2. Hay WW, Levin MJ, Sondheimer JM, Deterding RR. Disorders affecting the nervous system in infants & children. In: Hay WW, Levin MJ, Sondheimer JM, Deterding RR, eds. *CURRENT Diagnosis & Treatment: Pediatrics*. 20th ed. New York, NY: McGraw-Hill; 2011:Chapter 23. http://www.accessphysiotherapy.com/content/6585098. Accessed July 6, 2013.

ADDITIONAL REFERENCES

- Dutton M. The cervical complex. In: Dutton M, ed. *Dutton's Orthopedic Survival Guide: Managing Common Conditions*. New York, NY: McGraw-Hill; 2011:Chapter 11. http://www.accessphysiotherapy.com/content/8656096. Accessed July 6, 2013.
- Dutton M, ed. *Orthopaedic Examination, Evaluation, and Intervention*. 2nd ed. New York, NY: McGraw-Hill; 2008. http://www.accessphysiotherapy.com/resource/612. Accessed July 6, 2013.
- ICD9Data.com. http://www.icd9data.com. Accessed July 6, 2013.
- ICD10Data.com. http://www.icd10data.com/ICD10CM/Codes. Accessed July 6, 2013.
- Malone TR, Hazle C, Grey ML. Introduction to musculoskeletal imaging. In: Malone TR, Hazle C, Grey ML, eds. *Imaging in Rehabilitation*. New York, NY: McGraw-Hill; 2008:Chapter 1. http://www.accessphysiotherapy.com/content/5940000. Accessed July 6, 2013.
- Pattern 4E. Impaired joint mobility, motor function, muscle performance, and range of motion associated with localized inflammation. In: *Guide to Physical Therapist Practice*. 2nd ed. Alexandria, VA: American Physical Therapy Association; 2001. Revised 2003.
- Rapport AM. Acute treatment of migraine: established and emerging therapies. *Headache*. 2012;52(Suppl 2):60–64. doi: 10.1111/j.1526-4610.2012.02240.x.

110 FRACTURE, SKULL

Eric Shamus, PhD, DPT, PT, CSCS
Megan Samantha Rosga, DPT, MSPT, NCS
Mollie Venglar, DSc, MSPT, NCS

ICD-9-CM CODES[1]

- 803 Other and unqualified skull fractures
- 803.0 Other closed skull fracture without mention of intracranial injury
- 803.00 Other closed skull fracture without intracranial injury with state of consciousness unspecified
- 803.1 Other closed skull fracture with cerebral laceration and contusion
- 803.2 Other closed skull fracture with subarachnoid subdural and extradural hemorrhage
- 803.3 Closed skull fracture with other and unspecified intracranial hemorrhage
- 803.4 Closed skull fracture with intracranial injury of other and unspecified nature
- 803.5 Other open skull fracture without mention of intracranial injury
- 803.6 Other open skull fracture with cerebral laceration and contusion
- 803.7 Other open skull fracture with subarachnoid subdural and extradural hemorrhage
- 803.8 Other open skull fracture with other and unspecified intracranial hemorrhage
- 803.9 Other open skull fracture with intracranial injury of other and unspecified nature

ICD-10-CM CODES[2]

- S02.91XA Unspecified fracture of skull, initial encounter for closed fracture
- S02.91XB Unspecified fracture of skull, initial encounter for open fracture

PREFERRED PRACTICE PATTERN[3]

- 5C: Impaired Motor Function and Sensory Integrity Associated with Nonprogressive Disorders of the Central Nervous System—congenital origin or acquired in infancy or childhood
- 5D: Impaired Motor Function and Sensory Integrity Associated with Nonprogressive Disorders of the Central Nervous System—acquired in adolescence or adulthood

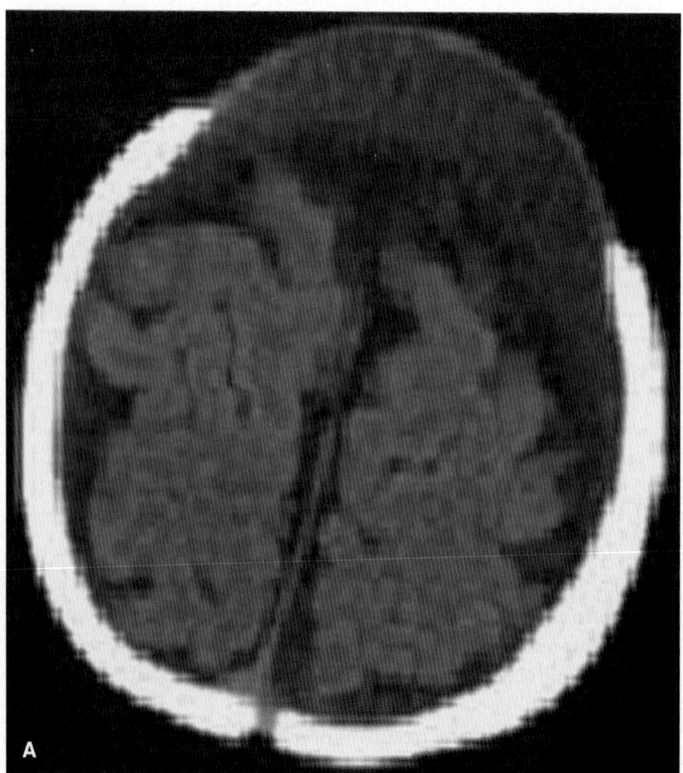

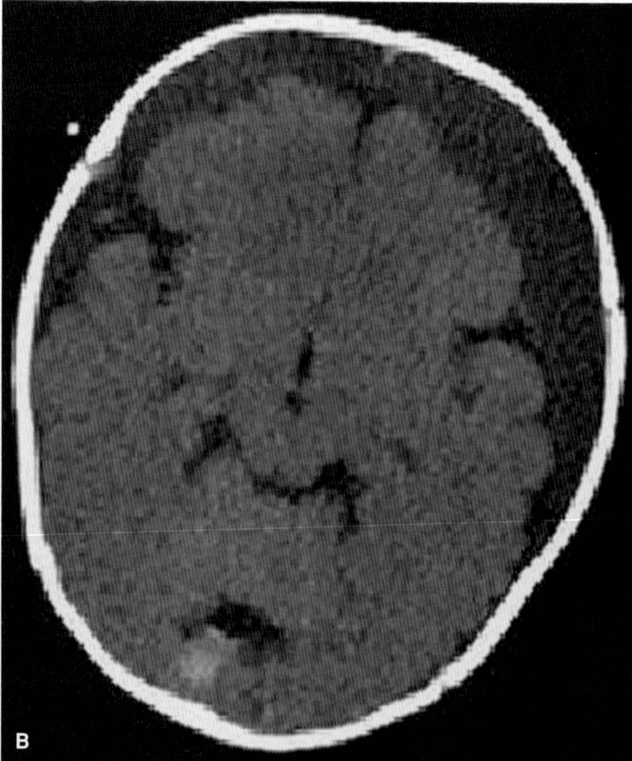

FIGURE 110-1 (**A**) Bifrontal chronic subdural hematoma extending through the anterior fontanelle in a 1-month-old child. (**B**) Second image, in the same child showing bifrontal chronic subdural hematoma as well as small, acute intraparenchymal hemorrhage in the posterior fossa. (From Tintinalli JE, Stapczynski J, Ma OJ, Cline D, Cydulka R, Meckler G. *Tintinalli's Emergency Medicine: A Comprehensive Study Guide*. 7th ed. http://www.accessmedicine.com. Copyright © The McGraw-Hill Companies, Inc. All rights reserved.)

PATIENT PRESENTATION

While riding his bicycle home from school, a 15-year-old boy veered off the side of the road to avoid an oncoming car. The front wheel of his bike hit a large rock, which stopped the bicycle suddenly. The boy was thrown over the handlebars and landed head first on the ground. He was not wearing a helmet. When the emergency medical team arrived (approximately 8 minutes after receiving a 911 call) the boy was unconscious and lying on his back. The back of his head was lying in a pool of blood due to a skull fracture.

KEY FEATURES

Description

- Defined as external trauma to the skull that results in damage to one or more parts of the brain.
- Fracture of the skull
  - Open head injury (penetrating): Fracture of the skull with brain injury.
  - Closed head injury (blunt, nonpenetrating): Skull remains intact, but brain injury is evident.
- Depressed skull fracture: Break in a cranial bone with depression toward the brain.
- Linear skull fracture: Break in a cranial bone, thin line without splintering, depression, or distortion of the bone.
- Initial presentation will range from comatose to ambulatory and verbal depending on the extent and location of damage.

Essentials of Diagnosis

- Damage to the brain may result in changes or dysfunction to any body functions including:
  - Motor loss
  - Sensory loss
  - Autonomic dysfunction
  - Perceptual changes
  - Cognitive, personality, and behavioral changes
  - Changes in consciousness
  - Communication difficulties
  - Eating, swallowing, bowel, and bladder changes

General Considerations

- Delayed effects of the trauma are common.
- Full extent of the injury is not known at the time of injury.
- Intracranial swelling must be addressed/controlled before the full extent of the damage can be identified.
- Swelling will cause secondary damage to parts of the brain that were not impacted by the initial trauma.
- Cerebral hypoxia and/or ischemia, cerebral hemorrhages, electrolyte imbalances, infections from open wounds/open head injury, and seizures are common.
- Physical activity is contraindicated until the full effects of the brain injury are known and the patient has stable intracranial pressures.

Demographics

- American Trauma Society[1] estimates approximately 500,000 people are admitted to the hospital each year in America due to cerebral trauma; 75,000 to 90,000 die from the cerebral trauma, and many others remain permanently disabled.
- Most commonly injured are between the ages of 15 and 24 years[4]

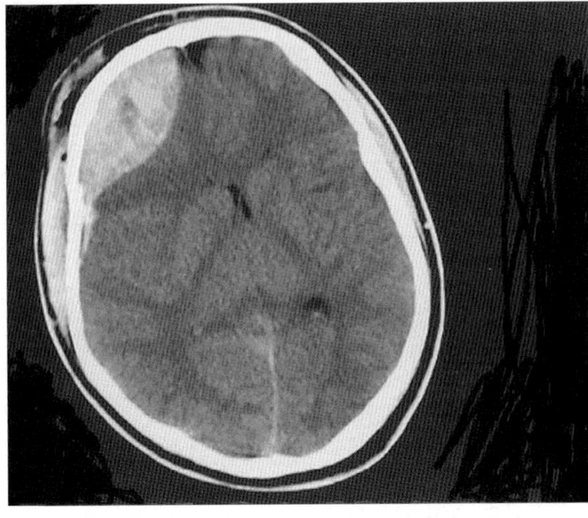

FIGURE 110-2 CT scan showing epidural bleeding. (From Patel DR, Greydanus DE, Baker RJ. *Pediatric Practice: Sports Medicine*. http://www.accesspediatrics.com. Copyright © The McGraw-Hill Companies, Inc. All rights reserved.)

- Men are twice as likely as women to suffer a brain injury.[4]
- Leading cause of brain injury in the young adult is motor vehicle crash.[4]
- Leading cause of brain injury in people over the age of 65 is fall.[4]

CLINICAL FINDINGS

SIGNS AND SYMPTOMS

- Signs and symptoms are dependent on the part(s) of the brain that are injured and the extent of the injury
- Common sequela treated by a PT include:
  - Behavioral changes
  - Cognitive function changes
  - Motor and motor planning deficits
  - Sensory deficits
  - Spasticity or hypertonicity

Functional Implications

- Loss of independence with all aspects of mobility, ADLs, and self-care
- Loss of ability to interact with others effectively
- Difficulty with cognitive processing, particularly executive function

Possible Contributing Causes

- Previous brain injury
- Falls
- Automobile accident
- Physical assault
- Sports
- Risk-taking behaviors

Differential Diagnosis

- The mechanism of injury indicates the diagnosis.

MEANS OF CONFIRMATION OR DIAGNOSIS

Laboratory Tests

- Intracranial pressure
- Oxygen saturation

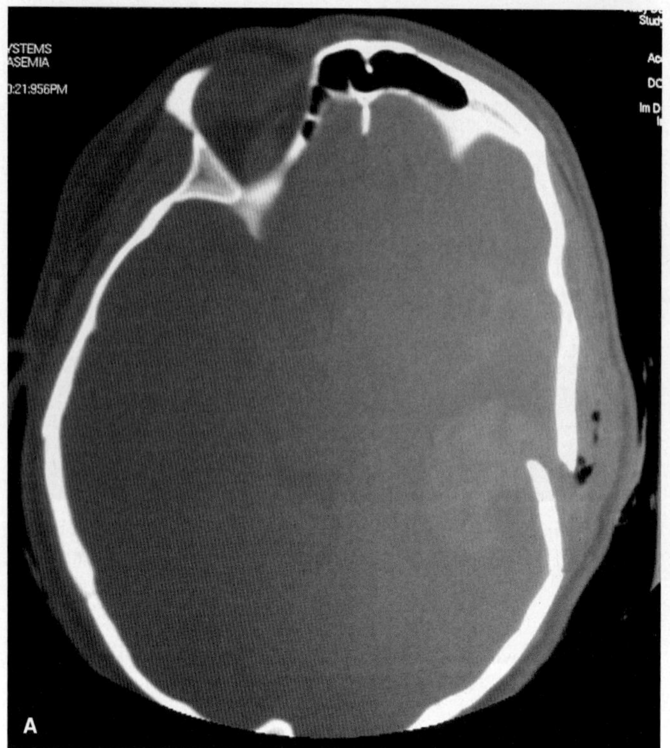

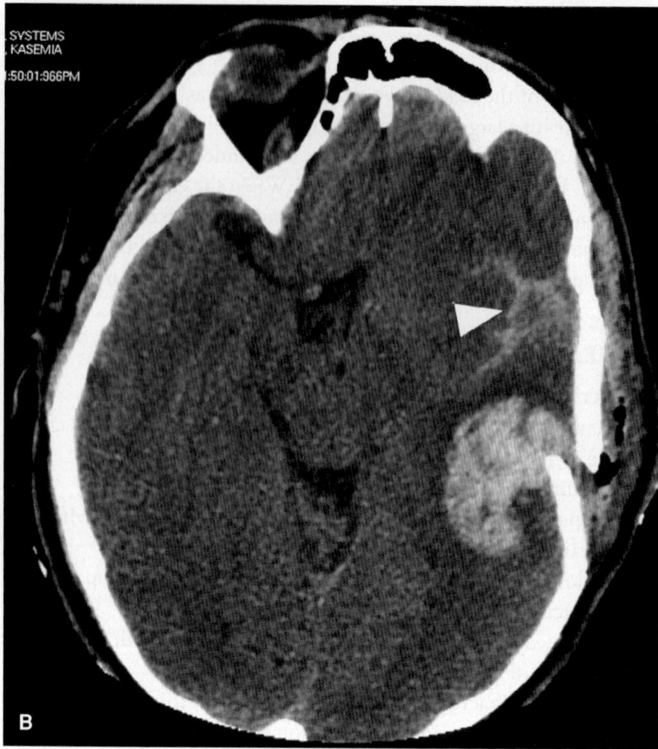

FIGURE 110-3 (**A**) Bone-window axial head computed tomography (CT) of a patient who presented aphasic after being struck with the bottom of a beer bottle. CT demonstrates a depressed skull fracture in the left posterior temporoparietal area. (**B**) Brain-window axial head CT demonstrating intraparenchymal hematoma caused by laceration of cortical vessels by the edge of the fractured bone. *Arrowhead* indicates traumatic subarachnoid hemorrhage in the sylvanian fissure. (From Brunicardi FC et al: *Schwartz's Principles of Surgery*. 9th ed. http://www.accessmedicine.com. Copyright © The McGraw-Hill Companies, Inc. All rights reserved.)

- Hemoglobin
- Electrolyte and acid-base levels

Imaging

- CT
- MRI
- Radiographs

Medications

- Hyperosmolar therapy
- Corticosteroids
- Blood pressure management
- Dantrolene sodium for general spasticity, botulinum toxin type A for specific muscle spasticity
- Carbamazepine or propranolol to treat aggression and agitation
- Gabapentin for intractable neurogenic pain
- Valproic acid for seizure control
- Antibiotics for nosocomial or opportunistic infections
- Oral baclofen for increased tone
- Baclofen pump

FINDINGS AND INTERPRETATION

- Fracture of the skull
  - Open head injury (penetrating): Fracture of the skull with brain injury
  - Closed head injury (blunt, nonpenetrating): Skull remains intact, but brain injury is evident

REFERRALS/ADMITTANCE

- To emergency room physician
- To neurologist or neurosurgeon as needed, based on location and severity of injury, management of medications, and management of future needs
- To neuropsychologist for cognitive testing
- To physiatrist for specific rehabilitation physician care. If not managed by a neurologist, the physiatrist will manage medications, symptoms, future needs, etc.
- To occupational therapist for ADLs, cognitive retraining, and fine motor tasks
- To speech/language pathologist for speech, cognition, and swallowing impairments
- To respiratory therapist as needed (depending on the respiratory impact of the brain injury)
- To support groups for patients and family/caregivers
- To case management or social work for assistance with coordination of care

IMPAIRMENTS

- Arousal
- Attention
- Behavior
- Cognition
- Cranial nerve integrity
- Peripheral nerve integrity, possibly from a comorbid diagnosis
- Gait

- Wheelchair mobility
- Balance
  - Static sit
  - Dynamic sit
  - Static stand
  - Dynamic stand
  - Moving base of support
- Muscle strength
- Muscle recruitment
- Coordination
- Postural control
- Posture
- ROM
- Reflexes
  - Deep tendon reflexes
  - Babinski
  - Clonus
- Muscle tone, anticipate hypertonicity or spasticity
- Sensation
- Motor planning
- Bed mobility
- Transfers
- Neglect: Evident in cases of primary damage to one side of the brain
- Endurance
- Aerobic capacity
- Self-care
- Home management
- Fine motor
- Respiratory compromise

TESTS AND MEASURES

- Glasgow Outcome Scale
- Glasgow Coma Scale
- Rancho Los Amigos Scale
- Modified Ashworth Scale
- Functional measures
  - Barthel Index
  - Functional Independence Measure
- Gait and balance measures
  - Tinetti
  - Motor Assessment Scale
  - Gait assessment rating scale
  - Rancho Los Amigo Observational Gait Analysis
  - 6-minute walk test
  - Multi-directional reach test
  - High-level mobility assessment tool (HiMAT) (if appropriate for patients who have appropriate scores on Berg Balance Scale and Dynamic Gait Index)
- Cognitive testing and cognitive behavioral level via Rancho Los Amigos
- Sensory testing, may be limited by cognition or consciousness
- Strength, includes speed of force production and ability to change force production
- Active and passive ROM, flexibility
- Bed mobility
- Transfers
- Cranial nerves, particularly vision
- Vestibular assessment

INTERVENTION

- ROM/Stretching/Positioning
- Tone management
- Orientation to vertical position
- Strengthening
- Balance training
- Gait training (if appropriate and with appropriate bracing and assistive devices)
- Transfer training
- Bed-mobility training
- Wheelchair-mobility training (curbs, ramps, various surfaces, negotiating obstacles)
- Cardiovascular and pulmonary endurance

FUNCTIONAL GOALS

Note: Goals below are based on the cognitive behavioral levels identified in the Rancho Los Amigos scale. These will have to be modified based on the likely comorbidities acquired concurrently with the brain injury.

- Rancho level 1 and 2
  - Patient will demonstrate a response to tactile or verbal stimulation 80% of the time to show improving brain function.
  - Patient's caregiver will demonstrate appropriate bed and wheelchair positioning to prevent skin breakdown.
- Rancho level 3
  - Patient will tolerate
    - Tilt table at 75% of upright position for 10 minutes with vital signs stable to increase tolerance and orientation to vertical position.
    - Sitting at the edge of the mat with minimal physical support and maximal verbal cues to attend to the task for 3 minutes without loss of balance.
- Rancho level 4
  - Patient will demonstrate escalation less than
    - 25% of treatment time during PT treatment in a closed environment.
    - 75% of treatment time during PT treatment in an open environment.
- Rancho level 5
  - Patient will ambulate 250 ft with minimal assistance for balance indoors over level surfaces in a nondistracting environment to increase safe functional independence and mobility
- Rancho level 6
  - Patient will ambulate indoors over level surfaces while negotiating obstacles ×500' with contact guard assist for safety and moderate verbal cues for path-finding and attention to task in order to increase safe functional independence and mobility.
- Rancho level 7
  - Patient will perform floor recovery with supervision and upper-extremity (UE) support on stable surface to increase safe functional independence.
- Rancho level 8
  - Patient will ambulate >500 ft indoors/outdoors over level and unlevel surfaces in a distracting environment with distant supervision and occasional cues for attention to task in order to increase safe and efficient functional mobility and independence.
- Rancho level 9
  - Patient will be completely independent with bilateral rolling, supine to/from sit, and scooting to ensure safe functional independence.

- Rancho level 10
  - Patient will
    - Increase BBS score ≥6 points to increase safe functional independence, increase balance, and decrease fall risk.
    - Tolerate assessment of HiMAT balance assessment to determine additional deficits in functional mobility to promote safe return to appropriate premorbid activities.

PROGNOSIS

- The following have been indicated to impact prognosis:
  - Age: Those older than 40 years tend to have a worse prognosis compared to people younger than 40.
  - Rehabilitation: Early rehabilitation (shorter time between brain injury and start of rehabilitation) has been shown to produce better outcomes.
  - Size of lesion: There is evidence to support that people suffering from smaller lesions will have better outcomes.
  - Type of lesion: Most patients with corpus callosum and dorsolateral brainstem lesions will not recover from a persistent vegetative state.
- Several factors contribute to the severity of an injury and the ability to access health care. Speed at which an individual receives emergency care following the head trauma will also impact prognosis.

PATIENT RESOURCE

- American Trauma Society. www.amtrauma.org. Accessed July 10, 2013.

REFERENCES

1. ICD9Data.com. http://www.icd9data.com. Accessed July 10, 2013.
2. ICD10Data.com. http://www.icd10data.com. Accessed July 10, 2013.
3. *Guide to Physical Therapist Practice*. 2nd ed. Alexandria, VA: American Physical Therapy Association; 2001. Revised 2003.
4. American Trauma Society. www.amtrauma.org. Accessed July 10, 2013.

ADDITIONAL REFERENCES

- Barthel Index. StrokEngine. http://www.medicine.mcgill.ca/strokengine-assess/module_bi_intro-en.html. Accessed July 10, 2013.
- Biros MH, Heegaard WE. Head injury. In: Marx JA, ed. *Rosen's Emergency Medicine: Concepts and Clinical Practice*. 7th ed. Philadelphia, PA: Mosby Elsevier; 2009.
- Components of the Gait Assessment Rating Score (GARS). University of Missouri. http://web.missouri.edu/~proste/tool/GARS.pdf. Accessed July 10, 2013.
- Dutton M, ed. *Orthopaedic Examination, Evaluation, and Intervention*. 2nd ed. New York, NY: McGraw-Hill; 2008. http://www.accessphysiotherapy.com/content/55601056. Accessed July 10, 2013.
- Functional Independence Measure (FIM). StrokEngine. http://www.medicine.mcgill.ca/strokengine-assess/module_fim_intro-en.html. Accessed July 10, 2013.
- Hay WW, Levin MJ, Sondheimer JM, Deterding RR. Rehabilitation medicine. In: Hay WW, Levin MJ, Sondheimer JM, Deterding RR, eds. *CURRENT Diagnosis & Treatment: Pediatrics*. 20th ed. New York, NY: McGraw-Hill; 2011:Chapter 26. http://www.accessphysiotherapy.com/content/6586370. Accessed July 10, 2013.
- Introduction to the Extended Glasgow Outcome Scale. The center for outcome measurement in brain injury. http://tbims.org/combi/gose/index.html. Accessed July 10, 2013.
- Introduction to the High Level Mobility Assessment Tool. The center for outcome measurement in brain injury. http://tbims.org/combi/himat/index.html. Accessed July 10, 2013.
- Leveque JC. Hoff JT. Neurosurgery. In: Greenfield LJ, Mulholland MW, Oldham KT, Zelenock GB, Lillemoe KD, eds. *Greenfield's Surgery: Scientific Principles and Practice*. 4th ed. Philadelphia, PA: Lippincott Williams & Wilkins; 2005.
- Malone TR, Hazle C, Grey ML. Imaging of the brain. In: Malone TR, Hazle C, Grey ML, eds. *Imaging in Rehabilitation*. New York, NY: McGraw-Hill; 2008:Chapter 2. http://www.accessphysiotherapy.com/content/5940267. Accessed July 10, 2013.
- Motor Assessment Scale (MAS). StrokEngine. http://www.medicine.mcgill.ca/strokengine-assess/module_mas_intro-en.html. Accessed July 10, 2013.
- Multidirectional Reach Test. Temple University Gait Study Center. http://podiatry.temple.edu/research/gait-study-center/techniques-and-methods/multi-directional-reach-test. Accessed May 14, 2014.
- Observational Gait Analysis. University of Oklahoma Health Sciences Center. http://moon.ouhsc.edu/dthompso/gait/knmatics/oga.htm. Accessed July 10, 2013.
- Panus PC, Jobst EE, Masters SB, Katzung B, Tinsley SL, Trevor AJ, eds. *Pharmacology for the Physical Therapist*. New York, NY: McGraw-Hill; 2009. http://www.accessphysiotherapy.com/content/6091942. Accessed July 10, 2013.
- Rancho Los Amigos Cognitive Scale Revised. Northeast Center for Special Care. http://www.northeastcenter.com/rancho_los_amigos_revised.htm. Accessed July 10, 2013.
- Ropper AL, Samuels MA. *Adams and Victor's Principles of Neurology*. 9th ed. New York, NY: McGraw-Hill; 2009:846–873.
- Shamus E, Stern DF. Content standardization/component requirements. In: Shamus E, Stern DF, eds. *Effective Documentation for Physical Therapy Professionals*. 2nd ed. New York, NY: McGraw-Hill; 2011:Chapter 4. http://www.accessphysiotherapy.com/content/55665293. Accessed July 10, 2013.
- Six-minute Walk Test (6MWT). StrokEngine. http://www.medicine.mcgill.ca/strokengine-assess/module_6mwt_intro-en.html. Accessed July 10, 2013.
- Testing Spasticity. The Modified Ashworth Scale. Advance for Physical Therapy and Rehab Medicine. http://physical-therapy.advanceweb.com/Article/Testing-Spasticity-The-Modified-Ashworth-Scale.aspx. Accessed July 10, 2013.
- Tinetti Balance and Gait Evaluation. http://www.bhps.org.uk/falls/documents/TinettiBalanceAssessment.pdf. Accessed July 10, 2013.
- Waxman SG. Imaging of the brain. In: Waxman SG, ed. *Clinical Neuroanatomy*. 26th ed. New York, NY: McGraw-Hill; 2010: Chapter 22. http://www.accessphysiotherapy.com/content/5275385. Accessed July 10, 2013.
- Winkler PA. Traumatic brain injury. In: Umphred DA, eds. *Neurological Rehabilitation*. 5th ed. St. Louis, MO: Mosby Elsevier; 2007: 532–566.

111 TEMPOROMANDIBULAR JOINT DISORDERS

Eric Shamus, PhD, DPT, PT, CSCS
Ilan Shamus, DDS

CONDITION/DISORDER SYNONYMS

- Costen syndrome
- Temporomandibular joint dysfunction (TMJD)
- Temporomandibular joint dysfunction syndrome
- Temporomandibular joint internal derangement
- Temporomandibular joint pain

ICD-9-CM CODES[1]

- 524.6 Temporomandibular joint disorders
- 524.60 Temporomandibular joint disorders, unspecified
- 524.61 Temporomandibular joint disorders, adhesions and ankylosis (bony or fibrous)
- 524.62 Temporomandibular joint disorders, arthralgia of temporomandibular joint
- 524.63 Temporomandibular joint disorders, articular disk disorder (reducing or nonreducing)
- 524.64 Temporomandibular joint disorders, temporomandibular joint sounds on opening and/or closing the jaw
- 524.69 Other specified temporomandibular joint disorders

ICD-10-CM CODES[2]

- M26.60 Temporomandibular joint disorder, unspecified
- M26.61 Adhesions and ankylosis of temporomandibular joint
- M26.62 Arthralgia of temporomandibular joint
- M26.63 Articular disk disorder of temporomandibular joint
- M26.69 Other specified disorders of temporomandibular joint

PREFERRED PRACTICE PATTERNS[3]

- 4D: Impaired Joint Mobility, Motor Function, Muscle Performance, and Range of Motion Associated with Connective Tissue Dysfunction
- 4E: Impaired Joint Mobility, Motor Function, Muscle Performance, and Range of Motion Associated with Localized Inflammation

PATIENT PRESENTATION

A 32-year-old female presents at the clinic with right lateral jaw pain. The patient states she thought she had an ear infection, but the family physician stated the ear was clear. She states she has been under a lot of stress. Her husband states she grinds her teeth at night. Patient has complaints of headaches and difficulty eating apples that are uncut. Upon opening of her jaw, it is noted that the mandible deviates to the left.

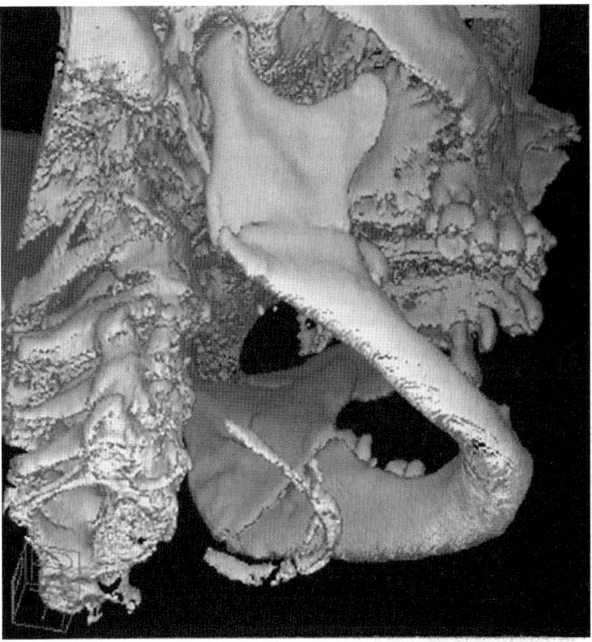

FIGURE 111-1 This three-dimensional CT image reveals fractures of the mandibular angles bilaterally. (From Malone TR, Hazle C, Grey ML. *Imaging in Rehabilitation*. http://accessphysiotherapy.com. Copyright © The McGraw-Hill Companies, Inc. All rights reserved.)

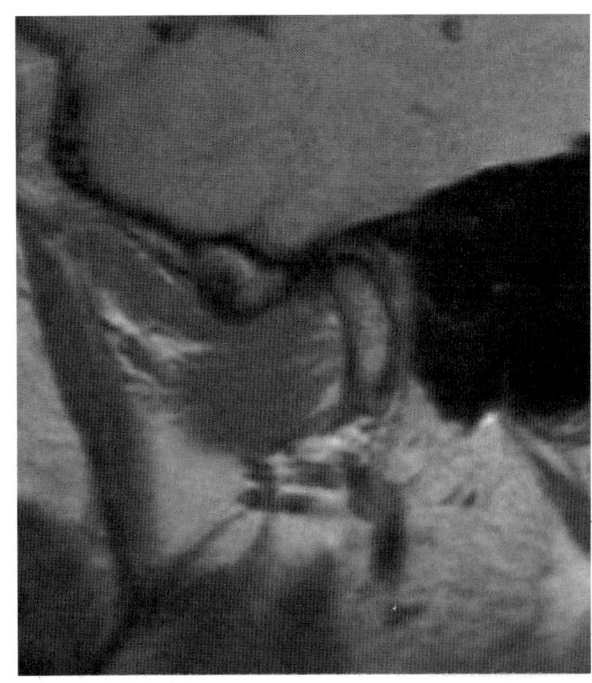

FIGURE 111-2 In this sagittal MRI of a 36-year-old female, the disk on the asymptomatic right is positioned normally in the fossa superior to the mandibular condyle. (From Malone TR, Hazle C, Grey ML. *Imaging in Rehabilitation*. http://accessphysiotherapy.com. Copyright © The McGraw-Hill Companies, Inc. All rights reserved.)

KEY FEATURES

Description

- Often referred to as TMJ (temporomandibular joint) which is the name of the joint, but does not describe any specific dysfunction
- Syndrome is an umbrella term describing acute or chronic inflammation of the TMJ
- Diagnosis covers an array or acute or chronic problems of the TMJ
- Originally described by James B. Costen in 1934 and initially known as Costen syndrome
- Five stages of disk displacement

Essentials of Diagnosis

- Dysfunction of the joint, muscle imbalances[4]
- Alignment problems between the temporal and mandible bones and the cervical spine

General Considerations

- The TMJ has two joints, allowing one to rotate and slide (translate)
- Ligament laxity and disk desiccation need to be assessed
- Wear of the bone and cartilage can lead to popping, clicking, and pain

Demographics

- Women more likely than men
- Age range: 20 to 40 years of age

CLINICAL FINDINGS

SIGNS AND SYMPTOMS

- Audible click/pop with opening and closing of the jaw
- Can involve one or more of the TMJ components such as the muscles, nerves, tendons, ligaments, bones, and teeth[4]
- Crepitus
- Deviation of the mandible with opening and closing
- Ear pain, ache (otalgia), and ear swelling
- Grinding
- Headaches/migraines
- Hypertonicity of the pterygoids and masseter muscles
- Inability to open/close jaw/locking
- Malalignment of the teeth
- Orofacial pain
- Reciprocal clip
- Swelling, heat, redness at the TMJ
- Tinnitus
- Trigeminal nerve issues, cranial nerve (CN) V
- Wearing of the teeth, flattening of the top of the teeth

Functional Implications

- Inability to bite/eat larger objects such as an apple
- Headaches that limit function
- Locking of the jaw

Possible Contributing Causes

- Blunt trauma, punch or hit to the face increased lateral movement of the mandible
- Degenerative joint disease
- Developmental abnormality
- Disorders to the teeth such as tooth mobility or loss
- Excessive gum chewing or nail biting
- Flattened mandible
- Grinding or clinching of the teeth, bruxism
- Jaw thrusting from tongue and speech problems

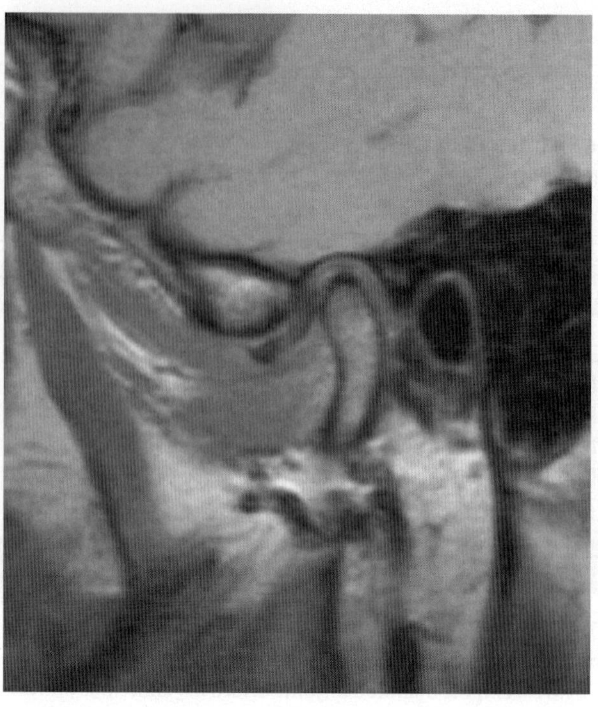

FIGURE 111-3 On the symptomatic left during closure, note the anterior position of the disk in comparison to the asymptomatic side. (From Malone TR, Hazle C, Grey ML. *Imaging in Rehabilitation*. http://accessphysiotherapy.com. Copyright © The McGraw-Hill Companies, Inc. All rights reserved.)

- Lack of an overbite
- Ligament laxity
- Malalignment, from bridge, overlay, or crown that alters bite and pressures
- Muscle imbalances; head, neck
- Opening jaw extra wide, over-opening such as when biting into an apple

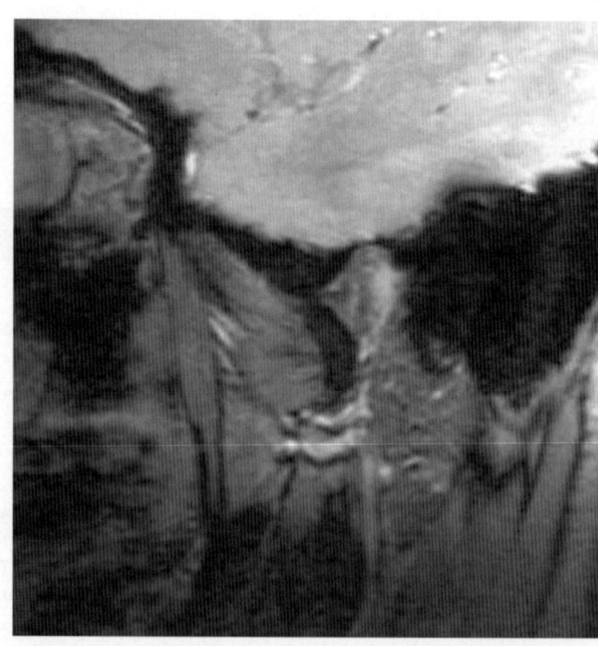

FIGURE 111-4 In this image, captured during opening movement, the disk on the asymptomatic right is properly positioned between the mandibular condyle and articular eminence. (From Malone TR, Hazle C, Grey ML. *Imaging in Rehabilitation*. http://accessphysiotherapy.com. Copyright © The McGraw-Hill Companies, Inc. All rights reserved.)

- Osteoarthritis
- Poor kyphotic posture with forward head
- Poor occlusion
- Previous orthodontic work, wisdom teeth extraction
- Rheumatoid arthritis
- Size of food eaten and bites eaten
- Stress
- Trauma
- Wearing of articular surfaces
- Whiplash

Differential Diagnosis

- Bells palsy
- Cavity
- Ear infection
- Gum disease
- Sinus infection/problem
- Tooth infection
- Trigeminal neuralgia

MEANS OF CONFIRMATION OF DIAGNOSIS

Imaging

- X-ray
- MRI
- CT scan

FINDINGS AND INTERPRETATION

- Osteoarthritis or rheumatoid arthritis in the joint
- Dislocation of the disc

TREATMENT

Medication

- NSAIDs
- Tricyclic antidepressants (muscle relaxants)

MEDICAL PROCEDURES

- Arthrocentesis (joint irrigation under anesthesia)
- Arthroscopic
- Reposition jaw or replace the disk
- Radio wave therapy

REFERRALS/ADMITTANCE

- To orthodontist for alignment issues of the teeth
- To oral surgeon for arthroscopic surgery

IMPAIRMENTS

- The temporomandibular joint can lock which limits eating, chewing, talking, and yawning.
- Restricted jaw function.

TESTS AND MEASURES

- Opening width measurement in millimeters
- Deviation measurement in millimeters
- Trigeminal nerve assessment
- Medical screening questionnaire

INTERVENTION

- Orthodontics
  - Occlusal splint, night guard

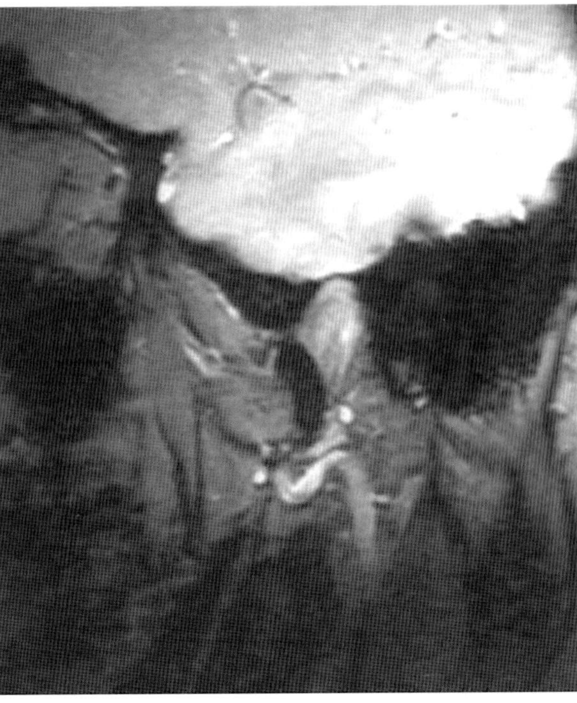

FIGURE 111-5 This image on the symptomatic left, also captured during opening movement, reveals a forwardly displaced disk which is folding and kinking. The findings of the images are consistent with disk displacement without reduction. (From Malone TR, Hazle C, Grey ML. *Imaging in Rehabilitation*. http://accessphysiotherapy.com. Copyright © The McGraw-Hill Companies, Inc. All rights reserved.)

  - Splint therapy: Mandibular repositioning devices
  - Restoring teeth position
- Elimination of parafunctional habits
  - Clenching, grinding, lip or cheek biting, forward jaw posturing
  - Biofeedback to relax the muscles and bruxism
  - Stress reduction
- Inflammation
  - Ice
  - Ultrasound
  - Iontophoresis
- Manual therapy
  - Joint mobilization for disk position
  - Release techniques for hypertonicity of muscles
  - Upper-cervical spine
  - Craniosacral therapy
  - Trigger point therapy

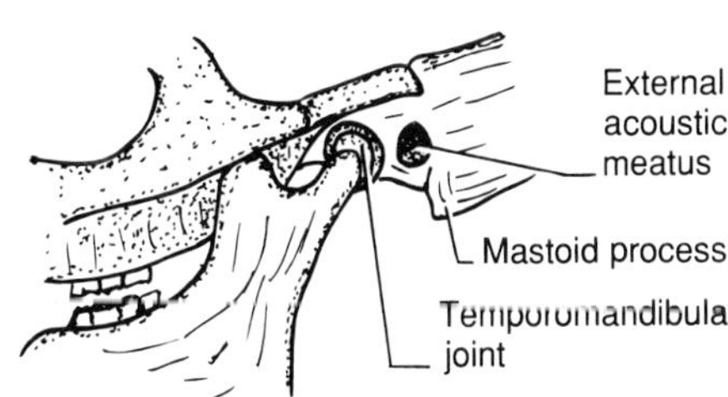

FIGURE 111-6 Anatomy of the TMJ. Note the nearness of the joint to the external acoustic meatus, so the joint may be palpated by a finger in the meatus. (From LeBlond RF, DeGowin RL, Brown DD. *DeGowin's Diagnostic Examination*. 9th ed. http://www.accessmedicine.com. Copyright © The McGraw-Hill Companies, Inc. All rights reserved.)

- Therapeutic procedure
  - Muscle balance training
  - Feldenkrais TMJ program
  - Isometric muscle balance strengthening
  - Postural training
  - Exercises; perform six times each at a frequency of six times per day
    - Tongue rest position and nasal breathing
    - Controlled opening
    - Rhythmic stabilization
    - Liberation of cervical extension
    - Axial neck extension
    - Shoulder retraction

FUNCTIONAL GOALS

- Patient will be able to
  - Identify appropriate foods and size to eat.
  - Control the amount of opening to limit disk slippage.
  - Eat, pain free.
  - Eliminate joint locking.

PROGNOSIS

- Good, with a combination of muscle relaxation, bite alignment, muscle balance, and avoidance of irritating activities.

PATIENT RESOURCE

- TMJ Disorder. The TMJ Association. http://www.tmj.org/site. Accessed July 14, 2013.

REFERENCES

1. ICD9Data.com. http://www.icd9data.com. Accessed July 14, 2013.
2. ICD10Data.com. http://www.icd10data.com. Accessed July 14, 2013.
3. *Guide to Physical Therapist Practice*. 2nd ed. Alexandria, VA: American Physical Therapy Association; 2001. Revised 2003.
4. Dutton M. The temporomandibular joint. In: Dutton M, ed. *Dutton's Orthopaedic Examination, Evaluation, and Intervention*. 3rd ed. New York, NY: McGraw-Hill; 2012:Chapter 24. http://www.accessphysiotherapy.com/content/55592810. Accessed July 14, 2013.

ADDITIONAL REFERENCES

- Carlsson SG, Gale EW. Biofeedback in the treatment of long-term temporomandibular joint pain: an outcome study. *Biofeedback Self Regul.* 1977;2(2):161–165.
- Clark GT, Adachi NY, Dornan MR. Physical medicine procedures affect temporomandibular disorders: a review. *J Am Dent Assoc.* 1990;121(1):151–161.
- Gardea MA, Gatchel RJ, Mishra KD. Long-term efficacy of biobehavioral treatment of temporomandibular disorders. *J Behav Med.* 2001;24(4):341–359.
- Kight M, Gatchel RJ, Wesley L. Temporomandibular disorders: evidence for significant overlap with psychopathology. *Health Psychol.* 1999;18(2):177–182.
- Korszun A, Papadopoulos E, Demitrack M, et al. The relationship between temporomandibular disorders and stress-associated syndromes. *Oral Surg Oral Med Oral Pathol Oral Radiol Endod.* 1998;86(4):416–420.

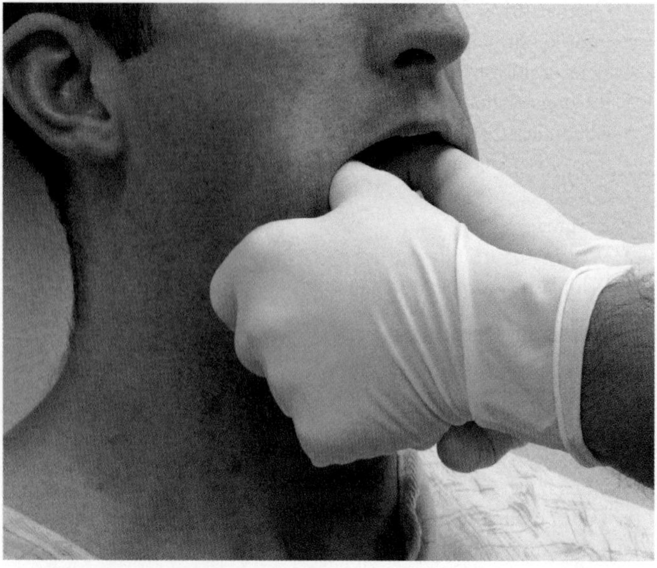

FIGURE 111-7 Reduction of dislocated mandible technique in a seated patient. The thumbs are placed over the molars, and pressure is applied downward and backward. (From Tintinalli JE, Stapczynski J, Ma OJ, Cline D, Cydulka R, Meckler G. *Tintinalli's Emergency Medicine: A Comprehensive Study Guide.* 7th ed. http://www.accessmedicine.com. Copyright © The McGraw-Hill Companies, Inc. All rights reserved.)

- Linde C, Isacsson G, Jonsson BG. Outcome of 6-week treatment with transcutaneous electric nerve stimulation compared with splint on symptomatic temporomandibular joint disk displacement without reduction. *Acta Odontol Scand.* 1995;53(2): 92–98.
- Malone TR, Hazle C, Grey ML. Imaging of the cervical spine and temporomandibular joint. In: Malone TR, Hazle C, Grey ML, eds. *Imaging in Rehabilitation*. New York, NY: McGraw-Hill; 2008:Chapter 3. http://www.accessphysiotherapy.com/content/5940352. Accessed July 14, 2013.
- Mohl ND, Ohrbach RK, Crow HC, et al. Devices for the diagnosis and treatment of temporomandibular disorders, III: thermography, ultrasound, electrical stimulation, and electromyographic biofeedback. *J Prosthet Dent.* 1990;(6395):472–477.
- Murphy GJ. Electrical physical therapy in treating TMJ patients. *J Craniomand Pract.* 1983;2(8341):67–73.
- Patel DR, Greydanus DE, Baker RJ. Maxillofacial and dental injuries. In: Patel DR, Greydanus DE, Baker RJ, eds. *Pediatric Practice: Sports Medicine*. New York, NY: McGraw-Hill; 2009: Chapter 33. http://www.accessphysiotherapy.com/abstract/6981877#6981877. Accessed July 14, 2013.
- Schiffman EL. The role of the randomized clinical trial in evaluating management strategies for temporomandibular disorders. In: Fricton JR, Dubner R, eds. *Orofacial pain and temporomandibular disorders* (advances in pain research and therapy, Vol 21). New York, NY: Raven Press; 1995:415–63.
- Simon EP, Lewis DM. Medical hypnosis for temporomandibular disorders: treatment efficacy and medical utilization outcome. *Oral Surg Oral Med Oral Pathol Oral Radiol Endod.* 2000;90 (1):54–63.
- Tegelberg A, Kopp S. Short-term effect of physical training on temporomandibular joint disorder in individuals with rheumatoid arthritis and ankylosing spondylitis. *Acta Odontol Scand.* 1988; 46(1):49–51.

SECTION B SPINE DISORDERS

112 ANKYLOSING SPONDYLITIS

Eric Shamus, PhD, DPT, PT, CSCS
Kathy Swanick, DPT, PT, OCS

CONDITION/DISORDER SYNONYMS

- Bekhterev disease
- Bekhterev syndrome
- Marie-Strümpell disease
- Rheumatoid spondylitis
- Spondylitis
- Spondyloarthropathy

ICD-9-CM CODE[1]

- 720.0 Ankylosing spondylitis

ICD-10-CM CODE[2]

- M45.9 Ankylosing spondylitis of unspecified sites in spine

PREFERRED PRACTICE PATTERNS[3]

- 4B: Impaired Posture
- 4E: Impaired Joint Mobility, Motor Function, Muscle Performance, and ROM Associated with Localized Inflammation
- 4F: Impaired Joint Mobility, Motor Function, Muscle Performance, Range of Motion, and Reflex Integrity Associated with Spinal Disorders

PATIENT PRESENTATION

A 33-year-old female presents with complaints of low back pain with insidious onset and duration of over 3 months. She reports that her neck is also stiff, and driving a car has been difficult. She works for a company that provides computer technical support to many local businesses and needs to drive for her work. She has morning stiffness that generally improves with activity and exercise. There has also been a recent onset of swelling in the left knee and heel pain. There are times when the pain wakes her from sleep in the middle of the night; however, if she gets up and walks around or takes a hot shower, her pain is relieved enough to be able to go back to sleep.

She is referred to physical therapy by her rheumatologist, and has the results of several tests. Pulmonary function tests show decreased vital capacity and total lung capacity, although residual and functional residual lung volumes were increased. Hematology tests showed a mild normocytic anemia, and a normal white count. Erythrocyte sedimentation rate and alkaline and creatinine phosphatase were elevated. There was no rheumatoid factor present. Posture shows a flattening of the lumbar lordosis and a dorsal stooping posture with an accentuation of the thoracic kyphosis. There is tenderness over the spinous processes of the lumbar and thoracic vertebrae. A bony spur is palpated at the right heel at the proximal insertion of the plantar fascia. AROM is severely diminished lateral flexion of the spine, forward flexion and extension are decreased by 50%. Left knee ROM is decreased both actively and passively by 10 degrees.

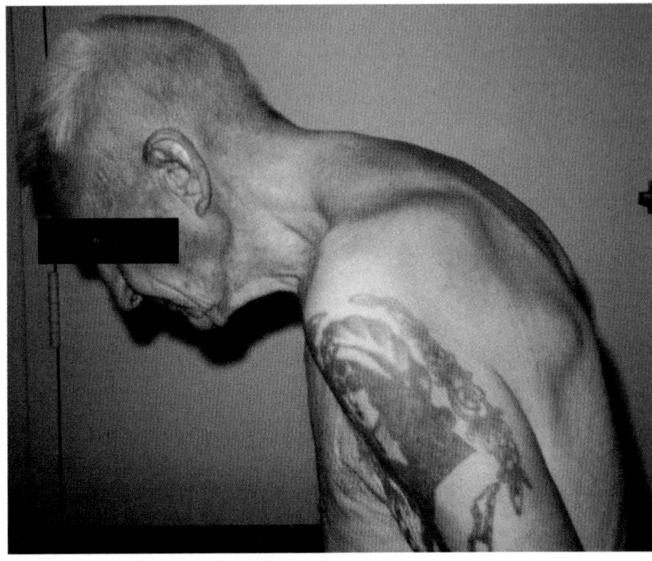

FIGURE 112-1 Ankylosing spondylitis: an immobile, curved spine with forward jutting of the head. It can be seen with atrioventricular block or aortic regurgitation. (From Fuster V, Walsh RA, Harrington RA. *Hurst's The Heart*. 13th ed. www.accessmedicine.com. Copyright © The McGraw-Hill Companies, Inc. All rights reserved.)

KEY FEATURES

Description

- Progressive inflammation of the spinal joints that leads to bone formation, natural fusion, and often increased kyphosis of the thoracic spine.
- *Ankylosing* means fusion; *spondylitis* means inflammation of the spine.

Essentials of Diagnosis[4]

- Characterized by SI joint pain and dysfunction[4]
- Etiology unknown
- Pain for >3 months
- Relief with NSAIDs

General Considerations

- Begins with intermittent low back pain
- Pain and stiffness at rest or sleep

- Improvement with low levels of activity
- May have rapid and severe onset
- Secondary problems include
  - Pulmonary fibrosis
  - Restrictive lung disease
  - Aortic heart valve (aortic insufficiency)
  - Heart rhythm problems

Demographics

- Disease onset between ages 20 and 40 years
- Male-to-female ratio: 10:1
- Caucasians afflicted more frequently than African Americans

CLINICAL FINDINGS

SIGNS AND SYMPTOMS

- Fatigue
- Decreased range of motion and joint play
- Intermittent back pain
- Eye inflammation
- Heel pain
- Hip pain and stiffness
- Joint pain and swelling in the shoulders, knees, and ankles
- Loss of appetite
- Slight fever
- Weight loss
- Morning stiffness
- Acute painful flare-ups and chronic, persistent pain
- Thoracic and Pulmonary involvement

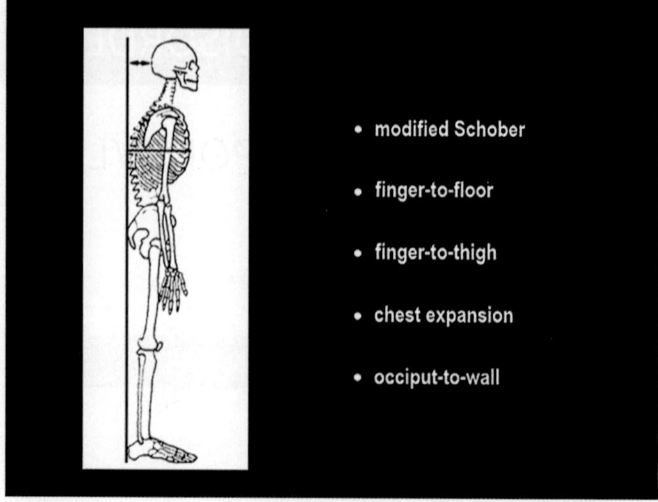

• modified Schober
• finger-to-floor
• finger-to-thigh
• chest expansion
• occiput-to-wall

FIGURE 112-2 Postural assessment parameters. (From Lawry GV. *Systematic Musculoskeletal Examinations*. www.accessmedicine.com. Copyright © The McGraw-Hill Companies, Inc. All rights reserved.)

Functional Implications

- Limited mobility
- Aerobic endurance limitation

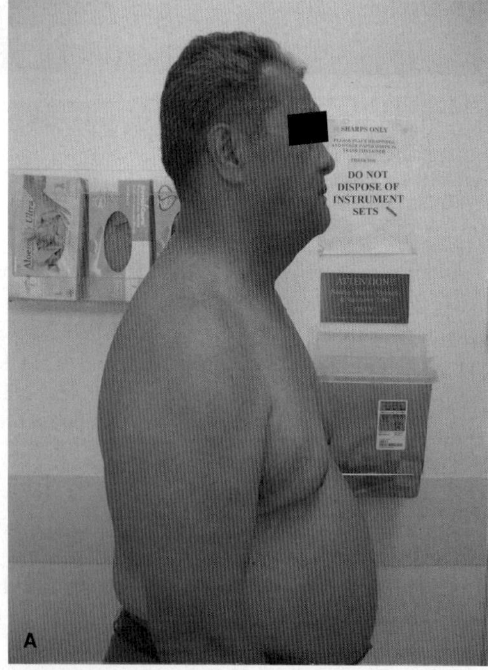

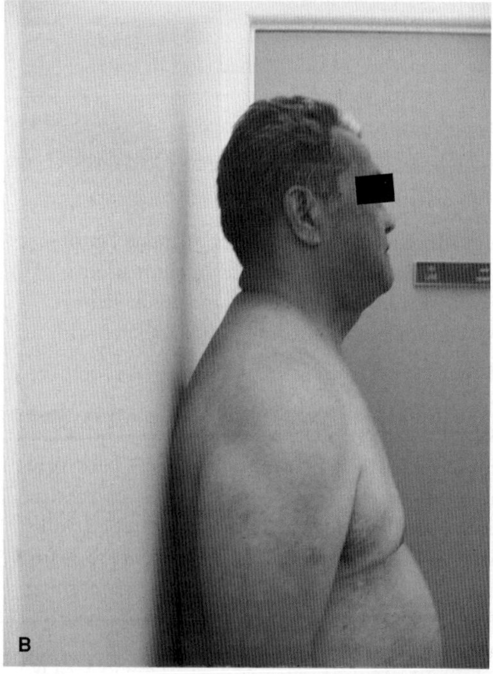

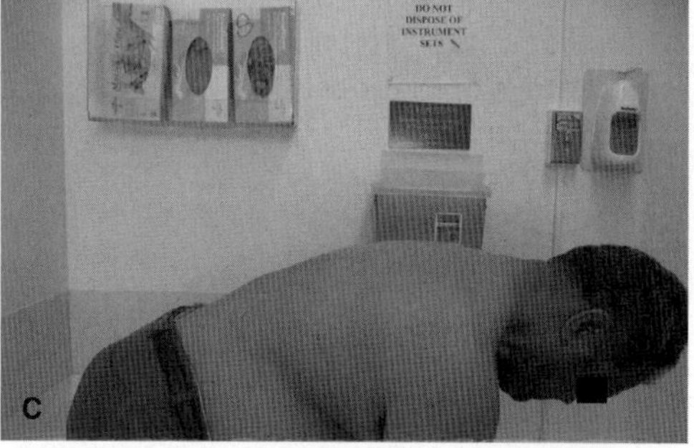

FIGURE 112-3 Long-standing ankylosing spondylitis. Despite extensive spinal involvement the patient has maintained an upright posture with only a slightly exaggerated thoracic kyphosis (**A**). The occiput-to-wall test, however, reveals marked reduction of cervical extension (**B**). Fusion of the lumbar spine causes straightening of the lower back and an inability to reverse the lumbar lordosis when the patient attempts to touch his toes with knees extended (**C**). (Courtesy of Dr. Lianne S. Wener, University of California, San Francisco.)

Possible Contributing Causes

- Family history of ankylosing spondylitis
- GI infections

Differential Diagnosis

- Spinal stenosis
- Disc herniation
- Crohn disease
- Forestier disease
- Reiter syndrome (reactive arthritis)
- Whipple disease
- Yersinia arthritis
- Facet joint arthritis
- Psoriatic arthritis
- Rheumatoid arthritis

MEANS OF CONFIRMATION OR DIAGNOSIS

Imaging

- X-ray of the spine and pelvis
- MRI of the spine

Laboratory Tests

- Complete blood count (CBC)
- ESR
- HLA-B27 antigen, genetic marker
- No single blood test
- Negative serologic tests for rheumatoid factor

FINDINGS AND INTERPRETATION

- Late stages affect C1-C2 segment with decreased range of motion[5]

TREATMENT

Medication

- NSAIDs
- TNF-inhibitors
- Corticosteroids
- Cytotoxic drugs
- Biologic medications

REFERRALS/ADMITTANCE

- Rheumatologist to assess underlying complications
- Surgical consult
- Ophthalmologist for eye symptoms

IMPAIRMENTS

- Mobility
- Functional rotation and bending

TESTS AND MEASURES

- Straight-leg raise
- Sit and reach test
- Trunk active range of motion (AROM)

INTERVENTION

- Education in gentle range of motion to maintain mobility
- Flexibility and stability strengthening exercises to decrease stress on the joints
  - Core stabilization
- Education on joint protection
- Postural training
- Warm shower or heat to increase mobility

FUNCTIONAL GOALS

- Patient will be able to.
  - Be independent with home exercise program.
  - Have decreased pain and be able to perform household activities, such as cleaning and laundry.
  - Have improved functional level sufficient for grocery shopping.

PROGNOSIS

- Disease progression is not specific; joints may become fused as disease becomes more severe.
- Symptoms may be intermittent.
- Patients function well until severe progression of joint fusion in the spine and hips occurs.

PATIENT RESOURCES

- Ankylosing Spondylitis. NIH, National Institute of Arthritis and Musculoskeletal and Skin Diseases. http://www.niams.nih.gov/health_info/Ankylosing_Spondylitis/default.asp. Accessed March 1, 2013.
- Spondylitis Association of America. http://www.spondylitis.org. Accessed January 14, 2013.
- Safety and Effectiveness of Adalimumab (Humira) in Patients with Ankylosing Spondylitis in Clinical Routine. http://clinicaltrialsfeeds.org/clinical-trials/show/NCT01079182. Accessed January 14, 2013.

REFERENCES

1. ICD-9-CM. http://www.icd9data.com. Accessed March 1, 2013.
2. ICD-10-CM. http://www.icd10data.com. Accessed March 1, 2013.
3. APTA Guide to Physical Therapist Practice. http://guidetoptpractice.apta.org./ Accessed March 1, 2013.
4. Dutton M. The sacroiliac joint. In: Dutton M, ed. *Dutton's Orthopaedic Examination, Evaluation, and Intervention*. 3rd ed. New York, NY: McGraw-Hill; 2012:Chapter 27. http://www.accessphysiotherapy.com/content/55597747. Accessed January 27, 2013.
5. Dutton M. Differential diagnosis. In: Dutton M, ed. *Dutton's Orthopaedic Examination, Evaluation, and Intervention*. 3rd ed. New York, NY: McGraw-Hill; 2012:Chapter 9. http://www.accessphysiotherapy.com/content/5545886. Accessed January 27, 2013.

ADDITIONAL REFERENCE

- Dutton M. Musculoskeletal physical therapy. In: Dutton M, ed. *McGraw-Hill's NPTE (National Physical Therapy Examination)*. 2nd ed. New York, NY: McGraw-Hill; 2012:Chapter 8. http://www.accessphysiotherapy.com/content/5397601. Accessed January 27, 2013.

113 CERVICAL FACET JOINT SYNDROME

Arie J. Van Duijn, EdD, MSc, PT, OCS
Eric Shamus, PhD, DPT, PT, CSCS

CONDITION/DISORDER SYNONYMS

- Facet joint syndrome, cervical spine
- Sprain of facet joint
- Arthritic changes in facet joint

ICD-9-CM CODE

- 847.0 Cervical sprain

ICD-10-CM CODE

- S13.8XXA Sprain of joints and ligaments of other parts of neck

PREFERRED PRACTICE PATTERN

- 4F: Impaired Joint Mobility, Motor Function, Muscle Performance, Range of Motion, and Reflex Integrity Associated With Spinal Disorders[1]

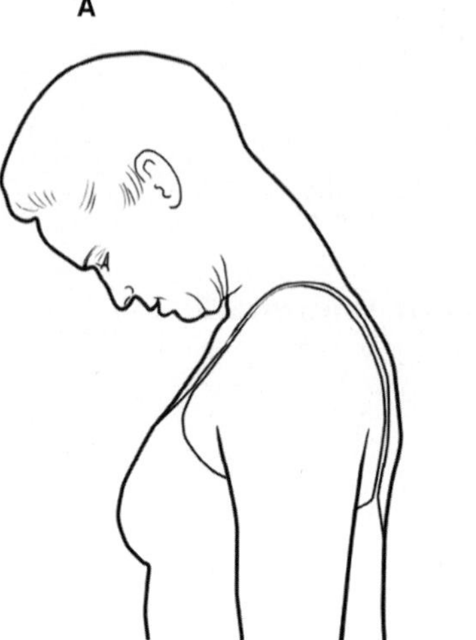

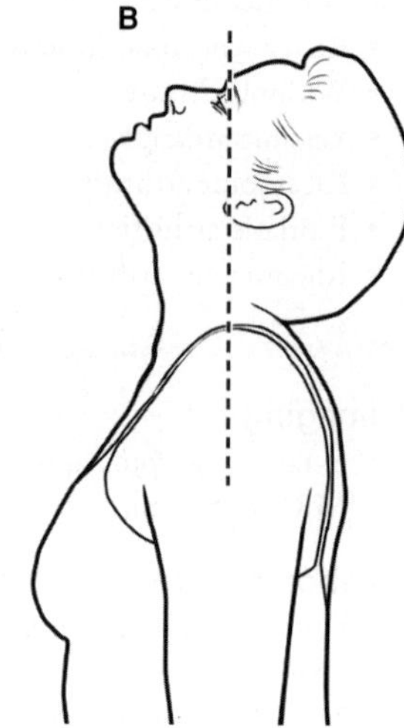

FIGURE 113-2 Flexion and extension of the cervical spine. Normal flexion brings the chin to within a fingerbreadth of the chest (**A**). With normal extension of the neck, an imaginary line should connect the eye, ear lobe, and shoulder (**B**). (From Imboden J, Hellmann DB, Stone JH. *Current Rheumatology Diagnosis & Treatment*. 2nd ed. www.accessmedicine.com. Copyright © The McGraw-Hill Companies, Inc. All rights reserved.)

PATIENT PRESENTATION

A 45-year-old male presents with pain and stiffness in the left cervical region. He reports waking up with this condition 3 days ago. The pain is located along the left C3-4 and C4-5 spinal segments, and is aggravated by looking over the left shoulder and looking up. Increased muscle tone is present in the left levator scapula and upper trapezius muscles. No pain, numbness, or tingling in the upper extremities is noted, and neurological examination is normal. Passive intervertebral motion (PIVM) testing reveals restriction in downglide mobility of the left C3-4 facet joint. Quadrant testing is positive when combining extension, left side bending, and left rotation. Point tenderness is noted upon palpation of the left C3-4 facet joint.

KEY FEATURES

Description

- Neck pain with primary involvement of cervical facet joint
- Upper limb symptoms might be present in a nondermatomal pattern as a result of referred pain

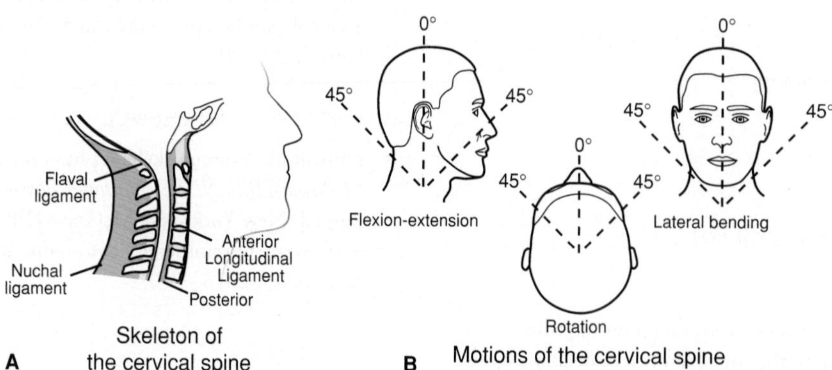

FIGURE 113-1 Anatomy and motions of the cervical spine. (**A**) The skeleton of the cervical spine. (**B**) Motions of the cervical spine: normal range of motion exceeds the angles, which are shown as points of reference. (From LeBlond RF, DeGowin RL, Brown DD. *DeGowin's Diagnostic Examination*. 9th ed. www.accessmedicine.com. Copyright © The McGraw-Hill Companies, Inc. All rights reserved.)

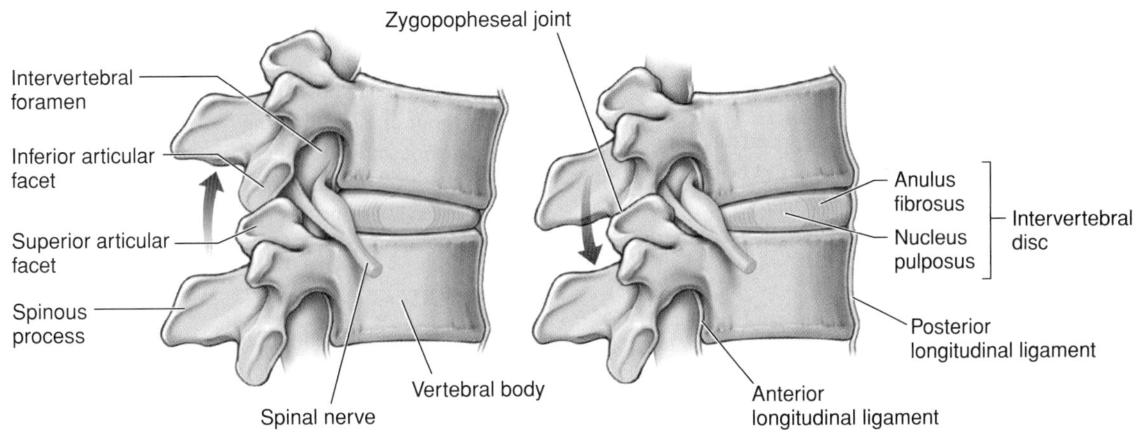

FIGURE 113-3 The intervertebral disk, articulations, ligaments, and neurologic structures. (Reproduced with permission from Morton, DA, Foreman KB, Albertine KH. *The Big Picture: Gross Anatomy,* McGraw-Hill; 2011.)

- No neurological findings
- Unilateral symptoms

Essentials of Diagnosis

- Diagnosis made by clinical examination
- Reproduction of symptoms when joint in closed-packed position (combination of extension, side bending, and rotation toward involved side)

General Considerations

- Presentation can vary based on anatomical structures and psychosocial factors.
- C0 to C3 facet joint dysfunction may be associated with cervicogenic headache or dizziness.

Demographics

- Variable, based on specific condition.

CLINICAL FINDINGS

SIGNS AND SYMPTOMS

- Pain in cervical area that can be reproduced mechanically
- Unilateral or bilateral referred pain in upper extremities possible in a nonradicular pattern
- Active range of motion (AROM) limited in a capsular pattern; rotation and side bending limited in same direction
- Cervical segmental hypomobility may be present in capsular pattern
- Can be associated with forward-head posture

Functional Implications

- May cause decreased ability to perform ADLs/IADLs.
- May impact ability to participate in sports and other recreational activities.

Possible Contributing Causes

- Congenital anomalies
- Obesity
- Occupational factors
- Physical condition
- Postural changes including forward-head posture
- Psychosocial and behavioral factors
- Smoking
- Socioeconomic factors

Differential Diagnosis

- Malignant spinal tumor or metastasis
- Peripheral nerve impairment
- Radiculopathy
- Referred pain from visceral structures
- Systematic autoimmune diseases (RA, Reiter's, etc.)

MEANS OF CONFIRMATION OR DIAGNOSIS

Imaging

- Not necessary in most cases; only with persistent symptoms that do not respond to conservative management or presence of red/yellow flags.

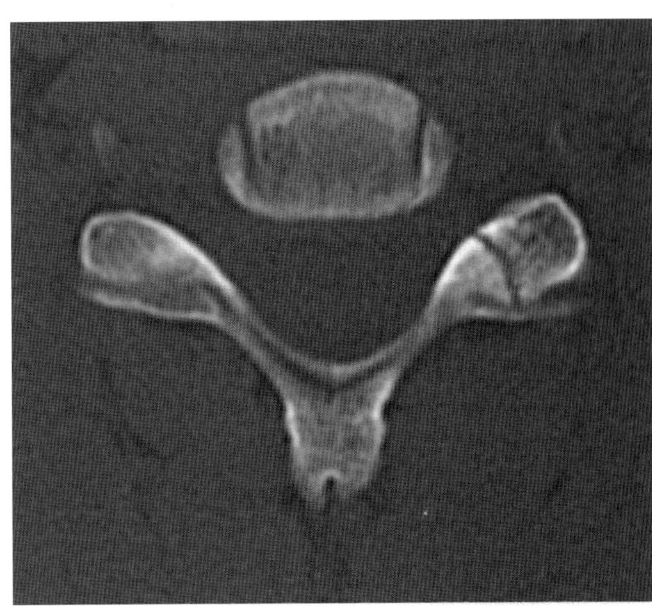

FIGURE 113-4 The axial CT image of the C6 vertebra in this image reveals a fracture of the zygapophysial joint surface. (From Malone TR, Hazle C, Grey ML. *Imaging in Rehabilitation*. www.accessphysiotherapy.com. Copyright © The McGraw-Hill Companies, Inc. All rights reserved.)

- MRI helps visualize compressed or inflamed nerve root/disc pathology in diagnosis[2]
- X-ray/Plain-film radiograph helps assess alignment, fractures, stability (flexion/extension radiograph)[3]
- CT scan to show herniation compressing the spinal canal or nerves[3]
- Electrodiagnostic/Nerve conduction testing can help determine a specific impaired nerve function[4]
- Doppler ultrasound to examine vascular function

Diagnostic Procedures

- Electrodiagnostic/Nerve conduction testing can help determine a specific impaired nerve function[4]

FINDINGS AND INTERPRETATION

- Physical Examination
  - Algorithm for examination of the cervical spine[4]

TREATMENT

Medication

- Nonsteroidal anti-inflammatory drugs (NSAIDs)
- Corticosteroids

REFERRALS/ADMITTANCE

- For imaging
- For surgical consult if myelopathy suspected (lumbar radiculopathy)
- For imaging and medical consult if disease suspected
- If vascular insufficiency suspected

IMPAIRMENTS

- Hypomobile cervical spine
- Weakness of deep neck flexors and upper-extremity stabilizers
- Shortening of upper trapezius, levator scapulae, pectoral muscles
- Postural changes
- Inability to rotate head

TESTS AND MEASURES

- Cervical spine AROM
- Sharp–Purser: Atlantoaxial instability
- Cervical passive intervertebral motion testing
- Sub-cranial translation instability testing
- Passive physiological intervertebral mobility testing (PPIVM)[5]
- Upper-extremity screening examination
- Postural examination
- Muscle length testing, including upper trapezius, levator scapulae, pectoral muscles
- Upper limb nerve tension test[6]
- Deep neck-flexor endurance test
- Upper-extremity neurological screen (dermatome, myotome, reflexes)

INTERVENTION

- Joint mobilization/manipulation
- Postural correction
- Initiate stabilization exercises after normalizing ROM (deep neck flexors)
- Stretching exercises and myofascial mobilization for shortened musculature
- Modalities for short-term pain control

FUNCTIONAL GOALS

- Patient will be able to
  - Sit with a cervicothoracic spine posture for more than 30 minutes with 0 out of 10 pain rating.
  - Sit at work station and perform computer work for 45 minutes with 0 out of 10 pain rating.
  - Rotate cervical spine 80 degrees to look over shoulder when driving without pain.

PROGNOSIS

- Fair to very good depending on specific impairments.
- Chronic cervical pain prognosis significantly less.

PATIENT RESOURCE

- Ray CD. Symptoms and diagnosis of facet joint problems. http://www.spine-health.com/conditions/arthritis/symptoms-and-diagnosis-facet-joint-problems. Accessed March 18, 2013.

REFERENCES

1. The American Physical Therapy Association. Pattern 4F: impaired joint mobility, motor function, muscle performance, range of motion, and reflex integrity associated with spinal disorders. *Interactive Guide to Physical Therapist Practice* 2003. doi: 10.2522/ptguide.3.1_6 http://guidetoptpractice.apta.org/content/1/SEC13.extract. Accessed May 21, 2014.
2. Dutton M. Imaging studies. In: Orthopaedics. *Dutton's Orthopaedic Examination, Evaluation, and Intervention*. 3rd ed. New York, NY: McGraw-Hill; 2012:Chapter 31. http://www.accessphysiotherapy.com/abstract/55601371#55601371. Accessed March 18, 2013.
3. Malone TR, Hazle C, Grey ML. Introduction to musculoskeletal imaging. *Imaging in Rehabilitation*. New York, NY: McGraw-Hill; 2008:Chapter 1. http://www.accessphysiotherapy.com/abstract/5940003#5940003. Accessed March 18, 2013.
4. Dutton M. The cervical complex. In: Dutton M, ed. *Dutton's Orthopedic Survival Guide: Managing Common Conditions*. New York, NY: McGraw-Hill; 2011:Chapter 11. http://www. accessphysiotherapy.com/abstract/8656044#8656333. Accessed March 18, 2013.
5. Dutton M. The lumbopelvic complex. In: Dutton M, ed. *Dutton's Orthopedic Survival Guide: Managing Common Conditions*. New York, NY: McGraw-Hill; 2011:Chapter 13. http://www. accessphysiotherapy.com/abstract/8656044#8656333. Accessed March 18, 2013.
6. Dutton M. Neurodynamic mobilizations. *Dutton's Orthopaedic Examination, Evaluation, and Intervention*. 3rd ed. New York, NY: McGraw-Hill; 2012:Chapter 12. http://www.accessphysiotherapy.com/abstract/55601371#55601371. Accessed March 18, 2013.

ADDITIONAL REFERENCES

- Fritz JM, Cleland JA, Childs JD. Subgrouping patients with low back pain: Evolution of a classification approach to physical therapy. *J Orthop Sports Phys Ther*. 2007;37(6):290–302.
- ICD9DATA web site. http://www.icd9data.com. Accessed January 21, 2013.
- ICD10DATA web site. http://www.icd10data.com. Accessed January 21, 2013.
- Liebenson C. *Rehabilitation of the Spine*. Baltimore MD: Lippincott, Williams & Wilkins; 2007.
- Olsen KA. *Manual Therapy of the Spine*. St. Louis, MI: Saunders Elsevier; 2009.

114 CERVICAL RADICULOPATHY

Eric J. Chaconas, DPT, PT, FAAOMPT
Eric Shamus, PhD, DPT, PT, CSCS

CONDITION/DISORDER SYNONYMS

- Herniated intervertebral disk
- Prolapsed intervertebral disk
- Slipped disk
- Ruptured disk
- Herniated nucleus pulposus

ICD-9-CM CODES

- 719.48 Pain in joint involving other specified sites
- 721.1 Cervical spondylosis with myelopathy
- 722.0 Displacement of cervical intervertebral disc without myelopathy
- 722.4 Degeneration of cervical intervertebral disc
- 722.71 Intervertebral disc disorder with myelopathy cervical region

ICD-10-CM CODES

- M47.12 Other spondylosis with myelopathy, cervical region
- M50.00 Cervical disc disorder with myelopathy, unspecified cervical region
- M50.30 Other cervical disc degeneration, unspecified cervical region

PREFERRED PRACTICE PATTERN

- 4F: Impaired Joint Mobility, Motor Function, Muscle Performance, Range of Motion, and Reflex Integrity Associated with Spinal Disorders[1]

PATIENT PRESENTATION

A 57-year-old female presents with reports of left-sided neck, shoulder, and arm pain persisting for the past eight months. She does not recall a specific injury and reports a gradual onset of pain. Symptoms are described as aching with burning and numbness into the arm and hand. She works as a medical billing specialist and reports increased symptoms after sitting at her desk for over an hour and driving her car for extended periods of time. Cervical left side bending and rotation movements increase arm pain and manual distraction provides symptom relief. Significant forward-head posture is noted along with weakness of the bilateral rhomboids, middle trapezius and serratus anterior. Diminished sensation is noted over the left thumb along with weakness of the left wrist extensors.

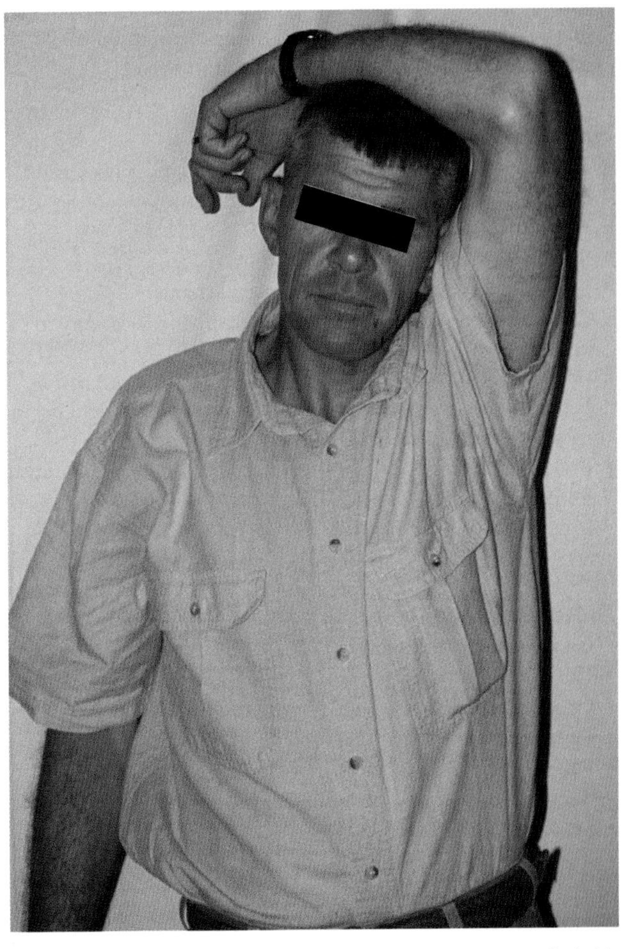

FIGURE 114-1 Cervical Radiculopathy. This is the classic position of relief for cervical radicular pain. This patient presented with severe pain in the neck with radiation to the extremity. The only way the patient was able to get relief was by holding his arm over his head in the position shown. This patient has a C5 to C6 herniated nucleus pulposus. (From Knoop KJ, Stack LB, Storrow AB, Thurman RJ. *The Atlas of Emergency Medicine.* 3rd ed. www.accessmedicine.com. Copyright © The McGraw-Hill Companies, Inc. All rights reserved. Photo contributor: Kevin J. Knoop, MD, MS.)

KEY FEATURES

Description

- Any disorder that affects the spinal nerve roots
- Lateral cervical spine nerve root compression
- Gradual or acute onset secondary to intervertebral disc or osteophyte formation in the intervertebral foramen[1]

Essentials of Diagnosis

- Diagnosis made by clinical examination
- Dermatome or myotome pattern
- Reproduction of symptoms

General Considerations

- Herniated disk is one cause
- Avoid positions that increase symptoms

Demographics

- Women at greater risk than men, middle-aged to geriatric

CLINICAL FINDINGS

SIGNS AND SYMPTOMS

- Neck, shoulder, upper-extremity pain, and parasthesia often radiating to hand[1]
- Pain in cervical spine worsens with cervical extension, side bending, and rotation to the involved side[1]
- Diminished sensation, motor control, and reflexes in the distribution of the involved nerve[1]

Functional Implications

- Difficulty sustaining sitting postures secondary to neck and arm pain
- Inability to sleep
- Weakness with upper-extremity lifting
- Loss of movement or feeling in upper extremity
- Difficulty with neck movements, as with driving, secondary to pain

Possible Contributing Causes

- Forward-head or rounded-shoulder posture due to tight pectoralis, weak periscapular, deep neck-flexor muscles
- Prolonged extension or position of cervical side bending toward impaired nerve
- Facet hypertrophy
- Size of spinal canal; can be congenital

Differential Diagnosis

- Carpal tunnel syndrome
- Chiari malformation
- Degenerative disk disease
- Peripheral nerve impairment
- Rhomboid/trapezius spams
- Shoulder pathology with radiating pain pattern
- Spinal tumor
- Thoracic outlet syndrome

MEANS OF CONFIRMATION OR DIAGNOSIS

Imaging

- MRI helps to visualize compressed or inflamed nerve root in diagnosis[2]
- X-ray/Plain-film radiograph helpful if osteophyte located in intervertebral foramen[3]
- CT scan to show herniation compressing the spinal canal/nerves[3]

Diagnostic Procedures

- Electrodiagnostic/nerve conduction testing can help determine a specific impaired nerve function[4]

FINDINGS AND INTERPRETATION

- Physical examination cluster to rule in cervical radiculopathy[3]
  - Spurling test[2]
  - Rotation limited to ipsilateral side
  - Upper limb nerve tension test[2]
  - Diminished brachioradialis reflex

TREATMENT

Medication

- Nonsteroidal anti-inflammatory drugs (NSAIDs)
- Corticosteroids

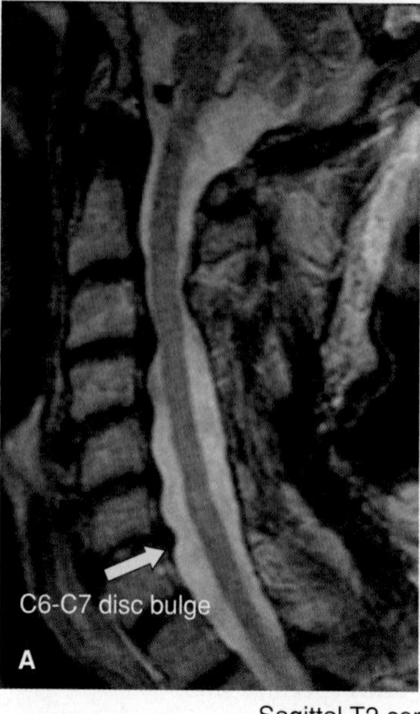

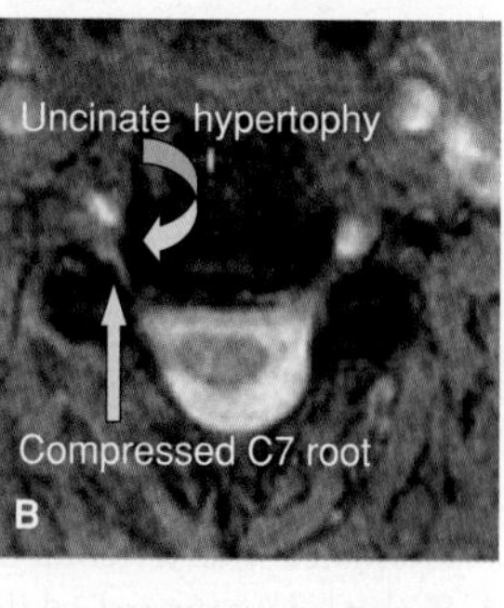

Sagittal T2 cervical spine

FIGURE 114-2 Right C7 radiculopathy **A.** Sagittal T2-weighted image shows mild disk bulging at C6–7 and a mildly narrowed spinal canal, but no visible nerve root compression. **B.** Axial T2-weighted image. The combination of uncinate hypertrophy and facet hypertrophy (ovoid dark space just lateral to the C7 root) narrows the right C6–7 intervertebral foramen resulting in right C7 nerve root compression. (From Longo DL, Fauci AS, Kasper DL, Hauser SL, Jameson JL, Loscalzo J, eds. *Harrison's Principles of Internal Medicine*. 18th ed. New York, NY: McGraw-Hill; 2012.)

REFERRALS/ADMITTANCE

- To hospital for imaging
- To physician for surgical consult if myelopathy suspected
- To hospital for imaging and medical consult if sinister disease suspected
  - Decompression[2]
  - Diskectomy[2]
  - Fusion[2]

TABLE 114-1 Nonmusculoskeletal Causes of Back Pain

Neoplasm	**Vascular Causes**
• Lung cancer	• Abdominal aortic aneurysm
• Liver metastasis	• Aortic dissection
• Pancreatic cancer	• Renal infarction
• Renal cancer	• Cardiac ischemia
• Prostate cancer	**Miscellaneous Causes**
• Testicular cancer	• Kidney stones
• Ovarian neoplasm	• Diabetic radiculopathy
• Uterine fibroids	• Osteoporosis
Infection	• Osteomalacia
• Pneumonia	• Gout and pseudogout
• Pleural effusion	• Prolapsed uterus
• Chronic prostatitis	• Endometriosis
• Pyelonephritis	• Pancreatitis
• Pelvic inflammatory disease	• Cholecystitis
	• Peptic ulcer disease
	• Herpes zoster

Source: Simon RR, Sherman SC. *Emergency Orthopedics*. 6th ed. http://www.accessemergencymedicine.com.

- Hemilaminectomy[2]
- Laminectomy[2]
- Laser diskectomy[2]
- Microdisectomy[2]
- Percutaneous diskectomy[2]

- To physician for corticosteroid injection if condition does not improve
- To physician for anti-inflammatory medication

IMPAIRMENTS

- Restricted mobility of the upper- or mid-thoracic spine and subcranial spine
- Hypermobile mid-cervical spine
- Tight pectoralis major and minor
- Weakness of longus colli and longus capitis
- Weakness of periscapular muscles

TESTS AND MEASURES

- Cervical spine AROM
- Sharp–Purser: Atlantoaxial instability
- Cervical passive intervertebral motion testing
- Sub-cranial translation instability testing
- Passive physiological intervertebral mobility testing (PPIVM)
- Upper-extremity screening examination
- Postural examination
- Muscle length testing, including upper trapezius, levator scapulae, pectoral muscles
- Upper limb nerve tension test
- Neck Disability Index (NDI)
- Deep neck-flexor endurance test
- Upper-extremity neurological screen (dermatome, myotome, reflexes)

INTERVENTION

- Rest
- Joint manipulation to the thoracic and upper-cervical spine
- Cervical distraction and traction to relieve nerve compression
- Cranio-cervical flexion exercises
- Periscapular strengthening
- Address pain
  - Electrical stimulation
  - Heat/Ice to increase mobility
- Address hypertonicity
  - Soft tissue massage
  - Heat
- Address muscle weakness
  - Deep neck-flexor training
  - Strengthening of lower/middle trapezius, rhomboids, rotator cuff
  - Serratus anterior, latissimus dorsi

FUNCTIONAL GOALS

- Patient will be able to
  - Sit with a neutral cervical and thoracic spine posture for >30 minutes with 0/10 pain rating.
  - Patient will be able to sit at work station and perform computer work for 45 minutes with 0/10 pain rating.
  - Patient will be able to rotate cervical spine 70 degrees to talk on phone with 0/10 pain rating in the neck or arm.

TABLE 114-2 Pain Distribution from Cervical Structures

Structure	Pain Area
Occipital condyles	Frontal
Occipitocervical tissues	Frontal
C1 posterior (dorsal) ramus	Orbit, frontal, and vertex
C1–2	Temporal and suboccipital
C3 posterior (dorsal) ramus	Occiput, mastoid, and frontal

Source: Data from Meadows J. A Rationale and Complete Approach to the Sub-Acute Post-MVA Cervical Patient. Calgary, AB: Swodeam Consulting, 1995.

PROGNOSIS

- Fair to very good depending on severity of nerve root compression and cervico/thoracic impairments.

PATIENT RESOURCE

- Cervical Radiculopathy. American Academy of Orthopeadic Surgeons. http://orthoinfo.aaos.org/topic.cfm?topic=A00332, Accessed January 2, 2013.

REFERENCES

1. American Physical Therapy Association. Pattern 4E: impaired joint mobility, motor function, muscle performance, and range of motion associated with localized inflammation. *Interactive Guide to Physical Therapist Practice by American Physical Therapy Association*. 2003. ISBN: 978-1-887759-87-8. doi : 10.2522/ptguide.978-1-931369-64-0.
2. Dutton M. *Orthopaedic Examination, Evaluation, and Intervention*. New York, NY: McGraw-Hill; 2008. http://www.accessphysiotherapy.com/resource/612. Accessed March 1, 2013.
3. Malone TR, Hazle C, Grey ML. *Imaging in Rehabilitation*. New York, NY: McGraw-Hill; 2008. http://www.accessphysiotherapy.com/resource/613. Accessed February 28, 2013.
4. Dutton M. *Dutton's Orthopedic Survival Guide: Managing Common Conditions*. New York, NY: McGraw-Hill; 2011. http://www.accessphysiotherapy.com/resource/685. Accessed March 1, 2013.

ADDITIONAL REFERENCES

- ICD9DATA web site. http://www.icd9data.com. Accessed January 21, 2013.
- ICD10DATA web site. http://www.icd10data.com. Accessed January 21, 2013.
- Prentice WE, Quillen WS, Underwood F. Principles of electrophysiologic evaluation and testing. In: Prentice WE, Quillen WS, Underwood F, eds. *Therapeutic Modalities in Rehabilitation, 4e*. http://www.accessphysiotherapy.com/content/8137409, Accessed January 2, 2013:Chapter 8.
- Wainner RS, Fritz JM, Irrgang JJ, Boninger ML, Delitto A, Allison S. Reliability and diagnostic accuracy of the clinical examination and patient self-report measures for cervical radiculopathy. *Spine*. 2003;28(1):52–62.

115 CERVICAL SPINAL STENOSIS

Arie J. Van Duijn, EdD, MSc, PT, OCS
Eric Shamus, PhD, DPT, PT, CSCS

CONDITION/DISORDER SYNONYMS

- Cervical spinal stenosis
- Cervical central stenosis
- Central stenosis
- Lateral stenosis

ICD-9-CM CODES

- 723.0 Spinal stenosis in cervical region
- 724.0 Spinal stenosis other than cervical

ICD-10-CM CODES

- M48.00 Spinal stenosis, site unspecified
- M48.02 Spinal stenosis, cervical region

PREFERRED PRACTICE PATTERN

- 4F: Impaired Joint Mobility, Motor Function, Muscle Performance, Range of Motion, and Reflex Integrity Associated with Spinal Disorders[1]

PATIENT PRESENTATION

A 72-year-old male presents with gradually increasing complaints of diffuse neck pain, cramping and pain in both the upper and lower extremities, and occasional loss of bladder control. These symptoms are aggravated with cervical extension and relieved with cervical flexion. A pronounced forward-head posture is noted, and there is a significant loss of active and passive cervical range of motion in all directions. Neurological examination revealed increased muscle tone bilaterally in the biceps brachii and gastrocnemius muscles with brisk deep tendon reflexes. A positive Babinski reflex was present bilaterally. MRI evaluation revealed

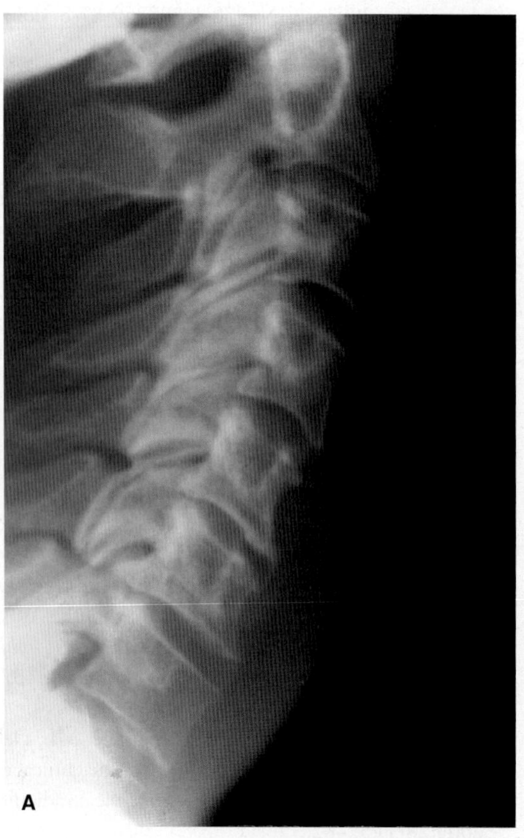

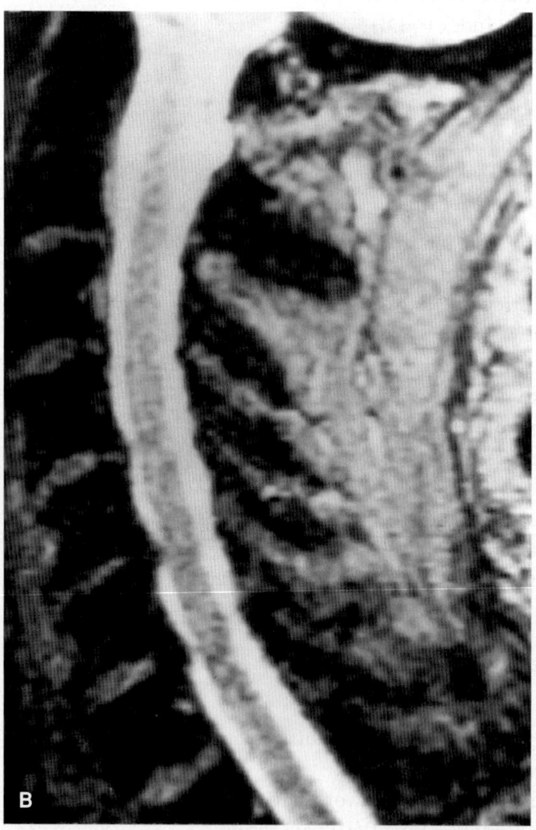

FIGURE 115-1 Imaging studies in a patient with cervical spondylosis and chronic neck pain. (**A**) Radiograph showing collapsed disk space between C5 and C6 and a large posterior osteophyte at the inferior endplate of C6. (**B**) MRI showing collapsed disk spaces, a mild stenosis of the spinal canal, and effacement of the spinal cord by an osteophyte at C6. (From Skinner HB. *Current Diagnosis & Treatment in Orthopedics*. 4th ed. www.accessmedicine.com. Copyright © The McGraw-Hill Companies, Inc. All rights reserved.)

narrowing of the central spinal canal in the lower cervical region, along with loss of disk height and significant osteophyte formation in this area.

KEY FEATURES

Description

- Common, degenerative spinal condition
- Associated with narrowing of the spinal canal (central stenosis) or foraminal canals (lateral stenosis)
- Caused by degenerative changes in intervertebral disks and facet joints
- Can result in spinal cord compression or nerve root compression

Essentials of Diagnosis

- Causes neurogenic claudication, with pain, cramping, and paresthesias in the upper extremity and lower extremity aggravated by cervical extension, relieved by cervical flexion
- Diagnosis made by clinical examination
- Differentiation between vascular and neurologic claudication
- Reproduction of symptoms in specific postures and activities

General Considerations

- Cervical spinal stenosis can result in spinal cord compression and resulting upper motor neuron signs
- Cervical central stenosis can give both upper- and lower-extremity symptoms

Demographics

- Prevalence increases with age.
- Primarily occurs after 65 years of age.

CLINICAL FINDINGS

SIGNS AND SYMPTOMS

- Bilateral leg pain
- Unilateral or bilateral upper limb pain and myelopathy with cervical stenosis
- Pain worse with walking, relieved by sitting
- Can be with or without neck pain
- Altered sensation, motor control, and reflexes in the distribution of the involved nerve roots

Functional Implications

- Difficulty with walking long distances
- Difficulty with standing activities
- Possible bowel or bladder dysfunction with cervical stenosis
- Difficulty looking up
- Difficulty reaching overhead, painting overhead

Possible Contributing Causes

- Postural changes
- Weakness of core musculature

Differential Diagnosis

- Degenerative disk disease
- Osteoarthritis
- Peripheral nerve impairment
- Peripheral neuropathy
- Spinal tumor
- Thoracic outlet syndrome
- Vascular insufficiency

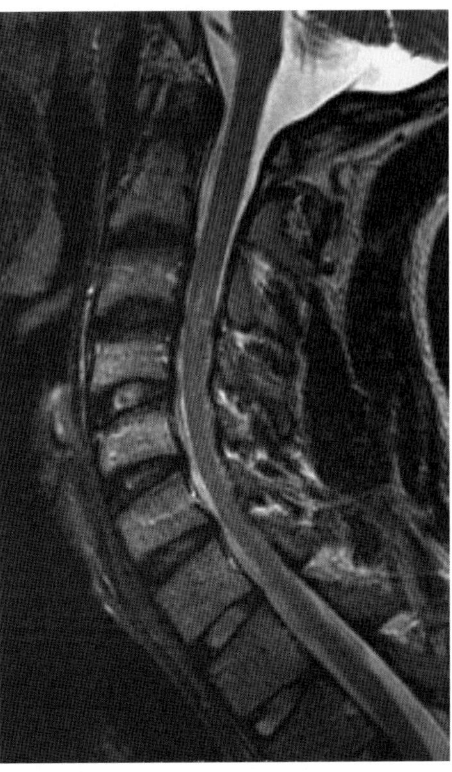

FIGURE 115-2 A sagittal section T2-weighted MRI of the cervical spine in a 21-year-old man. Note the signal change present within the spinal cord approximating the C3–4 levels, which is consistent with edema and a spinal cord contusion. This individual was particularly susceptible to injury because of congenital stenosis. (From Malone TR, Hazle C, Grey ML. *Imaging in Rehabilitation*. www.accessphysiotherapy.com. Copyright © The McGraw-Hill Companies, Inc. All rights reserved.)

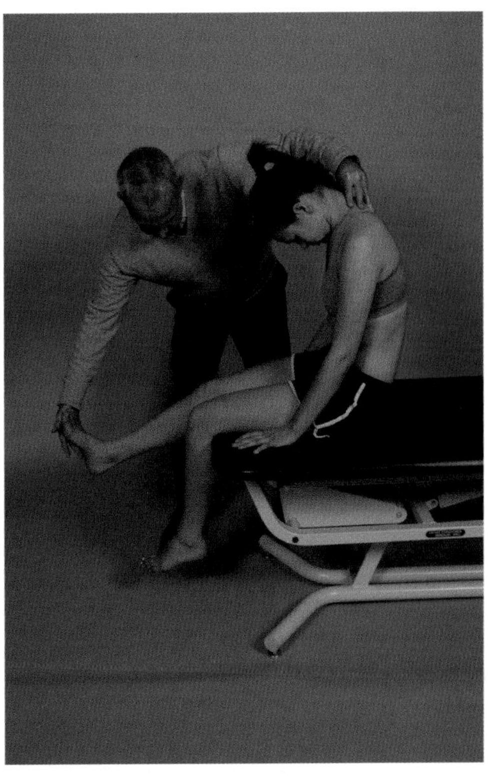

FIGURE 115-3 Cervical active range of motion with passive overpressure. (From Dutton M. *Dutton's Orthopaedic Examination, Evaluation, and Intervention*. 3rd ed. http://www.accessphysiotherapy.com. Copyright © The McGraw-Hill Companies, Inc. All rights reserved.)

MEANS OF CONFIRMATION OR DIAGNOSIS

Imaging

- MRI
- X-ray/Plain-film radiograph
- CT

Diagnostic Procedures

- Electrodiagnostic/nerve conduction testing can help determine a specific impaired nerve function.[2]
- Doppler ultrasound to examine vascular function.

FINDINGS AND INTERPRETATION

- MRI helps to visualize compressed or inflamed nerve root in diagnosis.[3]
- X-ray/Plain-film radiograph helpful if osteophyte located in intervertebral foramen.[4]
- CT scan to show herniation compressing the spinal canal/nerves.[4]

REFERRALS/ADMITTANCE

- To hospital for imaging
- To physician for surgical consult if myelopathy suspected
  - Fusion[3]
  - Decompression[3]
  - Laminectomy[3]
- To hospital for imaging and medical consult if disease suspected
- To vascular surgeon if suspected vascular insufficiency

IMPAIRMENTS

- Hypomobile cervical spine
- Weakness of core stabilizing muscles
- Inability to stand/walk for prolonged time
- Inability to look for prolonged time (visual fatigue)

TESTS AND MEASURES

- Cervical spine AROM
- Sharp–Purser: Atlantoaxial instability
- Cervical passive intervertebral motion testing
- Sub-cranial translation instability testing
- Passive physiological intervertebral mobility testing (PPIVM)
- Neck Disability Index (NDI)
- Postural examination
- Muscle length testing, including upper trapezius, levator scapulae, pectoral muscles
- Deep neck-flexor endurance test
- Upper-extremity neurological screen (dermatome, myotome, reflexes)
- Physical examination
  - Two-stage treadmill test
  - ABI to screen for PAD
  - Quadrant test[2]
  - Slump test[3]
  - Upper limb nerve tension test[3]
  - Deep tendon reflexes
  - Passive physiological intervertebral mobility testing (PPIVM)[2]

INTERVENTION

- Joint manipulation to the thoracic and lumbar spine when joint hypomobility is present.

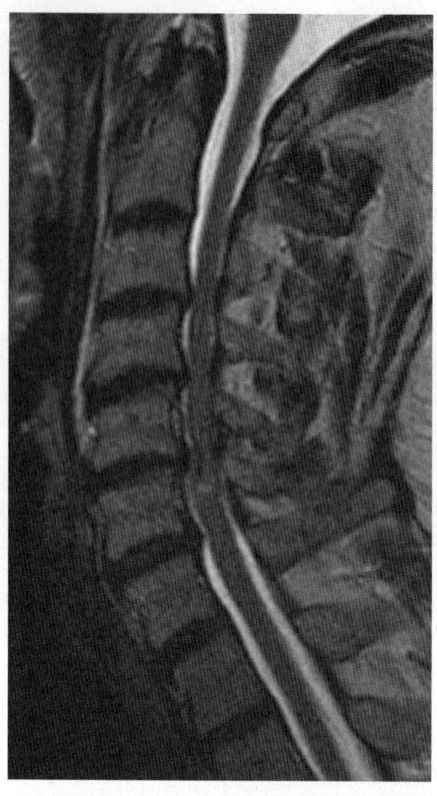

FIGURE 115-4 A sagittal view T2-weighted MRI revealing advanced degenerative change resulting in central spinal canal stenosis. Note the absence of signal from the cerebrospinal fluid in the areas of osteophytic growth and disk bulging. (From Malone TR, Hazle C, Grey ML. *Imaging in Rehabilitation*. www.accessphysiotherapy.com. Copyright © The McGraw-Hill Companies, Inc. All rights reserved.)

TABLE 115-1 Movement Restrictions of the Craniovertebral Joints and Their Probable Causes

Movement Restriction	Probable Causes
Flexion and right side bending	Left flexion hypomobility Extensor muscle tightness Posterior capsular adhesions Left subluxation (into extension)
Extension and right side bending	Right extension hypomobility Left flexor muscle tightness Anterior capsular adhesions Right subluxation (into flexion)
Flexion and right side bending motion greater than extension and left side bending	Left capsular pattern (arthritis and arthrosis)
Flexion and right side bending equal to extension and left side bending	Left arthrofibrosis (very hard capsular end-feel)
Right-side flexion in flexion and extension	Probably an anomaly

Source: Dutton M. *Dutton's Orthopaedic Examination, Evaluation, and Intervention*. 3rd ed. http://www.accessphysiotherapy.com. Copyright © The McGraw-Hill Companies, Inc. All rights reserved.

- Specific exercises in flexion when pain centralizes with repeated movement/posture into flexion
- Lumbar stabilization exercises to address core stability
- Stretching exercises and myofascial mobilization for shortened musculature
- Unweighted treadmill walking
- Aquatic exercise
- Mechanical traction in flexion position

FUNCTIONAL GOALS

- Patient will be able to
    - Walk for 30 minutes with 0/10 pain rating so as to grocery shop or walk in a mall.
    - Increase standing tolerance to >30 minutes without pain to fulfill recreational or work activity requirements.

PROGNOSIS

- Variable: Multimodal conservative management, including progressive exercise, unweighted walking, manual therapy show positive outcomes
- Severe cases of stenosis may require surgical intervention

PATIENT RESOURCE

- Spinal Stenosis. NIH, National Institute of Arthritis and Musculoskeletal and Skin Diseases. http://www.niams.nih.gov/health_info/Spinal_Stenosis/default.asp. Accessed March 18, 2013.

REFERENCES

1. American Physical Therapy Association. Pattern 4E: impaired joint mobility, motor function, muscle performance, and range of motion asssociated with localized inflammation. *Interactive Guide to Physical Therapist Practice by American Physical Therapy Association*. 2003. ISBN: 978-1-887759-87-8. doi : 10.2522/ptguide.978-1-931369-64-0.
2. Dutton M. *Dutton's Orthopedic Survival Guide: Managing Common Conditions*. New York, NY: McGraw-Hill; 2011. http://www.accessphysiotherapy.com/resource/685. Accessed March 18, 2013.
3. Dutton M. *Dutton's Orthopaedic Examination, Evaluation, and Intervention*. 3rd ed. New York, NY: McGraw-Hill; 2012. http://www.accessphysiotherapy.com/resource/612. Accessed March 1, 2013.
4. Malone TR, Hazle C, Grey ML. *Imaging in Rehabilitation*. New York, NY: McGraw-Hill; 2008. http://www.accessphysiotherapy.com/resource/613. Accessed March 18, 2013.

ADDITIONAL REFERENCES

- Fritz JM, Cleland JA, Childs JD. Subgrouping patients with low back pain: evolution of a classification approach to physical therapy. *J Orthop Sports Phys Ther*. 2007;37(6):290–302.
- ICD9DATA web site. http://www.icd9data.com. Accessed March 18, 2013.
- ICD10DATA web site. http://www.icd10data.com. Accessed March 18, 2013.
- Liebenson C. *Rehabilitation of the Spine*. Baltimore, MD: Lippincott, Williams & Wilkins; 2007.
- Olsen KA. *Manual Therapy of the Spine*. St. Louis, MI: Saunders Elsevier; 2009.

116 CERVICAL SPONDYLOLISTHESIS

Eric Shamus, PhD, DPT, PT, CSCS
Eric J. Chaconas, DPT, PT, FAAOMPT

CONDITION/DISORDER SYNONYM

- Cervical spondylolisthesis

ICD-9-CM CODES

- 738.4 Acquired spondylolisthesis
- 756.12 Spondylolisthesis congenital
- 805.02 Closed fracture of second cervical vertebra

ICD-10-CM CODES

- M43.10 Spondylolisthesis, site unspecified
- Q76.2 Congenital spondylolisthesis
- S12.100A Unspecified displaced fracture of second cervical vertebra, initial encounter for closed fracture
- S12.101A Unspecified nondisplaced fracture of second cervical vertebra, initial encounter for closed fracture

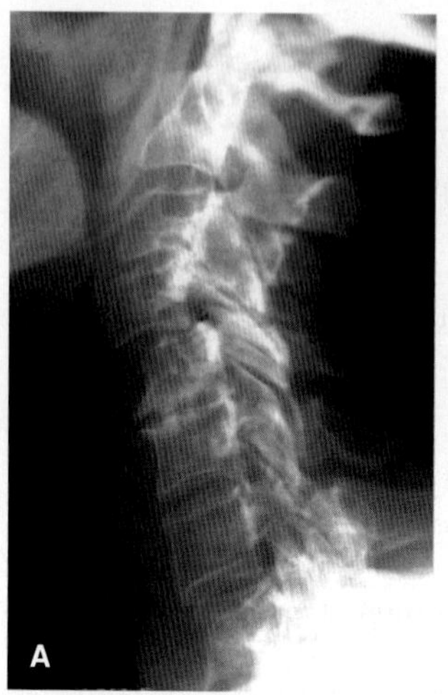

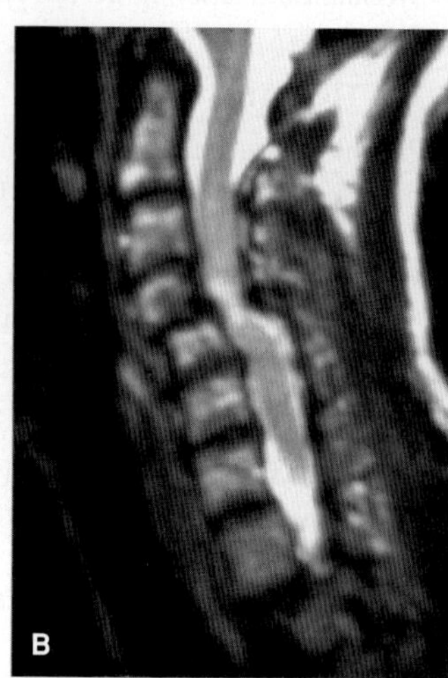

FIGURE 116-1 **A.** Lateral radiograph of a 50-year-old man with neck pain and myelopathy. **B.** Sagittal T2-weighted MRI showing spinal cord compression at C4–5 at the level of the spondylolisthesis. (From Doherty GM. Current Diagnosis & Treatment: Surgery. 13th ed. www.accessmedicine.com. Copyright © The McGraw-Hill Companies, Inc. All rights reserved.)

PREFERRED PRACTICE PATTERN

- 4E: Impaired Joint Mobility, Motor Function, Muscle Performance, and ROM Associated with Localized Inflammation[1]

PATIENT PRESENTATION

A 50-year-old man presents with a gradual onset of neck pain for 2 years. Plain-film radiographs reveal a low-grade spondylolisthesis of the C5 vertebrae. He reports the symptoms are worse while lying supine, cervical backward bending, and prolonged sitting postures. A palpable step is noted in the mid cervical spine along with increased paraspinal muscle tone. Neurologic signs and instability testing are all negative. Decreased motor control and endurance of the deep neck flexors are noted along with decreased joint mobility in the upper thoracic spine.

KEY FEATURES

Description

- Anterior (forward) translation of a vertebra
- Fracture of the pedicles on the vertebra below
- Slipping of the vertebra in relationship to the vertebra below
- Neurogenic claudication
- Fracture widens at the pars
- Hangman's fracture
- C2 vertebra anterior translated on C3 with fracture of C2 pedicles

Essentials of Diagnosis

- Made by X-ray
- May be acquired or congenital
- Clinical examination may find step deformity
- Dermatome/myotome pattern
- Low-grade isthmic spondylolisthesis: less than 50% displacement
- High-grade isthmic spondylolisthesis: greater than 50% displacement
- Four grades[2]
  - Grade 1: 0% to 25% slippage
  - Grade 2: 25% to 50% slippage
  - Grade 3: 50% to 75% slippage
  - Grade 4: 75% to 100% slippage
- Spondylolysis: Fracture without displacement

General Considerations

- Instability
- Avoid extension positions that increase symptoms
- Wiltse–Newman classification of spondylolisthesis[2]

Demographics

- May be congenital or acquired.

CLINICAL FINDINGS

SIGNS AND SYMPTOMS

- Cervical, shoulder, arm, and upper extremity pain and paresthesia, often radiating into the lower extremities if central cord involvement
- Constricted pupil (Horner sign)
- Stiffness along spine
- Headaches

TABLE 116-1 Examination Findings and the Possible Conditions Causing Them

Findings	Possible Condition
Dizziness	Upper cervical impairment, vertebrobasilar ischemia, and craniovertebral ligament tear; also may be relatively benign
Quadrilateral paresthesia	Cord compression and vertebrobasilar ischemia
Bilateral upper limb paresthesia	Cord compression and vertebrobasilar ischemia
Hyperreflexia	Cord compression and vertebrobasilar ischemia
Babinski or clonus sign	Cord compression and vertebrobasilar ischemia
Consistent swallow on transverse ligament stress tests	Instability, retropharyngeal hematoma, and rheumatoid arthritis
Nontraumatic capsular pattern	Rheumatoid arthritis, ankylosing spondylitis, and neoplasm
Arm pain lasting >6–9 mo	Neoplasm
Persistent root pain <30 y	Neoplasm
Radicular pain with coughing	Neoplasm
Pain worsening after 1 mo	Neoplasm
>1 level involved	Neoplasm
Paralysis	Neoplasm or neurologic disease
Trunk and limb paresthesias	Neoplasm
Bilateral root signs and symptoms	Neoplasm
Nontraumatic strong spasm	Neoplasm
Nontraumatic strong pain in elderly patient	Neoplasm
Signs worse than symptoms	Neoplasm
Radial deviator weakness	Neoplasm
Thumb flexor weakness	Neoplasm
Hand intrinsic weakness or atrophy	Neoplasm, thoracic outlet syndrome, and carpal tunnel syndrome
Horner syndrome	Superior sulcus tumor, breast cancer, cervical ganglion damage, and brain stem damage
Empty end-feel	Neoplasm
Severe posttraumatic capsular pattern	Fracture
Severe posttraumatic spasm	Fracture
Loss of ROM posttrauma	Fracture
Posttraumatic painful weakness	Fracture

Source: Meadows J. *Orthopaedic Differential Diagnosis in Physical Therapy*. New York, NY: McGraw-Hill; 1999.
ROM, range of motion.

- Pain in cervical spine worsens with extension
- Diminished sensation, motor control, and reflexes in the distribution of the involved nerve
- Neurogenic claudication

Functional Implications

- Difficulty sustaining standing postures secondary to neck and arm pain
- Inability to sleep flat on the back without a pillow
- Weakness with lifting
- Loss of movement or feeling in the upper extremity
- Difficulty with movements secondary to pain, especially reaching overhead
- Limited sports participation

Possible Contributing Causes

- Forceful extension from hit under the chin (sports)
- Congenital
- Car accident, hit from rear
- Hyperextension of the cervical spine
- Suicidal hanging
- Increased cervical lordosis posture

Differential Diagnosis

- Peripheral nerve impairment
- Spinal tumor
- Infection
- Peripheral neuropathy
- Paraspinal spasms
- Degenerative disk disease
- Stenosis

MEANS OF CONFIRMATION OR DIAGNOSIS

Imaging

- MRI helpful in diagnosis to visualize compressed or inflamed nerve root[3]

- X-ray/Plain-film radiograph to see vertebra position (Scottie dog collar)[2]
- CT scan to show herniation compressing the spinal canal or nerves[4]
- Electrodiagnostic/nerve conduction testing can help determine a specific impaired nerve function[5]

Diagnostic Procedure

- Electrodiagnostic/nerve conduction testing can help determine a specific impaired nerve function.[4]

FINDINGS AND INTERPRETATION

- Cervical vertebra anterior translated on the lower cervical vertebrae with fracture of pedicles

TREATMENT

Medication

- Nonsteroidal anti-inflammatory drugs (NSAIDs)
- Corticosteroids

REFERRALS/ADMITTANCE

- For imaging
- For surgical consult if myelopathy is suspected
  - Fusion[3]
  - Decompression[3]
  - Laminectomy[3]
  - Hemilaminectomy[3]
- For corticosteroid injection
- For anti-inflammatory medication
- For halo vest traction device, cervical bracing

IMPAIRMENTS

- Restricted mobility of the upper cervical spine
- Hypermobility
- Weakness of neck musculature

TESTS AND MEASURES

- Cervical spine AROM
- Sharp–Purser: Atlantoaxial instability
- Cervical passive intervertebral motion testing
- Subcranial translation instability testing
- Passive physiologic intervertebral mobility testing (PPIVM)
- Upper-extremity screening examination
- Postural examination
- Muscle length testing, including the upper trapezius, levator scapulae, and pectoral muscles
- Upper limb nerve tension test
- Deep neck flexor endurance test
- Upper-extremity neurologic screen (dermatome, myotome, reflexes)
- Neck Disability Index (NDI)

INTERVENTION

- Rest
- Bracing
- Address pain
  - Electrical stimulation
  - Heat/Ice[6]

TABLE 116-2 Wiltse–Newman Classification of Spondylolisthesis

I. Dysplastic
II. Isthmic
  (IIa) Disruption of the pars interarticularis due to stress fracture
  (IIb) Elongation of the pars without disruption due to repetitive healed microfractures
  (IIc) Acute fracture of the pars interarticularis
III. Degenerative
IV. Traumatic
V. Pathologic
VI. Post-Operative

Source: From Patel DR, Greydanus DE, Baker RJ. *Pediatric Practice: Sports Medicine.* http://www.accesspediatrics.com.

- Address hypertonicity
  - Soft-tissue massage
  - Heat
- Address muscle weakness
  - Stability exercises

FUNCTIONAL GOALS

- Patient will be able to
  - Sit with neutral cervical spine posture for >30 minutes with 0/10 pain rating.
  - Stand at work station and perform computer work for 45 minutes with 0/10 pain rating.
  - Rotate cervical spine 75 degrees to look over shoulder while driving the car with 0/10 pain rating.

PROGNOSIS

- Fair to good, depending on severity of vertebral translation, amount of nerve root compression, and upper/lower extremity impairments.
- Possible death from asphyxia.

PATIENT RESOURCE

- American Academy of Orthopaedic Surgeons. Spondylolysis and Spondylolisthesis. http://orthoinfo.aaos.org/topic.cfm?topic=A00053. Accessed August 8, 2014.

REFERENCES

1. The American Physical Therapy Association. Pattern 4E: Impaired joint mobility, motor function, muscle performance, and range of motion associated with localized inflammation. *Interactive Guide to Physical Therapist Practice.* 2003. DOI: 10.2522/ptguide.3.1_5. Accessed March 1, 2013.
2. Patel DR, Rowe D. Chapter 30. Thoracolumbar spine injuries. In: Patel DR, Greydanus DE, Baker RJ, eds. *Pediatric Practice: Sports Medicine.* New York, NY: McGraw-Hill; 2009. http://www.accessphysiotherapy.com/abstract/6981360. Accessed February 28, 2013.
3. Dutton M. *Orthopaedic Examination, Evaluation, and Intervention.* New York, NY: McGraw-Hill; 2008. http://www.accessphysiotherapy.com/resource/612. Accessed February 28, 2013.

4. Malone TR, Hazle C, Grey ML. *Imaging in Rehabilitation.* New York, NY: McGraw-Hill; 2008. http://www.accessphysiotherapy.com/resource/613. Accessed February 28, 2013.
5. Dutton M. *Dutton's Orthopedic Survival Guide: Managing Common Conditions.* New York, NY: McGraw-Hill; 2011. http://www. accessphysiotherapy.com/resource/685. Accessed January 6, 2013.
6. Prentice WE. Chapter 9. Cryotherapy and thermotherapy. In: Prentice WE, Quillen WS, Underwood F, eds. *Therapeutic Modalities in Rehabilitation.* 4th ed. New York, NY: McGraw-Hill; 2011. http://www.accessphysiotherapy.com/abstract/8138405 #8138406. Accessed March 1, 2013.

ADDITIONAL REFERENCES

- Curtis C, d'Hemecourt P. Diagnosis and management of back pain in adolescents. *Adolesc Med State Art Rev.* 2007;18: 140–164.
- Dutton M. Common orthopedic conditions. In: Dutton M, ed. *McGraw-Hill's NPTE (National Physical Therapy Examination).* 2nd ed. New York, NY: McGraw-Hill; 2012. http://www. accessphysiotherapy.com/content/5398559. Accessed January 27, 2013.
- ICD9DATA web site. http://www.icd9data.com. Accessed January 21, 2013.
- ICD10DATA web site. http://www.icd10data.com. Accessed January 21, 2013.
- Prentice WE, Quillen WS, Underwood F. Chapter 8. Principles of electrophysiologic evaluation and testing. In: Prentice WE, Quillen WS, Underwood F, eds. *Therapeutic Modalities in Rehabilitation.* 4th ed. http://www.accessphysiotherapy.com/ content/8137409. Accessed January 21, 2013.
- Wainner RS, Fritz JM, Irrgang JJ, et al. Reliability and diagnostic accuracy of the clinical examination and patient self-report measures for cervical radiculopathy. *Spine.* 2003;28(1):52–62. Accessed January 21, 2013.

117 CERVICAL SPONDYLOLYSIS

Eric Shamus, PhD, DPT, PT, CSCS
Eric J. Chaconas, DPT, PT, FAAOMPT

CONDITION/DISORDER SYNONYM

- Cervical spondylolysis

ICD-9-CM CODE

- 738.4 Acquired spondylolisthesis

ICD-10-CM CODE

- M43.00 Spondylolysis, site unspecified

PREFERRED PRACTICE PATTERN

- 4E: Impaired Joint Mobility, Motor Function, Muscle Performance, and ROM Associated with Localized Inflammation[1]

PATIENT PRESENTATION

A 29-year-old man presents with acute neck pain after trauma to the cervical spine during soccer practice. He was immobilized with a rigid cervical collar for 6 weeks after advanced imaging confirmed a pars defect at the C4 level. Currently, he presents with guarded movement in all directions and increased tone and tenderness in the cervical spine musculature. Significant weakness is noted in the longus colli, longus capitis, middle trapezius, and rhomboids. Neurological examination is negative, and the patient's goal is to return to playing soccer.

KEY FEATURES

Description

- Stress fracture of the pedicles on the vertebra below
- Tightness or pain in the neck region
- Often no symptoms
- Weakness in the pars

Essentials of Diagnosis

- Diagnosis made by X-ray
- Can be acquired or congenital
- Neck pain

General Considerations

- Instability
- Avoid extension positions that increase symptoms
- Thin vertebral bone: Pars

Demographics

- Teenagers with high-risk activities are more at risk
- Runs in families

CLINICAL FINDINGS

SIGNS AND SYMPTOMS

- Pain in the cervical spine, shoulder, arm, upper extremity
- Stiffness along the spine
- Headaches
- Pain in the cervical spine worsens with extension

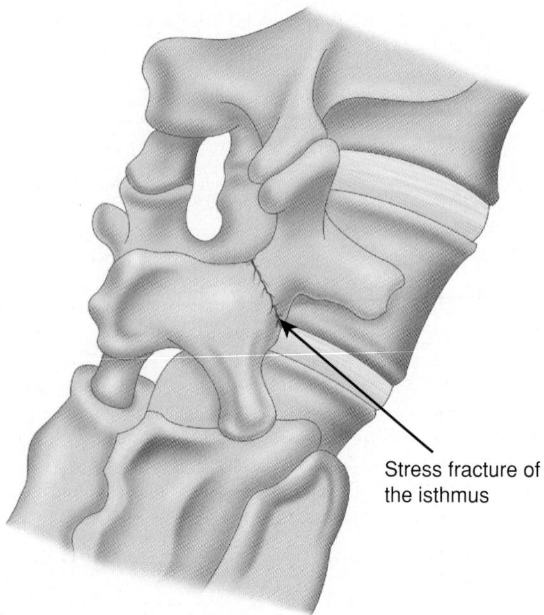

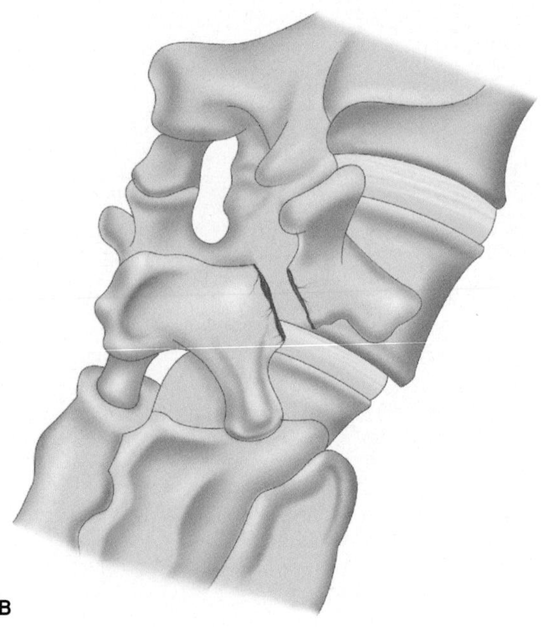

FIGURE 117-1 Schematic drawings of spondylolysis (**A**), and spondylolisthesis (**B**). (From Patel DR, Greydanus DE, Baker RJ. *Pediatric Practice: Sports Medicine.* www.accesspediatrics.com. Copyright © The McGraw-Hill Companies, Inc. All rights reserved.)

▶ Functional Implications

- Difficulty sustaining standing postures secondary to neck and arm pain
- Inability to sleep flat on the back without a pillow
- Difficulty with movements (reaching overhead) secondary to pain
- Limit sports participation

▶ Possible Contributing Causes

- Forceful extension from hit under the chin (sports)
- Congenital
- Car accident, hit from rear
- Hyperextension of the cervical spine
- Increased cervical lordosis posture

▶ Differential Diagnosis

- Peripheral nerve impairment
- Spinal tumor
- Peripheral neuropathy
- Paraspinal spasms
- Degenerative disk disease
- Stenosis

MEANS OF CONFIRMATION OR DIAGNOSIS

▶ Imaging

- MRI helps to visualize compressed or inflamed nerve root in diagnosis[2]
- X-ray/Plain-film radiograph to see vertebra position[3]
- CT scan to show herniation compressing the spinal canal/nerves[3]
- Electrodiagnostic/nerve conduction testing can help determine a specific impaired nerve function[4]

FINDINGS AND INTERPRETATION

- Stress fracture of the pars

TREATMENT

▶ Medication

- Nonsteroidal anti-inflammatory drugs (NSAIDs)
- Corticosteroids

REFERRALS/ADMITTANCE

- For imaging
- For surgical consult if myelopathy is suspected
  - Fusion[2]
  - Decompression[2]
  - Laminectomy[2]
  - Hemilaminectomy[2]
- For corticosteroid injection, anti-inflammatory medication
- For halo vest traction device, cervical bracing

IMPAIRMENTS

- Restricted mobility of the upper cervical spine
- Hypermobility
- Weakness noted in the neck musculature

TESTS AND MEASURES

- Cervical spine AROM
- Sharp–Purser: Atlantoaxial instability

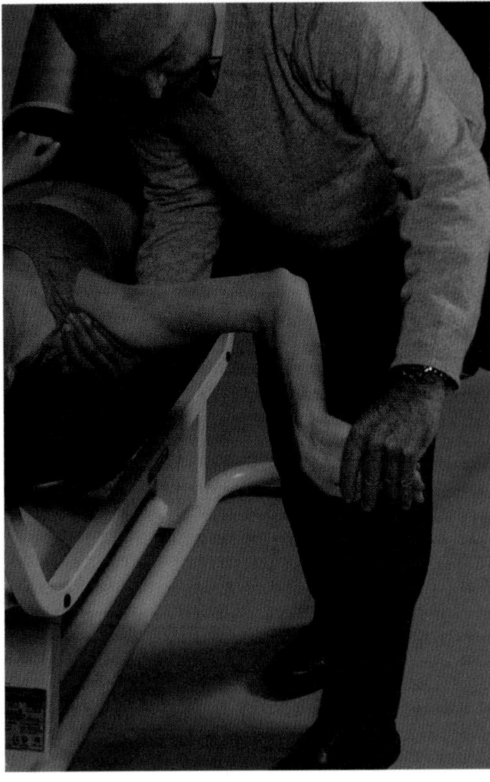

FIGURE 117-2 Upper limb neural tension test. (From Dutton M. *Dutton's Orthopedic Survival Guide: Managing Common Conditions*. www.accessphysiotherapy.com. Copyright © The McGraw-Hill Companies, Inc. All rights reserved.)

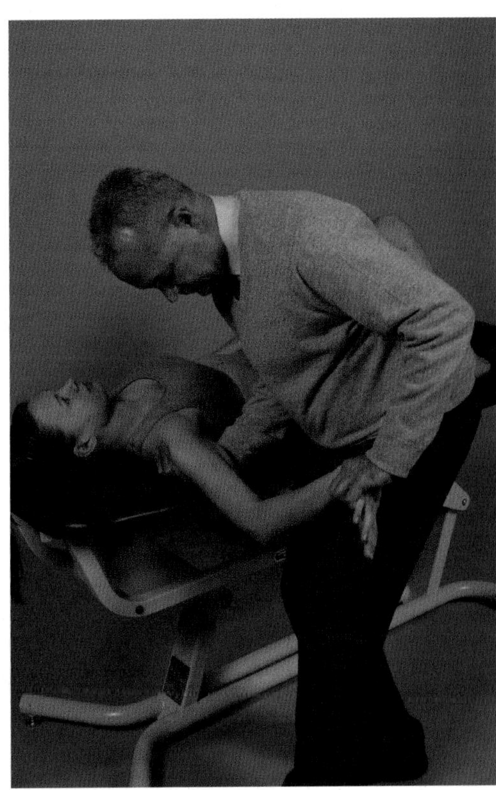

FIGURE 117-3 Upper limb neural tension test: radial nerve bias. (From Dutton M. *Dutton's Orthopedic Survival Guide: Managing Common Conditions*. www.accessphysiotherapy.com. Copyright © The McGraw-Hill Companies, Inc. All rights reserved.)

- Cervical passive intervertebral motion testing
- Subcranial translation instability testing
- Passive physiologic intervertebral mobility testing (PPIVM)[5]
- Upper-extremity screening examination
- Neck Disability Index (NDI)
- Postural examination
- Muscle length testing, including the upper trapezius, levator scapulae, pectoral muscles
- Upper limb nerve tension test[6]
- Deep neck flexor endurance test
- Upper-extremity neurologic screen (dermatome, myotome, reflexes)

INTERVENTION

- Rest
- Bracing
- Address Pain
  - Electrical stimulation
  - Heat/Ice[5]
- Address hypertonicity
  - Soft-tissue massage
  - Heat
- Address muscle weakness
  - Stability exercises

FUNCTIONAL GOALS

- Patient will be able to
  - Sit with neutral cervical spine posture for >30 minutes with 0 out of 10 pain rating.
  - Stand at work station and perform computer work for 45 minutes with 0 out of 10 pain rating.
  - Rotate cervical spine 75 degrees so as to look over the shoulder while driving the car with 0 out of 10 pain rating.

PROGNOSIS

- Fair to good, depending on severity of vertebral translation, amount of nerve-root compression, and upper/lower-extremity impairments.

PATIENT RESOURCE

- American Academy of Orthopaedic Surgeons. Spondylolysis and Spondylolisthesis. http://orthoinfo.aaos.org/topic.cfm?topic=A00053. Accessed April 28, 2013.

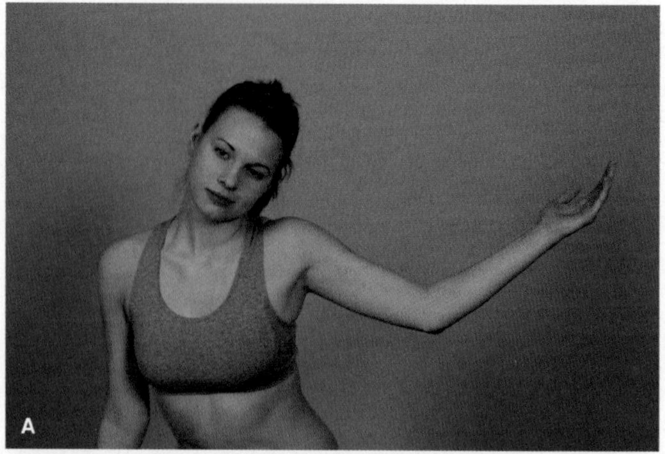

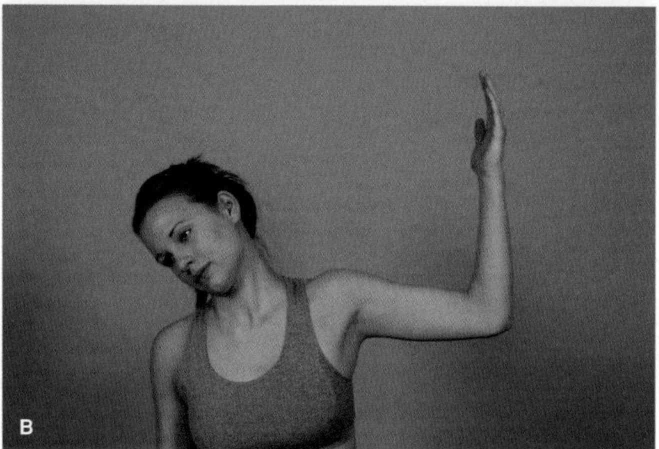

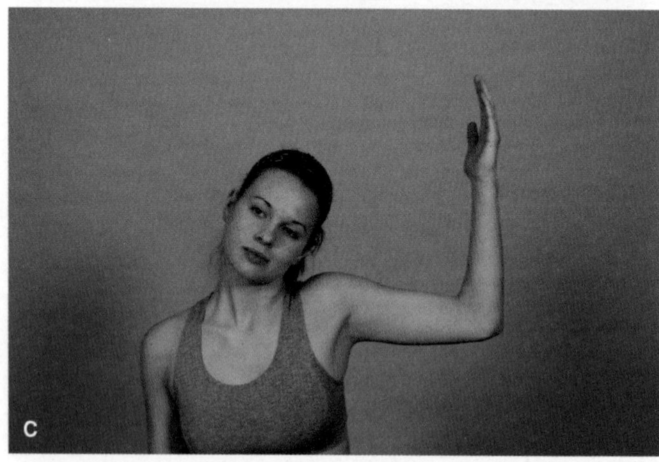

FIGURE 117-4 (A) step 1, (B) step 2, and (C) step 3 of generic self neural mobilization. (From Dutton M. *Dutton's Orthopedic Survival Guide: Managing Common Conditions*. www.accessphysiotherapy.com. Copyright © The McGraw-Hill Companies, Inc. All rights reserved.)

REFERENCES

1. The American Physical Therapy Association. Pattern 4E: Impaired joint mobility, motor function, muscle performance, and range of motion associated with localized inflammation. *Interactive Guide to Physical Therapist Practice*. 2003. DOI: 10.2522/ptguide.978-1-931369-64-0. Online February 28, 2012. Accessed April 28, 2013.
2. Dutton M. *Orthopaedic Examination, Evaluation, and Intervention*. New York, NY: McGraw-Hill; 2008. http://www.accessphysiotherapy.com/resource/612. Accessed April 28, 2013.
3. Malone TR, Hazle C, Grey ML. *Imaging in Rehabilitation*. New York, NY: McGraw-Hill; 2008. http://www.accessphysiotherapy.com/resource/613. Accessed April 28, 2013.
4. Dutton M. *Dutton's Orthopedic Survival Guide: Managing Common Conditions*. New York, NY: McGraw-Hill; 2011. http://www.accessphysiotherapy.com/resource/685. Accessed April 28, 2013.
5. Prentice WE. Chapter 9. Cryotherapy and thermotherapy. In: Prentice WE, Quillen WS, Underwood F, eds. *Therapeutic Modalities in Rehabilitation*. 4th ed. New York, NY: McGraw-Hill; 2011. http://www.accessphysiotherapy.com/content/8137995#8137995. Accessed April 28, 2013.

ADDITIONAL REFERENCES

- ICD9DATA web site. http://www.icd9data.com. Accessed April 28, 2013.
- ICD10DATA web site. http://www.icd10data.com. Accessed April 28, 2013.
- Prentice WE, Quillen WS, Underwood F. Chapter 8. Principles of electrophysiologic evaluation and testing. In: Prentice WE, Quillen WS, Underwood F, eds. *Therapeutic Modalities in Rehabilitation*. 4th ed. http://www.accessphysiotherapy.com/content/8137409. Accessed April 28, 2013.
- Wainner RS, Fritz JM, Irrgang JJ, et al. Reliability and diagnostic accuracy of the clinical examination and patient self-report measures for cervical radiculopathy. *Spine*. 2003;28(1):52–62. [PMID: 12544957]

118 CERVICAL SPONDYLOSIS

Eric Shamus, PhD, DPT, PT, CSCS
Eric J. Chaconas, DPT, PT, FAAOMPT

CONDITION/DISORDER SYNONYMS

- Cervical osteoarthritis
- Spinal osteoarthritis

ICD-9-CM CODES

- 721 Spondylosis and allied disorders
- 721.0 Cervical spondylosis without myelopathy
- 721.1 Cervical spondylosis with myelopathy
- 721.9 Spondylosis of unspecified site
- 721.90 Spondylosis of unspecified site without myelopathy
- 721.91 Spondylosis of unspecified site with myelopathy

ICD-10-CM CODES

- M47.12 Other spondylosis with myelopathy, cervical region
- M47.812 Spondylosis without myelopathy or radiculopathy, cervical region
- M47.819 Spondylosis without myelopathy or radiculopathy, site unspecified

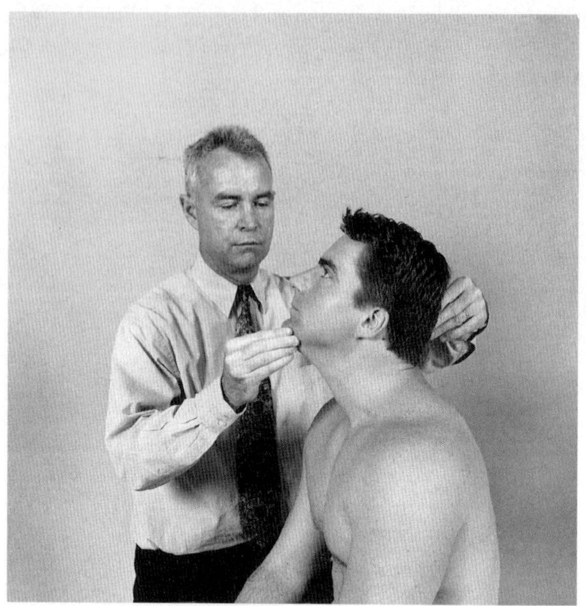

FIGURE 118-1 Short neck extension. (From Dutton M. *Dutton's Orthopedic Survival Guide: Managing Common Conditions.* http://www.accessphysiotherapy.com. Copyright © The McGraw-Hill Companies, Inc. All rights reserved.)

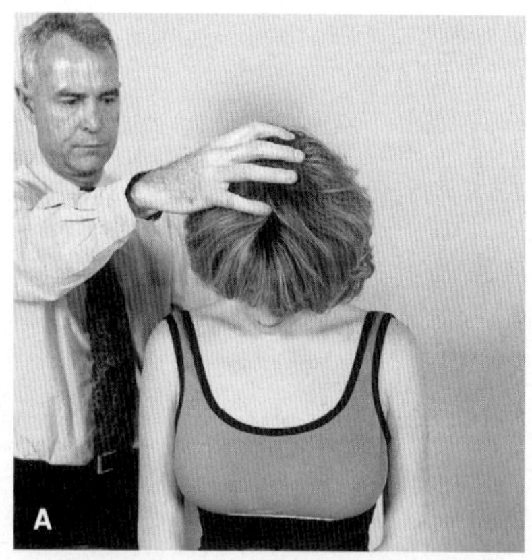

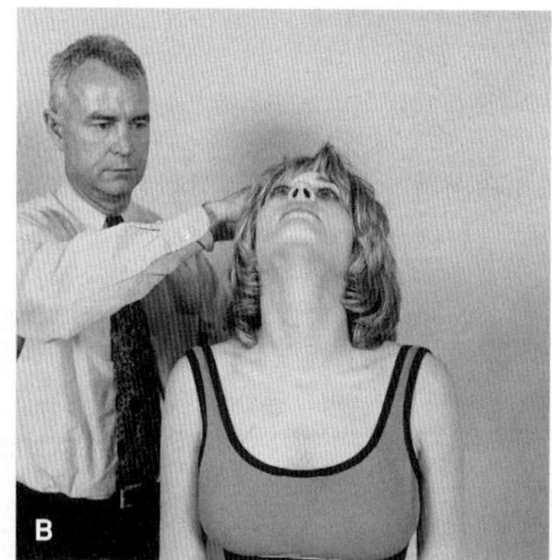

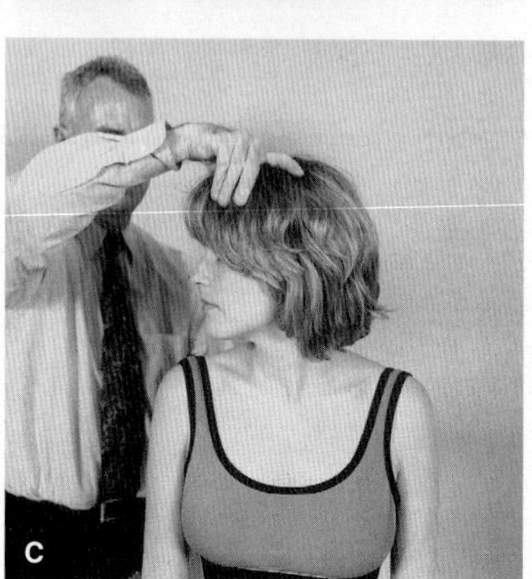

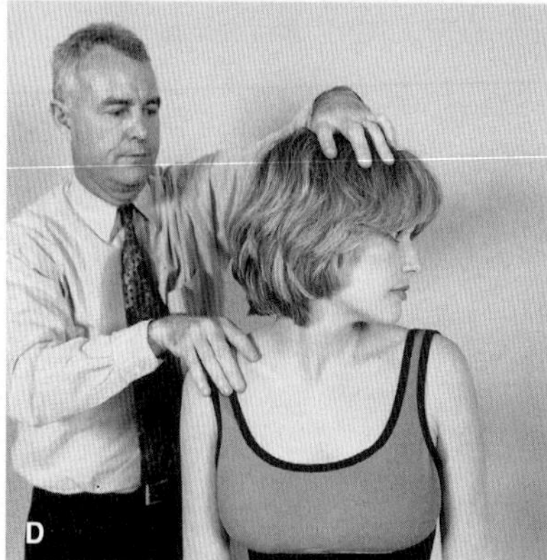

FIGURE 118-2 Cervical active range of motion with passive overpressure. (From Dutton M. *Dutton's Orthopedic Survival Guide: Managing Common Conditions.* http://www.accessphysiotherapy.com. Copyright © The McGraw-Hill Companies, Inc. All rights reserved.)

PREFERRED PRACTICE PATTERNS

- 4B: Impaired Posture[1]
- 4D: Impaired Joint Mobility, Motor Function, Muscle Performance, and Format Range of Motion Associated with Connective Tissue Dysfunction[2]
- 4E: Impaired Joint Mobility, Motor Function, Muscle Performance, and ROM Associated with Localized Inflammation[3]

PATIENT PRESENTATION

A 72-year-old woman presents with neck and bilateral upper extremity pain. She reports worsening of symptoms over the past 2 months and increased numbness into the bilateral hands. Magnetic resonance imaging (MRI) reveals stenosis of the spinal canal at the C6 level along with myelopathy. Diminished sensation is noted in the bilateral thumbs along with weakness of the wrist extensors. Balance impairments are noted, and the patient reports increasing difficulty with ambulation.

KEY FEATURES

Description

- Osteoarthritis of the cervical spine
- Chronic degeneration
- Progressive arthritis of the cervical spinal joints
- As space between the vertebrae decreases, there may be compression onto the nerve roots
- Arthritis can be central- or lateral-foramen based
  - Central: Usually bilateral symptoms
  - Lateral: Usually unilateral
- Pain, paresthesia, and weakness in the upper extremities, can affect lower extremities if central and severe
- Pressure on the nerve root can cause radiculopathy

Essentials of Diagnosis

- X-ray
- Acute painful flare-ups, chronic persistent pain
- Relief with nonsteroidal anti-inflammatory drugs (NSAIDs)
- Morning stiffness

General Considerations

- Begins with intermittent pain
- Pain and stiffness at rest/sleep
- Improved with low-level activity
- May have rapid and severe onset
- Vertebrobasilar insufficiency is secondary problem

Demographics

- Common in adults aged 60 years and older

CLINICAL FINDINGS

SIGNS AND SYMPTOMS

- Fatigue
- Stiffness
- Heaviness in the upper extremities
- Loss of range of motion and joint play
- Intermittent pain, increases with weight bearing
- Paresthesia
- Tingling sensation in the upper extremity
- Diminished reflexes

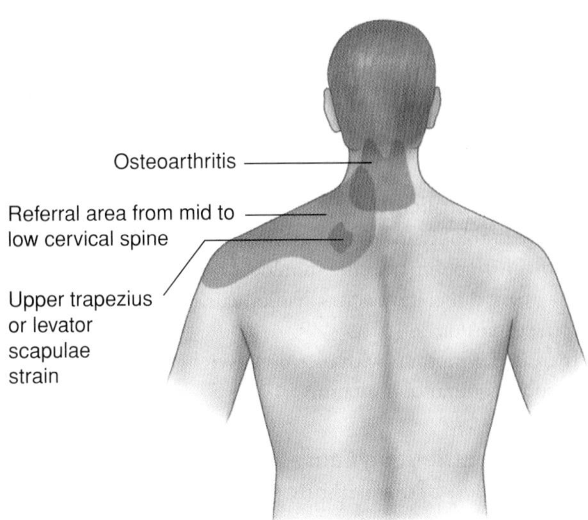

FIGURE 118-3 Pain location and possible diagnoses. (From Dutton M. *Dutton's Orthopedic Survival Guide: Managing Common Conditions.* http://www.accessphysiotherapy.com. Copyright © The McGraw-Hill Companies, Inc. All rights reserved.)

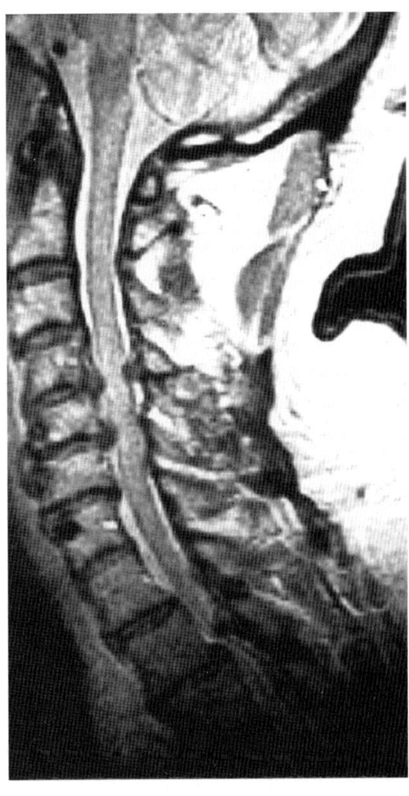

FIGURE 118-4 MRI in a patient with symptomatic cervical spondylosis. The spinal cord at C4-C5 and C5-C6 is flattened on its ventral surface by spondylotic bars and on its posterior surface by ligamentous hypertrophy. Axial images are required to confirm that the cord is truly compressed and that the subarachnoid space is nearly or completely obliterated. (From Ropper AH, Samuels MA. *Adams & Victor's Principles of Neurology.* 9th ed. www.accessmedicine.com. Copyright © The McGraw-Hill Companies, Inc. All rights reserved.)

- Lower motor neuron dysfunction
- Muscle weakness in the arm
- Radiculopathy
- Characteristics of the different syndromes of cervical spondylotic myelopathy[4]

Functional Implications
- Limited mobility in cervical motion
- Difficulty looking over the shoulder while driving
- May have difficulty washing hair at hair dresser due to cervical spine extension
- Increased symptoms with increased weight-bearing
- Aerobic endurance limitation

Possible Contributing Causes
- Family history of osteoarthritis
- Bone spurs
- Instability
- Weakness
- Poor posture
- Limited flexibility

Differential Diagnosis
- Spinal stenosis
- Disc herniation
- Reiter syndrome (reactive arthritis)
- Whipple disease
- Facet joint arthritis
- Rheumatoid arthritis

MEANS OF CONFIRMATION OR DIAGNOSIS

Imaging
- X-ray of the cervical spine[5]
- MRI of the cervical spine[6]

FINDINGS AND INTERPRETATION
- Decreased space between the cervical vertebrae on X-ray

TREATMENT

Medication
- NSAIDs
- Corticosteroids

REFERRALS/ADMITTANCE
- To rheumatologist to assess underlying complications
- To orthopedic surgeon for surgical consult

IMPAIRMENTS
- Mobility
- Functional rotation and bending

TESTS AND MEASURES
- Cervical spine AROM
- Sharp–Purser: Atlantoaxial instability
- Cervical passive intervertebral motion testing
- Subcranial translation instability testing
- Passive physiologic intervertebral mobility testing (PPIVM)[5]

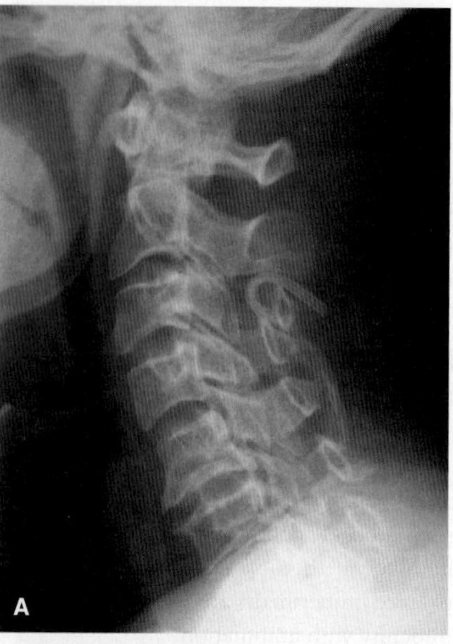

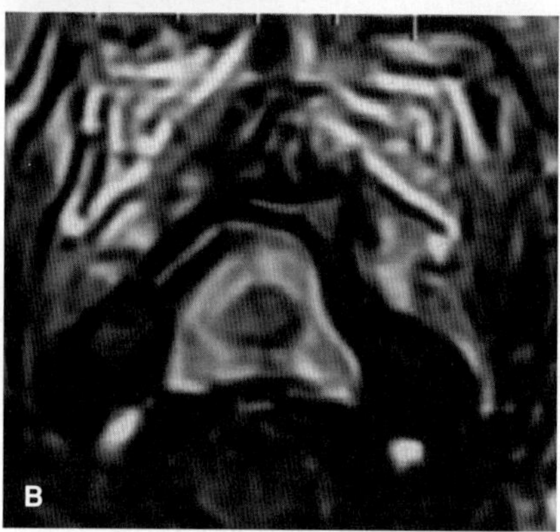

FIGURE 118-5 **A:** Lateral postoperative radiograph of a patient who had multisegmental cervical stenosis and myelopathy treated with canal expansive cervical laminoplasty from C3 to C7. **B:** Postoperative axial MRI image showing significant canal expansion after the procedure. (From Doherty GM. *Current Diagnosis & Treatment: Surgery.* 13th ed. www.accessmedicine.com. Copyright © The McGraw-Hill Companies, Inc. All rights reserved.)

- Upper-extremity screening examination
- Postural examination
- Neck Disability Index (NDI)
- Muscle length testing, including the upper trapezius, levator scapulae, and pectoral muscles
- Upper limb nerve tension test[6]
- Deep neck flexor endurance test
- Upper-extremity neurological screen (dermatome, myotome, reflexes)

INTERVENTION
- Education in gentle range of motion to maintain mobility
- Exercise: Flexibility and stability strengthening to decrease stress on the joints
- Joint protection education
- Postural training
- Joint manipulation to the thoracic and upper cervical spine
- Cervical distraction and traction to relieve nerve compression
- Craniocervical flexion exercises
- Periscapular strengthening

- Address Pain
  - Electrical stimulation
  - Heat/Ice to increase mobility
- Address hypertonicity
  - Soft-tissue massage
  - Heat
- Address muscle weakness
  - Deep neck flexor training
  - Strengthening of the lower/middle trapezius, rhomboids, rotator cuff
  - Serratus anterior, latissimus dorsi
- Heat or warm shower to increase mobility

FUNCTIONAL GOALS

- Patient will
  - Be independent with home exercise program.
  - Be have decreased pain to perform household activities such as cleaning and laundry.
  - Have improved functional level to look over the shoulder while driving.

PROGNOSIS

- Disease progression is not specific; joints may become limited and have increased compression as disease becomes more severe.
- Symptoms may be intermittent.
- Patients function well until severe progression of joint mobility.

PATIENT RESOURCE

- American Academy of Orthopeadic Surgeons. Cervical Spondylosis. http://orthoinfo.aaos.org/topic.cfm?topic=A00369. Accessed April 14, 2013.

REFERENCES

1. The American Physical Therapy Association. Pattern 4B: Impaired posture. *Interactive Guide to Physical Therapist Practice.* 2003. DOI: 10.2522/ptguide.3.1_2. Online February 28, 2012. Accessed April 1, 2013.
2. The American Physical Therapy Association. Pattern 4D: Impaired joint mobility, motor function, muscle performance, and range of motion associated with connective tissue dysfunction. *Interactive Guide to Physical Therapist Practice.* 2003. DOI: 10.2522/ptguide.3.1_4. Online February 28, 2012. Accessed April 1, 2013.
3. The American Physical Therapy Association. Pattern 4E: Impaired joint mobility, motor function, muscle performance, and range of motion associated with localized inflammation. *Interactive Guide to Physical Therapist Practice.* 2003. DOI: 10.2522/ptguide.978-1-931369-64-0. Online February 28, 2012. Accessed April 1, 2013.
4. Dutton M. Chapter 23. The cervical spine. In: Dutton M, ed. *Orthopaedic Examination, Evaluation, and Intervention.* 2nd ed. New York, NY: McGraw-Hill; 2008. http://www.accessphysiotherapy.com/content/55592048. Accessed April 24, 2013.
5. Malone TR, Hazle C, Grey ML. Chapter 9. The knee. In: Malone TR, Hazle C, Grey ML, eds. *Imaging in Rehabilitation.* New York, NY: McGraw-Hill; 2008. http://www.accessphysiotherapy.com/abstract/5941231. Accessed April 24, 2013.
6. Hamilton N, Weimar W, Luttgens K. Chapter 3. The Musculoskeletal System: The Musculature. In: Hamilton N, Weimar W, Luttgens K, eds. *Kinesiology: Scientific Basis of Human Motion.* New York, NY: McGraw-Hill; 2008. http://www.accessphysiotherapy.com/abstract/6150358#6150373. Accessed April 24, 2013.

ADDITIONAL REFERENCES

- Dutton M. Pattern 4D: Impaired joint mobility, motor function, muscle performance, and format range of motion associated with connective tissue dysfunction. In: Dutton M, ed. *Dutton's Orthopaedic Examination, Evaluation, and Intervention.* 3rd ed. New York, NY: McGraw-Hill; 2012. http://www.accessphysiotherapy.com/content/55592048. Accessed April 24, 2013.
- Friedenberg ZB, Miller WT. Degenerative disc disease of the cervical spine. *J Bone Joint Surg.* 1963;45:1171–1178.
- ICD9DATA web site. http://www.icd9data.com. Accessed April 21, 2013.
- ICD10DATA web site. http://www.icd10data.com. Accessed April 14, 2013.
- Jeffreys E. Cervical spondylosis. In: Jeffreys E, ed. *Disorders of the Cervical Spine.* Boston, MA: Butterworths. 1980:90–106. http://www.spondylitis.org. Accessed April 14, 2013.

119 COCCYDYNIA

Elizabeth R. Northrop, DPT, PT
Cynthia E. Neville, DPT, PT, WCS

CONDITION/DISORDER SYNONYM

- Coccydynia

ICD-9-CM CODES

- 724.7 Disorders of coccyx
- 724.70 Unspecified disorder of coccyx
- 724.71 Hypermobility of coccyx
- 724.79 Other disorders of coccyx
- 839.41 Closed dislocation, coccyx
- 839.42 Closed dislocation, sacrum
- 847.3 Sprain of sacrum
- 847.4 Sprain of coccyx

ICD-10-CM CODES

- M53.2X8 Spinal instabilities, sacral and sacrococcygeal region
- M53.3 Sacrococcygeal disorders, not elsewhere classified
- S33.2XXA Dislocation of sacroiliac and sacrococcygeal joint, initial encounter
- S33.8XXA Sprain of other parts of lumbar spine and pelvis, initial encounter

PREFERRED PRACTICE PATTERNS[1]

- 4B: Impaired Posture
- 4D: Impaired Joint Mobility, Motor Function, Muscle Performance, and Range of Motion Associated with Connective Tissue Dysfunction
- 4E: Impaired Joint Mobility, Motor Function, Muscle Performance, and Range of Motion Associated with Localized Inflammation
- 4G: Impaired Joint Mobility, Muscle Performance, and Range of Motion Associated with Fracture

PATIENT PRESENTATION

A 25-year-old woman delivered her first baby vaginally. She had epidural anesthesia during the delivery. During the delivery, she heard a loud "pop" noise. After the epidural wore off, she felt a severe pain in her rear end. She was unable to sit on the edge of the hospital bed and had severe pain when she attempted to sit in a chair.

KEY FEATURES

Description

- Tailbone pain
- Pain often increases with sitting, defecation, transitional movements, and palpation of the coccyx

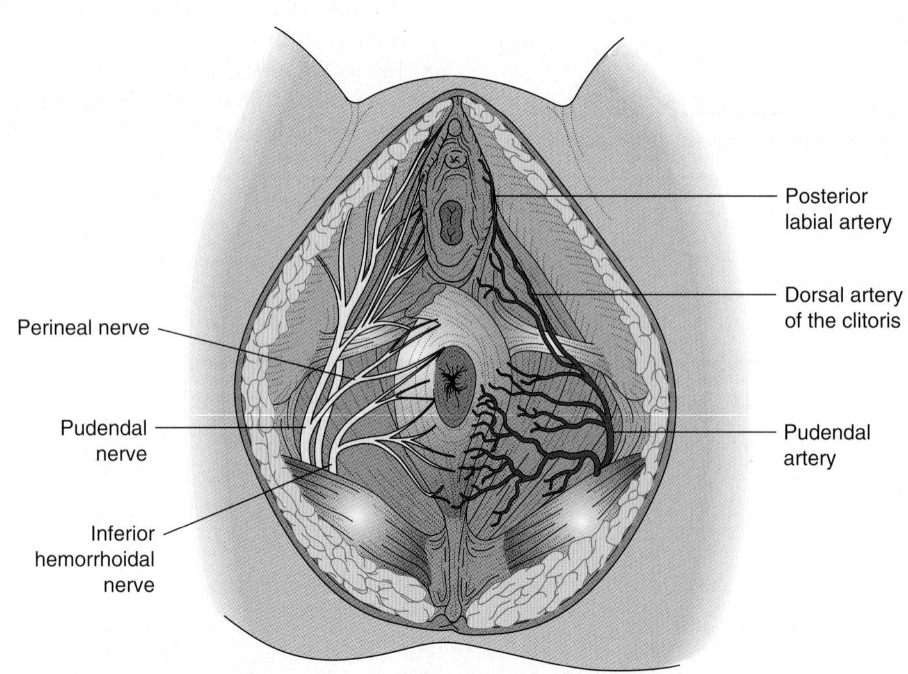

FIGURE 119-1 Arteries and nerves of the perineum. (From DeCherney AH, Nathan L, Goodwin TM, Laufer N, Roman AS. *Current Diagnosis & Treatment: Obstetrics & Gynecology.* 11th ed. www.accessmedicine.com. Copyright © The McGraw-Hill Companies, Inc. All rights reserved.)

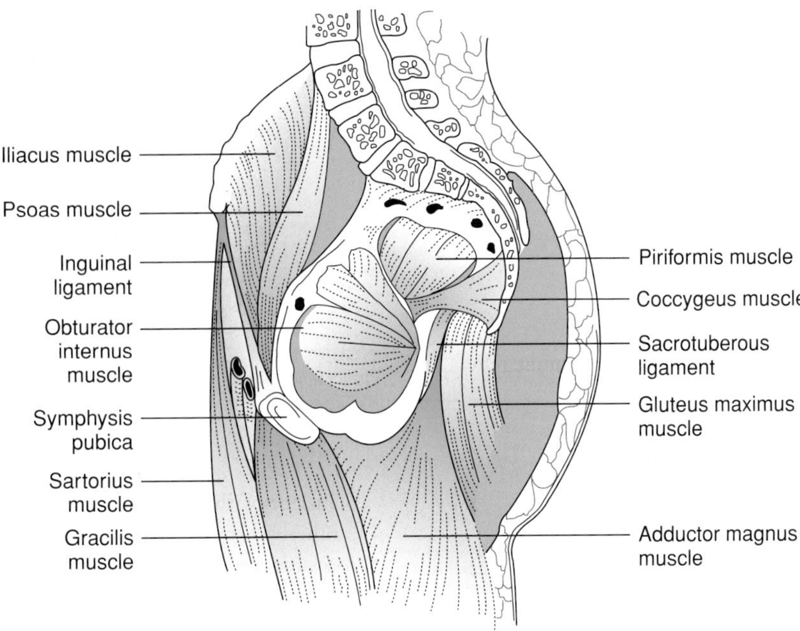

FIGURE 119-2 Pelvic muscles. (From DeCherney AH, Nathan L. *Current Diagnosis & Treatment: Obstetrics & Gynecology.* 10th ed. www.accessmedicine.com. Copyright © The McGraw-Hill Companies, Inc. All rights reserved.)

General Considerations

- Consider sacroiliac (SI) joint as potential cause of pain
- Ask patient about the history of falls; distant history can contribute to coccydynia
- Occupations requiring prolonged sitting may contribute to coccydynia
- Pain may be referred from muscles, including the obturator internus, levator ani, and gluteus maximus

Demographics

- Five times more common in women than in men
- Mean age of onset is 40 years
- Three times more common in obese patients

CLINICAL FINDINGS

SIGNS AND SYMPTOMS

- Pain in sitting position
- Pain with transition from sitting to standing
- Pain with standing, walking, forward flexion
- Pain with defecation, coughing
- Increased pain during menstruation
- Inflammation
- Poor sitting posture
- Frequent shifts in sitting position, sitting down carefully
- Luxation, hypermobility, hypomobility of the coccyx

Functional Implications

- Difficulty sitting, impacting ability to perform work and daily activities
- Difficulty or pain with defecation

Possible Contributing Causes

- Vaginal delivery
- Postpartum
- Direct trauma from fracture, fall, childbirth
- Poor sitting posture
- Prolonged sitting
- Anorectal infection
- Levator ani spasm
- Trigger points of obturator internus, levator ani, or gluteus maximus
- Overuse of levator ani
- Neoplasm
- Pelvic asymmetry
- Stretch or rupture of sacrococcygeal ligaments
- Soft-tissue damage

Differential Diagnosis

- Sacral chordoma
- Tarlov cyst
- Pilonidal cyst
- SI joint pain

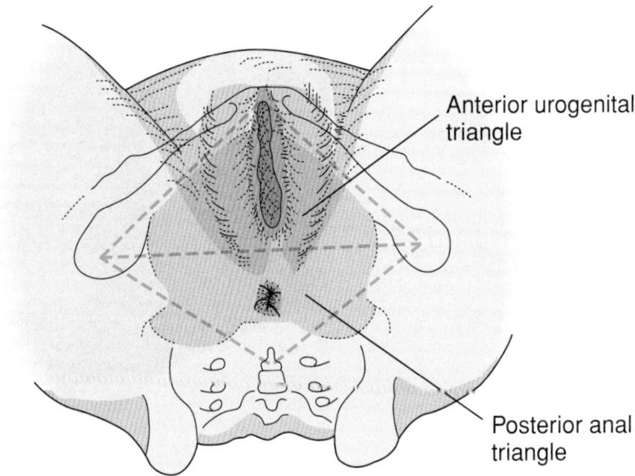

FIGURE 119-3 Urogenital and anal triangles. (From DeCherney AH, Nathan L. *Current Diagnosis & Treatment: Obstetrics & Gynecology.* 10th ed. www.accessmedicine. com. Copyright © The McGraw-Hill Companies, Inc. All rights reserved.)

MEANS OF CONFIRMATION OR DIAGNOSIS

Imaging

- Dynamic radiograph of coccyx position
- Dynamic radiography (stand vs. sit)

Diagnostic Procedures

- Joint injection at the coccyx–sacral junction
- Physical examination
- Diagnostic joint injection

FINDINGS AND INTERPRETATION

- Joint injection at the coccyx–sacral junction to determine relief

TREATMENT

Medications

- Muscle relaxants
- Oral analgesics
- Oral corticosteroids

MEDICAL PROCEDURES

- Trigger point injections
- Corticosteroid injection
- Local anesthetic injection
- Coccygectomy

REFERRALS/ADMITTANCE

- To physician/interventional radiologist for trigger point injections

IMPAIRMENTS

- Pain
- Overactive pelvic floor muscles
- Poor posture
- Limited joint mobility
- Obstructed defecation

TESTS AND MEASURES

- Palpation and mobility of the coccyx
  - Palpate the coccyx externally with single digit; attempt to move it 20 to 30 degrees.

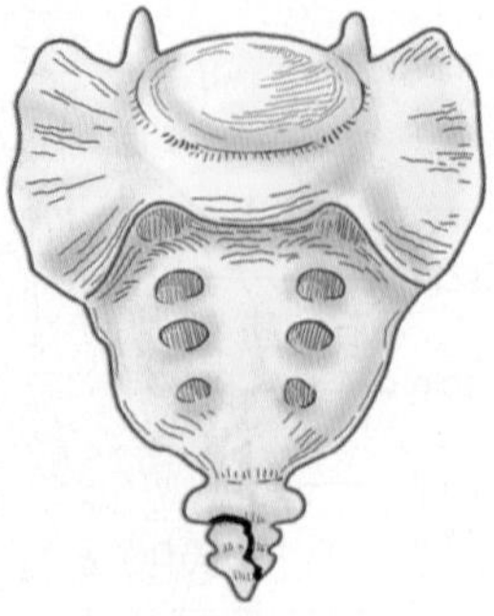

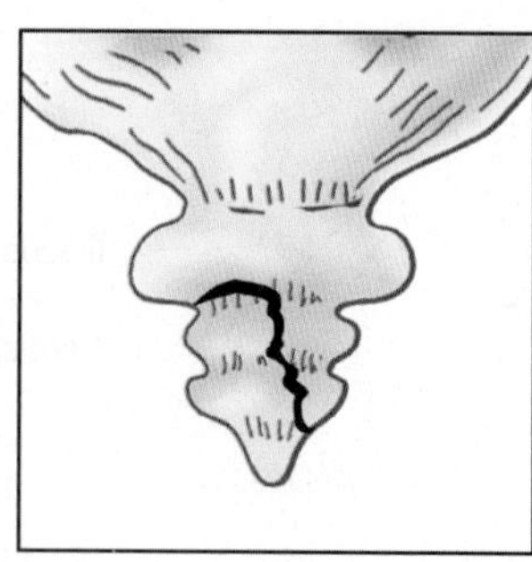

FIGURE 119-4 Coccyx fracture. (From Simon RR, Sherman SC. *Emergency Orthopedics.* 6th ed. www.accessemergencymedicine.com. Copyright © The McGraw-Hill Companies, Inc. All rights reserved.)

  - Patients with coccydynia often have pain with movement; otherwise, movement should be pain free.
- Assessment of the pelvic floor muscle
- Palpation of the coccygeus, levator ani, obturator internus, and gluteus maximus for trigger points
- Posture assessment
- Assessment of pelvic girdle with pain provocation test

INTERVENTION

- Seating adaptation: Coccyx cut-out wedge cushion ("donut" cushion)
- Postural instruction
- Education on normal defecation, to avoid constipation
- Education on stress management and relaxation for patients with anxiety
- Coccyx manipulation, sacrococcygeal joint manipulation or mobilization
- Joint mobilizations to address hypomobility of the SI joint, lumbar, hip, or pubic symphysis dysfunction
- Myofascial treatment to the coccygeus, levator ani, obturator internus, gluteus maximus, piriformis
- Transvaginal or transrectal myofascial release
- Vaginal or rectal electrical stimulation
- Coccyx taping
- Pelvic floor muscle exercise and training

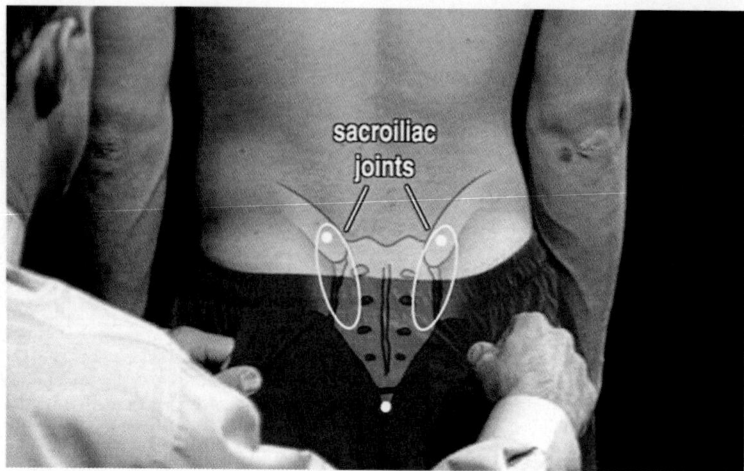

FIGURE 119-5 Sacrum and Coccyx position for palpation in standing. (From Lawry GV. *Systematic Musculoskeletal Examinations.* www.accessmedicine.com. Copyright © The McGraw-Hill Companies, Inc. All rights reserved.)

- Contraction
- Relaxation, "bulging"
- Motor control
- Endurance
- Power

- Surface electromyography (sEMG) biofeedback for down-training of pelvic floor muscles
- Exercises to address biomechanical dysfunction of the SI joint
  - Lumbosacral active ROM in quadruped
    - "Cat and camel"
    - Pelvic sway, "tail wag"
  - Isometric contract–relax exercises of gluteal and iliopsoas muscles and/or hip abductors and adductors

FUNCTIONAL GOALS

- Patients will be able to
  - Demonstrate proper posture to reduce pain and prevent reinjury of the coccyx.
  - Perform sit-to-stand transfers independently without increased pain.
  - Increase sitting tolerance to ____ minutes to be able to drive, ride in car, perform desk work.
  - Demonstrate independence with home exercise program, promoting relaxation and awareness of the pelvic floor muscle for long-term self-management.

PROGNOSIS

- Patients with normal coccyx mobility have 43% success rate with conservative treatment.[2]
- Patients with immobile coccyx have 16% success rate with conservative treatment.[2]
- Patients with hypermobility or subluxation of the coccyx have 85% success rate with combined manipulation and steroid/anesthetic injection.[2]

PATIENT RESOURCE

- Coccyx pain. www.coccyx.org. Accessed June 21, 2013.

REFERENCES

1. The American Physical Therapy Association. *Interactive Guide to Physical Therapist Practice*. Alexandria, VA: The American Physical Therapy Association; 2003. http://guidetoptpractice.apta.org/. Accessed June 21, 2013.
2. Patel R, Appannagari A, Whang PG. Coccydynia. *Curr Rev Musculoskelet Med*. 2008;1:223–226.

ADDITIONAL REFERENCES

- ICD9Data.com. http://www.icd9data.com. Accessed June 21, 2013.
- ICD10Data.com. http://www.icd10data.com. Accessed June 21, 2013.
- Dutton M. Pathology, Gynecology, and Psychology. In: Dutton M, ed. *McGraw-Hill's NPTE (National Physical Therapy Examination)*. 2nd ed. New York, NY: McGraw-Hill; 2012. http://www.accessphysiotherapy.com/content/5402528. Accessed June 21, 2013.
- Dutton M. The Sacroiliac Joint. In: Dutton M, ed. *Dutton's Orthopaedic Examination, Evaluation, and Intervention*. 3rd ed. New York, NY: McGraw-Hill; 2012. http://www.accessphysiotherapy.com/content/55598142. Accessed June 21, 2013.
- Simon RR, Sherman SC. Pelvis. In: Simon RR, Sherman SC, eds. *Emergency Orthopedics*. 6th ed. New York, NY: McGraw-Hill; 2011. http://www.accessphysiotherapy.com/content/7706610. Accessed June 21, 2013.

120 CERVICAL DYSTONIA

Ariel Diana Schumer, DPT
Eric Shamus, PhD, DPT, PT, CSCS

CONDITION/DISORDER SYNONYMS

- Acquired torticollis
- Adult torticollis
- Anterocollis
- Dystonia
- Focal dystonia
- Laterocollis
- Retrocollis
- Spasmodic torticollis
- Torticollis

ICD-9-CM CODES

- 333.83 Spasmodic torticollis
- 723.5 Torticollis unspecified

ICD-10-CM CODES

- G24.3 Spasmodic torticollis
- M43.6 Torticollis

PREFERRED PRACTICE PATTERN

- 4E: Impaired Joint Mobility, Motor Function, Muscle Performance, and ROM Associated with Localized Inflammation

PATIENT PRESENTATION

Patient is a 66-year-old woman who has complaints over the last 2 years of neck pain and a pulling to the right side. Over the last year, she has had head tremors. She has tried Botox injections, which gave her temporary relief. Her friend gave her a cervical collar to wear and feels that if she does not wear it her head falls to the side. Past medical history: Severe whiplash injury 3 years ago due to a car accident.

KEY FEATURES

Description

- Dystonia is a condition characterized by involuntary intermittent or prolonged muscular contractions (e.g., twisting, jerky, or repetitive movements) that may cause abnormal postures and movements.
- Dystonia may be generalized or focal.
- Cervical dystonia (CD) is the most common focal dystonia.
- CD is commonly referred to as spasmodic torticollis, which may be misleading.
  - Spasmodic describes movements that are intermittent or clonic and tremulous, though some patients with CD present with prolonged contractions.
  - Torticollis implies rotary impairment, though patients with CD often present with combined postures associated with flexion, extension, and side-bending.
- Further classification may be based on the head position or movement.[1]
  - Forward tilt is called anterocollis.
  - Backward tilt is called retrocollis.

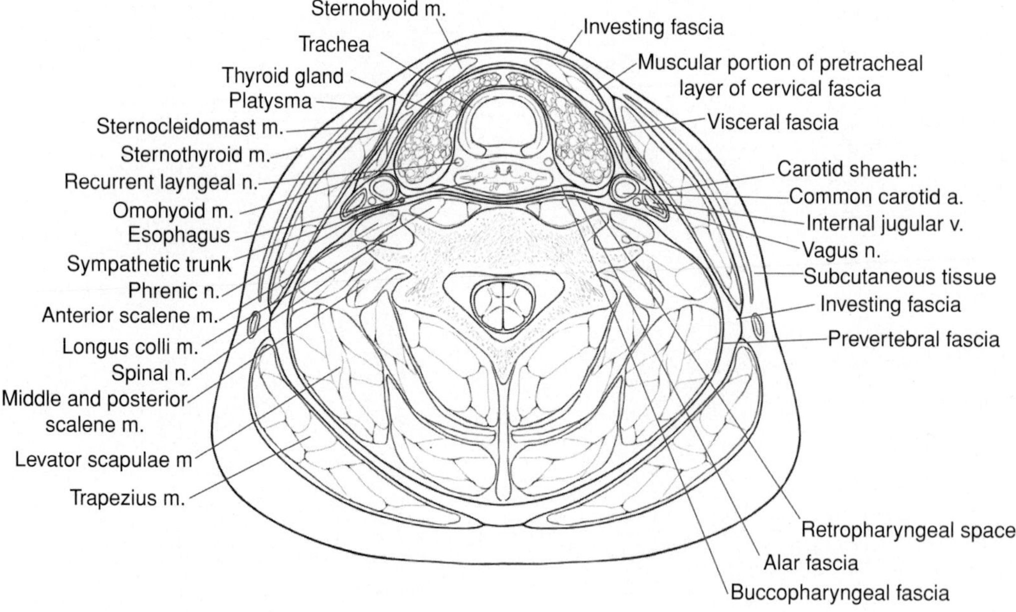

FIGURE 120-1 Fascial planes of the neck. (cross-section at C7). (From Lalwani AK. *Current Diagnosis & Treatment in Otolaryngology—Head & Neck Surgery.* 3rd ed. www.accesssurgery.com. Copyright © The McGraw-Hill Companies, Inc. All rights reserved.)

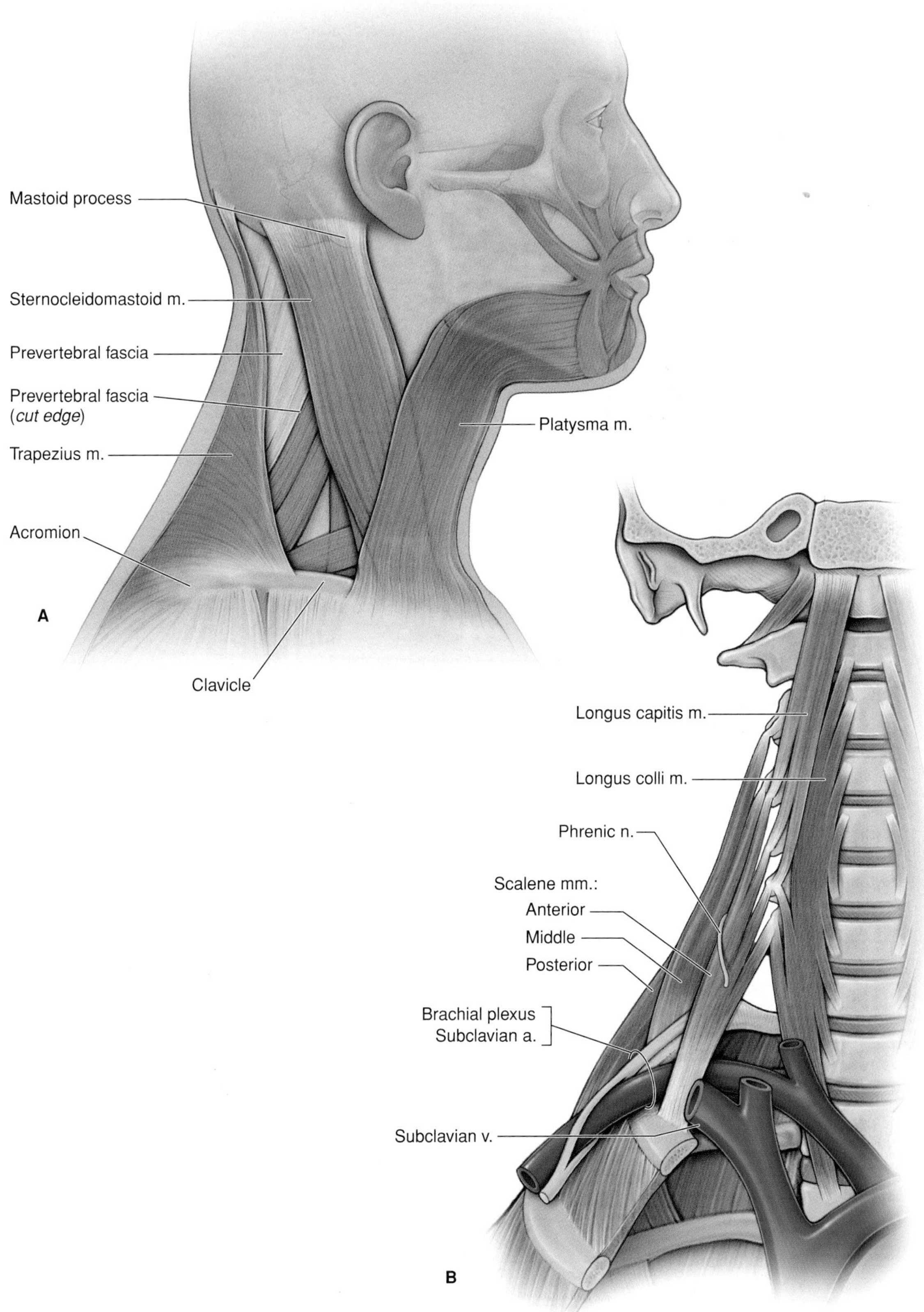

FIGURE 120-2 (**A**) Muscles of the neck. (**B**) Anterior view of the scalene and prevertebral muscles. (From Morton DA, Foreman KB, Albertine KH. *The Big Picture: Gross Anatomy.* http://www.accessmedicine.com. Copyright © The McGraw-Hill Companies, Inc. All rights reserved.)

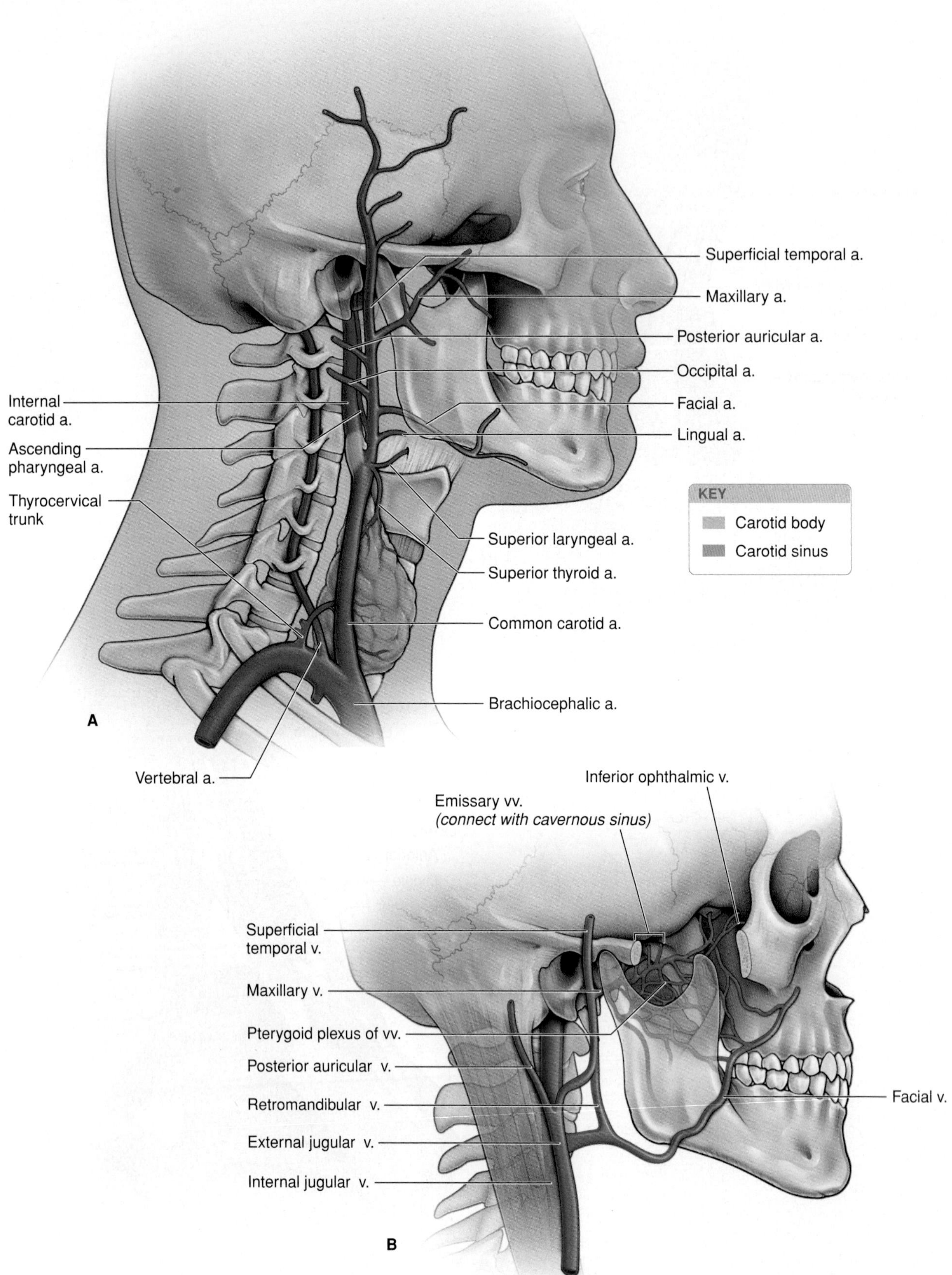

FIGURE 120-3 (**A**) The principal arteries of the head and neck. (**B**) The principal venous drainage of the head and neck. (From Morton DA, Foreman KB, Albertine KH. *The Big Picture: Gross Anatomy.* http://www.accessmedicine.com. Copyright © The McGraw-Hill Companies, Inc. All rights reserved.)

- Left or right tilt is called laterocollis.
- Moving from side to side is called rotational spasmodic torticollis.
- Turning and shaking of the head is called mixed torticollis.

Essentials of Diagnosis

- Traditional classification is based on etiology.
  - Primary (idiopathic)
  - Secondary (of known cause)
- Current classification describes each person based on the following characteristics:
  - Age of onset
  - Distribution of symptoms

General Considerations

- Most cases develop in adulthood.
- May begin in the neck and progress to the shoulders, usually stabilizes after a few years.
- A similar musculoskeletal condition during infancy is called congenital muscular torticollis.
- Patients with CD can show signs of self-consciousness and depression.

Demographics

- Incidence of CD is 8.9 per 100,000 people
- Occurrence in men to women ranges from 1 man to 1.4 to 2.2 women (1:1.4–2.2)
- Mean age of onset is 39.2 years for men and 42.9 years for women[2]
- Approximately 90% of cases are idiopathic and 10% to 20% are from a defined cause.

CLINICAL FINDINGS

SIGNS AND SYMPTOMS

- Common to patients with primary and secondary CD
  - Pain
  - Enlargement of the neck muscles
  - Shoulder elevation on the affected side
  - Ipsilateral head tilt and contralateral head rotation
  - Head tremor or spasmodic jerking
  - Tremors of the arm
  - Possible difficulty swallowing
- Unique to patients with posttraumatic CD
  - Marked limitation in range of motion
  - Lack of improvement after sleep
  - Lack of geste antagoniste, also known as sensory tricks, are physical positioning, such as touching the chin, which have been shown to temporarily reduce dystonia[3]

Functional Implications

- Postural control abnormalities
- Greater reliance on vision for maintaining postural stability[2]
- Reduced ability to perform activities of daily living involving head or neck movements
- Difficulty sleeping
- Reduced psychosocial functioning

Possible Contributing Causes

- Primary CD
  - Idiopathic cause
- Secondary CD
  - Drugs
    - Neuroleptics
    - Dopamine agonists
    - Anticonvulsants
    - Antimalarial drugs
  - Environmental toxins
    - Manganese
    - Carbon monoxide
    - Methanol
  - CNS lesions
    - Intramedullary lesions of the cervical cord
    - Focal brain lesions, such as vascular malformation, tumor, or abscess
    - Demyelinating lesions, such as with multiple sclerosis
    - Traumatic brain injury to the contralateral basal ganglia or thalamus
    - Encephalitis
    - After hemiplegia as a delayed reaction to stroke
  - Disease or condition
    - Parkinson disease
    - Huntington disease
    - Wilson' disease
    - Progressive supranuclear palsy
    - Multiple system atrophy
    - Cerebral palsy
    - Hypoparathyroidism[1]

Differential Diagnosis

- Diagnosis is by clinical examination; no standard laboratory tests are employed to diagnose CD
- Determining that there is no evidence for cause of secondary dystonia is essential in diagnosing primary dystonia
- In addition to the possible contributing causes listed, the following pathologies must be ruled out to diagnose primary CD:
  - Cervical disc disease
  - Spinal abnormalities
  - Epilepsy
  - Muscular dystrophy
  - Thyroiditis
  - Endocrine disease[4]

MEANS OF CONFIRMATION OR DIAGNOSIS

Imaging

- Imaging
  - X-ray
  - MRI
  - CT

Diagnostic Procedures

- Diagnosis is made by clinical observation
- Toronto Western Spasmodic Torticollis Rating Scale
- Torticollis Rating Scale of Tsui
- CD Impact Profile

FINDINGS AND INTERPRETATION

- Imaging (X-ray, MRI, CT) to rule out congenital deformities of the cervical spine, ocular anomalies, CNS pathology,[5] neoplasm, thyroiditis, and endocrine disease[4]

TREATMENT

▸ Medication[6,7]

- Botulinum toxin A
  - Most commonly used pharmacotherapy for CD
  - Two preparations, botox and dysport, are available
  - Injected into overactive musculature to weaken dystonic muscles
  - Injections often performed with Electromyography (EMG) to enhance accuracy
  - Average duration of benefit is 12 to 16 weeks
- For symptomatic relief and treatment of underlying causes, the following oral medications may be used
  - Analgesics
  - Benzodiazepines
  - Baclofen
  - Dopaminergic drugs
  - Anticholinergic agents
  - Tetrabenazine with lithium[2]

MEDICAL PROCEDURES

- Surgery is not to be considered unless all other options have failed and symptoms have remained stable over 12 months.[2]
  - Selective peripheral denervation.
  - For laterocollis, denervation of ipsilateral posterior cervical paraspinals, splenius capitis, and sternocleidomastoid muscles is performed.
  - For rotary torticollis, similar to laterocollis with the exception of denervation of the contralateral sternocleidomastoid.
  - Deep brain stimulation.
- Microelectrodes placed within the globus pallidus internus or subthalamic nucleus.
- Multiple follow-up visits required to properly program settings for the stimulator.
- Procedure is reversible, and microstimulator settings are adjustable.[2]

REFERRALS/ADMITTANCE

- To physician
  - If cervical subluxation is suspected
  - If patient does not respond to physical therapy
- To occupational and speech therapists as necessary
- To surgeon if alternatives have failed

IMPAIRMENTS

- Pain in the neck region
- Decreased cervical range of motion
- Decreased cervical strength
- Difficulty maintaining head in midline
- Dystonic posturing
- Poor postural alignment
- Balance deficits

INTERVENTION

- A thorough examination includes, but is not limited to head position, cervical range of motion, postural alignment and control, muscle length and strength throughout the spine and shoulder region, tone, and balance.[2]
- Functional abilities must be addressed, including stress management, energy conservation, adaptive equipment, mobility, splinting.[1]
- Heat
- Traction
- Massage
- Stretching
- Conservative strengthening
- Aquatic therapy
- Joint mobilization
- Inhibitory techniques to temporarily reduce spasm or tone[1]

FUNCTIONAL GOALS

- Patient will be able to
  - Maintain midline cervical posture for 3 minutes to enhance computer-related tasks.
  - Achieve 60 degrees of active, combined cervical rotation bilaterally to increase safety while operating a vehicle.
  - Reduce cervical pain to 2/10 or better 90% of the time.
  - Demonstrate supportive positioning of the cervical spine to decrease frequency of waking during the night.

PROGNOSIS

- Most often, CD progresses gradually over a period of months to years.
- Remissions have been reported, though most are temporary.
- Persistent CD can lead to restricted movements, postural deformity, degenerative osteoarthritis of the cervical spine, and spinal radiculopathies.

PATIENT RESOURCE

- National Spasmodic Torticollis Association. Spasmodic Torticollis/Cervical Dystonia. Torticollis.org. http://www.torticollis.org. Accessed June 20, 2013.

REFERENCES

1. Fuller KS, Corboy JR, Winkler PA. Degenerative diseases of the central nervous system. In: Goodman C, Boissonnault WG, Fuller KS, eds. *Pathology: Implications for the Physical Therapist.* 3rd ed. Philadelphia, PA: Saunders; 2007.
2. Crowner BE. Cervical dystonia: disease profile and clinical management. *Phys Therl.* 2007;87(11):1511–1526.
3. Martino D, Luizzi D, Macerollo A, Aniello MS, Livrea P, Defazio G. The phenomenology of the geste antagoniste in primary blepharospasm and cervical dystonia. *Movement Disorders.* 2010;25(4):407–412. doi: 10.1002/mds.23011.
4. Goodman CC, Snyder TEK. Screening the head, neck, and back. In: Goodman CC, Snyder TEK, eds. *Differential Diagnosis for Physical Therapists: Screening for Referral.* 4th ed. St. Louis, MO: Saunders; 2007:640.
5. Goodman CC, Glanzman A, Miedaner J. Genetic and developmental disorders. In: Goodman C, Boissonnault WG, Fuller KS, eds. *Pathology: Implications for the Physical Therapist.* 3rd ed. Philadelphia, PA: Saunders; 2007.
6. Torticollis. MDGuidelines. http://www.mdguidelines.com/torticollis. Accessed June 20, 2013.
7. Panus PC, Jobst EE, Masters SB, Katzung B, Tinsley SL, Trevor AJ. Skeletal muscle relaxants. In: Panus PC, Jobst EE, Masters SB, et al., eds. *Pharmacology for the Physical Therapist.* New York, NY: McGraw-Hill; 2009. http://www.accessphysiotherapy.com/content/6095617. Accessed June 20, 2013.

ADDITIONAL REFERENCES

- ICD9DATA web site. http://www.icd9data.com. Accessed June 16, 2013.
- ICD10DATA web site. http://www.icd10data.com. Accessed June 16, 2013.
- Ostrowski C, Ronan L, Sheridan R, Pearce V. An osteoporotic fracture mimicking cervical dystonia in idiopathic Parkinson's disease. *Age Ageing*. 2013;42(5):658–659.
- Pelosin E, Avanzino L, Marchese R, et al. Kinesio taping reduces pain and modulates sensory function in patients with focal dystonia: a randomized crossover pilot study. *Neurorehabil Neural Repair*. 2013;27(8):722–731.
- Queiroz MA, Chien HF, Sekeff-Sallem FA, Barbosa ER. Physical therapy program for cervical dystonia: a study of 20 cases. *Funct Neurol*. 2012;27(3):187–192.

121 FACET JOINT SYNDROME, LUMBAR

Arie J. Van Duijn, EdD, MSc, PT, OCS
Eric Shamus, PhD, DPT, PT, CSCS

CONDITION/DISORDER SYNONYMS

- Sprain of the facet joint, Lumbar
- Arthritic changes in the facet joint

ICD-9-CM CODE

- 847.2 Lumbar sprain

ICD-10-CM CODES

- S33 Dislocation and sprain of joints and ligaments of lumbar spine and pelvis
- S33.5 Sprain of ligaments of lumbar spine

PREFERRED PRACTICE PATTERN

- Pattern 4F: Impaired Joint Mobility, Motor Function, Muscle Performance, Range of Motion, and Reflex Integrity Associated with Spinal Disorders[1]

PATIENT PRESENTATION

A 35-year-old man presents with a sudden onset of low back pain (LBP) 5 days ago, following bending over to pick up an item from the floor. The pain is located along the right side of the lumbar spine, sometimes radiating to the buttock region. Muscle guarding is present along the right side of the lumbar spine. Pain and loss of active range of motion is noted with forward bending, left side bending, and right rotation. Passive intervertebral motion (PIVM) testing revealed significant loss of passive mobility in the same directions. Neurologic examination was unremarkable.

KEY FEATURES

Description

- LBP with primary involvement of the lumbar facet joint
- Lower limb symptoms might be present in a nondermatomal pattern as a result of referred pain
- Neurologic findings, minimal
- Unilateral symptoms

Essentials of Diagnosis

- Diagnosis made by clinical examination
- Use of treatment- (impairment) based classification system is useful to determine evidence-based practice (EBP) treatment plan

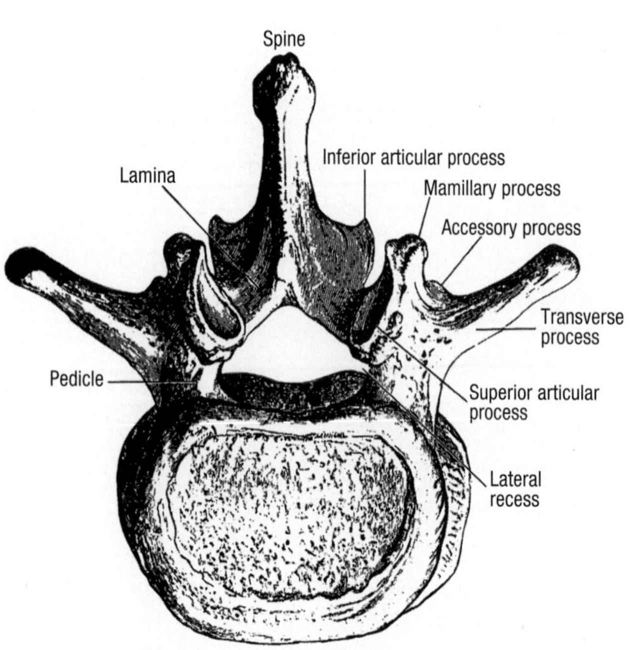

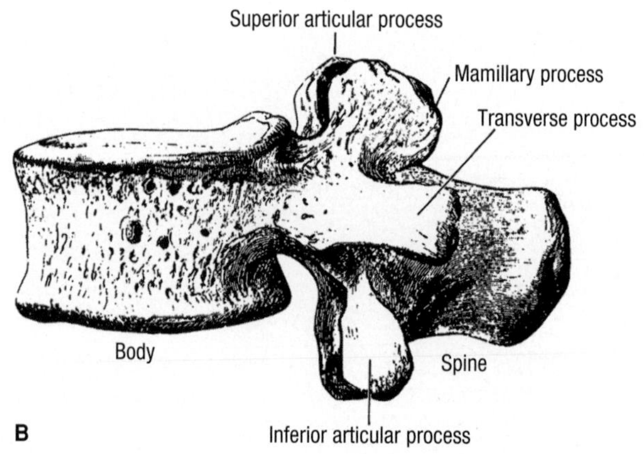

FIGURE 121-1 The fifth lumbar vertebra viewed from above (**A**) and from the side (**B**). (From Ropper AH, Samuels AH. *Adams & Victor's Principles of Neurology.* 9th ed. www.accessmedicine.com. Copyright © The McGraw-Hill Companies, Inc. All rights reserved.)

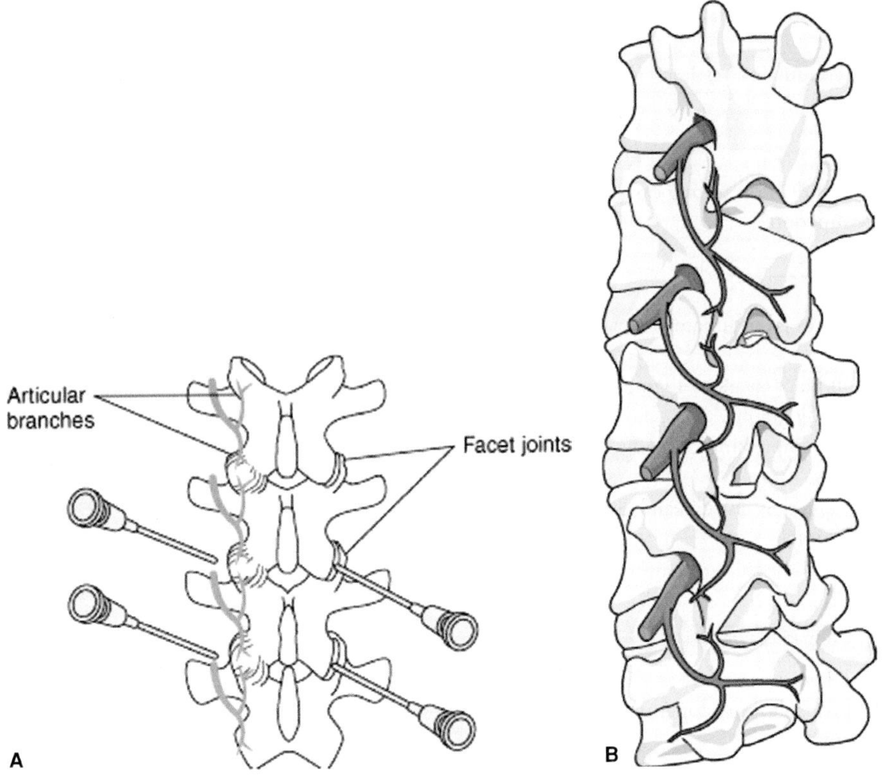

FIGURE 121-2 Lumbar medial branch nerve and facet blocks. (**A**) Posterior view. (**B**) 30-degree oblique posterior view. (From Morgan GE, Mikhail MS, Murray MJ. *Clinical Anesthesiology.* 4th ed. www.accessmedicine.com. Copyright © The McGraw-Hill Companies, Inc. All rights reserved.)

- Reproduction of symptoms when putting joint in a closed packed position (combination of extension, side-bending toward involved side, rotation away from involved site)

General Considerations

- Presentation can vary significantly based on anatomical structures and psychosocial factors.
- Often difficult to diagnose the cause of pain.

Demographics

- Variable, based on specific condition.

CLINICAL FINDINGS

SIGNS AND SYMPTOMS

- Pain in the lumbar or sacral area that can be mechanically reproduced
- Possible unilateral or bilateral referred pain, or pain in lower extremities
- ROM limited in a capsular pattern: rotation and side-bending limited in opposite direction
- Lumbar segmental hypomobility may be present in capsular pattern
- May be associated with poor core-muscle strength and postural deviations

Functional Implications

- Leading cause of occupational disability
- May cause decreased ability to perform activities of daily living (ADLs)/instrumental activities of daily living (IADL)
- May impact ability to participate in sports and other recreational activities

Possible Contributing Causes

- Congenital anomalies
- Obesity
- Occupational factors
- Physical condition
- Postural changes
- Psychosocial and behavioral factors
- Smoking
- Socioeconomic factors
- Tightness of the hip flexors, external rotators, hamstrings
- Weakness of the core musculature

Differential Diagnosis

- Abdominal aortic aneurism
- Ankylosing spondylitis
- Hip pathology with radiating pain pattern
- Malignant spinal tumor or metastasis
- Peripheral nerve impairment
- Radiculopathy
- Referred pain from visceral structures
- Systematic autoimmune diseases (rheumatoid arthrtitis [RA], Reiter syndrome, etc.)
- Vascular insufficiency

MEANS OF CONFIRMATION OR DIAGNOSIS

Imaging

- Not necessary in most cases; only with persistent symptoms that do not respond to conservative management or presence of red/yellow flags
- MRI[2]

- X-ray/Plain-film radiograph (flexion/extension radiograph)[3]
- CT scan[3]
- Electrodiagnostic/nerve conduction testing[4]
- Doppler ultrasound

Diagnostic Procedures

- Electrodiagnostic/nerve conduction testing can help determine a specific impaired nerve function.

FINDINGS AND INTERPRETATION

- MRI helps to visualize compressed or inflamed nerve root/disc pathology in diagnosis.[2]
- X-ray/Plain-film radiograph helps to assess alignment, fractures, stability (flexion/extension radiograph).[3]
- CT scan to show herniation compressing the spinal canal/nerves, rule out abdominal pathology.[3]
- Electrodiagnostic/nerve conduction testing can help determine a specific impaired nerve function.[4]
- Doppler ultrasound to examine vascular function.

REFERRALS/ADMITTANCE

- To hospital for imaging
- To physician for surgical consult if myelopathy is suspected (see Lumbar Radiculopathy)
- To hospital for imaging and medical consult if disease is suspected
- To physician if vascular insufficiency is suspected

IMPAIRMENTS

- Hypomobile lumbar spine
- Weakness of abdominals and other core-stabilizing muscles
- Shortening of hamstrings, hip flexors
- Postural changes
- Inability to walk for prolonged time
- Inability to stand for prolonged time

TESTS AND MEASURES

- Algorithm for examination of the lumbar spine[4]
- Passive physiologic intervertebral mobility testing (PPIVM)[5]
- Passive accessory intervertebral movement (PAIVM)
- Lower extremity screening examination
- Postural examination
- Muscle length testing, including hamstrings, hip flexors, calf muscles
- Quadrant test[6]
- Straight leg-raise test[7]
- Slump test[7]
- Lower limb nerve tension test[7]
- Prone instability test
- Lower extremity neurological screen (dermatome, myotome, reflexes)
- Repeated movement testing
- Fear-Avoidance Beliefs Questionnaire (FABQ)

INTERVENTION

- Joint manipulation indicated when, with:
  - Pain lasting <16 days
  - No radicular symptoms/pain distal to the knee
  - Fear avoidance beliefs questionaire (FABQ) score <19
  - Internal rotation of >35 degrees for at least one hip
  - Hypomobility of a least one level of the lumbar spine

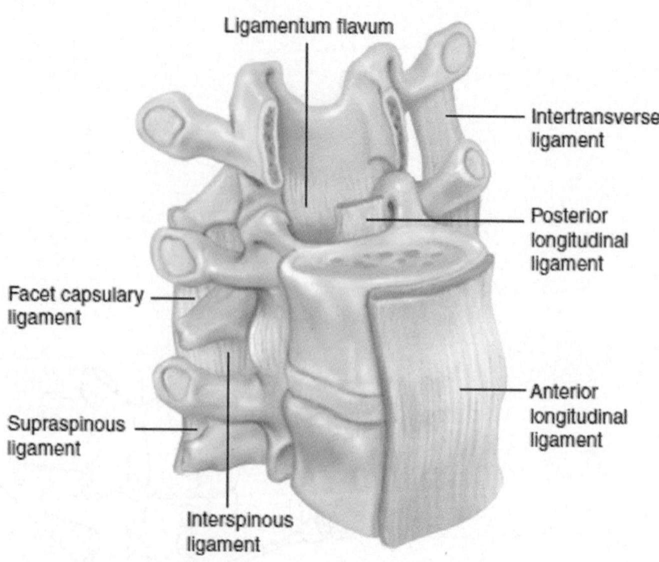

FIGURE 121-3 Ligament structures in the lumbar spine. (From McKean S, Ross JJ, Dressler DD, Brotman DJ, Ginsberg JS. *Principles and Practice of Hospital Medicine.* www.accessmedicine.com. Copyright © The McGraw-Hill Companies, Inc. All rights reserved.)

- Joint mobilization
- Lumbar stabilization exercises to address core stability when
  - Positive prone instability test
  - Presence of aberrant motion
  - Straight leg-raise >91 degrees
  - Age <41 years
- Initiate stabilization exercises after normalizing ROM
- Stretching exercises and myofascial mobilization for shortened musculature
- Unweighted treadmill walking
- Aquatic exercise
- Modalities for short-term pain control
- Cognitive behavioral therapy

FUNCTIONAL GOALS

- Patient will be able to
  - Sit with a neutral lumbar spine posture for greater than 30 minutes with 0/10 pain rating.
  - Sit at work station and perform computer work for 45 minutes with 0/10 pain rating.
  - Rotate lumbar spine 25 degrees with 0/10 pain rating in lower extremity to reach into the back seat in the car.
  - Walk for 30 minutes with 0/10 pain rating to go shopping.
  - Increase standing tolerance to >30 minutes without pain to fulfill recreational activity requirements.

PROGNOSIS

- Fair to very good, depending on specific impairments.
- Chronic LBP prognosis significantly less.

PATIENT RESOURCE

- American Academy of Orthopeadic Surgeons. Back Pain. http://orthoinfo.aaos.org/topic.cfm?topic=A00311 Accessed March 1, 2013.

REFERENCES

1. The American Physical Therapy Association. Pattern 4F: Impaired joint mobility, motor function, muscle performance, range of motion, and reflex integrity associated with spinal disorders. *Interactive Guide to Physical Therapist Practice*. 2003. DOI: 10.2522/ptguide.3.1_6. Accessed March 18, 2013.
2. Dutton M. Chapter 31. Imaging studies. In: Dutton M, ed. *Orthopaedic Examination, Evaluation, and Intervention*. New York, NY: McGraw-Hill; 2004. http://www.accessphysiotherapy.com/abstract/55601371#55601371. Accessed May 18, 2014.
3. Malone TR, Hazle C, Grey ML. Chapter 1. Introduction to musculoskeletal imaging. In: Malone TR, Hazle C, Grey ML, eds. *Imaging in Rehabilitation*. New York, NY: McGraw-Hill; 2008. http://www.accessphysiotherapy.com/abstract/5940003#5940003. Accessed May 18, 2014.
4. Dutton M. Chapter 11. The cervical complex. In: Dutton M, ed. *Dutton's Orthopedic Survival Guide: Managing Common Conditions*. New York, NY: McGraw-Hill; 2011. http://www.accessphysiotherapy.com/abstract/8656044#8656333. Accessed March 18, 2013.
5. Dutton M. Chapter 13. The lumbopelvic complex. In: Dutton M, ed. *Dutton's Orthopedic Survival Guide: Managing Common Conditions*. New York, NY: McGraw-Hill; 2011. http://www.accessphysiotherapy.com/abstract/8656044#8656333. Accessed March 18, 2013.
6. Dutton M. Chapter 8. The hip joint. In: Dutton M, ed. *Dutton's Orthopedic Survival Guide: Managing Common Conditions*. New York, NY: McGraw-Hill; 2011. http://www.accessphysiotherapy.com/abstract/8656044#8656333. Accessed March 18, 2013.
7. Dutton M. Chapter 12. Neurodynamic mobilizations. In: Dutton M, ed. *Orthopaedics. Orthopaedic Examination, Evaluation, and Intervention*. New York, NY: McGraw-Hill; 2004. http://www.accessphysiotherapy.com/abstract/55601371#55601371. Accessed May 18, 2014.

ADDITIONAL REFERENCES

- Fritz JM, Cleland JA, Childs JD. Subgrouping patients with low back pain: evolution of a classification approach to physical therapy. *J Orthop Sports Phys Ther*. 2007;37(6):290–302.
- ICD9DATA web site. http://www.icd9data.com. Accessed March 18, 2013.
- ICD10DATA web site. http://www.icd10data.com. Accessed March 18, 2013.
- Liebenson C. *Rehabilitation of the Spine*. Baltimore, MD: Lippincott, Williams & Wilkins; 2007.
- Olsen KA. *Manual Therapy of the Spine*. St. Louis, MI: Saunders Elsevier; 2009.

122 HANGMAN'S FRACTURE

Eric Shamus, PhD, DPT, PT, CSCS

CONDITION/DISORDER SYNONYM

- Cervical spondylolisthesis

ICD-9-CM CODES

- 738.4 Acquired spondylolisthesis
- 756.12 Spondylolisthesis congenital
- 805.02 Closed fracture of second cervical vertebra

ICD-10-CM CODES

- M43.10 Spondylolisthesis, site unspecified
- Q76.2 Congenital spondylolisthesis
- S12.100A Unspecified displaced fracture of second cervical vertebra, initial encounter for closed fracture
- S12.101A Unspecified nondisplaced fracture of second cervical vertebra, initial encounter for closed fracture

PREFERRED PRACTICE PATTERN

- 4E: Impaired Joint Mobility, Motor Function, Muscle Performance, and ROM Associated with Localized Inflammation[1]

PATIENT PRESENTATION

Patient is a 58-year-old woman involved in a motor vehicle accident. Patient had a bilateral C2 pars interarticularis fracture. The surgeon and patient agreed on conservative management. The patient presents 3 months later with decreased range of motion of the cervical spine and muscle spasms. The patient does not have any dizziness or upper or lower extremity symptoms.

KEY FEATURES

Description

- Anterior (forward) translation of a vertebra
- C2 vertebra anterior translated on C3 with a fracture of C2 pedicles
- Fracture of the pedicles on the C2 vertebra
- Slipping of the vertebra in relationship to the vertebra below
- Neurogenic claudication
- Fracture widens at the pars

Essentials of Diagnosis

- Diagnosis made by X-ray
- Clinical examination may find step deformity
- Dermatome/myotome pattern
- Stability of the cervical spine is critical
- Spondylolysis: Fracture without displacement

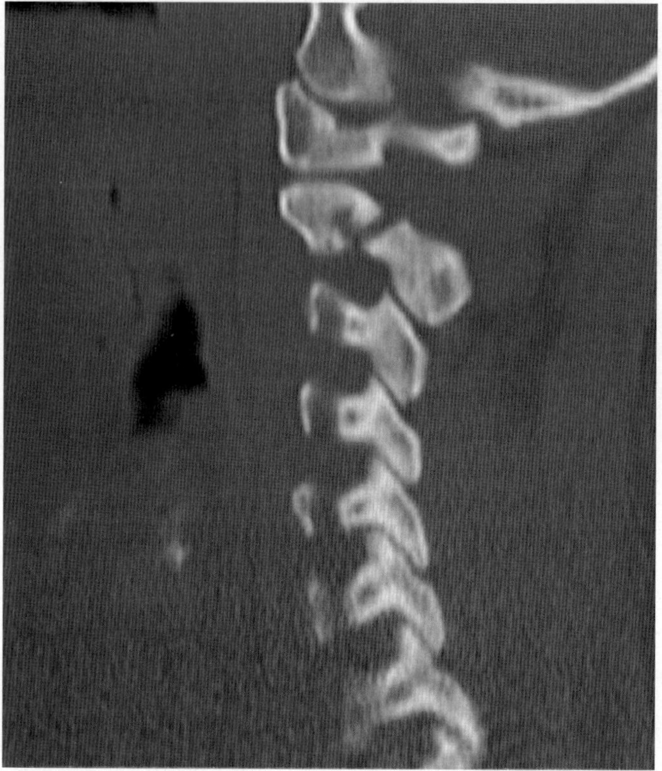

FIGURE 122-1 This sagittal CT reconstruction reveals injury to C2 known as a hangman's fracture. (From Malone TR, Hazle C, Grey ML. *Imaging in Rehabilitation.* http://www.accessphysiotherapy.com. Copyright © The McGraw-Hill Companies, Inc. All rights reserved.)

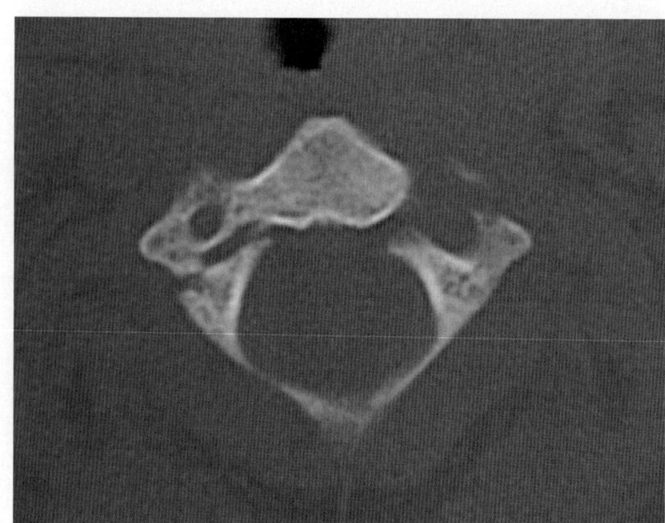

FIGURE 122-2 The axial image reveals the bilateral fracture pattern associated with a hangman's fracture. (From Malone TR, Hazle C, Grey ML. *Imaging in Rehabilitation.* http://www.accessphysiotherapy.com. Copyright © The McGraw-Hill Companies, Inc. All rights reserved.)

General Considerations

- Instability
- Individual may not know they have a fracture immediately following an accident
- Avoid extension positions that increase symptoms

Demographics

- After trauma
- Suicidal hanging

CLINICAL FINDINGS

SIGNS AND SYMPTOMS

- Cervical, shoulder, arm, and upper-extremity pain and paresthesia, often radiating into lower extremities if central cord involved
- Constricted pupil (Horner sign)
- Stiffness along the spine
- Headaches
- Pain in the cervical spine worsens with extension
- Diminished sensation, motor control, reflexes in the distribution of involved nerve
- Neurogenic claudication

Functional Implications

- May cause death
- Difficulty maintaining standing posture secondary to neck and arm pain
- Inability to sleep flat on the back without a pillow
- Weakness with lifting
- Loss of movement or feeling in the upper extremity
- Difficulty with movements (reaching overhead) secondary to pain
- Limited sports participation

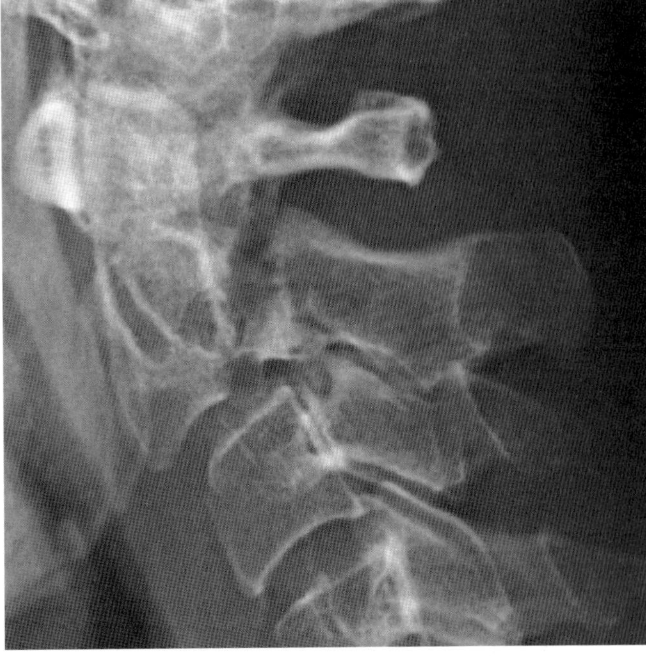

FIGURE 122-3 Hangman's fracture. (From Tintinalli JE, Stapczynski JS, Ma OJ, et al. *Tintinalli's Emergency Medicine: A Comprehensive Study Guide.* 7th ed. http://www.accessmedicine.com. Copyright © The McGraw-Hill Companies, Inc. All rights reserved.)

Possible Contributing Causes

- Forceful extension from hit under the chin (as in sports)
- Congenital
- Car accident, hit from rear
- Hyperextension of the cervical spine

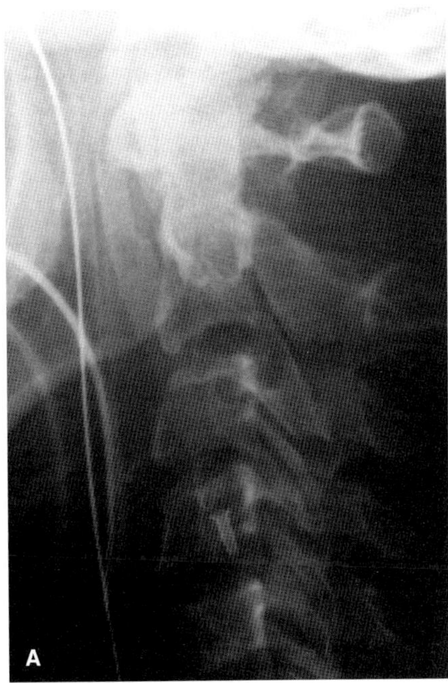

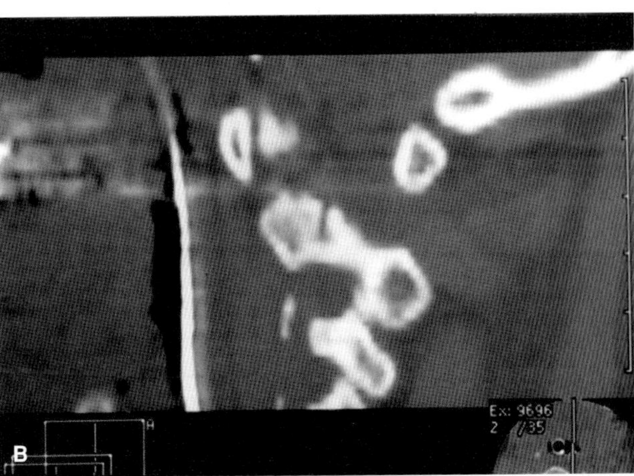

FIGURE 122-4 Imaging studies in a patient who was in a motor vehicle accident and sustained a hangman's fracture, or traumatic spondylolisthesis of C2. (**A**) Lateral radiographic view, which is largely unremarkable. (**B**) Sagittal reconstruction using CT scanning to better delineate the fracture site at the base of the posterior elements. The patient was treated nonoperatively. (From Skinner HB. *Current Diagnosis & Treatment in Orthopedics.* 4th ed. http://www.accessmedicine.com. Copyright © The McGraw-Hill Companies, Inc. All rights reserved.)

Differential Diagnosis

- Peripheral-nerve impairment
- Spinal tumor
- Peripheral neuropathy
- Paraspinal spasms
- Degenerative disc disease
- Stenosis

MEANS OF CONFIRMATION OR DIAGNOSIS

Imaging

- MRI helps visualize compressed or inflamed nerve root in diagnosis.[2]
- X-ray/Plain-film radiograph to see vertebral position[3]
  - Canadian C-Spine rule.
- CT to show herniation compressing the spinal canal/nerves.[3]
- Electrodiagnostic/nerve conduction testing can help determine a specific impaired nerve function.[4]

FINDINGS AND INTERPRETATION

- C2 vertebra anterior translated on C3 with a fracture of C2 pedicles

REFERRALS/ADMITTANCE

- To hospital for imaging
- To neurosurgeon for surgical consult if myelopathy suspected
  - Fusion[2]
- To physician for corticosteroid injection
- To physician for anti-inflammatory medication
- To orthopedist for halo vest traction device, cervical bracing

IMPAIRMENTS

- Restricted mobility of the upper cervical spine
- Hypermobility
- Noted weakness of the neck musculature

TESTS AND MEASURES

- Neck Disability Index score
- Cervical spine AROM
- Sharp–Purser: Atlantoaxial instability
- Cervical passive intervertebral motion testing
- Subcranial translation instability testing
- Passive physiologic intervertebral mobility (PPIVM) testing
- Upper-extremity screening examination
- Postural examination
- Muscle length testing, including the upper trapezius, levator scapulae, pectoral muscles
- Upper limb nerve tension test
- Deep neck flexor endurance test
- Upper-extremity neurologic screen (dermatome, myotome, reflexes)

INTERVENTION

- Rest
- Bracing
- Address pain
  - Electrical stimulation
  - Heat/Ice
- Address hypertonicity
  - Soft-tissue massage
  - Heat
- Address muscle weakness
  - Stability exercises

FUNCTIONAL GOALS

- Patient will be able to
  - Sit with neutral cervical-spine posture for >30 minutes with 0/10 pain rating.
  - Stand at work station and perform computer work for 45 minutes with 0/10 pain rating.
  - Rotate cervical spine 75 degrees in order to look over the shoulder while driving with 0/10 pain rating.

PROGNOSIS

- Fair to good depend on severity of vertebral translation, amount of nerve-root compression, upper/lower-extremity impairments.
- Possible death from asphyxiation.

PATIENT RESOURCE

- The Pediatric Orthopaedic Society of North America (POSNA). Cervical Spine Fractures. http://www.posna.org/education/StudyGuide/cervicalSpineFractures.asp. Accessed March 8, 2013.

REFERENCES

1. The American Physical Therapy Association. Pattern 4E: Impaired joint mobility, motor function, muscle performance, and range of motion associated with localized inflammation. *Interactive Guide to Physical Therapist Practice*. 2003. DOI: 10.2522/ptguide.3.1_5. http://guidetoptpractice.apta.org/content/1/SEC12.extract?sid=40ddc4d6-882c-4e24-9073-22045a162c05. Accessed May 22, 2014.
2. Dutton M. *Orthopaedic Examination, Evaluation, and Intervention*. New York, NY: McGraw-Hill; 2008. http://www.accessphysiotherapy.com/resource/612. Accessed March 3, 2013.
3. Malone TR, Hazle C, Grey ML. *Imaging in Rehabilitation*. New York, NY: McGraw-Hill; 2008. http://www.accessphysiotherapy.com/resource/613 . Accessed March 8, 2013.
4. Dutton M. *Dutton's Orthopedic Survival Guide: Managing Common Conditions*. New York, NY: McGraw-Hill; 2011. http://www.accessphysiotherapy.com/resource/685. Accessed March 8, 2013.

ADDITIONAL REFERENCES

- ICD9DATA web site. http://www.icd9data.com. Accessed March 6, 2013.
- ICD10DATA web site. http://www.icd10data.com. Accessed March 1, 2013.
- Prentice WE, Quillen WS, Underwood F. Chapter 8. Principles of electrophysiologic evaluation and testing. In: Prentice WE, Quillen WS, Underwood F, eds. *Therapeutic Modalities in Rehabilitation*. 4th ed. New York, NY: McGraw-Hill; 2011. http://www.accessphysiotherapy.com/abstract/8135087#8135091. Accessed March 8, 2013.
- Schneider RC, Livingston KE, Cave AJ, Hamilton G. Hangman's fracture of the cervical spine. *J Neurosurg*. 1965;22(2):141–154. http://thejns.org/doi/abs/10.3171/jns.1965.22.2.0141?journalCode=jns
- Wainner RS, Fritz JM, Irrgang JJ, et al. Reliability and diagnostic accuracy of the clinical examination and patient self-report measures for cervical radiculopathy. *Spine*. 2003;28(1):52–62. [PMID: 12544957]

123 IDIOPATHIC NECK PAIN

Eric Shamus, PhD, DPT, PT, CSCS
Lindsey (Davis) Hornecke, DPT

CONDITION/DISORDER SYNONYMS

- Simple neck pain
- Neck sprain/strain
- Mechanical neck pain

ICD-9-CM CODE

- 729.1 Myalgia and myositis unspecified

ICD-10-CM CODES

- M60.9 Myositis, unspecified
- M79.1 Myalgia

PREFERRED PRACTICE PATTERN

- 4D: Impaired joint mobility, motor function, muscle performance, and range of motion associated with connective tissue dysfunction[1]

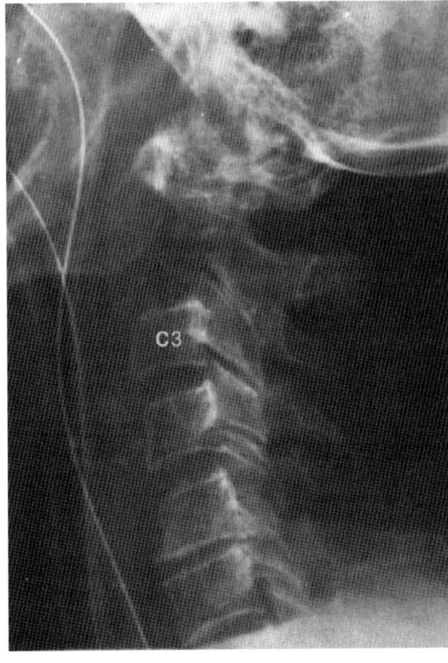

FIGURE 123-1 A 63-year-old man presents with severe upper neck pain not responding to anti-inflammatory medication. (From Chen MYM, Pope TL, Ott DJ. *Basic Radiology.* 2nd ed. www.accessmedicine.com. Copyright © The McGraw-Hill Companies, Inc. All rights reserved.)

PATIENT PRESENTATION

A 38-year-old female dental hygienist presents with complaints of neck pain with insidious onset 3 weeks ago. She reports she has pain while working on her dental patients and the pain gets worse throughout the day. She rates her pain at 8/10 at its worst. Her pain subsides with rest to a 3/10. She reports having approximately three to four headaches per week that typically arise in the middle of her workday. She also notes she is a very active cyclist and competes in many local races throughout the year.

Her primary care physician in order to evaluate and treat refers her for physical therapy. Physical therapy examination revealed decreased range of motion (ROM) in bilateral cervical rotation and cervical lateral flexion. Cervical and thoracic joint mobility was normal. On palpation, muscle tenderness was noted in the upper trapezius, sternocleidomastoid, scalene, and levator scapulae muscles bilaterally. She also has two active trigger points: one in her right upper trapezius and one in her right levator scapulae. Spurling test and upper limb nerve tension tests were negative for the reproduction of symptoms. There are no signs of muscle atrophy. Manual muscle testing revealed strength 4−/5 for bilateral shoulder elevation, 3/5 for scapular retraction, 3/5 for right cervical lateral flexion, 3+/5 for left cervical lateral flexion, and 3/5 for bilateral cervical rotation.

KEY FEATURES

Description

- Neck pain from unknown cause
- No underlying disease or specific disorder
- Usually acute
- Chronic, persistent, deep aching pains in the muscle, nonarticular in origin
- Usually caused by sudden overload, overstretching, repetitive/sustained muscle activities
- Pain associated with activities, generally relieved with rest
- Can be in localized area affecting any muscle or fascia

Essentials of Diagnosis

- Diagnosis made by clinical examination (generally palpation) with no medical diagnostic tests available
- Differentiated from fibromyalgia, as it can occur in a single area; fibromyalgia occurs in multiple locations, has specific tender points

General Considerations

- Very common, affects most people in their lifetimes.
- Latent trigger points are palpable, taut bands not tender to palpation, but may be converted into active trigger point.

Demographics

- In the United States, 14.4% of general population suffers from chronic musculoskeletal pain.
- 21% to 93% of patients reporting regional pain have myofascial pain.[2]
- 25% to 54% of asymptomatic individuals have latent trigger points.[2]

- No racial differences in incidence of myofascial pain have been described.
- Myofascial pain affects men and women equally.
- Likelihood of developing active trigger points increases with age and activity level.
- Sedentary individuals more prone to developing active trigger points than individuals who exercise vigorously on a daily basis.

CLINICAL FINDINGS

SIGNS AND SYMPTOMS

- Acute pain
- Difficulty sleeping
- Headaches
- Joint stiffness
- Limited ROM
- Muscle stiffness
- Pain with palpation of the trigger point
- Paresthesias
- Referred pain
- Vertigo
- Weakness without atrophy may be seen when performing manual muscle testing

▶ Functional Implications

- Pain with standing, ambulation, activities of daily living (ADLs)
- Limited ROM
- Weakness

▶ Possible Contributing Causes

- Anxiety
- Behavior
- Emotional/psychological stress
- Improper lifting, poor biomechanics
- Improper posture
- Inflammatory conditions affecting ligaments, muscles, tendons
- Lack of activity, immobility (cast)
- Obesity
- Overuse
- Poor muscular or ligamentous support
- Repetitive stress
- Traumatic events

▶ Differential Diagnosis

- Arnold–Chiari malformation
- Carpal tunnel syndrome
- Complex regional pain syndrome
- Degenerative disc disease
- Fibromyalgia
- Herniated disc
- Ligamentous sprain
- Muscle strain
- Peripheral nerve impairment
- Radiculopathy
- Rheumatoid arthritis
- Shoulder pathology with radiating pain pattern
- Spinal tumor
- Thoracic outlet syndrome

MEANS OF CONFIRMATION OR DIAGNOSIS

▶ Imaging

- Imaging not usually needed with nonspecific neck pain unless warranted for differential diagnosis.

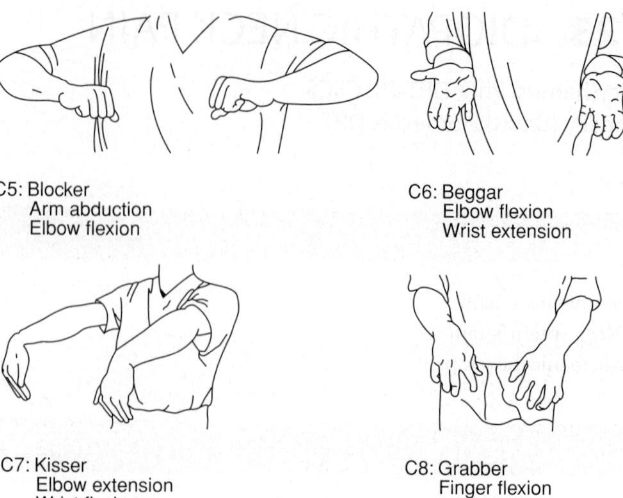

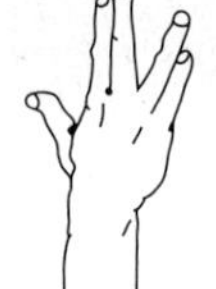

FIGURE 123-2 Upper extremity motor evaluation. (From South-Paul JE, Matheny SC, Lewis EL. *Current Diagnosis & Treatment in Family Medicine.* 3rd ed. www.accessmedicine.com. Copyright © The McGraw-Hill Companies, Inc. All rights reserved.)

  - MRI helps visualize compressed or inflamed nerve root in diagnosis.
  - X-ray/Plain-film radiograph helpful if osteophyte located in intervertebral foramen.
  - CT to show herniation compressing the spinal canal/nerves.
  - Electrodiagnostic/nerve conduction testing can help determine specific impaired nerve function.

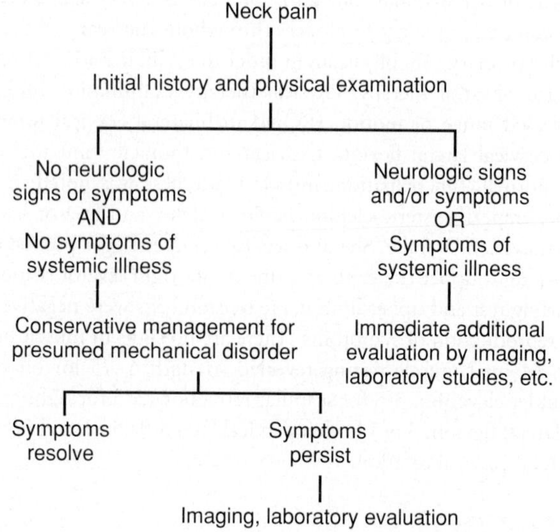

FIGURE 123-3 The initial evaluation of the patient with neck pain. (From Imboden J, Hellmann DB, Stone JH. *Current Rheumatology Diagnosis & Treatment.* 2nd ed. www.accessmedicine.com. Copyright © The McGraw-Hill Companies, Inc. All rights reserved.)

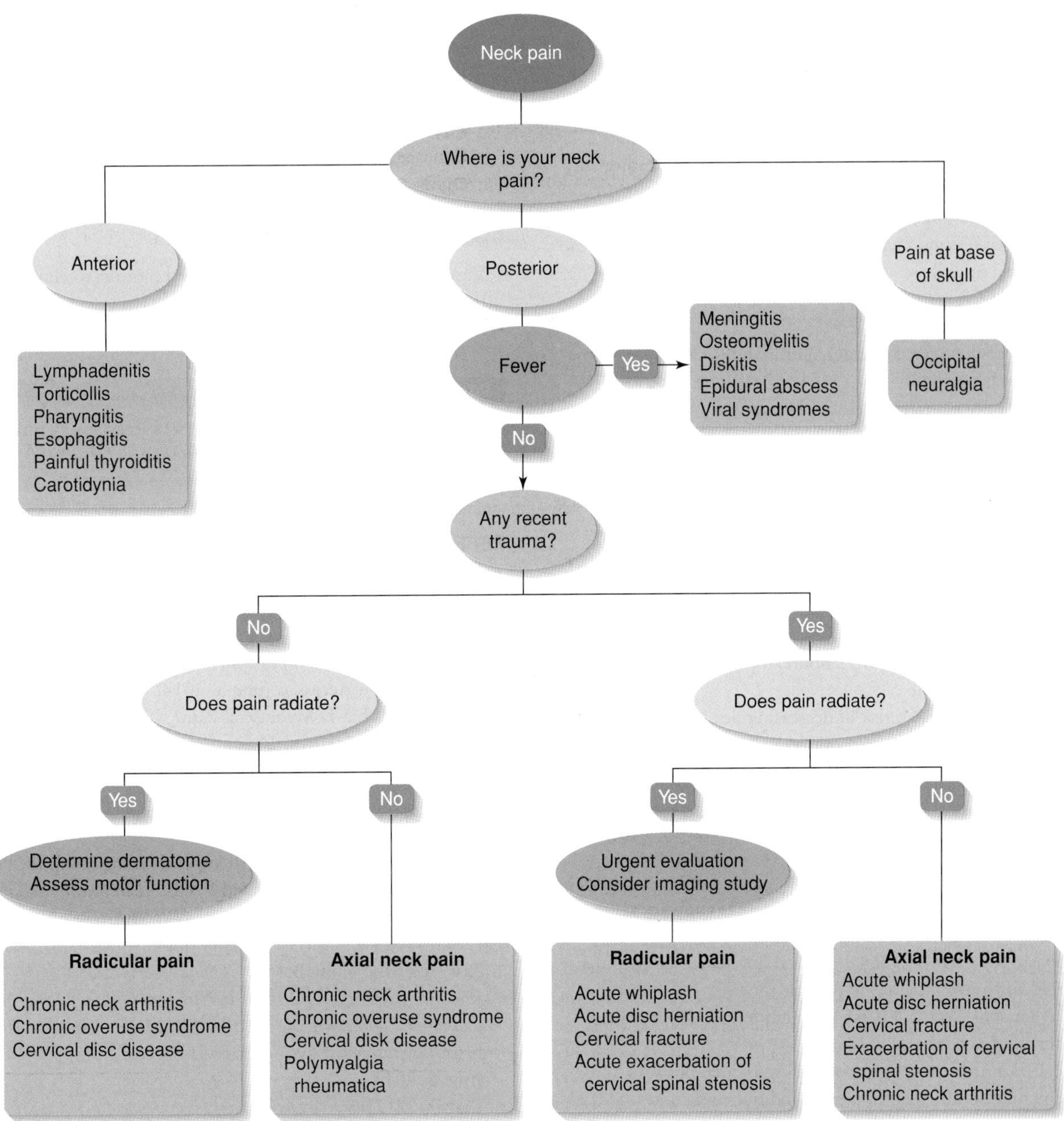

FIGURE 123-4 Diagnostic approach: Neck pain. (From Henderson MC, Tierney LM, Smetana GW. *The Patient History: An Evidence-Based Approach to Differential Diagnosis*. www.accessmedicine.com. Copyright © The McGraw-Hill Companies, Inc. All rights reserved.)

Diagnostic Procedures

- Palpation

FINDINGS AND INTERPRETATION

- Taut, fibrous band felt with palpation of the muscle
- Limited ROM may be common finding
- Physical examination cluster to rule in cervical radiculopathy
  - Spurling test
  - Rotation limited to ipsilateral side
  - Upper limb nerve tension test
  - Diminished brachioradialis reflex

REFERRALS/ADMITTANCE

- To psychologist for psychological counseling if appropriate
- To dietitian to address obesity if appropriate
- To massage therapist

IMPAIRMENTS

- Pain
- Limited function due to reduced ROM
- Mobility
- Ability to self-care diminished
- Role at home, school, work, and in community impacted
- Ability to participate in recreation, leisure, and sports impacted

TESTS AND MEASURES

- Cervical spine AROM
- Sharp–Purser: Atlantoaxial instability
- Cervical passive intervertebral motion testing
- Subcranial translation instability testing
- Passive physiologic intervertebral mobility (PPIVM) testing
- Upper-extremity screening examination
- Postural examination
- Muscle length testing, including the upper trapezius, levator scapulae, pectoral muscles
- Upper limb nerve tension test
- Deep neck flexor endurance test
- Disabilities of the Arm, Shoulder, and Hand (DASH) score to assess physical function
- Upper-extremity neurologic screen (dermatome, myotome, reflexes)

INTERVENTION

- Soft-tissue massage and joint oscillations to reduce pain or muscle guarding
- Address biomechanical factors: Improper posture, ergonomics, body mechanics during work, and leisure
- Spray and stretch technique
- Cryotherapy
  - In acute cases within 24 to 72 hours of injury to alleviate pain, reduce inflammation
  - Caution must be used; risk of decreasing flexibility or reinjury
- Thermotherapy: Hot packs or whirlpool after initial inflammation subsides to increase circulation and relaxation
- Hydrotherapy
- Ultrasound to minimize scarring, stimulate tissue healing, increase circulation to the area, relax musculature
- Electric stimulation
  - Microcurrent when inflammation is present and very acute
- Stimulates healing, decreases inflammation
  - Biphasic/Russian when inflammation not acute, fatigue muscle to minimize contractures, re-educate muscle
- Transcutaneous electrical nerve stimulation (TENS) for symptomatic relief of pain
- Desensitization of the trigger point with manual pressure
- Implementation of strength, power, endurance exercises
  - Risk of decreasing flexibility and reinjury
- Progress from active-assistive to active to resistive exercises, then task-specific performance training
- Posture education
  - Sitting: Select appropriate ergonomic chair with low-back support
  - Standing: Posture
  - Functional: Proper body mechanics
- Massage
  - Slow, light percussion to increase circulation, flush lactic acid out of the muscle tissues
  - Effleurage to relax the muscles
  - Deep tissue when desensitizing trigger points
- Joint mobilizations to eliminate bony restrictions

FUNCTIONAL GOALS

- Patient will be able to
  - Sit with neutral cervical and thoracic spine posture for more than 30 minutes with 0/10 pain rating.
  - Sit at work station and perform computer work for 45 minutes with 0/10 pain rating.
  - Rotate the cervical spine 70 degrees so as to talk on the telephone with 0/10 pain rating in the neck/arm
  - Decrease inflammation to enable repetitive movement.
  - Increase circulation to decrease inflammation and improve healing response.
  - Educate patient on proper body mechanics, work area ergonomics, relaxation techniques.

PROGNOSIS

- Very good, though it may take several months to eliminate trigger points.
- Pain may recur if biomechanical causes not addressed

PATIENT RESOURCE

- National Guideline Clearing House. Neck Pain, Clinical Practice. http://guideline.gov/content.aspx?id=14703. Accessed June 5, 2013.

REFERENCES

1. The American Physical Therapy Association. Pattern 4D: Impaired joint mobility, motor function, muscle performance, and range of motion associated with connective tissue dysfunction. *Interactive Guide to Physical Therapist Practice*. 2003. DOI: 10.2522/ptguide.3.1_4. Accessed June 5, 2013.
2. Eustice C. What Is Myofascial Pain? *About.com Arthritis and Joint Conditions.* http://arthritis.about.com/od/diseasesandconditions/a/myofascial_pain.htm. Accessed June 5, 2013.

ADDITIONAL REFERENCES

- Draper DO, Prentice WE. Therapeutic ultrasound. In: Prentice WE, Quillen WS, Underwood F, eds. *Therapeutic Modalities in Rehabilitation.* 4th ed. New York, NY: McGraw-Hill; 2011. http://www.accessphysiotherapy.com/abstract/8138751. Accessed June 5, 2013.
- Dutton M. *Dutton's Orthopedic Survival Guide: Managing Common Conditions.* New York, NY: McGraw-Hill; 2011. http://www.accessphysiotherapy.com/resource/685. Accessed June 5, 2013.
- Dutton M. *Dutton's Orthopaedic Examination, Evaluation, and Intervention.* New York, NY: McGraw-Hill; 2008. http://www.accessphysiotherapy.com/resource/612. Accessed June 5, 2013.
- Goodman CC, Fuller KS. *Pathology: Implications for the Physical Therapist.* 3rd ed. Philadelphia, PA: Saunders Elsevier; 2009.
- Hall SJ. The biomechanics of human bone growth and development. In: Hall SJ, ed. *Basic Biomechanics.* 5th ed. New York, NY: McGraw-Hill; 2007. http://www.accessphysiotherapy.com/content/6060744. Accessed June 5, 2013.
- Hooker DN, Prentice WE. Basic principles of electricity and electrical stimulating currents. In: Prentice WE, Quillen WS, Underwood F, eds. *Therapeutic Modalities in Rehabilitation.* 4th ed. New York, NY: McGraw-Hill; 2011. http://www.accessphysiotherapy.com/content/8136367#8136367. Accessed June 5, 2013.
- ICD10Data.com. http://www.icd10data.com. Accessed June 5, 2013.
- ICD9Data.com. http://www.icd9data.com. Accessed June 5, 2013.
- Kisner C, Colby LA. *Therapeutic Exercise: Foundations and Techniques.* 5th ed. Philadelphia, PA: F.A. Davis Company; 2007.

- Malone DJ, Bishop KL. *Physical Therapy in Acute Care: A Clinician's Guide*. Thorofare, NJ: Slack Inc.; 2006.
- Malone TR, Hazle C, Grey ML. *Imaging in Rehabilitation*. New York, NY: McGraw-Hill; 2008. http://www.accessphysiotherapy.com/resource/613. Accessed June 5, 2013.
- Martini FH, Timmons MJ, Tallitsch RB. *Human Anatomy*. 6th ed. San Francisco, CA: Pearson Education, Ltd; 2008.
- Prentice WE. Therapeutic massage. In: Prentice WE, Quillen WS, Underwood F, eds. *Therapeutic Modalities in Rehabilitation*. 4th ed. New York, NY: McGraw-Hill; 2011. http://www.accessphysiotherapy.com/abstract/8140838#8140936. Accessed June 5, 2013.
- Silva AG, Cruz AL. Standing balance in patients with whiplash-associated neck pain and idiopathic neck pain when compared with asymptomatic participants: a systematic review. *Physiother Theory Pract*. 2013;29(1):1–18.
- Simons DG, Travell JG, Simons LS, Cummings BD. *Travell & Simons' Myofascial Pain & Dysfunction: The Trigger Point Manual*. 2nd ed. Baltimore, MD: Lippincott Williams & Wilkins; 1999.
- Soep JB. Chapter 27. Rheumatic diseases. In: Hay WW, Levin MJ, Sondheimer JM, Deterding RR, eds. *CURRENT Diagnosis & Treatment: Pediatrics*. 20th ed. New York, NY: McGraw-Hill; 2011. http://www.accessphysiotherapy.com/abstract/6586584#6586588. Accessed June 5, 2013.
- Wainner RS, Fritz JM, Irrgang JJ, et al. Reliability and diagnostic accuracy of the clinical examination and patient self-report measures for cervical radiculopathy. *Spine*. 2003;28(1):52–62.

124 ILIOLUMBAR LIGAMENT SPRAIN

Eric Shamus, PhD, DPT, PT, CSCS
Arie J. Van Duijn, EdD, MSc, PT, OCS
Kristie Centner, DPT

CONDITION/DISORDER SYNONYMS

- Low back pain
- Mechanical low back pain
- Lumbar sprain

ICD-9-CM CODES

- 724.2 Lumbago
- 847.2 Sprain of lumbar

ICD-10-CM CODES

- M54.5 Low back pain
- S33.5 Sprain of ligaments of lumbar spine

PREFERRED PRACTICE PATTERN

- 4F: Impaired Joint Mobility, Motor Function, Muscle Performance, Range of Motion, and Reflex Integrity Associated with Spinal Disorders[1]

PATIENT PRESENTATION

A 15-year-old girl presents with complaints of unilateral pain along the left iliac crest up to the L5 vertebra. The patient states she has just recently joined a gymnastics team and has had this nonradiating pain since her last practice 5 days ago. She vaguely remembers feeling pain in this area of her left low back after landing a spotted back handspring incorrectly. The patient states she is unable to practice or sit for periods of 30 minutes or longer due to pain and a feeling of instability. Upon palpation, the patient complains of point tenderness along the left iliac crest running up to the transverse process of the L5 vertebra. Passive intervertebral motion testing indicates hypermobility at the L5-S1 segment. Manual muscle testing of lumbar extension and trunk flexion are both 3/5. The patient tests negative for the straight leg raise test and X-rays are negative for fractures.

KEY FEATURES

Description

- Iliolumbar ligament runs from transverse process of the L5 vertebra to the iliac crest.
- Strain can be unilateral or bilateral depending on mechanism of injury.
- Tenderness along the line of ligament or at attachments.
- Pain over the ligament that does not radiate.
- Most episodes are self-limiting.

Essentials of Diagnosis

- Diagnosis made by clinical examination.
- Use of treatment- or impairment-based classification system is useful to determine evidence-based treatment plan.
- Reproduction of symptoms in specific postures and activities.
- Rule out systemic disease (red and yellow flags).

General Considerations

- Presentation may vary significantly based on anatomical structures and psychosocial factors.
- Often difficult to determine pathoanatomical cause of pain.
- Poor spinal alignment can cause irritation of the ligament by altering the length–tension ratio.

Demographics

- Athletes and younger populations who are prone to extreme spinal movements.

CLINICAL FINDINGS

SIGNS AND SYMPTOMS

- Pain in the lumbar or sacral area that can be mechanically reproduced
- Unilateral or bilateral pain along the length of ligament or attachment

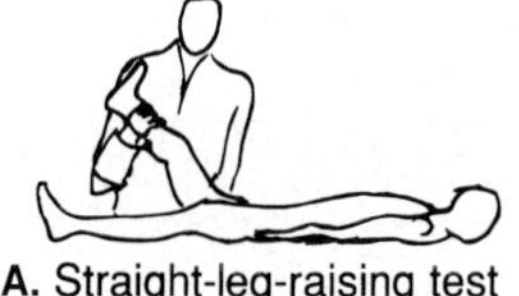

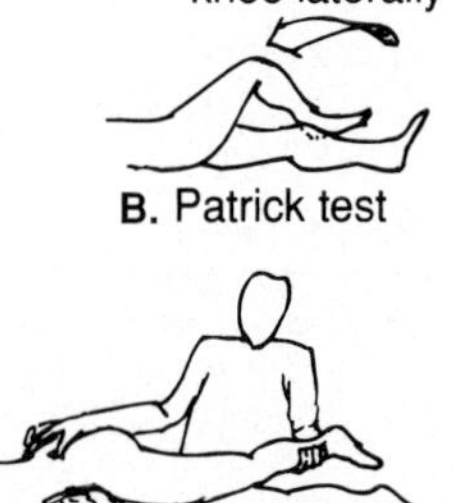

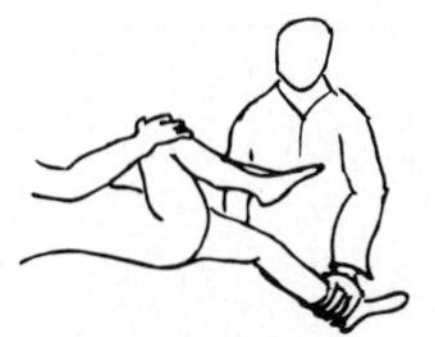

FIGURE 124-1 Tests at the hip and SI joint. (**A**) Straight-leg-raising test: The examiner lifts the supine patient's lower limb when the knee is held in extension. (**B**) Patrick test: Lateral rotation of the hip is assessed by having the knee flexed and the foot of that leg placed on the opposite patella. The examiner then pushes the flexed knee down and out to rotate the head of the femur. (**C**) Passive hyperextension of the thigh (Gaenslen test): While supine, the patient flexes the knee and femur on the affected side and holds the knee with the hands to eliminate lumbar lordosis. The examiner then hyperextends the unaffected thigh by letting it, sinks over the side of the table. In disease of the SI joint, this maneuver evokes pain. (**D**) Active hyperextension: With the patient prone and the abdomen resting on a pillow, the patient lifts the spine against the resistance offered by the examiner's hand; SI disease causes pain. (From LeBlond RF, DeGowin RL, Brown DD. *DeGowin's Diagnostic Examination.* 9th ed. www.accessmedicine.com. Copyright © The McGraw-Hill Companies, Inc. All rights reserved.)

- Lumbar segmental hypermobility may be present and indicates instability.
- Often associated with poor body mechanics, core-muscle weakness, and postural deviations.

Functional Implications

- May impede ability to perform activities of daily living (ADLs)/instrumental activities of daily living (IADL)
- May impede participation in sports and other social activities

Possible Contributing Causes

- Congenital anomalies
- Obesity
- Occupational factors
- Physical condition
- Postural changes
- Psychosocial and behavioral factors
- Smoking
- Socioeconomic factors
- Tightness of the hip flexors, hip external rotators, and hamstrings
- Weakness of the core musculature

Differential Diagnosis

- Erector spinae muscle strain
- Facet joint dysfunction
- Herniated disc
- Malignant spinal tumor or metastasis
- Myofascial pain syndrome
- Referred pain from visceral structures
- Sacral dysfunction
- Spinal misalignment
- Spondylitis
- Spondylolisthesis
- Spondylosis
- Systemic autoimmune disease (rheumatoid arthritis, Reiter syndrome)

MEANS OF CONFIRMATION OR DIAGNOSIS

Imaging

- Not necessary in most cases; only with persistent symptoms not responding to conservative management or if red/yellow flags are present.
- MRI helpful in diagnosis to visualize structure of the ligament, compressed or inflamed nerve root, or disc pathology.[2]
- X-ray/Plain-film radiograph helps assess alignment, fractures, and stability (flexion/extension radiograph).[3]
- CT to show ligament structure, herniation compressing the spinal canal/nerves, or to rule out abdominal pathology.[3]
- Electrodiagnostic/nerve conduction testing can help determine specific impaired nerve function.[4]
- Doppler ultrasound to examine vascular function.
- Diagnostic ultrasound to analyze fiber orientation.

FINDINGS AND INTERPRETATION

- Negative nerve-conduction tests
- Inflammation on MRI

REFERRALS/ADMITTANCE

- To hospital for imaging
- To physician for surgical consult if myelopathy suspected (see Lumbar Radiculopathy)
- To physician for imaging and medical consult if systemic disease suspected
- To other specialist if vascular insufficiency suspected

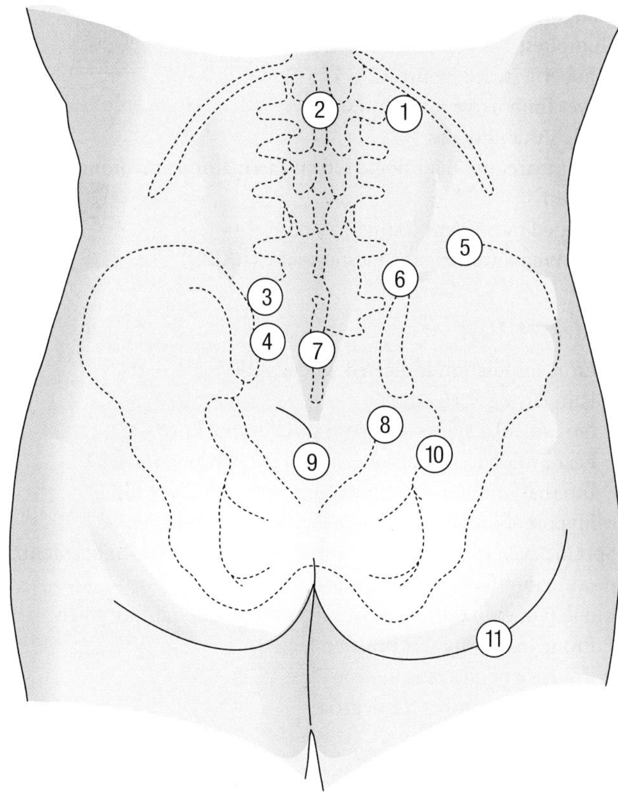

FIGURE 124-2 (*1*) Costovertebral angle. (*2*) Spinous process and interspinous ligament. (*3*) Region of articular facet (fifth lumbar to first sacral). (*4*) Dorsum of sacrum. (*5*) Region of iliac crest. (*6*) Iliolumbar angle. (*7*) Spinous processes of the fifth lumbar and first sacral vertebrae (tenderness = faulty posture or occasionally spina bifida occulta). (*8*) Region between the posterior superior and posteroinferior spines. Sacroiliac ligaments (tenderness = sacroiliac sprain, often tender, with the fifth lumbar or first sacral disc). (*9*) Sacrococcygeal junction (tenderness = sacrococcygeal injury; i.e., sprain or fracture). (*10*) Region of sacrosciatic notch (tenderness = fourth or fifth lumbar disc rupture and sacroiliac sprain). (*11*) Sciatic nerve trunk (tenderness = ruptured lumbar disc or sciatic nerve lesion). (From Ropper AH, Samuels MA. *Adams & Victor's Principles of Neurology*. 9th ed. www.accessmedicine.com. Copyright © The McGraw-Hill Companies, Inc. All rights reserved.)

IMPAIRMENTS

- Decreased lumbar stability
- Weakened abdominals and other core-stabilizing muscles
- Shortened hamstrings and hip flexors
- Postural changes
- Inability to walk, stand, sit for prolonged periods of time

TESTS AND MEASURES

- Passive physiologic intervertebral mobility (PPIVM) testing[4]
- Lower extremity screening examination
- Postural examination
- Muscle-length testing, including the hamstrings, hip flexors, and calf muscles
- Quadrant test

- Straight-leg raise test
- Slump test
- Schober test, see Figure 124-3
- Lower limb nerve tension test
- Prone instability test
- Lower extremity neurologic screen (dermatome, myotome, reflexes)
- Repeated movement testing
- Fear-Avoidance Beliefs Questionnaire (FABQ)

INTERVENTION

- Joint manipulation indicated when, with:
    - Pain lasting <16 days
    - No radicular symptoms/pain distal to the knee
    - Fear avoidance beliefs questionaire (FABQ) score <19
    - Internal rotation of >35 degrees for at least one hip
    - Hypomobility of a least one level of the lumbar spine
- Specific exercise when pain centralizes with repeated movement/ posture into flexion or extension
- Lumbar-stabilization exercises to address core stability when
    - Prone instability test positive
    - Presence of aberrant motion
    - Straight-leg raise >91 degrees
    - Age <41 years
- Traction when
    - Radiculopathy findings present
    - Positive crossed straight-leg raise
    - Pain peripheralized with repeated extension
- Stretching exercises, myofascial mobilization for shortened musculature
- Unweighted treadmill walking
- Aquatic exercise
- Modalities for short-term pain control
- Cognitive behavioral therapy

FUNCTIONAL GOALS

- Patient will be able to
    - Sit with neutral lumbar spine posture for >30 minutes with 0 out of 10 pain rating for computer work and desk activities
    - Sit at work station and perform computer work for 45 minutes with 0 out of 10 pain rating
    - Rotate lumbar spine 25 degrees so as to reach into the back seat of a car with 0 out of 10 pain rating in lower extremity
    - Walk for 30 minutes with 0 out of 10 pain rating so as to go shopping.
    - Increase standing tolerance to >30 minutes without pain so as to stand at work.

PROGNOSIS

- Fair to very good, depending on specific impairments.
- Chronic low back pain prognosis significantly lowered.

PATIENT RESOURCES

- Livestrong. Dynamic Lumbar Stabilization Exercises. http://www.livestrong.com/dynamic-lumbar-stabilization-exercises. Accessed July 6, 2013.

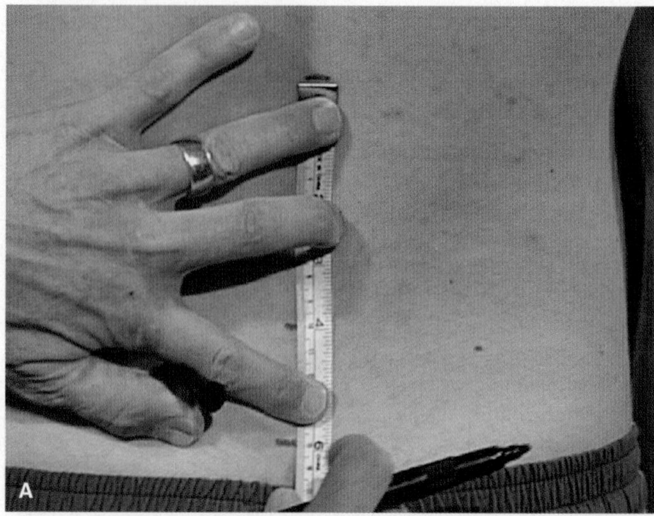

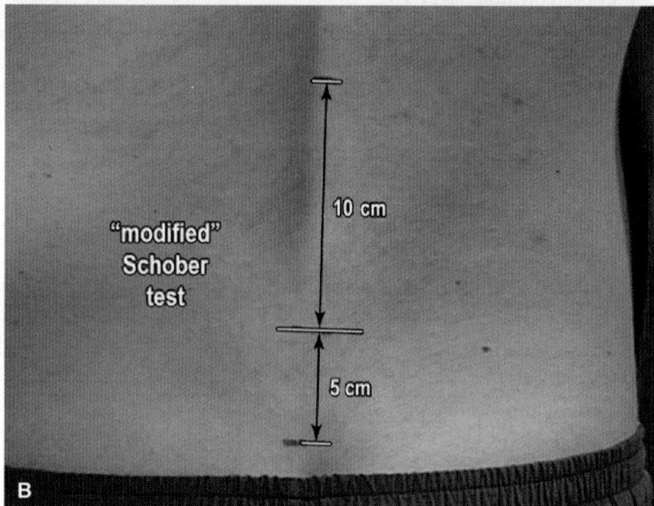

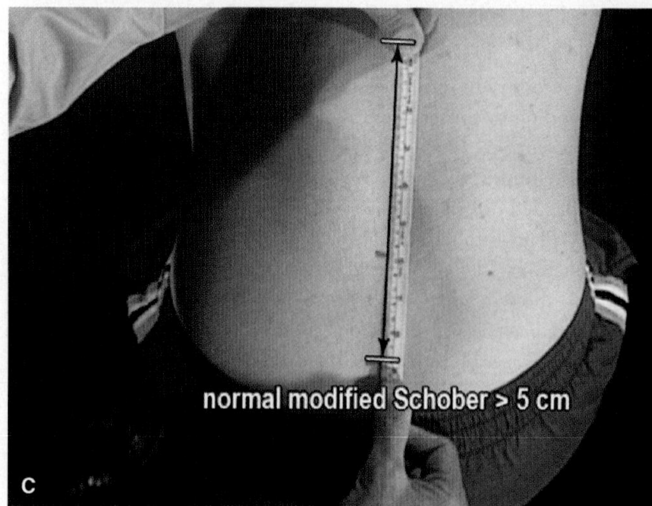

FIGURE 124-3 Modified Schober test (**A**) Mark at the 5th lumbar (L5) vertebrae (**B**) Mark 10 cm above L5 and 5 cm below L5 (**C**) The patient flexes forward and less than 5 cm of motion increase indicates reduced lumbar mobility. (From Lawry GV. *Systematic Musculoskeletal Examinations.* www.accessmedicine.com. Copyright © The McGraw-Hill Companies, Inc. All rights reserved.)

REFERENCES

1. The American Physical Therapy Association. Pattern 4F: Impaired joint mobility, motor function, muscle performance, range of motion, and reflex integrity associated with spinal disorders. *Interactive Guide to Physical Therapist Practice*. Alexandria, VA: The American Physical Therapy Association; 2003. http://guidetoptpractice.apta.org. Accessed July 6, 2013.
2. Dutton M. *Orthopaedic Examination, Evaluation, and Intervention*. New York, NY: McGraw-Hill; 2008. http://www.accessphysiotherapy.com/resource/612. Accessed July 6, 2013.
3. Malone TR, Hazle C, Grey ML. Imaging in Rehabilitation. New York, NY: McGraw-Hill; 2008. http://www.accessphysiotherapy.com/resource/613. Accessed July 6, 2013.
4. Dutton M. *Dutton's Orthopedic Survival Guide: Managing Common Conditions*. New York, NY: McGraw-Hill; 2011. http://www.accessphysiotherapy.com/content/8656264#8656264. Accessed July 6, 2013.

ADDITIONAL REFERENCES

- Fritz JM, Cleland JA, Childs JD. Subgrouping patients with low back pain: evolution of a classification approach to physical therapy. *J Orthop Sports Phys Ther*. 2007;37:290–302.
- Liebenson C. *Rehabilitation of the Spine: A Practitioner's Manual*. 2nd ed. Baltimore, MD: Lippincott, Williams & Wilkins; 2007.
- Pool-Goudzwaard A, Hoek van Dijke G, Mulder P, et al. The iliolumbar ligament: its influence on stability of the sacroiliac joint. *Clin Biomech* (Bristol, Avon). 2003;18(2):99–105.
- Olsen KA. *Manual Physical Therapy of the Spine*. St. Louis, MI: Saunders Elsevier; 2009.

125 JEFFERSON FRACTURE

Eric Shamus, PhD, DPT, PT, CSCS
Melissa Tabor, DO

ICD-9-CM CODES

- 738.4 Acquired spondylolisthesis
- 756.12 Spondylolisthesis congenital
- 805.01 Closed fracture of first cervical vertebra

ICD-10-CM CODES

- M43.10 Spondylolisthesis, site unspecified
- Q76.2 Congenital spondylolisthesis
- S12.000A Unspecified displaced fracture of first cervical vertebra, initial encounter for closed fracture
- S12.001A Unspecified nondisplaced fracture of first cervical vertebra, initial encounter for closed fracture

PREFERRED PRACTICE PATTERN

- 4E: Impaired Joint Mobility, Motor Function, Muscle Performance, and ROM Associated with Localized Inflammation[1]

PATIENT PRESENTATION

Patient is a 36-year-old construction worker who fell off a ladder and had a burst fracture of the atlas. The physician and patient decided to treat the fracture with immobilization with halo traction and halo vest. Patient achieved a union of his fracture. The patient presents with increased tone bilateral upper trapezius and scalenes with decreased range of motion of the cervical spine.

KEY FEATURES

Description

- Anterior (forward) translation of a vertebra
- Fracture of the anterior and posterior arches of the C1 vertebra
- Slipping of the vertebra in relationship to the vertebra below
- Ataxia
- Fracture widens at the pars
- Typically a four-part or "burst" fracture

Essentials of Diagnosis

- Diagnosis made by X-ray, children may require CT scan
- Clinical examination may find step deformity
- Axial load on top of the head
- Reports diving into a shallow pool

General Considerations

- Instability
- Avoid extension positions that increase symptoms

Demographics

- Usually from landing on head, as with diving into a shallow pool

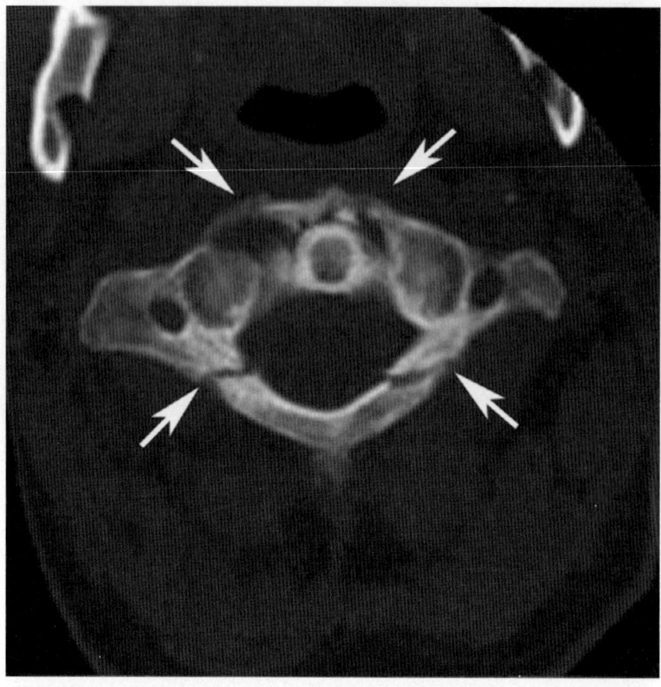

FIGURE 125-1 Axial CT demonstrates four fracture lines (*arrows*) separating C1 in four parts. Jefferson fracture is usually caused by axial impact to the head such as diving in shallow water. (From Longo DL, Fauci A, Kasper D, et al., eds. *Harrison's Principles of Internal Medicine.* 18th ed. http://www.accessmedicine.com. Copyright © The McGraw-Hill Companies, Inc. All rights reserved.)

CLINICAL FINDINGS

SIGNS AND SYMPTOMS

- Ataxia
- Injury to vertebral artery
- Cervical, shoulder, arm, and upper-extremity pain; often radiating into lower extremities if central cord involved
- Constricted pupil (Horner sign)
- Stiffness along spine
- Headaches
- Pain in the cervical spine worsens with extension

Functional Implications

- Difficulty maintaining standing postures secondary to neck pain
- Difficulty with movements (reaching overhead) secondary to pain
- Limited sports participation
- Can cause quadriplegia or death

Possible Contributing Causes

- Forceful extension from hit under the chin (as in sports)
- Car accident, hit from rear
- Hyperextension of the cervical spine
- Diving into a shallow pool

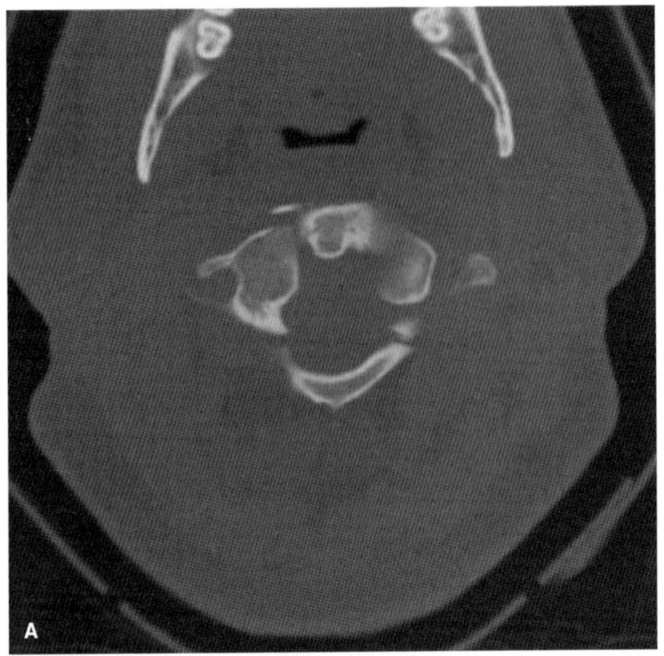

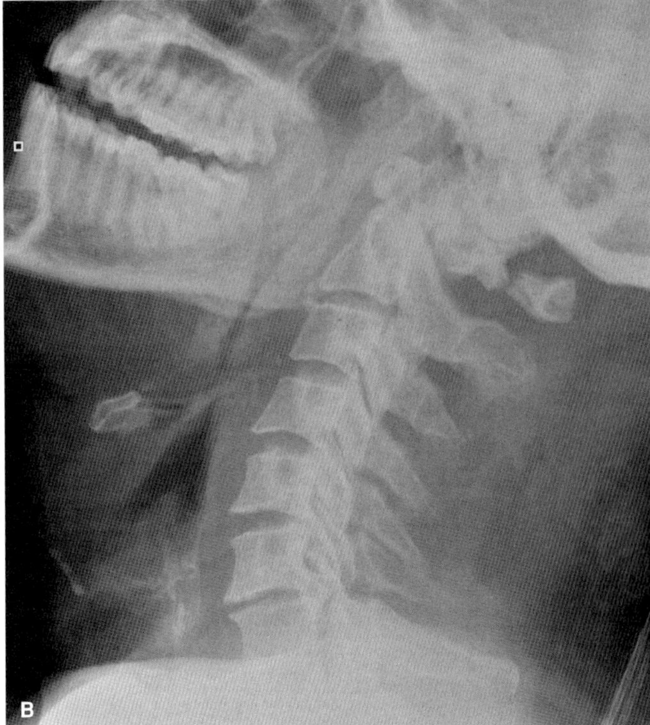

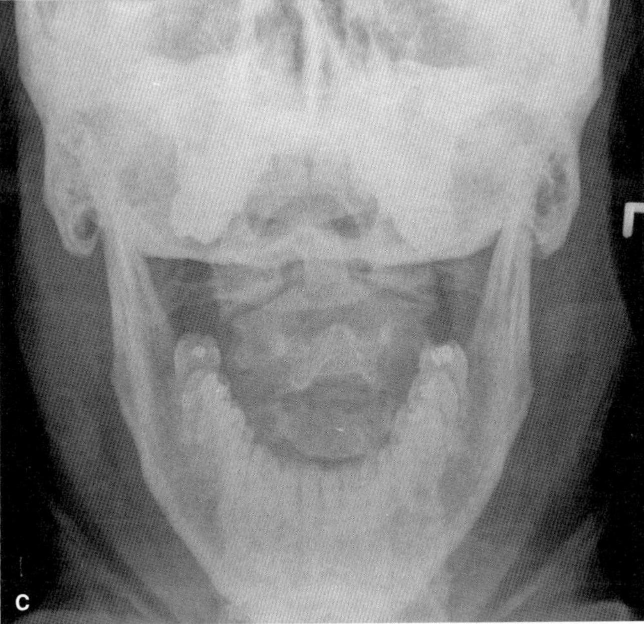

FIGURE 125-2 Jefferson fracture CT and radiographs show a Jefferson burst fracture in a 46-year-old man, who sustained injuries while body surfing. (**A**) Axial CT images viewed on bone windows show bilateral fractures of both the anterior and posterior arches of C1. (**B**) Lateral radiograph of the cervical spine shows the fracture of the posterior arch of C1, with slight distraction of the posterior fracture fragment. (**C**) Open-mouth view shows slight asymmetry of the dens in relation to the lateral masses of C1, with slight widening of the interval between C1 and the dens. The right lateral mass of C1 is slightly subluxed laterally at the right atlantoaxial joint. (From Tintinalli JE, Stapczynski J, John Ma O, et al. *Tintinalli's Emergency Medicine: A Comprehensive Study Guide.* 7th ed. http://www.accessmedicine.com. Copyright © The McGraw-Hill Companies, Inc. All rights reserved.)

Differential Diagnosis

- Peripheral nerve impairment
- Spinal tumor
- Peripheral neuropathy
- Paraspinal spasms
- Degenerative disc disease
- Hangman's fracture
- C2 vertebra anterior translated on C3 with fracture of C2 pedicles

MEANS OF CONFIRMATION OR DIAGNOSIS

Imaging

- MRI helps visualize compressed or inflamed nerve root in diagnosis.[2]
- X-ray/Plain-film radiograph to see vertebra position.[3]
- CT to show herniation compressing the spinal canal/nerves.[3]
- Electrodiagnostic/nerve conduction testing can help determine a specific impaired nerve function.[4]

FINDINGS AND INTERPRETATION

- Fracture of the anterior and posterior arches of the C1 vertebra

TREATMENT

- Rules of Spence
- Surgical fusion[2]

REFERRALS/ADMITTANCE

- To hospital for imaging
- To surgeon for surgical consult if myelopathy suspected
- To physician for anti-inflammatory medication
- To orthopedist for halo vest traction device, cervical bracing

IMPAIRMENTS

- Restricted mobility of the upper cervical spine
- Hypermobility
- Noted weakness of the neck musculature

TESTS AND MEASURES

- Cervical spine AROM
- Sharp–Purser: Atlantoaxial instability
- Cervical passive intervertebral motion testing
- Subcranial translation instability testing
- Passive physiologic intervertebral mobility (PPIVM) testing
- Upper-extremity screening examination
- Postural examination
- Muscle length testing, including the upper trapezius, levator scapulae, and pectoral muscles
- Upper limb nerve tension test
- Deep neck flexor endurance test
- Upper-extremity neurologic screen (dermatome, myotome, reflexes)

INTERVENTION

- Rest
- Bracing
- Address pain
  - Electrical stimulation
  - Heat/Ice[5]
- Address hypertonicity
  - Soft-tissue massage
  - Heat
- Address muscle weakness
  - Stability exercises

FUNCTIONAL GOALS

- Patient will be able to
  - Sit with neutral cervical-spine posture for >30 minutes with 0/10 pain rating.
  - Stand at work station and perform computer work for 45 minutes with 0/10 pain rating.
  - Rotate cervical spine 75 degrees to look over the shoulder while driving with 0/10 pain rating.

PROGNOSIS

- Fair to good, depending on severity of vertebral translation, amount of nerve-root compression, and upper/lower-extremity impairments.
- Possible death.

PATIENT RESOURCE

- The Pediatric Orthopaedic Society of North America (POSNA). Cervical Spine Fractures. http://www.posna.org/education/StudyGuide/cervicalSpineFractures.asp. Accessed July 7, 2013.

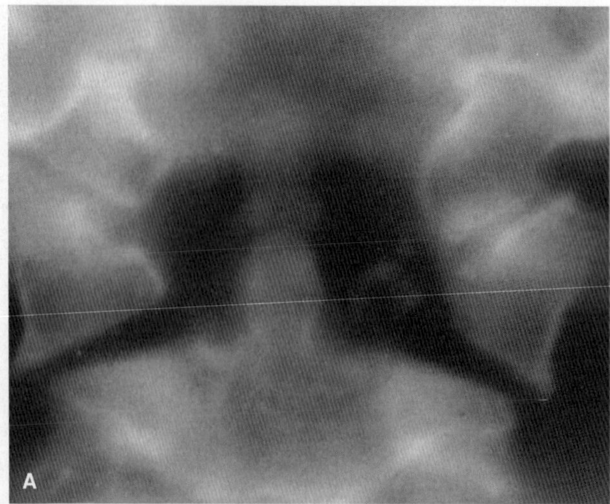

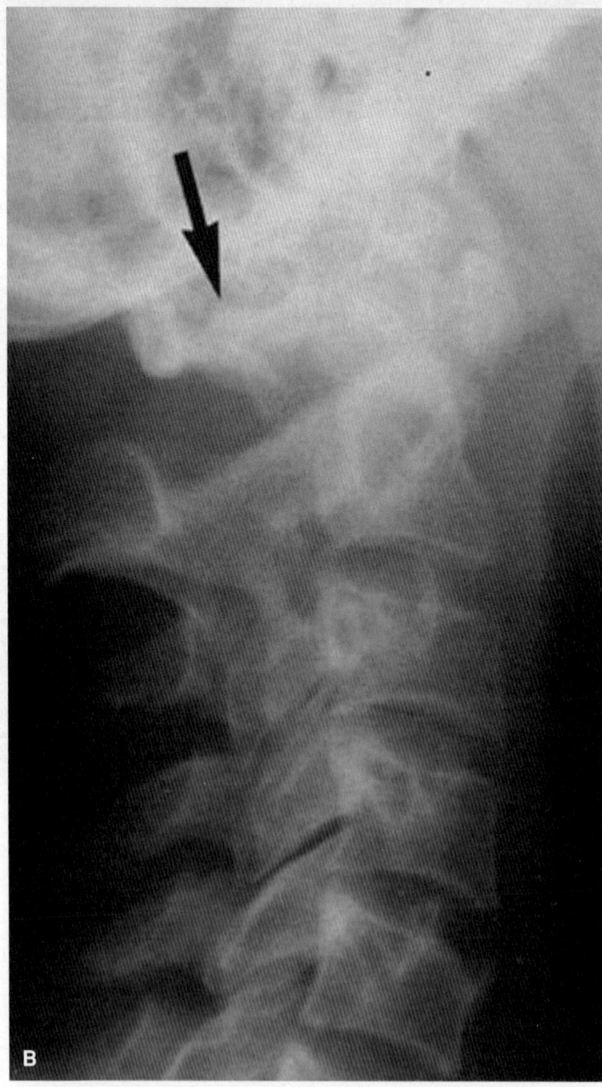

FIGURE 125-3 **A.** AP tomogram confirming an unstable Jefferson fracture with avulsion of the transverse ligament from the lateral mass of C1. **B.** Lateral view showing fracture of the posterior arch of C1 (*arrow*). (From Hall JB, Schmidt GA, Wood LDH. *Principles of Critical Care.* 3rd ed. http://www.accessmedicine.com. Copyright © The McGraw-Hill Companies, Inc. All rights reserved.)

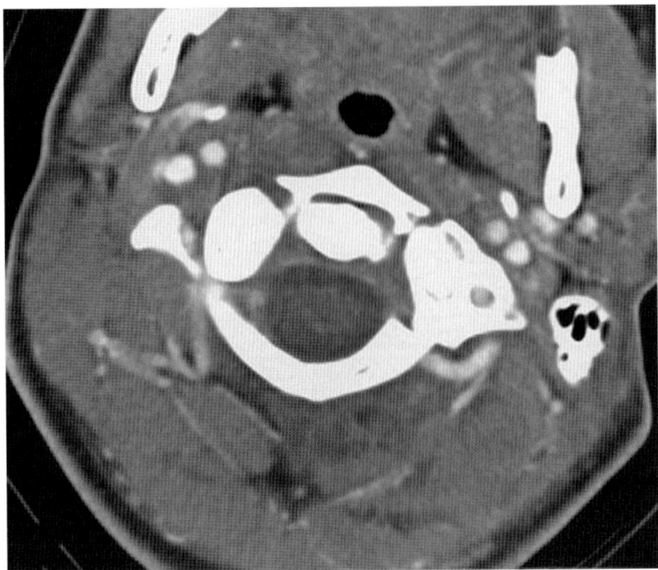

FIGURE 125-4 An axial CT bone windows view of a Jefferson fracture in a 15-year-old boy. Note the quadripartite configuration of the atlas with fractures anterior and posterior to the lateral masses bilaterally. (From Malone TR, Hazle C, Grey ML. *Imaging in Rehabilitation*. http://www.accessphysiotherapy.com.

REFERENCES

1. The American Physical Therapy Association. Pattern 4E: Impaired joint mobility, motor function, muscle performance, and range of motion associated with localized inflammation. *Interactive Guide to Physical Therapist Practice*. 2003. DOI: 10.2522/ptguide.3.1_5. Accessed July 7, 2013.
2. Dutton M. *Orthopaedic Examination, Evaluation, and Intervention*. New York, NY: McGraw-Hill; 2008. http://www.accessphysiotherapy.com/resource/612. Accessed July 7, 2013.
3. Malone TR, Hazle C, Grey ML. *Imaging in Rehabilitation*. New York, NY: McGraw-Hill; 2008. http://www.accessphysiotherapy.com/resource/613. Accessed July 7, 2013.
4. Dutton M. *Dutton's Orthopedic Survival Guide: Managing Common Conditions*. New York, NY: McGraw-Hill; 2011. http://www.accessphysiotherapy.com/resource/685. Accessed July 7, 2013.
5. Prentice WE. Chapter 9. Cryotherapy and thermotherapy. In: Prentice WE, Quillen WS, Underwood F, eds. *Therapeutic Modalities in Rehabilitation*. 4th ed. New York, NY: McGraw-Hill; 2011. http://www.accessphysiotherapy.com/content/8137995#8137995. Accessed July 7, 2013.

ADDITIONAL REFERENCES

- Dettling SD, Morscher MA, Masin JS, Adamczyk MJ. Cranial nerve IX and X impairment after a sports-related Jefferson (C1) fracture in a 16-year-old male: a case report. *J Pediatr Orthop*. 2013;33(3):e23–e27.
- ICD9DATA web site. http://www.icd9data.com. Accessed July 7, 2013.
- ICD10DATA web site. http://www.icd10data.com. Accessed July 7, 2013.
- Wainner RS, Fritz JM, Irrgang JJ,et al. Reliability and diagnostic accuracy of the clinical examination and patient self-report measures for cervical radiculopathy. *Spine*. 2003;28(1):52–62.

126 KYPHOSIS

Jennifer Cabrera, DPT, GCS
Eric Shamus, PhD, DPT, PT, CSCS

CONDITION/DISORDER SYNONYMS

- Scheuermann disease
- Juvenile disc disease
- Roundback
- Hunchback
- Postural kyphosis

ICD-9-CM CODES

- 737 Curvature of spine
- 737.0 Adolescent postural kyphosis
- 737.1 Kyphosis (acquired)
- 737.10 Kyphosis (acquired) (postural)
- 737.11 Kyphosis due to radiation
- 737.12 Kyphosis postlaminectomy
- 737.19 Other kyphosis acquired

ICD-10-CM CODES

- M40.00 Postural kyphosis, site unspecified
- M40.209 Unspecified kyphosis, site unspecified
- M96.2 Postradiation kyphosis
- M96.3 Postlaminectomy kyphosis
- M40.299 Other kyphosis, site unspecified

PREFERRED PRACTICE PATTERNS

- 4A: Primary Prevention/Risk Reduction for Skeletal Demineralization[1]
- 4B: Impaired Posture[2]
- 4E: Impaired Joint Mobility, Motor Function, Muscle Performance, and ROM Associated with Localized Inflammation[3]
- 6E: Impaired Ventilation and Respiration/Gas Exchange Associated with Ventilatory Pump Dysfunction or Failure[4]

PATIENT PRESENTATION

A 93-year-old woman and her family report she had declined in function throughout the last 1 to 2 months. She has extensive history of postmenopausal osteoporosis for 15 years. Despite the use of bisphosphonates, she has experienced vertebral compression fractures at T8 and T11. She reports chronic back pain, which is severely limiting her activity. She presents with a dowager hump deformity.

KEY FEATURES

Description

- Excessive posterior curvature of the thoracic spine
- Adult kyphosis: Scheuermann disease (juvenile disc disease) caused by wedging of several vertebrae[5]
- Postural kyphosis: From slouching or poor posture

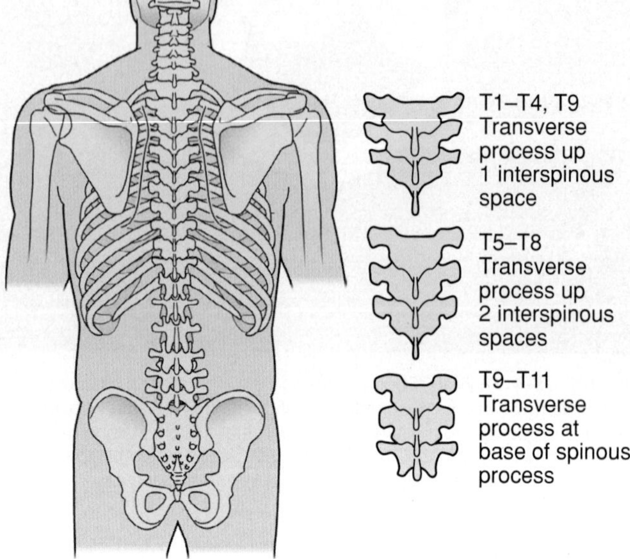

FIGURE 126-1 The rule of threes. (From Dutton M. *Dutton's Orthopaedic Examination, Evaluation, and Intervention*. 3rd ed. http://www.accessphysiotherapy.com. Copyright © The McGraw-Hill Companies, Inc. All rights reserved.)

- Congenital kyphosis: Under-development of the spinal column[6]
- Gibbus deformity: Structural kyphosis from tuberculosis
- Types of kyphotic deformities
  - Round back
    - Decreased pelvic inclination with thoracolumbar or thoracic kyphosis
    - Caused by tightness in soft tissues from prolonged postural change
    - Compensatory mechanism to maintain body's center of gravity
  - Hunchback (hump back)
    - Gibbus: Localized, sharp, posterior angulation
    - Structural cause
      - Anterior wedging of one to two thoracic vertebral bodies
      - Wedging may be caused by fracture, tumor, bone disease
    - Pelvic inclination usually normal
  - Flat back
    - Decreased pelvic inclination
    - Thoracic spine remains mobile
    - Kyphosis present
    - Does not have appearance of excessive kyphotic curve
  - Dowager hump
    - Secondary to postmenopausal osteoporosis
    - Anterior-wedge fractures of several upper or middle thoracic vertebrae
    - Contributes to decrease in height

Essentials of Diagnosis

- Diagnosis usually made by clinical examination
- Can be an independent diagnosis, not associated with a disease process
- Cobb angle for measurement of scoliosis[5]

▶ General Considerations

- Pain and stiffness at rest/sleep
- Inability to sleep supine
- Respiratory problems secondary to changes in rib-cage space

▶ Demographics

- Women affected more frequently than men due to postmenopausal alteration
- Can occur at any age

CLINICAL FINDINGS

SIGNS AND SYMPTOMS

- Pain in the upper and middle thoracic spine
- Tight pectoral, hamstring, hip flexor muscles
- Fatigue
- Overstretched and weak middle-/lower-trapezius and rhomboid muscles
- Local tenderness with palpation seen in vertebral compression fractures
- Scapular winging
- Forward head positioning
- Weak spinal extensors
- Tight cervical extensors
- Weak cervical flexors
- Respiratory problems
- Stiffness in the spine

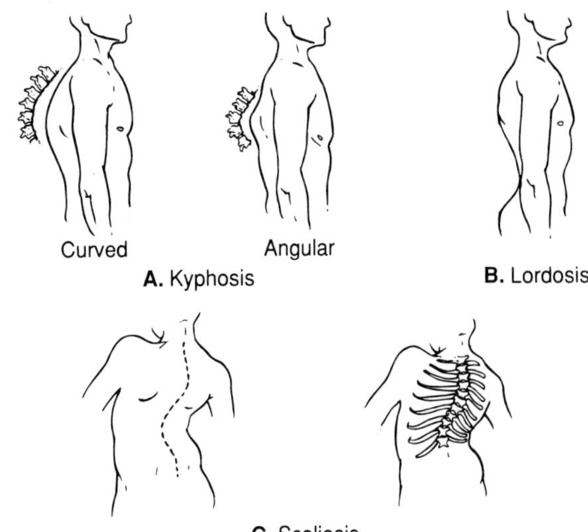

FIGURE 126-2 Curvatures of the spine affecting the thorax. **A.** Kyphotic thorax. **B.** Lordotic thorax. **C.** Scoliotic thorax. Note the narrowing of the rib interspaces on the right and the accentuation of the interspaces, posterior humping of the chest, and elevation of the shoulder on the left. (From LeBlond RF, DeGowin RL, Brown DD. *DeGowin's Diagnostic Examination*. 9th ed. http://www.accessmedicine.com. Copyright © The McGraw-Hill Companies, Inc. All rights reserved.)

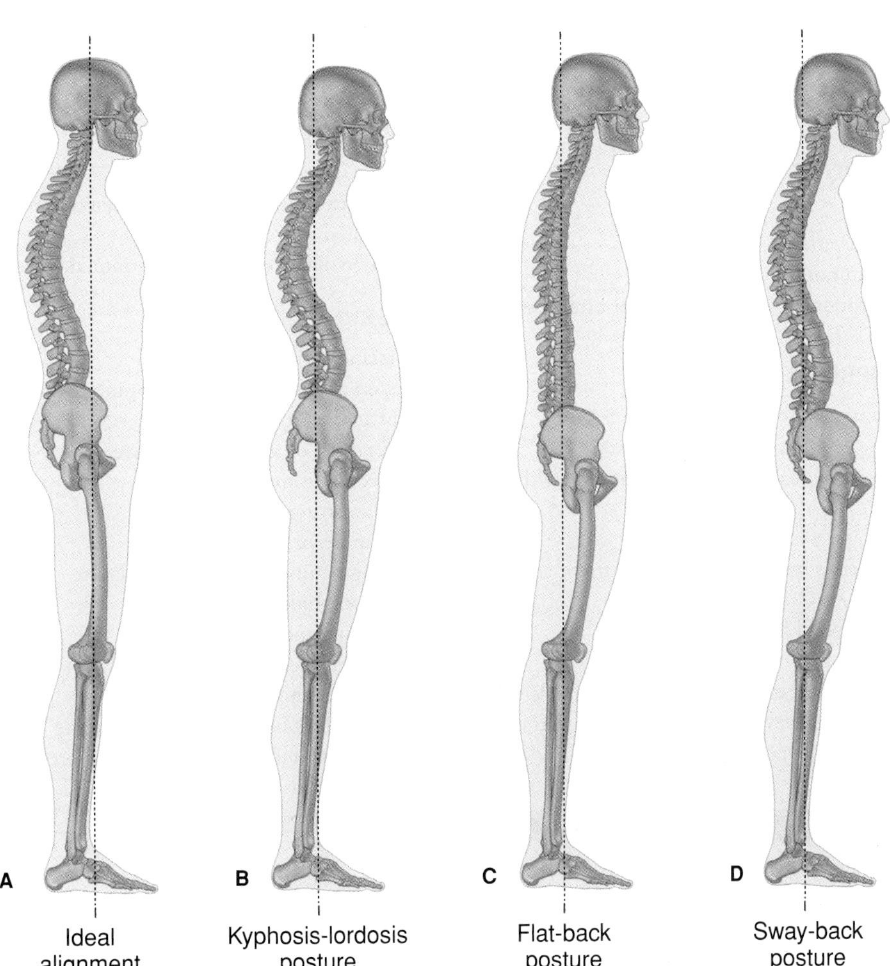

FIGURE 126-3 Common postural dysfunctions. (From Dutton M. *Dutton's Orthopaedic Examination, Evaluation, and Intervention*. 3rd ed. http://www.accessphysiotherapy.com. Copyright © The McGraw-Hill Companies, Inc. All rights reserved.)

Functional Implications

- Pain while in supine position without head-of-bed elevation
- Difficulty reaching overhead
- Decreased endurance secondary to impaired pulmonary capacity

Possible Contributing Causes

- Ankylosing spondylitis
- Arthritis
- Cerebral palsy (pediatric)
- Degeneration of intervertebral discs
- Endocrine disorders
- Infection
- Metastatic tumor
- Neurofibromatosis
- Osteoporosis
- Paget's disease
- Polio
- Poor nutrition: rickets[7]
- Poor posture
- Scheuermann disease
- Spina bifida
- Spondylolisthesis
- Tuberculosis
- Vertebral compression fractures

Differential Diagnosis

- Vertebral compression fracture
- Spinal stenosis
- Ehlers–Danlos syndrome
- Pott disease

MEANS OF CONFIRMATION OR DIAGNOSIS

Imaging

- X-ray for wedging of the vertebrae[8]
- MRI for neurologic or tumor[9]
- Dual-energy X-ray absorptiometry (DEXA) scan for osteoporosis[10]

FINDINGS AND INTERPRETATION

- Flexicurve assessment demonstrates kyphotic index >13
- Occiput-to-wall test
  - Positive finding indicated by inability to touch the wall with the back of the head
- Height loss
  - Difference between patient's recalled height and current actual height
  - Used for detection of vertebral fractures
- Rib-to-pelvic distance
  - Indicative of osteoporosis related to vertebral compression fractures
  - Distance of ≤2 finger widths between inferior margin of the ribs and superior surface of the pelvis

REFERRALS/ADMITTANCE

- To hospital for imaging, X-ray
- To physician for medication: Anti-inflammatory or opioid pain management
- To physician for endocrinology consult: Bone mineral density or osteoporosis treatment
- To physician for neurology consult
- To PT for bracing
  - Milwaukee brace
- To physician for surgical consult: Warranted in those with
  - Severe curves
  - Continuous progression of curve
  - Progressive neurologic symptoms
  - Unmanageable pain
  - Kyphoplasty[11]

IMPAIRMENTS

- Difficulty reaching overhead due to poor scapular positioning
- Flexed posture with ambulation due to structural positioning, weakness in spinal extensors, and tight hip flexors/hamstrings
- Difficulty picking up objects from floor secondary to inability to shift body weight posteriorly
- Forward-bending of the trunk during stance phase of gait secondary to tight hip flexor and weakness of hip extensor
- Decreased lung capacity

TESTS AND MEASURES

- Algorithm for examination of the lumbar spine
- Passive physiologic intervertebral mobility (PPIVM) testing
- Lower extremity screening examination
- Postural examination
- Muscle length testing, including the hamstrings, hip flexors, and calf muscles
- Quadrant test
- Straight-leg raise test
- Slump test
- Lower limb nerve tension test
- Prone instability test
- Lower extremity neurologic screen (dermatome, myotome, reflexes)
- Repeated movement testing
- Fear-Avoidance Beliefs Questionnaire (FABQ)

INTERVENTION

- Bracing: Milwaukee brace
- External postural supports: Spinomed
- Postural education
- Stretching of tight musculature
  - Pectoralis major and minor
  - Hamstrings
  - Hip flexors
- Strengthening postural musculature
  - Rhomboids
  - Middle and lower trapezius
  - Spinal extensors
- Soft-tissue mobilization
- Vertebral mobilizations if appropriate
  - Posteroanterior central-vertebral pressure
- Address pain
  - Ice
  - Massage
  - Electrical stimulation

FUNCTIONAL GOALS

- Patient will be able to
  - Demonstrate improved resting posture while standing as indicated by flexicurve assessment kyphotic index score of <13.

- Increase bilateral hip-extension to 0 degrees during mid and terminal stance of gait.
- Increase speed of gait to 1.2 m/sec to facilitate ability to safely cross the street.

PROGNOSIS

- Young adults with Scheuermann disease do well once growth plates close and stabilize.
- Elderly patients with osteoporotic fractures often need kyphoplasty surgery to correct deformity.

PATIENT RESOURCE

- Scoliosis Research Society. Traumatic Kyphosis. http://www.srs.org/patient_and_family/kyphosis. Accessed July 2, 2013.

REFERENCES

1. The American Physical Therapy Association. Pattern 4A: Primary prevention/risk reduction for skeletal demineralization. *Interactive Guide to Physical Therapist Practice*. 2003. DOI: 10.2522/ptguide.3.1_1. Accessed July 1, 2013.
2. The American Physical Therapy Association. Pattern 4B: Impaired posture. *Interactive Guide to Physical Therapist Practice*. 2003. DOI: 10.2522/ptguide.3.1_2. Accessed July 1, 2013.
3. The American Physical Therapy Association. Pattern 4E: Impaired joint mobility, motor function, muscle performance, and range of motion associated with localized inflammation. *Interactive Guide to Physical Therapist Practice*. 2003. DOI: 10.2522/ptguide.3.1_5. Accessed July 1, 2013.
4. The American Physical Therapy Association. Pattern 6E: Impaired ventilation and respiration/gas exchange associated with ventilatory pump dysfunction or failure. *Interactive Guide to Physical Therapist Practice*. 2003. DOI: 10.2522/ptguide.3.3_5. Accessed July 1, 2013.
5. Patel DR, Rowe D. Chapter 30. Thoracolumbar spine injuries. In: Patel DR, Greydanus DE, Baker RJ, eds. *Pediatric Practice: Sports Medicine*. New York, NY: McGraw-Hill; 2009. http://www.accessphysiotherapy.com/abstract/6981276#6981276. Accessed July 2, 2013.
6. Polousky JD. Chapter 24. Orthopedics: Growth disturbances of the musculoskeletal system. In: Hay WW, Levin MJ, Sondheimer JM, Detering RR, eds. *CURRENT Diagnosis & Treatment: Pediatrics*. New York, NY: McGraw-Hill; 2011. http://www.accessphysiotherapy.com/abstract/6585883#6585884. Accessed July 2, 2013.
7. Panus PC, Jobst EE, Masters SB, et al. Chapter 25. Drugs that affect bone mineral homeostasis. In: Panus PC, Jobst EE, Masters SB, eds. *Pharmacology for the Physical Therapist*. New York, NY: McGraw-Hill; 2009. http://www.accessphysiotherapy.com/abstract/6093763#6093775. Accessed May 22, 2014.
8. Hall SJ. Spinal curves. In: Hall SJ, ed. *Basic Biomechanics*. 5th ed. New York, NY: McGraw-Hill; 2007. http://www.accessphysiotherapy.com/content/6063126. Accessed July 7, 2013.
9. Hamilton N, Weimar W, Luttgens K. Chapter 3. The musculoskeletal system: the musculature. kinesiology: scientific basis of human motion. New York, NY: McGraw-Hill; 2008. http://www.accessphysiotherapy.com/abstract/6150358#6150373. Accessed July 2, 2013.
10. Baker RJ. Chapter 6. Sports nutrition. In: Patel DR, Greydanus DE, Baker RJ, eds. *Pediatric Practice: Sports Medicine*. New York, NY: McGraw-Hill; 2009. http://www.accessphysiotherapy.com/abstract/6973053#6973061. Accessed July 2, 2013.
11. Dutton M. Chapter 8. Musculoskeletal physical therapy. *NPTE (National Physical Therapy Examination)*. 2nd ed. New York, NY: McGraw-Hill; 2012. http://www.accessphysiotherapy.com/abstract/5398881#5398889. Accessed May 22, 2014.

ADDITIONAL REFERENCES

- Goodman CC, Boissonnault WG, Fuller KS. *Pathology: Implications for the Physical Therapist*. 2nd ed. Philadelphia, PA: Saunders; 2003.
- ICD9DATA web site. http://www.icd9data.com. Accessed July 2, 2013.
- ICD10DATA web site. http://www.icd10data.com. Accessed July 2, 2013.
- Magee DJ. *Orthopedic Physical Assessment*. 5th ed. St. Louis, MO: Saunders Elsevier; 2008.

127 LUMBAGO

Arie J. Van Duijn, EdD, MSc, PT, OCS
Eric Shamus, PhD, DPT, PT, CSCS
Kathy Swanick, DPT, PT, OCS

CONDITION/DISORDER SYNONYMS

- Low back pain
- Mechanical low back pain
- Nonspecific low back pain
- Lumbar sprain

ICD-9-CM CODES

- 724.2 Lumbago
- 847.2 Lumbar sprain

ICD-10-CM CODES

- M54.5 Low back pain
- S33.5 Sprain of ligaments of lumbar spine

PREFERRED PRACTICE PATTERN

- 4F: Impaired Joint Mobility, Motor Function, Muscle Performance, Range of Motion, and Reflex Integrity Associated with Spinal Disorders[1]

PATIENT PRESENTATION

A 27-year-old emergency room nurse presents with a low back injury while assisting in lowering a patient from an ambulance onto the pavement outside the hospital. Instead of facing the patient stretcher directly, she bent forward with a twist to one side and had to give a quick tug to lift along with the other personnel. It was much heavier than she expected, and it caught her off guard. She felt something "snap" in her back and experienced severe mid-lumbar pain. For several minutes she was unable to move from the semiflexed position and then gradually moved upright. The pain was intense for ~5 minutes, then eased off but increased again 30 minutes later and became progressively worse over the next few hours. This injury occurred 10 days ago.

Presently any movement causes pain, and bending forward is impossible. There is relief when lying supine or side lying, although prone lying and turning over in the bed aggravate the pain. Sitting relieves pain, although moving from sit to stand is very guarded, and she eases herself slowly down when returning to sit relying heavily on her arms for support. She identifies that the maximal site of the pain is in the L3-4 region.

There is point tenderness in the L4-5 region. Straight leg raise (SLR) is 80° bilaterally, and sacroiliac tests are negative. X-rays are negative for fracture and r/o spondylolisthesis.

KEY FEATURES

Description

- Pain in lumbar or sacral area that can be mechanically reproduced.
- Most episodes are self-limiting.
- Leading cause of disability for people under the age of 45 years.

Essentials of Diagnosis

- Diagnosis made by clinical examination
- Use of treatment- (impairment) based classification system is useful to determine evidence-based practice treatment plan

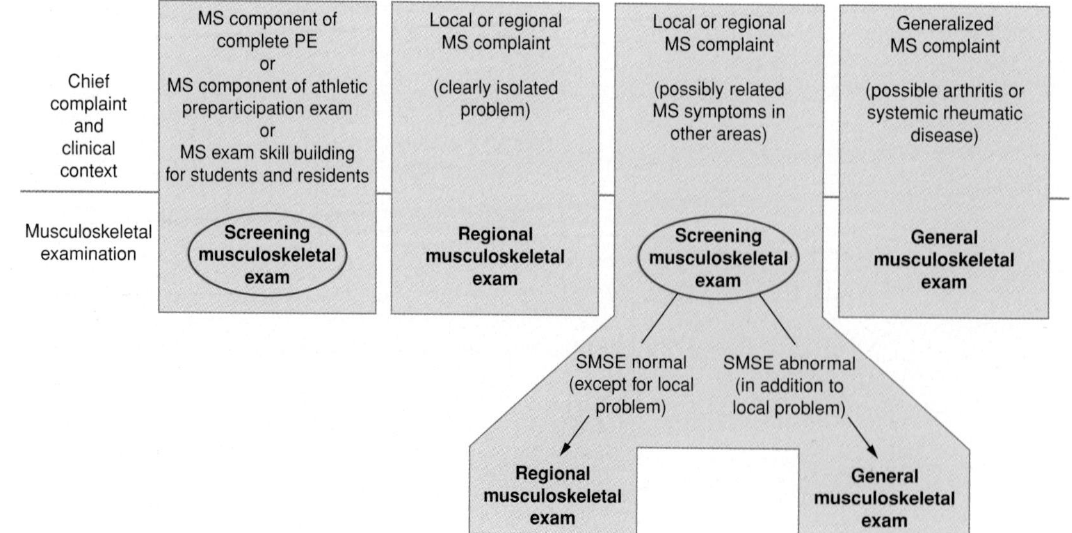

FIGURE 127-1 Low back pain: regional or general musculoskeletal exam. (From Lawry GV. *Systematic Musculoskeletal Examinations.* www.accessmedicine.com. Copyright © The McGraw-Hill Companies, Inc. All rights reserved.)

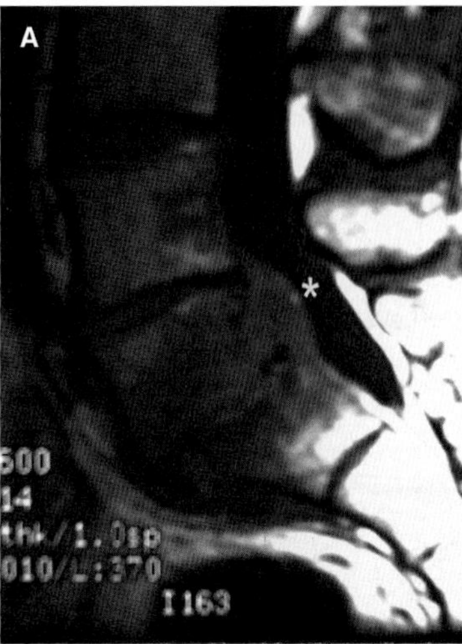

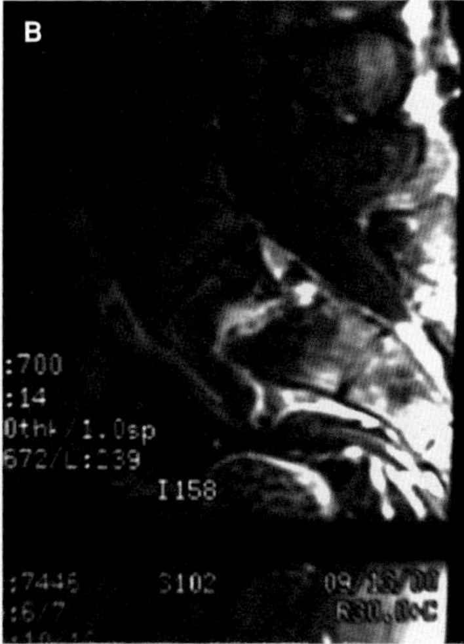

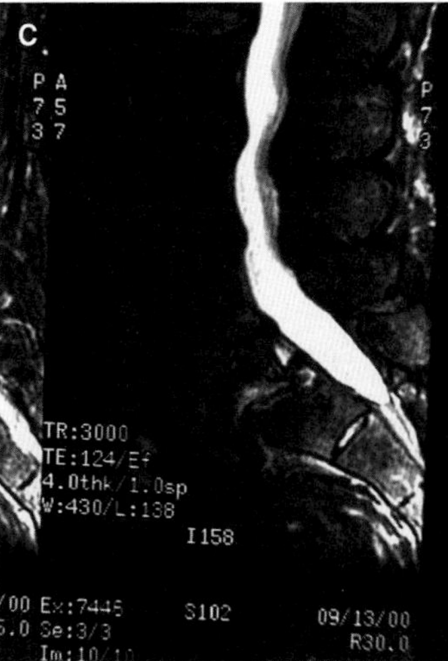

FIGURE 127-2 Sagittal MRI images of a patient with low back pain due to L5–S1 discitis, vertebral osteomyelitis, and a small anterior epidural abscess. (**A**) T1-weighted image. (**B**) T1-weighted image with gadolinium vascular contrast. (**C**) T2-weighted image. (From Doherty GM. *Current Diagnosis & Treatment: Surgery.* 13th ed. www.accessmedicine.com. Copyright © The McGraw-Hill Companies, Inc. All rights reserved.)

- Reproduction of symptoms in specific postures and activities
- Rule out disease (red and yellow flags)

General Considerations

- Presentation can vary significantly based on anatomical structures and psychosocial factors.
- Is often difficult to determine pathoanatomical cause of pain.

Demographics

- Occurs in up to 80% of population
- Variable, based on specific condition

CLINICAL FINDINGS

SIGNS AND SYMPTOMS

- Unilateral or bilateral referred or radiating pain in lower extremities possible
- Altered sensation, motor control, reflexes in the distribution of involved nerve roots indicate nerve-root compression (see Lumbar Radiculopathy)
- Pain may centralize or become peripheralized with repeated movement
- Lumbar segmental hypomobility may be present and indicates instability
- Often associated with poor core-muscle strength and postural deviations

Functional Implications

- Leading cause of occupational disability
- May impede ability to perform activities of daily living/instrumental activities of daily living
- May impede participation in sports and other social activities

Possible Contributing Causes

- Occupational factors
- Congenital anomalies
- Physical condition
- Smoking
- Obesity
- Socioeconomic factors
- Psychosocial and behavioral factors
- Postural changes
- Weakness of the core musculature
- Tightness of the hip flexors, external rotators, and hamstrings

Differential Diagnosis

- Abdominal aortic aneurism
- Ankylosing spondylitis
- Hip pathology with radiating pain pattern
- Malignant spinal tumor or metastasis
- Peripheral nerve impairment
- Referred pain from visceral structures
- Systematic autoimmune diseases (rheumatoid arthritis, Reiter syndrome)
- Vascular insufficiency

MEANS OF CONFIRMATION OR DIAGNOSIS

Imaging

- Not necessary in most cases; only with persistent symptoms that do not respond to conservative management or if red/yellow flags are present
- MRI[2]
- X-ray/Plain-film radiograph (flexion/extension radiograph)[3]

TABLE 127-1 Common Descriptors of Pain and Their Origin

Descriptor	Origin
Deep ache and boring	Bony tissues
Dull, achy, sore, burning, and cramping	Muscle/fascia
Sharp, life like, shooting, lancinating, tingling, burning, numbness, and weakness	Nerve
Burning, stabbing, throbbing, tingling, and cold	Vascular
Deep pain, cramping, and stabbing	Visceral

Source: From Dutton M. *Dutton's Orthopaedic Examination, Evaluation, and Intervention*. 3rd ed. http://www.accessphysiotherapy.com. Copyright © The McGraw-Hill Companies, Inc. All rights reserved.

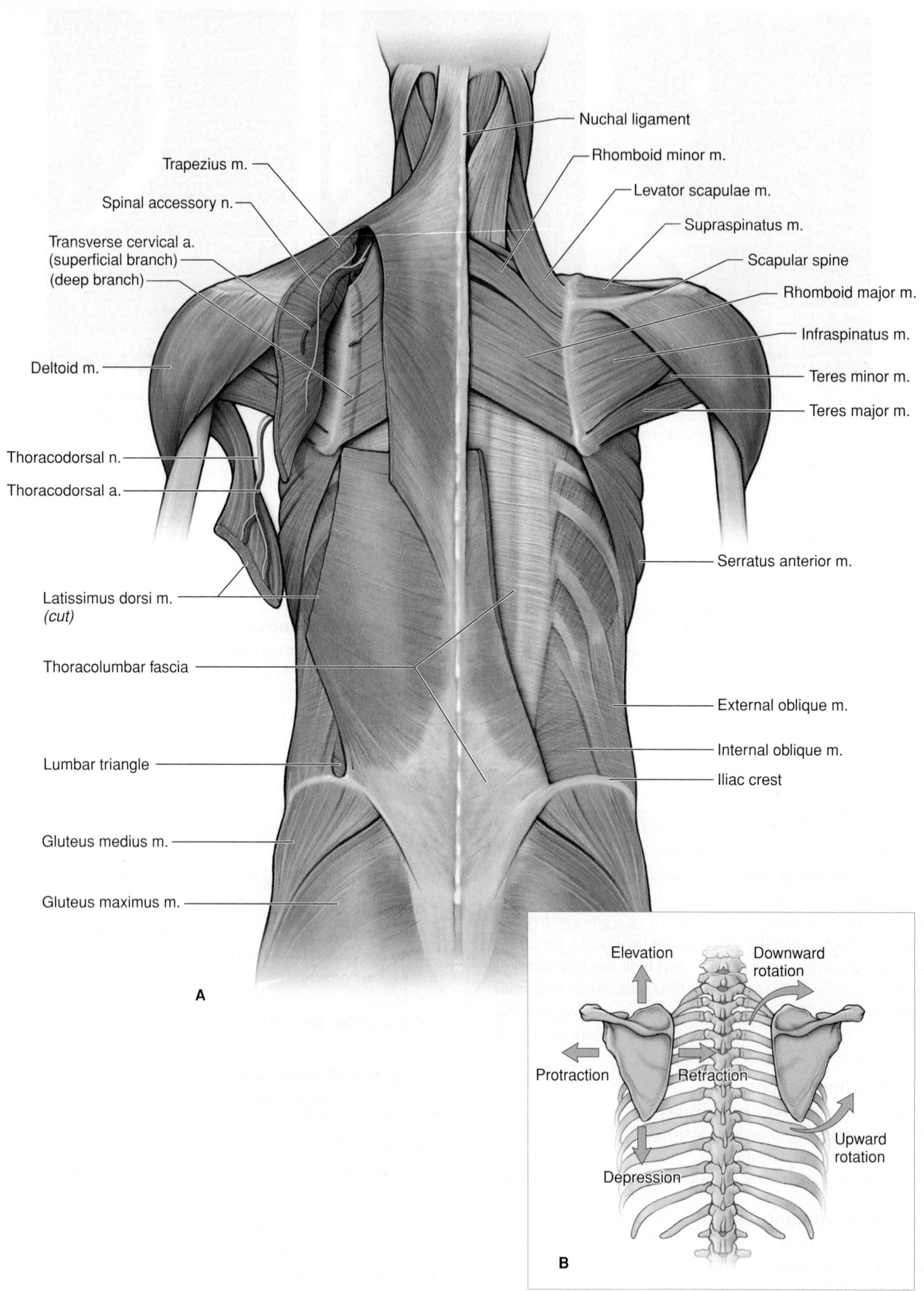

FIGURE 127-3 (**A**) Superficial muscles of the back. (**B**) Scapular actions. (From Morton DA, Foreman KB, Albertine KH. *The Big Picture: Gross Anatomy.* www.accessmedicine.com. Copyright © The McGraw-Hill Companies, Inc. All rights reserved.)

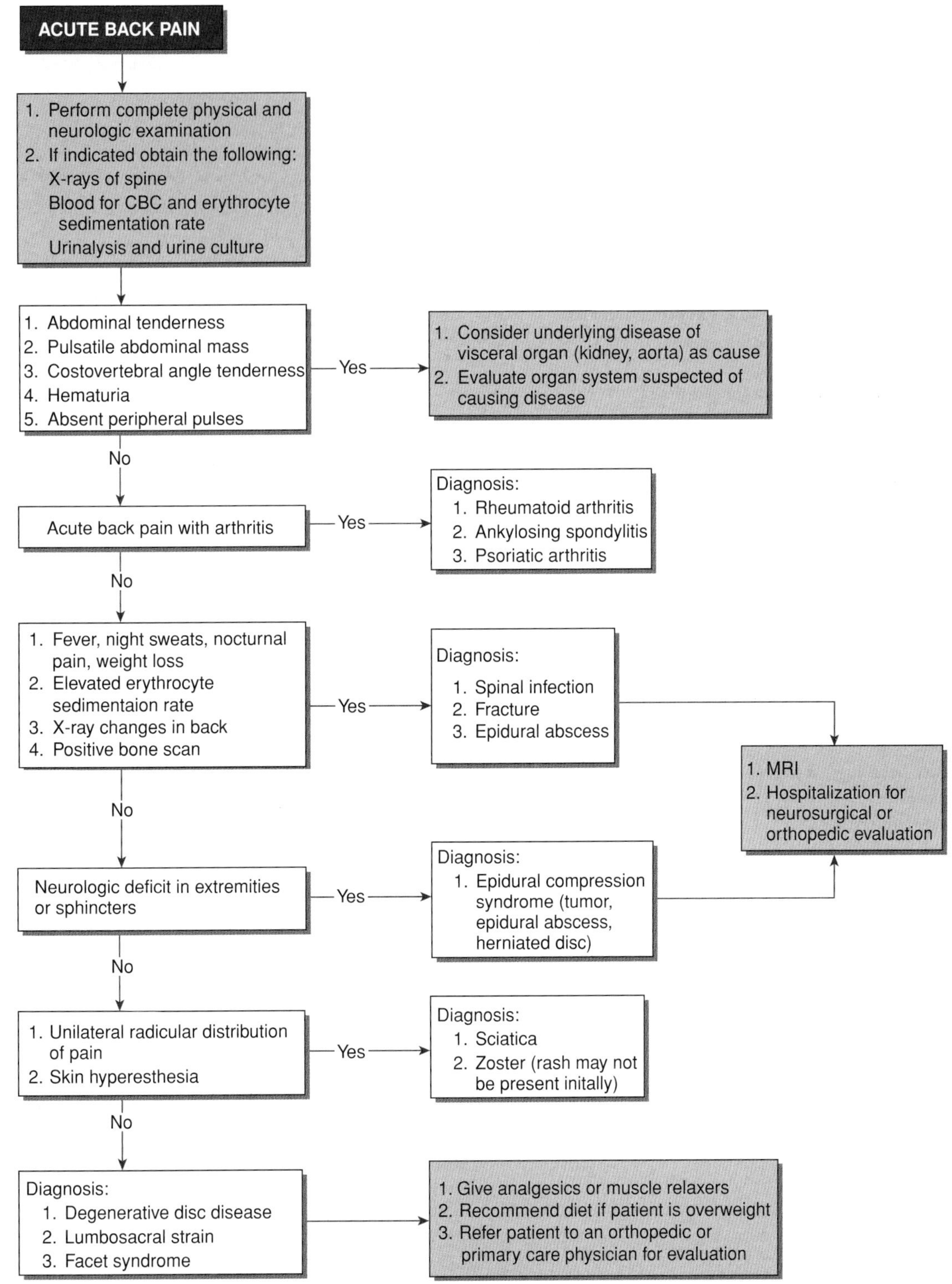

FIGURE 127-4 Assessment of patients with acute back pain. (From Stone CK, Humphries RL. *Current Diagnosis & Treatment: Emergency Medicine.* 7th ed. www.accessmedicine.com. Copyright © The McGraw-Hill Companies, Inc. All rights reserved.)

- CT[3]
- Electrodiagnostic/nerve conduction testing[4]
- Doppler ultrasound

FINDINGS AND INTERPRETATION

- MRI helps in diagnosis to visualize compressed or inflamed nerve root/disc pathology.[2]
- X-ray/Plain-film radiograph helps assess alignment, fractures, stability (flexion/extension radiograph).[3]
- CT helps show herniation compressing the spinal canal or nerves or rule out abdominal pathology.[3]
- Electrodiagnostic/nerve conduction testing can help determine specific impaired nerve function.[4]
- Doppler ultrasound helps examine vascular function.

REFERRALS/ADMITTANCE

- To hospital for imaging
- To physician for surgical consult if myelopathy suspected (see Lumbar Radiculopathy)
- To physician for imaging and medical consult if disease suspected
- To other specialist if vascular insufficiency suspected

IMPAIRMENTS

- Hypomobile lumbar spine
- Decreased lumbar stability
- Weakness of abdominals and other core-stabilizing muscles
- Shortened hamstrings and hip flexors
- Postural changes
- Inability to walk, stand, or sit for prolonged time

TESTS AND MEASURES

- Algorithm for examination of the lumbar spine
- Passive physiologic intervertebral mobility (PPIVM) testing
- Lower extremity screening examination
- Postural examination
- Muscle length testing, including the hamstrings, hip flexors, and calf muscles
- Quadrant test
- Straight-leg raise test
- Slump test
- Lower limb nerve tension test
- Prone instability test
- Lower extremity neurologic screen (dermatome, myotome, reflexes)
- Repeated movement testing
- Fear-Avoidance Beliefs Questionnaire (FABQ)

INTERVENTION

- Joint manipulation indicated when
  - Duration of current episode of low back pain <16 days
  - No radicular symptoms/pain distal to the knee
  - FABQ score less than 19
  - Hip Internal Rotation of greater than 35 degrees for at least one hip
  - Segemental hypomobility of at least one level of the lumbar spine
- Specific exercise when pain centralizes upon repeated movement/ posture into flexion or extension
- Lumbar stabilization exercises to address core stability when
  - Positive prone instability test
  - Presence of aberrant motion
  - Straight leg raise >91 degrees
  - Age <41 years
- Traction when
  - Radiculopathy findings present
  - Positive crossed SLR
  - Pain becomes peripheralized with repeated extension
- Stretching exercises, myofascial mobilization for shortened musculature
- Unweighted treadmill walking
- Aquatic exercise
- Modalities for short-term pain control
- Cognitive behavioral therapy

TABLE 127-2 Red Flags for the Low Back Region

Condition	Red Flags
Back-related tumor	Age over 50 yr History of cancer Unexplained weight loss Failure of conservative therapy
Back-related infection (spinal osteomyelitis)	Recent infection (e.g., urinary tract or skin infection) Intravenous drug user/abuser Concurrent immunosuppressive disorder
Cauda equina syndrome	Urine retention or incontinence Fecal incontinence Saddle anesthesia Global or progressive weakness in the lower extremities Sensory deficits in the feet (i.e., L4, L5, and S1 areas)

Source: Data from DuVall RE, Godges J. Introduction to physical therapy differential diagnosis: the clinical utility of subjective examination. In: Wilmarth MA, ed. *Medical Screening for the Physical Therapist. Orthopaedic Section Independent Study Course 14.1.1.* La Crosse, WI: Orthopaedic Section, APTA, Inc., 2003:1–44.

FUNCTIONAL GOALS

- Patient will be able to
  - Sit with neutral lumbar spine posture for >30 minutes with 0/10 pain rating.
  - Sit at work station and perform computer work for 45 minutes with 0/10 pain rating.
  - Rotate lumbar spine 25 degrees so as to reach into the back seat of the car with 0/10 pain rating in lower extremity.
  - Walk for 30 minutes with 0/10 pain rating so as to go shopping.
  - Increase standing tolerance to >30 minutes without pain so as to fulfill recreational activity requirements.

PROGNOSIS

- Fair to very good, depending on specific impairments.
- Chronic low back pain prognosis significantly less.

PATIENT RESOURCE

- American Academy of Orthopeadic Surgeons. Back Pain. http://orthoinfo.aaos.org/topic.cfm?topic=A00311. Accessed July 5, 2013.

REFERENCES

1. The American Physical Therapy Association. Pattern 4F: Impaired joint mobility, motor function, muscle performance, range of motion, and reflex integrity associated with spinal disorders. *Interactive Guide to Physical Therapist Practice*. 2003. DOI: 10.2522/ptguide.3.1_6. Accessed July 5, 2013.
2. Dutton M. *Dutton's Orthopaedic Examination, Evaluation, and Intervention*. 3rd ed. New York, NY: McGraw-Hill; 2012. http://www.accessphysiotherapy.com/resource/612. Accessed July 5, 2013.

3. Malone TR, Hazle C, Grey ML. *Imaging in Rehabilitation*. New York, NY: McGraw-Hill; 2008. http://www.accessphysiotherapy.com/resource/613. Accessed July 5, 2013.
4. Dutton M. *Dutton's Orthopedic Survival Guide: Managing Common Conditions*. New York, NY: McGraw-Hill; 2011. http://www.accessphysiotherapy.com/resource/685. Accessed July 5, 2013.

ADDITIONAL REFERENCES

- ICD-9-CM. http://www.icd9data.com. Accessed July 5, 2013.
- ICD-10-CM. http://www.icd10data.com. Accessed July 5, 2013.
- Fritz JM, Cleland JA, Childs JD. Subgrouping patients with low back pain: evolution of a classification approach to physical therapy. *J Orthop Sports Phys Ther*. 2007;37(6):290–302.
- Liebenson, C. *Rehabilitation of the Spine*. Baltimore, MD: Lippincott, Williams & Wilkins; 2007.
- Olsen KA. *Manual Therapy of the Spine*. St. Louis, MI: Saunders Elsevier; 2009.

128 RADICULOPATHY, LUMBAR SPINE

Eric Shamus, PhD, DPT, PT, CSCS
Kathy Swanick, DPT, PT, OCS

CONDITION/DISORDER SYNONYMS

- Herniated intervertebral disc
- Prolapsed intervertebral disc
- Slipped disc
- Ruptured disc
- Herniated nucleus pulposus

ICD-9-CM CODES

- 722.73 Intervertebral disc disorder with myelopathy lumbar region
- 724.4 Thoracic or lumbosacral neuritis or radiculitis, unspecified

ICD-10-CM CODES

- M54.16 Radiculopathy, lumbar region
- M54.17 Radiculopathy, lumbosacral region

PREFERRED PRACTICE PATTERN

- 4E: Impaired Joint Mobility, Motor Function, Muscle Performance, and ROM Associated with Localized Inflammation[1]

PATIENT PRESENTATION

A 40-year-old woman, employed as a nurse practitioner, presents with low back pain, left sciatica, and the following history. During the last three of her four pregnancies, she experienced left sciatica that resolved with continued low back pain. This persistent discomfort did not keep her from activities until approximately 8 months ago when she had greater pain than usual, which required 9 days of bed rest until symptoms decreased. Several weeks ago she experienced another bout of spontaneous back pain, but could not take any time off and continued to work. Pain is aggravated by sitting in a soft chair, bending, or lifting/straining activities. Pain is relieved by lying in recumbent position, sitting in a firm/straight back chair, and when walking. After about a week, the back pain diminished; however, there was a sudden onset of severe pain radiating down the left buttock, ischial tuberosity to the posterior thigh, and leg as well as the lateral aspect of the left foot.

She believes the pain started when she bent forward to lift a heavy box. There is a feeling of numbness in the left lateral foot. Presently sitting tolerance is poor, even for short durations. Driving is difficult. Pain is increased with sneezing, coughing, walking, and bending. Pain is diminished when lying supine with the left leg bent and supported by a pillow, although pain in the left leg is persistent in any position. There is a lateral shift to the left in the direction of the sciatica, which is diminished when she lies down. There is a significant flattening of the lumbar spine. There is no evidence of swelling. There is mild lumbosacral tenderness, pain at the intervertebral foramen, and no palpable step deformity. The paraspinals feel tight and in spasm.

She is able to walk tip toe, but unable to maintain plantar flexion on the left due to weakness (3–/5). She is able to heel walk on the lateral boarder of her foot, but not medial. There is mild weakness of the hamstring and gluteal muscles on the left; extensor hallucis longus is normal. Patella reflexes are equal and normal bilaterally; left ankle reflex is diminished when compared with right. Distal medial and lateral hamstring reflexes are diminished on the left. Unsustained clonus of the left ankle is noted.

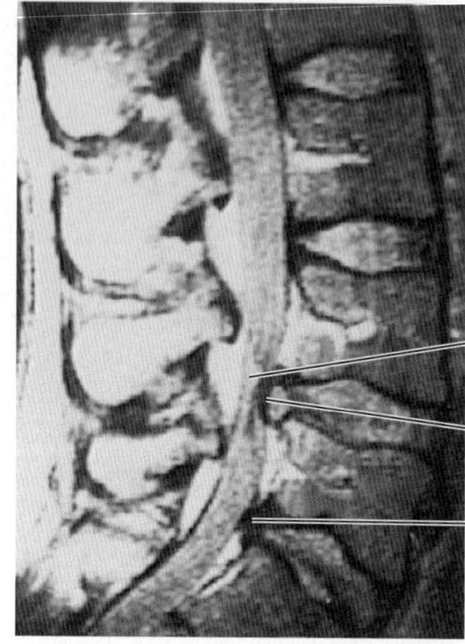

FIGURE 128-1 Magnetic resonance image (surface coil technique) of a sagittal section through the lower lumbar spine of a patient with low back pain. Note the herniation of the nucleus pulposus at L4–5 compressing the cauda equina. (From Waxman SG. *Clinical Neuroanatomy.* 26th ed. www.accessmedicine.com. Copyright © The McGraw-Hill Companies, Inc. All rights reserved.)

KEY FEATURES

Description

- Any disorder that affects the spinal nerve roots
- Lateral lumbar spine nerve-root compression
- Gradual or acute onset secondary to intervertebral disc or osteophyte formation in the intervertebral foramen[2]

Essentials of Diagnosis

- Diagnosis made by clinical examination
- Dermatome/myotome pattern
- Reproduction of symptoms

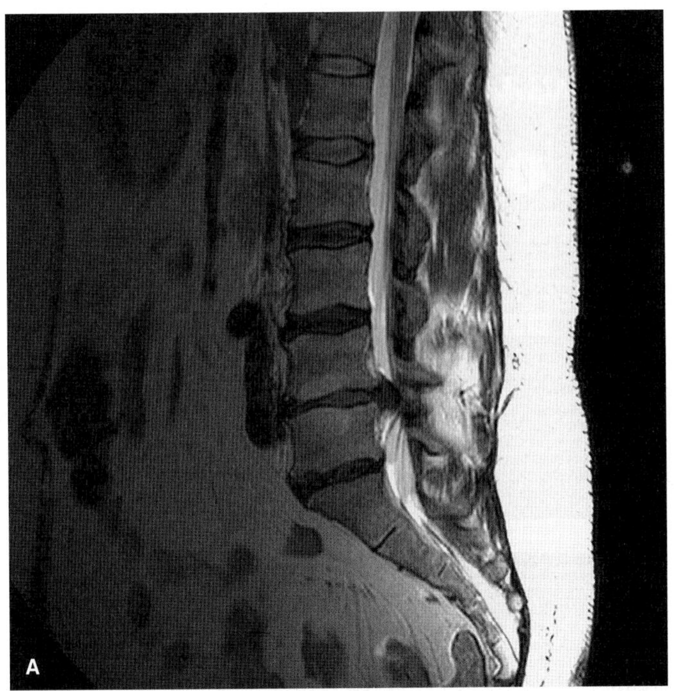

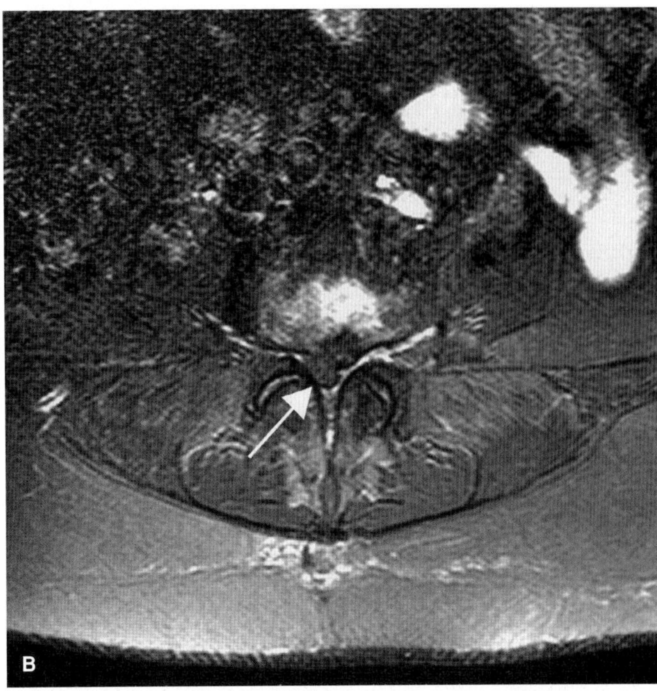

FIGURE 128-2 Lumbar radiculopathy. **A.** Sagittal T2-weighted image of the lumbar spine shows severe L4–L5 disc herniation with effacement of the thecal sac. **B.** Axial fat suppressed T2-weighted image at the L4–L5 level shows the disc herniation (*arrow*) obliterating the right lateral recess, impinging upon the right L5 nerve root. (From Tintinalli JE, J. Stephan Stapczynski, O. John Ma, et al. *Tintinalli's Emergency Medicine: A Comprehensive Study Guide.* 7th ed. www.accessmedicine.com.)

General Considerations

- Herniated disc is one cause of radiculopathy.
- Avoid positions that increase symptoms.

Demographics

- Women at greater risk than men
- Onset typically middle-aged to geriatric

CLINICAL FINDINGS

SIGNS AND SYMPTOMS

- Pain in the lumbar, hip, buttock, leg, and lower extremity; paresthesia often radiating into the foot[2]
- Pain in the lumbar spine worsens with extension, side bending, rotation to the involved side[2]
- Diminished sensation, motor control, and reflexes in the distribution of involved nerve[2]

Functional Implications

- Difficulty maintaining sitting postures secondary to back and leg pain
- Inability to sleep
- Weakness with lifting, prolonged standing
- Loss of movement or feeling in the lower extremity
- Loss of bowel and bladder control
- Difficulty with movements (driving, twisting) secondary to pain
- Prolonged walking may increase weakness (patients need to be cautious with their biomechanics: at heel strike the position may mimic a straight leg raise (SLR) that may cause increased nerve irritation

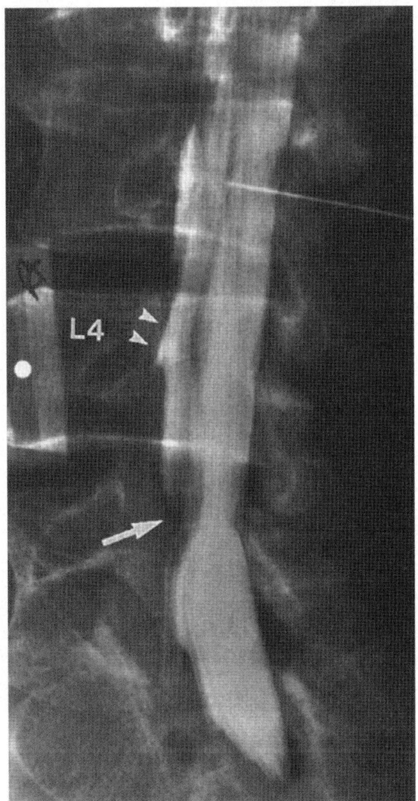

FIGURE 128-3 A 58-year-old man with right-sided L5 radiculopathy. A myelogram was performed, and an oblique view demonstrating the right-sided nerve roots is displayed. (From Chen MYM, Pope TL, Ott DL. *Basic Radiology.* 2nd ed. www.accessmedicine.com.)

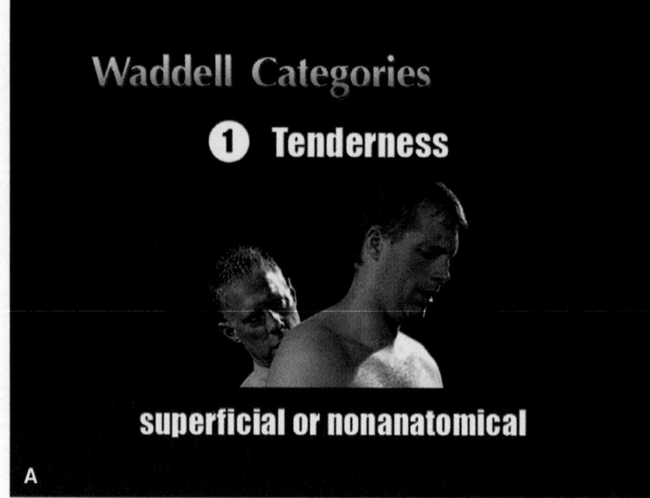

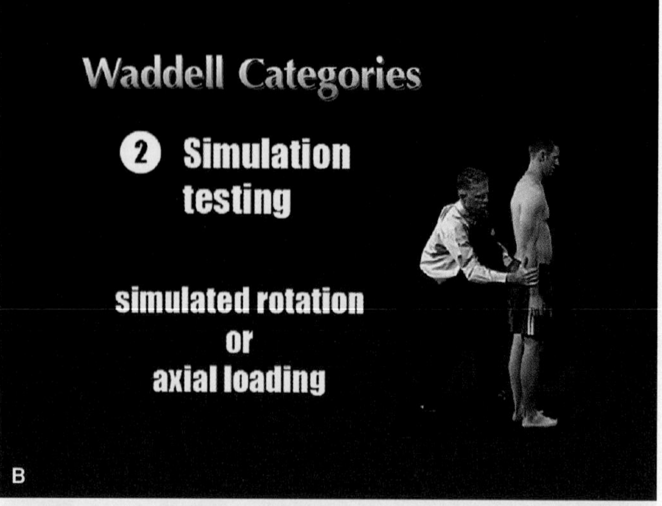

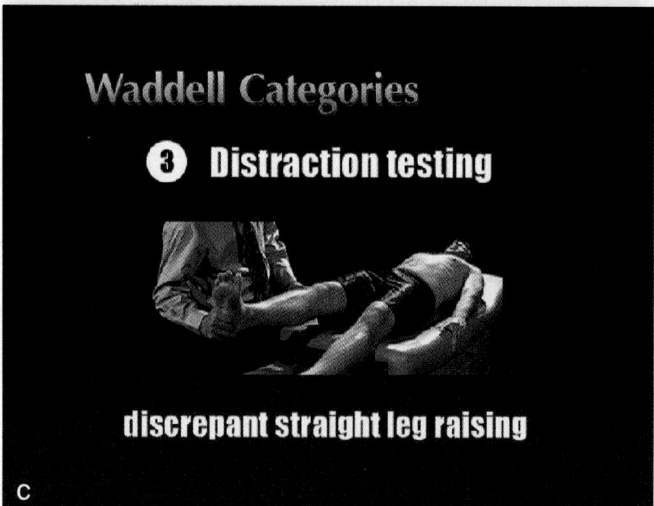

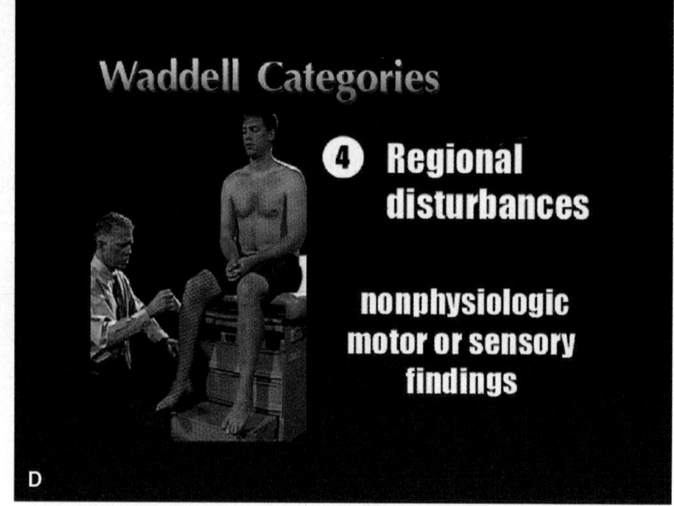

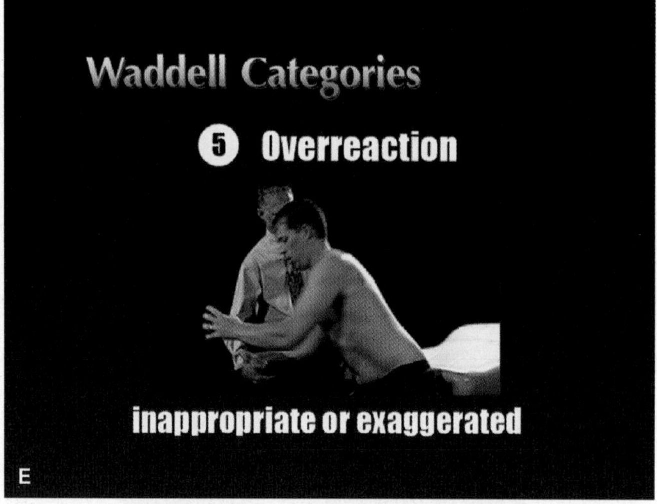

FIGURE 128-4 **A–E.** Waddell categories (From Lawry GV. *Systematic Musculoskeletal Examinations*. www.accessmedicine.com. Copyright © The McGraw-Hill Companies, Inc. All rights reserved.)

Possible Contributing Causes

- Decreased lumbar lordosis posture due to tight hamstrings, weak abdominal muscles
- Prolonged side-bending position toward impaired nerve or prolonged flexion
- Facet hypertrophy
- Size of the spinal canal, may be congenital

Differential Diagnosis

- Degenerative disc disease
- Hip pathology with radiating pain pattern
- Lyme disease
- Paraspinal spasms
- Peripheral nerve impairment
- Peripheral neuropathy
- Piriformis syndrome
- Sacral or pelvic dysfunction
- Sciatica
- Spinal tumor
- Spinal stenosis

MEANS OF CONFIRMATION OR DIAGNOSIS

Imaging

- MRI helps visualize compressed or inflamed nerve root in diagnosis.[3]
- X-ray/Plain-film radiograph helpful if osteophyte located in the intervertebral foramen.[4]
- CT to show herniation compressing the spinal canal or nerves.[4]
- Electrodiagnostic/nerve conduction testing can help determine specific impaired nerve function.[2, 5]

FINDINGS AND INTERPRETATION

Physical examination to rule in lumbar radiculopathy

TREATMENT

- Surgery
  - Fusion
  - Decompression
  - Laminectomy
  - Laser discectomy
  - Microdiscectomy
  - Percutaneous discectomy
  - Discectomy
  - Hemilaminectomy

REFERRALS/ADMITTANCE

- To hospital for imaging
- To physician for surgical consult if myelopathy suspected[3]
- To physician for imaging and medical consult if disease suspected
- To physician for corticosteroid injection if condition does not improve
- To physician for anti-inflammatory medication

IMPAIRMENTS

- Restricted mobility of the upper lumbar and lower thoracic spine
- Hypermobile lower lumbar (L5) spine

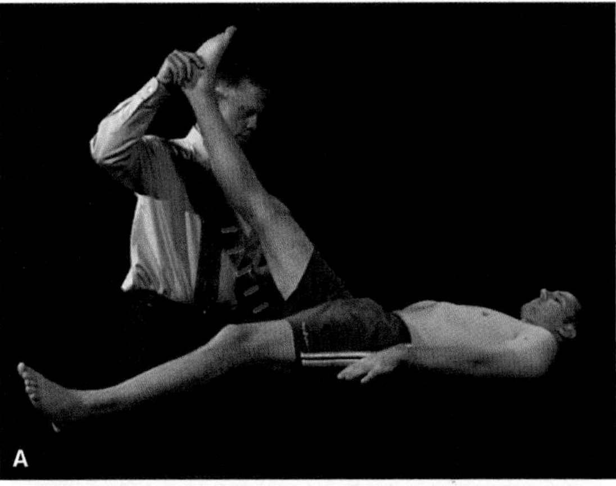

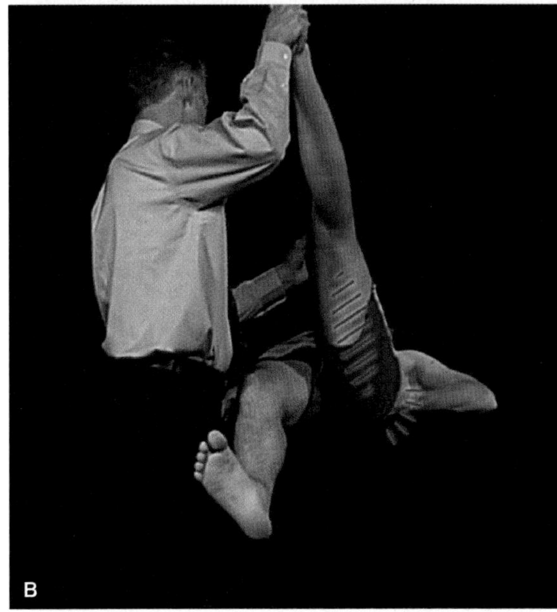

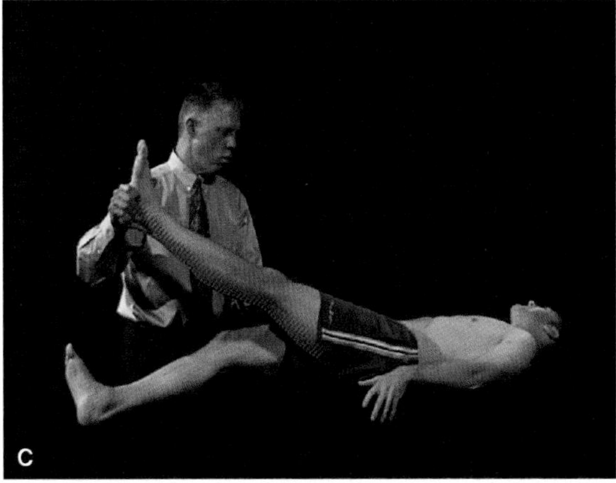

FIGURE 128-5 A–C. Straight leg raise test differential zones (From Lawry GV. *Systematic Musculoskeletal Examinations.* www.accessmedicine.com. Copyright © The McGraw-Hill Companies, Inc. All rights reserved.)

TABLE 128-1 Common Radicular Syndromes of the Lumbar Spine

Disc Level	Nerve Root	Motor Deficit	Sensory Deficit	Reflex Compromise
L3–L4	L4	Quadriceps (knee extension)	Anterolateral thigh Anterior knee Medial leg and foot	Patellar
L4–L5	L5	Extensor hallucis longus (great toe extension)	Lateral thigh Anterolateral leg Mid-dorsal foot	Medial hamstrings
L5–S1	S1	Gastrocnemius Soleus Flexor digitorum longus Tibialis posterior (ankle plantar flexion)	Posterior leg Lateral foot	Achilles

Source: From Patel DR, Greydanus DE, Baker RJ. *Pediatric Practice: Sports Medicine.* http://www.accesspediatrics.com. Copyright © The McGraw-Hill Companies, Inc. All rights reserved.

- Tight hamstring limiting stride-length during gait
- Noted weakness of abdominals and core stability

TESTS AND MEASURES

- Algorithm for examination of the lumbar spine
- FABER test[2]
- Fear-Avoidance Beliefs Questionnaire (FABQ)
- Lower extremity neurologic screen (dermatome, myotome, reflexes)
- Lower extremity screening examination
- Lower limb nerve tension test[3]
- Muscle length testing, including the hamstrings, hip flexors, and calf muscles
- Passive physiologic intervertebral mobility (PPIVM) testing[2]
- Patella, Achilles, hamstring reflexes[2]
- Postural examination
- Prone instability test
- Quadrant test[2]
- Radicular pattern[6]
- Repeated movement testing
- Slump test[3]
- SLR test[3]

INTERVENTION

- Rest
- Joint manipulation to the thoracic and lumbar spine in the absence of red flags
- Lower-extremity distraction and traction to relieve nerve compression
- Address pain
  - Electrical stimulation
  - Ice
- Address hypertonicity
  - Soft-tissue massage
  - Heat
- Address muscle weakness
  - Core stability exercises

FUNCTIONAL GOALS

- Patient will be able to:
  - Sit with neutral lumbar spine posture for >30 minutes with 0/10 pain rating.
  - Sit at work station and perform computer work for 45 minutes with 0/10 pain rating.
  - Rotate lumbar spine 25 degrees so as to reach into the back seat in the car with 0/10 pain rating in the lower extremity.

PROGNOSIS

Fair to very good, depending on severity of nerve-root compression and lumbar impairments.

PATIENT RESOURCE

- Lumbar Radiculopathy. http://www.aanem.org/Education/Patient-Resources/Disorders/Lumbar-Radiculopathy.aspx. Accessed July 5, 2013.

TABLE 128-2 Intradiscal Pressures and Forces Generated by Common Tasks

Task	Total Load (kg)[a]
Lying supine	25
Side lying	75
Standing	150
Bending at waist in standing position	200
Sitting	175
Bending at waist in sitting position	225

[a] Represents total load on the third lumbar disc in a 70-kg subject.
Source: Data from Nachemson A. Disc pressure measurements. *Spine.* 1981;6:93–97; Nachemson A, Morris JM. In vivo measurements of intradiscal pressure. *J Bone Joint Surg.* 1964;46:1077; Nachemson A. Lumbar intradiscal pressure. In: Jayson MIV, ed. *The Lumbar Spine and Back Pain.* Edinburgh: Churchill Livingstone; 1987:191–203.

REFERENCES

1. The American Physical Therapy Association. Pattern 4E: Impaired joint mobility, motor function, muscle performance, and range of motion associated with localized inflammation. *Interactive Guide to Physical Therapist Practice*. 2003. DOI: 10.2522/ptguide.3.1_5. Accessed July 5, 2013.
2. Dutton M. *Dutton's Orthopedic Survival Guide: Managing Common Conditions*. New York, NY: McGraw-Hill; 2011. http://www.accessphysiotherapy.com/resource/685. Accessed July 5, 2013.
3. Dutton M. *Dutton's Orthopaedic Examination, Evaluation, and Intervention*. 3rd ed. New York, NY: McGraw-Hill; 2012. http://www.accessphysiotherapy.com/resource/612. Accessed July 5, 2013.
4. Malone TR, Hazle C, Grey ML. *Imaging in Rehabilitation*. New York, NY: McGraw-Hill; 2008. http://www.accessphysiotherapy.com/resource/613. July 5, 2013.
5. Halle J, Greathouse D. Chapter 8. Principles of electrophysiologic evaluation and testing. In: Prentice WE, Quillen WS, Underwood F, eds. *Therapeutic Modalities in Rehabilitation*. 4th ed. New York, NY: McGraw-Hill; 2011. http://www.accessphysiotherapy.com/abstract/8137670. Accessed July 5, 2013.
6. Patel DR, Rowe D. Chapter 30. Thoracolumbar spine injuries. In: Patel DR, Greydanus DE, Baker RJ, eds. *Pediatric Practice: Sports Medicine*. New York, NY: McGraw-Hill; 2009. http://www.accessphysiotherapy.com/abstract/6981360. Accessed July 5, 2013.

ADDITIONAL REFERENCES

- ICD9DATA web site. http://www.icd9data.com. Accessed July 5, 2013.
- ICD10DATA web site. http://www.icd10data.com. Accessed July 5, 2013.
- Prentice WE, Quillen WS, Underwood F. Chapter 8. Principles of electrophysiologic evaluation and testing. In: Prentice WE, Quillen WS, Underwood F, eds. *Therapeutic Modalities in Rehabilitation*. 4th ed. New York, NY: McGraw-Hill; 2011. http://www.accessphysiotherapy.com/content/8137409. Accessed July 5, 2013.
- Wainner RS, Fritz JM, Irrgang JJ, et al. Reliability and diagnostic accuracy of the clinical examination and patient self-report measures for cervical radiculopathy. *Spine*. 2003;28(1):52–62.

129 SPINAL STENOSIS, LUMBAR

Arie J. Van Duijn, EdD, MSc, PT, OCS
Eric Shamus, PhD, DPT, PT, CSCS

CONDITION/DISORDER SYNONYMS

- Lumbar spinal stenosis (LSS)
- Lumbar central stenosis
- Lumbar lateral stenosis

ICD-9-CM CODES

- 724.02 Spinal stenosis, lumbar region, without neurogenic claudication
- 724.03 Spinal stenosis, lumbar region, with neurogenic claudication

ICD-10-CM CODES

- M48.06 Spinal stenosis, lumbar region
- M48.08 Spinal stenosis, sacral and sacrococcygeal region

PREFERRED PRACTICE PATTERN

- 4F: Impaired Joint Mobility, Motor Function, Muscle Performance, Range of Motion, and Reflex Integrity Associated with Spinal Disorders[1]

PATIENT PRESENTATION

A 64-year-old retired elementary school teacher presents with complaints of intermittent low back pain. She works with the elementary school-aged children, and she would often find herself in a posture of leaning forward to help the students with their work. She spends most of her day in a standing position.

Her pain is in the low back and buttock region and occurs primarily in the standing position. She has noticed that the pain occurs quicker now, and she is not able to stand as long as you used to. If she leans forward over a chair or a shopping cart, the pain is often relieved, but resumes after resuming normal work activities. She used to walk daily with her spouse; however, approximately 10 months ago she started experiencing buttock and calf pain bilaterally during prolonged walking. She is disappointed that she cannot exercise. When walking initially there is no pain, but after about 10 blocks she has low back pain, which gradually intensifies and migrates into both buttocks and thigh, but does not usually radiate into the foot. The pain forces her to sit down at any seat that is available, and she has avoided long shopping trips. Sometimes elevating one leg on a curb can help alleviate the symptoms enough to get back home; however, the pain cycle repeats. There is a flattened lumbar spine and is postured in –5° of hip extension. There is no region of point tenderness over the lumbar spine; there is no palpable gap over the spinous processes. Both feet feel warm. She is able to bend over and reach approximately 6[2] from the floor. Lateral flexion is 20° in each direction. Maintaining lumbar extension for more than 25 seconds replicates her lower extremity symptoms. ROM of the hip joints are WNL and painless. Generalized hypomobility of all lumbar segments in all directions of movement. Significant loss of movement at L5–S1 and L4–L5. Relative normal strength for age with decreased hamstring and gastroc/soleus flexibility bilaterally.

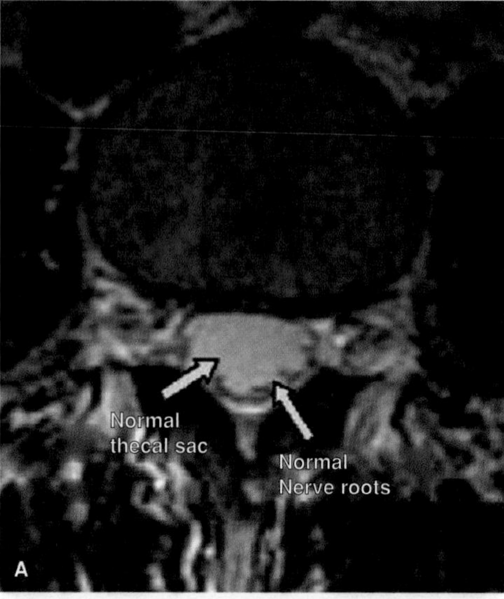

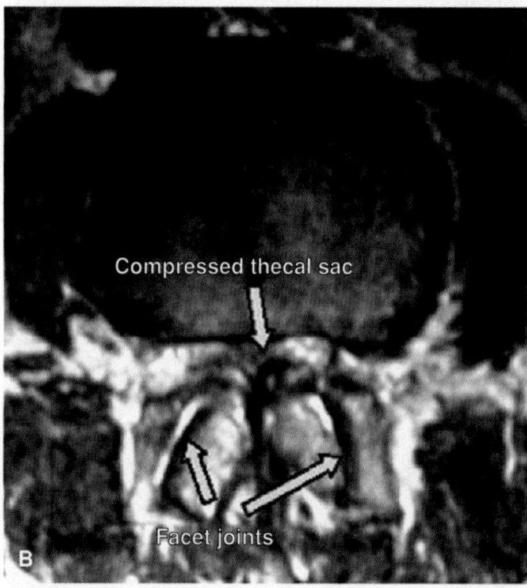

FIGURE 129-1 Axial T2-weighted images of the lumbar spine. (**A**) A normal thecal sac within the lumbar spinal canal. The thecal sac is bright. The lumbar roots are dark punctuate dots in the posterior thecal sac with the patient supine. (**B**) The thecal sac is not well visualized due to severe lumbar spinal canal stenosis, partially the result of hypertrophic facet joints. (From Longo DL, Fauci A, Kasper D, et al., eds. *Harrison's Principles of Internal Medicine.* 18th ed. New York, NY: McGraw-Hill; 2012.)

KEY FEATURES

Description

- Common, degenerative spinal condition
- Associated with narrowing of the spinal canal (central stenosis) or foraminal canals (lateral stenosis)

- Caused by degenerative changes to intervertebral discs and facet joints
- Can result in spinal cord compression, cauda equina compression, or nerve-root compression

Essentials of Diagnosis

- Can result in neurogenic claudication, with pain, cramping, paresthesias in the lower limbs aggravated by walking and relieved by sitting or flexion
- Diagnosis made by clinical examination
- Differentiation between vascular and neurologic claudication
- Reproduction of symptoms in specific postures and activities

General Considerations

- Lumbar spinal stenosis can result in spinal cord compression, loss of bowel and bladder control
- Cervical central stenosis can cause bilateral symptoms in lower extremity

Demographics

- Prevalence increases with age
- Primarily occurs in people aged 65 years or older

CLINICAL FINDINGS

SIGNS AND SYMPTOMS

- Unilateral or bilateral leg pain with lumbar stenosis
- Pain worsens with walking, relieved by sitting
- May be with or without low back pain or neck pain
- Altered sensation, motor control, reflexes in the distribution of involved nerve roots
- Loss of bladder and bowel control
- Neurogenic claudication

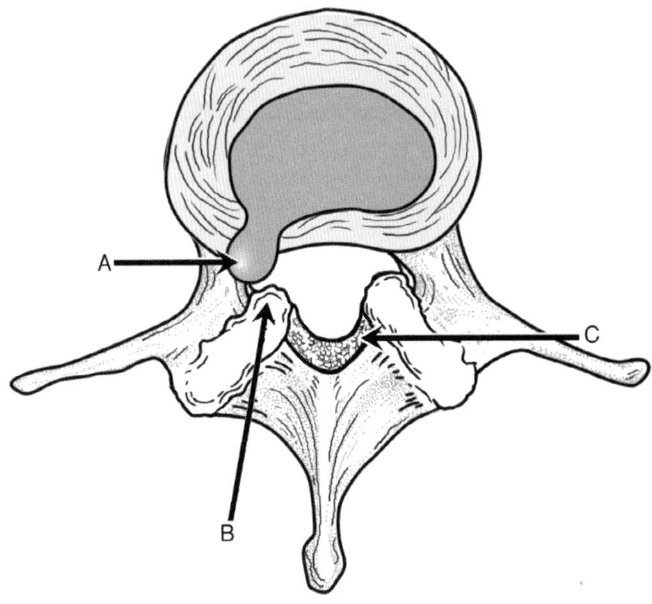

FIGURE 129-2 Spinal stenosis secondary to a combination of disc herniation (**A**), facet joint hypertrophy (**B**), and hypertrophy of the ligamentum flavum (**C**). (From Imboden J, Hellmann DB, Stone JH. *Current Rheumatology Diagnosis & Treatment.* 2nd ed. www.accessmedicine.com. Copyright © The McGraw-Hill Companies, Inc. All rights reserved.)

Functional Implications

- Difficulty walking longer distances
- Difficulty with standing activities
- Possible bowel or bladder dysfunction

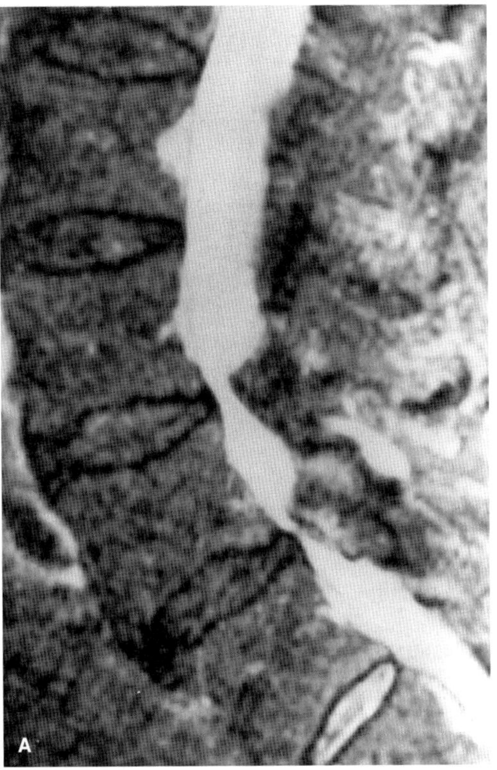

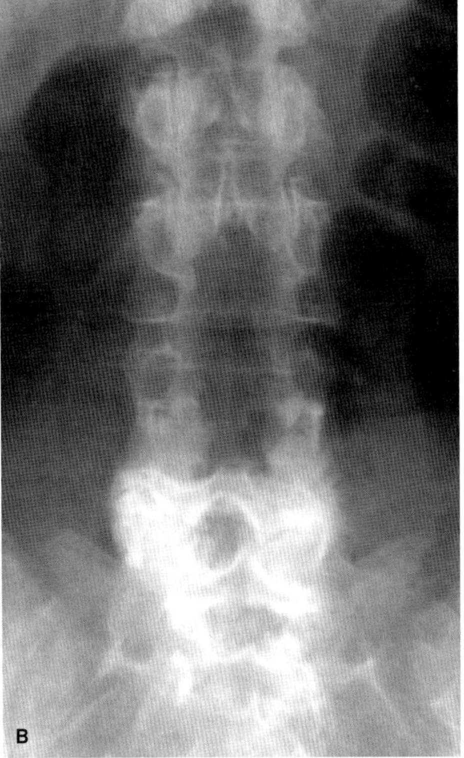

FIGURE 129-3 Imaging studies in a patient with stenosis of the lumbar spine and leg pain. (**A**) MRI showing stenosis at L3–L4. (**B**) Radiograph taken after two-level laminectomy, which led to resolution of the preoperative leg pain. (From Skinner HB. *Current Diagnosis & Treatment in Orthopedics.* 4th ed. www.accessmedicine.com. Copyright © The McGraw-Hill Companies, Inc. All rights reserved.)

Possible Contributing Causes

- Postural changes
- Weakness of the core musculature
- Tightness of the hip flexors, external rotators, and hamstrings
- Osteoporosis
- Spinal disc herniation
- Achondroplasia/Psuedoachondroplasia

Differential Diagnosis

- Degenerative disc disease
- Hip pathology with radiating pain pattern
- Osteoarthritis
- Peripheral nerve impairment
- Peripheral neuropathy
- Spinal tumor
- Vascular insufficiency/claudication

MEANS OF CONFIRMATION OR DIAGNOSIS

Imaging

- MRI[2]
- X-ray/Plain-film radiograph[3]
- CT scan[3]
- Electrodiagnostic/nerve conduction testing[4]
- Doppler ultrasound

FINDINGS AND INTERPRETATION

- MRI helpful in diagnosis to visualize compressed or inflamed nerve root[2]
- X-ray/Plain-film radiograph helpful if osteophyte located in intervertebral foramen[3]
- CT scan to show herniation compressing the spinal canal/nerves[3]
- Electrodiagnostic/nerve conduction testing can assist to determine a specific impaired nerve function[4]
- Doppler ultrasound to examine vascular function

TREATMENT

- Surgery
  - Fusion[2]
  - Decompression[2]
  - Laminectomy[2]

REFERRALS/ADMITTANCE

- To hospital for imaging
- To physician for surgical consult if myelopathy suspected
- To physician for imaging and medical consult if disease suspected
- To physician for if vascular insufficiency suspected

IMPAIRMENTS

- Hypomobile lumbar spine
- Noted weakness of abdominals and core-stabilizing muscles
- Shortening of hamstrings, hip flexors
- Inability to walk for prolonged time
- Inability to stand for prolonged time

TESTS AND MEASURES

- Algorithm for examination of the lumbar spine[4]
- Ankle-Brachial Pressure Index (ABPI) to screen for peripheral artery disease
- Crossed straight leg raise test
- Fear-Avoidance Beliefs Questionnaire (FABQ)
- Lower extremity neurologic screen (dermatome, myotome, reflexes)
- Lower limb nerve tension test[2]
- Muscle length testing, including the hamstrings, hip flexors, and calf muscles
- Passive physiologic intervertebral mobility (PPIVM) testing[4]
- Postural examination
- Prone instability test
- Quadrant test[4]
- Repeated movement testing
- Slump test[2]
- Straight leg raise test[2]
- Two-stage treadmill test

INTERVENTION

- Joint manipulation to the thoracic and lumbar spine when joint hypomobility is present
- Specific exercises in flexion when pain centralizes upon repeated movement/posture into flexion
- Lumbar stabilization exercises to address core stability
- Stretching exercises and myofascial mobilization for shortened musculature
- Unweighted treadmill walking
- Aquatic exercise
- Mechanical traction in flexion position

FUNCTIONAL GOALS

- Patient will be able to
  - Walk for 30 minutes with 0/10 pain rating to reach a grocery store or walk in a mall.
  - Increase standing tolerance to >30 minutes without pain so as to fulfill requirements for recreational and employment activity.

PROGNOSIS

- Variable: Multimodal, conservative management including progressive exercise, unweighted walking, and manual therapy have shown positive outcomes.
- Severe cases of stenosis may require surgical intervention.

PATIENT RESOURCES

- American Association of Neurological Surgeons. Lumbar Spinal Stenosis. http://www.aans.org/Patient%20Information/Conditions%20and%20Treatments/Lumbar%20Spinal%20Stenosis.aspx. Accessed July 7, 2013.
- NIH, National Institute of Arthritis and Musculoskeletal and Skin Diseases. Spinal Stenosis. http://www.niams.nih.gov/health_info/Spinal_Stenosis/default.asp. Accessed July 7, 2013.

REFERENCES

1. The American Physical Therapy Association. Pattern 4F: Impaired joint mobility, motor function, muscle performance, range of motion, and reflex integrity associated with spinal disorders. *Interactive Guide to Physical Therapist Practice*. 2003. DOI: 10.2522/ptguide.3.1_6. Accessed July 7, 2013.
2. Dutton M. *Orthopaedic Examination, Evaluation, and Intervention*. New York, NY: McGraw-Hill; 2008. http://www.accessphysiotherapy.com/resource/612. Accessed July 7, 2013.
3. Malone TR, Hazle C, Grey ML. *Imaging in Rehabilitation*. New York, NY: McGraw-Hill; 2008. http://www.accessphysiotherapy.com/resource/613. Accessed July 7, 2013.
4. Dutton M. *Dutton's Orthopedic Survival Guide: Managing Common Conditions*. New York, NY: McGraw-Hill; 2011. http://www.accessphysiotherapy.com/resource/685. Accessed July 7, 2013.

ADDITIONAL REFERENCES

- Fritz JM, Cleland JA, Childs JD. Subgrouping patients with low back pain: Evolution of a classification approach to physical therapy. *J Orthop Sports Phys Ther*. 2007;37(6):290–302.
- ICD9DATA web site. http://www.icd9data.com. Accessed July 7, 2013.
- ICD10DATA web site. http://www.icd10data.com. Accessed July 7, 2013.
- Liebenson C. *Rehabilitation of the Spine*. Baltimore, MD: Lippincott, Williams & Wilkins; 2007.
- Olsen KA. *Manual Therapy of the Spine*. St. Louis, MI: Saunders Elsevier; 2009.

130 SPONDYLOLISTHESIS, LUMBAR

Eric Shamus, PhD, DPT, PT, CSCS

CONDITION/DISORDER SYNONYMS

- Congenital spondylolisthesis
- Degenerative spondylolisthesis
- Isthmic spondylolisthesis
- Pathologic spondylolisthesis
- Spondylolisthesis acquisita
- Traumatic spondylolisthesis

ICD-9-CM CODES

- 738.4 Acquired spondylolisthesis
- 756.12 Spondylolisthesis congenital

ICD-10-CM CODES

- M43.10 Spondylolisthesis, site unspecified
- Q76.2 Congenital spondylolisthesis

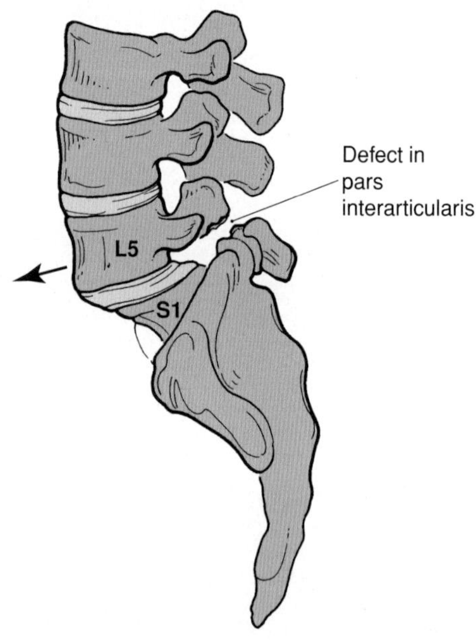

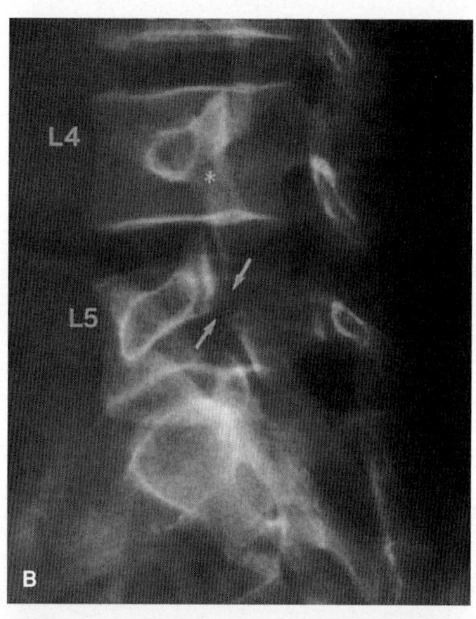

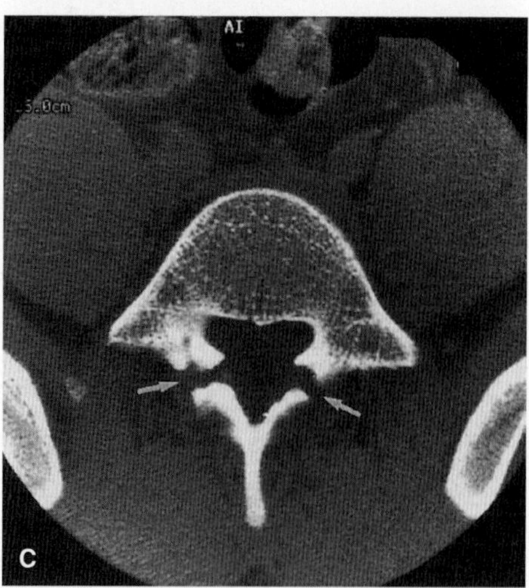

FIGURE 130-1 (**A**) Diagram of spondylolisthesis of L5 over S1 caused by spondylolysis of L5. (**B**) Oblique plain film of the lumbar spine demonstrates a spondylolysis or pars defect on the right side at L5 (arrows). Note the intact pars at L4 (*). (**C**) CT bone window of a different patient shows spondylolysis defects (arrows). Although these resemble facet joints, they are more horizontal in orientation and more irregular, lacking a smooth cortical margin. (From Chen MYM, Pope TL, Ott DL. *Basic Radiology*. 2nd ed. www.accessmedicine.com. Copyright © The McGraw-Hill Companies, Inc. All rights reserved.)

PREFERRED PRACTICE PATTERN

- 4E: Impaired Joint Mobility, Motor Function, Muscle Performance, and ROM Associated with Localized Inflammation[1]

PATIENT PRESENTATION

A 49-year-old man employed as a high school gym teacher and coach reports a long 15+ year history of generalized lumbosacral ache, which has been getting steadily worse over the past year. Lately, this has interfered with his job since the jarring motions associated with sports increase his symptoms. He recalls falling from a 12-foot wall and landing on his buttocks when he was a teenager and also recalls several sporting injuries. He recalls returning to normal activity within 6 weeks of the fall.

Up until his early 30s, he did not experience any significant back pain; however, after age 35 years, there was a steady increase in periodic low back pain. Presently, he has pain every day, which starts as a stiff ache every morning. Getting out of bed is difficult, and he must log roll to his side to get up from supine. After a hot shower and some simple exercises, he is able to move better. Coughing and jarring movements are painful. Walking is relatively pain free on level surfaces, but painful on hills and stairs. Sitting and lying relieve pain. Getting in and out of the car is difficult and many work postures, especially bending forward aggravate the pain and you must often support yourself by leaning on an arm. The pain has not radiated into the lower extremity and is confined to the low back and buttocks. There is tenderness at L4 and L5 spinous processes, with palpable step.

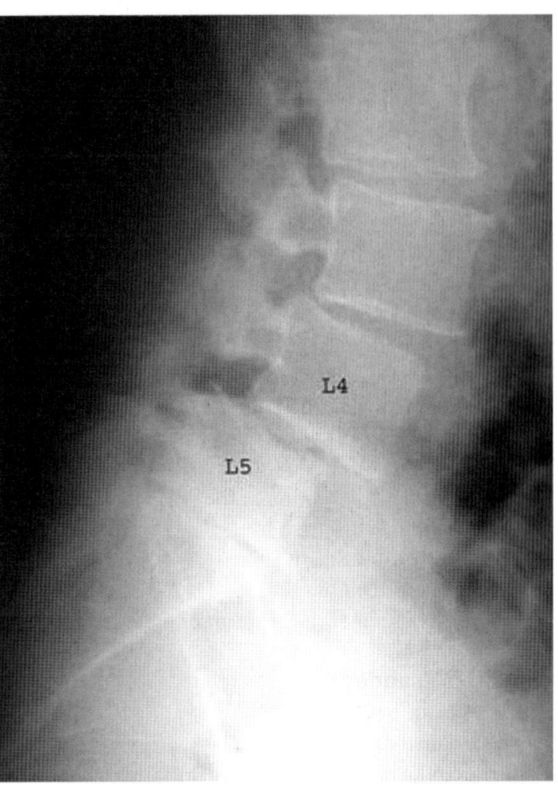

FIGURE 130-2 Lateral lumbar spine X-ray demonstrates a 25% anterior slippage of L4 on L5 due to a defect in the L4 pars interarticularis. This is called spondylolisthesis. (From Brunicardi FC, Andersen D, Billiar T, et al. *Schwartz's Principles of Surgery*. 9th ed. http://www.accessmedicine.com. Copyright © The McGraw-Hill Companies, Inc. All rights reserved.)

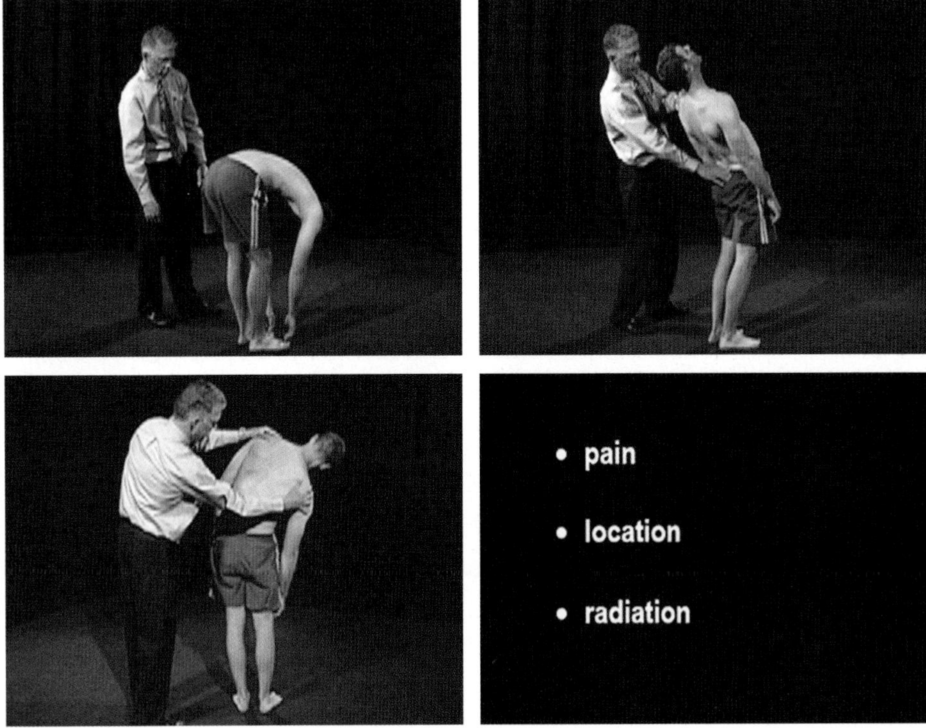

FIGURE 130-3 Repeated motion testing for directional preference. (From Lawry GV. *Systematic Musculoskeletal Examinations*. www.accessmedicine.com. Copyright © The McGraw-Hill Companies, Inc. All rights reserved.)

KEY FEATURES

Description

- Anterior (forward) translation of a vertebra
- Fracture of the pedicles on the vertebra below
- Slipping of the vertebra in relationship to the vertebra below
- Neurogenic claudication
- Fracture widens at the pars
- Congenital (Dysplastic) spondylolisthesis
  - Dysplasia of the L5 vertebra and sacral arches, malformation of the lumbosacral junction with incompetent facet joints
- Isthmic spondylolisthesis
  - Acute fracture, stress fracture, elongation of the pars
- Degenerative spondylolisthesis
  - Wear and tear to the L4–L5 vertebrae
- Traumatic spondylolisthesis
  - Fracture or acute dislocation of the zygapophyseal joint
- Pathologic spondylolisthesis
  - Systemic disease causing weakness
- Spondylolisthesis acquisita
  - Surgical disruption of the ligament or bone

Essentials of Diagnosis

- Diagnosis made by X-ray
- Can be acquired or congenital
- Clinical examination may find step deformity
- Dermatome/myotome pattern
- Meyerding classification of spondylolisthesis[2]
  - Grade 1: less than 25% slippage
  - Grade 2: 26% to 50% slippage
  - Grade 3: 51% to 75% slippage
  - Grade 4: 76% to 99% slippage
- Low-grade isthmic spondylolisthesis: Less than 50% displacement
- High-grade isthmic spondylolisthesis: Greater than 50% displacement
- Spondylolysis: Fracture without displacement
- Hangman's fracture
  - C2 vertebra anteriorly translated on C3 with a fracture of C2 pedicles

General Considerations

- Instability
- Herniated disc a cause of radiculopathy
- Avoid extension positions that increase symptoms
- Wiltse–Newman classification of spondylolisthesis[2]

Demographics

- Can be congenital or acquired

CLINICAL FINDINGS

SIGNS AND SYMPTOMS

- Pain in the lumbar, hip, buttock, leg, and lower extremity; parasthesia often radiating into the foot
- Stiffness along spine
- Pain in the lumbar spine worsens with extension
- Altered sensation, motor control, reflexes in the distribution of involved nerve roots
- Neurogenic claudication

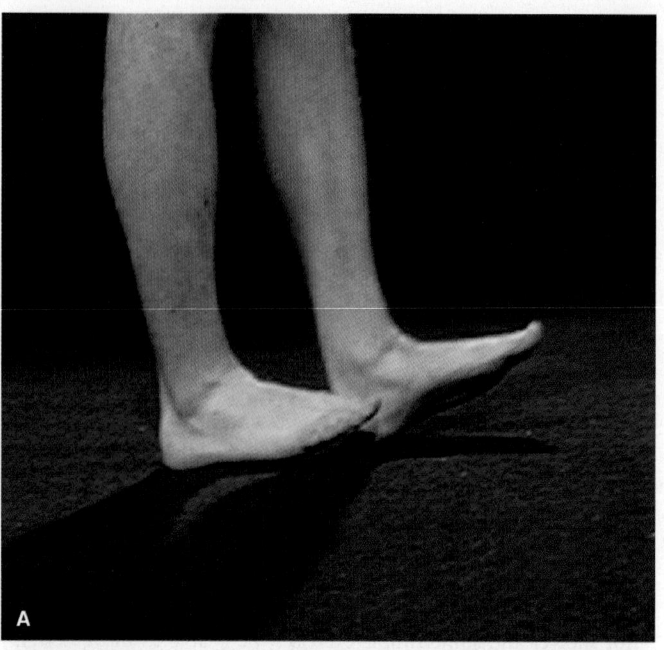

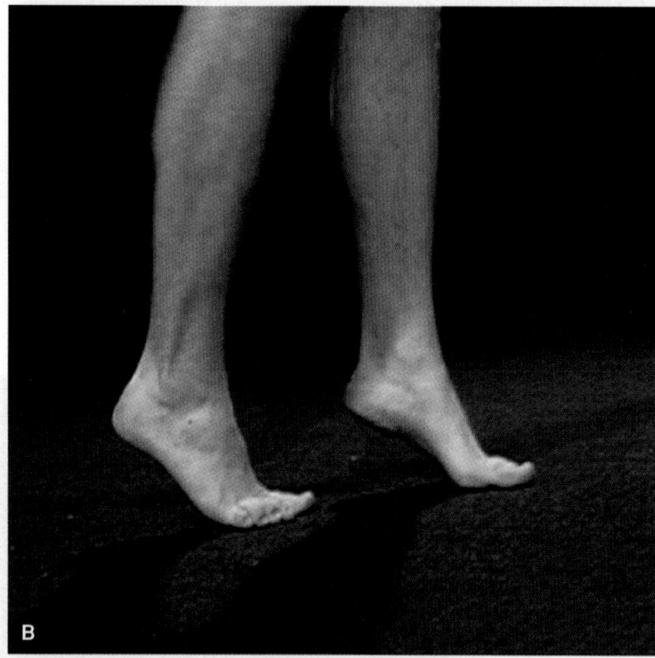

FIGURE 130-4 (**A**) Heel walking. (**B**) Toe walking. (From Lawry GV. *Systematic Musculoskeletal Examinations*. www.accessmedicine.com. Copyright © The McGraw-Hill Companies, Inc. All rights reserved.)

Functional Implications

- Difficulty maintaining standing postures secondary to back and leg pain
- Inability to sleep on the back
- Weakness with lifting, prolonged standing
- Loss of movement or feeling in lower extremity
- Loss of bowel and bladder control if severe
- Difficulty with movements (as with driving, twisting) secondary to pain
- Limit sports participation

Possible Contributing Causes

- Increased lumbar lordosis posture due to tight hip flexors, weak abdominal muscles
- Congenital
- Car accident, hit from rear

Differential Diagnosis

- Degenerative disc disease
- Hip pathology with radiating pain pattern
- Infection
- Paraspinal spasms
- Peripheral nerve impairment
- Peripheral neuropathy
- Piriformis syndrome
- Sacral or pelvic dysfunction
- Sciatica
- Spinal tumor

MEANS OF CONFIRMATION OR DIAGNOSIS

Imaging

- MRI[3]
- X-ray/Plain-film radiograph[2]
- CT[4]
- Electrodiagnostic/nerve conduction testing[5]

FINDINGS AND INTERPRETATION

- MRI helps visualize compressed or inflamed nerve root in diagnosis.[3]
- X-ray/Plain-film radiograph to see vertebra position (Scottie dog collar).[2]
- CT to show herniation compressing the spinal canal/nerves.[4]
- Electrodiagnostic/nerve conduction testing can help determine specific impaired nerve function.[5]
- Meyerding classification of spondylolisthesis, see Figure 130-7

REFERRALS/ADMITTANCE

- To hospital for imaging
- To physician for surgical consult if myelopathy suspected[3]
  - Fusion
  - Decompression
  - Laminectomy
  - Hemilaminectomy
- To physician for imaging and medical consult if disease suspected
- To physician for corticosteroid injection if condition does not improve
- To pharmacy for anti-inflammatory medication

IMPAIRMENTS

- Restricted mobility of the upper-lumbar and lower-thoracic spine
- Hypermobility of the L5 vertebra on the sacrum
- Tight hip flexors limiting stride length during gait
- Noted weakness of abdominals and core stability

TESTS AND MEASURES

- Algorithm for examination of the lumbar spine[5]
- FABER test[5]
- Fear-Avoidance Beliefs Questionnaire (FABQ)

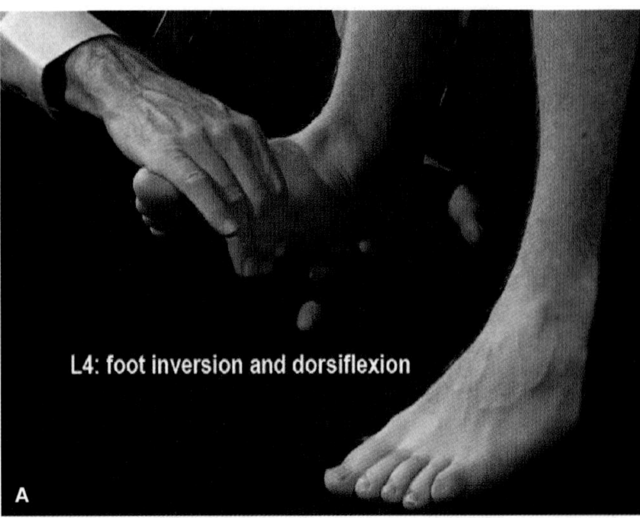

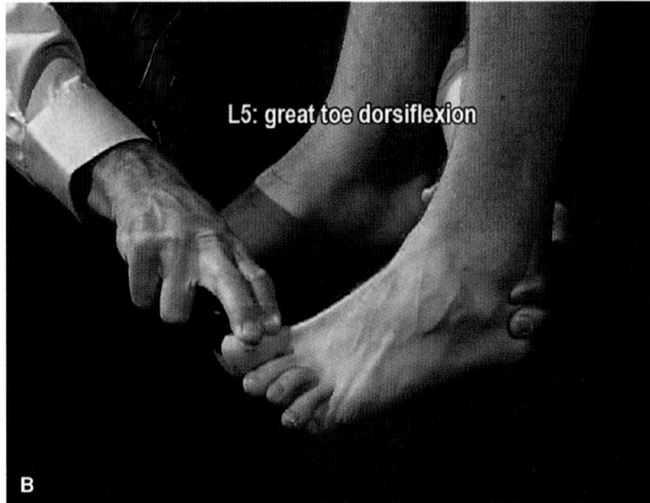

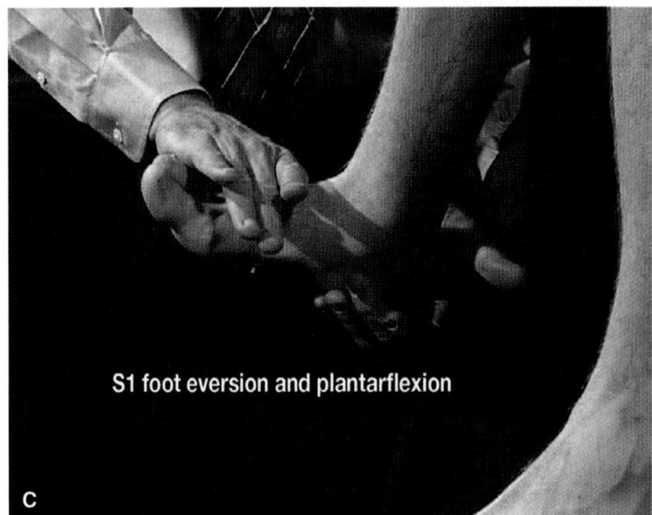

FIGURE 130-5 (**A**) L4 myotome testing. (**B**) L5 myotome testing. (**C**) S1 myotome testing. (From Lawry GV. *Systematic Musculoskeletal Examinations.* www.accessmedicine.com. Copyright © The McGraw-Hill Companies, Inc. All rights reserved.)

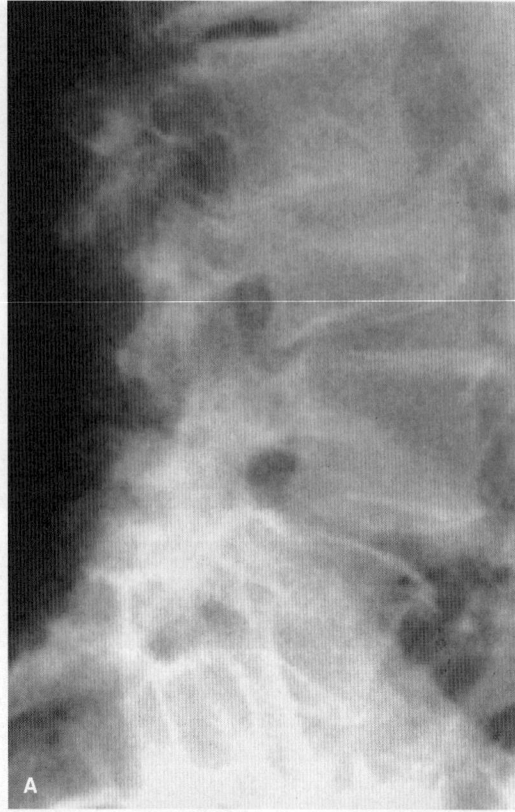

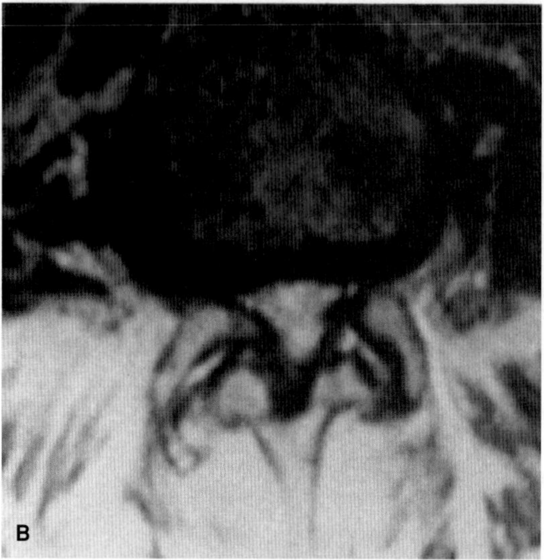

FIGURE 130-6 Imaging studies in a patient with degenerative stenosis of the lumbar spine. (**A**) Radiograph showing degenerative spondylolisthesis between L4 and L5, as well as an old compression fracture of L3. (**B**) MRI showing severe stenosis of the spinal canal at L4–L5, marked facet hypertrophy and ligamentous hypertrophy resulting in central canal stenosis, and lateral recess stenosis. (From Skinner HB. *Current Diagnosis & Treatment in Orthopedics.* 4th ed. www.accessmedicine.com.)

- Lower extremity neurologic screen (dermatome, myotome, reflexes)
- Lower limb nerve tension test[3]
- Muscle length testing, including the hamstrings, hip flexors, and calf muscles
- Passive physiologic intervertebral mobility (PPIVM) testing[5]
- Patella, Achilles, hamstring reflex[5]
- Postural examination
- Prone instability test
- Quadrant test[5]
- Repeated movement testing
- Slump test[3]
- Straight leg raise test[3]

INTERVENTION

- Rest
- Bracing
- Address pain
  - Electrical stimulation
  - Heat/ice[6]
- Address hypertonicity
  - Soft-tissue massage
  - Heat
- Address muscle weakness
  - Core stability exercises
- Abdominal drawing-in
- Multifidus activation
- Posterior pelvic tilts

FUNCTIONAL GOALS

- Patient will be able to
  - Sit with neutral lumbar spine posture for >30 minutes with 0/10 pain rating.
  - Stand at work station and perform computer work for 45 minutes with 0/10 pain rating.
  - Rotate lumbar spine 25 degrees, so as to reach into the back seat in the car, with 0/10 pain rating in the lower extremity.

PROGNOSIS

- Fair to very good, depending on severity of vertebral translation, amount of nerve-root compression, and lumbar impairments.

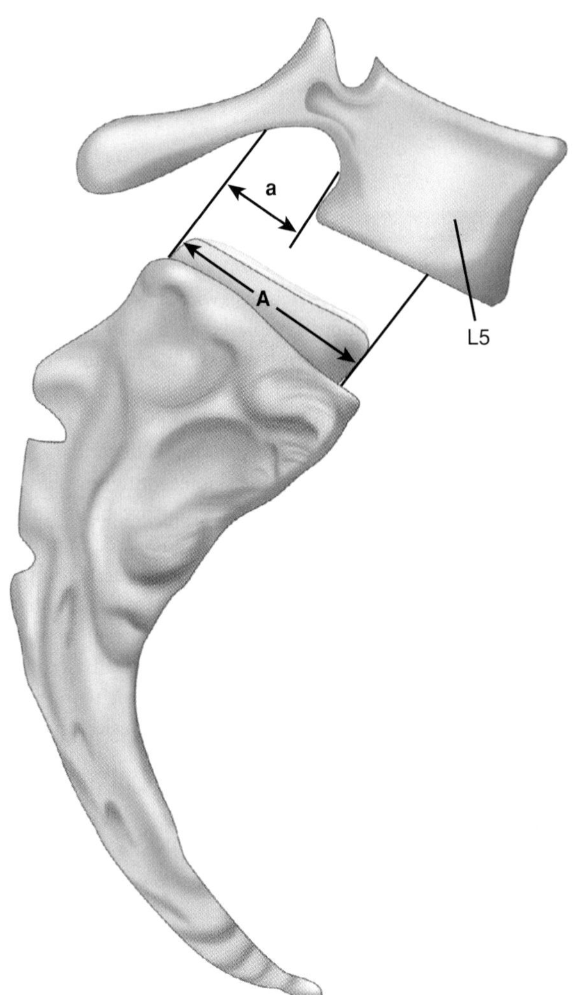

FIGURE 130-7 Meyerding classification of spondylolisthesis. Grade 1 is less than 25% slip, grade 2 is 26% to 50% slip, grade 3 is a 51% to 75% slip, and grade 4 is 76% to 99% slip. The percentage of the slip is determined based on the radiographic measurements (lateral view of the spine) using the formula $a/A \times 100$, where a is the distance between the posterior edge of the inferior endplate of the proximal vertebra and the posterior edge of the superior endplate of the vertebral below it and A is the distance between the anterior and posterior edge of the superior endplate of the distal vertebra. (From Patel DR, Greydanus DE, Baker RJ. *Pediatric Practice: Sports Medicine*. http://www.accesspediatrics.com. Copyright © The McGraw-Hill Companies, Inc. All rights reserved.)

PATIENT RESOURCE

- American Academy of Orthopaedic Surgeons. Spondylolysis and Spondylolisthesis. http://orthoinfo.aaos.org/topic.cfm?topic=A00053. Accessed July 7, 2013.

REFERENCES

1. The American Physical Therapy Association. Pattern 4E: Impaired joint mobility, motor function, muscle performance, and range of motion associated with localized inflammation. *Interactive Guide to Physical Therapist Practice*. 2003. DOI: 10.2522/ptguide.3.1_5. Accessed July 7, 2013.
2. Patel DR, Rowe D. Chapter 30. Thoracolumbar spine injuries. In: Patel DR, Greydanus DE, Baker RJ, eds. *Pediatric Practice: Sports Medicine*. New York, NY: McGraw-Hill; 2009. http://www.accessphysiotherapy.com/abstract/6981360. Accessed July 7, 2013.
3. Dutton M. *Dutton's Orthopaedic Examination, Evaluation, and Intervention*. 3rd ed. New York, NY: McGraw-Hill; 2012. http://www.accessphysiotherapy.com/resource/612. Accessed July 7, 2013.
4. Malone TR, Hazle C, Grey ML. *Imaging in Rehabilitation*. New York, NY: McGraw-Hill; 2008. http://www.accessphysiotherapy.com/resource/613. Accessed July 7, 2013.
5. Dutton M. *Dutton's Orthopedic Survival Guide: Managing Common Conditions*. New York, NY: McGraw-Hill; 2011. http://www.accessphysiotherapy.com/resource/685. Accessed July 7, 2013.
6. Prentice WE. Chapter 9. Cryotherapy and thermotherapy. In: Prentice WE, Quillen WS, Underwood F, eds. *Therapeutic Modalities in Rehabilitation*. 4th ed. New York, NY: McGraw-Hill; 2011. http://www.accessphysiotherapy.com/content/8137995#8137995. Accessed July 7, 2013.

ADDITIONAL REFERENCES

- Curtis C, d'Hemecourt P. Diagnosis and management of back pain in adolescents. *Adolesc Med State Art Rev*. 2007;18:140–164.
- Dutton M. Common orthopedic conditions. In: Dutton M, ed. *McGraw-Hill's NPTE (National Physical Therapy Examination)*. 2e. New York, NY: McGraw-Hill; 2012. http://www.accessphysiotherapy.com/content/5398559. Accessed July 7, 2013.
- Dutton M. Integration of Practice Patterns 4H and 4I: Impaired Joint Mobility, Motor Function, Muscle Performance, ROM Associated with Fractures, Joint Arthroplasty, and Soft Tissue Surgical Procedures. In: Dutton M, ed. *Dutton's Orthopaedic Examination, Evaluation, and Intervention*. 3rd ed. New York, NY: McGraw-Hill; 2012. http://www.accessphysiotherapy.com/content/55596694. Accessed July 7, 2013.
- ICD9DATA web site. http://www.icd9data.com. Accessed July 7, 2013.
- ICD10DATA web site. http://www.icd10data.com. Accessed July 7, 2013.
- Wainner RS, Fritz JM, Irrgang JJ, et al. Reliability and diagnostic accuracy of the clinical examination and patient self-report measures for cervical radiculopathy. *Spine*. 2003;28(1):52–62.

131 SPONDYLOLYSIS, LUMBAR

Eric Shamus, PhD, DPT, PT, CSCS
Jennifer Volz, DPT

CONDITION/DISORDER SYNONYMS

- Lumbosacral spondylolysis
- Lumbar pars fracture

ICD-9-CM CODE

- 738.4 Acquired spondylolisthesis

ICD-10-CM CODE

- M43.00 Spondylolysis, site unspecified

PREFERRED PRACTICE PATTERN

- 4E: Impaired Joint Mobility, Motor Function, Muscle Performance, and ROM Associated with Localized Inflammation[1]

PATIENT PRESENTATION

The patient is a 17-year-old high school football quarterback. He has been currently lifting weights twice a week for the past few months for conditioning. He played in a football game the other night and was tackled from behind. He felt pain and tightness across his low back that has not been relieved by stretching. Now he has complaints of pain with standing and has a hard time receiving the ball when hiked due to pain in his lower back. After standing for extended periods of time, he feels tingling sensation down both of his legs. The onset of tingling has been since he was tackled from behind. Because he had increased symptoms, his coach has placed him on injured reserve until further notice.

Since he was 15, he has had complaints of low back pain during football and weightlifting season, but it was never significant enough to limit his sporting interaction. He was advised to lift less weight during his dead lift, and this reduced his pain. He has found it difficult to sleep and only finds relief when sleeping on his back with a pillow under his knees.

After the game, the patient went to see a physical therapist and had a positive prone instability test and slump test and was hypermobile at the L4–L5 level during passive intervertebral motion testing.

The patient had a follow-up X-ray that showed a small stress fracture of the L4–L5 pars.

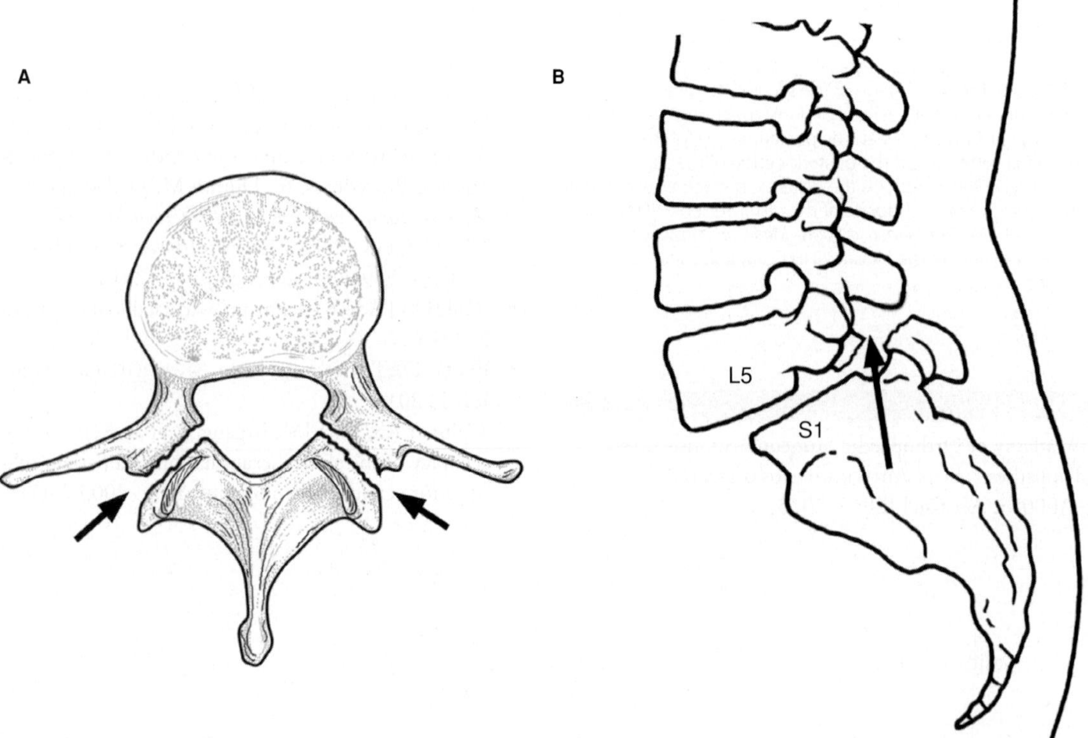

FIGURE 131-1 (**A**) Spondylolysis with bilateral defects in the pars interarticularis (*arrows*). (**B**) Spondylolysis of the L5 vertebra (*arrow*) resulting in isthmic spondylolisthesis at L5–S1. (From Imboden J, Hellmann DB, Stone JH. *Current Rheumatology Diagnosis & Treatment.* 2nd ed. www.accessmedicine.com. Copyright © The McGraw-Hill Companies, Inc. All rights reserved.)

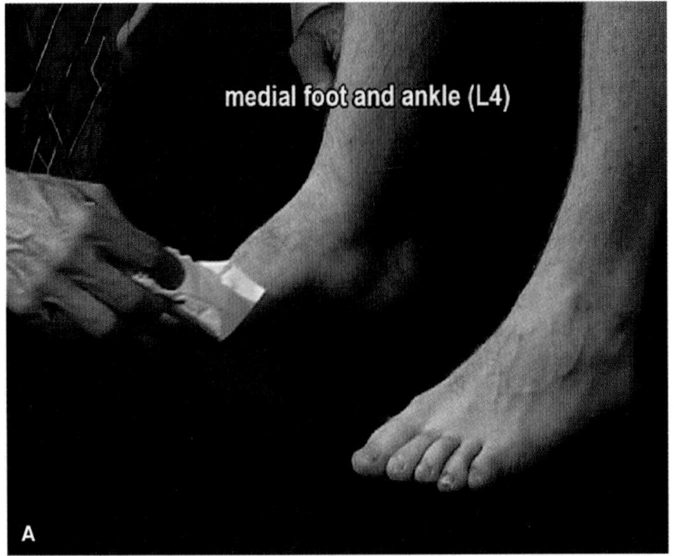

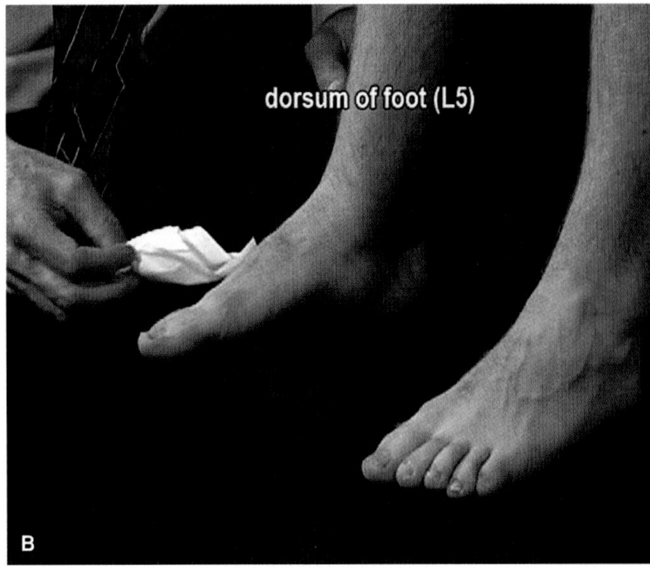

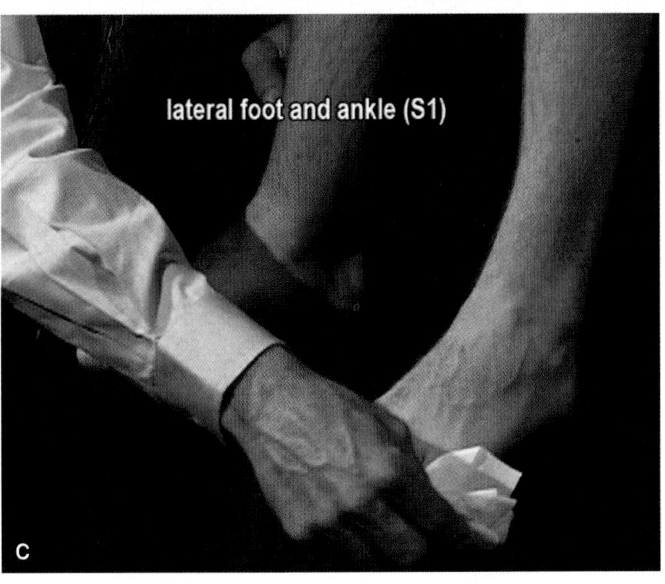

FIGURE 131-2 Sensation, light touch testing (**A**) L4 level (**B**) L5 level (**C**) S1 level (From Lawry GV. *Systematic Musculoskeletal Examinations.* www.accessmedicine.com.

KEY FEATURES

Description

- Stress fracture of the pedicles on the vertebra below
- Tightness or pain across the back region
- Often no symptoms
- Weakness in the pars

Essentials of Diagnosis

- Diagnosis made by X-ray
- Can be acquired or congenital
- Back pain

General Considerations

- Instability
- Avoid extension positions that increase symptoms
- Thin vertebral bone: Pars
- Most common at the L5 level

Demographics

- Onset most often during teenage years
- Runs in families

CLINICAL FINDINGS

SIGNS AND SYMPTOMS

- Back pain
- Stiffness along the spine
- Pain in the lumbar spine worsens with extension

Functional Implications

- Difficulty maintaining standing postures secondary to back pain
- Inability to sleep flat on the back without a pillow
- Difficulty with movements (bending over) secondary to pain
- Limit sports participation

Possible Contributing Causes

- Forceful extension as a result of a hit from behind (as in sports)
- Congenital
- Car accident, hit from rear
- Hyperextension of the lumbar spine
- Increased lordosis posture

Differential Diagnosis

- Peripheral nerve impairment
- Spinal tumor
- Peripheral neuropathy
- Paraspinal spasms
- Degenerative disc disease
- Stenosis

MEANS OF CONFIRMATION OR DIAGNOSIS

Imaging

- MRI helps visualize compressed or inflamed nerve root in diagnosis[2]
- X-ray/Plain-film radiograph to see vertebra position[3]
- CT to show herniation compressing the spinal canal/nerves[3]
- Electrodiagnostic/nerve conduction testing can help determine a specific impaired nerve function[4]

FINDINGS AND INTERPRETATION

- Stress fracture of the pars

REFERRALS/ADMITTANCE

- To hospital for imaging
- To physician for surgical consult if myelopathy suspected[2]
    - Fusion
    - Decompression
    - Laminectomy
    - Hemilaminectomy
- To physician for corticosteroid injection
- To physician for anti-inflammatory medication
- To orthopedist for lumbar bracing

IMPAIRMENTS

- Restricted mobility of the lumbar spine
- Hypermobility
- Noted weakness noted of core musculature

TESTS AND MEASURES

- Algorithm for examination of the lumbar spine
- Passive physiologic intervertebral mobility (PPIVM) testing
- Lower extremity screening examination
- Postural examination
- Muscle length testing, including the hamstrings, hip flexors, and calf muscles
- Quadrant test
- Straight-leg raise test
- Slump test
- Lower limb nerve tension test
- Prone instability test
- Lower extremity neurologic screen (dermatome, myotome, reflexes)
- Repeated movement testing
- Fear-Avoidance Beliefs Questionnaire (FABQ)

INTERVENTION

- Rest
- Bracing
- Ergonomic training

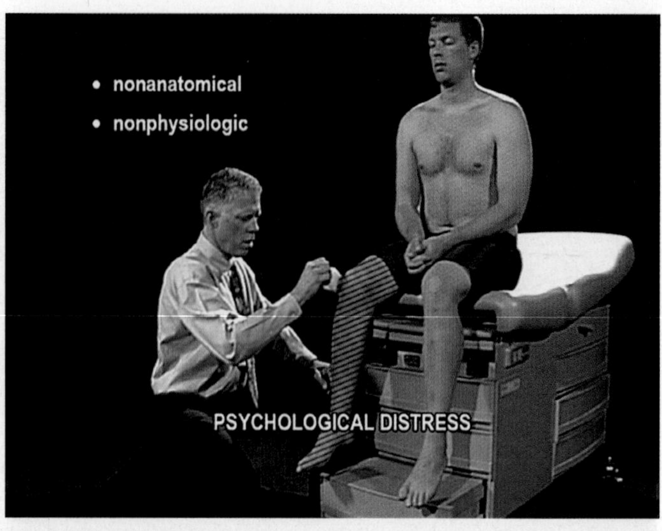

FIGURE 131-3 Non-anatomical and non-physiologic sensation testing results may indicate psychological stress. (From Lawry GV. *Systematic Musculoskeletal Examinations.* www.accessmedicine.com. Copyright © The McGraw-Hill Companies, Inc. All rights reserved.)

- Address pain
    - Electrical stimulation
    - Heat/ice[5]
- Address hypertonicity
    - Soft-tissue massage
    - Heat
- Address muscle weakness
    - Core stability exercises

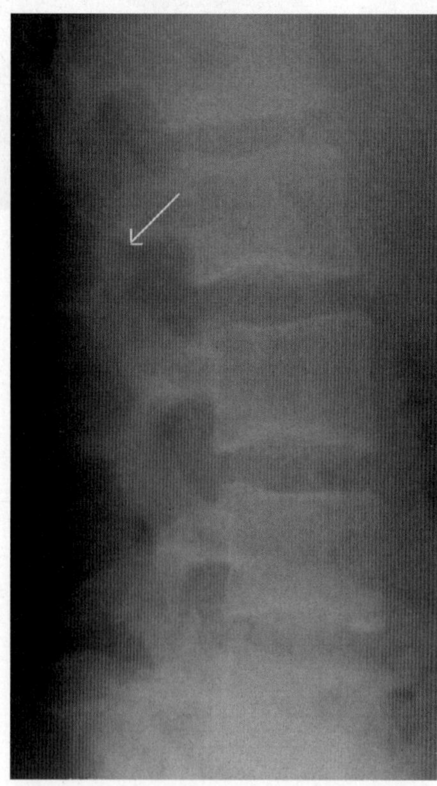

FIGURE 131-4 X-ray of spondylolysis. Note the pars defect at L2 on this lateral radiograph. (From Patel DR, Greydanus DE, Baker RJ. *Pediatric Practice: Sports Medicine.* http://www.accesspediatrics.com. Copyright © The McGraw-Hill Companies, Inc. All rights reserved.)

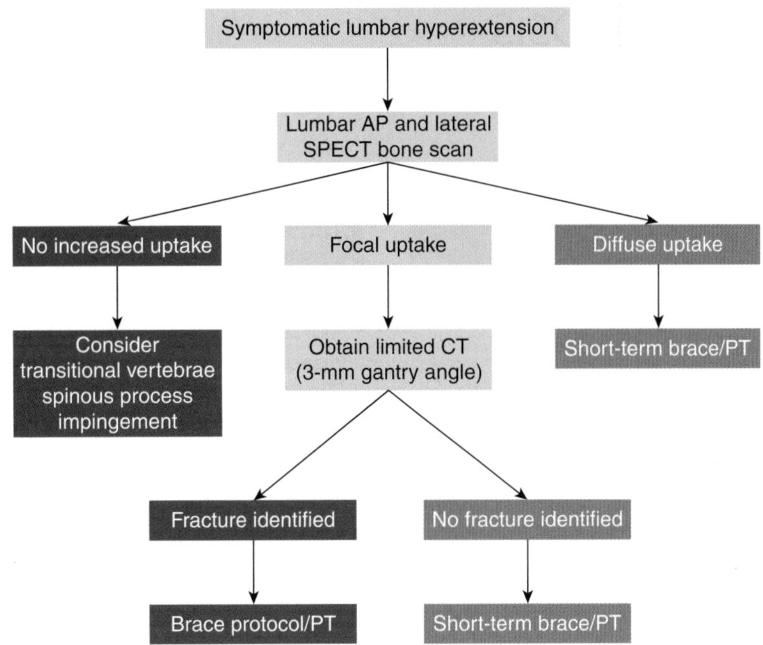

FIGURE 131-5 Boston Children Hospital Imaging Protocol for Spondylolysis. (From Patel DR, Greydanus DE, Baker RJ. *Pediatric Practice: Sports Medicine*. http://www.accesspediatrics.com. Copyright © The McGraw-Hill Companies, Inc. All rights reserved.)

- Bent-leg fall out
- Progressive limb loading 1
- Progressive limb loading 2

FUNCTIONAL GOALS

- Patient will be able to
  - Sit with neutral lumbar spine posture for >30 minutes with 0/10 pain rating.
  - Stand at work station and perform computer work for 45 minutes with 0/10 pain rating.
  - Rotate the lumbar spine in order to lift/pick up items off the floor with 0/10 pain rating.

PROGNOSIS

- Very good with proper ergonomic training, strengthening, and precautions

PATIENT RESOURCE

- American Academy of Orthopaedic Surgeons. Spondylolysis and Spondylolisthesis. http://orthoinfo.aaos.org/topic.cfm?topic=A00053. Accessed July 7, 2013.

REFERENCES

1. The American Physical Therapy Association. Pattern 4E: Impaired joint mobility, motor function, muscle performance, and range of motion associated with localized inflammation. *Interactive Guide to Physical Therapist Practice*. 2003. DOI: 10.2522/ptguide.3.1_5. Accessed July 7, 2013.
2. Dutton M. *Dutton's Orthopaedic Examination, Evaluation, and Intervention*. 3rd ed. New York, NY: McGraw-Hill; 2012. http://www.accessphysiotherapy.com/resource/612. Accessed July 7, 2013.
3. Malone TR, Hazle C, Grey ML. *Imaging in Rehabilitation*. New York, NY: McGraw-Hill; 2008. http://www.accessphysiotherapy.com/resource/613. Accessed July 7, 2013.
4. Dutton M. *Dutton's Orthopedic Survival Guide: Managing Common Conditions*. New York, NY: McGraw-Hill; 2011. http://www.accessphysiotherapy.com/resource/685. Accessed July 7, 2013.
5. Prentice WE. Chapter 9. Cryotherapy and thermotherapy. In: Prentice WE, Quillen WS, Underwood F, eds. *Therapeutic Modalities in Rehabilitation*. 4th ed. New York, NY: McGraw-Hill; 2011. http://www.accessphysiotherapy.com/content/8137995#8137995. Accessed July 7, 2013.

ADDITIONAL REFERENCES

- Halle J, Greathouse D. Chapter 8. Principles of electrophysiologic evaluation and testing. In: Prentice WE, Quillen WS, Underwood F, eds. *Therapeutic Modalities in Rehabilitation*. 4th ed. New York, NY: McGraw-Hill; 2011. http://www.accessphysiotherapy.com/content/8137409. Accessed July 7, 2013.
- ICD9DATA web site. http://www.icd9data.com. Accessed July 7, 2013.
- ICD10DATA web site. http://www.icd10data.com. Accessed July 7, 2013.
- Wainner RS, Fritz JM, Irrgang JJ, et al. Reliability and diagnostic accuracy of the clinical examination and patient self-report measures for cervical radiculopathy. *Spine*. 2003;28(1):52–62.

132 LUMBAR SPONDYLOSIS

Eric Shamus, PhD, DPT, PT, CSCS
Jennifer Volz, DPT

CONDITION/DISORDER SYNONYMS

- Degenerative conditions of the lumbar spine
- Spinal osteoarthritis

ICD-9-CM CODES[1]

- 721 Spondylosis and allied disorders
- 721.3 Lumbosacral spondylosis without myelopathy
- 721.4 Thoracic or lumbar spondylosis with myelopathy
- 721.42 Spondylosis with myelopathy, lumbar region
- 721.9 Spondylosis of unspecified site
- 721.90 Spondylosis of unspecified site, without myelopathy
- 721.91 Spondylosis of unspecified site, with myelopathy

ICD-10-CM CODES[2]

- M47.16 Other spondylosis with myelopathy, lumbar region
- M47.817 Spondylosis without myelopathy or radiculopathy, lumbosacral region
- M47.819 Spondylosis without myelopathy or radiculopathy, site unspecified

PREFERRED PRACTICE PATTERNS

- 4B: Impaired Posture
- 4D: Impaired Joint Mobility, Motor Function, Muscle Performance, and Format Range of Motion Associated with Connective Tissue Dysfunction
- 4E: Impaired Joint Mobility, Motor Function, Muscle Performance, and ROM Associated with Localized Inflammation

PATIENT PRESENTATION

The patient is a 72-year-old woman with complaints of low back pain that has been increasingly getting worse over the last few years. Patient reports tingling and numbness down her right leg. She is fairly active and has been a walker and a golfer for many years. She has recently noticed that during walking there is a decrease in distance due to her right leg feeling heavy and tired. She has stopped playing golf due to decreased power in her swing and wonders if it is from the weakness in her leg.

She reports that she is very stiff in the morning and loosens up after she gets ready for the day. Patient reports that she has relief with Motrin. The patient says that she does not like driving and cannot sit through watching her television shows at night anymore. She says that the pain is not bad as long as she keeps moving, and standing always seems to help alleviate her pain. She said

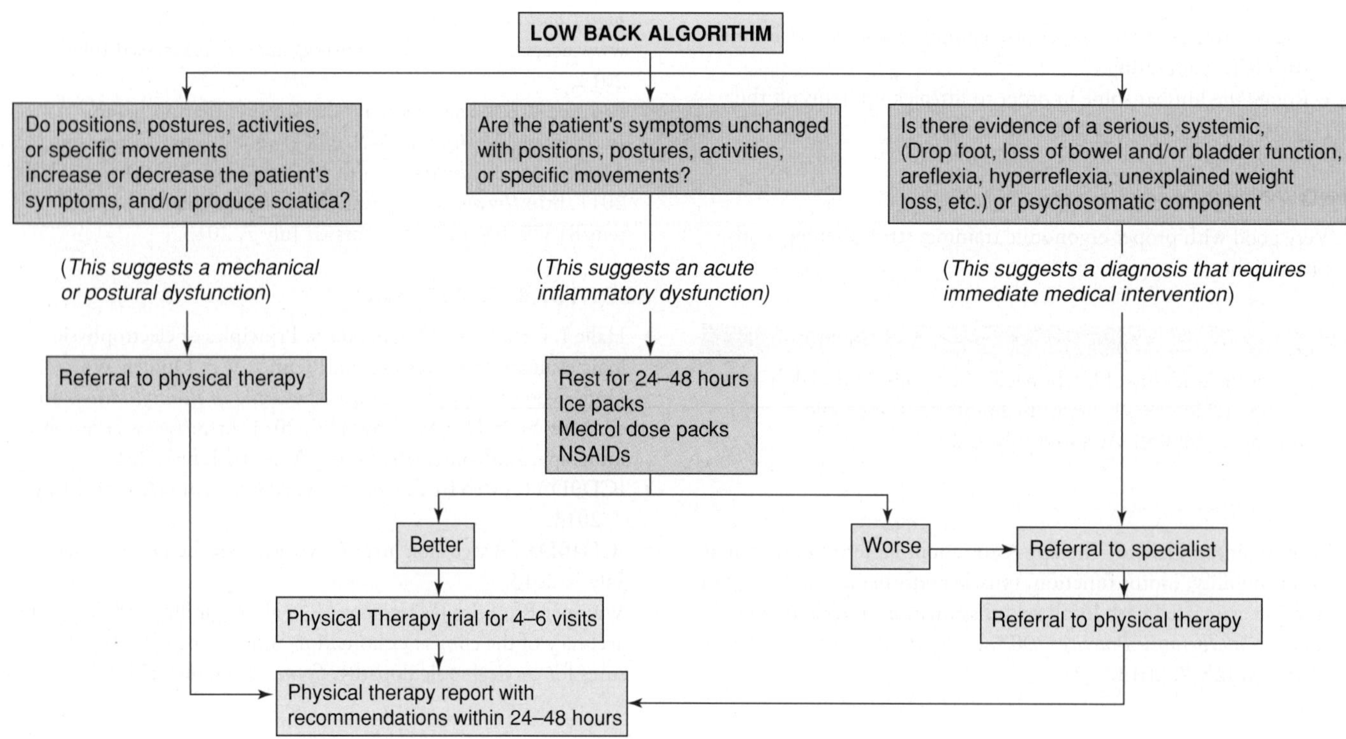

FIGURE 132-1 Examination algorithm for the low back. (From Dutton M. *Dutton's Orthopaedic Examination, Evaluation, and Intervention*. 3rd ed. http://www.accessphysiotherapy.com. Copyright © The McGraw-Hill Companies, Inc. All rights reserved.)

that she has to get her son to help her carry the groceries now because it hurts too much.

During the evaluation, there was hypomobility at L3/L4 and L4/L5 during passive intervertebral motion testing. She had a positive slump test and had a grade of +1 for right patella tendon reflex. She tested positive for straight leg raise test at 30 degrees.

Patient had imaging done and shows a narrowing of the spinal canal between L3–L4 and L4–L5.

KEY FEATURES

Description

- Osteoarthritis of the lumbar spine
- Chronic degeneration
- Progressive arthritis of the lumbar spinal joints
- As the space between the lumbar vertebrae decreases, there can be compression onto the nerve roots
- Arthritis can be central or lateral foramen based
  - Central: Usually bilateral symptoms in the lower extremities
  - Lateral: Usually unilateral symptoms in the leg
- Pain, paresthesia, and weakness in the lower extremities
- Pressure on the nerve root can cause radiculopathy

TABLE 132-1 Medical Screening Questionnaire for the Low Back Region

	Yes	No
Have you recently had a major trauma, such as a vehicle accident or a fall from a height?		
Have you ever had a medical practitioner tell you that you have osteoporosis?		
Do you have a history of cancer?		
Do you have pain at night that wakes you up?		
Does your pain ease when you rest in a comfortable position?		
Have you recently had a fever?		
Have you recently lost weight even though you have not been attempting to eat less or exercise more?		
Have you recently taken antibiotics or other medications for an infection?		
Have you been diagnosed as having an immunosuppressive disorder?		
Have you noticed a recent onset of difficulty with retaining your urine?		
Have you noticed a recent need to urinate more frequently?		
Have you noticed a recent onset of numbness in the area where you would sit on a bicycle seat?		
Have you recently noticed your legs becoming weak while walking or climbing stairs?		

Sources: Data from Bigos S, Bowyer O, Braen G, et al. *Acute Low Back Problems in Adults,* AHCPR Publication 95–0642. Rockville, MD: Agency for Health Care Policy and Research, Public Health Service, U.S. Department of Health and Human Services, 1994; DuVall RE, Godges J. Introduction to physical therapy differential diagnosis: the clinical utility of subjective examination. In: Wilmarth MA, ed. *Medical Screening for the Physical Therapist. Orthopaedic Section Independent Study Course 14.1.1.* La Crosse, WI: Orthopaedic Section, APTA, Inc., 2003:1–44. Permission from Orthopaedic Section, APTA.

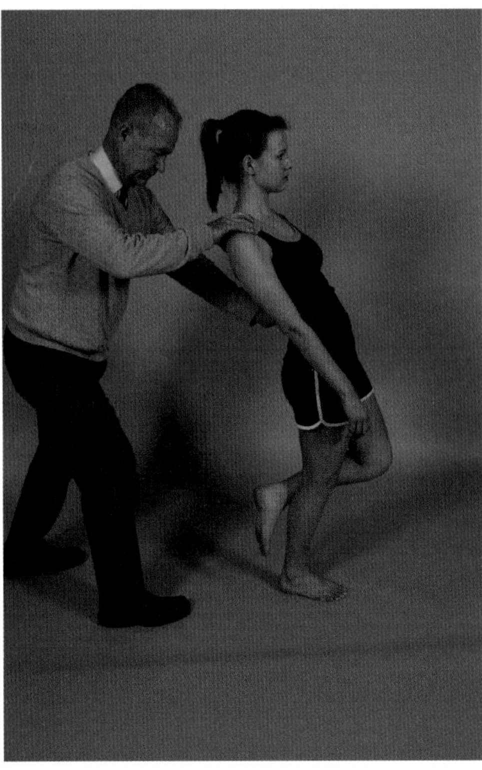

FIGURE 132-2 Single-legged hyperextension test. (From Dutton M. *Dutton's Orthopaedic Examination, Evaluation, and Intervention.* 3rd ed. http://www.accessphysiotherapy.com. Copyright © The McGraw-Hill Companies, Inc. All rights reserved.)

Essentials of Diagnosis

- X-ray
- Acute painful flare-ups, chronic persistent pain
- Relief with nonsteroidal anti-inflammatory drugs (NSAIDs)
- Morning stiffness

General Considerations

- Begins with pain that is intermittent
- Pain and stiffness at rest/sleep
- Improved with low-level activity
- Could have rapid and severe onset

Demographics

- Common in adults aged 60 years and older

TABLE 132-2 Relieving Positions or Movements

Relieving Position or Movement	Probable Cause
Flexion	Facet joint involvement Low back strain Lateral stenosis
Extension	Disk involvement Nerve root irritation (disk herniation)
Rest	Neurogenic claudication

Source: From Dutton M. *Dutton's Orthopaedic Examination, Evaluation, and Intervention.* 3rd ed. http://www.accessphysiotherapy.com. Copyright © The McGraw-Hill Companies, Inc. All rights reserved.

TABLE 132-3 Reliability of the Historical Examination[a]

Historical Question	Population	Kappa Value or % Agreement
Patient report of McCombe et al.[b]	Group 1:50 patients with low back pain	Interexaminer reliability
Foot pain		$K = 0.12, 0.73$
Leg pain		$K = 0.53, 0.96$
Thigh pain	Group 2:33 patients with low back pain	$K = 0.39, 0.78$
Buttock pain		$K = 0.34, 0.44$
Back pain		$K = 0.19, 0.16$
Pain ever below the knee	475 patients with back pain	Test–retest among patient questionnaire Agreement 100%
Pain ever into the foot		Agreement 92%
Numbness below knee (Waddell et al.)[c]		Agreement 95%
Increased pain with (Roach et al.)[d]	53 subjects with a primary complaint of low back pain	Test–retest among patient questionnaire
Sitting		$K = 0.46$
Standing		$K = 0.70$
Walking		$K = 0.67$
Increased pain with (Vroomen et al.)[e]	A random selection of 91 patients with low back pain	Interexaminer reliability
Sitting		$K = 0.49$
Standing		$K = 1.0$
Walking		$K = 0.56$
Lying down		$K = 0.41$
Pain with sitting (Van Dillen et al.)[f]	95 patients with low back pain	Interexaminer reliability $K = 0.99, 1.0$
Pain with bending (Van Dillen et al.)[f]		Interexaminer reliability $K = 0.98, 0.99$
Pain with bending (Roach et al.)[d]	53 subjects with a primary complaint of low back pain	Test–retest among patient questionnaire $K = 0.65$
Pain with bending (McCombe et al.)[b]	Group 1: 50 patients with low back pain Group 2: 33 patients with low back pain	Interexaminer reliability $K = 0.51, 0.56$
Increased pain with coughing/sneezing (Vroomen et al.)[e]	A random selection of 91 patients with low back pain	Interexaminer reliability $K = 0.64$
Increased pain with coughing (Roach et al.)[d]	53 subjects with a primary complaint of low back pain	Test–retest among patient questionnaire $K = 0.75$
Pain with pushing/lifting/carrying (Roach et al.)[d]		Test–retest among patient questionnaire $K = 0.77, 0.89$
Sudden or gradual onset of pain[c]	475 patients with back pain	Test–retest among patient questionnaire Agreement 79%

[a]Data from Cleland J. *Thoracolumbar Spine, Orthopaedic Clinical Examination: An Evidence-Based Approach for Physical Therapists*. Carlstadt, NJ: Icon Learning Systems, LLC, 2005:166–167.
[b]Data from McCombe PF, Fairbank JCT, Cockersole BC, et al. Reproducibility of physical signs in low back pain. *Spine.* 1989;14:908–918.
[c]Data from Waddell G, Main CJ, Morris EW, et al. Normality and reliability in the clinical assessment of backache. *BMJ.* 284:1519–1523, 1982.
[d]Data from Roach KE, Brown MD, Dunigan KM, et al. Test-retest reliability of patient reports of low back pain. *J Orthop Sports Phys Ther.* 1997;26:253–259.
[e]Data from Vroomen PC, de Krom MC, Knottnerus JA. Consistency of history taking and physical examination in patients with suspected lumbar nerve root involvement. *Spine.* 2000;25:91–96; discussion 97.
[f]Data from Van Dillen LR, Sahrmann SA, Norton BJ, et al. Reliability of physical examination items used for classification of patients with low back pain. *Phys Ther.* 1998;78:979–988.
Source: From Dutton M. *Dutton's Orthopaedic Examination, Evaluation, and Intervention*. 3rd ed. http://www.accessphysiotherapy.com.

CLINICAL FINDINGS

SIGNS AND SYMPTOMS

- Diminished reflexes
- Fatigue
- Heaviness in the legs
- Loss of range of motion (ROM) and joint play
- Lower motor neuron dysfunction
- Muscle weakness
- Pain that is intermittent, increased with weight-bearing activities
- Paresthesia
- Radiculopathy
- Stiffness
- Tingling sensation in the lower extremity

Functional Implications

- Limited mobility
- Increased symptoms with increased weight-bearing exercises
- Aerobic endurance limitation

Possible Contributing Causes

- Bone spurs
- Family history of osteoarthritis
- Instability
- Limited flexibility
- Poor posture
- Weakness

Differential Diagnosis

- Disc herniation
- Facet joint arthritis
- Forestier disease
- Psoriatic arthritis
- Reiter syndrome (reactive arthritis)
- Spinal stenosis
- Whipple disease
- Yersinia arthritis

MEANS OF CONFIRMATION OR DIAGNOSIS

Imaging

- X-ray of the spine and pelvis
- MRI of the spine

FINDINGS AND INTERPRETATION

- Decreased space on X-ray between the vertebrae

TREATMENT

Medication

- NSAIDs
- Corticosteroids
- Surgery[3]

REFERRALS/ADMITTANCE

- Rheumatologist to assess underlying complications
- Surgical consult
- Orthopedic surgeon

IMPAIRMENTS

- Mobility
- Functional rotation and bending

TESTS AND MEASURES

- Dermatomes
- Myotomes
- Neural tension test
- Reflexes
- Single-legged hyperextension test
- Sit and reach test
- Slump test
- Straight leg raise test
- Trunk active range of motion (AROM)

INTERVENTION

- Education in gentle ROM to maintain mobility
- Exercise, flexibility, and stability strengthening to decrease stress on the joints
- Joint protection education
- Postural training
- Warm shower or heat to increase mobility

FUNCTIONAL GOALS

- Patient will have
  - Independence in home exercise program.
  - Decreased pain to perform household activities such as cleaning and laundry.
  - Improved functional level to participate in grocery shopping.

PROGNOSIS

- The disease progression is not specific.
- As it becomes more severe joints, may become limited and increase compression.
- Symptoms can be intermittent.
- Patients function well until severe progression of joint mobility.

PATIENT RESOURCE

- Middleton K, Fish DE. Lumbar spondylosis: clinical presentation and treatment approaches. *Curr Rev Musculoskeletal Med.* 2009;2(2):94–104.

REFERENCES

1. ICD9Data.com. http://www.icd9data.com. Accessed July 7, 2013.
2. ICD10Data.com. http://www.icd10data.com. Accessed July 7, 2013.
3. Gibson JN, Grant IC, Waddell G. The Cochrane review of surgery for lumbar disc prolapse and degenerative lumbar spondylosis. *Spine.* 1999;24:1820–1832.

ADDITIONAL REFERENCES

- Dutton M. *Orthopaedic Examination, Evaluation, and Intervention Guide to Physical Therapist Practice.* 3rd ed. New York, NY: McGraw-Hill Education; 2012.
- Hamilton N, Weimar W, Luttgens K. Chapter 3. The musculoskeletal system: the musculature. In: Hamilton N, Weimar W, Luttgens K, eds. *Kinesiology: Scientific Basis of Human Motion.* New York, NY: McGraw-Hill; 2008. http://www.accessphysiotherapy.com/content/6150242. Accessed July 7, 2013.

- Malone TR, Hazle C, Grey ML. Knee: Standard conventional radiographs. In: Malone TR, Hazle C, Grey ML, eds. *Imaging in Rehabilitation*. New York, NY: McGraw-Hill; 2008. http://www.accessphysiotherapy.com/content/5941207. Accessed July 7, 2013.
- McAuley J, Farah N, van Gröningen R, Green C. A Questionnaire-based study on patients' experiences with rechargeable implanted programmable generators for spinal cord stimulation to treat chronic lumbar spondylosis pain. *Neuromodulation*. 2013; 16(2):142–146.
- Pedziwiatr H. Psychological attachment in patients with spondylosis of cervical and lumbar spine. *Adv Exp Med Biol.* 2013;755:357–363.
- Tan Y, Aghdasi BG, Montgomery SR, et al. Kinetic magnetic resonance imaging analysis of lumbar segmental mobility in patients without significant spondylosis. *Eur Spine J.* 2012;21(12): 2673–2679.

133 MYOFASCIAL PAIN SYNDROME

Eric Shamus, PhD, DPT, PT, CSCS
Mila Marhovich, DPT

CONDITION/DISORDER SYNONYM

- Chronic myofascial pain (CMP)

ICD-9-CM CODE

- 729.1 Myalgia and myositis unspecified

ICD-10-CM CODES

- M60.9 Myositis, unspecified
- M79.1 Myalgia

PREFERRED PRACTICE PATTERN

- 4D: Impaired Joint Mobility, Motor Function, Muscle Performance, and ROM Associated with Connective Tissue Dysfunction

PATIENT PRESENTATION

The patient is a 28-year-old woman who presents with complaints of an insidious onset of pain and tightness along the last lower rib on the left side that started 2 to 3 years ago and has been getting worse since. The pain is worse with rotation and side bending at the waist; with frequent exacerbations of pain in the morning after exercising the night before, after prolonged walking, and rollerblading. The pain is better with heat and rest. She states that performing her job as a group exercise instructor is becoming very difficult and she has had to take several days off this month. She denies any specific episode of trauma and any systemic symptoms or pain anywhere else in her body.

The patient is a direct access, self pay, without a physician's referral. Initial physical therapy examination did not reveal any systemic symptoms or signs of a sinister pathology. She demonstrated reduced lumbar curvature, a posterior pelvic tilt, and a slight left rotation at L4–5 in standing posture. Range of motion (ROM) testing revealed reduced left rotation (30 degrees) and left side bending (15 degrees) due to pain with soft tissue guarding along the left paraspinals, left thoracolumbar fascia, and left quadratus lumborum. Palpation examination revealed presence of a taut palpable band of tissue with a localized area of painful hypersensitivity 4/10 at the proximal insertion of the left quadratus lumborum. manual muscle test findings: thoracolumbar extension 5/5; left hip elevation 4+/5; left hip extension 5/5.

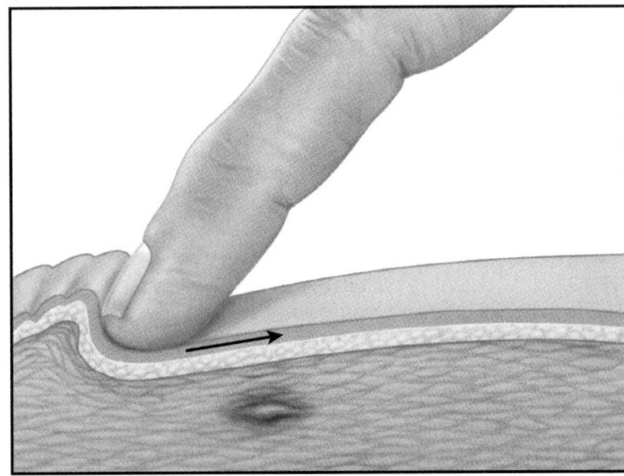

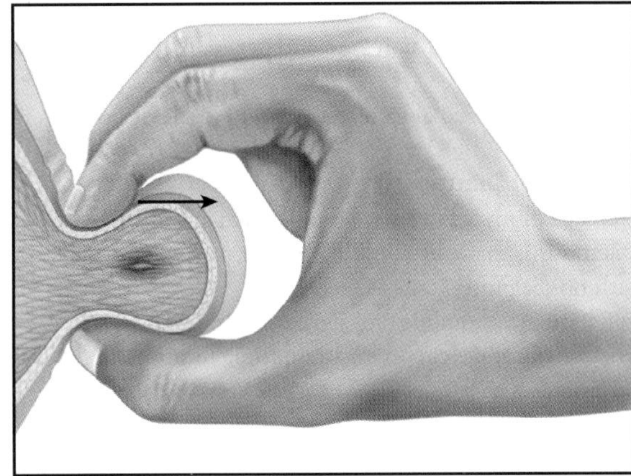

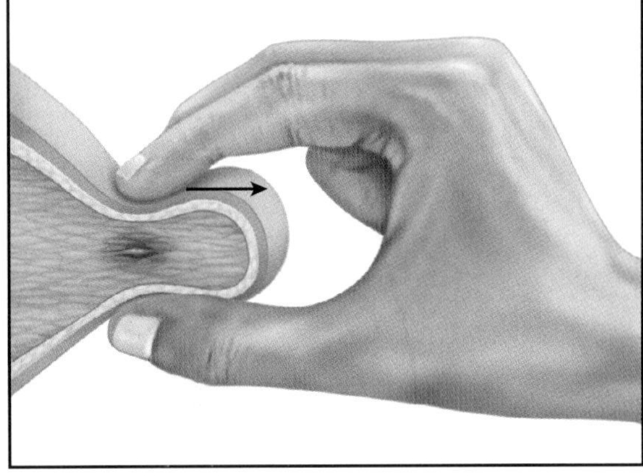

FIGURE 133-1 Techniques for trigger point palpation. (**A**) With flat palpation, fingertips stroke across the muscle surface. (**B**) With pincer palpation. The muscle is grasped and palpation for trigger points is completed as the muscle slips through the fingers. (From Hoffman BL, Schorge JO, Schaffer JI, et al. *Williams Gynecology*. 2nd ed. www.accessmedicine.com. Copyright © The McGraw-Hill Companies, Inc. All rights reserved.)

KEY FEATURES

Description

- Chronic, persistent, deep aching pains in the muscle; nonarticular in origin

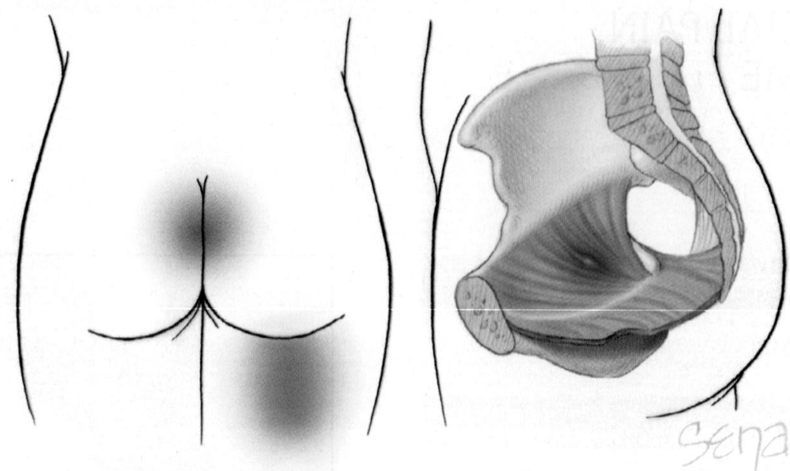

FIGURE 133-2 An extensive pattern of referred pain (*red shading in the left image*) can be created by trigger points in the obturator internus muscle (*right image*). (From Hoffman BL, Schorge JO, Schaffer JI, et al. *Williams Gynecology*. 2nd ed. www.accessmedicine.com. Copyright © The McGraw-Hill Companies, Inc. All rights reserved. Images contributed by Ms. Marie Sena.)

- Characterized by well-defined, highly sensitive tender spots (trigger points)
- Usually caused by sudden overload, overstretching and/or repetitive/sustained muscle activities
- Pain associated with activities, and generally relieved with rest
- Fascial restrictions
- Can be in localized areas affecting any muscle or fascia

Essentials of Diagnosis

- Presence of myofascial trigger points (MTrPs).
- Diagnosis is made by clinical assessment (generally palpation) with no diagnostic tests available.
- Differentiates from fibromyalgia as it can occur in a single area, whereas fibromyalgia occurs in multiple locations and has tender points.
- According to Simons,[1] the diagnosis of myofascial pain syndrome (MPS) can be made if five major criteria and at least one out of three minor criteria are met.
  - The major criteria are
    - Localized spontaneous pain.
    - Spontaneous pain or altered sensations in the expected referred pain area for a given trigger point.
    - Presence of a taut palpable band in an accessible muscle.
    - Exquisite localized tenderness in a precise point along the taut band.
    - Some degree of reduced range of movement when measurable.
  - Minor criteria include
    - Reproduction of spontaneously perceived pain and altered sensations by pressure on the trigger point.
    - Elicitation of a local twitch response of muscular fibers by "transverse" snapping palpation, or by needle insertion into the trigger point.
    - Pain relieved by muscle stretching or injection of the trigger point.

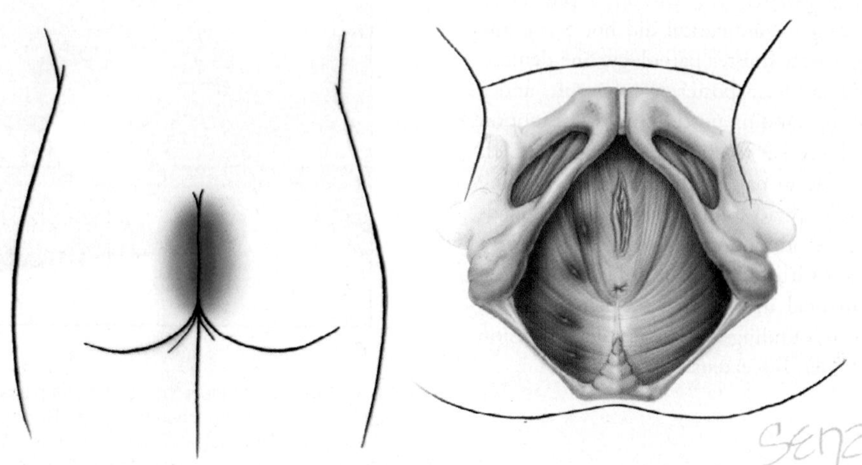

FIGURE 133-3 Pattern of referred pain (*red shading in the left image*) created by trigger points in the levator ani and coccygeus muscles (*right image*). (From Hoffman BL, Schorge JO, Schaffer JI, et al. *Williams Gynecology*. 2nd ed. www.accessmedicine.com. Copyright © The McGraw-Hill Companies, Inc. All rights reserved. Images contributed by Ms. Marie Sena.)

General Considerations
- Very common; affects most people during their lifetime
- Trigger points: Active trigger points are tender to palpation and have a characteristic referral pattern of pain when provoked
- Latent trigger points are palpable taut bands that are not tender to palpation, but can be converted into an active trigger point

Demographics
- In the United States, 14.4% of the general population suffers from chronic musculoskeletal pain.[1]
- 21% to 93% of patients with regional pain complaints have myofascial pain.[1]
- 25% to 54% of asymptomatic individuals have latent trigger points.[2]
- No racial differences in the incidence of myofascial pain have been described in the literature.
- Myofascial pain is distributed equally between men and women
- Myofascial trigger points can be found in persons/children of all ages.
- The likelihood of developing active trigger points increases with age and activity level.
- Sedentary individuals are more prone to develop active trigger points than are individuals who exercise vigorously on a daily basis.

CLINICAL FINDINGS

SIGNS AND SYMPTOMS
- Muscle stiffness
- Headaches
- Vertigo
- Paresthesias
- Referred pain
- Joint stiffness
- Limited ROM
- Deep aching pain that is constant
- Pain upon palpation of the trigger point
- Upon palpation of the trigger point, pain can be referred to other areas of the body
- Difficulty sleeping
- Weakness without atrophy may be seen when performing manual muscle testing

Functional Implications
- Pain with standing, ambulation, and activities of daily living
- Limited ROM
- Weakness

Possible Contributing Causes
- Improper posture
- Connective tissue disease
- Emotional/psychological stress
- Anxiety
- Behavioral
- Traumatic events
- Spinal discogenic disease
- Improper lifting/poor biomechanics
- Lack of activity (cast)
- Repetitive stress
- Overuse
- Poor muscular/ligamentous support
- Obesity
- Inflammatory conditions affecting the ligaments, muscles, and tendons

Differential Diagnoses
- Herniated disc
- Fibromyalgia
- Rheumatoid arthritis
- Complex regional pain syndrome
- Radiculopathy
- Ligamentous sprain
- Muscle strain

MEANS OF CONFIRMATION OR DIAGNOSIS

Imaging
- Can be used in looking for a differential diagnosis

Laboratory test
- Can be used in looking for a differential diagnosis

Diagnostic Procedure
- Palpation

FINDINGS AND INTERPRETATION
- A taut fibrous band will be felt upon palpation of the muscle.
- Band may be painful or not.
- Limited ROM may be a common finding.

REFERRALS/ADMITTANCE
- To psychologist, if counseling appropriate
- To dietitian to address obesity, if appropriate
- To massage therapist

IMPAIRMENTS
- Lower back pain
- Limited function due to limited ROM

TESTS AND MEASURES
- Palpation for the presence of MTrPs
- Algorithm for examination of the lumbar spine
- Passive physiologic intervertebral mobility (PPIVM) testing
- Lower extremity screening examination
- Postural examination
- Muscle length testing, including the hamstrings, hip flexors, and calf muscles
- Quadrant test
- Straight-leg raise test
- Slump test
- Lower limb nerve tension test
- Prone instability test
- Lower extremity neurologic screen (dermatome, myotome, reflexes)
- Repeated movement testing
- Fear-Avoidance Beliefs Questionnaire (FABQ)

INTERVENTIONS
- Soft-tissue massage techniques and joint oscillations to reduce pain and/or muscle guarding
- Address biomechanical factors: Improper posture, ergonomics, body mechanics at work and leisure
- Use of spray and stretch technique
- Cryotherapy may be used in acute cases within 24 to 72 hours of an injury to alleviate pain and reduce inflammation

- Thermotherapy: Hot packs, whirlpool after the initial inflammation has subsided to increase circulation and relaxation
- Hydrotherapy
- Ultrasound to minimize scarring, stimulate proper tissue healing, increase circulation to the area, relax the musculature
- Electric stimulation
  - Microcurrent when inflammation is present and is very acute
  - Microcurrent stimulates healing, decreases inflammation
  - Biphasic/Russian currents: When inflammation is not acute, fatiguing the muscle in order to minimize contractures, reeducate the muscle
- Transcutaneous electrical nerve stimulation (TENS) for symptomatic relief of pain
- Desensitization of trigger point with manual pressure
- Implementation of strength, power, and endurance exercises
  - Risk of decreased flexibility and reinjury
- Progress from active assistive to active to resistive exercises, then to task-specific performance training
- Gait training
  - Evaluate whether there is a dysfunction in lumbopelvic rhythm, hip flexors, hamstrings to alleviate compensation and low back stress
  - Consider foot orthotics if there is leg discrepancy
  - Teach proper postural alignment when walking, standing, etc.
- Posture education
  - Sitting: Selecting appropriate ergonomic chair with low back support
  - Standing: Posture
  - Functional: Proper body mechanics
- Massage
  - Slow, light percussion to increase circulation, flush lactic acid out of the muscle tissues
  - Effleurage to relax the muscles
  - Deep tissue treatments when desensitizing the trigger points
- Joint mobilizations: To eliminate bony restrictions

FUNCTIONAL GOALS

- The patient will be able to
  - Decrease inflammation to perform repetitive movement.
  - Relieve muscular contractions (spasms) to allow full trunk motion to reach to floor.
  - Increase circulation to decrease inflammation and improve healing response.
- Educate patient on proper body mechanics, work-area ergonomics, relaxation techniques

PROGNOSIS

- Very good, although may take several months to get rid of the trigger points.
- MPS may reoccur if biomechanical causes are not addressed.

PATIENT RESOURCE

- Myofascial Trigger Point Therapy. National Association of Mypfascial Trigger Point Therapy. http://www.myofascialtherapy.org/index.html. Accessed May 25, 2014.

REFERENCES

1. Simons DG. Muscular pain syndromes. In: Fricton JR, Awad E, eds. *Advances in Pain Research and Therapy*. New York, NY: Raven Press; 1990:1–41.
2. Eustice C. Myofascial Pain. http://arthritis.about.com/od/diseasesandconditions/a/myofascial_pain.htm. Accessed July 7, 2013.

ADDITIONAL REFERENCES

- APTA Guide to Physical Therapist Practice. http://guidetoptpractice.apta.org/. Accessed July 7, 2013.
- Bishop KL, Malone DJ, Lindsay KB. *Physical Therapy in Acute Care: A Clinician's Guide*. Thorofare, NJ: SLACK, Inc.; 2006.
- Dutton M. Complex disorders. In: Dutton M, ed. *McGraw-Hill's NPTE (National Physical Therapy Examination)*. 2nd ed. New York, NY: McGraw-Hill; 2012. http://www.accessphysiotherapy.com/content/5402428. Accessed July 7, 2013.
- Dutton M. Generalized body pain. In: Dutton M, ed. *Orthopaedic Examination, Evaluation, and Intervention*. 2nd ed. New York, NY: McGraw-Hill; 2008. http://www.accessphysiotherapy.com/content/5546970. Accessed July 7, 2013.
- Dutton M. Integration of Practice Patterns 4B, 4C, and 4F: Impaired Joint Mobility, Motor Function, Muscle Performance and Range of Motion Secondary to Impaired Posture, Systemic Dysfunction (Referred Pain Syndromes), Spinal Disorders, and Myofascial Pain Dysfunction. In: Dutton M, ed. *Orthopaedic Examination, Evaluation, and Intervention*. 2nd ed. New York, NY: McGraw-Hill; 2008. http://www.accessphysiotherapy.com/content/55593563. Accessed July 7, 2013.
- Dutton M. Neurophysiologic techniques. In: Dutton M, ed. *Orthopaedic Examination, Evaluation, and Intervention*. 2nd ed. New York, NY: McGraw-Hill; 2008. http://www.accessphysiotherapy.com/content/5550880. Accessed July 7, 2013.
- Goodman CC, Fuller KS. *Pathology Implications for the Physical Therapist*. 3rd ed. St. Louis, MO: Saunders Elsevier; 2009.
- ICD-9-CM. http://www.icd9data.com. Accessed July 7, 2013.
- ICD-10-CM. http://www.icd10data.com. Accessed July 7, 2013.
- Kisner C, Colby LA. *Therapeutic Exercise: Foundations and Techniques*. 5th ed. Philadelphia, PA: F.A. Davis Company; 2007.
- Martini FH, Timmons MJ, Tallitsch RB. *Human Anatomy*. San Francisco, CA: Pearson Education, Inc.; 2009.
- Simons D, Travell J, Simons P, Cummings, B. *Travell & Simons' Myofascial Pain and Dysfunction: The Trigger Point Manual* (Vols. 1–2). Baltimore, MD: Lippincott Williams & Wilkins; 1998.

134 OSTEOMALACIA

Eric Shamus, PhD, DPT, PT, CSCS
Lindsey (Davis) Hornecke, DPT

CONDITION/DISORDER SYNONYM

- Rickets

ICD-9-CM CODE[1]

- 268.2 Osteomalacia unspecified

ICD-10-CM CODE[2]

- M83.9 Adult osteomalacia, unspecified

PREFERRED PRACTICE PATTERNS[3]

- 4A: Primary Prevention/Risk Reduction for Skeletal Demineralization
- 4B: Impaired Posture
- 4C: Impaired Muscle Performance
- 4F: Impaired joint Mobility, Motor Function, Muscle Performance, ROM and Reflex Integrity Association with Spinal Disorders
- 4G: Impaired Joint Mobility, Muscle Performance, and ROM Associated with Fracture

PATIENT PRESENTATION

A 60-year-old female patient presents with right transfemoral hip fracture s/p ORIF. She reported the fracture occurred when she was walking down the stairs and she missed the last step. No fall occurred. Prior to the fracture she reports she was having bone pain in both lower extremities and that her legs were feeling weaker than normal.

Her orthopedic surgeon refers her to physical therapy. Her weight-bearing status is weight bearing as tolerated and she ambulates with a standard walker. On physical therapy examination, she has noticeable weakness and muscular atrophy in both lower extremities, right > left. She is a very thin woman with an increased thoracic kyphosis. Manual muscle testing revealed overall right hip strength 3/5, with the exception of 2+/5 for right hip abduction. Left hip strength is 3+/5.

KEY FEATURES

Description

- Softening of bone mass and density with a marked decrease in cortical thickness and cancellous bone trabeculae, leading to increased fragility, deformity, and/or fracture
- Osteomalacia is due to a lack or an inability to process of vitamin D
- Metabolic bone disease

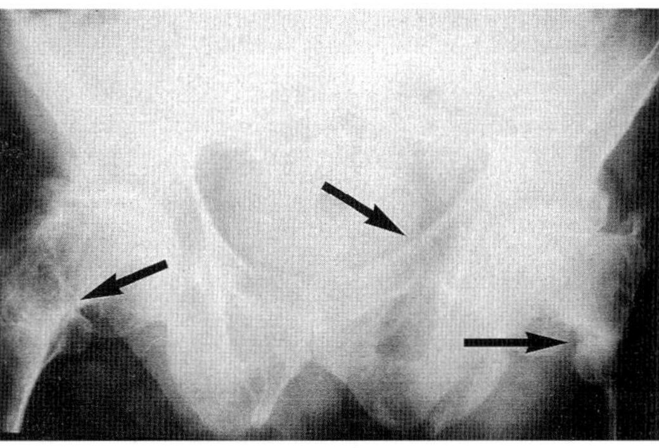

FIGURE 134-1 X-ray of the pelvis of an elderly woman with osteomalacia. Note marked bowing of both femoral necks, with pseudofractures of the medial aspect of the femoral necks and the superior aspect of the left pubic ramus (arrows). (From McPhee SJ, Papadakis MA. *Current Medical Diagnosis and Treatment 2011*. 50th edition. New York, NY: McGraw-Hill. Photograph courtesy of Dr. Harry Genant.)

- Inadequate or delayed mineralization of osteoid in mature cortical and spongy bone[1]
- Has normal amount of collagen
- Fracture with minimal injury
- Rickets in children affects mineralization of the growth plates

Essentials of Diagnosis

- Bone mineral density (BMD) measurements are related to both peak bone mass and bone loss.
- Decreased serum calcium levels
  - Low levels of serum 25-hydroxyvitamin D
- Bone Densitometry: Normal BMD within 1 SD of the mean, *T*-score at −1.0 and greater.
- Bone Densitometry: Low BMD (referred to as osteopenia) occurs between 1 and 2.5 SD below the mean, T-score between −1.0 and −2.5.
- Increased fracture propensity is due to demineralization secondary to osteoporosis that often occurs at the spine, hips, pelvis, or wrist.
- Accurate patient and family medical histories and early recognition through physical examination may lead to improved therapeutic outcomes.
- 10-year risk for fracture can be measured through FRAX® score and response to pharmacotherapy can be measured through changes in laboratory values.

General Considerations

- Widespread bone pain
- Persons with low bone density are at an increased risk for the development of osteoporosis; prevention is critical to reduce incidence
- According to the National Osteoporosis Foundation (NOF), over 10 million Americans have osteoporosis and another 34 million have low bone mass and therefore are at increased risks for the development of osteoporosis.

Demographics
- Children, disorder is rickets
- The elderly
- Individuals with absorption issues in the intestines

CLINICAL FINDINGS

SIGNS AND SYMPTOMS
- Known clinically as a "silent" disease, can be asymptomatic until fracture occurs
- Vertebral fractures may present as severe back pain or with no pain sensation noted
- Muscle weakness
- Hypocalcemia
- Bone pain, common in the hips
- Deformations of the vertebral spine and loss of height may present clinically as kyphosis or lordosis
- Hand and foot spasms
- Heart arrhythmia

Functional Implications
- Causes disability for aging and in elderly women and men.
- Approximately 20% of women and 30% to 50% of men with hip fractures secondary to osteoporosis die within 1 year of sustained fracture.[3,4]

Possible Contributing Causes
- Vitamin D deficiency
- Age (50 years and older)
- Gender (female > male)
- Kidney failure
- Liver disease
- Limited sun exposure
- Overuse of sun tan lotion with no sun exposure
- Cancer
- Menopause in women; low testosterone levels in men
- History of broken bones
- Consumption of alcohol or tobacco
- Poor dietary habits or eating disorders
- Lifestyle (sedentary versus active)
- Use of medications known to increase risk for fracture or bone mineral loss
- Certain comorbid diseases

Differential Diagnosis
- Trauma
- Pathologic fracture from neoplasm
- Osteogenesis imperfecta
- Inadequate mineralization of existing bone matrix (osteoid) or poor bone quality
- Paget disease
- Infections (such as tuberculosis)
- Fibrous dysplasia
- Peripheral neuropathy
- Repetitive stress fractures
- Multiple myeloma, lymphoma, or metastatic cancer
- Leukemia
- Renal osteodystrophy
- Hormone deficiency (estrogen in women; androgen in men)
- Cushing syndrome or glucocorticoid administration
- Hyperthyroidism
- Hyperparathyroidism
- History of drug abuse or misuse (alcohol, tobacco, excessive vitamin D/A)
- Juvenile osteoporosis occurs in children or young adults of both genders with normal gonadal function; onset typically occurs around age 8 to 14 years and hallmarks include rapid onset of bone pain and/or fracture secondary to trauma
- Type 1 (Postmenopausal Osteoporosis) typically occurs in women 50 to 65 years of age and is characterized by accelerated bone loss (trabecular bone)
- Type II (Age-Associated or Senile Osteoporosis) presents in women and men older than 70 years as a result of bone loss associated with the aging process; fractures occur in both cortical and trabecular bone

MEANS OF CONFIRMATION OR DIAGNOSIS

Laboratory Tests
- Blood calcium levels
- 24-hour urine calcium measurement
- Thyroid function test
- Parathyroid hormone levels
- Testosterone level (men)
- 25-Hydroxyvitamin D test
- Biochemical markers

Imaging
- Spinal and pelvic radiographs may demonstrate demineralization and vertebral compression and are commonly utilized to assess pathologies.
- Posterior, anterior, and lateral radiographs of affected areas of the spine are utilized to identify location and severity of fracture(s).
- Other modalities include single energy x-ray absorptiometry (SEXA), quantitative computed tomography (QCT), and radiographic absorptiometry.

Diagnostics Procedures
- Dual-energy X-ray absorptiometry (DEXA) is used to diagnose and confirm osteoporosis at both the axial and appendicular skeletons; DEXA delivers negligible radiation with a high degree of precision.
- Qualitative CT delivers more radiation but is also accurate in conformation.

FINDINGS AND INTERPRETATION
- Disability for aging and elderly women and men.
- Improved rates of screenings may help identify persons at an increased risk for fracture or low bone mineral density, which enables health care providers to educate the patient on healthy lifestyle changes and preventative strategies.

TREATMENT

Medication: Pain Management
- Nonsteroidal anti-inflammatory drugs (NSAIDs)
- Narcotics
- Topical pain relieving agents
- Nerve blocking injections

Medication: Stimulation of Bone Formation
- Bisphosphonates
- Vitamin D, phosphorus, and calcium supplement

▶ **Medication: Reduction of Bone Resorption**
- Bisphosphonates
- Estrogens
- Selective estradiol receptor modulators (SERMs)
- Calcitonin
- Calcium
- Human Monoclonal Antibody (Denosumab®)
- Thiazide diuretics
- Anabolic agents (Teriparatide®) if failed bisphosphonate therapy
- Parathyroid hormone

MEDICAL PROCEDURES

- Kyphoplasty
- Vertebroplasty
- Surgical (repair of fracture): Utilized to control pain

REFERRALS/ADMITTANCE

- Endocrinologists
- Family physicians or general practitioners
- Geriatricians
- Occupational therapists for ADL training
- Orthopedists for joint assessment
- Pharmacists for bone supplements
- Registered Dietitians for Nutrition
- Rheumatologists

IMPAIRMENTS

- Physical impairment
  - Chronic or recurrent pain or discomfort
  - Difficulty gripping or holding objects
  - Incomplete use of arms or fingers
  - Incomplete use of feet or legs
  - Disfigurement or deformity
- Activity limitations
  - Self-care
  - Mobility
  - Physical transport
  - Activities of Daily Living (ADLs)
  - Socialization and social activities
  - Work loss or employment restrictions
- Quality of Life (QoL) and Health-Related Quality of Life (HQoL)
- Environment and adjustments
  - Assistive devices
  - Home and occupational modifications
  - Family assistance

TESTS AND MEASURES

- X-ray
- Computer-assisted tomography (CT)
- Vertebral fracture assessment (VFA)
- Bone scan or radiography
- Diagnostic ultrasound (mobile community-based screening)

INTERVENTION

- Fall Risk Assessments: FRAX® score (10-year risk assessment)
- Therapeutic Exercise
- Progressive weight-bearing exercises, i.e., aquatic therapy
- Patient Education and Lifestyle Changes
- Moist heat/cryotherapy
- Ultrasound/phonophoresis/iontophoresis
- Transcutaneous electric nerve stimulation (TENS)
- Manual therapy/joint mobilization with precaution of bone density
- Soft-tissue massage
- Orthotics to decrease flexion forces and reduce pain or dysfunction

FUNCTIONAL GOALS

- Reduction in calcium loss
- Prevention of future fractures
- Adequate control of pain
- Prevention of disability
- Improves strength, flexibility, posture, and balance
- Decreases risks for falls

PROGNOSIS

- Reductions in bone pain may occur within 2 to 4 weeks of therapy, depending on appropriateness of pharmacologic therapy.
- High-risk patients are recommended to receive a DEXA scan every 2 to 3 years if the baseline is found to be normal; every 1 to 2 years if currently on pharmacotherapy.
- If from vitamin deficiency, can be reversible in 4 to 8 months for increased bone calcium.

PATIENT RESOURCE

- NIH Osteoporosis and Related Bone Diseases. Osteoporosis Handout on Health. Bethesda, MD: National Resource Center; 2011. http://www.niams.nih.gov/Health_Info/Bone/Osteoporosis/osteoporosis_hoh.asp. Accessed June 5, 2013.

REFERENCES

1. ICD9data. http://www.icd9data.com/2012/Volume1/710-739/730-739/733/733.00.htm. Accessed June 5, 2013.
2. APTA Guide to Physical Therapy Practice. http://guidetoptpractice.apta.org/search?fulltext=osteoporosis&submit=yes&x=0&y=0. Accessed July 7, 2013.
3. National Osteoporosis Foundation. *Clinician's Guide to Prevention and Treatment of Osteoporosis*. Washington, DC: National Osteoporosis Foundation; 2010. http://www.nof.org/professionals. Accessed June 5, 2013.
4. Jacobs-Kosmin D. Osteoporosis. In: Diamond HS, ed. 23 Sept. *2011 Medscape*. http://emedicine.medscape.com/article/330598-overview. Accessed June 5, 2013.
5. International Osteoporosis Foundation. Osteoporosis. http://www.iofbonehealth.org. Accessed June 5, 2013.

ADDITIONAL REFERENCES

- Chandrasoma P, Taylor CR. Metabolic bone disease. In: Chandrasoma P, Taylor CR, eds. *Concise Pathology*. 3rd ed. New York, NY: McGraw-Hill; 2011. http://www.accessphysiotherapy.com/content/193568. Accessed June 5, 2013.

- Dutton M. Metabolic disease. In: Dutton M, ed. *Orthopaedic Examination, Evaluation, and Intervention*. 2nd ed. New York, NY: McGraw-Hill; 2008. http://www.accessphysiotherapy.com/content/5546939. Accessed June 5, 2013.
- McPhee SJ, Hammer GD. Pathophysiology of selected disorders of calcium metabolism. In: McPhee SJ, Hammer GD, eds. *Pathophysiology of Disease*. 6th ed. New York, NY: McGraw-Hill; 2010. http://www.accessphysiotherapy.com/content/5370820. Accessed June 5, 2013.
- Rahman N, Bhatia K. Impairments and disability associated with arthritis and osteoporosis. Arthritis series No4. Cat. no. PHE 90. Canberra: AIHW. 2007 http://www.aihw.gov.au/publication-detail/?id=6442468025. Accessed June 5, 2013.

135 OSTEOPOROSIS

Angela S. Garcia, PharmD, MPH, CPh
Eric Shamus, PhD, DPT, PT, CSCS

CONDITION/DISORDER SYNONYM

- Brittle Bones

ICD-9-CM CODES

- 733.0 Osteoporosis
- 733.00 Osteoporosis unspecified
- 733.01 Senile osteoporosis
- 733.02 Idiopathic osteoporosis
- 733.03 Disuse osteoporosis
- 733.09 Other osteoporosis

ICD-10-CM CODES

- M81.0 Age-related osteoporosis without current pathologic fracture
- M81.8 Other osteoporosis without current pathologic fracture

PREFERRED PRACTICE PATTERNS

- 4A: Primary Prevention/Risk Reduction for Skeletal Demineralization
- 4B: Impaired Posture
- 4C: Impaired Muscle Performance
- 4F: Impaired Joint Mobility, Motor Function, Muscle Performance, ROM and Reflex Integrity Association with Spinal Disorders
- 4G: Impaired Joint Mobility, Muscle Performance, and ROM Associated with Fracture

PATIENT PRESENTATION

The patient is a 72-year-old woman who is having mid-thoracic pain after a coughing bout. The patient is having a dull ache pain that is constant. Upon X-rays, thoracic compression fractures are found. The patient received kyphoplasty surgery. Physical therapy treatment followed by progressive weight-bearing exercises.

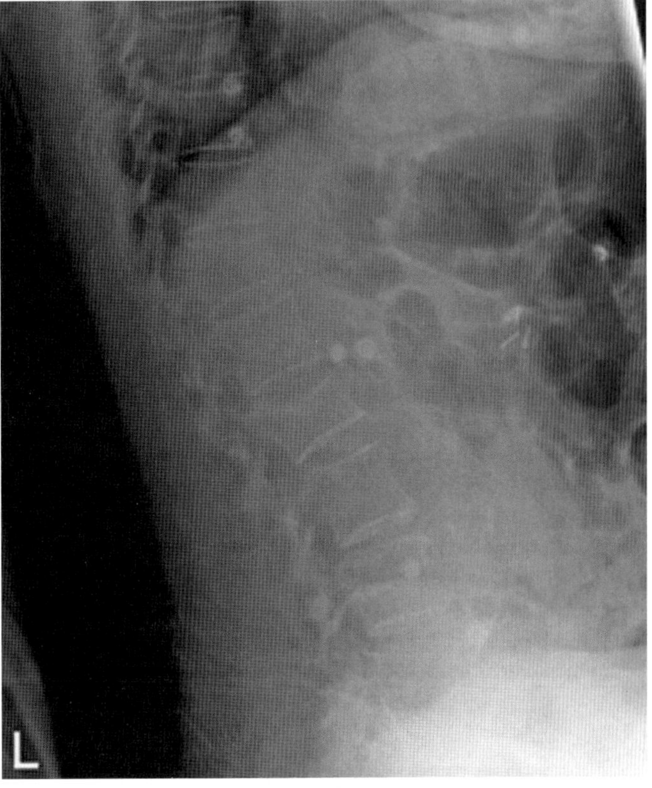

FIGURE 135-1 A lateral view radiograph in this 75-year-old woman reveals significant loss of bone density as the upper lumbar and lower thoracic vertebral bodies are almost radiolucent. Also note the compression fractures present at T12 and L2. (From Malone TR, Hazle C, Grey ML. *Imaging in Rehabilitation.* www.accessmedicine.com. Copyright © The McGraw-Hill Companies, Inc. All rights reserved.)

KEY FEATURES

- Deterioration of bone mass and density with a marked decrease in cortical thickness and cancellous bone trabeculae, which leads to increased fragility, deformity, and/or fracture.
- Osteoporosis is initially categorized by etiology and skeletal localization then further divided into primary and secondary classifications.
- Considered both a progressive and chronic disease with primary prevention tied to childhood bone health and reduced risk factors (skeletal and nonskeletal).
- Primary osteoporosis
  - Type 1: Postmenopausal osteoporosis
  - Type 2: Age-associated (senile) osteoporosis
  - Idiopathic osteoporosis (juvenile, premenopausal women, middle-aged men)
- Secondary osteoporosis (identifiable cause of bone loss)
  - Underlying disease, deficiency, or drug induced
- The operational definition of osteoporosis by the World Health Organization (WHO) is bone density that falls 2.5 standard deviations (SDs) or more below the mean for a young healthy same sex adult; referred to as a *T*-score of −2.5.
- Bone mineral density (BMD) measurements are related to both peak bone mass and bone loss.
- Bone densitometry: Normal BMD within 1 SD of the mean; *T*-score at −1.0 and greater.
- Bone densitometry: Low BMD (referred to as osteopenia) occurs between 1 and 2.5 SDs below the mean; *T*-score between −1.0 and −2.5.
- Increased fracture propensity due to demineralization secondary to osteoporosis; often occurs at the spine, hips, pelvis, or wrist.
- As a comorbid condition, low levels of serum 25-hydroxyvitamin D are noted.
- Accurate patient and family medical histories and early recognition through physical examination may lead to improved therapeutic outcomes.

- 10-year risk for fracture can be measured through Fracture Risk Assessments (FRAX® score).
- Pharmacotherapy can be measured through changes in laboratory values.
- Osteoporosis is considered a major public health problem of the elderly, especially postmenopausal women.
- Lifetime osteoporosis-related fracture will be experienced by 50% of all women and 25% of all men over age 50.[1–4]
- Persons with low BMD are at an increased risk for the development of osteoporosis; prevention is critical to reduce incidence.
- According to the National Osteoporosis Foundation (NOF), over 10 million Americans have osteoporosis and another 34 million have low BMD, and therefore at increased risks for the development of osteoporosis.[1–4]
- Osteoporosis is the cause of approximately 1.5 million fractures per year, with 80% occurring in women and 20% occurring in men.
- Recovery to prefracture levels of activity and function are estimated to be only 33% of all sustained fractures.
- More than 50% of fractures among postmenopausal women, including hip fractures, are secondary to low BMD.
- Juvenile osteoporosis occurs in children or young adults of both genders with normal gonadal function; onset typically occurs around age 8 to 14 years and hallmarks include rapid onset of bone pain and/or fracture secondary to trauma.
- Type I (postmenopausal osteoporosis) typically occurs in women 50 to 65 years of age and is characterized by accelerated bone loss (trabecular bone).
- Type II (age-associated or senile osteoporosis) presents in women and men older than 70 years as a result of bone loss associated

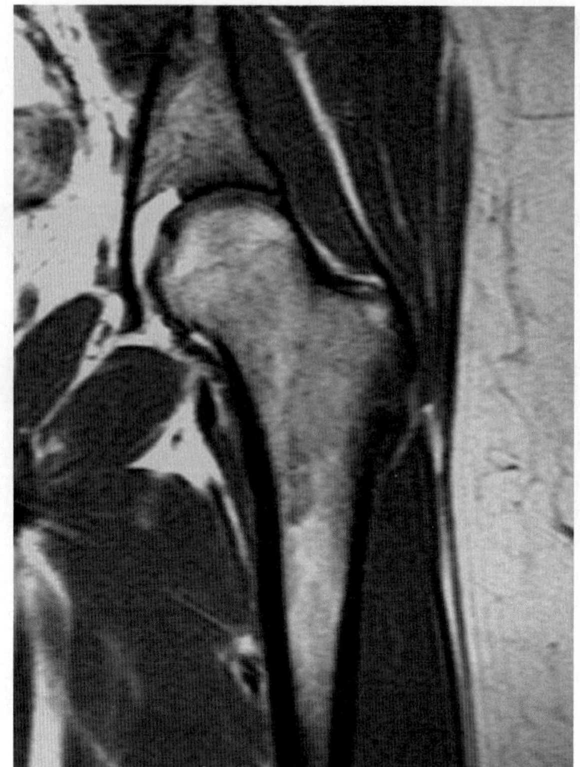

FIGURE 135-2 A coronal section of a T1-weighted MRI revealing decreased signal intensity consistent with transient osteoporosis in a 23-year-old woman. (From Malone TR, Hazle C, Grey ML. *Imaging in Rehabilitation*. www.accessmedicine.com. Copyright © The McGraw-Hill Companies, Inc. All rights reserved.)

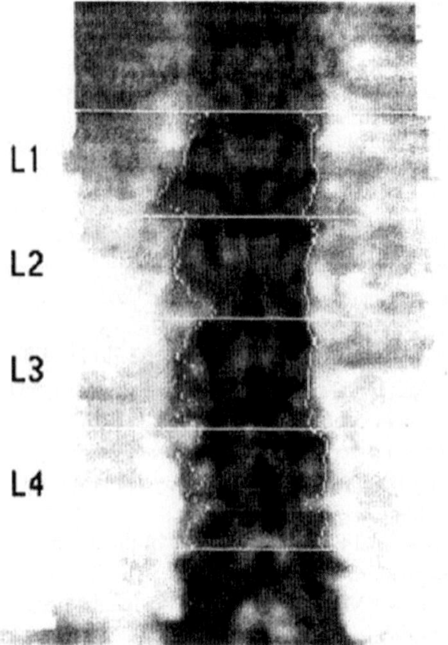

Image not for diagnosis
3.00ma:Hi-Res Fast DPXIQ 0.6x1.2mm 1.68mm
743381:435225 276.30:205.49:146.42
%Fat = 30.2(1.332)

L2-L4 Comparison to Reference

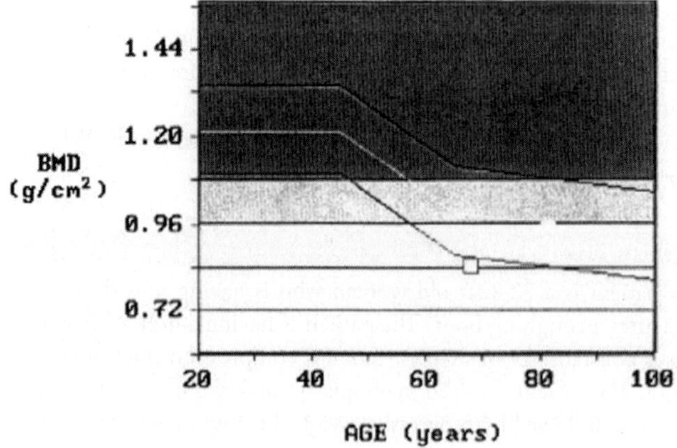

Region	BMD[1,7] g/cm²	Young-Adult[2] %	Young-Adult[2] T	Age-Matched[3] %	Age-Matched[3] Z
L2-L4	0.844	70	-3.0	86	-1.2

FIGURE 135-3 An example of a dual-energy X-ray absorptiometry (DEXA) report. Note the *T*-score value of 3.0, which is categorized as osteoporosis according to the World Health Organization definition. (From Malone TR, Hazle C, Grey ML. *Imaging in Rehabilitation*. www.accessmedicine.com. Copyright © The McGraw-Hill Companies, Inc. All rights reserved.)

with the aging process; fractures occur in both cortical and trabecular bones.
- Although osteoporosis occurs in all races and ethnicities, increased risk and incidence are documented for whites and Asians; approximately 20% are estimated to have osteoporosis and another 52% to have low BMD.
- Approximately 1:3 women and 1:5 men over the age of 50 years will experience osteoporotic fractures, with worldwide estimates projected to increase over 200-fold by 2050.

CLINICAL FINDINGS

SIGNS AND SYMPTOMS

- Known clinically as a "silent" disease, osteoporosis is asymptomatic until fracture occurs.
- Vertebral fractures may present as severe back pain or with no pain sensation noted.
- Deformations of the vertebral spine and loss of height may present clinically as kyphosis or lordosis.

Functional Implications

- One of the leading causes of disability for aging and elderly women and men.
- Approximately 20% of women and 30% to 50% of men with hip fractures secondary to osteoporosis die within 1 year of sustained fracture.[1–3]

Possible Contributing Causes

- Age (50 years and greater)
- Gender (female > male)
- Menopause in women; low testosterone levels in men
- History of broken bones or osteoporosis (personal and family)
- Consumption of alcohol or tobacco
- Poor dietary habits or eating disorders
- Lifestyle (sedentary vs. active)
- Use of medications known to increase risk for fracture or bone mineral loss
- Certain comorbid diseases

Differential Diagnoses

- Trauma
- Pathologic fracture from neoplasm
- Osteomalacia or rickets
- Osteogenesis imperfecta
- Inadequate mineralization of existing bone matrix (osteoid) or poor bone quality
- Paget disease
- Infections, such as tuberculosis
- Fibrous dysplasia
- Peripheral neuropathy
- Repetitive stress fractures
- Multiple myeloma, lymphoma, or metastatic cancer
- Leukemia
- Renal osteodystrophy
- Hormone deficiency (estrogen in women; androgen in men)
- Cushing syndrome or glucocorticoid administration
- Hyperthyroidism
- Hyperparathyroidism
- History of drug abuse or misuse (alcohol, tobacco)
- Excessive vitamin D/A

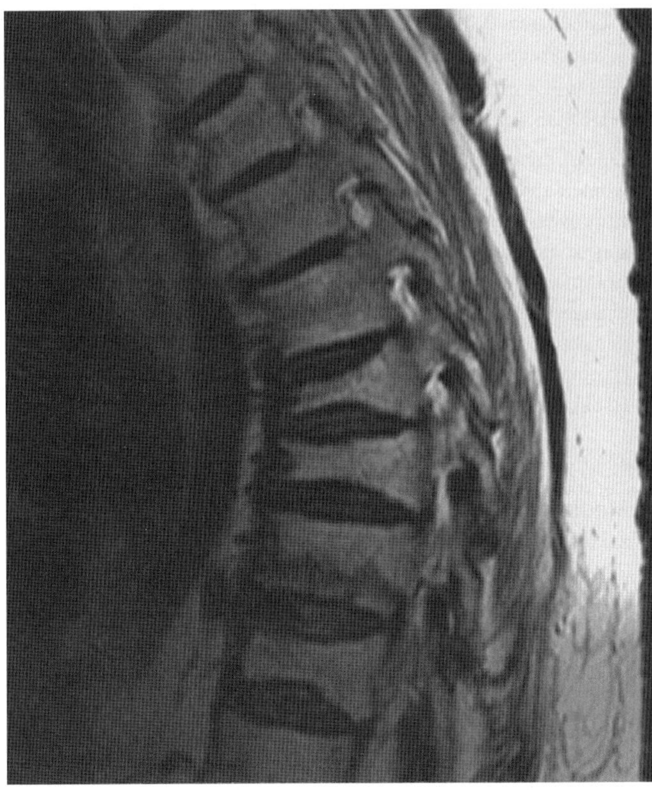

FIGURE 135-4 This T1-weighted MR demonstrates collapse of the vertebrae as associated with osteoporotic fractures. (From Malone TR, Hazle C, Grey ML. *Imaging in Rehabilitation.* www.accessmedicine.com. Copyright © The McGraw-Hill Companies, Inc. All rights reserved.)

MEANS OF CONFIRMATION OR DIAGNOSIS

Laboratory Tests

- 24-hour urine calcium measurement
- 25-Hydroxyvitamin D test
- Biochemical markers
- Blood calcium levels
- Parathyroid hormone levels
- Testosterone level (men)
- Thyroid function test

Imaging

- X-ray
- Computer-assisted tomography (CT)
- Vertebral fracture assessment (VFA)
- Bone scan
- Diagnostic Ultrasound (mobile community-based screening)
- Spinal and pelvic X-rays may demonstrate demineralization, vertebral compression
- Posterior, anterior, and lateral X-rays of affected areas of the spine are utilized to identify location and severity of fracture(s)
- MRI of the area of possible infection
- Single-energy X-ray absorptiometry (SXA); quantitative computed tomography (QCT); radiographic absorptiometry (RA)

Diagnostic Procedures

- Dual-energy X-ray absorptiometry (DEXA) is used to diagnose and confirm osteoporosis at both the axial and appendicular skeleton; delivers negligible radiation with a high degree of precision

- Qualitative CT delivers more radiation, but is also accurate in conformation.

FINDINGS AND INTERPRETATION

- One of the leading causes of disability for aging and elderly women and men.
- Improved rates of osteoporosis screenings may help identify persons at an increased risk for fracture or low BMD, which enables health care providers to educate the patient on healthy lifestyle changes and preventative strategies to decrease the onset of osteopenia and eventual development osteoporosis.
- Normal values are usually found for serum parathyroid hormone (PTH), calcium, phosphorus, and alkaline phosphatase.

TREATMENT

Medication

- Pain management
  - NSAIDs
  - Narcotics
  - Topical pain relieving agents
  - Nerve blocking injections
- Stimulation of bone formation
  - Bisphosphonates
  - Vitamin D
- Reduction of bone resorption
  - Bisphosphonates
  - Estrogens
  - Selective estrogen receptor modulators (SERMs)
  - Calcitonin
  - Calcium
  - Human monoclonal antibody (Denosumab)
  - Thiazide diuretics
  - Anabolic agents (Teriparatide*) if failed bisphosphonate therapy
  - PTH

MEDICAL PROCEDURES

- Kyphoplasty
- Vertebroplasty
- Surgical (repair of fracture): Utilized for pain control

REFERRALS/ADMITTANCE

- To endocrinologist
- To general practitioner
- To geriatrician
- To orthopedist for joint assessment
- To rheumatologist
- To pharmacist for bone supplements
- To occupational therapist for ADL training
- To registered dietitian for nutrition education

IMPAIRMENTS

- Physical impairments
  - Chronic or recurrent pain or discomfort
  - Difficulty gripping or holding objects
  - Incomplete use of arms or fingers
  - Incomplete use of feet or legs
  - Disfigurement or deformity

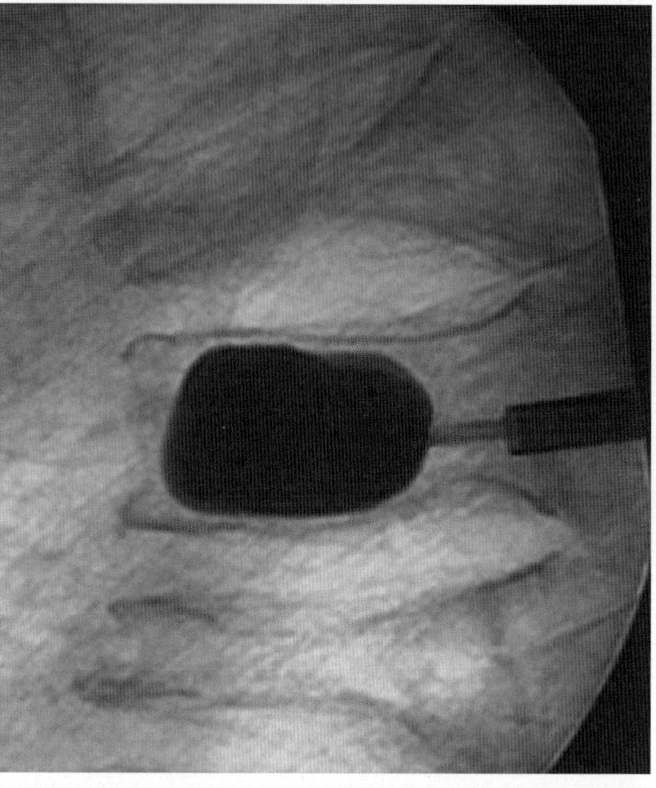

FIGURE 135-5 In this image, captured during the kyphoplasty procedure, a balloon is enlarged within the vertebral body to reverse the wedging. The vertebral body is then stabilized by injection of polymethyl methacrylate within the cavity formed by the balloon. Note the reduction in wedging with expansion of the balloon. (From Malone TR, Hazle C, Grey ML. *Imaging in Rehabilitation*. www.accessmedicine.com. Copyright © The McGraw-Hill Companies, Inc. All rights reserved.)

- Activity limitations
  - Self-care
  - Mobility
  - Physical transport
  - ADLs
  - Socialization and social activities
  - Work loss or employment restrictions
- Environment and adjustments
  - Assistive devices
  - Home and occupational modifications
  - Family assistance

TESTS AND MEASURES

- Fall Risk Assessment Tool: FRAT
- Quality of Life (QoL) and Health-Related Quality of Life (HQoL)

INTERVENTION

- Therapeutic exercise
- Progressive weight-bearing exercises, for example, aquatic therapy
- Patient education and lifestyle changes
- Moist heat/cryotherapy
- Ultrasound/phonophoresis/iontophoresis
- Transcutaneous electric nerve stimulation (TENS)
- Cervical and lumbar traction
- Manual therapy/joint mobilization with precaution of bone density
- Soft-tissue massage
- Orthotics to decrease flexion forces and reduce pain or dysfunction

FUNCTIONAL GOALS

- Reduction in bone loss for the prevention of future fractures
- Adequate control of pain in the prevention of disability
- Improves strength, flexibility, posture, and balance to decrease the risks for falls

PROGNOSIS

- Osteoporosis is not curable, but has a good prognosis when fracture is decreased through pharmacotherapy and reduction in risk factors.
- Progressive osteopenia can be reversed if caught early through screenings and assessment of risk factors, which may lead to a decrease in the incidence of osteoporosis.
- Reductions in bone pain may occur within 2 to 4 weeks of therapy, depending on appropriateness of pharmacologic therapy (combinations of pain and antiresorptive agents).
- Approximately 20% of women and 30% to 50% of men with hip fractures secondary to osteoporosis die within 1 year of sustained fracture.
- High-risk patients are recommended to receive a DEXA scan every 2 to 3 years (if the baseline is found to be normal); every 1 to 2 years if currently on pharmacotherapy.

PATIENT RESOURCES

- National Osteoporosis Foundation. *Clinician's Guide to Prevention and Treatment of Osteoporosis.* Washington, DC: National Osteoporosis Foundation; 2010. http://www.nof.org/professionals. Accessed July 7, 2013.
- Osteoporosis Handout on Health (NIH Publication No. 11-5158). NIH Osteoporosis and Related Bone Diseases Resource Center; 2011. Bethesda, MD. http://www.niams.nih.gov/Health_Info/Bone/Osteoporosis/osteoporosis_hoh.asp. Accessed July 7, 2013.

REFERENCES

1. National Osteoporosis Foundation. *Clinician's Guide to Prevention and Treatment of Osteoporosis.* Washington, DC: National Osteoporosis Foundation; 2010. http://www.nof.org/professionals. Accessed July 7, 2013.
2. Jacobs-Kosmin D, Shanmugam S. Osteoporosis. In: Diamond HS, ed. *eMedicine Medscape Reference website.* Published 23 September 2011. http://emedicine.medscape.com/article/330598-overview. Accessed July 7, 2013.
3. Osteoporosis Handout on Health (NIH Publication No. 11-5158). NIH Osteoporosis and Related Bone Diseases Resource Center; 2011. Bethesda, MD. http://www.niams.nih.gov/Health_Info/Bone/Osteoporosis/osteoporosis_hoh.asp. Accessed July 7, 2013.
4. Osteoporosis. MDGuidelines website. http://www.mdguidelines.com/osteoporosis. Published 2008. Accessed July 7, 2013.

ADDITIONAL REFERENCES

- APTA Guide to Physical Therapy Practice. http://guidetoptpractice.apta.org/search?fulltext=osteoporosis&submit=yes&x=0&y=0. Accessed July 7, 2013.
- ICD9DATA.com. http://www.icd9data.com/2012/Volume1/710-739/730-739/733/733.00.htm. Accessed July 7, 2013.
- International Osteoporosis Foundation website. About osteoporosis. http://www.iofbonehealth.org/health-professionals/about-osteoporosis.html. Accessed July 7, 2013.
- Rahman N, Bhatia K. Impairments and disability associated with arthritis and osteoporosis. Arthritis Series No. 4. Cat. no. PHE 90. Canberra: Australian Institute of Health and Welfare (AIHW); 2007. http://www.aihw.gov.au/publication-detail/?id=6442468025. Accessed July 7, 2013.

136 PIRIFORMIS SYNDROME

Stephen A. Black, DSc, MEd, PT, ATC, CSCS
Eric Shamus, PhD, DPT, PT, CSCS

CONDITION/DISORDER SYNONYMS

- Deep gluteal syndrome
- Fat wallet syndrome
- Hip lateral rotator tendinitis
- Hip lateral rotator tendinosis
- Sciatic nerve impingement with (out) inflammation
- Wallet sciatica

ICD-9-CM CODE

- 355.0 Lesion of sciatic nerve

ICD-10-CM CODE

- G57.00 Lesion of sciatic nerve, unspecified lower limb

PREFERRED PRACTICE PATTERN

- 4E: Impaired Joint Mobility, Motor Function, Muscle Performance, and ROM Associated with Localized Inflammation

PATIENT PRESENTATION

A 27-year-old woman presenting with complaints of left ischial/hip pain with sciatic radiation of the pain. She reports that the pain has been present for approximately 5 months with onset following a 13-mile run in older running shoes. Since the onset of symptoms, the ischial/hip pain has not decreased in intensity. The sciatic pain radiation has also not improved, however has not progressed or moved further distally.

Since the onset of symptoms she has had extensive medical workup, including an MRI and CT scan that were both negative for lumbar radiculopathy. Her primary complaints of pain are with sitting (especially while driving) or prolonged standing. There is relief of symptoms when lying down. She has modified but continued her daily workouts including 30 minutes on the stair master and runs of 6 miles or less, despite her persistent pain. She admits poor or absent stretching habits and frequently returns to her sedentary work routine immediately following exercise. Observation of lower extremity alignment reveals excessive femoral external rotation, lateral tibial torsion, and excessive pronation of both feet. There is tenderness in the left buttock region between the sacrum and the greater trochanter. Active range of motion (AROM) is within normal limits (WNL) for the lumbar spine. Hip AROM is limited in internal rotation.

KEY FEATURES

Description

- Neuropathic pain from compression of the sciatic nerve as it courses through the piriformis muscle or myofascial pain from a

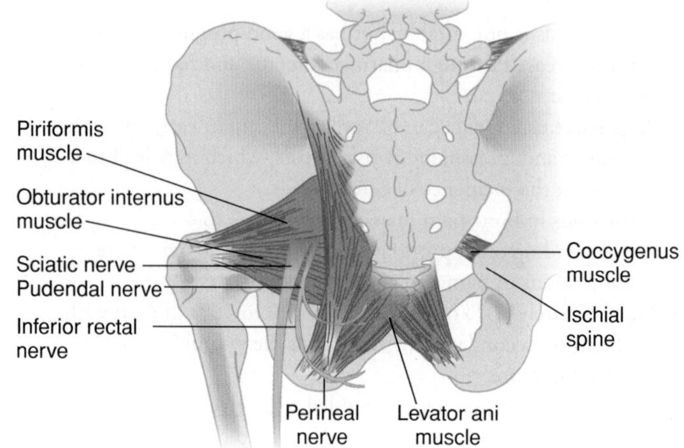

FIGURE 136-1 Proximity of the piriformis muscle and the sciatic nerve. (Reproduced with permission from Simon RR, Sherman SC, Koenigsknecht SJ. *Emergency Orthopedics, The Extremities*. 5th ed. © 2007, McGraw-Hill Inc., New York.)

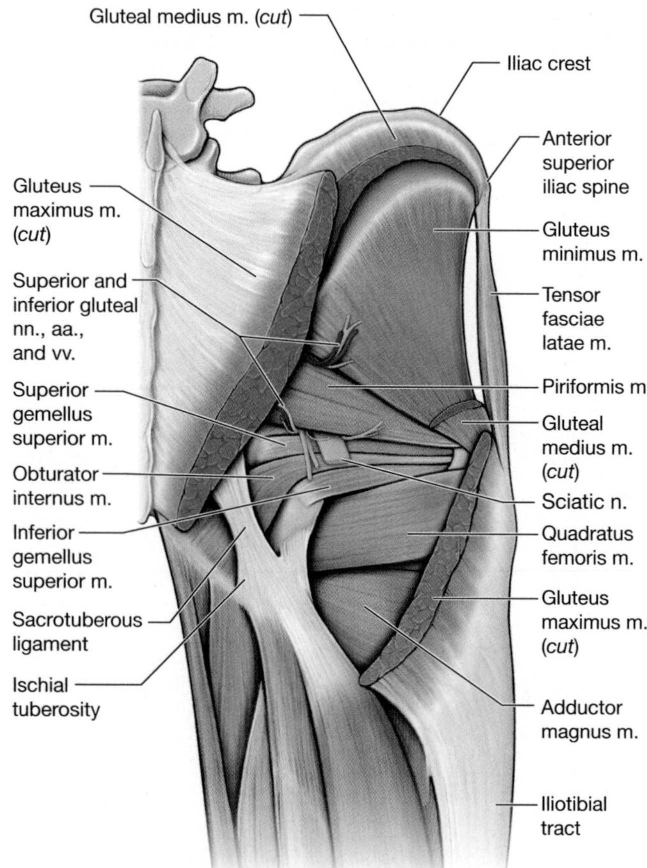

FIGURE 136-2 Deeper muscles of the posterior hip. (Reproduced, with permission, from Morton DA, Foreman KB, Albertine KH. *The Big Picture: Gross Anatomy*. McGraw-Hill, 2011.)

tight, hypertrophic, and tender piriformis without nerve entrapment
- Major muscles at the posterior hip function together based on how much the hip is flexed
  - Gluteals
  - Piriformis
  - Gemelli
  - Obturator internus
  - Quadratus femoris
- These muscles are usually involved whenever there is low back pain or a lower extremity problem that requires compensation of motion
- The sciatic nerve may even pass through the piriformis (17% of an assumed normal population)

Essentials of Diagnosis

- Diagnosis usually made by patient history and clinical examination
- Most often an independent diagnosis
- Must be isolated from gluteus medius, other hip lateral rotators, and sciatic nerve impingement
- Positive FAIR test

General Considerations

- Anatomic variations of the divisions of the sciatic nerve above, below, and through the belly of the piriformis muscle may be causative factors.
- The piriformis is routinely implicated in cases of sciatica, although it is only one of several muscles in this area that cause sciatica.

Demographics

- Higher incidence in females (6:1)

CLINICAL FINDINGS

SIGNS AND SYMPTOMS

- Pain and instability are often imprecise, but often present in the hip, coccyx, buttock, groin, or distal part of the affected leg.
- Tingling/numbness in the affected buttock: May be present with sitting on the toilet, bleachers, or narrow bicycle seat.
- Pain with forced hip external rotation.

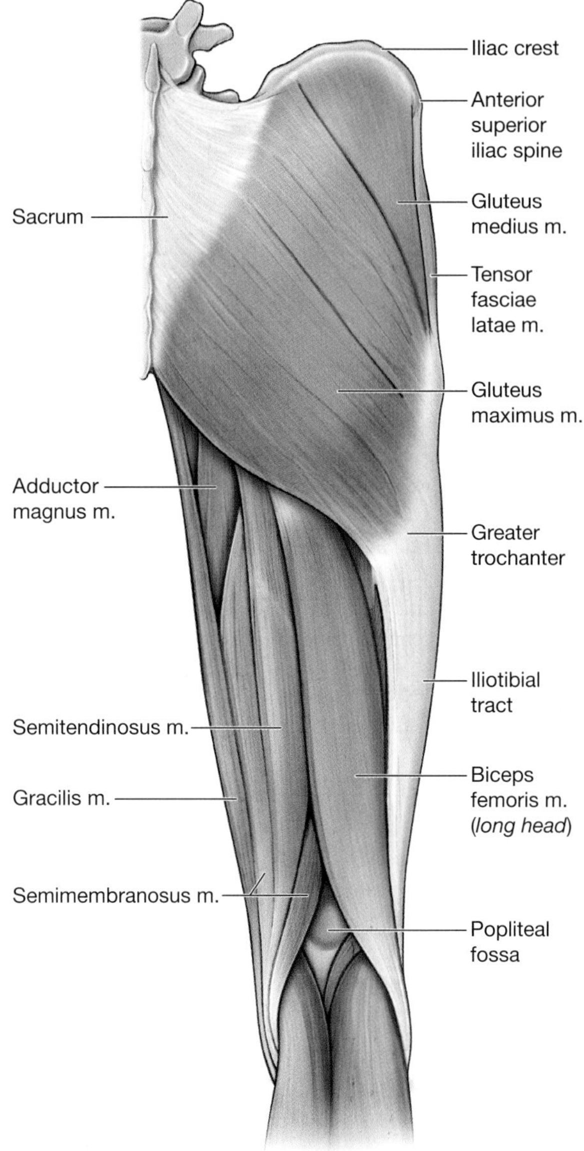

FIGURE 136-3 Superficial muscles of the posterior hip. (Reproduced, with permission, from Morton DA, Foreman KB, Albertine KH. *The Big Picture: Gross Anatomy*. McGraw-Hill, 2011.)

Functional Implications

- Pain on ambulation/running with uncompensated pronation
- Increased pain with increased activity or prolonged sitting

Possible Contributing Causes

- Prolonged sitting (occupational, driving, flying, etc., for long periods)
- Activities requiring extensive and repetitive lateral hip rotation
- Compensatory foot biomechanics (increased locomotor pronation)
- Athletes
  - Skiers (Classic Nordic or skate skiing)
  - Long-distance cyclists
  - Tennis players
- Spinal stenosis (can lead to bilateral piriformis tenderness)
- Shortened sacrotuberous and or sacrospinous/iliolumbar ligaments
- Trauma to the buttocks or gluteal region
- Pregnancy
  - Postural changes
  - Increased weight
  - Change in foot biomechanics during ambulation
- Accessory piriformis muscle fibers
- Attachment of the piriformis to the sacrotuberous ligament
- Hypertrophy of the piriformis
- Muscle imbalance of strength and flexibility of hip internal rotators and external rotators
- Obturator internus dysfunction
- Trauma
- Anatomical anomalies

Differential Diagnoses

- Spinal disc herniation
- Ischial bursitis
- Sacroiliitis
- Gluteal/Hip pain
- Pseudosciatica
- Spinal stenosis

MEANS OF CONFIRMATION OR DIAGNOSIS

Imaging

- CT scan
- X-ray or leg length
- EMG
- MRI to identify anatomical anomalies that may lead to sciatic or lumbosacral nerve root compression
- Diagnostic ultrasound to reveal nerve entrapment of the sciatic nerve either:
  - Where the sciatic nerve passes through the piriformis muscle
  - Where the sciatic nerve passes under the piriformis muscle and over the gemellus superior muscle

Diagnostic Procedures

- Nerve block to determine involvement and relief of symptoms

FINDINGS AND INTERPRETATION

- MRI can show
  - Accessory piriformis muscle fibers
  - Attachment of the piriformis to the sacrotuberous ligament
  - Hypertrophy of the piriformis
  - Tumor
- X-ray: Ipsilateral short leg

TREATMENT

Medication

- Oral: Analgesic, nonsteroidal anti-inflammatory drugs (NSAIDs)
- Injection: Corticosteroid, botulinum toxin

MEDICAL PROCEDURES

- Guided/unguided injection
  - Fluoroscopy
  - Diagnostic ultrasound

REFERRALS/ADMITTANCE

- To radiologist for X-ray

IMPAIRMENTS

- Antalgic gait secondary to
  - Weak gluteus medius, hip lateral rotators
  - Decreased flexibility of the hip lateral rotators
  - Decreased flexibility of the hip flexors, adductors, and internal rotators
  - Increased compensatory pronation
- Inability to ambulate distances of ≥100 yards secondary to pain
- Inability to sit for more than >30 minutes secondary to pain
- Inability to participate in sports/activities of choice

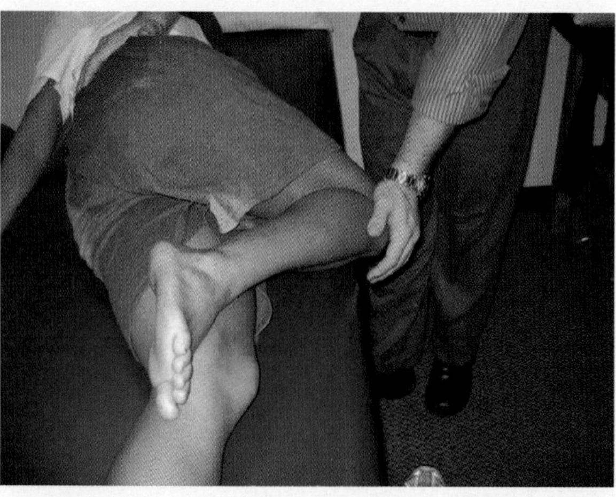

FIGURE 136-4 Piriformis test. The athlete lies on the side with affected leg up. The hip is flexed to 60 degrees with knee flexed. The examiner stabilizes the hip with one hand while applying downward stress to the knee. Pain deep in the buttock or sciatica-type symptoms will be elicited in piriformis syndrome. (From Patel DR, Greydanus DE, Baker RJ. *Pediatric Practice: Sports Medicine.* www.accesspediatrics.com. Copyright © The McGraw-Hill Companies, Inc. All rights reserved.)

TESTS AND MEASURES

- Beatty maneuver: Raising of the knee several centimeters off the table while side-lying on the contralateral side
- FABER (Patrick) test: Positive
- FAIR test: Supine passive flexion, adduction, and internal rotation (FAIR) position by the examiner reproduces symptoms[1]
- Freiberg sign/maneuver: Pain with forced internal rotation of the flexed thigh
- Mirkin test: Pressure into the buttocks where the sciatic nerve crosses the piriformis muscle while the patient slowly bends to the floor
- Pace sign/maneuver: Abduction of the affected leg while sitting
- Piriformis test
- Reflexes
- Sensory
- Weak gluteus maximus, gluteus medius, biceps femoris

INTERVENTION

- Modified activity relative to frequency, intensity, and duration
- Dry needling
- Advise patient to carry billfold or large objects in side pocket, if carried at all
- Orthotics derived for subtalar neutral impression to accommodate compensatory pronation
- Kinesio taping techniques to facilitate hip flexion and lateral rotation
- Modalities inclusive of ultrasound, electric stimulation, cold laser, ice/cryotherapy
- Addressing lack of flexibility
  - Modified yoga pose (pigeon)
  - Yoga "frog" pose
  - Supine FAIR stretch either by the patient as a home exercise or by the clinician to increase mobility of the piriformis
  - Addressing additional shortening found through manual examination
- Addressing mobilization
  - Active release techniques for
    - Piriformis
    - Gemellus superior

        - Gluteus medius
        - Psoas
        - Iliolumbar/sacrotuberous and sacrospinous ligaments
    - Nerve glides for all points of sciatic encroachment
    - Graston technique to the piriformis and related structures
    - Mobilization techniques for the sacroiliac joint
    - Advise patient in the use of self-mobilization devices
- Foam roller
- The® Stick
- Appropriate size/density ball (e.g., tennis ball)
- Addressing weakness
    - Side-lying abduction with the hip and knee in 90-degree flexion
    - Quadruped hydrant exercise
    - Supine bridge bilateral
    - Progressive limb loading 2
    - Progressive limb loading 3
    - Unilateral supine bridge with progression to physioball bilateral to unilateral

FUNCTIONAL GOALS

- Patient will be able to
    - Stand and ambulate with symmetrical weight-bearing for 30 minutes
    - Drive pain free for 1 hour
    - Mount/dismount the toilet pain-free.
    - Actively perform the supine FAIR position pain-free.

PROGNOSIS

- Very good, although without comprehensive care may result in severe pain, secondary complication, and require surgical intervention.

PATIENT RESOURCE

- Boyajian-O'Neill LA, McClain Rl, Coleman MK, Thomas PP. Diagnosis and Management of piriformis syndrome: an osteopathic approach. *J Am Osteopath Assoc.* 2008;108:657–664.

REFERENCE

1. Kean Chen C, Nizar AJ. Prevalence of piriformis syndrome in chronic low back pain patients. A clinical diagnosis with modified FAIR test. *Pain Pract.* 2013;13(4):276–281.

ADDITIONAL REFERENCES

- Betts A. Combined fluoroscopic and nerve stimulator techniques for injection of the piriformis muscle. *Pain Physician.* 2004;7(2):279–281.
- Dutton M. Common orthopedic conditions. In: Dutton M, ed. *Dutton's Orthopedic Survival Guide: Managing Common Conditions.* New York, NY: McGraw-Hill; 2011. http://www.accessphysiotherapy.com/content/8654096. Accessed July 1, 2013.
- Dutton M. Muscle length tests. In: Dutton M, ed. *McGraw-Hill's NPTE (National Physical Therapy Examination)2e.* New York, NY: McGraw-Hill; 2012. http://www.accessphysiotherapy.com/content/5398271. Accessed July 1, 2013.
- Dutton M. Muscles. In: Dutton M, ed. *Dutton's Orthopaedic Examination, Evaluation, and Intervention.* 3rd ed. New York, NY: McGraw-Hill; 2012. http://www.accessphysiotherapy.com/content/55597817. Accessed July 1, 2013.
- Fishman LM, Dombi GW, Michaelson C, et al. Piriformis syndrome: diagnosis, treatment and outcome—a 10-year study. *Arch Phys Med Rehab.* 2002;83(3):295–301.
- Kirschner JS, Foye PM, Cole JL. Piriformis syndrome, diagnosis, and treatment. *Muscle Nerve.* 2009;40(1);10–18.
- Patel DR, Lyne ED, Bancroft S. Chapter 25. Overuse Injuries of the Hip, Pelvis, and Thigh. In: Patel DR, Greydanus DE, Baker RJ, eds. *Pediatric Practice: Sports Medicine.* New York, NY: McGraw-Hill; 2009. http://www.accessphysiotherapy.com/content/6979587. Accessed July 6, 2013.
- Robinson DR. Piriformis syndrome: the relation to sciatic pain. *Am J Surg.* 1947;73(3):355–358.

137 PUBALGIA-OSTEITIS PUBIS

Patrick Pabian, DPT, SCS, OCS

CONDITION/DISORDER SYNONYMS

- Pubalgia
- Athletic pubalgia
- Pelvic sprain
- Osteitis pubis

ICD-9-CM CODE[1]

- 848.5 Sprain of pelvic

ICD-10-CM CODE[2]

- S33.8XXA Sprain of other parts of lumbar spine and pelvis, initial encounter

PREFERRED PRACTICE PATTERN[3]

- 4E: Impaired Joint Mobility, Motor Function, Muscle Performance, and Range of Motion Associated with Localized Inflammation

PATIENT PRESENTATION

A 23-year-old woman presents with pain in her lower abdomen and groin that has been present for the past week. She reports initiation of kickboxing classes 2 months ago. She notes pain increases with participation in the classes and some relief with rest. She has difficulty rising from deep squat positions and rising from a chair when there is pain and weakness. She has also noted an inability to perform sit-ups when the pain is present. The patient has tenderness to palpation of the pubic tubercles bilaterally, and adductor insertions on the superior pubic rami. She has negative tenderness to McBurney point, and no palpable masses in the lower abdomen or along the inguinal ligament bilaterally.

KEY FEATURES

Description

- Pubalgia-osteitis pubis is a collective term that refers to disorders causing chronic pubic pain.
- Pubalgia-osteitis pubis includes osteitis pubis and athletic pubalgia, which are overuse conditions involving stress to the pubic symphysis.
- All conditions result in abnormal stress to the pubic bone, pubic tubercle, or pubic symphysis.
- Symptoms due to increased mechanical stress in the pubic region due to abnormalities or stress from osseous, ligamentous, or muscular structures.
- Symptoms typically reduce with light activity, but worsen with exertion.

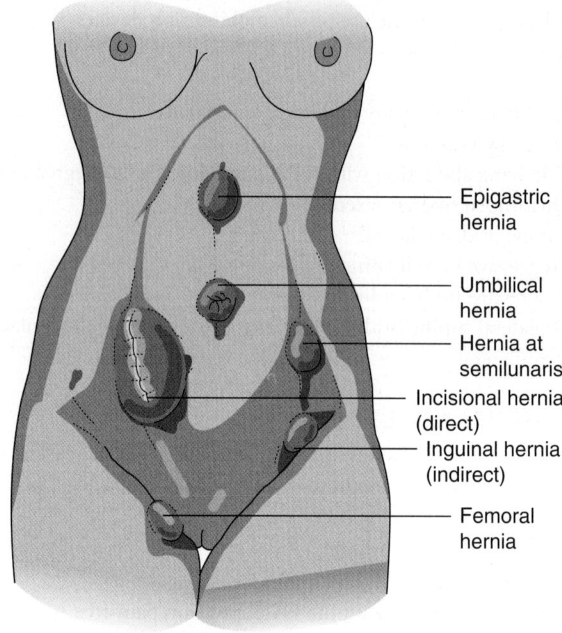

FIGURE 137-1 Hernia sites. (From DeCherney AH, Nathan L, Murphy Goodwin T, Laufer N, Roman AS. *Current Diagnosis & Treatment: Obstetrics & Gynecology*. 11th ed. www.accessmedicine.com. Copyright © The McGraw-Hill Companies, Inc. All rights reserved.)

Essentials of Diagnosis

- Diagnosed primarily through signs and symptoms, and exclusion of other pathologies typical to the region.
- Clustering of special tests/signs and symptoms is most accurate, as there are no confirmatory special tests.
- Injury typically due to chronic, repetitive stress to the pubic region during exertional sports.
- Often result of repetitive stress such as kicking, sprinting, or twisting at high speeds during sports.
- Stresses from hip adductor insertion or rectus abdominis precipitate symptoms.
- Weight-bearing forces with athletic activity result in stress to pubic symphysis.
- Palpation of pubic tubercles, inferior pubic rami, rectus abdominis and adductor tendons elicit pain.
- Differential diagnosis from other orthopedic (pubic, spine) or medical (intra-abdominal pathology, hernia) pathologies that may warrant a more immediate surgical or medical intervention is essential.

General Considerations

- Pubalgia-osteitis pubis is collective term and often refers to several possible conditions.
- Caused by repeated trauma from exertional activities that over-stress the pubic bone or tendons that insert upon it, and shearing of the pubic symphysis.
- Diagnosis often made through exclusion of other pathologies.

- Full history of symptoms, medical history screening, and differential pelvic/lower abdominal orthopedic and medical screening examination will ensure appropriate diagnosis.

Demographics

- Common in participants in exertional sports or distance running

CLINICAL FINDINGS

SIGNS AND SYMPTOMS

- Lower abdominal pain or anterior pelvic pain with exertion, responds to rest
- Lower abdominal pain or anterior pelvic pain with sit-ups, kicking, running, sprinting, or squats
- Tenderness over the pubic tubercles
- Possible tenderness over the proximal insertions of the adductor tendons or insertion of the rectus abdominis.
- Possible pain and ROM limitation with passive hip flexion or abduction
- Possible weakness of lower abdominals or any components of the hip musculature

Functional Implications

- Pain/limitation with running
- Pain/limitation with squatting into or rising from chair
- Pain/limitation with getting up from floor
- Pain/limitation with sitting up from supine positions

Possible Contributing Causes

- Limited hip ROM
- Increased tone or shortening of iliopsoas, rectus abdominis, or hip adductors
- Participation in exertional sports (e.g., hockey, soccer, track)
- Pubic instability

Differential Diagnosis

- Bladder infection
- Femoral neck stress fracture
- Groin (adductor) strain
- Iliopsoas abscess
- Inguinal hernia
- Lower abdominal (rectus abdominis) strain
- Osteomyelitis
- Pelvic inflammatory disease
- Prostatitis
- Pubic stress fracture
- Sacral dysfunction
- Sports hernia

MEANS OF CONFIRMATION OR DIAGNOSIS

Imaging

- Radiographs
  - Articular erosion at pubic symphysis
  - Subarticular sclerosis at pubic symphysis
- MRI
  - MRI could confirm suspicion of tendinous involvement, with edema in insertion of adductor musculature or rectus abdominis.
- Nuclear bone scan

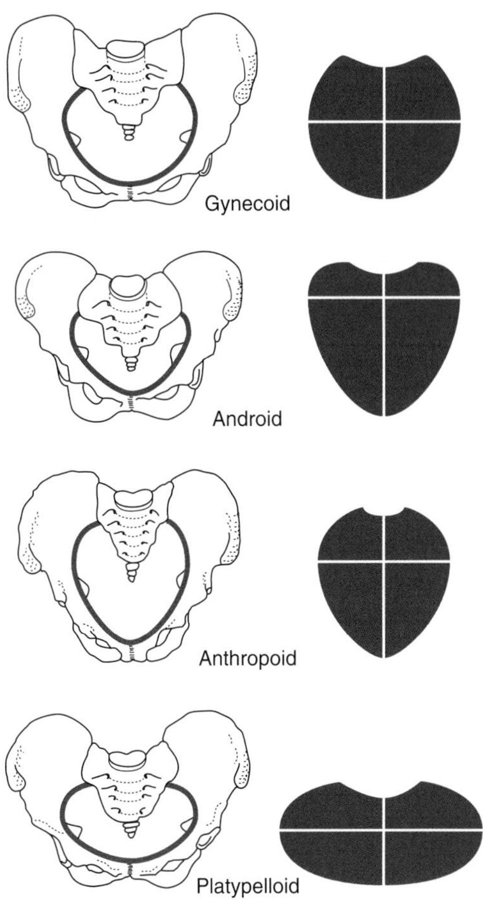

FIGURE 137-2 Types of pelves. White lines in the diagrams at right (after Steele) show the greatest diameters of the pelves at left. (Reproduced, with permission, from Benson RC. *Handbook of Obstetrics & Gynecology*. 8th ed. Los Altos, CA: Lange; 1983.)

Diagnostic Procedures

- Diagnosis based on patient history, signs and symptoms, and exclusion of alternate orthopedic and medical conditions

FINDINGS AND INTERPRETATION

- Radiographs can be normal, but likely have positive findings when present for chronic duration.
  - Articular erosion at pubic symphysis.
  - Subarticular sclerosis at pubic symphysis.
- MRI may show increased bone edema in pubic rami.
  - MRI could confirm suspicion of tendinous involvement, with edema in insertion of adductor musculature or rectus abdominis.
- Nuclear bone scan can show increased uptake of isotope over pubic symphysis or pubic rami.

TREATMENT

Medication

- NSAIDs
- Antibiotics if infection confirmed
- Prolotherapy

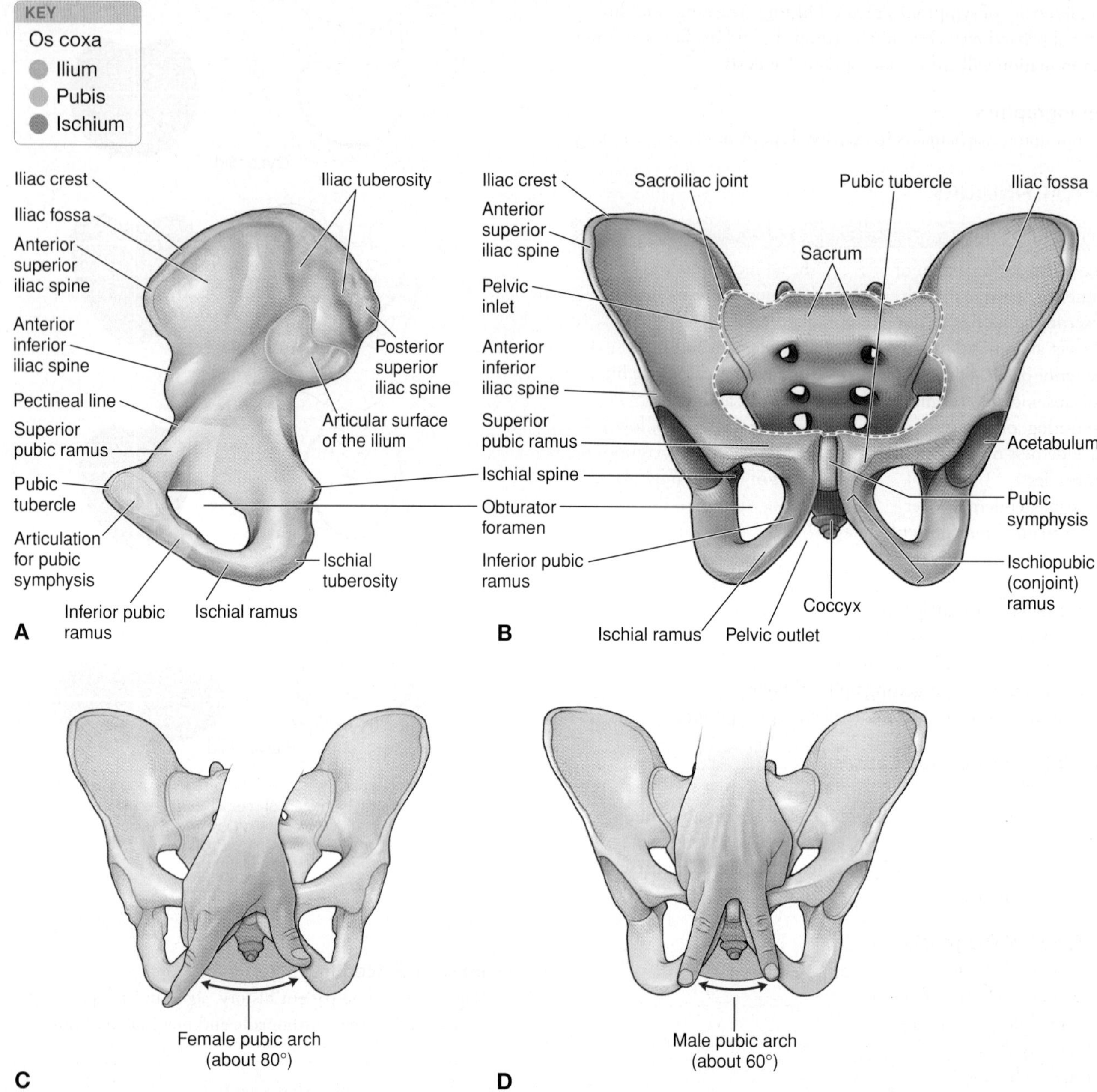

FIGURE 137-3 (**A**) Medial view of the os coxa. (**B**) Anterior view of the pelvis. (**C**) Female pelvis. (**D**) Male pelvis. (From Morton DA, Foreman KB, Albertine KH. *The Big Picture: Gross Anatomy*. http://www.accessmedicine.com. Copyright © The McGraw-Hill Companies, Inc. All rights reserved.)

MEDICAL PROCEDURES

- Surgical intervention for associated or related injuries
- Tendinous tears, hernia repair
- Arthrodesis
- Curettage
- Wedge resection

REFERRALS/ADMITTANCE

- To radiologist for imaging: X-ray, MRI, bone scan
- To primary care for laboratory studies for suspected rheumatic disorder or infection
- To orthopedist for surgical consult for failed conservative treatment

IMPAIRMENTS

- Weakness or pain with squatting down to perform dressing activities or household chores
- Weakness or pain with rising from squat positions, or ascending/descending stairs
- Muscle imbalances
  - Iliopsoas, rectus abdominis, adductor tightness
  - Weakness of proximal hip musculature (possible in all planes)

TESTS AND MEASURES

- Pain, visual analog scale (VAS)
  - 24-hour pain

- Worst average pain
- Best average pain

- Functional independence measure
  - Locomotion
- Cardiovascular integrity
  - Blood pressure at rest and after activity
  - Heart rate at rest and after activity
- Neurologic examination
  - Sensation
    - Light touch
    - Pin prick
  - Lower extremity deep tendon reflexes
  - Proprioception at the hip
  - Kinesthetic awareness at the hip
  - Coordination
- Trunk active and passive ROM
- Hip and knee active and passive ROM
- Flexibility testing
  - Hamstrings
  - Iliopsoas
  - Quadriceps
  - Iliotibial band
  - Abductors
  - Adductors
- Joint integrity of the spine
- Sacroiliac joint integrity
- Hip joint integrity
  - Hip scour
  - Flexion abduction external rotation (FABER) test
  - Flexion induction internal rotation (FAIR) test
- Limb strength
  - Manual muscle test (MMT)
    - Hamstrings
    - Quadriceps
    - Iliopsoas
    - Gluteus maximus
    - Gluteus medius
    - Gluteus minimus
    - Adductors
- LE contralateral limb strength
- Balance
  - Static single-leg standing (eyes open, eyes closed)
    - Contralateral LE
  - Dynamic standing
    - Berg Balance Scale
    - Functional gait assessment
- Gait assessment
  - Observational analysis
  - Gait speed via the 10-m walk test
  - Two-minute walk test
  - Six-minute walk test
  - Retro running

INTERVENTION

- Intervention will vary depending upon the severity of the symptoms.
- Modification/avoidance of activities
  - Running, jumping, squatting, kicking
  - Sports participation
- Exercise interventions
  - Muscle flexibility and strengthening per presenting deficits
  - Progressive weight-bearing activities and then progressive stresses for exertion to return to athletic participation
- Modalities
  - Rest
  - Ice
  - Transcutaneous electrical nerve stimulation (TENS) for pain control
  - Ultrasound
  - Cryotherapy or thermotherapy (per patient presentation)

FUNCTIONAL GOALS

- Patient will be able to
  - Rise from squatting positions without pain.
  - Squat to don/doff shoes without pain or weakness.
  - Sit up without assistance of upper extremities.
  - Perform variable effort running activities without pain or compensatory patterns.
  - Perform twisting and pivoting athletic activities without pain or compensatory patterns.

PROGNOSIS

- Fair.
- Dependent on the underlying cause of the inflammation and the ability of the patient to control exacerbating activities and perform the optimal dosage of therapeutic exercise.

PATIENT RESOURCES

- American Orthopaedic Society for Sports Medicine. Sports Hernia (Athletic Pubalgia). http://orthoinfo.aaos.org/topic.cfm?topic=A00573. Accessed July 3, 2013.
- The Canadian Society of Orthopaedic Technologists. What is Osteitis Pubis? http://www.pappin.com/csot/summer-2009-rounds.html. Accessed July 3, 2013.

REFERENCES

1. ICD9Data.com. http://www.icd9data.com. Accessed July 6, 2013.
2. ICD10Data.com. http://www.icd10data.com. Accessed July 3, 2013.
3. American Physical Therapy Association. Pattern 4E: Impaired joint mobility, motor function, muscle performance, and range of motion associated with localized inflammation. In: *Guide to Physical Therapist Practice*. 2nd ed. Alexandria, VA: American Physical Therapy Association; 2001. Revised 2003.

ADDITIONAL REFERENCES

- Anderson J, Read J. The pelvis, hip and thigh. In: Anderson J, Read J, eds. *Atlas of Imaging in Sports Medicine*. 2nd ed. Australia: McGraw-Hill; 285–390.
- Bradshaw C, Holmich P. Longstanding groin pain. In: *Clinical Sports Medicine*. 3rd ed. Australia: McGraw-Hill; 2009:405–426.
- Choi H, McCartney M, Best TM. Treatment of osteitis pubis and osteomyelitis of the pubic symphysis in athletes: a systematic review. *Br J Sports Med*. 2011;45(1):57–64.
- Dutton M. The hip joint. In: Dutton M, ed. *Dutton's Orthopedic Survival Guide: Managing Common Conditions*. New York, NY: McGraw-Hill; 2011:589–592.

- Dutton M. The hip joint. In: Dutton M, ed. *Dutton's Orthopaedic Examination, Evaluation, and Intervention.* 3rd ed. New York, NY: McGraw-Hill; 2012. New York, NY: McGraw-Hill; 2008: 841–931.
- Jarosz BS. Individualized multi-modal management of osteitis pubis in an Australian Rules footballer. *J Chiropr Med.* 2011; 10(2):105–110.
- Kavroudakis E, Karampinas PK, Evangelopoulos DS, Vlamis J. Treatment of osteitis pubis in non-athlete female patients. *Open Orthop J.* 2011;5:331–334.
- Prentice WE. The thigh, hip, groin, and pelvis. In: Prentice WE, ed. *Principles of Athletic Training: A Competency-Based Approach.* New York, NY: McGraw-Hill; 2011:604–638.
- Sudarshan A. Physical therapy management of osteitis pubis in a 10-year-old cricket fast bowler. *Physiother Theory Pract.* 2013; 29(6):476–486.

138 MUSCLE STRAIN, QUADRATUS LUMBORUM

Eric Shamus, PhD, DPT, PT, CSCS
Gina DiBagno-Moreno, DPT, CSCS

CONDITION/DISORDER SYNONYMS

- Low back pain
- Lumbar sprain
- Mechanical low back pain

ICD-9-CM CODES

- 724.2 Lumbago
- 847.2 Sprain of lumbar

ICD-10-CM CODES

- M54.5 Low back pain
- S33.5 Sprain of ligaments of lumbar spine

PREFERRED PRACTICE PATTERN[1]

- Pattern 4F: Impaired Joint Mobility, Motor Function, Muscle Performance, Range Of Motion, and Reflex Integrity Associated with Spinal Disorders

PATIENT PRESENTATION

A 35-year-old man presents with complaints of unilateral low back pain on his right side. He explains that the pain increases when he inhales deeply, but cannot recall a mechanism of injury. Upon palpation to the lumbar region, the patient complains of tenderness along the 12th rib running inferiorly to the posterior superior iliac crest. The patient has palpable muscle guarding in this region as well. Postural assessment of the patient indicates slight right lateral flexion. The patient tests negative in straight-leg raise test. The patient's radiograph, which was ordered by the referring physician, is negative for any fractures or foreign bodies.

KEY FEATURES

Description

- Quadratus lumborum muscle runs from the posterior superior iliac crest to the 12th rib.
- Can be unilateral or bilateral depending on mechanism of injury.
- Tenderness along origin, insertion, and line of muscle.
- Pain over muscle that radiates with trigger point pattern.
- May cause respiratory issues due to insertion of the muscle on the 12th rib.
- Most episodes are self-limiting.

Essentials of Diagnosis

- Diagnosis made by clinical examination.
- Use of treatment- or impairment-based classification system is useful to determine evidence-based treatment plan.

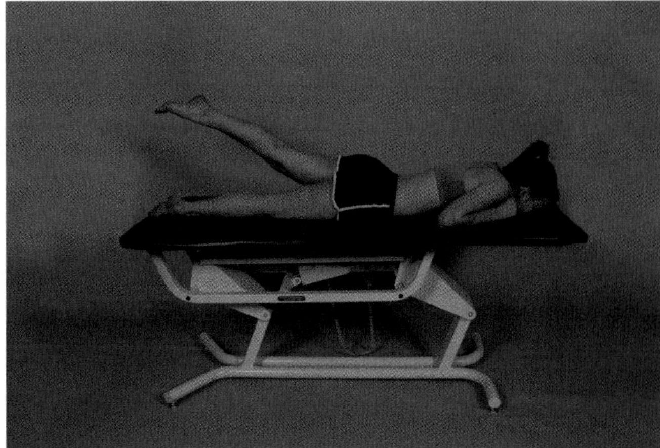

FIGURE 138-1 Prone progression. (From Dutton M. *Dutton's Orthopaedic Examination, Evaluation, and Intervention*. 3rd ed. http://www.accessphysiotherapy.com. Copyright © The McGraw-Hill Companies, Inc. All rights reserved.)

- Reproduction of symptoms in specific postures and activities.
- Rule out systemic disease (red and yellow flags).

General Considerations

- Presentation may vary significantly based on anatomical structures and psychosocial factors.
- Often difficult to determine pathoanatomical cause of pain.
- Poor spinal alignment, scoliosis, and 12th-rib dysfunction can cause irritation of muscle by altering the length–tension ratio.

Demographics

- May be specific to athletes, younger populations prone to extreme spinal movements.

CLINICAL FINDINGS

SIGNS AND SYMPTOMS

- Pain lateral to lumbar spine between 12th rib and iliac crest that can be mechanically reproduced
- Unilateral or bilateral pain along length of muscle or attachment
- Lumbar segmental and 12th-rib hypomobility
- Respiratory limitations
- Difficulty with lumbar spine ROM
- Often associated with poor body mechanics, core-muscle weakness, and postural deviations

Functional Implications

- May be a leading cause of occupational disability
- May impede ability to perform ADLs/IADLs
- May impede participation in sports and other social activities

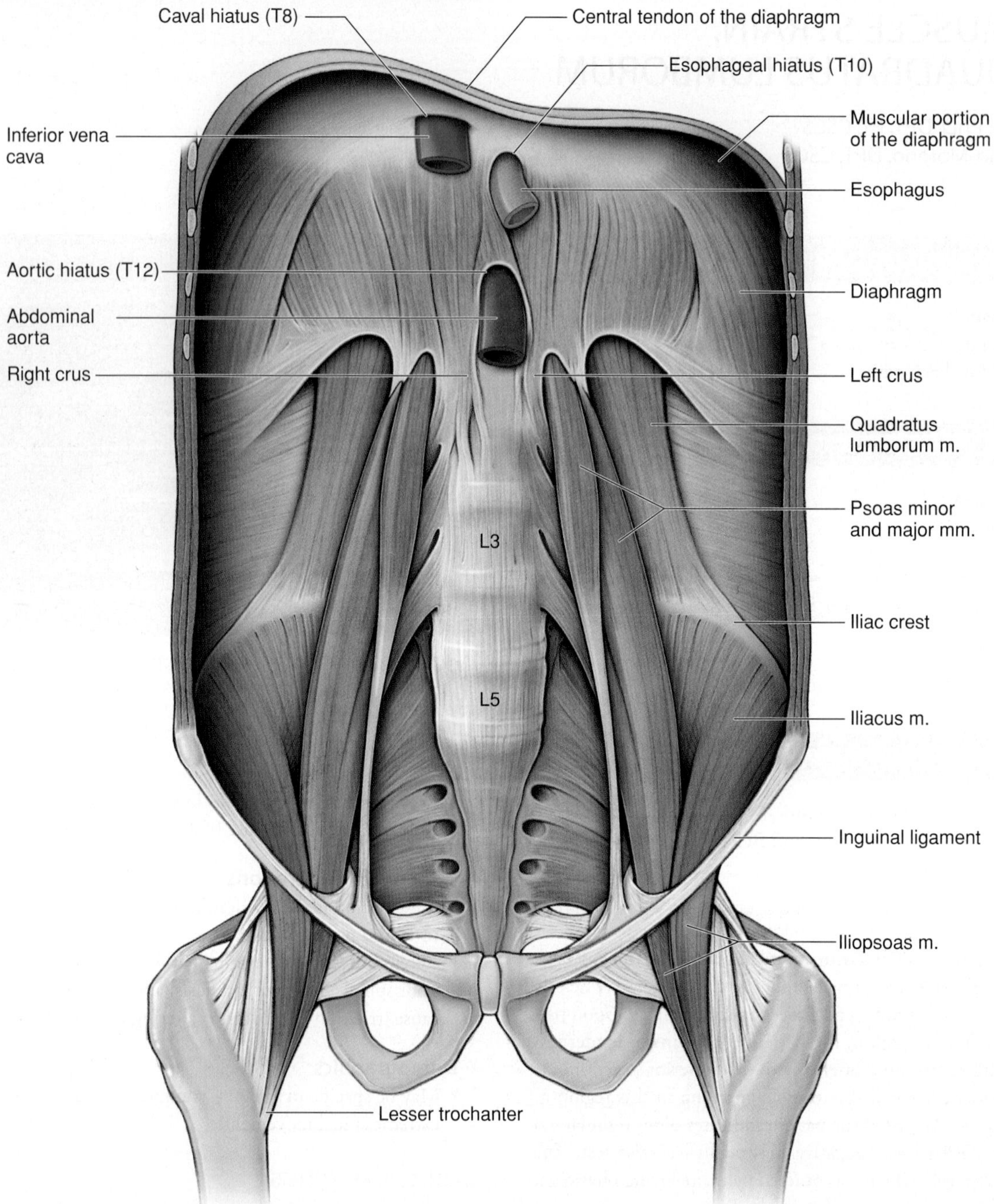

FIGURE 138-2 Muscles of the posterior abdominal wall. (From Morton DA, Foreman KB, Albertine KH. *The Big Picture: Gross Anatomy.* http://www.accessmedicine.com. Copyright © The McGraw-Hill Companies, Inc. All rights reserved.)

▸ Possible Contributing Causes

- Congenital anomalies
- Obesity
- Occupational factors
- Physical condition
- Postural changes
- Psychosocial and behavioral factors
- Smoking
- Socioeconomic factors
- Tightness of hip flexors, external rotators, hamstrings
- Weakness of core musculature

▸ Differential Diagnosis

- 12th-rib dysfunction
- 12th-rib fracture
- Erector spinae muscle strain
- Facet joint dysfunction
- Herniated disc
- Leg-length discrepancy
- Malignant spinal tumor or metastasis
- Myofascial pain syndrome
- Referred pain from visceral structures
- Respiratory problems

- Sacral dysfunction
- Scoliosis
- Spinal misalignment
- Spondylitis
- Spondylolisthesis
- Spondylosis
- Systemic autoimmune disease (rheumatoid arthritis, Reiter syndrome)

MEANS OF CONFIRMATION OR DIAGNOSIS

Imaging

- Not necessary in most cases; only with persistent symptoms not responding to conservative management or if red/yellow flags are present
- MRI helpful in diagnosis to visualize structure of muscle, compressed or inflamed nerve root, or disc pathology
- X-ray/Plain-film radiograph helps to assess alignment, fractures, stability (flexion/extension radiograph)
- CT to show muscle structure, herniation compressing the spinal canal/nerves, or to rule out abdominal pathology
- Electrodiagnostic/nerve conduction testing can help determine specific impaired nerve function
- Doppler ultrasound to examine vascular function
- Diagnostic ultrasound to analyze fiber orientation

FINDINGS AND INTERPRETATION

- X-ray test will be negative for pathology.

REFERRALS/ADMITTANCE

- To hospital for imaging
- To physician for surgical consult if myelopathy suspected
- To physician for imaging and medical consult if systemic disease suspected
- To other specialist if vascular insufficiency suspected

IMPAIRMENTS

- Hyper- or hypomobile lumbar spine
- Decreased lumbar stability
- Weakened abdominals and other core-stabilizing muscles
- Shortened hamstrings and hip flexors
- Postural changes
- Inability to walk, stand, sit for prolonged periods of time

TESTS AND MEASURES

- Algorithm for examination of the lumbar spine
- Passive physiological intervertebral mobility testing (PPIVM)
- Lower-extremity screening examination
- Postural examination
- Muscle length testing, including hamstrings, hip flexors, calf muscles
- Quadrant test
- Straight-leg raise test
- Slump test
- Lower limb nerve tension test
- Prone instability test
- Lower extremity neurological screen (dermatome, myotome, reflexes)
- Repeated movement testing
- Fear-Avoidance Beliefs Questionnaire (FABQ)

INTERVENTION

- Joint manipulation of lumbar spine indicated when[2]
  - Duration of symptoms less than 16 days
  - Hypomobility upon PIVM testing
  - No pain past the knee
  - FABQ work subscale score greater than 19 points
  - Less than 35 degrees internal rotation in at least one hip joint
- Specific exercise when pain centralizes with repeated movement/posture into flexion or extension
- Lumbar-stabilization exercises to address core stability when[3]
  - Prone instability test positive
  - Presence of aberrant motion
  - Straight-leg raise greater than 91 degrees
  - Age younger than 40 years
- Traction when
  - Radiculopathy findings present
  - Positive crossed straight-leg raise
  - Pain peripheralized with repeated extension
- Stretching exercises, myofascial mobilization for shortened musculature
- Unweighted treadmill walking
- Aquatic exercise
- Modalities for short-term pain control
- Stretching of quadratus lumborum
- Manual therapy for release of quadratus lumborum

FUNCTIONAL GOALS

- Patient will be able to
  - Sit with neutral lumbar spine posture for >30 minutes with 0/10 pain rating for computer work and desk activities.
  - Sit at work station and perform computer work for 45 minutes with 0/10 pain rating.
  - Rotate lumbar spine 25 degrees so as to reach into back seat of car with 0/10 pain rating in lower extremity.
  - Walk for 30 minutes with 0/10 pain rating so as to go shopping.
  - Increase standing tolerance to >30 minutes without pain so as to stand at work.

PROGNOSIS

- Fair to very good, depending on specific impairments.
- Chronic low back pain (LBP) prognosis significantly lowered.

PATIENT RESOURCE

- Back Pain. American Academy of Orthopeadic Surgeons. http://orthoinfo.aaos.org/topic.cfm?topic=A00311. Accessed July 5, 2013.

REFERENCES

1. The American Physical Therapy Association. Pattern 4F: impaired joint mobility, motor function, muscle performance, range of motion, and reflex integrity associated with spinal disorders. *Interactive Guide to Physical Therapist Practice* 2003. http://guidetoptpractice.apta.org/content/1/SEC13.extract. Accessed May 25, 2014.
2. Flynn T, Fritz J, Whitman J, , et al. A clinical prediction rule for classifying patients with low back pain who demonstrate short-

term improvement with spinal manipulation. *Spine.* 2002;27(24): 2835–2843.
3. Hicks GE, Fritz JM, Delitto A, McGill SM. Preliminary development of a clinical prediction rule for determining which patients with low back pain will respond to a stabilization exercise program. *Arch Phys Med Rehabil.* 2005;86(9):1753–1762.

ADDITIONAL REFERENCES

- Dutton M. *Dutton's Orthopedic Survival Guide: Managing Common Conditions.* New York, NY: McGraw-Hill; 2011. http://www.accessphysiotherapy.com/resource/685. Accessed July 2, 2013.
- Dutton M. *Dutton's Orthopaedic Examination, Evaluation, and Intervention.* 3rd ed. New York, NY: McGraw-Hill; 2012. http://www.accessphysiotherapy.com/resource/612. Accessed July 2, 2013.
- Fritz JM, Cleland JA, Childs JD. Subgrouping patients with low back pain: evolution of a classification approach to physical therapy. *J Orthop Sports Phys Ther.* 2007;37(6):290–302.
- ICD-9-CM. http://www.icd9data.com. Accessed July 2, 2013.
- ICD-10-CM. http://www.icd10data.com. Accessed July 2, 2013.
- Liebenson C. *Rehabilitation of the Spine: A Practitioner's Manual.* Baltimore, MD: Lippincott, Williams & Wilkins; 2007.
- Malone TR, Hazle C, Grey ML. *Imaging in Rehabilitation.* New York, NY: McGraw-Hill; 2008. http://www.accessphysiotherapy.com/resource/613. Accessed July 2, 2013.
- Olsen KA. *Manual Physical Therapy of the Spine.* St. Louis, MI: Saunders Elsevier; 2008.

139 SCIATICA

Arie J. Van Duijn, EdD, MSc, PT, OCS
Eric Shamus, PhD, DPT, PT, CSCS

CONDITION/DISORDER SYNONYM

- Lumbosacral radicular syndrome

ICD-9-CM CODES[1]

- 355.0 Lesion of sciatic nerve
- 722.73 Intervertebral disc disorder with myelopathy lumbar region
- 724.3 Sciatica
- 724.4 Thoracic or lumbosacral neuritis or radiculitis unspecified

ICD-10-CM CODES[2]

- G57.00 Lesion of sciatic nerve, unspecified lower limb
- M54.16 Radiculopathy, lumbar region
- M54.17 Radiculopathy, lumbosacral region
- M54.3 Sciatica

PREFERRED PRACTICE PATTERNS

- 4F: Impaired Joint Mobility, Motor Function, Muscle Performance, Range of Motion, and Reflex Integrity Associated with Spinal Disorders[3]
- 4E: Impaired Joint Mobility, Motor Function, Muscle Performance, and ROM Associated with Localized Inflammation[3]

PATIENT PRESENTATION

A 32-year-old female presents with complaints of left ischial pain with sciatic radiation of the pain. She reports that the pain has been present for approximately 5 months. Since the onset of symptoms, the ischial pain has not decreased in intensity. The sciatic pain radiation has also not improved, however, has not progressed or moved further distally. She recalls a fall approximately 2 months prior to the onset of symptoms when she fell on her left buttock along the edge of a carted stairway. She was carrying a heavy object at the time, and reports a significant black and blue on her left buttock that lasted for about 3 weeks.

Since the onset of symptoms she had extensive medical workup, including an MRI and CT scan that were both negative for lumbar radiculopathy. The primary complaints of pain are with sitting or standing, there is relief of symptoms when lying. There is significant point tenderness over the piriformis muscle. Stretching of this muscle reproduces the complaints.

KEY FEATURES

Description

- Low back pain radiating into the lower extremity (LE)
- Can result from lateral lumbar/sacral spine nerve root compression or piriformis syndrome

Essentials of Diagnosis

- Diagnosis made by clinical examination
- Dermatome/myotome pattern compared to peripheral nerve distribution
- Reproduction of symptoms

General Considerations

- Presence of leg pain significantly increases the odds of condition becoming persistent

Demographics

- Nonspecific
- Most individuals will have sciatica symptoms at least once in their lifetime

CLINICAL FINDINGS

SIGNS AND SYMPTOMS

- Pain radiating down the leg(s), below the knee, along the distribution of the sciatic nerve
- Usually related to mechanical pressure and/or inflammation of lumbosacral nerve roots
- Can be with or without low back pain (LBP)
- Diminished sensation, motor control, and reflexes in the distribution of the involved nerve

Functional Implications

- Difficulty maintaining sustained sitting postures secondary to back and leg pain
- Inability to sleep
- Weakness with lifting, prolonged standing
- Loss of movement or feeling in the LE
- Difficulty with movements secondary to pain such as driving or twisting

Possible Contributing Causes

- Postural changes including weakness of core musculature and tightness of hip flexors, external rotators, and hamstrings
- Prolonged occupational stresses
- Pregnancy
- Disk pathology, other sources of nerve root compression
- Smoking

Differential Diagnosis

- Peripheral nerve impairment
- Hip pathology with radiating pain pattern
- Spinal tumor
- Lyme disease
- Peripheral neuropathy
- Paraspinal muscle hypertonicity
- Degenerative disk disease
- Sacral or pelvis dysfunction

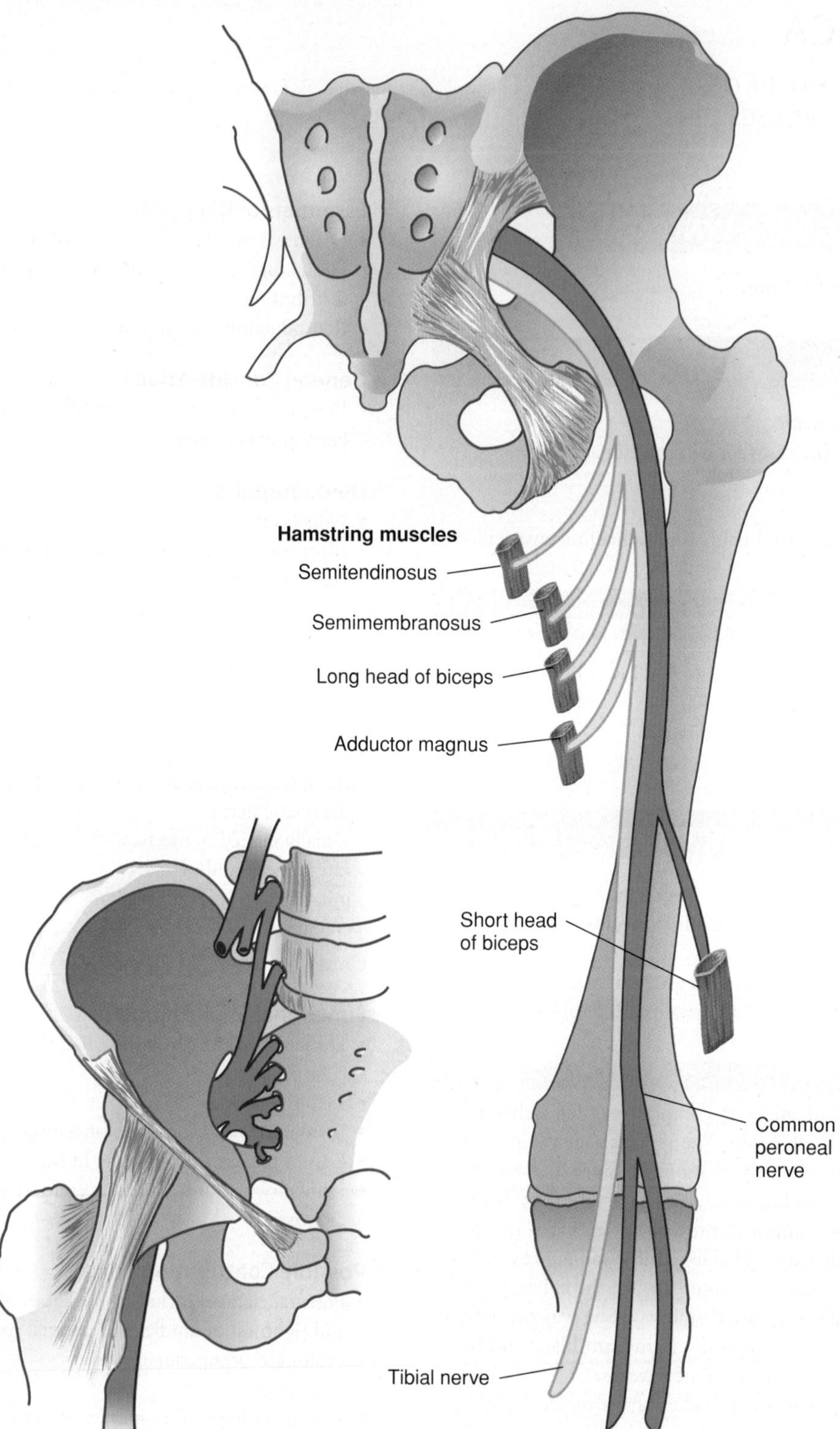

FIGURE 139-1 The sciatic nerve (L4, 5; S1–3). (From Waxman SG. *Clinical Neuroanatomy*. 26th ed. http://www.accessmedicine.com. Copyright © The McGraw-Hill Companies, Inc. All rights reserved.)

MEANS OF CONFIRMATION OR DIAGNOSIS

Imaging

- MRI
- X-ray/Plain-film radiograph
- CT scan
- Electrodiagnostic/nerve conduction testing

FINDINGS AND INTERPRETATION

- MRI helpful in diagnosis to visualize compressed or inflamed nerve root
- X-ray/Plain-film radiograph helpful if osteophyte located in intervertebral foramen
- CT scan to show herniation compressing the spinal canal/nerves

- Electrodiagnostic/nerve conduction testing can assist to determine a specific impaired nerve function

TREATMENT

Medication

- Anti-inflammatory medication
- Corticosteroid injection if condition does not improve
- Epidural

MEDICAL PROCEDURES

- Decompression
- Diskectomy
- Fusion
- Hemilaminectomy
- Laminectomy
- Laser diskectomy
- Microdiskectomy
- Percutaneous diskectomy

REFERRALS/ADMITTANCE

- For imaging
- For surgical consult if myelopathy is suspected
- For medication

IMPAIRMENTS

- Hypermobile or hypomobile lower lumbar spine
- Inability to sit for prolonged time
- Inability to stand for prolonged time
- Restricted mobility of the upper lumbar and lower thoracic spine
- Weakness noted of abdominals and core stabilizing muscles

TESTS AND MEASURES

- Physical examination
  - Algorithm for examination of the lumbar spine
  - Quadrant test
  - FABER test
  - Rotation limited to ipsilateral side
  - Straight-leg raise test
  - Crossed straight-leg raise test
  - Slump test
  - Lower limb nerve tension test
  - Patella, Achilles, hamstring reflex
  - Lower limb sensation testing
  - Radicular pattern
  - Passive physiological intervertebral mobility testing (PPIVM)
  - Repeated lumbar movements
  - Prone instability test

INTERVENTION

- Joint manipulation to the thoracic and lumbar spine when joint hypomobility is present
- Specific exercise in extension when pain centralizes with repeated movement into extension
- Traction if pain does not centralize with repeated movements, and/or peripheralizes with repeated movements into extension
- Lumbar stabilization exercises to address core stability
- Stretching exercises and myofascial mobilization for shortened musculature

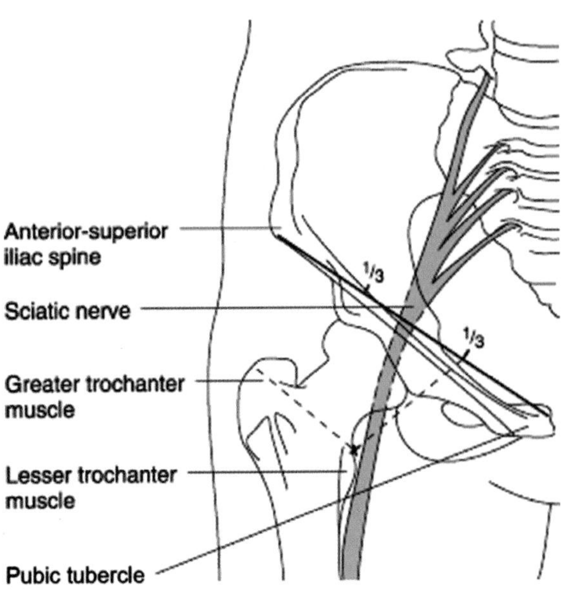

FIGURE 139-2 Sciatic nerve block, anterior approach. (From Morgan GE, Mikhail MS, Murray MJ. *Clinical Anesthesiology*. 4th ed. www.accessmedicine.com. Copyright © The McGraw-Hill Companies, Inc. All rights reserved.)

- Modalities to provide short-term pain relief
  - Electrical stimulation
  - Heat/ice

FUNCTIONAL GOALS

- Patient will be able to
  - Sit with a neutral lumbar spine posture for >30 minutes with 0/10 pain.
  - Sit at work station and perform computer work for 45 minutes with 0/10 pain.

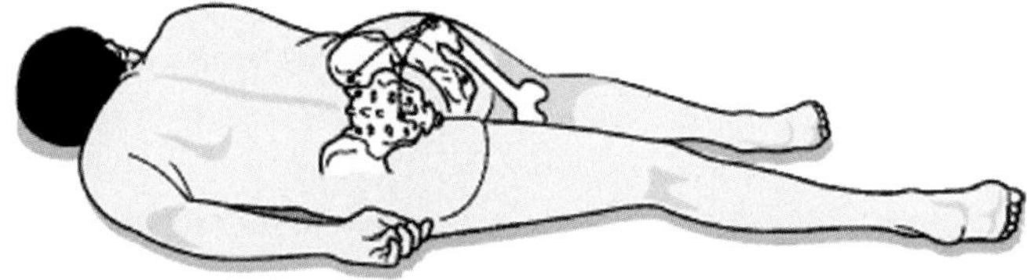

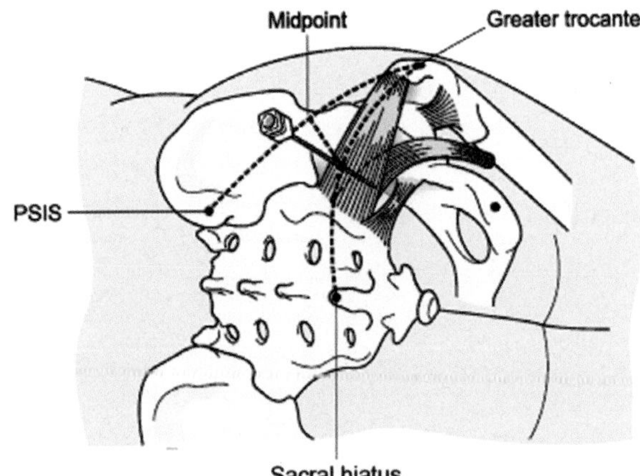

FIGURE 139-3 Sciatic nerve block, posterior approach. PSIS, posterior superior iliac spine. (From Morgan GE, Mikhail MS, Murray MJ. *Clinical Anesthesiology*. 4th ed. www.accessmedicine.com. Copyright © The McGraw-Hill Companies, Inc. All rights reserved.)

- Increase standing tolerance to >30 minutes without pain to fulfill work requirements.

PROGNOSIS

- Fair to good: Presence of lower limb radicular symptoms increases the odds of condition becoming chronic.

ADDITIONAL INFORMATION

- For more information, please review Case Study: *Right Buttock Pain* on AccessPhysiotherapy.com.

PATIENT RESOURCES

- Sciatica. AAOS, American Academy of Orthopeadic Surgeons. 2007. http://orthoinfo.aaos.org/topic.cfm?topic=A00351. Accessed July 17, 2013.
- Sciatica. MedlinePlus. US Library of Medicine, NIH National Institutes of Health. 2012. http://www.nlm.nih.gov/medlineplus/sciatica.html. Access July 17, 2013.

REFERENCES

1. *Guide to Physical Therapist Practice*. 2nd ed. Alexandria, VA: American Physical Therapy Association; 2001. Revised 2003.
2. ICD9Data.com. http://www.icd9data.com. Accessed July 6, 2013.
3. ICD10Data.com. http://www.icd10data.com. Accessed July 6, 2013.

ADDITIONAL REFERENCES

- Dutton M. *Dutton's Orthopedic Survival Guide: Managing Common Conditions*. New York, NY: McGraw-Hill; 2011. http://www.accessphysiotherapy.com/resource/685. Accessed July 6, 2013.
- Dutton M. *Dutton's Orthopaedic Examination, Evaluation, and Intervention*. 3rd ed. New York, NY: McGraw-Hill; 2012. http://www.accessphysiotherapy.com/resource/612. Accessed July 6, 2013.
- Fritz JM, Cleland JA, Childs JD. Subgrouping patients with low back pain: evolution of a classification approach to physical therapy. *J Orthop Sports Phys Ther*. 2007;37(6):290–302. doi:10.2519/jospt.2007.2498.
- Halle J, Greathouse D. Principles of electrophysiologic evaluation and testing. In: Prentice WE, Quillen WS, Underwood F, eds. *Therapeutic Modalities in Rehabilitation*. 4th ed. New York, NY: McGraw-Hill; 2011. http://www.accessphysiotherapy.com/content/8137409. Accessed July 6, 2013.
- Jewell DV, Riddle DL. Interventions that increase or decrease the likelihood of a meaningful improvement in physical health in patients with sciatica. *Phys Ther*. 2005;85(11):1139–1150.
- Malone TR, Hazle C, Grey ML. Introduction to musculoskeletal imaging. In: Malone TR, Hazle C, Grey ML, eds. *Imaging in Rehabilitation*. New York, NY: McGraw-Hill; 2008. http://www.accessphysiotherapy.com/content/5940000. Accessed July 6, 2013.
- Patel DR, Rowe D. Thoracolumbar spine injuries. In: Patel DR, Greydanus DE, Baker RJ, eds. *Pediatric Practice: Sports Medicine*. New York, NY: McGraw-Hill; 2009. http://www.accessphysiotherapy.com/popup.aspx?aID=6981371. Accessed July 6, 2013.

140 SCOLIOSIS (KYPHOSCOLIOSIS) IDIOPATHIC

Doris Newman, DO, PT, FAAO
Eric Shamus, PhD, DPT, PT, CSCS

CONDITION/DISORDER SYNONYM

- Kyphoscoliosis

ICD-9-CM CODE

- 737.30 Scoliosis (and kyphoscoliosis) idiopathic

ICD-10-CM CODE

- M41.20 Other idiopathic scoliosis, site unspecified

PREFERRED PRACTICE PATTERN

- 4B: Impaired Posture

PATIENT PRESENTATION

A 16-year-old girl is referred to your outpatient physical therapy clinic. The patient comes with her mom. The patient states she has been going to cheerleading practice and is having back pain. The referring physician told her she had scoliosis with a Cobb angle of 27 degrees. They do a lot of stretching in cheerleading practice, but she is having difficulty with the backward bends. She is starting to have some instability in the thoracic spine with localized pain and erector spinae spasms.

KEY FEATURES

Description

- Three-dimensional curvatures of the spine and trunk
  - Lateral curve is an S- or C-shaped curve in the sagittal plane
  - Torsional component with vertebrae rotating toward the convexity
  - Anteroposterior distortion leads to hyperkyphosis and/or hyperlordosis in the coronal plane
- Functional lateral curvature of the spine, typically reversible
- Structural lateral curvature of the spine, fixed
  - Most commonly idiopathic
  - May be present in conjunction with another condition
  - 80% to 85% are idiopathic
  - Congenital
    - Hemi-vertebrae malformation
- Infantile onset: Younger than 3 years
- Juvenile onset 3 to 9 years old
- Adolescent idiopathic scoliosis (AIS) onset 10 to 18 years old
- Adult onset: Older than 18 years
- AIS is the most common form and occurs in otherwise healthy children during puberty (80%–85% of cases)
- Relatively benign condition

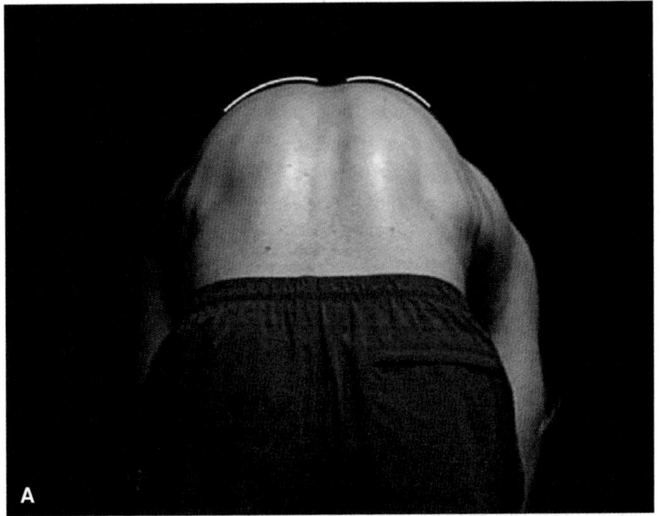

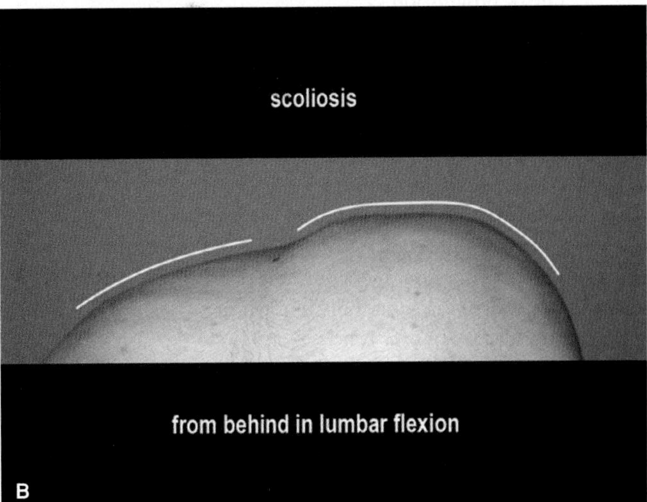

FIGURE 140-1 Adam's forward bending test. (**A**) No visible rib hump, negative test. (**B**) Visible rub hump, positive test. (From Lawry GV. *Systematic Musculoskeletal Examinations*. www.accessmedicine.com. Copyright © The McGraw-Hill Companies, Inc. All rights reserved.)

- Named for the side of the convexity of the lateral curve (right, dextroscoliosis; left, levoscoliosis)
- Degree of curvature most commonly defined by the Cobb method, radiographically
- Increased risk of curve progression during growth spurts in adolescents

Essentials of Diagnosis

- Adam's forward bending test
  - Patient stands with back to the clinician and then actively bends forward toward the floor.

- Examination reveals a rib hump, which represents the posteriorly displaced rib angles due to vertebral rotation on the convex side of the curve.
  - Functional: During forward bending, the rib hump disappears with ipsilateral side bending.
  - Structural: During forward bending, the rib hump persists with ipsilateral side bending.
- Inclinometer measuring device may be utilized to clinically document progression or regression of curve without radiation exposure.
- X-rays (occiput to sacrum) used to define severity of curve.
  - Anteroposterior view with Cobb angle measurements
    - A perpendicular line at the top of the vertebral body of the superior most acutely angles vertebral segment intersecting a similar line at the inferior most acutely angles segment.
    - The angle of intersection of two lines placed perpendicular to the above two lines is considered the Cobb angle for that lateral spine curvature.
  - Lateral view to identify hyperkyphosis and/or lordosis.
  - Also used to rule out primary structural or mass deformities causing a secondary scoliotic curvature.
  - Cobb angle measurements: Limited in ability to determine spinal flexibility and the three-dimensional aspect of the condition. Tends to overestimate the curve.
  - Cobb Angle measurements
    - <10 degrees is a normal variation and unlikely to progress.
    - 10 to 35 degrees often treated conservatively, depending on rate of progression.
    - >35 degrees considered for surgical intervention but guidelines and outcomes vary.
    - >50 degrees considered surgical to prevent cardiopulmonary compromise, rib motion restriction, pain, cosmetic deformity.
- Skeletal maturity
- MRI
  - Used to identify spinal cord and brain stem abnormalities.
- Three-dimensional computerized modeling techniques
  - Advanced computer modeling able to create three-dimensional images can reduce the number of X-rays needed to monitor scoliosis over time.

General Considerations

- Occurs frequently in the general population

Demographics

- 2% to 3% of the population[1]
- 10% of adolescents have some degree of scoliosis but only 1% need treatment[1]
- Runs in families, with a 20% chance of developing the condition among relatives[1]
- Girls:boys is an 8:1 ratio[1]
- Greater participation in gymnastics[1]

CLINICAL FINDINGS

SIGNS AND SYMPTOMS

- Typically painless in early stages
- Head tilt
- Uneven shoulders
- Unlevel hips
- Clothes appear uneven (neckline; hemlines)
- Breasts appear unequal in size
- Protruding shoulder blade

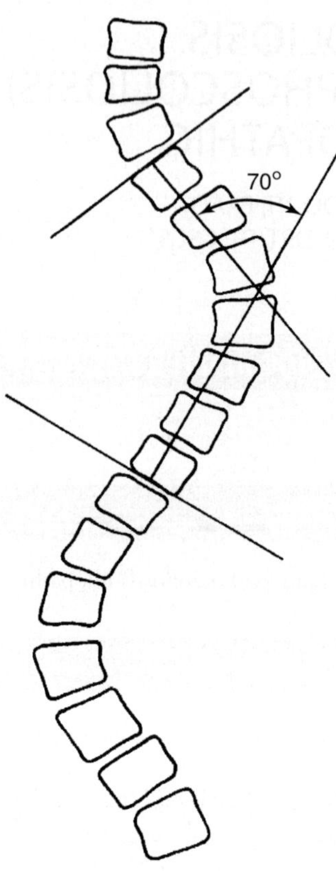

FIGURE 140-2 Use of the Cobb method to measure the scoliotic curve. First, lines are drawn along the endplates of the upper and lower vertebrae that are maximally tilted into the concavity of the curve. Next, a perpendicular line is drawn to each of the earlier-drawn lines. The angle of intersection is the Cobb angle. (Reproduced with permission from Day LJ, Bovill EG, Trafton PG. Orthopedics. In: Way LW, ed. *Current Surgical Diagnosis & Treatment*. 9th ed. Stamford: Appleton & Lange; 1991.)

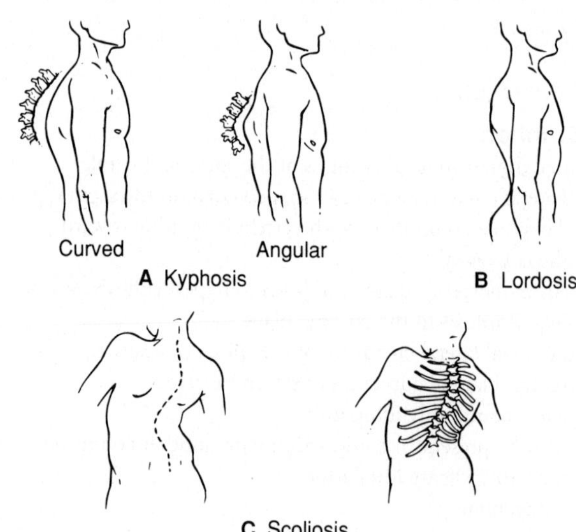

FIGURE 140-3 Curvatures of the spine affecting the thorax. (**A**) Kyphotic thorax. (**B**) Lordotic thorax. (**C**) Scoliotic thorax. Note the narrowing of the rib interspaces on the right and the accentuation of the interspaces, posterior humping of the chest, and elevation of the shoulder on the left. (From LeBlond RF, DeGowin RL, Brown DD. *DeGowin's Diagnostic Examination*. 9th ed. www.accessmedicine.com. Copyright © The McGraw-Hill Companies, Inc. All rights reserved.)

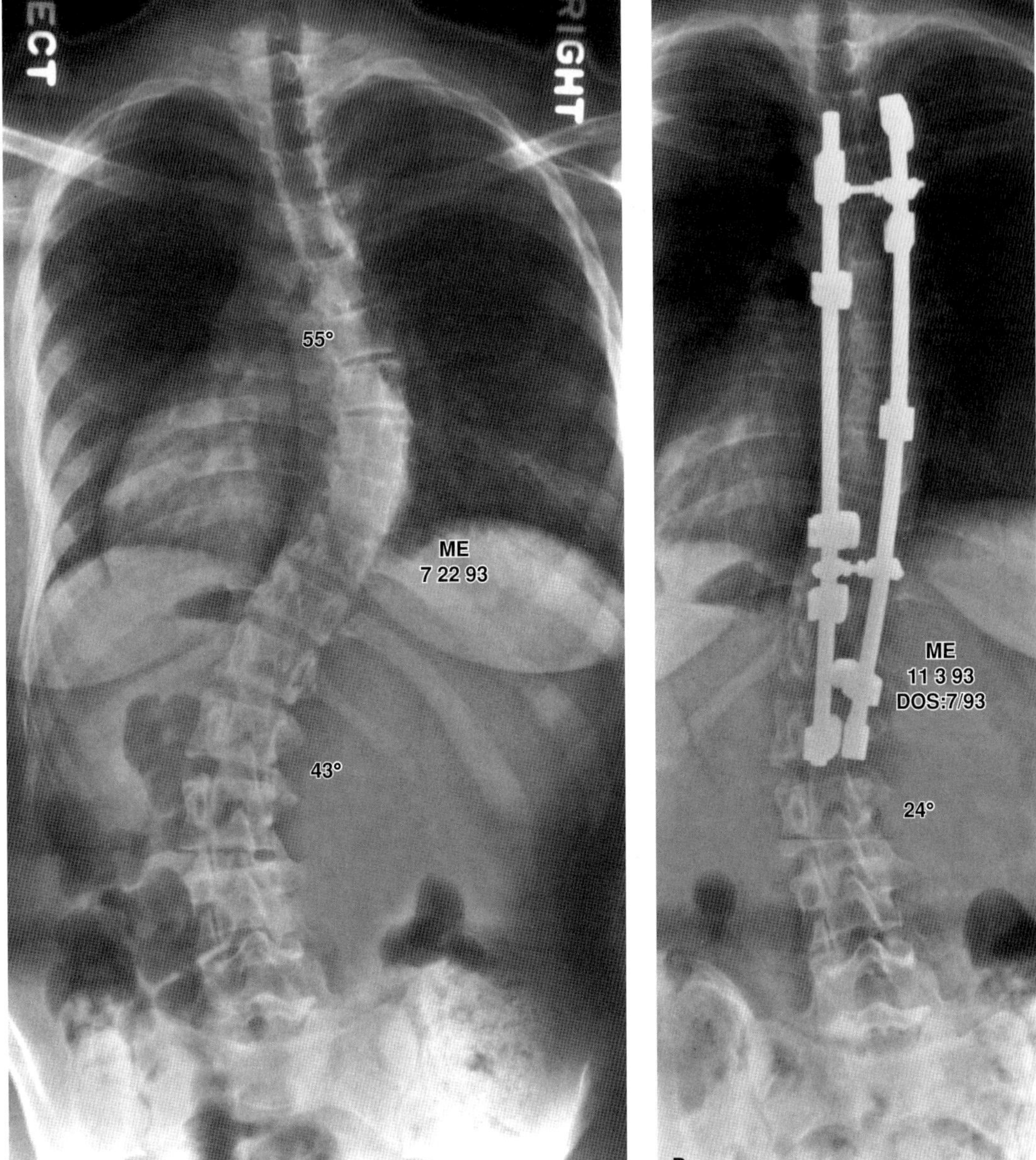

FIGURE 140-4 Imaging studies in a patient with scoliosis. (**A**) Radiograph showing preoperative curvature. (**B**) Radiograph taken after treatment using Cotrel–Dubousset instrumentation. (From Skinner HB. *Current Diagnosis & Treatment in Orthopedics*. 4th ed. www.accessmedicine.com.)

- Psychological issues due to cosmetic appearance
- Functional issues due to asymmetric reaching and twisting ability
- Rib mobility limited
- Pain

▶ Functional Implications

- Cardiopulmonary compromise in advanced curves

▶ Possible Contributing Causes

- Functional
  - Muscle spasms
  - Leg length discrepancy
  - Viscerosomatic reflexes from inflammatory conditions such as appendicitis
- Structural or fixed curves
  - Associated with
    - Cardiopulmonary diseases
    - Neurofibromatosis
    - Osteitis deformans
    - Osteoporosis
    - Muscular dystrophy
    - Radiation therapy
    - Rickets
    - Tuberculosis

FINDINGS AND INTERPRETATION

- Cobb angle
- Risser grades (0–V) define the extent of ossification of the apophysis from the anterolateral to the posteromedial aspect of the iliac

crest. Define boney maturity and may be obtained from X-ray or ultrasound to reduce long-term radiation exposure.
- Risser grade 0: Absence of ossification of the iliac crest
- Risser grade I: Ossification within the first quarter (0%–25%)
- Risser grade II: Ossification of the second quarter of the iliac crest (25%–50%)
- Risser grade III: Ossification of the third quarter (50%–75%)
- Risser grade IV: Ossification within the fourth quarter (>75%)
- Risser grade V: Complete fusion of the apophysis to the ilium

REFERRALS/ADMITTANCE

- For imaging
  - X-rays for initial Cobb angle and Risser grade
  - US for follow-up Risser grading
  - MRI as indicated
- For bracing
  - Milwaukee brace: Has a neck ring and can be used with any level curve
  - Boston brace (thoracolumbosacral [TLSO] or lumbosacral [LSO]): An underarm brace that can only be used with apex of the curve below eighth thoracic vertebral segment
- For manual therapy (manual therapy specialist, osteopathic physicians, chiropractors)
  - Inconclusive evidence on efficacy of manual therapy due to lack of scientific data
- For acupuncture
  - Shown to influence spinal curvatures less than 35 degrees[1]
- For Surgical consult
  - Generally, indications for surgery are Cobb Angle curves greater than 50 degrees[1]
  - May be performed for cosmetic reasons only, but outcomes vary

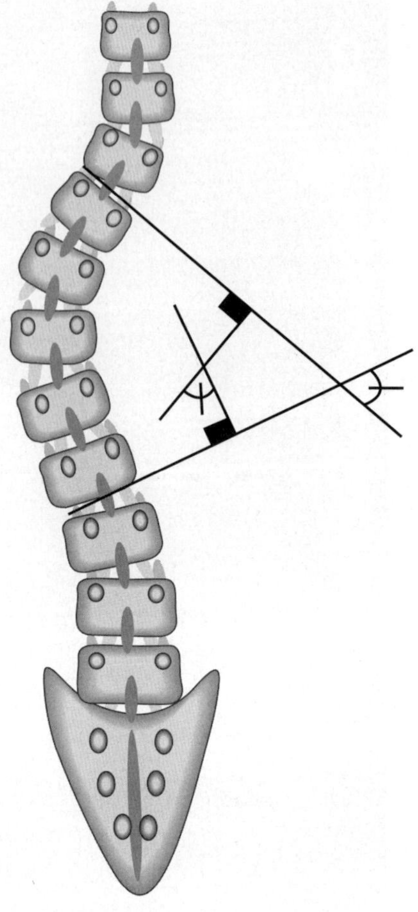

FIGURE 140-5 Measurement of spinal deformity using the Cobb method. (From Doherty GM. *Current Diagnosis & Treatment: Surgery*. 13th ed. www.accessmedicine.com. Copyright © The McGraw-Hill Companies, Inc. All rights reserved.)

IMPAIRMENTS

- Dependent upon degree of curvature and boney maturity at onset
- Chronic pain
- Cardiopulmonary compromise with reduction in vital capacity function

TESTS AND MEASURES

- Algorithm for examination of the lumbar spine
- Passive physiological intervertebral mobility testing (PPIVM)
- Lower-extremity screening examination
- Postural examination
- Muscle length testing, including hamstrings, hip flexors, calf muscles
- Quadrant test
- Straight-leg raise test
- Slump test
- Lower limb nerve tension test
- Prone instability test
- Lower-extremity neurological screening (dermatome, myotome, reflexes)
- Repeated movement testing
- Fear-Avoidance Beliefs Questionnaire (FABQ)

INTERVENTION

- Address motor weakness and lack of flexibility
  - Sequential stretching and strengthening exercises: Standard therapeutic exercise approach isolating muscle groups, plane by plane (e.g., one exercise to correct in the frontal plane, a second exercise to correct in the transversal plane, and a third exercise to correct in the sagittal plane)
  - Scoliosis-specific exercises in three-dimensions: More recent approach whereby patient will try, with and without external assistance, to achieve the best possible frontal, transversal, and physiological sagittal alignment before producing any active muscle activation to stabilize the correction. The three-dimensional correction must be performed in combination and synchronized in all three planes.
  - Core strengthening: Isolated versus three-dimensional techniques
- Posture education addressing all three dimensions
  - Used to prevent asymmetric compressive forces
- Pain control
  - Ice
  - Therapeutic massage
  - Electric stimulation
  - Ultrasound
- Address articular restrictions
  - Joint mobilization of involved spinal segments, ribs, and other areas as indicated
- Address sacral base unleveling, if present
- Monitor bracing for curve response and complications such as skin irritation and comfort

- Training in ADLs
- Multi-disciplinary team approach
  - Physician (MD or DO), PT, orthotist, psychologist
- Reduce secondary muscle imbalance
- Prevent asymmetric torsional forces from gait

FUNCTIONAL GOALS

- Patient will
  - Have improved measurement on spinal inclinometer.
  - Be independent with home exercise program.
  - Have decreased pain to be able to perform household activities such as cleaning and laundry.
  - Have improved functional level to participate in grocery shopping.
  - Prevent curve progression to limit respiratory dysfunction.

PROGNOSIS

- Depends upon severity of Cobb angle, rate of progression, and boney maturity at onset.
  - The lower the Cobb angle and the higher the Risser grade (boney maturity), the better the prognosis

PATIENT RESOURCE

- *Scoliosis.* National Institute of Arthritis and Musculoskeletal and Skin Diseases. July 2008. http://www.niams.nih.gov/Health_Info/Scoliosis/. Accessed June 12, 2013.

REFERENCE

1. Homnick DN. Chest and pulmonary conditions. In: Patel DR, Greydanus DE, Baker RJ, eds. *Pediatric Practice: Sports Medicine.* New York, NY: McGraw-Hill; 2009:Chapter 12. http://www.accessphysiotherapy.com/content/6974869#6974869. Accessed June 12, 2013.

ADDITIONAL REFERENCES

- Dutton M. Gait, posture, ergonomics, and occupational health. In: Dutton M, ed. *McGraw-Hill's NPTE (National Physical Therapy Examination).* New York, NY: McGraw-Hill; 2009:Chapter 7. http://www.accessphysiotherapy.com/content/5396959. Accessed June 12, 2013.
- Dutton M. The lumbar spine. In: Dutton M, ed. *Orthopaedic Examination, Evaluation, and Intervention.* 2nd ed. New York, NY: McGraw-Hill; 2008:Chapter 26. http://www.accessphysiotherapy.com/content/55595190. Accessed June 12, 2013.
- Fusco C, Zaina F, Atanasio S, Romano M, Negrini A, Negrini S. Physical exercises in the treatment of adolescent idiopathic scoliosis: an updated systematic review. *Physiother Theory Pract.* 2011;27(1):80–114. doi:10.3109/09593985.2010.533342.
- Hamilton N, Weimar W, Luttgens K. The musculoskeletal system: the musculature. In: Hamilton N, Weimar W, Luttgens K, eds. *Kinesiology: Scientific Basis of Human Motion.* New York, NY: McGraw-Hill; 2008:Chapter 3. http://www.accessphysiotherapy.com/content/6150242. Accessed June 12, 2013.
- ICD9Data.com. http://www.icd9data.com. Accessed June 12, 2012.
- ICD10Data.com. http://www.icd10data.com/ICD10CM/Codes. Accessed June 12, 2013.
- Lange JE, Steen H, Brox JI. Long-term results after Boston brace treatment in adolescent idiopathic scoliosis. *Scoliosis.* 2009;26:4–17. doi:10.1186/1748-7161-4-17.
- Negrini S, Grivas TB, Kotwicki T, Rigo M, Zaina F. Guidelines on "Standards of management of idiopathic scoliosis with "corrective braces in everyday clinics and in clinical research": SOSORT Consensus 2008. *Scoliosis.* 2009;4:2. doi:10.1186/1748-7161-4-2.
- Patel DR, Greydanus DE, Baker RJ. Thoracolumbar spine injuries. In: Patel DR, Greydanus DE, Baker RJ, eds. *Pediatric Practice: Sports Medicine.* New York, NY: McGraw-Hill; 2009:Chapter 30. http://www.accessphysiotherapy.com/popup.aspx?aID=6981371. Accessed June 12, 2013.
- Pattern 4B: Impaired posture. In: *Guide to Physical Therapist Practice.* 2nd ed. Alexandria, VA: American Physical Therapy Association; 2001. Revised 2003.
- Prentice WE, Quillen WS, Underwood F, eds. *Therapeutic Modalities in Rehabilitation.* 4th ed. New York, NY: McGraw-Hill; 2011. http://www.accessphysiotherapy.com/content/8137872. Accessed June 12, 2013.
- Romano M, Negrini S. Manual therapy as a conservative treatment for adolescent idiopathic scoliosis: a systematic review. *Scoliosis.* 2008;3:2. doi:10.1186/1748-7161-3-2.
- Scoliosis—Treatment for Adult Scoliosis. Baltimore Washington Medical Center. May 2009. http://health.bwmc.umms.org/patiented/articles/what_surgical_procedures_scoliosis_000068_10.htm. Accessed June 12, 2013.
- Thaler M, Kaufmann G, Steingruber I, Mayr E, Liebensteiner M, Bach C. Radiographic versus ultrasound evaluation of the Risser Grade in adolescent idiopathic scoliosis: a prospective study of 46 patients. *Eur Spine J.* 2008;17(9):1251–1255. doi: 10.1007/s00586-008-0726-6.
- Weiss HR, Bohr S, Jahnke A, Pleine S. Acupuncture in the treatment of scoliosis - a single blind controlled pilot study. *Scoliosis.* 2008;3:4. doi:10.1186/1748-7161-3-4.

141 SPONDYLITIS

Eric Shamus, PhD, DPT, PT, CSCS
Shallen (McClain) Flory, DPT

CONDITION/DISORDER SYNONYMS

- Bekhterev syndrome
- Marie-Strümpell disease
- Pott disease
- Rheumatoid spondylitis
- Spondyloarthropathy

ICD-9-CM CODE

- 720.81 Inflammatory spondylopathies in diseases classified elsewhere

ICD-10-CM CODE

- M49.80 Spondylopathy in diseases classified elsewhere, site unspecified

PREFERRED PRACTICE PATTERNS

- 4B: Impaired Posture[1]
- 4E: Impaired Joint Mobility, Motor Function, Muscle Performance, and ROM Associated with Localized Inflammation[2]
- 4F: Impaired Joint Mobility, Motor Function, Muscle Performance, Range of Motion, and Reflex Integrity Associated with Spinal Disorders[3]

PATIENT PRESENTATION

A 45-year-old female presents with complaints of low back pain with insidious onset and duration of 4 months. She reports that she has pain while trying to sleep and is very stiff in the morning after waking up. As she walks around and gets ready for work, she notes that the stiffness subsides. She notes that the pain comes and goes throughout the day, and at the worst it is a 7/10 and at best it is a 1/10. She mentions that she works as a secretary for a local business and sits at her desk answering phones most of the day. She also notes that her daily walks of 3 miles with her dog are becoming more difficult even though the back pain is not present on the walks. Finally, she mentions pain in her right heel and a stiff right hip.

She is referred to physical therapy by her primary care physician. The physician tested her pulmonary function and noted that she showed decreased vital capacity and total lung capacity, while residual and functional residual lung volumes showed an increase. The PT examination revealed decreased ROM in the lumbar spine with flexion and extension. Mobility scale of 2 at T10 to T12 and 2 at L3 to S1 was revealed during joint play assessment. Tenderness at the SI joint was noted with palpation. MMT of the lower extremity (LE) reveals strength 5/5 in the left LE and the right hip adductors, 4/5 in the right hip flexors, right hip extensors, right hip abductors, and right dorsiflexors, and 4-/5 in the right plantarflexors.

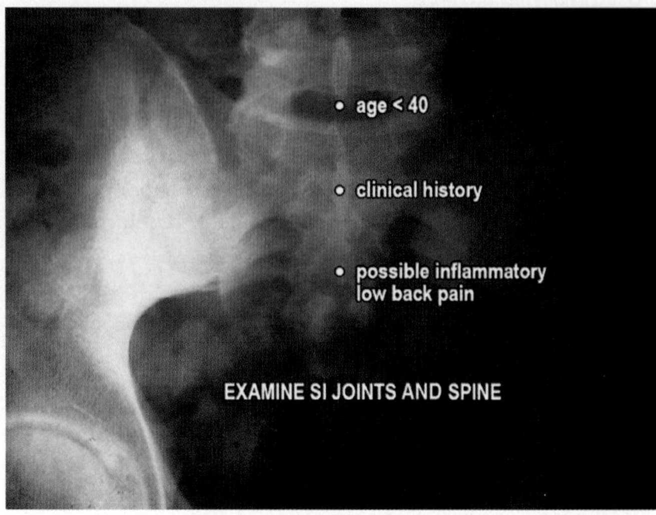

FIGURE 141-1 X-ray of Spondylitis/Spondyloarthritis. (From Lawry GV. *Systematic Musculoskeletal Examinations*. www.accessmedicine.com. Copyright © The McGraw-Hill Companies, Inc. All rights reserved.)

KEY FEATURES

Description

- Inflammation of one or more spinal vertebrae
- Can be localized due to infection of a certain spinal area, degenerative arthritis, or following a traumatic injury

Essentials of Diagnosis

- Most characterized with sacroiliac (SI) joint pain and dysfunction
- Etiology unknown
- Acute, painful flare-ups
- Chronic, persistent pain
- Pain for longer than 3 months
- Relief with nonsteroidal anti-inflammatory drugs (NSAIDs)
- Morning stiffness

General Considerations

- Begins with intermittent low back pain
- Improved with low-level activity
- May have rapid and severe onset
  - Secondary problems
    - Pulmonary fibrosis
    - Restrictive lung capacity

Demographics

- Begins ages 18 to 45
- Can affect any age or gender

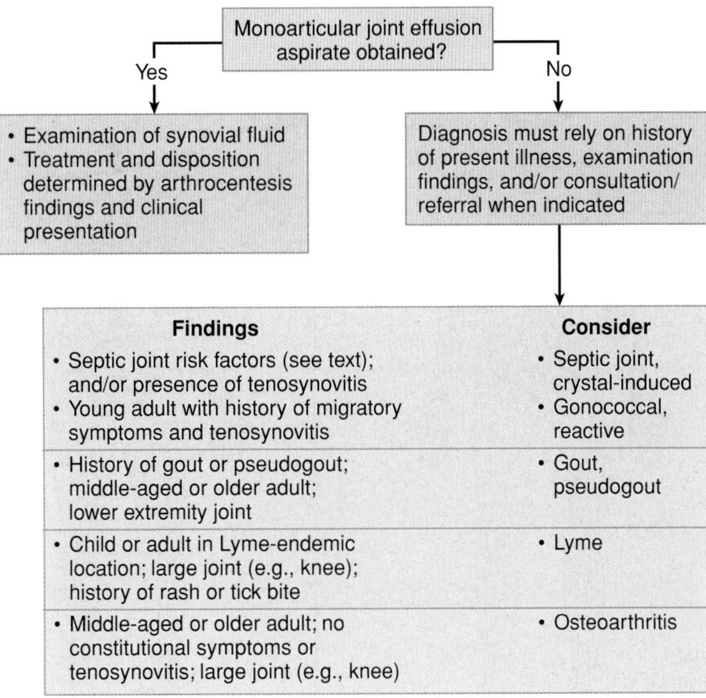

FIGURE 141-2 Diagnostic algorithm for the nontraumatic, acute monoarticular arthritis patient. Common, acute diagnoses and disease presentations are included in this algorithm. Patients may have uncommon disease presentation, overlapping diagnoses (e.g., gout and septic joint), or illnesses not included in the algorithm. (From Tintinalli JE, Stapczynski J, Ma OJ, Cline D, Cydulka R, Meckler G. *Tintinalli's Emergency Medicine: A Comprehensive Study Guide*. 7th ed. www.accessmedicine.com. Copyright © The McGraw-Hill Companies, Inc. All rights reserved.)

CLINICAL FINDINGS

SIGNS AND SYMPTOMS

- Loss of ROM and joint play
- Intermittent back pain
- Pain and stiffness during rest/sleep
- Heel pain
- Hip pain and stiffness
- Joint pain and swelling in shoulders, knees, ankles
- Thoracic and pulmonary involvement

Functional Implications

- Limited mobility
- Aerobic endurance limitation
- May impede ability to perform ADLs/IADLs
- May impede participation in sports and other social activities

Possible Contributing Causes

- Congenital anomalies
- Degenerative arthritis
- Gastrointestinal infections
- Obesity
- Occupational factors
- Physical condition
- Postural changes
- Psychosocial and behavioral factors
- Smoking
- Socioeconomic factors
- Tightness of hip flexors, hip external rotators, hamstrings
- Trauma
- Weakness of core musculature

Differential Diagnosis

- Ankylosing spondylitis
- Crohn disease
- Disc herniation
- Erector spinae muscle strain
- Facet joint arthritis
- Forestier disease
- Myofascial pain syndrome
- Psoriatic arthritis
- Reiter syndrome (reactive arthritis)
- Rheumatoid arthritis
- Sacral dysfunction
- Spinal alignment
- Spinal stenosis
- Spondylolisthesis
- Spondylosis
- Systemic autoimmune diseases (rheumatoid arthritis, Reiter syndrome)
- Whipple disease
- Yersinia arthritis

MEANS OF CONFIRMATION OR DIAGNOSIS

Laboratory Tests

- To rule out systemic disease, differential diagnosis
  - Complete blood count (CBC)
  - Erythrocyte sedimentation rate (ESR)
  - HLA-B27 antigen, genetic marker for ankylosing spondylitis
  - No single blood test can determine spondylitis
  - Negative serologic tests for rheumatoid factor

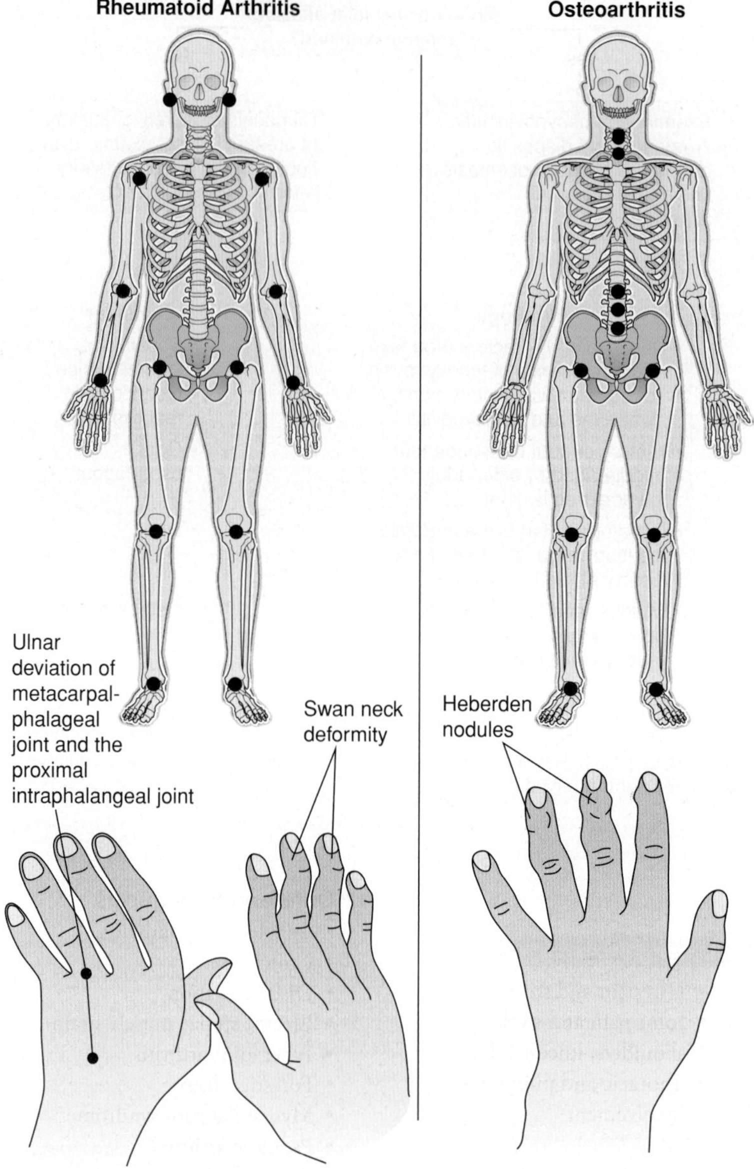

FIGURE 141-3 Rheumatoid arthritis versus osteoarthritis. (From Toy EC, Patlan JT. *Case Files: Internal Medicine*. 3rd ed. www.accessmedicine.com. Copyright © The McGraw-Hill Companies, Inc. All rights reserved.)

Imaging

- MRI helpful in diagnosis to visualize structure of ligament, compressed or inflamed nerve root, disc pathology
- X-ray/Plain-film radiograph helps to assess alignment, fractures, stability (flexion/extension radiograph)
- CT to show structure of ligament, herniation compressing the spinal canal/nerves, or to rule out abdominal pathology
- Electrodiagnostic/Nerve conduction testing can help determine specific impaired nerve function
- Doppler ultrasound to examine vascular function
- Diagnostic ultrasound to analyze fiber orientation

FINDINGS AND INTERPRETATION

- Single segmental problem
- Multi-level "bamboo spine": Ankylosing spondylitis
- Late stages affect segmental loss of ROM

TREATMENT

Medication

- NSAIDs
- Corticosteroids

REFERRALS/ADMITTANCE

- To rheumatologist to assess underlying complications
- To surgeon for consult
- To orthopedic surgeon if nerve entrapment exists

Impairments

- Mobility limitations
- Functional rotation and bending limitations
- Weakened abdominals and other core-stabilizing muscles
- Shortened hamstrings and hip flexors
- Postural changes
- Inability to walk, stand, sit for prolonged periods of time

TESTS AND MEASURES

- Passive physiological intervertebral mobility testing (PPIVM)
- LE screening examination
- Postural examination
- Muscle length testing, including hamstrings, hip flexors, calf muscles
- Quadrant test
- Straight-leg raise test
- Slump test
- Lower limb nerve tension test
- Prone instability test
- LE neurological screening (dermatome, myotome, reflexes)
- Repeated movement testing
- Fear-Avoidance Beliefs Questionnaire (FABQ)

INTERVENTION

- Education in gentle ROM to maintain mobility
- Exercise: Flexibility and stability strengthening to decrease stress on joints
- Joint protection education
- Postural training
- Warm shower or heat to increase mobility
- Joint manipulation indicated when
    - Duration of current episode of low back pain less than 16 days
    - No radicular symptoms/pain distal to the knee
    - FABQ score less than 19
    - Hip Internal Rotation of greater than 35 degrees for at least one hip
    - Segemental hypomobility of at least one level of the lumbar spine
- Specific exercise when pain centralizes upon repeated movement/ posture into flexion or extension
- Lumbar stabilization exercises to address core stability when
    - Prone instability test positive
    - Presence of aberrant motion
    - Straight-leg raise greater than 91 degrees
    - Age younger than 41 years
- Traction when
    - Radiculopathy findings present
    - Positive crossed straight-leg raise
    - Pain becomes peripheralized with repeated extension
- Stretching exercises, myofascial mobilization for shortened musculature
- Unweighted treadmill walking
- Aquatic exercise
- Modalities for short-term pain control
- Cognitive behavioral therapy

FUNCTIONAL GOALS

- Patient will be independent with home exercise program.
- Patient will have 2/10 pain rating while performing household activities.
- Patient will have improved functional level so as to grocery shop.
- Patient will be able to
    - Sit with neutral lumbar spine posture for >30 minutes with 0 out of 10 pain rating for computer work and desk activities.
    - Sit at work station and perform computer work for 45 minutes with 0/10 pain rating.
    - Rotate lumbar spine 25 degrees so as to reach into back seat of car with 0/10 pain rating in LE.
    - Walk for 30 minutes with 0/10 pain rating so as to go shopping.
    - Increase standing tolerance to >30 minutes without pain so as to stand at work.

PROGNOSIS

- Disease progression is not specific; joints may create encroachment on neural structures as disease becomes more severe.
- Symptoms may be intermittent.
- Patients function well until severe progression of osteophytes and spinal joint fusion.

PATIENT RESOURCE

- Spondylitis Association of America. http://www.spondylitis.org. Accessed July 10, 2013.

REFERENCES

1. The American Physical Therapy Association. Pattern 4B: impaired posture. *Interactive Guide to Physical Therapist Practice.* 2003. http://guidetoptpractice.apta.org/content/1/SEC9.extract. Accessed May 25, 2014.
2. The American Physical Therapy Association. Pattern 4E: impaired joint mobility, motor function, muscle performance, and range of motion associated with localized inflammation. *Interactive Guide to Physical Therapist Practice.* 2003. http://guidetoptpractice.apta.org/content/1/SEC12.extract. Accessed May 25, 2014.
3. The American Physical Therapy Association. Pattern 4F: impaired joint mobility, motor function, muscle performance, range of motion, and reflex integrity associated with spinal disorders. *Interactive Guide to Physical Therapist Practice.* 2003. http://guidetoptpractice.apta.org/content/1/SEC13.extract. Accessed May 25, 2014.

ADDITIONAL REFERENCES

- ClinicalTrialsFeeds.org. *Safety and Effectiveness of Adalimumab (Humira) in Patients with Ankylosing Spondylitis in Clinical Routine.* http://clinicaltrialsfeeds.org/clinical-trials/show/NCT01079182. Accessed July 10, 2013.
- Dutton M. Musculoskeletal physical therapy. In: Dutton M, ed. *McGraw-Hill's NPTE (National Physical Therapy Examination).* 2nd ed. New York, NY: McGraw-Hill; 2012. http://www.accessphysiotherapy.com/content/5397601. Accessed July 10, 2013.
- Dutton M. *Orthopaedic Examination, Evaluation, and Intervention.* New York, NY: McGraw-Hill; 2008. http://www.accessphysiotherapy.com/resource/612. Accessed July 10, 2013.
- Dutton M. *Dutton's Orthopedic Survival Guide: Managing Common Conditions.* New York, NY: McGraw-Hill; 2011. http://www.accessphysiotherapy.com/resource/685. Accessed July 10, 2013.
- Fritz JM, Cleland JA, Childs JD. Subgrouping patients with low back pain: evolution of a classification approach to physical therapy. *J Orthop Sports Phys Ther.* 2007;37:290-302.
- ICD-9-CM. http://www.icd9data.com. Accessed July 10, 2013.
- ICD-10-CM. http://www.icd10data.com. Accessed July 10, 2013.
- Liebenson C. *Rehabilitation of the Spine: A Practitioner's Manual.* Baltimore, MD: Lippincott, Williams & Wilkins; 2007.
- Malone TR, Hazle C, Grey ML. *Imaging in Rehabilitation.* New York, NY: McGraw-Hill; 2008. http://www.accessphysiotherapy.com/resource/613. Accessed July 10, 2013.
- Olsen KA. *Manual Physical Therapy of the Spine.* St. Louis, MI: Saunders Elsevier; 2009.

142 SWAYBACK

Eric Shamus, PhD, DPT, PT, CSCS
Shallen (McClain) Flory, DPT

CONDITION/DISORDER SYNONYMS

- Lumbar hyperlordosis
- Saddle back

ICD-9-CM CODES

- 737.2 Lordosis (acquired)
- 754.2 Congenital musculoskeletal deformities of spine

ICD-10-CM CODES

- Q67.5 Congenital deformity of spine
- Q76.3 Congenital scoliosis due to congenital bony malformation
- Q76.425 Congenital lordosis, thoracolumbar region
- Q76.426 Congenital lordosis, lumbar region
- Q76.427 Congenital lordosis, lumbosacral region

PREFERRED PRACTICE PATTERNS

- 4B: Impaired Posture[1]
- 4E: Impaired Joint Mobility, Motor Function, Muscle Performance, and ROM Associated With Localized Inflammation[2]
- 4F: Impaired Joint Mobility, Motor Function, Muscle Performance, Range of Motion, and Reflex Integrity Associated With Spinal Disorders[3]

PATIENT PRESENTATION

A 38-year-old female was referred to physical therapy by her primary care physician. She presents with low back pain (LBP) that began in her seventh month of pregnancy. She reports that her baby is 3 months old, but the pain is still present. She notes that the pain is worse after standing for long periods of time at work as a middle school teacher. She notes that the pain is worse when she rotates her back to write on the board. She mentions that it is becoming difficult to carry her baby due to the pain.

The PT examination revealed the following information. Posture showed an increase in lumbar lordosis with an anterior pelvic tilt. Pain was reproduced during the lower quarter screening during lumbar extension. MMT revealed hamstring strength bilaterally 4-/5, with all other bilateral lower extremity (LE) muscles 5/5. PIVM showed mobility in the spine to be 5 at L2 to L4 and 4 at L5 to S1. Patient had a positive quadrant test to the right side, a positive prone instability test, and a positive Thomas test.

KEY FEATURES

Description

- Excessive lumbar lordosis curvature
- Increased extension of the lumbar spine compresses the facets

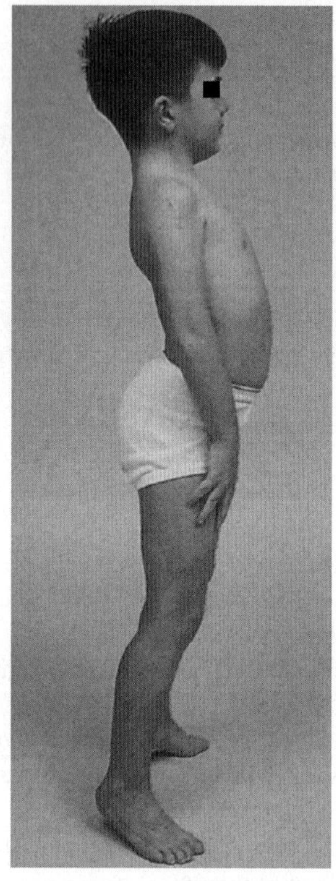

FIGURE 142-1 Lordotic posture, exaggerated by standing on toes, associated with trunk and hip weakness. (From Longo DL, Fauci AS, Kasper DL, Hauser SL, Jameson JL, Loscalzo J, eds. *Harrison's Principles of Internal Medicine*. 18th ed. New York, NY: McGraw-Hill; 2012.)

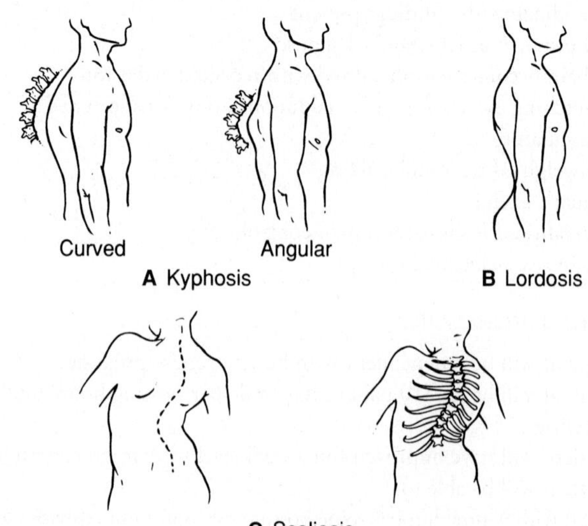

FIGURE 142-2 Curvatures of the spine affecting the thorax. (**A**) Kyphotic thorax. (**B**) Lordotic thorax. (**C**) Scoliotic thorax. Note the narrowing of the rib interspaces on the right and the accentuation of the interspaces, posterior humping of the chest, and elevation of the shoulder on the left. (From LeBlond RF, DeGowin RL, Brown DD. *DeGowin's Diagnostic Examination*. 9th ed. www.accessmedicine.com. Copyright © The McGraw-Hill Companies, Inc. All rights reserved.)

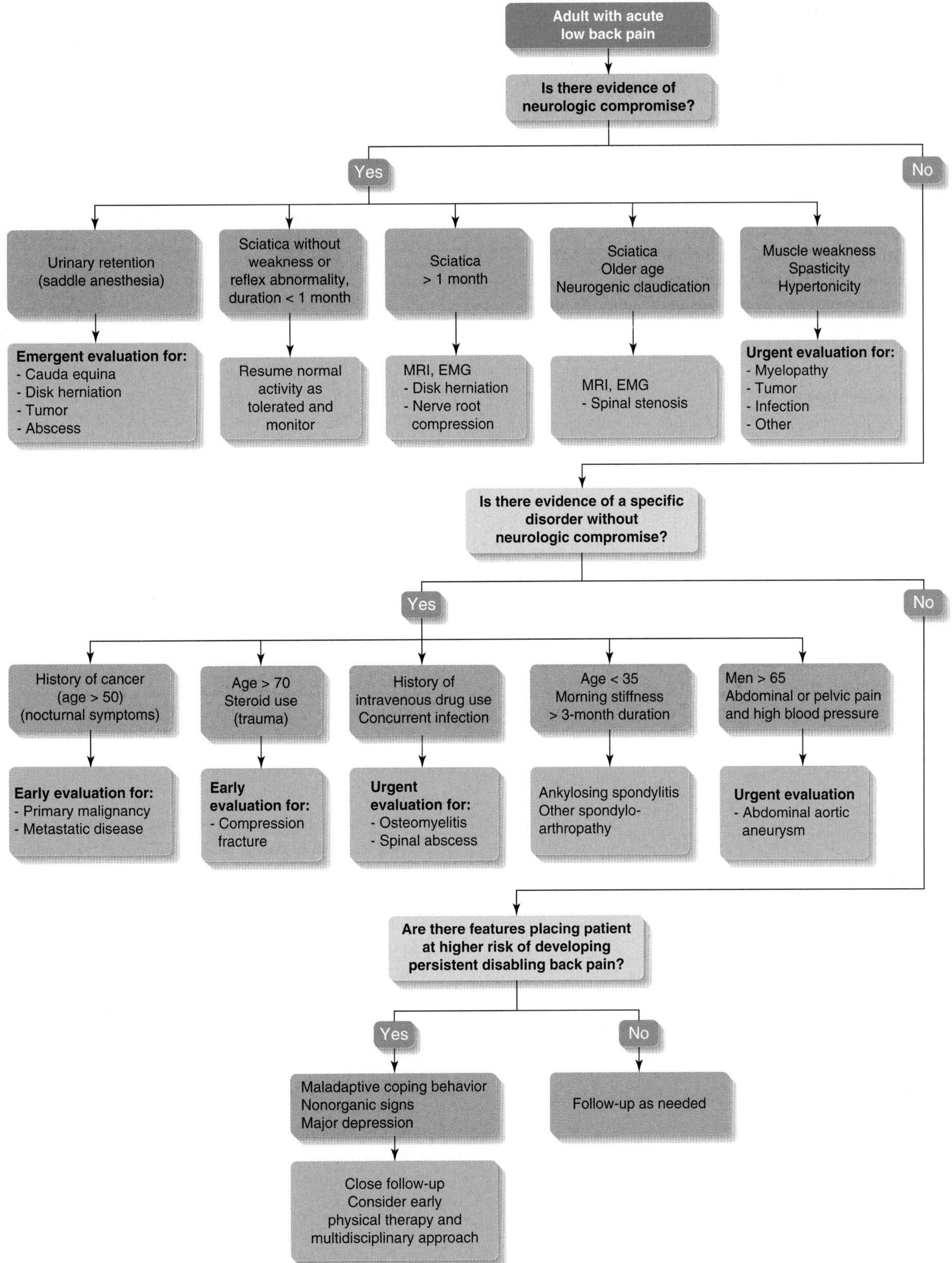

FIGURE 142-3 Diagnostic approach: low back pain. EMG, electromyography; MRI, magnetic resonance imaging. (From Henderson MC, Tierney LM, Smetana GW. *The Patient History: An Evidence-Based Approach to Differential Diagnosis*. http://www.accessmedicine.com. Copyright © The McGraw-Hill Companies, Inc. All rights reserved.)

- Anterior pelvic tilt
- LBP with primary involvement of lumbar facet joint
- Lower limb symptoms might be present in a nondermatomal pattern as a result of referred pain
- Neurological findings, minimal
- Bilateral symptoms

▶ Essentials of Diagnosis

- Symptoms are depending if the curve reverses when flexed
- Diagnosis made by clinical examination
- Use of treatment (impairment) based classification system is useful to determine EBP based treatment plan
- Reproduction of symptoms when putting the joint in closed packed position (combination of extension, side bending toward involved side, rotation away from involved site

▶ General Considerations

- Presentation can vary significantly in presentation based upon anatomical structures
- Tight lumbar spine musculature and tight quadriceps
- Associated with thoracic kyphosis

▶ Demographics

- Can be postural or hereditary

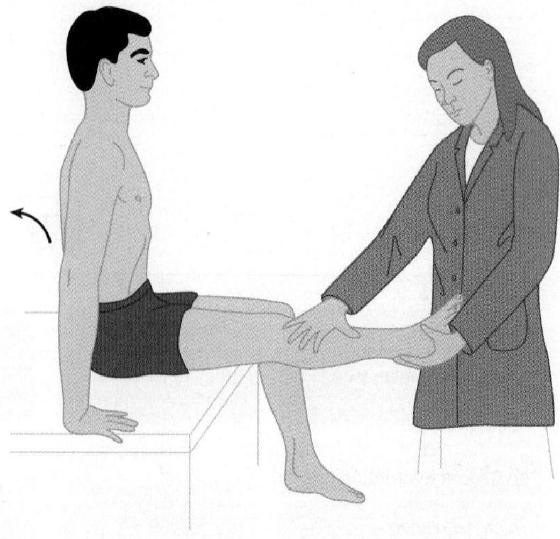

FIGURE 142-4 Sitting knee extension test. With the patient sitting on a table, both hip and knees flexed at 90 degrees, slowly extend the knee as if evaluating the patella or bottom of the foot. This maneuver stretches nerve roots as much as a moderate degree of supine straight-leg raising. (From Tintinalli JE, Stapczynski J, Ma OJ, Cline D, Cydulka R, Meckler G. *Tintinalli's Emergency Medicine: A Comprehensive Study Guide*. 7th ed. www.accessmedicine.com. Copyright © The McGraw-Hill Companies, Inc. All rights reserved.)

CLINICAL FINDINGS

SIGNS AND SYMPTOMS

- Pain in lumbar/sacral area that can be mechanically reproduced
- Bilateral referred or pain in LE possible
- ROM limited in a capsular pattern: Rotation and side bending limited in opposite direction
- Lumbar segmental hypomobility may be present in capsular pattern
- Can be associated with poor core-muscle strength and postural deviations

▶ Functional Implications

- Prolonged standing can cause compression pain.
- May cause decreased ability to perform ADLs/IADLs.
- May impact ability to participate in sports and other social activities.

▶ Possible Contributing Causes

- Occupational factors
- Rickets
- Vitamin D deficiency
- Congenital anomalies
- Physical condition
- Obesity
- Postural changes
- Weakness of core musculature
- Tightness of hip flexors

▶ Differential Diagnosis

- Peripheral nerve impairment
- Hip pathology with radiating pain pattern
- Malignant spinal tumor or metastasis
- Referred pain from visceral structures
- Systematic autoimmune diseases (RA, Reiter's, etc.)
- Ankylosing spondylitis
- Abdominal aortic aneurism
- Radiculopathy

MEANS OF CONFIRMATION

▶ Imaging

- In most cases not necessary, only with persistent symptoms that do not respond to conservative management or presence of red/yellow flags
- Computed tomography (CT)
- Doppler ultrasound
- Electrodiagnostic/nerve conduction testing
- Magnetic resonance imaging (MRI)
- X-ray/Plain-film radiograph

FINDINGS AND INTERPRETATION

- CT scan to show herniation compressing the spinal canal/nerves, r/o abdominal pathology
- Doppler ultrasound to examine vascular function
- Electrodiagnostic/nerve conduction testing can assist to determine a specific impaired nerve function
- MRI helpful in diagnosis to visualize compressed or inflamed nerve root/disc pathology
- X-ray/Plain-film radiograph helpful to assess alignment, fractures, stability (flexion/extension radiograph)

REFERRALS/ADMITTANCE

- For imaging
- For surgical consult if myelopathy is suspected (see Lumbar Radiculopathy, Chapter 128)
- For imaging and medical consult if disease is suspected

IMPAIRMENTS

- Hypomobile lumbar spine
- Inability to stand for prolonged time
- Inability to walk for prolonged time
- Postural changes
- Shortening of hip flexors
- Weakness of abdominals and other core stabilizing muscles

TESTS AND MEASURES

- Passive physiological intervertebral mobility testing (PPIVM)
- LE screening examination
- Postural examination
- Muscle length testing, including hamstrings, hip flexors, calf muscles
- Quadrant test
- Straight-leg raise test
- Slump test
- Lower limb nerve tension test
- Prone instability test
- LE neurological screening (dermatome, myotome, reflexes)
- Repeated movement testing
- Fear-Avoidance Beliefs Questionnaire (FABQ)
- Algorithm for examination of the lumbar spine

INTERVENTION

- Joint manipulation indicated when[4]
  - Duration of current episode of low back pain less than 16 days
  - No radicular symptoms/pain distal to the knee
  - Fear avoidance beliefs questionaire (FABQ) score less than 19
  - Hip Internal Rotation of greater than 35 degrees for at least one hip
  - Segemental hypomobility of at least one level of the lumbar spine
- Joint mobilization
- Lumbar stabilization exercises to address core stability when[4]
  - Positive prone instability test
  - Presence of aberrant motion
  - Straight-leg raise greater than 91 degrees
  - Age younger than 41 years
- Initiate stabilization exercises after normalization of ROM
- Stretching exercises and myofascial mobilization for shortened musculature, hip flexors
- Unweighted treadmill walking
- Strengthen hamstrings and hip extensors
- Posterior pelvic tilts
- Aquatic exercise
- Modalities for short-term pain control
- Cognitive behavioral therapy

FUNCTIONAL GOALS

- Patient will be able to
  - Stand with a neutral lumbar spine posture for >30 minutes with 0/10 pain.
  - Stand at work station and perform computer work for 45 minutes with 0/10 pain.
  - Rotate lumbar spine 25 degrees with 0/10 LE pain to reach into the back seat in the car.
  - Walk for 30 minutes with 0/10 pain to go shopping.
  - Increase standing tolerance to >30 minutes without pain to fulfill recreational activity requirements.

PROGNOSIS

- Fair to very good, depending on specific impairments.
- Chronic LBP prognosis is significantly less.

PATIENT RESOURCE

- Hyper-lordosis. Seattle Children's Hospital, Research and Foundation. http://www.seattlechildrens.org/medical-conditions/bone-joint-muscle-conditions/spinal-conditions-treatment/scoliosis/lordosis. Accessed May 25, 2014.

REFERENCES

1. The American Physical Therapy Association. Pattern 4B: impaired posture. *Interactive Guide to Physical Therapist Practice*. 2003. http://guidetoptpractice.apta.org/content/1/SEC9.extract. Accessed May 25, 2014.
2. The American Physical Therapy Association. Pattern 4E: impaired joint mobility, motor function, muscle performance, and range of motion associated with localized inflammation. *Interactive Guide to Physical Therapist Practice*. 2003. http://guidetoptpractice.apta.org/content/1/SEC12.extract. Accessed May 25, 2014.
3. The American Physical Therapy Association. Pattern 4F: impaired joint mobility, motor function, muscle performance, range of motion, and reflex integrity associated with spinal disorders. *Interactive Guide to Physical Therapist Practice*. 2003. http://guidetoptpractice.apta.org/content/1/SEC13.extract. Accessed May 25, 2014.
4. Fritz JM, Cleland JA, Childs JD. Subgrouping patients with low back pain: evolution of a classification approach to physical therapy. *J Orthop Sports Phys Ther*. 2007;37:290–302.

ADDITIONAL REFERENCES

- Dutton M. The lumbopelvic complex. In: Dutton M, ed. *Dutton's Orthopedic Survival Guide: Managing Common Conditions*. New York, NY: McGraw-Hill; 2011:Chapter 13. http://www.accessphysiotherapy.com/content/8657033. Accessed July 6, 2013.
- ICD-9-CM. http://www.icd9data.com. Accessed July 10, 2013.
- ICD-10-CM. http://www.icd10data.com. Accessed July 10, 2013.
- Liebenson C. *Rehabilitation of the Spine: A Practitioner's Manual*. Baltimore, MD: Lippincott, Williams & Wilkins; 2007.
- Malone TR, Hazle C, Grey ML. *Imaging in Rehabilitation*. New York, NY: McGraw-Hill; 2008. http://www.accessphysiotherapy.com/resource/613. Accessed July 10, 2013.
- Olsen KA. *Manual Physical Therapy of the Spine*. St. Louis, MI: Saunders Elsevier; 2009.
- Schuler TC, Subach BR, Branch CL, Foley KT, Burkus JK, Lumbar Spine Study Group. Segmental lumbar lordosis: manual versus computer-assisted measurement using seven different techniques. *J Spinal Disord Tech*. 2004;17(5):372–379.

143 SPINAL FRACTURE

Jennifer Cabrera, DPT, GCS
Eric Shamus, PhD, DPT, PT, CSCS

CONDITION/DISORDER SYNONYM

- Vertebral compression fracture

ICD-9-CM CODES[1]

- 805.0 Closed fracture of cervical vertebra without mention of spinal cord injury
- 805.1 Open fracture of cervical vertebra without mention of spinal cord injury
- 805.2 Closed fracture of dorsal (thoracic) vertebra without spinal cord injury
- 805.3 Open fracture of dorsal (thoracic) vertebra without spinal cord injury
- 805.4 Closed fracture of lumbar vertebra without spinal cord injury
- 805.5 Open fracture of lumbar vertebra without spinal cord injury
- 805.6 Closed fracture of sacrum and coccyx without spinal cord injury
- 805.7 Open fracture of sacrum and coccyx without spinal cord injury
- 805.8 Closed fracture of unspecified part of vertebral column without spinal cord injury
- 805.9 Open fracture of unspecified part of vertebral column without spinal cord injury

ICD-10-CM CODES[2]

- S12.9XXA Fracture of neck, unspecified, initial encounter
- S22.009A Unspecified fracture of unspecified thoracic vertebra, initial encounter for closed fracture
- S22.009B Unspecified fracture of unspecified thoracic vertebra, initial encounter for open fracture
- S32.009A Unspecified fracture of unspecified lumbar vertebra, initial encounter for closed fracture
- S32.009B Unspecified fracture of unspecified lumbar vertebra, initial encounter for open fracture
- S32.10XA Unspecified fracture of sacrum, initial encounter for closed fracture
- S32.2XXA Fracture of coccyx, initial encounter for closed fracture
- S32.10XB Unspecified fracture of sacrum, initial encounter for open fracture
- S32.2XXB Fracture of coccyx, initial encounter for open fracture

PREFERRED PRACTICE PATTERN[3]

- 4G: Impaired Joint Mobility, Muscle Performance, and Range of Motion Associated with Fracture

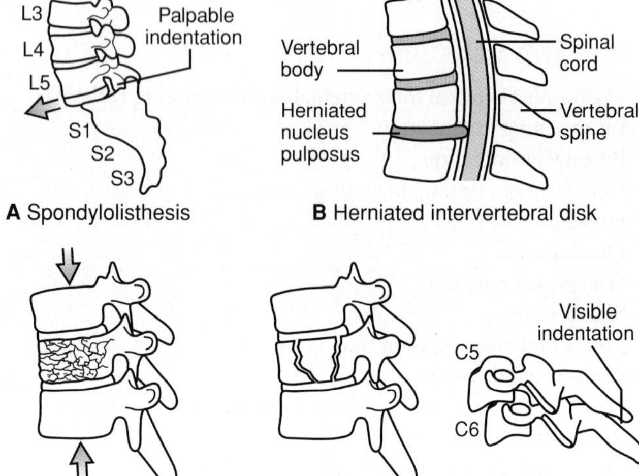

FIGURE 143-1 Lesions of a single vertebra. (**A**) Spondylolisthesis. (**B**) Herniated intervertebral disk. (**C**) Stable compression vertebral fracture. (**D**) Unstable compression vertebral fracture. (**E**) Interlocking or subluxation of vertebra. (From LeBlond RF, DeGowin RL, Brown DD. *DeGowin's Diagnostic Examination*. 9th ed. www.accessmedicine.com. Copyright © The McGraw-Hill Companies, Inc. All rights reserved.)

PATIENT PRESENTATION

A 78-year-old man lost his balance and fell while ambulating at home with his four-wheeled rolling walker. He reports he hit his back on the sofa as he was falling and landed in a sitting position. He reports immediate pain with inability to stand up, so emergency services are contacted. He has a history of chronic obstructive pulmonary disease for which he has had prolonged exposure to steroids for management. He presents with increased pain with all movements and his only position of mild comfort is lying supine. Radiographs showed T12-L1 acute compression fractures. There was anterior vertebral body wedging deformity noted on the lateral view and decreased vertebral height noted on the posterior view.

KEY FEATURES

▶ Description

- Fracture
- Any defect in the continuity of the end plate or vertebral body
- Types of spinal fractures
  - Compression fracture
    - Wedge deformity
    - Anterior vertebral body fractures, with loss of height greater anteriorly than posteriorly
    - Usually stable
    - Rarely associated with neurologic symptoms
  - Axial burst fracture
    - Anterior and posterior vertebral body fracture
    - Mechanism of injury is usually fall from height

- Flexion/Distraction fracture
    - Vertebra is pulled apart
    - Such as in a motor vehicle accident
- Transverse process fracture
    - Uncommon
    - Results from rotation or extreme lateral bending
- Fracture–dislocation
    - Unstable injury
    - Involves bone and soft tissue injury
    - Vertebra becomes displaced from adjacent vertebra
    - Results in serious spinal cord compression

Essentials of Diagnosis

- Diagnosis is usually made by clinical examination.
- Can be an independent diagnosis and not associated with a disease process.

General Considerations

- Most common fractures of the spine occur in the thoracic and lumbar spine.

Demographics

- Men experience these fractures four times more often than women.
- Increased risk of spinal fracture in the elderly secondary to osteoporosis.
    - Occurs in approximately 700,000 individuals yearly.

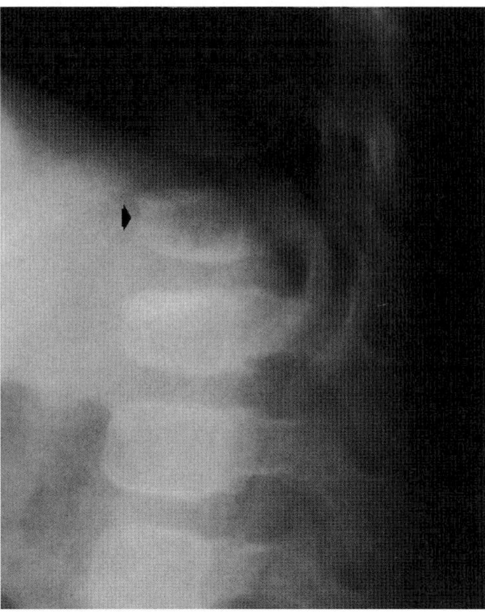

FIGURE 143-2 Compression fracture. The wedging of T-12 (*arrows*) and probably L1 indicates vertebral compression fractures. These fractures are the result of significant forces applied to the spinal column and are often indicative of child abuse. (From Knoop KJ, Stack LB, Storrow AB, Thurman RJ. *The Atlas of Emergency Medicine*. 3rd ed. www.accessmedicine.com. Copyright © The McGraw-Hill Companies, Inc. All rights reserved. Photo contributor: Alan E. Oestreich, MD.)

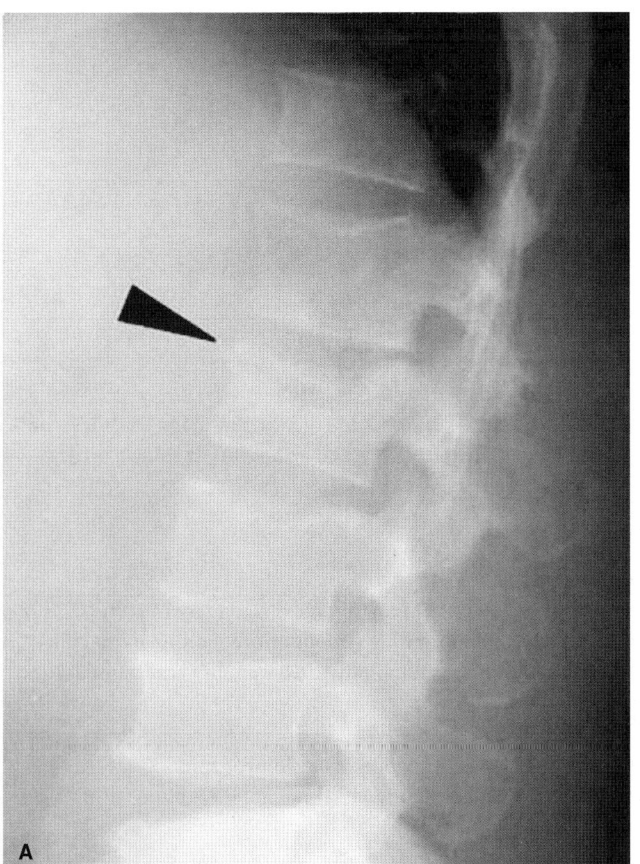

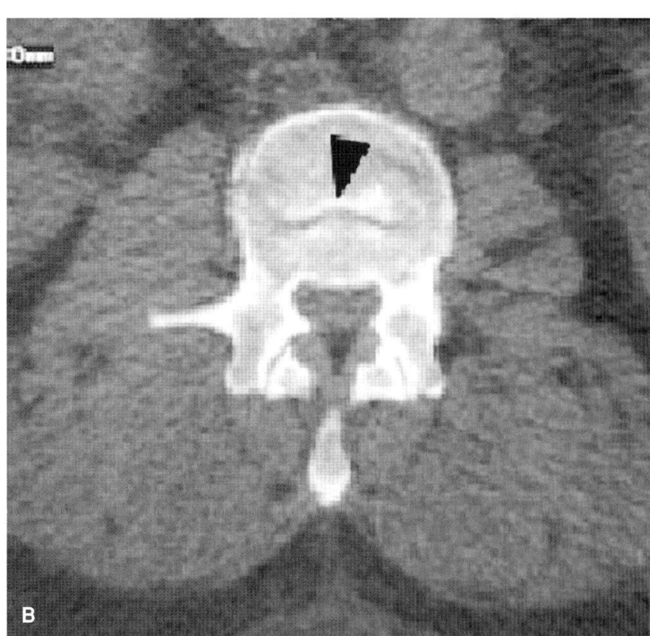

FIGURE 143-3 (**A**) Lateral lumbar spine X-ray showing a compression fracture of L2. *Arrowhead* points to anterior wedge deformity. Note that the posterior wall of the vertebral body has retained normal height and alignment. (**B**) Axial computed tomography scan through the same fracture. *Arrowhead* demonstrates a transverse discontinuity in the superior endplate of the L2 body. (From Brunicardi FC et al. *Schwartz's Principles of Surgery*. 9th ed. http://www.accessmedicine.com. Copyright © The McGraw-Hill Companies, Inc. All rights reserved.)

CLINICAL FINDINGS

SIGNS AND SYMPTOMS

- Moderate to severe back pain
- Pain is exacerbated with movement
- Loss of height
- Constipation
- Respiratory problems
- Some pain relief with lying down
- Deformity of the spine
- If spinal cord is involved, individual presents with
  - Numbness and tingling in lower extremities (LEs)
  - LE weakness
  - Alterations in bowel and bladder function

Functional Implications

- Pain with all movements
- Impaired functional mobility
- Pain with lifting items: Groceries

Possible Contributing Causes

- Osteoporosis
- Tumor
- Osteogenesis imperfecta
- High-velocity accident
  - Motor vehicle accident
  - Fall from height
  - Athletic accident
- Gun shot wound
- Metastatic tumor

Differential Diagnosis

- Muscle strain
- Cancer
- Facet impingement

MEANS OF CONFIRMATION OR DIAGNOSIS

Imaging

- X-ray for fracture, often limited view
- CT scan: Image
- MRI

FINDINGS AND INTERPRETATION

- Pain with all movements and positions
- Inability to tolerate prolonged sitting positions
- Inability to find a position of comfort
- If neurologic structures are involved, the individual will report numbness and decreased ability to move the foot and/or toes

TREATMENT

- Compression fracture
  - Brace (such as thoracic-lumbar-sacral orthosis [TLSO] or lumbar-sacral orthosis [LSO]) for 6 to 12 weeks
  - Kyphoplasty
- Axial burst fracture
  - Stable will have a brace for 6 to 12 weeks
  - Unstable will undergo a laminectomy (surgical decompression) with stabilization of the fracture
- Flexion/Distraction fracture
  - Only vertebral body involvement will require brace or cast for 12 months
  - If posterior ligaments or disks are involved, will undergo surgery to stabilize fracture

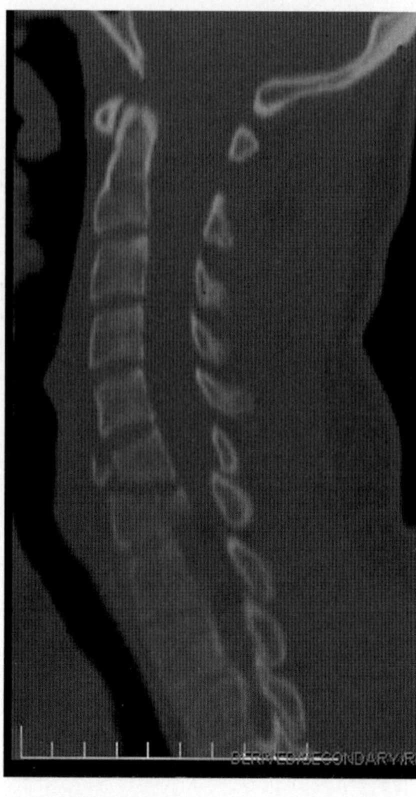

FIGURE 143-4 Sagittal reconstruction of a cervical CT scan demonstrating a C6–7 traumatic fracture. (From Doherty GM. *Current Diagnosis & Treatment: Surgery*. 13th ed. www.accessmedicine.com. Copyright © The McGraw-Hill Companies, Inc. All rights reserved.)

- Transverse process fracture
  - May or may not require bracing
- Fracture–dislocation
  - Requires surgical stabilization due to serious spinal cord damage

REFERRALS/ADMITTANCE

- For imaging, X-ray or CT
- For medication: NSAID or opioid for pain management, Denosumab
- For emergency orthopedic consult
- Lumbar–sacral orthosis: Emergency neurology consult if individual demonstrates signs and symptoms of spinal cord involvement

IMPAIRMENTS

- Antalgic gait secondary to pain
- Inability to ambulate long distances secondary to pain
- Inability to stand for long periods of time secondary to pain
- Decreased functional mobility: Bed mobility and transfers

TESTS AND MEASURES

- Algorithm for examination of the lumbar spine
- Passive physiological intervertebral mobility testing (PPIVM)
- LE screening examination
- Postural examination
- Muscle length testing, including hamstrings, hip flexors, calf muscles
- Treadmill test
- Quadrant test
- Straight-leg raise test

- Slump test
- Lower limb nerve tension test
- Prone instability test
- LE neurological screening (dermatome, myotome, reflexes)
- Repeated movement testing
- Fear-Avoidance Beliefs Questionnaire (FABQ)

INTERVENTION

- Monitor for signs/symptoms of deep vein thrombosis (DVT) in the LE
  - Positive Homans sign
  - Edema
  - Pain
  - Calor
  - Erythema
- Maintain back precautions
  - Log rolling
  - No lifting
  - No bending
  - No twisting
- Address pain
  - Ice/Cryotherapy
  - Massage
  - Electrical stimulation
- Address lack of flexibility via stretching
  - Hip flexors
  - Rectus femoris
  - Hamstrings
  - Gastrocnemius
  - Pectoralis
- Address neural mobility
  - Sciatic nerve
  - Tibial nerve
  - Sural nerve
  - Common peroneal nerve
- Address weakness via strengthening activities
  - Open chain in all planes while maintaining back precautions
  - Closed-chain activities (e.g., mini squats, heel raises, side stepping while maintaining back precautions)
  - Core strengthening
    - Transabdominal bracing
  - Postural re-education
- Address functional mobility
  - Bed-mobility training while maintaining back precautions
  - Transfer training with use of assistive device (e.g., rolling walker)
  - Body mechanics training
- Address scar mobility
  - Scar tissue mobilization progressing from parallel to perpendicular upon wound closure
- Address proprioception
  - Standing balance on level surface eyes open/closed
  - Standing balance activities with use of foam
    - Eyes open
    - Eyes closed
  - Standing balance activities on balance machines
- Gait training
  - Promote normal gait pattern
  - Promote advancement of gait speed
  - Promote postural awareness while ambulating

FUNCTIONAL GOALS

- Patient will be able to
  - Independently perform bed mobility while maintaining back precautions to decrease burden of care.
  - Ambulate 50 ft with a rolling walker with supervision to get from bedroom to the bathroom.
  - Increase the Tinetti performance-oriented mobility assessment (POMA) score to 24 in order to decrease fall risk.
  - Independently maintain proper body mechanics while lifting a grocery bag.

PROGNOSIS

- Depends upon the underlying cause of the fracture.
- Success with Kyphoplasty surgery for a single level.

PATIENT RESOURCES

- American Academy of Orthopaedic Surgeons. *Fractures of the Thoracic and Lumbar Spine.* http://orthoinfo.aaos.org/topic.cfm?topic=A00368. Accessed July 10, 2013.
- American Academy of Orthopaedic Surgeons. *Osteoporosis and Spinal Fractures.* http://orthoinfo.aaos.org/topic.cfm?topic=A00538. Accessed July 10, 2013.

REFERENCES

1. ICD9Data.com. http://www.icd9data.com. Accessed August 8, 2014.
2. ICD10Data.com. http://www.icd10data.com. Accessed August 8, 2014.
3. Pattern 4G: impaired joint mobility, muscle performance, and range of motion associated with fracture. In: *Guide to Physical Therapist Practice.* 2nd ed. Alexandria, VA: American Physical Therapy Association; 2001. Revised 2003.

ADDITIONAL REFERENCES

- Dutton M, ed. *Orthopaedic Examination, Evaluation, and Intervention.* 2nd ed. New York, NY: McGraw-Hill; 2008. http://www.accessphysiotherapy.com/resource/612. Accessed August 8, 2014.
- Goodman CC, Boissonnault WG, Fuller KS. *Pathology: Implications for the Physical Therapist.* 2nd ed. Philadelphia, PA: Saunders; 2003.
- Hall SJ. The biomechanics of human bone growth and development. In: Hall SJ, ed. *Basic Biomechanics.* 5th ed. New York, NY: McGraw-Hill; 2007:Chapter 4. http://www.accessphysiotherapy.com/content/6060744. Accessed August 8, 2014.
- Kisner C, Colby LA. *Therapeutic Exercise: Foundations and Techniques.* 5th ed. Philadelphia, PA: F.A. Davis Company; 2007.
- Magee DJ. *Orthopedic Physical Assessment.* 5th ed. St. Louis, MO: Saunders Elsevier; 2008.
- Malone TR, Hazle C, Grey ML. Introduction to musculoskeletal imaging. In: Malone TR, Hazle C, Grey ML, eds. *Imaging in Rehabilitation.* New York, NY: McGraw-Hill; 2008:Chapter 1. http://www.accessphysiotherapy.com/content/5940000. Accessed August 8, 2014.
- Prentice WE, Quillen WS, Underwood F, eds. *Therapeutic Modalities in Rehabilitation.* 4th ed. New York, NY: McGraw-Hill; 2011. http://www.accessphysiotherapy.com/resource/675. Accessed August 8, 2014.

144 WHIPLASH

Eric J. Chaconas, DPT, PT, FAAOMPT
Eric Shamus, PhD, DPT, PT, CSCS

CONDITION/DISORDER SYNONYMS

- Cervical acceleration–deceleration injury (CAD)
- Neck sprain
- Neck strain
- Whiplash associated disorders (WAD)

ICD-9-CM CODE

- 847.0 Sprain of neck

ICD-10-CM CODES

- S13.4XXA Sprain of ligaments of cervical spine, initial encounter
- S13.8XXA Sprain of joints and ligaments of other parts of neck, initial encounter

PREFERRED PRACTICE PATTERNS

- 4D: Impaired Joint Mobility, Motor Function, Muscle Performance, And Range Of Motion Associated with Connective Tissue Dysfunction[1]
- 4E: Impaired Joint Mobility, Motor Function, Muscle Performance, and Range of Motion Associated with Localized Inflammation

PATIENT PRESENTATION

A 43-year-old male presents with reports of generalized neck pain and stiffness 9 days post motor vehicle accident. The patient was traveling approximately 30 miles per hour when his vehicle collided with another vehicle. The patient received cervical spine and open mouth radiographs in the hospital emergency department revealing no abnormalities. Currently, cervical range of motion is limited in all directions with axial cervical spine pain. Hypertonicity is noted in the cervical musculature particularly bilateral sternocleidomastoid and scalenes. Instability testing is negative but craniocervical flexion testing reveals impaired longus colli and capitis control with movement generated by anterior scalene and sternocleidomastoid. Encouragement and education appears to help the patient increase cervical spine movement.

KEY FEATURES

Description

- WAD: Injury dysfunction and symptoms
- Cervical acceleration–deceleration injury (CAD): Mechanism of injury
- Traumatic neck pain from being hit from behind
- Quick movement through a S curve causing upper cervical flexion and lower cervical hyperextension[2]

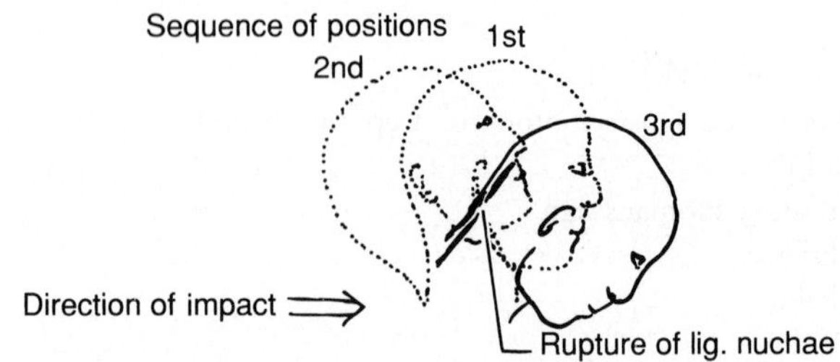

FIGURE 144-1 Extension injury (Whiplash) of the cervical spine. Violent impact from behind produces rapid translation between three sequential positions, causing rupture of the ligamentum nuchae. (From LeBlond RF, DeGowin RL, Brown DD. *DeGowin's Diagnostic Examination*. 9th ed. www.accessmedicine.com. Copyright © The McGraw-Hill Companies, Inc. All rights reserved.)

- Post-traumatic mechanism of injury to the head/neck, most commonly secondary to motor vehicle accident[3]
- Injury to the soft tissues, joint capsule and ligaments, zygapophyseal joint, central or peripheral neurologic systems, intervertebral disk, posterior (dorsal) root ganglia, vascular structures (verterbrobasilar arteries), and visceral structures (secondary to ruptures or contusions)[3]

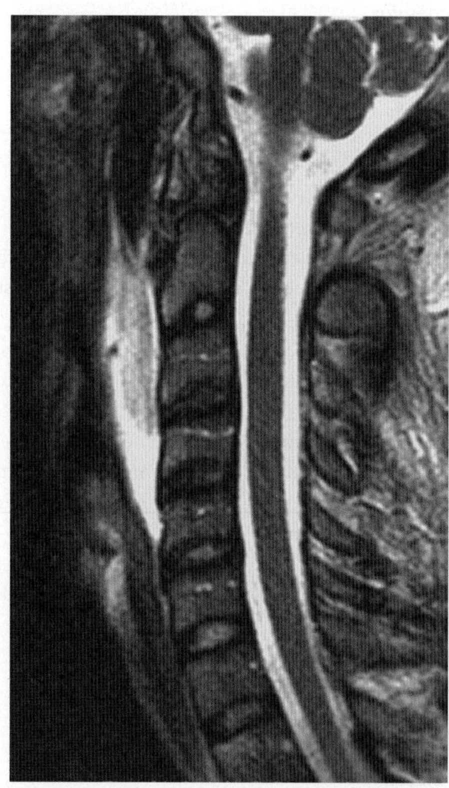

FIGURE 144-2 The outstanding feature of this sagittal section T2-weighted MR image is the increased signal intensity consistent with edema from soft tissue injury. The presence of such findings warrants particular caution to examine scrupulously for the presence of fractures. (From Malone TR, Hazle C, Grey ML. *Imaging in Rehabilitation*. www.accessmedicine.com. Copyright © The McGraw-Hill Companies, Inc. All rights reserved.)

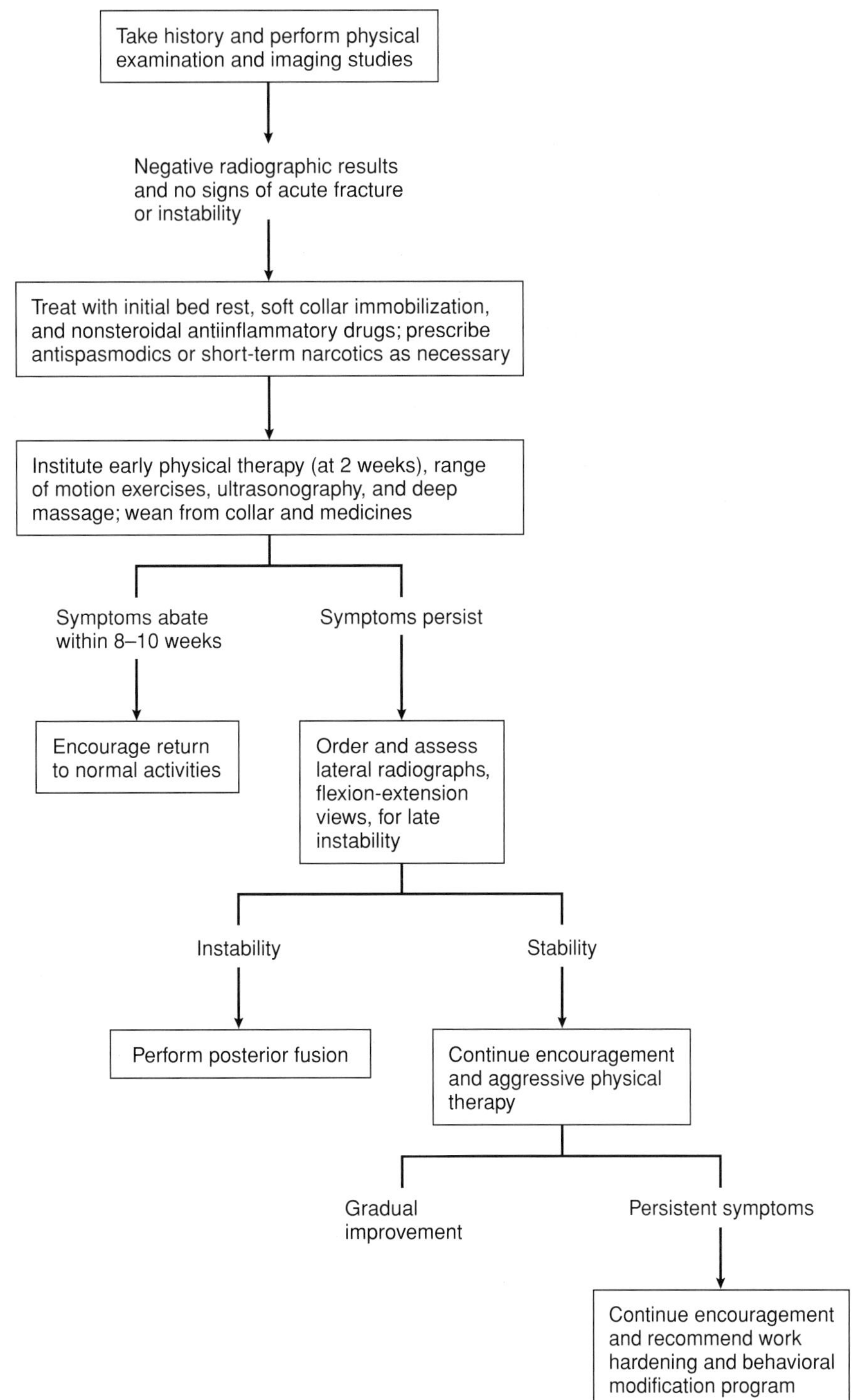

FIGURE 144-3 Algorithm for management of patients with cervical strain. (From Skinner HB. *Current Diagnosis & Treatment in Orthopedics*. 4th ed. www.accessmedicine.com. Copyright © The McGraw-Hill Companies, Inc. All rights reserved.)

Essentials of Diagnosis

- Symptoms maybe delayed for 24 hours[2]
- Diagnosis made by clinical examination and patient history
- Quebec task force grade levels[4]
  - Grade 0
    - No complaint of neck pain
    - No physical signs
  - Grade 1
    - Neck complaint of pain
    - Stiffness or tenderness only
    - No physical signs
  - Grade 2
    - Neck complaint
    - Musculoskeletal signs including decreased range of motion and point tenderness

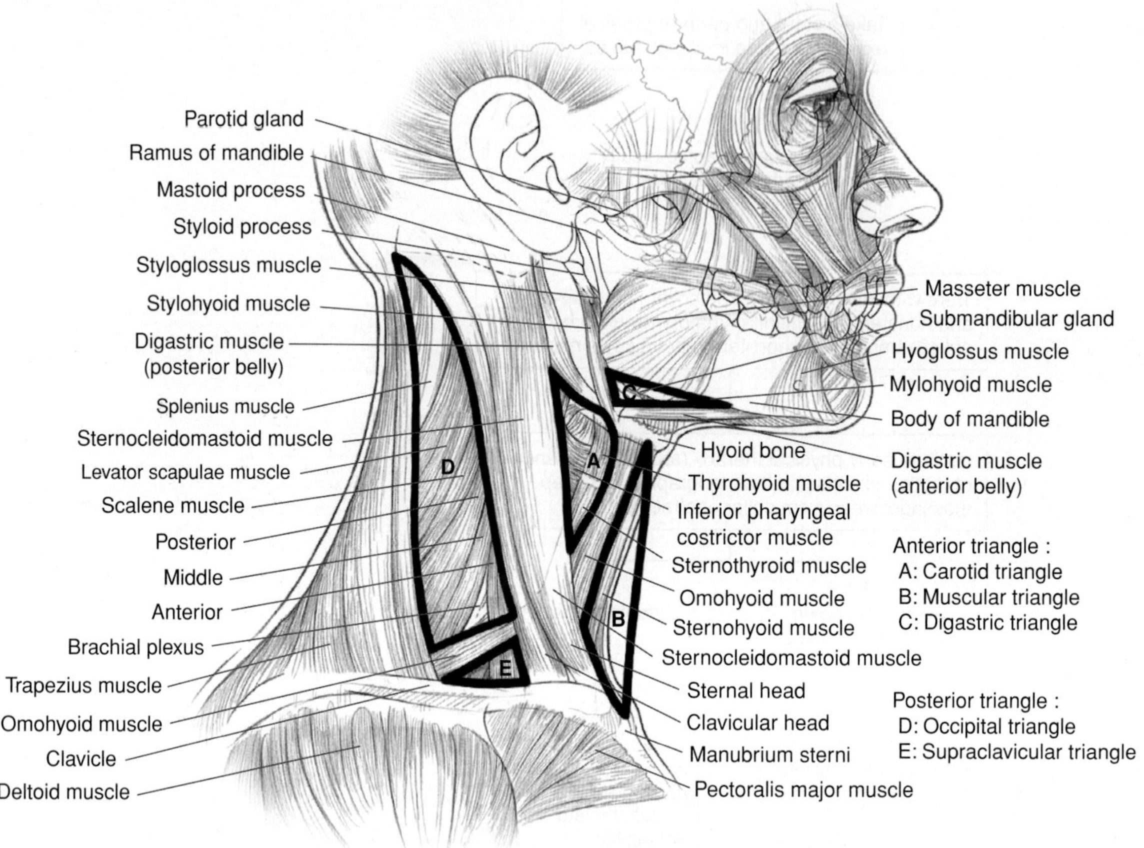

FIGURE 144-4 Muscles and triangles of the neck. (From Lalwani AK. *Current Diagnosis & Treatment in Otolaryngology—Head & Neck Surgery*. 3rd ed. www.accessurgery.com. Copyright © The McGraw-Hill Companies, Inc. All rights reserved.)

- Grade 3
  - Neck complaint
  - Musculoskeletal signs including decreased or absent deep tendon reflexes, muscle weakness, and sensory deficits
- Grade 4
  - Neck complaint and fracture or dislocation

General Considerations

- More common in women than men, possibly from neck muscle strength and stability.
- Pain may become chronic if musculature strength not regained.

Demographics

- Women appear to be at greater risk secondary to less stiffness of the cervical structures.[5]

CLINICAL FINDINGS

SIGNS AND SYMPTOMS

- Neck pain[6]
- Soft tissue injury
- Muscle pain[6]
- Stiffness
- Headaches, 50% to 60%[6]
- Dizziness
- Generalized neck and upper back pain, typically absent of radiculopathy
- Ringing in the ears
- Blurred vision
- Sleep disturbance
- Guarded and limited active motion of the cervical spine
- Hypertonic surrounding musculature
- Compensatory neck motion initiated by global cervical musculature, including sternocleidomastoid and scalenes
- Potential sympathetic symptoms
- Post-traumatic psychosocial impairments

Functional Implications

- Difficulty maintaining sustained sitting postures

Possible Contributing Causes

- Motor vehicle accident
- Horseback riding falls
- Pull on the arms
- Trauma from physical abuse or contact sports

Differential Diagnosis

- Cervical fracture including C2 hangman's fracture
- Odontoid process fracture
- Examine for complete loss of neck movement, pain with gentle compression/traction, and severe muscle spasm
- Subcranial instability
- Cervical radiculopathy

MEANS OF CONFIRMATION OR DIAGNOSIS

Imaging

- Plain-film open-mouth radiograph essential to rule out odontoid fracture

- CT imaging essential to rule out odontoid fracture
- Radiograph and CT helpful to rule out c-spine factures
- MRI often negative in the presence of clinical impairments and significant pain with the absence of neurologic involvement[7]

FINDINGS AND INTERPRETATION

- MRI is performed if there are signs and symptoms of radiculopathy or cord injury.[6]
- Severe muscle spasm, muscle weakness, or pain upon gentle compression of the cervical spine may indicate fracture.[1]

TREATMENT

Medication

- Nonsteroidal anti-inflammatory drugs (NSAIDs)
- Corticosteroids

REFERRALS/ADMITTANCE

- For imaging and surgical consult if fracture/instability is suspected
- For pain medication if self-care measures insufficient
- For psychological consult if post-traumatic stress suspected

IMPAIRMENTS

- Guarded active cervical spine motion secondary to hypertonic musculature
- Hypermobile cervical spine
- Weakness noted of longus colli and longus capitis
- Weakness noted of periscapular muscles

TESTS AND MEASURES

- Cervical spine AROM
- Sharp–Purser: Atlantoaxial instability
- Cervical passive intervertebral motion testing
- Sub-cranial translation instability testing
- Passive physiological intervertebral mobility testing (PPIVM)[6]
- Upper-extremity screening examination
- Neck Disability Index (NDI)
- Postural examination
- Muscle length testing, including upper trapezius, levator scapulae, pectoral muscles
- Upper limb nerve tension test[7]
- Deep neck flexor endurance test
- Upper-extremity neurological screening (dermatome, myotome, reflexes)

INTERVENTION

- Pain-free active movement exercises
- Postural training and positioning
- Quebec task force recommends manipulation, mobilization, and ROM exercises for grades 1 to 3
- Soft collar use if indicated early, first 72 hours
- Addressing pain
  - Electrical stimulation
  - Thermal modalities: Heat/ice
- Addressing hypertonicity
  - Soft tissue massage
  - Soft tissue manipulation to decrease tone
  - Heat
- Addressing muscle weakness
  - Craniocervical flexion exercises
  - Periscapular strengthening
  - Deep neck flexor training
  - Strengthening of lower/middle trapezius, rhomboids, rotator cuff serratus anterior, latissimus dorsi

FUNCTIONAL GOALS

- Patient will be able to
  - Sit with a neutral cervical and thoracic spine posture for >30 minutes with 0/10 pain while at a desk at work.
  - Drive an automobile for 45 minutes with 0/10 pain.
  - Rotate cervical spine 70 degrees to look over shoulder while backing automobile out of a parking space.

PROGNOSIS

- Fair to very good, depending upon severity of trauma and prior cervicothoracic impairments.
- History of previous cervical spine impairment worsens prognosis.
- Pre-existing headaches and degenerative changes in the cervical spine are predictive of unfavorable outcome past 6 months.[1]

PATIENT RESOURCES

- Clinical guidelines for the nest practice management of acute and chronic whiplash-associated disorders. Australian Government, National Health and Medical Research Council. http://www.nhmrc.gov.au/_files_nhmrc/publications/attachments/cp112.pdf. Accessed July 14, 2013.
- Motor Accidents Authority. *Guidelines for the Management of Whiplash-Associated Disorders.* 2nd ed. 2007. http://www.clinicalguidelines.gov.au/browse.php?treePath=C.D009422.D009461&pageType=2&fldglrID=1306&. Accessed July 14, 2013.

REFERENCES

1. The American Physical Therapy Association. *Interactive Guide to Physical Therapist Practice.* Alexandria, VA: The American Physical Therapy Association; 2003. http://guidetoptpractice.apta.org. Accessed July 14, 2013.
2. Hamilton N, Weimar W, Luttgens K. Common injuries of the neck, back, and thorax. In: Hamilton N, Weimar W, Luttgens K, eds. *Kinesiology: Scientific Basis of Human Motion.* 11st ed. New York, NY: McGraw-Hill; 2008. http://www.accessphysiotherapy.com/content/6153367. Accessed July 14, 2013.
3. Dutton M. The cervical spine. In: Dutton M, ed. *Dutton's Orthopaedic Examination, Evaluation, and Intervention.* 3rd ed. New York, NY: McGraw-Hill; 2008. http://www.accessphysiotherapy.com/content/56551567. Accessed July 14, 2013.
4. Sterling M. A proposed new classification system for whiplash associated disorders-implications for assessment and management. *Man Ther.* 2004;9(2):60–70. doi:10.1016/j.math.2004.01.006.
5. Stemper BD, Yoganandan N, Pintar FA. Gender dependent cervical spine segmental kinematics during whiplash. *J Biomech.* 2003;36(9):1281–1289.
6. Hall SJ. Common injuries of the back and neck. In: Hall SJ, ed. *Basic Biomechanics.* 5th ed. New York, NY: McGraw-Hill; 2007. http://www.accessphysiotherapy.com/content/6063178. Accessed July 14, 2013.

7. Malone TR, Hazle C, Grey ML. Magnetic resonance imaging. In: Malone TR, Hazle C, Grey ML, eds. *Imaging in Rehabilitation*. New York, NY: McGraw-Hill; 2008. http://www.accessphysiotherapy.com/content/5940460. Accessed July 14, 2013.

ADDITIONAL REFERENCES

- American Physical Therapy Association. *Guide to Physical Therapist Practice*. 2nd ed. Alexandria, VA: American Physical Therapy Association; 2001. Revised 2003.
- Atlas SJ, Deyo RA, Patrick DL, Convery K, Keller RB, Singer DE. The Quebec Task Force classification for Spinal Disorders and the severity, treatment, and outcomes of sciatica and lumbar spinal stenosis. *Spine (Phila Pa 1976)*. 1996;21(24):2885-2892.
- Dutton M. The cervical complex. In: Dutton M, ed. *Dutton's Orthopedic Survival Guide: Managing Common Conditions*. New York, NY: McGraw-Hill; 2011. http://www.accessphysiotherapy.com/content/8656027. Accessed July 14, 2013.
- Dutton M, ed. *Dutton's Orthopaedic Examination, Evaluation, and Intervention*. 2nd ed. New York, NY: McGraw-Hill; 2008. http://www.accessphysiotherapy.com/resource/612. Accessed July 14, 2013.
- Eck JC, Hodges SD, Humphreys SC. Whiplash: a review of a commonly misunderstood injury. *Am J Med*. 2001;110(8):651–656.
- Hamilton N, Weimar W, Luttgens K. The spinal column and thorax. In: Hamilton N, Weimar W, Luttgens K, eds. *Kinesiology: Scientific Basis of Human Motion*. 11th ed. New York, NY: McGraw-Hill; 2008. http://www.accessphysiotherapy.com/content/6153367. Accessed July 14, 2013.
- ICD9Data.com. http://www.icd9data.com. Accessed July 14, 2013.
- ICD10Data.com. http://www.icd10data.com. Accessed July 14, 2013.
- Malone TR, Hazle C, Grey ML. Imaging of the cervical spine and temporomandibular joint. In: Malone TR, Hazle C, Grey ML, eds. *Imaging in Rehabilitation*. New York, NY: McGraw-Hill; 2008. http://www.accessphysiotherapy.com/content/5940352. Accessed July 14, 2013.
- Prentice WE, Quillen WS, Underwood F, eds. *Therapeutic Modalities in Rehabilitation*. 4th ed. New York, NY: McGraw-Hill; 2011. http://www.accessphysiotherapy.com/resource/675. Accessed July 14, 2013.
- Stemper BD, Yoganandan N, Pintar FA. Kinetics of the head-neck complex in low-speed rear impact. *Biomed Sci Instrum*. 2003;39:245–250.

SECTION C RIBCAGE AND ABDOMINAL DISORDERS

145 COSTOCHONDRITIS

Eric Shamus, PhD, DPT, PT, CSCS

CONDITION/DISORDER SYNONYM

- Costochondral junction syndrome

ICD-9-CM CODE

- 733.6 Tietze disease

ICD-10-CM CODE

- M94 Other disorders of cartilage

PREFERRED PRACTICE PATTERN

- 4E: Impaired Joint Mobility, Motor Function, Muscle Performance, and ROM Associated with Localized Inflammation

PATIENT PRESENTATION

A 22-year-old young man presents with right chest pain and heart burn. He states that pain began suddenly after reaching behind from the front seat to the back seat in the car. He also states that the pain gets worse when he coughs or sneezes. He complains of difficulty with sleeping at night when there is pressure on the lateral portion of the ribs. Palpable tenderness and reproduction of pain are localized at the right fourth rib costosternal junction. The patient also complains of discomfort in the fourth rib laterally.

KEY FEATURES

Description

- Local palpable pain at the costal cartilage between the sternum and the ribs

Essentials of Diagnosis

- Can be reproduced with compression of the cartilage that attaches the ribs to the sternum
- Pain may be provoked by certain movements like overhead reaching
- Usually caused by exercise, upper respiratory infection, or minor trauma
- Most common sites: Second to fifth ribs[1]
- Tietze syndrome now thought to be a progression from costochondritis or of severity level
- Benign

General Considerations

- Rule out myocardial infarction
- Need to rule out a heart attack until proven otherwise
- Stabbing or twinging pain, but no radicular or systemic symptoms
- Inflammation, tenderness
- Relatively harmless

Demographics

- Children and adolescents, 10 to 20 years of age[2]
- Females > males

CLINICAL FINDINGS

SIGNS AND SYMPTOMS

- Acute or chronic upper anterior chest pain
- Stabbing pain, but no radicular or systemic symptoms
- No radicular pain, helps to differentiate with Tietze syndrome
- Pain increases with respiration or activity with rib movement
- Nausea
- Tenderness along the costal cartilage and the sternum (breastbone)

Functional Implications

- Aerobic/breathing limitations
- Pain with sleeping and lying on the ribs
- Inability to carry bags of groceries by one's side
- Inability to turn the steering wheel in a car
- Inability to carry heavy items
- Inability to dig in the garden

Possible Contributing Causes

- Physical strain
- Repetitive coughing
- Injury to chest and breast tissue
- Impact form airbag/steering wheel in a car accident
- Injury during exercise (dips, chest fly, exercises that open the chest wall)
- Viral infection

Differential Diagnosis[3]

- Myocardial infarction (heart attack) can have identical symptoms with acute pain and pain in the shoulder and arm.
- Costochondritis is different in that no electrical heart change and no damage to the organs occurs.
- Costochondritis pain occurs during muscle exertion or deep breathing, whereas myocardial infarction can present at rest or after an activity.
- Tietze syndrome is different in that there is swelling of the costal cartilage and radiating arm pain.

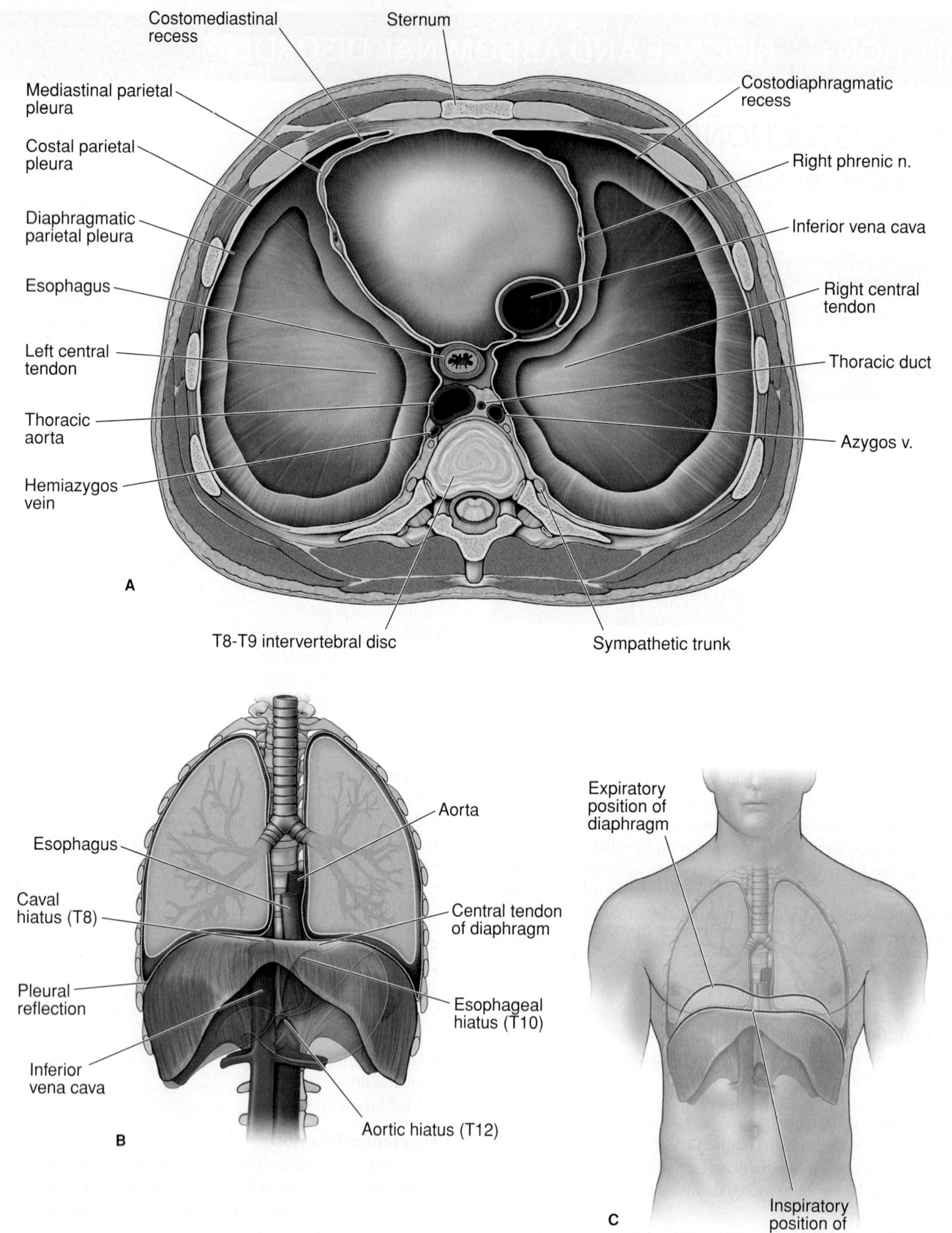

FIGURE 145-1 (**A**) Superior view of the axial section of the thorax above the diaphragm. (**B**) Anterior view of the diaphragm and its relationship to the lungs. (**C**) Position of the diaphragm during inspiration and expiration. (From Morton DA, Foreman KB, Albertine KH. *The Big Picture: Gross Anatomy.* http://www.accessmedicine.com. Copyright © The McGraw-Hill Companies, Inc. All rights reserved.)

- Bruised ribs
- Broken ribs
- Pleurisy
- Pneumothorax
- Shingles
- Pneumonia
- Viral respiratory infection

MEANS OF CONFIRMATION OR DIAGNOSIS

Laboratory Tests

- Blood testing for heart damage (cardiac enzymes and troponin levels), negative for inflammation
- Sedimentation rate
- C-reactive protein test (CRP test)

Imaging

- Chest X-ray used to rule out parenchymal lung disease and rib fracture[1]

Diagnostic Procedure

- ECG

FINDINGS AND INTERPRETATION

- Tenderness, palpable at costal cartilage
- No X-ray findings

TREATMENT

Medications

- Aspirin
- Nonsteroidal, anti-inflammatory
- Analgesics

REFERRALS/ADMITTANCE

- Rule out myocardial infarction
- Difficulty breathing
- Fever
- Increased pain even with medication
- Signs of infection, pus

IMPAIRMENTS

- Debilitating pain
- Inability for gas exchange
- Limiting movement and exertion

TESTS AND MEASURES

- Thoracic and rib mobility
- Diaphragm doming
- Trunk rotation

INTERVENTION

- Cryotherapy[4]
- Cortisone injection/lidocaine patch
- Joint mobilization to the costovertebral articulations, thoracic and rib mobilization
- Myofascial release to the diaphragm[5]
- Taping for support of ribs or costal cartilage

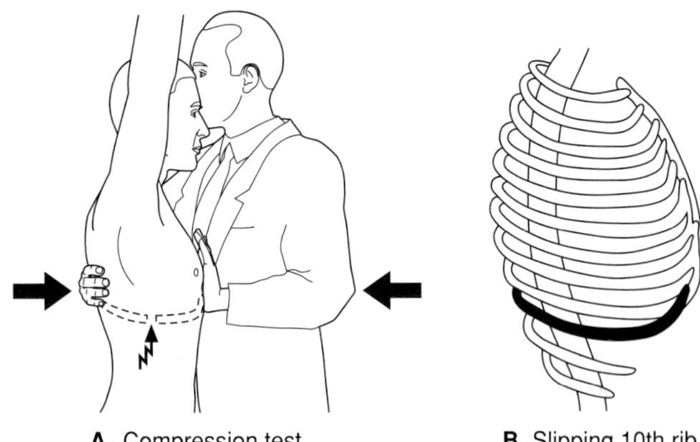

FIGURE 145-2 Examining for rib pain. (**A**) Compression test for rib fracture. When the site of suspected rib fracture is located by point tenderness, the sternum is pushed toward the spine with one hand while the other hand supports the patient's back. The maneuver will elicit pain at the untouched fracture site. (**B**) Slipping tenth rib. When the tenth rib lacks an anterior attachment, it can slip forward upon the ninth rib during respiratory movements and cause pain. (From LeBlond RF, DeGowin RL, Brown DD. *DeGowin's Diagnostic Examination.* 9th ed. www.accessmedicine.com. Copyright © The McGraw-Hill Companies, Inc. All rights reserved.)

FUNCTIONAL GOALS

- Pain-free full deep breath
- To carry bags of groceries by patient's side
- Pain-free driving, to turn the steering wheel in a car
- Pain-free lifting, to carry heavy items
- Pain-free yard work, to dig in the garden

PROGNOSIS

- Symptoms usually resolve in a year.[6]
- Can last from hours to weeks or months, depending on the ability to rest and limit movement of the area.

ADDITIONAL INFORMATION

- See case study in chapter 27, Right Anterior Chest Pain, in Dutton's Orthopaedic Examination, Evaluation, and Intervention, 3rd ed.

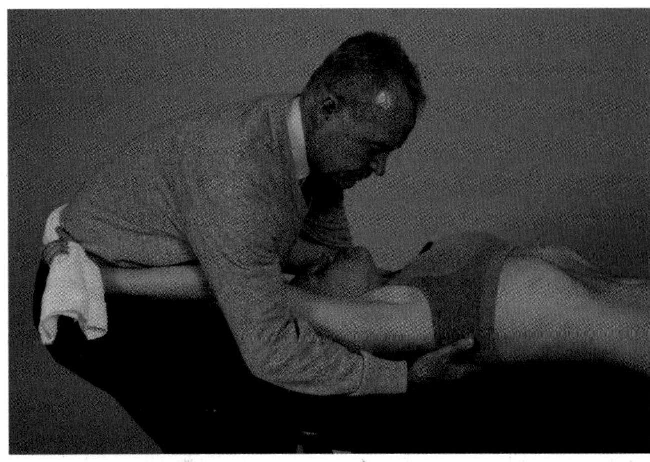

FIGURE 145-3 Supine myofascial stretch into extension. (From Dutton M. *Dutton's Orthopaedic Examination, Evaluation, and Intervention.* 3rd ed. http://www.accessphysiotherapy.com. Copyright © The McGraw-Hill Companies, Inc. All rights reserved.)

TABLE 145-1 Chest Pain Patterns

Origin of Pain	Site of Referred Pain	Type of Disorder
Substernal or retrosternal	Neck, jaw, back, left shoulder and arm, and abdomen	Angina
Substernal, anterior chest	Neck, jaw, back, and bilateral arms	Myocardial infarction
Substernal or above the sternum	Next, upper back, upper trapezius, supraclavicular area, left arm, and costal margin	Pericarditis
Anterior chest (thoracic aneurysm); abdomen (abdominal aneurysm)	Posterior thoracic, chest, neck, shoulders, interscapular, or lumbar region	Dissecting aortic aneurysm
Variable	Variable, depending on structures involved	Musculoskeletal
Costochondritis (inflammation of the costal cartilage): sternum and rib margins	Abdominal oblique trigger points: pain referred up into the chest area	
Upper rectus abdominis trigger points (left side), pectoralis, serratus anterior, and sternalis muscles: precordial pain	Pectoralis trigger points: pain referred down medial bilateral arms along ulnar nerve distribution (fourth and fifth fingers)	
Precordium region (upper central abdomen and diaphragm)	Sternum, axillary lines, and either side of vertebrae; lateral and anterior chest wall; occasionally to one or both arms	Neurologic
Substernal, epigastric, and upper abdominal quadrants	Around chest area, shoulders, and upper back region	Gastrointestinal
Within breast tissue; may be localized in pectoral and supraclavicular regions	Chest area, axilla, mid-back, and neck and posterior shoulder girdle	Breast pain
Commonly substernal and anterior chest region	No referred pain	Anxiety

Source: Data from Donato EB. Physical examination procedures to screen for serious disorders of the head, neck, chest, and upper quarter. In: Wilmarth MA, ed. *Medical Screening for the Physical Therapist. Orthopaedic Section Independent Study Course 14.1.1.* La Crosse, WI: Orthopaedic Section, APTA, Inc., 2003:1–43; Goodman CC, Boissonnault WG. *Pathology: Implications for the Physical Therapist.* Philadelphia, PA: WB Saunders, 1998.

PATIENT RESOURCES

- MedlinePlus, US National Library of Medicine, NIH. Costochondritis. http://www.nlm.nih.gov/medlineplus/ency/article/000164.htm. Accessed June 8, 2013.
- Wisniewski A. Taking a closer look at costochondritis. *Critic Care.* 2006;36(11):64cc1–64cc2.

REFERENCES

1. Homnick DN. Chest and Pulmonary Conditions. In: Patel DR, Greydanus DE, Baker RJ, eds. *Pediatric Practice: Sports Medicine.* New York, NY: McGraw-Hill; 2009. http://www.accessphysiotherapy.com/content/6974842#6974842. Accessed May 8, 2013.
2. Dutton M. The Thoracic Spine and Rib Cage. In: Dutton M, ed. *Orthopaedic Examination, Evaluation, and Intervention.* 2nd ed. New York, NY: McGraw-Hill; 2012. http://www.accessphysiotherapy.com/content/55594726#55594726. Accessed May 8, 2013.
3. Miyamoto SD, Sondheimer HM, Fagan TE, Collins KK. Cardiovascular Diseases. In: Hay WW, Levin MJ, Sondheimer JM, Deterding RR, eds. *CURRENT Diagnosis & Treatment: Pediatrics.* 20th ed. New York, NY: McGraw-Hill; 2009. http://www.accessphysiotherapy.com/content/6582856#6582856. Accessed May 8, 2013.
4. Prentice WE. Cryotherapy and Thermotherapy. In: Prentice WE, Quillen WS, Underwood F, eds. *Therapeutic Modalities in Rehabilitation.* 4th ed. New York, NY: McGraw-Hill; 2011. http://www.accessphysiotherapy.com/content/8137995#8137995. Accessed May 8, 2013.
5. Prentice WE. Therapeutic Massage. In: Prentice WE, Quillen WS, Underwood F, eds. *Therapeutic Modalities in Rehabilitation.* 4th ed. New York, NY: McGraw-Hill; 2011. http://www.accessphysiotherapy.com/content/8140971#8140971. Accessed May 8, 2013.
6. Dutton M. Causes of Thoracic Pain. In: Dutton M, ed. *Dutton's Orthopaedic Examination, Evaluation, and Intervention.* 3rd ed. New York, NY: McGraw-Hill; 2012. http://www.accessphysiotherapy.com/content/56525737. Accessed May 8, 2013.

ADDITIONAL REFERENCES

- Aspegren D, Hyde T, Miller M. Conservative treatment of a female collegiate volleyball player with costochondritis. *J Manipulative Physiol Ther.* 2007;30(4):321–325.
- Cubos J, Cubos A, Di Stefano F. Chronic costochondritis in an adolescent competitive swimmer: a case report. *J Can Chiropr Assoc.* 2012;54(4):271–275.
- Erwin WM, Jackson PC, Homonko DA. Innervation of the human costovertebral joint: implications for clinical back pain syndromes. *J Manipulative Physiol Ther.* 2000;23(6):395–403.
- Freeston J, Karim Z, Lindsay K, Gough A. Can early diagnosis and management of costochondritis reduce acute chest pain admissions? *J Rheumatol.* 2004;31(11):2269–2271.
- Hudes K. Low-tech rehabilitation and management of a 64-year-old male patient with acute idiopathic onset of costochondritis. *J Can Chiropr Assoc.* 2008;52(4):224–228.
- Jensen S. Musculoskeletal causes of chest pain. *Aust Fam Physician.* 2001;30(9):834–839.
- Proulx AM, Zryd TW. Costochondritis: diagnosis and treatment. *Am Fam Physician.* 2009;80(6):617–620.

146 DIASTASIS RECTI

Stephanie Boren Baker, MS, PT, CSCS
Eric Shamus, PhD, DPT, PT, CSCS

CONDITION/DISORDER SYNONYMS

- Diastasis recti abdominis (DRA)
- Abdominal separation

ICD-9-CM CODE

- 728.84 Diastasis of muscle

ICD-10-CM CODE

- M62.00 Separation of muscle (nontraumatic), unspecified site

PREFERRED PRACTICE PATTERNS

- 4C: Impaired muscle performance[1]
- 4E: Impaired joint mobility, motor function, muscle performance, and range of motion associated with localized inflammation

PATIENT PRESENTATION

A 34-year-old woman 12 weeks s/p C-section presents with complaints of low back pain. The patient has two children with less than 18 months between deliveries, first was a C-section due to larger gestational size followed by a repeat C-section. Her weight gain with each pregnancy was approximately 40 lbs. No episodes of urinary incontinence reported since delivery. She is experiencing pain during childcare activities, especially lifting, bending, and prolonged sitting.

Pain is described as a constant dull ache across the center of the low back with no radicular symptoms or sensory involvement. Pain is increased when lifting or carrying her oldest child and when bending or leaning forward while bathing or changing a diaper. She reports intermittent pain when breastfeeding in a sitting position for more than 15 minutes. Increased lumbar lordosis is noted with forward head and rounded shoulders posture. A palpable diastasis of approximately 3 cm is noted just superior to umbilicus, and there is tenderness to palpation over the lumbar paraspinals. Prone instability test is positive and Thomas test is positive bilaterally. Lumbar AROM is WFL, but painful after 50% of flexion and after 75% of extension. Hip ROM is WNL. Hip flexion and extension strength are 4/5, and transverse abdominis and multifidus strength are diminished.

KEY FEATURES

Description

- Midline separation of the rectus abdominis muscle at the linea albea
- Usually greater than two fingertips in width

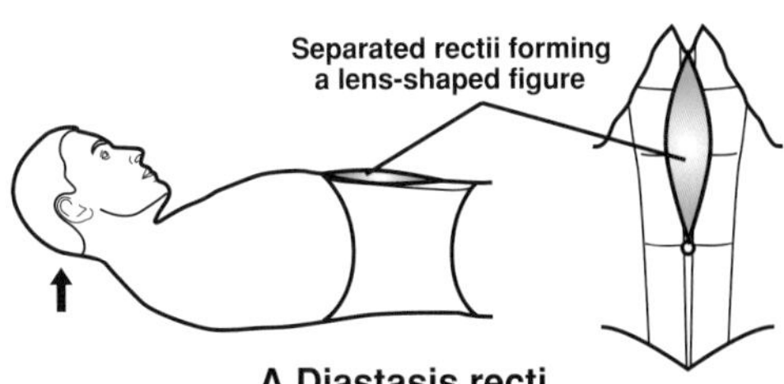

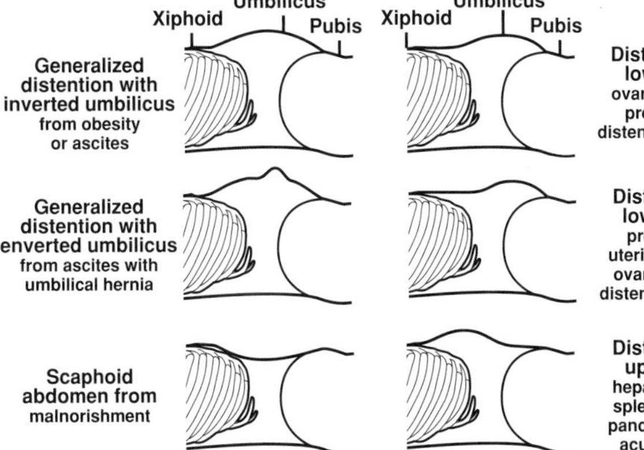

FIGURE 146-1 Visible abdominal signs. (**A**) Diastasis recti. This is abnormal separation of the abdominal rectus muscles. It is frequently not detected when the patient is supine unless the patient's head is raised from the pillow so that the abdominal muscles are tensed. (**B**) Abdominal profiles. Careful inspection from the side may give the first clue to abnormality, directing attention to a specific region and prompting search for more signs. (From LeBlond RF, DeGowin RL, Brown DD. *DeGowin's Diagnostic Examination.* 9th ed. www.accessmedicine.com. Copyright © The McGraw-Hill Companies, Inc. All rights reserved.)

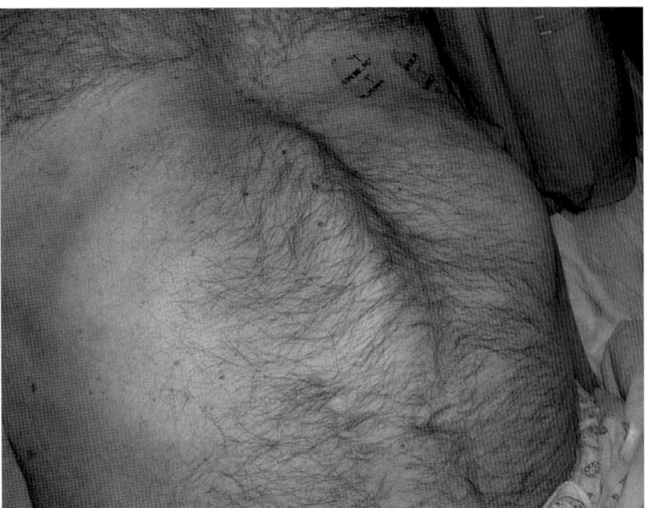

FIGURE 146-2 Diastasis recti visible in the midepigastrium with Valsalva maneuver. The edges of the rectus abdominis muscle, rigid with voluntary contraction, are palpable along the entire length of the bulging area. This should not be mistaken for a ventral hernia. (From Brunicardi FC, Andersen D, Billiar T, et al. *Schwartz's Principles of Surgery.* 9th ed. http://www.accessmedicine.com. Copyright © The McGraw-Hill Companies, Inc. All rights reserved.)

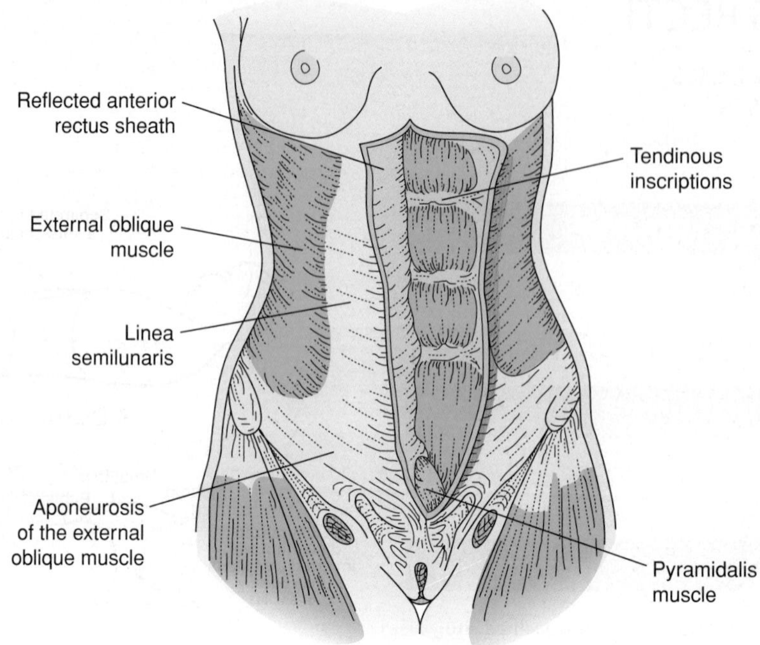

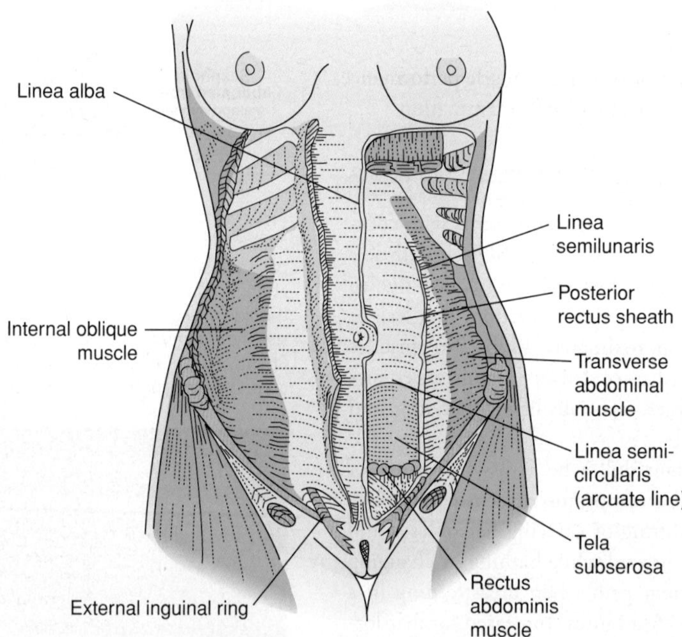

FIGURE 146-3 Musculature of abdominal wall. (From DeCherney AH, Nathan L. *Current Diagnosis & Treatment Obstetrics & Gynecology.* 10th ed. www.accessmedicine.com. Copyright © The McGraw-Hill Companies, Inc. All rights reserved.)

Essentials of Diagnosis

- Rectus abdominis muscle
  - Originates from the pubis, with insertion into xiphoid process and fifth to seventh costal cartilages.
  - Acts to flex the vertebral column.
  - Is separated by a midline band of connective tissue known as the linea alba.
- Diagnosis is usually made by clinical examination due to the superficial position of the rectus abdominis.

General Considerations

- Limited research, but significant relationship between DRA and pregnancy has been established.
- Incidence of DRA diminishes post-partum, but thinning of rectus abdominis and increased inter-recti distance may persist.
- DRA is considered a cosmetic condition by most insurance carriers.

Demographics

- Usually occurs during pregnancy or delivery.
- Highest incidence of DRA in second and third trimesters.
- Most common location of diastasis at the umbilicus, then superior to the umbilicus; least common location is inferior to the umbilicus.
- Research indicates increased incidence of DRA in nonexercising pregnant women versus pregnant women who exercise.

CLINICAL FINDINGS

SIGN AND SYMPTOMS

- Separation of rectus abdominis at midline, resulting in protrusion and palpable gap between the borders
- Abdominal pain

▶ Functional Implications

- Increased prevalence of DRA in patients with support-related pelvic floor dysfunction (urinary incontinence, fecal incontinence, pelvic organ prolapse)
- Lumbopelvic pain related to diminished contribution of rectus abdominis or altered mechanics of spinal muscles

▶ Possible Contributing Causes

- Hormonal changes and uterine growth during pregnancy causing stretching of rectus abdominis
- Postural changes during pregnancy, including anterior pelvic tilt and increased lumbar lordosis, changes angle of insertion and muscle's line of action
- Pregnancy/Multiple-birth pregnancy[2]
- Large gestational size
- Excess uterine fluid
- Obesity or excessive weight gain during pregnancy
- Previous DRA

▶ Differential Diagnosis

- Umbilical hernia
- Ventral hernia

MEANS OF CONFIRMATION OR DIAGNOSIS

▶ Laboratory Tests

- Patient positioned in supine with the hips and knees flexed to 90 degrees, and contracts rectus abdominis to flex trunk.[3]
- Measurements should be taken at the umbilicus and 4.5 cm superior and inferior to the umbilicus.
- Palpable separation of ≥2.5 cm considered diastasis.

▶ Imaging

- Ultrasonography accurate in measuring DRA
- CT and MRI utilized more frequently to diagnose hernia

FINDINGS AND INTERPRETATIONS

- Infants can present with a raised area above the umbilicus, more common in premature newborns

TREATMENTS

▶ Medications

- Nonsteroidal anti-inflammatory drugs (NSAIDs)

MEDICAL INTERVENTION

- Repair of DRA often performed in conjunction with abdominoplasty (tummy tuck)

REFERRALS/ADMITTANCE

- To women's health physical therapist for treatment of incontinence
- To physician or surgical referral if poor response to conservative treatment

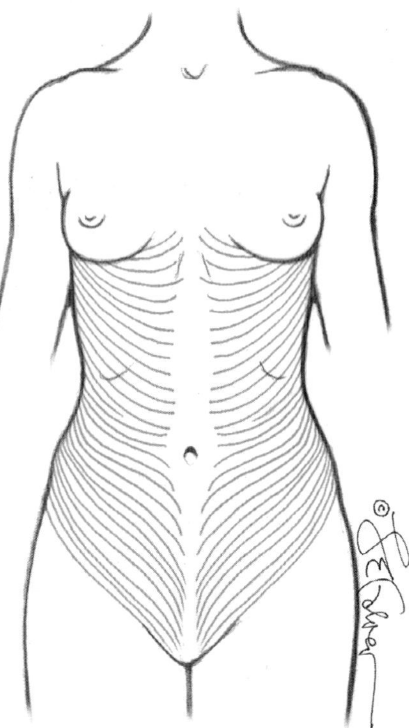

FIGURE 146-4 Langer lines of skin tension. (From Hoffman BL, Schorge JO, Schaffer JI, et al. *Williams Gynecology.* 2nd ed. www.accessmedicine.com. Copyright © The McGraw-Hill Companies, Inc. All rights reserved.)

IMPAIRMENTS

- Lumbopelvic pain
- Urogynecologic dysfunction
- Increased risk of hernia
- Appearance/cosmetic of abdominal region

TESTS AND MEASURES

- Postural examination
- Muscle length testing, including the hamstrings, hip flexors, and calf muscles
- Quadrant test
- Straight-leg raise test
- Slump test
- Prone instability test
- Lower-extremity neurologic screen (dermatome, myotome, reflexes)
- Repeated movement testing
- Fear-Avoidance Beliefs Questionnaire (FABQ)

INTERVENTION

- Post-partum core strengthening program
  - Initial emphasis on transverse abdominis and multifidus stabilization exercises
  - Progress to movement-related global muscle strengthening, emphasizing proper posture/alignment without compensatory motion of the pelvis
- Patients with C-section must wait 6 weeks or until physician clearance to begin program
- Exercise may begin when separation is <2 cm

FUNCTIONAL GOALS

- Patient will have
  - Reduced DRA to <2.5 cm in order to support internal structures.

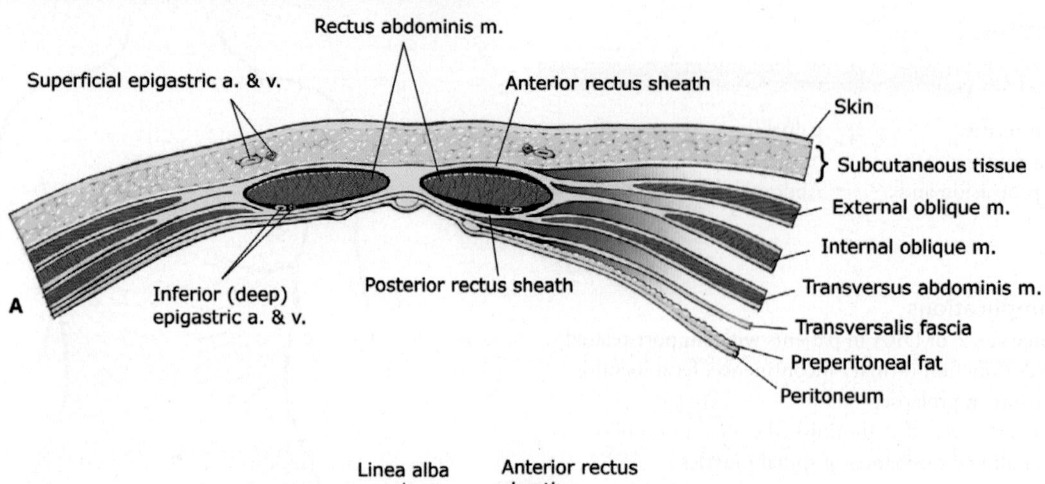

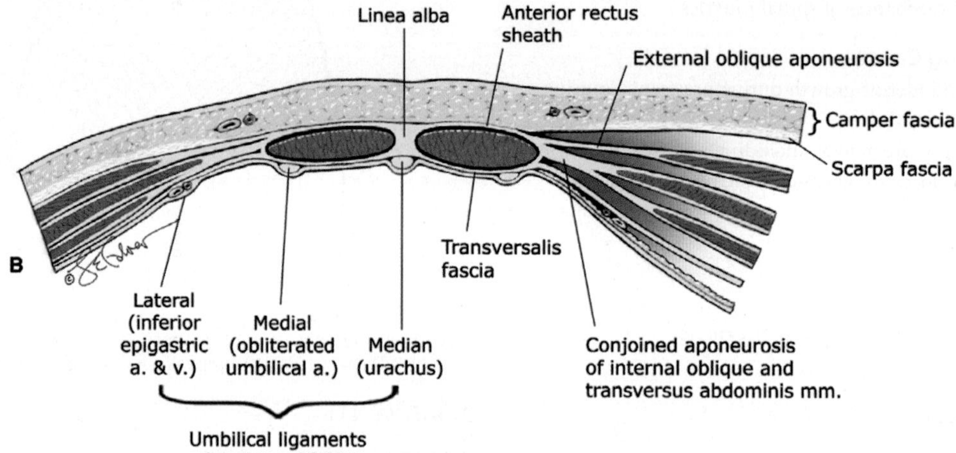

FIGURE 146-5 Transverse sections of the anterior abdominal wall above (**A**) and below (**B**) the arcuate line. (From Hoffman BL, Schorge JO, Schaffer JI, et al. *Williams Gynecology.* 2nd ed. www.accessmedicine.com. Copyright © The McGraw-Hill Companies, Inc. All rights reserved.)

- Strengthened deep and superficial musculature to perform infant care giving activities pain-free.
- Improved posture and body mechanics with overhead reaching.

PROGNOSIS

- DRA improves during initial post-partum period, but exercise beneficial in decreasing inter-recti distance and improving both pelvic-floor strength and lumbopelvic function.

PATIENT RESOURCE

- MedlinePlus, NIH National Institutes of Health. Diastasis Recti. http://www.nlm.nih.gov/medlineplus/ency/article/001602.htm Accessed May 12, 2013.

REFERENCES

1. The American Physical Therapy Association. Pattern 4C: Impaired muscle performance. *Interactive Guide to Physical Therapist Practice.* 2003. DOI: 10.2522/ptguide.3.1_3. Accessed May 12, 2013.
2. Dutton M. Practice Pattern 4E: Impaired joint mobility, motor function, muscle performance, and ROM associated with localized inflammation. In: Dutton M, ed. *Dutton's Orthopaedic Examination, Evaluation, and Intervention.* 3rd ed. New York, NY: McGraw-Hill; 2012. http://www.accessphysiotherapy.com/content/56555501. Accessed May 12, 2013.
3. Dutton M. Pathology, Gynecology, and Psychology. In: Dutton M, ed. *McGraw Hill's NPTE (National Physical Therapy Examination).* 2nd ed. New York, NY: McGraw-Hill; 2012. http://www.accessphysiotherapy.com/content/5402549#5402549. Accessed May 12, 2013.

ADDITIONAL REFERENCES

- Boxer S, Jones S. Intra-rater reliability of rectus abdominis diastasis measurement using dial calipers. *Aust J Physiother.* 1997;43(2):109–114.
- Chiarello CM, Falzone LA, McCaslin KE, Patel MN, Ulery KR. The effects of an exercise program on diastasis recti abdominis in pregnant women. *J Women's Health Phys Ther.* 2005;29(1):11–16.
- Coldron Y, Stokes MJ, Newham DJ, Cook K. Postpartum characteristics of rectus abdominis on ultrasound imaging. *Man Ther.* 2008;13(2):112–121.
- Gilleard WL, Brown JM. Structure and function of the abdominal muscles in primigravid subjects during pregnancy and the immediate postbirth period. *Phys Ther.* 1996;76(7):750–762.
- ICD9Data.com. http://www.icd9data.com. Accessed May 12, 2013.
- ICD10Data.com. http://www.icd10data.com. Accessed May 12, 2013.
- Mendes DA, Nahas FX, Veiga DF, et al. Ultrasonography for measuring rectus abdominis muscles diastasis. *Acta Cir Bras.* 2007;22(3):182–186.
- Spitznagle TM, Leong FC, Van Dillen LR. Prevalence of diastasis recti abdominis in a urogynecological patient population. *Int Urogynecol J Pelvic Floor Dysfunct.* 2007;18(3):321–328.
- Wang SM, Dezinno P, Maranets I, et al. Low back pain during pregnancy: Prevalence, risk factors, and outcomes. *Obstet Gynecol.* 2004;104:65–70.

147 SNAPPING SCAPULA SYNDROME

Eric Shamus, PhD, DPT, PT, CSCS
Ana Marcelina Moura, PT (Brazil)
Daniel Curtis, DPT, PT, MTC

CONDITION/DISORDER SYNONYMS

- Scapulothoracic crepitus
- Scapulocostal syndrome
- Scapulothoracic syndrome

ICD-9-CM CODE[1]

- 726.10 Disorders of bursae and tendons in shoulder region unspecified

ICD-10-CM CODE[2]

- M75.50 Bursitis of unspecified shoulder

PREFERRED PRACTICE PATTERN

- 4E: Impaired Joint Mobility, Motor Function, Muscle Performance, and Range of Motion Associated with Localized Inflammation[3]

PATIENT PRESENTATION

A 19-year-old male semi-professional tennis player presents with a chief complaint of a grinding sensation when he moves his right shoulder, especially with overhead and reaching motions. Other symptoms include pain in the lateral and anterior shoulder and crepitus about the scapula. The patient's primary concern is that his tennis serve is limited due to the grinding and posterior shoulder pain.

Examination reveals significant scapular protraction and increased thoracic kyphosis (combination of structural and postural), positive impingement test on the right, muscle weakness of the serratus anterior, middle and lower trapezius as well as gross weakness of the rotator cuff musculature. Examination of flexibility reveals shortening of anterior chest musculature, especially pectoralis minor on the right. Joint mobility of the thoracic spine is moderately hypomobile, and the glenohumeral (GH) joint is mildly limited in inferior glide and moderately limited in posterior glide. Joint mobility of the ribcage reveals a bucket handle exhaled fifth rib. There is a positive scapular retraction test on the right, negative on the left. During functional activities, he demonstrates overuse of scapula upward rotators during GH elevation. Activities such as performing a overhead tennis serve reproduce his symptoms of both crepitus and shoulder pain. Patient's score on the DASH Sports/Performing Arts Module is 50. Your screening examination is negative for neurologic causes and the cervical spine is cleared.

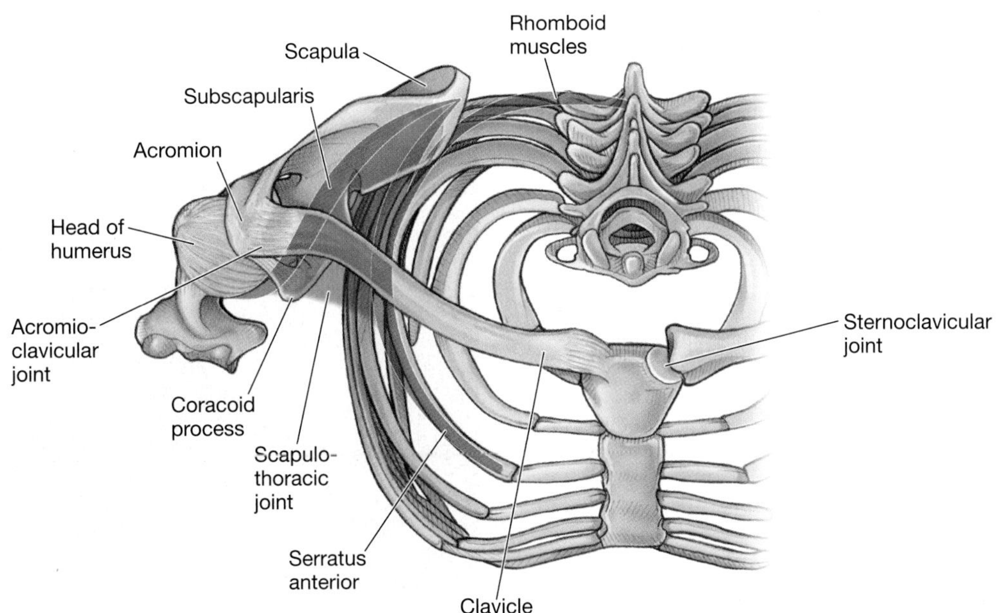

FIGURE 147-1 Superior aspect of the shoulder showing angle of scapula. (Reproduced with permission from Morton DA, Foreman KB, Albertine KH. *The Big Picture: Gross Anatomy*. New York, NY: McGraw-Hill, 2011.)

KEY FEATURES

Description

- Scapulothoracic joint is not a true synovial joint
- Scapulothoracic motion produces a snapping, popping, crepitus sound
- Scapula has the greatest number of muscles attached to it than any other bone
- Scapula dysrhythmia can cause friction along the muscles and ribs
- Can be a result of serratus anterior muscle dysfunction
- Injury to the long thoracic nerve

Essentials of Diagnosis

- Often asymptomatic
- Winging can help identify a dysfunction possibly occurring in the shoulder
- Symptoms of pain and weakness
- Can be a result of a brachial plexus injury
- Parsonage–Turner syndrome (brachial neuritis) underlying

General Considerations

- Postural changes of the thoracic spine and ribcage: Scoliosis
- 2:1 ratio of GH elevation to scapulothoracic elevation[4]
- Loss of serratus anterior muscle
- Weakness of trapezius strength, scapular stabilizers
- Commonly associated with presence of other orthopedic pathologies such as subacromial impingement syndrome, rotator cuff pathology, and labral pathology
- Creates an abnormal scapulothoracic rhythm
- Commonly associated with repeated overhead or overuse activities
- Full history of symptoms, medical history screening, and differential shoulder orthopedic examination will ensure appropriate diagnosis

Demographics

- Nonspecific
- Overhead athletes

CLINICAL FINDINGS

SIGNS AND SYMPTOMS

- Pain
- Symptoms of bursitis
- Crepitus
- Muscle spasm along the rib cage
- Weakness is commonly noted with functional reaching tasks
- Scapula instability, moving away from the rib cage

Functional Limitations

- Inability to raise or lower arms without the scapula's inferior angle tilting away from the rib cage
- Pain/limitation with:
  - Overhead activities
  - Reaching
  - Lifting
  - Dressing and grooming
  - Sustained or repetitive shoulder activities

Possible Contributing Causes

- GH joint dysfunction[5]
- Osseous abnormalities[5]

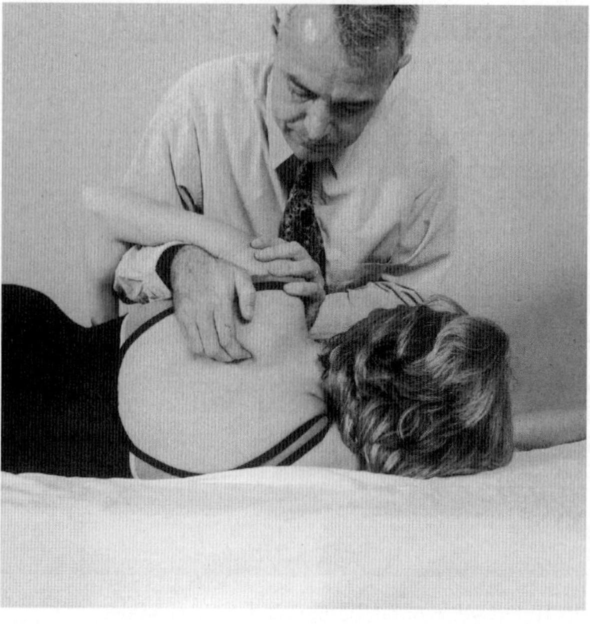

FIGURE 147-2 The clinician gently brings both hands together, lifting the scapula. (From Dutton M. *Dutton's Orthopedic Survival Guide: Managing Common Conditions.* http://www.accessphysiotherapy.com. Copyright © The McGraw-Hill Companies, Inc. All rights reserved.)

- Subscapularis muscle atrophy
- Increased thoracic kyphosis and suboptimal posture
- Luschka tubercle
- Sprengel deformity
- Abnormally shaped rib cage: Scoliosis
- Repetitive overhead activities
- Posterior shoulder capsule tightness
- Inferior angle tilting of the scapula
- Instability of the scapula to the thoracic wall
- Muscle atrophy
- Pectoralis minor tightness
- Poor neuromuscular control: Nerve injury
- Nontraumatic injury to the long thoracic nerve
  - Influenza
  - Drug overdose

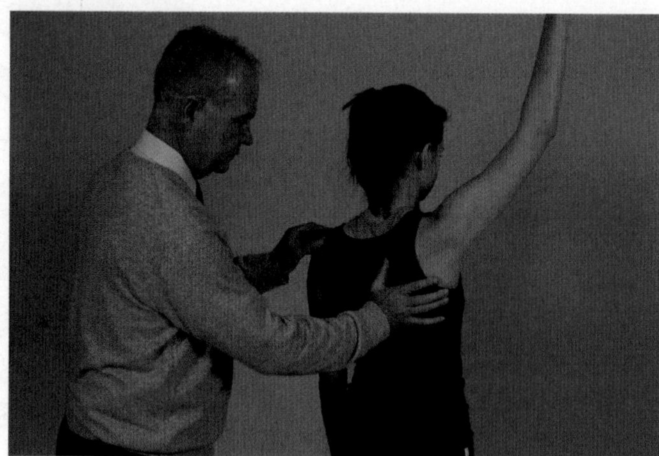

FIGURE 147-3 Scapular assist. (From Dutton M. *Dutton's Orthopaedic Examination, Evaluation, and Intervention.* 3rd ed. http://www.accessphysiotherapy.com. Copyright © The McGraw-Hill Companies, Inc. All rights reserved.)

- Traumatic injury to the long thoracic nerve
  - Impact injury
  - Stretch to cervical spine
  - Electrical shock
  - Mastectomy with axillary node dissection
- Brachial neuritis (Parsonage–Turner syndrome)

Differential Diagnosis

- Scapulothoracic bursitis
- Winging scapula
- Scapula alata
- Facioscapulohumeral (FSH) muscular dystrophy
- Serratus anterior palsy
- Cervical radiculopathy, C5-8
- Referred pain from the lungs or diaphragm
- Rotator cuff pathology (tendonitis, full- or partial-thickness tear)
- GH instability
- Labral tear
- Rib fracture
- Neuropathy
- Internal impingement
- Chondrosarcoma
- Elastofibroma

MEANS OF CONFIRMATION OR DIAGNOSIS

- Diagnosis made based on orthopedic special tests, signs and symptoms, imaging studies, and exclusion of differential diagnosis
- X-ray of the thoracic spine and rib cage
- Three-dimensional CT

FINDINGS AND INTERPRETATION

- Atrophy of the subscapularis muscle
- Bone abnormalities of the ribs
- Bursitis subscaula

TREATMENTS

Medications

- Nonsteroidal anti-inflammatory drugs (NSAIDs)

MEDICAL INTERVENTION

- Injection of scapulothoracic bursae[6]
- Partial scapulectomy[6]
- Resection of the superomedial angle of the scapula[6]
- Open bursal resection[6]
- Arthroscopic bursectomy[6]

REFERRALS/ADMITTANCE

- To radiologist for imaging, X-ray
- For MRI for differential diagnosis

IMPAIRMENTS

- Weakness and pain limiting overhead activities or activities involving arm out to side or across body, including dressing or grooming daily activities
- Impaired (suboptimal) posture
- Muscle imbalances

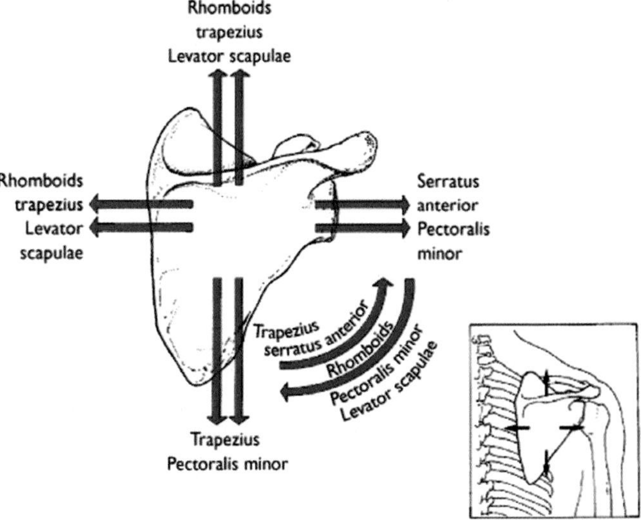

FIGURE 147-4 Actions of the scapular muscles. (From Hall SJ. *Basic Ciomechanics*. 5th ed. http://www.accessmedicine.com. Copyright © The McGraw-Hill Companies, Inc. All rights reserved.)

  - Periscapular muscle weakness (particularly upward rotators and depressors/retractors)
  - Pectoralis minor tightness
- Decreased thoracic ROM (particularly extension)
- Rotator cuff overuse/fatigue
- Neuropathy and subsequent muscle weakness
- Hypermobility at the GH joint and or scapulothoracic articulations
- Pain with active elevation

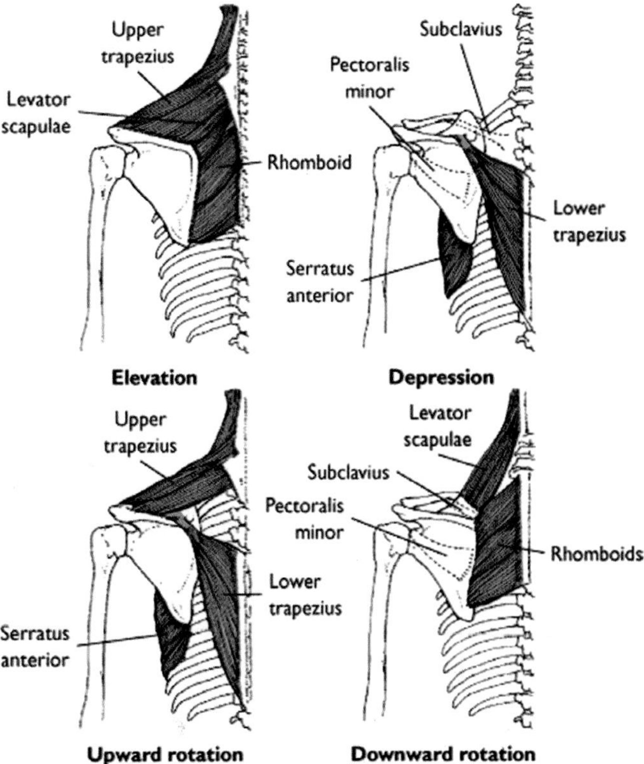

FIGURE 147-5 The muscles of the scapula. (From Hall SJ. *Basic Ciomechanics*. 5th ed. http://www.accessmedicine.com. Copyright © The McGraw-Hill Companies, Inc. All rights reserved.)

TESTS AND MEASURES

- Diagnosis based on orthopedic special tests, signs and symptoms, imaging studies, and exclusion of differential diagnosis
- Disabilities of the Arm, Shoulder, and Hand (DASH) score to assess physical function
- Special tests
  - Push-up test
  - Serratus wall test
  - Scapular retraction test

INTERVENTION

- Address muscle imbalances
  - Rotator cuff strength and endurance exercises
  - Muscle length of pectoralis major and minor
  - Postural education
- Strengthening of scapular musculature
  - Lower trap
  - Serratus anterior
  - Other scapular stabilizers
  - Shoulder lateral and medial rotation
  - Isometric
  - Thera-Band resisted
  - Handheld weight resisted
  - Progression through higher ranges of elevation
  - Scapular strength/stabilization
    - Retraction
    - Prone shoulder extension, scapular plane elevation
- Functional activities (depending on work/recreational desires
- Joint mobilization
  - Scapular mobility
  - Rib cage mobility
  - Clavicle mobility
- Addressing pain and inflammation
  - Ice
  - Rest
  - Activity modification (avoiding impingement positions)
  - Ultrasound
  - Electric stimulation

FUNCTIONAL GOALS

- Patient will be able to:
  - Reach into overhead cabinets in kitchen without pain or restriction while maintaining scapular control.
  - Lift a gallon milk carton from refrigerator at shoulder level, pain free, while maintaining scapular control.
  - Turn steering wheel, pain free, while maintaining scapular control.
  - Perform all dressing and grooming activities (tuck in shirt behind back, wash hair, etc.) without pain or compensation while maintaining scapular control.

PROGNOSIS

- If neurologically based, control may not be regained.
- Good to control symptoms.
- Prognosis is dependent on:
  - Underlying cause.
  - Presence of concomitant shoulder pathology.
  - Quality of the tissues involved.
  - Ability of the patient to control exacerbating activities and perform the optimal dosage of therapeutic exercise.

PATIENT RESOURCE

- A Patient's Guide to Snapping Scapula Syndrome. eOrthopod, n.d. Web. December 5, 2011. http://www.eorthopod.com/content/snapping-scapula-syndrome. Accessed July 2, 2013.

REFERENCES

1. ICD9Data.com. http://www.icd9data.com. Accessed July 3, 2013.
2. ICD10Data.com. http://www.icd10data.com. Accessed July 3, 2013.
3. American Physical Therapy Association. Pattern 4E: Impaired joint mobility, motor function, muscle performance, and range of motion associated with localized inflammation. In: *Guide to Physical Therapist Practice.* 2nd ed. Alexandria, VA: American Physical Therapy Association; 2001. Revised 2003.
4. Prentice WE. The Shoulder Complex. In: Prentice WE, ed. *Principles of Athletic Training: A Competency-Based Approach.* New York, NY: McGraw-Hill; 2011:639-680.
5. Lazar MA, Kwon YW, Rokito AS. Snapping scapula syndrome. *J Bone Joint Surg Am.* 2009;91(9):2251–2262.
6. Conduah AH, Backer CL 3rd, Backer CL Jr. Clinical management of scapulothoracic bursitis and the snapping scapula. *Sports Health.* 2012;2(20):147–155.

ADDITIONAL REFERENCES

- Dutton M. Chapter 8. Musculoskeletal Physical Therapy. In: Dutton M, ed. *McGraw-Hill's NPTE (National Physical Therapy Examination).* 2nd ed. New York, NY: McGraw-Hill; 2012. http://www.accessphysiotherapy.com/content/5397601. Accessed July 5, 2013.
- Dutton, M. Chapter 14. The Shoulder Complex. In: Dutton M, ed. *Orthopaedic Examination, Evaluation, and Intervention.* 2nd ed. New York, NY: McGraw-Hill; 2008. http://www.accessphysiotherapy.com/content/5552983. Accessed July 2, 2013.
- Dutton M. Chapter 5. The Shoulder Complex. In: Dutton M, ed. *Dutton's Orthopedic Survival Guide: Managing Common Conditions.* New York, NY: McGraw-Hill; 2011. http://accessphysiotherapy.com/content18651960. Accessed July 3, 2013.
- Gaskill T, Millett PJ. Snapping scapula syndrome: diagnosis and management. *J Am Acad Orthop Surg.* 2013;21(4):214–224.
- Hamilton N, Weimar W, Luttgens K, eds. *Kinesiology: Scientific Basis of Human Motion.* New York, NY: McGraw-Hill; 2008. http://www.accessphysiotherapy.com/content/6150577. Accessed July 4, 2013.
- Kuhne M, Boniquit N, Ghodadra N, Romeo AA, Provencher MT. The snapping scapula: diagnosis and treatment. *Arthroscopy.* 2009;25(11):1298–1311.
- Manske RC, Reiman MP, Stovak ML. Nonoperative and operative management of snapping scapula. *Am J Sports Med.* 2004;32(6):1554–1565.
- U.S National Library of Medicine NIH National Institutes of Health. Medline Plus. Tendinitis. http://www.nlm.nih.gov/medlineplus/ency/article/001229.htm. Accessed July 4, 2013.

148 TIETZE SYNDROME

Eric Shamus, PhD, DPT, PT, CSCS
Colin Brooks, MBA, SPHR

CONDITION/DISORDER SYNONYM

- Tietze disease

ICD-9-CM CODE

- Tietze disease

ICD-10-CM CODE

- M94.0 Chondrocostal junction syndrome [Tietze]

PREFERRED PRACTICE PATTERN

- 4E: Impaired Joint Mobility, Motor Function, Muscle Performance, and Range of Motion Associated with Localized Inflammation

PATIENT PRESENTATION

The patient is a 30-year-old man who presents with anterior rib pain. The patient states that his 3-year-old daughter jumped up and landed on his chest while he was lying on his back on the floor. He had pain along the anterior rib cage. The patient had a positive sedimentation rate and C-reactive protein test for inflammation. There is localized pain with palpation of the upper ribs at the rib cartilage. The patient said when he coughs or sneezes the pain increases.

KEY FEATURES

Description

- Described in 1921 by Alexander Tietze, a German surgeon
- Benign nonsuppurative inflammation of the costal cartilage

Essentials of Diagnosis

- Unknown cause
- Localized nonsuppurative nodule, usually located at the second or third costochondral junction[1]

General Considerations

- Inflammation, tenderness, and swelling
- Need to rule out a heart attack until proven otherwise, as symptoms very similar and can cause anxiety attacks, hyperventilation

Demographics

- More common in teens than in adults

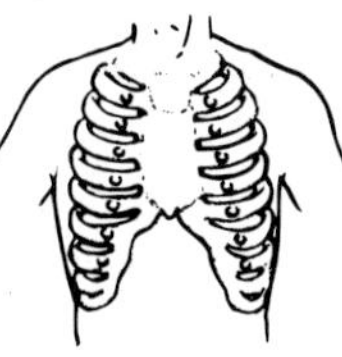
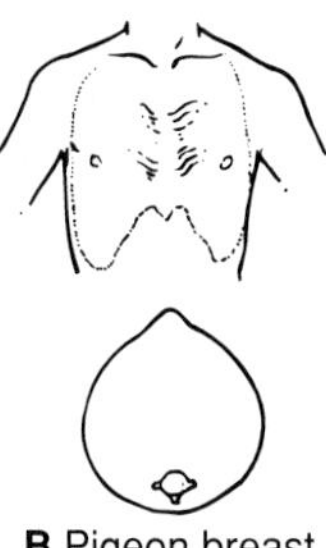
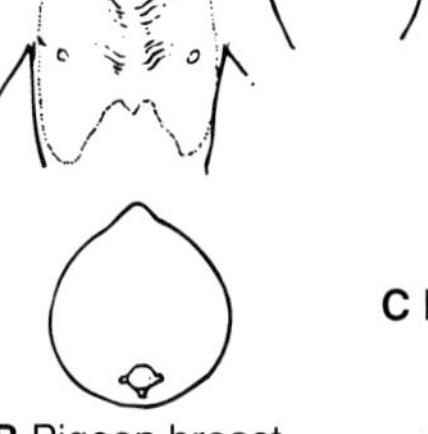
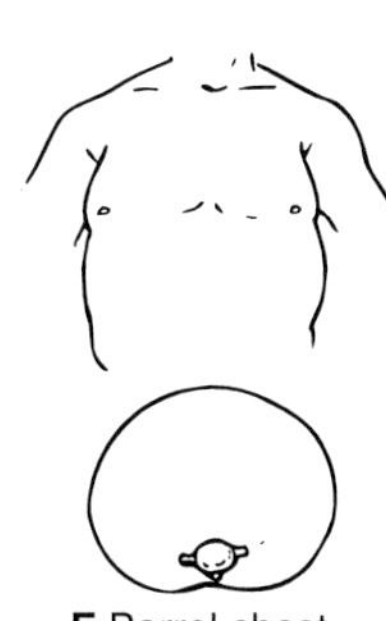

FIGURE 148-1 Deformities of the thorax. (A) Rachitic rosary. (B) Pigeon breast. (C) Harrison grooves. (D) Funnel breast. (E) Barrel chest. (From LeBlond RF, DeGowin RL, Brown DD. *DeGowin's Diagnostic Examination.* 9th ed. www.accessmedicine.com. Copyright © The McGraw-Hill Companies, Inc. All rights reserved.)

CLINICAL FINDINGS

SIGNS AND SYMPTOMS

- Tenderness and swelling along costal cartilage along the sternum (breast bone)
- Acute chest pain, anterior-upper
- Pain radiating into the shoulder and arm
- Pain increased with respiration (deep inspiration), coughing, sneezing

Functional Implications

- Breathing limitations, hyperventilation
- Pain with sleeping and lying on the ribs
- Inability to carry bags of groceries by one's side
- Inability to turn the steering wheel in a car
- Inability to carry heavy items
- Inability to dig in the garden

Possible Contributing Causes

- Excessive laughing
- Impact from airbag/steering wheel in a car accident
- Injury to chest and breast tissue
- Physical strain
- Psychological stress
- Radiation to the chest region
- Repetitive coughing

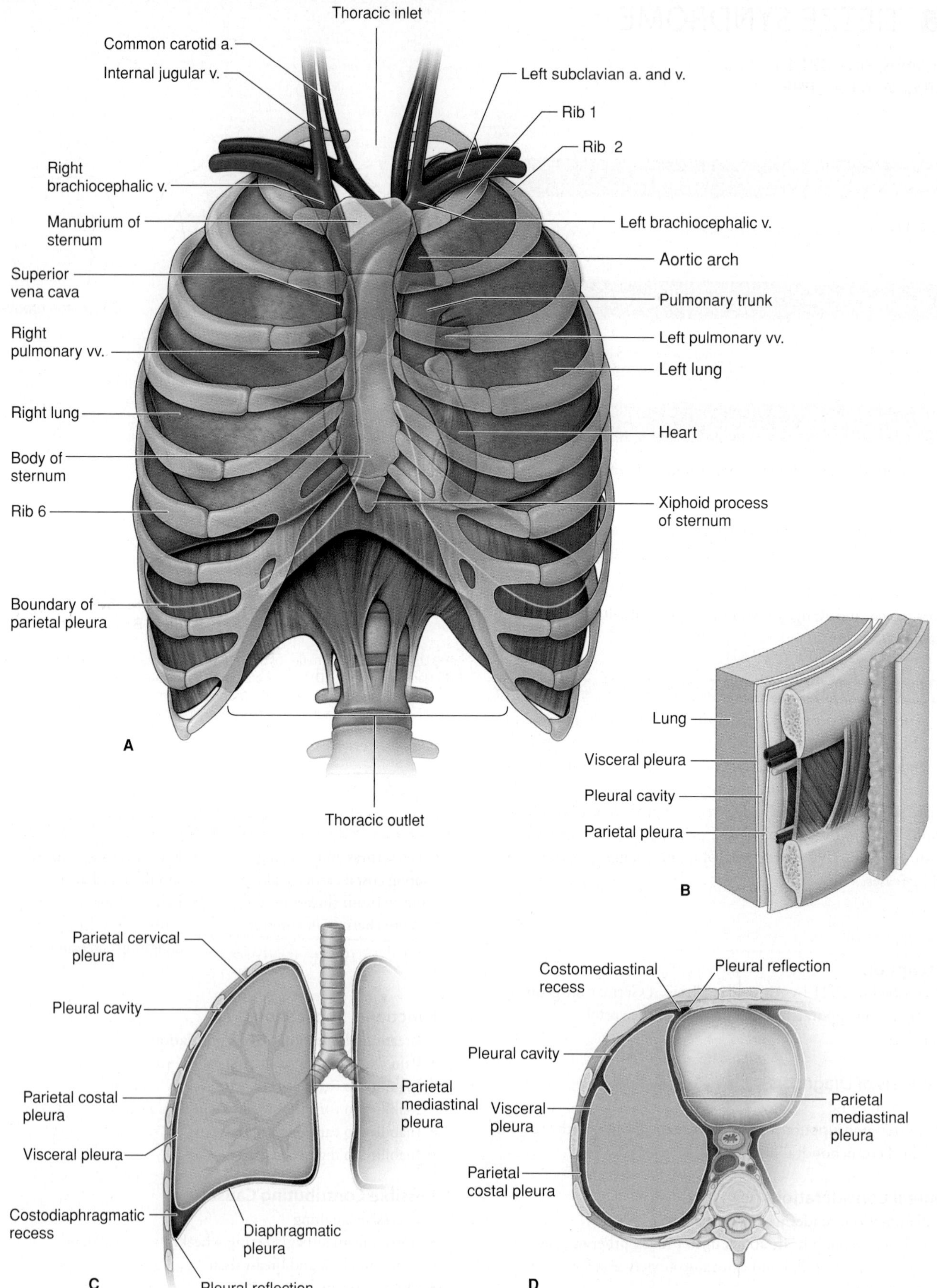

FIGURE 148-2 Components of the respiratory system. (Reproduced with permission from Morton DA, Foreman KB, Albertine KH. *The Big Picture: Gross Anatomy.* New York, NY: McGraw-Hill, 2011.)

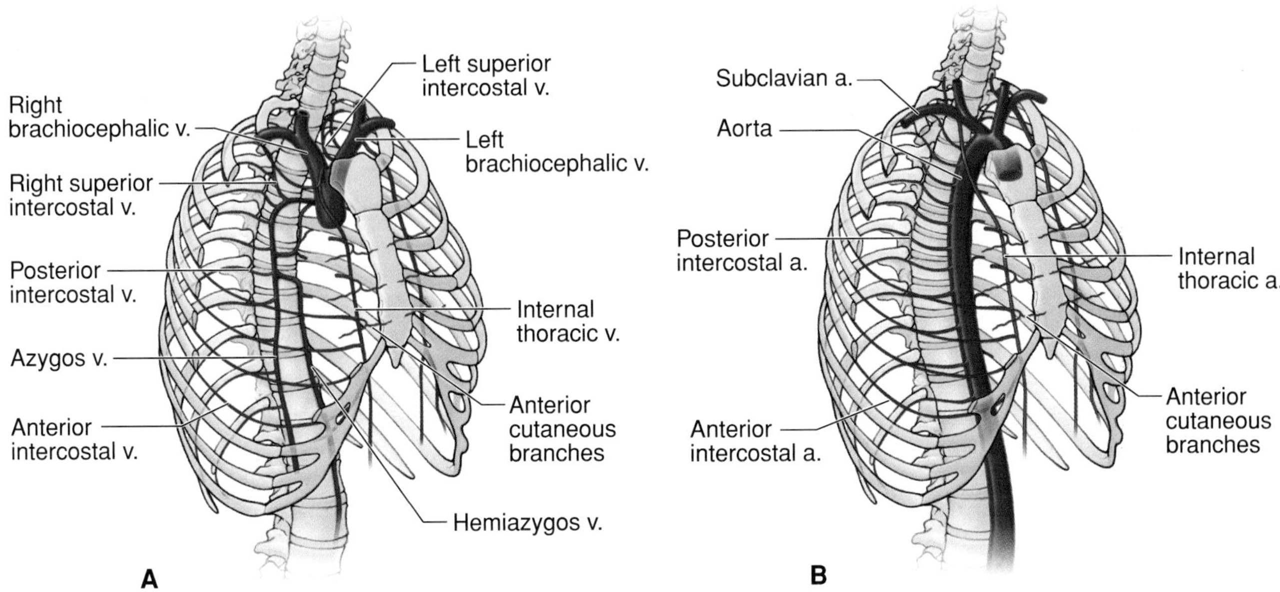

FIGURE 148-3 Vasculature of the thoracic region. (Reproduced with permission from Morton DA, Foreman KB, Albertine KH. *The Big Picture: Gross Anatomy.* New York, NY: McGraw-Hill, 2011.)

Differential Diagnosis

- Myocardial infarction (heart attack): Identical symptoms with acute pain and pain into the shoulder and arm, different in terms of no electrical heart change and no damage to the organs
- Costochondritis (different in that there is no swelling of the costal cartilage)
- Bruised ribs
- Broken ribs
- Pleurisy
- Pneumothorax
- Shingles
- Pneumonia

MEANS OF CONFIRMATION OR DIAGNOSIS

Laboratory Tests

- To rule out other diagnoses
- Blood test for heart damage (cardiac enzymes and troponin levels), negative for inflammation
- Sedimentation rate for inflammation
- C-reactive protein (CRP) test

Imaging

- ECG
- Bone scintigraphy
- Chest CT
- X-ray usually not helpful for cartilage, useful for pneumonia
  - Rule out parenchymal lung disease and rib fracture

FINDINGS AND INTERPRETATION

- Localized tenderness and swelling, palpable coastal cartilage

TREATMENT

Medication

- Acetylsalicylic acid
- Anti-inflammatory

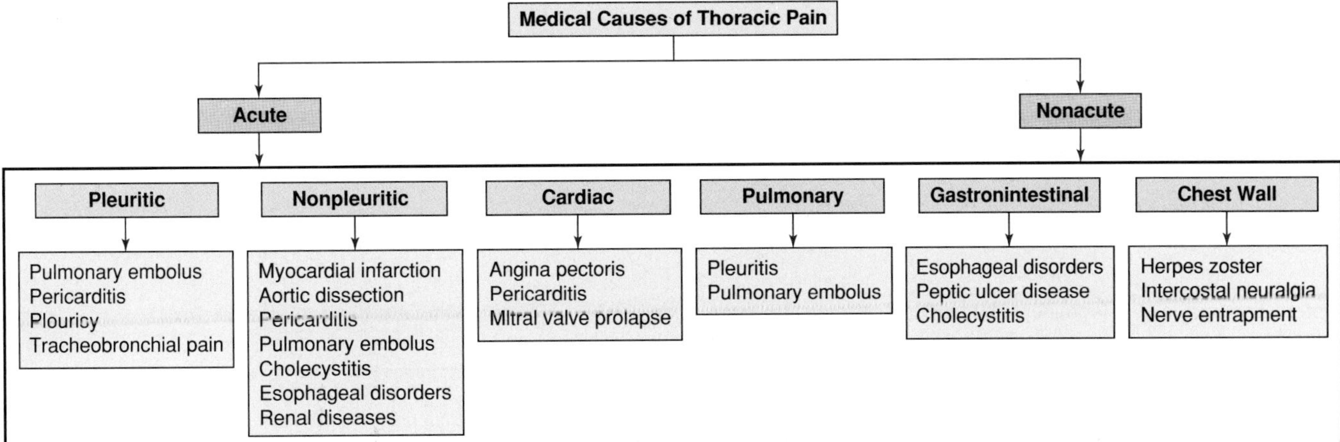

FIGURE 148-4 Medical causes of thoracic symptoms. (From Dutton M. *Dutton's Orthopaedic Examination, Evaluation, and Intervention.* 3rd ed. http://www.accessphysiotherapy.com.)

TABLE 148-1 Biomechanics of the Thorax

Motions	Z Joint	Rib Motion	Costotransverse Joint
Vertebromanubrial (T1–2)			
Flexion	Superoanterior glide	Anterior rotation	NA
Extension	Inferoposterior glide	Posterior rotation	NA
Latexion	Ipsilateral coupling	NA	NA
Rotexion	Ipsilateral coupling	NA	NA
Inspiration	NA	Elevation	NA
Expiration	NA	Depression	NA
Vertebrosternal (T3–7)			
Flexion	Superoanterior glide	Varies (very mobile) anteroposterior rotation	Superior–inferior glide (varies)
Extension	Posteroinferior glide	Varies (very mobile) anteroposterior rotation	Superior–inferior glide (varies)
Latexion	Ipsilateral side bend and contralateral rotation	Ipsilateral—anterior rotation Contralateral—posterior rotation	Ipsilateral—superior glide Contralateral—inferior glide
Rotexion	Ipsilateral side bend and ipsilateral rotation	Ipsilateral—posterior rotation Contralateral—anterior rotation	Ipsilateral—inferior glide Contralateral—superior glide
Inspiration	NA	Posterior rotation bilaterally	Inferior glide
Expiration	NA	Anterior rotation bilaterally	Superior glide
Vertebrochonral (T8–10)			
Flexion	Superoanterior glide	Anterior rotation	SMP glide
Extension	Inferoposterior glide	Posterior rotation	ILA glide
Latexion	Varies	NA	Apex in line with trochanter Ipsilateral—SMP Contralateral—ILA If not, the reverse occurs
Rotexion	Ipsilateral—inferior glide Contralateral—superior glide	NA	Ipsilateral—ILA, then anteromedial Contralateral—SMP, then posterolateral glide
Inspiration	NA	NA	ILA glide
Expiration	NA	NA	SMP glide

NA, not applicable; SMP, superior medial posterior; ILA, inferior lateral anterior.

Source: From Dutton M. *Dutton's Orthopaedic Examination, Evaluation, and Intervention.* 3rd ed. http://www.accessphysiotherapy.com.

TABLE 148-2 Rib Dysfunctions

Dysfunction	Rib Angle	Intercostal Space	Anterior Rib	Thoracic Findings
Anterior subluxation	Less prominent	Tender	NA	More prominent
Posterior subluxation	More prominent	Tender	NA	Less prominent
External rib torsion	Prominent and tender superior border	Wide above and narrow below	ERS, ipsilateral at the level above	NA
Internal rib torsion	Prominent and tender inferior border	Narrow above and wide below	FRS, contralateral at the level above	NA

ERS, extended, rotated, and side flexed; FRS, flexed, rotated, and side flexed; NA, not applicable.

Source: Data from Bookhout MR. Evaluation of the thoracic spine and rib cage. In: Flynn TW, ed. *The Thoracic Spine and Rib Cage: Musculoskeletal Evaluation and Treatment.* Boston, MA: Butterworth-Heinemann, 1996:147–167.

- Cortisone injection
- Lidocaine patch

REFERRALS/ADMITTANCE

- Rule out myocardial infarction

IMPAIRMENTS

- Debilitating pain, limiting movement and exertion
- Respiratory issues

TESTS AND MEASURES

- Thoracic and rib mobility
- Diaphragm doming
- Trunk rotation strength and range of motion

INTERVENTION

- Ice
- Joint mobilization to the costovertebral articulations
- Rib mobilization
- Diaphragm mobilization
- Breathing training
- Trunk rotation exercises

FUNCTIONAL GOALS

- Patient should be able to
  - Take a pain-free, full, deep breath.
  - Carry bags of groceries by their side.
  - Turn the steering wheel in a car.
  - Carry heavy items.
  - Dig in the garden.

PROGNOSIS

- Can last from hours to weeks.
- Generally resolves in 12 weeks.

ADDITIONAL INFORMATION

- See Case Study: Right Anterior Chest Pain on AccessPhysiotherapy.com for more information

PATIENT RESOURCE

- American Academy of Family Physicians. Tietze Syndrome. http://www.aafp.org/afp/viewRelatedDocumentsByMesh.htm?meshId=D013991. Accessed June 12, 2013.

REFERENCE

1. Dutton M. Chapter 25. The Thoracic Spine and Rib Cage. In: Dutton M, ed. *Orthopaedic Examination, Evaluation, and Intervention.* 2nd ed. New York, NY: McGraw-Hill; 2008. http://www.accessphysiotherapy.com/content/55593869. Accessed June 12, 2013.

ADDITIONAL REFERENCES

- Aeschlimann A, Kahn MF. Tietze's syndrome: a critical review. *Clin Exp Rheumatol.* 1990;8(4):407–412.
- Dutton M. Chapter 25. The Thoracic Spine and Rib Cage. In: Dutton M, ed. *Orthopaedic Examination, Evaluation, and Intervention.* 2nd ed. New York, NY: McGraw-Hill; 2008. http://www.accessphysiotherapy.com/content/55593869. Accessed June 12, 2013.
- Dutton M. Common Orthopedic Conditions. In: Dutton M, ed. *Dutton's Orthopedic Survival Guide: Managing Common Conditions.* New York, NY: McGraw-Hill; 2011. http://www.accessphysiotherapy.com/content/8656843. Accessed June 12, 2013.
- Homnick DN. Chapter 12. Chest and Pulmonary Conditions. In: Patel DR, Greydanus DE, Baker RJ, eds. *Pediatric Practice: Sports Medicine.* New York, NY: McGraw-Hill; 2009. http://www.accessphysiotherapy.com/abstract/6974839#6974842. Accessed June 12, 2013.
- ICD9Data.com. http://www.icd9data.com. Accessed June 12, 2013.
- ICD10Data.com. http://www.icd10data.com/ICD10CM/Codes. Accessed June 12, 2013.
- Jensen S. Musculoskeletal causes of chest pain. *Aust Fam Physician.* 2001;30(9):834–839.
- Kamel M, Kotob H. Ultrasonographic assessment of local steroid injection in Tietze's syndrome. *Br J Rheumatol.* 1997;36(5):547–550.
- American Physical Therapy Association. Pattern 4E: Impaired joint mobility, motor function, muscle performance, and range of motion associated with localized inflammation. In: *Guide to Physical Therapist Practice.* 2nd ed. Alexandria, VA: American Physical Therapy Association; 2001. Revised 2003.
- Volterrani L, Mazzei MA, Giordano N, et al. Magnetic resonance imaging in Tietze's syndrome. *Clin Exp Rheumatol.* 2008;26(5):848–853.

SECTION D SHOULDER DISORDERS

149 ACROMIOCLAVICULAR JOINT SEPARATION

Eric Shamus, PhD, DPT, PT, CSCS
Jennifer Shamus, PhD, DPT, COMT, CSCS

CONDITION/DISORDER SYNONYMS

- Separated Shoulder
- AC separation
- AC dislocation
- Shoulder Separation

ICD-9-CM CODES

- 840.0 Acromioclavicular (joint or ligament) sprain
- 831.04 Closed dislocation of acromioclavicular (joint)
- 831.14 Open dislocation of acromioclavicular (joint)

ICD-10-CM CODES

- S43.109A Unspecified dislocation of unspecified acromioclavicular joint, initial encounter
- S43.50XA Sprain of unspecified acromioclavicular joint, initial encounter

PREFERRED PRACTICE PATTERN

- 4E: Impaired Joint Mobility, Motor Function, Muscle Performance, and Range of Motion Associated with Localized Inflammation[1]

PATIENT PRESENTATION

A 53-year-old woman presents with 8/10 pain in the left shoulder after a bicycle accident 2 days ago. The patient states she fell off of her bike onto her outstretched arm during the "sprint" phase of interval training on the road. The patient complains of pain in the top aspect of her left shoulder and is unable to lift her left arm. The patient also states she hears a snapping sound if attempting to move her shoulder. Upon palpation, the patient reports severe pain in the acromioclavicular joint and a significant step deformity is present. Inflammation is present throughout the entire acromioclavicular joint. The Full Can/Empty Can, Neer, and Yergason tests are negative. The Acromioclavicular Resisted Extension Test is positive.

KEY FEATURES

Description

- Inflammation, irritation, or separation of the joint between the clavicle and acromion (AC joint)[2]
- Three ligaments of stability:
  - Acromioclavicular ligament[2]
  - Coracoacromial ligament
  - Coracoclavicular ligament: Made up of the conoid ligament and trapezoid ligament[2]

Essentials of Diagnosis

- Patient history and clinical examination
- X-ray
- Occurs most often from falling on an outstretched arm or hand
- AC separation occurs when the ligaments are completely torn and there is a dislocation of the joint
- Look for separation of the clavicle and acromion
- Step deformity often noticed when the clavicle is raised due to ligament tearing
- Six grades of sprain to separation: Rockwood Scale
  - Grade I
    - Slight displacement of the joint
    - Partially torn AC ligament
    - Separation <4 mm
  - Grade II
    - Partial dislocation of the joint
    - Complete disruption tear of the AC ligament
    - Partial disruption of the coracoclavicular ligament
    - Separation >5 mm
  - Grade III
    - Partial dislocation of the joint
    - Complete disruption tear of the AC ligament
    - Complete disruption/rupture of the coracoclavicular ligament
  - Grade IV
    - Dislocation of the joint
    - Posterior displacement
    - Requires surgery
  - Grade V
    - Dislocation of the joint
    - Superior displacement
    - Requires surgery
  - Grade VI
    - Dislocation of the joint
    - Inferior displacement
    - Requires surgery

General Considerations

- Not a synovial joint.
- Osteoarthritis is common without treatment or with prolonged instability.

Demographics

- Predominately in individuals with a history of activities involving overhead reach: Swimming, tennis, and baseball as well as with occupational activities involving repetitive overhead activity

CLINICAL FINDINGS

SIGNS AND SYMPTOMS

- Ache in the anterior top aspect of the shoulder
- Frequently worsens with overhead lifting or activity
- Pain with palpation at the AC joint
- Step deformity of the clavicle and acromion
- Occasional sound or sensation of snapping
- Pain with traction on the arm

Functional Implications

- May limit overhead activities, especially lifting
- May limit throwing and other rapid arm movements

Possible Contributing Causes

- Trauma
- Direct blow on the lateral tip of the acromion
- Rotator cuff weakness
- Shoulder instability
- Fall on outstretched hand

Differential Diagnosis

- AC joint arthritis
- Bicep tear
- Clavicle fracture
- Labral tear[3]
- Rotator cuff impingement
- Rotator cuff tear
- Shoulder instability

MEANS OF CONFIRMATION OR DIAGNOSIS

Imaging

- Radiographs while a patient holds a weight at his or her side
- MRI

Findings and Interpretation

- Radiographs will show a gap/step deformity between the clavicle and acromion.
- MRI will help evaluate ligament for structural changes or rupture.[4]
- Swelling may be minimal with Grade I separation.

TREATMENT

Medication

- Nonsteroidal anti-inflammatory drugs (NSAIDs)[3]
- Steroid injection

MEDICAL PROCEDURES

- Surgical repair of Grades IV through VI
- Mumford procedure
- Weaver–Dunn procedure

REFERRALS/ADMITTANCE

- To hospital for imaging
- To physician for surgery
- To physician for injection

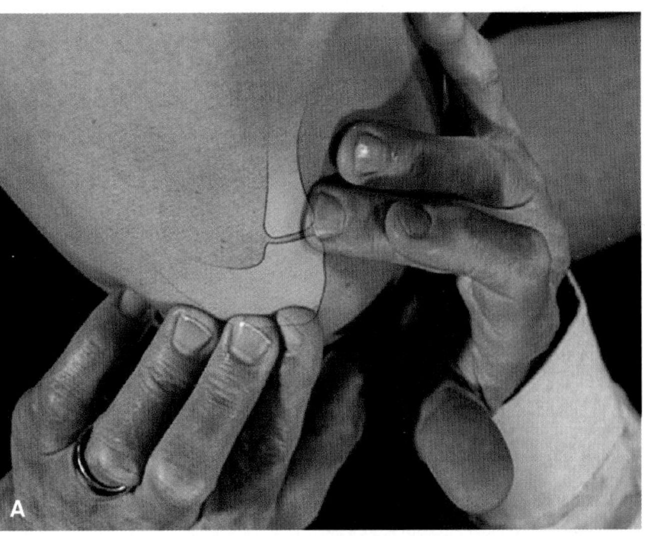

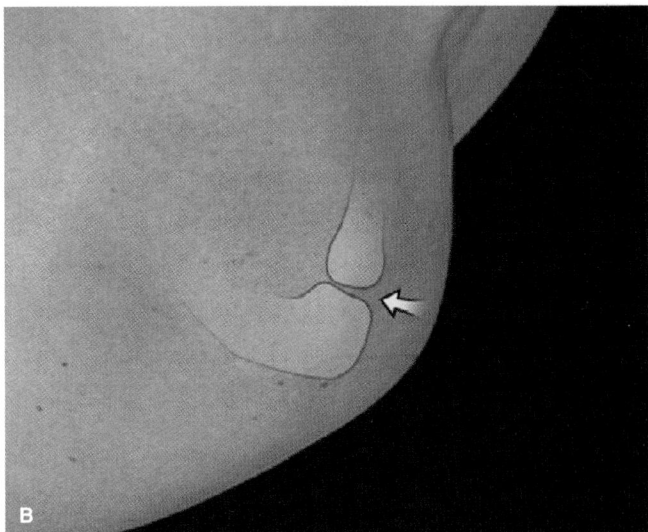

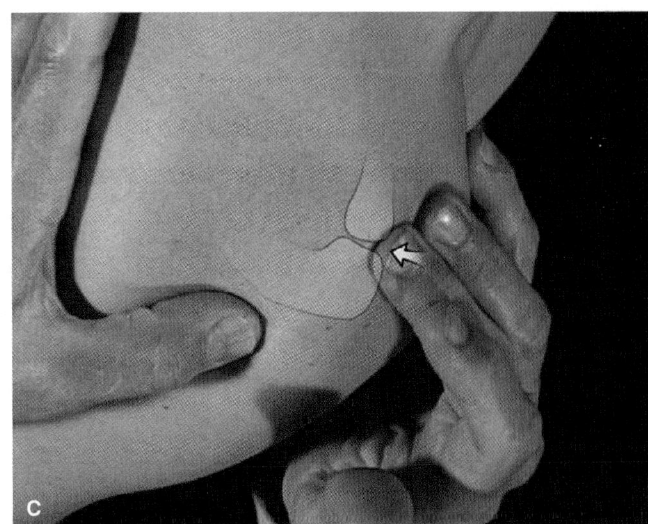

FIGURE 149-1 **A.** Palpation of the AC joint with the shoulder in neutral. **B** and **C.** Demonstrating increased space of the AC joint with the shoulder in internal rotation. (From Lawry GV. *Systematic Musculoskeletal Examinations*. www.accessmedicine.com. Copyright © The McGraw-Hill Companies, Inc. All rights reserved.)

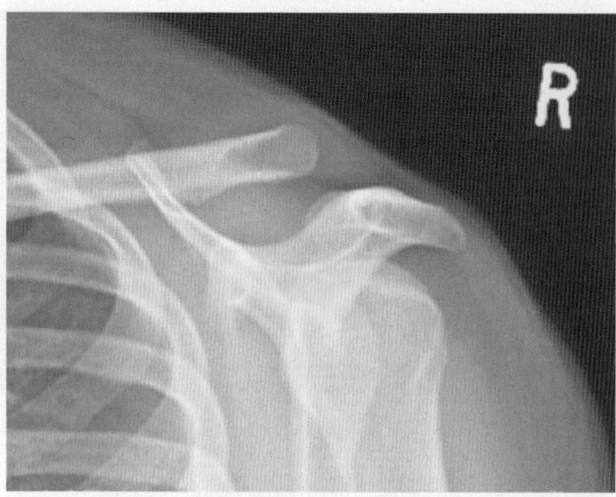

FIGURE 149-2 Acromioclavicular joint separation (third degree) with a wide AC joint and the clavicle displaced from the acromion. (From Simon RR, Sherman SC, Koenigsknecht SJ. *Emergency Orthopedics the Extremities,* p. 297, fig. 11-54, McGraw-Hill, Copyright 2007.)

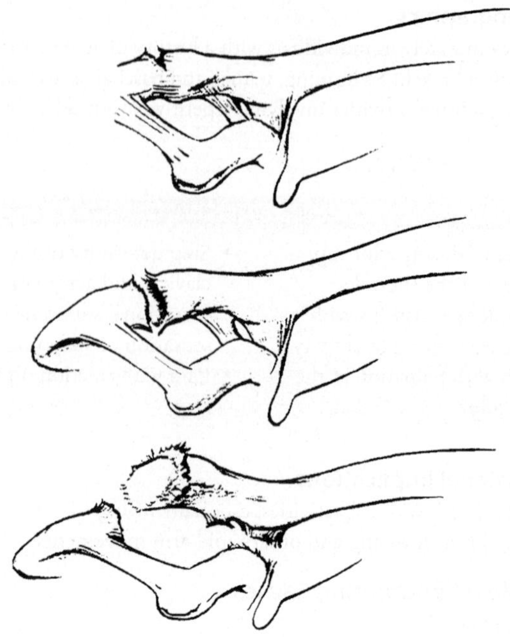

FIGURE 149-3 Grades of acromioclavicular joint separations. (From Skinner HB. *Current Diagnosis & Treatment in Orthopedics.* 4th ed. www.accessmedicine.com. Copyright © The McGraw-Hill Companies, Inc. All rights reserved.)

IMPAIRMENTS

- Inability to carry a briefcase due to the traction on the arm
- Inability to perform overhead activities such as swimming, baseball, or tennis
- Inability to perform jobs involving repetitive overhead reaching, lifting, or carrying

TESTS AND MEASURES

- Acromioclavicular shear test[3]
- O'Brien test[3]
- Acromioclavicular resisted extension test[3]
- Crossover impingement/horizontal adduction test[3]
- Pain provocation test[3]
- Disabilities of the Arm, Shoulder, and Hand (DASH) score to assess physical function
- Shoulder Pain and Disability Index[3]

INTERVENTION

- Acute
  - Rest
  - Electrotherapeutic modalities
  - Ice[5]
  - Transverse friction massage
  - Gentle stretching and AROM
  - Hemiplegic sling that draws the humeral head upward without keeping the shoulder internally rotated
  - Taping of the AC joint to unload weight of the arm[6]
- Post-acute
  - Once pain and inflammation are controlled, progress through further active exercises in pain-free ranges

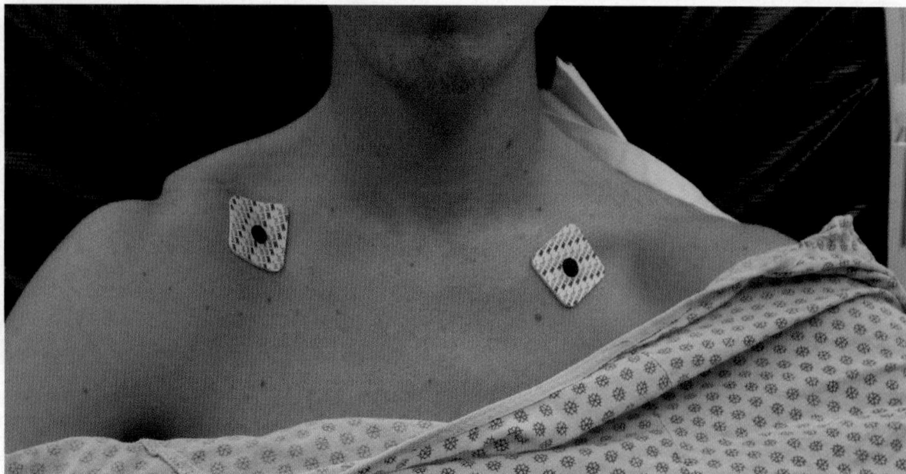

FIGURE 149-4 AC joint separation. Large deformity at the right distal clavicle suggesting complete ligament disruption. (From Knoop KJ, Stack L, Storrow A, Jason Thurman R. *The Atlas of Emergency Medicine.* 3rd ed. www.accessmedicine.com. Copyright © The McGraw-Hill Companies, Inc. All rights reserved. Photo contributor: R. Jason Thurman, MD.)

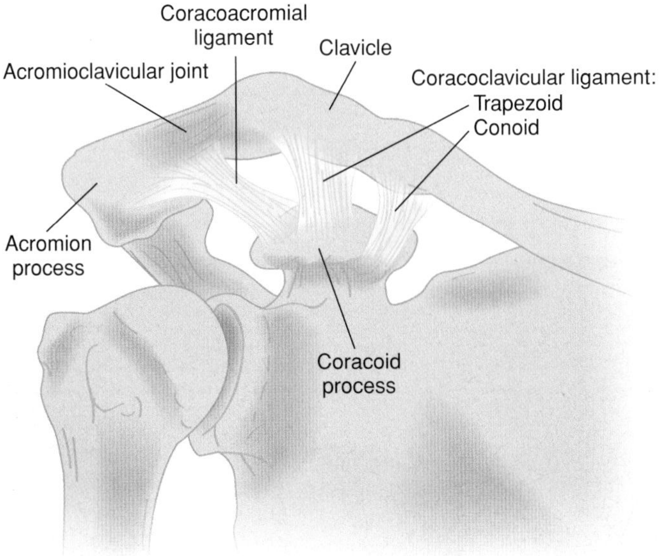

FIGURE 149-5 Anatomy of the acromioclavicular joint. (From Tintinalli JE, Stephan Stapczynski J, John Ma O, et al. *Tintinalli's Emergency Medicine: A Comprehensive Study Guide.* 7th ed. www.accessmedicine.com. Copyright © The McGraw-Hill Companies, Inc. All rights reserved.)

  - Posterior glenohumeral glides
  - Progressive closed-chain strengthening once pain-free
- Injury prevention
  - Avoid activities that involve repetitive or excessive overhead movement

FUNCTIONAL GOALS

- Patient will be able to
  - Carry a brief case pain-free.
  - Resume all overhead activities and ADLs without exacerbating inflammation.
  - Resume all sports activities as prior to onset.
  - Resume all reach activities without symptoms or limitation.
  - Resume all lifting activities without limitations due to pain or weakness of the upper extremities.
  - Drive without return of anterior shoulder pain.

PROGNOSIS

- Patients with Grade III separation require 4 to 5 months of rehabilitation, but do not always need surgery.
- Symptoms improve and resolve with treatment, rest, and unloading of weight on the arm.

PATIENT RESOURCE

- American Academy of Orthopaedic Surgeons. Shoulder Separation. http://orthoinfo.aaos.org/topic.cfm?topic=A00033, Accessed January 25, 2013.

REFERENCES

1. The American Physical Therapy Association. Pattern 4E: Impaired joint mobility, motor function, muscle performance, and range of motion associated with localized inflammation. *Interactive Guide to Physical Therapist Practice.* 2003. DOI: 10.2522/ptguide.3.1_5. Accessed January 25, 2013.
2. Hamilton N, Weimar W, Luttgens K. *Kinesiology: Scientific Basis of Human Motion.* New York, NY: McGraw-Hill; 2008. http://www.accessphysiotherapy.com/resource/618. Accessed January 25, 2013.
3. Dutton M. *Orthopaedic Examination, Evaluation, and Intervention.* New York, NY: McGraw-Hill; 2008. http://www.accessphysiotherapy.com/resource/612. Accessed January 25, 2013.
4. Malone TR, Hazle C, Grey ML. *Imaging in Rehabilitation.* New York, NY: McGraw-Hill; 2008. http://www.accessphysiotherapy.com/resource/613. Accessed January 25, 2013.
5. Prentice WE. Chapter 9. Cryotherapy and thermotherapy. In: Prentice WE, Quillen WS, Underwood F, eds. *Therapeutic Modalities in Rehabilitation.* 4th ed. New York, NY: McGraw-Hill; 2011. http://www.accessphysiotherapy.com/content/8137995#8137995. Accessed January 25, 2013.
6. Shamus J, Shamus E. A taping technique for the treatment of acromioclavicular joint sprains: A case study. *J Orthop Sports Phys Ther.* 1997;25(6):390-394.

ADDITIONAL REFERENCES

- ICD9DATA web site. http://www.icd9data.com. Accessed January 25, 2013.
- ICD10DATA web site. http://www.icd10data.com. Accessed January 25, 2013.

150 ACROMIOCLAVICULAR LIGAMENT SPRAIN

Eric Shamus, PhD, DPT, PT, CSCS
Jennifer Shamus, PhD, DPT, COMT, CSCS

CONDITION/DISORDER SYNONYMS

- Separated shoulder
- AC separation
- AC dislocation
- Shoulder separation

ICD-9-CM CODE

- 840.0 Acromioclavicular (joint, ligament) sprain

ICD-10-CM CODE

- S43.50XA Sprain of unspecified acromioclavicular joint, initial encounter

PREFERRED PRACTICE PATTERN

- 4E: Impaired Joint Mobility, Motor Function, Muscle Performance, and Range of Motion Associated with Localized Inflammation[1]

PATIENT PRESENTATION

A 42-year-old man presents with right shoulder pain due to a fall he sustained on his outstretched arm while walking his dog one week ago. The patient complains of an ache in the top, anterior aspect of the right shoulder and reports that he cannot lift his arm to wash his hair or complete other overhead activities without a significant increase in pain. Upon palpation, the patient reports pain and tenderness in the acromioclavicular joint, most notably along the acromioclavicular ligament. A step deformity of 5 mm is present with elevation of the clavicle. The Full Can/Empty Can, Neer, and Yergason tests are negative. The Acromioclavicular Resisted Extension Test is positive.

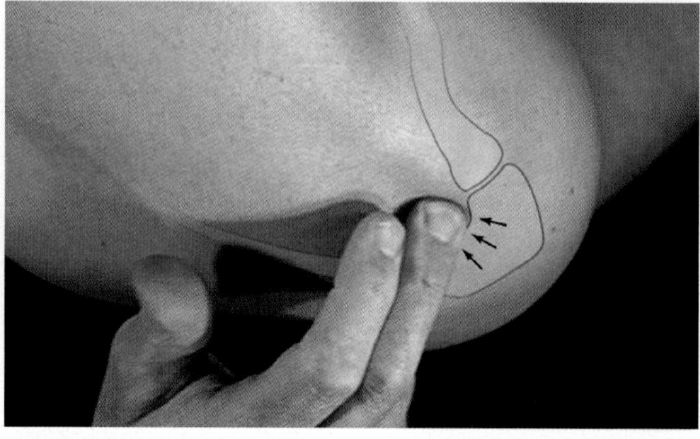

FIGURE 150-1 Palpation of the supraspinatus fossa. (From Lawry GV. *Systematic Musculoskeletal Examinations.* www.accessmedicine.com. Copyright © The McGraw-Hill Companies, Inc. All rights reserved.)

KEY FEATURES

Description

- Inflammation, irritation, or separation of the joint between the clavicle and acromion (AC joint)[2]
- Three ligaments of stability:
  - Acromioclavicular ligament[2]
  - Coracoacromial ligament
  - Coracoclavicular ligament: Made up of the Conoid ligament and trapezoid ligament[2]

Essentials of Diagnosis

- Patient history and clinical examination
- X-ray
- Occurs most often from falling on an outstretched arm or hand
- Occurs when the ligaments are completely torn and there is a dislocation of the joint
- Look for separation of the clavicle and acromion
- Step deformity often noticed when the clavicle is raised due to ligament tearing
- Six grades of sprain to separation: Rockwood Scale
  - Grade I
    - Slight displacement of the joint
    - Partially torn AC ligament
    - Separation <4 mm
  - Grade II
    - Partial dislocation of the joint
    - Complete disruption tear of the AC ligament
    - Partial disruption of the coracoclavicular ligament
    - Separation >5 mm
  - Grade III
    - Partial dislocation of the joint
    - Complete disruption tear of the AC ligament
    - Complete disruption/rupture of the coracoclavicular ligament
  - Grade IV
    - Dislocation of the joint
    - Posterior displacement
    - Requires surgery
  - Grade V
    - Dislocation of the joint
    - Superior displacement
    - Requires surgery
  - Grade VI
    - Dislocation of the joint
    - Inferior displacement
    - Requires surgery

General Considerations

- No synovial joint
- Osteoarthritis is common without treatment or with prolonged instability

Demographics

- Predominately in individuals with a history of activities involving overhead reach: Swimming, tennis, and baseball as well as with occupational activities involving repetitive overhead activity

CLINICAL FINDINGS

SIGNS AND SYMPTOMS

- Ache in the anterior top aspect of the shoulder
- Frequently worsens with overhead lifting or activity
- Pain with palpation at the AC joint
- Step deformity of the clavicle and acromion
- Occasional sound or sensation of snapping
- Pain with traction on the arm

Functional Implications

- May limit overhead activities, especially lifting
- May limit throwing and other rapid arm movements

Possible Contributing Causes

- Frequent and prolonged overhead activity
- Prolonged repetitive use of the involved arm
- Poor posture (i.e., rounded shoulders)
- Anterior displacement of the humeral head
- Rotator cuff weakness
- Fall on outstretched hand
- Landing on lateral tip of the acromion

Differential Diagnosis

- Bicep tear
- Bicep tendinopathy
- Labral tear[3]
- Rotator cuff impingement
- Rotator cuff tear
- Rotator cuff tendinitis
- Subacromial bursitis

MEANS OF CONFIRMATION OR DIAGNOSIS

Imaging

- Radiographs while patient holds a weight at his or her side
- MRI

FINDINGS AND INTERPRETATION

- Radiographs will show a gap between the clavicle and acromion
- MRI images to evaluate ligament for structural changes or rupture[4]
- Swelling may be minimal with Grade I separation

TREATMENT

Medication

- Nonsteroidal anti-inflammatory drugs (NSAIDs)[3]
- Steroid injection

MEDICAL PROCEDURES

- Surgical repair of Grades IV through VI
- Mumford procedure
- Weaver–Dunn procedure

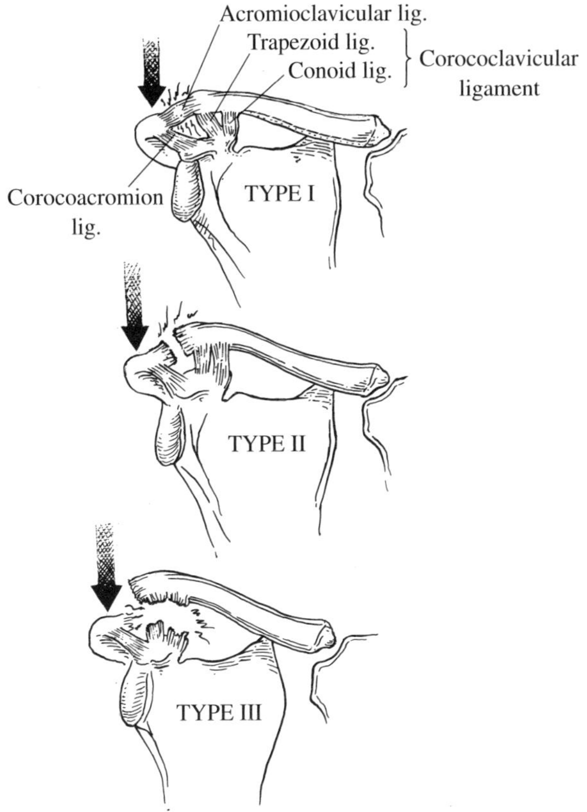

FIGURE 150-2 Acromioclavicular joint injuries. Types of acromioclavicular joint injuries. Classification schemes may subdivide type III injuries into III through VI depending on the position of the clavicle. (From Knoop KJ, Stack L, Storrow A, Jason Thurman R. *The Atlas of Emergency Medicine.* 3rd ed. www.accessmedicine.com. Copyright © The McGraw-Hill Companies, Inc. All rights reserved.)

REFERRALS/ADMITTANCE

- To hospital for imaging (MRI)[4]
- To physician for surgery
- To physician for injection

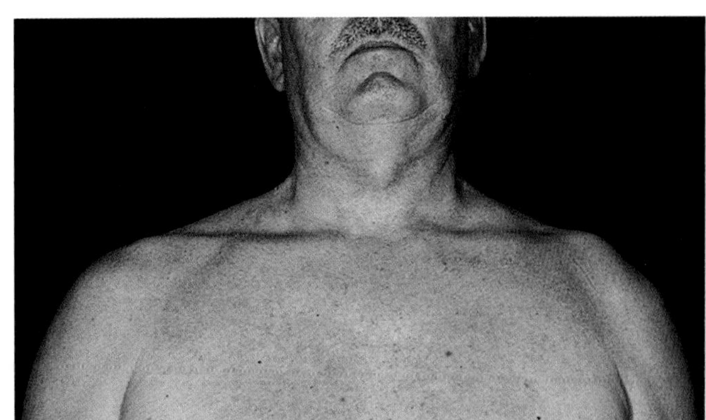

FIGURE 150-3 AC joint separation. Subtle prominence of the left distal clavicle. The upward displacement of the clavicle is due to stretching or disruption of the suspending ligaments. (From Knoop KJ, Stack L, Storrow A, Jason Thurman R. *The Atlas of Emergency Medicine.* 3rd ed. www.accessmedicine.com. Copyright © The McGraw-Hill Companies, Inc. All rights reserved. Photo contributor: Frank Birinyi, MD.)

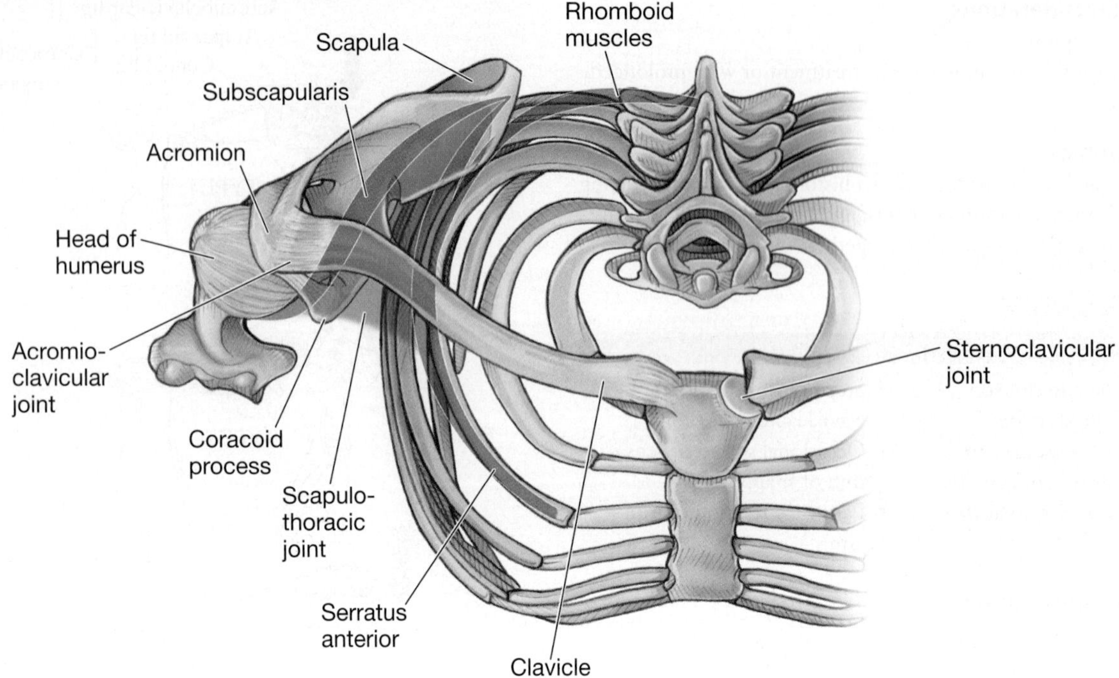

FIGURE 150-4 Superior aspect of shoulder showing angle of scapula. (Reproduced with permission from Morton DA, Foreman KB, Albertine KH. *The Big Picture: Gross Anatomy.* New York, NY: McGraw-Hill; 2011.)

IMPAIRMENTS

- Inability to carry a briefcase due to traction on the arm
- Inability to perform overhead activities such as swimming, baseball, or tennis
- Inability to perform jobs involving repetitive overhead reaching or lifting

TESTS AND MEASURES

- Acromioclavicular shear test[3]
- O'Brien test[3]
- Acromioclavicular resisted extension test[3]
- Crossover impingement/horizontal adduction test[3]
- Pain provocation test[3]
- Disabilities of the Arm, Shoulder, and Hand (DASH) score to assess physical function
- Shoulder Pain and Disability Index[3]

INTERVENTION

- Acute
  - Rest
  - Reduce inflammation with NSAIDs and electrotherapeutic modalities
  - Ice/heat[5]
  - Transverse friction massage
  - Gentle stretching and AROM
  - Hemiplegic sling that draws the humeral head upward without keeping the shoulder in internally rotated
  - Taping of the AC joint to unload weight of the arm[6]
- Post-acute
  - Once pain and inflammation are controlled, progress through further active exercises in pain-free ranges
  - Posterior glenohumeral glides
  - Progressive closed-chain strengthening once pain-free
- Injury prevention
  - Avoid activities that involve repetitive or excessive overhead movement

FUNCTIONAL GOALS

- Patient will be able to
  - Carry a brief case pain-free.
  - Resume all overhead activities and ADLs without exacerbating inflammation.
  - Resume all sports activities as prior to onset.
  - Resume all reach activities without symptoms or limitation.
  - Resume all lifting activities without limitations due to pain or weakness of the upper extremities.
  - Drive without return of anterior shoulder pain.

PROGNOSIS

- Patients with Grade III separation require 4 to 5 months of rehabilitation, but do not always need surgery.
- Symptoms improve and resolve with treatment, rest, and unloading of weight on the arm.
- If the injury is the result of overuse, a change in activity and work habits may be needed.

PATIENT RESOURCE

- American academy of orthopaedic surgeons. Shoulder Separation. http://orthoinfo.aaos.org/topic.cfm?topic=A00033. Accessed January 25, 2013

REFERENCES

1. The American Physical Therapy Association. Pattern 4E: Impaired joint mobility, motor function, muscle performance, and range of motion associated with localized inflammation. *Interactive Guide to Physical Therapist Practice*. 2003. DOI: 10.2522/ptguide.3.1_5. Accessed March 1, 2013.
2. Hamilton N, Weimar W, Luttgens K. Kinesiology: scientific basis of human motion. New York, NY: McGraw-Hill; 2008. http://www.accessphysiotherapy.com/resource/618. Accessed March 1, 2013.
3. Dutton M. *Dutton's Orthopaedic Examination, Evaluation, and Intervention*. 3rd ed. New York, NY: McGraw-Hill; 2012. http://www.accessphysiotherapy.com/resource/612. Accessed March 1, 2013.
4. Malone TR, Hazle C, Grey ML. *Imaging in Rehabilitation*. New York, NY: McGraw-Hill; 2008. http://www.accessphysiotherapy.com/resource/613. Accessed March 1, 2013.
5. Prentice WE. Chapter 9. Cryotherapy and Thermotherapy. In: Prentice WE, Quillen WS, Underwood F, eds. *Therapeutic Modalities in Rehabilitation.* 4th ed. New York, NY: McGraw-Hill; 2011. http://www.accessphysiotherapy.com/content/8137995#8137995. Accessed March 1, 2013.
6. Shamus JL, Shamus EC. A Taping Technique for the Treatment of Acromioclavicular Joint Sprains: A Case Study. *J Orthop Sports Phys Ther*. 1997;25(6):390–394.

ADDITIONAL REFERENCES

- ICD9DATA web site. http://www.icd9data.com. Accessed March 1, 2013.
- ICD10DATA web site. http://www.icd10data.com. Accessed March 1, 2013.

151 ADHESIVE CAPSULITIS (FROZEN SHOULDER)

Matthew Daugherty, DPT, MOT, OCS, FAAOMPT

CONDITION/DISORDER SYNONYM

- Frozen shoulder syndrome

ICD-9-CM CODE[1]

- 726.0 Adhesive capsulitis of shoulder

ICD-10-CM CODE[2]

- M75.00 Adhesive capsulitis of unspecified shoulder

PREFERRED PRACTICE PATTERN[3]

- 4E: Impaired Joint Mobility, Motor Function, Muscle Performance, and ROM Associated with Localized Inflammation

PATIENT PRESENTATION

A 48-year-old woman, whom is employed as an insurance agent, comes to your outpatient physical therapy clinic self-referred with a 3-month history of right shoulder pain. She first noticed general pain around her glenohumeral joint when putting on her seat belt and fastening her bra. She denies any mechanism of injury and feels that the symptoms are gradually worsening. In addition to the pain, she reports an inability to reach overhead or behind her back and is unable to sleep on her right side.

Her right shoulder passive range of motion (PROM) is limited to 115 degrees of flexion, 100 degrees of abduction, 35 degrees of extension, 30 degrees of external rotation, and 50 degrees of internal rotation. Her left shoulder PROM is 175 degrees of flexion, 175 degrees of abduction, 40 degrees of extension, 90 degrees of external rotation, and 70 degrees of internal rotation. When testing her right glenohumeral joint mobility you determine global hypomobility with a very firm end feel and local discomfort reported during motion testing. She has palpable tenderness at the coracoid process, intertubercular groove, and the greater tuberosity of the humerus. Functionally she has difficulty finding a position of comfort.

KEY FEATURES

Description

- Self-limiting shoulder pain and dysfunction due to:
  - Localized inflammation of the glenohumeral joint capsule
  - Paucity of synovial fluid
  - Fibrosis of the capsule causing adherence to the humeral head
- Three pathologic pathways
  - Primary (idiopathic)

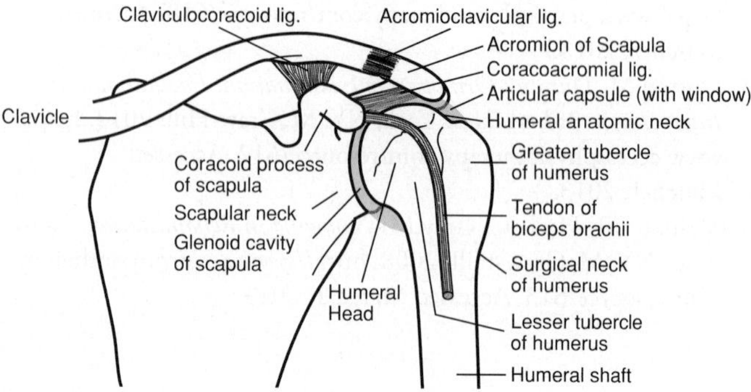

FIGURE 151-1 Anatomy of the shoulder joint. The anterior window in the joint capsule exposes the inner attachment of the biceps brachii muscle. (From LeBlond RF, DeGowin RL, Brown DD. *DeGowin's Diagnostic Examination*. 9th ed. www.accessmedicine.com. Copyright © The McGraw-Hill Companies, Inc. All rights reserved.)

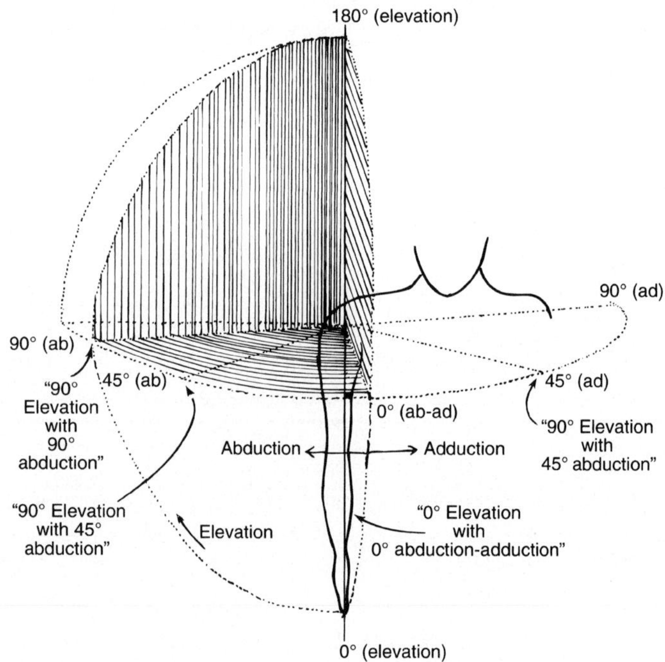

FIGURE 151-2 Motions at the shoulder. There has been much confusion in terminology about shoulder motion. The system presented here leaves no room for misinterpretation. Elevation is a movement of the arm along any meridian, measured from position at the south pole. Elevation along the meridian in the parasagittal plane passing through the shoulder joint are flexion (forward) and extension (backwards). Movement medial to this is adduction; movement lateral to the plane is abduction. When the arm is elevated in any meridian other than the parasagittal one, the motion is expressed as "elevation in abduction" or "elevation in abduction." The amount of deviation from the parasagittal plane is noted in degrees, for example, "elevation in 70 degrees of abduction." (From LeBlond RF, DeGowin RL, Brown DD. *DeGowin's Diagnostic Examination*. 9th ed. www.accessmedicine.com. Copyright © The McGraw-Hill Companies, Inc. All rights reserved.)

- Secondary: Can be attributed to a known intrinsic, extrinsic, or systemic cause
- Tertiary: Postoperative or post-fracture
- Adhesive capsulitis can be divided into four stages
  - Stage 1: "Preadhesive"
    - Near normal range of motion (ROM), pain at end points of motion and mild synovitis
  - Stage 2: "Freezing"
    - Marked loss of motion, pain at end points with thickened read synovitis
  - Stage 3: "Frozen"
    - Marked loss of motion, painless ROM with capsule fibrosis and adhesions
  - Stage 4: "Thawing"
    - Improved glenohumeral motion, painless ROM; no synovitis present

Essentials of Diagnosis

- Extrinsic factors
  - Cardiopulmonary disease
  - Cervical disc
  - CVA
  - Humerus fractures
  - Parkinson disease
- Intrinsic factors
  - Dupuytren disease
  - Rotator cuff tendinitis
  - Rotator cuff tears
  - Biceps tendinitis
  - Calcific tendinitis
- Systemic factors
  - Diabetes mellitus
  - Hypothyroidism
  - Hyperthyroidism
  - Hypoadrenalism
  - Dupuytren disease

Demographics

- Affects 2% to 5% of the general population
- Affects 10% to 38% of patients with thyroid disease or diabetes mellitus
- Primary AC generally affects individuals aged 40 to 65 years
- Greater incidence in females than in males
- Occurrence in one shoulder increases the risk of contralateral shoulder involvement from 5% to 34%

CLINICAL FINDINGS

SIGNS AND SYMPTOMS

- Pain in the anterior lateral shoulder described as achy at rest and sharp with end-range motion
- Symptoms typically present for <3 months if stage 1
- Nighttime pain and pain when reaching behind the back are common
- Active and passive ROM are equally limited

Functional Implications

- Pain/Limitation with overhead activities
- Pain/Limitation with reaching
- Pain/Limitation with lifting

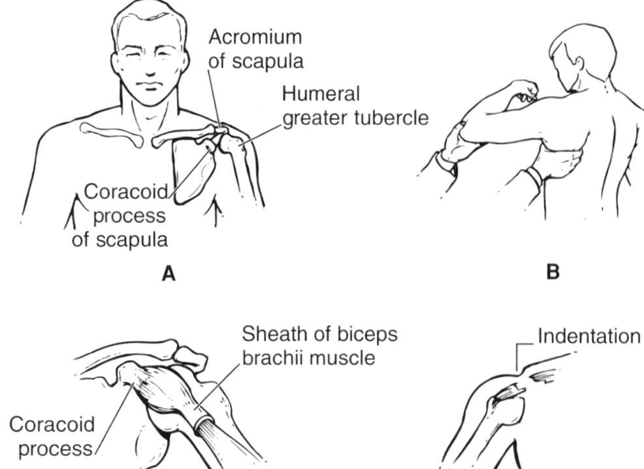

FIGURE 151-3 Examination of the shoulder joint. (**A**) Topography of the shoulder: The bony prominences of the humeral greater tubercle and the coracoid and acromial processes of the scapula form a right-angled triangle. (**B**) Immobilization of the scapula to test shoulder motion. (**C**) Fluid in the shoulder joint: The heavily stippled structures are the joint capsules distended with fluid. (**D**) Rupture of the supraspinatus tendon. (From LeBlond RF, DeGowin RL, Brown DD. *DeGowin's Diagnostic Examination.* 9th ed. www.accessmedicine.com. Copyright © The McGraw-Hill Companies, Inc. All rights reserved.)

- Pain/Limitation while dressing
- Pain/Limitation with sustained or repetitive shoulder activities
- Pain at night disrupting sleep

Possible Contributing Causes

- Degenerative changes at the acromioclavicular (AC) joint
- Rotator cuff tendinopathy
- Bicipital tendinopathy
- Humeral fracture
- Capsular tightness
- Increased thoracic kyphosis and suboptimal posture
- History of trauma
- Diabetes mellitus
- Treatment with antiretroviral therapy

Differential Diagnosis

- Cervical radiculopathy
- Full-thickness rotator cuff tear
- Glenohumeral arthritis
- Glenohumeral contracture
- Internal impingement
- Labral tear
- Neuropathy (suprascapular nerve)
- Referred pain from the lungs or diaphragm
- Subacromial impingement

MEANS OF CONFIRMATION OR DIAGNOSIS

Imaging

- Radiograph
  - Glenohumeral joint space
  - OA
  - Allows for secondary causes to be viewed
  - Views: AP, axillary lateral, scapular Y-view

- MRI
  - Not required to make the diagnosis of adhesive capsulitis
  - Usually will demonstrate decreased hydration
  - Tissue quality
  - Capsulolabral and biceps labral pathology

Diagnostic Procedure

- Subacromial injection with lidocaine

Findings and Interpretations

- Subacromial injection with lidocaine: If pain decreases and motion improves, cuff pathology is present

TREATMENT

Medication

- Anti-inflammatory
- Corticosteroid injection
  - Short-term symptom improvement only

MEDICAL PROCEDURE

- Surgery warranted if conservative management ≥6 months yields no change in symptoms
- Arthroscopic surgical release of the capsule
- Manipulation under anesthesia
- Capsular distention

REFERRALS/ADMITTANCE

- To physician or radiologist for imaging
- To physician or pharmacist for medication
- To orthopedic surgeon for surgical consult if conservative treatment unsuccessful, possible manipulation under anesthesia

IMPAIRMENTS

- Limited AROM/PROM
- Capsular pattern of accessory hypomobility
- Impaired or suboptimal posture
- Muscle imbalances
  - Rotator cuff weakness
  - Periscapular muscle weakness (particularly upward rotators and depressors/retractors)
  - Pectoralis minor/major, tightness in latissimus
- Decreased thoracic ROM
- Pain with active movements away from the body and reaching hand behind back

TESTS AND MEASURES

- Disabilities of the Arm, Shoulder, and Hand (DASH) score to assess physical function
- Inferior glenohumeral glide

INTERVENTION

- Acute stage
  - Rest, ice/cryotherapy, and activity modification (avoid aggravating positions)
  - Specific home exercise plan with short stretches (1–5 seconds)
  - Low-grade (I and II) mobilizations
  - Intra-articular steroid injections by physician if highly irritable and severe functional limitations
- Sub-acute and chronic stages
  - Address joint impairments
    - GH hypomobility (mobilization grades I–IV)
    - Thoracic spine hypomobility (mobilization/manipulation)
  - Address muscle imbalances
    - Rotator cuff strength and endurance exercises
    - Muscle length of pectoralis major, minor, latissimus, and other muscles with decreased length
  - Strengthening of scapular musculature
    - Lower trapezius
    - Serratus anterior
    - Other scapular stabilizers
  - Functional activities such as dressing (depending on work or recreational desires)
  - Address pain and inflammation
    - Ice/Cryotherapy
    - Rest
    - Activity modification (avoiding impingement positions)
    - Ultrasound, phonophoresis, iontophoresis
    - Electrical stimulation
  - Address lack of flexibility through stretching
    - Posterior capsule/posterior cuff
    - Pectoralis minor
    - Pectoralis major
    - Latissimus dorsi
  - Address joint mobility
    - Posterior humeral glides
    - Inferior humeral glides
    - Anterior humeral glides
    - Thoracic mobilization/manipulation
    - Scapulothoracic mobility
      - Distraction
      - Retraction
      - Upward rotation
      - Posterior tip

FUNCTIONAL GOALS

- Patient will be able to
  - Move upper extremity through full range of elevation without pain while reaching in the cabinet for a cup.
  - Reach back pocket (or fasten brassier, if female) without pain
  - Reach for a gallon of milk without pain.

PROGNOSIS

- Dependent on current stage of condition.
- Patient's ability to control exacerbating activities and perform the optimal dosage of therapeutic exercise.

PATIENT RESOURCES

- American Academy of Orthopaedic Surgeons. Frozen Shoulder. http://orthoinfo.aaos.org/topic.cfm?topic=A00071. Accessed May 5, 2013.
- MedlinePlus. NIH, National Institutes of Health. Frozen Shoulder. http://www.nlm.nih.gov/medlineplus/ency/article/000455.htm. Accessed May 5, 2013.

REFERENCES

1. ICD-9-CM. http://www.icd9data.com. Accessed May 1, 2013.
2. ICD-10-CM. http://www.icd10data.com. Accessed May 1, 2013.
3. APTA Guide to Physical Therapist Practice. http://guidetoptpractice.apta.org/. Accessed May 1, 2013.

ADDITIONAL REFERENCES

- Dutton M. *Orthopedic Examination, Evaluation, and Intervention*. 3rd ed. New York, NY: McGraw-Hill; 2004:420–519.
- Dutton M. The Shoulder Complex. In: Dutton M, ed. *Dutton's Orthopedic Survival Guide: Managing Common Conditions*. New York, NY: McGraw Hill; 2011. http://www.accessphysiotherapy.com/content/8652400#8652400. Accessed May 13, 2013.
- Griesser MJ, Harris J, Campbell J, Jones G. Adhesive capsulitis of the shoulder: a systematic review of the effectiveness of intra-articular corticosteroid injections. *J Bone Joint Surg Am*. 2011;93:1727–1733.
- Kisner C, Colby LA. *Therapeutic Exercise*. 5th ed. Philadelphia, PA: FA Davis; 2007:502–511.
- Krabak BJ, Banks NL. Adhesive capsulitis. In: Frontera WR, Silver JK, eds. *Essentials of Physical Medicine and Rehabilitation*. 2nd ed. Philadelphia, PA: Saunders Elsevier; 2008:chap 10.
- Miller RH, Dlabach JA. Shoulder and elbow injuries. In: Canale ST, Beatty JH, eds. *Campbell's Operative Orthopaedics*. 11th ed. Philadelphia, PA: Mosby Elsevier; 2007:chap 44.
- Neviaser A, Neviaser R. Adhesive capsulitis of the shoulder. *J Am Acad Orthop Surg*. 2011;19:536–542.
- Skirven T, Osterman A, Fedorczyk J, Amadio P. *Rehabilitation of the Hand and Upper Extremity*. 6th ed. Philadelphia, PA: Elsevier Mosby; 2011:1174–1188.

152 BICEPS RUPTURE

Jesse Solotoff, DPT
Tiffany M. Barber, DPT
Eric Shamus, PhD, DPT, PT, CSCS

CONDITION/DISORDER SYNONYMS

- Biceps distal tear
- Biceps proximal tear

ICD-9-CM CODES

- 727.62 Nontraumatic rupture of the tendons of biceps (long head)
- 840.8 Sprains and strains of other specified sites of shoulder and upper arm

ICD-10-CM CODES

- M66.829 Spontaneous rupture of other tendons, unspecified upper arm
- S46.119A Strain of muscle, fascia and tendon of long head of biceps, unspecified arm, initial encounter

PREFERRED PRACTICE PATTERNS

- 4D: Impaired joint mobility, motor function, muscle performance, and range of motion associated with connective tissue dysfunction
- 4E: Impaired Joint Mobility, Motor Function, Muscle Performance, and Range of Motion Associated with Localized Inflammation[1]

PATIENT PRESENTATION

A 42-year-old man presents with upper arm pain and decreased ability to flex or extend the arm. The patient is a construction worker and tried to catch a falling piece of heavy metal. The patient states he heard a loud pop in the upper arm. Upon observation he has an abnormal biceps appearance with limited strength in elbow flexion. The patient smokes two packs of cigarettes a day.

KEY FEATURES

Description

- Rupture of the biceps brachii tendon either complete or partial
- Distal rupture will cause swelling, bruising, and a gap in front of elbow created by absence of tendon
  - Avulsion of the tendon from the radial tuberosity
- Proximal rupture will cause bulging, bruising, and gathering of the muscle ("Popeye" sign may indicate rupture)
  - Avulsion of the long head of the biceps brachii from the superior rim of the anterior glenoid labrum

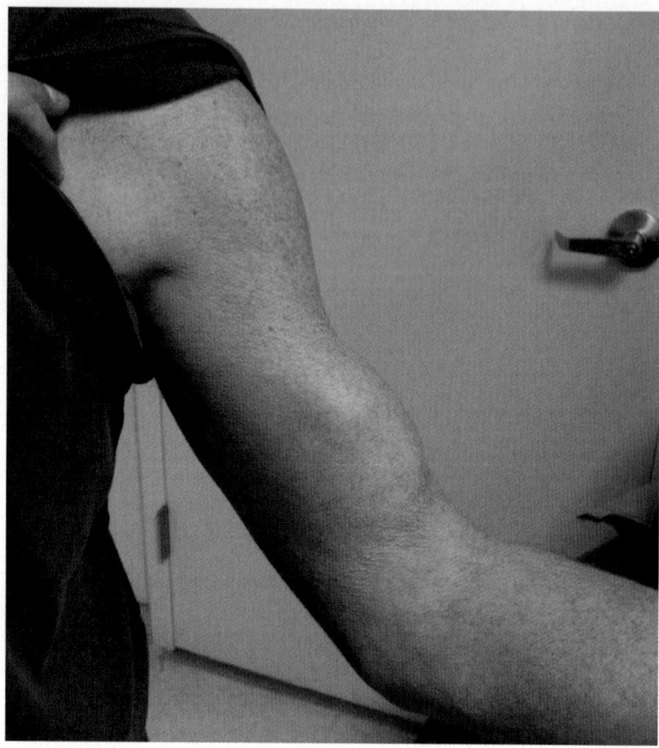

FIGURE 152-1 A patient with rupture of the biceps tendon. Note the "Popeye" appearance of the muscle. (From Simon RR, Sherman SC. *Emergency Orthopedics.* 6th ed. www.accessemergencymedicine.com. Copyright © The McGraw-Hill Companies, Inc. All rights reserved.)

Essentials of Diagnosis

- History and clinical examination
- Diagnosis of proximal tear often easily visible with observation due to bulge left by deformed muscle ("Popeye sign")
- Diagnosis of distal tear
  - Palpation of gap at the elbow
  - Manually testing supination strength compared with uninvolved side
  - Sudden event trauma
- Partial tears harder to diagnose and may require manually testing bicep muscle for signs of pain with activation of muscle
- Occurs from a sudden high force, typically with weightlifting (i.e., biceps curls or activities with elbow flexion), eccentric force
- May arise from a repetitive type activity that leads to a gradual degeneration
- MRI to show both partial and complete tendon tears

General Considerations

- History of repetitive motion, especially activities overhead
- Common in swimming, tennis, baseball, and with occupational activities involving repetitive or overhead activity due to microtrauma

- Smoking affects overall nutrition of tendon due to nicotine side effects
- Corticosteroid medications has been linked to decreased muscle and tendon strength

Demographics

- Predominately individuals involved in repetitive activities in sports or work
- Long head tears are seen in the fourth decade of life

CLINICAL FINDINGS

SIGNS AND SYMPTOMS

- Patient will describe an audible pop or snap associated with injury
- Sharp pain occurring suddenly in the upper arm
- Ecchymosis, swelling, bulging of the upper arm
- Pain and tenderness with palpation of the shoulder and elbow
- Diminished strength of elbow flexion and supination
- Appearance of bulge ("Popeye muscle") with indentation closer to shoulder for proximal tear
- Distal tear will result in bulge in upper part of arm due to recoiled, shortened tendon
- Distal tear will result in gap at elbow due to severed tendon

Functional Implications

- For proximal long head tear mild weakness can persist in elbow flexion
- For distal tears significant loss of supination will limit patient from performing activities that include motions involving rotating forearm from palm down to palm up
- Overhead activities may be limited
- Inability to lift heavy objects

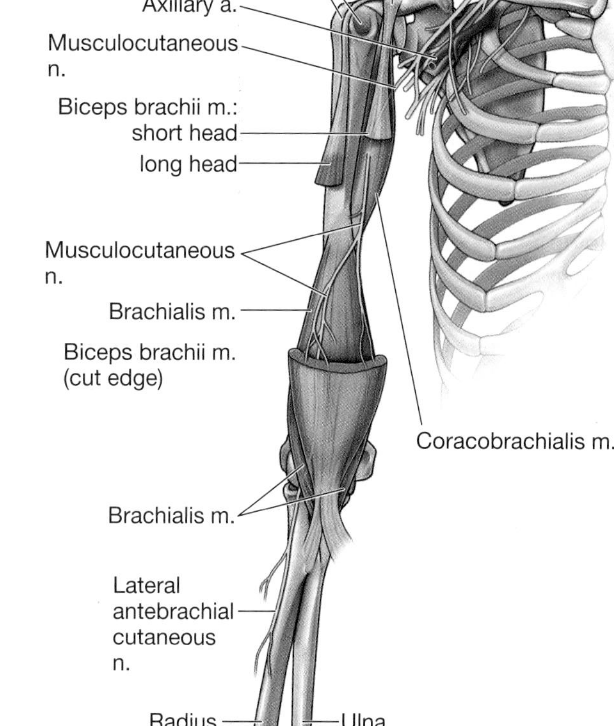

FIGURE 152-2 The brachialis muscle. (Reproduced with permission from Morton DA, Foreman KB, Albertine KH. *Gross Anatomy: The Big Picture.* New York, NY: McGraw-Hill, 2011.)

Possible Contributing Causes

- Frequent and prolonged overhead activity
- Prolonged repetitive use of the involved arm
- Poor posture (rounded shoulders)
- Anteriorly displaced humeral head
- Rotator cuff weakness
- Steroid use
- Aging
- Systemic diseases, such a rheumatoid arthritis or diabetes
- Previous bicipital injury

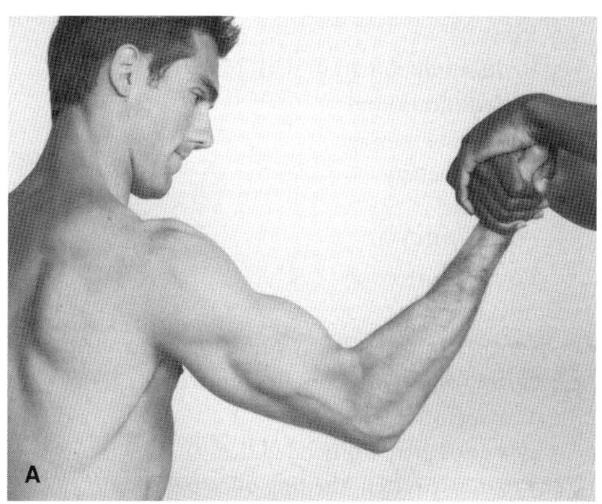

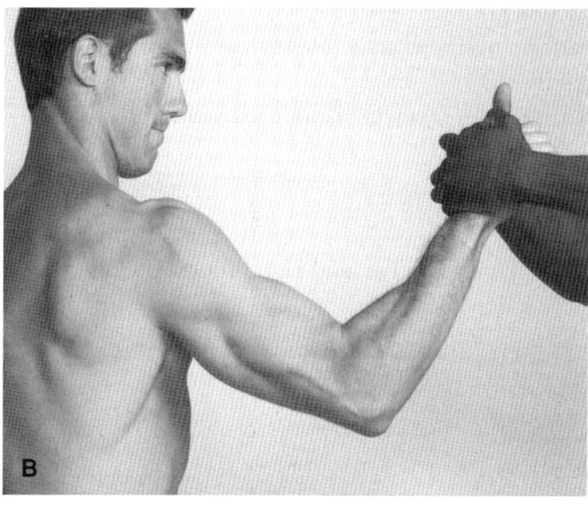

FIGURE 152-3 Flexion of the forearm. (**A**) in a position of supination; (**B**) in a position of pronation. The biceps brachii is less active when the forearm is pronated than when it is supinated. (From Hamilton N, Weimar W, Luttgens K. *Kinesiology: Scientific Basis of Human Motion.* 11th ed. http://www.accessphysiotherapy.com. Copyright © McGraw-Hill Education. All rights reserved.)

▸ **Differential Diagnosis**
- Bicep tendinopathy
- Labral tear[2]
- Pectoralis muscle tear
- Rotator cuff impingement
- Rotator cuff tear
- Rotator cuff tendonitis
- Subacromial bursitis
- Upper anterior arm compartment syndrome

MEANS OF CONFIRMATION OR DIAGNOSIS

▸ **Imaging**
- Diagnostic ultrasound
- Radiographs
- MRI[3]

FINDINGS AND INTERPRETATION

- Radiographs may show calcification or other bony abnormalities of the shoulder
- MRI to evaluate soft tissue for structural changes or rupture[3]
- Acute tears will demonstrate hemorrhage and edema and chronic tears will demonstrate fibrosis and scarring

TREATMENT

▸ **Medication**
- NSAIDs[2]
- Steroid injection

MEDICAL PROCEDURE

- Surgery to repair tendon

REFERRALS/ADMITTANCE

- For imaging: Orthopedist, family physician, radiologist
- For surgery: Orthopedic surgeon
  - Prompt assessment as muscle shortening occurs
- For injection: Orthopedist, family physician

IMPAIRMENTS

- Debilitating pain, limiting movement and exertion
- Decreased torque and work/repetition, especially with shoulder adduction
- Inability to perform overhead activities, such as swimming, baseball, or tennis
- Inability to perform jobs involving repetitive overhead reaching or lifting

TESTS AND MEASURES

- Disabilities of the Arm, Shoulder, and Hand (DASH) score to assess physical function
- Functional reach test
- Yergason test[2]
- Speed test[2]
- Clunk test[2]
- O'Brien test[2]
- Anterior slide test[2]
- Biceps load test[2]
- Compression–rotation test[2]

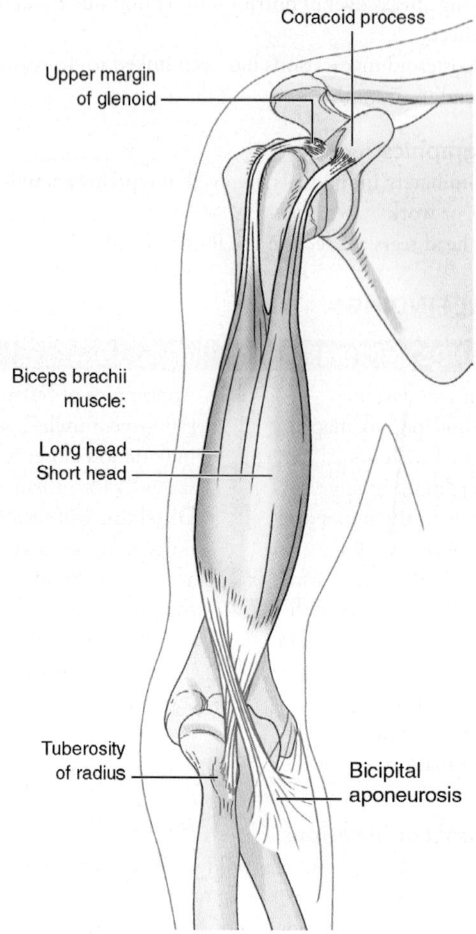

FIGURE 152-4 The anatomy of the biceps brachii muscle. (From Simon RR, Sherman SC. *Emergency Orthopedics.* 6th ed. www.accessemergencymedicine.com.)

- Pronated load test[2]
- Pain provocation test[2]
- Resisted supination external rotation test[2]
- Shoulder pain and disability index[2]

INTERVENTION

- Acute
  - Rest
  - Reduce inflammation with NSAIDs
  - Pulsed ultrasound
  - Soft-tissue massage
  - Electrotherapy
  - Ice/Heat[4]
  - Gentle AROM
  - Posture correction
- Post-acute
  - Once pain and inflammation are controlled, progress through further active exercises in pain-free ranges
  - Progress stretching
  - Posterior glenohumeral glides
  - Progressive strengthening once pain-free
- Injury prevention
  - Avoid activities that place repetitive, excessive stress on the tendon
  - Cross-training

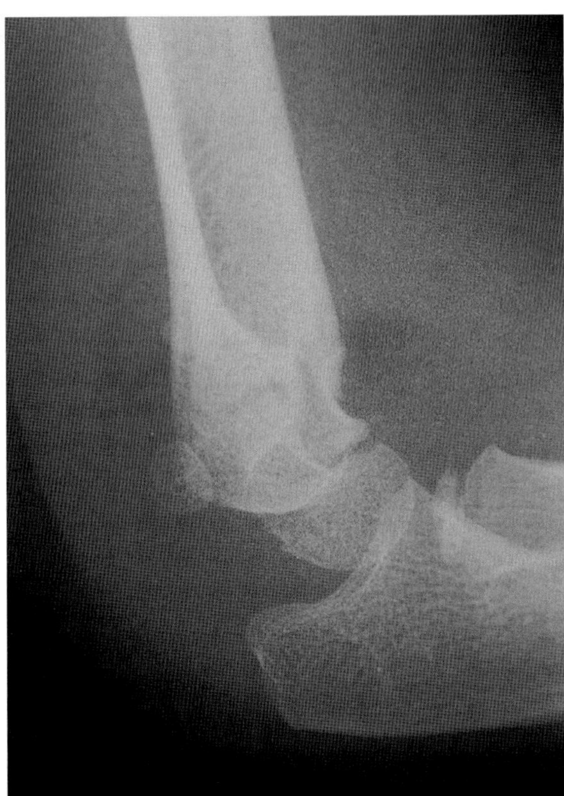

FIGURE 152-5 Biceps tendon rupture. The biceps tendon is noted to contract within the arm after rupture. (From Knoop KJ, Stack L, Storrow A, Jason Thurman R. *The Atlas of Emergency Medicine.* 3rd ed. www.accessmedicine.com. Copyright © The McGraw-Hill Companies, Inc. All rights reserved. Photo contributor: Daniel L. Savitt, MD.)

- Warm-up and stretching prior to activity
- Use proper ergonomics
- Keep muscles strong and flexible

FUNCTIONAL GOALS

- Patient will be able to resume
  - All overhead activities and ADLs without exacerbating inflammation.
  - All sport activities as prior to onset.
  - All reach activities without symptoms or limitation.
  - All lifting activities without limitation from pain or weakness in upper extremities.
  - Driving without return of anterior shoulder pain.

PROGNOSIS

- For proximal long head bicep tears surgery is rarely performed.
  - Older, less active patient will resume prior activities with only slight decrease in overall strength.
  - For athletes and younger patients, surgery may be to attempt restoring full return to activity and prior strength levels.
- Distal tendon tears are generally more uncommon; however, surgery is required to prevent severe loss of prior strength, especially supination.
- Symptoms should improve and resolve with treatment and rest.
- If injury is the result of overuse, changes in activity and work habits may be needed.

PATIENT RESOURCES

- Cleveland Clinic. Biceps Tendon Injuries. http://my.clevelandclinic.org/disorders/musculoskeletal_pain/hic_bicep. Accessed June 17, 2013.
- Mayo Clinic Staff. Tendinitis. http://www.mayoclinic.com/health/tendinitis/DS00153. Accessed June 17, 2013.
- Biceps Tendon Tear at the Elbow. American Academy of Orthopaedic Surgeons. http://orthoinfo.aaos.org/topic.cfm?topic=A00376. Accessed June 17, 2013.
- Biceps Tendon Tear at the Shoulder. American Academy of Orthopaedic Surgeons. http://orthoinfo.aaos.org/topic.cfm?topic=A00031. Accessed June 17, 2013.

REFERENCES

1. The American Physical Therapy Association. Pattern 4E: Impaired joint mobility, motor function, muscle performance, and range of motion associated with localized inflammation. *Interactive Guide to Physical Therapist Practice*. 2003. DOI: 10.2522/ptguide.3.1_5. Accessed March 1, 2012.
2. Dutton M. *Orthopaedic Examination, Evaluation, and Intervention*. New York, NY: McGraw-Hill; 2008. http://www.accessphysiotherapy.com/resource/612. Accessed June 17, 2013.
3. Malone TR, Hazle C, Grey ML. *Imaging in Rehabilitation*. New York, NY: McGraw-Hill; 2008. http://www.accessphysiotherapy.com/resource/613. Accessed June 17, 2013.
4. Prentice WE. Chapter 9. Cryotherapy and Thermotherapy. In: Prentice WE, Quillen WS, Underwood F, eds. *Therapeutic Modalities in Rehabilitation*. 4th ed. New York, NY: McGraw-Hill; 2011. http://www.accessphysiotherapy.com/content/8137995#8137995. Accessed June 17, 2013.

ADDITIONAL REFERENCES

- Cope MR, Ali A, Bayliss NC. Biceps rupture in body builders: Three case reports of rupture of the long head of the biceps at the tendon-labrum junction. *J Shoulder Elbow Surg*. 2004;13(5):580-582.
- ICD9DATA web site. http://www.icd9data.com. Accessed June 17, 2013.
- ICD10DATA web site. http://www.icd10data.com. Accessed June 17, 2013.
- Simon RR, Sherman SC. Upper Arm Soft-Tissue Injury and Dislocations. In: Simon RR, Sherman SC, eds. *Emergency Orthopedics*. 6th ed. New York, NY: McGraw-Hill; 2011. http://www.accessphysiotherapy.com/content/7705284. Accessed June 17, 2013.
- Vidal AF, Drakos MC, Allen AA. Biceps tendon and triceps tendon injuries. *Clin Sports Med*. 2004;23(4):707–722.

153 BICIPITAL TENDINOSIS

E. Thomas Pitney, DPT, PT, SCS, ATC
Eric Shamus, PhD, DPT, PT, CSCS

CONDITION/DISORDER SYNONYMS

- Biceps tendinitis
- Biceps tendonitis
- Bicep tenosynovitis
- Bicipital tenosynovitis

ICD-9-CM CODE

- 726.12 Bicipital tenosynovitis

ICD-10-CM CODE

- M75.20 Bicipital tendinitis, unspecified shoulder

PREFERRED PRACTICE PATTERN

- 4E: Impaired joint mobility, motor function, muscle performance, and range of motion associated with localized inflammation[1]

PATIENT PRESENTATION

This patient is a 45-year-old male who recently returned to a fitness center exercise program. He began to experience pain in the anterior shoulder and upper one-third of the arm after significantly increasing resistance with his upper body program, especially taking preacher curls to fatigue failure and doubling his weight over a 2-week period. The patient has specific tenderness over the bicipital groove and the long head of the bicep tendon to the musculotendinous junction. Resistive elbow flexion is painful in the same region and is 4-/5 compared to 5/5 through the remainder of the shoulder girdle. A/PROM is full and symmetrical with the uninvolved side. Speed's test is positive and Neer and Hawkins-Kennedy tests are negative. There is no visible deformity, swelling, or asymmetry of appearance.

KEY FEATURES

Description

- Irritation of the long head of biceps tendon
- Occurs most often from repetitive motion injuries or impingement syndrome, but can occur with sudden strain/stress to the tendon, or with rotator cuff tendonitis or pathology
- Early stages
  - Tendon becomes swollen and red
  - As tendinosis develops, the tendon sheath may thicken
- Late stages
  - Chronic irritation may result in fraying of the tendon or necrosis
  - May progress to rupture

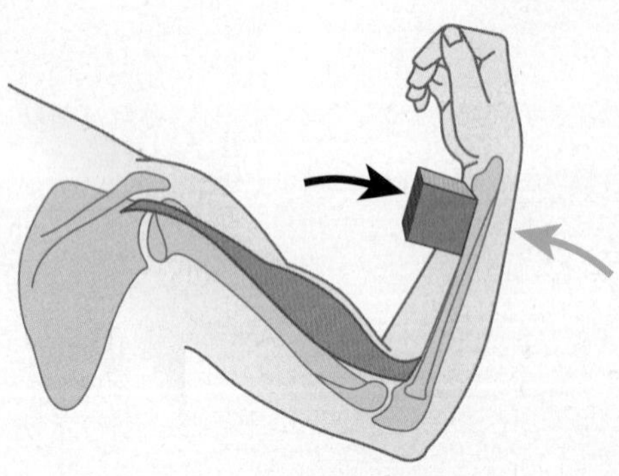

FIGURE 153-1 Biceps (C5, 6; musculocutaneous nerve). The supinated forearm is flexed against resistance. (From Waxman SG. *Clinical Neuroanatomy*. 26th ed.. www.accessmedicine.com. Copyright © The McGraw-Hill Companies, Inc. All rights reserved.)

- Rupture will cause bulging, bruising, and gathering of the muscle ("Popeye" sign may indicate rupture)

Essentials of Diagnosis

- History and clinical examination
- Look for signs of pain with A/PROM, resistance, palpation, and specific tests for the bicep tendon
- Pain with palpation of the bicipital groove with arm at 10 degrees of internal rotation
- Pain with passive stretch of the bicep

General Considerations

- History of repetitive motion, especially activities overhead
- Common in swimming, tennis, baseball, and with occupational activities involving repetitive or overhead activity due to micro trauma
- Can be seen in individuals with other system-wide diseases such as rheumatoid arthritis or diabetes
- Often occurs secondary to impingement syndrome or rotator cuff injury

Demographics

- Predominately individuals involved in repetitive activities in sports or work

CLINICAL FINDINGS

SIGNS AND SYMPTOMS

- Ache in the anterior medial or anterior lateral aspect of the shoulder that may travel down the anterior upper arm
- Frequently worsens with overhead lifting or activity
- Pain or ache with palpation at the bicipital groove
- Occasional snapping sound or sensation often alleviated with active scapular retraction

- Full A/PROM, though pain may occur at the end ROM
- Pain with resisted elbow-flexion or resisted forward-flexion of the shoulder
- Pain with passive stretch of the bicep
- Positive special tests for the biceps

Functional Implications

- Limited overhead activities, especially lifting
- Limited throwing and other rapid arm movements

Possible Contributing Causes

- Frequent and prolonged overhead activity
- Prolonged repetitive use of the involved arm
- Poor posture (rounded shoulders)
- Anteriorly displaced humeral head
- Rotator cuff weakness
- Aging
- Systemic diseases, such as rheumatoid arthritis or diabetes
- Previous bicipital or FOOSH injury
- Labral tears

Differential Diagnosis

- Biceps calcific tendinitis
- Bicep tear
- Labral tear[2]
- Pectoralis tendonitis
- Rotator cuff impingement
- Rotator cuff tear
- Rotator cuff tendonitis
- Sub-acromial bursitis

MEANS OF CONFIRMATION OR DIAGNOSIS

Imaging

- Radiographs looking for calcification or boney abnormalities
- Ultrasound
- MRI[3]

FINDINGS AND INTERPRETATION

- Radiographs may show calcification or other boney abnormalities of the shoulder
- MRI to evaluate soft tissue for structural changes or rupture[3]
- Swelling may be apparent

TREATMENT

Medication

- NSAIDs[2]
- Steroid injection

MEDICAL PROCEDURES

- Arthroscopic debridement of chronic fraying
- Biceps tenodesis in severe chronic cases
- Tenotomy

REFERRALS/ADMITTANCE

- For MRI[3]
- For surgery
- For injection

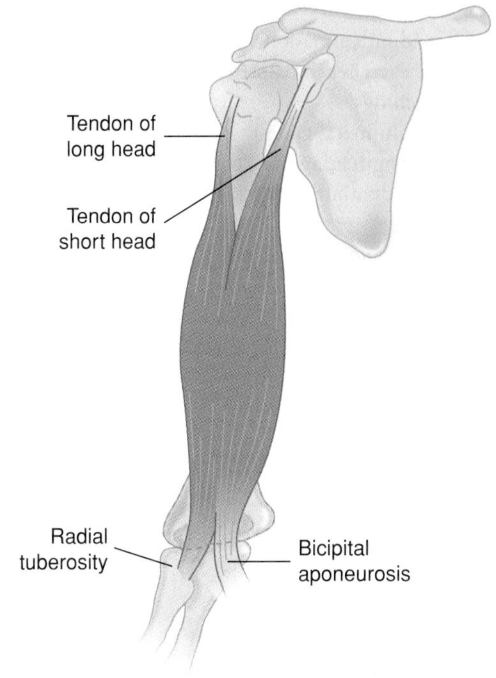

FIGURE 153-2 Biceps muscle anatomy. (From Tintinalli JE, Stapczynski JS, John Ma O, et al. *Tintinalli's Emergency Medicine: A Comprehensive Study Guide.* 7th ed.. www.accessmedicine.com. Copyright © The McGraw-Hill Companies, Inc. All rights reserved.)

IMPAIRMENTS

- Inability to perform overhead activities, such as in swimming, baseball, or tennis
- Inability to perform jobs involving repetitive overhead reaching or lifting

TESTS AND MEASURES

- Disabilities of the Arm, Shoulder, and Hand (DASH) score to assess physical function
- Functional reach test
- Yergason's test[2]
- Speed's test[2]
- Clunk test[2]
- O'Brien's test[2]
- Anterior slide test[2]
- Biceps load test[2]
- Compression–rotation test[2]
- Pronated load test[2]
- Pain provocation test[2]
- Resisted supination external rotation test[2]
- Shoulder pain and disability index[2]

INTERVENTION

- Acute
  - Rest
  - Reduce inflammation with NSAIDs and electrotherapeutic modalities
  - Ice/Heat[4]
  - Transverse friction massage
  - Gentle stretching and AROM

- Post-acute
  - Once pain and inflammation are controlled, progress through further active exercises in pain-free ranges
  - Progress stretching
  - Posterior glenohumeral glides
  - Progressive strengthening once pain-free
  - Painful eccentric training for 12 weeks
- Injury prevention
  - Avoid activities that place repetitive, excessive stress on the tendon
  - Cross-training
  - Improve technique
  - Warm-up and stretching prior to activity
  - Use proper ergonomics
  - Keep muscles strong and flexible

FUNCTIONAL GOALS

- Patient will be able to resume
  - All overhead activities and ADLs without exacerbating inflammation.
  - All sport activities as prior to onset.
  - All reach activities without symptoms or limitation.
  - All lifting activities without limitation from pain or weakness in upper extremities.
  - Driving without return of anterior shoulder pain.

PROGNOSIS

- Symptoms should improve and resolve with treatment and rest.
- If injury is the result of overuse, changes in activity and work habits may be needed.

PATIENT RESOURCES

- Mayo Clinic Staff. *Tendinitis*. Available at: http://www.mayoclinic.com/health/tendinitis/DS00153. Accessed June 17, 2013.
- NIH National Institutes of Health. *U.S National Library of Medicine*. Medline Plus. Available at: http://www.nim.nih.gov/medlineplus/ency/article/001229.htm. Accessed June 17, 2013.
- Tendonitis of the Long Head of the Biceps. American Academy of Orthopaedic Surgeons. http://orthoinfo.aaos.org/topic.cfm?topic=A00026. Accessed June 17, 2013.

REFERENCES

1. The American Physical Therapy Association. Pattern 4E: Impaired joint mobility, motor function, muscle performance, and range of motion associated with localized inflammation. *Interactive Guide to Physical Therapist Practice*. 2003. doi: 10.2522/ptguide.3.1_5. Accessed June 17, 2013.
2. Dutton M. *Orthopaedic Examination, Evaluation, and Intervention*. New York, NY: McGraw-Hill; 2008. http://www.access-physiotherapy.com/resource/612. Accessed June 17, 2013.
3. Malone TR, Hazle C, Grey ML. *Imaging in Rehabilitation*. New York, NY: McGraw-Hill; 2008. http://www.accessphysiotherapy.com/resource/613. Accessed June 17, 2013.
4. Prentice WE. Cryotherapy and thermotherapy, Chapter 9. In: Prentice WE, Quillen WS, Underwood F, eds. *Therapeutic Modalities in Rehabilitation*.4th ed. New York, NY: McGraw-Hill; 2011. http://www.accessphysiotherapy.com/content/8137995#8137995. Accessed June 17, 2013.

ADDITIONAL REFERENCES

- Cleveland Clinic. *Biceps Tendon Injuries*. Available at: http://my.clevelandclinic.org/disorders/musculoskeletal_pain/hic_bicep. Accessed June 17, 2013.
- ICD9DATA web site. http://www.icd9data.com. Accessed June 17, 2013.
- ICD10DATA web site. http://www.icd10data.com. Accessed June 17, 2013.

154 BURSITIS, SUBACROMIAL

Patrick S. Pabian, DPT, PT, SCS, OCS, CSCS

CONDITION/DISORDER SYNONYM

- Shoulder bursitis

ICD-9-CM CODE[1]

- 726.19 Other specified disorders of bursae and tendons in shoulder region

ICD-10-CM CODE[2]

- M75.80 Other shoulder lesions, unspecified shoulder

PREFERRED PRACTICE PATTERN[3]

- 4E: Impaired Joint Mobility, Motor Function, Muscle Performance, and Range of Motion Associated with Localized Inflammation

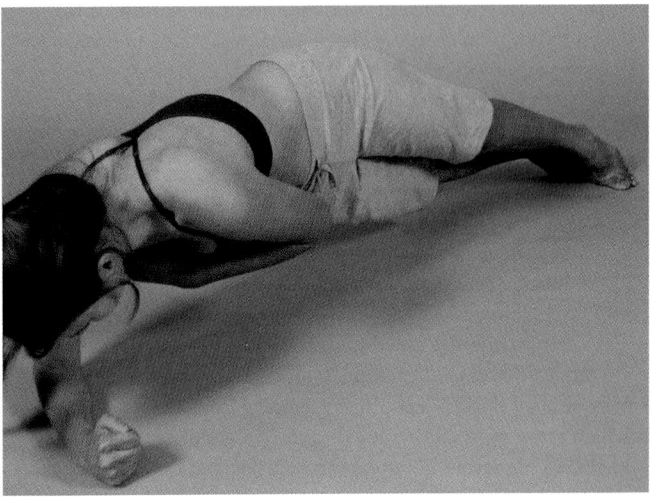

FIGURE 154-1 Side planks for shoulder stability. (From Dutton M. *Dutton's Orthopaedic Examination, Evaluation, and Intervention*. 3rd ed.. http://www.accessphysiotherapy.com. Copyright © The McGraw-Hill Companies, Inc. All rights reserved.)

PATIENT PRESENTATION

A 40-year-old male carpenter presents with right shoulder pain that has been present for the past 2 months. The patient complains of a dull ache at the anterolateral shoulder that is worsened after working. He reports pain is increasing and he now has difficulty with washing his hair or reaching up into overhead cabinets. He also notes weakness with holding objects out away from his body and lifting a gallon of milk out of refrigerator. He has protracted scapular posture. Posterior capsular tightness is evident. The patient has positive Hawkins Kennedy, Neer, and Painful Arc tests, and negative Drop Arm and ER Lag tests.

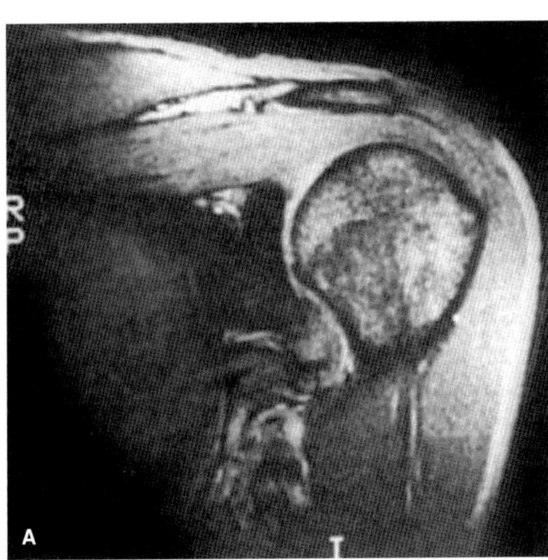

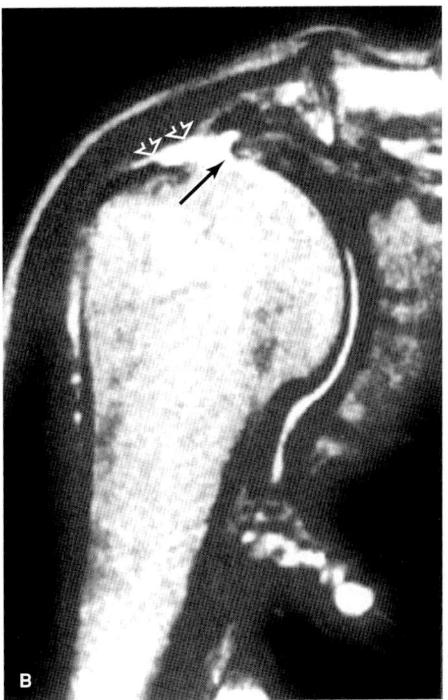

FIGURE 154-2 MRI demonstrating (**A**) normal shoulder anatomy and (**B**) cystic changes at the greater tuberosity with rotator cuff tear (*arrow*). (From Skinner HB. *Current Diagnosis & Treatment in Orthopedics*. 4th ed. www.accessmedicine.com. Copyright © The McGraw-Hill Companies, Inc. All rights reserved.)

KEY FEATURES

Description

- Shoulder pain and dysfunction due to compression and abrasion of the subacromial bursa beneath the coracoacromial arch.
- The coracoacromial arch consists of the undersurface of the acromion, coracoacromial ligament as well as the undersurface of the acromioclavicular (AC) joint.
- Subacromial bursa lies beneath the acromion and serves to cushion the rotator cuff tendons from the osseous undersurface of the acromion.
- Subacromial bursitis results when the subacromial bursa fills with blood and serous fluid as response to either acute or repeated micro-trauma (compression and/or abrasion).
  - Fibrotic changes in the bursa can result from chronic impingement or stress.
  - Increase in bursa size decreases volume of subacromial space and can lead to subacromial impingement syndrome.
- Subacromial bursitis leads to subacromial impingement syndrome, which is the most commonly diagnosed shoulder problem and likely has numerous potential mechanisms that can impact both treatment and prognosis.

Essentials of Diagnosis

- Compression or abrasion of the subacromial bursa can be either acute, involving a fall, usually on a flexed elbow, or chronic, which can be more multifactorial in nature
- Chronic (repeated micro-trauma) mechanism thought to be related to intrinsic and/or extrinsic mechanisms
  - Extrinsic mechanisms (extratendinous, cause decreased subacromial space and subsequent micro-trauma with repetitive movements)
    - Mechanical wear under the coracoacromial arch
    - Aberrant movement patterns due to rotator cuff and or periscapular muscular dysfunction
    - Capsular abnormalities
    - Capsular tightness (particularly posterior capsule)
    - Capsular laxity (poor humeral head dynamic control)
    - Suboptimal posture
    - Muscle imbalances
    - Overuse/repetitive motions occurring at more than 90 degrees of elevation
  - Intrinsic factors (directly associated with the narrowing of the subacromial space)
    - Vascular supply/changes to the cuff tendons
    - Acromial morphology (structural variations)
      - Type I (flat)
      - Type II (curved)
      - Type III hooked)
    - Degenerative and/or structural changes to the AC joint
- Other trophic changes in the coracoacromial arch or humeral head
- Differential diagnosis from other shoulder pathologies that may warrant surgical intervention is essential (rotator cuff tear, superior labral tear)

General Considerations

- Commonly diagnosed and associated with presence of other orthopedic pathologies: subacromial impingement syndrome, rotator cuff pathology, labral pathology
- Commonly associated with repeated overhead or overuse activities.
- Full history of symptoms, medical history screening, and differential shoulder orthopedic examination will ensure appropriate diagnosis

Demographics

- Occurs primarily in adults but can occur in teenagers participating in overhead athletics or with trauma
- Similar demographics as subacromial impingement syndrome
  - Primary impingement (generally occurs in patients ages 40 and older)
  - Secondary impingement (generally occurs in younger patients ages 15 to 35)

CLINICAL FINDINGS

SIGNS AND SYMPTOMS

- Pain in anterior lateral shoulder with active movement involving primarily overhead activities and motions across the body (horizontal abduction)
- Painful arc commonly present in the mid-range of shoulder elevation
- Pain to palpation of the subacromial bursa
- Weakness is commonly noted with functional reaching tasks
- Weakness primarily in shoulder abduction and external rotation

Functional limitations

- Pain/Limitation with overhead activities
- Pain/Limitation with reaching
- Pain/Limitation with lifting
- Pain/Limitation dressing and grooming
- Pain/Limitation with sustained or repetitive shoulder activities
- Pain at night (sleep disruption)

Possible Contributing Causes

- Acromion morphology
  - Type I
  - Type II
  - Type III
- Degenerative changes at the AC joint
- Rotator cuff pathology
- Bicipital pathology
- Capsular laxity, glenohumeral (GH) hypermobility
- Capsular tightness
- Increased thoracic kyphosis and suboptimal posture
- Repetitive overhead activities
- Poor neuromuscular control

Differential Diagnosis

- AC separation
- Adhesive capsulitis
- Cervical radiculopathy
- Fluid can be aspirated to rule out septic bursitis
- GH arthritis
- GH instability
- Internal impingement
- Labral tear
- Neuropathy (suprascapular nerve)
- Referred pain from lungs or diaphragm

- Rotator cuff pathology (tendonitis, full- or partial-thickness tear)
- Subacromial impingement syndrome (per another origin)

MEANS OF CONFIRMATION OR DIAGNOSIS

- Diagnosis made based on orthopedic special tests, signs and symptoms, imaging studies, and exclusion of differential diagnosis.
- Special tests
  - Neer test
  - Horizontal adduction test
  - Painful arc test
  - Hawkins–Kennedy test
  - Yocum test
- Tests can be repeated post-injection of analgesic into bursa to confirm diagnosis.
- Imaging
  - Radiographs are usually normal.
    - May show osseous abnormalities of acromion, clavicle, or subacromial space, and may lead to suspicion of diagnosis.
  - MRI will show increased fluid/edema isolated within the subacromial bursa.
    - T2-weighted MRI would best visualize and result in increased signal intensity within subacromial bursa.
    - MRI will help visualize other potential soft tissue sources of patient symptoms.
- Laboratory studies for suspected rheumatoid disorders
  - Aspirated fluid can be cultured and evaluated for crystals to rule out gout.

TREATMENT

▶ Medication

- NSAIDs
- Corticosteroid injection
- Antibiotics if infection confirmed

MEDICAL PROCEDURES

- Surgical intervention
  - Surgical intervention via arthroscopy to restore subacromial space and address other concomitant pathologies.
  - Could potentially involve:
    - Subacromial decompression: debridement of subacromial bursa, resection of the coracoacromial ligament
    - Acromioplasty
    - Distal clavicle excision

REFERRALS/ADMITTANCE

- Radiologist for imaging: X-ray, MRI
- Primary care for aspiration and laboratory studies
- Orthopedist for surgical consult for injection or subacromial decompression, acromioplasty

IMPAIRMENTS

- Weakness and pain limiting overhead activities or activities involving arm out to side or across body including dressing or grooming daily activities
- Impaired (suboptimal) posture
- Muscle imbalances
  - Rotator cuff weakness
  - Periscapular muscle weakness (particularly upward rotators and depressors/retractors)
  - Pectoralis minor tightness
- Decreased thoracic ROM (particularly extension)
- Rotator cuff overuse/fatigue
- Neuropathy and subsequent muscle weakness
- Hypermobility at the GH joint and or scapulothoracic articulations
- Pain with active elevation
- Hypo- or hypermobility at the GH, scapulothoracic, AC, or sternoclavicular (SC) joints

TEST AND MEASURES

- Selective tissue tension tests
- Neer impingement test
- Drop arm (Codman) test
- External rotation lag sign (ERLS)/dropping arm sign
- Empty can test
- Hawkins–Kennedy impingement sign/test
- Passive horizontal adduction test
- Pain with resisted abduction
- Painful arc sign/test
- C5–6 dermatome/myotome testing
- Infraspinatus muscle test[1]
- Diagnostic test properties for subacromial impingement
- Yergason test
- Speed test
- Clunk test
- O'Brien test
- Anterior slide test
- Biceps load test
- Compression–rotation test
- Pronated load test
- Pain provocation test
- Resisted supination external rotation test
- Disabilities of the Arm, Shoulder, and Hand (DASH) score to assess physical function
- Shoulder pain and disability index

INTERVENTION

- Intervention will vary depending upon the severity of impingement and presence of concomitant pathologies such as rotator cuff or labral pathology.
- Acute Phase
  - PRICE: Protection, rest, ice compression, elevation
  - Activity modification: To avoid positions that elicit pain.
  - Low-level cold laser
  - Ice massage
  - Ultrasound
- Subacute to chronic stages (addressing specific impairments associated with the impingement)
  - Address joint impairments
    - GH hypomobility (mobilization)
    - GH hypermobility (stabilization)
    - Thoracic spine hypomobility (mobilization/manipulation)
  - Address muscle imbalances
    - Rotator cuff strength and endurance exercises
    - Muscle length of pectoralis (pec) major and minor, latissimus dorsi (lats) and other muscles with decreased length

- Strengthening of scapular musculature
  - Lower trap
  - Serratus anterior
  - Other scapular stabilizers
- Functional activities (depending on work/recreational desires)
- Addressing pain and inflammation
  - Ice
  - Rest
  - Activity modification (avoiding impingement positions)
  - Ultrasound, phonophoresis, iontophoresis
  - Electronic stimulation
- Addressing weakness, joint hypermobility
  - Shoulder lateral and medial rotation
    - Isometric
    - Thera-Band resisted
    - Handheld-weight resisted
    - Progression through higher ranges of elevation
  - Scapular strength/stabilization
    - Retraction
    - Prone shoulder extension, abduction, scapular plane elevation
- Addressing lack of flexibility
  - Stretching
    - Posterior capsule/posterior cuff
    - Pectoralis minor
    - Pectoralis major
    - Lats
- Addressing joint mobility
  - Posterior humeral glides
  - Inferior humeral glides
  - Thoracic mobilization/manipulation
  - Scapulothoracic mobility
    - Distraction
    - Retraction
    - Upward rotation
    - Posterior tip

FUNCTIONAL GOALS

- Patient will be able to:
  - Reach into overhead cabinets in kitchen without pain or restriction.
  - Lift a gallon milk carton from refrigerator at shoulder level, pain free.
  - Turn steering wheel, pain free.
  - Perform all dressing and grooming activities (tuck in shirt behind back, wash hair, etc.) without pain or compensation.

PROGNOSIS

- Good. A prolonged period of healing can last several months.
- Prognosis is dependent on the underlying cause of the bursitis.
  - Presence of concomitant shoulder pathology.
  - Quality of the tissues involved.
  - Ability of the patient to control exacerbating activities and perform the optimal dosage of therapeutic exercise.

PATIENT RESOURCE

- Pathway Guidelines for Subacromial Shoulder Pain. Draft V14, September 2012. British Orthopaedic Association. http://www.boa.ac.uk/PP/Documents/Subacromial%20Pain%20Guidelines%20V14.pdf. Accessed June 3, 2013.

REFERENCES

1. ICD9Data.com. http://www.icd9data.com. Accessed March 3, 2013.
2. ICD10Data.com. http://www.icd10data.com. Accessed March 3, 2013.
3. Pattern 4E: Impaired joint mobility, motor function, muscle performance, and range of motion associated with localized inflammation. In: *Guide to Physical Therapist Practice*. 2nd ed. Alexandria, VA: American Physical Therapy Association; 2001. Revised 2003.

ADDITIONAL REFERENCES

- Cleland JA, Koppenhaver SK. Shoulder. In: Cleland JA, Koppenhaver SK, eds. *Netter's Orthopaedic Clinical Examination: An Evidence-Based Approach*. Philadelphia, PA: Saunders Elsevier; 2011: 377–438.
- Dutton M. The Shoulder Complex. In: Dutton M, ed. *Dutton's Orthopaedic Examination, Evaluation, and Intervention*. 3rd ed. New York, NY: McGraw-Hill; 2012. New York, NY: McGraw-Hill; 2008: 489–653.
- Hamilton N, Weimar W, Luttgens K. The upper extremity: The shoulder region, Chapter 5. In: Hamilton N, Weimar W, Luttgens K, eds. *Kinesiology: Scientific Basis of Human Motion*. New York, NY: McGraw-Hill; 2008. http://www.accessphysiotherapy.com/content/6150569. Accessed March 11, 2013.
- Prentice WE. The shoulder complex. In: Prentice WE, ed. *Principles of Athletic Training: A Competency-Based Approach*. New York, NY: McGraw-Hill; 2011: 639–680.

155 PECTORAL MUSCLE TEAR

Kelley Henderson, MEd, ATC
Eric Shamus, PhD, DPT, PT, CSCS

CONDITION/DISORDER SYNONYMS

- Torn pectoral
- Pectoral rupture

ICD-9-CM CODE

- 840.8 Sprains and strains of other specified sites of shoulder and upper arm

ICD-10-CM CODES

- S43.499A Other sprain of unspecified shoulder joint, initial encounter
- S46.819A Strain of other muscles, fascia and tendons at shoulder and upper arm level, unspecified arm, initial encounter

PREFERRED PRACTICE PATTERNS

- 4D: Impaired Joint Mobility, Motor Function, Muscle Performance, and Range of Motion Associated with Connective Tissue Dysfunction
- 4E: Impaired Joint Mobility, Motor Function, Muscle Performance, and Range of Motion Associated with Localized Inflammation

PATIENT PRESENTATION

A 23-year-old male college gymnast presents with right shoulder pain and significant ecchymosis that spreads down to the elbow. He reports that he over-rotated during a flip on the parallel bars and he caught himself with his right arm. He felt a sudden sharp pain in his right shoulder and then a cramp-like contraction in his right arm and chest. He later noticed discoloration in his chest and right arm and a depression in the right anterior portion of his chest. He states that he feels a constant pain in his right shoulder along with noticeable weakness.

KEY FEATURES

Description

- Partial or complete rupture of the pectoral muscles
- Grades of tear[1,2]
  - Grade 1: Contusion or strain
  - Grade 2: Partial tear
  - Grade 3: Complete rupture
  - Grade 3A: Tear muscle origin
  - Grade 3B: Tear muscle belly
  - Grade 3C: Musculotendinous junction
  - Grade 3D: Muscle tendon itself

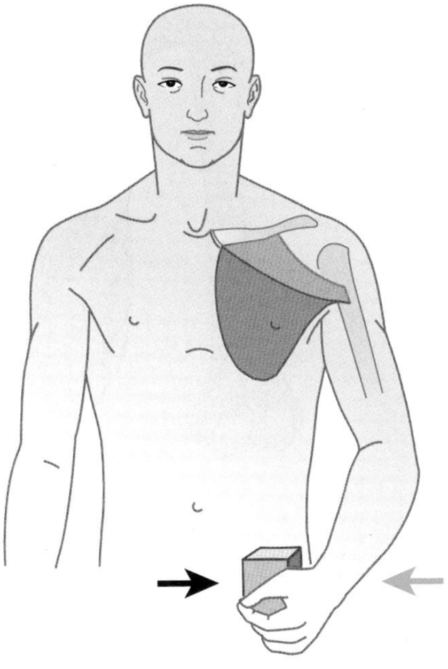

FIGURE 155-1 Pectoralis major, lower portion (C5–8; T1; lateral and medial pectoral nerves). The arm is adducted from a forward position below the horizontal level against resistance. (From Waxman SG: *Clinical Neuroanatomy*. 26th ed.. www.accessmedicine.com. Copyright © The McGraw-Hill Companies, Inc. All rights reserved.)

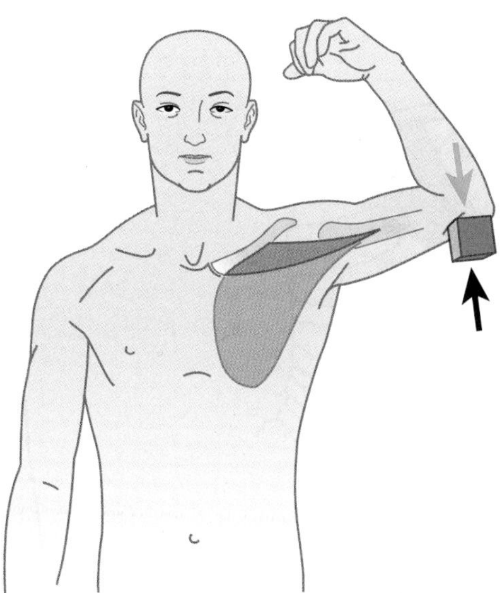

FIGURE 155-2 Pectoralis major, upper portion (C5–8; T1; lateral and medial pectoral nerves). The arm is adducted from an elevated or horizontal and forward position against resistance. (From Waxman SG. *Clinical Neuroanatomy*. 26th ed. www.accessmedicine.com. Copyright © The McGraw-Hill Companies, Inc. All rights reserved.)

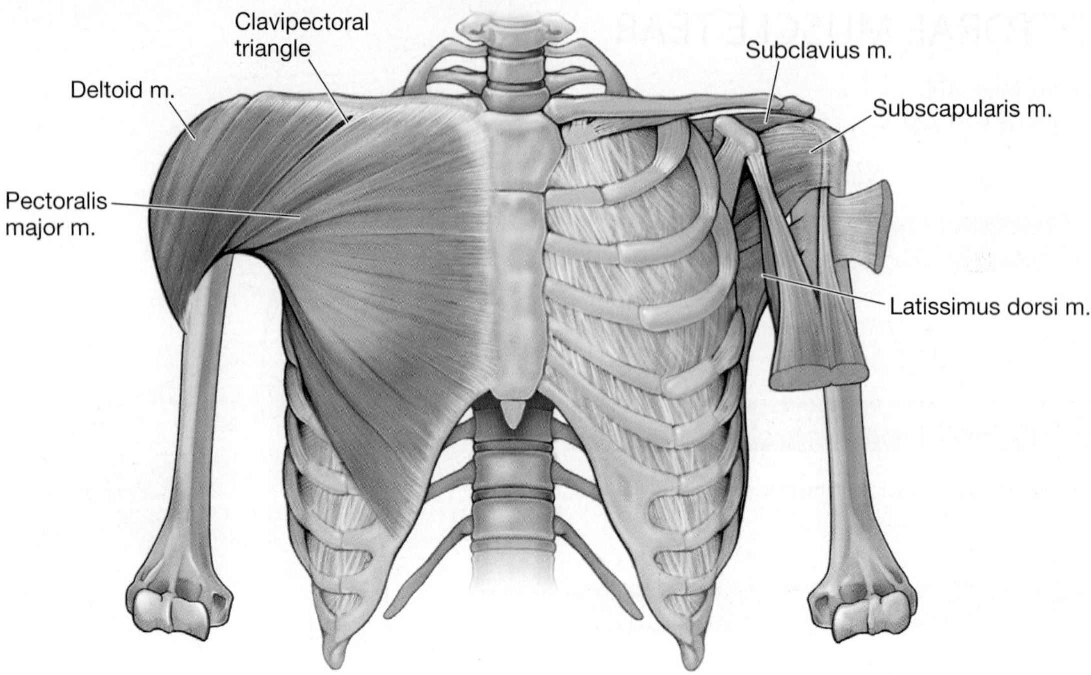

FIGURE 155-3 Pectoralis major muscle. (Reproduced with permission from Morton DA, Foreman KB, Albertine KH. *The Big Picture: Gross Anatomy*. McGraw-Hill, 2011.)

- Four common locations
  - Rupture at the humeral insertion
  - Rupture at the musculotendinous junction
  - Rupture at the muscle belly
  - Muscle torn off the sternum
- Commonly affects the pectoralis major muscle

Essentials of Diagnosis

- Rare condition
- Diagnosis is made by history and clinical examination with MRI for confirmation of location
- Occurs from a sudden high force, typically with weightlifting (i.e., bench or chest press)
- May arise from a repetitive type activity that leads to a gradual degeneration
- Sudden pain or tearing sensation in the chest may be experienced

General Considerations

- Swelling, ecchymosis, and functional pain
- Treatment may depend on location of rupture with tendon avulsion from the humerus treated with prompt surgical repair

Demographics

- More common in men between the ages of 20 and 50 that participate in contact sports and weight lifting

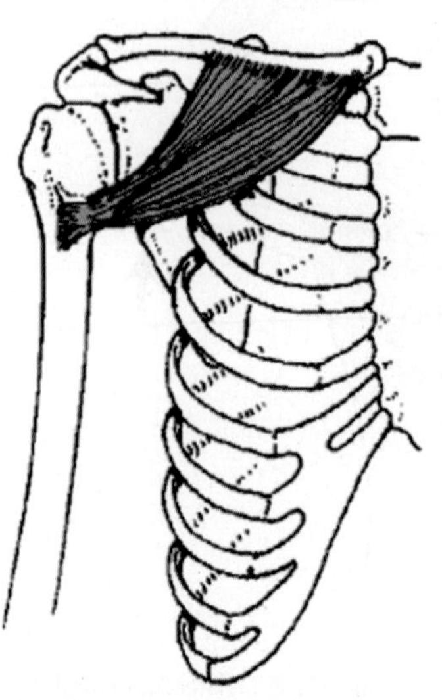

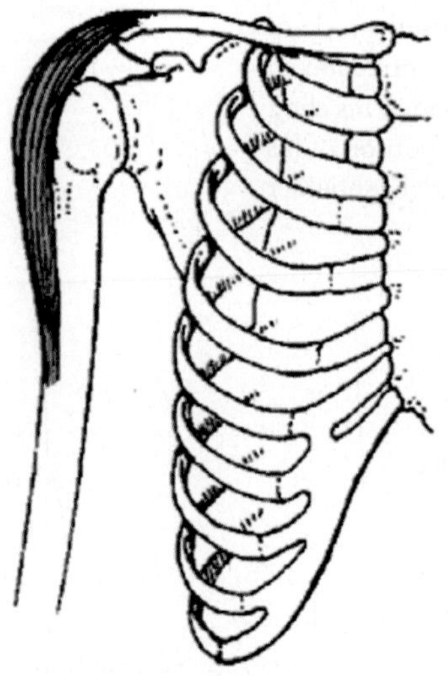

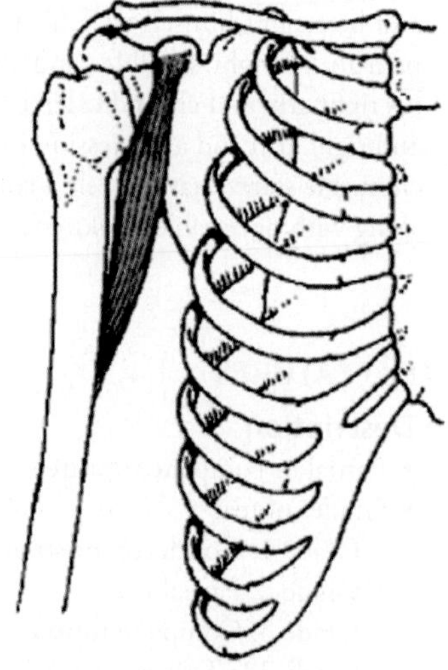

FIGURE 155-4 The major flexor muscles of the shoulder. (From Hall SJ. *Basic Biomechanics*. 5th ed. www.accessphysiotherapy.com. Copyright © The McGraw-Hill Companies, Inc. All rights reserved.)

CLINICAL FINDINGS

SIGNS AND SYMPTOMS

- Audible snap or pop at the time of injury
- Sudden pain or tearing sensation in chest
- Mild swelling and ecchymosis over anterior lateral chest wall or in proximal arm
- Loss of normal pectoralis contour
- Weakness with horizontal shoulder adduction

▶ Functional Implications

- Pushing activities
- Weight training with overload eccentric contractions: Such as bench press, push ups, chin ups, dips, and chest flys can cause a rupture
- Overhead activities may be limited
- Inability to lift heavy objects

▶ Possible Contributing Causes

- Abnormal biomechanics
- Muscle weakness or imbalance
- Muscle tightness
- Poor posture with change in humeral head position
- Excessive or inappropriate activity
- Inadequate warm up
- Steroid use
- Forceful eccentric activity (i.e., bench pressing)
- Often seen in football and rugby injuries

▶ Differential Diagnosis

- Long head of biceps tendon rupture
- Shoulder dislocation
- Proximal humerus fracture
- Rotator cuff tendon tear
- Medial Pectoral nerve entrapment

MEANS OF CONFIRMATION OR DIAGNOSIS

▶ Imaging

- Radiographs
- MRI
- Diagnostic ultrasound

▶ Findings and Interpretation

- Radiographs may show avulsion from humerus
- MRI can be useful in assessing location and severity of tear
- Acute tears will demonstrate hemorrhage and edema and chronic tears will demonstrate fibrosis and scarring

TREATMENT

▶ Medication

- NSAIDs
- Steroid injection

MEDICAL PROCEDURES

- Surgical repair of tendon rupture for site 1 and type 2 ruptures
- Ruptures at site 3 and 4 are not surgically repaired

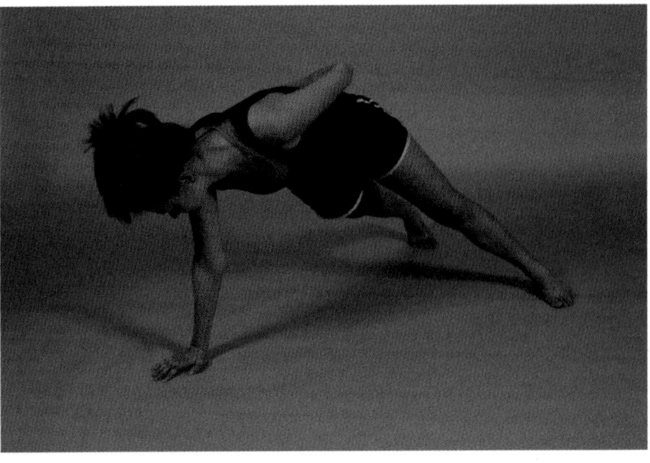

FIGURE 155-5 One arm push-up position. (From Dutton M. *Dutton's Orthopaedic Examination, Evaluation, and Intervention*. 3rd ed. http://www.access-physiotherapy.com. Copyright © The McGraw-Hill Companies, Inc. All rights reserved.)

REFERRALS/ADMITTANCE

- For imaging: Orthopedist, family physician, radiologist
- For surgery: Orthopedic surgeon
- For injection: Orthopedist, family physician

IMPAIRMENTS

- Debilitating pain, limiting movement and exertion
- Inability to perform overhead activities, such as in swimming, baseball, or tennis
- Inability to perform jobs involving repetitive overhead reaching or lifting
- Decreased torque and work/repetition, especially with shoulder adduction

TESTS AND MEASURES

- Anterior slide test
- Biceps load test
- Clunk test
- Compression–rotation test
- Disabilities of the Arm, Shoulder, and Hand (DASH) score to assess physical function
- Functional reach test
- O'Brien test
- Pain provocation test
- Pronated load test
- Resisted supination external rotation test
- Shoulder pain and disability index[2]
- Speed test
- Yergason test

INTERVENTION

- Acute
  - Rest
  - Reduce inflammation with NSAIDs
  - Ultrasound
  - Soft tissue massage
  - Electrotherapy
  - Ice/Heat

  - Gentle AROM
  - Posture correction
- Post-acute
  - Once pain and inflammation are controlled, progress through further active exercises in pain-free ranges
  - Progress stretching
  - Posterior glenohumeral glides
  - Progressive strengthening once pain-free
- Injury prevention
  - Avoid activities that place repetitive, excessive stress on the tendon
  - Cross-training
  - Improve technique
  - Warm-up and stretching prior to activity
  - Use proper ergonomics
  - Keep muscles strong and flexible

FUNCTIONAL GOALS

- Patient will be able to resume
  - All overhead activities and ADLs without exacerbating inflammation.
  - All sports activities as prior to onset.
  - All push activities without symptoms or limitation.
  - All lifting activities without limitations due to pain or weakness of the upper extremities.

PROGNOSIS

- Grade 1 and 2 tears: Rest, immobilization and therapy.
- Grade 3 tear: Depends on the location.
- Grade 3A, 3B, and 3C tears: Immobilization and rehabilitation.
- Conservative treatment: Several weeks to months but may not regain normal strength.
- Grade 3D[1] is a good surgical candidate depending on location.
- Type 1 has a good success rate with surgery, to return to prior level of function.
- Post surgery: 12 to 16 weeks for treatment; weightlifters may be limited with some activities for 6 months following surgery.

PATIENT RESOURCE

- Pectoralis Major Rupture Rehabilitation Protocol. Shady Grove Orthopaedic Associates. http://www.shadygroveortho.com/forms/Pectoral_Rehab.pdf. Accessed July 7, 2013.

REFERENCES

1. Tietjen R. Closed injuries of the pectoralis major muscle. *J Trauma.* 1980;20(3):262-264.
2. Bak K, Cameron EA, Henderson IJ. Rupture of the Pectoralis major: a meta-analysis of 112 cases. *Knee Surg Sports Traumatol Athrosc.* 2000;8(2):113–119.

ADDITIONAL REFERENCES

- Aarimaa V, Rantanen J, Heikkila J, Helttula L, Orava S. Rupture of the pectoralis major muscle. *Am J Sports Med.* 2004;32(5):1256–1262.
- Cline S. Acute injuries of the shoulder complex and arm. In: Patel DR, Greydanus DE, Baker RJ, eds. *Pediatric Practice: Sports Medicine.* New York, NY: McGraw-Hill; 2009. http://www.accessphysiotherapy.com/content/6977968. Accessed July 7, 2013.
- Connell DA, Potter HG, Sherman MF, Wickiewicz TL. Injuries of the pectoralis major muscle: evaluation with MR imaging. *Radiology.* 1999;210(3):785–791.
- Manske RC, Prohaska D. Pectoralis major tendon repair post surgical rehabilitation. *N Am J Sports Phys Ther.* 2007;2(1):22–23. http://www.ncbi.nlm.nih.gov/pmc/articles/PMC2953288/. Accessed July 7, 2013.
- McMahon PJ, Kaplan LD. Sports medicine, Chapter 4 In: Skinner HB, ed. *CURRENT Diagnosis & Treatment in Orthopedics.* 4th ed. New York, NY: McGraw-Hill; 2006. http://www.accessmedicine.com/content.aspx?aID=2318624. Accessed July 7, 2013.
- Park JY, Espiniella JL. Rupture of pectoralis major muscle: A case report and review of literature. *J Bone Joint Surg Am.* 1970;52(3):577–581.
- Petilon J, Carr DR, Sekiya JK, Unger DV. Pectoralis muscle injuries: evaluation and management. *J Am Acad Orthop Surg.* 2005;13 (1):59–68.

156 ROTATOR CUFF TENDINITIS

Eric Shamus, PhD, DPT, PT, CSCS
W. Justin Jones, DPT, PT, OCS

CONDITION/DISORDER SYNONYMS

- Supraspinatus tendonitis
- Infraspinatus tendonitis

ICD-9-CM CODES

- 726.10 Disorders of bursae and tendons in shoulder region, unspecified
- 840.3 Infraspinatus (muscle) (tendon) sprain
- 840.4 Rotator cuff (capsule) sprain
- 840.5 Subscapularis (muscle) sprain
- 840.6 Supraspinatus (muscle) (tendon) sprain

ICD-10-CM CODES

- S43.429A Sprain of unspecified rotator cuff capsule, initial encounter
- S43.80XA Sprain of other specified parts of unspecified shoulder girdle, initial encounter

PREFERRED PRACTICE PATTERN

- 4E: Impaired Joint Mobility, Motor Function, Muscle Performance, and Range of Motion Associated with Localized Inflammation

PATIENT PRESENTATION

A 20-year-old right hand dominant male college student who recently started painting houses for his summer employment. He reports working 5 consecutive days painting primarily with his right arm for 10+ hours each day. He subsequently developed progressive pain in the anterior/lateral aspect of his shoulder and had difficulty using his right arm for work activities. In addition, he reports currently experiencing pain reaching behind his back to tuck in his shirt, and with any reaching out to the side which is impacting his ability to perform his normal ADLs. He consulted with his PCP who started him on an oral NSAID and referred him to PT. Some of his examination findings include pain provocation with resisted isometric lateral rotation, and abduction, positive Neer and Hawkins Kennedy Impingement signs, and tenderness to palpation over the greater tuberosity. His cervical range of motion is WNL and Spurlings test is negative. In addition, his drop arm and external rotation lag signs were negative.

KEY FEATURES

Description

- Inflammation, irritation, swelling of one or more of the rotator cuff tendons.

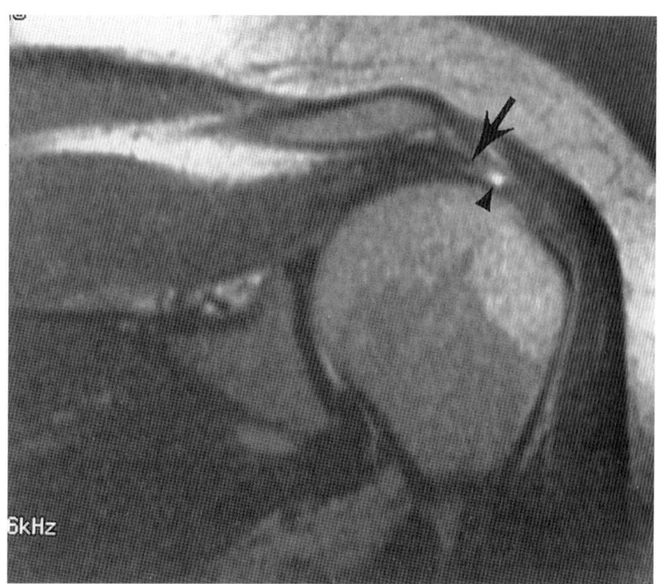

FIGURE 156-1 Rotator cuff tear. MRI coronal image of the shoulder reveals a tear in the supraspinatus tendon (*arrow*) with edema (*arrowhead*). (From Tintinalli JE, Stapczynski JS, John Ma O, et al. *Tintinalli's Emergency Medicine: A Comprehensive Study Guide*. 7th ed. www.accessmedicine.com. Copyright © The McGraw-Hill Companies, Inc. All rights reserved.)

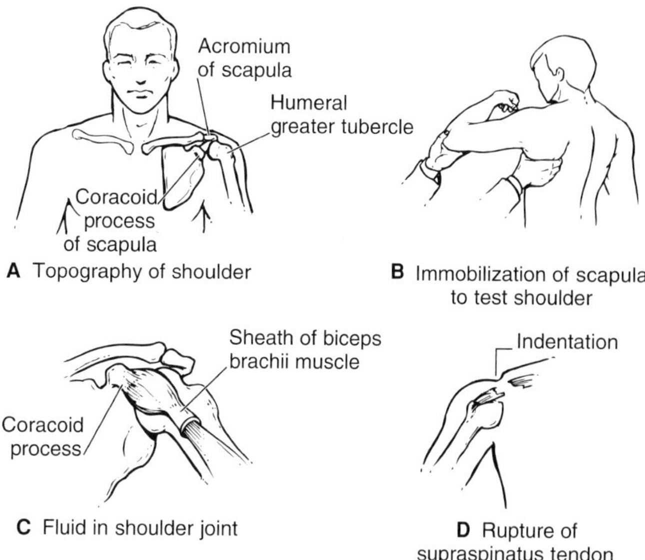

FIGURE 156-2 Examination of the shoulder joint. (**A**) Topography of the shoulder. The bony prominences of the humeral greater tubercle and the coracoid and acromial processes of the scapula form a right-angled triangle. (**B**) Immobilization of the scapula to test shoulder motion. (**C**) Fluid in the shoulder joint. The heavily stippled structures are the joint capsules distended with fluid. (**D**) Rupture of supraspinatus tendon. (From LeBlond RF, DeGowin RL, Brown DD. *DeGowin's Diagnostic Examination*. 9th ed. www.accessmedicine.com. Copyright © The McGraw-Hill Companies, Inc. All rights reserved.)

- Supraspinatus muscle
- Infraspinatus muscle
- Teres minor muscle
- Subscapularis muscle
- Occurs most often from repetitive motion injuries or impingement syndrome but can occur with a sudden strain/stress to the tendon.
- Early stages: The tendon becomes swollen and red, and as the tendonitis develops, the tendon sheath may thicken.
- Late stages: Chronic inflammation may result in fraying of the tendon (tendinosis) and could progress to rupture with long-term inflammation.
- Shoulder pain and dysfunction due to compression and abrasion of one or more of the rotator cuff tendons.
- Impingement is the most commonly diagnosed shoulder problem and likely has numerous potential mechanisms, which can impact both treatment and prognosis.

Essentials of Diagnosis

- Multifactorial and thought to be related to intrinsic and/or extrinsic mechanisms.
  - Extrinsic mechanisms (extratendinous, caused by decreased sub-acromial space and subsequent micro-trauma with repetitive movements)
    - Mechanical wear under the coracoacromial arch
    - Aberrant movement patterns due to rotator cuff and/or periscapular muscular dysfunction
    - Capsular abnormalities
      - Capsular tightness (particularly posterior capsule)
      - Capsular laxity (poor humeral head dynamic control)
    - Sub-optimal posture
      - Muscle imbalances
    - Overuse/repetitive motions occurring at more than 90 degrees of elevation
  - Intrinsic factors (directly associated with the narrowing of the sub-acromial space)
    - Vascular supply/changes to the cuff tendons
    - Acromial morphology (structural variations)
      - Type I (flat)
      - Type II (curved)
      - Type III hooked)
    - Degenerative and/or structural changes to the AC joint
    - Other trophic changes in the coracoacromial arch or humeral head
- Classification
  - Primary impingement is usually associated with degenerative changes to any of the following tissues:
    - Rotator cuff tendons
    - Acromioclavicular (AC) joint
    - Coracoacromial arch
  - Secondary impingement is the result of muscle imbalances and/or joint instability, which can result in altered dynamics and subsequent secondary impingement.
  - A third class of impingement, not sub-acromial in nature, is referred to as internal impingement and occurs between the undersurface (articular side) of the rotator cuff tendons and the posterior/superior surface of the labrum in the position of abduction and external rotation that occurs with throwing.
  - Regardless of the specific classification, all types of impingement are proposed to be mechanisms of rotator cuff and biceps tendinopathy.

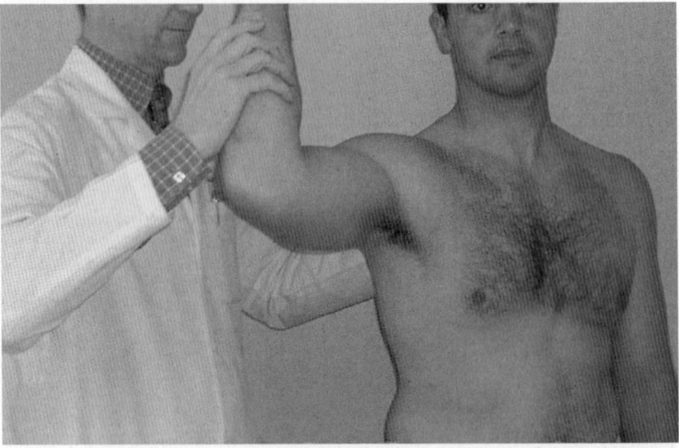

FIGURE 156-3 Hawkins impingement sign. (From Imboden J, Hellmann DB, Stone JH. *Current Diagnosis & Treatment in Rheumatology*. 2nd ed. http://www.accessmedicine.com. Copyright © The McGraw-Hill Companies, Inc. All rights reserved.)

General Considerations

- The rotator cuff stabilizes and steers the head of the humerus in the glenoid of the scapular at the glenohumeral (GH) joint.
- Rotator cuff and possibly the biceps are thought to compresses the head of the humerus into the glenoid to allow for the deltoid muscle to elevate the humerus in synchronicity with the scapula known as scapulohumeral rhythm.

Demographics

- History of repetitive motion and activities, especially overhead

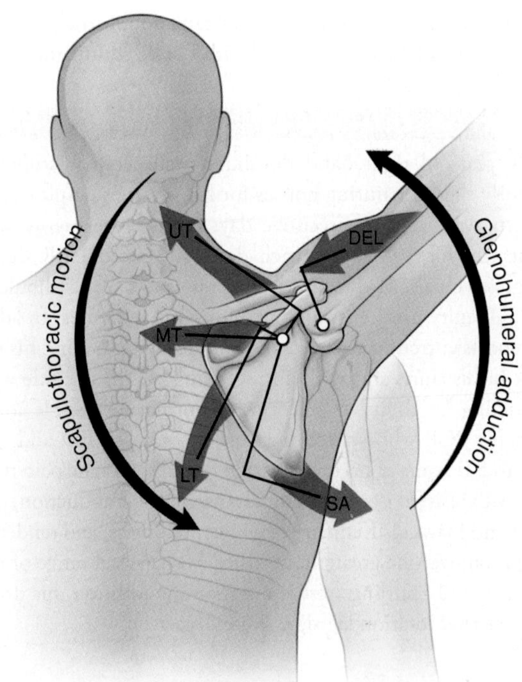

FIGURE 156-4 The scapulohumeral rhythm. (From Dutton M. *Dutton's Orthopaedic Examination, Evaluation, and Intervention* 3rd ed. http://www.access-physiotherapy.com. Copyright © The McGraw-Hill Companies, Inc. All rights reserved.)

- Common in swimming, tennis, and baseball as well as with occupational activities involving repetitive or overhead activity due to micro-trauma.
- Predominately in individuals involved in repetitive activities in sports or work.
- Can be seen in individuals with other system-wide diseases such as rheumatoid arthritis and diabetes.
- Primary impingement (generally occurs in patients ages 40 and older).
- Secondary impingement (generally occurs in younger patients ages 15 to 35).

CLINICAL FINDINGS

SIGNS AND SYMPTOMS

- Pain anterior lateral shoulder with active movement and overhead activities
- Deep ache in the shoulder
- Painful arc commonly present in the mid-range of shoulder elevation
- Weakness is commonly noted with functional reaching tasks
- Scapular dyskinesis may be present
- Acute pain with the inability to elevate the arm

Functional Implications

- Pain/Limitation with overhead activities
- Pain/Limitation with reaching
- Pain/Limitation with lifting
- Pain/Limitation dressing
- Pain/Limitation with sustained or repetitive shoulder activities
- Pain at night (sleep disruption)
- May limit throwing and other rapid arm movements

Possible Contributing Causes

- Acromion morphology
  - Type I
  - Type II
  - Type III
- Degenerative changes at the AC joint
- Instability of the GH capsule
- Frequent and prolonged overhead activity
- Prolonged repetitive use of the involved arm
- Poor posture, rounded shoulders
- Anteriorly displaced humeral head
- Rotator cuff weakness
- Aging
- Systemic diseases such as rheumatoid arthritis or diabetes
- Bicipital tendinopathy or previous biceps injury
- Capsular laxity
- Capsular tightness
- Increased thoracic kyphosis and sub-optimal posture
- Repetitive overhead activities
- Poor neuromuscular control

Differential Diagnosis[1]

- AC separation
- Adhesive capsulitis
- Cervical radiculopathy
- Full-thickness rotator cuff tear
- GH arthritis
- GH instability

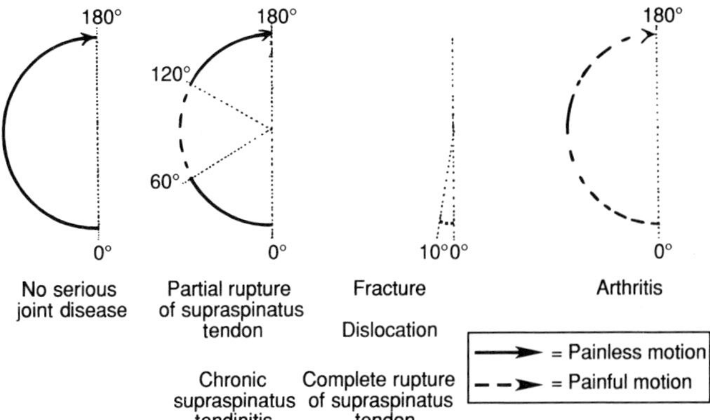

FIGURE 156-5 Causes of pain and limited motion with elevation of the arm in abduction. (From LeBlond RF, DeGowin RL, Brown DD. *DeGowin's Diagnostic Examination*. 9th ed. www.accessmedicine.com. Copyright © The McGraw-Hill Companies, Inc. All rights reserved.)

- Internal impingement
- Labral tear
- Neuropathy (suprascapular nerve)
- Referred pain from lungs or diaphragm
- Sub-acromial bursitis
- Tendonitis of the long head of the bicep tendon

Means of Confirmation or Diagnosis

- Sub-acromial injection (lidocaine) to see if impingement signs reduce

Imaging

- Radiograph
  - Acromion type
  - Spurs
  - Humeral head position
  - Osteoarthritis
  - Sclerotic changes
  - Views
  - Anteroposterior
  - Lateral
  - Supraspinatus outlet view
- Diagnostic Ultrasound
- MRI
  - Rotator cuff tear
  - Tissue quality

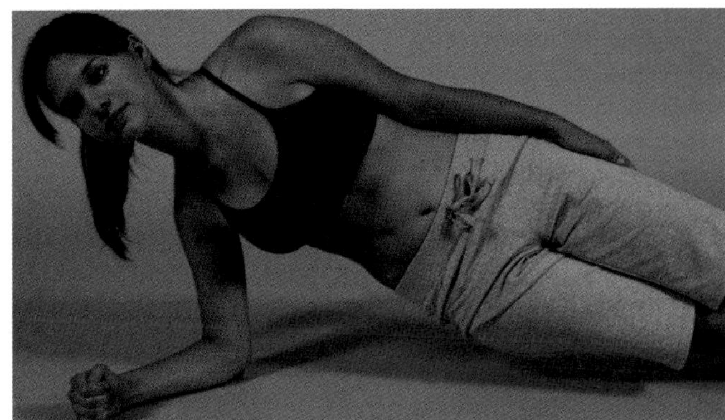

FIGURE 156-6 Side planks for shoulder and core strengthening. (From Dutton M. *Dutton's Orthopaedic Examination, Evaluation, and Intervention*. 3rd ed. http://www.accessphysiotherapy.com. Copyright © The McGraw-Hill Companies, Inc. All rights reserved.)

- Capsulolabral and biceps labral pathology
- Acromion
- AC joint
- Labrum

Findings and Interpretation

- Imaging to diagnose additional pathology
- Diagnostic ultrasound
  - Maybe helpful in diagnosing moderate to large cuff tear
  - Less effective in diagnosing small tears or tendonitis

TREATMENT

Medication

- Anti-inflammatory
- Corticosteroid injection

MEDICAL PROCEDURE

- Surgery
  - Acromioplasty is commonly performed on patients who have not responded to conservative care including activity modification, PT, NSAIDs, and injections and have imaging evidence of intrinsic changes to the acromion, rotator cuff, or AC joint (minimum 6 months).
  - If the condition has progressed to a full-thickness rotator cuff tear, acromioplasty is often performed concomitantly with a cuff repair.
  - If the biceps tendon has changes associated with wear, then a tenotomy or tenodesis are often performed.

REFERRALS/ADMITTANCE

- Orthopedic surgeon or radiologist for imaging
- Physician or pharmacist for medication
- Orthopedic surgeon for surgical consult if failed conservative treatment
- When to refer to a specialist

IMPAIRMENTS

- Impaired (sub-optimal) posture
- Muscle imbalances
  - Rotator cuff weakness
  - Periscapular muscle weakness (particularly upward rotators and depressors/retractors)
  - Pectoralis minor tightness
- Decreased thoracic ROM (particularly extension)
- Rotator cuff overuse/fatigue
- Neuropathy and subsequent muscle weakness
- Hypomobile posterior GH capsule
- Hypermobility at the GH and or scapulothoracic articulations
- Pain with active elevation
- Hypo- or hypermobility at the GH, scapulothoracic, AC, or sternoclavicular (SC) joints

TESTS AND MEASURES

- Diagnosis is usually made by clinical examination and often accompanies three or more special tests[1]
  - Anterior slide test
  - Biceps load test
  - C5–6 dermatome/myotome testing
  - Clunk test
  - Compression–rotation test
  - Diagnostic test properties for sub-acromial impingement
  - Disabilities of the Arm, Shoulder, and Hand (DASH) score to assess physical function
  - Drop arm (Codman's) test
  - Empty can test
  - External rotation lag sign (ERLS)/dropping arm sign
  - Hawkins–Kennedy impingement sign/test
  - Infraspinatus muscle test[1]
  - Neer impingement test
  - O'Brien test
  - Pain provocation test
  - Pain with resisted abduction
  - Painful arc sign/test
  - Passive horizontal adduction test
  - Pronated load test
  - Resisted supination external rotation test
  - Shoulder pain and disability index
  - Speed test
  - Yergason test

INTERVENTION

- This will vary depending on the type of impingement, causes, stage of healing, and tissue quality but generally involve portions of the following.
  - Acute stage
    - Rest, ice, and activity modification (avoiding impinging positions)
  - Sub-acute–chronic stages (addressing specific impairments associated with the impingement)
    - Address joint impairments
      - GH hypomobility (mobilization)
      - GH hypermobility (stabilization)
      - Thoracic spine hypomobility (mobilization/manipulation)
    - Address muscle imbalances
      - Rotator cuff strength and endurance exercises
      - Muscle length of pectoralis major, minor, latissimus, and other muscles with decreased length
    - Strengthening of scapular musculature
      - Lower trapezius
      - Serratus anterior
      - Other scapular stabilizers
    - Functional activities (depending on work/recreational desires)
  - Addressing pain and inflammation
    - Ice
    - Rest
    - Activity modification (avoiding impingement positions)
    - Ultrasound, phonophoresis, ionophoresis
    - Electric stimulation
  - Addressing weakness, joint hypermobility
    - Shoulder lateral and medial rotation
      - Isometric
      - Painful eccentric exercises
      - Thera-Band resisted
      - Handheld weight resisted
      - Progression through higher ranges of elevation
    - Scapular strength/stabilization
    - Retraction
    - Prone shoulder extension, abduction, scapular plane elevation

- Front and side plank exercises
- Closed chain stability exercises
- Addressing lack of flexibility
  - Stretching
    - Posterior capsule/posterior cuff
    - Pectoralis minor
    - Pectoralis major
    - Latissimus dorsi
- Addressing joint mobility
  - Posterior humeral glides
  - Inferior humeral glides
  - Thoracic mobilization/manipulation
  - Scapulothoracic mobility
    - Distraction
    - Retraction
    - Upward rotation
    - Posterior tip
- Addressing tendinopathy
  - Eccentric cuff exercises

FUNCTIONAL GOALS

- Patient will be able to:
  - Move upper extremity through full range of elevation without pain to reach in the cabinet.
  - Reach back pocket (or fasten brassiere for female) without pain
  - Reach for a gallon of milk without pain.

PROGNOSIS

- Prognosis is dependent on the underlying cause, the quality of the tissues involved as well as the patient's ability to control exacerbating activities and perform the optimal dosage of therapeutic exercise.
- Some tendonitis can progress to a tear/rupture if untreated.

PATIENT RESOURCE

- Tanji J. Rotator Cuff Tendonitis. American Medical Society for Sports Medicine. http://www.newamssm.org/Handouts/RotatorCuff.pdf. Accessed July 8, 2013.

REFERENCE

1. Park HB, Yokota A, Gill HS, et al. Diagnostic accuracy of clinical tests for the different degrees of subacromial impingement syndrome. *J Bone Joint Surg Am.* 2005;87:1446–1455.

ADDITIONAL REFERENCES

- Bang MD, Deyle GD. Comparison of supervised exercise with and without manual physical therapy for patients with shoulder impingement syndrome. *J Orthop Sports Phys Ther.* 2000; 30(3):26–137.
- Bigliani LU, Levine WN. Current Concepts Review: Subacromial Impingement Syndrome. *J Bone Joint Surg Am.* 1997; 79(12):1854–1868.
- Dutton M, ed. *Dutton's Orthopaedic Examination, Evaluation, and Intervention.* 3rd ed. New York, NY: McGraw-Hill; 2012. http://www.accessphysiotherapy.com/content/5552983. Accessed July 7, 2013.
- Dutton M. Common orthopedic conditions. In: Dutton M, ed. *Dutton's Orthopedic Survival Guide: Managing Common Conditions.* New York, NY: McGraw-Hill; 2011. http://www.accessphysiotherapy.com/content/8652285. Accessed July 7, 2013.
- Hamilton N, Weimar W, Luttgens K. The upper extremity: The shoulder region, Chapter 5. In: Hamilton N, Weimar W, Luttgens K, eds. *Kinesiology: Scientific Basis of Human Motion.* New York, NY: McGraw-Hill; 2008. http://www.accessphysiotherapy.com/content/6150569. Accessed July 8, 2013.
- ICD9Data.com. http://www.icd9data.com. Accessed July 3, 2013.
- ICD10Data.com. http://www.icd10data.com. Accessed July 3, 2013.
- Kisner C, Colby LA. *Therapeutic Exercise.* 5th ed. Philadelphia, PA: F.A. Davis Company; 2007:502–511.
- Ludewig PM, Braman JP. Shoulder impingement: biomechanical considerations in rehabilitation. *Man Ther.* 2011;16(1):33–39. doi:10.1016/j.math.2010.08.004. [PMID: 20888284]
- Malone TR, Hazle C, Grey ML. Shoulder complex, Chapter 5. In: Malone TR, Hazle C, Grey ML, eds. *Imaging in Rehabilitation.* New York, NY: McGraw-Hill; 2008. http://www.accessphysiotherapy.com/content/5940757. Accessed July 7, 2013.
- Patel DR, Greydanus DE, Baker RJ. Overuse injuries of the shoulder, Chapter 21. In: Patel DR, Greydanus DE, Baker RJ, eds. *Pediatric Practice.* NEW York, NY: McGraw-Hill, 2009. http://www.accessphysiotherapy.com/popup.aspx?aID=6978348. Accessed July 8, 2013.
- Pattern 4E: Impaired joint mobility, motor function, muscle performance, and range of motion associated with localized inflammation. In: *Guide to Physical Therapist Practice.* 2nd ed. Alexandria, VA: American Physical Therapy Association; 2001. Revised 2003.
- Prentice WE, Quillen WS, Underwood F, eds. *Therapeutic Modalities in Rehabilitation.* 4th ed. New York, NY: McGraw-Hill; 2011. http://www.accessphysiotherapy.com/content/8138750. Accessed July 8, 2013.
- Theisen C, van Wagensveld A, Timmesfeld N, et al. Co-occurrence of outlet impingement syndrome of the shoulder and restricted range of motion in the thoracic spine–a prospective study with ultrasound-based motion analysis. *BMC Musculoskelet Disord.* 2010;11:135. doi:10.1186/1471-2474-11-135.
- Wilk KE, Reinold MM, Andrews JR, eds. *The Athlete's Shoulder.* 2nd ed. New York, NY: Churchill Livingstone; 2009:115–140.

157 SCAPULA WINGING

Eric Shamus, PhD, DPT, PT, CSCS
Mae L. Yahara, MS, PT, ATC

CONDITION/DISORDER SYNONYMS

- Facioscapulohumeral muscular dystrophy (FSH)
- Scapula alata
- Serratus anterior palsy
- Winging scapula

ICD-9-CM CODE[1]

- 736.89 Other acquired deformity of other parts of limb

ICD-10-CM CODE[2]

- M21.80 Other specified acquired deformities of unspecified limb

PREFERRED PRACTICE PATTERN[3]

- 4E: Impaired Joint Mobility, Motor Function, Muscle Performance, and Range of Motion Associated with Localized Inflammation

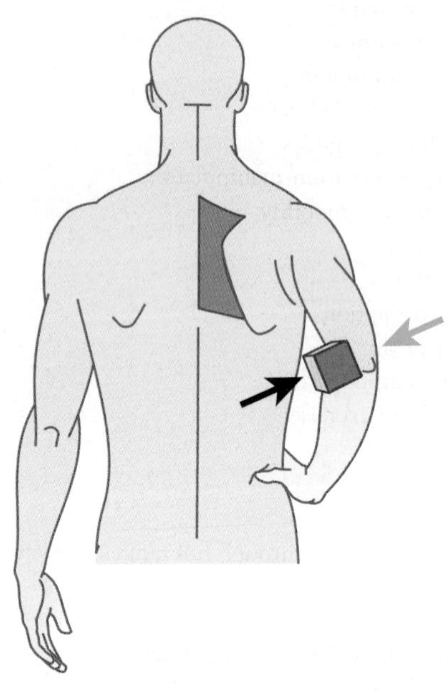

FIGURE 157-1 Rhomboids (C4, 5; dorsal scapular nerve). The shoulder is thrust backward against resistance. (From Waxman SG: *Clinical Neuroanatomy*. 26th ed. www.accessmedicine.com. Copyright © The McGraw-Hill Companies, Inc. All rights reserved.)

PATIENT PRESENTATION

Patient is a 35-year-old male immigrant farm worker who does not speak English. He had an accident at work in which he sustained fractures to the left tibia and fibula which required ORIF. Postoperatively he used a walker with a non-weight bearing gait pattern. As his weight bearing was progressed, he began to utilize one axillary crutch on the right side. He did not receive any instruction with the crutch. He began to notice symptoms in his right shoulder approximately one month later. He states that his girlfriend noticed his shoulder blade "sticking out" and he reported it to the doctor. He is complaining of weakness in the right upper extremity with overhead activities and pain in the right peri-scapular region.

KEY FEATURES

Description

- Inferior angle tilting of the scapula
- Instability of the scapula to the thoracic wall
- Scapula has the greatest number of muscles attached to it than any other bone
- Scapula dysrhythmia
- Result of serratus anterior muscle dysfunction
- Injury to long thoracic nerve

Essentials of Diagnosis

- Often asymptomatic
- Winging can help identify a dysfunction possibly occurring in the shoulder
- Symptoms of pain and weakness
- Can be a result of a brachial plexus injury
- Parsonage–Turner syndrome (brachial neuritis) underlying

General Considerations

- Loss of serratus anterior muscle
- Weakness of trapezius strength
- Weakness of scapular stabilizers
- Commonly associated with presence of other orthopedic pathologies: subacromial impingement syndrome, rotator cuff pathology, labral pathology
- Creates an abnormal scapulothoracic rhythm
- Commonly associated with repeated overhead or overuse activities
- Full history of symptoms, medical history screening, and differential shoulder orthopedic examination will ensure appropriate diagnosis

Demographics

- Non-specific

CLINICAL FINDINGS

SIGNS AND SYMPTOMS

- Pain
- Weakness is commonly noted with functional reaching tasks
- Scapula instability, moving away from rib cage

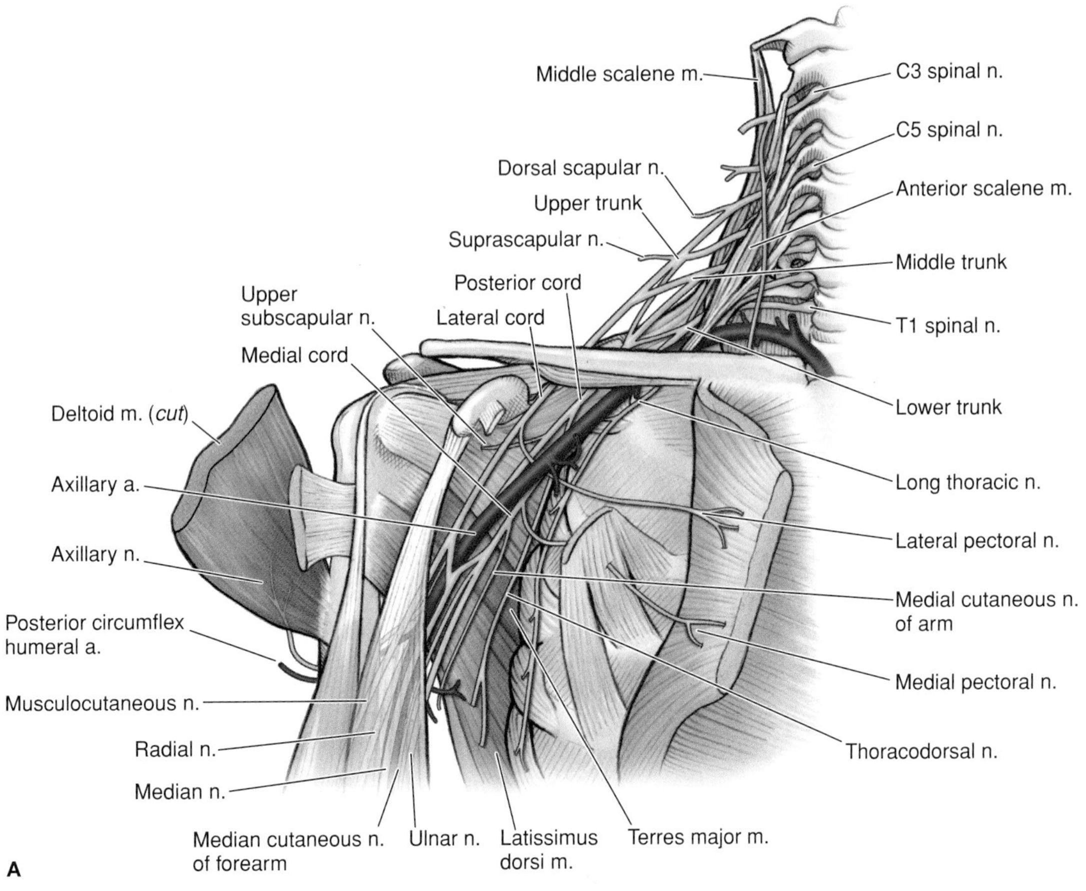

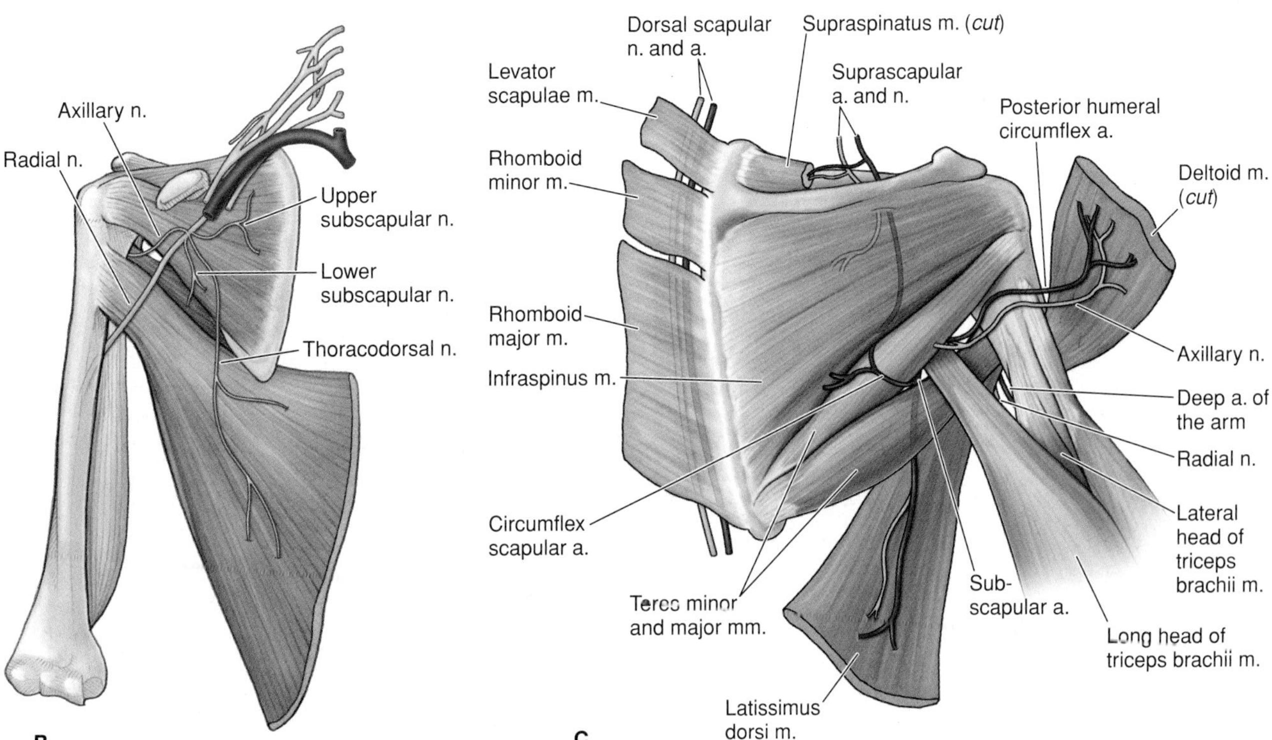

FIGURE 157-2 (**A**) Brachial plexus and topography of the axillary artery. (**B**) Posterior division of the brachial plexus. (**C**) Posterior view of the shoulder joint. (Reproduced with permission from Morton DA, Foreman KB, Albertine KH: *The Big Picture: Gross Anatomy*. McGraw-Hill, 2011.)

Functional Limitations

- Inability to raise or lower the arms without the scapula's inferior angle tilting away from the rib cage
- Pain/Limitation with overhead activities
- Pain/Limitation with reaching
- Pain/Limitation with lifting
- Pain/Limitation dressing and grooming
- Pain/Limitation with sustained or repetitive shoulder activities

Possible Contributing Causes

- Serratus anterior palsy
- Trapezius palsy
- Increased thoracic kyphosis and sub-optimal posture
- Repetitive overhead activities
- Posterior shoulder capsule tightness
- Pectoralis minor tightness
- Poor neuromuscular control
- Non-traumatic injury to the long thoracic nerve
  - Influenza
  - Drug overdose
- Traumatic injury to the long thoracic nerve
  - Impact injury
  - Stretch to cervical spine
  - Electrical shock
  - Mastectomy with axillary node dissection
- Clavicle fracture
- Rupture of the lower trapezius and Rhomboid major[4]
- Brachial neuritis (Parsonage–Turner syndrome)

Differential Diagnosis

- Cervical radiculopathy, C7
- Referred pain from lungs or diaphragm
- Rotator cuff pathology (tendonitis, full- or partial-thickness tear)
- Glenohumeral (GH) instability
- Labral tear
- Neuropathy
- Internal impingement

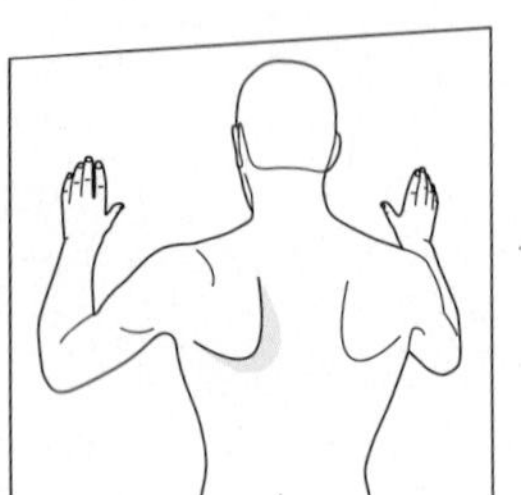
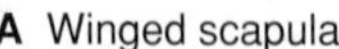

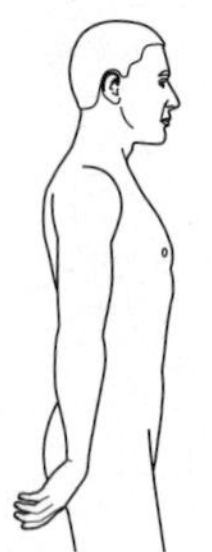
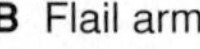

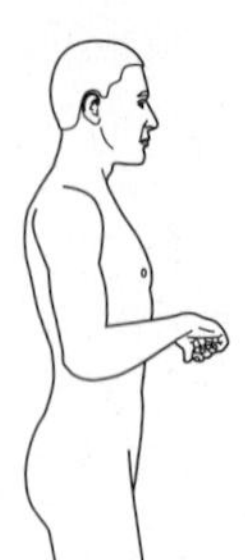

FIGURE 157-3 Disorders of the intact shoulder. (**A**) Winged scapula. When the patient pushes the hands against a wall the involved scapula protrude posteriorly, forming a winged scapula. (**B**) Flail arm. The arm hangs limply at the side with palm posterior and fingers partially flexed. (**C**) Spastic arm. The arm assumes flexion at the elbow with the upper arm at elevation, flexion at the wrist and fingers, with slight adduction of the humerus; the forearm is in pronation. (From LeBlond RF, DeGowin RL, Brown DD: *DeGowin's Diagnostic Examination*. 9th ed. www.accessmedicine.com. Copyright © The McGraw-Hill Companies, Inc. All rights reserved.)

Means of Confirmation or Diagnosis

- Diagnosis based on orthopedic special tests, signs and symptoms, imaging studies, and exclusion of differential diagnosis
- Special tests
  - Push-ups test
  - Serratus wall test

TREATMENT

Medications

- NSAIDs

MEDICAL PROCEDURE

- Surgery: intercostal nerve transfer

REFERRALS/ADMITTANCE

- Radiologist for imaging: X-ray, MRI for differential diagnosis
- Nerve conduction test

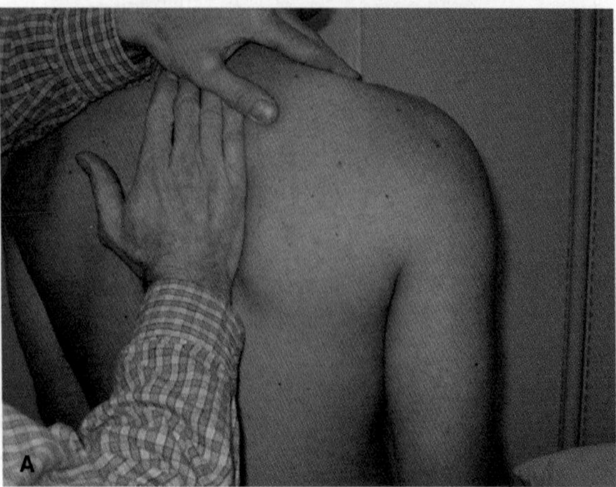

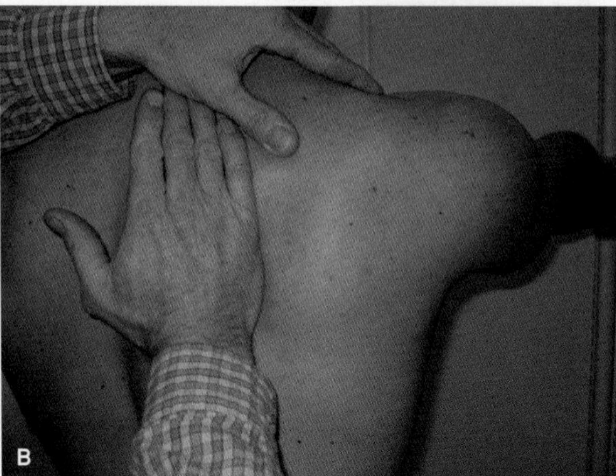

FIGURE 157-4 Scapular retraction test. From behind the athlete the examiner stabilizes the medial border of the scapula as the athlete elevates the arm. A positive test is indicated by relief of rotator cuff impingement pain and suggests a role of the periscapular muscles in the pathophysiology and rehabilitation of the impingement syndrome. (From Patel DR, Greydanus DE, Baker RJ: *Pediatric Practice: Sports Medicine*. http://www.accesspediatrics.com. Copyright © The McGraw-Hill Companies, Inc. All rights reserved.)

IMPAIRMENTS

- Weakness and pain limiting overhead activities or activities involving arm out to side or across body including, dressing or grooming daily activities
- Impaired (sub-optimal) posture
- Muscle imbalances
  - Periscapular muscle weakness (particularly upward rotators and depressors/retractors)
  - Pectoralis minor tightness
- Decreased thoracic ROM (particularly extension)
- Rotator cuff overuse/fatigue
- Neuropathy and subsequent muscle weakness
- Hypermobility at the GH joint and or scapulothoracic articulations
- Pain with active elevation

TESTS AND MEASURES

- Diagnosis made based on orthopedic special tests, signs and symptoms, imaging studies, and exclusion of differential diagnosis.
- Disabilities of the Arm, Shoulder and Hand (DASH) score to assess physical function
- Special tests
  - Push-ups
  - Serratus wall test

INTERVENTION

- Address muscle imbalances
  - Rotator cuff strength and endurance exercises
  - Muscle length of pectoralis major and minor
- Strengthening of scapular musculature
  - Lower trap
  - Serratus anterior
  - Other scapular stabilizers
  - Shoulder lateral and medial rotation
  - Isometric
  - Thera-Band resisted
  - Handheld weight resisted
  - Progression through higher ranges of elevation
  - Scapular strength/stabilization
    - Retraction
    - Prone shoulder extension, HABD, scapular plane elevation
- Functional activities (depending on work/recreational desires)
- Addressing pain and inflammation
  - Ice
  - Rest
  - Activity modification (avoiding impingement positions)
  - Ultrasound
  - E-stimulation

FUNCTIONAL GOALS

- Patient will be able to:
  - Reach into overhead cabinets in kitchen without pain or restriction while maintaining scapular control.
  - Lift a gallon milk carton from refrigerator at shoulder–level, pain free, while maintaining scapular control.
  - Turn steering wheel, pain free, while maintaining scapular control
  - Perform all dressing and grooming activities (tuck in shirt behind back, wash hair, etc.) without pain or compensation while maintaining scapular control.

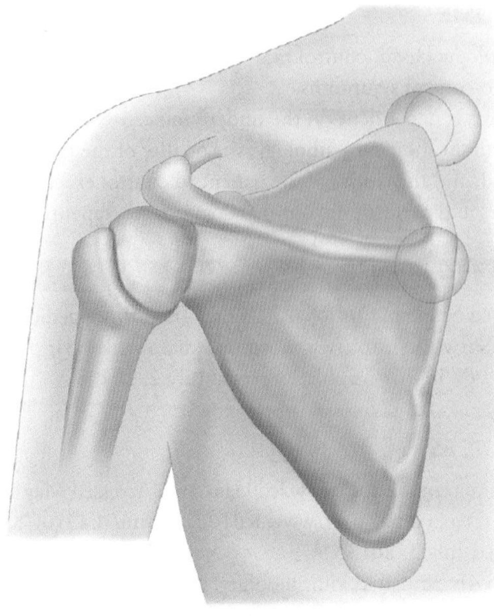

FIGURE 157-5 Various scapulothoracic bursae locations. Symptomatic bursitis may affect the infraserratus bursae at the inferior angle of the scapula as well as the superomedial angle. A small bursa over the base of the spine of the scapula, called the trapezoid bursa may also be affected. (From Patel DR, Greydanus DE, Baker RJ: *Pediatric Practice: Sports Medicine.* http://www.accesspediatrics.com.)

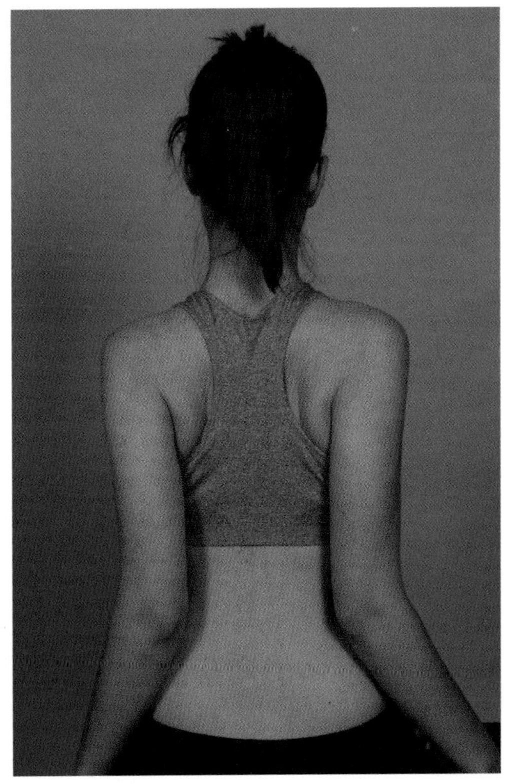

FIGURE 157-6 Scapular pinch. (From Dutton M: *Dutton's Orthopaedic Examination, Evaluation, and Intervention.* 3rd ed. http://www.accessphysiotherapy.com.)

PROGNOSIS

- If neurologic based, control may not be regained.
- Good to control symptoms.
- Prognosis is dependent on the underlying cause, the presence of concomitant shoulder pathology, the quality of the tissues involved, and the ability of the patient to control exacerbating activities and perform the optimal dosage of therapeutic exercise.

PATIENT RESOURCE

- Winged Scapula. OrthopaedicsOne, The Orthopaedic Knowledge Network. http://www.orthopaedicsone.com/display/Review/Winged+Scapula. Accessed July 2, 2013.

REFERENCES

1. ICD9Data.com. http://www.icd9data.com. Accessed May 25, 2014.
2. ICD10Data.com. http://www.icd10data.com/ICD10CM/Codes. Accessed July 3, 2013.
3. Pattern 4E: Impaired joint mobility, motor function, muscle performance, and range of motion associated with localized inflammation. In: *Guide to Physical Therapist Practice*. 2nd ed. Alexandria, VA: American Physical Therapy Association; 2001. Revised 2003.
4. Lee SG, Kim JH, Lee SY, Choi IS, Moon ES. Winged scapula caused by rhomboideus and trapezius muscles rupture associated with repetitive minor trauma: A case report. *J Korean Med Sci*. 2006;21(3):581–584. doi: 10.3346/jkms.2006.21.3.581. [PMID 16778411]

ADDITIONAL REFERENCES

- Atasoy E, Majd M. Scapulothoracic stabilization for wining of the scapula using strips of autogenous fascia lata. *J Bone Joint Surg Br*. 2000;82(6):813–817. [PMID 10990302]
- Dutton M. Chapter 8. Musculoskeletal physical therapy. In: Dutton M, ed. *McGraw-Hill's NPTE (National Physical Therapy Examination)2e*. New York, NY: McGraw-Hill; 2012.
- Dutton M, ed. *Orthopaedic Examination, Evaluation, and Intervention*. 2nd ed. New York, NY: McGraw-Hill; 2008.http://www.accessphysiotherapy.com/content/5552983. Accessed July 2, 2013.
- Dutton M. Chapter 5. The shoulder complex. In: Dutton M, ed. *Dutton's Orthopedic Survival Guide: Managing Common Conditions*. New York, NY: McGraw-Hill; 2011. http://accessphysiotherapy.com/content18651960. Accessed January 3, 2013.
- Hamilton N, Weimar W, Luttgens K. The Shoulder Girdle (Acromioclavicular and Sternoclavicular Articulations). In: Hamilton N, Weimar W, Luttgens K, eds. *Kinesiology: Scientific Basis of Human Motion*. New York, NY: McGraw-Hill; 2008. http://www.accessphysiotherapy.com/content/6150577. Accessed July 1, 2013.
- Marin R. Scapula winger's brace: a case series of the management of long thoracic nerve palsy. *Arch Phys Med Rehabil*. 1998;79(10):1226–1230. doi: 10.1016/S0003-9993(98)90266-0. [PMID 9779675]
- Martin RM, Fish DE. Scapular winging: anatomical review, diagnosis, and treatments. *Curr Rev Musculoskelet Med*. 2008;1(1):1–11. doi: 10.1007/s12178-007-9000-5. [PMID 19468892]
- Novak CB, Mackinnon SE. Surgical treatment of a long thoracic nerve palsy. *Ann Thorac Surg*. 2002;73(5):1643–1645. doi: 10.1016/S0003-4975(01)03372-0. [PMID 12022573]
- Prentice WE. The shoulder complex. In: Prentice WE, ed. *Principles of Athletic Training: A Competency-Based Approach*. New York, NY: McGraw-Hill; 2011:639–680.
- Vinson EN. Clinical images: Scapular winging. *Arthritis Rheum*. 2006;54(12):4027. doi: 10.1002/art.22274. [PMID 17133539]
- Waxman SG. Appendix B. Testing Muscle Function. In: Waxman SG, ed. *Clinical Neuroanatomy*. 26th ed. New York, NY: McGraw-Hill; 2010. http://www.accessphysiotherapy.com/popup.aspx?aID=5276476. Accessed July 2, 2013.

158 SHOULDER DISLOCATION

Eric Shamus, PhD, DPT, PT, CSCS
Marangela Obispo, MSPT, GCS

CONDITION/DISORDER SYNONYMS

- Shoulder dislocation
- Humerus dislocation

ICD-9-CM CODES

- 831 Dislocation of shoulder
- 831.0 Closed dislocation of shoulder
- 831.00 Closed dislocation of shoulder, unspecified
- 831.01 Closed anterior dislocation of humerus
- 831.02 Closed posterior dislocation of humerus
- 831.03 Closed inferior dislocation of humerus
- 831.09 Closed dislocation of shoulder, other
- 831.1 Open dislocation of shoulder
- 831.10 Open dislocation of shoulder, unspecified
- 831.11 Open anterior dislocation of humerus
- 831.12 Open posterior dislocation of humerus
- 831.13 Open inferior dislocation of humerus
- 831.19 Open dislocation of shoulder, other

ICD-10-CM CODES

- S43.006A Unspecified dislocation of unspecified shoulder joint, initial encounter
- S43.016A Anterior dislocation of unspecified humerus, initial encounter
- S43.026A Posterior dislocation of unspecified humerus, initial encounter
- S43.036A Inferior dislocation of unspecified humerus, initial encounter
- S43.086A Other dislocation of unspecified shoulder joint, initial encounter
- S43.109A Unspecified dislocation of unspecified acromioclavicular joint, initial encounter

PREFERRED PRACTICE PATTERN

- 4D: Impaired Joint Mobility, Motor Function, Muscle Performance, and Range of Motion Associated with Connective Tissue Dysfunction

PATIENT PRESENTATION

A 57-year-old male arrived with a complaint of right shoulder pain. Patient reports sudden onset of pain 2 days ago after falling on his outstretched right arm while playing soccer. He reports has been in "extreme" pain since then for which has been taking ibuprofen. He reports enjoys playing soccer at least once a week. Patient's PMH includes HTN, appendectomy, tonsillectomy, and right humeral fracture as a child due to a fall. He reports feeling concerned due to his current inability to work as a plumber as well as his inability to perform some ADLs. Patient lives with his wife, who has been helping him mainly to get dressed and shower. He was unable to sleep on his right side (as usual) due to increased pain. Upon examination, patient appears in pain with a guarded posture to his right arm which is in mild abduction and external rotation. ROM and strength of the right shoulder were unable to assess due to pain. MMT of the right hand and elbow were decreased. Sensation on the right anterior shoulder area was diminished to light touch. Special tests were positive for the Sulcus sign on the right shoulder. Right shoulder Anterior Drawer, Load and Shift, and Apprehension tests were unable to assess due to pain (which were expected to be positive). Right shoulder x-rays showed anterior dislocation of the humeral head. Right shoulder MRI showed tear of the anterior inferior labrum.

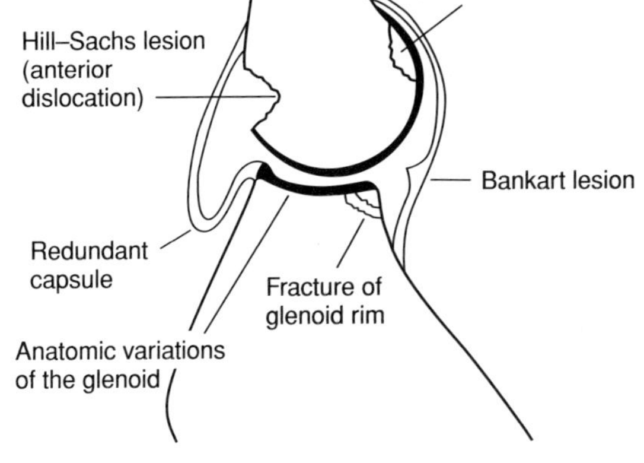

FIGURE 158-1 Anatomic lesions producing shoulder instability. (From Skinner HB: *Current Diagnosis & Treatment in Orthopedics.* 4th ed. www.accessmedicine.com. Copyright © The McGraw-Hill Companies, Inc. All rights reserved.)

KEY FEATURES

Description

- Humerus can dislocate anteriorly, posteriorly or inferiorly out of the socket.
- Excessive translation of the humeral head in one or more directions.
- The instability may be associated with dislocation or subluxation associated with a trauma event.
- GH instability may also be secondary to atraumatic factors associated with structural, postural, or movement dysfunction and possibly from recurrent minor injury to the structures of the glenohumeral joint.[1–3]
- Symptomatology and management is different depending on the onset, degree, frequency, direction, associated pathology, neuromuscular control, and premorbid activity level.[3]

- Anterior or anterior inferior instability.
  - Mechanism
    - 95% of traumatic shoulder instabilities.[3]
    - Can result in dislocation or subluxation.
    - The humerus is forced into extreme abduction and external rotation and/or horizontal abduction.
    - Associated pathology includes Bankart lesion (anterior), humeral avulsion of GH ligaments (HAGL), and Hill–Sachs lesion.[4]
  - Symptoms
    - Anterior and inferior shoulder pain
    - Instability and apprehension to abduction, external rotation and horizontal abduction motions.
- Posterior Instability
  - Mechanism
    - 5% of traumatic shoulder instabilities.[3]
    - Can result in dislocation or subluxation.
    - A fall on an outstretched arm of movements of extreme horizontal adduction or internal rotation.
    - Associated pathology includes disruption of the posterior capsule, tearing of the teres minor, and reverse Hill–Sachs lesion.[5]
  - Symptoms
    - Posterior shoulder pain
    - Instability and apprehension to flexion, horizontal adduction, and internal rotation.
- Multidirectional instability
  - Mechanism
    - May occur without episode of trauma, however, patient may have a history of traumatic dislocation.[6]
    - Can result in dislocation or subluxation.
    - Instability and apprehension are present in multiple directions, although one direction may be the primary direction of instability.
    - Associated pathology depends on the primary direction of instability, duration of instability, and history of trauma.[3,6]
  - Symptoms
    - Pain and instability are often determined by the direction of primary instability and can vary based on activity.

Essentials of Diagnosis

- Diagnosis is made primarily by clinical examination; however, imaging is often necessary to rule in or out associated pathology.
- Anterior instability is the most common followed by multidirectional and then posterior instability.

General Considerations

- Dislocation can tear ligaments, cartilage, and cause vascular or nerve (brachial plexus) injuries.
- Onset, degree, frequency, direction, associated pathology, neuromuscular control, and premorbid activity level dictate the diagnosis and management.[3]
- The GH, scapulothoracic, acromioclavicular, and sternoclavicular joint interaction must be examined to determine the optimal treatment plan.[7,8]

Demographics

- Young athletes are most commonly affected.[6]
- Males are more affected than females by traumatic instability; inconclusive evidence for atraumatic or multidirectional.

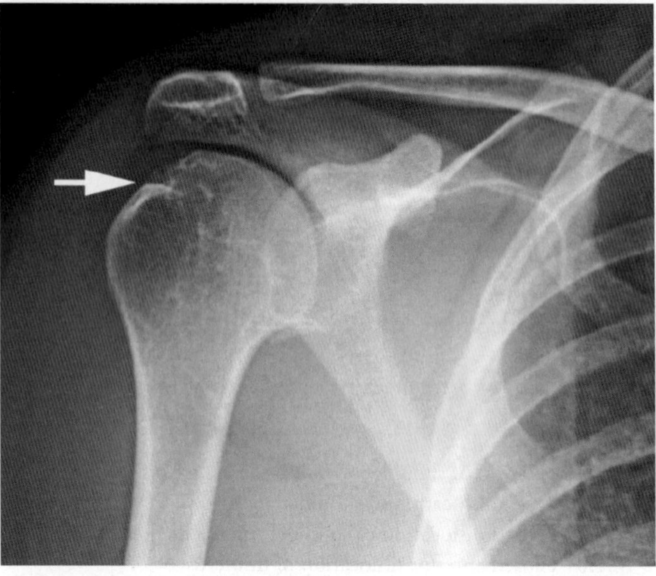

FIGURE 158-2 *Arrow* points to the Hill–Sachs deformity, resulting from a prior anterior shoulder dislocation. (Reproduced with permission from Simon RR, Sherman SC, Koenigsknecht SJ: *Emergency Orthopedics, The Extremities.* 5th ed. © 2007, McGraw-Hill Inc., New York.)

- Multidirectional instability may be associated with gymnastics, swimming, and weightlifting, and the individual may have increased joint laxity throughout the body.[6]

CLINICAL FINDINGS

SIGNS AND SYMPTOMS

- Specific signs and symptoms depend on the onset, degree, frequency, direction, and associated pathology of the injury
- Pain in the shoulder, location is often dependent on the primary direction of instability
- Feelings of instability and apprehension that are direction dependent to the primary direction of instability
- Hypermobility of the GH joint that is direction specific to the primary direction of instability[1]
- Clicking and popping may be present in the shoulder with movement
- Decreased upward rotation and increased internal rotation and protraction of the scapula
- Special tests for instability specific to the primary direction of instability
- In multidirectional instability, the patient may have higher scores on the Beighton scale for assessing generalized joint hypermobility
- Numbness for brachial plexus injury
- Vascular tearing or impingement

Functional Implications

- Difficulty with overhead activities
- Pain with end range motions of the shoulder
- Pain and difficulty with pushing and pulling activities
- Pain and difficulty with weight-bearing activities on the arm
- Pain with sleeping on the affected side

Possible Contributing Causes

- Poor posture: Specifically forward-shoulder posture and downwardly rotated, internally rotated, and/or protracted scapula
- Athletes, specifically swimmers, gymnasts, and overhead athletes[3,6]
- Increased joint laxity elsewhere in the body (high Beighton scale scores)
- Atraumatic instability may be increased by prior traumatic instability injury or a history of other shoulder injury[9]
- Genetic laxity
- Trauma

Differential Diagnosis

- Bankart lesion (anterior)
- Differential diagnosis may be direction specific
- Ehlers–Danlos
- Hill–Sachs lesion (anterior)
- Humeral avulsion of glenohumeral ligaments (HAGL) (anterior)
- Marfan syndrome
- Osteogenesis imperfect
- Reverse Hill–Sachs lesion (posterior)
- Tearing of the posterior capsule (posterior)
- Tearing of the Teres minor (posterior)

Means of Confirmation or Diagnosis

- Special tests[10,11]
  - Anterior instability
    - Apprehension test
    - Apprehension–relocation test
    - Sulcus sign
    - Anterior slide (drawer) test
    - Load and shift test
    - Crank test
  - Posterior instability
    - Posterior apprehension test
    - Posterior drawer
    - Load and shift test
    - Sulcus sign
  - Multidirectional instability
    - Sulcus sign
    - All tests for anterior and posterior instability are appropriate and may be indicated
  - Beighton scale

Imaging

- MRI and MR arthrography are the images of choice for instability.[9,12]
  - Conventional-traumatic
  - Arthrography-chronic
- CT
- Conventional radiograph

FINDINGS AND INTERPRETATION

- Physical examination is the current accepted means of diagnosis.
- Imaging to diagnose additional pathology.
- Hypermobility of the GH joint that may be direction specific.[1]
- Decreased upward rotation of the scapula and/or increased medial winging (internal rotation) of the scapula with humeral elevation.
- Increased scapulohumeral rhythm.
- Direction-specific positive special tests.
- Increased joint laxity throughout the body may be present.

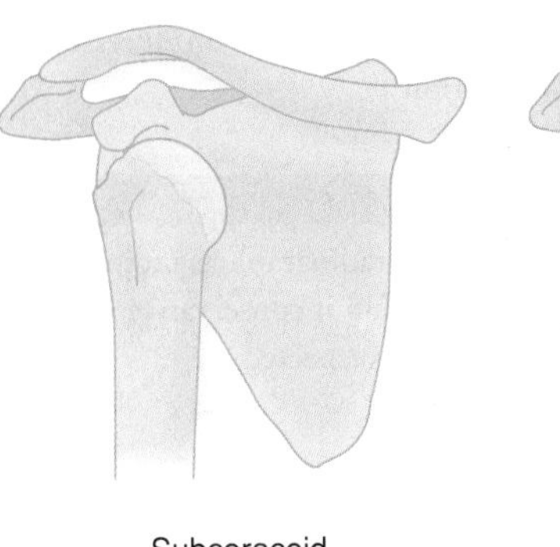

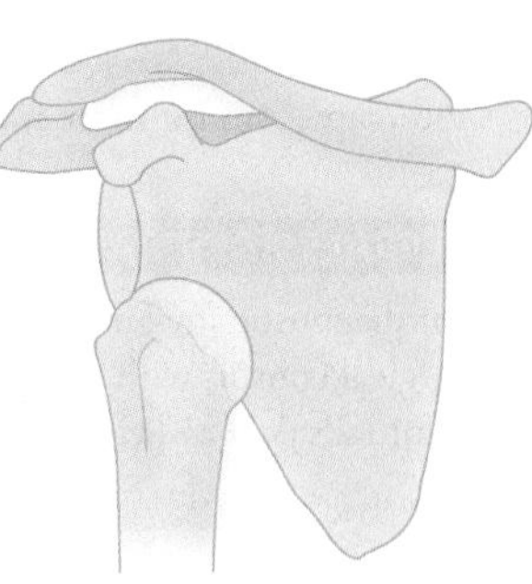

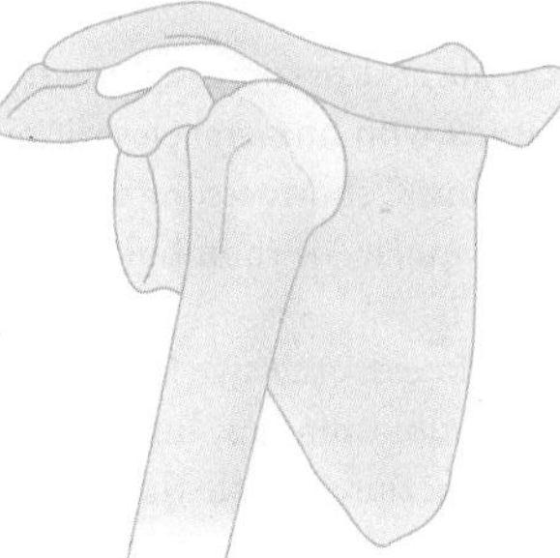

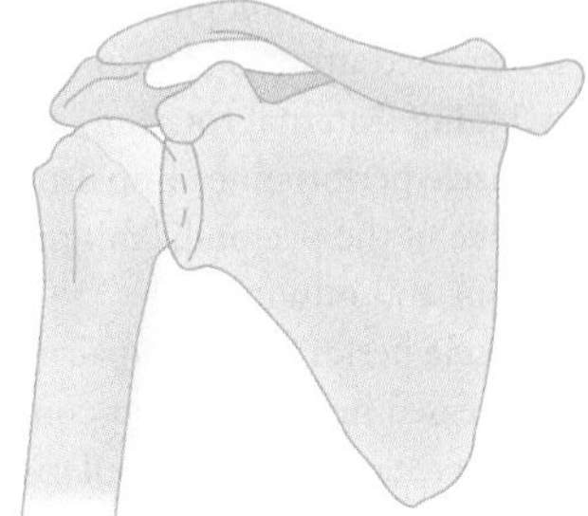

FIGURE 158-3 Types of anterior shoulder dislocations. (From Tintinalli JE et al: *Tintinalli's Emergency Medicine: A Comprehensive Study Guide.* 7th ed. www.accessmedicine.com. Copyright © The McGraw-Hill Companies, Inc. All rights reserved.)

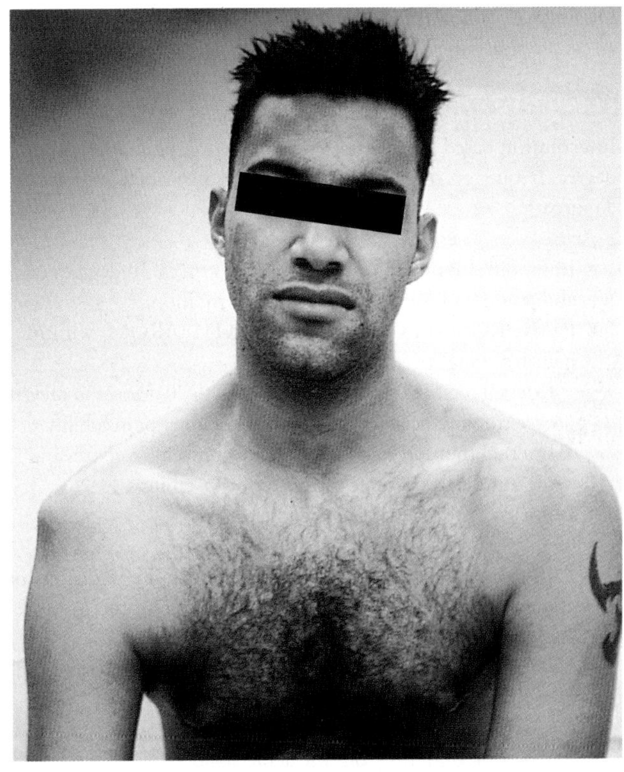

FIGURE 158-4 Anterior shoulder dislocation. This right anterior shoulder dislocation occurred when the patient fell while playing basketball. There is an obvious contour deformity as well as prominence of the acromion. (From Knoop KJ et al: *The Atlas of Emergency Medicine.* 3rd ed. www.accessmedicine.com. Copyright © The McGraw-Hill Companies, Inc. All rights reserved. Photo contributor: Kevin J. Knoop, MD, MS.)

- See Case Study: Neck Pain and Arm Paresthesia on AccessPhysiotherapy.com for more information

REFERRALS/ADMITTANCE

- For diagnostic imaging, MRI, CT, or radiograph as indicated
- Surgical consult with orthopedic surgeon if conservative treatment fails or if associated pathology is suspected

IMPAIRMENTS

- Hypermobility of the GH joint that may be direction specific;[1]
- Excessive, direction-specific accessory motions of the humeral head with physiologic shoulder movements;
- Decreased upward rotation of the scapula and/or increased medial winging (internal rotation) of the scapula with humeral elevation;
- Muscle performance impairment of stiffness, shortness, or dominance of the pectoralis minor, levator scapulae, or rhomboid major and minor;
- Muscle performance impairment of weakness, excessive length, or decreased neuromuscular control of the supraspinatus, infraspinatus, teres minor, subscapularis, upper trapezius, middle trapezius, lower trapezius, and serratus anterior;
- Structural impairments of the humerus or glenoid, such as flattening of the glenoid may be present;
- Pain with direction-specific shoulder motions. Range of motion may initially be excessive; however, the shoulder ROM may be limited by pain once symptomatic.

TESTS AND MEASURES

- Disabilities of the Arm, Shoulder and Hand (DASH) score to assess physical function

INTERVENTION

- Intervention based on the type (traumatic or atraumatic), onset, degree, frequency, direction, and potential associated pathology.[3]
- Traumatic
  - Acute
    - Immobilization may be used with the arm in 30 degrees of abduction and 30 degrees of external rotation.[13]
    - Passive ROM (PROM) and active ROM (AROM) within pain-free ranges.
      - External rotation may be limited to 65 to 70 degrees to prevent overstressing the anterior structures for anterior instability.
      - Internal rotation may be limited to prevent overstressing the anterior structures for posterior instability.
    - Isometric, pain-free strengthening.
    - Gentle, pain-free weight bearing on the arm.
    - Pain-free dynamic stabilization with the arm in 30 degrees of abduction, neutral rotation and 30 degrees into the scapular plane.
    - Modalities as needed to control pain, inflammation, and muscle guarding.
  - Intermediate
    - Progression of items from the acute stage.
    - Isotonic strengthening may be initiated with emphasis on rotator cuff musculature to promote stability.
    - Progression of weight-bearing exercise such as modified push-ups with an emphasis on maintaining correct scapular alignment may be initiated to promote stability.

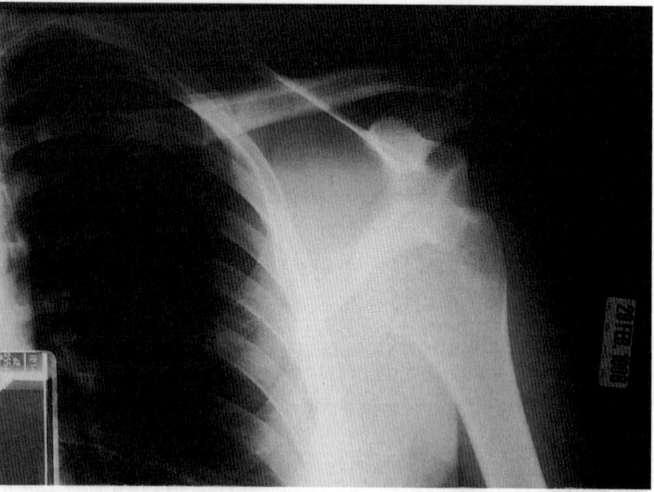

FIGURE 158-5 Anterior shoulder dislocation. Radiographic evaluation demonstrates that the humeral head is not in the glenoid fossa but is located anterior and inferior to it. (From Knoop KJ et al: *The Atlas of Emergency Medicine.* 3rd ed. www.accessmedicine.com. Copyright © The McGraw-Hill Companies, Inc. All rights reserved. Photo contributor: Kevin J. Knoop, MD, MS.)

    - Trunk stabilization exercise may be initiated to enhance correct movement patterns and reduce abnormal stress to the GH joint.
    - Neuromuscular electrical stimulation (NMES) to the muscles of the rotator cuff during exercise to improve muscle fiber recruitment.
  - Advanced
    - Progression of all items from intermediate stage.
    - Unilateral weight-bearing stability exercise, such as wall stabilization drills with medicine or stability balls.
    - Proper alignment of the scapula should be maintained during all stabilization exercise.
    - Plyometric exercise progressing to overhead and then unilateral may be indicated if the patient is returning to sport.
- Atraumatic
  - Intervention is very similar to that used following traumatic instability.
  - Progression may be slower than with traumatic.
  - Care should be taken to prevent stretching of capsular tissues.
  - Exercise that emphasizes co-contraction and proprioception is indicated.

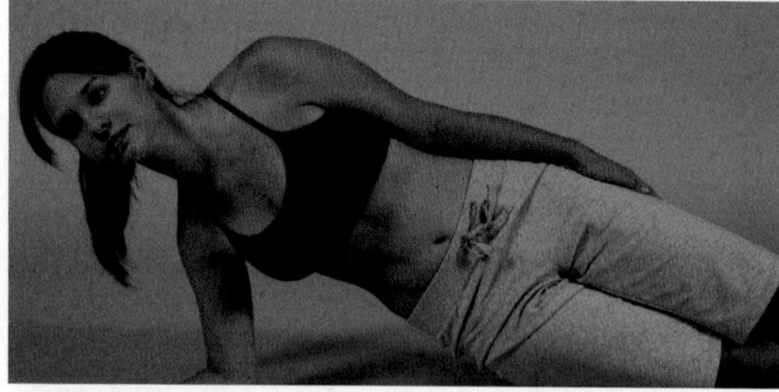

FIGURE 158-6 Side planks for shoulder and core stability. (From Dutton M: *Dutton's Orthopaedic Examination, Evaluation, and Intervention.* 3rd ed. http://www.accessphysiotherapy.com. Copyright © The McGraw-Hill Companies, Inc. All rights reserved.)

- Exercise with an emphasis on muscle balance about the shoulder girdle with correct positioning and movement of the scapula should be performed.
- Trunk-stability exercise to improve stability during functional tasks should be initiated once patient is able to stabilize the GH joint.

FUNCTIONAL GOALS

Note: The duration portion of the goals will be dependent on the onset, degree, frequency, direction, associated pathology, neuromuscular control, and premorbid activity level.[3]

- Patient will be able to
  - Dress without pain or instability 95% of the time.
  - Perform all self-care activities without pain or instability 95% of the time.
  - Sleep through the night without being woken by pain 95% of the time.
  - Bear full weight through the arms without pain or instability 95% of the time.
  - Lift 10 pounds overhead without pain or instability 95% of the time.
  - Perform all daily activities without pain or instability 95% of the time.
  - Return to recreational tasks without pain or instability 95% of the time.

PROGNOSIS

- Return to function may be anywhere from 2 weeks to 6 months and rehabilitation visits may range from 3 to 36 visits, dependent on the onset, degree, frequency, direction, associated pathology, neuromuscular control, and premorbid activity level.[3,14]
- Recurrence is common in the younger population, while additional pathology is often seen in individuals more than 40 years of age.[15]

PATIENT RESOURCE

- Traumatic shoulder dislocation. AOSSM Sports Tips. http://www.sportsmed.org/uploadedFiles/Content/Patient/Sports_Tips/ST%20Traumatic%20Shoulder%2008.pdf. Accessed July 9, 2013.

REFERENCES

1. Cameron KL, Duffey ML, DeBerardino TM, Stoneman PD, Jones CJ, Owens BD. Association of generalized joint hypermobility with a history of glenohumeral joint instability. *J Athl Train*. 2010;45(3):253–258. [PMID: 20446838]
2. Owens BD, Duffey ML, Nelson BJ, DeBerardino TM, Taylor DC, Mountcastle SB. The incidence and characteristics of shoulder instability at the United States Military Academy. *Am J Sports Med*. 2007;35(7):1168–1173. doi: 10.1177/0363546506295179. [PMID: 17581976]
3. Wilk KE, Macrina LC, Reinold MM. Non-operative rehabilitation for traumatic and atraumatic glenohumeral instability. *N Am J Sports Phys Ther*. 2006;1(1):16–31. [PMID: 21522197]
4. Pope EJ, Ward JP, Rokito AS. Anterior shoulder instability - a history of arthroscopic treatment. *Bull NYU Hosp Jt Dis*. 2011;69(1):44–49. [PMID: 21332438]
5. Hottya GA, Tirman PF, Bost FW, Montgomery WH, Wolf EM, Genant HK. Tear of the posterior shoulder stabilizers after posterior dislocation: MR imaging and MR arthrographic findings with arthroscopic correlation. *AJR Am J Roentgenol*. 1998;171(3):763–768. [PMID: 9725313]
6. Cordasco FA. Understanding multidirectional instability of the shoulder. *J Athl Train*. 2000;35(3):278–285. [PMID: 16558641]
7. Kikuchi K, Itoi E, Yamamoto N, et al. Scapular inclination and glenohumeral joint stability: a cadaveric study. *J Orthop Sci*. 2008;13(1):72–77. doi: 10.1007/s00776-007-1186-2. [PMID: 18274859]
8. Ludewig PM, Reynolds JF. The association of scapular kinematics and glenohumeral joint pathologies. *J Orthop Sports Phys Ther*. 2009;39(2):90–104. doi: 10.2519/jospt.2009.2808. [PMID: 19194022]
9. Jana M, Gamanagatti S. Magnetic resonance imaging in glenohumeral instability. *World J Radiol*. 2011;3(9):224–232. doi: 10.4329/wjr.v3.i9.224. [PMID: 22007285]
10. Cook CE, Hegedus EJ. *Orthopedic Physical Examination Tests: An Evidence-Based Approach*. Upper Saddle River, NJ: Prentice Hall; 2008.
11. Magee DJ. *Orthopedic physical assessment*. 5th ed. St. Louis, MO: Saunders Elsevier; 2008.
12. Waldt S, Rummeny EJ. [Magnetic resonance imaging of glenohumeral instability]. *Rofo*. 2006;178(6):590–599. doi: 10.1055/s-2006-926745. [PMID: 16703494]
13. Itoi E, Hatakeyama Y, Kido T, et al. A new method of immobilization after traumatic anterior dislocation of the shoulder: a preliminary study. *J Shoulder Elbow Surg*. 2003;12(5):413–415. doi:10.1016/S1058-2746(03)00171-X. [PMID: 14564258]
14. American Physical Therapy Association. Guide to Physical Therapists Practice 2nd Ed. *Phys Ther*. 2002;81:9–744. [PMID: 11175682]
15. Sonnabend DH. Treatment of primary anterior shoulder dislocation in patients older than 40 years of age. Conservative versus operative. *Clin Orthop Relat Res*. 1994;(304):74–77. [PMID: 8020237]

ADDITIONAL REFERENCES

- Dutton M, ed. *Dutton's Orthopaedic Examination, Evaluation, and Intervention*. 3rd ed. New York: McGraw-Hill; 2012. http://www.accessphysiotherapy.com/content/55598900. Accessed July 9, 2013.
- Dutton M, Dutton M, eds. *Dutton's Orthopedic Survival Guide: Managing Common Conditions*. New York, NY: McGraw-Hill; 2011. http://www.accessphysiotherapy.com/content/8656027. Accessed August 9, 2014.
- ICD9Data.com. http://www.icd9data.com. Accessed July 3, 2013.
- ICD10Data.com. http://www.icd10data.com. Accessed July 3, 2013.
- Malone TR, Hazle C, Grey ML. Chapter 1. Introduction to Musculoskeletal Imaging. In: Malone TR, Hazle C, Grey ML, eds. *Imaging in Rehabilitation*. New York, NY: McGraw-Hill; 2008. http://www.accessphysiotherapy.com/content/5940000. Accessed August 9, 2014.
- Pattern 4D: Impaired joint mobility, motor function, muscle performance, and range of motion associated with connective tissue dysfunction. In: *Guide to Physical Therapist Practice*. 2nd ed. Alexandria, VA: American Physical Therapy Association; 2001. Revised 2003.

159 SHOULDER FRACTURE

Jennifer Cabrera, DPT, GCS
Eric Shamus, PhD, DPT, PT, CSCS

CONDITION/DISORDER SYNONYMS

- Proximal humeral fracture
- Shoulder fracture

ICD-9-CM CODES[1]

- 812.00 Fracture of unspecified part of upper end of humerus closed
- 812.01 Fracture of surgical neck of humerus closed
- 812.02 Fracture of anatomical neck of humerus closed
- 812.03 Fracture of greater tuberosity of humerus closed
- 812.09 Other closed fractures of upper end of humerus
- 812.10 Fracture of unspecified part of upper end of humerus open
- 812.11 Fracture of surgical neck of humerus open
- 812.12 Fracture of anatomical neck of humerus open
- 812.13 Fracture of greater tuberosity of humerus open
- 812.19 Other open fractures of upper end of humerus

ICD-10-CM CODES[2]

- S42.209A Unspecified fracture of upper end of unspecified humerus, initial encounter for closed fracture
- S42.209B Unspecified fracture of upper end of unspecified humerus, initial encounter
- S42.213A Unspecified displaced fracture of surgical neck of unspecified humerus, initial encounter for closed fracture
- S42.213B Unspecified displaced fracture of surgical neck of unspecified humerus, initial encounter for open fracture
- S42.216A Unspecified nondisplaced fracture of surgical neck of unspecified humerus, initial encounter for closed fracture
- S42.216B Unspecified nondisplaced fracture of surgical neck of unspecified humerus, initial encounter for open fracture
- S42.253A Displaced fracture of greater tuberosity of unspecified humerus, initial encounter for closed fracture
- S42.253B Displaced fracture of greater tuberosity of unspecified humerus, initial encounter for open fracture
- S42.256A Nondisplaced fracture of greater tuberosity of unspecified humerus, initial encounter for closed fracture
- S42.256B Nondisplaced fracture of greater tuberosity of unspecified humerus, initial encounter for open fracture
- S42.293A Other displaced fracture of upper end of unspecified humerus, initial encounter for closed fracture
- S42.293B Other displaced fracture of upper end of unspecified humerus, initial encounter for open fracture
- S42.295A Other nondisplaced fracture of upper end of left humerus, initial encounter for closed fracture
- S42.296A Other nondisplaced fracture of upper end of unspecified humerus, initial encounter for closed fracture or open fracture
- S42.296B Other nondisplaced fracture of upper end of unspecified humerus, initial encounter for open fracture

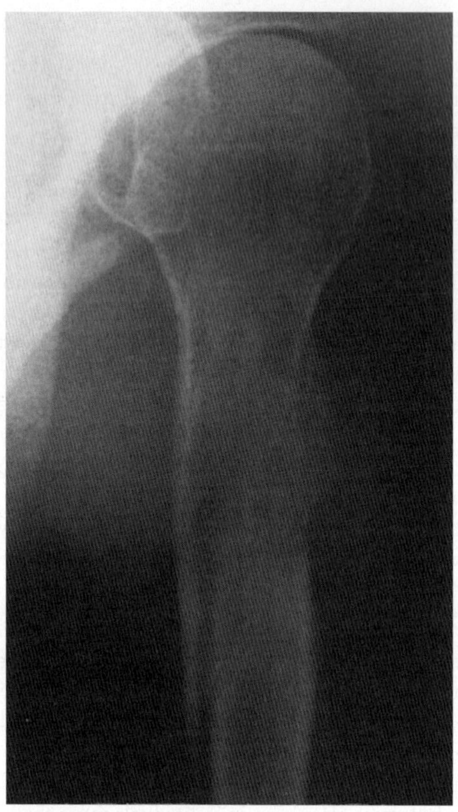

FIGURE 159-1 AP view of the proximal left humerus. An acute fracture has occurred through an area of bone destruction caused by metastatic carcinoma. Conventional radiographs are used to identify bony metastases that have destroyed enough bone to make a pathologic fracture likely. (From Chen MYM, Pope TL, Ott DJ. *Basic Radiology*. 2nd ed. http://www.accessmedicine.com. Copyright © The McGraw-Hill Companies, Inc. All rights reserved.)

PREFERRED PRACTICE PATTERN

- 4G: Impaired Joint Mobility, Muscle Performance, and Range of Motion Associated with Fracture[3]

PATIENT PRESENTATION

An 83-year-old woman went to use the restroom, slipped and hit her right arm against the sink. She felt immediate pain in her arm and was unable to move her shoulder. Patient has diagnosed osteoporosis × 10 years for which she does not take bisphosphonates. She presented with pain and swelling throughout the upper extremity (UE) with visible deformity. She demonstrated increased tenderness upon palpation of humerus and shoulder. Radiograph showed a displaced transverse fracture of the proximal humerus.

KEY FEATURES

▶ Description

- Fracture
- Any defect in continuity of the proximal humerus

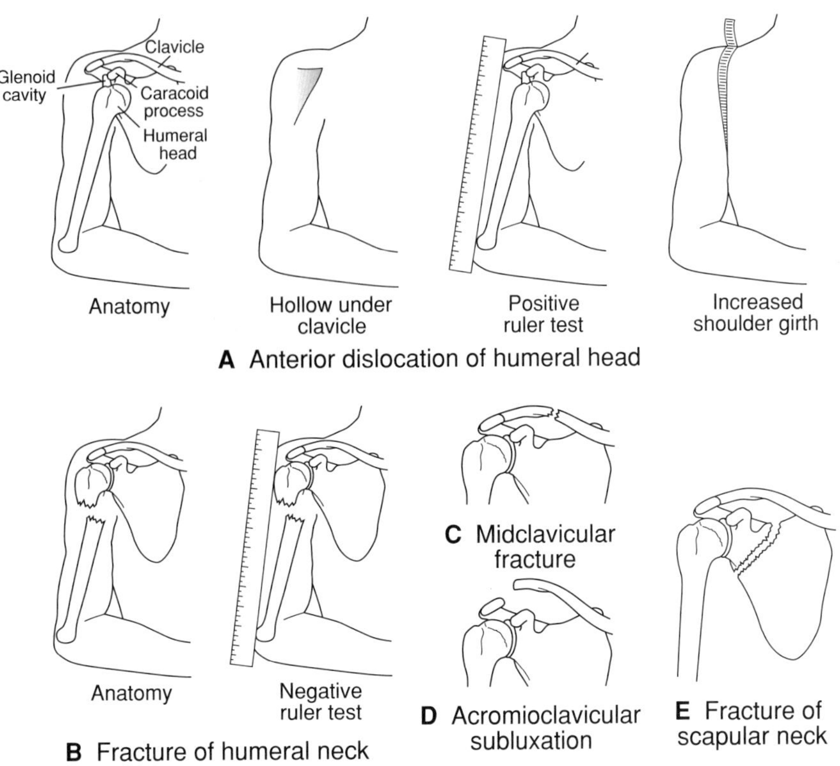

FIGURE 159-2 Traumatic disorders of the shoulder. (**A**) Anterior dislocation of the humeral head. (**B**) Fracture of the humeral neck. (**C**) Midclavicular fracture. (**D**) Acromioclavicular subluxation. (**E**) Fracture of the scapular neck. (From LeBlond RF, DeGowin RL, Brown DD. *DeGowin's Diagnostic Examination*. 9th ed. http://www.accessmedicine.com. Copyright © The McGraw-Hill Companies, Inc. All rights reserved.)

- Displaced (proximal humerus is moved on either side of the fracture) or nondisplaced (proximal humerus has not moved)
- Closed (skin is intact) or open (skin is breached)

Essentials of Diagnosis

- Diagnosis is usually made by clinical examination
- May not be a fracture, but a dislocation, an acromioclavicular (AC) sprain, or a rotator cuff strain

General Considerations

- Accounts for 5% of all fractures

Demographics

- Occurs primarily in older patients

CLINICAL FINDINGS

SIGNS AND SYMPTOMS

- Pain
- Point tenderness
- Edema
- Ecchymosis
- Loss of general function
- Loss of active mobility
- Muscle guarding with passive movement

Functional Implications

- Patient will present with involved UE in position of protection: Shoulder adduction, internal rotation, and elbow flexion.
- Patient will be unable to tolerate any functional use of involved UE secondary to pain.

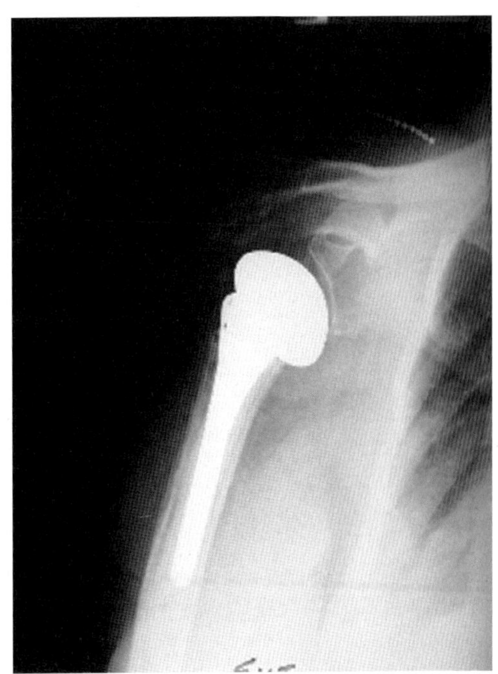

FIGURE 159-3 Surgical reconstruction with hemiarthroplasty. (From Doherty GM. *Current Diagnosis & Treatment: Surgery*. 13th ed. http://www.accessmedicine.com. Copyright © The McGraw-Hill Companies, Inc. All rights reserved.)

Possible Contributing Causes

- Osteoporosis
- Mechanism of injury
  - Fall on outstretched hand
  - High-energy trauma (younger children)
  - Violent muscle contractions (seizure, athletic activity)
  - Direct blow to proximal humerus
- Impaired standing balance
- Polypharmacy

Differential Diagnosis

- Shoulder dislocation
- Scapular fracture
- AC sprain
- Rotator cuff strain or tear

MEANS OF CONFIRMATION OR DIAGNOSIS

Imaging

- X-ray for fracture, often limited view
- Computerized tomography (CT) scan for detailed imaging

FINDINGS AND INTERPRETATION

- Involved UE in position of protection: Shoulder adduction and internal rotation and elbow flexion secondary to glenohumeral (GH) capsular pattern (external rotation, abduction, internal rotation).
- Unable to tolerate active ROM (AROM)/passive ROM (PROM) of involved UE secondary to pain.
- If vascular structures are involved, the UE will appear cool and pale, with diminished palpable pulses.
- If neurologic structures are involved, the individual will report numbness and decreased ability to move the involved UE (e.g., axillary nerve).

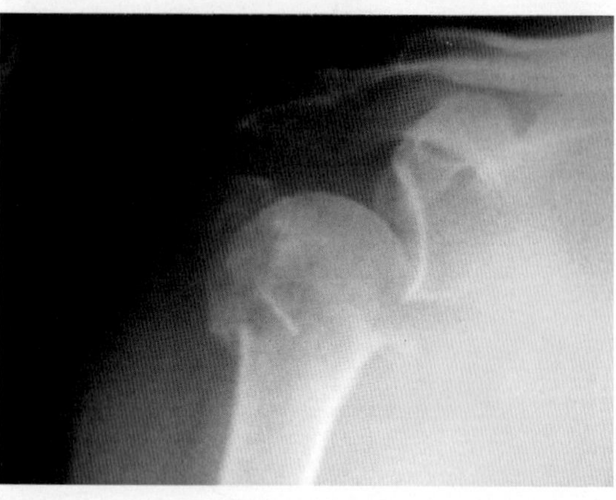

FIGURE 159-4 Four-part proximal humerus fracture, impacted on inferior glenoid rim. (From Doherty GM. *Current Diagnosis & Treatment: Surgery*. 13th ed. http://www.accessmedicine.com. Copyright © The McGraw-Hill Companies, Inc. All rights reserved.)

REFERRALS/ADMITTANCE

- For imaging, X-ray or CT
- For medication, NSAID or opioid for pain management
- For orthopedic consult
  - Nondisplaced fractures are treated nonoperatively
    - Immobilization via sling/sling and swathe/shoulder immobilizer
  - Displaced fractures are treated operatively
    - Open reduction with internal fixation
    - Closed reduction with percutaneous fixation
    - Humeral head replacement

IMPAIRMENTS

- Inability to
  - Perform self-care needs secondary to pain and impaired ROM
  - Reach overhead secondary to pain

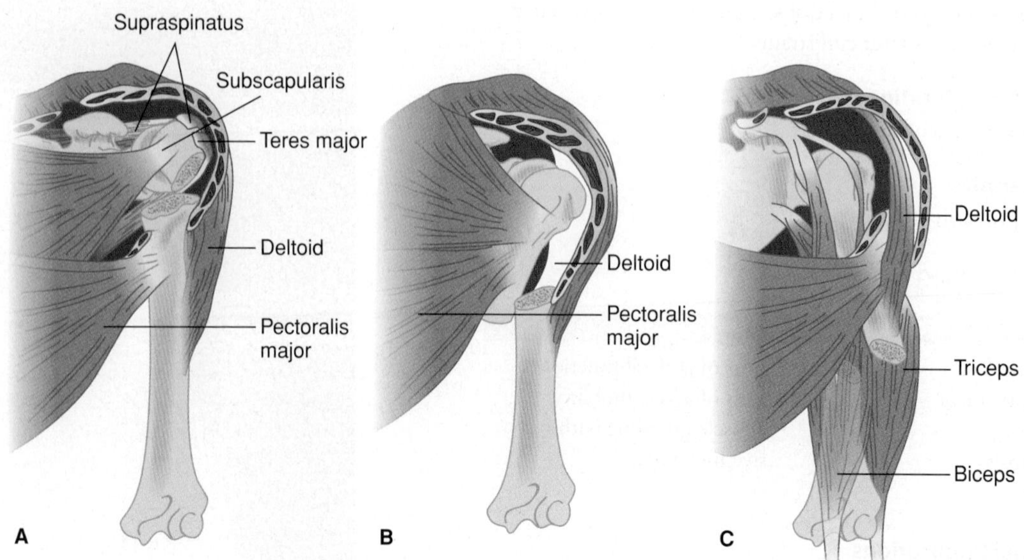

FIGURE 159-5 Humeral fractures anterior view. The actions of the muscles inserting on the humeral shaft determine fracture angulation and displacement. (**A**) Angulation of fragments with fracture line distal to rotator cuff insertion. (**B**) Angulation of fragments with fracture line distal to pectoralis major insertion. (**C**) Angulation of fragments with fracture line distal to deltoid insertion. (From Tintinalli JE, Stapczynski J, Ma OJ, Cline D, Cydulka R, Meckler G. *Tintinalli's Emergency Medicine: A Comprehensive Study Guide*. 7th ed. www.accessmedicine.com. Copyright © The McGraw-Hill Companies, Inc. All rights reserved.)

- ◦ Bear weight on involved UE secondary to pain
- ◦ Carry groceries secondary to pain and muscle weakness

TESTS AND MEASURES

- Aerobic endurance
- Functional strength, manual muscle testing (MMT)
- Upper-extremity ROM
- Posture
- Structural (shoulder complex, cervical, thoracic)
- Disabilities of the Arm, Shoulder and Hand (DASH) score to assess physical function
- Sensory integrity

INTERVENTION

- Address swelling
  - Ice/cryotherapy
  - Compression
  - Elevation
  - Electrical stimulation
- Address pain
  - Ice/cryotherapy
  - Massage
  - Electrical stimulation
- Address lack of flexibility via stretching
  - Long head of the biceps
  - Pectoralis
  - Wand exercises for increased joint ROM
- Address mobilization upon healing of fracture site (after 6 weeks postoperative)
  - GH distraction
  - GH caudal glide for abduction
  - GH posterior glide for flexion and internal rotation
  - GH anterior glide for extension and external rotation
- Address weakness via strengthening activities
  - Closed-chain weight-bearing activities
  - Isometric exercises (initially submaximal)
  - Open chain via use of free weights and resistance bands
- Address functional mobility if applicable
  - Bed-mobility training
  - Transfer training with use of assistive device (such as hemi walker, quad cane, straight cane)
- Address scar mobility
  - Scar tissue mobilization progressing from parallel to perpendicular upon wound closure

FUNCTIONAL GOALS

- Patient will
  - Demonstrate decreased QuickDASH (disability of the arm, shoulder, and hand) score to 18 in order to exhibit diminishing disability.
  - Increase shoulder internal rotation to 70 degrees in order to don/doff brassiere.
  - Increase shoulder abduction to 112 degrees in order to comb hair.
  - Increase arm curl test repetitions to 24 in order to increase UE strength for household chores.

PROGNOSIS

- Shoulder fracture as a whole requires 1 year of recovery.
- Major cause of morbidity in the elderly population.
- Individuals who undergo an open reduction internal fixation.
  - 9% implant related complications.
  - 35% nonimplant related complications.

PATIENT RESOURCE

- Frankle M. *Proximal Humerus Fractures*. Medscape Reference. Available at: http://emedicine.medscape.com/article/1261320-overview#aw2aab6b2b1aa. Accessed on July 2, 2013.

REFERENCES

1. ICD9Data.com. http://www.icd9data.com. Accessed July 3, 2013.
2. ICD10Data.com. http://www.icd10data.com. Accessed July 3, 2013.
3. Pattern 4G: impaired joint mobility, muscle performance, and range of motion associated with fracture. In: *Guide to Physical Therapist Practice*. 2nd ed. Alexandria, VA: American Physical Therapy Association; 2001. Revised 2003.

ADDITIONAL REFERENCES

- Goodman CC, Boissonnault WG, Fuller KS. *Pathology: Implications for the Physical Therapist*. 2nd ed. Philadelphia, PA: Saunders; 2003.
- Hall SJ. The biomechanics of human bone growth and development. In: Hall SJ, ed. *Basic Biomechanics*. 5th ed. New York, NY: McGraw-Hill; 2007:Chapter 4. http://www.accessphysiotherapy.com/content/6060744. Accessed July 9, 2013.
- Kisner C, Colby LA. *Therapeutic Exercise: Foundations and Techniques*. 5th ed. Philadelphia, PA: F.A. Davis Company; 2007.
- Magee DJ. *Orthopedic Physical Assessment*. 5th ed. St. Louis, MO: Saunders Elsevier; 2008.
- Malone TR, Hazle C, Grey ML. Introduction to musculoskeletal imaging. In: Malone TR, Hazle C, Grey ML, eds. *Imaging in Rehabilitation*. New York, NY: McGraw-Hill; 2008:Chapter 1. http://www.accessphysiotherapy.com/content/5940000. Accessed July 9, 2013.
- Maxey L, Magnusson J. *Rehabilitation for the Postsurgical Orthopedic Patient*. 2nd ed. St. Louis, MO: Mosby Elsevier; 2007.
- Prentice WE, Quillen WS, Underwood F, eds. *Therapeutic Modalities in Rehabilitation*. 4th ed. New York, NY: McGraw-Hill; 2011. http://www.accessphysiotherapy.com/content/8137872. Accessed July 9, 2013.

160 SUBACROMIAL IMPINGEMENT SYNDROME

W. Justin Jones, DPT, PT, OCS
Eric Shamus, PhD, DPT, PT, CSCS

CONDITION/DISORDER SYNONYMS

- Impingement syndrome shoulder
- Shoulder impingement
- Subacromial compression

ICD-9-CM CODE[1]

- 726.19 Other specified disorders of bursae and tendons in shoulder region

ICD-10-CM CODE[2]

- M75.80 Other shoulder lesions, unspecified shoulder

PREFERRED PRACTICE PATTERN[3]

- Pattern 4E: Impaired Joint Mobility, Motor Function, Muscle Performance, and Range of Motion Associated with Localized Inflammation

PATIENT PRESENTATION

A 43-year-old male presents to the OP PT clinic with complaints of right shoulder pain. The patient states it has been bothering him for about 4 weeks. He describes the pain as more of a discomfort. He denies any cervical pain and any radicular symptoms in the arms. He thinks it began when he was throwing a Nerf football with his 10-year-old son. The football does not weigh very much and he says he has to throw the ball hard when passing. If he does not use the arm overhead the shoulder does not bother him much. The patient has good strength throughout the shoulder and is negative for an empty can test and acromioclavicular (AC) compression test.

KEY FEATURES

Description

- Shoulder pain and dysfunction due to compression and abrasion of one or more of the rotator cuff tendons, the long head of the bicep tendon, and/or the subacromial bursa beneath the coracoacromial arch due to an abnormal mechanical relationship.
- The coracoacromial arch consists of the undersurface of the acromion, coracoacromial ligament as well as the undersurface of the AC joint.
- Impingement is the most commonly diagnosed shoulder problem and likely has numerous potential mechanisms, which can impact both treatment and prognosis.

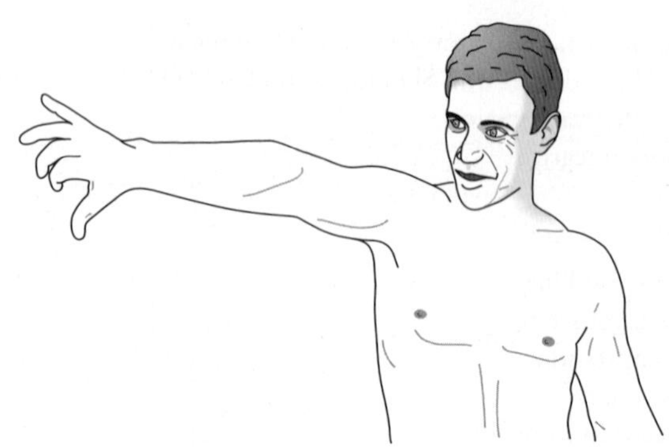

FIGURE 160-1 Evaluating for impingement of the supraspinatus tendon with the "empty can" test. (From Skinner HB. *Current Diagnosis & Treatment in Orthopedics*. 4th ed. www.accessmedicine.com. Copyright © The McGraw-Hill Companies, Inc. All rights reserved.)

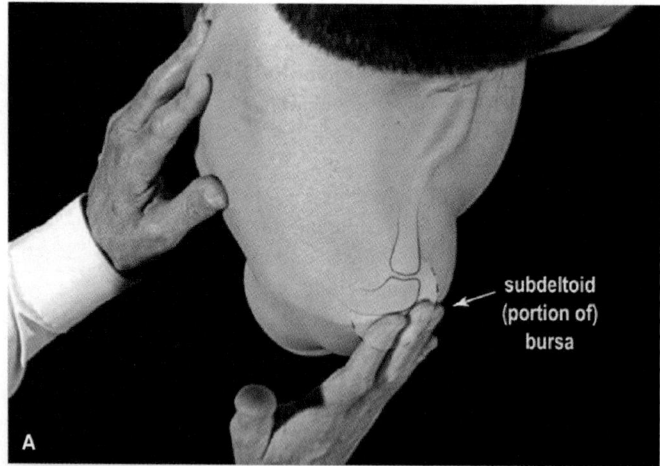

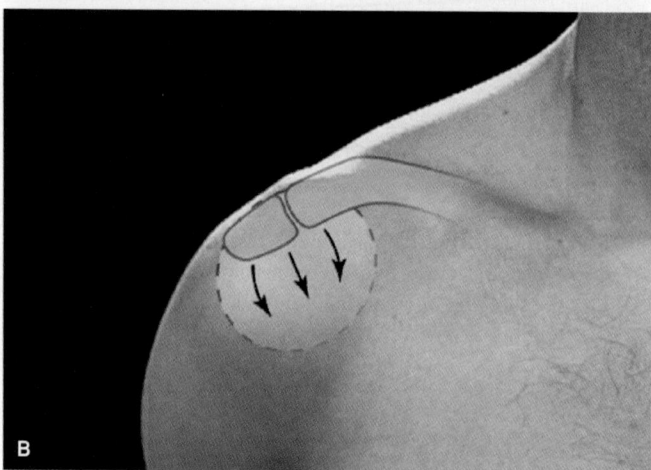

FIGURE 160-2 **A** and **B**. Palpation and location of the subdeltoid portion of the bursa. (From Lawry GV. *Systematic Musculoskeletal Examinations*. www.accessmedicine.com. Copyright © The McGraw-Hill Companies, Inc. All rights reserved.)

Essentials of Diagnosis

- Multifactorial and thought to be related to intrinsic and/or extrinsic mechanisms
  - Extrinsic mechanisms (extratendinous, cause decreased subacromial space and subsequent microtrauma with repetitive movements)
    - Mechanical wear under the coracoacromial arch
    - Aberrant movement patterns due to rotator cuff and or periscapular muscular dysfunction
    - Capsular abnormalities
      - Capsular tightness (particularly posterior capsule)
      - Capsular laxity (poor humeral head dynamic control)
    - Suboptimal posture
      - Muscle imbalances
    - Overuse/repetitive motions occurring above 90 degrees of elevation
  - Intrinsic factors (directly associated with the narrowing of the subacromial space)
    - Vascular supply/changes to the cuff tendons
    - Acromial morphology (structural variations)
      - Type I (flat)
      - Type II (curved)
      - Type III (hooked)
    - Degenerative and/or structural changes to the AC joint
    - Other trophic changes in the coracoacromial arch or humeral head
- Classification
  - Primary impingement is usually associated with degenerative changes to any of the following tissues:
    - Rotator cuff tendons
    - AC joint
    - Coracoacromial arch
  - Secondary impingement is the result of muscle imbalances and/or joint instability, which can result in altered dynamics and subsequent secondary impingement.
  - Neer stages
    - Stage I: Edema and hemorrhage of the subacromial bursa; patient is generally younger than 25 years of age
    - Stage II: Histologic changes of tendinosis to the effected tendons; patient usually between 25 and 40 years of age
    - Stage III: Partial or complete rupture of the cuff and or bicep tendons and potential associated changes to the acromion and AC joint; patient usually older than 40 years of age
      - Third class of impingement, not subacromial in nature: Internal impingement occurs between the undersurface (articular side) of the rotator cuff tendons and the posterior/superior surface of the labrum in the position of abduction and external rotation that occurs with throwing.
  - Regardless of classification, all types of impingement are proposed to be mechanisms of rotator cuff and biceps tendinopathy
  - Treatment varies based on impingement type, contributing factors, and associated tissue quality
  - Diagnosis is usually made by clinical examination and often accompanies three or more special tests[4]
    - Neer's impingement test
    - Hawkins–Kennedy impingement sign/test
    - Passive horizontal adduction test
    - Pain with resisted abduction
    - Painful arc sign/test
    - Pain in the C5–C6 dermatome region
    - Infraspinatus muscle test[1]
    - Diagnostic test properties for subacromial impingement

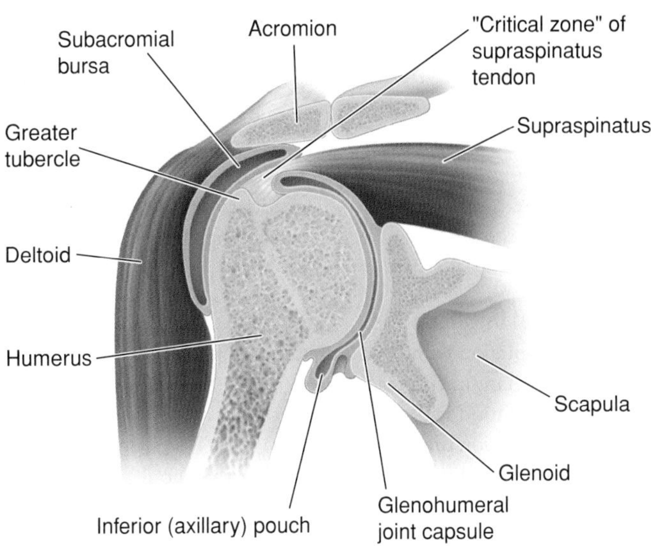

FIGURE 160-3 Coronal section of the shoulder illustrating the relationships of the glenohumeral joint, the joint capsule, the subacromial bursa, and the rotator cuff (supraspinatus tendon). (From F Kozin. In: WJ Koopman, ed. *Arthritis and Allied Conditions*. 13th ed. Baltimore, Williams & Wilkins; 1997, with permission.)

General Considerations

- Most common orthopedic shoulder problem
- Thought to often precipitate cuff and biceps tendinopathy

Demographics

- Primary impingement (generally occurs in patients aged 40 and older)
- Secondary impingement (generally occurs in younger patients aged 15 to 35)

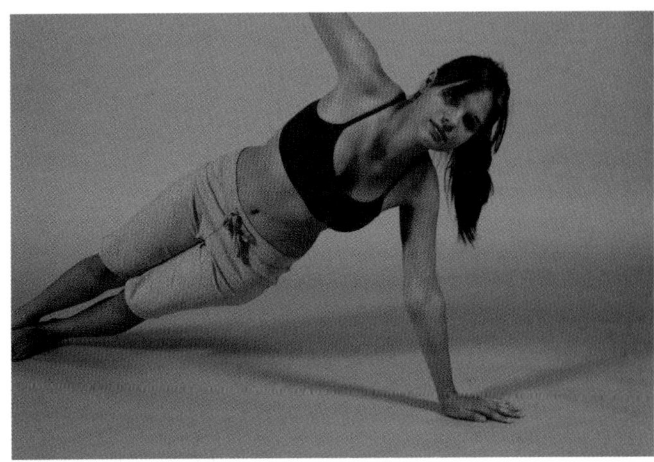

FIGURE 160-4 Straight arm side planks for increased difficulty of shoulder and core training. (From Dutton M. *Dutton's Orthopaedic Examination, Evaluation, and Intervention*. 3rd ed. http://www.accessphysiotherapy.com. Copyright © The McGraw-Hill Companies, Inc. All rights reserved.)

CLINICAL FINDINGS

SIGNS AND SYMPTOMS

- Pain in anterior lateral shoulder with active movement and overhead activities
- Painful arc commonly present in the midrange of shoulder elevation
- Weakness is commonly noted with functional reaching tasks

Functional Implications

- Pain/Limitation with overhead activities
- Pain/Limitation with reaching
- Pain/Limitation with lifting
- Pain/Limitation dressing
- Pain/Limitation with sustained or repetitive shoulder activities
- Pain at night (sleep disruption)

Possible Contributing Causes

- Acromion morphology
  - Type I
  - Type II
  - Type III
- Degenerative changes at the AC joint
- Rotator cuff tendinopathy
- Bicipital tendinopathy
- Capsular laxity
- Capsular tightness
- Increased thoracic kyphosis and suboptimal posture
- Repetitive overhead activities
- Poor neuromuscular control

Differential Diagnosis[1]

- AC separation
- Cervical radiculopathy
- Referred pain from lungs or diaphragm
- Full-thickness rotator cuff tear
- Glenohumeral (GH) arthritis
- GH instability
- Labral tear
- Adhesive capsulitis
- Neuropathy (suprascapular nerve)
- Internal impingement

MEANS OF CONFIRMATION OR DIAGNOSIS

Imaging

- Diagnostic ultrasound
  - Maybe helpful in diagnosing moderate to large cuff tear
  - Less effective in diagnosing small tears or tendonitis
- Radiograph
  - Acromion type
  - Spurs
  - Humeral head position
  - Osteoarthritis
  - Sclerotic changes
  - Views
  - Anteroposterior
  - Lateral
  - Supraspinatus outlet view
- MRI
  - Rotator cuff tear
  - Tissue quality
  - Capsulolabral and biceps labral pathology
  - Acromion
  - AC joint
  - Labrum

TREATMENT

Medication

- Anti-inflammatory
- Corticosteroid injection

MEDICAL PROCEDURES

- Subacromial injection (lidocaine) to see if impingement signs reduce.
- Surgery
  - Acromioplasty for patients who have not responded to conservative care including activity modification, PT, NSAIDs, and injections and have imaging evidence of intrinsic changes to the acromion, rotator cuff, or AC joint (minimum 6 months).
  - If the condition has progressed to a full-thickness rotator cuff tear, acromioplasty is often performed concomitantly with a cuff repair.
  - If the biceps tendon has changes associated with wear, tenotomy, or tenodesis are often performed.

REFERRALS/ADMITTANCE

- For imaging
- For medication
- For surgical consult if failed conservative treatment
- Other instances

IMPAIRMENTS

- Impaired (suboptimal) posture
- Muscle imbalances
  - Rotator cuff weakness
  - Periscapular muscle weakness (particularly upward rotators and depressors/retractors)
  - Pectoralis (pec) minor tightness
- Decreased thoracic ROM (particularly extension)
- Rotator cuff overuse/fatigue
- Neuropathy and subsequent muscle weakness
- Hypomobile posterior GH capsule
- Hypermobility at the GH and or scapulothoracic articulations
- Pain with active elevation
- Hypo- or hypermobility at the GH, scapulothoracic, AC, or sternoclavicular (SC) joints

TEST AND MEASURES

- AC compression test
- Anterior slide test
- Biceps load test
- C5–C6 dermatome/myotome testing
- Clunk test
- Compression–rotation test
- Diagnostic test properties for subacromial impingement

- Disabilities of the Arm, Shoulder, and Hand (DASH) score to assess physical function
- Drop arm (Codman) test
- Empty can test
- External rotation lag sign (ERLS)/dropping arm sign
- Hawkins–Kennedy impingement sign/test
- Infraspinatus muscle test[1]
- Neer impingement test
- O'Brien test
- Pain provocation test
- Pain with resisted abduction
- Painful arc sign/test
- Passive horizontal adduction test
- Pronated load test
- Resisted supination external rotation test
- Shoulder pain and disability index
- Speed test
- Yergason test

INTERVENTION

Note: Varies depending on the type of impingement, causes, stage of healing, and tissue quality but generally involves portions of the following:

- Acute stage
  - Rest, ice, and activity modification (avoiding impinging positions)
- Subacute/Chronic stages (addressing specific impairments associated with the impingement)
  - Address joint impairments
    - GH hypomobility (mobilization)
    - GH hypermobility (stabilization)
    - Thoracic spine hypomobility (mobilization/manipulation)
  - Address muscle imbalances
    - Rotator cuff strength and endurance exercises
    - Muscle length of pec major/minor, latissimus dorsi (lats), and other muscles with decreased length
  - Strengthening of scapular musculature
    - Lower trap
    - Serratus anterior
    - Other scapular stabilizers
  - Functional activities (depending on work/recreational desires)
- Addressing pain and inflammation
  - Ice
  - Rest
  - Activity modification (avoiding impingement positions)
  - Ultrasound, phonophoresis, iontophoresis
  - Electronic stimulation
- Addressing weakness, joint hypermobility
  - Shoulder lateral and medial rotation
    - Isometric
    - Thera-Band resisted
    - Handheld weight resisted
    - Progression through higher ranges of elevation
  - Scapular strength/stabilization
  - Retraction
  - Prone shoulder extension, abduction, scapular plane elevation
- Addressing lack of flexibility
  - Stretching
    - Posterior capsule/posterior cuff
    - Pectoralis minor
    - Pectoralis major
    - Latissimus dorsi
- Addressing joint mobility
  - Posterior humeral glides
  - Inferior humeral glides
  - Thoracic mobilization/manipulation
  - Scapulothoracic mobility
    - Distraction
    - Retraction
    - Upward rotation
    - Posterior tip
- Addressing tendinopathy
  - Eccentric cuff exercises

FUNCTIONAL GOALS

- Patient will be able to:
  - Move upper extremity (UE) through full range of elevation without pain to reach in the cabinet.
  - Reach back pocket (or fasten bra for female) without pain.
  - Reach for a gallon of milk without pain.

PROGNOSIS

- Prognosis depends on the underlying cause of the impingement, the quality of the tissues involved as well as the patient's ability to control exacerbating activities and perform the optimal dosage of therapeutic exercise.
- The stage of the impingement according to Neer can be prognostic with Stage I generally having a better prognosis than Stage III.

PATIENT RESOURCE

- A Musculoskeletal Medicine Approach to Subacromial Impingement Syndrome. Australian Association of Musculoskeletal Medicine. http://www.musmed.com/Subacromial%20impingement.pdf. Accessed June 14, 2013.

REFERENCES

1. ICD9Data.com. http://www.icd9data.com. Accessed June 14, 2013.
2. ICD10Data.com. http://www.icd10data.com. Accessed June 14, 2013.
3. Pattern 4E: impaired joint mobility, motor function, muscle performance, and range of motion associated with localized inflammation. In: *Guide to Physical Therapist Practice*. 2nd ed. Alexandria, VA: American Physical Therapy Association; 2001. Revised 2003.
4. Park HB, Yokota A, Gill HS, et al. Diagnostic accuracy of clinical tests for the different degrees of subacromial impingement syndrome. *J Bone Joint Surg Am*. 2005;87:1446–1455. doi:10.2106/JBJS.D.02335.

ADDITIONAL REFERENCES

- Bang MD, Deyle GD. Comparison of supervised exercise with and without manual physical therapy for patients with shoulder impingement syndrome. *J Orthop Sports Phys Ther*. 2000;30(3):26–137.
- Bigliani LU, Levine WN. Current Concepts Review: Subacromial Impingement Syndrome. *J Bone Joint Surg Am*. 1997;79:1854–1868.

- Dutton M. The shoulder complex. In: Dutton M, ed. *Dutton's Orthopaedic Examination, Evaluation, and Intervention*. 3rd ed. New York, NY: McGraw-Hill; 2012:Chapter 14; Orthopaedic Examination, Evaluation, and Intervention. 2nd ed. New York, NY: McGraw-Hill; 2008. http://www.accessphysiotherapy.com/content/5552983. Accessed August 9, 2014.
- Dutton M, Dutton M. The shoulder complex. In: Dutton M, Dutton M, eds. *Dutton's Orthopedic Survival Guide: Managing Common Conditions*. New York, NY: McGraw-Hill; 2011:Chapter 5. http://www.accessphysiotherapy.com/content/8651960. Accessed August 9, 2014.
- Hamilton N, Weimar W, Luttgens K. The upper extremity: the shoulder region. In: Hamilton N, Weimar W, Luttgens K, eds. *Kinesiology: Scientific Basis of Human Motion*. New York, NY: McGraw-Hill; 2008:Chapter 5. http://www.accessphysiotherapy.com/content/6150569. Accessed August 9, 2014.
- Kisner C, Colby LA. *Therapeutic Exercise: Foundations and Techniques*. 5th ed. Philadelphia, PA: FA Davis; 2007:502–511.
- Ludewig PM, Braman JP. Shoulder impingement: Biomechanical considerations in rehabilitation. *Man Ther*. 2011;16(1):33–39. doi:10.1016/j.math.2010.08.004.
- Malone TR, Hazle C, Grey ML. Chapter 5. Shoulder complex. In: Malone TR, Hazle C, Grey ML, eds. *Imaging in Rehabilitation*. New York, NY: McGraw-Hill; 2008. http://www.accessphysiotherapy.com/content/5940757. Accessed August 9, 2014.
- Patel DR, Greydanus DE, Baker RJ. Overuse injuries of the shoulder. In: Patel DR, Greydanus DE, Baker RJ, eds. *Pediatric Practice: Sports Medicine*. New York, NY: McGraw-Hill; 2009:Chapter 21. http://www.accessphysiotherapy.com/popup.aspx?aID=6978348. Accessed June 14, 2013.
- Theisen C, van Wagensveld A, Timmesfeld N, et al. Co-occurrence of outlet impingement syndrome of the shoulder and restricted range of motion in the thoracic spine–a prospective study with ultrasound-based motion analysis. *BMC Musculoskelet Disord*. 2010;11:135. doi:10.1186/1471-2474-11-135.
- Wilk KE, Reinold MM, Andrews JR. *The Athletes Shoulder*. 2nd ed. Philadelphia, PA: Churchill Livingstone Elsevier; 2009; 115–140.

SECTION E ELBOW AND FOREARM DISORDERS

161 OLECRANON BURSITIS

Patrick S. Pabian, DPT, PT, SCS, OCS, CSCS

CONDITION/DISORDER SYNONYMS

- Elbow bursitis
- Student's elbow[1]
- Draftsman's elbow[1]
- Miner's elbow

ICD-9-CM CODE

- 726.33 Olecranon bursitis

ICD-10-CM CODE

- M70.20 Olecranon bursitis, unspecified elbow

PREFERRED PRACTICE PATTERN

- 4E: Impaired Joint Mobility, Motor Function, Muscle Performance, and Range of Motion Associated with Localized Inflammation

PATIENT PRESENTATION

A 54-year-old male bartender presents with posterior elbow pain that has been present for the past 2 weeks. The patient complains of dull pain with difficulty bending and straightening the elbow for dressing activities and weakness with pushing heavy items at work. He has marked pain when leaning his weight on his elbow when bent, especially on hard surfaces. The patient has focal swelling at the posterior elbow over the olecranon, which he notes varies in size when he leans on his elbow at work. The patient has had plain film x-rays which were negative for fracture.

KEY FEATURES

Description

- Localized inflammation of the olecranon bursa, which is a subcutaneous bursa at the olecranon process of the elbow
- Bursa fills with blood and serous fluid as a response to either acute or repeated microtrauma
- Presents as pronounced, local swelling, isolated to the posterior elbow

Essentials of Diagnosis

- Olecranon bursitis (OB) is a result of single episode of trauma or repeat trauma to the posterior elbow when the elbow is in a flexed position.
- Commonly related to occupation or specific activity that causes rubbing or pressure on the posterior elbow from a hard surface.
- Swelling is contained to olecranon bursa which results in the visualization of an "egg" appearance at the posterior elbow.
- Patients often note focal pain to palpation of swollen bursa, decreased range of motion, or inability to don a long-sleeved shirt.
- Laboratory evaluation of the bursal aspirate.[1]

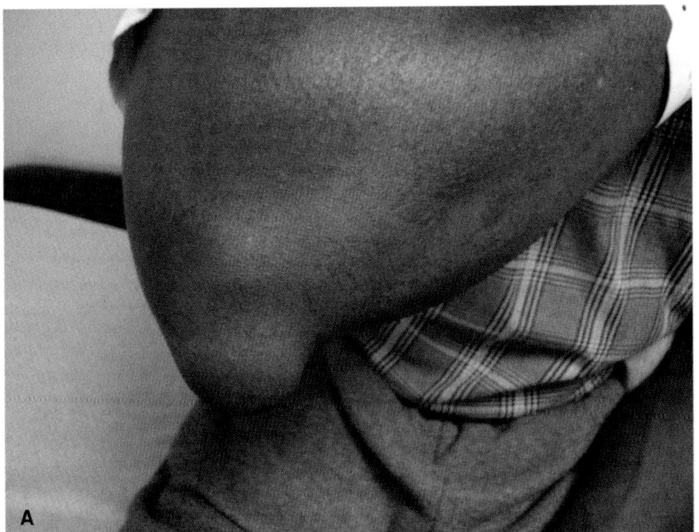

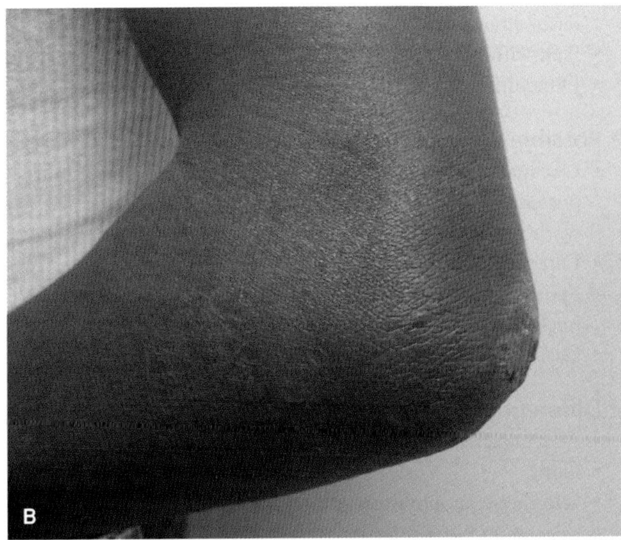

FIGURE 161-1 Olecranon bursitis. (**A**) Noninfectious. (**B**) The significant swelling and erythema suggested an infectious etiology. (From Simon RR, Sherman SC: *Emergency Orthopedics*, 6th ed www.accessemergencymedicine.com. Copyright © The McGraw-Hill Companies, Inc. All rights reserved.)

General Considerations

- Isolated diagnosis related to acute or chronic activity (pressure to the posterior elbow by a hard surface) and focal swelling/pain to the olecranon bursa
- Marked tenderness or swelling with acute onset may signal underlying fracture
- Exquisite swelling, marked tenderness, and redness or heat may be indicative of infection

Demographics

- No reports identifying or limiting demographics. Incidence related to activity
- Occurs primarily in adults, but can occur in children and athletes of any age
- Chronic cases often associated with occupation (miner) or prolonged activity (student), which places posterior elbow on hard surface
- Acute cases often associated with acute blow to the posterior elbow when flexed (athletes) [1]

CLINICAL FINDINGS

SIGNS AND SYMPTOMS

- Point tenderness to the posterior elbow
- Focal swelling to the posterior elbow
- Stiffness of elbow
- Pain with rubbing or light pressure to posterior elbow (wearing long-sleeved shirt)
- Pain with focal pressure (leaning on desk with bent elbow)
- Elbow range of motion can be reduced, either flexion, extension, or both
- Pain and swelling can be either insidious or acute
- Occasionally, swelling can be spontaneous and without pain
- Possible reduction in strength due to pain and inflammation

Functional Limitations

- Difficulty with dressing, grooming, reaching due to decreased elbow range of motion
- Pain with sitting or leaning postures due to contact on the posterior elbow
- Pain with movements of the hand and wrist
- Difficulties with reaching, grasping, or pushing activities

Possible Contributing Causes

- Occupations or activities that involve repeated contact of the posterior elbow on hard surface (e.g., bartender, office work, student)
- Direct trauma to the posterior elbow with elbow flexed
- Sporting activities involving direct blow to posterior elbow (e.g., hockey, basketball, football)
- Olecranon bursa infection

Differential Diagnoses

- Acute olecranon fracture
- Gout
- Olecranon apophysitis/avulsion fracture
- Olecranon bursa infection
- Rheumatoid arthritis
- Triceps tendinitis

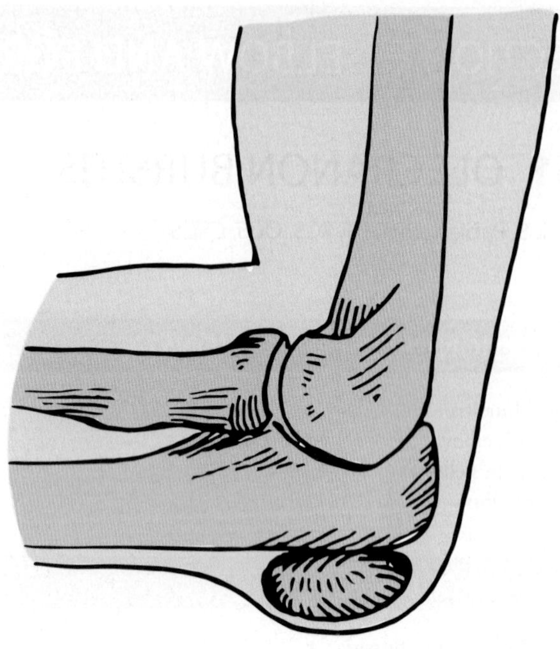

FIGURE 161-2 Olecranon bursitis. (Reproduced, with permission, from Simon RR, Koenigsknecht SJ: *Emergency Orthopedics: The Extremities,* 3rd ed. Originally published by Appleton & Lange. Copyright © 1995 by The McGraw-Hill Companies, Inc.)

MEANS OF CONFIRMATION OR DIAGNOSIS

Laboratory Tests

- Aspirated fluid can be cultured and evaluated for crystals to rule out gout and septic bursitis
- Laboratory studies for suspected rheumatoid disorders

Imaging

- Radiographs usually taken to rule out olecranon fracture
- MRI

FINDINGS AND INTERPRETATION

- MRI will show increased fluid/edema isolated within the olecranon bursa
- T2-weighted MRI would best visualize and result in increased signal intensity within olecranon bursa

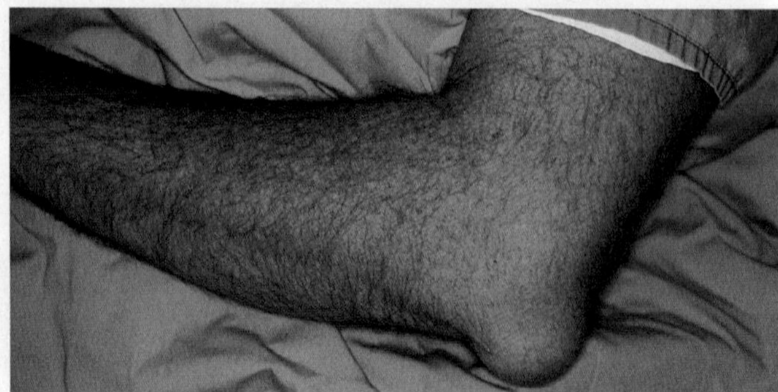

FIGURE 161-3 Olecranon bursitis. Olecranon bursitis is evident in this flexed elbow. (From Knoop KJ, Stack LB, Storrow AB, Thurman RJ. *The Atlas of Emergency Medicine.* 3rd ed. www.accessmedicine.com. Copyright © The McGraw-Hill Companies, Inc. All rights reserved. Photo contributor Selim Suner, MD, MS.)

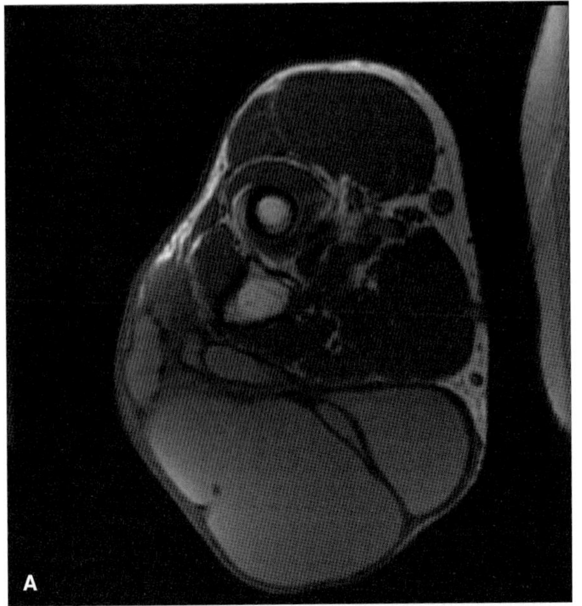

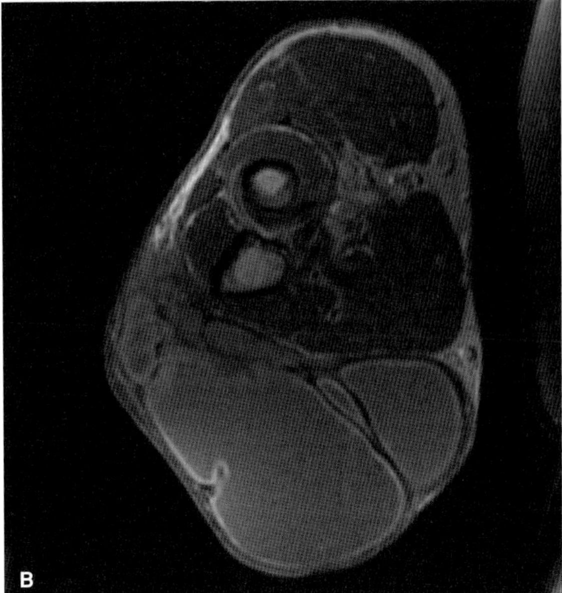

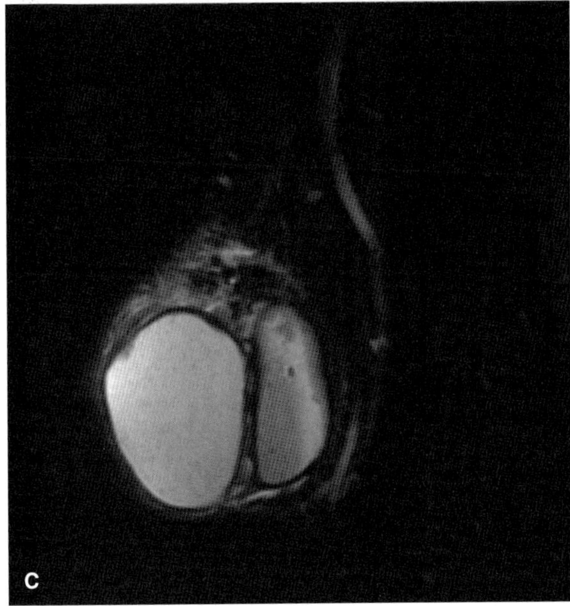

FIGURE 161-4 Olecranon bursitis in the setting of gout. Axial T1 (**A**) and T1 post-contrast (**B**) images and a coronal (**C**) T2 fat saturated image of the elbow demonstrate a large, multiloculated fluid collection posterior to the olecranon with an irregular, enhancing wall and internal debris, consistent with olecranon bursitis in this patient with gout. (From Imboden JB, Hellmann DB, Stone JH [eds]: *Current Diagnosis & Treatment Rheumatology,* 3rd ed. New York, McGraw-Hill, 2013.)

TREATMENT

Medication

- NSAIDs
- Corticosteroid injection
- Antibiotics, if infection confirmed

MEDICAL PROCEDURES

- Aspiration may assist in recovery
- Surgical excision

REFERRALS/ADMITTANCE

- To radiologist for imaging; X-ray
- To primary care physician for aspiration and lab studies
- To orthopedist for surgical consult for injection or excision

IMPAIRMENTS

- Restricted range of motion in elbow for reaching activities
- Decreased strength for pushing activities

TESTS AND MEASURES

- Disabilities of the Arm, Shoulder, and Hand (DASH) score to assess physical function
- Selective tissue tension tests
- Circumference
- Shine a pen light to see if fluid is clear or how it lights up, that is, blood

INTERVENTION

- Acute phase
  - PRICE: Protection, Rest, Ice Compression, Elevation
  - Bracing and padding to reduce pressure to posterior elbow

  - Low-level cold laser
  - Ice massage
  - Pulsed ultrasound
  - Active movement during the day with prevention of direct pressure to area from external hard surfaces
- Chronic phase
  - Gradually increase workload as pain and discomfort diminish
  - Continue padding/bracing to reduce contact to area
  - Addressing pain
    - Ice
    - High-Voltage Pulsed Stimulation (HVPS)
    - Iontophoresis
    - Ultrasound
    - Extracorporeal Shock Wave Therapy (ESWT)
  - Addressing swelling
    - Ice
    - Elevation
    - Iontophoresis
    - Increased focus on compression
  - Addressing weakness; joint instability
    - As symptoms improve, gradually resume activities
    - Establish full, pain-free elbow range of motion
    - Incorporate stretching and progressive strengthening exercises as warranted to restore full mobility and strength

FUNCTIONAL GOALS

- Patient will be able to
  - Press up from seated position with use of upper extremities without pain.
  - Reach into overhead cabinets in kitchen without pain or restriction.
  - Lift a gallon milk carton from refrigerator at shoulder level without pain.
  - Turn steering wheel without pain.
  - Use garden tools without pain.
  - Turn a door knob without pain.

PROGNOSIS

- Good. A prolonged period of healing can last several months.
- Slower recovery for those with infection.
- Aspiration may hasten recovery, but risk of infection exists.

PATIENT RESOURCE

- A closer look at bursitis. American Academy of Orthopaedic Surgeons. http://www.aaos.org/news/aaosnow/jul11/clinical10.asp. Accessed March 27, 2013.

REFERENCE

1. Dutton M. Common orthopedic conditions. In: Dutton M, ed. *Dutton's Orthopedic Survival Guide: Managing Common Conditions.* New York, NY: McGraw-Hill; 2011. http://www.accessphysiotherapy.com/content/8652850. Accessed March 27, 2013.

ADDITIONAL REFERENCES

- Bell S. Elbow and arm pain. In: Brukner P, Khan K, eds. *Clinical Sports Medicine*. 3rd ed. North Ryde, NSW, Australia: McGraw-Hill Book Company Australia; 2006:289–307.
- Dutton M. Practice Pattern 4E: impaired joint mobility, motor function, muscle performance, and range of motion associated with localized inflammation. In: Dutton M, ed. *Dutton's Orthopaedic Examination, Evaluation, and Intervention*. 3rd ed. New York, NY: McGraw-Hill; 2012. http://www.accessphysiotherapy.com/content/55576376. Accessed March 27, 2013.
- Dutton M. The elbow complex. In: Dutton M, ed. *Orthopaedic Examination, Evaluation, and Intervention*. 2nd ed. New York, NY: McGraw-Hill; 2008:653–733.
- Prentice WE. The elbow. In: Prentice WE, ed. *Principles of Athletic Training: A Competency-Based Approach*. New York, NY: McGraw-Hill; 2011:681–701.
- Simon RR, Sherman SC. Elbow soft-tissue injury and dislocations. In: Simon RR, Sherman SC, eds. *Emergency Orthopedics: The Extremities*. 6th ed. New York, NY: McGraw-Hill; 2011. http://www.accessphysiotherapy.com/content/7704994. Accessed March 27, 2013.

162 ELBOW DISLOCATION

Patrick S. Pabian, DPT, PT, SCS, OCS, CSCS

CONDITION/DISORDER SYNONYMS

- Elbow subluxation
- Nursemaid's elbow

ICD-9-CM CODES

- 832 Dislocation of elbow
- 832.0 Closed dislocation of elbow
- 832.00 Closed dislocation of elbow, unspecified
- 832.01 Closed anterior dislocation of elbow
- 832.02 Closed posterior dislocation of elbow
- 832.03 Closed medial dislocation of elbow
- 832.04 Closed lateral dislocation of elbow
- 832.09 Closed dislocation of elbow, other
- 832.1 Open dislocation of elbow
- 832.10 Open dislocation of elbow, unspecified
- 832.11 Open anterior dislocation of elbow
- 832.12 Open posterior dislocation of elbow
- 832.13 Open medial dislocation of elbow
- 832.14 Open lateral dislocation of elbow
- 832.19 Open dislocation of elbow, other
- 832.2 Nursemaid's elbow

ICD-10-CM CODES

- S53.016A Anterior dislocation of unspecified radial head, initial encounter
- S53.116A Anterior dislocation of unspecified ulnohumeral joint, initial encounter
- S53.146A Lateral dislocation of unspecified ulnohumeral joint, initial encounter
- S53.136A Medial dislocation of unspecified ulnohumeral joint, initial encounter
- S53.033A Nursemaid's elbow, unspecified elbow, initial encounter
- S53.096A Other dislocation of unspecified radial head, initial encounter
- S53.196A Other dislocation of unspecified ulnohumeral joint, initial encounter
- S53.026A Posterior dislocation of unspecified radial head, initial encounter
- S51.009A Unspecified open wound of unspecified elbow, initial encounter
- S53.006A Unspecified dislocation of unspecified radial head, initial encounter
- S53.106A Unspecified dislocation of unspecified ulnohumeral joint, initial encounter

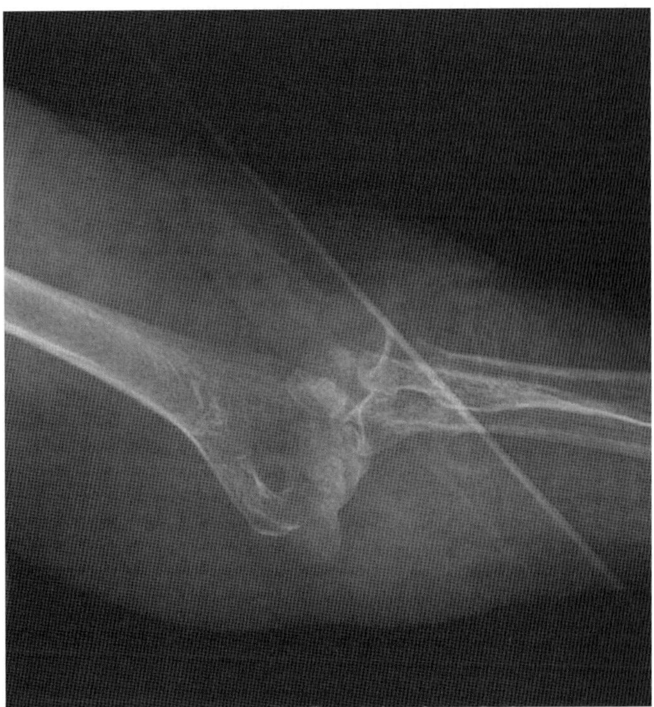

FIGURE 162-1 This oblique view radiograph reveals a frank dislocation of the elbow. (From Malone TR, Hazle C, Grey ML. *Imaging in Rehabilitation*. http://www.accessphysiotherapy.com. Copyright © The McGraw-Hill Companies, Inc. All rights reserved.)

PREFERRED PRACTICE PATTERN

- 4D: Impaired Joint Mobility, Motor Function, Muscle Performance, and Range of Motion (ROM) Associated with Connective Tissue Dysfunction

PATIENT PRESENTATION

A 17-year-old male presents with elbow pain, weakness, and lack of mobility. Patient sustained an elbow dislocation 2 weeks ago due to a fall on an extended elbow while playing football. He reports immediate pain and inability to move his elbow, necessitating transport to urgent care for relocation. He reports that pre-and postreduction X-rays did not reveal a fracture. He was placed in a hinged brace with ROM limits as set by the orthopedic physician.

He currently presents with moderate global swelling and bruising into his forearm. The patient has difficulty with writing while at school and dressing, grooming, and eating due to decreased mobility. He also notes weakness with carrying objects due to diminished grip strength. He has negative varus and valgus stress tests. Patient has normal capillary refill and no sensory deficits in hand.

KEY FEATURES

Description

- Traumatic injury to the elbow
- Displacement of the ulna and radius in a posterior, anterior, or lateral direction
- Mechanism of injury is a forced hyperextension
- Typically from fall on outstretched elbow
- Traumatic unidirectional blow to the elbow
- Forceful twisting of the elbow while in a flexed position
- Nursemaid's elbow
    - Subluxation of the radial head

Essentials of Diagnosis

- Injury warrants *immediate* medical referral for imaging studies, relocation (often under anesthesia), and evaluation of neurovascular structures around the elbow.
- Traumatic event/mechanism of injury, resulting in obvious deformity, pain, and acute inflammatory response.
- Injury commonly observed in contact sport athletics, but also in other situations where traumatic blow or fall occurs.

General Considerations

- Most common direction is posterior dislocation of ulna and radius.
- Comprehensive evaluation of all neurovascular structures around the elbow is necessary after relocation.
- Examination of all ulnar and lateral collateral ligament branches is necessary after relocation to assess for possible injury.
- Postreduction radiographs and other possible advanced imaging techniques are required to evaluate for associated fractures or additional soft tissue injuries.
- Humeroulnar joint is generally stable once reduced but often results in elbow flexion contracture that needs to be managed by rehabilitation provider.
- "Dislocation" can also refer to isolated radius dislocation
    - Injury can be result of similar trauma.
    - Dislocation of radial head is termed "pulled elbow syndrome," which results in radial head slipping under the annular ligament due to tractional force through the radius.[1]
    - Fibers of interosseous membrane are not aligned to optimally resist distraction force, as they do to compression force.

Demographics

- No reports identifying or limiting demographics
- Incidence related to traumatic incident
- Injury commonly observed in contact sport athletics as well as situations where traumatic blow or fall occurs

CLINICAL FINDINGS

SIGNS AND SYMPTOMS

- Prereduction
    - Visual deformity
    - Severe pain
    - Immediate swelling
- Postreduction
    - Gross effusion
    - Reduced ROM in all planes of motion
    - Commonly results in elbow flexion contracture
    - Reduced elbow strength in all planes of motion
    - Reduced grip strength
    - Potential laxity or pain in collateral ligaments
    - Potential neurovascular symptoms to distal forearm or hand if traumatized in initial injury or if moderate effusion present

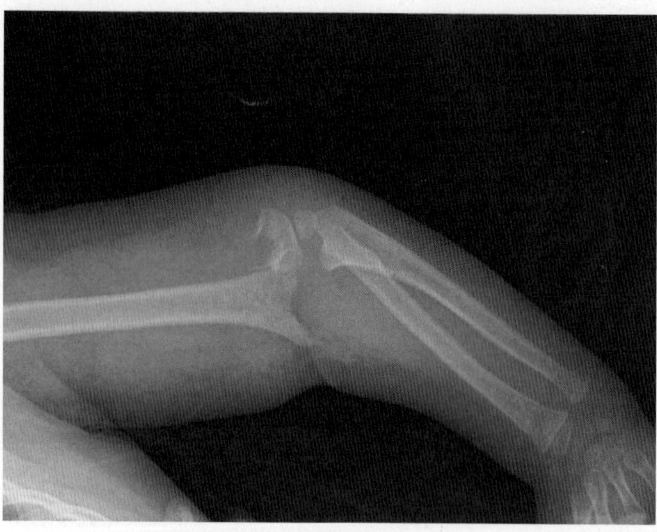

FIGURE 162-2 In this radiograph, a fracture dislocation of the elbow is demonstrated in a 3-year-old. The fracture evident on this image is consistent with a Salter–Harris type I epiphyseal fracture. (From Malone TR, Hazle C, Grey ML. *Imaging in Rehabilitation*. http://www.accessphysiotherapy.com. Copyright © The McGraw-Hill Companies, Inc. All rights reserved.)

Functional Limitations

- Difficulty dressing, grooming, or reaching due to decreased elbow ROM
- Difficulty reaching, grasping, or pushing activities
- Difficulty, pain, or weakness when grasping and pulling for dressing activities

Possible Contributing Causes

- Ligamentous laxity
- Participation in contact or high-velocity sports

Differential Diagnosis

- Elbow or distal humerus fractures
- Brachial plexus injury
- Muscle rupture

MEANS OF CONFIRMATION OR DIAGNOSIS

Laboratory Tests

- No special tests noted
- Tuning fork for vibration irritation
- Suspicion of neurologic or vascular compromise warrants immediate medical referral

Imaging

- Pre- and postreduction radiographs necessary to evaluate for presence of associated fractures
- CT scan possible for further evaluation of suspected fractures
    - Axial CT, ORIF
- MRI possible for evaluation of ligamentous integrity or other soft tissue injuries

Findings and Interpretation

- Fracture with displacement of the proximal ulna
- Elbow fracture dislocation, Salter–Harris type I epiphyseal fracture
- Supracondylar fracture
- Lateral view, radial head fracture
- Fracture of the tip of the olecranon
- Radial head fracture
- Oblique view, frank dislocation of the elbow
- Avulsion fracture of the medial epicondyle

TREATMENT

Medication

- Nonsteroidal anti-inflammatory drugs (NSAIDs) as prescribed by physician
- Pain medication as prescribed by physician

MEDICAL PROCEDURES

- Surgical intervention possible for fracture presence or with associated soft tissue injury (collateral ligament tear)
- Bracing for protection of soft tissues

REFERRALS/ADMITTANCE

- Immediate medial referral for evaluation, imaging, and reduction.
- To radiologist for imaging, X-ray.
- To orthopedist for surgical consult if associated injuries present.

IMPAIRMENTS

- Restricted ROM in elbow for reaching activities
- Decreased strength for pushing activities

TESTS AND MEASURES

- Neurologic examination
- ROM
- Strength assessment
- Disabilities of the Arm, Shoulder, and Hand (DASH) score to assess physical function

INTERVENTION

- Acute phase
  - Brace/splint until acute pain subsides
  - PRICE: protection, rest, ice compression, elevation
  - Low-level cold laser
  - Ice massage
  - Pulsed ultrasound
  - Active and passive movement allowed, but protect from varus/valgus stresses due to potential associated injury to collateral ligaments
- Chronic phase
  - Gradually increase workload as pain and discomfort diminish
  - Gradually progress to aggressive stretching/ROM to establish normal mobility. May require dynamic splinting to obtain full ROM.
  - Addressing pain
    - Ice
    - High-voltage pulsed stimulation
    - Ultrasound
    - Extracorporeal shockwave therapy

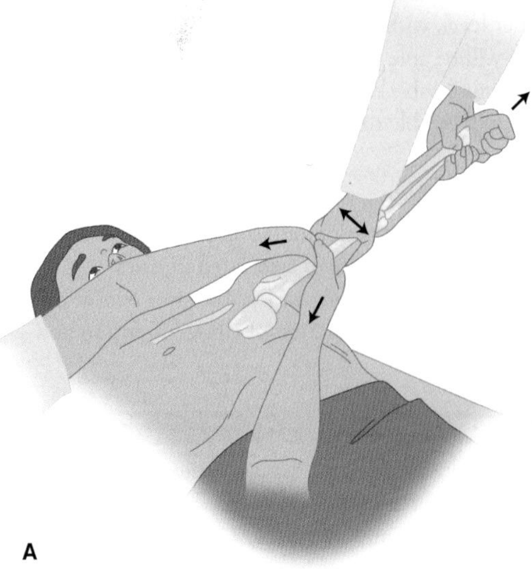

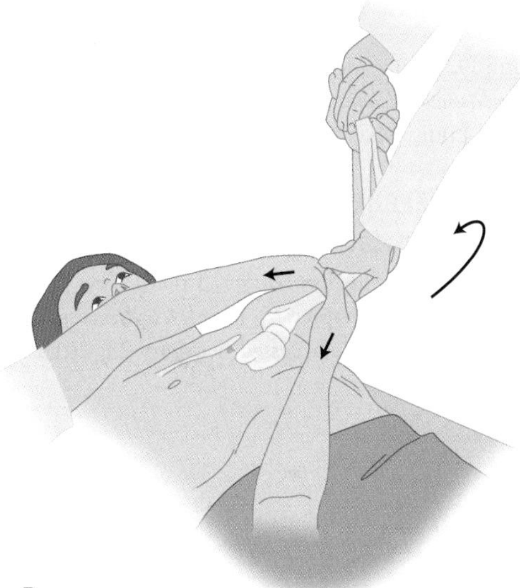

FIGURE 162-3 **A** and **B.** Reduction of a posterior elbow dislocation. (From Tintinalli JE, Stapczynski J, Ma OJ, Cline D, Cydulka R, Meckler Geds. *Tintinalli's Emergency Medicine: A Comprehensive Study Guide*. 7th ed. http://www.accessmedicine.com. Copyright © The McGraw-Hill Companies, Inc. All rights reserved.)

  - Addressing swelling
    - Ice
    - Elevation
  - Addressing weakness and joint instability
    - As symptoms improve, gradually resume activities
    - Establish full, pain-free elbow ROM
    - Incorporate stretching and progressive strengthening exercises as warranted to restore full mobility and strength
  - Medical intervention
    - May be necessary if associated neurovascular or soft tissue injury is present

FUNCTIONAL GOALS

- Patient will be able to reach into overhead cabinets in kitchen without pain or restriction

- Patient will be able to lift a gallon milk carton from refrigerator at shoulder level, without pain
- Patient will be able to turn steering wheel, without pain
- Patient will be able to use garden tools, without pain
- Patient will be able to turn a door knob, without pain

PROGNOSIS

- Good. A prolonged period of healing can last several months, especially in the presence of associated injuries
- Humeroulnar joint usually very stable after relocation, but often results in significant limitation of elbow extension and supination ROM

PATIENT RESOURCE

- Elbow Dislocations and Fracture-Dislocations. American Academy of Orthopaedic Surgeons. http://orthoinfo.aaos.org/topic.cfm?topic=a00029, Accessed February 23, 2013.

REFERENCE

1. Neumann D. Elbow and Forearm. In: Neumann D, ed. *Kinesiology of the Musculoskeletal System: Foundations for Rehabilitation.* 2nd ed. St. Louis, MO: Mosby; 2010:173–215.

ADDITIONAL REFERENCES

- Dutton M. The elbow complex. In: *Dutton's Orthopaedic Examination, Evaluation, and Intervention.* 3rd ed. New York, NY: McGraw-Hill; 2012:Chapter 15. http://www.accessphysiotherapy.com/content/55575512. Accessed February 23, 2013.
- Hall SJ. Common joint injuries and pathologies. In: Hall SJ, ed. *Basic Biomechanics.* 5th ed. New York, NY: McGraw-Hill; 2007. http://www.accessphysiotherapy.com/content/6061136. Accessed February 23, 2013.
- Hay WW, Levin MJ, Sondheimer JM, Deterding RR. Trauma. In: Hay WW, Levin MJ, Sondheimer JM, Deterding RR, eds. *CURRENT Diagnosis & Treatment: Pediatrics.* 20th ed. New York, NY: McGraw-Hill; 2011. http://www.accessphysiotherapy.com/content/6585929. Accessed February 23, 2013.
- ICD9Data.com. http://www.icd9data.com. Accessed February 23, 2013.
- ICD10Data.com. http://www.icd10data.com. Accessed February 23, 2013.
- Malone TR, Hazle C, Grey ML. The elbow. In: Malone TR, Hazle C, Grey ML, eds. *Imaging in Rehabilitation.* New York, NY: McGraw-Hill; 2008:Chapter 6. http://www.accessphysiotherapy.com/content/5940841. Accessed February 23, 2013.
- Pattern 4D: impaired joint mobility, motor function, muscle performance, and range of motion associated with connective tissue dysfunction. In: *Guide to Physical Therapist Practice.* 2nd ed. Alexandria, VA: American Physical Therapy Association; 2001. Revised 2003.
- Prentice WE. The Elbow. In: Prentice WE, ed. *Arnheim's Principles of Athletic Training: A Competency-Based Approach.* New York, NY: McGraw-Hill; 2011:681–701.
- Ryan J, Salvo J. Elbow injuries. In: Starkey C, Johnson G, eds. *Athletic Training and Sports Medicine.* 4th ed. Rosemont, IL: American Academy of Orthopaedic Surgeons; 2006:337–385.

163 ELBOW, RADIAL HEAD/ NECK FRACTURE

Jennifer Cabrera, DPT, GCS
Eric Shamus, PhD, DPT, PT, CSCS

ICD-9-CM CODES[1]

- 813.05 Fracture of head of radius closed
- 813.06 Fracture of neck of radius closed
- 813.15 Fracture of head of radius open
- 813.16 Fracture of neck of radius open

ICD-10-CM CODES[2]

- S52.123A Displaced fracture of head of unspecified radius, initial encounter for closed fracture
- S52.126A Nondisplaced fracture of head of unspecified radius, initial encounter for closed fracture
- S52.133A Displaced fracture of neck of unspecified radius, initial encounter for closed fracture
- S52.136A Nondisplaced fracture of neck of unspecified radius, initial encounter for closed fracture
- S52.123B Displaced fracture of head of unspecified radius, initial encounter for open fracture type I or II
- S52.123C Displaced fracture of head of unspecified radius, initial encounter for open fracture type IIIA, IIIB, or IIIC
- S52.126B Nondisplaced fracture of head of unspecified radius, initial encounter for open fracture type I or II
- S52.126C Nondisplaced fracture of head of unspecified radius, initial encounter for open fracture type IIIA, IIIB, or IIIC
- S52.133B Displaced fracture of neck of unspecified radius, initial encounter for open fracture type I or II
- S52.133C Displaced fracture of neck of unspecified radius, initial encounter for open fracture type IIIA, IIIB, or IIIC
- S52.136B Nondisplaced fracture of neck of unspecified radius, initial encounter for open fracture type I or II
- S52.136C Nondisplaced fracture of neck of unspecified radius, initial encounter for open fracture type IIIA, IIIB, or IIIC

PREFERRED PRACTICE PATTERN

- 4G: Impaired Joint Mobility, Muscle Performance, and Range of Motion Associated with Fracture[3]

PATIENT PRESENTATION

A 38-year-old woman arrives to the emergency room complaining of 10/10 elbow pain. She reports she was running in the street, did not see a hole in the road and experienced a "hard" fall against the concrete. She continued to report putting out her arm to attempt to dampen the fall, but felt immediate sharp pain in her elbow upon impact. The woman demonstrated increased upper extremity (UE) guarding with any attempted elbow movements

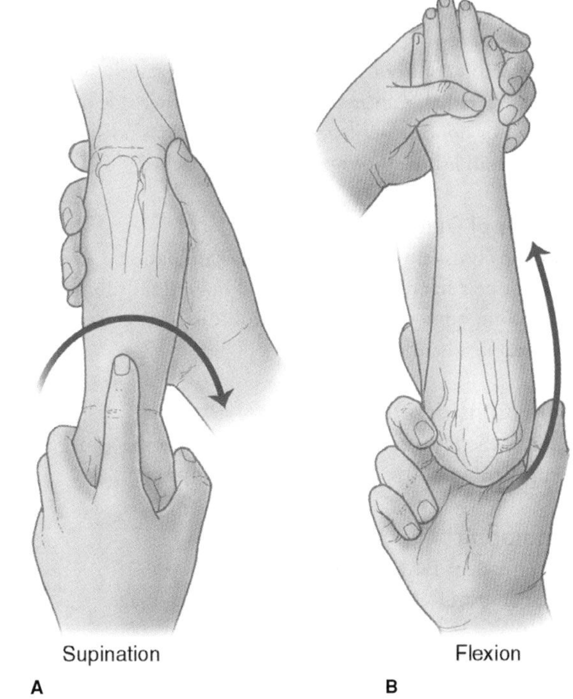

FIGURE 163-1 (**A**) Supination and (**B**) flexion techniques for radial head subluxation reduction. (From Simon RR, Sherman SC. *Emergency Orthopedics.* 6th ed. http://www.accessemergencymedicine.com. Copyright © The McGraw-Hill Companies, Inc. All rights reserved.)

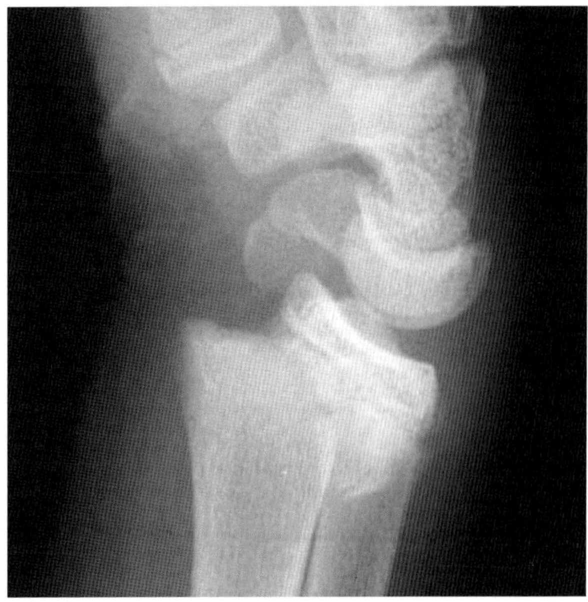

FIGURE 163-2 Salter II fracture of the distal radius in a child. This fracture requires reduction in the emergency department. (From Simon RR, Sherman SC. *Emergency Orthopedics.* 6th ed. http://www.accessemergencymedicine. com. Copyright © The McGraw-Hill Companies, Inc. All rights reserved.)

and visible deformity at the distal elbow with edema. Upon palpation, patient demonstrated tenderness directly over radial head. Crepitus was noted with forearm supination. X-rays were performed and patient was found to have a displaced proximal radial head fracture.

KEY FEATURES

Description

- Fracture
- Any defect in continuity of the radial head or neck
- Displaced (radial head/neck is moved on either side of the fracture) or nondisplaced (radial head/neck has not moved)
- Closed (skin is intact) or open (skin is breached)

Essentials of Diagnosis

- Diagnosis is usually made by clinical examination.
- May not be a fracture but a proximal radioulnar subluxation/dislocation, humeroradial subluxation/dislocation, radial collateral ligament sprain.

General Considerations

- Radius is the most commonly broken bone in the arm.
- Occurs in about 20% of all acute elbow injuries.

Demographics

- More frequent in women than in men
- Occurs most often between 30 and 40 years of age

CLINICAL FINDINGS

SIGNS AND SYMPTOMS

- Pain on the outside of the elbow
- Point tenderness
- Edema
- Ecchymosis
- Loss of general function
- Loss of active elbow movement
- Loss of active forearm movement (supination/pronation)
- Muscle guarding with passive movement
- Crepitus

Functional Implications

- Pain with weight-bearing activities on involved UE
- Pain with vertical positioning of arm at side
- Pain with all elbow and forearm movements (passive or active)

Possible Contributing Causes

- Mechanism of injury
- Fall on outstretched hand
- Blunt or penetrating trauma is a rare cause

Differential Diagnosis

- Proximal radioulnar subluxation/dislocation
- Humeroradial subluxation/dislocation
- Radial collateral ligament sprain

MEANS OF CONFIRMATION

Imaging

- X-ray for fracture, often limited view
- CT scan for detailed imaging

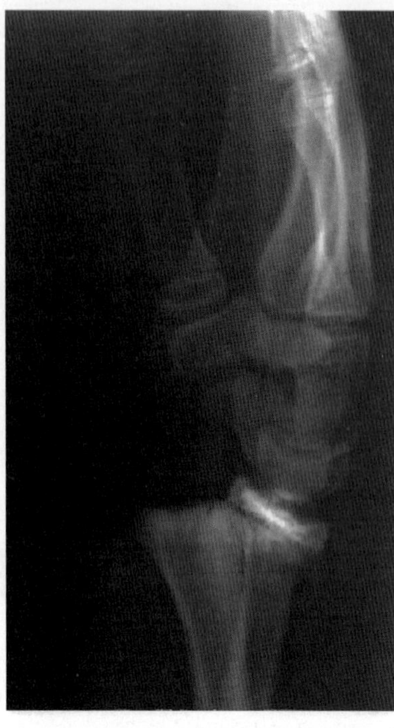

FIGURE 163-3 Fracture of the radial epiphysis with displacement. (From Simon RR, Sherman SC. *Emergency Orthopedics*. 6th ed. http://www.accessemergency-medicine.com. Copyright © The McGraw-Hill Companies, Inc. All rights reserved.)

FINDINGS AND INTERPRETATION

- Pain and crepitus with passive/active ROM of the elbow and forearm.
- UE held in protective positioning in order to avoid gravity's distraction of the joint.

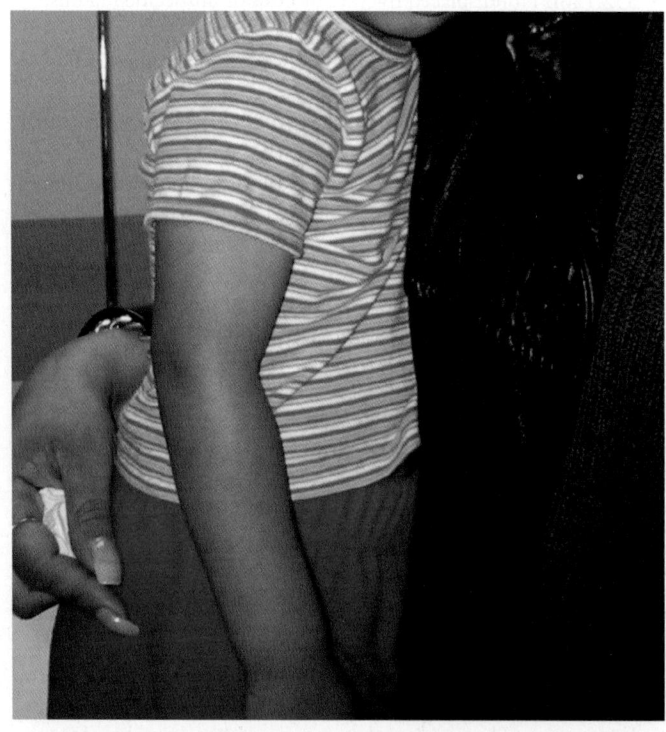

FIGURE 163-4 Radial head subluxation. The arm is held in slight flexion and pronation. Any movement from this position is resisted by the patient. (From Simon RR, Sherman SC. *Emergency Orthopedics*. 6th ed. http://www.accessemergencymedicine.com. Copyright © The McGraw-Hill Companies, Inc. All rights reserved.)

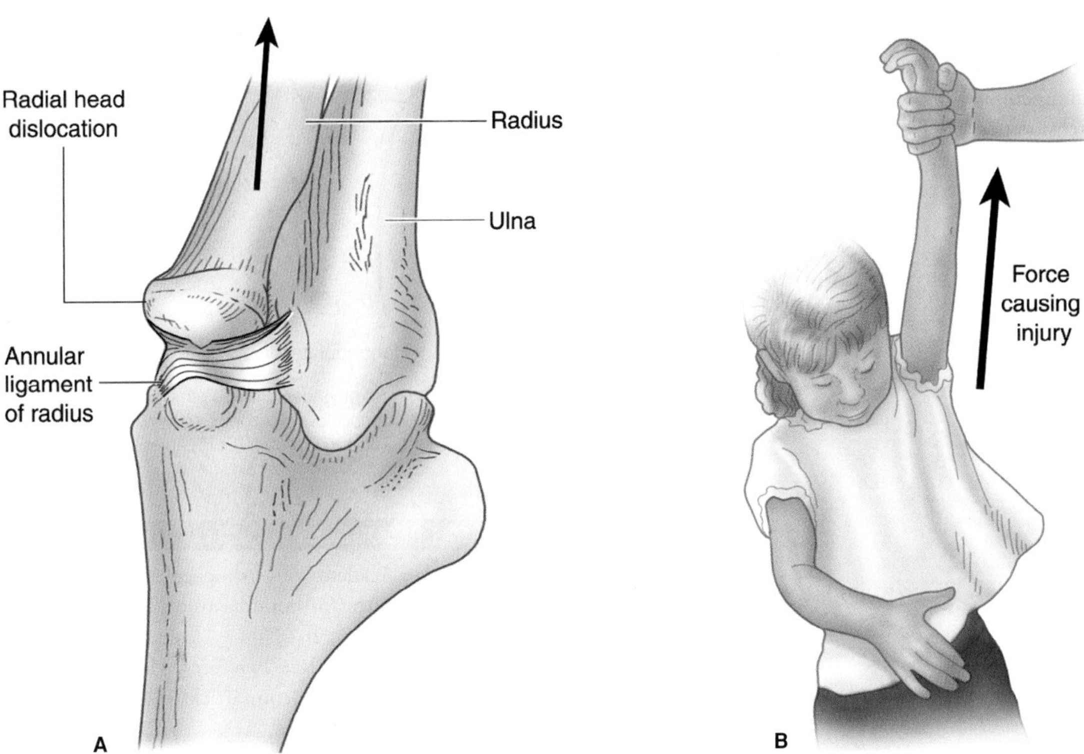

FIGURE 163-5 Radial head subluxation (nursemaid's elbow). **A.** Drawing demonstrating direction of pull. **B.** Example of some tractioning the arm that can cause a dislocation of the radial head. (From Simon RR, Sherman SC. *Emergency Orthopedics.* 6th ed. http://www.accessemergencymedicine.com. Copyright © The McGraw-Hill Companies, Inc. All rights reserved.)

- Muscle guarding with all movements.
- Inability to actively perform elbow movements or forearm pronation/supination secondary to pain.
- If vascular structures are involved, the involved forearm and hand will appear cool and pale with diminished palpable pulses.
- If neurologic structures are involved, the individual will report numbness and decreased ability to move the involved forearm and hand.
- If patient reports severe pain, the individual may be suffering from compartment syndrome.

REFERRALS/ADMITTANCE

- For imaging, X-ray or CT
- For medication, NSAIDs or opiod for pain management
- For immediate orthopedic consult
  - Nondisplaced fractures or displaced fractures that may be reduced are treated nonoperatively
    - Immobilization splint or sling
  - Severely displaced fractures are treated operatively via
    - Open reduction internal fixation
    - Radial head resection
    - Insertion of radial head prosthesis if elbow instability is severe

IMPAIRMENTS

- Inability to perform ADLs with involved UE
- Inability to bear weight on involved forearm and hand
- Inability to use involved hand to write (especially if it is the patient's dominant hand)
- Inability to grab a cup secondary to pain and muscle weakness

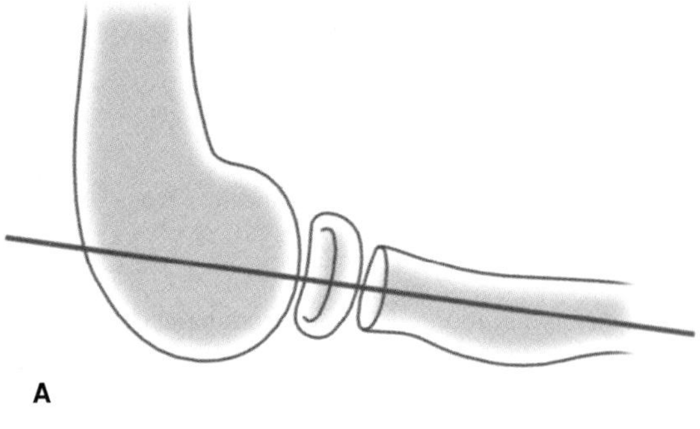

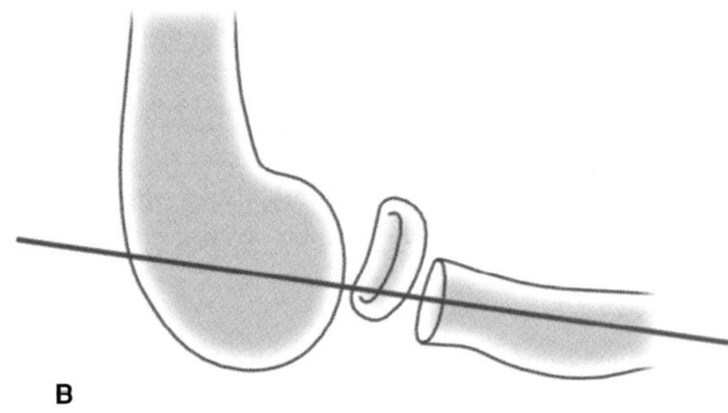

FIGURE 163-6 (**A**) The radiocapitellar line drawn through the center of the radius should pass through the center of the capitellum of the humerus on the lateral view. (**B**) It is useful in making the diagnosis in patients with a fracture of the radial neck in whom the epiphysis has not closed. (From Simon RR, Sherman SC. *Emergency Orthopedics.* 6th ed. http://www.accessemergencymedicine.com. Copyright © The McGraw-Hill Companies, Inc. All rights reserved.)

TESTS AND MEASURES

- Disabilities of the Arm, Shoulder, and Hand (DASH) score to assess physical function
- Upper limb tension test (ULTT), radial nerve dominant
- Sensory loss may include diminished two-point discrimination, decreased vibration sense, increased threshold in Semmes–Weinstein monofilament test

INTERVENTION

- Address swelling
  - Ice/Cryotherapy
  - Compression
  - Elevation
  - Electrical stimulation
- Address pain
  - Ice/Cryotherapy
  - Massage
  - Electrical stimulation
- Address lack of flexibility via stretching
  - Wrist flexors
  - Wrist extensors
  - Elbow flexors
- Address mobilization upon healing of fracture site (6 weeks postoperative)
  - Humeroulnar distraction for pain management
  - Humeroulnar distal glide to increase elbow flexion
  - Humeroradial dorsal glide for elbow extension
  - Humeroradial volar glide for elbow flexion
  - Proximal radioulnar joint dorsal glide for pronation
  - Proximal radioulnar joint volar glide for supination
  - Distal radioulnar joint dorsal glide for supination
  - Distal radioulnar joint volar glide for pronation
- Address weakness via strengthening activities
  - Closed chain weight-bearing activities
  - Isometric exercises (initially submaximal)
  - Open chain via use of free weights and resistance bands
  - Grip strengthening
- Address scar mobility
  - Scar tissue mobilization progressing from parallel to perpendicular upon wound closure

FUNCTIONAL GOALS

- Patient will:
  - Increase grip strength to 30 kg in order to facilitate opening jars.
  - Increase forearm supination to 55 degrees in order to facilitate eating with a fork.
  - Increase arm curl test of the involved UE to 24 repetitions in order to facilitate carrying groceries.
  - Increase proximal radioulnar joint mobility to three in order to allow the individual to turn the knob of a door.

PROGNOSIS

- Good, if there is mechanical stability with reduction and stable internal fixation.
- Some residual loss of elbow extension is expected.

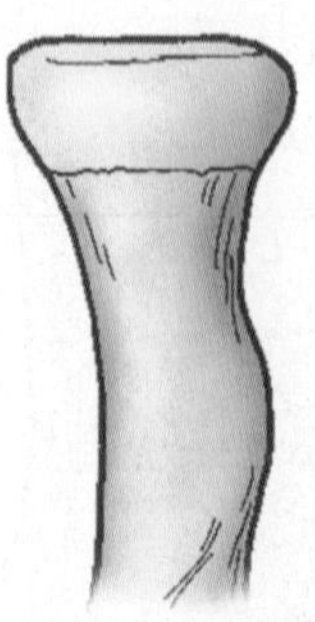

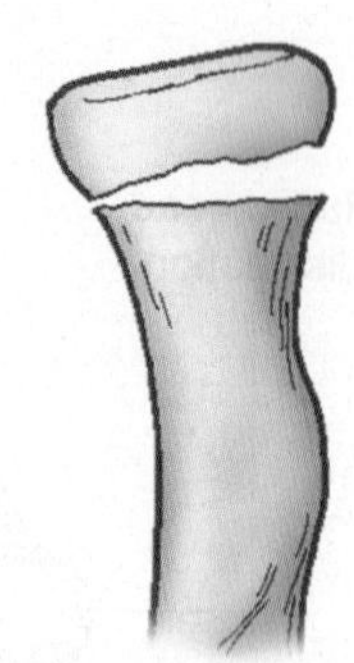

FIGURE 163-7 Epiphyseal radial head fractures. (From Simon RR, Sherman SC. *Emergency Orthopedics*. 6th ed. http://www.accessemergencymedicine.com. Copyright © The McGraw-Hill Companies, Inc. All rights reserved.)

PATIENT RESOURCES

- American Academy of Orthopaedic Surgeons. Radial Head Fractures. http://orthoinfo.aaos.org/topic.cfm?topic=A00073. Accessed April 6, 2013.
- Rabin SI. Radial Head Fractures. Medscape Reference. http://emedicine.medscape.com/article/1240337-overview#showall. Accessed April 6, 2013.

REFERENCES

1. ICD9Data.com. http://www.icd9data.com. Accessed April 6, 2013.
2. ICD10Data.com. http://www.icd10data.com/ICD10CM/Codes. Accessed April 6, 2013.
3. Pattern 4G: impaired joint mobility, muscle performance, and range of motion associated with fracture. In: *Guide to Physical Therapist Practice*. 2nd ed. Alexandria, VA: American Physical Therapy Association; 2001. Revised 2003.

ADDITIONAL REFERENCES

- Goodman CC, Fuller KS. *Pathology Implications for the Physical Therapist*. 3rd ed. St. Louis, MO: Saunders Elsevier; 2009.
- Hall SJ. The biomechanics of human bone growth and development. In: Hall SJ, ed. *Basic Biomechanics*. 5th ed. New York, NY: McGraw-Hill; 2007:Chapter 4. http://www.accessphysiotherapy.com/content/6060744. Accessed March 7, 2013.
- Kisner C, Colby LA. *Therapeutic Exercise: Foundations and Techniques*. 5th ed. Philadelphia, PA: F.A. Davis Company; 2007.
- Magee DJ. *Orthopedic Physical Assessment*. 5th ed. St. Louis, MO: Saunders Elsevier; 2008.
- Malone TR, Hazle C, Grey ML, eds. *Imaging in Rehabilitation*. New York, NY: McGraw-Hill; 2008. http://www.accessphysiotherapy.com/content/5940000. Accessed March 7, 2013.
- Prentice WE, Quillen WS, Underwood F, eds. *Therapeutic Modalities in Rehabilitation*. 4th ed. New York, NY: McGraw-Hill; 2011. http://www.accessphysiotherapy.com/content/8137872. Accessed August 9, 2014.

164 LATERAL EPICONDYLITIS

Kenneth Lee, DPT, PT
Eric Shamus, PhD, DPT, PT, CSCS

CONDITION/DISORDER SYNONYMS

- Lateral tendon injury
- Lateral tendonitis
- Lateral humeral epicondylitis
- Tennis elbow
- Lateral tennis elbow

ICD-9-CM CODE

- 726.32 Lateral epicondylitis

ICD-10-CM CODE

- M77.10 Lateral epicondylitis, unspecified elbow

PREFERRED PRACTICE PATTERN

- 4E: Impaired Joint Mobility, Motor Function, Muscle Performance, and Range of Motion Associated with Localized Inflammation[1]

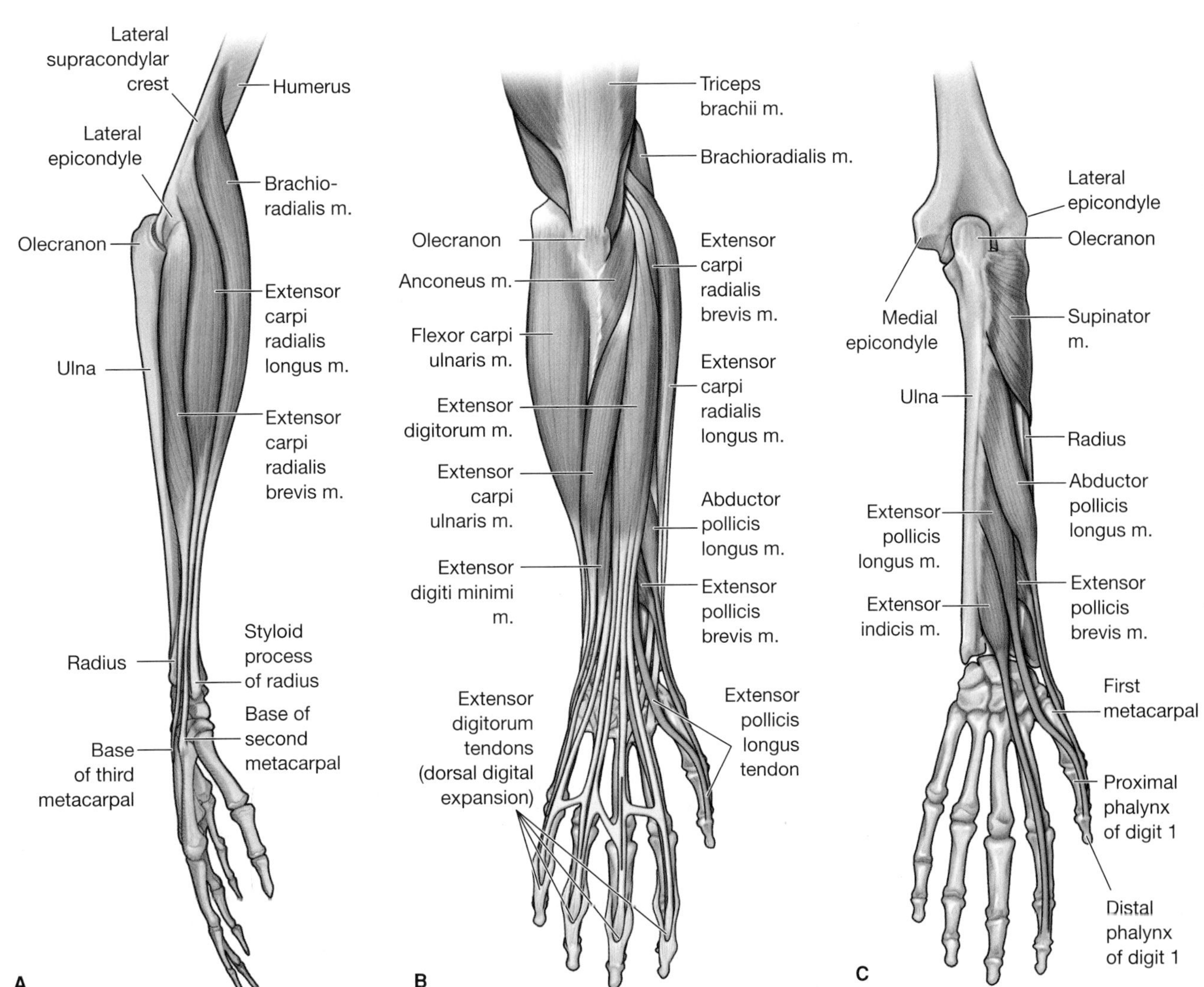

FIGURE 164-1 (**A**) Lateral view of the forearm, superficial (**B**) and deep (**C**) muscles of the posterior forearm. (From Morton DA, Foreman KB, Albertine KH. *The Big Picture: Gross Anatomy*. www.accessmedicine.com. Copyright © The McGraw-Hill Companies, Inc. All rights reserved.)

PATIENT PRESENTATION

A 42-year-old female has come to the physical therapy out-patient clinic for an evaluation of her right upper extremity. As a part of her initial history, the patient states that she is a police officer and an amateur bodybuilder. The patient states that the pain in her arm started suddenly and was noticeable when turning the ignition key of her police cruiser. She points to pain along the lateral aspect of her right elbow. She has point tenderness with palpation of area with increased pain in elbow with wrist and elbow extension. Imaging radiographs are normal. Physical inspection reveals that rubor and warmth are present in the muscle bellies of extensor digitorum and extensor carpi radialis longus.

KEY FEATURES

Description

- Tendinosis of wrist extensor tendons that attach at the lateral humeral epicondyle.[2]
- Normal collagen response is disrupted by fibroblastic, immature vascular response and an incomplete reparative phase.
- Early stages may display inflammatory or synovitic characteristics.
- Later stages may demonstrate microtearing, tendon degeneration with or without calcification, or incomplete vascular response.
- Pain in lateral elbow with resisted wrist extension and radial deviation with elbow extended.

Essentials of Diagnosis

- Tendonitis of the elbow is rarely caused by acute trauma except in sports-related events, such as tennis.[3]
- Usually affects middle-aged clients; aging process leads to decreased mucopolysaccharide chondroitin sulfate within tissues, making tendons less extensible.
- Age-related tissue changes for tennis elbow appear in patients aged 35 years and older.

General Considerations

- Tendinosis affecting the elbow is rarely acute unless by direct trauma (then considered tendonitis).
- Pain usually is associated with activity, more so afterward.
- Onset of pain is associated with wrist extension, elbow extension, and forearm pronation activities.
- Direct blows to lateral epicondyle can initiate symptoms.[2]

Demographics

- People aged 40 to 50 years[4]
- Accounts for 7% of all sports injuries[4]
- Males and females equally affected[4]
- 75% of patients are symptomatic in their dominant arm[4]

CLINICAL FINDINGS

SIGNS AND SYMPTOMS

- Pain of insidious onset
- Active movement may reproduce pain
- Passive movement of full wrist flexion with pronation and elbow extension reproduces pain at the lateral epicondyle
- Resistive isometric: Resisted wrist extension and elbow extension reproduces pain at lateral epicondyle
- Elbow-joint movements should be full and painless

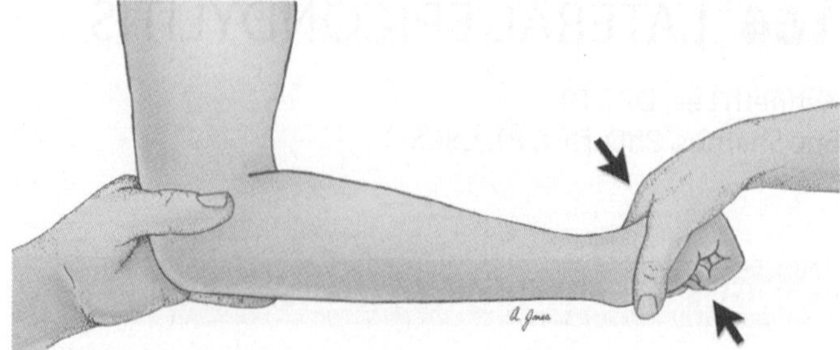

FIGURE 164-2 Tennis elbow can be diagnosed when pain over the lateral epicondyle is exacerbated when the patient extends the wrist and supinates the forearm against resistance. (From Simon RR, Sherman SC. *Emergency Orthopedics*. 6th ed. www.accessemergencymedicine.com. Copyright © The McGraw-Hill Companies, Inc. All rights reserved.)

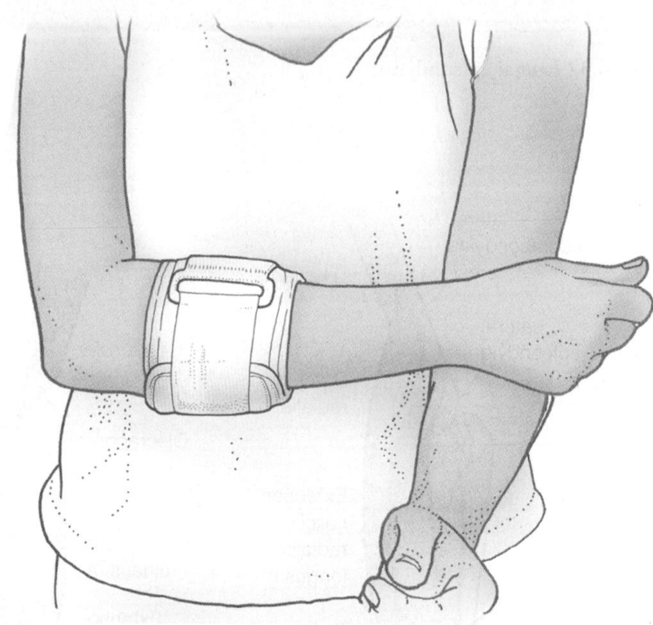

FIGURE 164-3 Placement of a tennis elbow band. The proximal edge of the band should be placed 2 to 3 cm distal to the lateral epicondyle, over the bulk of the extensor muscles. (From Simon RR, Sherman SC. *Emergency Orthopedics*. 6th ed. www.accessemergencymedicine.com. Copyright © The McGraw-Hill Companies, Inc. All rights reserved.)

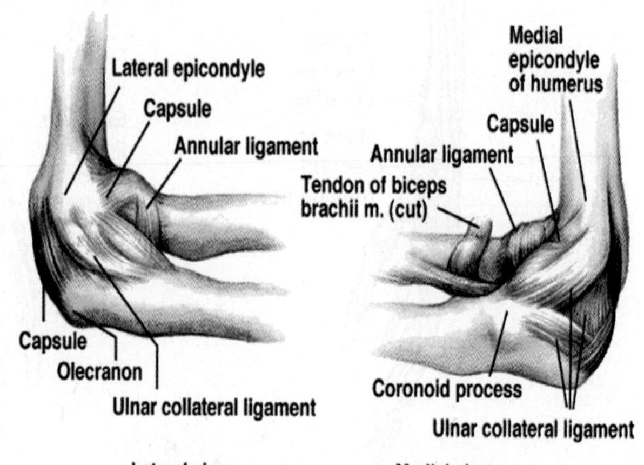

FIGURE 164-4 Elbow anatomy. (Used with permission from Van De, Graaff KM. *Human Anatomy*. 6th ed. New York, NY: McGraw Hill; 2002: Figure 8-27, p 218.)

- Palpation tenderness at lateral epicondyle within musculature of extensor digitorum and extensor carpi radialis longus; rarely involves extensor carpi ulnaris or extensor carpi radialis brevis (ECRB)
- Rubor and warmth may be present over lateral epicondyle or associated muscle belly
- Pain and tenderness over the lateral epicondyle
- Pain response varies between dull ache, no pain at rest, sharp pain with activities

Functional limitations

- Pain with pinching, squeezing, holding heavy objects, wringing
- Pain with movements of the hand and wrist
- Loss of strength
- Difficulty with grasping activities

Possible Contributing Causes

- Occupations requiring repetitive use of hands for excessive periods of time
- Direct trauma to tendon or wrist
- Sports or occupational activities
  - Tennis, golf, bowling, football, archery, weightlifting
  - Carpentry, plumbing, mechanic
- Most commonly results from repetitive forearm, wrist, hand motions

Differential Diagnosis

- Radial nerve entrapment
- Bicipital tendonitis
- Rheumatoid arthritis
- Radiocapitellar arthritis
- Posterior interosseous nerve compression (radial tunnel syndrome)
- Osteochondritis dissecans of the capitellum
- Carpal tunnel syndrome
- Triceps tendonitis
- Pronator syndrome

MEANS OF CONFIRMATION OR DIAGNOSIS

Laboratory Tests

- Laboratory studies for suspected rheumatoid disorders

Imaging

- Radiographs
- Electromyography (EMG) for patients with neurologic alterations[5]
- MRI can show inflammation/edema and microtearing

FINDINGS AND INTERPRETATION

- Radiographs
  - Usually normal
  - Can show calcification of ECRB: Anteroposterior and lateral views

TREATMENT

Medication

- Anti-inflammatory
- Corticosteroid injection
- NSAIDs[6]

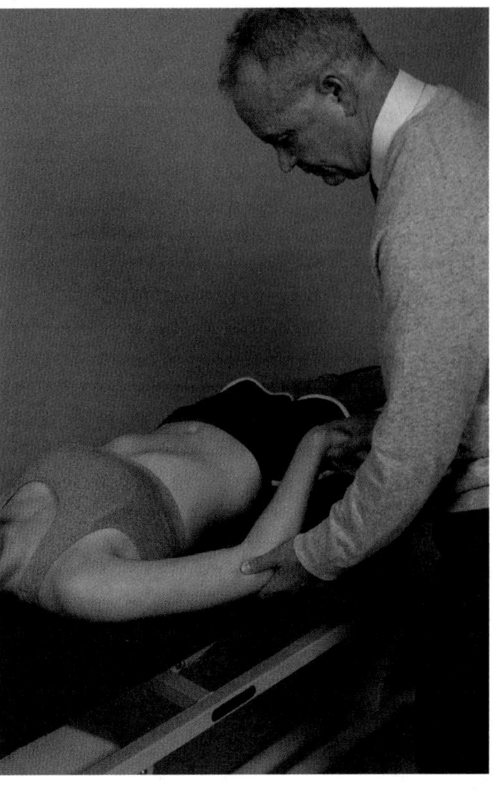

FIGURE 164-5 Mill's test. (Dutton M. *Dutton's Orthopaedic Examination, Evaluation, and Intervention*. 3rd ed. www.accessphysiotherapy.com. Copyright © The McGraw-Hill Companies, Inc. All rights reserved.)

REFERRALS/ADMITTANCE

- To radiologist for imaging, X-ray
- To orthopedist for surgical consult, injection

IMPAIRMENTS

- Hand weakness with grasping, squeezing, pinching
- Restricted ROM in elbow and wrist

TESTS AND MEASURES

- Cozen test
- Mill test
- Tinel sign at elbow
- Disabilities of the Arm, Shoulder, and Hand (DASH) score to assess physical function
- Froment sign

INTERVENTION

- Acute phase
  - Rest
  - Immobilization
  - Taping, bracing: Inhibit painful muscles or facilitate muscle activity
  - Low-level cold laser[7]
  - Active movement during day with prevention of high-strain loading of tissue
  - Address swelling
    - Ice[8]
    - Elevation
    - Iontophoresis[9]

- Chronic phase
  - Gradually increase workload as pain and discomfort diminish
  - Elbow and wrist brace to limit motion
  - Counterforce brace to reduce acceleration force
  - Address pain
    - Ice[8]
    - High-voltage pulsed stimulation
    - Iontophoresis
    - Ultrasound[10]
    - Extracorporeal shockwave therapy[11]
  - Address weakness, joint instability[12]
    - Gradually resume normal activity as symptoms improve
    - Establish full, pain-free wrist and elbow ROM
    - Incorporate stretching and progressive isometric exercise
    - Painful eccentric exercises
    - Progress to concentric and eccentric resistive exercise as flexibility and strength returns
    - Grip exercises and progressive strengthening of extensor and flexors using high-repetition/low-weight ratio
    - Concentrate on ECRB, extensor digitorum, and extensor carpi radialis longus
  - Address mobilization, radial head mobility

FUNCTIONAL GOALS

- Patient will be able to
  - Turn a door knob without pain.
  - Turn on faucet without pain.
  - Lift a gallon carton of milk from refrigerator at shoulder level without pain.
  - Grip steering wheel without pain.
  - Use a screw driver without pain.
  - Use garden tools without pain.

PROGNOSIS

- Good; prolonged period of healing can last up to 1 year.
- Recalcitrant cases and individuals with prolonged pain not resolved after 1 year may require surgical intervention.

ADDITIONAL INFORMATION

For additional information, please see the Case Study in Chapter 15 of *Orthopaedic Examination, Evaluation, and Intervention* on www.accessphysiotherapy.com[5]

PATIENT RESOURCE

- Tennis Elbow/Lateral Epicondylitis. American Society for Surgery of the Hand. http://www.assh.org/Public/HandConditions/Pages/TennisElbow.aspx. Accessed March 9, 2013.

REFERENCES

1. The American Physical Therapy Association. Pattern 4E: impaired joint mobility, motor function, muscle performance, and range of motion associated with localized inflammation. *Interactive Guide to Physical Therapist Practice*. 2003. doi: 10.2522/ptguide.3.1_5. http://guidetoptpractice.apta.org/content/1/SEC12.extract. Accessed May 26, 2014.
2. American Physical Therapy Association. Anatomy and physiology revealed. McGraw-Hill; 2007. http://anatomy.mcgraw-hill.com/apt.html?login=1319535274396&system=Skeletal§ion=Dissection&topic=Elbow%20joint&topicAbbr=Elj&view=Anterior&viewAbbr=Ant&catAbbr=Oth&grpAbbr=San&structure=Surface%20projection%20of%20lateral%20epicondyle%20of%20humerus. Accessed March 9, 2013.
3. Dutton M. *McGraw Hill's NPTE (National Physical Therapy Examination)*. 2nd ed. New York, NY: McGraw-Hill; 2012. http://www.accessphysiotherapy.com/resource/611. Accessed Accessed March 9, 2013.
4. Hertling D, Kessler R M. The elbow and forearm. In: *Management of Common Musculoskeletal Disorders: Physical Therapy Principles and Methods*. 4th ed. New York, NY: Lippincott Williams & Wilkins; 2006:Chapter 12.
5. Prentice WE. Biofeedback. In: Prentice WE, Quillen WS, Underwood F, eds. *Therapeutic Modalities in Rehabilitation*. 4th ed. New York, NY: McGraw-Hill; 2011:Chapter 7. http://www.accessphysiotherapy.com/abstract/8137184#8137184. Accessed March 9, 2013.
6. Dutton M. Orthopaedic examination, evaluation, and intervention. New York, NY: McGraw-Hill; 2008. http://www.accessphysiotherapy. com/resource/612. Accessed March 9, 2013.
7. Houghton PE. The role of therapeutic modalities in wound healing. In: Prentice WE, Quillen WS, Underwood F, eds. *Therapeutic Modalities in Rehabilitation*. 4th ed. New York, NY: McGraw-Hill; 2011:Chapter 3. http://www.accessphysiotherapy.com/abstract/8135453#8135453. Accessed March 9, 2013.
8. Prentice WE. Cryotherapy and thermotherapy. In: Prentice WE, Quillen WS, Underwood F, eds. *Therapeutic Modalities in Rehabilitation*. 4th ed. New York, NY: McGraw-Hill; 2011: Chapter 9. http://www.accessphysiotherapy.com/content/8137995#8137995. Accessed March 9, 2013.
9. Prentice WE. Iontophoresis. In: Prentice WE, Quillen WS, Underwood F, eds. *Therapeutic Modalities in Rehabilitation*. 4th ed. New York, NY: McGraw-Hill; 2011:Chapter 6. http://www.accessphysiotherapy.com/abstract/8136925. Accessed March 9, 2013.
10. Draper DO, Prentice WE. Therapeutic ultrasound. In: Prentice WE, Quillen WS, Underwood F, eds. *Therapeutic Modalities in Rehabilitation*. 4th ed. New York, NY: McGraw-Hill; 2011: Chapter 10. http://www.accessphysiotherapy.com/abstract/8138751. Accessed March 9, 2013.
11. Thigpen C. Extracorporeal shockwave therapy. In: Prentice WE, Quillen WS, Underwood F, eds. *Therapeutic Modalities in Rehabilitation*. 4th ed. New York, NY: McGraw-Hill; 2011: Chapter 11. http://www.accessphysiotherapy.com/abstract/8139510#8139510. Accessed Accessed March 9, 2013.
12. Dutton M. *Dutton's Orthopedic Survival Guide: Managing Common Conditions*. New York, NY: McGraw-Hill; 2011. http://www.accessphysiotherapy.com/resource/685. Accessed March 9, 2013.

ADDITIONAL REFERENCES

- Brulhart L, Gabay C. The differential diagnosis of tenosynovitis. *Rev Med Suisse*. 2011;7(286):587–588, 590, 592–593.
- ICD9DATA web site. http://www.icd9data.com. Accessed March 9, 2013.
- ICD10DATA web site. http://www.icd10data.com. Accessed March 9, 2013.

165 MEDIAL EPICONDYLITIS

Kenneth Lee, DPT, PT
Eric Shamus, PhD, DPT, PT, CSCS

CONDITION/DISORDER SYNONYMS

- Medial tendon injury
- Medial tendonitis
- Golfer's elbow
- Bowler's elbow
- Little leaguer's elbow

ICD-9-CM CODE

- 726.31 Medial epicondylitis

ICD-10-CM CODE

- M77.00 Medial epicondylitis, unspecified elbow

PREFERRED PRACTICE PATTERN

- 4E: Impaired Joint Mobility, Motor Function, Muscle Performance, and Range of Motion Associated with Localized Inflammation[1]

PATIENT PRESENTATION

A 37-year-old male has come to the physical therapy out-patient clinic for an evaluation of his left upper extremity. As a part of his initial history, the patient states that he is a carpenter and enjoys recreational golf with friends on most weekends. The patient states that he has a high pain tolerance, but his current pain became more evident after a vigorous round of golf this weekend. He points to pain along the medial aspect of his left elbow. He has point tenderness with palpation of area with increased pain in elbow with wrist flexion and pronation of forearm. Imaging reveals calcification of medical collateral ligament of elbow. Rubor and warmth are present in the muscle bellies of flexor carpi ulnaris, pronator teres, palmaris longus, flexor digitorum superficialis, and flexor carpi radialis.

KEY FEATURES

Description

- Tendinosis of wrist flexor tendons that attach at medial humeral epicondyle[2]
- Involvement of common flexor origin, flexor carpi radialis, and humeral head of the pronator teres
- Normal collagen response is disrupted by fibroblastic, immature vascular response and incomplete reparative phase
- Early stages may display inflammatory or synovitic characteristics
- Later stages may demonstrate microtearing, tendon degeneration with or without calcification, or incomplete vascular response
- Pain in medial elbow with resisted wrist flexion[2]

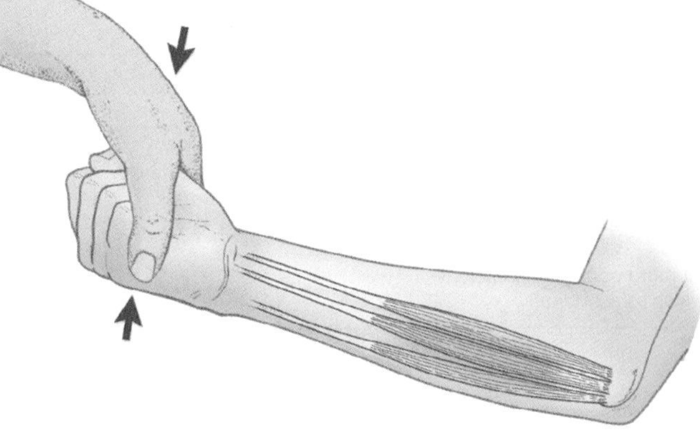

FIGURE 165-1 A test for medial epicondylitis. Forced flexion of the wrist will cause pain over the medial epicondyle. (From Simon RR, Sherman SC. *Emergency Orthopedics*. 6th ed. www.accessemergencymedicine.com. Copyright © The McGraw-Hill Companies, Inc. All rights reserved.)

Essentials of Diagnosis

- Caused by medial tension overload of the elbow associated with repetitive microtrauma of flexor–pronator musculature at its origin on medial epicondyle[2]
- Usually affects middle-aged clients; aging process leads to decreased mucopolysaccharide chondroitin sulfate within tissues, making tendons less extensible

General Considerations

- Tendinosis affecting the elbow is rarely acute unless by direct trauma (then characterized as tendonitis.)[3]
- Pain is usually associated with activity, more so afterward.
- Onset of pain is associated with wrist flexion.
- Direct blows to the medial epicondyle can initiate symptoms.

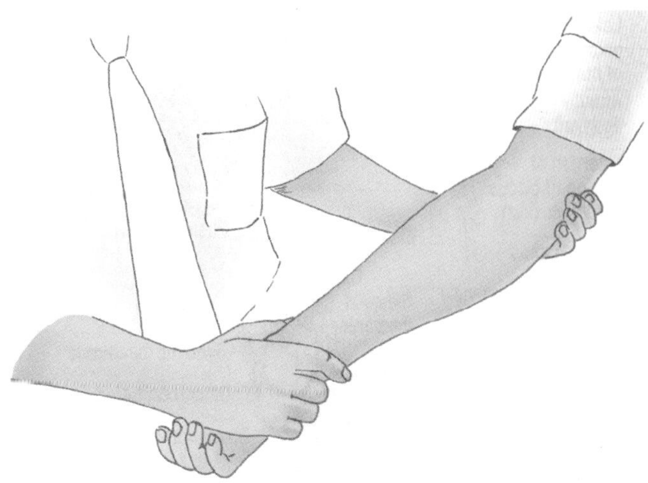

FIGURE 165-2 Stress test of the collateral ligaments of the elbow. (From Simon RR, Sherman SC. *Emergency Orthopedics*. 6th ed. www.accessemergencymedicine.com. Copyright © The McGraw-Hill Companies, Inc. All rights reserved.)

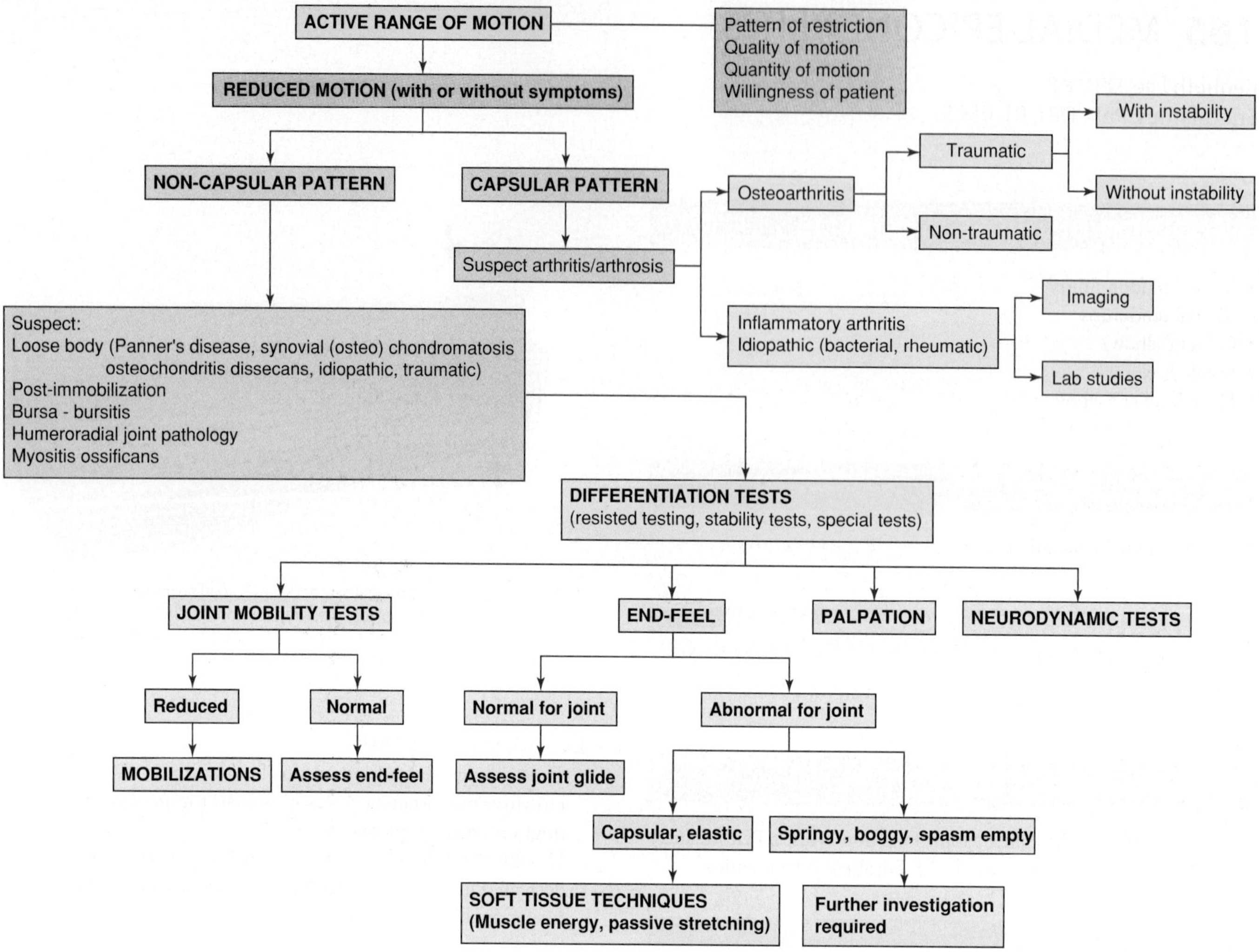

ACTIVE RANGE OF MOTION
- Pattern of restriction
- Quality of motion
- Quantity of motion
- Willingness of patient

REDUCED MOTION (with or without symptoms)

NON-CAPSULAR PATTERN

Suspect:
Loose body (Panner's disease, synovial (osteo) chondromatosis osteochondritis dissecans, idiopathic, traumatic)
Post-immobilization
Bursa - bursitis
Humeroradial joint pathology
Myositis ossificans

CAPSULAR PATTERN

Suspect arthritis/arthrosis
- Osteoarthritis
  - Traumatic
    - With instability
    - Without instability
  - Non-traumatic
- Inflammatory arthritis Idiopathic (bacterial, rheumatic)
  - Imaging
  - Lab studies

DIFFERENTIATION TESTS
(resisted testing, stability tests, special tests)

- JOINT MOBILITY TESTS
  - Reduced → MOBILIZATIONS
  - Normal → Assess end-feel
- END-FEEL
  - Normal for joint → Assess joint glide
  - Abnormal for joint
    - Capsular, elastic → SOFT TISSUE TECHNIQUES (Muscle energy, passive stretching)
    - Springy, boggy, spasm empty → Further investigation required
- PALPATION
- NEURODYNAMIC TESTS

FIGURE 165-3 Examination sequence in the presence of painful flexion and/or extension at the elbow. (From Dutton M. *Dutton's Orthopaedic Examination, Evaluation, and Intervention*. 3rd ed. www.accessphysiotherapy.com. Copyright © The McGraw-Hill Companies, Inc. All rights reserved.)

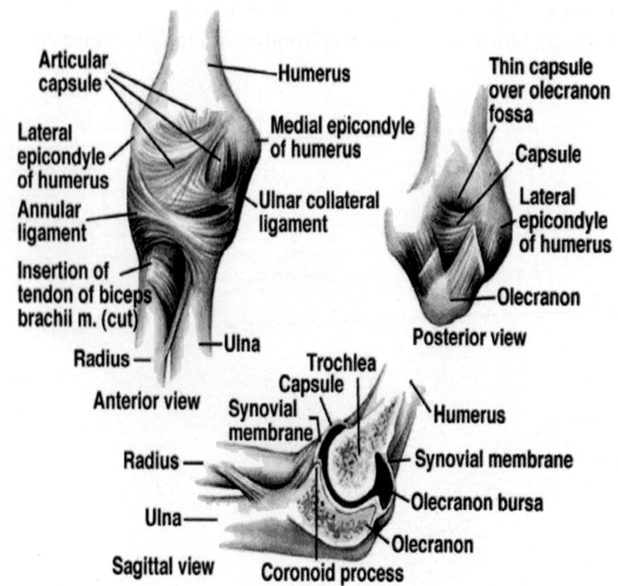

FIGURE 165-4 Elbow anatomy. (Used with permission from Van De, Graaff KM. *Human Anatomy*. 6th ed. New York, NY: McGraw Hill; 2002: Figure 8-27, p 218.)

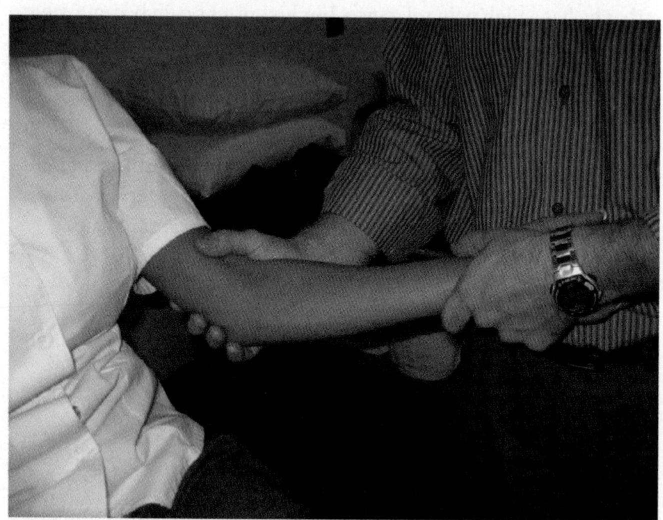

FIGURE 165-5 Elbow ulnar collateral ligament stress test. With forearm in pronation elbow flexed approximately 30 degrees, a valgus stress is applied to the forearm. Pain or increased laxity is indicative of sprained medial or ulnar collateral ligament of the elbow. (From Patel DR, Greydanus DE, Baker RJ. *Pediatric Practice: Sports Medicine*. www.accesspediatrics.com. Copyright © The McGraw-Hill Companies, Inc. All rights reserved.)

Demographics
- People aged 12 to 80 years[4]
- More common during fourth and fifth decade of life[4]
- Males and females equally affected[4]
- 75% of patients are symptomatic in their dominant arm[4]

CLINICAL FINDINGS

SIGNS AND SYMPTOMS
- Pain of insidious onset
- Pain and tenderness over medial epicondyle
- Pain may be related to wrist flexion and pronation
- Pain response varies between dull ache, no pain at rest, and sharp pain with activities
- Active movement may reproduce pain
- Passive movement of full wrist extension with supination and elbow extension reproduces pain at medial epicondyle
- Resistive isometric: resisted wrist flexion and resisted wrist pronation reproduces pain at medical epicondyle
- Elbow-joint movements should be full and painless
- Palpation tenderness at medial epicondyle within the musculature of flexor carpi ulnaris, pronator teres, palmaris longus, flexor digitorum superficialis, and flexor carpi radialis
- Rubor and warmth may be present over medial epicondyle or proximal 5 to 10 mm of associated muscle belly

Functional limitations
- Pain with pinching, squeezing, holding heavy objects, wringing
- Pain with movements of the hand and wrist
- Loss of strength
- Difficulty with grasping activities

Possible Contributing Causes
- Occupations requiring repetitive use of hands for excessive periods of time
- Direct trauma to tendon or wrist
- Sports or occupational activities
  - Tennis, golf, bowling, football, archery, weightlifting
  - Carpentry, plumbing, mechanic
- Most commonly results from repetitive forearm, wrist, hand motions

Differential Diagnosis
- Medial ulnar collateral ligamentous instability
- Ulnar neuritis
- Compression or entrapment of ulnar nerve
- Rheumatoid arthritis
- Medial elbow intra-articular pathology
- Carpal tunnel syndrome
- Pronator syndrome

MEANS OF CONFIRMATION OR DIAGNOSIS

Laboratory Tests
- Laboratory studies for suspected rheumatoid disorders

Imaging
- Radiographs and electromyography (EMG) for patients with neurologic alterations[5]
- MRI for throwing athletes to evaluate ulnar collateral ligament
- MRI may show inflammation/edema or microtearing

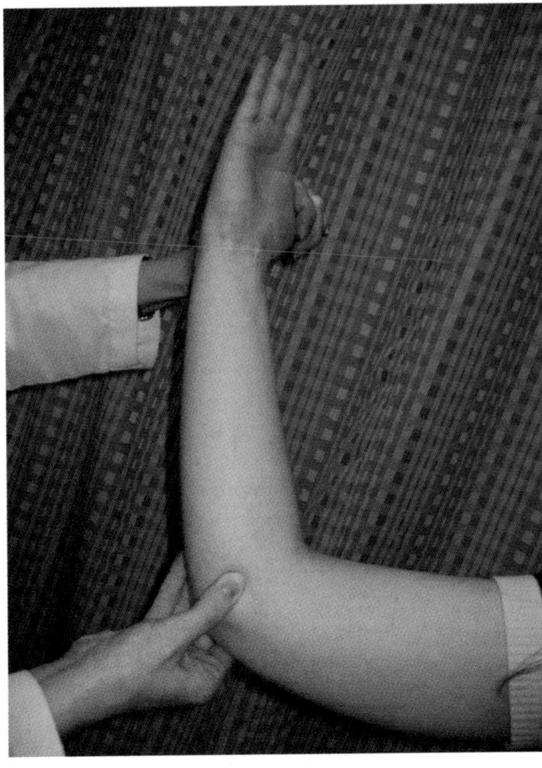

FIGURE 165-6 Milking maneuver. The elbow is held at 90-degree flexion with shoulder in 90-degree abduction. The examiner places one hand over the medial elbow and with the other hand grasps the athlete's hand and thumb. The arm is supinated and externally rotated while maintaining a valgus stress at the elbow. Assess for pain or instability of the medial elbow. (From Patel DR, Greydanus DE, Baker RJ. *Pediatric Practice: Sports Medicine.* www.accesspediatrics.com. Copyright © The McGraw-Hill Companies, Inc. All rights reserved.)

FINDINGS AND INTERPRETATION
- Radiographs usually normal, used to rule out arthritis or osteochondral loose bodies
- Throwing athletes may have ulnar traction spurs and medial collateral calcification

TREATMENT

Medication
- Anti-inflammatory
- Corticosteroid injection
- NSAIDs[6]

REFERRALS/ADMITTANCE
- To radiologist for imaging, X-ray
- To orthopedist for surgical consult, injection

IMPAIRMENTS
- Hand weakness with grasping, squeezing, pinching
- Restricted ROM in elbow and wrist

TESTS AND MEASURES
- Cozen test
- Mill test
- Disabilities of the Arm, Shoulder, and Hand (DASH) score to assess physical function
- Tinel sign at elbow
- Froment sign

INTERVENTION

- Acute phase
  - Rest
  - Immobilization
  - Taping, bracing to inhibit painful muscles or facilitate muscle activity
  - Low-level cold laser[7]
  - Active movement during the day with prevention of high-strain loading of tissue
  - Address swelling
    - Ice[8]
    - Elevation
    - Iontophoresis[9]
- Chronic phase
  - Gradually increase workload as pain and discomfort diminish
  - Elbow and wrist brace to limit motion
  - Counterforce brace to reduce acceleration force
  - Address pain
    - Ice[8]
    - High-voltage pulsed stimulation
    - Iontophoresis
    - Ultrasound[10]
    - Extracorporeal shockwave therapy[11]
  - Address weakness, joint instability
    - Gradually resume normal activity as symptoms improve; establish full, pain-free wrist and elbow ROM
    - Incorporate stretching and progressive isometric exercise
    - Painful eccentric exercises
    - Progress to concentric and eccentric resistive exercise as flexibility and strength returns
    - Grip exercises and progressive strengthening of extensor and flexors using high-repetition/low-weight ratio
    - Concentrate on flexor carpi ulnaris and flexor digitorum superficialis
  - Address mobilization
    - Lateral tilt of the humeroulnar joint

FUNCTIONAL GOALS

- Patient will be able to
  - Turn a door knob without pain.
  - Turn on faucet without pain.
  - Lift a gallon carton of milk from refrigerator at shoulder level without pain.
  - Grip steering wheel without pain.
  - Use a screw driver without pain.
  - Use garden tools without pain.

PROGNOSIS

- Good; prolonged period of healing can last up to 1 year.
- Recalcitrant cases and individuals with prolonged pain not resolved after 1 year may require surgical intervention.

PATIENT RESOURCE

- Golf Injuries to the Hand, Wrist and Elbow. American Society for Surgery of the Hand, ASSH. http://www.assh.org/Public/HandConditions/Pages/Golf.aspx. Accessed June 16, 2013.

REFERENCES

1. The American Physical Therapy Association. Pattern 4E: Impaired joint mobility, motor function, muscle performance, and range of motion associated with localized inflammation. *Interactive Guide to Physical Therapist Practice*. 2003. doi: 10.2522/ptguide.3.1_5. Accessed June 16, 2013.
2. Wolf JM, Mountcastle S, Burks R, Sturdivant RX, Owens BD. Epidemoiology of Lateral and Medial Epicondylitis in a Military Population. *Mil Med.* 2010;175(5):336–339.
3. Dutton M. *McGraw Hill's NPTE (National Physical Therapy Examination)*. 2nd ed. New York, NY: McGraw-Hill; 2012. http://www.accessphysiotherapy.com/resource/611. Accessed June 16, 2013.
4. Ciccotti MC, Schwartz MA, Ciccotti MG. Diagnosis and treatment of Medial Epicondylitis of the elbow. *Clinics in Sports Medicine*. Elsevier Saunders; 693–705:2004.
5. Prentice WE. Biofeedback. In: Prentice WE, Quillen WS, Underwood F, eds. *Therapeutic Modalities in Rehabilitation*. 4th ed. New York, NY: McGraw-Hill; 2011:Chapter 7. http://www.accessphysiotherapy.com/abstract/8137184#8137184. Accessed June 16, 2013.
6. Dutton M. *Orthopaedic Examination, Evaluation, and Intervention*. New York, NY: McGraw-Hill; 2008. http://www.accessphysiotherapy.com/resource/612. Accessed June 16, 2013.
7. Houghton PE. The role of therapeutic modalities in wound healing. In: Prentice WE, Quillen WS, Underwood F, eds. *Therapeutic Modalities in Rehabilitation*. 4th ed. New York, NY: McGraw-Hill; 2011:Chapter 3. http://www.accessphysiotherapy.com/abstract/8135453#8135453. Accessed June 16, 2013.
8. Prentice WE. Cryotherapy and thermotherapy. In: Prentice WE, Quillen WS, Underwood F, eds. *Therapeutic Modalities in Rehabilitation*. 4th ed. New York, NY: McGraw-Hill; 2011:Chapter 9. http://www.accessphysiotherapy.com/content/8137995#8137995. Accessed June 16, 2013.
9. Prentice WE. Iontophoresis. In: Prentice WE, Quillen WS, Underwood F, eds. *Therapeutic Modalities in Rehabilitation*. 4th ed. New York, NY: McGraw-Hill; 2011:Chapter 6. http://www.accessphysiotherapy.com/abstract/8136925. Accessed June 16, 2013.
10. Draper DO, Prentice WE. Therapeutic ultrasound. In: Prentice WE, Quillen WS, Underwood F, eds. *Therapeutic Modalities in Rehabilitation*. 4th ed. New York, NY: McGraw-Hill; 2011:Chapter 10. http://www.accessphysiotherapy.com/abstract/8138751. Accessed June 16, 2013.
11. Thigpen C. Extracorporeal shockwave therapy. In: Prentice WE, Quillen WS, Underwood F, eds. *Therapeutic Modalities in Rehabilitation*. 4th ed. New York, NY: McGraw-Hill; 2011: Chapter 11. http://www.accessphysiotherapy.com/abstract/8139510#8139510. Accessed June 16, 2013.

ADDITIONAL REFERENCES

- Hertling D, Kessler RM. The Elbow and Forearm. *Management of Common Musculoskeletal Disorders: Physical Therapy Principles and Methods*. 4th ed. New York, NY: Lippincott Williams & Wilkins; 2006:Chapter 12.
- ICD9DATA. http://www.icd9data.com. Accessed June 16, 2013.
- ICD10DATA. http://www.icd10data.com. Accessed June 16, 2013.

166 GLENOHUMERAL JOINT INSTABILITY

Steven B. Ambler, DPT, PT, OCS

CONDITION/DISORDER SYNONYMS

- GH instability
- Anterior or anterior-inferior GH instability
- Posterior GH instability
- Multidirectional GH instability

ICD-9-CM CODE[1]

- 831.00 Closed dislocation of shoulder

ICD-10-CM CODES

- S43.006 Unspecified dislocation of unspecified shoulder joint
- M25.311 Other instability, right shoulder

PREFERRED PRACTICE PATTERN

- 4D: Impaired Joint Mobility, Motor Function, Muscle Performance, and Range of Motion Associated with Connective Tissue Dysfunction[2]

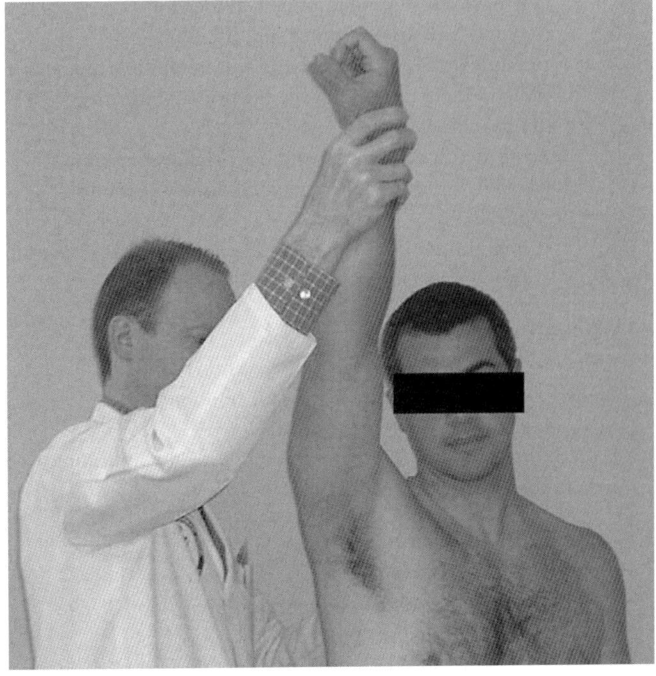

FIGURE 166-1 The apprehension test. (From Imboden J, Hellmann DB, Stone JH. *Current Diagnosis & Treatment in Rheumatology.* 2nd ed. http://www.accessmedicine.com. Copyright © The McGraw-Hill Companies, Inc. All rights reserved.)

PATIENT PRESENTATION

A 19-year-old patient is being seen in the clinic with a chief complaint of right anterior shoulder pain that began after a shoulder dislocation 1 week ago. He states that he injured the shoulder while sustaining a direct blow to the arm playing semipro football and that the dislocation did require relocation in the emergency room. Patient has been wearing a sling since the injury and was given a shoulder stabilizer brace to wear during football. The patient is taking Naproxen and has no pain at rest at this time. He does have 4–5/10 pain when he wakes in the morning and when he has to reach overhead. He denies numbness and tingling and has no other complaints at this time. The patient is currently not practicing and is keeping the arm in the sling. He is left handed and would like to be able to return to his team this season where he plays quarterback.

KEY FEATURES

▶ Description

- Excessive and symptomatic translation of the humeral head in one or more directions
- Instability may be associated with dislocation or subluxation associated with trauma
- Glenohumeral instability may be secondary to atraumatic factors associated with structural, postural, or movement dysfunction or from recurrent minor injury to the structures of the glenohumeral joint[3,4]
- Symptomatology and management vary based on onset, degree, frequency, direction, associated pathology, neuromuscular control, and premorbid activity level[4]
  - Anterior or anterior-inferior instability
    - Mechanism
      - 95% of traumatic shoulder instabilities[4]
      - May result in dislocation or subluxation
      - The humerus is forced into extreme abduction and external rotation, or horizontal abduction
      - Associated pathology includes Bankart lesion (anterior), humeral avulsion of glenohumeral ligaments (HAGL), and Hill–Sachs lesion[5]
    - Symptoms
      - Anterior and inferior shoulder pain
      - Instability and apprehension to abduction, external rotation, horizontal abduction motions
  - Posterior instability
    - Mechanism
      - 5% of traumatic shoulder instabilities4
      - May result in dislocation or subluxation
      - Fall on an outstretched arm, movements of extreme horizontal adduction or internal rotation
      - Associated pathology includes disruption of the posterior capsule, tearing of the teres minor, reverse Hill–Sachs lesion[6]

- Symptoms
  - Posterior shoulder pain
  - Instability and apprehension to flexion, horizontal adduction, internal rotation
- Multidirectional instability
  - Mechanism
    - May occur without episode of trauma, though patient may have a history of traumatic dislocation[7]
    - May result in dislocation or subluxation
    - Instability and apprehension present in multiple directions, though one direction may be the primary direction of instability
    - Associated pathology depends on primary direction of instability, duration of instability, history of trauma[4,7]
  - Symptoms
    - Pain and instability are often determined by the direction of primary instability and can vary based on activity

Essentials of Diagnosis

- Diagnosis made primarily by clinical examination, though imaging often necessary to rule in or out associated pathology
- Anterior instability is most common, followed by multidirectional, then posterior instability

General Considerations

- Onset, degree, frequency, direction, associated pathology, neuromuscular control, and premorbid activity level dictate the diagnosis and management[4]
- Interaction between glenohumeral, scapulothoracic, acromioclavicular, and sternoclavicular joints must be examined to determine optimal treatment plan[8,9]

Demographics

- Young athletes most commonly affected[7]
- Males more often affected than females by traumatic instability; inconclusive evidence for atraumatic or multidirectional
- Multidirectional instability may be associated with gymnastics, swimming, weightlifting, and the individual may have increased joint laxity throughout the body[7]

CLINICAL FINDINGS

SIGNS AND SYMPTOMS

- Specific signs and symptoms depend on onset, degree, frequency, direction, and associated pathology of the injury
- Pain in shoulder; location often depend on the primary direction of instability
- Direction-dependent feelings of instability and apprehension toward the primary direction of instability
- Direction-specific hypermobility of the glenohumeral joint toward the primary direction of instability[3]
- Clicking and popping in the shoulder with movement
- Decreased upward rotation, increased internal rotation and protraction of the scapula
- Special tests for instability specific to the primary direction of instability
- In multidirectional instability, patient may have higher scores on the Beighton scale for assessing generalized joint hypermobility

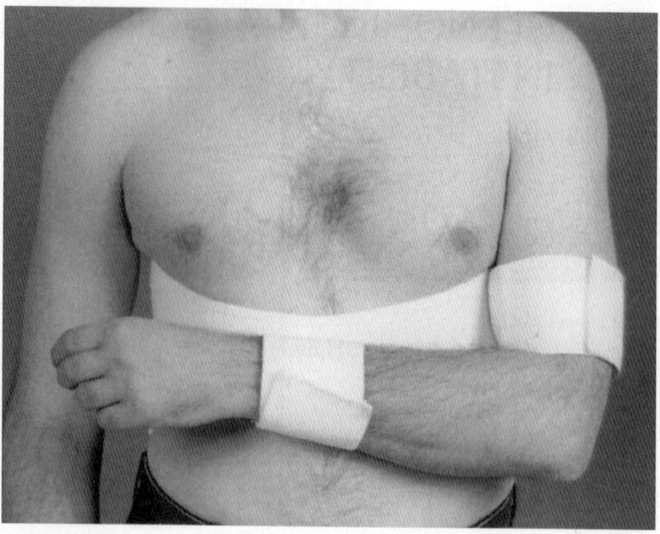

FIGURE 166-2 Shoulder immobilizer. (From Tintinalli JE et al. *Tintinalli's Emergency Medicine: A Comprehensive Study Guide.* 7th ed. www.accessmedicine.com. Copyright © The McGraw-Hill Companies, Inc. All rights reserved.)

Functional Implications

- Difficulty with overhead activities
- Pain with end-range motions of the shoulder
- Pain and difficulty with pushing/pulling activities
- Pain and difficulty with weight-bearing on the arm
- Pain with sleeping on affected side

Possible Contributing Causes

- Poor posture: Forward-shoulder and downwardly rotated, internally rotated, or protracted scapula
- Athletes: Swimmers, gymnasts, and overhead athletes[4,7]

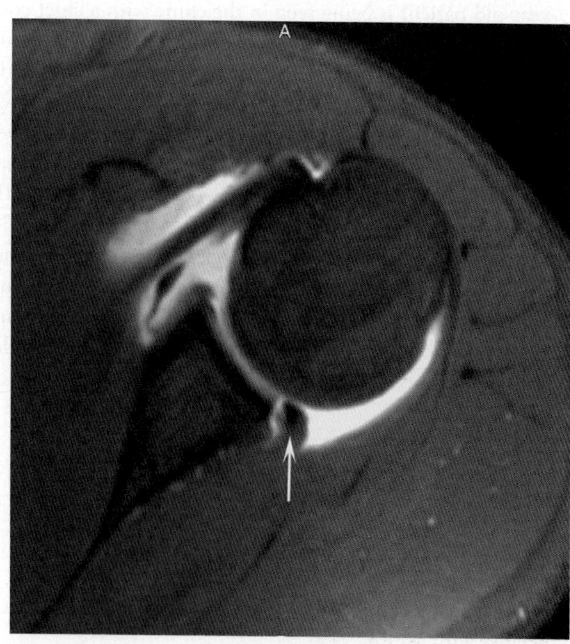

FIGURE 166-3 Axial T1-weighted fat-saturated MR image of the shoulder in a patient with a previous posterior dislocation revealing detachment of the posterior labrum (*arrow*). (From Chen MYM, Pope TL, Ott DJ. *Basic Radiology.* 2nd ed. http://www.accessmedicine.com. Copyright © The McGraw-Hill Companies, Inc. All rights reserved.)

- Increased joint laxity elsewhere in the body (high Beighton scale scores)
- Atraumatic instability may be increased by prior traumatic instability injury or history of other shoulder injury[4]

Differential Diagnosis

- Differential diagnosis may be direction-specific
  - Bankart lesion (anterior)[10]
  - Humeral avulsion of glenohumeral ligaments (HAGLs), anterior
  - Hill–Sachs lesion (anterior)[10]
  - Reverse Hill–Sachs lesion (posterior)[11]
  - Tearing of posterior capsule (posterior)
  - Tearing of teres minor (posterior)
  - Marfan syndrome
  - Osteogenesis imperfecta
  - Ehlers–Danlos syndrome

MEANS OF CONFIRMATION OR DIAGNOSIS

Imaging

- MRI and MR arthrography[10] are images of choice for instability[12,13]
  - Conventional-traumatic
  - Arthrography-chronic
- CT[14]
- Conventional radiograph[10]

Diagnostic Procedures

- Arthroscopy

FINDINGS AND INTERPRETATION

- Imaging to diagnose additional pathology
- Hypermobility of the glenohumeral joint, may be direction-specific[3]
- Decreased upward rotation of the scapula or increased medial winging (internal rotation) of the scapula with humeral elevation
- Increased scapulohumeral rhythm[10]
- Direction-specific positive special tests
- Increased joint laxity throughout the body may be present
- Sample case study[10]

TREATMENT

Medication

- Anti-inflammatory

MEDICAL PROCEDURES

- Surgery
- Bankart repair
- Thermocapsular shift

REFERRALS/ADMITTANCE

- To hospital for diagnostic imaging: MRI, CT, or radiograph as indicated
- To orthopedic surgeon for surgical consult if conservative treatment fails or associated pathology suspected

IMPAIRMENTS

- Hypermobility of the glenohumeral joint, may be direction-specific[3]
- Excessive, direction-specific accessory motions of the humeral head with physiologic shoulder movements
- Decreased upward rotation of the scapula or increased medial winging (internal rotation) of the scapula with humeral elevation
- Muscle performance impairment: Stiffness, shortness, dominance of the pectoralis minor, levator scapulae, rhomboid major and minor
- Muscle performance impairment: Weakness, excessive length, or decreased neuromuscular control of the supraspinatus, infraspinatus, teres minor, subscapularis, upper trapezius, middle trapezius, lower trapezius, and serratus anterior
- Structural impairments of the humerus or glenoid, such as flattening of the glenoid, may be present
- Pain with direction-specific shoulder motions; range of motion may be excessive initially, but limited by pain once symptomatic

TESTS AND MEASURES

- Anterior instability[15,16]
  - Apprehension test
  - Apprehension-relocation test
  - Sulcus sign[10]
  - Anterior slide (drawer) test[10]
  - Load and shift test[10]
  - Crank test[10]
- Posterior instability[15,16]
  - Posterior apprehension test
  - Posterior drawer
  - Load and shift test
  - Sulcus sign
- Multidirectional instability[15,16]
  - Sulcus sign
  - All tests for anterior and posterior instability are appropriate and may be indicated
- Crossover impingement/horizontal adduction test
- Pain provocation test
- Disabilities of the Arm, Shoulder, and Hand (DASH) score to assess physical function
- Shoulder Pain and Disability Index

INTERVENTION

- Intervention based on type (traumatic or atraumatic), onset, degree, frequency, direction, and potential associated pathology[4,17]
- Traumatic
  - Acute
    - Immobilization may be used with the arm in 30 degrees of abduction and 30 degrees of external rotation[18]
    - PROM and AROM within pain-free ranges
      - External rotation may be limited to 65 to 70 degrees to prevent overstressing the anterior structures for anterior instability
      - Internal rotation may be limited to prevent overstressing the anterior structures for posterior instability
    - Isometric, pain-free strengthening
    - Gentle, pain-free weight-bearing on the arm
    - Pain-free dynamic stabilization with the arm in 30 degrees of abduction, neutral rotation, and 30 degrees into the scapular plane
    - Modalities as needed to control pain, inflammation, and muscle guarding
  - Intermediate

        - Progression of items from the acute stage
        - Isotonic strengthening may be initiated with emphasis on rotator cuff musculature to promote stability
        - Progression of weight-bearing exercise, such as modified push-ups, may be initiated to promote stability with emphasis on maintaining correct scapular alignment
        - Trunk-stabilization exercise may be initiated to enhance correct movement patterns and reduce abnormal stress to the glenohumeral joint
        - Neuromuscular electrical stimulation (NMES) to muscles of the rotator cuff during exercise to improve muscle fiber recruitment
    - Advanced
        - Progression of all items from intermediate stage
        - Unilateral weight-bearing stability exercise, such as wall stabilization drills with medicine or stability balls
        - Proper alignment of the scapula should be maintained during all stabilization exercise
        - Plyometric exercise, progressing to overhead then unilateral, may be indicated if the patient is returning to sports[17]
- Atraumatic
    - Intervention similar to that used for traumatic instability
    - Progression may be slower than with traumatic
    - Care should be taken to prevent stretching of capsular tissues
    - Exercise that emphasizes co-contraction and proprioception is indicated
    - Exercise with emphasis on muscle balance around the shoulder girdle with correct positioning and movement of the scapula
    - Trunk-stability exercise to improve stability during functional tasks should be initiated once patient is able to stabilize the glenohumeral joint

FUNCTIONAL GOALS

Note: Duration of the goals will depend on the onset, degree, frequency, direction, associated pathology, neuromuscular control, and premorbid activity level.[4]

- Patient will be able to
    - Dress without pain or instability 100% of the time
    - Perform all self-care activities without pain or instability 100% of the time.
    - Sleep through the night without waking from pain 100% of the time.
    - Bear full weight through the arms without pain or instability 100% of the time.
    - Lift 10 pounds overhead without pain or instability 100% of the time.
    - Perform all daily activities without pain or instability 100% of the time.
    - Resume recreational tasks without pain or instability 100% of the time.

PROGNOSIS

- Return to full function may be anywhere from 2 weeks to 6 months; rehabilitation visits may range from 3 to 36 visits depending on onset, degree, frequency, direction, associated pathology, neuromuscular control, and premorbid activity level.[4,19]
- Recurrence is common in younger populations, while additional pathology often seen in individuals over 40 years of age.[20]

PATIENT RESOURCE

- Shoulder Instability. Newsletter of the American Orthopaedic Society for Sports Medicine. November/December 2008. http://www.sportsmed.org/uploadedFiles/Content/Medical_Professionals/Professional_Educational_Resources/Publications_and_Resources/Sports_Medicine_Update/SMU_2008/SMU%20Nov%20Dec%2008.pdf. Accessed March 1, 2013.

REFERENCES

1. ICD9DATA web site. http://www.icd9data.com. Accessed March 6, 2013.
2. The American Physical Therapy Association. Pattern 4D: Impaired joint mobility, motor function, muscle performance, and range of motion associated with connective tissue dysfunction. *Interactive Guide to Physical Therapist Practice*. 2003. DOI: 10.2522/ptguide.3.1_4. Accessed March 1, 2013.
3. Cameron KL, Duffey ML, DeBerardino TM, et al. Association of generalized joint hypermobility with a history of glenohumeral joint instability. *J Athl Train*. 2010;45(3):253–258.
4. Owens BD, Duffey ML, Nelson BJ, et al. The incidence and characteristics of shoulder instability at the United States Military Academy. *Am J Sports Med*. 2007;35(7):1168–1173.
5. Wilk KE, Macrina LC, Reinold MM. Non-operative rehabilitation for traumatic and atraumatic glenohumeral instability. *N Am J Sports Phys Ther*. 2006;1(1):16–31.
6. Pope EJ, Ward JP, Rokito AS. Anterior shoulder instability—a history of arthroscopic treatment. *Bull NYU Hosp Jt Dis*. 2011;69(1):44–49.
7. Hottya GA, Tirman PF, Bost FW, et al. Tear of the posterior shoulder stabilizers after posterior dislocation: MR imaging and MR arthrographic findings with arthroscopic correlation. *AJR Am J Roentgenol*. 1998;171(3):763–768.
8. Cordasco FA. Understanding multidirectional instability of the shoulder. *J Athl Train*. 2000;35(3):278–285.
9. Kikuchi K, Itoi E, Yamamoto N, et al. Scapular inclination and glenohumeral joint stability: a cadaveric study. *J Orthop Sci*. 2008;13(1):72–77.
10. Ludewig PM, Reynolds JF. The association of scapular kinematics and glenohumeral joint pathologies. *J Orthop Sports Phys Ther*. 2009;39(2):90–104.
11. Dutton M. *Orthopaedic Examination, Evaluation, and Intervention*. New York, NY: McGraw-Hill; 2008. http://www.accessphysiotherapy.com/resource/612. Accessed March 3, 2013.
12. Dutton M. *McGraw Hill's NPTE (National Physical Therapy Examination)*. 2nd ed. New York, NY: McGraw-Hill; 2012. http://www.accessphysiotherapy.com/resource/611. Accessed March 9, 2013.
13. Jana M, Gamanagatti S. Magnetic resonance imaging in glenohumeral instability. *World J Radiol*. 2011;3(9):224–232.
14. Waldt S, Rummeny EJ. Magnetic resonance imaging of glenohumeral instability. *Rofo*. 2006;178(6):590–599.
15. Malone TR, Hazle C, Grey ML. *Imaging in Rehabilitation*. New York, NY: McGraw-Hill; 2008. http://www.accessphysiotherapy.com/resource/613. Accessed February 28, 2013.
16. Cook C, Hegedus EJ. *Orthopedic physical examination tests: an evidence-based approach*. Upper Saddle River, NJ: Pearson Prentice Hall; 2008.
17. Magee DJ. *Orthopedic physical assessment*. 5th ed. St. Louis, MO: Saunders Elsevier; 2008.

18. Dutton M. *Dutton's Orthopedic Survival Guide: Managing Common Conditions*. New York, NY: McGraw-Hill; 2011. http://www.accessphysiotherapy.com/resource/685. Accessed March 8, 2013.
19. Itoi E, Hatakeyama Y, Kido T, et al. A new method of immobilization after traumatic anterior dislocation of the shoulder: a preliminary study. *J Shoulder Elbow Surg*. 2003;12(5):413–415.
20. American Physical Therapy Association. *Guide to Physical Therapists Practice*. 2nd ed. *Phys Ther*. 2002;81:9–744.

ADDITIONAL REFERENCE

- ICD10DATA web site. http://www.icd10data.com. Accessed March 1, 2013.
- Sonnabend DH. Treatment of primary anterior shoulder dislocation in patients older than 40 years of age. Conservative versus operative. *Clin Orthop Relat Res*. 1994;(304):74–77.

167 GLENOHUMERAL JOINT OSTEOARTHRITIS

Eric Shamus, PhD, DPT, PT, CSCS
Reuben Escorpizo, DPT, MSc, PT

CONDITION/DISORDER SYNONYM

- Glenohumeral joint osteoarthritis (OA)

ICD-9-CM CODES

- 715 Osteoarthrosis and allied disorders
- 715.11 Osteoarthrosis localized primary involving shoulder region
- 715.21 Osteoarthrosis localized secondary involving shoulder region
- 715 .9 Osteoarthrosis unspecified whether generalized or localized

ICD-10-CM CODES

- M19.019 Primary osteoarthritis, unspecified shoulder
- M19.219 Secondary osteoarthritis, unspecified shoulder

PREFERRED PRACTICE PATTERNS

- 4D: Impaired Joint Mobility, Motor Function, Muscle Performance, and Range of Motion Associated with Connective Tissue Dysfunction[1]
- 4F: Impaired Joint Mobility, Motor Function, Muscle Performance, Range of Motion, and Reflex Integrity Associated with Spinal Disorders[2]
- 4H: Impaired Joint Mobility, Motor Function, Muscle Performance, and Range of Motion Associated with Joint Arthroplasty[3]
- 4I: Impaired Joint Mobility, Motor Function, Muscle Performance, and Range of Motion Associated with Bony or Soft Tissue Surgery[4]

PATIENT PRESENTATION

A 48-year-old man who formerly played high school and collegiate football presents with chronic right shoulder pain with progressive loss of function. The patient describes the pain as a deep ache. The patient has all shoulder motions limited. He is slightly weaker on the right side. He denies any neck pain and has full cervical spine range of motion (ROM). The patient had an X-ray that showed decreased joint space at the glenohumeral joint.

KEY FEATURES

Description

- Most common form of arthritis
- Degenerative joint disease
- Commonly affects weight-bearing joints
- Associated with increased age, obesity, previous trauma, previous surgery
- Associated with abnormal loading of joints
- Characterized by joint pain
- Arthrosis
- Osteoarthrosis
- Polyarthrosis

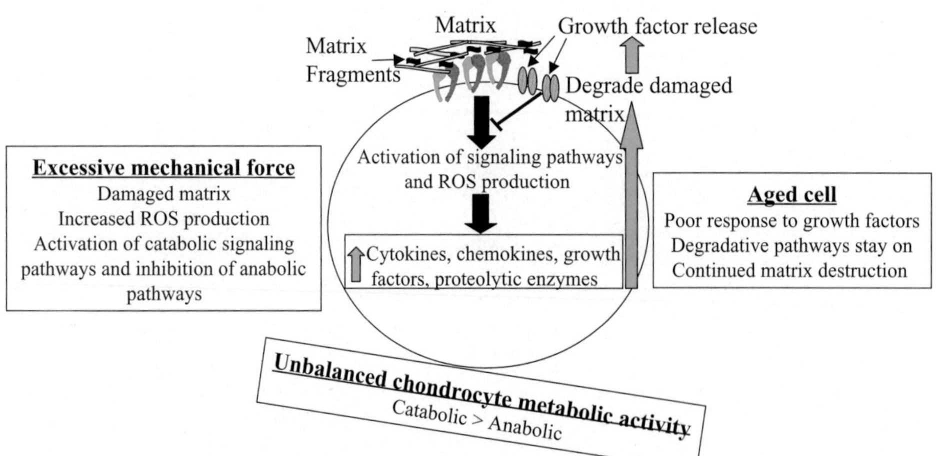

FIGURE 167-1 Theoretical model for pathways involved in cartilage destruction during the development of osteoarthritis. Excessive mechanical forces stimulate the chondrocyte directly or indirectly through signals generated by matrix damage including generation of matrix fragments. The resultant activation of signaling pathways, including ROS generation, results in increased production of cytokines, chemokines, and proteolytic enzymes. This catabolic response to injury serves to degrade the damaged matrix. Matrix degradation results in release of growth factors stored in the matrix, which would normally feedback on the cell and shut down the catabolic pathways. But aged chondrocytes have an insufficient response to growth factor stimulation, resulting in continued matrix destruction from unbalanced catabolic and anabolic activity. (Reproduced with permission from Loeser RF. Molecular mechanisms of cartilage destruction: mechanics, inflammatory mediators and aging collide. *Arthritis Rheum.* 2006;54:1357.)

Essentials of Diagnosis

- Radiography is standard method for diagnosis
- Kellgren and Lawrence (KL) grade ≥2 (definite radiographic OA)[5]
- Osteophytes, joint-space narrowing, sclerosis
- Cartilage lesions, bone marrow lesions, synovitis, effusion, and subchondral bone attrition/sclerosis
- Erosion of articular cartilage
- Synovial hyperplasia
- Fibrosis
- Inflammatory cell infiltration
- Conventional radiograph is most commonly used tool in OA[6]
- Diagnosis is based on a careful history, physical examination, imaging studies, laboratory examination, and exclusion of other possible diseases

General Considerations

- Low bone-mineral density (BMD)
- Repetitive joint use or loading
- Joint alignment
- Bone or joint morphology
- Calcification of the biceps tendon
- Bone formation, cyst formation
- Thickening of subchondral bone plate, osteosclerosis
- Overall joint dysfunction
- Joint swelling and inflammation (in certain, severe cases)
- Joint pain
- Morning stiffness
- Long-term disease
- Secondary problems
  - Muscle atrophy and weakness
  - Bony protrusion or prominence
  - Joint deformity
  - Difficulty with ADLs

Demographics

- More common in middle- to older-aged populations
- Women more commonly affected than men
- More common in African Americans than other ethnic groups
- May affect approximately 12% of the population in the United States and other developed countries[7]

CLINICAL FINDINGS

SIGNS AND SYMPTOMS

- Joint pain, aching
- Joint stiffness
- Muscle weakness
- Muscle atrophy
- Crepitus
- Bony enlargement
- Limited ROM in joint
- Joint-line tenderness
- Joint deformity in severe cases
- Activity limitation

Functional Implications

- Limited mobility
- Household and work-related activity limitations/restrictions
- Decreased overall activity and participation

Possible Contributing Causes

- Chronic factors affecting the joint (obesity, BMD, LLD)
- Aging

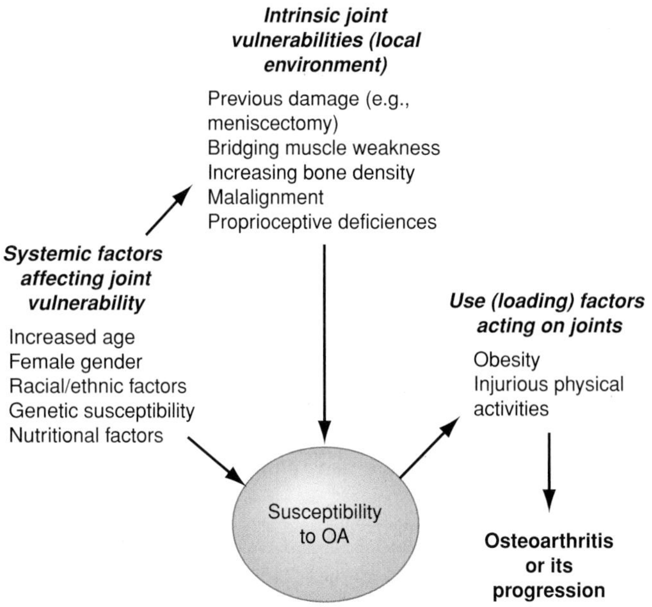

FIGURE 167-2 Risk factors for osteoarthritis either contribute to the susceptibility of the joint (systemic factors or factors in the local joint environment) or increase risk by the load they put on the joint. Usually a combination of loading and susceptibility factors is required to cause disease or its progression. (From Longo DL, Fauci A, Kasper D, et al., eds. *Harrison's Principles of Internal Medicine.* 18th ed. New York, NY: McGraw-Hill, 2012.)

- Chronic and vigorous joint-loading
- Previous chronic joint injury (e.g., accident, trauma); secondary OA

Differential Diagnosis

- Rheumatoid arthritis
- Gout
- Cervical radiculopathy
- Rotator cuff tear
- Bursitis
- Biceps tendinitis
- Adhesive capsulitis
- Fibromyalgia syndrome
- Spondyloarthropathy

MEANS OF CONFIRMATION

Laboratory Tests

- Synovial fluid examination (optional, not required)
- Other laboratory tests can be done to rule out other conditions

Imaging

- Conventional radiograph of the joint
- MRI of the joint
- Diagnostic ultrasound of the joint and synovium[8]

FINDINGS AND INTERPRETATION

- OA is a clinical diagnosis, which can be based on
  - Persistent usage-related pain in joint or joints
  - Age ≥45 years[7]
  - Morning stiffness ≤30 minutes[7]
- Imaging studies (e.g., radiograph):
  - Osteophytes, joint-space narrowing, sclerosis

- Cartilage lesions, bone marrow lesions, synovitis, effusion, subchondral bone attrition/sclerosis
- Erosion of articular cartilage

TREATMENT

- Surgery: Total joint replacement, joint lavage, and debridement
- Medication
  - NSAIDs (including topical NSAIDs, capsaicin)[8]
  - Acetaminophen
  - Opioids
  - Glucosamine and chondroitin sulfate
  - Glucocorticoids or corticosteroids
  - Intra-articular injections (corticosteroids, hyaluronic acid)
  - Emerging drugs: Anti-tumor necrosis factor (anti-TNF), calcitonin, growth factors, nerve growth factor antibodies

REFERRALS/ADMITTANCE

- To rheumatologist for assessment of underlying complications
- To internal medicine specialist
- To orthopedic specialist
- To surgeon for surgical consult
- To dietician/nutritionist for dietary counseling

IMPAIRMENTS

- Mobility
- Self-care
- Overhead reaching
- Sleeping on affected side
- Role at home and in community
- School and work
- Recreation, leisure, sports

TESTS AND MEASURES

- Pain provocation test
- Disabilities of the Arm, Shoulder, and Hand (DASH) score to assess physical function
- Shoulder Pain and Disability Index

INTERVENTION

- Exercises (resistance, endurance, flexibility)
  - Aquatic exercises
- Training on ADLs
- Use of assistive or adaptive devices
- Heat therapy
- Weight management
- Rest
- Orthoses, shoulder sling
- Ice[9]
- Diet
- Acupuncture
- Pain management
- Energy conservation techniques
- Joint protection
- Ultrasound[10]
- Electric stimulation[11]
- Patient education

FUNCTIONAL GOALS

- Patient will have
  - Improved joint mobility and stability to reach overhead.
  - Improved muscle strength to lift dishes into cabinet.
  - Improved muscle and aerobic endurance.
  - Improved activity and participation at home, at work, and in the community.
- Patient will be able to
  - Resume ADLs pain-free.
  - Turn a key or doorknob pain-free.
  - Lift a baby from crib without pain, maintaining neutral wrist posture.

PROGNOSIS

- No definite cure for OA.
- Treatment is for symptom-management, though emerging drugs may modify OA disease mechanism.
- Joint damage is irreversible.
- Recovery or relief from symptoms may depend on disease duration and timely intervention.
- OA is a chronic disease, may mean long-term burden.
- Factors affecting prognosis: Demographics, severity and natural history of disease, medical comorbidities, behavioral comorbidities (fear avoidance, catastrophizing, central sensitization).
- General endurance, good muscle strength, and mobile joints are good prognosticating factors.
- Motivation and compliance with physical therapy intervention (e.g., home exercise program) and support from family and environment could also improve treatment outcomes.

PATIENT RESOURCE

- Osteoarthritis Research Society International. OARSI Primer; 2010. Last updated 2011. http://primer.oarsi.org. Accessed June 20, 2013.

REFERENCES

1. The American Physical Therapy Association. Pattern 4D: Impaired joint mobility, motor function, muscle performance, and range of motion associated with connective tissue dysfunction. *Interactive Guide to Physical Therapist Practice*. 2003. DOI: 10.2522/ptguide.3.1_4. Accessed June 20, 2013.
2. The American Physical Therapy Association. Pattern 4F: Impaired joint mobility, motor function, muscle performance, range of motion, and reflex integrity associated with spinal disorders. *Interactive Guide to Physical Therapist Practice*. 2003. DOI: 10.2522/ptguide.3.1_6. Accessed June 20, 2013.
3. The American Physical Therapy Association. Pattern 4H: Impaired joint mobility, motor function, muscle performance, and range of motion associated with joint arthroplasty. *Interactive Guide to Physical Therapist Practice*. 2003. DOI: 10.2522/ptguide.3.1_8. Accessed June 20, 2013.
4. The American Physical Therapy Association. Pattern 4I: Impaired joint mobility, motor function, muscle performance, and range of motion associated with bony or soft tissue surgery. *Interactive Guide to Physical Therapist Practice* 2003. DOI: 10.2522/ptguide.3.1_9. Accessed June 20, 2013.
5. Kellgren JH, Lawrence JS. *Atlas of Standard Radiographs*. Oxford, UK: Oxford University Press; 1963.

6. McKinnis L. *Fundamentals of Musculoskeletal Imaging (Contemporary Perspectives in Rehabilitation)*. Philadelphia, PA: F.A. Davis; 2005.
7. Royal College of Physicians. *Osteoarthritis: National Clinical Guideline and Management in Adults*. London, UK: Royal College of Physicians; 2008.
8. Dutton M. *Orthopaedic Examination, Evaluation, and Intervention*. New York, NY: McGraw-Hill; 2008. http://www.accessphysiotherapy.com/resource/612. Accessed June 20, 2013.
9. Prentice WE. Chapter 9. Cryotherapy and thermotherapy. In: Prentice WE, Quillen WS, Underwood F, eds. *Therapeutic Modalities in Rehabilitation, 4e*. New York: McGraw-Hill; 2011. http://www.accessphysiotherapy.com/content/8137995#8137995. Accessed June 20, 2013.
10. Draper DO, Prentice WE. Chapter 10. Therapeutic ultrasound. In: Prentice WE, Quillen WS, Underwood F, eds. *Therapeutic Modalities in Rehabilitation.* 4th ed. New York, NY: McGraw-Hill; 2011. http://www.accessphysiotherapy.com/abstract/ 8138751. Accessed June 20, 2013.
11. Dutton M. *McGraw Hill's NPTE (National Physical Therapy Examination)2e*. New York, NY: McGraw-Hill; 2012. http://www.accessphysiotherapy.com/resource/611. Accessed June 20, 2013.

ADDITIONAL REFERENCES

- ICD9DATA web site. http://www.icd9data.com. Accessed June 20, 2013.
- ICD10DATA web site. http://www.icd10data.com. Accessed June 20, 2013.

168 VOLKMANN ISCHEMIC CONTRACTURE

Stacey L. Frazee, DPT
Eric Shamus, PhD, DPT, PT, CSCS

CONDITION/DISORDER SYNONYMS

- Forearm, anterior compartment syndrome
- Volkmann contracture
- Volkmann ischemic contracture

ICD-9-CM CODE[1]

- 958.6 Volkmann ischemic contracture

ICD-10-CM CODE[2]

- T79.6 Traumatic ischemia of muscle

PREFERRED PRACTICE PATTERN[3]

- 4E: Impaired Joint Mobility, Motor Function, Muscle Performance, and Range of Motion Associated with Localized Inflammation

PATIENT PRESENTATION

A 38-year-old man with a recent supracondylar humerus fracture presents with disproportionate unilateral forearm pain. He is currently experiencing tingling in the area. His radial pulse is absent. Distal phalanges are blanched tint and are cool to the touch. His wrist and fingers are in a flexed position and he has diminished sensation on the volar side of his hand.

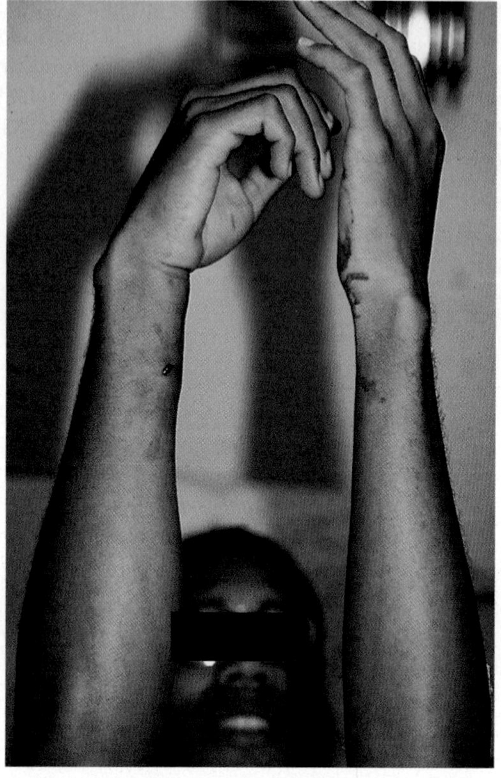

FIGURE 168-1 Compartment syndrome. Volkmann contracture is a serious late complication of unrelieved compartment syndrome. (From Knoop KJ, Stack L, Storrow A, Jason Thurman R. *The Atlas of Emergency Medicine*. 3rd ed. http://www.accessmedicine.com. Copyright © The McGraw-Hill Companies, Inc. All rights reserved. Photo contributor: Lawrence B. Stack, MD.)

KEY FEATURES

Description

- Flexion contracture of the wrist, resulting in claw-like deformity
- Obstruction of brachial artery near the elbow
  - Obstruction commonly caused by compartment syndrome or fracture
- Three levels of severity
  - Mild: Contracture of two or three fingers only, only limited sensation deficit
  - Moderate: All fingers (including thumb) contracted in flexed position; wrist may be in flexion and slight sensation loss
  - Severe: All muscles in the forearm affected (flexors and extensors)
- Arteriolar compression occurs and causes muscle and nerve ischemia
  - Acute, sensory changes develop after 30 minutes of ischemia
  - Acute, irreversible nerve damage in 12 to 24 hours
  - Acute, irreversible muscle changes (i.e., necrosis) in 3 to 8 hours

Essentials of Diagnosis

- Diagnosis is typically made by clinical examination and compartment pressure measurement
- Severe pain that is not alleviated by elevation or pain medication
  - Pain increases with passive/active range of motion and compression
- Distal pulses are diminished/absent
- Strength and sensation are diminished
- Edema in affected limb

General Considerations

- Occurs in the flexor/volar compartment of the forearm
  - Flexor digitorum profundus becomes fibrotic and shortened
  - Flexor pollicis longus becomes fibrotic and shortened
- Classic P's
  - Pain
  - Pallor
  - Pulselessness
  - Paresthesias
  - Paralysis

- Complications
  - Infection
  - Contractures
  - Deformity
  - Amputation
  - Acidosis
  - Hyperkalemia
  - Myoglobinuria
  - Acute renal failure and shock

Demographics

- Younger age, high-energy/high-velocity trauma, and systemic hypotension associated with an increased risk of traumatic accident
- More common in children
- High-risk patients include:
  - Soft-tissue injury in males aged <35 years with bleeding disorder or receiving anticoagulants
  - Crush injury patients
  - Patients with prolonged limb compression
- Individuals using circumferential wraps, restrictive dressings, casts, or immobilizer are at an increased risk

CLINICAL FINDINGS

SIGNS AND SYMPTOMS

- Swollen and tense tender compartment
- Severe pain that does not go away with pain medicine or raising the affected area
- Passive extension of fingers is limited and painful
  - Flexor digitorum profundus and flexor pollicis longus often effected
- First signs
  - Decreased sensation, numbness
  - Tingling, parethesias
- Paresis
- Decreased palpable pulses (radial pulse is absent)
- Pallor of skin overlying compartment, paleness of skin
- Motor weakness or paralysis
- Pain when the area is squeezed
- Extreme pain when moving affected area
  - Deep, throbbing pressure out of proportion to that expected from the injury

Functional Implications

- Flexion contractures in wrist and fingers
- Pain out of proportion top that expected from the injury
- Decreased strength in affected limb
- Loss of sensation and 2-point discrimination deficits
- Inability to use upper extremity
- Fatigue

Possible Contributing Causes

- Traumatic compartment syndrome
  - Car accident
  - Crush injury
  - Hematoma
  - Surgery
  - Complex fractures
    - Supracondylar fracture of humerus
    - Radial fracture

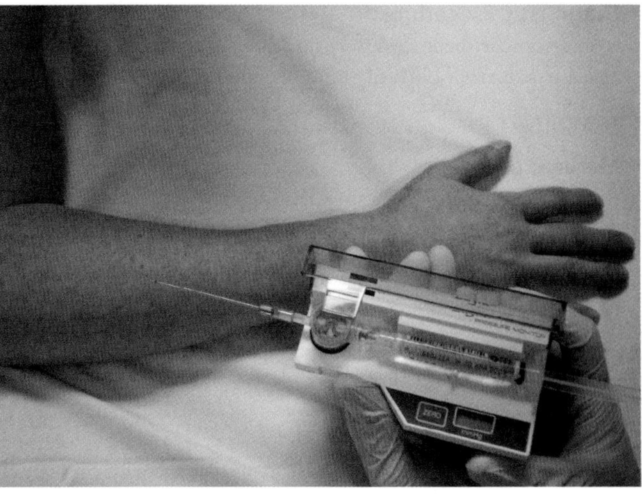

FIGURE 168-2 Forearm extensor compartment pressure measurement. (From Tintinalli JE, Stephan Stapczynski J, John Ma O, et al., eds. *Tintinalli's Emergency Medicine: A Comprehensive Study Guide.* 7th ed. http://www.accessmedicine.com. Copyright © The McGraw-Hill Companies, Inc. All rights reserved.)

- Chronic compartment syndrome
  - Repetitive activities
  - Poor upper extremity biomechanics
- Vascular conditions
  - Arterial or venous injuries with hemorrhage
  - Deep vein thrombosis
  - Constrictive casts or dressings
  - Tourniquets
  - Bleeding disorders (i.e., hemophilia)
- Soft-tissue injuries
  - Burns
  - Crush injury
  - Contusion
  - Snakebite
  - Prolonged limb compression
- Anabolic steroids
- Creatine supplementation[5]

Differential Diagnosis

- Forearm compartment syndrome
- Rhabdomyolysis
- Carpal tunnel syndrome
- Fracture
- Periostitis
- Tumor
- Nerve entrapment
- Muscle tear
- Necrotizing fasciitis
- Cellulitis
- Cnidaria Envenomation
- Gas Gangrene
- Peripheral vascular injuries

MEANS OF CONFIRMATION OR DIAGNOSIS

Imaging

- Radiographs, bone scans, CT scans, or MRI can be used to rule out fractures and/or muscle tears
- Doppler ultrasound used to evaluated arterial flow and rule out DVT

Diagnostic Procedure

- Intracompartmental pressure measurements
- Pulse oximetry to identify limb hypoperfusion

TREATMENT

Medication

- Non-steriodal anti-inflammatory drugs (NSAIDs)

MEDICAL PROCEDURES

- Restoration of blood flow
- Subcutaneous fasciotomy to reduce compartmental pressure
- Surgery to release fixed tissues and improve function of hand
- Hyperbaric oxygen therapy

FINDINGS AND INTERPRETATION

- Emergency surgery to prevent permanent damage with pressure measurements of ≥30 mm Hg

REFERRALS/ADMITTANCE

- For imaging: X-ray, CT, or MRI
- For surgery if fasciotomy is required

IMPAIRMENTS

- Weakness
- Numbness and tingling
- Severe pain

TESTS AND MEASURES

- Pain, visual analog scale (VAS)
  - 24-hour pain
  - Worst average pain
  - Best average pain
  - Tenderness on palpation
- Cardiovascular integrity
  - Blood pressure at rest and after activity
  - Palpation of distal pulses
  - Capillary refill
- Skin integrity
  - Associated skin assessment
    - Edema (linear girth measurements, palpation)
    - Color
    - Temperature
- Neurologic examination
  - Sensation
    - Light touch
    - Pin prick Limb sensation
    - 2-point discrimination
  - Upper extremity deep tendon reflexes
  - Proprioception
  - Kinesthetic awareness
  - Coordination
- Limb strength
  - Manual muscle test (MMT)

INTERVENTION

- Avoid external pressure
  - If cast or bandage is causing the problem it should be loosened or removed.
  - Avoid splints, tight wound dressing.
- Rest
- Address swelling
- Address pain
- Wound care
- Laser therapy

FUNCTIONAL GOALS

- The patient will be able to:
  - Regain full ROM in upper extremity (UE).
  - Return to activities such as computer use, writing, and driving.

PROGNOSIS

- Determined by severity and stage of disease at the time treatment was initiated.
- Determined by injury leading to the syndrome.
- Permanent injury can occur to nerves or muscles if diagnosis is delayed.
- Complete recovery if there is good collateral circulation.[5]

PATIENT RESOURCE

- MedlinePlus, NIH National Institutes of Health. Compartment Syndrome. http://www.ncbi.nlm.nih.gov/pubmedhealth/PMH0002204/. Accessed July 4, 2013.

REFERENCES

1. ICD-9-CM. http://www.icd9data.com. Accessed July 4, 2013.
2. ICD-10-CM. http://www.icd10data.com. Accessed July 4, 2013.
3. The American Physical Therapy Association. *Guide to Physical Therapist Practice*. Alexandria, VA: The American Physical Therapy Association; 2003. http://guidetoptpractice.apta.org./ Accessed July 4, 2013.
4. Hile AM, Anderson JM, Fiala KA, et al. Creatine supplementation and anterior compartment pressure during exercise in the heat in dehydrated men. *J Athl Train*. 2006;41(1):30–35.
5. Simon RR, Sherman SC. Chapter 4. Complications. In: Simon RR, Sherman SC, eds. *Emergency Orthopedics*. 6th ed. New York, NY: McGraw-Hill; 2011. http://www.accessphysiotherapy.com/content/7701649. Accessed July 17, 2013.

ADDITIONAL REFERENCES

- Botte MJ, Gelberman RH. Acute compartment syndrome of the forearm. *Hand Clin*. 1998;14(3):391–403.
- Dutton M. Vascular disorders. In: Dutton M, ed. *Dutton's Orthopaedic Examination, Evaluation, and Intervention*. 3rd ed. New York, NY: McGraw-Hill; 2012. http://www.accessphysiotherapy.com/content/56526316. Accessed July 17, 2013.
- France RC. *Introduction to Sports Medicine & Athletic Training*. 2nd ed. Independence, KY: Cengage Learning. 2011. ISBN 1435464362.
- Geiderman JM, Katz D. General principles of orthopedic injuries. In: Marx J, ed. *Emergency Medicine: Concepts and Clinical Practice*. 7th ed. Philadelphia, PA: Mosby Elsevier; 2009: Chapter 46.
- Goodman CC, Fuller KS. *Pathology Implications for the Physical Therapist*. 3rd ed. Philadelphia, PA: Saunders Elsevier; 2009.
- Gourgiotis S, Villias C, Germanos S, Foukas A, Ridolfini MP. Acute limb compartment syndrome: a review. *J Surg Educ*. 2007;64(3):178–186.

- Hensinger RN. Complications of fractures in children. In: Green NE, Swiontkowski MF, eds. *Skeletal Trauma in Children*. 4th ed. Philadelphia, PA: Saunders Elsevier; 2008: Chapter 6.
- Jobe MT. Compartment syndromes and Volkmann contracture. In: Canale ST, Beaty JH, eds. *Campbell's Operative Orthopaedics*. 11th ed. Philadelphia, PA: Mosby Elsevier; 2007: Chapter 71.
- Konstantakos EK, Dalstrom DJ, Nelles ME, Laughlin RT, Prayson MJ. Diagnosis and management of extremity compartment syndromes: an orthopaedic perspective. *Am Surg*. 2007;73(12): 1199–1209.
- Marshall ST, Browner BD. Emergency care of musculoskeletal injuries. In: Townsend CM Jr, Beauchamp RD, Evers BM, Mattox KL, eds. *Sabiston Textbook of Surgery*. 19th ed. Philadelphia, PA: Saunders Elsevier; 2012: Chapter 20.
- Naidu SH, Heppenstall RB. Compartment syndrome of the forearm and hand. *Hand Clin*. 1994;10(1):13–27.
- O'Neil D, Sheppard JE. Transient compartment syndrome of the forearm resulting from venous congestion from a tourniquet. *J Hand Surg Am*. 1989;14(5):894–896.
- Otsuka NY, Kasser JR. Supracondylar fractures of the humerus in children. *J Am Acad Orthop Surg*. 1997;5(1):19–26.
- Raimer L, McCarthy RA, Raimer D, Colome-Grimmer M. Congenital Volkmann ischemic contracture: a case report. *Pediatr Dermatol*. 2008;25(3):352–354.
- Rasul AT, Lorenzo CT, Agnew S. Acute compartment syndrome. 2001. http://emedicine.medscape.com/article/307668-overview. Accessed July 4, 2013.
- Rios M, Ribeiro C, Soares P, et al. Volkmann ischemic contracture in a newborn. *BMJ Case Rep*. 2011. DOI: pii: bcr0520114201.
- Twaddle BC, Amendola A. Compartment syndrome. In: Browner BD, Jupiter JB, Levine AM, Trafton PG, Krettek C, eds. *Skeletal Trauma*. 4th ed. Philadelphia, PA: Saunders Elsevier; 2008: Chapter 13.
- Wall CJ, Lynch J, Harris IA, et al. Clinical practice guidelines for the management of acute limb compartment syndrome following trauma. *ANZ J Surg*. 2010;80(3):151–156.
- Yamaguchi S, Viegas SF. Causes of upper extremity compartment syndrome. *Hand Clin*. 1998;14(3):365–370, viii.

SECTION F WRIST AND HAND DISORDERS

169 BOUTONNIÈRE DEFORMITY

Tiffany M. Barber, DPT
Eric Shamus, PhD, DPT, PT, CSCS
Jesse Solotoff, DPT
Linda M. Martin, PhD, OTR/L, FAOTA

CONDITION/SYNONYM

- BD

ICD-9-CM CODE

- 736.21 Boutonnière deformity

ICD-10-CM CODES

- M20.02 Boutonnière deformity
- M20.021 Boutonnière deformity of right finger(s)
- M20.022 Boutonnière deformity of left finger(s)
- M20.029 Boutonnière deformity of unspecified finger(s)

PREFERRED PRACTICE PATTERN

- 4E: Impaired joint mobility, motor function, muscle performance, and ROM associated with localized inflammation[1]

PATIENT PRESENTATION

The patient is a 42-year-old man who owns a landscaping business. He reports he was injured approximately 2 months ago while trying to clear grass from around a lawnmower blade, resulting in the loss of skin on the top of his middle finger. On examination in the emergency room, he was found to have full thickness skin loss of about 2.5 cm in diameter from the dorsum of the proximal interphalangeal (PIP) joint of the R middle finger; damage to the central tendon was also apparent. The surgeon debrided the wound and covered the joint using a pedicle flap from the radial side of the adjacent ring finger, and a partial thickness graft to the donor site. The doctor positioned the finger near full extension; subsequent release of the flap from the adjacent finger was done and healing occurred without complication.

Though cautioned against PIP flexion, or use of the hand that involved the finger, the patient reported he had resumed his work out of necessity, though on a limited basis. He presents with a stiff, enlarged PIP joint held in flexion at 40 degrees, and DIP joint at 10 degree hyperextension. He is unable to actively extend his PIP, and passive motion is limited to 10 degree extension from the initial measurement after treatment. Active and passive flexion of the DIP is limited to 5 degrees.

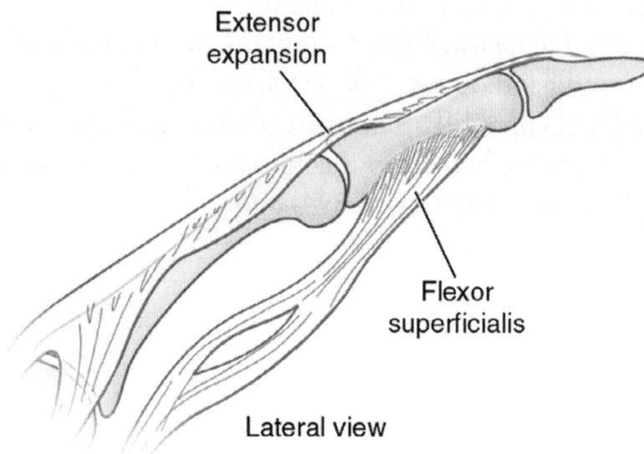

FIGURE 169-1 The tendons attaching to the middle phalanx. (From Simon RR, Sherman SC. *Emergency Orthopedics*. 6th ed. www.accessemergencymedicine.com. Copyright © The McGraw-Hill Companies, Inc. All rights reserved.)

KEY FEATURES

Description

- Generally from a forceful blow to a flexed finger
- Severed central slip tendon
- Signs and symptoms may develop in acute to subacute phase of injury
- Flexion of the PIP joint and extension of the distal interphalangeal (DIP) joint[2]
- Injury to the central slip tendon and often damage to the volar plate
- Volar displacement of the lateral bands
- Shortening of the oblique retinacular ligament

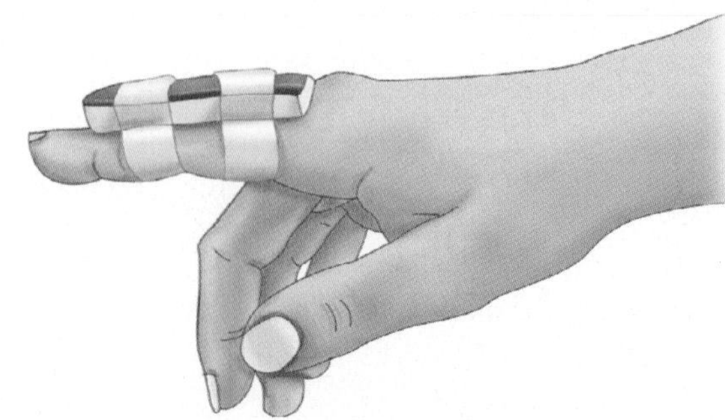

FIGURE 169-2 Boutonnière splint. The finger is splinted with the proximal interphalangeal joint held in extension. (From Patel DR, Greydanus DE, Baker RJ. *Pediatric Practice: Sports Medicine*. www.accesspediatrics.com. Copyright © The McGraw-Hill Companies, Inc. All rights reserved.)

Essentials of Diagnosis

- Diagnosis is usually made by clinical examination or x-ray
- Assess finger ROM
- Boutonnière classification
  - I: Mild extension lag, passively correctable
  - II: Moderate extension lag, passively correctable
  - III: Mild flexion contracture
  - IV: Advanced flexion contracture

General Considerations

- Symptoms can occur up to a few weeks after trauma
- Inflammation around the joint
- Can be associated with trauma (forceful blow or cut of the tendon)
- Rheumatoid arthritis

Demographics

- Adults
  - Hit or blow onto the finger, basketball[3]

CLINICAL FINDINGS

SIGNS AND SYMPTOMS

- Pain with grasping
- Flexion of the PIP joint and extension of the DIP joint
- Inflammation around the joint
- Joint redness and pain

Functional Implications

- Pain with grasping, holding objects
- Inability to fully extend the finger

Possible Contributing Causes

- Trauma
- Rheumatoid arthritis
- Central slip tendon injury
- Joint arthritis/injury
- Nerve damage
- Burns
- Infection
- Osteoarthritis

Differential Diagnosis

- Fracture
- Gout
- Mallet finger
- PIP joint flexion contracture

MEANS OF CONFIRMATION

- Imaging
  - X-ray

FINDINGS AND INTERPRETATION

- X-ray may show a bone spur
  - Location
  - Size

TREATMENT

Medication

- Anti-inflammatory
- Corticosteroid injection

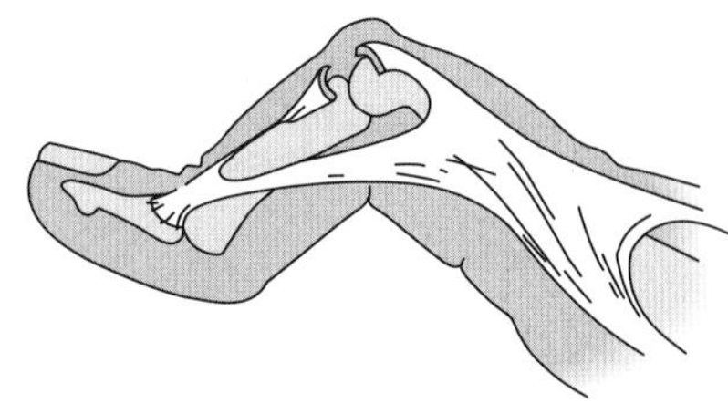

FIGURE 169-3 Boutonnière deformity caused by loss of active proximal interphalangeal extension secondary to loss of the central slip insertion on the proximal dorsal middle phalanx. (Reproduced, with permission, from Way LW, ed. *Current Surgical Diagnosis & Treatment*. 10th ed. Appleton & Lange, 1994.)

MEDICAL PROCEDURES

- Surgery in the case of RA, severed tendon, or minimal improvement with splinting
- Repair of the extensor tendon

REFERRALS/ADMITTANCE

- For imaging, X-ray
- For corticosteroid injection
- For surgical consult
- For occupational therapist to provide splints and instruct patient in joint protection techniques

IMPAIRMENTS

- Pain with grasping objects for work and daily activities

TESTS AND MEASURES

- Haines–Zancolli test
- Thenar muscle strength test (lateral pinch dynamometry)
- Manipulative ability test (nine-hole peg test)

INTERVENTION

- Rest, to reduce inflammation
- Bracing/Splinting

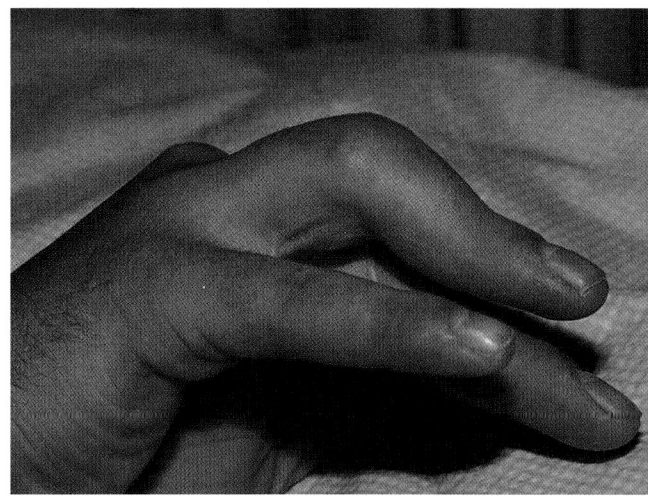

FIGURE 169-4 Boutonnière deformity. A boutonnière deformity of the fourth digit. Note the flexion of the PIP joint and the extension of the DIP joint. (From Knoop KJ, Knoop K, Stack L, Storrow A, Jason Thurman R. The Atlas of *Emergency Medicine*. 3rd ed. http://www.accessmedicine.com. Copyright © The McGraw-Hill Companies, Inc. All rights reserved. Photo contributor: E. Lee Edstrom, MD.)

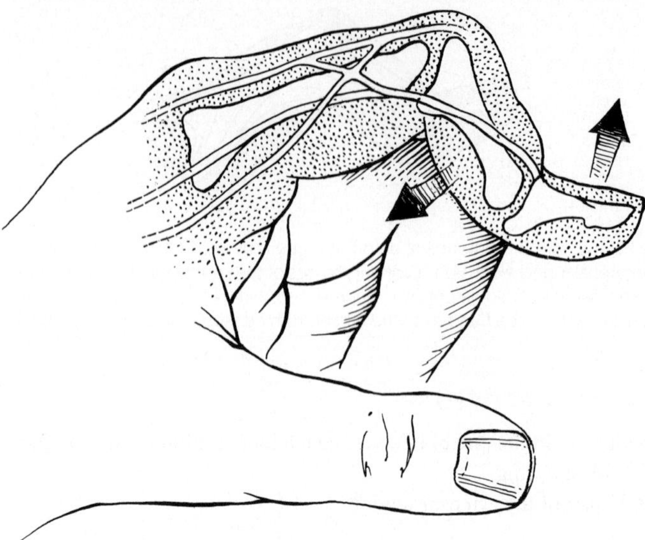

FIGURE 169-5 Boutonnière deformity. This depiction of a boutonnière deformity illustrates the rupture of the central slip and the resultant subluxation of the lateral bands. The subluxation exerts a pull on the middle phalanx resulting in the deformity. (From Knoop KJ, Knoop K, Stack L, Storrow A, Jason Thurman R. *The Atlas of Emergency Medicine.* 3rd ed. http://www.accessmedicine.com. Copyright © The McGraw-Hill Companies, Inc. All rights reserved.)

- Safety pin splinting is applied for approximately 4 to 6 weeks to help straighten the finger
- Taping techniques
- Address swelling and pain
  - Ice
- Address pain
  - Ice
  - Massage
  - Joint mobilization
  - Electric stimulation
  - Infrared
- Address weakness and joint instability
  - Strengthening of extensors
- Address lack of flexibility
  - Stretching
    - Intrinsic flexor stretching
    - Fluidotherapy
- Address joint mobilization
  - DIP glides and rotation
- Address soft tissue mobilization

FUNCTIONAL GOALS

- Patient will be able to
  - Open hand to place around a jar to open.
  - Fully extend the finger to don/doff gloves.

PROGNOSIS

- Good if early treatment; focus on stretching out the flexors.
- Surgery may be indicated if the flexion becomes severe.
- If associated with fragment fracture, 1 to 6 weeks of immobilization.

PATIENT RESOURCE

- AAOS, American Academy of Orthopaedic Surgeons. Boutonnière Deformity. http://orthoinfo.aaos.org/topic.cfm?topic=a00004. Accessed May 7, 2013.

REFERENCES

1. The American Physical Therapy Association. Pattern 4E: Impaired joint mobility, motor function, muscle performance, and range of motion associated with localized inflammation. Interactive Guide to Physical Therapist Practice. *The American Physical Therapy Association.* 2003. http://guidetoptpractice.apta.org/content/1/SEC12.extract?sid=ccb92104-9626-443e-ab17-b2a32a7792b7. DOI: 10.2522/ptguide.978-1-931369-64-0. Accessed May 7, 2013.
2. Dutton M. Finger injuries. In: Dutton M, ed. *McGraw-Hill's NPTE (National Physical Therapy Examination).* 2nd ed. New York, NY: McGraw-Hill; 2012. http://www.accessphysiotherapy.com/content/56504934. Accessed May 7, 2013.

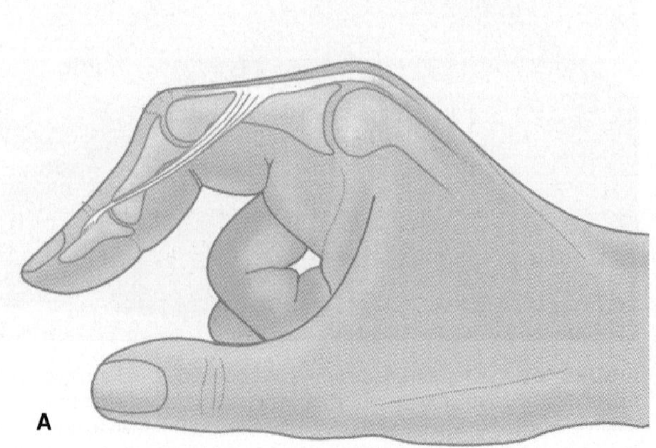

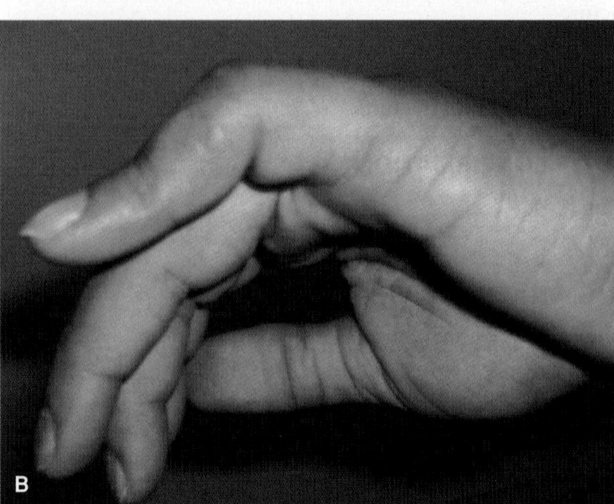

FIGURE 169-6 Boutonnière deformity. (**A**) The lateral bands of the extensor tendon slip volarly and cause PIP flexion and DIP extension. (**B**) Clinical photograph. (From Simon RR, Sherman SC. *Emergency Orthopedics.* 6th ed: www.accessemergencymedicine.com. Copyright © The McGraw-Hill Companies, Inc. All rights reserved.)

3. Cline S. Chapter 22. Acute injuries of elbow, forearm, wrist, and hand. In: Patel DR, Greydanus DE, Baker RJ, eds. *Pediatric Practice: Sports Medicine*. New York, NY: McGraw-Hill; 2009. http://www.accessphysiotherapy.com/content/6978574. Accessed May 7, 2013.

ADDITIONAL REFERENCES

- Burton RI, Eaton RG. Common hand injuries in the athlete. *Orthop Clin North Am*. 1973;4:809–838.
- Churchill M, Citron N. Isolated subluxation of the extensor pollicis longus tendon. A cause of 'boutonniere' deformity of the thumb. *J Hand Surg Br*. 1997;22(6):790–792.
- Dutton M. Tendon ruptures. In: Dutton M, ed. *Dutton's Orthopaedic Examination, Evaluation, and Intervention*. 3rd ed. New York, NY: McGraw-Hill; 2012. http://www.accessphysiotherapy.com/content/56540484. Accessed May 7, 2013.
- El-Sallakh S, Aly T, Amin O, Hegazi M. Surgical management of chronic boutonniere deformity. *Hand Surg*. 2012;17(3):359–364.
- Fox A, Kang N. Reinserting the central slip—a novel method for treating boutonniere deformity in rheumatoid arthritis. *J Plast Reconstr Aesthet Surg*. 2009;62(5):e91–e92.
- Haerle M, Lotter O, Mertz I, Buschmeier N. [The traumatic boutonnière deformity]. *Orthopade*. 2008;37(12):1194–1201.
- Hooker DN, Prentice WE. Basic principles of electricity and electrical stimulating currents. In: Prentice WE, Quillen WS, Underwood F, eds. *Therapeutic Modalities in Rehabilitation*. 4th ed. New York, NY: McGraw-Hill; 2011. http://www.accessphysiotherapy.com/content/8136367#8136367. Accessed May 7, 2013.
- ICD9Data.com. http://www.icd9data.com. Accessed May 7, 2013.
- ICD10Data.com. http://www.icd10data.com. Accessed May 7, 2013.
- Izadpanah A, Izadpanah A, Sinno H, Williams B. Pediatric boutonniere deformity after blunt closed traumatic injury. *Pediatr Emerg Care*. 2011;27(11):1069–1071.
- Massengill JB. The boutonniere deformity. *Hand Clin*. 1992; 8(4):787–801.
- Prentice WE. Cryotherapy and thermotherapy. In: Prentice WE, Quillen WS, Underwood F, eds. *Therapeutic Modalities in Rehabilitation*. 4th ed. New York, NY: McGraw-Hill; 2011. http://www.accessphysiotherapy.com/content/8137995#8137995. Accessed May 7, 2013.
- Silva PG, Lombardi I Jr, Breitschwerdt C, Poli Araújo PM, Natour J. Functional thumb orthosis for type I and II boutonniere deformity on the dominant hand in patients with rheumatoid arthritis: a randomized controlled study. *Clin Rehabil*. 2008;22(8):684–689.
- Simon RR, Sherman SC. Closed tendon injuries. In: Simon RR, Sherman SC, eds. *Emergency Orthopedics*. 6th ed. New York, NY: McGraw-Hill; 2011. http://www.accessphysiotherapy.com/content/7703566. Accessed May 7, 2013.
- Yoshino N, Watanabe N, Fujita N, et al. Boutonniere deformity of the second toe after planter dislocation of proximal interphalangeal joint: a case report. *Arch Orthop Trauma Surg*. 2009; 129(11):1527–1529.
- Zhang X, Yang L, Shao X, et al. Treatment of bony boutonniere deformity with a loop wire. *J Hand Surg Am*. 2011;36(6): 1080–1085.

170 THUMB CARPOMETACARPAL JOINT OSTEOARTHRITIS

Eric Shamus, PhD, DPT, PT, CSCS
Reuben Escorpizo, DPT, MSc, PT

ICD-9-CM CODES

- 715 Osteoarthrosis and allied disorders
- 715.14 Osteoarthrosis localized primary involving hand
- 715.24 Osteoarthrosis localized secondary involving hand
- 715.9 Osteoarthrosis unspecified whether generalized or localized
- 715.94 Osteoarthrosis unspecified whether generalized or localized involving hand

ICD-10-CM CODES

- M18.9 Osteoarthritis of first carpometacarpal joint, unspecified
- M19.049 Primary osteoarthritis, unspecified hand
- M19.249 Secondary osteoarthritis, unspecified hand

PREFERRED PRACTICE PATTERNS

- 4D: Impaired Joint Mobility, Motor Function, Muscle Performance, and Range of Motion Associated with Connective Tissue Dysfunction
- 4F: Impaired Joint Mobility, Motor Function, Muscle Performance, Range of Motion, and Reflex Integrity Associated with Spinal Disorders
- 4H: Impaired Joint Mobility, Motor Function, Muscle Performance, and Range of Motion Associated with Joint Arthroplasty
- 4I: Impaired Joint Mobility, Motor Function, Muscle Performance, and Range of Motion Associated with Bony or Soft Tissue Surgery

PATIENT PRESENTATION

The patient is a 67-year-old woman who presents with pain at the base of the right thumb with decreased ability to knit. It is affecting her grip and ability to manipulate small objects. She complains of a constant pain, but feels better in warm water when she washes the dishes. The patient has an X-ray that showed an osteophyte with degenerative changes at the carpometacarpal joint. The opposite side is starting to bother her. There is visual enlargement of the joint.

KEY FEATURES

Description

- Most common form of osteoarthritis (OA)
- Degenerative
- Commonly affects hand and weight-bearing joints
- Can also affect interphalangeal joints and first metatarsophalangeal joint
- Associated with increasing age, obesity, sex, and race/ethnicity
- Associated with abnormal loading of the joints

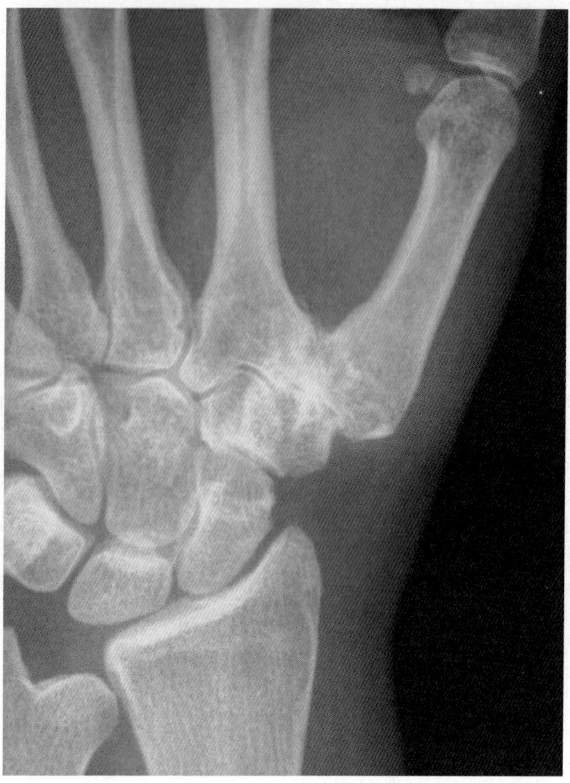

FIGURE 170-1 Radiograph of thumb basilar osteoarthritis. There is irregular loss of the joint space between the proximal thumb metacarpal and the trapezium bone, together with bony sclerosis and bony cysts. There is also proximal and radial subluxation of the thumb metacarpal, indicative of carpometacarpal joint ligament laxity, caused by the progressive arthritis. (From Imboden J, Hellmann DB, Stone JH. *Current Diagnosis & Treatment in Rheumatology.* 2nd ed. http://www.accessmedicine.com. Copyright © The McGraw-Hill Companies, Inc. All rights reserved.)

- Characterized by joint pain
- Arthrosis
- Osteoarthrosis
- Polyarthrosis
- Degenerative joint disease

Essentials of Diagnosis

- Radiography is a standard method for diagnosis
- Kellgren and Lawrence (KL) grade ≥2 (definite radiographic OA)[1]
- Osteophytes, joint-space narrowing, sclerosis
- Also cartilage lesions, bone marrow lesions, synovitis, effusion, and subchondral bone attrition/sclerosis
- Erosion of articular cartilage
- Synovial hyperplasia
- Fibrosis
- Inflammatory cell infiltration
- Conventional radiograph is the most commonly used tool in OA
- Diagnosis is made based on a careful history taking, physical examination, imaging studies, laboratory examination, and exclusion of other possible diseases

General Considerations

- Low bone mineral density (BMD)
- Repetitive joint use or loading
- Joint alignment

- Bone or joint morphology
- Calcification (e.g., of the knee meniscus)
- Bone formation, cyst formation
- Thickening of subchondral bone plate, osteosclerosis
- Overall joint dysfunction
- Joint swelling and inflammation (in certain cases, severe cases)
- Joint pain
- Morning stiffness
- Long-term disease
    - Secondary problems
        - Muscle atrophy and weakness
        - Bony protrusion/prominence
        - Joint deformity
        - Grasping difficulty
        - Difficulty with activities of daily living (ADLs)

Demographics

- Increase in age (middle to older age)
- Women are more affected than men
- Affects African Americans and Caucasians
- May affect about 12% of the population (United States and other developed countries)[2]

CLINICAL FINDINGS

SIGNS AND SYMPTOMS

- Aching joint
- Activity limitation
- Bony enlargement
- Crepitus
- Heberden nodes
- Joint deformity in severe cases
- Joint line tenderness
- Joint pain
- Joint stiffness
- Limited joint range of motion
- Muscle atrophy
- Muscle weakness

Functional Implications

- Limited mobility
- Household- and work-related activity limitation/restriction
- Decreased overall activity and participation

Possible Contributing Causes

- Chronic factors affecting the joint
    - Obesity
    - BMD
    - Leg length discrepancy (LLD)
- Aging
- Chronic and vigorous joint loading
- Previous chronic joint injury (e.g., accident, trauma), hence secondary OA

Differential Diagnosis

- Carpal tunnel syndrome
- Cervical radiculopathy
- Fibromyalgia syndrome
- Gout
- Rheumatoid arthritis
- Spondyloarthropathy

MEANS OF CONFIRMATION OR DIAGNOSIS

Laboratory Tests

- Not required: Synovial fluid examination
- Other laboratory tests can be performed to rule out other conditions

Imaging

- Conventional radiograph of the joint
- MRI of the joint
- Diagnostic ultrasound of the joint and synovium

FINDINGS AND INTERPRETATION

- OA is a clinical diagnosis that can be based on:
    - Persistent usage-related pain in the joint(s)
    - Age ≥ 45 years[2]
    - Morning stiffness equal or less than 30 minutes[2]
    - Imaging studies (e.g., radiograph)
        - Osteophytes, joint-space narrowing, sclerosis
        - Also cartilage lesions, bone marrow lesions, synovitis, effusion, and subchondral bone attrition/sclerosis
    - Erosion of articular cartilage

TREATMENT

Medication

- NSAIDs (including topical NSAIDs, capsaicin)
- Acetaminophen
- Opioids
- Glucosamine and chondroitin sulfate
- Glucocorticoids or corticosteroids
- Intra-articular injections (corticosteroids, hyaluronic acid)
- Emerging drugs such as anti-TNF, calcitonin, growth factors, and nerve growth factor antibodies

MEDICAL PROCEDURE

- Surgery: Total joint replacement, joint lavage and debridement

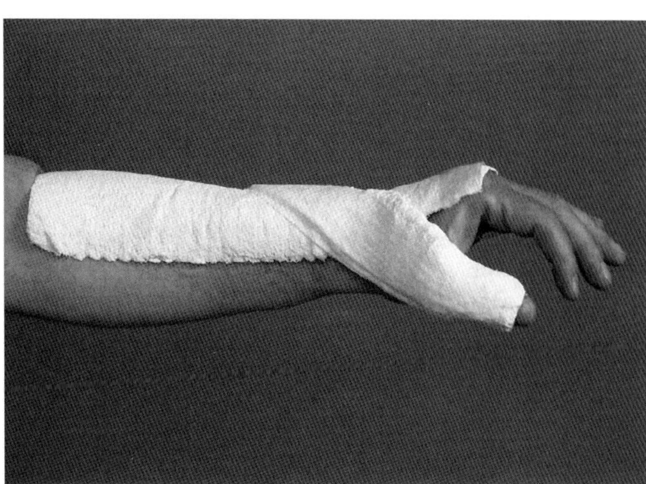

FIGURE 170-2 Thumb spica splint. (From Tintinalli JE, Stephan Stapczynski J, John Ma O, et al., eds. *Tintinalli's Emergency Medicine: A Comprehensive Study Guide.* 7th ed. http://www.accessmedicine.com. Copyright © The McGraw-Hill Companies, Inc. All rights reserved.)

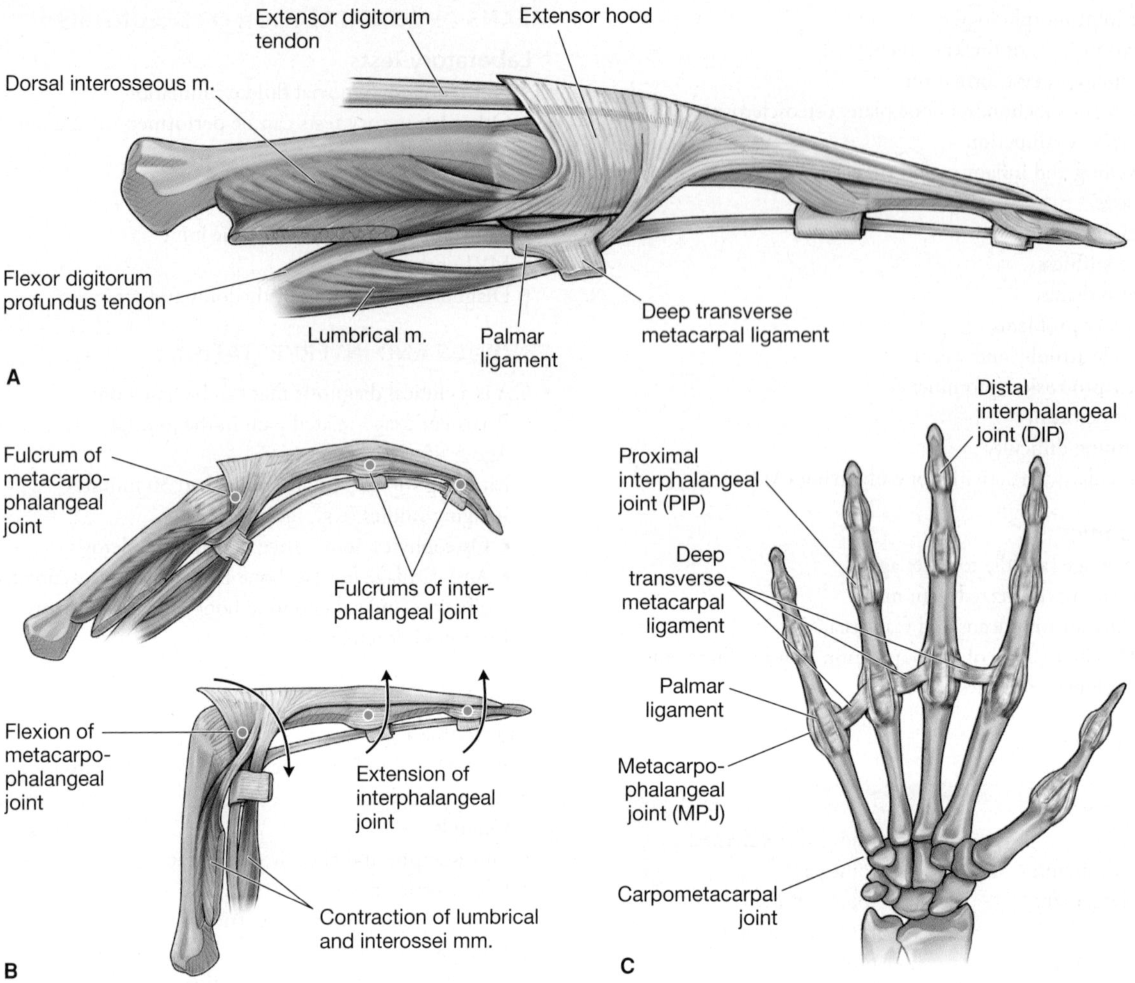

FIGURE 170-3 (**A**) Extensor expansion. (**B**) Movements of the lumbrical and interossei muscles. (**C**) Ligaments and joints of the hand. (From Morton DA, Foreman KB, Albertine KH. *The Big Picture: Gross Anatomy.* http://www.accessmedicine.com. Copyright © The McGraw-Hill Companies, Inc. All rights reserved.)

REFERRALS/ADMITTANCE

- Rheumatologist to assess underlying complications
- Internal medicine specialist
- Orthopedic specialist
- Surgical consult
- Dietician/nutritionist

IMPAIRMENTS

- Mobility
- Self-care
- Role at home and in the community
- School and work
- Recreation, leisure, and sports

TESTS AND MEASURES

- Disabilities of the Arm, Shoulder, and Hand (DASH) score to assess physical function
- Resisted isometric testing
- Finkelstein test

INTERVENTION

- Exercises (resistance, endurance, and flexibility)

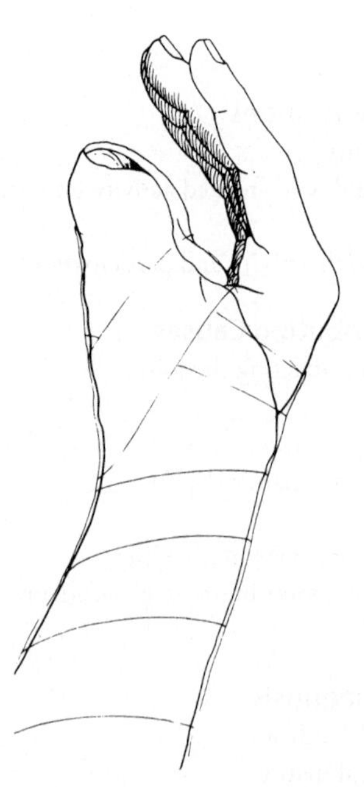

FIGURE 170-4 Thumb spica splint: a slab of plaster is applied over adequate padding and secured with a loose elastic bandage. (From Stone CK, Humphries RL. *Current Diagnosis & Treatment: Emergency Medicine.* 7th ed. http://www.accessmedicine.com. Copyright © The McGraw-Hill Companies, Inc. All rights reserved.)

- Training on ADLs
- Use of assistive or adaptive devices
- Heat therapy
- Rest
- Orthoses, splints
- Ice
- Acupuncture
- Pain management
- Energy conservation techniques
- Joint protection
- Ultrasound
- Electric stimulation
- Patient education

FUNCTIONAL GOALS

- Patient will be able to
  - Improve joint mobility and stability to improve grasping.
  - Improve muscle and general (aerobic) endurance.
  - Improve activity and participation related to role at home, at work, and in the community.
  - Return to pain-free ADL, sweeping, mopping.
  - Turn a key or door knob, pain free.
  - Lift baby crib without pain and maintain a neutral wrist posture.

PROGNOSIS

- No definite cure for OA.
- Treatment is for symptoms, but emerging drugs may modify OA disease mechanism.
- Joint damage is irreversible.
- Recovery or relief from symptoms may depend on disease duration and timely intervention.
- OA is a chronic disease and may mean long-term burden.
- May affect prognosis: Demographics, severity and natural history of the disease, medical comorbidities, and behavioral comorbidities such as fear avoidance, catastrophization, and central sensitization.
- Competent general endurance, good muscle strength, and mobile joints are good prognosticating factors.
- Motivation and compliance with PT intervention (e.g., home exercise program) and family and environmental support could also improve PT treatment outcomes.

PATIENT RESOURCE

- Osteoarthritis Research Society International. OARSI Primer. http://primer.oarsi.org. Accessed March 3, 2013.

REFERENCES

1. Kellgren JH, Lawrence JS, eds. *The Epidemiology of Chronic Rheumatism: Atlas of Standard Radiographs of Arthritis.* Oxford, UK: Blackwell Scientific; 1963.
2. National Collaborating Centre for Chronic Conditions at the Royal College of Physicians. *Osteoarthritis: National Clinical Guideline for Care and Management in Adults.* London, UK: Royal College of Physicians of London; 2008.

ADDITIONAL REFERENCES

- American Physical Therapy Association. *Guide to Physical Therapist Practice.* 2nd ed. Alexandria, VA: American Physical Therapy Association; 2001. Revised 2003.
- Dutton M, ed. *Orthopaedic Examination, Evaluation, and Intervention.* 2nd ed. New York, NY: McGraw-Hill; 2008. http://www.accessphysiotherapy.com/resource/612. Accessed March 13, 2013.
- Dutton M. Chapter 18. Adjunctive interventions. In: Dutton M, ed. *McGraw-Hill's NPTE (National Physical Therapy Examination).* 2nd ed. New York, NY: McGraw-Hill; 2012. http://www.accessphysiotherapy.com/content/5405918. Accessed March 13, 2013.
- ICD9Data.com. http://www.icd9data.com. Accessed March 3, 2013.
- ICD10Data.com. http://www.icd10data.com/ICD10CM/Codes. Accessed March 3, 2013.
- McKinnis LN. *Fundamentals of Musculoskeletal Imaging.* 2nd ed. Philadelphia, PA: F.A. Davis Company; 2005.
- Prentice WE, Quillen WS, Underwood F, eds. *Therapeutic Modalities in Rehabilitation.* 4th ed. New York, NY: McGraw-Hill; 2011. http://www.accessphysiotherapy.com/resource/675. Accessed March 13, 2013.

171 COLLES FRACTURE

Jennifer Cabrera, DPT, GCS
Eric Shamus, PhD, DPT, PT, CSCS

CONDITION/DISORDER SYNONYM

- Colles' fracture

ICD-9-CM CODES

- 813.41 Colles fracture closed
- 813.51 Colles fracture open

ICD-10-CM CODES

- S52.539A Colles fracture of unspecified, radius, initial encounter for closed fracture
- S52.539B Colles fracture of unspecified radius, initial encounter for open fracture type I or II
- S52.539C Colles fracture of unspecified radius, initial encounter for open fracture type IIIA, IIIB, or IIIC

PREFERRED PRACTICE PATTERN

- 4G: Impaired Joint Mobility, Muscle Performance, and Range of Motion Associated with Fracture[1]

PATIENT PRESENTATION

A 65-year-old woman tripped on a rug in her home and fell on her outstretched hand with her wrist dorsiflexed (extended). She felt immediate pain in her wrist and has difficulty moving her wrist or hand. She has been postmenopausal for 15 years and has never taken hormone replacement therapy or bisphosphonates. She presented with pain and swelling in her wrist. Her arm had a "dinner fork" deformity. Radiographs showed a distal radius fracture (Colles fracture). There was dorsal angulation seen on the lateral view.[2]

KEY FEATURES

Description

- Fracture[3]
- Any defect in continuity of the distal radius
- Displaced (distal radius is moved on either side of the fracture) or nondisplaced (distal radius has not moved)
- Closed (skin intact) or open (skin breached)

Essentials of Diagnosis

- Diagnosis usually made by clinical examination
- May not be fracture, but distal radioulnar subluxation/dislocation, wrist sprain

General Considerations

- Radius is the most commonly broken bone in the arm
- Most common fracture site in children (35.8%–45% of all pediatric fractures)

Demographics

- In pediatric population, higher frequency among boys than girls

CLINICAL FINDINGS

SIGNS AND SYMPTOMS

- Pain
- Point tenderness
- Edema
- Ecchymosis
- Visual wrist deformity
- Loss of general function
- Loss of active mobility
- Muscle guarding with passive movement
- Crepitus

Functional Implications

- Pain with weight bearing on involved forearm and hand
- Pain with vertical positioning of arm at side
- Pain with all movements (passive, active)

Possible Contributing Causes

- Osteoporosis
- Mechanisms of injury
  - Fall on outstretched hand with the wrist in extension
  - Direct impact

Differential Diagnosis

- Distal radioulnar subluxation or dislocation
- Wrist sprain

MEANS OF CONFIRMATION OR DIAGNOSIS

Imaging

- X-ray for fracture, often limited view[4]

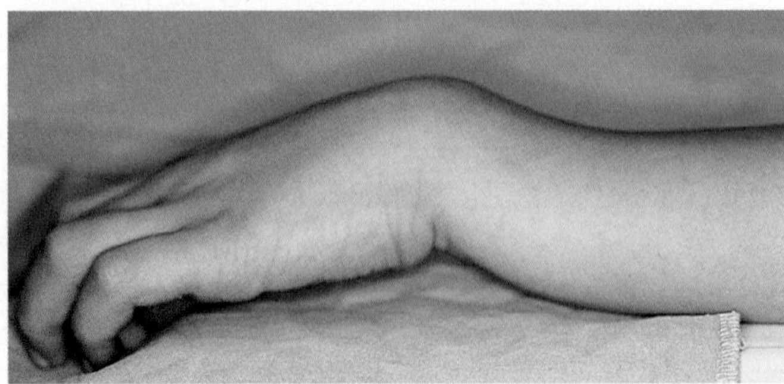

FIGURE 171-1 Colles fracture. The classic dinner-fork deformity is demonstrated in this photograph. The distal forearm is displaced dorsally. (From Knoop KJ, Stack L, Storrow A, Jason Thurman R. *The Atlas of Emergency Medicine.* 3rd ed. http://www.accessmedicine.com. Copyright © The McGraw-Hill Companies, Inc. All rights reserved. Photo contributor: Cathleen M. Vossler, MD.)

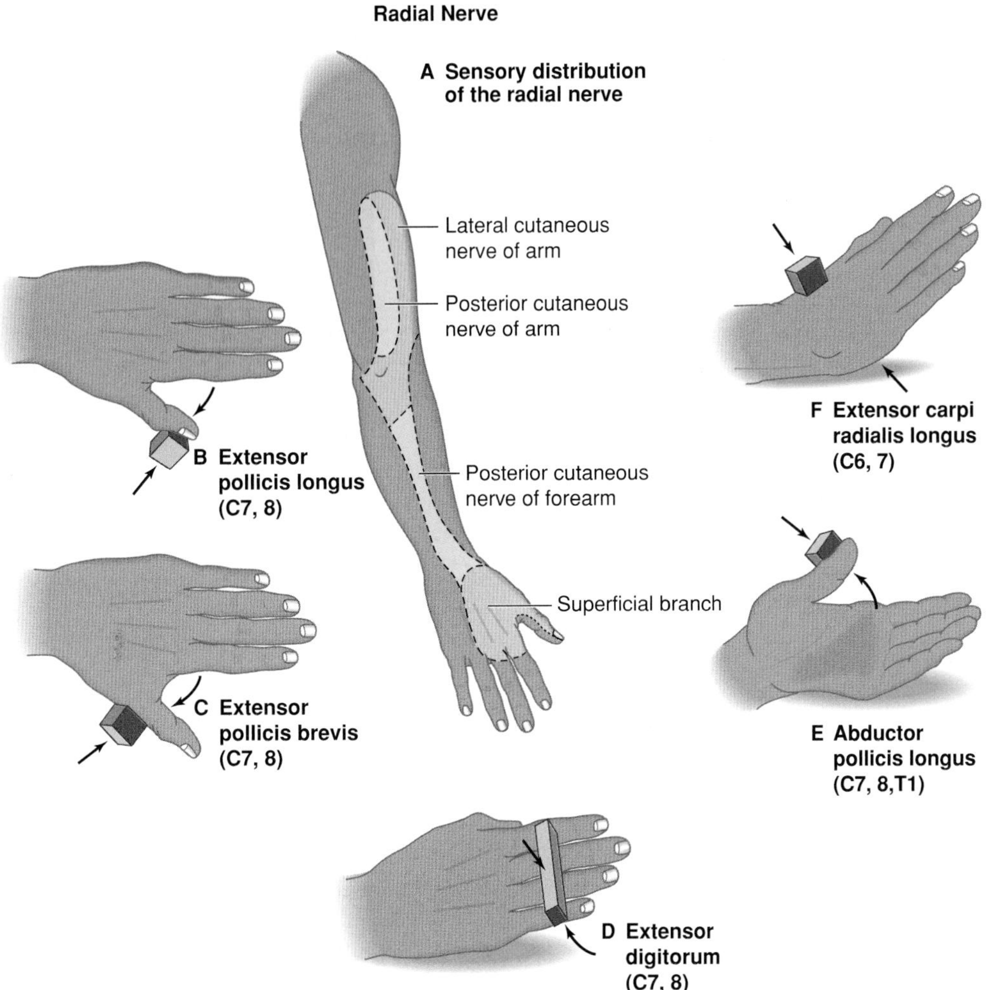

FIGURE 171-2 Testing the radial nerve. (**A**) Sensory distribution. The radial nerve supplies the dorsolateral surface of the upper arm, forearm, wrist, and hand; the dorsal surface of the thumb; the dorsal surface of the index and middle fingers above the distal interphalangeal joints; and the lateral half of the dorsal surface of the ring finger above the distal interphalangeal joint. (**B**) Extensor pollicis longus. The thumb is extended at the interphalangeal joint against resistance. (**C**) Extensor pollicis brevis. The thumb is extended at the metacarpophalangeal joint against resistance. (**D**) Extensor digitorum. The fingers are extended at the metacarpophalangeal joints against resistance. (**E**) Abductor pollicis longus. The thumb is abducted (elevated in a plane at 90 degrees to the palm) at the carpometacarpal joint against resistance. (**F**) Extensor carpi radialis longus. The wrist is extended toward the radial (thumb) side against resistance. (From Greenberg DA, Aminoff MJ, Simon RP. *Clinical Neurology.* 8th ed. http://www.accessmedicine.com. Copyright © The McGraw-Hill Companies, Inc. All rights reserved.)

- CT for detailed imaging[4]
- MRI
- Ultrasonography may be used in pediatric population

FINDINGS AND INTERPRETATION

- Pain and crepitus with passive or active ROM in the wrist and forearm
- Visible wrist deformity
- Upper extremity held in protective position to avoid gravitational distraction of the joint
- Muscle guarding with all movements
- Inability to actively perform wrist movements or forearm pronation/supination secondary to pain
- If vascular structures involved, affected hand will appear cool, pale, diminished palpable pulse
- If neurologic structures involved, individual will report numbness, decreased ability to move the affected hand

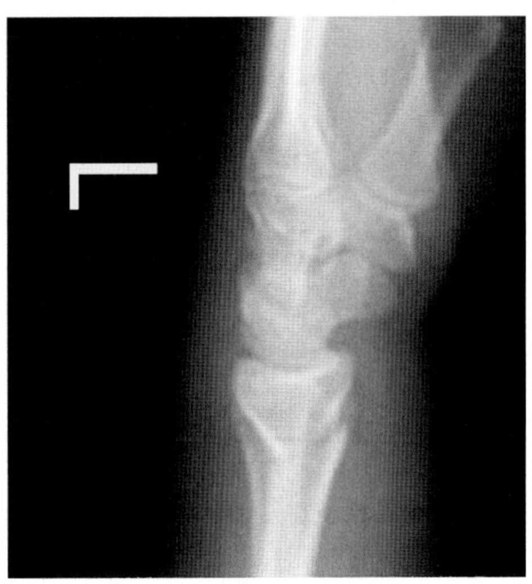

FIGURE 171-3 Lateral view of left wrist shows the dorsal angulation that gives the arm the "dinner fork" deformity. (From Simon RR, Sherman SC, Koenigsknecht SJ. *Emergency Orthopedics, the Extremities.* 5th ed. p. 204, Fig. 8-30 [right side], Copyright 2007, McGraw-Hill.)

REFERRALS/ADMITTANCE

- To hospital for imaging: X-ray or CT[4]
- To physician for medication: NSAIDs or opioid for pain management
- To orthopedist for immediate consult if
  - Nondisplaced fractures or displaced fractures that may be reduced are treated nonoperatively
    - Immobilization splint, casting
  - Severely displaced fractures treated operatively via
    - Open reduction internal fixation
    - External fixation

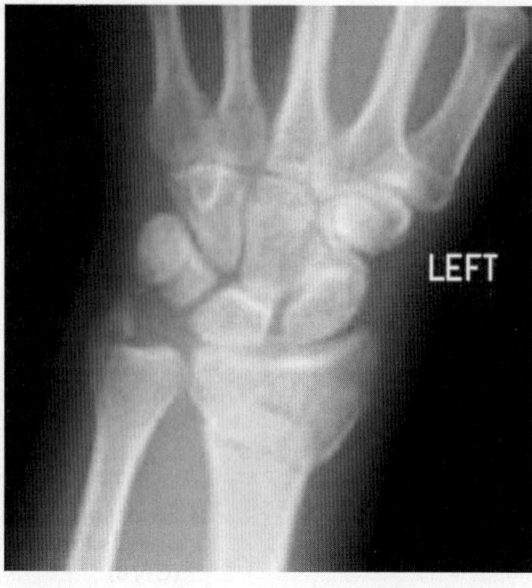

FIGURE 171-4 Anterior–posterior view demonstrating a transverse distal radius fracture (Colles fracture). (From Simon RR, Sherman SC, Koenigsknecht SJ. *Emergency Orthopedics, the Extremities.* 5th ed. p. 204, Fig. 8-30 [left side], Copyright 2007, McGraw-Hill.)

IMPAIRMENTS

- Inability to
  - Perform ADLs with involved upper extremity
  - Bear weight on involved forearm and hand
  - Write with involved hand (especially if dominant hand affected)
  - Grab a cup secondary to pain and muscle weakness

TESTS AND MEASURES

- Disabilities of the Arm, Shoulder, and Hand (DASH) score to assess physical function
- Joint mobility
- Strength assessment
- Sensory testing
- Reflex testing
- Vascular assessment

INTERVENTION

- Address swelling
  - Ice/cryotherapy[5]
  - Compression
  - Elevation
  - Electrical stimulation[6]
- Address pain
  - Ice/cryotherapy[5]
  - Massage
  - Electrical stimulation[6]
- Address lack of flexibility via stretching
  - Wrist flexors
  - Wrist extensors
  - Elbow flexors
- Address mobilization upon healing of fracture site (after 6 weeks postoperative)
  - Distal radioulnar joint dorsal glide for supination
  - Distal radioulnar joint volar glide for pronation
  - Radiocarpal joint distraction for pain management
  - Radiocarpal joint dorsal glide for wrist flexion
  - Radiocarpal joint volar glide for wrist extension
  - Radiocarpal joint radial glide for wrist ulnar deviation
  - Radiocarpal joint ulnar glide for wrist radial deviation
- Address weakness via strengthening activities
  - Closed chain weight-bearing activities
  - Isometric exercises (submaximal initially)
  - Open chain with free weights and resistance bands
  - Grip strengthening
- Address scar mobility
  - Scar tissue mobilization progressing from parallel to perpendicular upon wound closure

FUNCTIONAL GOALS

- Patient will have increased
  - Grip strength to 30 kg in order to open jars.
  - Forearm supination to 55 degrees in order to facilitate eating with fork.
  - Wrist-flexor strength to 4 out of 5 muscle strength score to carry a briefcase.
  - Distal radioulnar joint mobility to 3 in order to open doors.

PROGNOSIS

- Good, though recovery takes approximately 1 year.
- Some residual stiffness and ache expected for up to 2 years or permanently; more common among the following populations.
  - High-energy impact trauma (e.g., motorcycle accident).
  - Individuals aged 50 years or older.
  - Individuals with osteoarthritis (OA).

PATIENT RESOURCE

- American Academy of Orthopaedic Surgeons. Distal Radius Fracture. *OrthoInfo.* http://orthoinfo.aaos.org/topic.cfm?topic=A00412. Accessed June 10, 2013.

REFERENCES

1. The American Physical Therapy Association. Pattern 4G: Impaired joint mobility, muscle performance, and range of motion associated with fracture. *Interactive Guide to Physical Therapist Practice.* 2003. DOI: 10.2522/ptguide.3.1_7. Accessed June 10, 2013.
2. Chumley H. Chapter 97. Distal Radial Fracture. In: Usatine RP, Smith MA, Chumley H, Mayeaux E Jr, Tysinger J, eds. *The Color Atlas of Family Medicine.* New York, NY: McGraw-Hill; 2009. http://www.accessmedicine.com/content.aspx?aID=8204067. Accessed June 10, 2013.

3. Hall SJ. Chapter 4. The biomechanics of human bone growth and development. In: Hall SJ ed. *Basic Biomechanics.* 5th ed. New York, NY: McGraw-Hill; 2007. http://accessphysiotherapy.mhmedical.com/content.aspx?bookid=445&Sectionid=41288112. Accessed May 27, 2014.
4. Malone TR, Hazle C, Grey ML. *Imaging in Rehabilitation*. New York, NY: McGraw-Hill; 2008. http://www.accessphysiotherapy.com/resource/613. Accessed June 10, 2013.
5. Prentice WE. Chapter 9. Cryotherapy and thermotherapy. In: Prentice WE, Quillen WS, Underwood F, eds. *Therapeutic Modalities in Rehabilitation.* 4th ed. New York, NY: McGraw-Hill; 2011. http://www.accessphysiotherapy.com/content/8137995#8137995. Accessed June 10, 2013.
6. Hooker DN, Prentice WE. Chapter 5. Basic principles of electricity and electrical stimulating currents. In: Prentice WE, Quillen WS, Underwood F, eds. *Therapeutic Modalities in Rehabilitation.* 4th ed. New York, NY: McGraw-Hill; 2011. http://www.accessphysiotherapy.com/content/8136367#8136367. Accessed June 10, 2013.

ADDITIONAL REFERENCES

- Goodman CC, Boissonnault WG, Fuller KS. *Pathology: Implications for the Physical Therapist.* 2nd ed. Philadelphia, PA: Saunders; 2003.
- ICD9DATA web site. http://www.icd9data.com. Accessed June 10, 2013.
- ICD10DATA web site. http://www.icd10data.com. Accessed June 10, 2013.
- Kisner C, Colby LA. *Therapeutic Exercise: Foundations and Techniques.* 5th ed. Philadelphia, PA: F.A. Davis Company; 2007.
- Magee DJ. *Orthopedic Physical Assessment.* 5th ed. Louis, MO: Saunders Elsevier. St; 2008.
- Riego de Dios R. Distal Radial Fracture Imaging. Medscape Reference. http://emedicine.medscape.com/article/398406-overview#showall. Accessed June 10, 2013.

172 DE QUERVAIN TENOSYNOVITIS

Abby Lopez, LMT, CT, NCTMB
Eric Shamus, PhD, DPT, PT, CSCS
Mae L. Yahara, MS, PT, ATC

CONDITION/DISORDER SYNONYMS

- Washerwoman's sprain
- Radial styloid tenosynovitis
- de Quervain tenosynovitis
- de Quervain disease
- de Quervain stenosing tenosynovitis
- Mother's wrist
- Mommy thumb

ICD-9-CM CODE

- 727.04 Radial styloid tenosynovitis

ICD-10-CM CODE

- M65.4 Radial styloid tenosynovitis [de Quervain]

PREFERRED PRACTICE PATTERN

- 4E: Impaired Joint Mobility, Motor Function, Muscle Performance, and ROM Associated with Localized Inflammation[1]

PATIENT PRESENTATION

The patient is a 48-year-old woman who started a new job 6 months ago as a bookkeeper. She has been experiencing pain in the right wrist for approximately 1 month. The pain and tenderness are in the region of the styloid process of the radius. She states that the pain radiates into the forearm and thumb as her day progresses. She states that the pain began as a dull ache at the end of the day, but has progressed to the point of inability to complete her morning activities because of the discomfort. Her daily routine includes counting bills and receipts in the morning using her right hand with a repetitive pronation to supination movement. In the afternoon, her work is primarily done utilizing a keyboard. She has no hobbies, but does routine housework and cooking for herself and her spouse.

KEY FEATURES

Description

- Inflammation and thickening of the abductor pollicis longus and extensor pollicis brevis synovial tendon sheaths and extensor retinaculum[2]
- Named after Swiss surgeon, Fritz de Quervain
- Chronic tendinosis

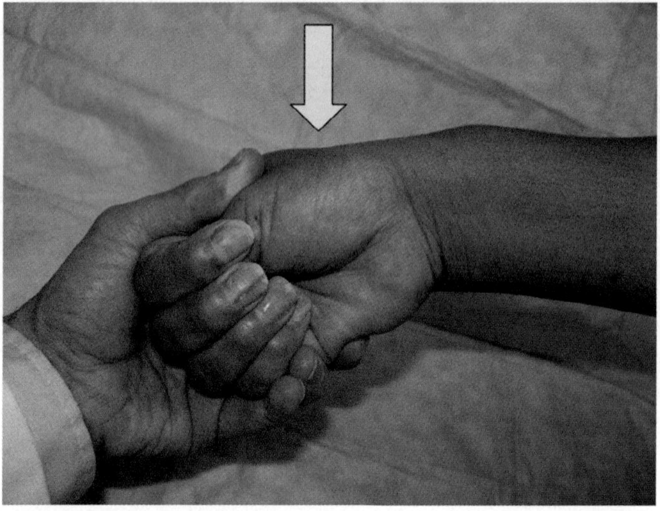

FIGURE 172-1 Finkelstein test. The patient places the thumb in the palm and makes a loose fist. The examiner then ulnarly deviates the patient's wrist (as indicated by the *arrow*). Pain at the first dorsal compartment with this maneuver is a positive response. (From Brunicardi FC, Andersen D, Billiar T, et al., eds. *Schwartz's Principles of Surgery.* 9th ed. http://www.accessmedicine.com. Copyright © The McGraw-Hill Companies, Inc. All rights reserved.)

Essentials of Diagnosis

- Tenderness with palpation
- Positive resisted isometric test in thumb abduction and extension
- Finkelstein test is best for diagnosis[3]

General Considerations

- Entrapment tendonitis, tendon friction
- Often a direct result of repetitive stress or chronic overuse of extensor and abductor muscles causing excessive friction to tendon sheath
- Patients likely to develop adhesions and irritation between tendons and their sheaths

Demographics

- Mostly found in women aged 30 to 50 years, possibly due to great angle of the styloid process
- Common among individuals who perform any activity requiring repetitive hand and wrist movement
- At-risk populations include
  - Massage therapists
  - Musicians
  - Milliners
  - Gardeners
  - Office workers
  - Pregnant and postpartum women

CLINICAL FINDINGS

SIGNS AND SYMPTOMS

- Forearm pain
- Crepitus of tendons within the extensor sheath
- Unilateral palmer pain and swelling
- Tendon friction rub
- Upper-extremity pain[4]
- Weak thumb abduction
- Decreased grip strength
- Wrist pain and swelling
- Decreased abduction ROM of the carpometacarpal (CMC) joint, thumb
- Pain with thumb activity, worsens when combined with wrist radial or ulnar deviation

Functional Implications

- Pain with pinching, grasping, squeezing, holding heavy objects, wringing
- Pain with movements of the hand and wrist
- Loss of strength
- Tendon rupture

Possible Contributing Causes

- Occupations that require repetitive use of hands for excessive periods of time
- A direct trauma to the tendon or wrist
- Inflammatory arthritis, such as rheumatoid arthritis

Differential Diagnosis

- Rheumatoid arthritis
- Carpal tunnel
- Osteoarthritis
- Intersection syndrome: Pain 2 to 3 inches proximal to the wrist
- Infection
- Dorsal wrist ganglion (tumor)
- Trigger finger
- Scaphoid fracture (history of trauma, tenderness over snuffbox)
- Wartenberg syndrome: Radial nerve entrapment at the forearm

MEANS OF CONFIRMATION OR DIAGNOSIS

Imaging

- X-ray to rule out arthritis at the thumb CMC joint
- MRI

FINDINGS AND INTERPRETATION

- MRI will often show acute inflammation or chronic tendinosis

TREATMENT

Medication

- NSAIDs[4]
- Cortisone injection

REFERRALS/ADMITTANCE

- To primary or secondary healthcare provider for corticosteroid injection to sheath
- To orthopedist for wrist/thumb splint allowing movement at the thumb interphalangeal (IP) joint only[5]

IMPAIRMENTS

- Hand weakness with grasping, squeezing, pinching
- Restricted ROM in thumb abduction and extension

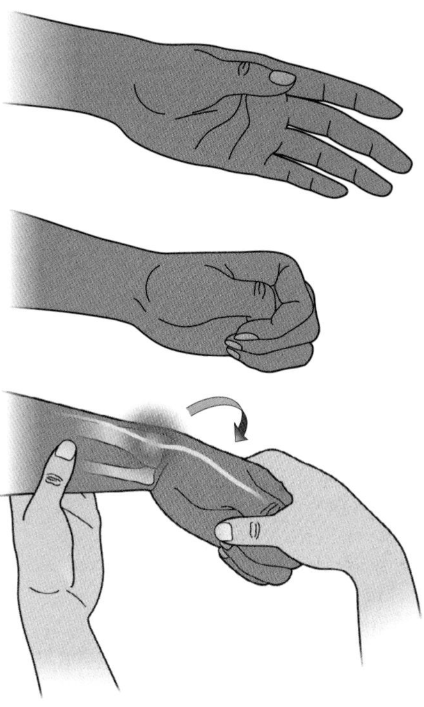

FIGURE 172-2 Finkelstein test. (From Dutton D. *Dutton's Orthopaedic Examination, Evaluation, and Intervention.* 3rd ed. http://accessphysiotherapy.mhmedical.com/ViewLarge.aspx?figid=40799084. Copyright © The McGraw-Hill Companies, Inc. All rights reserved.)

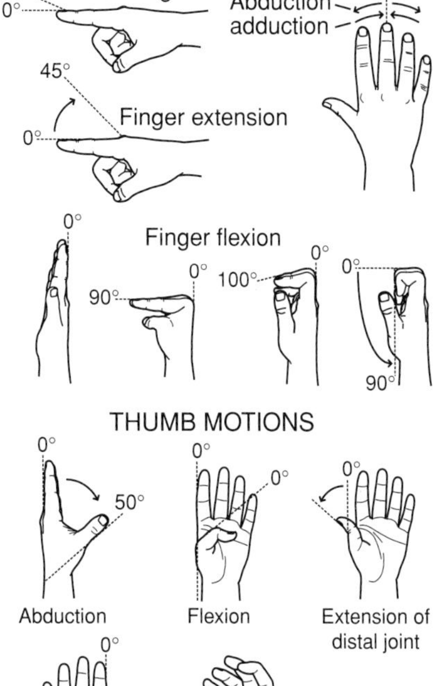

FIGURE 172-3 Motions of the fingers and thumb. (From LeBlond RF, DeGowin RL, Brown DD. *DeGowin's Diagnostic Examination.* 9th ed. http://www.accessmedicine.com. Copyright © The McGraw-Hill Companies, Inc. All rights reserved.)

TESTS AND MEASURES

- Disabilities of the Arm, Shoulder, and Hand (DASH) score to assess physical function
- Resisted isometric testing
- Finkelstein test[2]

INTERVENTION

- Acute stage
  - Rest
  - Cold laser[6]
  - Ultrasound[7]
  - Ice to reduce inflammation and swelling[8]
  - Wrist/thumb splint 3 to 4 weeks, early splint compliance essential
- Subacute stage
  - Stretching exercises
  - Eccentric exercises
- Chronic stage
  - Surgery only after conservative treatment has been exhausted
- Address weakness
  - Stretching and strengthening program
  - Hand coordination exercises, such as gripping and pinching
  - Ensure patient knowledge regarding home exercise program
  - Educate patient in postural awareness and proper body mechanics
  - Hand/wrist-joint protection strategies

FUNCTIONAL GOALS

- Patient will be able to
  - Grasp a gallon of milk pain-free with both hands.
  - Resume pain-free ADLs, sweeping, mopping.
  - Turn a key or door knob pain-free.
  - Lift baby from crib without pain, maintaining neutral wrist posture.

PROGNOSIS

- Most cases last between 4 and 8 months.
- Prognosis is very good.

PATIENT RESOURCES

- American Academy of Orthopeadic Surgeons. de Quervain's Contracture. http://orthoinfo.aaos.org/topic.cfm?topic=A00008 Accessed March 13, 2013.
- Mayo Clinic. De Quervain's Tenosynovitis. http://www.mayoclinic.com/health/de-quervains-tenosynovitis/DS00692/DSECTION=causes. Online April 3, 2010. Accessed March 13, 2013.
- Wesley Hand Centre. Fact Sheet: De Quervain's Tenosynovitis. http://www.wesleyhandcentre.com.au/pdf/de-quervains-tenosynovitis.pdf. Accessed March 13, 2013.

REFERENCES

1. The American Physical Therapy Association. Pattern 4E: Impaired joint mobility, motor function, muscle performance, and range of motion associated with localized inflammation. *Interactive Guide to Physical Therapist Practice*. 2003. DOI: 10.2522/ptguide.3.1_5. Accessed March 1, 2013.
2. Patel DR, Lyne ED. Chapter 23. Overuse injuries of elbow, forearm, wrist, and hand. In: Patel DR, Greydanus DE, Baker RJ, eds. *Pediatric Practice: Sports Medicine*. New York, NY: McGraw-Hill; 2009. http://www.accessphysiotherapy.com/abstract/6979237#6979237. Accessed March 13, 2013.
3. Dutton M. *Dutton's Orthopedic Survival Guide: Managing Common Conditions*. New York, NY: McGraw-Hill; 2011. http://www.accessphysiotherapy.com/resource/685. Accessed March 13, 2013.
4. Dutton M. *Orthopaedic Examination, Evaluation, and Intervention*. New York, NY: McGraw-Hill; 2008. http://www.accessphysiotherapy.com/resource/612. Accessed March 13, 2013.
5. *Anatomy and Physiology Revealed*. McGraw-Hill; 2007. http://anatomy.mcgraw-hill.com/apt.html?login=1318935388357&system=Muscular§ion=Dissection&topic=Forearm%20and%20hand&topicAbbr=For&view=Posterior&viewAbbr=Pos&catAbbr=Oth&grpAbbr=San&structure=Surface%20projection%20of%20interphalangeal%20joint%20of%25. Accessed March 13, 2013.
6. Houghton PE. Chapter 3. The role of therapeutic modalities in wound healing. In: Prentice WE, Quillen WS, Underwood F, eds. *Therapeutic Modalities in Rehabilitation.* 4th ed. New York, NY: McGraw-Hill; 2011. http://www.accessphysiotherapy.com/abstract/8135453#8135453. Accessed March 13, 2013.
7. Draper DO, Prentice WE. Chapter 10. Therapeutic ultrasound. In: Prentice WE, Quillen WS, Underwood F, eds. *Therapeutic Modalities in Rehabilitation.* 4th ed. New York, NY: McGraw-Hill; 2011. http://www.accessphysiotherapy.com/abstract/8138751. Accessed March 13, 2013.
8. Prentice WE. Chapter 9. Cryotherapy and thermotherapy. In: Prentice WE, Quillen WS, Underwood F, eds. *Therapeutic Modalities in Rehabilitation.* 4th ed. New York, NY: McGraw-Hill; 2011. http://www.accessphysiotherapy.com/content/8137995#8137995. Accessed March 13, 2013.

ADDITIONAL REFERENCES

- Brulhart L, Gabay C. The differential diagnosis of tenosynovitis. *Rev Med Suisse.* 2011;7(286):587–588, 590, 592–593.
- Car-Blanchard M. *Dequervain's Tenosynovitis—Wrist Tendonitis.* 2011. http://www.nyphysicaltherapy.net/Home/PatientEducation/tabid/3433/ctl/View/mid/5695/Default.aspx?ContentPubID=219. Accessed March 13, 2013.
- *Disease comparison results for de Quervain's tendonitis and gout.* Retrieved from http://en.diagnosispro.com/disease_comparison-for/dequervain-s-tendonitis-thumb-versus-gout/12970-14414.html. Accessed March 13, 2013.
- Drexel University. *Drummin' Doc.* http://www.pages.drexel.edu/~ak57/healthcare.html#intro. Accessed March 13, 2013.
- ICD9DATA web site. http://www.icd9data.com. Accessed March 6, 2013.
- ICD10DATA web site. http://www.icd10data.com. Accessed March 6, 2013.
- Lowe W. *Functional Assessment in Massage Therapy.* 3rd ed. Sisters, OR: Orthopedic Massage Education and Research Institute (OMERI); 1997.
- Pho C, Godges J. Hand muscle power deficits. Loma Linda University. http://xnet.kp.org/socal_rehabspecialists/ptr_library/04WristandHand%20Region/06Hand-MusclePowerDeficits.pdf. Accessed March 13, 2013.
- Zingas C, Failla JM, Van Holsbeeck M. Injection accuracy and clinical relief of de Quervain's tendinitis. *J Hand Surg Am.* 1998;23(1):89–96.

173 DUPUYTREN CONTRACTURE

Eric Shamus, PhD, DPT, PT, CSCS
George Hanbury, PhD

CONDITION/DISORDER SYNONYMS

- Morbus Dupuytren
- Dupuytren disease
- Palmar fasciitis
- Palmar fibromatosis

ICD-9-CM CODE

- 728.6 Contracture of palmar fascia

ICD-10-CM CODE

- M72.0 Palmar fascial fibromatosis [Dupuytren]

PREFERRED PRACTICE PATTERN

- 4D: Impaired Joint Mobility, Motor Function, Muscle Performance, and Range of Motion Associated with Connective Tissue Dysfunction[1]

PATIENT PRESENTATION

A 53-year-old man presents with stiffness in his hands. He says his hand began to feel stiff several years ago, and now he finds that he cannot straighten many of his fingers. He delayed seeing a physician because he did not feel any pain in his hands. He recently began having difficulty holding his woodworking tools and wants to regain the function he has lost in his hands.[2]

KEY FEATURES

Description

- Usually painless thickening of the fascia, contraction of palmar fascia (aponeurosis)
- Nodules develop along longitudinal tension lines
- Characterized by development of nodules in the palmar and digital fascia
- Can be associated with other fascial contractures
  - Feet (Ledderhose disease), callus under foot with curling of toes
  - Penis (Peyronie disease), curvature
  - Garrod knuckles, pads on back of finger knuckles
- Named after Baron Guillaume Dupuytren
- Viking disease

Essentials of Diagnosis

- Classified into three biologic stages:
  - First stage (proliferative stage): Intense proliferation of myofibroblasts (cells believed to generate the contractile forces responsible for tissue contraction) and formation of nodules
  - Second stage (involutional stage): Represented by alignment of the myofibroblasts along lines of tension
  - Third stage (residual stage): Tissue becomes mostly acellular and devoid of myofibroblasts, only thick bands of collagen remain

General Considerations

- Not usually associated with trauma, but can develop after surgery
- Unknown etiology, possibly autoimmune
- Usually bilateral with one side more severely affected
- Early stages based on palpable nodule, characteristic skin changes, changes in fascia, progressive joint contracture
- Skin changes caused by a retraction of skin, creating dimples or pits

Demographics

- Caucasian with Scandinavian/Northern European decent
- Usually associated with family history
- Rare with children
- Men 7 to 15 times more likely than women to require surgery
- Females develop less severe cases
- Incidence increases with age >40 years
- Higher incidence among people with alcoholism, diabetes, epilepsy

CLINICAL FINDINGS

SIGNS AND SYMPTOMS

- Thickening and shortening of fascia of the hand
- Contractures form at metacarpophalangeal (MCP), proximal interphalangeal (PIP), and occasionally distal interphalangeal (DIP) joints
- Fifth finger involved in 70% of cases

Functional Implications

- Limitation in opening hand, extending fingers fully
- Can limit ability to shake hands

Possible Contributing Causes

- Smoking may decrease vascular changes in the hands
- Alcoholism[3]
- Epilepsy[4]
- Pulmonary tuberculosis[5]

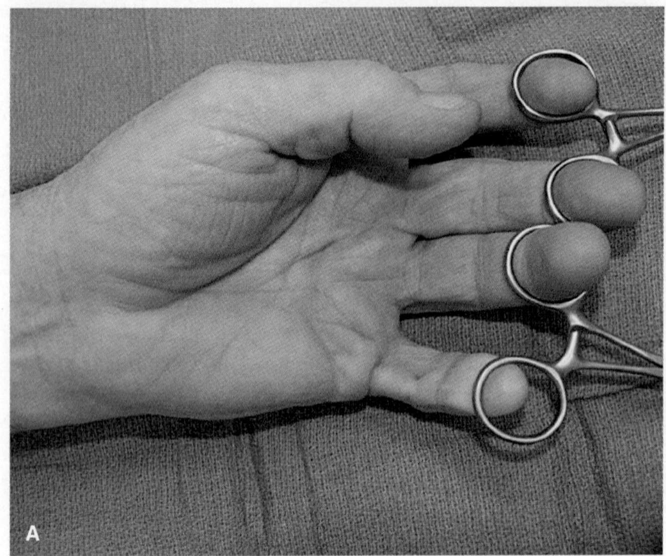

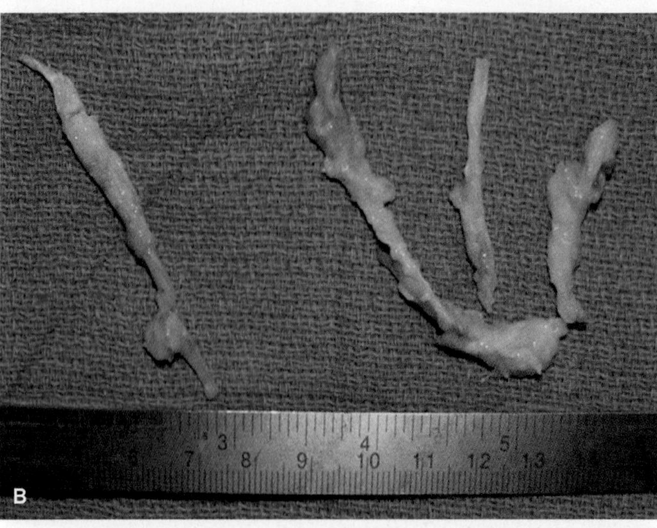

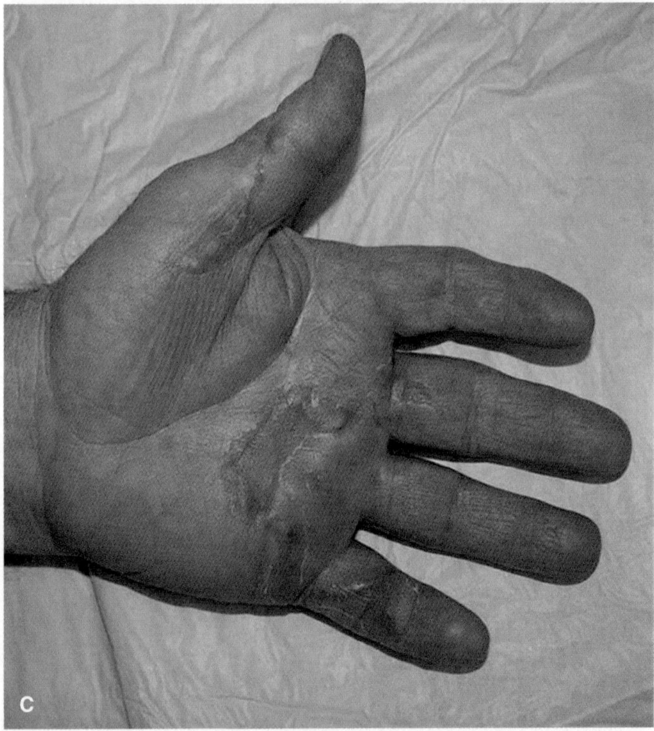

FIGURE 173-1 Dupuytren disease. (**A**) This patient has cords affecting the thumb, middle, ring, and small fingers. (**B**) The resected specimens are shown. (**C**) Postoperatively, the patient went on to heal all his incisions and, with the aid of weeks of hand therapy, recovered full motion. (From Brunicardi FC, Andersen DK, Billiar TR, et al., eds. *Schwartz's Principles of Surgery.* 9th ed. http://www.accessmedicine.com. Copyright © The McGraw-Hill Companies, Inc. All rights reserved.)

- Diabetes
- Liver disease or cirrhosis
  - Heredity: heterogeneous
  - Higher expression levels of the fibroblast growth factor 9 gene
- Effect androgen receptors in males
- Genetic association with chromosomes[6,11,16]

Differential Diagnosis

- Dupuytren contracture; a fixed-flexion contracture of the hand

MEANS OF CONFIRMATION OR DIAGNOSIS

Diagnostic Procedures

- Imaging not usually necessary

FINDINGS AND INTERPRETATION

- Cord-like thickening of the skin around the fourth and fifth fingers

TREATMENT

Surgery

- Surgery to skin graft and remove contracture
  - Return of fibrosis is common

Medication

- Enzyme injection

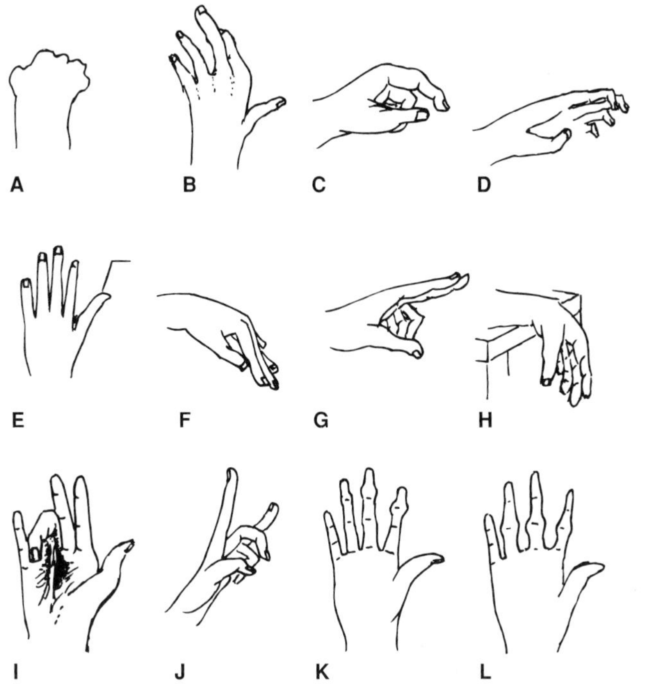

A B C D

E F G H

I J K L

FIGURE 173-2 Deformities of the hand. (**A**) Clubhand. This is a congenital lesion in which the hand development is rudimentary; the stub may be surmounted by rudimentary or normal digits. (**B**) Ulnar deviation. Also called ulnar drift. (**C**) Position of anatomic rest. (**D**) Clawhand. (**E**) Ape hand. (**F**) Carpal spasm. (**G**) Benediction hand. (**H**) Wrist-drop. (**I**) Dupuytren contracture. (**J**) Athetoid hand. (**K**) Heberden nodes. (**L**) Haygarth nodes. The spindle-shaped enlargements of the middle interphalangeal joints occur in RA. (From LeBlond RF, DeGowin RL, Brown DD. *DeGowin's Diagnostic Examination.* 9th ed. http://www.accessmedicine. com. Copyright © The McGraw-Hill Companies, Inc. All rights reserved.)

  - Triamcinolone
  - Collagenase clostridium
- Histolyticum (Xiaflex) to soften and break down taut bands

REFERRALS/ADMITTANCE

- Hospital for surgery to release fascia
- Acupuncture
- Physician for enzyme injection of the collagen-eroding enzyme, collagenase
- Physician for radiotherapy, radiation therapy (low-energy X-rays)

IMPAIRMENTS

- Restricted movement of the hand and fingers
- Hand deformity
- Difficulty wearing gloves or placing hand in pockets due to the inability to straighten fingers

TESTS AND MEASURES

- Visual and palpation for thickened scar tissue (fibrosis)
- Tabletop test; negative if able to lay hand flat on a table, palm down
- Skin pliability

INTERVENTION

- Scar management
- Stretching, massage, heat, paraffin
- Splinting
- Breaking apart the cords
  - Dry needling/acupuncture
  - Surgery[6]

FUNCTIONAL GOALS

- Patient will be able to
  - Open fingers and hand so as to put on gloves.
  - Lay hand flat on a table, palm down.

PROGNOSIS

- Can remain functional with treatment.
- Does not progress at any specific rate.
- Develops slowly over decades.

PATIENT RESOURCES

- ASSH, American Society for Surgery of the Hand. Dupuytren's Disease. http://www.assh.org/Public/HandConditions/Pages/DupuytrensDisease.aspx. Accessed June 20, 2013.
- International Dupuytren Society. Dupuytren's Disease. http://www.dupuytren-online.info/dupuytrens_contracture.html. Accessed June 20, 2013.

REFERENCES

1. The American Physical Therapy Association. Pattern 4D: Impaired joint mobility, motor function, muscle performance, and range of motion associated with connective tissue dysfunction. *Interactive Guide to Physical Therapist Practice.* 2003. DOI: 10.2522/ptguide.3.1_4. Accessed June 20, 2013.
2. Chumley H. Chapter 101. Dupuytren's disease. In: Usatine RP, Smith MA, Chumley H, Mayeaux E Jr, Tysinger J, eds. *The Color Atlas of Family Medicine.* New York, NY: McGraw-Hill; 2009. http://www.accessmedicine.com/content.aspx?aID=8204224. Accessed June 20, 2013.
3. US National Library of Medicine. Alcoholism and alcohol abuse. PubMed Health. http://www.ncbi.nlm.nih.gov/pubmedhealth/PMH0001940/. Online March 3, 2011. Accessed June 20, 2013.
4. US National Library of Medicine. Epilepsy. PubMed Health. http://www.ncbi.nlm.nih.gov/pubmedhealth/PMH0001714/. Online March 28, 2011. Accessed June 20, 2013.
5. US National Library of Medicine. Pulmonary tuberculosis. PubMed Health. http://www.ncbi.nlm.nih.gov/pubmedhealth/PMH0001141/. Online December 6, 2011. Accessed June 20, 2013.
6. Dutton M. Common orthopedic conditions. In: Dutton M, ed. *McGraw-Hill's NPTE (National Physical Therapy Examination).* 2nd ed. New York, NY: McGraw-Hill; 2012. http://www.accessphysiotherapy.com/content/5398559. Accessed June 20, 2013.

ADDITIONAL REFERENCES

- Al-Qattan MM. Factors in the pathogenesis of Dupuytren's contracture. *J Hand Surg Am.* 2006;31:1527–1534. doi: 10.1016/j.jhsa.2006.08.012.
- Dutton M. Observation. In: Dutton M, ed. *Dutton's Orthopedic Survival Guide: Managing Common Conditions.* New York, NY: McGraw-Hill; 2011. http://www.accessphysiotherapy.com/content/8653105. Accessed June 20, 2013.
- Dutton M. Practice Pattern 4D: Impaired joint mobility, motor function, muscle performance, and range of motion associated with connective tissue dysfunction. In: Dutton M, ed. *Orthopaedic Examination, Evaluation, and Intervention.* 2nd ed. New York, NY: McGraw-Hill; 2008. http://www.accessphysiotherapy.com/content/55578994. Accessed June 20, 2013.
- ICD9DATA web site. http://www.icd9data.com. Accessed June 20, 2013.
- ICD10DATA web site. http://www.icd10data.com. Accessed June 20, 2013.
- Michou L, Lermusiaux JL, Teyssedou JP, Bardin T, Beaudreuil J, Petit-Teixeira E. Genetics of Dupytren. *Joint Bone Spine.* January 2012;79(1):7–12.

174 GAMEKEEPER'S THUMB

Patrick S. Pabian, DPT, PT, SCS, OCS, CSCS
Linda M. Martin, PhD, OTR/L, FAOTA
Eric Shamus, PhD, DPT, PT, CSCS

CONDITION/DISORDER SYNONYMS

- Thumb ulnar collateral ligament (UCL) tear
- Thumb UCL sprain
- Skier's thumb
- Breakdancer's thumb

ICD-9-CM CODE[1]

- 842.12 Sprains and strains of metacarpophalangeal (joint) of hand

ICD-10-CM CODES[2]

- S63.649A Sprain of metacarpophalangeal joint of unspecified thumb, initial encounter
- S63.659A Sprain of metacarpophalangeal joint of unspecified finger, initial encounter

PREFERRED PRACTICE PATTERN[3]

- 4D: Impaired Joint Mobility, Motor Function, Muscle Performance, and ROM Associated with Connective Tissue Dysfunction

PATIENT PRESENTATION

The patient is a 22-year-old competitive downhill skier who injured herself during a fall on the slopes. She reports that her thumb was forced outward by the ski pole as she fell. She was taken to the emergency complaining of pain and inability to use the thumb. It was determined that a partial rupture of the UCL of her L thumb at its proximal insertion had occurred, and that conservative treatment was indicated. She was provided with a cast to the hand which held the thumb midway between radial and palmar abduction, and in approximately 5 degrees MP flexion, with the IP joint free. She presents to the clinic 3 weeks later.

The patient has focal swelling and tenderness at the medial aspect of the first metacarpophalangeal (MCP) joint. She is having difficulty with grasping kitchen utensils and drinking cups and difficulty turning doorknobs due to pain and weakness of the thumb. The patient presents with grade II laxity during a valgus stress test at 30 degrees of the first MCP joint.

KEY FEATURES

Description

- Injury involving the UCL of the MCP joint in the first ray (thumb)
- Acute or repeated forceful abduction (valgus force) to the proximal phalanx results in ligamentous disruption
- Instability of the MCP joint
- Forced extension or abduction of the proximal phalanx of the thumb

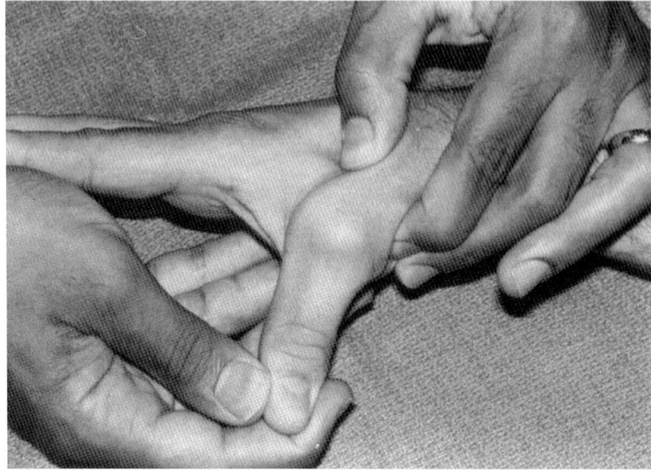

FIGURE 174-1 Gamekeeper's thumb. Laxity of 30 to 40 degrees more than the uninjured thumb measured in neutral and 30 degrees of flexion are strongly suggestive of a complete ulnar collateral ligament tear. There is no "endpoint" to the radial deviation of the phalanx. (Used with permission from Brunicardi FC, Anderson DK, Billar TR, et al. *Schwartz's Principles of Surgery*, 8th ed. © 2005 McGraw-Hill, New York, NY.)

Essentials of Diagnosis

- Gamekeeper's thumb is ligamentous disruption of the UCL of the first MCP joint due to acute or repeated valgus stress to the thumb.
- Presents as instability and/or pain with valgus forces to the thumb or pain and weakness with opposition or pinching.
- Tenderness or swelling may be present at medial aspect of the thumb.
- Valgus stress to the UCL of the first MCP joint will result in asymmetric laxity compared to uninvolved side or lack of an end point.

General Considerations

- Injury can be either acute or chronic and is common in athletics (especially skiing and football).
- Injury involves valgus force to the proximal phalanx of the thumb.
- Injury can also involve an avulsion fracture of the base of the proximal phalanx, which is termed "gamekeeper's fracture."
- Plain-film radiographs are beneficial to rule out fracture.
- Manage surgically or nonsurgically depending upon severity of signs and symptoms and orthopedic physician recommendations.

Demographics

- Common in athletes, typically involving a fall (football), impact from a ball (basketball), or repeated stress (skiing)
- Seen in fowl hunters

CLINICAL FINDINGS

SIGNS AND SYMPTOMS

- Pain over medial MCP joint
- Palpable tenderness and possible swelling over the medial MCP joint line/ UCL of the thumb
- Instability and/or pain with valgus stress to the MCP joint of the thumb
- Weakness with pinching or opposition
- Repeat subluxation of the MCP joint resulting in medial angulation of the proximal phalanx with valgus stress or force

Functional Limitations

- Difficulty and/or pain when
  - Grasping dishes, utensils, or drinking cups due to pain and weakness
  - Grasping and turning steering wheel
  - Turning doorknob

Possible Contributing Causes

- Participation in activities or sporting events that involve repeated valgus stress to the proximal phalanx in the thumb
- Participation in contact sports
- Generalized ligamentous laxity

Differential Diagnosis

- Gamekeeper's fracture
- Fracture of the base of the first metacarpal bone (Bennett fracture)
- Distal metacarpal fracture
- Proximal phalanx fracture
- Extensor tendon rupture (boutonnière deformity)

MEANS OF CONFIRMATION OR DIAGNOSIS

Imaging

- Radiographs to rule out fracture
- MRI

FINDINGS AND INTERPRETATION

- MRI may show increased fluid/edema at the medial MCP joint and can assess integrity of the UCL

TREATMENT

Medication

- NSAIDs
- Corticosteroid injection

MEDICAL PROCEDURES

- Recommended for grade II tears and avulsion fractures
- Involves open reduction internal fixation if displaced fracture present
- Involves repairing UCL or allograft replacement

REFERRALS/ADMITTANCE

- To radiologist for imaging, X-ray
- To orthopedist for surgical consult
- To occupational therapist to provide splints and instruct patient in joint protection techniques

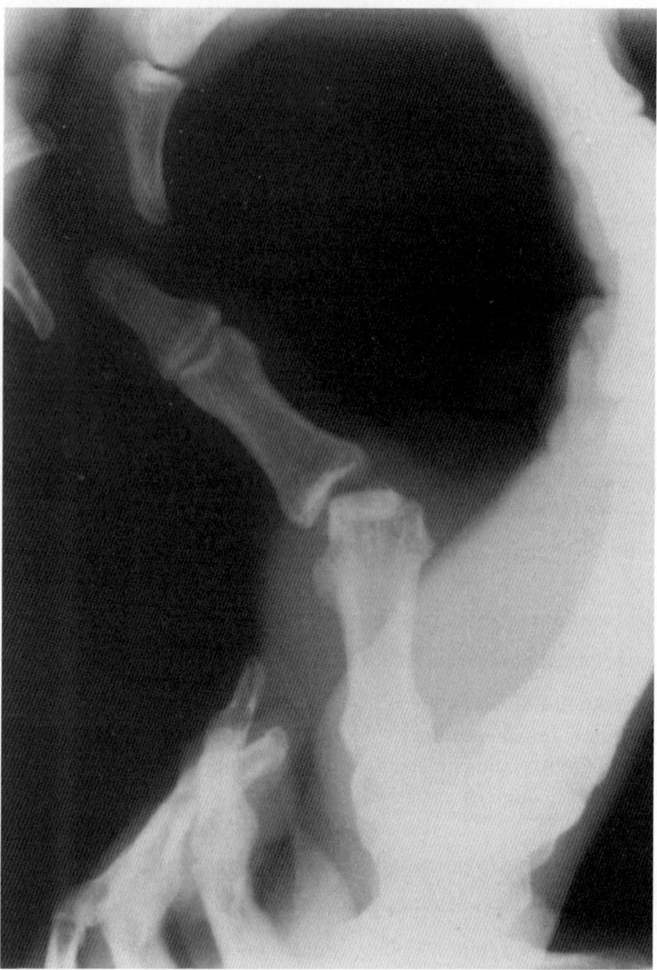

FIGURE 174-2 Gamekeeper's thumb. Stress x-ray of a thumb with a complete ulnar collateral ligament tear demonstrates marked instability of the ulnar side of the MP joint and radial deviation of the proximal phalanx. (Used with permission from Brunicardi FC, Anderson DK, Billar TR, et al. *Schwartz's Principles of Surgery.* 8th ed. © 2005 McGraw-Hill, New York, NY.)

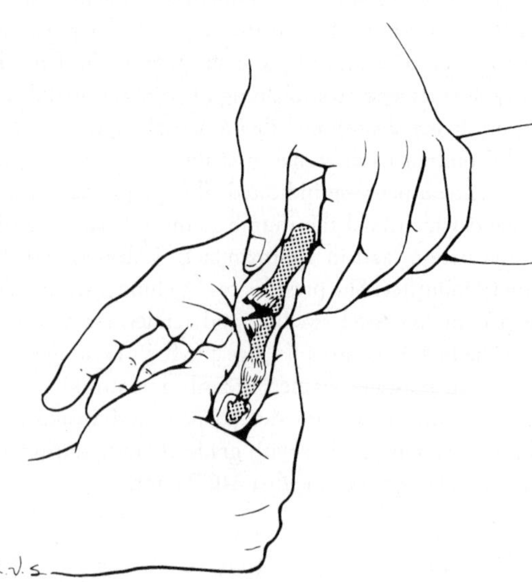

FIGURE 174-3 Stress examination of the thumb metacarpophalangeal collateral ligament. The ulnar side is injured more frequently. Test both sides in extension and 30 degrees of flexion. Compare the injured digit with the uninjured thumb. Feel for a firm end point and absence of excessive laxity. (From Stone CK, Humphries RL. *Current Diagnosis & Treatment: Emergency Medicine.* 7th ed. www.accessmedicine.com. Copyright © The McGraw-Hill Companies, Inc. All rights reserved.)

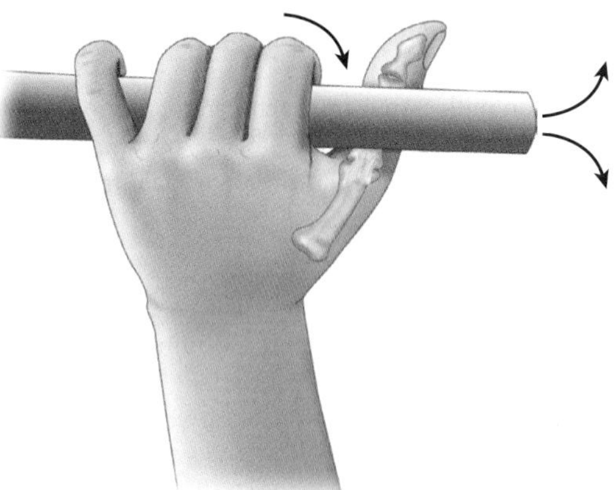

FIGURE 174-4 Mechanism of sprain of the ulnar collateral ligament of the thumb metacarpophalangeal joint. (From Patel DR, Greydanus DE, Baker RJ. *Pediatric Practice: Sports Medicine.* www.accesspediatrics.com. Copyright © The McGraw-Hill Companies, Inc. All rights reserved.)

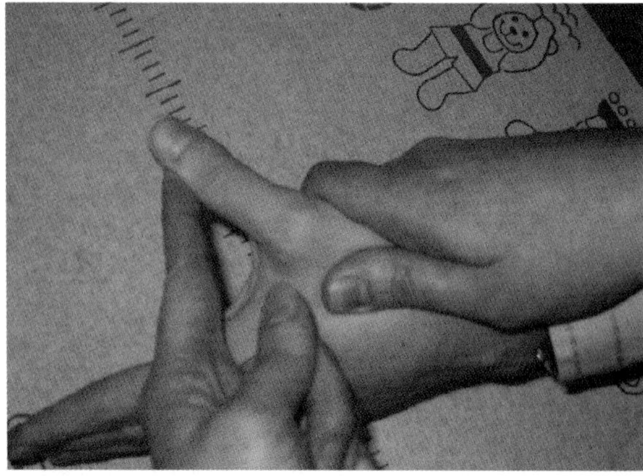

FIGURE 174-5 Stress test for ulnar collateral ligament of the MCP joint of the thumb. With thumb held in extension, the metacarpal is stabilized with one hand and a gentle stress is applied on the ulnar side of the proximal phalanx. Pain or increased laxity at the metacarpophalangeal joint will be elicited with ulnar collateral ligament sprain. (From Patel DR, Greydanus DE, Baker RJ. *Pediatric Practice: Sports Medicine.* www.accesspediatrics.com. Copyright © The McGraw-Hill Companies, Inc. All rights reserved.)

IMPAIRMENTS

- Decreased strength and pain for grasping activities (e.g., dressing and eating)
- Decreased strength, pain, and/or instability of the MCP joint with pinching activities (e.g., turning a key)

TESTS AND MEASURES

- Upper limb tension test (ULTT)
- Valgus stress to the UCL of the first MCP joint
  - Valgus stress test to the proximal phalanx at 0 degrees of extension and 30 degrees of flexion to test the accessory collateral ligament and UCL, respectively
- Self-reported symptoms on the Katz hand diagram[5]
- Sensory loss may include diminished two-point discrimination, decreased vibration sense, increased threshold in Semmes-Weinstein monofilament test
- Flick sign
- Thenar muscle strength test (lateral pinch dynamometry)
- Manipulative ability test (nine-hole peg test)

INTERVENTION

- Acute phase
  - PRICE: Protection, Rest, Ice Compression, Elevation
  - Splinting (thumb spica)
  - Ice massage
  - Pulsed ultrasound
  - Avoiding activities that provide valgus stress to the thumb
- Chronic phase
  - Gradually increase workload as pain and discomfort diminish

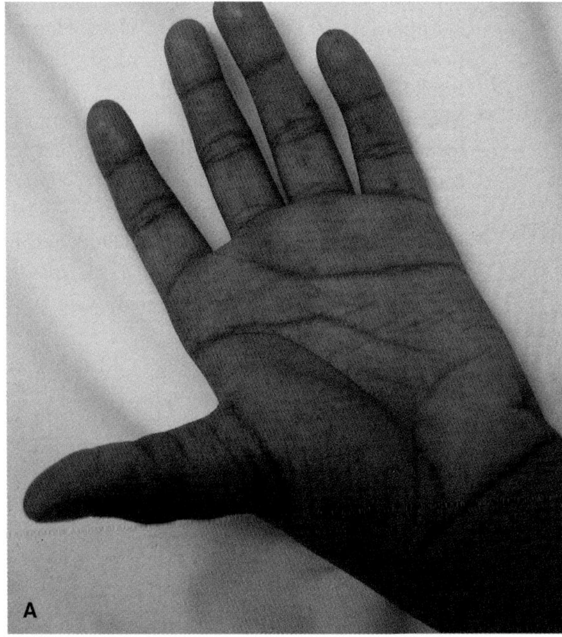

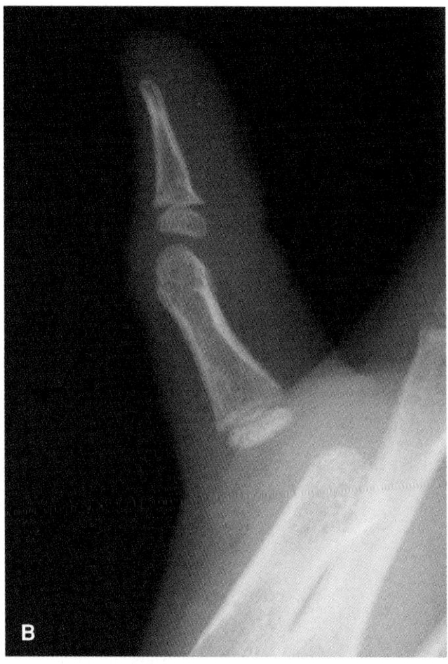

FIGURE 174-6 MCP dislocation of the thumb. (**A**) Clinical photograph. (**B**) Radiograph. (From Simon RR, Sherman SC. *Emergency Orthopedics.* 6th ed. www.accessemergencymedicine.com. Copyright © The McGraw-Hill Companies, Inc. All rights reserved.)

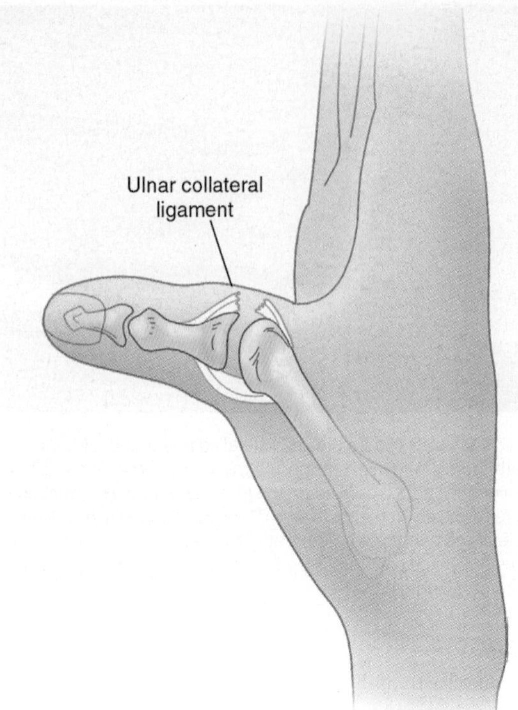

FIGURE 174-7 Examining for disruption of the ulnar collateral ligament of the thumb at the MCP joint. (From Simon RR, Sherman SC. *Emergency Orthopedics.* 6th ed. www.accessemergencymedicine.com. Copyright © The McGraw-Hill Companies, Inc. All rights reserved.)

- Continue taping or splinting when patient returns to sport participation
- Addressing pain
  - Ice
  - High-voltage pulsed stimulation
  - Iontophoresis
  - Ultrasound
  - Extracorporeal shockwave therapy
- Addressing swelling
  - Ice
  - Elevation
- Addressing Weakness, joint instability
  - As symptoms improve, gradually resume activities, with thumb spica taping for sports activities
  - Establish full, pain-free thumb ROM
  - Taping/splinting for sports participation thereafter until valgus stress is pain-free and stable
  - Incorporate stretching and progressive strengthening exercises as warranted to restore full mobility and strength.

FUNCTIONAL GOALS

- Patient will be able to
  - Turn doorknob and key without weakness, instability, or pain.
  - Use all kitchen and dining utensils without weakness, instability, or pain.
  - Lift a gallon milk carton from refrigerator at shoulder level, pain free.
  - Turn the key in her car and front door, pain free.
  - Use garden tools, pain free.

PROGNOSIS

- Good. Healing can be prolonged if rest/immobilization period is inadequate due to sports participation.
- Time periods of immobilization may vary depending upon degree of UCL injury.
- Immobilization period common, typically 3 weeks.

PATIENT RESOURCE

- Game Keeper's Thumb. Wheeless' Textbook of Orthopeadics. http://www.wheelessonline.com/ortho/gamekeepers_thumb. Accessed March 3, 2013.

REFERENCES

1. ICD9Data.com. http://www.icd9data.com. Accessed March 3, 2013.
2. ICD10Data.com. http://www.icd10data.com/ICD10CM/Codes. Accessed March 3, 2013.
3. American Physical Therapy Association. Pattern 4D: Impaired joint mobility, motor function, muscle performance, and range of motion associated with connective tissue dysfunction. In: *Guide to Physical Therapist Practice.* 2nd ed. Alexandria, VA: American Physical Therapy Association; 2001. Revised 2003.

ADDITIONAL REFERENCES

- Dutton M. The Forearm, Wrist, and Hand. In: Dutton M, ed. *Dutton's Orthopaedic Examination, Evaluation, and Intervention.* 3rd ed. New York, NY: McGraw-Hill; 2012. New York, NY: McGraw-Hill; 2008:735–838.
- Garnham A, Ashe M, Gropper P. Wrist, Hand, and Finger Injuries. In: *Clinical Sports Medicine.* 3rd ed. Australia: McGraw-Hill Book Company; 2009:308–339.
- Michaud EJ, Flinn S, Seitz WH Jr. Treatment of grade III thumb metacarpophalangeal ulnar collateral ligament injuries with early controlled motion using a hinged splint. *J Hand Ther.* 2010; 23(1):77–82.
- Prentice WE. The Forearm, Wrist, Hand, and Fingers. In: Prentice WE, ed. *Arnheim's Principles of Athletic Training: A Competency-Based Approach.* 13th ed. New York, NY: McGraw-Hill; 2011:722–723.
- Ritting AW, Baldwin PC, Rodner CM. Ulnar collateral ligament injury of the thumb metacarpophalangeal joint. *Clin J Sport Med.* 2010;20(2):106–112.

175 MALLET FINGER

Eric Shamus, PhD, DPT, PT, CSCS
Linda M. Martin, PhD, OTR/L, FAOTA

CONDITION/SYNONYMS

- Baseball finger
- Dropped finger

ICD-9-CM CODE

- 736.1 Mallet finger

ICD-10-CM CODE

- M20.019 Mallet finger of unspecified finger(s)

PREFERRED PRACTICE PATTERN

- 4E: Impaired joint mobility, motor function, muscle performance, and ROM associated with localized inflammation[1]

PATIENT PRESENTATION

The patient is a 46-year-old man who injured his middle finger while playing a casual game of basketball with friends. He reports that he attempted to catch a rebound, and the ball struck his outstretched finger, forcibly bending it. Examination revealed a characteristically flexed distal interphalangeal (DIP) joint and patient's inability to actively extend the DIP joint; X-ray revealed no bony disruption; mild swelling was present.

KEY FEATURES

Description

- Distal joint of the finger is bent into a claw-like position
- Usually due to trauma from impact on tip of the finger[2]
- Flexor muscles, fascia, tendons shorten
- Disruption of the extensor tendon, 15 to 20 degree loss of DIP finger extension
- Flexion of the DIP joint

Essentials of Diagnosis

- Diagnosis is usually made by clinical examination or x-ray
- Finger extension strength, often extensor digitorum communis injury

General Considerations

- Swelling
- Inflammation around the joint
- Can be associated with fracture, children type IV epiphyseal fracture[3]
- Altered joint position

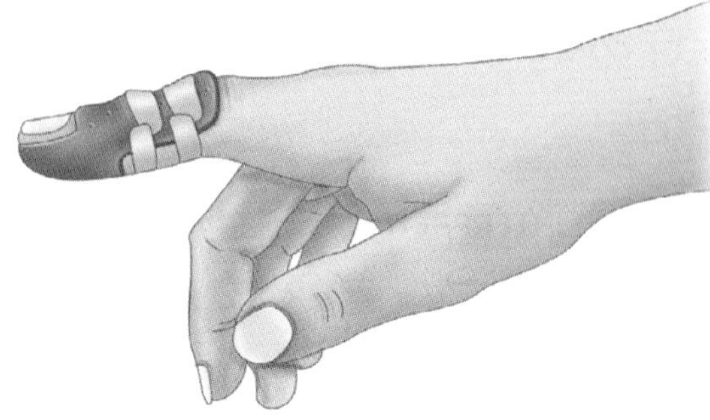

FIGURE 175-1 Mallet splint. The finger is splinted with distal interphalangeal joint held in extension. (From Patel DR, Greydanus DE, Baker RJ. *Pediatric Practice: Sports Medicine*. www.accesspediatrics.com.)

Demographics

- Adults
  - Hit or blow onto the finger tip from sports, i.e., basketball[3]

CLINICAL FINDINGS

SIGNS AND SYMPTOMS

- Pain with grasping
- Decreased extension of the finger, extensor lag
- Joint redness and pain

Functional Implications

- Pain with grasping, holding objects
- Inability to extend the finger
- At risk of injury in factories as finger not in alignment with the others and can get caught or injured

Possible Contributing Causes

- Muscle imbalance
- Extensor digitorum communis injury
- Trauma
- Joint arthritis/injury
- Muscle atrophy
- Nerve damage

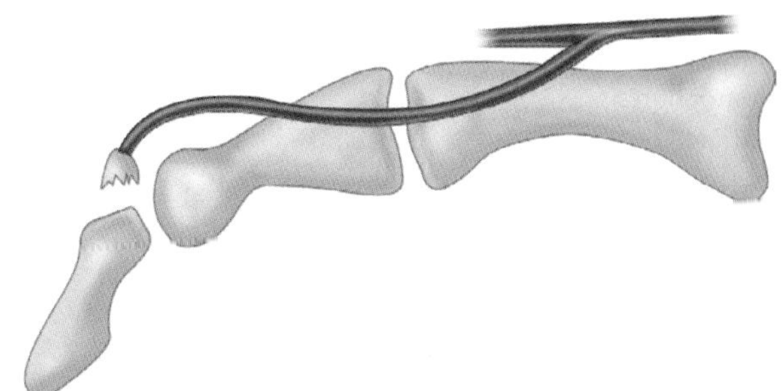

FIGURE 175-2 Mechanism of mallet finger injury. (From Patel DR, Greydanus DE, Baker RJ. *Pediatric Practice: Sports Medicine*. www.accesspediatrics.com.)

- Osteoarthritis
- Rheumatoid arthritis

▶ **Differential Diagnosis**
- Gout
- Boutonnière deformity
- Stress fracture

MEANS OF CONFIRMATION

- Imaging
  - X-ray

FINDINGS AND INTERPRETATION

- Bone spur, location and size

TREATMENT

▶ **Medication**
- Anti-inflammatory
- Surgery to straighten out the finger and lengthen ligaments/tendons

REFERRALS/ADMITTANCE

- For imaging, X-ray
- For corticosteroid injection
- For surgical consult
- For occupational therapist to provide splints and instruct patient in joint protection techniques

IMPAIRMENTS

- Pain with grasping objects for work and daily activities

TESTS AND MEASURES

- Thenar muscle strength test (lateral pinch dynamometry)
- Manipulative ability test (nine-hole peg test)

INTERVENTION

- Rest, to reduce inflammation
- Bracing/splinting for 6 weeks until extensor lag at the PIP joint is resolved
- Taping techniques
- Address swelling and pain
  - Ice
- Address pain
  - Ice
  - Massage
  - Joint mobilization
  - Electric stimulation
  - Iontophoresis
  - Infrared
- Address weakness and joint instability
  - Strengthening of extensors
- Address lack of flexibility
  - Stretching
    - Intrinsic flexor stretching
    - Fluidotherapy
- Address joint mobilization
  - DIP glides and rotation
- Address soft-tissue mobilization

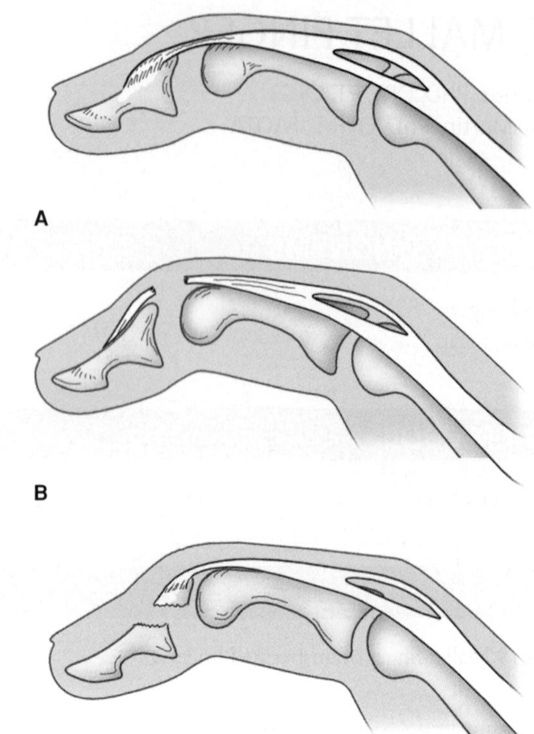

FIGURE 175-3 Three ways the extensor tendon can be disrupted. (**A**) A stretch of the tendon without division of the tendon. (**B**) When the tendon is ruptured from its insertion on the distal phalanx, there is a 40-degree flexion deformity present, and the patient cannot actively extend the tendon at the DIP joint. (**C**) A fragment of the distal phalanx can be avulsed with the tendon. (From Simon RR, Sherman SC. *Emergency Orthopedics.* 6th ed. www.accessemergencymedicine.com. Copyright © The McGraw-Hill Companies, Inc. All rights reserved.)

FUNCTIONAL GOALS

- Patient will be able to
  - Unclench hand to place around a jar to open.
  - Fully extend the finger to don/doff gloves.

PROGNOSIS

- Good; focus on stretching out the flexors.

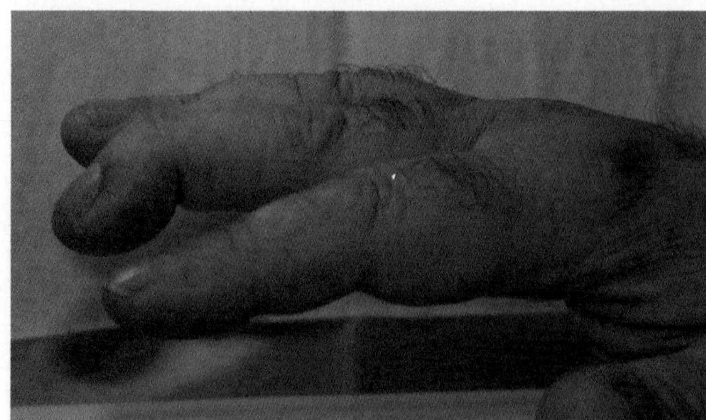

FIGURE 175-4 Flexion deformity the DIP of a mallet finger. (From Simon RR, Sherman SC. *Emergency Orthopedics.* 6th ed. www.accessemergencymedicine.com. Copyright © The McGraw-Hill Companies, Inc. All rights reserved.)

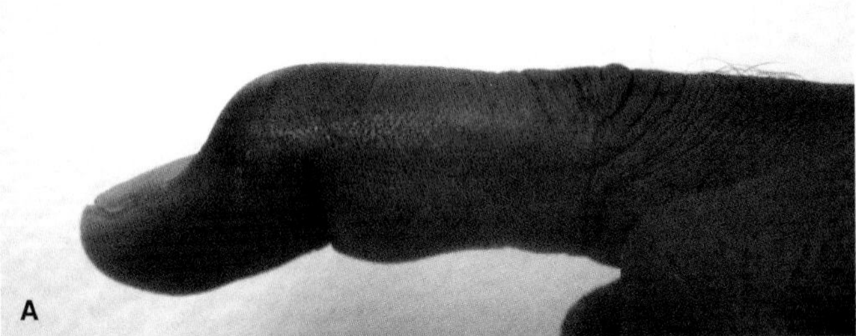

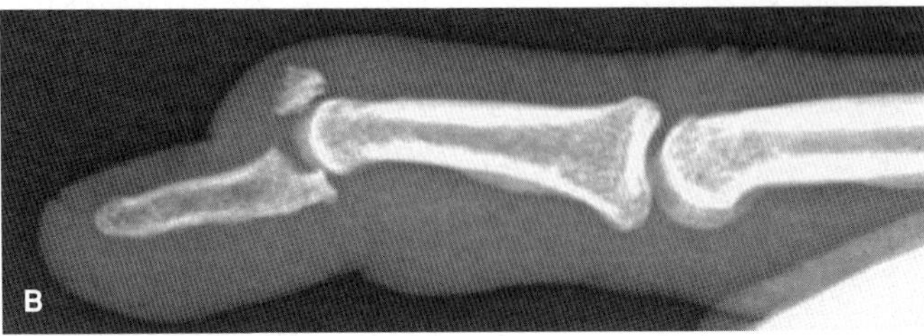

FIGURE 175-5 Mallet finger with fracture. (From Knoop KJ, Stack L, Storrow A, Jason Thurman R. *The Atlas of Emergency Medicine.* 3rd ed. www.accessmedicine.com. Copyright © The McGraw-Hill Companies, Inc. All rights reserved. Photo contributor: Matthew Kopp, MD.)

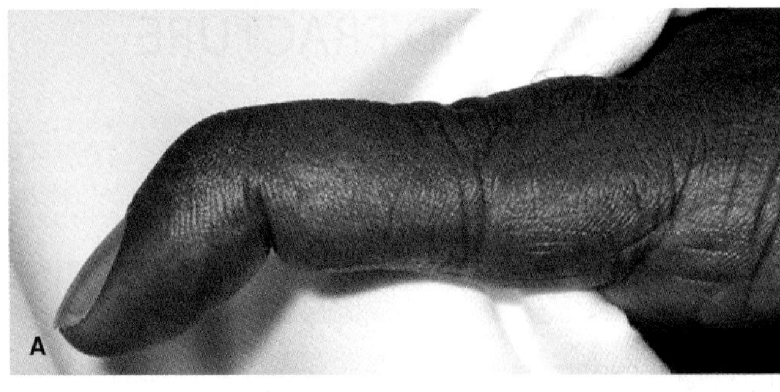

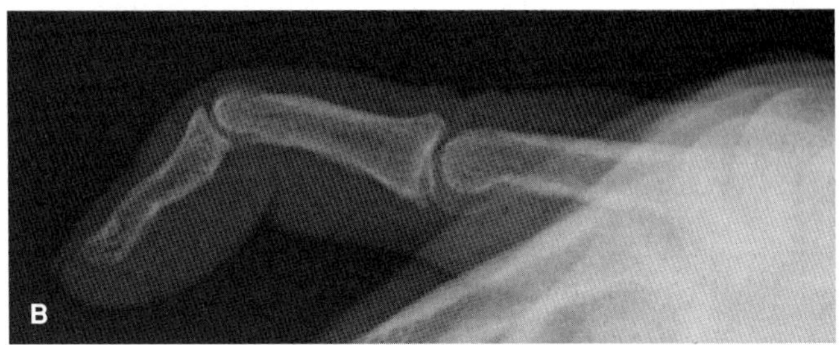

FIGURE 175-6 Mallet finger without fracture. (From Simon RR, Sherman SC. *Emergency Orthopedics.* 6th ed. www.accessemergencymedicine.com. Copyright © The McGraw-Hill Companies, Inc. All rights reserved.)

- Surgery may be indicated if the flexion becomes severe
- If associated with fragment fracture, 1 to 6 weeks of immobilization.

PATIENT RESOURCE

- American Academy of Orthopaedic Surgeons. Mallet Finger (Baseball Finger). http://orthoinfo.aaos.org/topic.cfm?topic=A00018. Accessed July 6, 2013.

REFERENCES

1. The American Physical Therapy Association. Pattern 4E: Impaired joint mobility, motor function, muscle performance, and range of motion associated with localized inflammation. interactive guide to physical therapist practice. *The American Physical Therapy Association.* 2003. http://guidetoptpractice.apta.org/content/1/SEC12.extract?sid=ccb92104-9626-443e-ab17-b2a32a7792b7. DOI: 10.2522/ptguide.978-1-931369-64-0. Accessed July 6, 2013.
2. Dutton M. Finger injuries. In: Dutton M, ed. *McGraw-Hill's NPTE (National Physical Therapy Examination).* 2nd ed. New York, NY: McGraw-Hill; 2012. http://www.accessphysiotherapy.com/content/56504934. Accessed July 6, 2013.
3. Cline S. Chapter 22. Acute Injuries of Elbow, Forearm, Wrist, and Hand. In: Patel DR, Greydanus DE, Baker RJ, eds. *Pediatric Practice: Sports Medicine.* New York, NY: McGraw-Hill; 2009. http://www.accessphysiotherapy.com/content/6978574. Accessed July 6, 2013.

ADDITIONAL REFERENCES

- Burton RI, Eaton RG. Common hand injuries in the athlete. *Orthop Clin North Am.* 1973;4:809–838.
- Dutton M. Tendon ruptures. In: Dutton M, ed. *Dutton's Orthopaedic Examination, Evaluation, and Intervention.* 3rd ed. New York, NY: McGraw-Hill; 2012. http://www.accessphysiotherapy.com/content/56540484. Accessed July 6, 2013.
- Hamilton N, Weimar W, Luttgens K. *Kinesiology: Scientific Basis of Human Motion.* 11th ed. New York, NY: McGraw-Hill; 2008. http://www.accessphysiotherapy.com/resource/618. Accessed July 6, 2013.
- Hooker DN, Prentice WE. Basic principles of electricity and electrical stimulating currents. In: Prentice WE, Quillen WS, Underwood F, eds. *Therapeutic Modalities in Rehabilitation.* 4th ed. New York, NY: McGraw-Hill; 2011. http://www.accessphysiotherapy.com/content/8136367#8136367. Accessed July 6, 2013.
- ICD9Data.com. http://www.icd9data.com. Accessed July 6, 2013.
- ICD10Data.com. http://www.icd10data.com. Accessed July 6, 2013.
- Malone TR, Hazle C, Grey ML. The ankle and foot. In: Malone TR, Hazle C, Grey ML, eds. *Imaging in Rehabilitation.* New York, NY: McGraw-Hill; 2008. http://www.accessphysiotherapy.com/content/5940160. Accessed July 6, 2013.
- Prentice WE. Cryotherapy and thermotherapy. In: Prentice WE, Quillen WS, Underwood F, eds. *Therapeutic Modalities in Rehabilitation.* 4th ed. New York, NY: McGraw-Hill; 2011. http://www.accessphysiotherapy.com/content/8137995#8137995. Accessed July 6, 2013.
- Simon RR, Sherman SC. Closed tendon injuries. In: Simon RR, Sherman SC, eds. *Emergency Orthopedics.* 6th ed. New York, NY: McGraw-Hill; 2011. http://www.accessphysiotherapy.com/content/7703566. Accessed July 6, 2013.

176 SCAPHOID FRACTURE

Jennifer Cabrera, DPT, GCS
Eric Shamus, PhD, DPT, PT, CSCS

CONDITION/DISORDER SYNONYM

- Navicular fracture of the hand

ICD-9-CM CODES[1]

- 814.01 Closed fracture of navicular (scaphoid) bone of wrist
- 814.11 Open fracture of navicular (scaphoid) bone of wrist

ICD-10-CM CODES[2]

- S62.009A Unspecified fracture of navicular (scaphoid) bone of unspecified wrist, initial encounter for closed fracture
- S62.009B Unspecified fracture of navicular (scaphoid) bone of unspecified wrist, initial encounter for open fracture

PREFERRED PRACTICE PATTERN[3]

- 4G: Impaired Joint Mobility, Muscle Performance, and Range of Motion Associated with Fracture

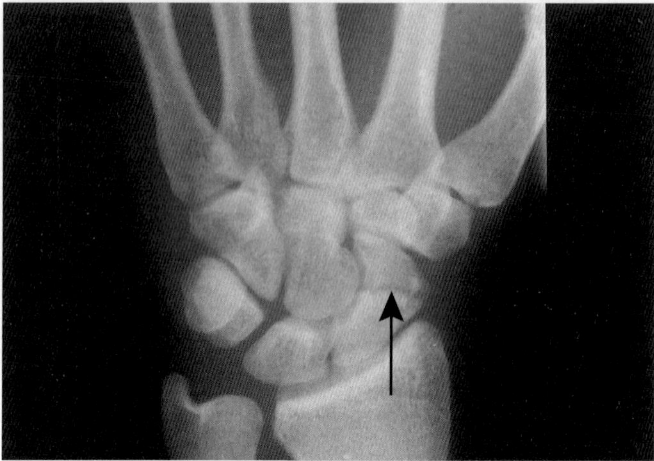

FIGURE 176-1 Scaphoid fracture in the middle third or waist (*arrow*). (From Tintinalli JE, Stapczynski JS, John Ma O, et al. *Tintinalli's Emergency Medicine: A Comprehensive Study Guide*. 7th ed. http://www.accessmedicine.com. Copyright © The McGraw-Hill Companies, Inc. All rights reserved.)

PATIENT PRESENTATION

A 25-year-old woman tripped while exiting her tub and fell onto her outstretched hand with her wrist extended. She felt immediate pain, but waited until the next day to seek medical attention. She presented with difficulty moving her wrist in all directions and difficulty gripping objects secondary to worsening pain. She demonstrated mild edema in the wrist and hand. Radiographs showed were negative for a distal scaphoid fracture. Patient was placed in a wrist immobilizer for 3 weeks secondary to pain with a tuning fork and as a precaution. Upon re-examination after 3 weeks patient continued with point tenderness in the snuff box and was sent for a follow-up X-ray. Follow-up X-ray demonstrated a healing fracture line of the scaphoid.

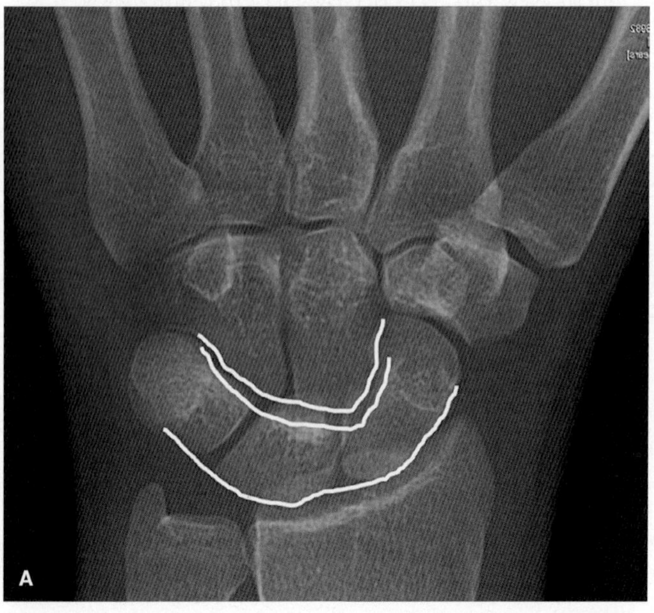

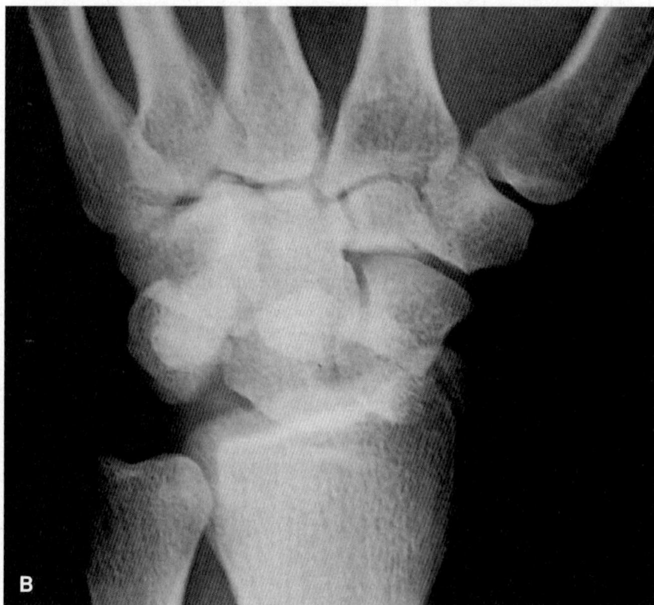

FIGURE 176-2 Gilula's arcs are seen shown in this normal patient (**A**) and in a patient with a scaphoid fracture and perilunate dislocation (**B**). (From Brunicardi FC, Andersen DK, Billiar TR, et al. *Schwartz's Principles of Surgery*. 9th ed. http://www.accessmedicine.com. Copyright © The McGraw-Hill Companies, Inc. All rights reserved.)

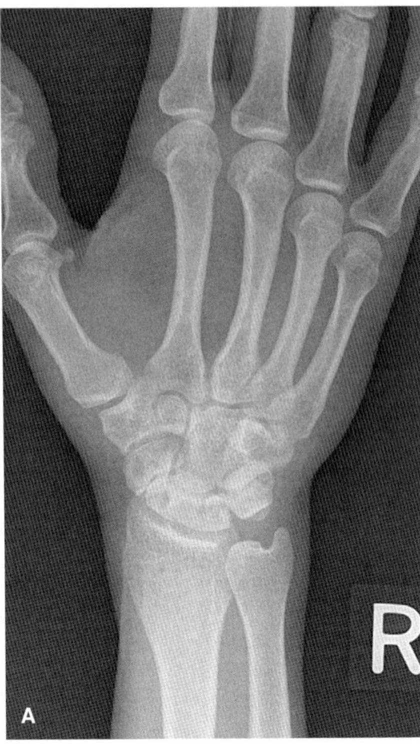

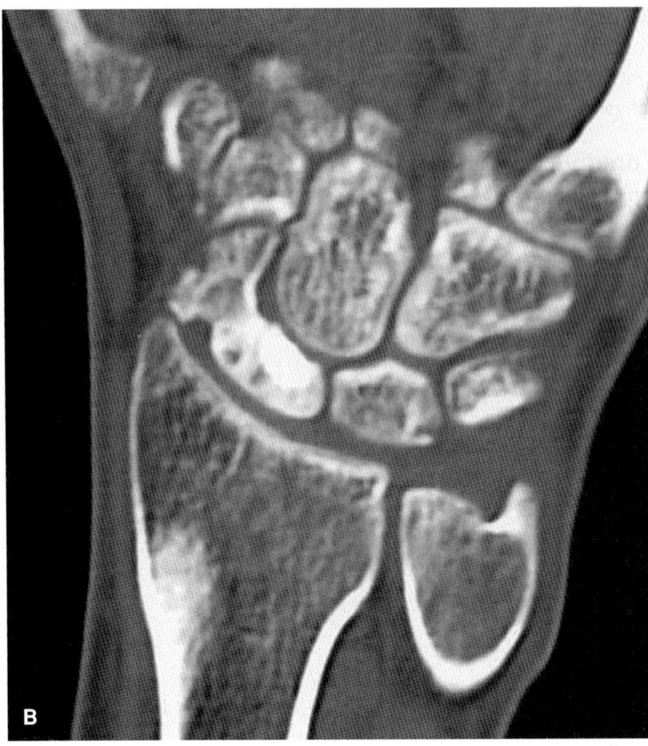

FIGURE 176-3 **A.** Preoperative images demonstrate a nonunion of a scaphoid fracture sustained 4 years earlier. **B.** Postoperatively, cross-sectional imaging with a computed tomography scan in the coronal plan demonstrates bone crossing the previous fracture line. This can be difficult to discern on plain x-rays due to overlap of bone fragments. (From Brunicardi FC, Andersen DK, Billiar TR, et al. *Schwartz's Principles of Surgery*. 9th ed. http://www.accessmedicine.com. Copyright © The McGraw-Hill Companies, Inc. All rights reserved.)

KEY FEATURES

Description

- Any defect in continuity of the scaphoid (carpal bone)
- Displaced (scaphoid is moved on either side of the fracture) or nondisplaced (scaphoid has not moved)
- Closed (skin is intact) or open (skin is breached)

Essentials of Diagnosis

- Diagnosis is usually made by clinical examination
- May not be a fracture but a wrist sprain, Colles fracture, distal radioulnar subluxation/dislocation, or fracture of any other carpal bone

General Considerations

- Most frequently fractured carpal bone (71% of all carpal bone fractures)

Demographics

- Occurs in young and middle-aged adults 15 to 60 years of age
- Men aged 20 to 30 years are most likely to suffer from a scaphoid fracture

CLINICAL FINDINGS

SIGNS AND SYMPTOMS

- Pain at the base of the thumb
- Point tenderness within the snuff box
- Edema
- Loss of general function
- Loss of active wrist and/or thumb mobility
- Muscle guarding with passive movement

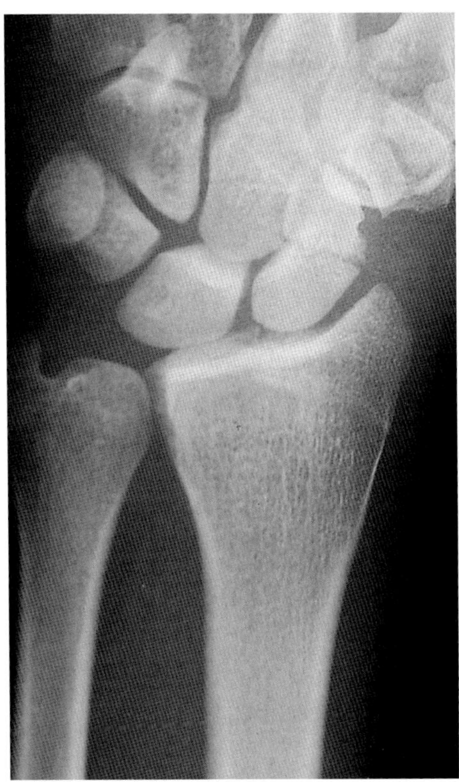

FIGURE 176-4 Scaphoid fracture. Fracture of the waist, or middle third, of the scaphoid. These injuries can be associated with delayed healing and avascular necrosis. (From Knoop KJ, Stack LB, Storrow AB, Thurman RJ. *The Atlas of Emergency Medicine*. 3rd ed. http://www.accessmedicine.com. Copyright © The McGraw-Hill Companies, Inc. All rights reserved. Photo contributor: Alan B. Storrow, MD.)

Functional Implications

- Pain with weight-bearing activities on involved hand
- Pain with wrist and thumb movements (passive or active)
- Pain when gripping something

Possible Contributing Causes

- Mechanism of injury
    - Fall on outstretched hand
    - Direct impact (i.e., athletic activity, motor vehicle accident)

Differential Diagnosis

- Colles fracture
- Distal radioulnar subluxation/dislocation
- Wrist sprain

MEANS OF CONFIRMATION OR DIAGNOSIS

Imaging

- X-ray for fracture, often limited view
- Computed tomography (CT) scan for detailed imaging
- MRI

FINDINGS AND INTERPRETATION

- Pain with passive/active ROM of the wrist and thumb
- Wrist will often be held in radial deviation
- Muscle guarding with all movements
- Inability to actively perform wrist or thumb movements secondary to pain
- Pain with gripping activities

REFERRALS/ADMITTANCE

- For imaging, x-ray or CT
- For medication: NSAIDs or opioid for pain management
- For immediate orthopedic consult
    - Distal scaphoid pole fractures are treated nonoperatively
        - Immobilization casting of hand and may or may not include thumb
    - Waist or proximal scaphoid pole fractures may be treated:
        - Nonoperatively, immobilization cast of hand and thumb
        - Operatively, open reduction internal fixation

IMPAIRMENTS

- Inability to perform activities of daily living with involved hand
- Inability to bear weight on involved hand
- Inability to use involved hand to write (especially if it is patient's dominant hand)
- Inability to grab a cup or open a door secondary to pain and muscle weakness

TESTS AND MEASURES

- Grip strength
- Flick sign
- Thenar muscle strength test (lateral pinch dynamometry)
- Disabilities of the Arm, Shoulder, and Hand (DASH) score to assess physical function
- Manipulative ability test (nine-hole peg test)
- Watson test

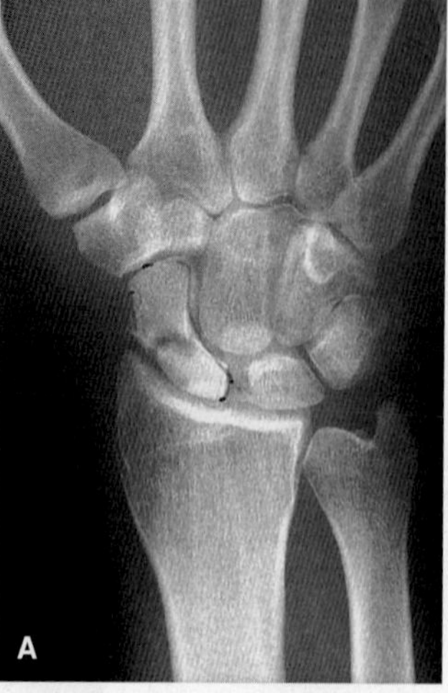

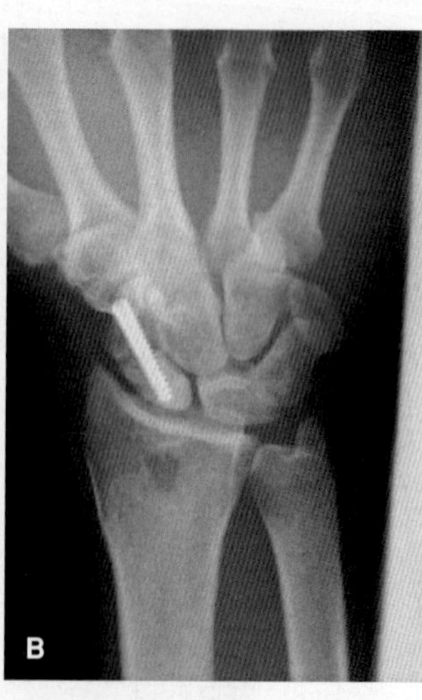

FIGURE 176-5 Scaphoid fracture. (**A**) Scaphoid fracture nonunion. (**B**) Open reduction and internal fixation of scaphoid nonunion. (From Doherty GM. *Current Diagnosis & Treatment in Surgery*. 13th ed. http://www.accessmedicine.com.)

INTERVENTION

- Address swelling
    - Ice/Cryotherapy
    - Compression
    - Elevation
    - Electrical stimulation
- Address pain
    - Ice/cryotherapy
    - Massage
    - Electrical stimulation
    - Address lack of flexibility via stretching
    - Wrist flexors
    - Wrist extensors
    - Thumb carpometacarpal extensors
    - Thumb metacarpophalangeal joint extensors
- Address mobilization upon healing of fracture site (6 weeks postoperative)

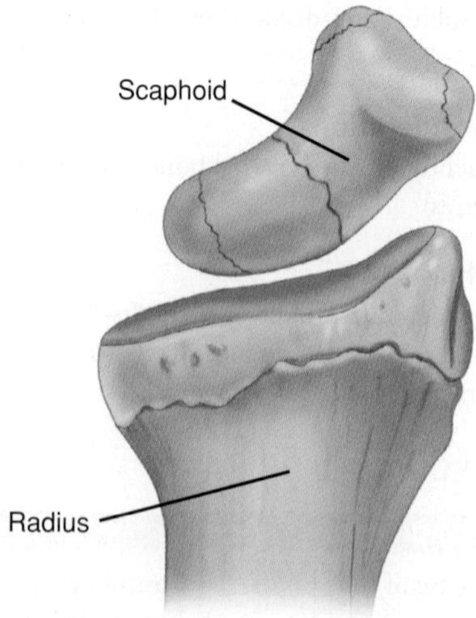

FIGURE 176-6 Line diagram showing scaphoid fracture sites. (From Patel DR, Greydanus DE, Baker RJ. *Pediatric Practice: Sports Medicine*. http://www.accesspediatrics.com.)

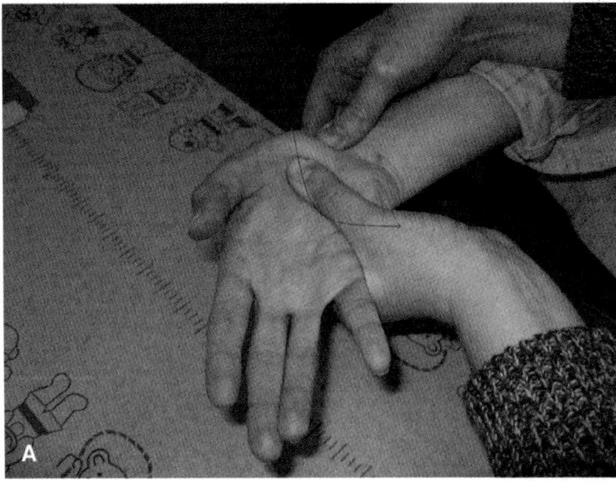

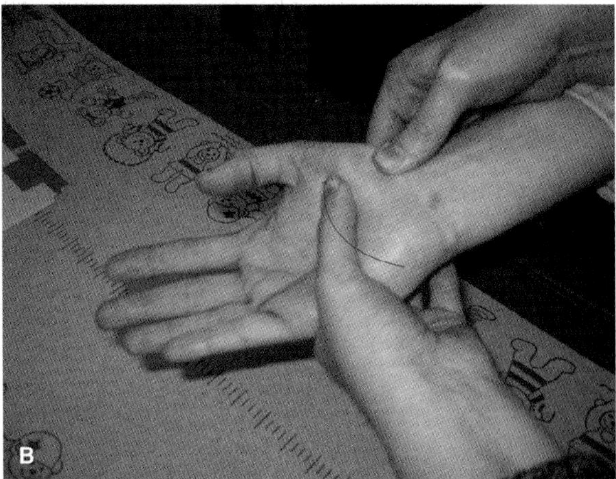

FIGURE 176-7 Watson test of scapholunate instability. Pain or a click or clunk in the wrist is felt when stabilizing the scaphoid with one hand and moving wrist from a position of radial deviation (**A**) to ulnar deviation (**B**) as pressure is applied on the scaphoid with the thumb of the other hand. (From Patel DR, Greydanus DE, Baker RJ. *Pediatric Practice: Sports Medicine*. http://www.accesspediatrics.com. Copyright © The McGraw-Hill Companies, Inc. All rights reserved.)

- Radiocarpal joint distraction for pain management
    - Radiocarpal joint dorsal glide for wrist flexion
    - Radiocarpal joint volar glide for wrist extension
    - Radiocarpal joint radial glide for wrist ulnar deviation
    - Radiocarpal joint ulnar glide for wrist radial deviation
    - Carpal gliding
- Address weakness via strengthening activities
    - Closed chain weight-bearing activities
    - Isometric exercises (initially submaximal)
    - Open chain via use of free weights and resistance bands
    - Grip-strengthening activities
- Address scar mobility
    - Scar tissue mobilization progressing from parallel to perpendicular upon wound closure
- Address functional use of hand
    - Finger opposition
    - Finger dexterity
    - Gripping cups/doorknobs/jars

FUNCTIONAL GOALS

- Patient will
    - Increase grip strength to 30 kg in order to facilitate bringing a glass to the mouth.
    - Increase wrist extension to 45 degrees in order to facilitate turning a doorknob.
    - Increase wrist flexor strength to 4/5 in order to facilitate carrying groceries.
    - Increase scapholunate joint mobility to 3 in order to allow the individual to use the telephone.

PROGNOSIS

- Good; however recovery varies based on length of time for fracture to heal.
- Some individuals report residual wrist stiffness and ache even after the fracture has healed.
- Nonunion is more common in scaphoid fractures secondary to poor blood supply.

PATIENT RESOURCES

- American Academy of Orthopaedic Surgeons. *Scaphoid Fracture of the Wrist*. Available at: http://orthoinfo.aaos.org/topic.cfm?topic=A00012. Accessed July 2, 2013.
- Boles CA. *Scaphoid Fracture Imaging*. Medscape Reference. Available at: http://emedicine.medscape.com/article/397230-overview#showall. Accessed July 2, 2013.

REFERENCES

1. ICD9Data.com. http://www.icd9data.com. Accessed July 3, 2013.
2. ICD10Data.com. http://www.icd10data.com/ICD10CM/Codes. Accessed July 3, 2013.
3. Pattern 4G: Impaired joint mobility, muscle performance, and range of motion associated with fracture. In: *Guide to Physical Therapist Practice*. 2nd ed. Alexandria, VA: American Physical Therapy Association; 2001. Revised 2003.

ADDITIONAL REFERENCES

- Goodman CC, Boissonnault WG, Fuller KS. *Pathology: Implications for the Physical Therapist*. 2nd ed. Philadelphia, PA: Saunders; 2003.
- Kisner C, Colby LA. *Therapeutic Exercise*. 5th ed. Philadelphia, PA: F.A. Davis Company; 2007.
- Magee DJ. *Orthopedic Physical Assessment*. 5th ed. St. Louis, MO: Saunders Elsevier; 2008.
- Malone TR, Hazle C, Grey ML, eds. *Imaging in Rehabilitation*. New York, NY: McGraw-Hill; 2008. http://www.accessphysiotherapy.com/content/5940000. Accessed July 8, 2013.
- Prentice WE, Quillen WS, Underwood F, eds. *Therapeutic Modalities in Rehabilitation*. 4th ed. New York, NY: McGraw-Hill; 2011. http://www.accessphysiotherapy.com/content/8137872. Accessed July 8, 2013.

177 SWAN-NECK DEFORMITY

Eric Shamus, PhD, DPT, PT, CSCS
Jesse Solotoff, DPT
Tiffany M. Barber, DPT
Linda M. Martin, PhD, OTR/L, FAOTA

CONDITION/DISORDER SYNONYMS

- Duck-bill deformity
- Recurvatum deformity
- Volar plate injury

ICD-9-CM CODE[1]

- 736.22 Swan-neck deformity

ICD-10-CM CODES[2]

- M20.03 Swan-neck deformity
- M20.031 Swan-neck deformity of right finger(s)
- M20.032 Swan-neck deformity of left finger(s)
- M20.039 Swan-neck deformity of unspecified finger(s)

PREFERRED PRACTICE PATTERN[3]

- 4D: Impaired Joint Mobility, Motor Function, Muscle Performance, and Range of Motion Associated with Connective Tissue Dysfunction

PATIENT PRESENTATION

Patient is a 32-year-old woman diagnosed with rheumatoid arthritis 3 years ago. She experienced an exacerbation of symptoms, with increased pain and inflammation in both hands 2 months ago, and was seen by her rheumatologist for medical management. Although pain and inflammation have subsided, she now reports difficulty in her job as a music teacher at the local high school. Her chief complaint is that she is unable to demonstrate playing instruments because her "fingers won't cooperate." When trying to straighten the fingers, "the middle joint bends backwards and gets in the way."

When asked to extend her fingers, the patient moved the index, long, and ring fingers of her right hand into a position involving proximal interphalangeal (PIP) joint hyperextension and distal interphalangeal (DIP) joint flexion; the small finger moved normally into extension. After demonstrating this, the patient then had mild difficulty returning to a flexed position (unintended slight hesitation). The MP joints were slightly swollen, but appeared to be in good alignment and functioning properly. Wrist motion was within normal limits (WNL).

KEY FEATURES

Description

- Injury or loosening of the volar plate (ligament connecting proximal and middle phalanx that prevents hyperextension of the PIP)

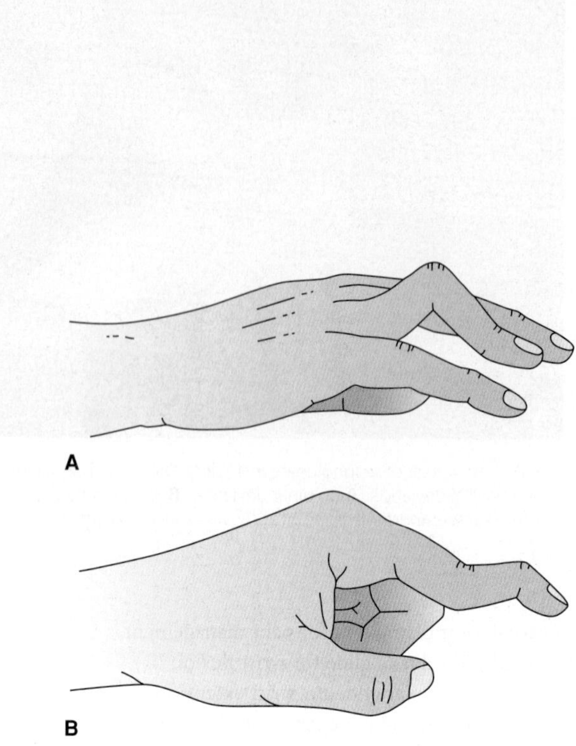

FIGURE 177-1 Boutonnière (**A**) and swan-neck (**B**) deformities. (From Toy EC, Patlan JT. *Case Files: Internal Medicine*. 3rd ed. www.accessmedicine.com. Copyright © The McGraw-Hill Companies, Inc. All rights reserved.)

- Hyperextension of the PIPjoint and flexion of the DIP joint
- Duck-bill deformity is the same issue in the thumb less one joint

Essentials of Diagnosis

- RA most common cause of swan-neck deformity
- Chronic inflammation loosens the volar plate and disrupts ligaments and other connective tissues making PIP susceptible to hyperextension
- Migration of the lateral bands of the extensor hood dorsally, to become extensor forces at the PIP
  - This neutralizes the oblique retinacular ligaments' ability to influence extension of the DIP, resulting in imbalance between the flexors and extensors which results in flexion of the DIP
- As a result, extensor tendon tightens causing DIP to pull into flexed position
- Swan-neck classification by Nalebuff[4]
  - I: PIP joint flexible in all positions
  - II: PIP motion limited only by tenodesis effect
  - III: Fixed PIP joint contracture, x-ray normal
  - IV: X-ray shows arthritic changes

General Considerations

- Pain and swelling of the PIP
- Can be managed surgically or nonsurgically depending upon signs and symptom severity, response to conservative treatment, and orthopedic physician recommendations
- Disruption of the hood and joint capsules results in a cascade of deformities

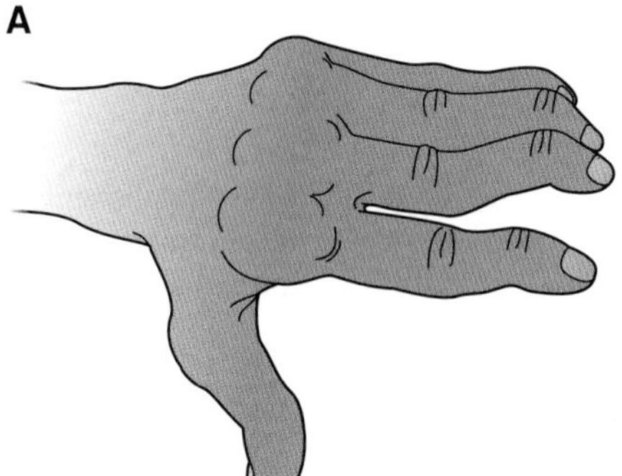

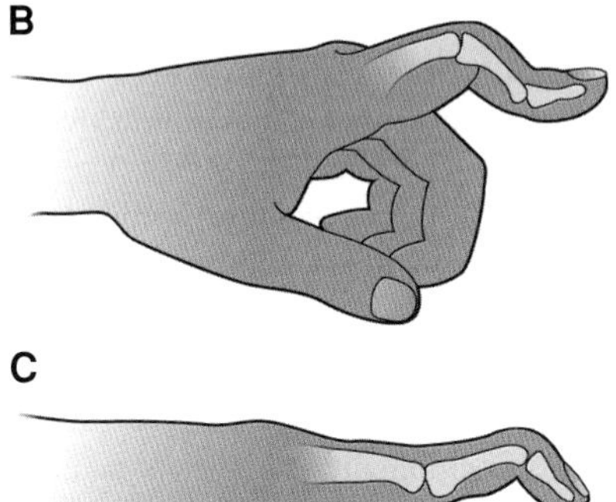

FIGURE 177-2 Finger deformities. (From Dutton M. *Dutton's Orthopaedic Examination, Evaluation, and Intervention*. 3rd ed. http://accessphysiotherapy.mhmedical.com/ViewLarge.aspx?figid=40799382. Copyright © The McGraw-Hill Companies, Inc. All rights reserved.)

- ◦ Ulnar drift can result from the EDC losing its dorsal position over the MP, volar subluxation of the MP (the result of the absence of extensor forces, leaving intrinsics and finger flexors unopposed in flexion)
  - ◦ Wrist radial deviation as a result of the patients attempt to bring the ulnarly deviated fingers into axial alignment for function
- Other causes include trauma, nerve injury such as cerebral palsy, Parkinson's disease, or stroke

Demographics

- Adults
- 50% of population with RA[4]
- Associated in population with neurological disorders (cerebral palsy, Parkinson's disease, CVA)

CLINICAL FINDINGS

SIGNS AND SYMPTOMS

- Pain and swelling of the PIP joint
- Laxity of the volar plate
- Snapping and locking of the fingers
- Hyperextension of the PIP and flexion of the DIP
- Signs of 11's (parallel course of lateral bands on the dorsum of the joint is clearly seen under the skin)

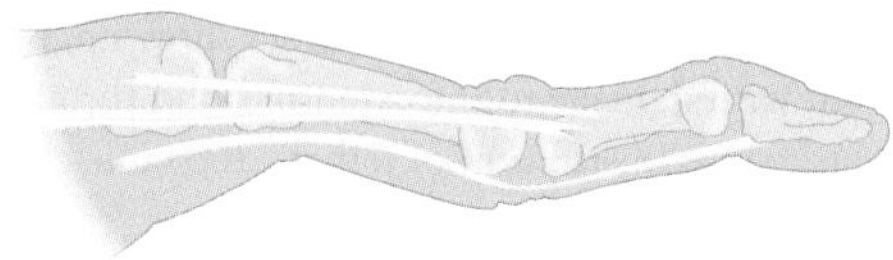

FIGURE 177-3 Swan-neck deformity. (From Tintinalli JE, Stapczynski JS, John Ma O, et al. *Tintinalli's Emergency Medicine: A Comprehensive Study Guide*. 7th ed. www.accessmedicine.com. Copyright © The McGraw-Hill Companies, Inc. All rights reserved.)

Functional Implications

- For patients with RA, pain is really only a problem in the inflammatory phase; do not report pain otherwise, just dysfunction
- Difficulty and/or pain with opening and closing hand in preparation for grasping or reaching
- Difficulty and/or pain with grasping dishes, utensils, or drinking cups due to pain and weakness
- Difficulty and/or pain with grasping and turning steering wheel
- Difficulty and/or pain with turning doorknob

Possible Contributing Causes

- Cerebral palsy
- Ehlers–Danlos syndrome
- Neurological disorders
- Overuse activity of the hand and fingers
- Parkinson disease
- Rheumatoid arthritis, or other rheumatic or connective tissue disorders
- Trauma
- Untreated mallet finger

Differential Diagnosis

- Ganglion of tendon sheath
- Loose body in the MCP joint
- Subluxation of the extensor digitorum communis

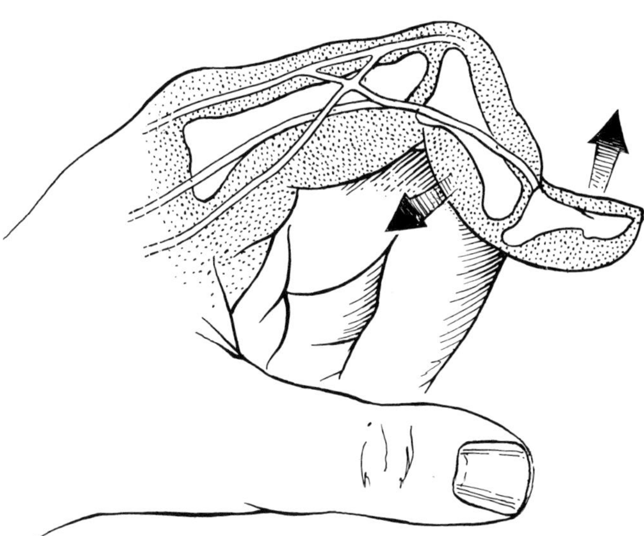

FIGURE 177-4 Swan-neck deformity. A swan-neck deformity of the index finger. Note the hyperextension of the PIP joint and the flexion of the DIP joint. (From Knoop KJ, Stack LB, Storrow AB, Thurman RJ. *The Atlas of Emergency Medicine*. 3rd ed. www.accessmedicine.com. Copyright © The McGraw-Hill Companies, Inc. All rights reserved. Photo contributor: Cathleen M. Vossler, MD.)

- May occur before swan-neck deformities show up, but usually, concurrent with damage to the extensor hood through inflammation/stretching/disruption of tethers, the same as happens at the PIP

MEANS OF CONFIRMATION OR DIAGNOSIS

Imaging

- X-ray to rule out fracture

TREATMENT

Medication

- NSAIDs
- Corticosteroid injection

MEDICAL PROCEDURES

- Surgical options possible after failed conservative care
- Soft tissue repair
- PIP arthroplasty (PIP replaced with metal implant)
- Interphalangeal arthrodesis

FINDINGS AND INTERPRETATION

- Classification III: Fixed PIP joint contracture, X-ray normal[4]
- Classification IV: X-ray shows arthritic changes[4]

REFERRALS/ADMITTANCE

- To radiologist for imaging, x-ray to rule out other pathology
- To primary care to rule out rheumatic causes or other connective tissue disorders
- To orthopedist for corticosteroid injection or surgical consult
- To occupational therapist to provide silver ring splints and instruct patient in joint protection techniques

IMPAIRMENTS

- Decreased strength and pain for grasping activities such as dressing and eating
- Pain with opening hand to reach for objects
- Decreased ability to open or close hand due to joint stiffness

TESTS AND MEASURES

- Start with a full fist, and then ask patient to open the hand and extend the fingers
- Lateral pinch dynamometry
- Disabilities of the Arm, Shoulder, and Hand (DASH) score to assess physical function
- Manipulative ability test (nine-hole peg test)

INTERVENTION

- Objective of treatment is to restore balance of the extensor tendon and volar plate
- Instruct in joint protection techniques and modify habits to delay/prevent associated joint deformity and dysfunction in the hands
- Acute phase
  - PRICE: Protection, rest, ice compression, elevation
  - Immobilization/splint
  - Taping to reduce exacerbating activities
  - Ice massage
  - Pulsed ultrasound
- Chronic phase
  - Gradually increase workload as pain and discomfort diminish
  - Continue intermittent taping or splinting to reduce repeated motions that may exacerbate symptoms
  - Addressing pain
    - Ice
    - High-voltage pulsed stimulation
    - Ultrasound
  - Addressing swelling
    - Ice
    - Massage
  - Addressing weakness, joint instability
    - As symptoms improve, gradually resume activities
    - Establish full, pain-free finger ROM
    - Incorporate stretching and progressive strengthening exercises as warranted to restore full mobility and strength

FUNCTIONAL GOALS

- Patient will be able to
  - Use all kitchen and dining utensils without pain, or restricted mobility.
  - Lift half gallon of milk with both hands.
  - Reach for kitchen and household items without pain or catching.
  - Use garden tools, pain free.

PROGNOSIS

- Symptoms reduction can be slower if associated with connective tissue disorders, rheumatoid arthritis, or in the presence of patient inability to control exacerbating activities.

PATIENT RESOURCE

- Arthritis: Rheumatoid Arthritis. American Society for Surgery of the Hand. http://www.assh.org/Public/HandConditions/Pages/ArthritisRheumatoidArthritis.aspx. Accessed July 7, 2013.

REFERENCES

1. ICD9Data.com. http://www.icd9data.com. Accessed July 7, 2013.
2. ICD10Data.com. http://www.icd10data.com. Accessed July 7, 2013.
3. Pattern 4D: impaired joint mobility, motor function, muscle performance, and range of motion associated with connective tissue dysfunction. In: *Guide to Physical Therapist Practice*. 2nd ed. Alexandria, VA: American Physical Therapy Association; 2001. Revised 2003.
4. Nalebuff EA. The rheumatoid swan-neck deformity. *Hand Clin.* 1989;5(2):203–214.

ADDITIONAL REFERENCES

- de Bruin M, van Vliet DC, Smeulders MJ, Kreulen M. Long-term results of lateral band translocation for the correction of swan neck deformity in cerebral palsy. *J Pediatr Orthop.* 2010;30(1):67–70. doi: 10.1097/BPO.0b013e3181c6c363.

- Dutton M. The forearm, wrist, and hand. In: Dutton M, ed. *Dutton's Orthopedic Survival Guide: Managing Common Conditions*. New York, NY: McGraw-Hill; 2011:Chapter 7. http://www.accessphysiotherapy.com/content/8653078. Accessed July 7, 2013.
- Dutton M. The forearm, wrist, and hand. In: Dutton M, ed. *Orthopaedic Examination, Evaluation, and Intervention*. 2nd ed. New York, NY: McGraw-Hill; 2008.
- Ercocen AR, Yenidunya MO, Yilmaz S, Ozbek MR. Dynamic swan neck defomity in a patient with ehlers-danlos syndrome. *J Hand Surg Eur*. 1997;22(1):128–130. doi: 10.1016/S0266-7681(97)80039-3.
- Garnham A, Ashe M, Gropper P. Wrist, hand, and finger injuries. In: *Clinical Sports Medicine*. 3rd ed. Australia: McGraw-Hill; 2009:308–339.
- Nalebuff EA, Feldon PG, Millender LH. Rheumatoid arthritis in the hand and wrist. In: Green DP, ed. *Green's Operative Hand Surgery*. 2nd ed. New York, NY: Churchill Livingstone; 1988.
- Prentice WE. The forearm, wrist, hand, and fingers. In: Prentice WE, ed. *Principles of Athletic Training: A Competency-Based Approach*. New York, NY: McGraw-Hill; 2011: 702–732.
- Prentice WE, Quillen WS, Underwood F, eds. *Therapeutic Modalities in Rehabilitation*. 4th ed. New York, NY: McGraw-Hill; 2011. http://www.accessphysiotherapy.com/content/8136922. Accessed July 7, 2013.
- Sirotakova M, Figus A, Jarrett P, Mishra A, Elliot D. Correction of swan neck deformity in rheumatoid arthritis using a new lateral extensor band technique. *J Hand Surg Eur Vol*. 2008;33(6):712–716. doi: 10.1177/1753193408092787.

178 TRIGGER FINGER

Patrick S. Pabian, DPT, PT, SCS, OCS, CSCS

CONDITION/DISORDER SYNONYMS

- Flexor tenosynovitis
- Locked finger
- Stenosing tenosynovitis
- Trigger digit
- Trigger thumb

ICD-9-CM CODE[1]

- 727.03 Trigger finger (acquired)

ICD-10-CM CODE[2]

- M65.30 Trigger finger, unspecified finger

PREFERRED PRACTICE PATTERN[3]

- 4D: Impaired Joint Mobility, Motor Function, Muscle Performance, and Range of Motion Associated with Connective Tissue Dysfunction

PATIENT PRESENTATION

A 45-year-old female receptionist presents with pain over the volar aspect of her second metacarpophalangeal (MCP) joint that has been present for the past 5 months. She reports the pain is worsening and now noting "catching" or feeling that her finger "gets stuck" when bending and straightening. The patient has a palpable nodule over the volar aspect of the first MCP, which is painful to palpation and has crepitus during finger flexion. She notes that she is having difficulty grasping dishes or utensils when eating or cooking due to pain and weakness. She has also recently been in consultation with a rheumatologist for other medical concerns unrelated to this specified hand pain.

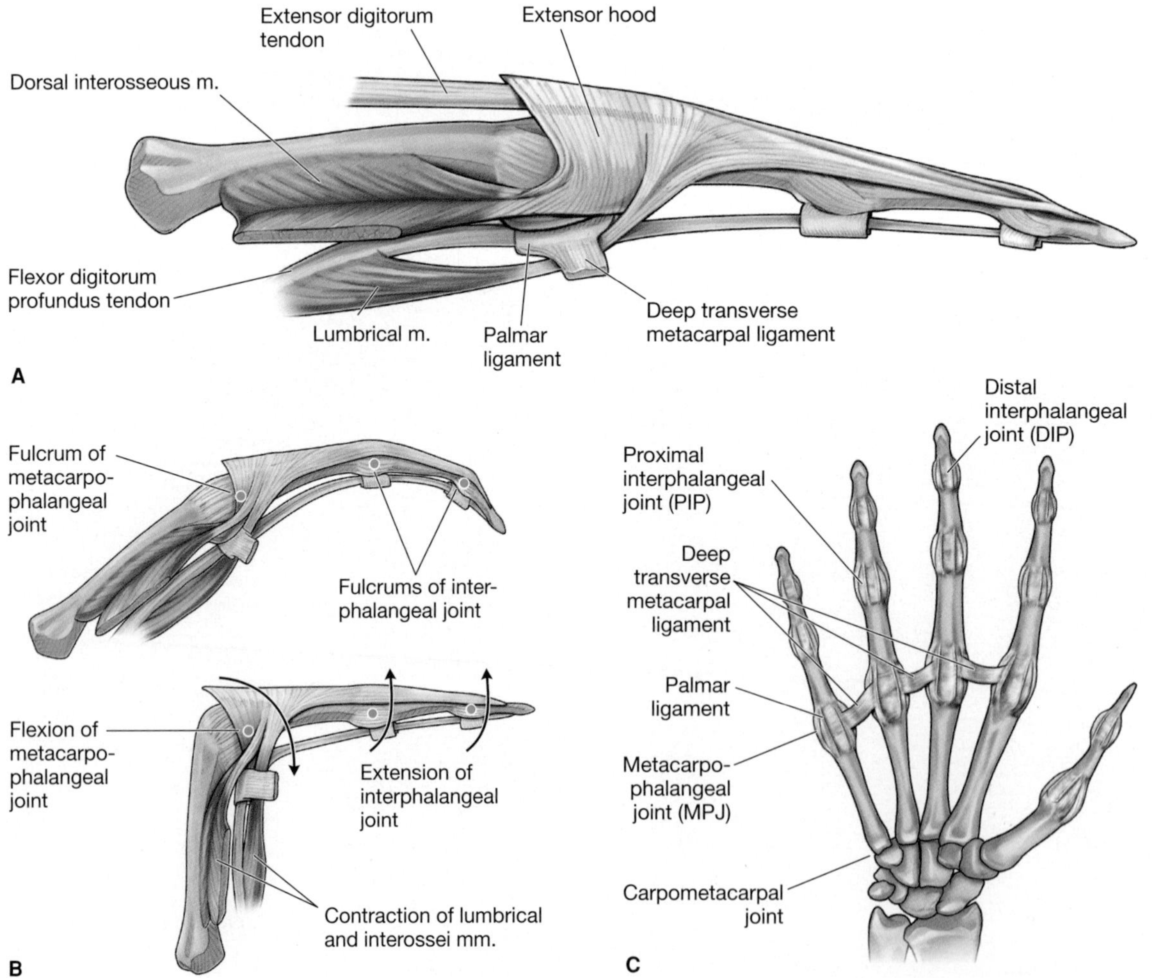

FIGURE 178-1 (**A**) Extensor expansion. (**B**) Movements of the lumbrical and interossei muscles. (**C**) Ligaments and joints of the hand. (From Morton DA, Foreman KB, Albertine KH. *The Big Picture: Gross Anatomy*. www.accessmedicine.com. Copyright © The McGraw-Hill Companies, Inc. All rights reserved.)

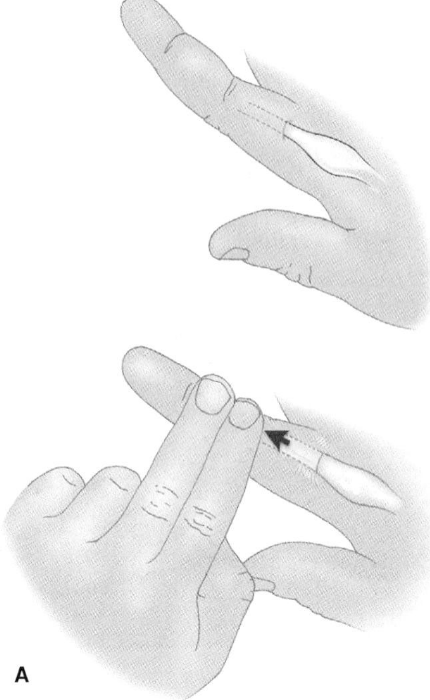

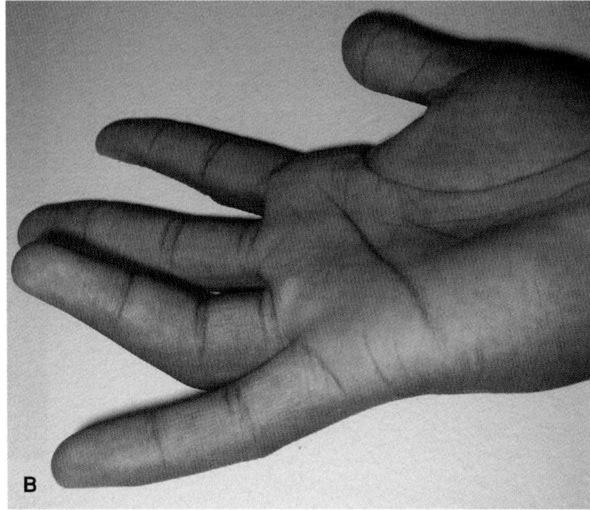

FIGURE 178-2 (**A**) Trigger finger occurs when a fibrous thickening of the tendon does not allow it to slide through the pulley. (**B**) Clinical photo of a finger locked in place due to trigger finger. (From Simon RR, Sherman SC. *Emergency Orthopedics*. 6th ed. www.accessemergencymedicine.com. Copyright © The McGraw-Hill Companies, Inc. All rights reserved.)

KEY FEATURES

Description

- Painful snapping or catching/locking of finger or thumb
- Inflammation of the fluid-filled sheath (tenosynovitis) surrounding the flexor tendons of the phalanges
- Painful nodule at the distal flexion crease
- Inflammation causes interference with gliding of tendon at the location of the A1 pulleys

Essentials of Diagnosis

- Thickening of sheath or tendon leads to constriction of the sliding tendon, and nodules can develop
- Crepitus and nodules may be palpable at location of A1 pulley
- Cause is typically nonspecific overuse
- Pain with digit motion precedes triggering or locking sensations

General Considerations

- Pain may precede symptoms of triggering.
- Mechanical symptoms exacerbate condition, leading to increased pain and decreased motion of the digit.
- Can be managed surgically or nonsurgically depending upon signs and symptom severity, response to conservative treatment, and orthopedic physician recommendations.

Demographics

- Unknown etiology, idiopathic
- Middle-aged women
- Increased incidence with diabetic population, young children, and menopausal women
- Associated in population with rheumatic disease/changes in the hand

CLINICAL FINDINGS

SIGNS AND SYMPTOMS

- Pain in palmar MCP joint region with digit motion, especially flexion
- Nodule along the A1 pulley
- Crepitus
- Palpable tenderness and possible swelling over palmar MCP joint
- Palpable crepitus over the palmar MCP joint
- Catching, locking, triggering with flexion of the digit

Functional Implications

- Difficulty and/or pain with opening and closing hand in preparation for grasping or reaching
- Difficulty and/or pain with grasping dishes, utensils, or drinking cups due to pain and weakness
- Difficulty and/or pain with grasping and turning steering wheel
- Difficulty and/or pain with turning doorknob

Possible Contributing Causes

- Rheumatoid arthritis, or other rheumatic or connective tissue disorders
- Diabetes mellitus
- Infection: *Mycobacterium kansasii*
- Carpal tunnel syndrome
- Psoriatic arthritis
- Gout
- Sarcoidosis
- Tuberculosis
- De Quervain's stenosing tenosynovitis
- Overuse activity of the hand and fingers

Differential Diagnosis

- Rheumatoid arthritis
- Ganglion of tendon sheath
- Dupuytren disease
- Loose body in the MCP joint
- Subluxation of the extensor digitorum communis
- Diabetes mellitus

MEANS OF CONFIRMATION OR DIAGNOSIS

Imaging

- No indication

Diagnostic Procedures

- Start with a full fist, and then ask patient to open the hand and extend the fingers

FINDINGS AND INTERPRETATION

- Radiographs can be taken to rule out fracture

TREATMENT

Medication

- NSAIDs
- Corticosteroid injection into flexor sheath

MEDICAL PROCEDURE

- Surgical release possible after failed conservative care

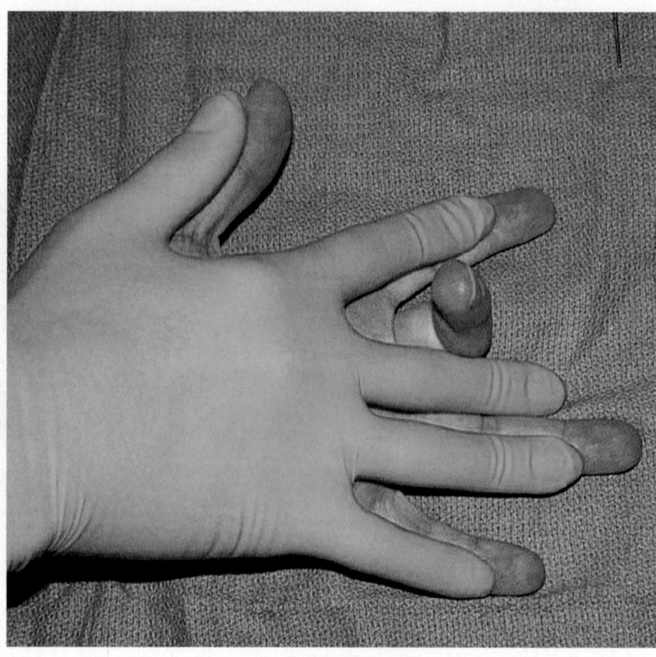

FIGURE 178-3 The examiner holds the untested fingers in full extension, preventing contracture of the flexor digitorum profundus. In this position, the patient is asked to flex the finger, and only the flexor digitorum superficialis will be able to fire. (From Brunicardi FC, Andersen DK, Billiar TR, et al. *Schwartz's Principles of Surgery*. 9th ed. www.accessmedicine.com. Copyright © The McGraw-Hill Companies, Inc. All rights reserved.)

REFERRALS/ADMITTANCE

- To radiologist for imaging, X-ray to rule out other pathology
- To primary care to rule out rheumatic causes or other connective tissue disorders
- To orthopedist for corticosteroid injections or surgical consult

IMPAIRMENTS

- Decreased strength and pain for grasping activities such as dressing and eating
- Pain, and locking or catching with opening hand to reach for objects
- Decreased ability to open or close hand due to joint stiffness

TESTS AND MEASURES

- Thenar muscle strength test (lateral pinch dynamometry)
- Manipulative ability test (nine-hole peg test)

INTERVENTION

- Objective of treatment is to reduce inflammation in the flexor tendon sheath and restore mobility of the tendon under the A1 pulley at the MCP joint
- Acute phase
  - PRICE: Protection, rest, ice compression, elevation
  - Immobilization/splint
  - Buddy taping to reduce exacerbating activities
  - Ice massage
  - Pulsed ultrasound
- Chronic phase
  - Gradually increase workload as pain and discomfort diminish
  - Continue intermittent taping or splinting to reduce repeated motions that may exacerbate symptoms
  - Addressing pain
    - Ice
    - High-voltage pulsed stimulation
    - Iontophoresis
    - Ultrasound
    - Extracorporeal shockwave therapy
  - Addressing swelling
    - Ice
    - Massage
  - Addressing weakness, joint instability
    - As symptoms improve, gradually resume activities
    - Establish full, pain-free finger ROM
    - Incorporate stretching and progressive strengthening exercises as warranted to restore full mobility and strength

FUNCTIONAL GOALS

- Patient will be able to

Use all kitchen and dining utensils without catching symptoms, pain, or restricted mobility.

- Lift a gallon milk carton from refrigerator at shoulder level, without pain.
- Reach for kitchen and household items without pain or catching.
- Garden tools, without pain.

PROGNOSIS

- Good.
- Symptoms reduction can be slower if associated with connective tissue disorders, rheumatoid arthritis, or in the presence of patient inability to control exacerbating activities.

ADDITIONAL INFORMATION

- For more information, please review the Iontophoresis Case Study 6-2 on AccessPhysiotherapy.com.

PATIENT RESOURCE

- Trigger Finger. American Society for Surgery of the Hand. http://www.assh.org/Public/HandConditions/Pages/TriggerFinger.aspx. Accessed July 7, 2013.

REFERENCES

1. ICD9Data.com. http://www.icd9data.com. Accessed July 7, 2013.
2. ICD10Data.com. http://www.icd10data.com. Accessed July 7, 2013.
3. Pattern 4D: Impaired joint mobility, motor function, muscle performance, and range of motion associated with connective tissue dysfunction. In: *Guide to Physical Therapist Practice*. 2nd ed. Alexandria, VA: American Physical Therapy Association; 2001. Revised 2003.

ADDITIONAL REFERENCES

- Dutton M. The forearm, wrist, and hand. In: Dutton M, ed. *Dutton's Orthopedic Survival Guide: Managing Common Conditions*. New York, NY: McGraw-Hill; 2011:Chapter 7. http://www.accessphysiotherapy.com/content/8653078. Accessed July 7, 2013.
- Dutton, M. The forearm, wrist, and hand. In: Dutton M, ed. *Dutton's Orthopaedic Examination, Evaluation, and Intervention*. 3rd ed. New York, NY: McGraw-Hill; 2012.
- Finsen V, Hagen S. Surgery for trigger finger. *Hand Surg.* 2003; 8(2):201–203.
- Garnham A, Ashe M, Gropper P. Wrist, hand, and finger injuries. In: *Clinical Sports Medicine*. 3rd ed. Australia: McGraw-Hill; 2009:308–339.
- Hwang M, Kang YK, Shin JY, Kim DH. Referred pain pattern of the abductor pollicis longus muscle. *Am J Phys Med Rehabil.* 2005;84(8):593–597.
- Prentice, WE. The forearm, wrist, hand, and fingers. In: Prentice WE, ed. *Principles of Athletic Training: A Competency-Based Approach*. New York, NY: McGraw-Hill; 2011:702–732.
- Prentice WE, Quillen WS, Underwood F, eds. *Therapeutic Modalities in Rehabilitation*. 4th ed. New York, NY: McGraw-Hill; 2011. http://www.accessphysiotherapy.com/content/8136922. Accessed July 7, 2013.
- Zingas C, Failla JM, Van Holsbeeck M. Injection accuracy and clinical relief of de Quervain's tendinitis. *J Hand Surg Am.* 1998;23(1):89–96.

SECTION G HIP DISORDERS

179 AVASCULAR NECROSIS, FEMORAL HEAD (AVN)

Stephanie Boren Baker, MS, PT, CSCS
Eric Shamus, PhD, DPT, PT, CSCS

CONDITION/DISORDER SYNONYMS

- Bone infarction
- Ischemic bone necrosis
- Osteonecrosis

ICD-9-CM CODES

- 733.4 Aseptic necrosis of bone
- 733.42 Aseptic necrosis of femoral head and neck

ICD-10-CM CODES

- M87 Osteonecrosis
- M87.1 Osteonecrosis due to drugs
- M87.2 Osteonecrosis due to previous trauma
- M87.3 Other secondary osteonecrosis
- M87.8 Other osteonecrosis
- M87.9 Osteonecrosis, unspecified

PREFERRED PRACTICE PATTERNS

- 4H: Impaired Joint Mobility, Motor Function, Muscle Performance, and Range of Motion Associated with Joint Arthroplasty[1]
- 4I: Impaired Joint Mobility, Motor Function, Muscle Performance, and Range of Motion Associated with Bony or Soft Tissue Surgery[2]

PATIENT PRESENTATION

Patient is a 48-year-old male who was hit by a car while riding his bicycle. Patient has a fractured pelvis and subluxed hip. After 6 weeks, patient began walking increased distances and was starting to feel better. Six months later, his hip began to become painful and stiff. Patient noticed an increase limp and difficulty putting weight onto his leg. Physician ordered an X-ray, which showed avascular necrosis (AVN) changes in the hip bone.

KEY FEATURES

Description

- AVN results from disrupted or lost blood flow to a joint or bone, resulting in damage to or death of bone tissue

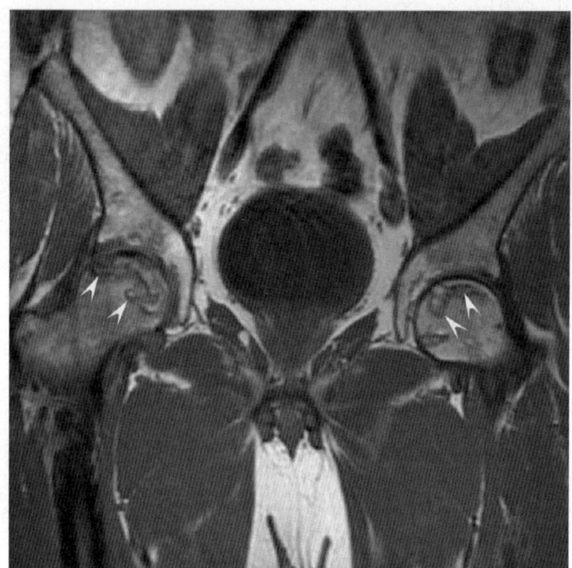

FIGURE 179-1 Coronal T1-weighted MR image of the pelvis in a patient with bilateral hip avascular necrosis. Note the serpiginous low signal abnormality in the subchondral regions of the femoral heads (*arrowheads*). (From Chen MYM, Pope TL, Ott DJ. *Basic Radiology*. 2nd ed. http://www.accessmedicine.com. Copyright © The McGraw-Hill Companies, Inc. All rights reserved.)

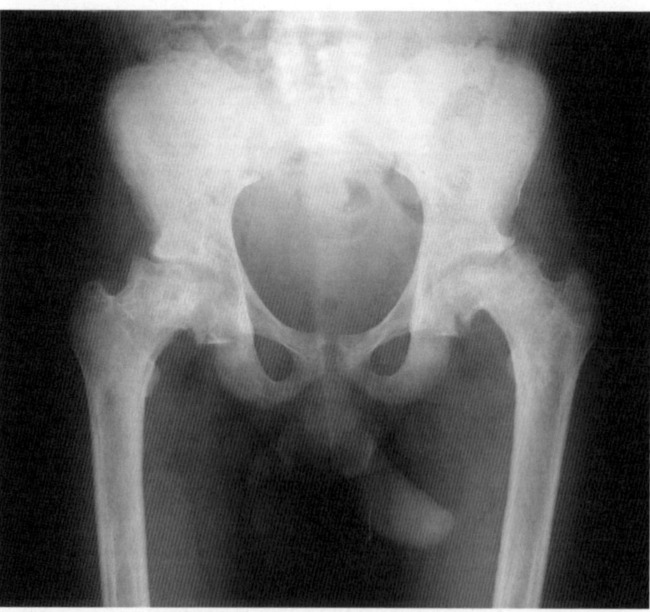

FIGURE 179-2 Avascular necrosis, bilateral hips (Stage 4). (Reproduced with permission from Simon RR, Sherman SC, Koenigsknecht SJ. *Emergency Orthopedics, The Extremities*. 5th ed. © 2007, McGraw-Hill Inc., New York, NY.)

- Femoral head is the most vulnerable site for development of AVN
  - Anterolateral aspect is particularly vulnerable as it is the principal weight-bearing region and site of greatest mechanical stress

Essentials of Diagnosis

- Known causes can be traumatic or atraumatic, including:
  - Corticosteroid use
  - Alcohol abuse
  - Intravascular coagulation from marrow fat enlargement, vessel wall injury, or thromboembolic event
- Early imaging with MRI is imperative as success of conservative treatment correlates with earlier stages

General Considerations

- AVN of the hip in children is known as Legg–Calvé–Perthes syndrome
- Can be idiopathic
- Clinical AVN affects the ends of long bones
- May result from local edema (compartment syndrome), occlusive vessel disease, fat embolism, or hypertrophy of fat cells, which block blood supplies and result in necrosis/death of marrow cells and osteocytes
- In femoral head AVN, weakened and necrotic bony trabeculae fail under compressive loading, resulting in subchondral and articular collapse

Demographics

- Estimated 15,000 to 20,000 new cases of femoral head AVN each year in the United States
- Accounts for 20% of joint replacements in the United States annually
- Most common in young males; male–female ratio 8:1
- Typical age of onset between 30 and 50 years
- Can occur in children (Legg–Calvé–Perthes syndrome)

CLINICAL FINDINGS

SIGNS AND SYMPTOMS

- Patients are asymptomatic early in disease process; diagnosis may result from incidental findings on imaging test
- Characterized by pain, stiffness in hip region, low back pain, or radiating pain to knee
- Antalgic gait
- Pain in groin
- Throbbing deep hip pain
- Rate of progression is variable
- Restricted hip internal rotation, flexion, abduction

Functional Implications

- Patients must avoid impact activities to preserve joint integrity
- Limited mobility
- Limited/restricted household and work-related activity
- Decreased overall activity and participation
- Loss of normal joint ROM results in compensatory movement patterns with potential for injury in other regions
- Restricted weight bearing may be prescribed during periods of symptom exacerbation
- Joint replacement often necessary, carries postsurgical ROM and weight-bearing restrictions

TABLE 179-1 Conditions Associated with Avascular Necrosis of the Femoral Head

Traumatic
Femoral neck fracture
Hip dislocation
Occult or minor trauma
Nontraumatic
Sickle cell disease
Collagen vascular diseases
Alcohol abuse
Renal transplant
Systemic lupus erythematosus
Dysbarism
Chronic pancreatitis
Exogenous steroid administration
Cushing disease
Caisson disease
Gaucher disease
Renal osteodystrophy
Idiopathic

Source: Tintinalli JE, Stapczynski JS, John Ma O, et al. *Tintinalli's Emergency Medicine: A Comprehensive Study Guide.* 7th ed. www.accessmedicine.com.

Possible Contributing Causes

- Strong association of nontraumatic AVN with corticosteroid use and alcoholism
  - Both believed to affect breakdown of fatty substances and disrupt blood flow
- Trauma
- Intravascular coagulation from marrow fat enlargement
- Vessel wall injury
- Thromboembolic event
- Cushing syndrome
- Gaucher disease
- Systemic lupus
- Pancreatitis
- Chemotherapy
- Radiation treatment
- Decompression diseases
- Blood disorders
- Steroid use
- Sickle cell anemia

Differential Diagnosis

- Ankylosing spondylitis
- Arthritis or advanced degenerative joint disease
- Bursitis
- Fibromyalgia syndrome
- Gout
- Hip fracture (femoral neck)
- Lumbar disk herniation
- Malignancy
- Osteomyeltis
- Rheumatoid arthritis
- Sacral dysfunction
- Septic arthritis
- Spondyloarthropathy

- Transient osteoporosis of the hip
- Visceral pathology

MEANS OF CONFIRMATION OR DIAGNOSIS

Imaging

- Contributes to accurate staging: Size and location of necrotic segment, absence/presence of collapse, degree of femoral head depression, evidence of acetabular involvement with signs of secondary osteoarthritis
- Hip CT[3]
- Plain-film radiography has high specificity for advanced AVN, low sensitivity in earlier stages
  - Progressively there is sclerosis surrounding an area of osteopenia, central radiolucency with sclerotic border, subchondral lucency (crescent sign), and flattening or collapse of femoral head with or without joint-space narrowing
- MRI preferred, imperative for early diagnosis
  - Signs include low subchondral intensity, margin of low signal, double-line sign, and joint fluid

FINDINGS AND INTERPRETATION

- Stage 1: X-ray normal, MRI abnormal[3]
- Stage 2: X-ray and MRI abnormal, no subchondral lucency, femoral head still spherical[3]
- Stage 3: X-ray and MRI abnormal, radioluscent crescent sign visible, femoral head still spherical[3]
- Stage 4: X-ray and MRI abnormal, flattening of femoral head; preventative surgery no longer a consideration, total joint replacement only surgical option[3]
- Stage 5: X-ray features may include osteophytes and decreased joint space
- Stage 6: Extensive joint destruction, total hip replacement if possible

TREATMENT

Medication

- Statin therapy with corticosteroids may reduce risk of developing AVN
- Biphosphonates (Fosamax) may delay femoral head collapse, especially in earlier stages, but more long-term studies are needed
- NSAIDs for pain management

MEDICAL PROCEDURES

- Core decompression
  - Involves removing a core of necrotic bone and replacing with bone graft to relieve pressure in femoral head and promote revascularization
- Bone marrow aspirate concentrate (BMAC)
  - Bone marrow stem cells from ASIS injected into necrotic bone to stimulate new bone growth
- Total joint replacement is the only surgical option in stages 4 and greater

REFERRALS/ADMITTANCE

- To physical and rehabilitation medicine specialist
- To physician for orthopedic or surgical consult, pharmaceutical management, surgical intervention
- To dietician/nutritionist for consult
- To support groups for assistance with long-term physical and psychological impact

IMPAIRMENTS

- Mobility
- Pain-limited functional activities
- Loss of joint ROM
- Abnormal gait, restricted weight bearing, use of assistive device
- Self-care limitation
- Restricted role at home, work, school, community
- Recreation, leisure, sports limitations

TEST AND MEASURES

- Hip joint integrity
  - Hip scour
  - Flexion, abduction, and external rotation (FABER) test
  - Flexion, adduction, and internal rotation (FAIR) test
- Limb strength
  - Functional strength testing
    - Five-times-sit-to-stand test
  - Manual muscle test (MMT)
    - Hamstrings
    - Quadriceps
    - Iliopsoas
    - Gluteus maximus
    - Gluteus medius
    - Gluteus minimus
    - Adductors
- LE contralateral limb strength
- Balance
  - Static single-leg standing (eyes open, eyes closed)
    - Contralateral LE
  - Dynamic standing
    - Berg Balance Scale
    - Functional Gait Assessment
- Gait assessment
  - Observational analysis
  - Gait speed via the 10-m walk test
  - 2-minute walk test
  - 6-minute walk test

INTERVENTION

- Physical therapy indicated in most stages to preserve functional mobility and for postsurgical rehabilitation
- Exercises (resistance, endurance, flexibility)
  - Aquatic exercises
- ADL training
- Assistive or adaptive devices
- Heat therapy
- Weight management
- Rest
- Orthoses, splints
- Walking aids
- Ice[4]
- Diet modification
- Acupuncture
- Pain management

- Energy conservation techniques
- Joint protection
- Footwear
- Psychosocial support
- Ultrasound[5]
- Electric stimulation[6]
- Patient education

FUNCTIONAL GOALS

- Patient will have improved activity and participation at home, work, and in community.
- Patient will be able to
  - Walk 0.5 miles pain-free without assistive device.
  - Resume pain-free ADLs, sweeping, mopping.
  - Maintain activity modification to preserve joint integrity.
  - Maintain joint ROM and muscle strength during disease progression.
  - Use assistive device(s) during periods of restricted weight bearing.
- Patient will have restored joint ROM/proprioception, increased muscle strength, and normal gait pattern postsurgery.

Note: Goals in Stage-3 cases are to minimize pain, preserve functional mobility, delay total joint replacement.

PROGNOSIS

- Success of conservative surgical intervention corresponds to stage of disease progression.
- Beyond Stage 3, 70% of patients will have femoral collapse within 3 years of diagnosis, and conservative surgical intervention is not effective.
  - Goals include pain minimization, preserved functional mobility, and delay need for total joint replacement.
- Elimination of pain and return to normal activity is possible with successful postsurgical rehab course and adherence to hip-joint replacement precautions.

PATIENT RESOURCE

- Minimally Invasive Total Hip Replacement. http://orthoinfo.aaos.org/topic.cfm?topic=A00404. Accessed January 20, 2013.

REFERENCES

1. The American Physical Therapy Association. Pattern 4H: Impaired joint mobility, motor function, muscle performance, and range of motion associated with joint arthroplasty. *Interactive Guide to Physical Therapist Practice*. 2003. doi: 10.2522/ptguide.3.1_8. http://guidetoptpractice.apta.org/content/1/SEC15.extract?sid=1863f521-e876-4b8e-bcb4-4ad56c0ed422. Accessed May 27, 2014.
2. The American Physical Therapy Association. Pattern 4I: Impaired joint mobility, motor function, muscle performance, and range of motion associated with bony or soft tissue surgery. *Interactive Guide to Physical Therapist Practice*. 2003. doi: 10.2522/ptguide.3.1_9. http://guidetoptpractice.apta.org/content/1/SEC16.extract?sid=096651b3-d918-4599-9b2b-3d4adeb20595. Accessed May 27, 2014.
3. Simon RR, Sherman SC. *Emergency Orthopedics: The Extremities*. 6th ed. New York, NY: McGraw-Hill; 2011. http://www.accessphysiotherapy.com/resource/665. Accessed January 20, 2013.
4. Prentice WE. Cryotherapy and thermotherapy. In: Prentice WE, Quillen WS, Underwood F, eds. *Therapeutic Modalities in Rehabilitation*. 4th ed. New York, NY: McGraw-Hill; 2011:Chapter 9. http://www.accessphysiotherapy.com/content/8137995#8137995. Accessed January 20, 2013.
5. Draper DO, Prentice WE. Therapeutic ultrasound. In: Prentice WE, Quillen WS, Underwood F, eds. *Therapeutic Modalities in Rehabilitation*. 4th ed. New York, NY: McGraw-Hill; 2011: Chapter 10. http://www.accessphysiotherapy.com/abstract/8138751. Accessed January 20, 2013.
6. Dutton M. *McGraw Hill's NPTE (National Physical Therapy Examination)*. 2nd ed. New York, NY: McGraw-Hill; 2012. http://www.accessphysiotherapy.com/resource/611. Accessed January 20, 2013.

ADDITIONAL REFERENCES

- Abramowitz AJ, Healy WL, Pfeifer BA, Richard I. Clinical outcome and survivorship analysis of core decompression for early osteonecrosis of the femoral head. Department of Orthopaedic Surgery, Lahey Hitchcock Medical Center, Burlington, Massachusetts USA; 18 June 2004.
- Agarwala S, Jain D, Joshi VR, Sule A. Efficacy of alendronate, a bisphosphonate, in the treatment of AVN of the hip. A prospective open-label study. *Rheumatology (Oxford)*. 2005;44(3):352–359.
- Agarwala S, Shah S, Joshi VR. The use of alendronate in the treatment of avascular necrosis of the femoral head: follow up to eight years. *J Bone Joint Surg BR*. 2009;91(8):1013–1018.
- DiGiovanni CW, Patel A, Calfee R, Nickisch F. Osteonecrosis in the foot. *J AM Acad Orthop Surg*. 2007;15(4):208–217.
- Gross GW, Articolo GA, Bowen JR. Legg-Calve-Perthes Disease: Imaging Evaluation and Management. *Semin Musculoskelet Radiol*. 1999;3(4):379–391.
- Malizos KN, Karantanas AH, Varitimidis SE, Dailiana ZH, Bargiotas K, Maris T. Osteonecrosis of the Femoral Head: Etiology, Imaging, and Treatment. *Eur J Radiol*. 2007;63(1):16–28.
- ICD9DATA. http://www.icd9data.com. Accessed January 20, 2013.
- ICD10DATA. http://www.icd10data.com. Accessed January 20, 2013.
- Pritchett JW. Statin therapy decreases the risk of osteonecrosis in patients receiving steroids. *Clin Orthop Relat Res*. 2001;386: 173–178.
- Osteoarthritis Research Society International. OARSI Primer; 2010. Last updated 2011. http://primer.oarsi.org. Accessed January 20, 2013.

180 GREATER TROCHANTERIC BURSITIS

Jason C. Craddock, EdD, ATC, CSCS
Eric Shamus, PhD, DPT, PT, CSCS

CONDITION/DISORDER SYNONYMS

- Hip greater trochanteric bursitis
- Greater trochanteric pain syndrome (GTPS)
- Hip abductor pain syndrome

ICD-9-CM CODE

- 726.5 Enthesopathy of the hip region

ICD-10-CM CODE

- M70.6 Trochanteric bursitis

PREFERRED PRACTICE PATTERN

- 4E: Impaired Joint Mobility, Motor Function, Muscle Performance, and Range of Motion Associated with Localized Inflammation[1]

PATIENT PRESENTATION

A 15-year-old female soccer player complains of left hip pain. After taking a thorough history, it is noted that formal team conditioning practice started 2 weeks ago and she has been running on the road in the evenings after practice in efforts to get into "shape." The athlete complains of pain at the beginning of practice that somewhat dissipates during practice but then returns with greater intensity after practice is over. She also mentioned that there is increased pain when she puts more weight on the left leg.

KEY FEATURES

Description

- Pain over the greater trochanter, lateral thigh pain[2]
- Differs from hip pointer (iliac crest contusion) based on location of injury/trauma
- Pain on transition between standing and lying down
- Direct trauma
  - Fall onto lateral hip
  - Direct blow
- Idiopathic[2]

Essentials of Diagnosis

- Diagnostic ultrasound can detect bursitis verse gluteal tendinosis, gluteal tears and thickening of the ITB tendon
- Friction between iliotibial band (ITB), bursa, and trochanter
  - Pressure from greater trochanter and overlying muscles compress bursa into the trochanter, creating pain and discomfort

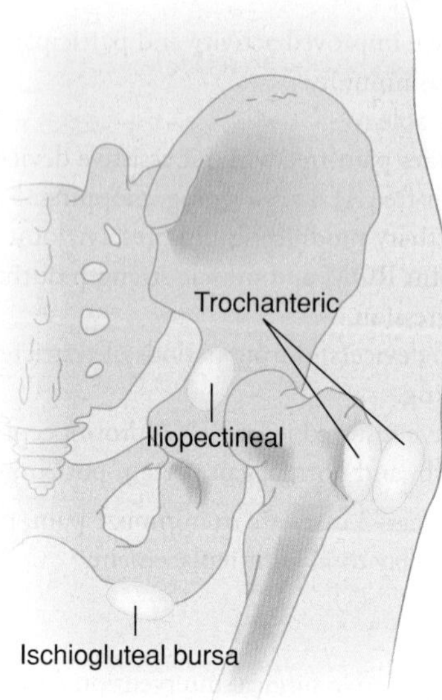

FIGURE 180-1 The bursae of the hip. (Reproduced with permission from Simon RR, Sherman SC, Koenigsknecht SJ. *Emergency Orthopedics, The Extremities*. 5th ed. © 2007, McGraw-Hill Inc., New York.)

  - Bursa is next to femur, between insertion of the gluteus medius and gluteus minimus
    - Functions as a shock absorber

General Considerations

- Concern regarding possible slipped growth plate in younger children

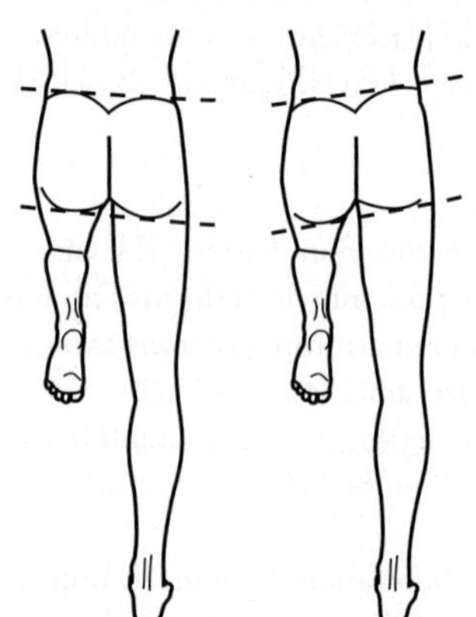
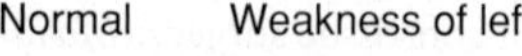

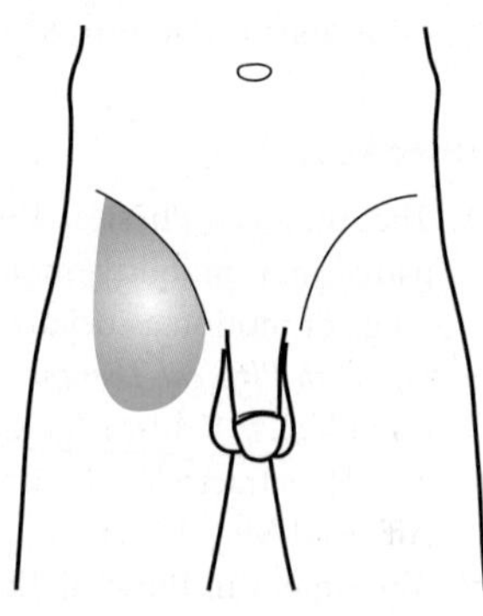

FIGURE 180-2 Lesions of the Hip and Groin. (**A**) Trendelenburg sign. When the patient stands on one foot, the buttock falls. (**B**) Subinguinal painless swelling. Swelling below the inguinal ligament may be either a psoas abscess or an effusion in the psoas bursa. (From LeBlond RF, DeGowin RL, Brown DD. *DeGowin's Diagnostic Examination*. 9th ed. http://www.accessmedicine.com. Copyright © The McGraw-Hill Companies, Inc. All rights reserved.)

- Stress fractures or blood-supply disruption to the hip may appear later

Demographics

- Common in runners

CLINICAL FINDINGS

SIGNS AND SYMPTOMS

- Audible or palpable snapping over lateral hip[3]
- Burning sensation
- Point tender with palpation
- Radicular pain into buttock, down leg into knee
- Limited motion adduction and internal rotation
- Pain with rising up and down from chair
- Swelling
- Redness
- Ecchymosis, if caused by direct trauma[3]
- During static weight bearing, patient may rotate femur to clear ITB from the greater trochanter
- Painful resisted hip external rotation
- Painful passive stretching of ITB, hip extension/flexion
- Weakness in hip abduction

Functional Implications

- Antalgic gait
- Painful end-ranges during ambulation
- Patient may increase weight bearing on the unaffected extremity
- Pain and weakness as ITB passes over greater trochanter
- Pain-limited functional activities (ADLs, physical and athletic activities)
- Difficulty sleeping on affected side

Possible Contributing Causes

- Trauma
- Poor lower-extremity mechanics (e.g., running mechanics, pronators)
- Tight hip adductors
- Hip musculature imbalance
- ITB tightness
- Weak hip abductors
- Sacral dysfunction
- OA of hip or lumbar spine
- Degenerative disk disease/low back pain
- Rheumatoid arthritis
- Leg-length discrepancy (true or perceived)
- Fibromyalgia
- Obesity
- Total hip arthroplasty
- Pes planus

Differential Diagnosis

- Abductor muscle strain
- Femoral head osteonecrosis
- Femoral-neck stress fracture
- Hip arthritis
- Hip avascular necrosis
- Inguinal and femoral hernia
- Ischial or iliopectineal bursitis
- ITB syndrome
- Lumbar degenerative disc disease
- Lumbar disk herniation
- Lumbar facet syndrome
- Lumbar spinal stenosis
- Lumbar spine compression fracture
- Metastatic tumor
- Osteoarthritis (OA)
- Sciatica

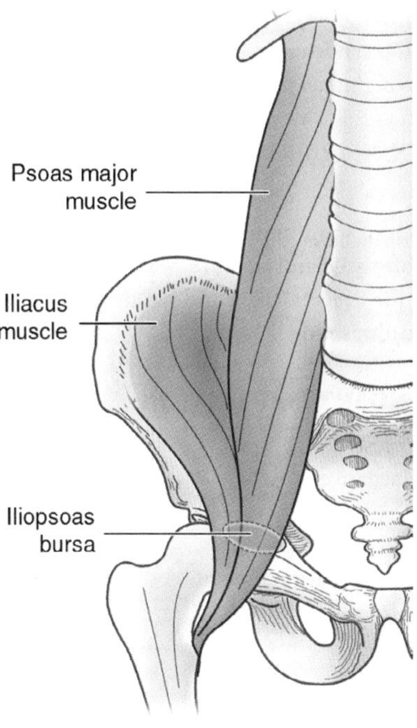

FIGURE 180-3 Internal snapping hip syndrome. Internal snapping hip syndrome occurs when the iliopsoas tendon snaps over the iliopectineal eminence of the pelvic brim as it proceeds to its insertion on the lesser tuberosity. (Reproduced with permission from Simon RR, Sherman SC. *Emergency Orthopedics, The Extremities*. 6th ed. © 2011, McGraw-Hill Inc., New York.)

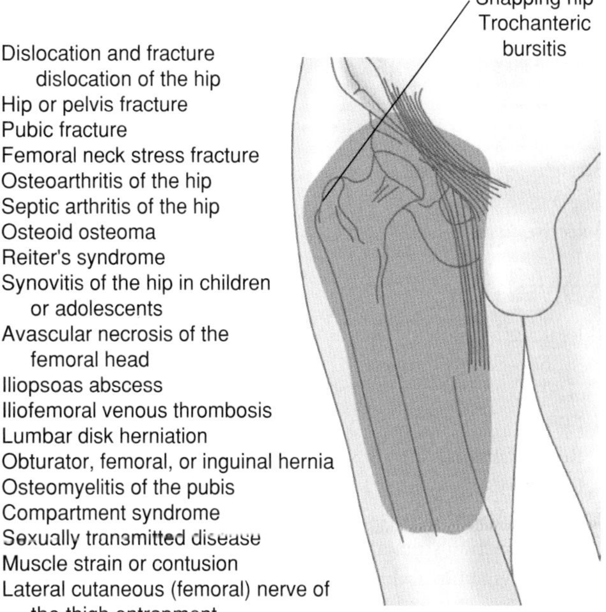

FIGURE 180-4 Potential causes of trochanteric, pubic, and anterior thigh pain. (From Dutton M. *Dutton's Orthopedic Survival Guide: Managing Common Conditions*. http://www.accessphysiotherapy.com. Copyright © The McGraw-Hill Companies, Inc. All rights reserved.)

- Septic arthritis
- Snapping hip syndrome
- Tendinitis of gluteus medius, gluteus maximus

MEANS OF CONFIRMATION

Imaging

- Radiographs of spine and hip
- MRI for soft tissue and fracture
- Bone scan for stress fracture and hip necrosis
- Diagnostic ultrasound[4]

FINDINGS AND INTERPRETATION

- Positive Ober test[2]
- Radiographs negative

TREATMENT

Medications

- Corticosteroid injection[5]
- NSAIDs
- Acetaminophen

REFERRALS/ADMITTANCE

- To hospital for imaging
- To physician for medication, anti-inflammatory, corticosteroid injection[5]
- To surgeon for surgical consult in advanced cases, arthroscopic bursectomy

IMPAIRMENTS

- Limited activity, especially with transition from hip flexion and extension (e.g., in and out of chair)
- Unable to sleep secondary to pain with lying on affected side
- Painful hip motion limiting ambulation or running
- Limitations in school, work, recreation, leisure, sports

TESTS AND MEASURES

- Ober test[2]
- FABER test[2]
- Straight leg raise test[2]
- Leg-length assessment
- Selective tissue tension tests

INTERVENTION

- If leg-length problem, heel-lift on unaffected side to shift
- Rest, non–weight-bearing
- Flexibility
  - ITB
  - Rectus femoris
  - Piriformis
- Strengthening
  - Hip abduction strengthening[4]
    - Side-lying hip abduction, progression to side-lying planks with hip abduction
    - Lateral lunges
- Manual therapy
  - If not acute condition or painful, cross-friction massage may loosen adhesions formed secondary to bursal inflammation

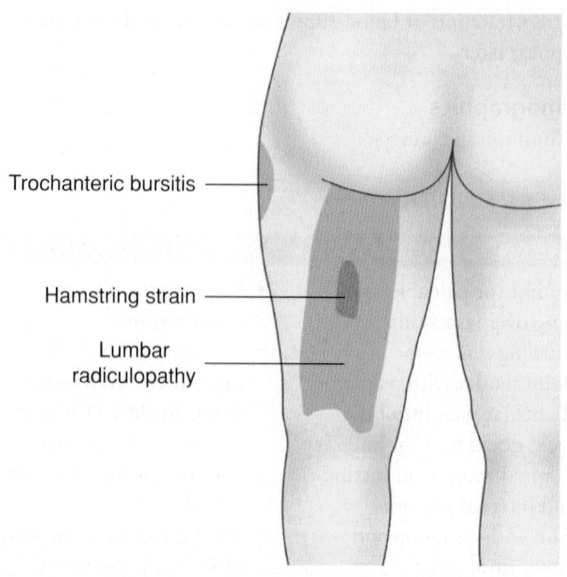

FIGURE 180-5 Potential causes of posterior thigh pain. (From Dutton M. *Dutton's Orthopedic Survival Guide: Managing Common Conditions.* http://www.accessphysiotherapy.com. Copyright © The McGraw-Hill Companies, Inc. All rights reserved.)

- Modalities
  - Swelling
    - Ice[6]
    - Electric stimulation[3]
  - Pain
    - Ice[6]
    - Electric stimulation[3]

FUNCTIONAL GOALS

- Patient will be able to
  - Rise up and down from chair without pain.
  - Sleep on ipsilateral side without pain.
  - Run without pain.
  - Get in and out of car with full hip ROM.

PROGNOSIS

- Condition usually responds well to conservative treatment.[2]
- Injection may be necessary if conservative treatment fails.

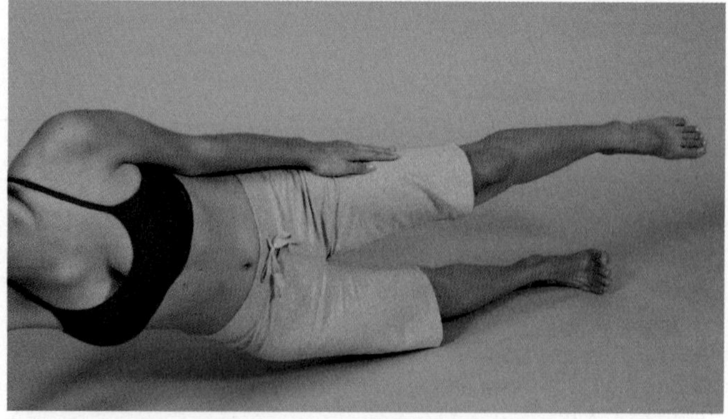

FIGURE 180-6 Side plank with hip abduction exercise. (From Dutton M. *Dutton's Orthopaedic Examination, Evaluation, and Intervention.* 3rd ed. http://www.accessphysiotherapy.com. Copyright © The McGraw-Hill Companies, Inc. All rights reserved.)

PATIENT RESOURCE

- Shbeeb MI, Matteson EL. Trochanteric Bursitis (greater trochanter pain syndrome). *Mayo Clinic Proceedings.* 1996;71(6):565–569. http://www.mayoclinicproceedings.org/article/S0025-6196(11)64113-X/fulltext

REFERENCES

1. The American Physical Therapy Association. Pattern 4E: Impaired joint mobility, motor function, muscle performance, and range of motion associated with localized inflammation. *Interactive Guide to Physical Therapist Practice.* 2003. doi: 10.2522/ptguide.3.1_5. http://guidetoptpractice.apta.org/content/1/SEC12.extract?sid=a3440a97-102f-4f1f-9273-34f60416f5ad. Accessed May 27, 2014.
2. Dutton M. *Dutton's Orthopedic Survival Guide: Managing Common Conditions.* New York, NY: McGraw-Hill; 2011. http://www.accessphysiotherapy.com/resource/685. Accessed March 8, 2013.
3. Dutton M. *McGraw Hill's NPTE (National Physical Therapy Examination).* 2nd ed. New York, NY: McGraw-Hill; 2012. http://www.accessphysiotherapy.com/resource/611. Accessed March 8, 2013.
4. Dutton M. *Orthopaedic Examination, Evaluation, and Intervention.* New York, NY: McGraw-Hill; 2008. http://www.accessphysiotherapy.com/resource/612. Accessed March 8, 2013.
5. Dionko E. Appendix B. Soft tissue injections, joint injections, and aspiration. In: Patel DR, Greydanus DE, Baker RJ, eds. *Pediatric Practice: Sports Medicine.* New York, NY: McGraw-Hill; 2009. http://www.accessphysiotherapy.com/abstract/6983351#6983400. Accessed March 8, 2013.
6. Prentice WE. Cryotherapy and Thermotherapy. In: Prentice WE, Quillen WS, Underwood F, eds. *Therapeutic Modalities in Rehabilitation.* 4th ed. New York, NY: McGraw-Hill; 2011:Chapter 9. http://www.accessphysiotherapy.com/content/8137995#8137995. Accessed March 8, 2013.

ADDITIONAL REFERENCES

- Long SS, Surrey DE, Nazarian LN. Sonography of greater trochanteric pain syndrome and the rarity of primary bursitis. *AJR Am J Roentgenol.* 2013;201(5);1083–1086.
- ICD9DATA. http://www.icd9data.com. Accessed May 27, 2014.
- ICD10DATA. http://www.icd10data.com. Accessed May 27, 2014.
- Segal NA, Felson DT, Torner JC, Zhu Y, et al. Greater trochanteric pain syndrome: epidemiology and associated factors. *Arch Phys Med Rehabil* 2007;88(8):988–992.

181 ILIAC CREST CONTUSION

Jason C. Craddock, EdD, ATC, CSCS
Eric Shamus, PhD, DPT, PT, CSCS

CONDITION/DISORDER SYNONYMS

- Hip pointer
- Subcutaneous contusion of the iliac crest

ICD-9-CM CODE

- 924.01 Contusion of hip

ICD-10-CM CODE

- S70.00XA Contusion of unspecified hip, initial encounter

PREFERRED PRACTICE PATTERN

- 4E: Impaired Joint Mobility, Motor Function, Muscle Performance, and Range of Motion Associated With Localized Inflammation

PATIENT PRESENTATION

Patient is a 17-year-old high school football player. He was tackled from the right side 1 week ago from a direct blow of the helmet onto the iliac crest. He said he had pain going down his right leg to the knee. He presents with a hematoma at the iliac crest and bruising from the iliac crest down the iliotibial band (ITB). He has a positive Ober test and weakness in hip abduction. He is ambulating with a wide gait pattern and does not like to lay on his right side.

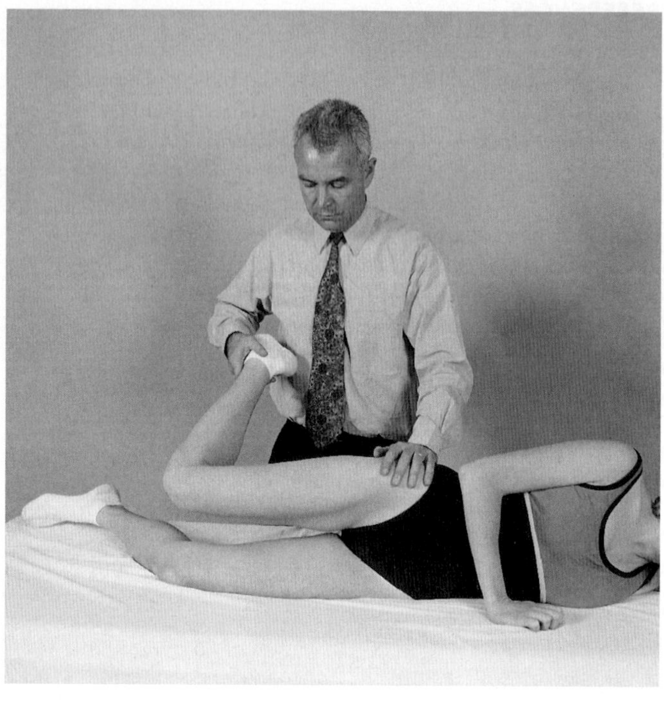

FIGURE 181-1 Ober test. (From Dutton M. *Dutton's Orthopedic Survival Guide: Managing Common Conditions*. http://www.accessphysiotherapy.com. Copyright © The McGraw-Hill Companies, Inc. All rights reserved.)

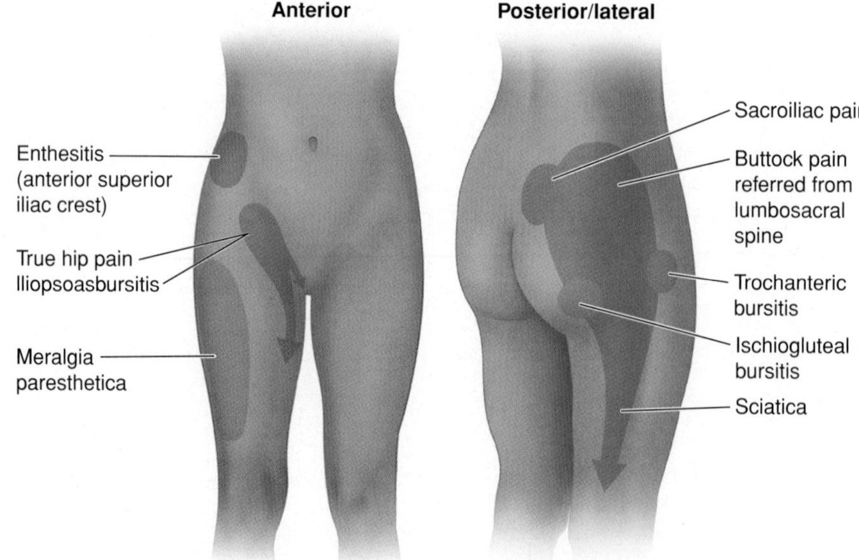

FIGURE 181-2 Origins of hip pain and dysesthesias. (From Cush JJ, Kavanaugh A, Stein CM. Evaluation of musculoskeletal complaints. In: JJ Cush, Kavanaugh A, Stein CM, eds. *Rheumatology: Diagnosis and Therapeutics*. 2nd ed. Philadelphia, PA: Lippincott Williams & Wilkins; 2005:pp. 3–20, with permission.)

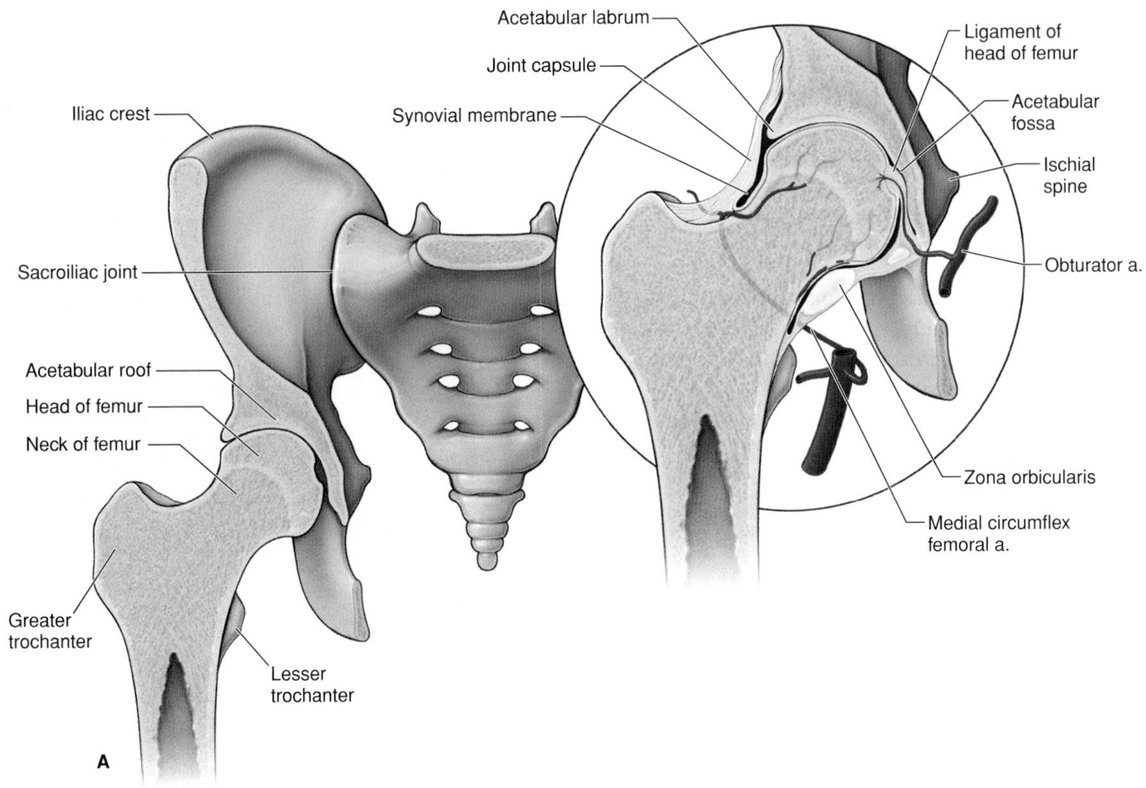

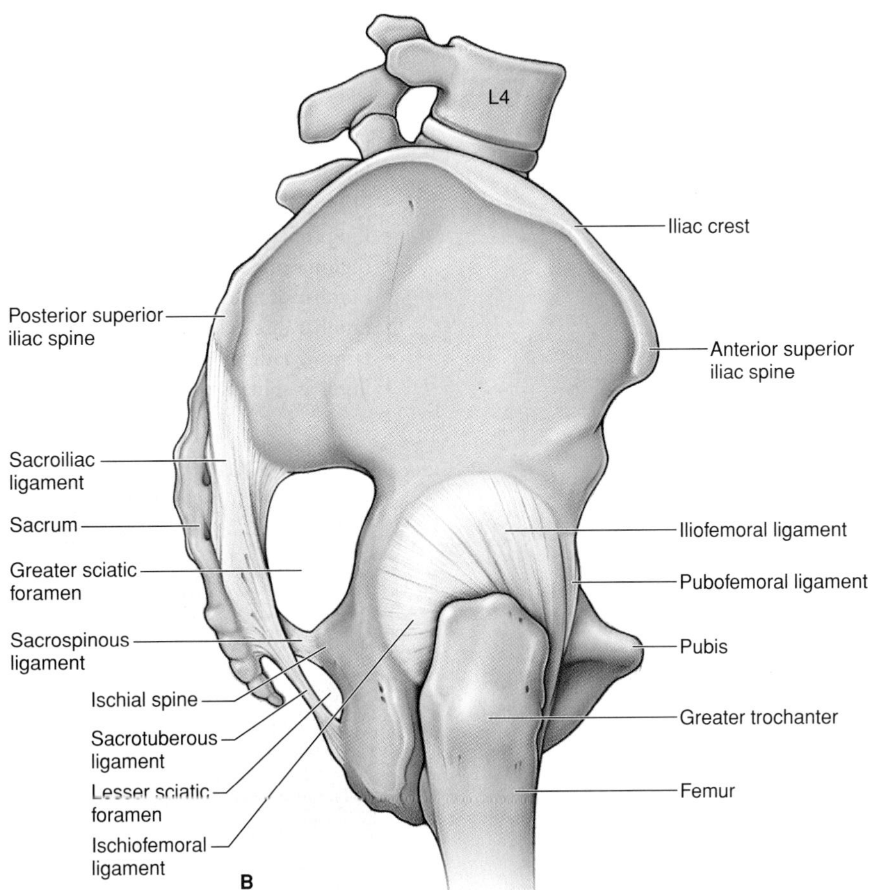

FIGURE 181-3 (**A**) Structure of the hip joint. (**B**) The right hip illustrating the lateral view of the ligaments of the hip joint. (From Morton DA, Foreman KB, Albertine KH. *The Big Picture: Gross Anatomy*. http://www.accessmedicine.com. Copyright © The McGraw-Hill Companies, Inc. All rights reserved.)

KEY FEATURES

Description

- Pain along the iliac crest where multiple muscle attachments occur
- Direct trauma/blow to iliac crest causing immediate pain and debilitation[1]

Essentials of Diagnosis

- Acute onset from initial trauma
  - Internal muscular bleeding and swelling can/will occur within minutes or hours of the injury
  - Pain radiating into the internal and external oblique muscles
  - Possible paresthesia over anterolateral thigh
  - Acute traumatic event; direct blow to unprotected ilium
  - Subcutaneous contusion, graded I to III

General Considerations

- In younger children, concern must be on a slipped growth plate or avulsion of the iliac apophysis
- Wearing of a hip pad in sports, to limit contusion
- Can lead to myositis ossificans[2]
- Stress fractures or blood supply disruption to the hip may show up later

Demographics

- Younger, athletic population
- Can be seen in older adults secondary to a fall or car accident

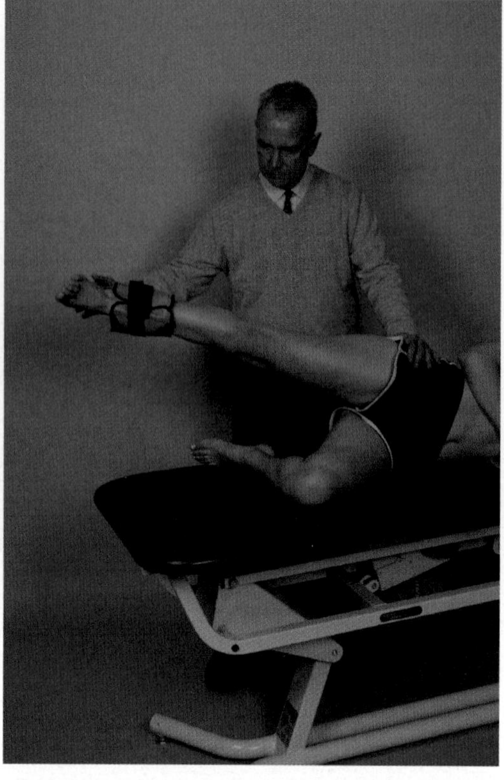

FIGURE 181-4 Gluteus medius strengthening. (From Dutton D. *Dutton's Orthopaedic Examination, Evaluation, and Intervention*. 3rd ed. www.accessphysiotherapy.com. Copyright © The McGraw-Hill Companies, Inc. All rights reserved.)

CLINICAL FINDINGS

SIGNS AND SYMPTOMS

- Hematoma[1]
- Point tender with palpation over iliac crest and associated muscles
- Crepitus felt during palpation
- Muscle spasm noted
- Pain with active range of motion (AROM) hip flexion, trunk rotation, trunk flexion
- Manual muscle test (MMT): Painful with associated muscles
- Swelling
- Redness
- Ecchymosis: If caused by direct trauma

Functional Implications

- Antalgic gait
- Painful end ranges during ambulation
- Decreased weight bearing on the involved side with increased weight bearing on the unaffected extremity
- Pain and weakness as the ITB passes over greater trochanter
- Pain limiting functional activities (ADLs, physical and athletic activities)
- Difficulty sleeping on affected side

Possible Contributing Causes

- Trauma, impact
- Fall on side
- Blood thinner medication, increases internal bleeding

Differential Diagnosis

- Avascular necrosis
- Avulsion fracture of the iliac apophysis
- Femoral neck stress fracture
- Greater trochanteric bursitis
- Hip arthritis
- Hip labral tear
- ITB syndrome
- Ilium fracture
- Inguinal and femoral hernia
- Lumbar degenerative disc disease
- Lumbar disc herniation
- Lumbar radiculopathy
- Lumbar spinal stenosis

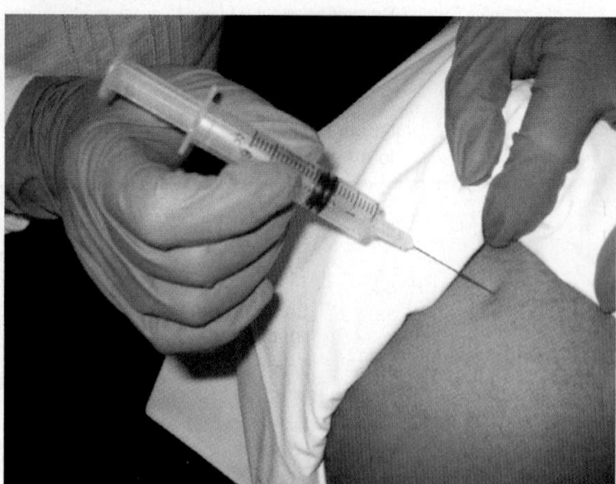

FIGURE 181-5 Site for injection or aspiration of trochanteric bursa. (From Patel DR, Greydanus DE, Baker RJ. *Pediatric Practice: Sports Medicine*. www.accesspediatrics.com. Copyright © The McGraw-Hill Companies, Inc. All rights reserved.)

- Metastatic tumor
- Muscle strain (gluteus minimus, internal oblique, external oblique)
- Piriformis syndrome
- Sacral iliac dysfunction
- Sciatica
- Septic arthritis
- Snapping hip syndrome
- Tendinitis of gluteus medius, gluteus maximus

MEANS OF CONFIRMATION OR DIAGNOSIS

Imaging

- Radiographs of ilium
- Radiographs of spine and hip
- MRI for soft tissue damage and for fracture
- Bone scan for stress fracture and hip necrosis
- Diagnostic ultrasound

FINDINGS AND INTERPRETATION

- Imaging unremarkable except for bruising

TREATMENT

Medications

- Corticosteroid injection at the trochanteric bursae[3]
- NSAIDs, acetaminophen

REFERRAL/ADMITTANCE

- To orthopedic physician for imaging and medications

IMPAIRMENTS

- Limited activity, especially with transition from hip flexion/extension (in/out of chair)
- Unable to sleep secondary to pain with lying on the affected side
- Painful hip motion limiting ambulation or running

TESTS AND MEASURES

- Ober test
- FABER (Patrick test)
- Lower-extremity screening examination
- Postural examination
- Hip examination
- MMT: Painful with associated muscles
- Muscle length testing, including hamstrings, hip flexors, calf muscles
- Quadrant test
- Straight-leg raise test
- Slump test
- Lower limb nerve tension test
- Prone instability test
- Leg-length assessment
- Lower-extremity neurological screening (dermatome, myotome, reflexes)
- Sensory check of the involved lower leg
- Repeated movement testing
- Fear-Avoidance Beliefs Questionnaire (FABQ)

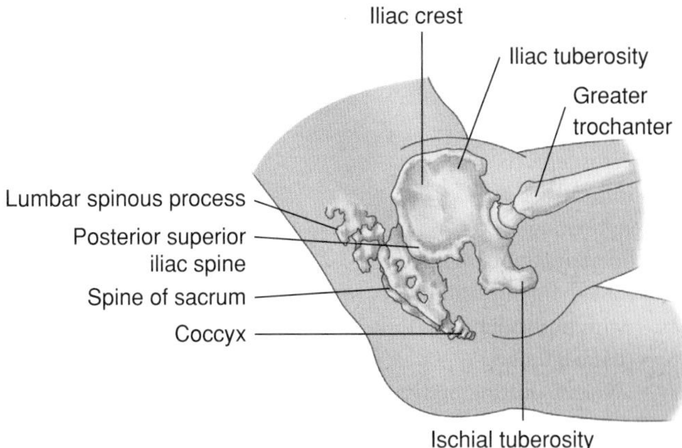

FIGURE 181-6 Bony landmarks—posterior and lateral view. (From Dutton M. *Dutton's Orthopedic Survival Guide: Managing Common Conditions*. http://www.accessphysiotherapy.com. Copyright © The McGraw-Hill Companies, Inc. All rights reserved.)

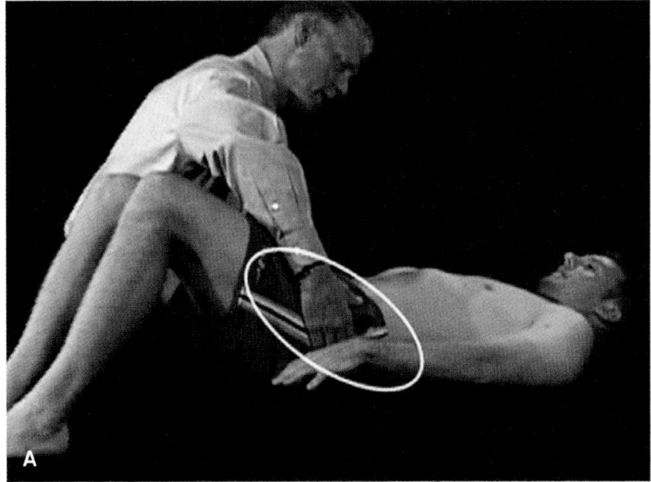

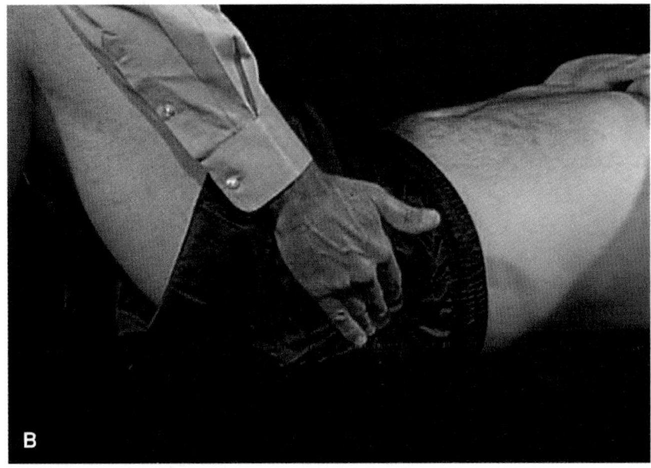

FIGURE 181-7 Palpation of the greater trochanter. (From Lawry GV. *Systematic Musculoskeletal Examinations*. www.accessmedicine.com. Copyright © The McGraw-Hill Companies, Inc. All rights reserved.)

INTERVENTION

- Rest, nonweight bearing
- Flexibility
  - ITB
  - Rectus femoris
  - Piriformis
- Strengthening
  - Hip abduction strengthening
    - Side-lying hip abduction, progression to side-lying planks with hip abduction
    - Lateral lunges
    - Weight shifting on fitter
    - Unilateral balancing
- If leg-length problem, heel lift on unaffected side to shift
- Manual therapy
  - Not acute condition or painful: Cross-friction massage may loosen adhesions formed secondary to the bursal inflammation
- Modalities
  - Swelling
    - Ice
    - Electric stimulation
  - Pain
    - Ice
    - Electric stimulation

FUNCTIONAL GOALS

- Patient will to be able to
  - Rise up and down from chair pain free.
  - Sleep on the ipsilateral side pain free.
  - Tolerate sitting for >1 hour.
  - Run pain free.

PROGNOSIS

- Responds well to conservative treatment.
- Grade I hip contusion functionally limits the patient 5 to 14 days.[4]
- Grade II and III hip contusion functionally limits the patient 14 to 21 days.[4]
- Injection may be necessary if conservative treatments fail.

PATIENT RESOURCE

- Hip-pointer contusion. McGraw-Hill Concise Dictionary of Modern Medicine. The McGraw-Hill Companies, Inc. 2002.

REFERENCES

1. Cline S. Acute injuries of the hip, pelvis, and thigh. In: Patel DR, Greydanus DE, Baker RJ, eds. *Pediatric Practice: Sports Medicine*. New York, NY: McGraw-Hill; 2009:Chapter 24. http://www.accessphysiotherapy.com/content/6979297. Accessed June 16, 2013.
2. Melamed H, Hutchinson M. Soft tissue problems of the hip in athletes. *Sports Med Arthroscopy Rev*. 2002;10:168–175.
3. Diokno E. Appendix B. Soft tissue injections, joint injections, and aspiration. In: Patel DR, Greydanus DE, Baker RJ, eds. *Pediatric Practice: Sports Medicine*. New York, NY: McGraw-Hill; 2009. http://www.accessphysiotherapy.com/content/6983400#6983400. Accessed June 16, 2013.
4. Dutton M. Practice pattern 4E: impaired joint mobility, motor function, muscle performance, and rom associated with localized inflammation. In: Dutton M, ed. *Dutton's Orthopaedic Examination, Evaluation, and Intervention*. 3rd ed. New York, NY: McGraw-Hill; 2012. http://www.accessphysiotherapy.com/content/56542444. Accessed June 16, 2013.

ADDITIONAL REFERENCES

- Dutton M. Fundamentals and core concepts. In: Dutton M, ed. *McGraw-Hill's NPTE. (National Physical Therapy Examination)*. 2nd ed. New York, NY: McGraw-Hill; 2012. http://www.accessphysiotherapy.com/content/5396134#5396134. Accessed June 16, 2013.
- Dutton M. The hip joint. In: Dutton M, ed. *Dutton's Orthopedic Survival Guide: Managing Common Conditions*. New York, NY: McGraw-Hill; 2011. http://www.accessphysiotherapy.com/content/8654377#8654377. Accessed June 16, 2013.
- Dutton M. The hip joint. In: Dutton M. *Orthopaedic Examination, Evaluation, and Intervention*. 2nd ed. New York, NY: McGraw-Hill; 2012. http://www.accessphysiotherapy.com/content/55581507#55581507. Accessed June 16, 2013.
- Hall M, Anderson J. Hip pointers. *Clin Sports Med*. 2013;32(2):325–330. doi: 10.1016/j.csm.2012.12.010.
- ICD9DATA. http://www.icd9data.com. Accessed June 16, 2013.
- ICD10DATA. http://www.icd10data.com. Accessed June 16, 2013.
- The American Physical Therapy Association. Pattern 4E: impaired joint mobility, motor function, muscle performance, and range of motion associated with localized inflammation. *Interactive Guide to Physical Therapist Practice*. 2003.doi: 10.2522/ptguide.3.1_5. http://guidetoptpractice.apta.org/content/1/SEC12.extract?sid=a3440a97-102f-4f1f-9273-34f60416f5ad. Accessed May 27, 2014.

182 HIP/FEMORAL NECK FRACTURE

Jennifer Cabrera, DPT, GCS
Eric Shamus, PhD, DPT, PT, CSCS

CONDITION/DISORDER SYNONYM

- Intertrochanteric fracture of the fermoral neck

ICD-9-CM CODES

- 820.00 Closed fracture of intracapsular section of neck of femur, unspecified
- 820.01 Closed fracture of epiphysis (separation) (upper) of neck of femur
- 820.02 Closed fracture of midcervical section of neck of femur
- 820.03 Closed fracture of base of neck of femur
- 820.09 Other closed transcervical fracture of neck of femur
- 820.10 Open fracture of intracapsular section of neck of femur, unspecified
- 820.11 Open fracture of epiphysis (separation) (upper) of neck of femur
- 820.12 Open fracture of midcervical section of neck of femur
- 820.13 Open fracture of base of neck of femur
- 820.19 Other open transcervical fracture of neck of femur
- 820.20 Closed fracture of trochanteric section of neck of femur
- 820.21 Closed fracture of intertrochanteric section of neck of femur
- 820.22 Closed fracture of subtrochanteric section of neck of femur
- 820.30 Open fracture of trochanteric section of neck of femur, unspecified
- 820.31 Open fracture of intertrochanteric section of neck of femur
- 820.32 Open fracture of subtrochanteric section of neck of femur
- 820.8 Closed fracture of unspecified part of neck of femur
- 820.9 Open fracture of unspecified part of neck of femur

ICD-10-CM CODES

- S72.019A Unspecified intracapsular fracture of unspecified femur, initial encounter for closed fracture
- S72.023A Displaced fracture of epiphysis (separation) (upper) of unspecified femur, initial encounter for closed fracture
- S72.026A Nondisplaced fracture of epiphysis (separation) (upper) of unspecified femur, initial encounter for closed fracture
- S72.033A Displaced midcervical fracture of unspecified femur, initial encounter for closed fracture
- S72.036A Nondisplaced midcervical fracture of unspecified femur, initial encounter for closed fracture
- S72.043A Displaced fracture of base of neck of unspecified femur, initial encounter for closed fracture
- S72.046A Nondisplaced fracture of base of neck of unspecified femur, initial encounter for closed fracture
- S72.099A Other fracture of head and neck of unspecified femur, initial encounter for closed fracture

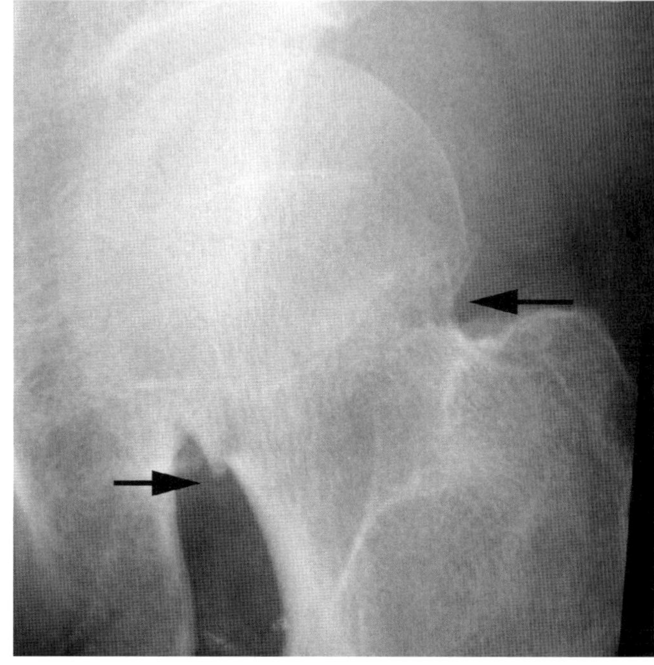

FIGURE 182-1 Nondisplaced, complete, femoral neck fracture (*black arrows*). Nondisplaced fractures can be incomplete (fracture through part of the femoral neck) or complete (fracture through the entire femoral neck). (From Simon RR, Sherman SC, Koenigsknecht SJ. *Emergency Orthopedics, the Extremities*. 5th ed. p. 358, Fig. 13-8, Copyright 2007, McGraw-Hill.)

- S72.019B Unspecified intracapsular fracture of unspecified femur, initial encounter for open fracture type I or II
- S72.019C Unspecified intracapsular fracture of unspecified femur, initial encounter for open fracture type IIIA, IIIB, or IIIC
- S72.023B Displaced fracture of epiphysis (separation) (upper) of unspecified femur, initial encounter for open fracture type I or II
- S72.023C Displaced fracture of epiphysis (separation) (upper) of unspecified femur, initial encounter for open fracture type IIIA, IIIB, or IIIC
- S72.026B Nondisplaced fracture of epiphysis (separation) (upper) of unspecified femur, initial encounter for open fracture type I or II
- S72.026C Nondisplaced fracture of epiphysis (separation) (upper) of unspecified femur, initial encounter for open fracture type IIIA, IIIB, or IIIC
- S72.033B Displaced midcervical fracture of unspecified femur, initial encounter for open fracture type I or II
- S72.033C Displaced midcervical fracture of unspecified femur, initial encounter for open fracture type IIIA, IIIB, or IIIC
- S72.036B Nondisplaced midcervical fracture of unspecified femur, initial encounter for open fracture type I or II
- S72.036C Nondisplaced midcervical fracture of unspecified femur, initial encounter for open fracture type IIIA, IIIB, or IIIC
- S72.043B Displaced fracture of base of neck of unspecified femur, initial encounter for open fracture type I or II

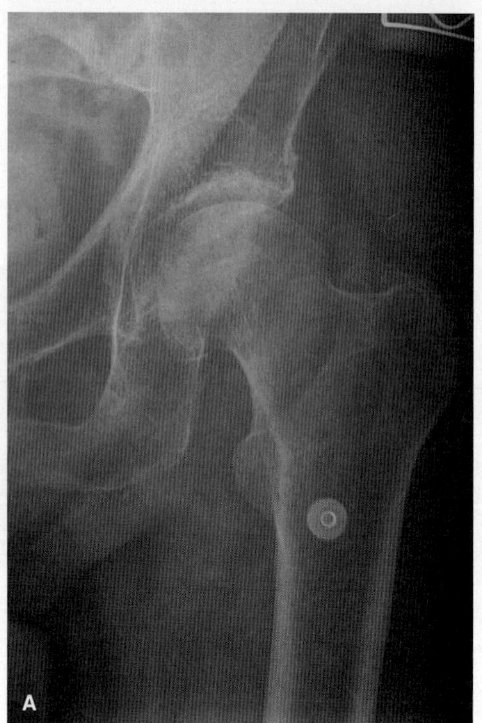

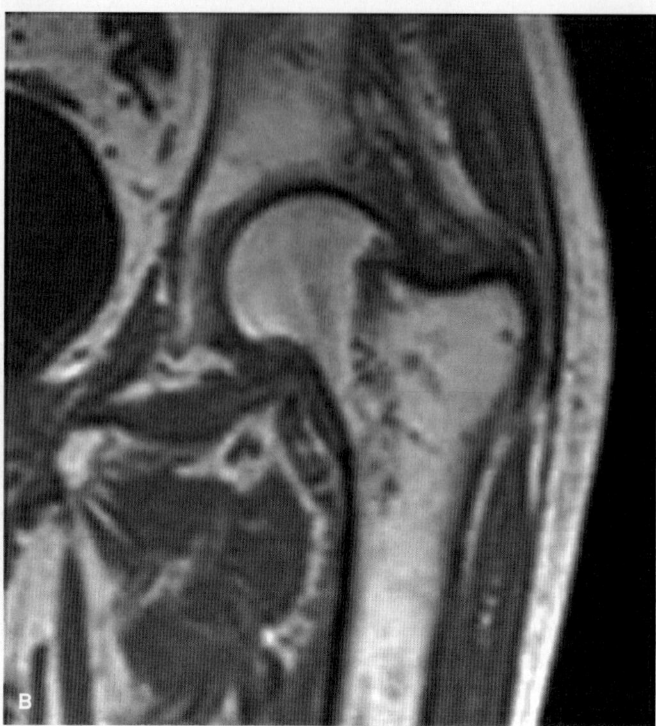

FIGURE 182-2 Occult femoral neck fracture. (**A**) Anteroposterior radiograph of a 78-year-old man who had left hip pain after a fall. No fracture is evident. (**B**) Coronal T1-weighted image of the left hip clearly demonstrates a nondisplaced femoral neck fracture. (From Tintinalli JE, Stapczynski J, Ma OJ, Cline D, Cydulka R, Meckler G, eds. *Tintinalli's Emergency Medicine: A Comprehensive Study Guide*. 7th ed. http://www.accessmedicine.com. Copyright © The McGraw-Hill Companies, Inc. All rights reserved.)

- S72.043C Displaced fracture of base of neck of unspecified femur, initial encounter for open fracture type IIIA, IIIB, or IIIC
- S72.046B Nondisplaced fracture of base of neck of unspecified femur, initial encounter for open fracture type I or II
- S72.046C Nondisplaced fracture of base of neck of unspecified femur, initial encounter for open fracture type IIIA, IIIB, or IIIC
- S72.099B Other fracture of head and neck of unspecified femur, initial encounter for open fracture type I or II
- S72.099C Other fracture of head and neck of unspecified femur, initial encounter for open fracture type IIIA, IIIB, or IIIC
- S72.109A Unspecified trochanteric fracture of unspecified femur, initial encounter for closed fracture
- S72.143A Displaced intertrochanteric fracture of unspecified femur, initial encounter for closed fracture
- S72.146A Nondisplaced intertrochanteric fracture of unspecified femur, initial encounter for closed fracture
- S72.23XA Displaced subtrochanteric fracture of unspecified femur, initial encounter for closed fracture
- S72.26XA Nondisplaced subtrochanteric fracture of unspecified femur, initial encounter for closed fracture
- S72.109B Unspecified trochanteric fracture of unspecified femur, initial encounter for open fracture type I or II
- S72.109C Unspecified trochanteric fracture of unspecified femur, initial encounter for open fracture type IIIA, IIIB, or IIIC
- S72.143B Displaced intertrochanteric fracture of unspecified femur, initial encounter for open fracture type I or II
- S72.143C Displaced intertrochanteric fracture of unspecified femur, initial encounter for open fracture type IIIA, IIIB, or IIIC
- S72.146B Nondisplaced intertrochanteric fracture of unspecified femur, initial encounter for open fracture type I or II
- S72.146C Nondisplaced intertrochanteric fracture of unspecified femur, initial encounter for open fracture type IIIA, IIIB, or IIIC
- S72.23XB Displaced subtrochanteric fracture of unspecified femur, initial encounter for open fracture type I or II
- S72.23XC Displaced subtrochanteric fracture of unspecified femur, initial encounter for open fracture type IIIA, IIIB, or IIIC
- S72.26XB Nondisplaced subtrochanteric fracture of unspecified femur, initial encounter for open fracture type I or II
- S72.26XC Nondisplaced subtrochanteric fracture of unspecified femur, initial encounter for open fracture type IIIA, IIIB, or IIIC
- S72.009A Fracture of unspecified part of neck of unspecified femur, initial encounter for closed fracture
- S72.009B Fracture of unspecified part of neck of unspecified femur, initial encounter for open fracture type I or II

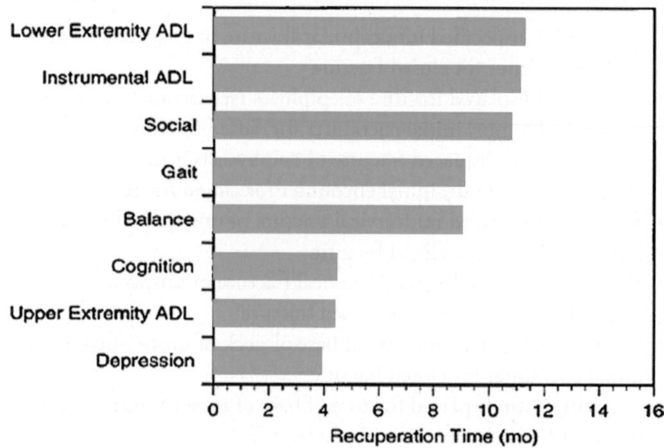

FIGURE 182-3 Time to recuperation following hip fracture in eight areas of function. (Magaziner et al. *J Gerontol Med Sci*. 2000;55A(9):M498–M507.)

- S72.009C Fracture of unspecified part of neck of unspecified femur, initial encounter for open fracture type IIIA, IIIB, or IIIC

PREFERRED PRACTICE PATTERN

- 4G: Impaired Joint Mobility, Muscle Performance, and Range of Motion Associated With Fracture

PATIENT PRESENTATION

A 75-year-old woman with moderate dementia is brought to the office by her family because she is refusing to walk for the past 2 days. Her caretakers are not aware of a fall, but states she seemed unsteady since beginning a new depression medication 4 weeks ago. She has a nondisplaced, complete, femoral neck fracture. Undoubtedly she fell when unobserved approximately 3 days ago. She is referred to orthopedics for management of her hip fracture. Unfortunately, the dementia is a bad prognostic sign for recovery of ambulation.[1]

KEY FEATURES

Description

- Fracture
- Any defect in continuity of the femoral neck, stress fracture[2]
- Displaced (femoral neck is moved on either side of the fracture) or nondisplaced (femoral neck has not moved)
- Closed (skin is intact) or open (skin is breached)

Essentials of Diagnosis

- Diagnosis is usually made by clinical examination.
- May not be a fracture, but a hip sprain or hip contusion.

General Considerations

- Common characteristics of those at risk of hip fracture
  - Family history of fracture later in life, especially in Caucasians and Asians
  - Low-calcium dietary intake
  - Smoking or excessive alcohol intake
  - Dementia
  - Physical frailty
- 24% of individuals over the age of 50 who experience a hip fracture will die within 12 months of injury secondary to complications.
- 51% of individuals over the age of 65 who suffer a hip fracture will be discharged from the hospital to a long-term care facility.

Demographics

- Rate of hip fractures increases in individuals age 65 or older
- Occurrence of hip fractures: Two to three times more in women than men
- White, postmenopausal women have one in seven chance of sustaining a hip fracture

CLINICAL FINDINGS

SIGNS AND SYMPTOMS

- Pain in the outer upper thigh and in the groin[2]
- Point tenderness
- Night pain[1]
- Increased pain on weight bearing

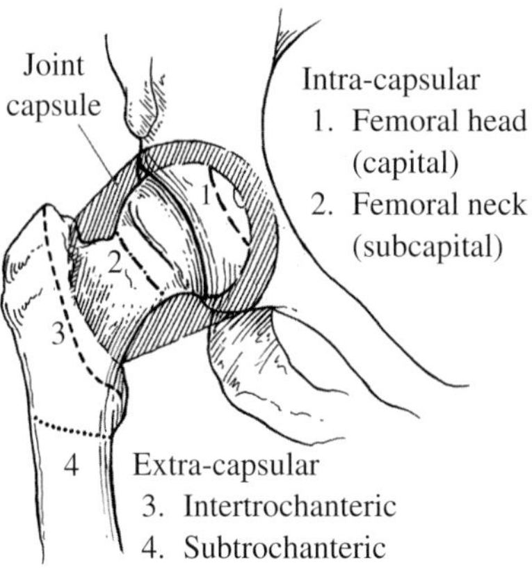

FIGURE 182-4 Hip fractures. This illustration depicts the different types of proximal femoral fractures. (From Knoop KJ, Stack LB, Storrow AB, Thurman RJ. *The Atlas of Emergency Medicine*. 3rd ed. http://www.accessmedicine.com. Copyright © The McGraw-Hill Companies, Inc. All rights reserved.)

- Edema
- Ecchymosis
- Loss of general function
- Loss of active mobility
- Muscle guarding with passive movement

Functional Implications

- Pain with standing.
- Inability to weight bear on injured lower extremity (LE).
- If patient has fallen and experienced a hip fracture, patient will have great difficulty transferring off of the floor.

Possible Contributing Causes

- Osteoporosis
- History of falls
- Impaired standing balance
- Polypharmacy

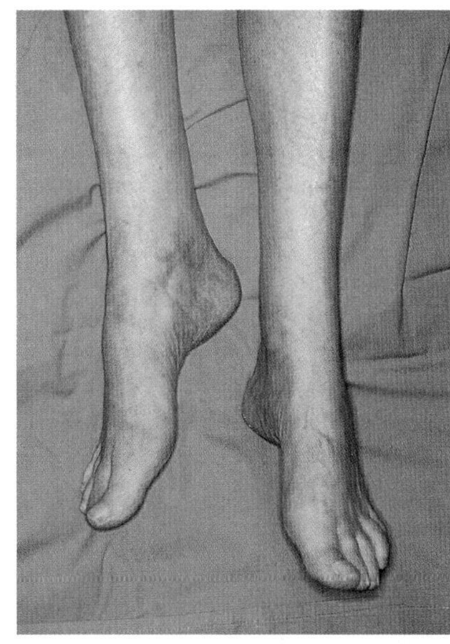

FIGURE 182-5 Hip fracture. Patients with hip fractures often present with the affected extremity shortened, externally rotated, and abducted. Note the rotation and shortening in this patient with a right intertrochanteric fracture. (From Knoop KJ, Stack LB, Storrow AB, Thurman RJ. *The Atlas of Emergency Medicine*. 3rd ed. http://www.accessmedicine.com. Copyright © The McGraw-Hill Companies, Inc. All rights reserved. Photo contributor: Cathleen M. Vossler, MD.)

Differential Diagnosis

- Hip sprain
- Hip contusion

MEANS OF CONFIRMATION OR DIAGNOSIS

Imaging

- X-ray for fracture, often limited view
- Computed tomography (CT) scan for detailed imaging
- Magnetic resonance imaging (MRI) for hidden fractures

FINDINGS AND INTERPRETATION

- Inability to ambulate
- Pain with passive flexion or rotation of the hip
- Exposed bone in case of an open and displaced fracture
- Possible integumentary deformity over underlying fracture
- If vascular structures are involved the LE will appear cool and pale
- If neurologic structures are involved the individual will report numbness and decreased ability to move the involved LE
- Patient demonstrates leg-length discrepancy as involved LE appears shorter
- Patient holds involved LE in external rotation and immobile

REFERRALS/ADMITTANCE

- For imaging, X-ray or CT
- For medication: NSAID or opioid for pain management
- For orthopedic consult
  - Fracture reduction via surgical intervention: Open reduction internal fixation or hip joint replacement
  - Nonsurgical treatment is only pursued in cases in which the individual is too ill to undergo surgery or if the patient is confined to a bed or wheelchair
    - Orthopedist follows the case closely to monitor for complications

IMPAIRMENTS

- Antalgic gait secondary to pain, which causes a decreased ability to weight shift onto involved LE
- Inability to ambulate long distances secondary to pain and/or likelihood of decreased weight-bearing status that makes ambulating a taxing activity
- Decreased stance time on the involved LE during ambulation
- Inability to stand for long periods of time secondary to pain
- Decreased mid/terminal stance during gait secondary to tight hip flexors
- Decreased functional mobility: Bed mobility and transfers

TESTS AND MEASURES

- Fulcrum test
- Auscultatory patellar-pubic percussion test
- Resisted straight-leg raising maneuver
- Pain, visual analog scale (VAS)
  - 24-hour pain
  - Worst average pain
  - Best average pain
- Functional independence measure
  - Locomotion
- Cardiovascular integrity
  - Blood pressure at rest and after activity
  - Heart rate at rest and after activity
- Skin Integrity
  - Scar
    - Approximation
    - Mobility/pliability
  - Associated skin assessment
    - Edema (linear girth measurements, palpation)
    - Color
    - Signs of infection
    - Mobility/turgor
    - Temperature
- Neurologic examination
  - Sensation
    - Light touch
    - Pin prick
  - LE deep tendon reflexes
  - Proprioception at the hip
  - Kinesthetic awareness at the hip
  - Coordination
- Trunk active and passive ROM
- Hip and knee active and passive ROM
- Flexibility testing
  - Hamstrings
  - Iliopsoas
  - Quadriceps
  - Iliotibial band
  - Abductors
  - Adductors
- Joint integrity of the spine
- Sacroiliac joint integrity
- Hip joint integrity
  - Hip scour
  - Flexion, abduction, external rotation (FABER) test
  - Flexion, adduction, internal rotation (FAIR) or (FADIR) test
- Limb strength
  - Functional strength testing
    - Five-times sit-to-stand test
  - Manual muscle test (MMT)
    - Hamstrings
    - Quadriceps
    - Iliopsoas
    - Gluteus maximus
    - Gluteus medius
    - Gluteus minimus
    - Adductors
- LE contralateral limb strength
- Balance
  - Static single-leg standing (eyes open, eyes closed)
    - Contralateral LE
  - Dynamic standing
    - Berg Balance Scale
    - Functional Gait Assessment
- Gait assessment
  - Observational analysis
  - Gait speed via the 10-m walk test
  - 2-minute walk test
  - 6-minute walk test
  - Retro running

INTERVENTION

- Monitor for signs/symptoms of deep vein thrombosis (DVT)
  - Positive Homans sign
  - Edema
  - Pain
  - Calor
  - Errythema
- If patient underwent a total hip replacement follow total hip precautions
  - Anterior approach
    - No hip extension
    - No hip external rotation
    - No hip adduction passed neutral
  - Posterior approach
    - No hip flexion greater than 90 degrees
    - No hip internal rotation
    - No hip adduction passed neutral
- Address swelling
  - Ice/cryotherapy
  - Compression
  - Elevation
  - Electrical stimulation
- Address pain
  - Ice/cryotherapy
  - Massage
  - Electrical stimulation
- Address lack of flexibility via stretching
  - Hip flexors with posterior approach
  - Rectus femoris
- Address weakness via strengthening activities
  - Open chain in all planes while maintaining total hip precautions (if applicable)
  - Closed chain activities (i.e., mini squats, heel raises, side stepping while maintaining total hip precautions if applicable)
- Address functional mobility
  - Bed-mobility training while maintaining total hip precautions is applicable
  - Transfer training with use of assistive device (i.e., rolling walker)
- Address scar mobility
  - Scar tissue mobilization progressing from parallel to perpendicular upon wound closure
- Address proprioception
  - Standing balance on level surface, eyes open/closed
  - Standing balance activities with use of foam
    - Eyes open
    - Eyes closed
  - Standing balance activities on balance machines
- Gait training
  - Lateral weight shifting to promote stance time on injured LE
  - Promote push off and heel strike
  - Promote increased hip extension during mid/terminal stance
    - Only with posterior approach, total hips if applicable

FUNCTIONAL GOALS

- Patient will be able to
  - Perform bed mobility independently to decrease burden of care.
  - Increase gait speed to 1.0 m/s to promote safe community ambulation.
  - Increase Timed Up and Go test performance to 20 seconds to decrease fall risk.
  - Active hip extension to 0 degrees to promote normal gait pattern during mid/terminal stance.

PROGNOSIS

- Good; individual should regain strength and independence within 3 months.

PATIENT RESOURCES

- American Academy of Orthopaedic Surgeons. *Live It Safe.* http://orthoinfo.aaos.org/topic.cfm?topic=A00245. Accessed February 10, 2013.
- American Academy of Orthopaedic Surgeons. *Live It Safe: Prevent Broken Hips.* http://orthoinfo.aaos.org/topic.cfm?topic=A00305. Accessed February 10, 2013.
- American Academy of Orthopaedic Surgeons. *Hip Fractures.* http://orthoinfo.aaos.org/topic.cfm?topic=A00392. Accessed February 10, 2013.

REFERENCES

1. Chumley H. Hip fracture. In: Usatine RP, Smith MA, Chumley H, Mayeaux E Jr, Tysinger J, eds. *The Color Atlas of Family Medicine.* New York, NY: McGraw-Hill; 2009:Chapter 99. http://www.accessmedicine.com/content.aspx?aID=8204140. Accessed February 10, 2013.
2. Dutton M. The hip joint. In: Dutton M, ed. *Dutton's Orthopedic Survival Guide: Managing Common Conditions.* New York, NY: McGraw-Hill; 2011. http://www.accessphysiotherapy.com/content/8654096. Accessed February 10, 2013.

ADDITIONAL REFERENCES

- Goodman CC, Boissonnault WG, Fuller KS. *Pathology: Implications for the Physical Therapist.* 2nd ed. Philadelphia, PA: Saunders; 2003.
- Kisner C, Colby LA. *Therapeutic Exercise: Foundations and Techniques.* 5th ed. Philadelphia, PA: F.A. Davis Company; 2007.
- Magee DJ. *Orthopedic Physical Assessment.* 5th ed. St. Louis, MO: Saunders Elsevier; 2008.

183 FEMUR FRACTURE

Jennifer Cabrera, DPT, GCS
Eric Shamus, PhD, DPT, PT, CSCS

CONDITION/DISORDER SYNONYM

- Femoral fracture

ICD-9-CM CODES

- 821 Fracture of other and unspecified parts of femur
- 821.0 Fracture of shaft or unspecified part of femur closed
- 821.00 Fracture of unspecified part of femur closed
- 821.01 Fracture of shaft of femur closed
- 821.1 Fracture of shaft or unspecified part of femur open
- 821.10 Fracture of unspecified part of femur open
- 821.11 Fracture of shaft of femur open
- 821.2 Fracture of lower end of femur closed
- 821.20 Fracture of lower end of femur unspecified part closed
- 821.21 Fracture of femoral condyle closed
- 821.22 Fracture of lower epiphysis of femur closed
- 821.23 Supracondylar fracture of femur closed
- 821.29 Other fracture of lower end of femur closed
- 821.3 Fracture of lower end of femur open
- 821.30 Fracture of lower end of femur unspecified part open
- 821.31 Fracture of femoral condyle open
- 821.32 Fracture of lower epiphysis of femur open
- 821.33 Supracondylar fracture of femur open
- 821.39 Other fracture of lower end of femur open

ICD-10-CM CODES

- S72.90XA Unspecified fracture of unspecified femur, initial encounter for closed fracture
- S72.309A Unspecified fracture of shaft of unspecified femur, initial encounter for closed fracture
- S72.90XB Unspecified fracture of unspecified femur, initial encounter for open fracture type I or II
- S72.90XC Unspecified fracture of unspecified femur, initial encounter for open fracture type IIIA, IIIB, or IIIC
- S72.309B Unspecified fracture of shaft of unspecified femur, initial encounter for open fracture type I or II
- S72.309C Unspecified fracture of shaft of unspecified femur, initial encounter for open fracture type IIIA, IIIB, or IIIC
- S72.409A Unspecified fracture of lower end of unspecified femur, initial encounter for closed fracture
- S72.413A Displaced unspecified condyle fracture of lower end of unspecified femur, initial encounter for closed fracture
- S72.416A Nondisplaced unspecified condyle fracture of lower end of unspecified femur, initial encounter for closed fracture
- S72.443A Displaced fracture of lower epiphysis (separation) of unspecified femur, initial encounter for closed fracture
- S72.446A Nondisplaced fracture of lower epiphysis (separation) of unspecified femur, initial encounter for closed fracture

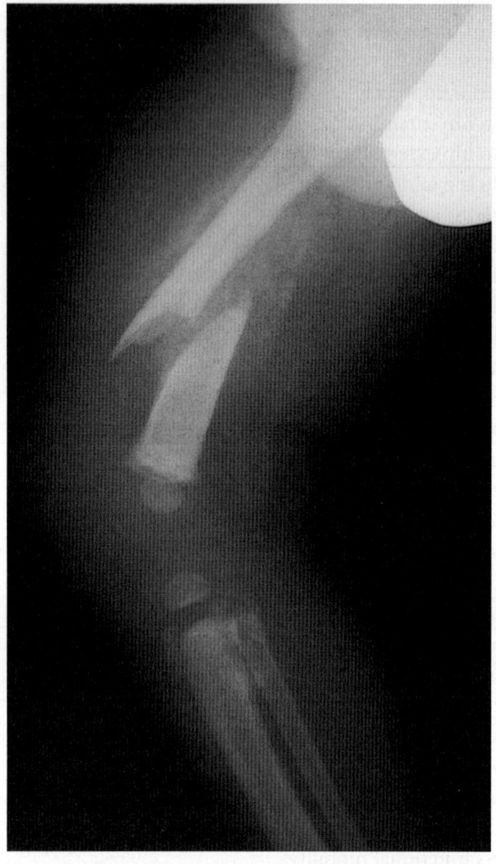

FIGURE 183-1 Spiral femur and proximal tibia fracture. Note displaced spiral femur fracture with faint callus formation and more solid (older) periosteal reaction of the proximal tibia. Child abuse is likely because there are two injuries which occurred at different times and no treatment was obtained. (From Knoop KJ, Stack LB, Storrow AB, Thurman RJ. *The Atlas of Emergency Medicine.* 3rd ed. http://www.accessmedicine.com. Copyright © The McGraw-Hill Companies, Inc. All rights reserved. Photo contributor: Alan E. Oestreich, MD.)

- S72.453A Displaced supracondylar fracture without intracondylar extension of lower end of unspecified femur, initial encounter for closed fracture
- S72.456A Nondisplaced supracondylar fracture without intracondylar extension of lower end of unspecified femur, initial encounter for closed fracture
- S72.499A Other fracture of lower end of unspecified femur, initial encounter for closed fracture
- S72.409B Unspecified fracture of lower end of unspecified femur, initial encounter for open fracture type I or II
- S72.409C Unspecified fracture of lower end of unspecified femur, initial encounter for open fracture type IIIA, IIIB, or IIIC
- S72.413B Displaced unspecified condyle fracture of lower end of unspecified femur, initial encounter for open fracture type I or II
- S72.413C Displaced unspecified condyle fracture of lower end of unspecified femur, initial encounter for open fracture type IIIA, IIIB, or IIIC

- IS72.416B Nondisplaced unspecified condyle fracture of lower end of unspecified femur, initial encounter for open fracture type I or II
- S72.416C Nondisplaced unspecified condyle fracture of lower end of unspecified femur, initial encounter for open fracture type IIIA, IIIB, or IIIC
- S72.443B Displaced fracture of lower epiphysis (separation) of unspecified femur, initial encounter for open fracture type I or II
- S72.443C Displaced fracture of lower epiphysis (separation) of unspecified femur, initial encounter for open fracture type IIIA, IIIB, or IIIC
- S72.446B Nondisplaced fracture of lower epiphysis (separation) of unspecified femur, initial encounter for open fracture type I or II
- S72.446C Nondisplaced fracture of lower epiphysis (separation) of unspecified femur, initial encounter for open fracture type IIIA, IIIB, or IIIC
- S72.453B Displaced supracondylar fracture without intracondylar extension of lower end of unspecified femur, initial encounter for open fracture type I or II
- S72.453C Displaced supracondylar fracture without intracondylar extension of lower end of unspecified femur, initial encounter for open fracture type IIIA, IIIB, or IIIC
- S72.456B Nondisplaced supracondylar fracture without intracondylar extension of lower end of unspecified femur, initial encounter for open fracture type I or II
- S72.456C Nondisplaced supracondylar fracture without intracondylar extension of lower end of unspecified femur, initial encounter for open fracture type IIIA, IIIB, or IIIC
- S72.499B Other fracture of lower end of unspecified femur, initial encounter for open fracture type I or II
- S72.499C Other fracture of lower end of unspecified femur, initial encounter for open fracture type IIIA, IIIB, or IIIC

PREFERRED PRACTICE PATTERN

- 4G: Impaired Joint Mobility, Muscle Performance, and Range of Motion Associated with Fracture[1]

PATIENT PRESENTATION

Patient is a 26-year-old male who was in a motorcycle accident. Patient had an intermedullary rod placed in the right femur to stabilize the femoral fracture. Patient presents to therapy with decreased weight bearing, gait dysfunction, and decreased strength. Patient is having discomfort over the scar incision.

KEY FEATURES

Description

- Fracture: Defect in continuity of the femur within the shaft[2]
- Displaced (femur moved on either side of the fracture) or non-displaced (femur has not moved)
- Closed (skin is intact) or open (skin is breached)
- Proximal femur fracture: Subtrochanteric to femoral head (with hip fractures)
- Distal femur fracture: Supracondylar to condylar (with knee fractures)
- Winquist and Hansen classification for degree of comminution[3]
  - Grade 1: Transverse or short oblique with less than 25% comminution

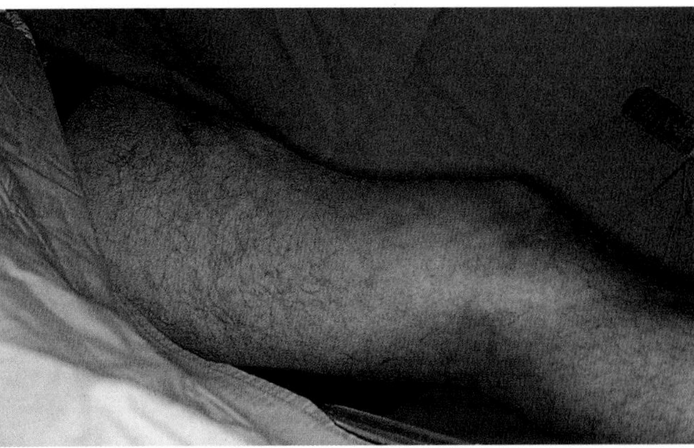

FIGURE 183-2 Midshaft femur fracture. A closed midshaft femoral fracture. Note the deformity in the middle of the thigh, consistent with this injury. (From Knoop KJ, Stack LB, Storrow AB, Thurman RJ. *The Atlas of Emergency Medicine*. 3rd ed. http://www.accessmedicine.com. Copyright © The McGraw-Hill Companies, Inc. All rights reserved. Photo contributor: Daniel L. Savitt, MD.)

  - Grade 2: Fractures have between 25% and 50% shaft-width comminution
  - Grade 3: Fractures have between 50% and 100% shaft-width comminution
  - Grade 4: Fractures have segmental comminution

Essentials of Diagnosis

- Usually made by clinical examination
- May not be a fracture, but muscle strain or contusion
- Three types of femoral shaft fractures
  - Type 1: Spiral or transverse
  - Type 2: Comminuted
  - Type 3: Open

General Considerations

- Occur from fall or direct blow to the leg (e.g., motor vehicle accident)
- Stabilization is critical with trauma to prevent further vascular or neurologic damage
- A leg fracture can mask the findings of a hip dislocation

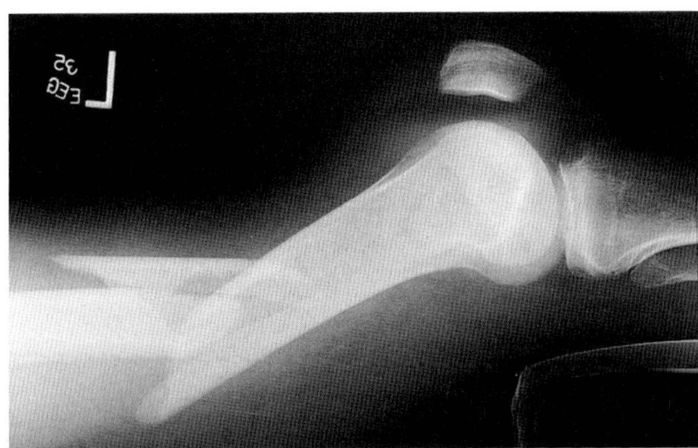

FIGURE 183-3 Femur fracture. Radiographic examination reveals a comminuted displaced distal femoral fracture. (From Knoop KJ, Stack LB, Storrow AB, Thurman RJ. *The Atlas of Emergency Medicine*. 3rd ed. http://www.accessmedicine.com. Copyright © The McGraw-Hill Companies, Inc. All rights reserved. Photo contributor: Cathleen M. Vossler, MD.)

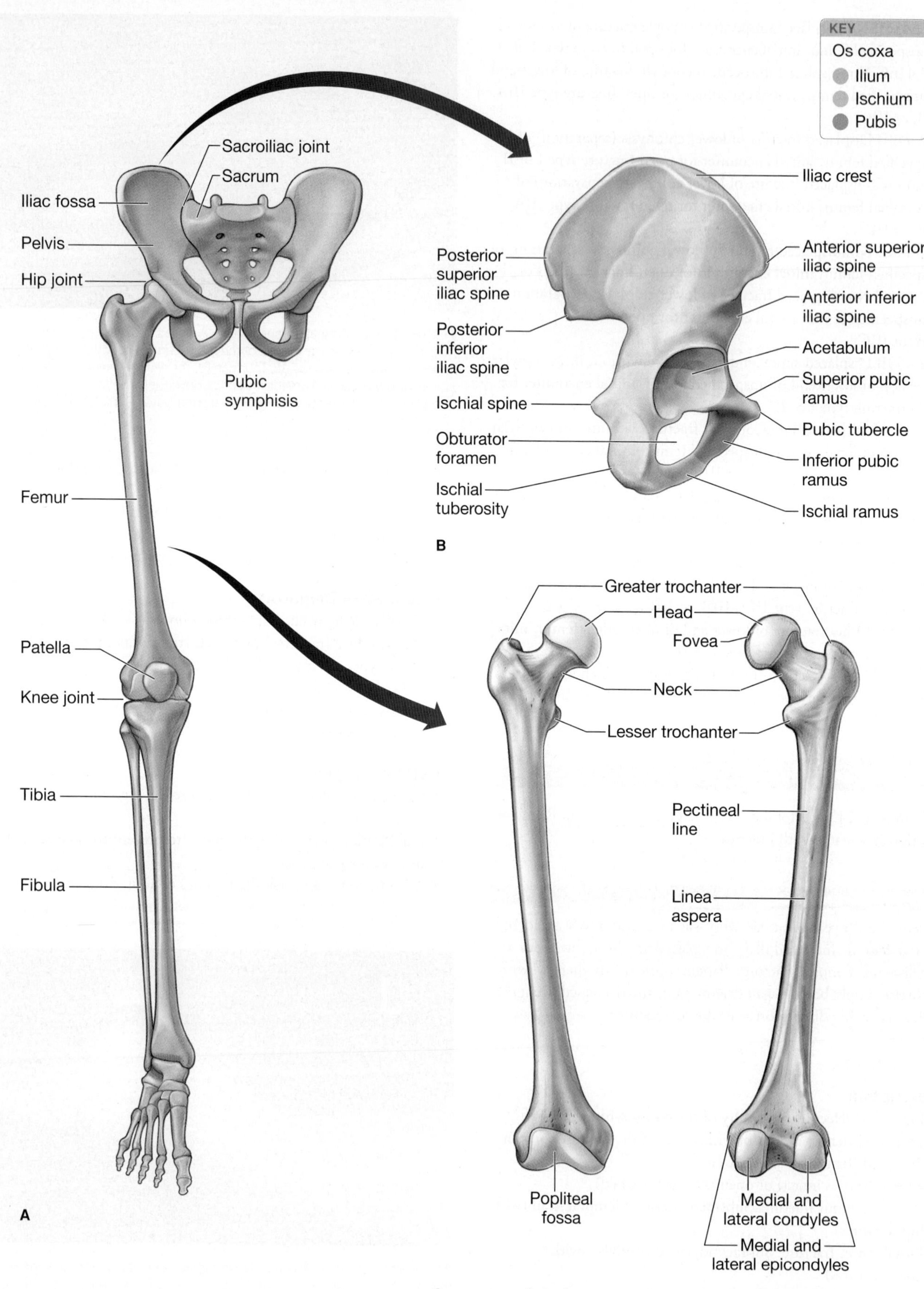

FIGURE 183-4 (**A**) Skeleton of the lower limb. (**B**) Osteology of the os coxa (pelvic bone). (**C**) Femur. (From Morton DA, Foreman KB, Albertine KH. *The Big Picture: Gross Anatomy*. http://www.accessmedicine.com. Copyright © The McGraw-Hill Companies, Inc. All rights reserved.)

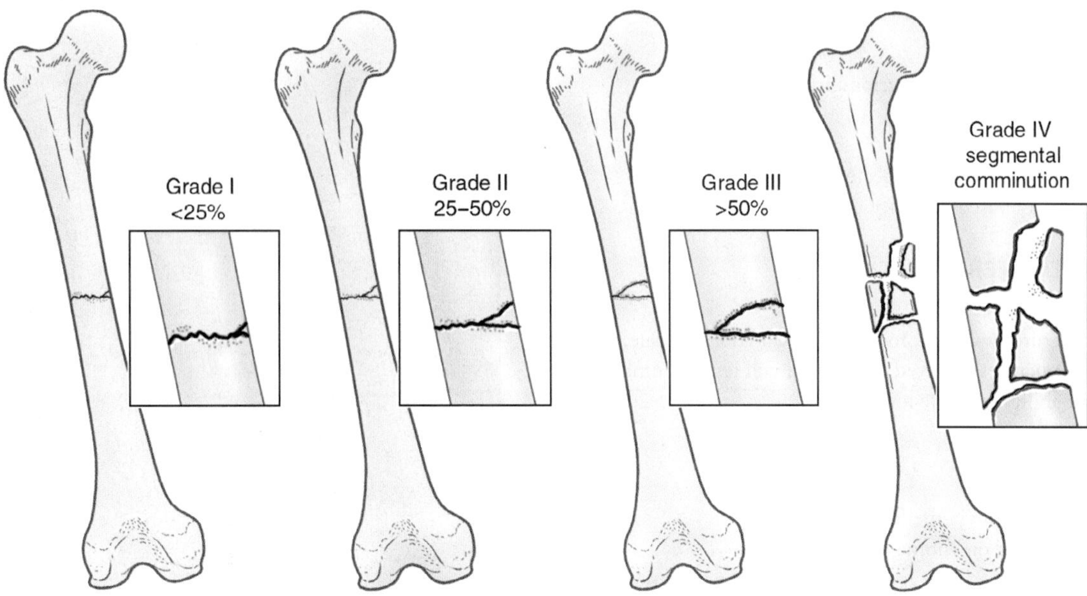

FIGURE 183-5 Comminuted femoral shaft fractures. (From Simon RR, Sherman SC. *Emergency Orthopedics*. 6th ed. http://www.accessemergencymedicine.com.)

Demographics

- Trauma with extreme force more common in younger population
- Fracture from falls or associated with osteoporosis more common in older population

CLINICAL FINDINGS

SIGNS AND SYMPTOMS

- Calor
- Ecchymosis
- Edema
- Erythema
- Exposed bone in cases of open and displaced fracture
- Inability to ambulate
- Increased pain on weight bearing
- Loss of active mobility
- Loss of general function
- Muscle guarding with passive movement
- Neurologic symptoms
- Pain and muscle guarding with lower-extremity (LE) movement
- Patient holds involved LE immobile
- Patient may demonstrate length discrepancy between legs with involved LE appearing shorter
- Point tenderness
- Possible integumentary deformity over underlying fracture
- Vascular symptoms

Functional Implications

- Pain with standing
- Inability to bear weight on injured LE
- If patient has fallen and sustained femoral fracture, will have great difficulty transferring off of the floor.

Possible Contributing Causes

- Bone cyst
- Cancer metastasis
- History of falls
- Impaired standing balance
- Osteoporosis
- Paget disease
- Polypharmacy
- Trauma, major force

Differential Diagnosis

- Muscle strain (e.g., quadriceps)
- Thigh contusion

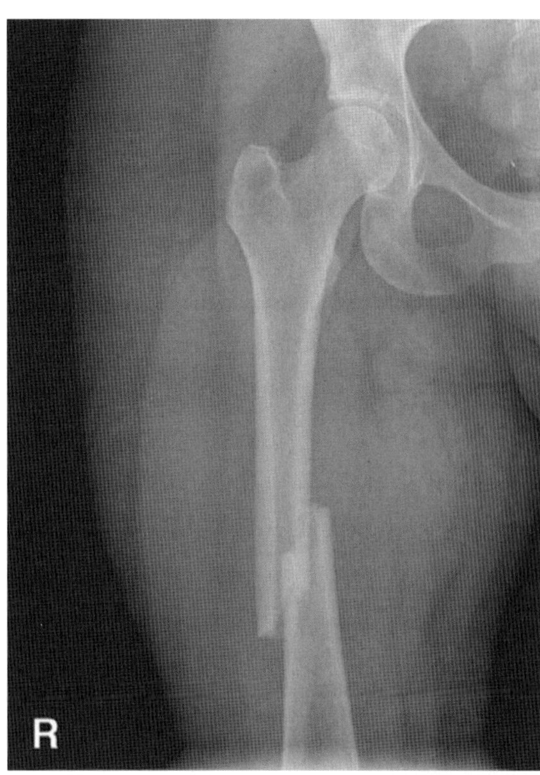

FIGURE 183-6 Oblique fracture of femur. This AP radiograph demonstrates an oblique fracture of the femur. A combination of compressive and bending loads typically cause these fracture orientations. (From Malone TR, Hazle C, Grey ML. *Imaging in Rehabilitation*. http://www.accessphysiotherapy.com.)

MEANS OF CONFIRMATION OR DIAGNOSIS

Imaging

- X-ray for fracture: Anteroposterior and lateral views[4]
- MRI
- CT for detailed imaging[4]
- Bone scan if stress fracture suspected[5]
- Arteriography for vascular injury

FINDINGS AND INTERPRETATION

- Positive Homans sign
- If vascular structures involved, foot will appear cool and pale.
- If neurologic structures involved, individual will report numbness and decreased ability to move foot or toes.

Treatment

- Surgery
  - Fracture reduction via the following
    - Traction: Hare or Thomas traction splints
    - Surgical intervention: Open reduction internal fixation (ORIF) or external fixation
    - Intramedullary rod

REFERRALS/ADMITTANCE

- To hospital for imaging, X-ray, CT[4]
- To physician for medication: NSAID or opiod for pain management
- To physician for orthopedic consult
  - Nonsurgical treatment only in cases of young children who may be placed in body spica casts

IMPAIRMENTS

- Antalgic gait secondary to pain causing decreased ability to shift weight onto involved LE
- Inability to ambulate long distances secondary to pain; decreased weight-bearing status makes ambulating taxing
- Decreased stance time on involved LE during ambulation
- Inability to stand for long periods of time secondary to pain
- Decreased knee flexion during swing phase of involved LE
- Decreased functional mobility (bed mobility and transfers)

TESTS AND MEASURES

- Pain, visual analog scale (VAS)
  - 24-hour pain
  - Worst average pain
  - Best average pain
- Functional independence measure
  - Locomotion
- Cardiovascular integrity
  - Blood pressure at rest and after activity
  - Heart rate at rest and after activity
- Skin Integrity
  - Scar
    - Approximation
    - Mobility/pliability
  - Associated skin assessment
    - Edema (linear girth measurements, palpation)
    - Color
    - Signs of infection

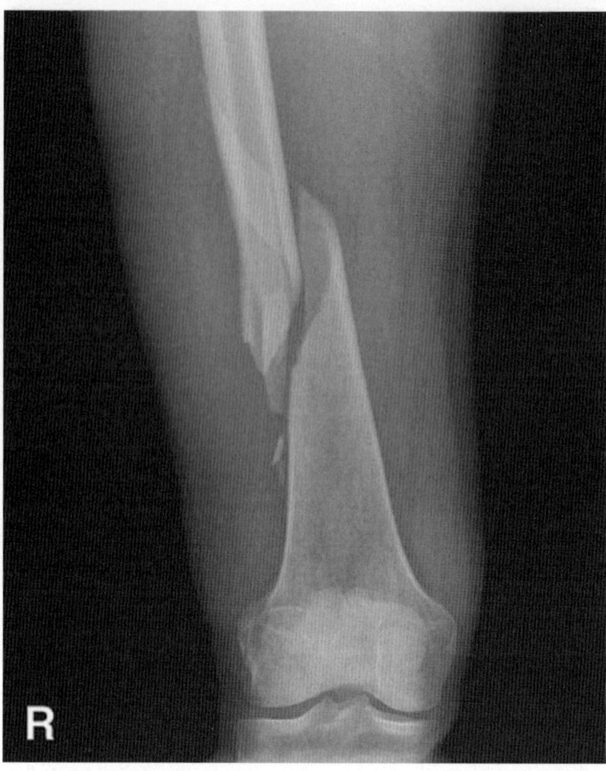

FIGURE 183-7 Spiral fracture of femur. Torsional loading, perpendicular to the long axis of the bone, is usually the cause of a spiral fracture as it appears in this anteroposterior (AP) radiograph. (From Malone TR, Hazle C, Grey ML. *Imaging in Rehabilitation*. http://www.accessphysiotherapy.com. Copyright © The McGraw-Hill Companies, Inc. All rights reserved.)

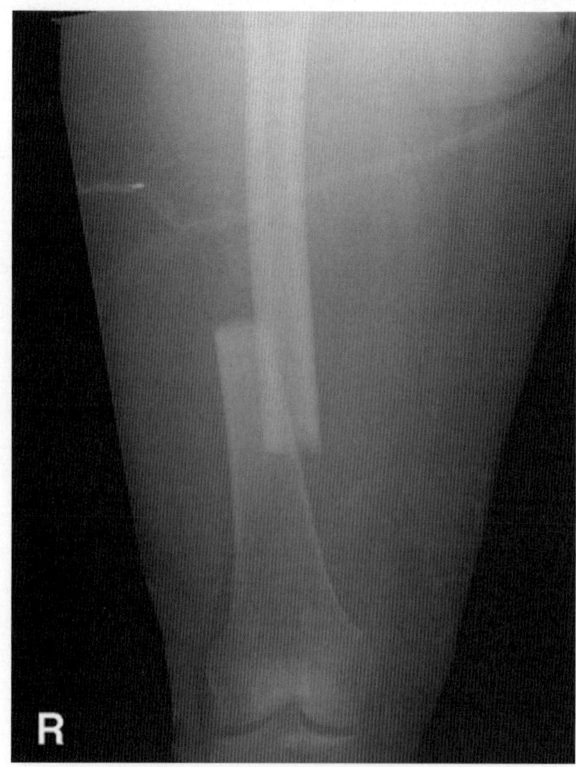

FIGURE 183-8 Transverse fracture of femur. Bending forces imposed on long bones will typically result in a transverse fracture line across the long axis of the bone as shown on this radiograph. (From Malone TR, Hazle C, Grey ML. *Imaging in Rehabilitation*. http://www.accessphysiotherapy.com. Copyright © The McGraw-Hill Companies, Inc. All rights reserved.)

- Mobility/turgor
- Temperature

- Neurologic examination
  - Sensation
    - Light touch
    - Pin prick
  - LE deep tendon reflexes
  - Proprioception at the hip
  - Kinesthetic awareness at the hip
  - Coordination
- Trunk active and passive ROM
- Hip and knee active and passive ROM
- Flexibility testing
  - Hamstrings
  - Iliopsoas
  - Quadriceps
  - Iliotibial band
  - Abductors
  - Adductors
- Joint integrity of the spine
- Sacroiliac joint integrity
- Hip joint integrity
  - Hip scour
  - Flexion abduction external rotation (FABER) test
  - Flexion adduction internal rotation (FAIR) or (FADIR) test
- Limb strength
  - Functional strength testing
    - Five-times sit-to-stand test
  - Manual muscle test (MMT)
    - Hamstrings
    - Quadriceps
    - Iliopsoas
    - Gluteus maximus
    - Gluteus medius
    - Gluteus minimus
    - Adductors
- LE contralateral limb strength
- Balance
  - Static single-leg standing (eyes open, eyes closed)
    - Contralateral LE
  - Dynamic standing
    - Berg Balance Scale
    - Functional Gait Assessment
- Gait assessment
  - Observational analysis
  - Gait speed via the 10-m walk test
  - 2-minute walk test
  - 6-minute walk test (6MWT)
  - Retro running

INTERVENTION

- Monitor for symptoms of deep vein thrombosis (DVT)
- Address swelling
  - Ice/cryotherapy[6]
  - Compression
  - Elevation
- Address pain
  - Ice/cryotherapy[6]
  - Massage
  - Electrical stimulation[7]
- Address lack of flexibility via stretching
  - Hip flexors
  - Rectus femoris
  - Hamstrings
  - Hip internal rotators
- Address weakness via strengthening activities
  - Open-chain hip and knee movements in all planes
  - Closed-chain activities: Mini squats, heel raises, side stepping, step-ups and -downs
- Address functional mobility
  - Bed-mobility training
  - Transfer training with use of assistive device: Rolling walker, bilateral axillary crutches
- Address scar mobility
  - Scar tissue mobilization progressing from parallel to perpendicular upon wound closure
- Address proprioception[4]
  - Standing balance activities on level surface
    - Eyes open
    - Eyes closed
  - Standing balance activities with use of foam
    - Eyes open
    - Eyes closed
  - Standing balance activities on balance machines
    - Gait training[8]
  - Lateral weight shifting to improve stance time on injured LE
  - Promote push-off and heel strike
  - Promote increased hip extension during mid/terminal stance
  - Promote knee flexion during swing phase of gait

FUNCTIONAL GOALS

- Patient will be able to
  - Perform bed mobility independently so as to decrease burden of care.
  - Improve 6MWT to 1150 ft so as to enhance community mobility.
  - Increase Berg Balance Score to 47/56 to decrease fall risk.
  - Increase active knee flexion to 100 degrees to ascend and descend a flight of stairs.

PROGNOSIS

- Good, though speed of recovery varies depending on age of the individual.
- Individuals older than 60 years have a 17% mortality rate and 54% complication rate.[9]

PATIENT RESOURCE

- Keany JE. Femur Fracture Follow-up: Prognosis. Medscape Reference. http://emedicine.medscape.com/article/824856-followup#a2650. Accessed July 1, 2013.

REFERENCES

1. The American Physical Therapy Association. Pattern 4G: impaired joint mobility, muscle performance, and range of motion associated with fracture. *Interactive Guide to Physical Therapist Practice*. 2003. doi: 10.2522/ptguide.3.1_7. http://guidetoptpractice.apta.org/content/1/SEC14.extract?sid=59a2cf68-8568-4df8-87e4-749de05c23bb. Accessed May 27, 2014.

2. Hall SJ. The biomechanics of human bone growth and development. In: *Basic Biomechanics*.4th ed. New York, NY: McGraw-Hill; 2007:Chapter 4. http://www.accessphysiotherapy.com/abstract/6060836#6060838. Accessed July 5, 2013.
3. Stannard JP, Schmidt AH, Kregor PJ. *Surgical Treatment of Orthopaedic Trauma*. New York, NY: Thieme; 2007.
4. Malone TR, Hazle C, Grey ML. Imaging in Rehabilitation. New York, NY: McGraw-Hill; 2008. http://www.accessphysiotherapy.com/resource/613. Accessed July 5, 2013.
5. Dutton M. Orthopaedic examination, evaluation, and intervention. New York, NY: McGraw-Hill; 2008. http://www.accessphysiotherapy.com/resource/612. Accessed July 5, 2013.
6. Prentice WE. Cryotherapy and thermotherapy. In: Prentice WE, Quillen WS, Underwood F, eds. *Therapeutic Modalities in Rehabilitation*. 4th ed. New York, NY: McGraw-Hill; 2011:Chapter 9. http://www.accessphysiotherapy.com/content/8137995#8137995. Accessed July 5, 2013.
7. Hooker DN, Prentice WE. Chapter 5. Basic principles of electricity and electrical stimulating currents. In: Prentice WE, Quillen WS, Underwood F, eds. *Therapeutic Modalities in Rehabilitation*. 4th ed. New York, NY: McGraw-Hill; 2011. http://www.accessphysiotherapy.com/content/8136367#8136367. Accessed July 2, 2013.
8. Dutton M. *McGraw Hill's NPTE (National Physical Therapy Examination)*. 2nd ed. New York, NY: McGraw-Hill; 2012. http://www.accessphysiotherapy.com/resource/611. Accessed July 1, 2013.
9. Keany JE. Femur fracture follow-up: prognosis. *Medscape Reference*. http://emedicine.medscape.com/article/824856-followup#a2650. Accessed July 1, 2013.

ADDITIONAL REFERENCES

- Goodman CC, Boissonnault WG, Fuller KS. *Pathology: Implications for the Physical Therapist*. 2nd ed. Philadelphia, PA: Saunders; 2003.
- ICD-9-CM. http://www.icd9data.com. Accessed July 1, 2013.
- ICD-10-CM. http://www.icd10data.com. Accessed July 1, 2013.
- Kisner C, Colby LA. *Therapeutic Exercise: Foundations and Techniques*. 5th ed. Philadelphia, PA: F.A. Davis Company; 2007.
- Magee DJ. *Orthopedic Physical Assessment*. 5th ed. St. Louis, MO: Saunders Elsevier; 2008.

184 HIP ADDUCTOR STRAIN

Eric Shamus, PhD, DPT, PT, CSCS
Patricia M. Tripp, PhD, ATC

CONDITION/DISORDER SYNONYM

- Groin (adductor) strain

ICD-9-CM CODES

- 843 Sprains and strains of hip and thigh
- 843.8 Sprain of other specified sites of hip and thigh
- 843.9 Sprain of unspecified site of hip and thigh

ICD-10-CM CODES

- S73.109A Unspecified sprain of unspecified hip, initial encounter
- S73.199A Other sprain of unspecified hip, initial encounter
- S76.919A Strain of unspecified muscles, fascia and tendons at thigh level, unspecified thigh, initial encounter

PREFERRED PRACTICE PATTERN

- 4E: Impaired Joint Mobility, Motor Function, Muscle Performance, and Range of Motion Associated with Localized Inflammation[1]

PATIENT PRESENTATION

A 65-year-old physically active and otherwise healthy female (5'7 in, 160 lb) slipped on ice while exiting the passenger side of a car. She described the scenario such that as she attempted to leave the vehicle and stood on her right leg, her foot slipped out beneath her. Although she grabbed onto the door for support and did not fall, she reported feeling a "pulling" sensation and immediate pain over her right inner thigh. She reported to the clinic for assessment—4 days postinjury. She states her inner thigh became "bruised" (black-and-blue) over the past 2 days and the pain has caused difficulty sleeping and performing activities of daily living. As she entered the clinic, she had a slight limp, with shortened stance time noted during right limb ambulation. Her chief complaint is pain. She presented with palpable pain and muscular defect over the mid-muscle belly of her adductor magnus. Active range of motion for hip flexion and extension is within normal limits (WNL), but she reports pain with hip adduction, abduction, and internal/external rotation. Passive ROM elicits pain during hip abduction and external rotation. She has 5/5 strength with hip flexion, extension, external rotation, and abduction; and 4/5 with hip adduction and internal rotation.

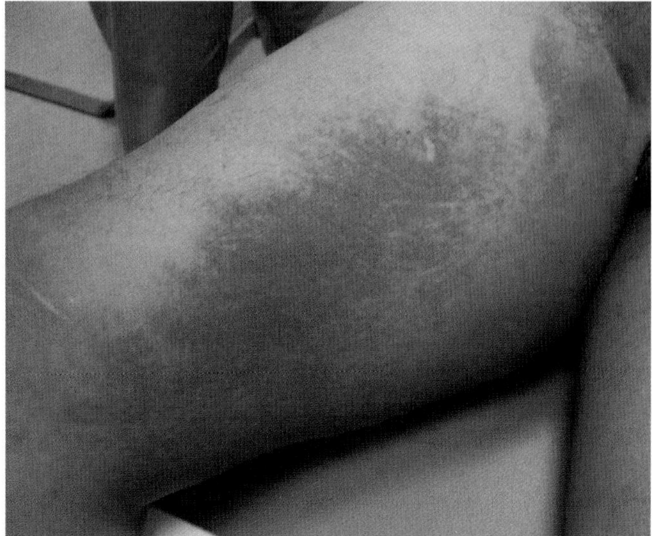

FIGURE 184-1 Adductor muscle strain/rupture is heralded in this patient by the degree of ecchymosis present. (From Simon RR, Sherman SC. *Emergency Orthopedics*. 6th ed. http://www.accessemergencymedicine.com.)

KEY FEATURES

Description

- Partial or complete tearing of the adductor muscles
  - Pectineus
  - Adductor brevis
  - Adductor longus
  - Adductor magnus
  - Gracilis
- May report feeling a pop/pulling sensation in the muscle
- Condition may result in abnormal stress to the pubic bone, pubic tubercle, or pubic symphysis
- Pubalgia–osteitis pubis: A collective term referring to disorders that cause chronic pubic pain
- Symptoms from increased mechanical stress in pubic region due to abnormalities or stress from osseous, ligamentous, or muscular structures

Essentials of Diagnosis

- Diagnosed primarily through signs and symptoms, exclusion of other pathologies typical to the region
- Defect of muscle fibers likely on palpation
- Grade 1: Minor stretch or tear of less than 10% of fibers
- Grade 2: 10% to 90% of fibers torn
- Grade 3: Full tear, rupture
- Can result from chronic, repetitive stress/exertion during sport (kicking, sprinting, or twisting at high speeds) (dynamic overloading)
- May be acute tear with sudden movement of hip abduction (overstretching)
- Rule out referred pain from other orthopedic (pelvis, spine) or medical (intra-abdominal pathology, hernia) pathologies

General Considerations

- Pubalgia–osteitis pubis: A collective term referring to disorders that cause chronic pubic pain

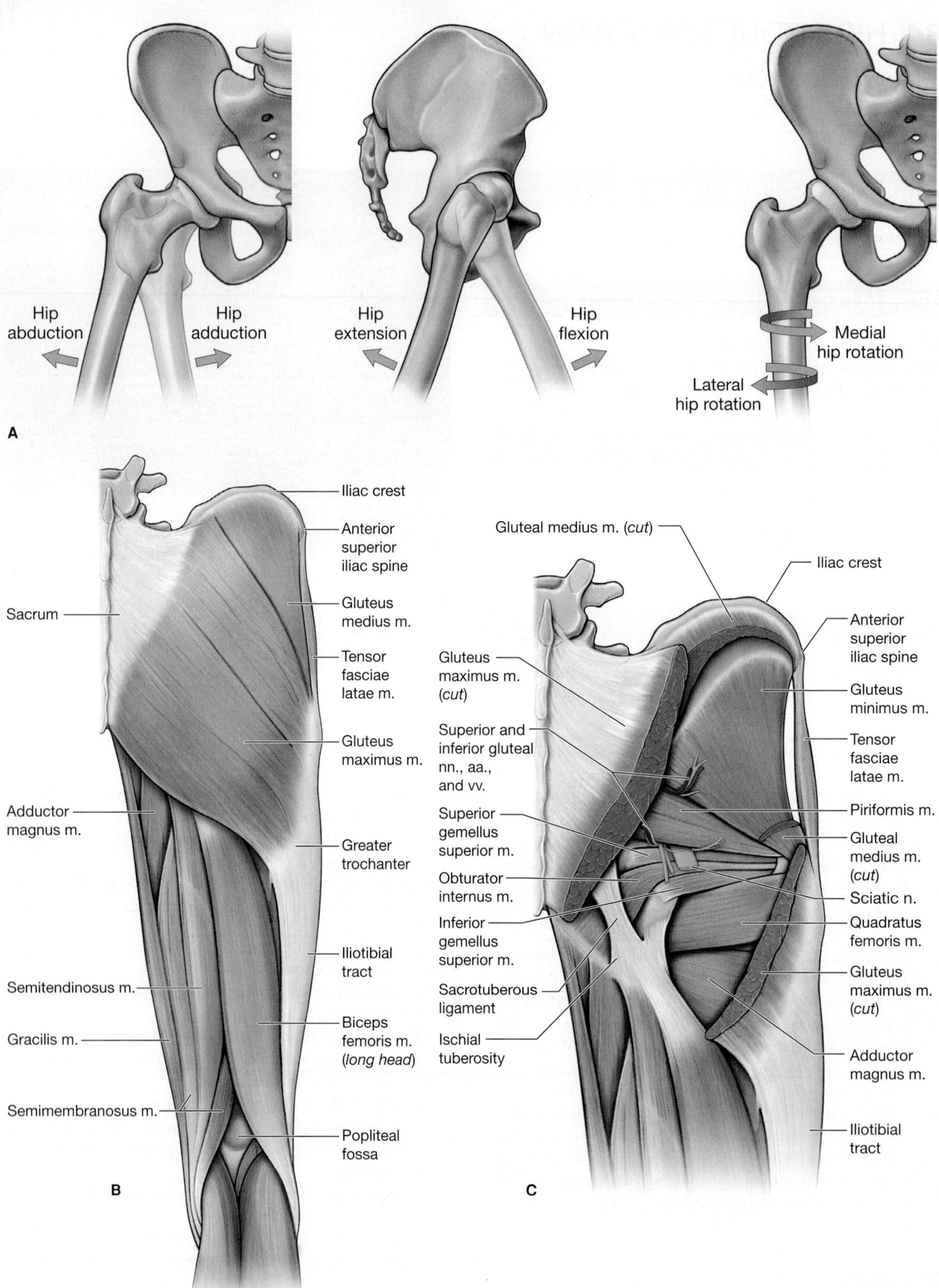

FIGURE 184-2 (**A**) Actions of the hip joint. The right gluteal region illustrating the posterior view of the superficial gluteal muscles (**B**) and the deep gluteal muscles (**C**). (From Morton DA, Foreman KB, Albertine KH. *The Big Picture: Gross Anatomy*. http://www.accessmedicine.com. Copyright © The McGraw-Hill Companies, Inc. All rights reserved.)

- Caused by repeated trauma from activities that over stress the pubic bone or tendons, causing shearing of the pubic symphysis
- Diagnosis often made through exclusion of other pathologies
- Full history, medical screening, and differential examination of pelvic/lower abdominal ensure appropriate diagnosis
- Treatment based on severity, duration of symptoms, associated pathology, physician preference

Demographics

- Common in participants of exertional sports/dynamic loading or shearing of pelvis or abduction of thigh
- Often a result of slip and fall

CLINICAL FINDINGS

SIGNS AND SYMPTOMS

- Medial thigh pain during functional activities requiring pelvic stabilization (i.e., kicking, running, sprinting, squats)
- Tenderness over the muscle belly or myotendinous junction
- Possible tenderness over proximal insertions of the adductor tendons or insertion of the rectus abdominus at pubic bone
- Possible pain and limited ROM with passive hip abduction or external rotation
- Possible weakness of lower abdominals or any components of hip musculature

Functional Limitations

- Pain/Limitation with ambulation, exacerbated with running
- Pain/Limitation between sitting and rising from chair
- Pain/Limitation with getting up from floor
- Pain/Limitation with rising from supine positions

Possible Contributing Causes

- Hip and/or pelvic muscle imbalance
- Forceful trauma or slipping of leg into abduction
- Limited ROM in hip/femoral acetabular impingement
- Increased tone or shortening of iliopsoas, rectus abdominus, or hip adductors
- Participation in exertional sports (i.e., hockey, soccer, track)
- Pubic instability

Differential Diagnosis

- Athletic pubalgia
- Bladder infection
- Femoral neck stress fracture
- Iliopsoas abscess
- Inguinal hernia
- Lower abdominal (rectus abdominus) strain
- Osteitis pubis
- Osteosarcoma
- Osteomyelitis
- Pelvic inflammatory disease
- Pelvic sprain
- Prostatitis
- Pubalgia
- Pubic stress fracture
- Sacral dysfunction

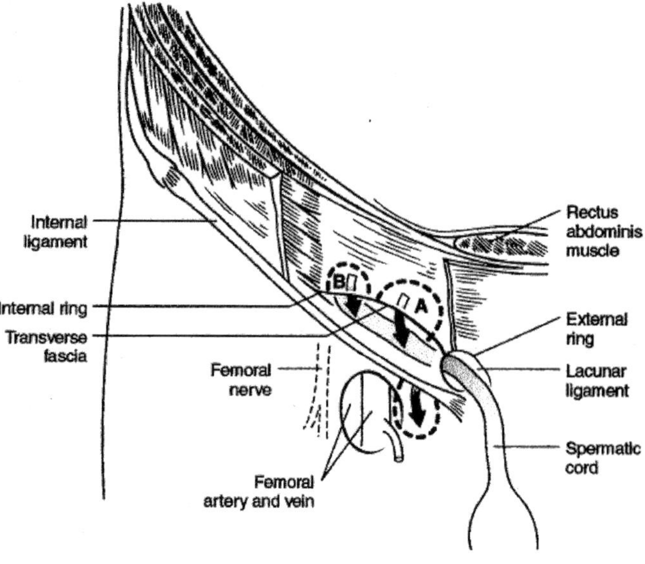

FIGURE 184-3 Anatomic location of groin hernias. Direct hernia (**A**), indirect hernia (**B**), femoral hernia (right groin from an anterior view) (**C**). (From Toy EC, Liu TH, Campbell AR. *Case Files: Surgery*. 3rd ed. www.accesssurgery.com. Copyright © The McGraw-Hill Companies, Inc. All rights reserved.)

MEANS OF CONFIRMATION OR DIAGNOSIS

Imaging

- None required for diagnosis
- Radiographs (X-rays), typically normal with positive osteotic changes noted with chronic or comorbid conditions
- MRI may show inflammation (i.e., pubic rami) or torn fibers and rule in or rule out comorbid condition(s)
- Bone scan to rule out differentials like bone cancer or osteocarcinoma

Diagnostic Procedures

- Diagnosis based on patient history, signs and symptoms, exclusion of alternate orthopedic and medical conditions

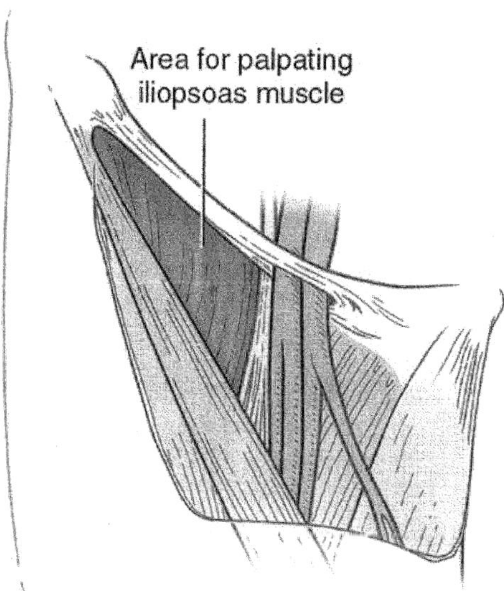

FIGURE 184-4 Shenton line extends from the inferior border of the femoral neck to the inferior border of the pubic ramus. Interruption of this line suggests an abnormally positioned femoral head. (Reproduced with permission from Simon RR, Sherman SC. *Emergency Orthopedics*. 6th ed. http://www.accessemergencymedicine.com. Copyright © The McGraw-Hill Companies, Inc. All rights reserved.)

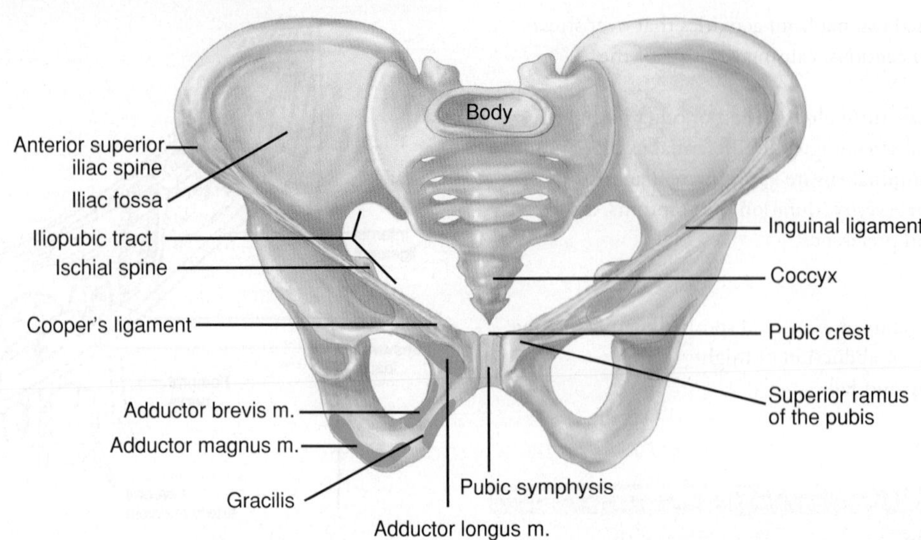

FIGURE 184-5 Ligaments that contribute to the inguinal canal include the inguinal ligament, which spans the anterior superior iliac spine to the pubic bone. Cooper ligament is seen as the lateral extension of the lacunar ligament, which is the fanning out of the inguinal ligament as it joins the pubic tubercle. The iliopubic tract originates and inserts in a similar fashion to the inguinal ligament, yet it is deep to it. m., muscle. (From Brunicardi FC et al. *Schwartz's Principles of Surgery*. 9th ed. http://www.accessmedicine.com. Copyright © The McGraw-Hill Companies, Inc. All rights reserved.)

FINDINGS AND INTERPRETATION

- Radiographs may be normal, but likely have positive findings with chronic duration.
  - Articular erosion at pubic symphysis
  - Subarticular sclerosis at pubic symphysis
- MRI may show inflammation or torn fibers
  - May confirm suspicion of comorbid condition (i.e., athletic pubalgia tendinous involvement with edema in insertion of adductor musculature or rectus abdominus)

TREATMENT

Medication

- NSAIDs

MEDICAL PROCEDURES

- Surgical intervention for associated injuries
  - Tendinous tears, hernia repair, athletic pubalgia (pelvic floor reconstruction surgery), etc.

REFERRALS/ADMITTANCE

- To radiologist for imaging: X-ray, MRI, bone scan[2]
- To primary care for laboratory tests, evaluate for rheumatic disorder or infection
- To orthopedist for surgical consult for failed conservative treatment

IMPAIRMENTS

- Pain with ADLs (sitting and/or rising from a seated position, gait initiation from a seated position)
  - Muscle imbalances and/or muscle length changes to hip abductors/external rotators versus adductors/internal rotators

TESTS AND MEASURES

- Pain, visual analog scale (VAS) or PQRST method for pain assessment
- Functional independence measure
  - Locomotion
- Neurologic examination
  - Proprioception at the hip
  - Kinesthetic awareness at the hip
  - Coordination
- Trunk active and passive ROM
- Hip and knee active and passive ROM
- Flexibility testing
  - Hamstrings
  - Iliopsoas
  - Quadriceps
  - Iliotibial band
  - Abductors
  - Adductors
  - Internal rotators
  - External rotators
- Joint integrity of the lumbar spine
- Sacroiliac joint integrity
- Selective tissue tension tests
- Hip joint integrity
  - Hip scour
  - Flexion, abduction, external rotation (FABER) test
  - Flexion, adduction, internal rotation (FAIR) or (FADIR) test
- Limb strength
  - Manual muscle test (MMT)
    - Hamstrings
    - Quadriceps
    - Iliopsoas
    - Gluteus maximus
    - Gluteus medius
    - Gluteus minimus
    - Adductors
    - Internal rotators
    - External rotators
- LE contralateral limb strength

- Balance
  - Static single-leg standing (eyes open, eyes closed)
    - Contralateral LE
  - Dynamic standing
    - Berg Balance Scale
    - Functional Gait Assessment
- Gait assessment
  - Observational analysis
  - Gait speed via the 10-m walk test
  - Lateral running drill
  - 6-minute walk test
  - Retro running

INTERVENTION

- Intervention will vary on the basis of the severity of symptoms
- Rest and inflammation reduction in early stages of treatment
- Restoration of muscular flexibility and strength in subacute stages of treatment
- Progressive weight bearing and exertion to so as to resume activities in advanced stages
- Modification/avoidance of
  - Running, jumping, squatting, kicking
  - Sports participation
- Exercise interventions
  - Muscle flexibility
  - Strengthening: Eccentric training
  - Progressive weight-bearing activities, then progressive exertion to resume athletic participation
  - Therapeutic modalities (i.e., massage, ultrasound, ice/heat, electrical stimulation, etc.)

FUNCTIONAL GOALS

- Patient will be able to
  - Rise from squatting positions without pain.
  - Perform variable-effort running activities without pain or compensatory patterns.
  - Resume twisting and pivoting athletic activities without pain or compensatory patterns.

PROGNOSIS

- Good, if first-time injury and proper therapy with eccentric training.
- Prognosis depends on underlying cause of the inflammation and patient's ability to control exacerbating activities and perform optimal dosage of therapeutic exercise.

PATIENT RESOURCE

- American Physical Therapy Association. *Physical Therapist's Guide to Groin Strain.* August 17, 2012. http://www.moveforwardpt.com/SymptomsConditionsDetail.aspx?cid=a718efd4-8b6c-4b7b-af9c-adeb8a5e7745. Accessed July 6, 2013.

REFERENCES

1. The American Physical Therapy Association. Pattern 4E: impaired joint mobility, motor function, muscle performance, and range of motion associated with localized inflammation. *Interactive Guide to Physical Therapist Practice.* 2003. doi: 10.2522/ptguide. 3.1_5. http://guidetoptpractice.apta.org/content/1/SEC12.extract?sid=abc7296a-dada-4fa6-baea-b4b8cd1517df. Accessed May 27, 2014.
2. Dutton M. The hip joint. In: Dutton M, ed. *Orthopaedic Examination, Evaluation, and Intervention.* 2nd ed. New York, NY: McGraw-Hill; 2008:841–931. http://www.accessphysiotherapy.com/resource/612. Accessed July 1, 2013.

ADDITIONAL REFERENCES

- Anderson J, Read J. The pelvis, hip and thigh. In: Anderson J, Read J, eds. *Atlas of Imaging in Sports Medicine.* 2nd ed. Australia: McGraw Hill; 285–390.
- Atkins JM, Taylor JC, Kane SF. Acute and overuse injuries of the abdomen and groin in athletes. *Curr Sports Med Rep.* 2010;9(2):115–120.
- Bradshaw C, Holmich P. Longstanding groin pain. In: *Clinical Sports Medicine.* 3rd ed. Australia: McGraw-Hill; 2009: 405–426.
- Dutton M. The hip joint. In: Dutton M, ed. *Dutton's Orthopedic Survival Guide: Managing Common Conditions.* New York, NY: McGraw Hill; 2011:589–592.
- Emery CA, Meeuwisse WH. Risk factors for groin injuries in hockey. *Med Sci Sports Exerc.* 2001;33(9):1423–1433.
- Holmich P, Larsen K, Krogsgaard K, Gluud C. Exercise program for prevention of groin pain in football players: a cluster-randomized trial. *Scand J Med Sci Sports.* 2010;20(6):814–821.
- Hureibi KA, McLatchie GR. Groin pain in athletes. *Scott Med J.* 2010;55(2):8–11.
- ICD9DATA. http://www.icd9data.com. Accessed July 6, 2013.
- ICD10DATA. http://www.icd10data.com. Accessed July 6, 2013.
- Maffey L, Emery C. What are the risk factors for groin strain injury in sport: a systematic review of the literature. *Sports Med.* 2007;37(10):881–894.
- Morelli V, Smith V. Groin Injuries in Athletes. *Am Fam Physician.* 2001;64(8):1405–1414.
- Nicholas SJ, Tyler TF. Adductor muscle strains in sport. *Sports Med.* 2002;32(5):339–344.
- Prentice WE. The thigh, hip, groin, and pelvis. In: Prentice WE, ed. *Principles of Athletic Training: A Competency-Based Approach.* New York, NY: McGraw-Hill; 2011: 604–638.

185 HIP DISLOCATION, ACQUIRED

Patrick S. Pabian, DPT, PT, SCS, OCS, CSCS

CONDITION/DISORDER SYNONYM

- Hip subluxation

ICD-9-CM CODES

- 835 Dislocation of hip
- 835.0 Closed dislocation of hip
- 835.00 Closed dislocation of hip, unspecified site
- 835.01Closed posterior dislocation of hip
- 835.02 Closed obturator dislocation of hip
- 835.03 Other closed anterior dislocation of hip
- 835.1 Open dislocation of hip
- 835.10 Open dislocation of hip, unspecified site
- 835.11 Open posterior dislocation of hip
- 835.12 Open obturator dislocation of hip
- 835.13 Other open anterior dislocation of hip

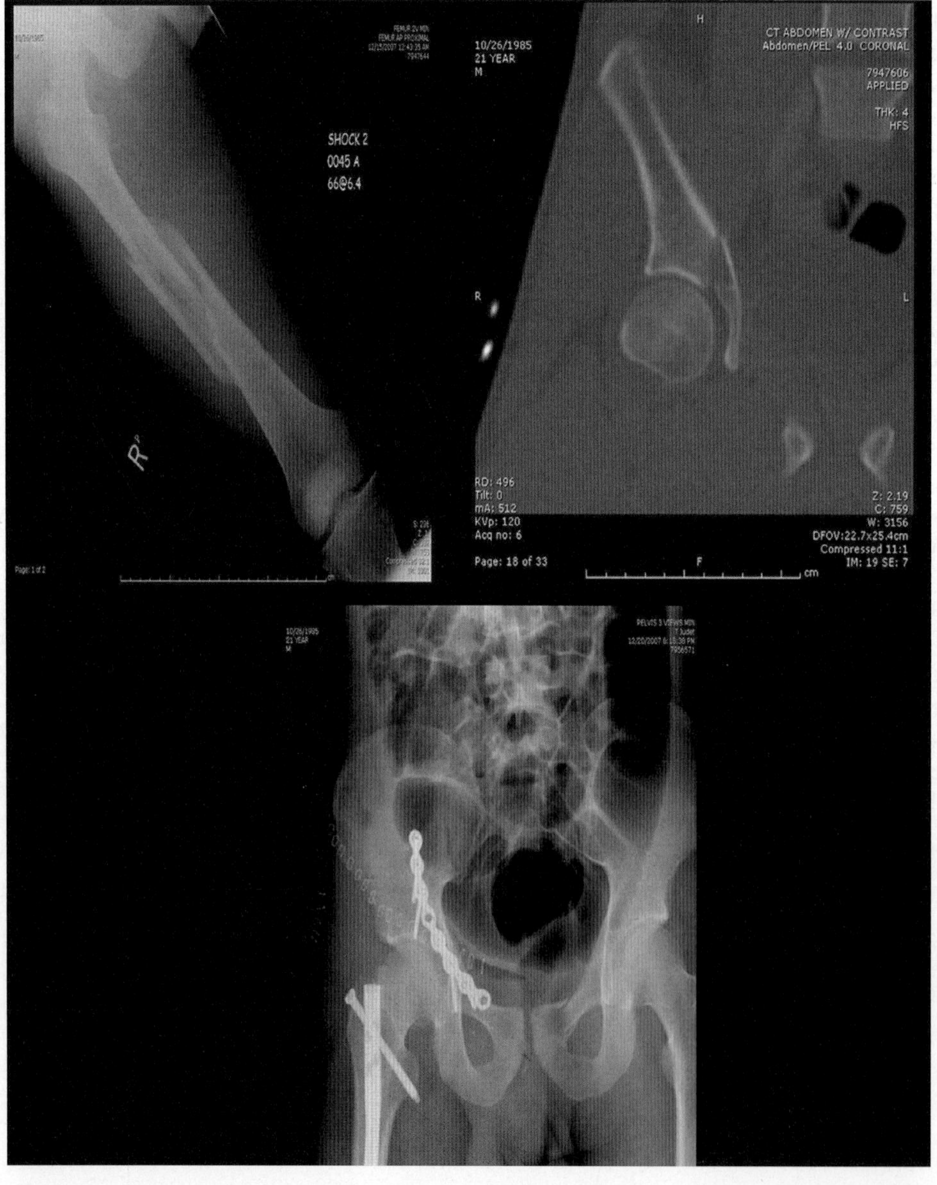

FIGURE 185-1 Computed tomographic image (*top*) and x-ray (*bottom*) of a patient with a spiral fracture of the right femur with an ipsilateral acetabular fracture. X-ray images postoperatively demonstrate the reamed nail with locking screw that internally fixes the femur, as well as the acetabular plate fixation. Note also the pubic ramus fracture that did not require surgical treatment. (From Brunicardi FC et al. *Schwartz's Principles of Surgery*. 9th ed. http://www.accessmedicine.com. Copyright © The McGraw-Hill Companies, Inc. All rights reserved.)

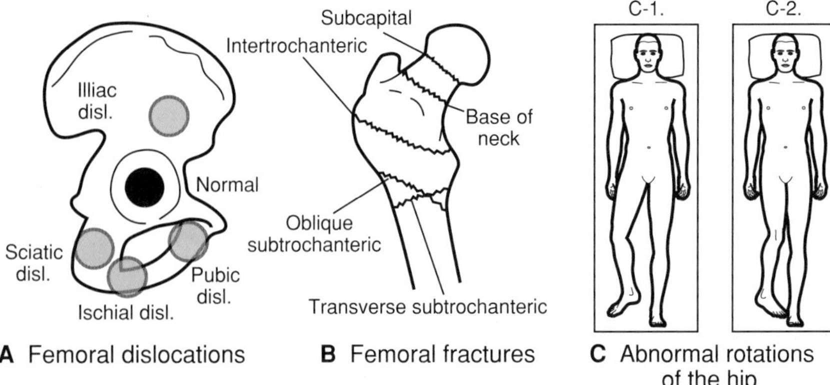

FIGURE 185-2 Femoral dislocations and fractures. (From LeBlond RF, DeGowin RL, Brown DD. *DeGowin's Diagnostic Examination*. 9th ed. http://www.accessmedicine.com. Copyright © The McGraw-Hill Companies, Inc. All rights reserved.)

ICD-10-CM CODES

- S71.009A Unspecified open wound, unspecified hip, initial encounter
- S73.00 Unspecified subluxation and dislocation of hip
- S73.006A Unspecified dislocation of unspecified hip, initial encounter
- S73.016A Posterior dislocation of unspecified hip, initial encounter
- S73.026A Obturator dislocation of unspecified hip, initial encounter
- S73.036A Other anterior dislocation of unspecified hip, initial encounter

PREFERRED PRACTICE PATTERN

- 4D: Impaired Joint Mobility, Motor Function, Muscle Performance, and Range of Motion Associated with Connective Tissue Dysfunction

PATIENT PRESENTATION

A 35-year-old female presents with global hip pain and dysfunction after a posterior hip dislocation 2 weeks ago. The patient sustained a hip dislocation when the car she was riding in rear-ended another vehicle. The patient reports her knee pressed into the dashboard during accident, resulting in immediate pain in her posterior hip. As EMS arrived, it was noted that her lower extremity (LE) appeared shorter than her uninvolved. After emergency transport to the ER, pre-reduction X-rays revealed posterior dislocation of the femoral head from the acetabulum. Pre- and post-reduction X-rays did not show evidence of associated fractures of acetabulum or femur.

The patient currently presents with an inability to ambulate without assistive device secondary to pain, weakness and loss of balance. The patient has an inability to don/doff shoes and socks or perform dressing without assistance due to diminished hip mobility. The patient has global weakness of hip musculature and reduced range of motion in all planes of motion. The patient is negative for neurovascular deficits in the involved LE. The physician has ordered follow up X-rays in 6 weeks to see if there are any avascular necrosis signs.

KEY FEATURES

Description

- Disarticulation between the femoral head and acetabulum
- Can occur as a result of trauma in an adult, or congenital in an infant
- Severe hip pain
- Adult presentation
  - Result of traumatic incident often involving force along long axis of femur
  - Typically when the knee is bent (typical to car accident)
  - Resulting in posterior displacement of the femoral head
  - Inability to bear weight on the extremity or move
  - LE appears shortened
  - Femur in an adducted, internally rotated and slightly flexed position
- Infant presentation (Developmental Dysplasia of the Hip)
  - More difficult to detect until child is of ambulatory age
  - Developmental dislocation of the hip

Essentials of Diagnosis

- Emergency, usually associated acetabular and femoral neck fracture

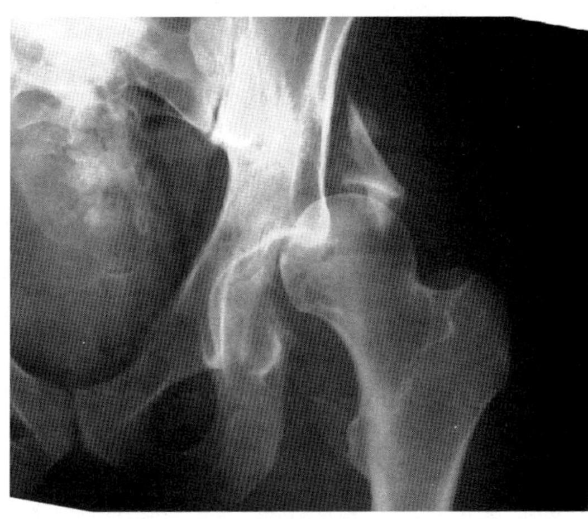

FIGURE 185-3 Posterior hip dislocation with concomitant fracture of the posterior wall and weight-bearing dome of the acetabulum. (From Doherty GM. *Current Diagnosis & Treatment: Surgery*. 13th ed. http://www.accessmedicine.com. Copyright © The McGraw-Hill Companies, Inc. All rights reserved.)

- Adult presentation
  - Patient often has inability to even move the LE
  - Immediate medical referral warranted via activation of EMS
  - Diagnosis confirmed with radiography

General Considerations

- Adult dislocation is traumatic event, result of high velocity incident, and warrants immediate medical notification
  - Dislocation most commonly in the posterior direction
  - Potential exists for injury to the sciatic nerve
  - Avascular necrosis
  - Nerve damage
  - Postreduction neurovascular screening is mandatory

Demographics

- Traumatic is typical for the adult population

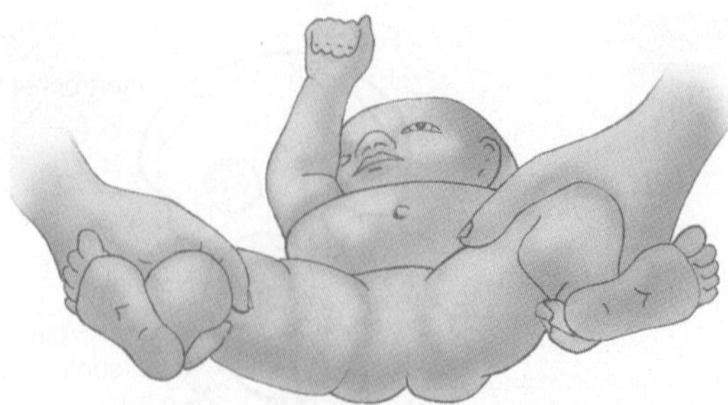

FIGURE 185-4 The Ortolani click test. In subluxation or dislocation, abduction is restricted and the involved hip is unable to be abducted as far as the opposite one, producing an audible or palpable click as the femoral head slips over the acetabular rim. (From Simon RR, Sherman SC. *Emergency Orthopedics*. 6th ed. http://www.accessemergencymedicine.com. Copyright © The McGraw-Hill Companies, Inc. All rights reserved.)

CLINICAL FINDINGS

SIGNS AND SYMPTOMS

- Adult prior to reduction
  - Patient has inability to move hip or bear weight
  - Hip appears shortened and in an adducted, internally rotated, and slightly flexed position
  - Femoral head may be palpable posterior to the acetabulum in the gluteal region
  - Severe bleeding
- Adult postreduction
  - Patient will have pain bearing weight, limited ROM, and gross muscle weakness

Functional Limitations

- Pain/Limitation with walking and running
- Pain/Limitation with squatting into or rising from chair
- Pain/Limitation with getting up from floor

Possible Contributing Causes

- Adult
  - Injury related to traumatic event

Differential Diagnosis

- Proximal femur or pelvic fracture
- Legg–Calvé–Perthes disease
- Slipped femoral capital epiphysis

MEANS OF CONFIRMATION OR DIAGNOSIS

Imaging[1]

- Adult
  - Plain-film radiographs
  - Ultrasonography
  - CT
  - MRI

FINDINGS AND INTERPRETATION

- Plain-film radiographs, trauma series for the hip will confirm diagnosis. Plain-film radiographs will reveal disarticulation
- Ultrasonography, visualization of the cartilage
- CT, sensitive to osteochondral defects
- MRI, subtle occult fractures

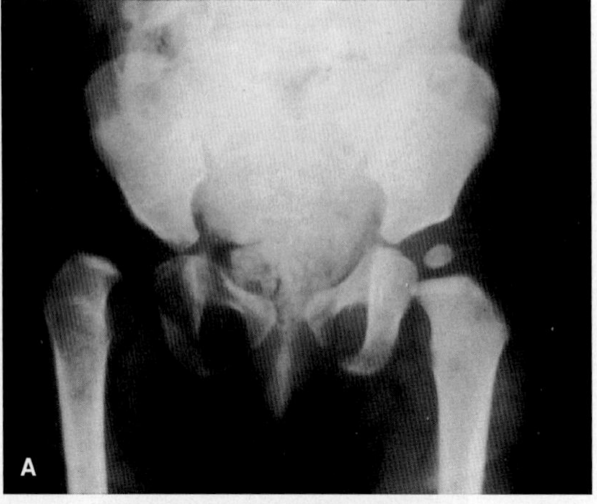

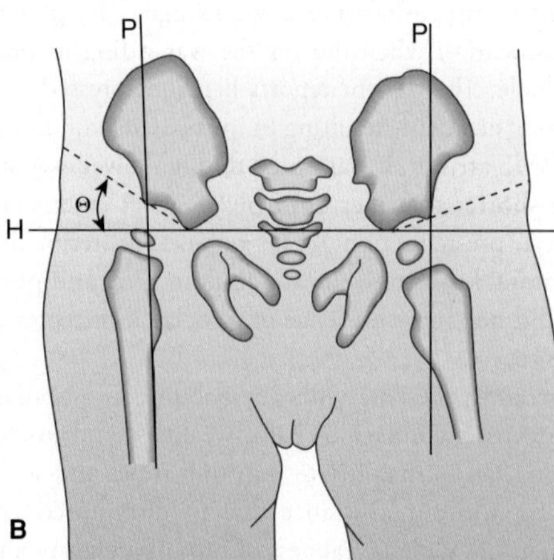

FIGURE 185-5 (**A**) X-ray of congenital dislocation of the right hip. (**B**) Analysis of hip radiographs presupposes adequately exposed films of a properly positioned patient. Hilgenreiner horizontal line is drawn through both triradiate cartilages (H), and Perkins vertical line is drawn through the outer margin of each acetabulum (P). If the hip is located, the proximal femoral epiphysis will lie in the inferomedial quadrant formed by the two intersecting lines. Proximal or lateral displacement indicates dislocation. Abnormal acetabular development is suggested by lack of obvious concavity and by an acetabular index (Θ) greater than 30 degrees. (From Doherty GM. *Current Diagnosis & Treatment: Surgery*. 13th ed. http://www.accessmedicine.com. Copyright © The McGraw-Hill Companies, Inc. All rights reserved.)

TREATMENT

- Adult
  - Immobilization and bed rest, per physician guidelines, and then weight-bearing exercises with assistive devices over the course of several weeks
  - Treatment based on severity, duration or symptoms, associated pathology, and physician preference

REFERRALS/ADMITTANCE

- Adult
  - Traumatic dislocation warrants immediate medical care

IMPAIRMENTS

- Inability to ambulate due to pain and LE dysfunction
- Weakness or pain with squatting down to perform dressing activities or household chores
- Weakness or pain with rising from squat positions, or ascending/descending stairs

TEST AND MEASURES

- Pain, visual analog scale (VAS)
  - 24-hour pain
  - Worst average pain
  - Best average pain
- Functional independence measure
  - Locomotion
- Cardiovascular integrity
  - Blood pressure at rest and after activity
  - Heart rate at rest and after activity
- Skin integrity
  - Scar
    - Approximation
    - Mobility/Pliability
  - Associated skin assessment
    - Edema (linear girth measurements, palpation)
    - Color
    - Signs of infection
    - Mobility/turgor
    - Temperature
- Neurologic examination
  - Sensation
    - Light touch
    - Pin prick
  - LE deep tendon reflexes
  - Proprioception at the hip
  - Kinesthetic awareness at the hip
  - Coordination
- Trunk active and passive ROM
- Hip and knee active and passive ROM
- Flexibility testing
  - Hamstrings
  - Iliopsoas
  - Quadriceps
  - Iliotibial band
  - Abductors
  - Adductors
- Joint integrity of the spine
- Sacroiliac joint integrity

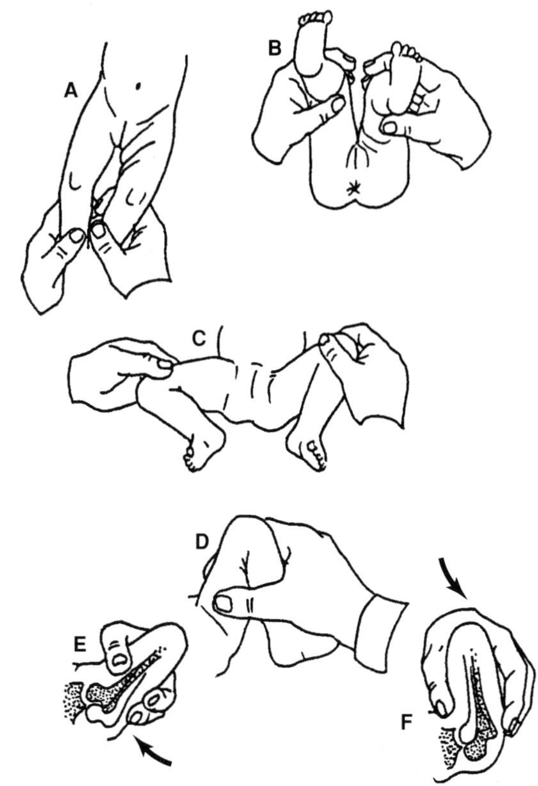

FIGURE 185-6 Clinical examination of developmental dislocation of the hip. In all pictures, the child's left hip is the abnormal side. (**A**) Asymmetric skin folds. (**B**) Galeazzi test. (**C**) Limitation of abduction. (**D–E–F**) Ortolani and Barlow tests (see text). (From Skinner HB. *Current Diagnosis & Treatment in Orthopedics*. 4th ed. http://www.accessmedicine.com. Copyright © The McGraw-Hill Companies, Inc. All rights reserved.)

- Hip joint integrity
  - Hip scour
  - Flexion, abduction, external rotation (FABER) test
  - Flexion, adduction, internal rotation (FAIR) or (FADIR) test
- Limb strength
  - Functional strength testing
    - Five-times sit-to-stand test
  - Manual muscle test (MMT)
    - Hamstrings
    - Quadriceps
    - Iliopsoas
    - Gluteus maximus
    - Gluteus medius
    - Gluteus minimus
    - Adductors
- LE contralateral limb strength
- Balance
  - Static single-leg standing (eyes open, eyes closed)
    - Contralateral LE
  - Dynamic standing
    - Berg Balance Scale
    - Functional Gait Assessment
- Gait assessment
  - Observational analysis
  - Gait speed via the 10-m walk test
  - 2-minute walk test
  - 6-minute walk test
  - Retro running

INTERVENTION

- Adult: Post reduction interventions will focus on restoration of joint mobility, strength/stability, and progression of weight-bearing activities
  - Acute
    - Progressive ambulation with assistive devices
    - ROM
    - Muscle flexibility and strengthening per presenting deficits
    - Rest
    - Ice
    - TENS for pain control
    - Cryotherapy
  - Chronic
    - Progressive weight-bearing activities to restore to prior level of function
    - Restoration of preinjury strength, muscular flexibility, and joint mobility
    - Functional training to restore prior level of function

FUNCTIONAL GOALS

- Patient will be able to
  - Squat to don/doff shoes without pain or weakness.
  - Sit up without assistance of upper extremities.
  - Rise from squatting positions without pain.
  - Perform variable effort running activities without pain or compensatory patterns.
  - Perform twisting and pivoting athletic activities without pain or compensatory patterns.

PROGNOSIS

- Good prognosis.
- Prognosis is dependent on the underlying cause of the dislocation and associated injuries from the incident.

PATIENT RESOURCE

- American Academy of Orthopaedic Surgeons. *Live It Safe: Prevent Broken Hips.* http://orthoinfo.aaos.org/topic.cfm?topic=A00305. Accessed June 10, 2013.

REFERENCE

1. McKinnis L. Radiologic evaluation of the pelvis and hip. In: McKinnis L, ed. *Fundamentals of Musculoskeletal Imaging.* 2nd ed. Philadelphia, PA: F.A. Davis Company; 2005.

ADDITIONAL REFERENCES

- Bradshaw C, Holmich P. Longstanding groin pain. In: *Clinical Sports Medicine.* 3rd ed. Australia: McGraw-Hill; 2009: 405–426.
- Dutton M. Differential diagnosis. In: Dutton M, ed. *Orthopaedic Examination, Evaluation, and Intervention.* 2nd ed. New York, NY: McGraw-Hill; 2008:Chapter 9. http://www.accessphysiotherapy.com/content/5545886. Accessed June 28, 2013.
- Dutton M. The hip joint. In: Dutton M, ed. *Dutton's Orthopedic Survival Guide: Managing Common Conditions.* New York, NY: McGraw-Hill; 2011:Chapter 8. http://www.accessphysiotherapy.com/content/8653838. Accessed June 28, 2013.
- Hay WW, Levin MJ, Sondheimer JM, Deterding RR. Hip injuries. In: Hay WW, Levin MJ, Sondheimer JM, Deterding RR, eds. *CURRENT Diagnosis & Treatment: Pediatrics.* 20th ed. New York, NY: McGraw-Hill; 2011. http://www.accessphysiotherapy.com/content/6586266. Accessed June 23, 2013.
- ICD9Data.com. http://www.icd9data.com. Accessed June 3, 2013.
- ICD10Data.com. http://www.icd10data.com/ICD10CM/Codes. Accessed June 13, 20123.
- Pattern 4D: Impaired joint mobility, motor function, muscle performance, and range of motion associated with connective tissue dysfunction. In: *Guide to Physical Therapist Practice.* 2nd ed. Alexandria, VA: American Physical Therapy Association; 2001. Revised 2003.
- Prentice WE. The thigh, hip, groin, and pelvis. In: Prentice WE, ed. *Principles of Athletic Training: A Competency-Based Approach.* New York, NY: McGraw-Hill; 2011:604–638.

186 HIP OSTEOARTHRITIS

Eric Shamus, PhD, DPT, PT, CSCS
Reuben Escorpizo, DPT, MSc, PT

CONDITION/DISORDER SYNONYMS

- Hip arthritis
- Hip degenerative joint disease

ICD-9-CM CODES

- 715 Osteoarthrosis and allied disorders
- 715.15 Osteoarthrosis localized primary involving pelvic region and thigh
- 715.25 Osteoarthrosis localized secondary involving pelvic region and thigh
- 715.35 Osteoarthrosis localized not specified whether primary or secondary involving pelvic region and thigh
- 715.9 Osteoarthrosis unspecified whether generalized or localized
- 715.95 Osteoarthrosis unspecified whether generalized or localized involving pelvic region and thigh

ICD-10-CM CODES

- M16.10 Unilateral primary osteoarthritis, unspecified hip
- M16.7 Other unilateral secondary osteoarthritis of hip
- M16.9 Osteoarthritis of hip, unspecified

PREFERRED PRACTICE PATTERNS

- 4D: Impaired Joint Mobility, Motor Function, Muscle Performance, and Range of Motion Associated With Connective Tissue Dysfunction[1]
- 4F: Impaired Joint Mobility, Motor Function, Muscle Performance, Range of Motion, and Reflex Integrity Associated with Spinal Disorders[2]
- 4H: Impaired Joint Mobility, Motor Function, Muscle Performance, and Range of Motion Associated with Joint Arthroplasty[3]
- 4I: Impaired Joint Mobility, Motor Function, Muscle Performance, and Range of Motion Associated with Bony or Soft Tissue Surgery[4]

PATIENT PRESENTATION

Patient is a 58-year-old male with insidious onset of groin pain on the right that has worsen over the years. It bothers him with walking, squatting, and going up and down stairs. He has an x-ray that showed arthritis. He has no complaints of low back pain. There is no other prevalent PMH.

Patient has limited hip range of motion (ROM) on the right with marked limitation in internal rotation. General weakness of all hip musculature 4/5 except adductors are 5/5. Sensation is intact and patient has capsular tightness. States when the hip is "acting up" his walking changes. Today, he has decreased stance time on the right with a wide gait pattern and bilateral decreased step length.

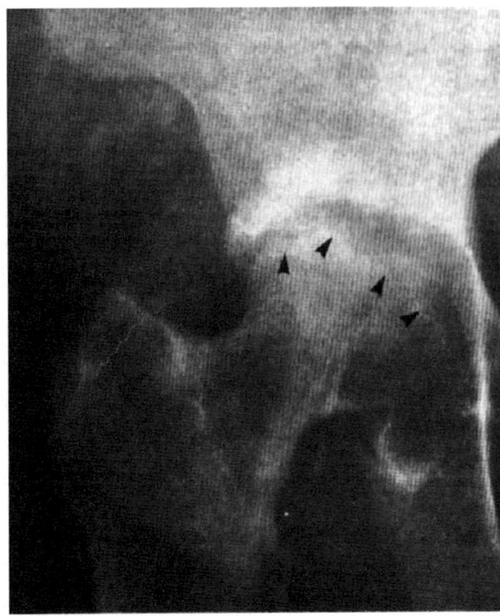

FIGURE 186-1 Frontal view of the right hip in a 59-year-old woman with renal failure and a long history of hemodialysis who was seen in the emergency department having experienced 2 days of intense right hip pain and fever. She had a fall 8 days ago. She has substantial limitation of motion in the right hip on physical examination. (From Chen MYM, Pope TL, Ott DJ. *Basic Radiology*. 2nd ed. http://www.accessmedicine.com. Copyright © The McGraw-Hill Companies, Inc. All rights reserved.)

KEY FEATURES

Description

- Most common form of arthritis
- Degenerative
- Commonly affects hip and knee joints (weight-bearing joints)
- May also affect spinal facet joints
- Associated with increased age, obesity, female sex, race/ethnicity
- Associated with abnormal loading of joints
- Characterized by joint pain
- Arthrosis
- Osteoarthrosis
- Degenerative joint disease

Essentials of Diagnosis

- Radiography is standard method for diagnosis
- Kellgren and Lawrence (KL) grade ≥ 2 (definite radiographic osteoarthritis [OA])[5]
- Osteophytes, joint-space narrowing, sclerosis
- Cartilage lesions, bone marrow lesions, synovitis, effusion, subchondral bone attrition or sclerosis
- Erosion of articular cartilage
- Synovial hyperplasia
- Fibrosis
- Inflammatory cell infiltration
- With or without OA symptoms
- Conventional radiograph is most commonly used tool for diagnosing OA

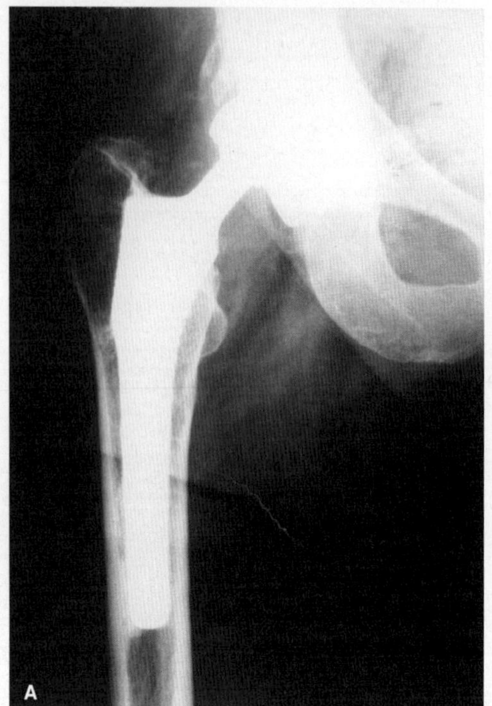

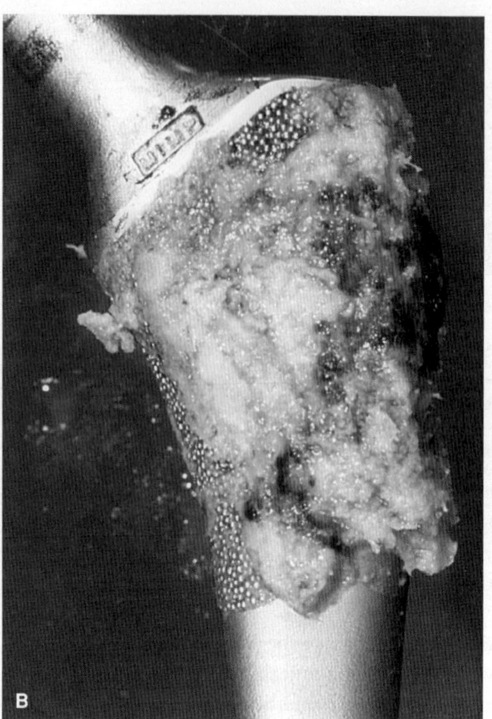

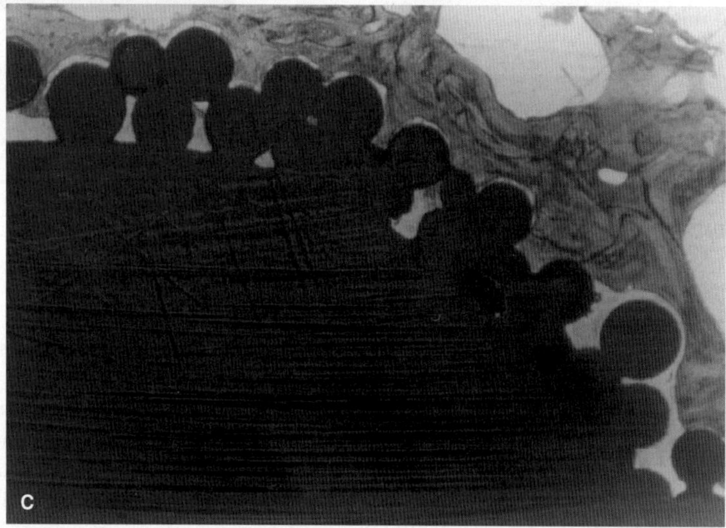

FIGURE 186-2 Four years after implantation, an uncemented porous-coated femoral stem was removed for revision because the patient suffered persistent thigh pain and limp. (**A**) The radiograph taken prior to stem removal showed a relatively poor fit, without subsidence but with the presence of nonanatomic remodeling, as evidenced by the so-called pedestal sign. (**B**) Gross specimen (posterior aspect) analysis suggested that the component was well fixed, as demonstrated by large amounts of bone. (**C**) Histologic examination demonstrated extensive bone ingrowth (basic fuchsin and toluidine blue stain; original magnification × 24). (From Skinner HB. *Current Diagnosis & Treatment in Orthopedics*. 4th ed. http://www.accessmedicine.com.)

General Considerations

- Low bone-mineral density (BMD)
- Bone or joint morphology
- Calcification (e.g., of the knee meniscus)
- Bone formation, cyst formation
- Thickening of subchondral bone plate, osteosclerosis
- Overall joint dysfunction
- Morning stiffness
- Long-term disease
- Secondary problems
  - Muscle atrophy and weakness
  - Bony protrusion or prominence
  - Joint deformity
  - Difficulty walking
  - Difficulty with ADLs

Demographics

- Increased age (middle- to older-age)
- Women more commonly affected than men
- African American and Caucasian more commonly affected than other ethnicities
- May affect approximately 12% of population in United States and other developed countries[6]

CLINICAL FINDINGS

SIGNS AND SYMPTOMS

- Joint pain or aching
- Joint swelling and inflammation (in severe cases)
- Joint stiffness
- Muscle weakness
- Muscle atrophy
- Crepitus
- Bony enlargement
- Limited joint ROM
- Joint-line tenderness
- Joint deformity in severe cases

Functional Implications

- Activity limitation
- Limited mobility
- Limited household and work-related activity
- Decreased overall activity and participation

Possible Contributing Causes

- Chronic factors affecting the joint, such as obesity, BMD
- Joint alignment
- Leg-length discrepancy (LLD)
- Ageing
- Repetitive joint use
- Chronic, vigorous joint loading
- Previous chronic joint injury (e.g., accident, trauma): Secondary OA

Differential Diagnosis

- Ankylosing spondylitis
- Bursitis
- Fibromyalgia syndrome
- Gout
- Polyarthrosis
- Rheumatoid arthritis
- Spondyloarthropathy

MEANS OF CONFIRMATION OR DIAGNOSIS

Laboratory Tests

- Synovial fluid examination (not required)
- Other laboratory tests can be done to rule out other conditions

Imaging

- Conventional radiograph of joint
- MRI of joint
- Diagnostic ultrasound of the joint and synovium[7]

FINDINGS AND INTERPRETATION

- OA is a clinical diagnosis, can be based on
  - Persistent usage-related pain in joint(s)
  - Age 45 years or older[6]
  - Morning stiffness ≤30 minutes[6]
- Imaging studies (e.g., radiograph)
  - Osteophytes, joint-space narrowing, sclerosis
  - Cartilage lesions, bone marrow lesions, synovitis, effusion, subchondral bone attrition or sclerosis
  - Erosion of articular cartilage

TREATMENT

Medication

- NSAIDs (including topical NSAIDs, capsaicin)[7]
- Acetaminophen

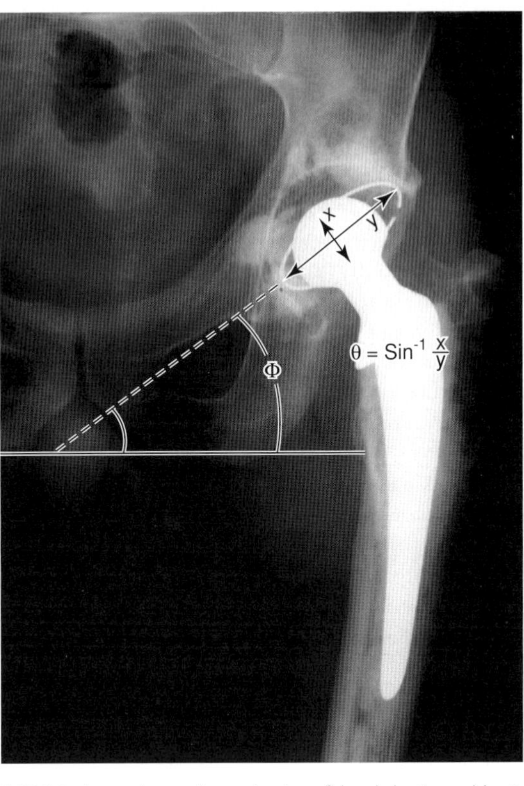

FIGURE 186-3 Approximate determination of the abduction-adduction angle and angle of anteversion of the cup. Exact measurement requires careful control of the direction of the x-ray beam. (From Skinner HB. *Current Diagnosis & Treatment in Orthopedics*. 4th ed. http://www.accessmedicine.com. Copyright © The McGraw-Hill Companies, Inc. All rights reserved.)

- Opioids
- Glucosamine and chondroitin sulfate
- Glucocorticoids or corticosteroids
- Intra-articular injections (corticosteroids, hyaluronic acid)
- Emerging drugs: Anti-tumor necrosis factors (TNF), calcitonin, growth factors, nerve growth factor antibodies

MEDICAL PROCEDURE

- Surgery: Total joint replacement, joint lavage, and debridement

REFERRALS/ADMITTANCE

- To rheumatologist for assessment of underlying complications
- To internal medicine specialist
- To orthopedic specialist
- To physical and rehabilitation medicine specialist
- To surgeon for surgical consult
- To dietician or nutritionist for dietary consult/counseling

IMPAIRMENTS

- Mobility
- Self-care
- Role at home and in community
- School, work, recreation, leisure, sports

TESTS AND MEASURES

- Self-report patient-specific measures of health-related quality of life[3]
  - Patient-specific functional scale (PSFS)

- Pain, visual analog scale (VAS)
  - 24-hour pain
  - Worst average pain
  - Best average pain
- Functional independence measure
  - Bed mobility
  - Transfers
  - Locomotion
- Cardiovascular integrity
  - Blood pressure at rest and after activity
  - Blood pressure in response to position changes
  - Heart rate at rest and after activity
  - Oxygen saturation
  - Presence of lower-extremity (LE) pulses
- Skin Integrity
  - Associated skin assessment
    - Edema (linear girth measurements, palpation)
    - Color
    - Mobility/turgor
    - Temperature
- Neurologic examination
  - Sensation
    - Light touch
    - Pin prick
    - Protective sensation
  - LE deep tendon reflexes
  - Proprioception at the hip/knee
  - Kinesthetic awareness at the hip/knee
  - Coordination
- Trunk active and passive ROM
- Hip and knee active and passive ROM
- Flexibility testing
  - Hamstrings
  - Iliopsoas
  - Quadriceps
  - Iliotibial band
  - Abductors
  - Adductors
- Joint integrity of the spine
- Sacroiliac joint integrity
- Hip joint integrity
  - Hip scour
  - Flexion, abduction, external rotation (FABER) test
  - Flexion, adduction, internal rotation (FAIR) or (FADIR) test
  - FADDIR test: Anterior hip impingement test
- Limb strength
  - Functional strength testing
    - Five-times-sit-to-stand test
  - Manual muscle test (MMT)
    - Hamstrings
    - Quadriceps
    - Iliopsoas
    - Gluteus maximus
    - Gluteus medius
    - Gluteus minimus
    - Adductors
    - Abdominals
    - Multifidus
- LE contralateral limb strength
- Balance

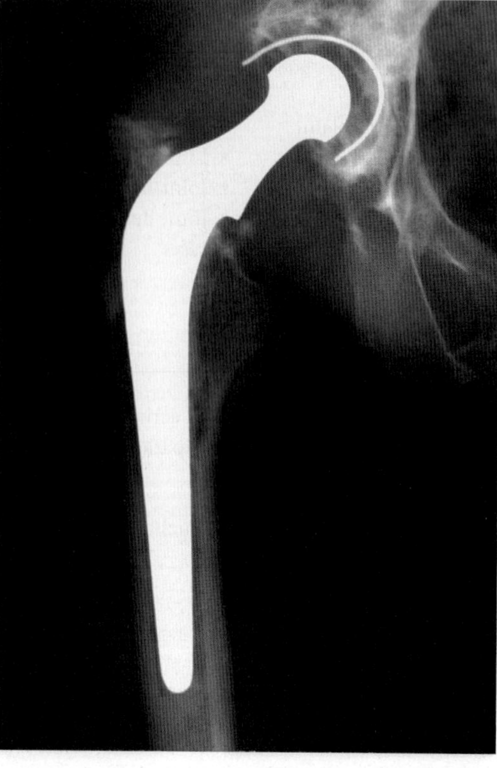

FIGURE 186-4 Radiograph of a Charnley arthroplasty. (From Skinner HB. *Current Diagnosis & Treatment in Orthopedics*. 4th ed. http://www.accessmedicine.com. Copyright © The McGraw-Hill Companies, Inc. All rights reserved.)

  - Static single-leg standing (eyes open, eyes closed)
    - Contralateral LE
  - Dynamic standing
    - Berg Balance Scale
    - Functional Gait Assessment
- Gait assessment
  - Observational analysis
  - Timed Up and Go test
  - Gait speed via the 10-m walk test
  - 2-minute walk test
  - 6-minute walk test
  - Dual task assessment
    - Timed Up and Go: Manual, cognitive
    - Walking while talking test: Simple, complex

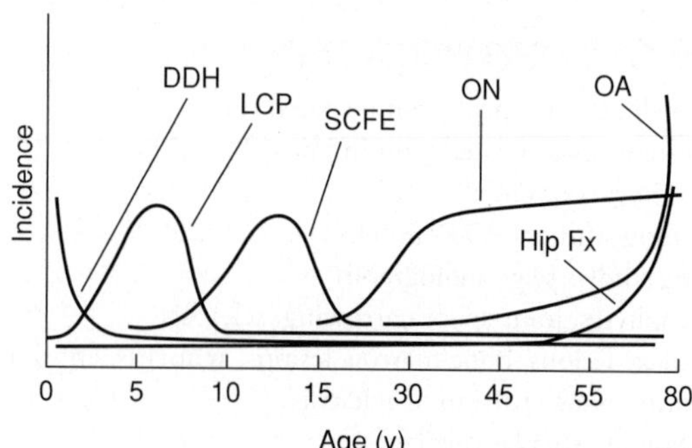

FIGURE 186-5 The age distribution of hip disorders is given in a schematic representation. DDH, developmental dysplasia of the hip; LCP, Legg–Calvé–Perthes disease; SCFE, slipped capital femoral epiphysis; ON, osteonecrosis; OA, osteoarthrosis; and Hip Fx, hip fracture. (From Skinner HB. *Current Diagnosis & Treatment in Orthopedics*. 4th ed. http://www.accessmedicine.com. Copyright © The McGraw-Hill Companies, Inc. All rights reserved.)

- Fall risk
  - Dynamic gait assessment
  - Functional gait assessment
- Fear of falling
  - Activities-specific balance confidence scale
  - Falls Efficacy Scale

INTERVENTION

- Exercises (resistance, endurance, flexibility)
  - Aquatic exercises
- Training on ADLs
- Use of assistive or adaptive devices
- Heat therapy
- Weight management
- Rest
- Orthoses, splints
- Walking aids
- Ice[8]
- Diet
- Acupuncture
- Pain management
- Energy conservation techniques
- Joint protection
- Footwear
- Psychosocial support
- Ultrasound in surrounding areas[9]
- Electric stimulation[10]
- Patient education

FUNCTIONAL GOALS

- Patient will have improved
  - Joint mobility and stability to improve balance.
  - Muscle strength so as to climb stairs.
  - Muscle and general (aerobic) endurance.
  - Level of activity and participation in home, work, community.
- Patient will be able to
  - Walk 0.5 miles pain free without assistive device.
  - Walk 1 mile pain free with assistive device.
  - Resume ADLs (e.g., sweeping, mopping) pain free.

PROGNOSIS

- No definite cure for OA: Chronic disease, may mean long-term burden
- Treatment primarily for symptom management, though emerging drugs may modify disease mechanism
- Joint damage is irreversible
- Recovery or relief from symptoms may depend on disease duration and timely intervention
- Factors affecting prognosis include: Demographics, severity and natural history of the disease, medical and behavioral comorbidities (fear avoidance, catastrophization, central sensitization)
- General endurance, muscle strength, and mobile joints are good prognosticating factors
- Motivation, compliance with PT intervention (e.g., home exercise program), support from family and environmental factors can improve outcomes

PATIENT RESOURCE

- Osteoarthritis. Arthritis Today. Arthritis Foundation. http://www.arthritistoday.org/conditions/osteoarthritis/index.php. Accessed June 16, 2013.

REFERENCES

1. The American Physical Therapy Association. Pattern 4D: impaired joint mobility, motor function, muscle performance, and range of motion associated with connective tissue dysfunction. *Interactive Guide to Physical Therapist Practice.* 2003. doi: 10.2522/ptguide.3.1_4. http://guidetoptpractice.apta.org/content/1/SEC11.extract?sid=0b3fde98-638b-4011-bec0-11cdb7628ea4. Accessed May 27, 2014.
2. The American Physical Therapy Association. Pattern 4F: impaired joint mobility, motor function, muscle performance, range of motion, and reflex integrity associated with spinal disorders. *Interactive Guide to Physical Therapist Practice.* 2003. doi: 10.2522/ptguide.3.1_6. http://guidetoptpractice.apta.org/content/1/SEC13.extract?sid=8ea6cb20-1ac4-4f60-9e10-5d19f24435bd. Accessed May 27, 2014.
3. The American Physical Therapy Association. Pattern 4H: impaired joint mobility, motor function, muscle performance, and range of motion associated with joint arthroplasty. *Interactive Guide to Physical Therapist Practice.* 2003. doi: 10.2522/ptguide.3.1_8. http://guidetoptpractice.apta.org/content/1/SEC15.extract?sid=deeed317-b53a-425c-9b59-d91d44ca6154. Accessed May 27, 2014.
4. The American Physical Therapy Association. Pattern 4I: impaired joint mobility, motor function, muscle performance, and range of motion associated with bony or soft tissue surgery. *Interactive Guide to Physical Therapist Practice.* 2003. doi: 10.2522/ptguide.3.1_9. http://guidetoptpractice.apta.org/content/1/SEC16.extract?sid=3bcbfe6d-e7b3-4af8-8b74-4db2092934a6. Accessed May 27, 2014.
5. Kellgren JH. Lawrence JS. *Atlas of standard radiographs.* Oxford, UK: Oxford University Press; 1963.
6. Royal College of Physicians. Osteoarthritis: national clinical guideline for care and management in adults. In: *Osteoarthritis: national clinical guideline and management in adults.* London, UK: Royal College of Physicians; 2008.
7. Dutton M. The nervous system. In: *Orthopaedic Examination, Evaluation, and Intervention.* New York, NY: McGraw-Hill; 2008:Chapter 2. http://www.accessphysiotherapy.com/abstract/5541168#5541193. Accessed June 16, 2013.
8. Prentice WE. Chapter 9. Cryotherapy and thermotherapy. In: Prentice WE, Quillen WS, Underwood F, eds. *Therapeutic Modalities in Rehabilitation.* 4th ed. New York, NY: McGraw-Hill; 2011. http://www.accessphysiotherapy.com/content/8137995#8137995. Accessed June 16, 2013.
9. Draper DO, Prentice WE. Therapeutic ultrasound. In: Prentice WE, Quillen WS, Underwood F, eds. *Therapeutic Modalities in Rehabilitation.* 4th ed. New York, NY: McGraw-Hill; 2011:Chapter 10. http://www.accessphysiotherapy.com/abstract/8138751. Accessed June 16, 2013.
10. Dutton M. *McGraw Hill's NPTE (National Physical Therapy Examination).* 2nd ed. New York, NY: McGraw-Hill; 2012. http://www.accessphysiotherapy.com/resource/611. Accessed June 16, 2013.

ADDITIONAL REFERENCES

- ICD9DATA. http://www.icd9data.com. Accessed June 16, 2013.
- ICD10DATA. http://www.icd10data.com. Accessed June 16, 2013.
- Osteoarthritis Research Society International. OARSI Primer; 2010 (last updated 2011). http://primer.oarsi.org. Accessed June 16, 2013.

187 ILIOTIBIAL BAND SYNDROME

Shawn D. Felton, EdD, ATC
Eric Shamus, PhD, DPT, PT, CSCS

CONDITION/DISORDER SYNONYMS

- Tensor fascia latae syndrome (TFLS)
- Iliotibial band friction syndrome (ITBFS)

ICD-9-CM CODE

- 728.89 Other disorders of muscle ligament and fascia

ICD-10-CM CODE

- M62.89 Other specified disorders of muscle

PREFERRED PRACTICE PATTERN

- 4D: Impaired Joint Mobility, Motor Function, Muscle Performance, and ROM Associated With Connective Tissue Dysfunction[1]

PATIENT PRESENTATION

A 19-year-old female cross-country athlete is being seen in the clinic complaining of intense right lateral knee pain when she runs. She notes that she has been a cross-country athlete for approximately 5 years, but this is her first season participating in Division IA competition. She states that her practices are more intense than she remembered as a high school athlete. With her moving from the southern United States to the Northeast region of the United States, she is running more on hills. The athlete mostly complains of pain 5 miles into the run and it forces her to stop running.

KEY FEATURES

Description

- Original presumed model of repetitive stress injury due to friction between the iliotibial band (ITB)[2,3] and lateral femoral condyle, occurring at approximately 30 degrees of knee flexion[4]
  - Acute inflammation begins at ITB's insertion and where friction develops between the ITB and lateral femoral condyle[1]
- Newer proposed model of the ITB being a thickness within the lateral fascia
  - Tightening is a result of the repetitive stress
  - Lateral extension of the knee synovial capsule, lateral synovial recess
  - Cyst formation
  - Osseous edema with out evidence of fascial inflammation
  - Bursitis that develops deep within the ITB as it crosses the lateral femoral condyle[3]

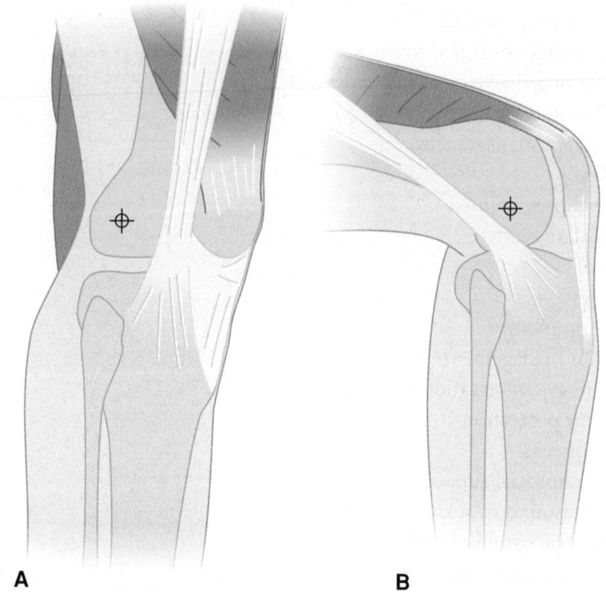

FIGURE 187-1 Iliotibial band site. (**A**) The iliotibial band lies anterior to the lateral femoral epicondyle when the knee is in extension and passes posterior to it with flexion. (**B**) The coursing back and forth over this bony prominence is the cause of a symptom complex referred to as the *iliotibial band syndrome.* (Reproduced with permission from Simon RR, Sherman SC, Koenigsknecht SJ. *Emergency Orthopedics, The Extremities.* 5th ed. © 2007, McGraw-Hill Inc., New York, NY.)

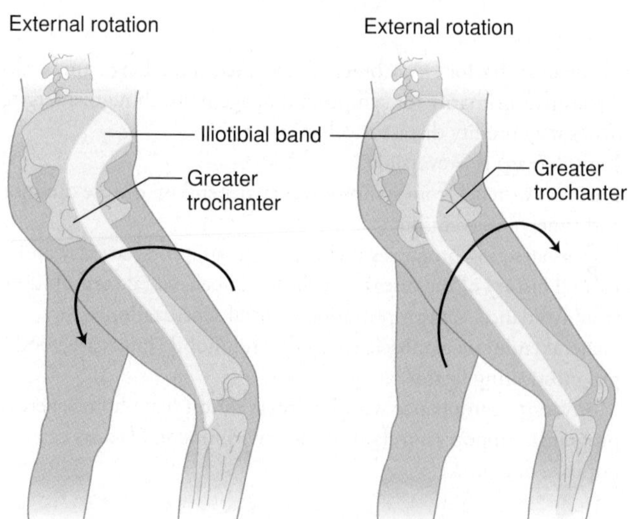

FIGURE 187-2 External snapping hip syndrome. In the snapping hip syndrome, the iliotibial band courses over the greater trochanter. (Reproduced with permission from Simon RR, Sherman SC, Koenigsknecht SJ. *Emergency Orthopedics, The Extremities.* 5th ed. © 2007, McGraw-Hill Inc., New York, NY.)

Essentials of Diagnosis

- Diagnosis usually made by clinical examination
- Progression of symptoms often associated with changes in training practice (e.g., increased running mileage or change in training surfaces, especially downhill running[1])
- Pain from ITBFS so severe that activity must be discontinued

General Considerations

- Most common overuse injury of the knee, especially in long-distance runners
- Frequently develops in people with inadequate warm-up or stretching program before exercise
- Associated with leg-length discrepancies, tensor fascia latae contractures, excessive pronation, tight heel cords[1,6]
- Though most common in runners, may occur with any activity requiring constant knee flexion and extension[1]

Demographics

- Men and women equally affected
- Distance runners, exacerbated with downhill running
- Cyclists
- Repetitive knee flexion, extension
- Training on uneven terrain or graded slopes
- Change in Q-angle as a result of leg-length discrepancy[4]

CLINICAL FINDINGS

SIGNS AND SYMPTOMS

- Localized tenderness and pain along lateral aspect of knee, especially with repetitive knee motion
- Pain may be diffuse and general at onset, becoming more specific and intense as ITBFS progresses
  - Specific pain localized approximately 2 cm above joint line over the lateral femoral condyle with knee flexed 30 degrees[3]
  - Pain will radiate to lateral joint line and distally to proximal tibia[1]
- Pain typically begins after completion of activity, but may occur during activity or periods of rest as condition progresses[7]
- Crepitus upon palpation over lateral condyle[3]
- Specific swelling over lateral condyle[3]
- Increased pain after long periods of sitting[4]

Functional Implications

- Pain with running (especially on downhill terrain) and cycling
- Pain with walking and other activities that elicit knee flexion, especially as the condition persists
- Pain with sitting for prolong periods

Possible Contributing Causes

- Biomechanical abnormalities
  - Leg-length discrepancies
  - Tensor fasciae latae contracture
  - Gluteus maximus contractures
  - Hamstring and quadriceps tightness
  - Excessive pronation leading to increased tibial torsion
  - Tight heel cords
  - Hip abductor/multifidus weakness
  - Pes cavus
  - Usually with genu varum and pronated feet[5]

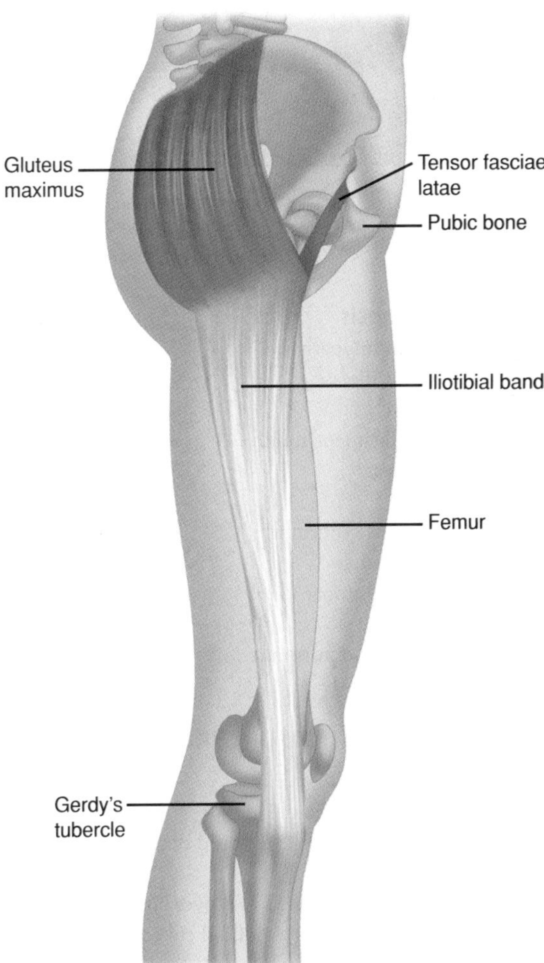

FIGURE 187-3 Iliotibial band causing snapping hip. (From Patel DR, Greydanus DE, Baker RJ. *Pediatric Practice: Sports Medicine*. http://www.accesspediatrics.com. Copyright © The McGraw-Hill Companies, Inc. All rights reserved.)

- Lumbar spine dysfunction
- Sudden change in training regimen
- History of poor training techniques[1]
- In cyclists, excessive bike-seat height or internal rotation of foot on the pedal

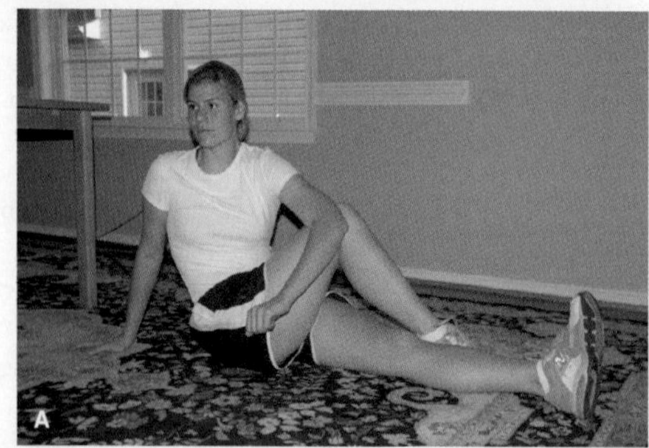

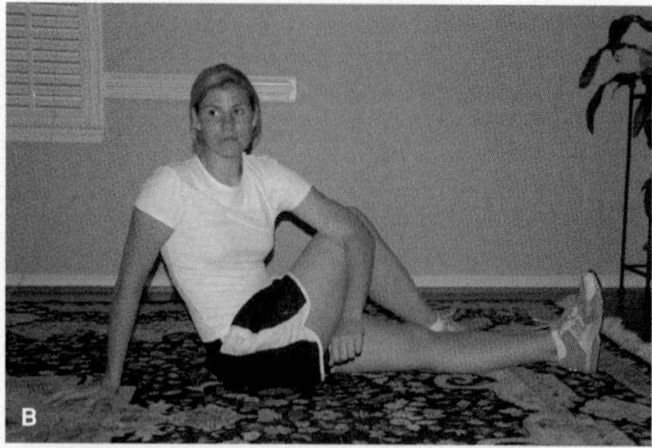

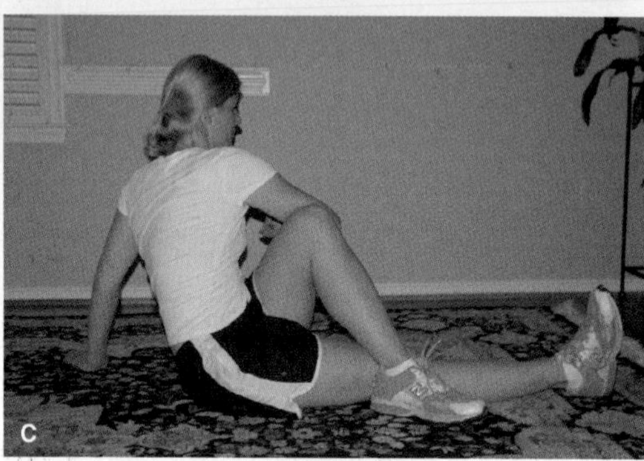

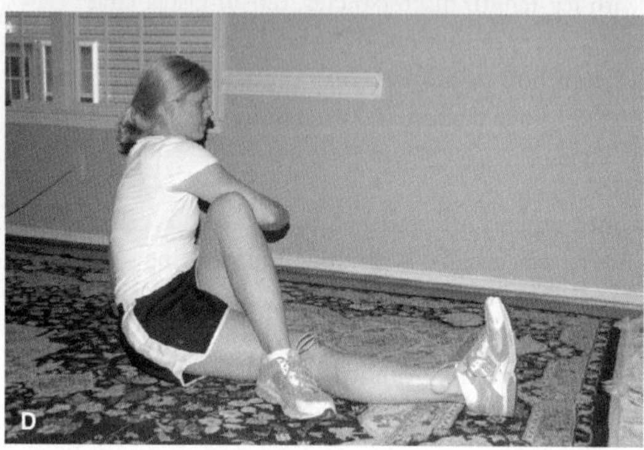

FIGURE 187-4 Iliotibial band stretch: Sit up with one knee bent over the other leg as shown (**A** and **C**). Twist to the right and push your knee with your left arm (**B** and **D**). You should feel a stretch on the outer side of your thigh. Hold it for a few seconds. Repeat — sets of —. (From Patel DR, Greydanus DE, Baker RJ. *Pediatric Practice: Sports Medicine*. http://www.accesspediatrics.com. Copyright © The McGraw-Hill Companies, Inc. All rights reserved.)

Differential Diagnosis

- Biceps femoris tendinopathy
- Degenerative joint disease
- Knee synovial cyst[8]
- Lateral collateral ligament sprain
- Lateral meniscal tear
- Myofascial pain
- Patellofemoral stress syndrome
- Popliteal tendinopathy
- Referred pain from lumbar spine
- Stress fracture
- Superior tibiofibular joint sprain
- Trochanteric hip bursitis

MEANS OF CONFIRMATION OR DIAGNOSIS

Imaging

- X-ray to rule out stress fracture
- Diagnostic ultrasound of ITB for fluid detection at insertion and pain site[4]
- MRI to demonstrate thickened ITB over lateral femoral condyles; will frequently detect a fluid collection

FINDINGS AND INTERPRETATION

- Increased pain when gait stride is lengthened
- Development of bursitis due to friction between ITB and lateral femoral condyle

TREATMENT

Medical Procedures

- Surgery for removal of cyst
- Corticosteroid injection

REFERRALS/ADMITTANCE

- To hospital for imaging, X-ray, MRI
- To physician for medication
  - Corticosteroid injection
- To surgeon for consult

IMPAIRMENTS

- Antalgic gait secondary to gluteus-medius weakness, which increases thigh adduction and internal rotation of the leg at mid-stance
- Antalgic gait secondary to increased knee pain with 30 degrees of knee flexion
- Inability to sit for long periods
- Inability to run on a downhill grade
- Trochanteric bursitis secondary to altered gait
- Limitations in recreation, leisure, sports

TESTS AND MEASURES

- Orthopedic tests considered positive if elicit pain or crepitus is felt[4]
  - Ober test[9]
  - Noble compression test[4]
  - Creak test[9]

INTERVENTION

- Rest, activity modification, address contributing factors
  - For example, decrease running mileage, replace running shoes, change bike-seat position
- Avoid repetitive knee flexion/extension exercises initially
- Initial goal of alleviating inflammation
- Orthotics may reduce pronation

- Address biomechanical factors contributing to the problem
- Surgical release of the posterior 2 cm of the ITB as it passes over the lateral epicondyle of the femur
- Address swelling/bursitis
  - Ice
  - Rest
  - Massage
  - Ultrasound[10]
- Address pain
  - Ice[11]
  - Massage
    - ITB massage with foam roller
    - Transverse friction massage to increase response
  - Electrical stimulation
  - Ultrasound[10]
- Address weakness, joint instability
  - Strengthening, eccentric exercises
    - Four-way hip, straight-leg raises
    - Gluteus medius
    - Other hip adductors
    - Quadriceps setting
- Address lack of flexibility
  - Myofascial release
  - Stretching[12]
    - Tensor fascia latae
    - Iliopsoas
    - Heel cords
- Address mobilization
  - Proximal and distal tibiofibular joint
  - L2 to L4 lumbar spine
  - Patellar mobilization
    - Medial glide
  - Medial tipping of the patella with friction massage along lateral border[13]

FUNCTIONAL GOALS

- Patient will be able to
  - Initiate pain-free closed kinetic chain (CKC) exercises progressed through all planes of motion to be able to climb stairs.[9]
  - Perform singe-leg mini squat on balance disc for 30 seconds.
  - Move pain free through 30 degrees of knee flexion for pain-free sit-to-stand.
  - Resume prior exercise routine free of pain.

PROGNOSIS

- Very good: Most patients improve within 3 to 6 weeks with use of proper modalities, rehabilitative exercise, and activity modifications.
- Surgical intervention should be considered for individuals who do not see improvement.[11]

PATIENT RESOURCE

- Iliotibial Band Syndrome. NIH, National Institute of Arthritis and Musculoskeletal and Skin Diseases. http://www.niams.nih.gov/health_info/knee_problems. Accessed July 6, 2013.

REFERENCES

1. Prentice WE. The knee and related structures. In: Prentice WE, ed. *Principles of Athletic Training: A Competency Based Approach.* 14th ed. New York, NY: McGraw-Hill; 2010:Chapter 20.
2. The American Physical Therapy Association. Pattern 4D: impaired joint mobility, motor function, muscle performance, and range of motion associated with connective tissue dysfunction. *Interactive Guide to Physical Therapist Practice.* 2003. doi: 10.2522/ptguide.3.1_4. Accessed July 6, 2013.
3. *Anatomy and Physiology Revealed.* McGraw-Hill; 2007. http://anatomy.mcgraw-hill.com/apt.html?login=1319025349139&system=Skeletal§ion=Dissection&topic=Femur&topicAbbr=Feb&view=Anterior%20and%20posterior&viewAbbr=Apo&catAbbr=Ske&grpAbbr=Fef&structure=Lateral%20condyle%20of%20femur. Accessed July 6, 2013.
4. Dutton M. *Orthopaedic Examination, Evaluation, and Intervention.* New York, NY: McGraw-Hill; 2008. http://www.accessphysiotherapy.com/resource/612. Accessed July 6, 2013.
5. Polousky JD. Orthopedics. In: Hay W, Levin MJ, Sondheimer JM, Detering RR, eds. *CURRENT Diagnosis & Treatment: Pediatrics.* New York, NY: McGraw-Hill; 2011:Chapter 24. http://www.accessphysiotherapy.com/abstract/6585905#6585905. Accessed July 6, 2013.
6. Hamilton N, Weimar W, Luttgens K. *Kinesiology: Scientific Basis of Human Motion.* New York, NY: McGraw-Hill; 2008. http://www.accessphysiotherapy.com/resource/618. Accessed July 6, 2013.
7. Khaund RM, Flynn SH. Iliotibial band syndrome: a common source of knee pain. *Am Fam Physician.* 2005;71(8):1545–1550.
8. Costa ML, Marshall T, Donell ST, Phillips H. Knee synovial cyst presenting as iliotibial band friction syndrome. *Knee.* 2004;11(3):247–248.
9. Dutton M. *Dutton's Orthopedic Survival Guide: Managing Common Conditions.* New York, NY: McGraw-Hill; 2011. http://www.accessphysiotherapy.com/resource/612. Accessed July 6, 2013.
10. Draper DO, Prentice WE. Therapeutic ultrasound. In: Prentice WE, Quelled WS, Underwood F, eds. *Therapeutic Modalities in Rehabilitation.*4th ed. New York, NY: McGraw-Hill; 2011:Chapter 10. http://www.accessphysiotherapy.com/abstract/8138751. Accessed July 6, 2013.
11. Prentice WE. Cryotherapy and thermotherapy. In: Prentice WE, Quillen WS, Underwood F, eds. *Therapeutic Modalities in Rehabilitation.* 4th ed. New York, NY: McGraw-Hill; 2011:Chapter 9. http://www.accessphysiotherapy.com/content/8137995#8137995. Accessed July 6, 2013.
12. Padua DA, Boling MC, Prentice WE. Rehabilitation of knee injuries. In: Prentice WE, ed. *Rehabilitation Techniques for Sports Medicine and Athletic Training.* 5th ed. New York, NY: McGraw-Hill; 2011:Chapter 21.
13. Kisner C, Colby L. The knee. In: Kisner C, Colby L. *Therapeutic Exercises: Foundations and Techniques.* 5th ed. Philadelphia, PA: F.A. Davis Company; 2007:Chapter 21.

ADDITIONAL REFERENCES

- ICD-9-CM. http://www.icd9data.com. Accessed July 6, 2013.
- ICD-10-CM. http://www.icd10data.com. Accessed July 6, 2013.
- Khaund R, Flynn SH. Iliotibial band syndrome: a common source of knee pain. *Am Fam Physician.* 2005;71(8):1545–1550. http://www.aafp.org/afp/2005/0415/p1545.html
- Lavine R. Iliotibial band friction syndrome. *Curr Rev Musculoskelet Med.* 2010;3(1-4):18–22. doi: 10.1007/s12178-010-9061-8.

SECTION H KNEE AND LOWER LEG DISORDERS

188 ANTERIOR CRUCIATE LIGAMENT TEAR

Eric Shamus, PhD, DPT, PT, CSCS
B. James Massey, DPT, OCS, FAAOMPT

CONDITION/DISORDER SYNONYMS

- ACL sprain
- ACL partial tear
- ACL full-thickness tear

ICD-9-CM CODES

- 717.83 Old disruption of anterior cruciate ligament
- 844.2 Sprain of cruciate ligament of knee

ICD-10-CM CODES

- M23.50 Chronic instability of knee, unspecified knee
- S83.509A Sprain of unspecified cruciate ligament of unspecified knee, initial encounter

PREFERRED PRACTICE PATTERN

- 4I: Impaired Joint Mobility, Motor Function, Muscle Performance, and Range of Motion (ROM) Associated with Bony or Soft Tissue Surgery

PATIENT PRESENTATION

Patient is a 17-year-old high school soccer player who injured her left knee in a noncontact injury. She was assessed on the field with a positive Lachman and anterior drawer test. The patient went the next day for follow-up with the physician and the MRI showed a completely torn anterior cruciate ligament (ACL). The patient was referred to physical therapy to decrease swelling and increase ROM. The patient had a negative varus and valgus stress tests and a negative McMurray test. The patient has 3 mm of anterior laxity on her right knee and 9 mm of laxity of the left using a KT-1000 at 20 lbs. The patient is scheduled for a consult for a possible autograft surgery in 4 weeks.

KEY FEATURES

Description

- ACL made up of two bundles
  - Anteromedial (AM) bundle: Anteromedially on the tibia and more proximal on the femoral side
  - Posterolateral (PL) bundle: Relatively PL
  - Parallel orientation in extension
  - Crossed orientation in flexion

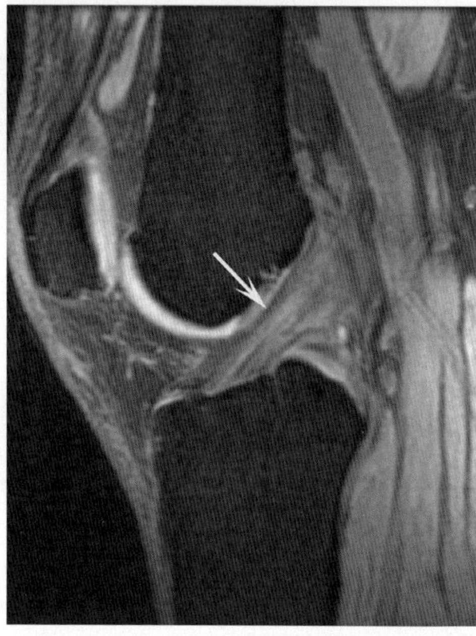

FIGURE 188-1 Sagittal T2-weighted fat-saturated MR image of the knee showing a normal ACL (*arrow*). Notice the fascicular arrangement. (From Chen MYM, Pope TL, *Ott DJ. Basic Radiology.* 2nd ed. www.accessmedicine.com. Copyright © The McGraw-Hill Companies, Inc. All rights reserved.)

- American Medical Association (AMA) has developed standard nomenclature for athletic injuries to ligamentous structures[1]
  - First-degree sprain: Minor tear of ligament fibers
  - Second-degree sprain: Partial tear of ligament structure
  - Third-degree sprain: Complete tear of ligament

Essentials of Diagnosis

- Clinical diagnosis of a partial tear[1]
  - Asymmetric Lachman test
  - Negative pivot-shift test
  - KT-1000 arthrometer test ≤3 mm
  - Confirming arthroscopic observation
- Medial and lateral menisci and medial collateral ligament (MCL) are commonly injured with the ACL[2]
- History
  - Contact injuries: Typically due to application of varus or valgus force to the knee imposing a shear force on the joint
  - Risk for injury increased by[2]
    - Sudden deceleration
    - Abrupt change in direction
    - Hyperextension of the knee

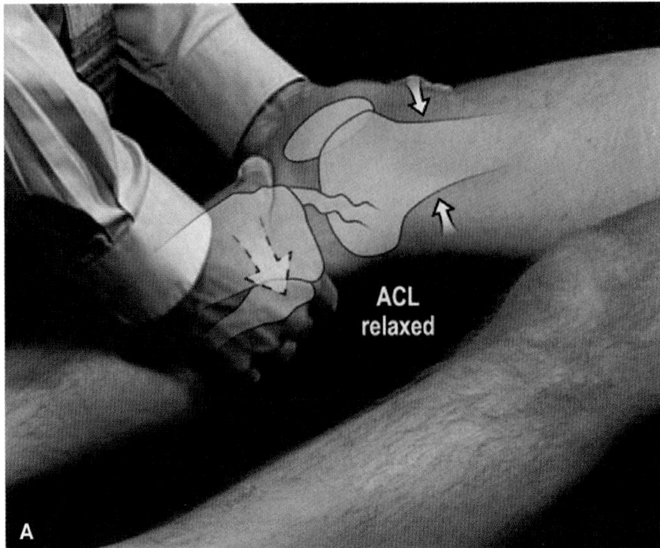

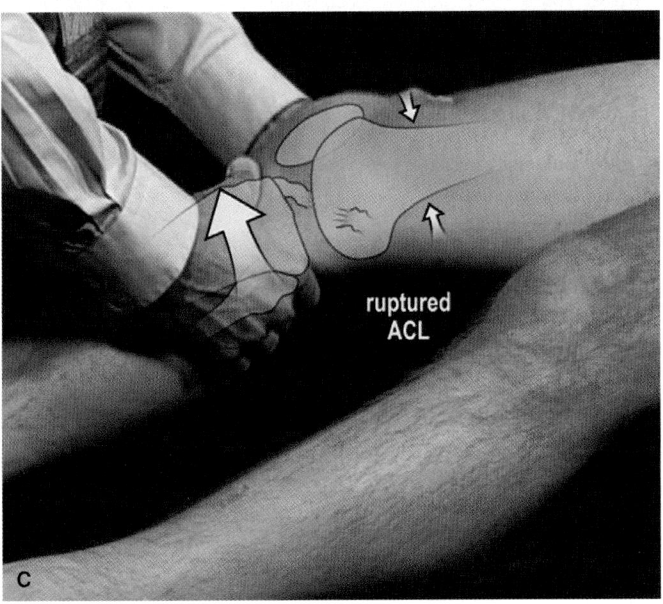

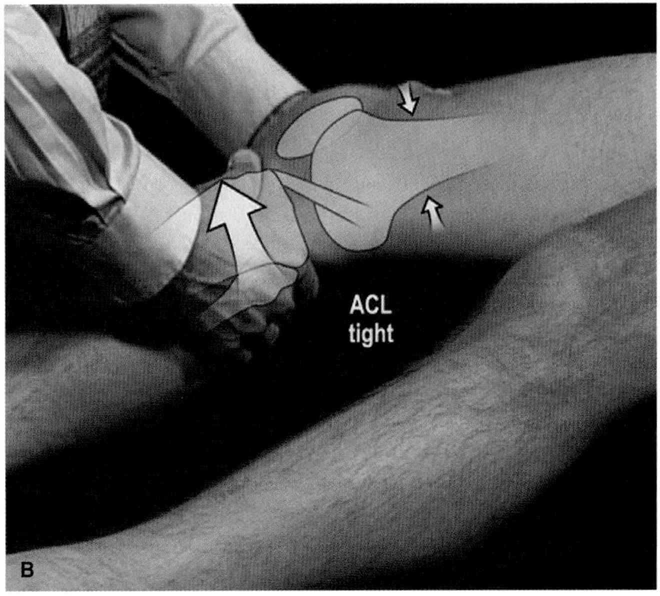

FIGURE 188-2 Lachman test (**A**) Start position of the Lachman test (**B**) Anterior glide of the tibia increases tension on the ACL and there should be a firm end feel (**C**) If the ACL is torn there will not be a firm end feel and there will be increased laxity (From Lawry GV. *Systematic Musculoskeletal Examinations.* www.accessmedicine.com. Copyright © The McGraw-Hill Companies, Inc. All rights reserved.)

- Noncontact injuries (70% of ACL injuries[3]) typically due to[4]
- Deceleration and change in direction (cutting maneuvers)
- Landing from a jump in full knee extension
- Pivoting with planted foot and extended knee
- Hyperextension/Flexion of the knee

General Considerations

- It is estimated that more than 250,000 ACL injuries occur in the United States each year.[2]
- Approximately 50% of ACL injuries occur in combination with other structural damage.
- Seventy percent occur noncontact.
- 75,000 to 100,000 ACL reconstructions performed annually.[5]

Demographics

- ACL injuries reported to be two to nine times more likely in females than in males.[3,6]

CLINICAL FINDINGS

SIGNS AND SYMPTOMS

- Feelings of instability in the knee[7]
- Severe pain at the time of injury[7]
- Audible pop at the time of injury[7]
- Immediate swelling at the time of injury (effusion)

Functional Implications

- Instability of the knee during weight-bearing tasks
- Ambulation distance
- Squatting
- Activities requiring single-leg stance (donning lower extremity [LE] clothing)
- Mobility on uneven terrain

Possible Contributing Causes

- Female sex
  - Tendency of females to land from a jump and change direction in a more erect posture, characterized with increased knee and hip extension[4,8]
  - Tendency of females to land with increased knee valgus[4,8]
  - Pelvic structure and LE alignment that result in a varied Q-angle[9]
  - More narrow intercondylar notch[4,9]
  - Smaller ACLs[4,9]
  - Increased estrogen levels and related increase in laxity[4] (This is controversial in research literature.)
- Increased duration of activity and fatigue[10]
- Athletic activities in dry weather conditions or playing on artificial turf[4]
- Increased body mass index (BMI)
- Decreased hamstring strength relative to quadriceps[3]
- Decreased core strength and proprioception[4]

Differential Diagnosis[2,11,12]

- ACL cyst
- Avulsion at the insertion of the ACL
- Fractures (including growth plate fractures)
- Lateral meniscus injury
- MCL injury
- Medial meniscus injury
- Osteochondral damage (bruise or avulsion)
- Posteriolateral corner injuries
- Posterior cruciate ligament (PCL) damage
- Terrible triad

MEANS OF CONFIRMATION

Imaging[1,13]

- Arthroscopy
- MRI
- Double-contrast arthrography if MRI is contraindicated

FINDINGS AND INTERPRETATION

- Degree of ACL tear and surrounding structure damage
  - Terrible triad
  - Meniscus
  - Articular cartilage
  - Bone bruise
  - Other ligaments

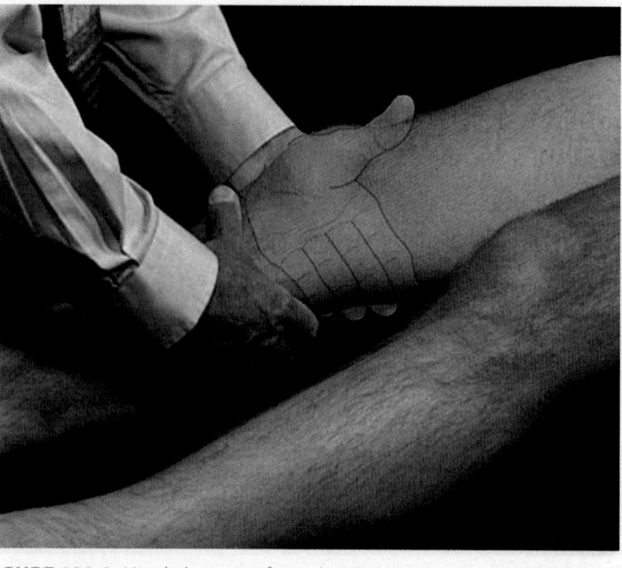

FIGURE 188-3 Hand placement for Lachman test. (From Lawry GV. *Systematic Musculoskeletal Examinations.* www.accessmedicine.com. Copyright © The McGraw-Hill Companies, Inc. All rights reserved.)

TREATMENT

- Ligament reconstruction
  - Traditionally a single-bundle ACL reconstruction is a single graft replicating the AM bundle
  - Double bundle technique utilizing two separate grafts one for the AM bundle and one for the PM bundle
  - Autograft
  - Allograft
  - Xenograft
- Arthroscopic debridement
- Nonsurgical rehabilitation

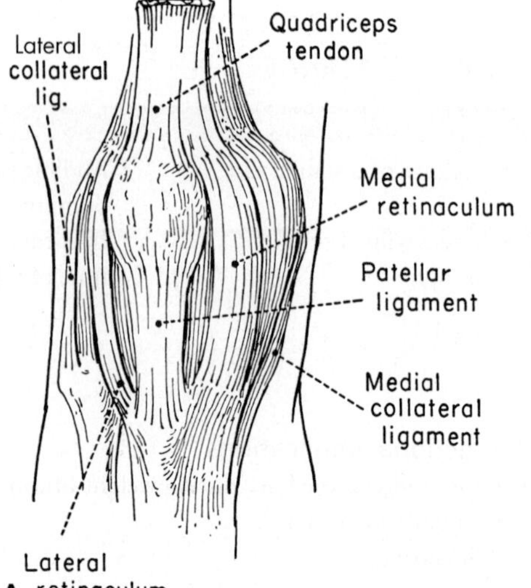

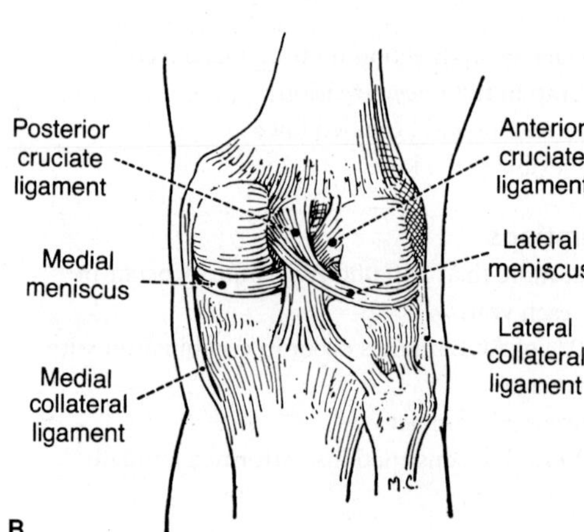

FIGURE 188-4 Anterior view of knee joint showing ligaments (**A**). Posterior view of knee joint showing cruciate ligaments (**B**). (From Hamilton N, Weimar W, Luttgens K. *Kinesiology: Scientific Basis of Human Motion.* 11th ed. http://www.accessphysiotherapy.com. Copyright © McGraw-Hill Education. All rights reserved.)

REFERRALS/ADMITTANCE

- For imaging
- For bracing
- For medication
- For surgical consult

IMPAIRMENTS

- Swelling/effusion
- Diminished AROM and PROM
- Muscle guarding of knee to provide stability to the joint (implications on ROM)
- Instability of the knee
- Gait deviations (antalgic)

TESTS AND MEASURES

- Lachman test
  - Sensitivity: 85% (95% CI, 83–87)
  - Specificity: 94% (95% CI, 92–95)
  - + Likelihood Ratio (LR): 10.2 (95% CI, 4.6–22.7)
  - LR of 0.2 (95% CI, 0.1–0.3)
- Pivot-shift test
  - Sensitivity: 32% (95% CI, 25–38)
  - Specificity: 98% (95% CI, 96–99)
  - + LR: 8.5 (95% CI, 4.7–15.5)
  - – LR: 0.9 (95% CI, 0.8–1.0)
- Anterior Drawer test
  - Sensitivity: 49% (95% CI, 43–55)
  - Specificity: 58% (95% CI, 39–76)
- KT-1000 arthrometer test
- Pain, visual analog scale (VAS)
  - 24-hour pain
  - Worst average pain
  - Best average pain
- Functional independence measure
  - Locomotion
- Cardiovascular integrity
  - Blood pressure at rest and after activity
  - Heart rate at rest and after activity
- Skin integrity
  - Scar
    - Approximation
    - Mobility/pliability
  - Associated skin assessment
    - Edema (linear girth measurements, palpation)
    - Color
    - Signs of infection
    - Mobility/turgor
    - Temperature
- Neurologic examination
  - Sensation
    - Light touch
    - Pin prick
  - LE deep tendon reflexes
  - Proprioception at the hip
  - Kinesthetic awareness at the hip
  - Coordination
- Trunk active and passive ROM
- Hip and knee active and Passive ROM

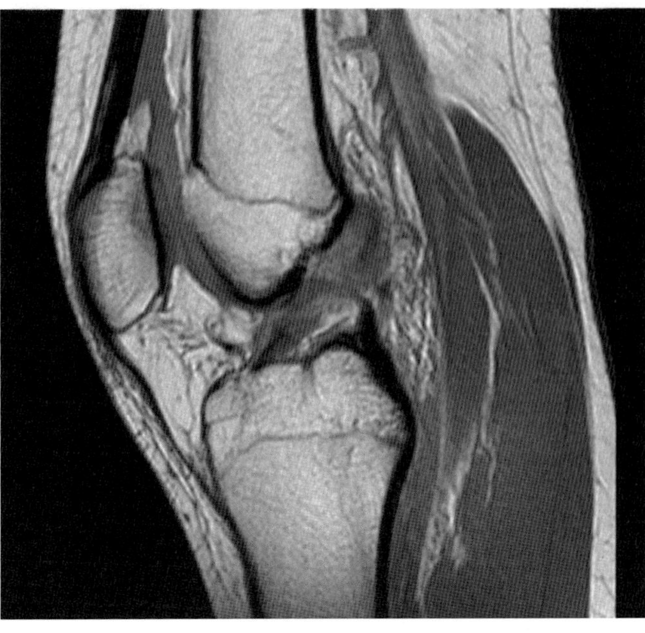

FIGURE 188-5 In this sagittal view MRI slice, rupture of the anterior cruciate ligament is demonstrated approximating the tibial attachment. This image is from a 16-year-old female; note the incompletely closed epiphyseal plates. (From Malone TR, Hazle C, Grey ML. *Imaging in Rehabilitation.* http://accessphysiotherapy.com. Copyright © The McGraw-Hill Companies, Inc. All rights reserved.)

- Flexibility testing
  - Hamstrings
  - Iliopsoas
  - Quadriceps
  - Iliotibial band
  - Abductors
  - Adductors
- Joint integrity of the spine
- Sacroiliac joint integrity
- Hip joint integrity
  - Flexion, adduction, internal rotation (FAIR) (FADIR) (FADDIR) test
- Limb strength
  - Functional strength testing
    - Five times sit-to-stand test
  - Biodex testing, comparison of bilateral quadriceps and quadricep to hamstring ratio
  - Manual muscle test (MMT)
    - Hamstrings
    - Quadriceps
    - Iliopsoas
    - Gluteus maximus
    - Gluteus medius
    - Gluteus minimus
    - Adductors
- LE contralateral limb strength
- Balance
  - Static single-leg standing (eyes open, eyes closed)
    - Contralateral LE
  - Dynamic standing
    - Berg Balance Scale
    - Functional gait assessment

TABLE 188-1 West Point Grading of Ankle Sprains

Criterion	Grade 1	Grade 2	Grade 3
Location of tenderness	ATFL	ATFL, CFL	ATFL, CFL, PTFL
Edema, ecchymosis	Slight, local	Moderate, local	Significant, diffuse
Weight-bearing ability	Full or partial	Difficult without crutches	Impossible without significant pain
Ligament damage	Stretched	Partial tear	Complete tear
Instability	None	None or slight	Definite

(From Patel DR, Greydanus DE, Baker RJ: *Pediatric Practice: Sports Medicine*. http://www.accesspediatrics.com. Copyright © The McGraw-Hill Companies, Inc. All rights reserved.)

- Gait assessment
  - Observational analysis
  - Gait speed via the 10-m walk test
  - Two-minute walk test
  - Six-minute walk test
  - Retro running

INTERVENTION

- Immobilization and rest to protect damaged tissue
  - Hinged brace
  - Casts
  - Removable splints
  - Soft dressing
  - Note: Prolonged (8 months) immobilization has been reported to decrease strength and energy absorption at failure with ACLs in primates[14]
- Address swelling
  - Elevation
  - Ice/Cryotherapy
  - Electrical stimulation
- Address pain
  - Ice/Cryotherapy
  - Manual therapy
  - Electrical stimulation
- Address proprioception
  - Standing balance on level surface
    - Eyes open
    - Eyes closed
  - Standing balance activities with use of foam
    - Eyes open
    - Eyes closed
  - Standing balance activities on balance machines
- Address neuromuscular coordination
  - Therapeutic exercise
  - Focus on decreasing dynamic genu valgus/ "kissing knees"
  - Electrical stimulation
- Address weakness and joint stability
  - Strength training
  - Special emphasis should be placed on strengthening the hamstrings,[15] as the hamstrings provide restraint from anterior translation of the proximal tibia
- Address soft tissue mobility/flexibility
  - Triceps surae
  - Quadriceps femoris
  - Hamstring
- Activity/sports: Specific training

FUNCTIONAL GOALS

- The primary goal of conservative and surgical intervention is to return functional stability to the affected knee to reduce the risk of radiographic osteoarthritis (estimated to be as high as 78% within 14 years of ACL injury).[16]
  - Single-leg hop for distance: ≥85% of nonaffected leg
  - Figure-of-eight running test
  - Return to full level sports
  - Isokinetic 100% hamstring strength, 85% quadricep strength

PROGNOSIS

- Good short- and mid-term prognoses with conservative intervention for rupture as measured by subjective and objective functional performance.[17]
- Individuals who have undergone conservative care for ACL rupture have demonstrated a 21% decline in activity levels postinjury.[17]
- Prognostic factors of conservative intervention include[17]
  - Age
  - Gender
  - Occupation
  - Sports participation level
  - Radiographic findings
  - KT-1000 arthrometric measurement
  - Knee function scores
  - Presence of additional knee injuries[17]

PATIENT RESOURCE

- Anterior Cruciate Ligament Injuries. American Academy of Orthopaedic Surgeons. http://orthoinfo.aaos.org/topic.cfm?topic=a00549. Accessed March 1, 2014.

REFERENCES

1. DeFranco MJ, Bach BR. A comprehensive review of partial anterior cruciate ligament tears. *J Bone Joint Surg Am*. 2009; 91(1):198–208.
2. Childs SG. Pathogenesis of anterior cruciate ligament injury. *Orthop Nurs*. 2002;21(4):35–40.

3. Prodromas CC, Han Y, Rogowski J, Joyce B. A Meta-analysis of the Incidence of Anterior Cruciate Ligament Tears as a Function of Gender, Sport, and a Knee Injury–Reduction Regimen. *Arthroscopy*. 2007;23(12):1320–1325.
4. Alentorn-Geli E, Myer GD, Silvers HJ, Samitier G. Prevention of non-contact anterior cruciate ligament injuries in soccer players. Part 1: Mechanisms of injury and underlying risk factors. *Knee Surg Sports Traumatol Arthrosc*. 2009;17(7):705–729.
5. Crawford C, Nyland J, Landes S, et al. Anatomic double bundle ACL reconstruction: a literature review. *Knee Surg Sports Traumatol Arthrosc*. 2007;15(8):946–964.
6. Arendt E, Dick R. Knee injury patterns among men and women in collegiate basketball and soccer. NCAA data and review of literature. *Am J Sports Med*. 1995;23(6):694–701.
7. Cabaud HE. Biomechanics of the anterior cruciate ligament. *Clin Orthop Relat Res*. 1983;172:26–31.
8. Yoo JH, Lim BO, Ha M, et al. A meta-analysis of the effect of neuromuscular training on the prevention of the anterior cruciate ligament injury in female athletes. *Knee Surg Sports Traumatol Arthrosc*. 2010;18(6):824–830.
9. Hewette TE, Lindenfield TN, Riccobene JV, Noyes FR. The effect of neuromuscular training on the incidence of knee injury in female athletes. A prospective study. *Am J Sports Med*. 1999;27(6):699–706.
10. Borotikar BS, Newcomer R, Koppes R, McLean SG. Combined effects of fatigue and decision making on female lower limb landing postures: central and peripheral contributions to ACL injury risk. *Clin Biochem*. 2008;32(1):81–92.
11. Bahk MS, Cosgarea AJ. Physical examination and imaging of the lateral collateral ligament and posterolateral corner of the knee. *Sports Med Arthrosc*. 2006;14(1):12–19.
12. Benjaminse A, Gokeler A, van der Schans CP. Clinical Diagnosis of an Anterior Cruciate Ligament Rupture: A Meta-analysis. *J Orthop Sports Phys Ther*. 2006;36(5):267–288.
13. Moore SL. Imaging the anterior cruciate ligament. *Orthop Clin North Am*. 2002;33:663–674.
14. Noyes FR. Functional properties of knee ligaments and alterations induced by immobilization: A correlative biomechanical and histological study in primates. *Clin Orthop Related Res*. 1977;123:210–242.
15. Hertling D, Kessler RM. *Management of Common Musculoskeletal Disorders: Physical Therapy Principles and Methods*. Philadelphia, PA: Lippincott Williams & Wilkins; 2006.
16. Murray MM. Current status and potential of primary ACL repair. *Clin Sports Med*. 2009;28:51–61.
17. Muaidi QI, Nicholson LL, Refshauge KM, Herbert RD, Maher CG. Prognosis of conservatively managed anterior cruciate ligament injury. *Sports Med*. 2007;37(8):703–716.

ADDITIONAL RESOURCES

- Dutton M. Ligaments. In: Dutton M, ed. *Dutton's Orthopaedic Examination, Evaluation, and Intervention*. 3rd ed. New York, NY: McGraw-Hill; 2012.
- Dutton M. Stress testing. In: Dutton M, ed. *Dutton's Orthopedic Survival Guide: Managing Common Conditions*. New York, NY: McGraw-Hill; 2011.
- Shamus E, Shamus J. *Sports Injury Prevention and Rehabilitation*. New York, NY: McGraw-Hill; 2001.

189 PREPATELLAR BURSITIS

Eric Shamus, PhD, DPT, PT, CSCS
Erika Albertini, DPT, PT, ATC
Oseas Florencio de Moura Filho, PT (Brazil), MSc

CONDITION/DISORDER SYNONYMS

- Infrapatellar bursitis
- Housemaid's knee

ICD-9-CM CODE[1]

- 726.65 Prepatellar bursitis

ICD-10-CM CODE[2]

- M70.40 Prepatellar bursitis, unspecified knee

PREFERRED PRACTICE PATTERN[3]

- 4E: Impaired Joint Mobility, Motor Function, Muscle Performance, and Range of Motion Associated with Localized Inflammation

PATIENT PRESENTATION

Patient is a 58-year-old male who decided to put tile down in his bathroom. His regular job is a salesman with limited physical activity. After 2 days on his hands and knees installing floor tile, he began having knee pain. He was unable to finish the installation. He has tried to ice the knee and stay off of it. He is having difficulty bending the knee and going down the stairs as his house. The patient has tenderness just above the tibial tubercule.

KEY FEATURES

Description

- Localized inflammation of the prepatellar bursa.
- Bursa fills with blood and serous fluid as response to either acute or repeated micro trauma.
- Presents as pronounced, local swelling isolated to the anterior knee.

Essentials of Diagnosis

- Result of single episode of trauma or repeat trauma to the anterior knee when in a flexed position.
- Bursitis is commonly related to occupation or specific activity that causes rubbing or pressure on the anterior knee from a hard surface.
- Swelling is contained to bursa which results in the visualization of a swollen appearance on both sides of the patella tendon.
- Patients often note focal pain to palpation of swollen bursa, decreased range of motion, or inability to bear weight on the flexed knee.
- Differential diagnosis is essential due to presence of infections to this area.
- Exquisite swelling, marked tenderness, and redness or heat may be indicative of differential diagnosis.

General Considerations

- Full history of symptoms and medical history screening will ensure appropriate diagnosis.
- Isolated diagnosis related to acute or chronic activity (pressure to the anterior flexed knee by a hard surface) and focal swelling/pain

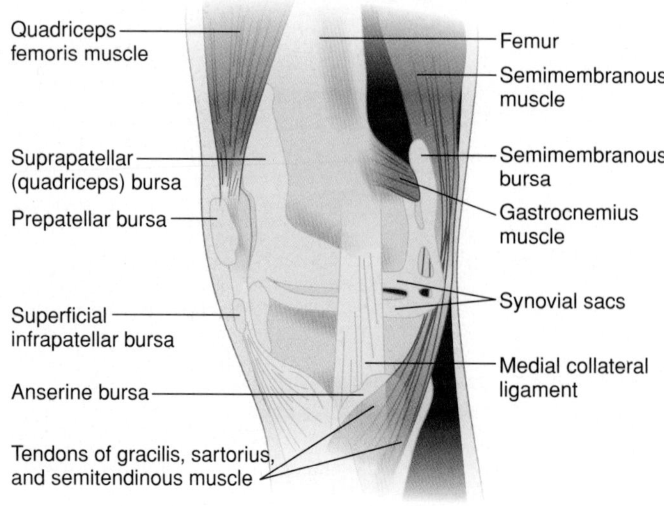

FIGURE 189-1 Knee bursa. (Reproduced with permission from Reichman EF, *Simon RR: Emergency Medicine Procedures.* © 2004.)

- Marked tenderness or swelling with acute onset may signal underlying fracture.
- Redness or heat may be indicative of infection.

Demographics

- No reports identifying or limiting demographics. Incidence related to activity.
- Occurs primarily in adults but can occur in children and athletes of any age.
- When chronic, often associated with occupation (maid) or prolonged activity (tile installer) which places flexed knee on hard surface.
- When acute, often associated with acute blow or fall when the knee is flexed (athletes).

CLINICAL FINDINGS

SIGNS AND SYMPTOMS

- Point tenderness to the anterior knee
- Focal swelling
- Stiffness with flexion
- Pain with rubbing or light pressure to the anterior knee
- Pain with focal pressure
- Knee ROM can be reduced, usually flexion
- Pain and swelling can be either insidious or acute.
- Occasionally, swelling can be spontaneous and without pain.
- Possible reduction in strength due to pain and inflammation.
- Pain in anterior knee
- Tenderness changes position with tendon movement during extension
- Increased swelling throughout the day
- Thickening of the tendon
- Decreased extension strength

Functional Implications

- Inability to climb stairs or ladder
- Inability to push-off during ambulation
- Decreased ability to kneel
- Decreased squat depth

Possible Contributing Causes

- Intrinsic risk factors
  - Decreased knee flexion ROM
  - Decreased quadriceps strength
  - Greater pronation/calcaneal varus and faster rate of maximum pronation
  - Obesity
- Extrinsic risk factors
  - Occupational factors with kneeling and weight bearing on the anterior knee
  - Fall or traumatic blow to the anterior potion of the knee

Differential Diagnosis

- ACL ligament instability
- Bone spur
- Chondromalacia
- Gout
- Knee infection
- L4 radiculopathy
- Meniscus tear
- Osgood–Schlatter disease

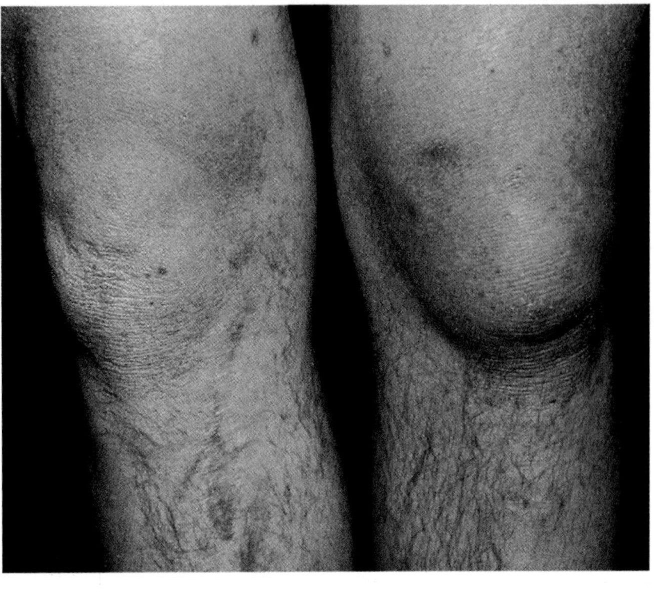

FIGURE 189-2 Prepatellar bursitis. Photograph reveals local bursal swelling of the left knee. (Reproduced with permission from Knoop K, Stack L, Storrow A, Thurman RJ: *Atlas of Emergency Medicine.* 3rd ed. © 2010. New York, NY: McGraw-Hill,)

- Osteoarthritis
- Patella fracture
- Sinding–Larsen–Johansson disease
- Tendinitis
- Tendon partial tear
- Tendon rupture

MEANS OF CONFIRMATION OR DIAGNOSIS

Laboratory Tests

- Fluid can be aspirated to rule out septic bursitis.
- Aspirated fluid can be cultured and evaluated for crystals to rule out gout.
- Laboratory studies for suspected rheumatoid disorders.

Imaging

- Ultrasonography
- X-ray
- Radiographs are usually normal taken to rule out fracture.
- MRI will show increased fluid/edema isolated within the bursa.
- T2-weighted MRI would best visualize and result in increased signal intensity within bursa.

FINDINGS AND INTERPRETATION

- Hypertrophic tendon
- Hyperechoic mass at midtendon
- Irregular tendon structure

TREATMENT

Medication

- NSAIDs
- Prolotherapy: Sclerotic injection (most common dextrose)
- Corticosteroid injection
- Antibiotics if infection confirmed

MEDICAL PROCEDURES

- Tendon debridement
- Extracorpeal shock wave therapy (ESWT)

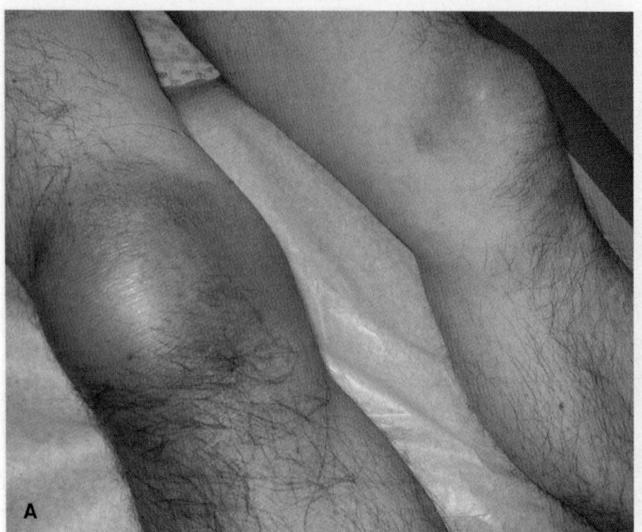

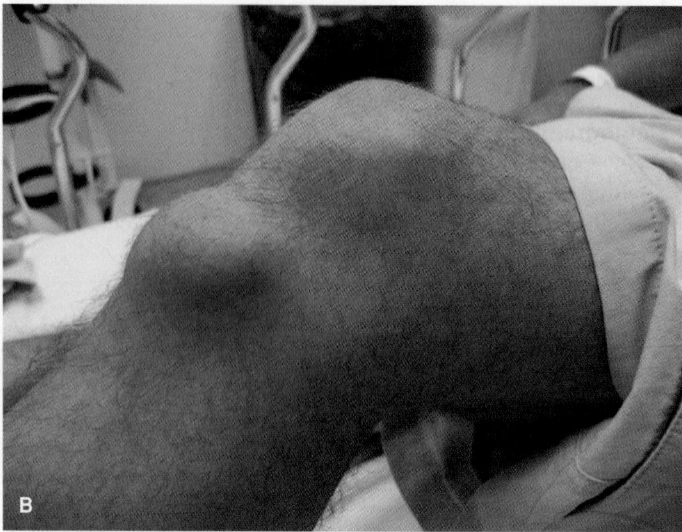

FIGURE 189-3 (**A**) Infected prepatellar bursitis. (**B**) Noninfected infrapatellar bursitis. (From Simon RR, Sherman SC. *Emergency Orthopedics*, 6th ed. Copyright © The McGraw-Hill Companies, Inc. All rights reserved.)

REFERRALS/ADMITTANCE

- To radiologist for imaging, X-ray
- To primary care for aspiration and lab studies
- To orthopedist for surgical consult for injection or excision

IMPAIRMENTS

- Restricted ROM
- Decreased knee extension strength
- Pain with movement after prolonged immobility with the knee flexed (e.g., after sitting at a desk, driving, or movies) that improves with activity

TESTS AND MEASURES

- Thomas test
- Modified Thomas test
- Ober test
- Anterior draw test
- Ballotable patella test
- Selective tissue tension tests
- Decreased performance of:
  - Hopping
  - Jumping
  - Squatting

INTERVENTION

- Acute phase
  - PRICE: Protection, rest, ice compression, elevation
  - Bracing and padding to reduce pressure
  - Low-level cold laser
  - Ice massage
  - Pulsed ultrasound
  - Active movement during the day with prevention of direct pressure to area from external hard surfaces
- Chronic phase
  - Gradually increasing workload as pain and discomfort diminish
  - Padding/Bracing to reduce contact to area.
  - Addressing pain
    - Ice
    - High-voltage pulsed stimulation
    - Iontophoresis
    - Ultrasound
  - Addressing swelling
    - Ice
    - Elevation
    - Iontophoresis
  - Addressing weakness, joint instability
    - As symptoms improve, gradually resume activities.
    - Establish full, pain-free ROM.
    - Incorporate stretching and progressive strengthening exercises as warranted to restore full mobility and strength.

FUNCTIONAL GOALS

- Patient will be able to
  - Kneel down and place pressure on the knee to lift an object.
  - Demonstrate and maintain neutral calcaneal alignment with heel strike through toe-off phases of gait.
  - Stand and walk without limitation due to pain after sitting for longer than 1 hour.
  - Demonstrate 5/5 manual muscle testing of quadriceps without limitation due to pain.
  - Squat with proper knee mechanics.
  - Demonstrate 50% speed running for 1 mile without limitation due to pain.
  - Demonstrate single-leg hopping on involved side without limitation due to pain.

PROGNOSIS

- Acute to sub-chronic
  - Good, nonsurgical.
  - Significant pain and impairment reduction.
  - Should be able to return pain free.

PATIENT RESOURCE

- Prepatellar (Kneecap) Bursitis. AAOS, American Academy of Orthopaedic Surgeons. http://orthoinfo.aaos.org/topic.cfm?topic=a00338. Accessed June 10, 2013.

REFERENCES

1. ICD9Data.com. http://www.icd9data.com. Accessed June 10, 2013.
2. ICD10Data.com. http://www.icd10data.com/ICD10CM/Codes. Accessed June 10, 2013.
3. American Physical Therapy Association. Pattern 4E: Impaired joint mobility, motor function, muscle performance, and range of motion associated with localized inflammation. In: *Guide to Physical Therapist Practice*. 2nd ed. Alexandria, VA: American Physical Therapy Association; 2001. Revised 2003.

ADDITIONAL REFERENCES

- Balasubramaniam P, Prathap K. The effect of injection of hydrocortisone into rabbit calcaneal tendons. *J Bone Joint Surg Br*. 1972;54(4):729–734.
- Carcia C, Martin R, Houck J, et al. Achilles pain, stiffness, and muscle power deficits: Achilles tendonitis. *J Orthop Sports Phys Ther*. 2010:40(9):A1–A26. doi:10.2519/jospt.2010.0305.
- Dutton M. Common orthopedic conditions. In: Dutton M, ed. *McGraw-Hill's NPTE (National Physical Therapy Examination)*. 2nd ed. New York, NY: McGraw-Hill; 2012. http://www.access-physiotherapy.com/content/5398559. Accessed April 10, 2013.
- Dutton M. *Dutton's Orthopedic Survival Guide: Managing Common Conditions*. New York, NY: McGraw-Hill. http://www.accessphysiotherapy.com/content/8655360. Accessed June 10, 2013.
- Dutton M. *Orthopaedic Examination, Evaluation, and Intervention, 2e*. New York, NY: McGraw-Hill. http://www.accessphysiotherapy.com/content/55586274. Accessed June 10, 2013.
- Hay WW, Levin MJ, Sondheimer JM, et al. Anterior knee pain. In: Hay WW, Levin MJ, Sondheimer JM, Deterding RR, eds. *CURRENT Diagnosis & Treatment: Pediatrics*. 20th ed. New York, NY: McGraw-Hill; 2011. http://www.accessphysiotherapy.com/content/6586302. Accessed June 10, 2013.
- James SL, Bates BT, Ostering LR. Injuries to runner. *Am J Sports Med*. 1978;6:40–45. doi: 10.1177/036354657800600202.
- Maffulli N, Sharma P, Luscombe KL. Achilles tendinopathy: aetiology and management. *J R Soc Med*. 2004;97(10):472–476. doi: 10.1258/jrsm.97.10.472
- Prentice WE, Quillen WS, Underwood F, eds. *Therapeutic Modalities in Rehabilitation*. 4th ed. New York, NY: McGraw-Hill; 2011. http://www.accessphysiotherapy.com/content/ 8136922. Accessed June 10, 2013.
- Ohberg L, Alfredson H. Effects on neovascularisation behind the good results with eccentric training in chronic mid-portion Achilles tendinosis? *Knee Surg Sports Traumatol Arthrosc*. 2004;12(5):465–470. doi: 10.1007/s00167-004-0494-8.
- Rompe JD, Furia J, Maffulli N. Eccentric loading compared with shock wave therapy for chronic insertional Achilles tendinopathy. *J Bone Joint Surg Am*. 2008;90(1):52–61. doi: 10.2106/JBJS.F.01494. [PMID: 18171957]
- Voorn R. Case report: Can sacroiliac joint dysfunction cause chronic Achilles tendinitis? *J Orthop Sports Phys Ther*. 1998;27(6): 436–443.
- Woodley BL, Newsham-West RJ, Baxter GD. Chronic tendinopathy: effectiveness of eccentric exercise. *Br J Sports Med*. 2007;41(4): 188–198. doi: 10.1136/bjsm.2006.029769.

190 CHONDROMALACIA PATELLAE

John Leschitz, DPT, PT, OCS
Eric Shamus, PhD, DPT, PT, CSCS
Erin N. Pauley, DPT, MS, ATC, CSCS

CONDITION/DISORDER SYNONYMS

- Chondromalacia
- Chondropathy
- Anterior knee pain
- Patellofemoral dysfunction
- Patellofemoral stress syndrome
- Patellofemoral lateral tracking
- Patellofemoral pain syndrome (PFPS)
- Patellofemoral arthralgia
- Patellofemoral compression syndrome
- Lateral patellar compression syndrome
- Excessive lateral pressure syndrome
- Patellar misalignment syndrome
- Patellalgia

ICD-9-CM CODES

- 717.7 Chondromalacia of patella
- 733.92 Chondromalacia

ICD-10-CM CODES

- M22.40 Chondromalacia patellae, unspecified knee
- M94.20 Chondromalacia, unspecified site

PREFERRED PRACTICE PATTERN

- Pattern 4E: Impaired Joint Mobility, Motor Function, Muscle Performance, and Range of Motion Associated with Localized Inflammation[1]

PATIENT PRESENTATION

Patient is a 14-year-old ballet dancer. Patient presents with medial knee pain. She has been training 2 hours a day for the last 3 weeks as the spring show is approaching. The pain is anterior and along the medial knee cap. The patient has very good flexibility with decreased quadriceps control. The patient received a knee brace with a patella buttress to stabilize the patella. The patient has a muscular imbalance from the vastus medialis to the vastus lateralis.

KEY FEATURES

Description

- Chondromalacia: Softening of cartilage on articular surface of patella at the patellofemoral joint.

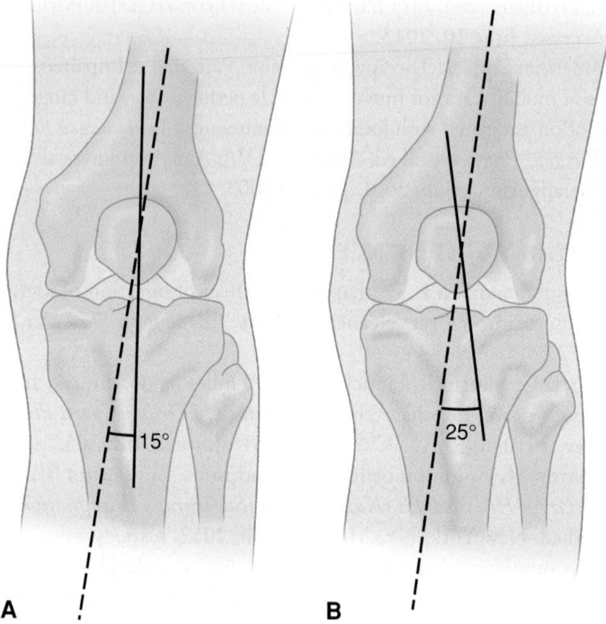

FIGURE 190-1 Measuring the Q angle. (**A**) The normal Q angle is approximately 15 degrees. (**B**) A Q angle of >20 degrees is considered to be abnormal. Patellar malalignment is determined clinically by measuring the *Q angle*. The Q angle is formed by a line drawn from the midpoint of the patella through the midpoint of the femoral shaft and a second line, drawn from the midpoint of the patella through the tibial tuberosity. (Reproduced with permission from Simon RR, Sherman SC, Koenigsknecht SJ. *Emergency Orthopedics, The Extremities.* 5th ed. © 2007. New York, NY: McGraw-Hill Inc.)

- Retropatellar knee pain with patellar cartilage damage.[2]
- Insidious onset typically defined by pain in the retropatellar or peripatellar region.[3]
- Also known as patellofemoral pain syndrome (PFPS), "anterior knee pain syndrome."[2]

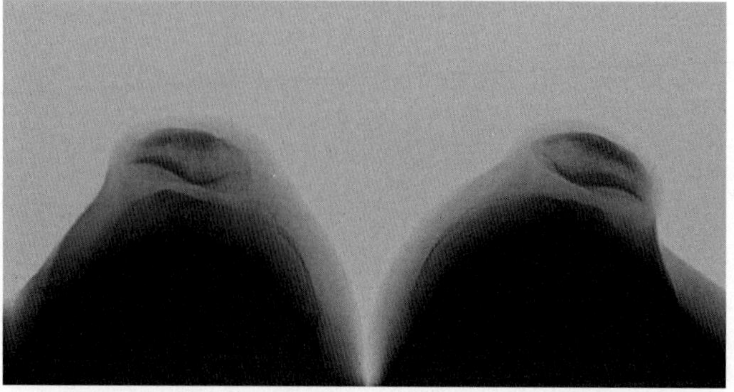

FIGURE 190-2 In this bilateral sunrise or skyline view, note the difference in positioning of the patellae. The image on the right shows much more lateral positioning. (From Malone TR, Hazle C, Grey ML. *Imaging in Rehabilitation.* www.accessphysiotherapy.com. Copyright © The McGraw-Hill Companies, Inc. All rights reserved.)

  - PFPS applies to patients with retropatellar pain and no cartilage damage; chondromalacia applies to patients with patellar damage.[2]
- Structures most likely to generate patellofemoral pain: Anterior synovium, infrapatellar fat pad, subchondral bone, medial or lateral retinaculum.[4,5]

▶ Essentials of Diagnosis

- Insidious onset aggravated by repetitive impact[6]
- Decreased hip stability due to muscular weakness, especially gluteus medius, may affect patellofemoral joint[7,8]
- Q-Angle greater than 20 degrees generally considered a structural abnormality, can put patient at risk for excessive lateral-patellar forces[7]
- Intermittent pain and swelling[6]
- Greater pronated foot posture in relaxed stance[3]

▶ General Considerations

- Patellofemoral joint dysfunction includes
  - Decreased quadriceps flexibility
  - Hypermobile patella
  - Altered vastus medialis oblique (VMO) response
  - Diminished quadriceps explosive strength[7]

▶ Demographics

- Chondral lesions more common, more severe in patients aged 30 years and older, and those who sustained ACL injury >5 years prior[6]
- Frequently occurs among physically active populations, aged 18 to 40 years[9]
- Higher incidence in women than in men[9]

CLINICAL FINDINGS

SIGNS AND SYMPTOMS

- Quadriceps weakness
- Patella maltracking[5]
- Anterior knee pain with deep squatting, descending stairs, prolonged sitting[7]

▶ Functional Implications

- Decreased sitting tolerance
- Difficulty descending stairs
- Decreased ability to squat

▶ Possible Contributing Causes

- Presence of excessively pronated foot posture is then hypothesized intrinsic risk factor[3]
  - Restrictions of first metatarsophalangeal joint (MTPJ) and ankle dorsiflexion reported to increase and prolong rearfoot eversion, respectively[3]
  - Greater foot mobility and greater pronated foot posture during static stance[3]
- PFPS results from increased or altered patellofemoral joint loading secondary to poor patellar tracking[3]
  - Excessive lateral translation or lateral tilt of the patella[10]
- Patella alta[11]
- Patella shape[12]
- Anterior knee pain within 3 months of beginning tennis lessons[7]
- Tight lateral knee structures: Iliotibial band, lateral knee capsule

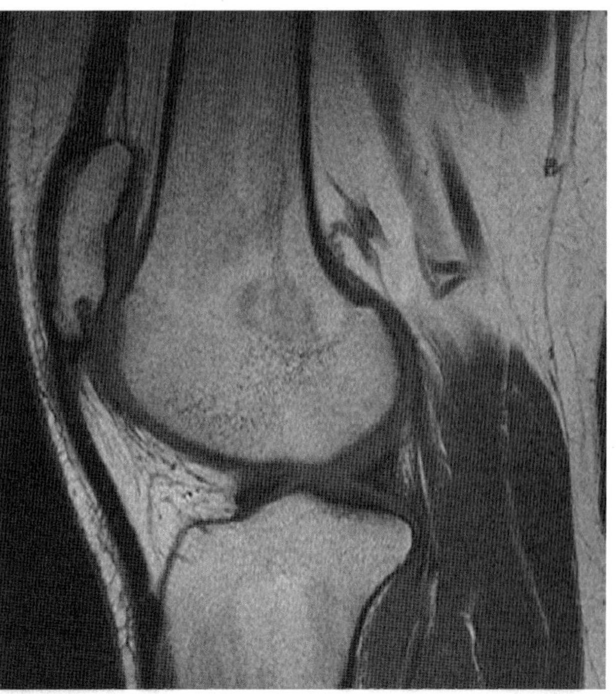

FIGURE 190-3 In addition to the patella alta present, note the sequelae of partial or attempted avulsion of the pole of the patella in this image. The posterior surface of the patella also suggests considerable chondromalacia. (From Malone TR, Hazle C, Grey ML. *Imaging in Rehabilitation.* www.accessphysiotherapy.com.)

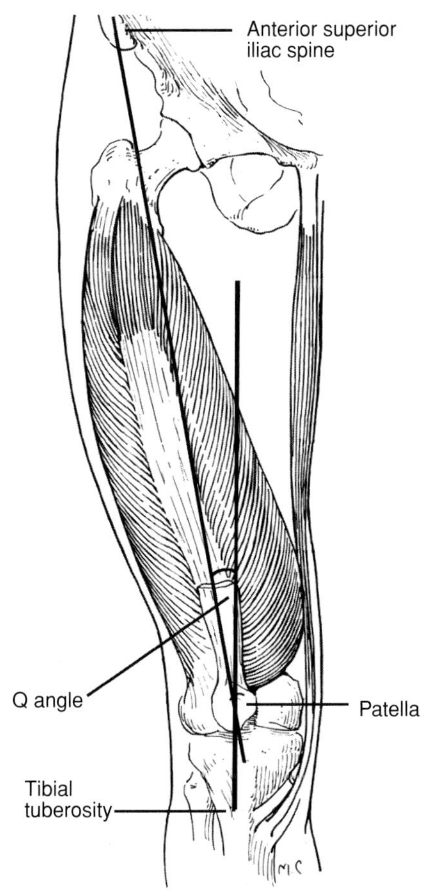

FIGURE 190-4 Q angle. (From Hamilton N, Weimar W, Luttgens K. *Kinesiology: Scientific Basis of Human Motion,* 11th ed. http://www.accessphysiotherapy.com.)

- Weak knee extensors: Quadriceps
- Eccentric under-activation of the hamstrings[13]

Differential Diagnosis

- Patellofemoral arthritis, subluxation, instability[6]
- Plica syndrome[6]
- Anterior knee pain[6]
  - Patellar subluxation, dislocation
  - Tibial apophysitis (Osgood–Schlatter lesion)
  - Jumper's knee (patellar tendonitis)
  - Posterior cruciate ligament (PCL) injury[7]
- Referred pain to low back (L4), sacroiliac joint, hip[7]
- Nonspecific knee, thigh, leg symptoms[6]
  - Arthrofibrosis
  - Deep vein thrombosis
  - Dislocation
  - Fracture
  - Neurovascular compromise
  - Osteoarthritis
  - Septic arthritis

MEANS OF CONFIRMATION OR DIAGNOSIS

Imaging

- Definitive diagnosis of chondromalacia patellae (CMP) requires objective confirmation of retropatellar cartilage disorder, usually by arthroscopy[14]
- X-ray for patella height and position: Sunrise/merchant view[15]

FINDINGS AND INTERPRETATION

- Common to see patella alta along with chondromalacia on radiograph[15]

REFERRALS/ADMITTANCE

- For imaging to rule out fracture in traumatic injury
  - Ottawa Knee rule: Knee radiograph series required in patients with any of the following criteria: [5,6]
    - Age 55 years or older
    - Isolated tenderness of patella (no bone tenderness of knee other than patella)
    - Tender head of fibula
    - Inability to flex knee to 90 degrees
    - Inability to bear weight immediately and in ER for four steps regardless of limping

IMPAIRMENTS

- Abnormal patellar mobility
- Patella alta/baja
- Tightness or weakness in quadriceps
- Tightness in hamstring, gastrocnemius, iliotibial band, iliopsoas
- Weakness with hip external rotation or abduction
- Decreased neuromuscular control of lower extremities

TESTS AND MEASURES

- Step-down test
- Retinacula test[16]
- Fairbank's apprehension test for patella stability[16]
- Ober test[16]
- McConnell test[16]

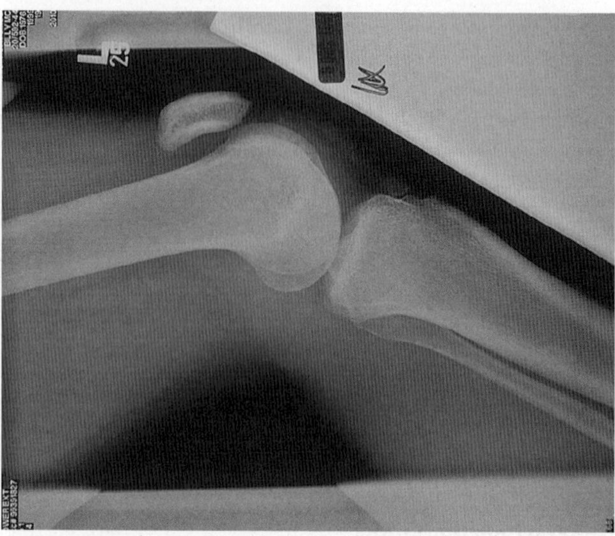

FIGURE 190-5 Patellar dislocation. An obvious lateral deformity of the right patella in a patient with patellar dislocation. (From Knoop K, Stack L, Storrow A, et al. *Atlas of Emergency Medicine,* 3rd ed. © 2010. New York, NY: McGraw-Hill. Photo contributor: Cathleen M. Vossler, MD.)

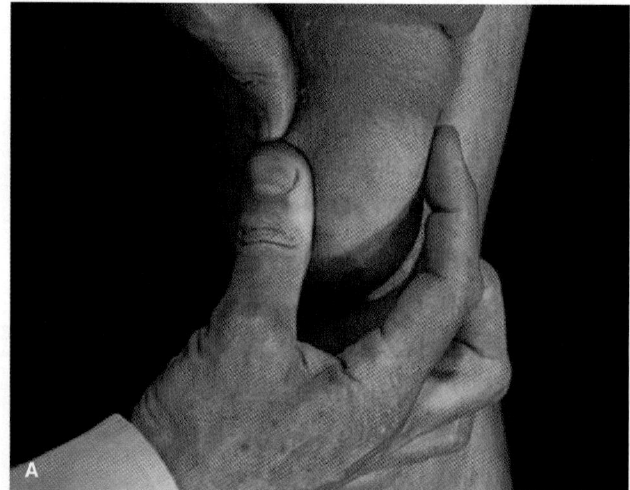

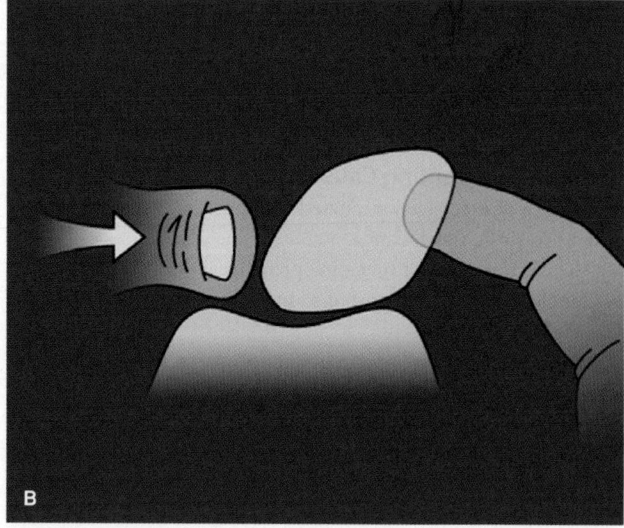

FIGURE 190-6 (**A**) Lateral patellar glide. (**B**) Lateral patellar glide with associated tilt. (From Lawry GV. *Systematic Musculoskeletal Examinations.* www.accessmedicine.com. Copyright © The McGraw-Hill Companies, Inc. All rights reserved.)

- Clarke sign[17]
  - Likelihood ratio for positive test: 1.18
  - Likelihood ratio for negative test: 0.91
  - Positive predictive value: 0.25
  - Negative predictive value: 0.80

INTERVENTION

- Nonoperative treatment is initial treatment of choice, appears effective in most patients[7]
  - Quadriceps strengthening in pain-free range
  - Biofeedback to enhance VMO, vastus lateralis timing[18]
  - Lower-extremity flexibility exercises
  - Orthotics and proper shoewear[5,7]
  - Strengthening, neuromuscular re-education: Hip abductor, external rotators
  - Patellar taping to decrease symptoms[7]
  - Manual therapy at regions proximal to patellofemoral joint have been found to decrease anterior knee pain[19]
- Education to reduce patellofemoral joint stress: avoiding terminal 30 degrees of knee extension during non–weight-bearing exercise, minimizing flexion beyond 90 degrees during weight-bearing activity[7]
- Surgical options (offered after bracing, non-operative PT, and corticosteroid injections have failed)[7]
  - Lateral release, chondroplasty, major proximal and distal realignments, injections[20]
  - Synovectomy (smaller plica resection or larger synovial removal), lateral retinacular release, realignment procedures[7]

FUNCTIONAL GOALS

- Patient will be able to:
  - Descend eight steps without anterior knee pain.
  - Run 1 mile without symptoms.
  - Sit 2 hours in class without pain.
- Patient will improve lower-extremity neuromuscular control during single-leg squat, demonstrated by lack of ipsilateral pelvic elevation, hip internal rotation, adduction.

PROGNOSIS

- Condition may persist in approximately 25% of individuals for average 16 years following initial presentation.[3]
- Four weeks of exercises 3 times per week resulted in pain reduction and improved function.[14]
- Most patients with PFPS respond well to conservative intervention; evidence supports use of exercise for PFPS treatment.[9]

ADDITIONAL INFORMATION

- Patellofemoral Rehabilitation Video[21]
- Anterior knee pain case study[5]

PATIENT RESOURCES

- Chondromalacia. NIH, National Institute of Arthritis and Musculoskeletal and Skin Diseases. http://www.niams.nih.gov/health_info/knee_problems. Accessed March 1, 2013.
- Rehabilitation for Patellofemoral Syndrome "Chondromalacia Patella". http://www.sportmed.com/pdf/Chondromalacia.pdf. Accessed February 12, 2013.

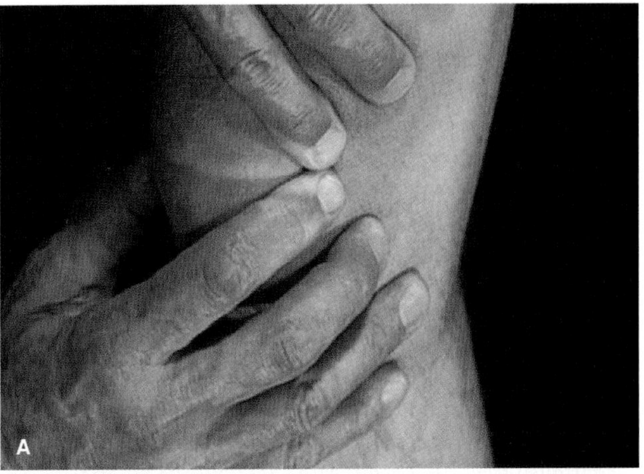

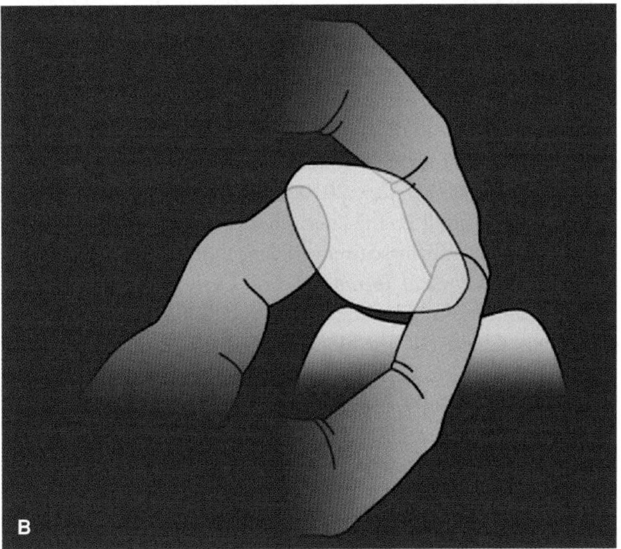

FIGURE 190-7 **A.** Mid patella position. **B.** Patellar tilt. (From Lawry GV. *Systematic Musculoskeletal Examinations.* www.accessmedicine.com. Copyright © The McGraw-Hill Companies, Inc. All rights reserved.)

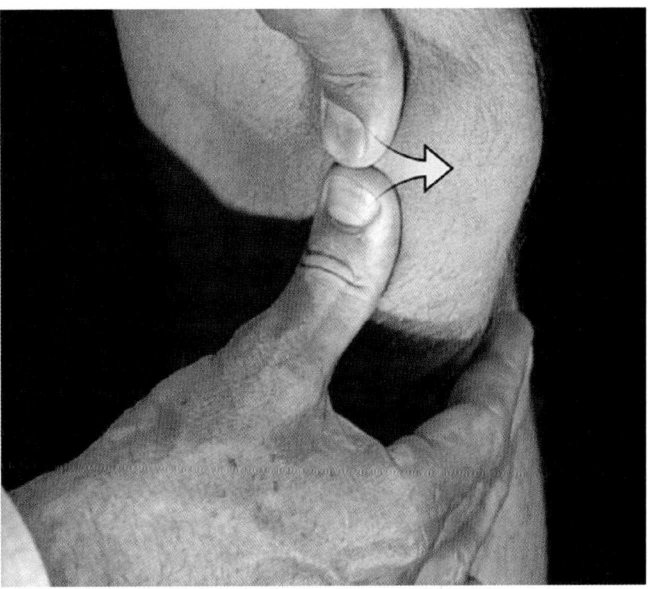

FIGURE 190-8 Assessment of lateral patellar mobility. (From Lawry GV. *Systematic Musculoskeletal Examinations.* www.accessmedicine.com. Copyright © The McGraw-Hill Companies, Inc. All rights reserved.)

REFERENCES

1. American Physical Therapy Association. Pattern 4E: Impaired joint mobility, motor function, muscle performance, and range of motion associated with localized inflammation. *Interactive Guide to Physical Therapist Practice*. 2003. doi: 10.2522/ptguide.3.1_5. Accessed March 1, 2013.
2. Heintjes E, Berger MY, Bierma-Zeinstra SM, et al.. Exercise therapy for patellofemoral pain syndrome. *Cochrane Database Syst Rev*. 2003;(4):CD003472.
3. Barton CJ, Bonanno D, Levinger P, et al. Foot and ankle characteristics in patellofemoral pain syndrome: A case control and reliability study. *J Orthop Sports Phys Ther*. 2010;40(5):286–296.
4. Crossley K, Bennell K, Green S, et al. Physical therapy for patellofemoral pain a randomized, double-blinded, placebo-controlled trial. *Am J Sports Med*. 2002;30(6):857–865.
5. Dutton M. *Orthopaedic Examination, Evaluation, and Intervention*. New York, NY: McGraw-Hill; 2008. http://www.accessphysiotherapy.com/resource/612. Accessed March 15, 2013.
6. Logerstedt DS, Snyder-Mackler L, Orthopedic Section of the American Physical Therapy Association, et al. Knee Pain and Mobility Impairments: meniscal and articular cartilage lesions. *J Orthop Sports Phys Ther*. 2010;40(6):A1–A35.
7. Manal TJ, Sturgill L. The knee: Physical therapy patient management utilizing current evidence. In: *Current Concepts of Orthopaedic Physical Therapy*. 2nd ed. Orthopedic section of the American Physical Therapy Association; 2006.
8. Hall SJ. Chapter 4. The biomechanics of human bone growth and development. *Basic Biomechanics*.4th ed. New York, NY: McGraw-Hill; 2007. http://www.accessphysiotherapy.com/abstract/6060836#6060838. Accessed August 9, 2014.
9. Fukuda TY, Rossetto FM, Magalhães E,et al. Short-term effects of hip abductors and lateral rotators strengthening in females with patellofemoral pain syndrome: A randomized controlled clinical trial. *J Orthop Sports Phys Ther*. 2010;40(11):736–742.
10. Draper CE, Besier TF, Santos JM, et al. Using real-time MRI to quantify altered joint kinematics in subjects with patellofemoral pain and to evaluate the effects of a patellar brace or sleeve on joint motion. *Journal of Orthopaedic Research*. 2009;27(5): 571–577.
11. Pal S, Besier TF, Beaupre GS, et al. Patellar maltracking is prevalent among patellofemoral pain subjects with patella alta: an upright, weightbearing MRI study. *Journal of Orthopaedic Research*. 2013;31(3):448–457. http://nmbl.stanford.edu/publications/pdf/Pal2012.pdf
12. Connolly KD, Ronsky JL, Westover LM, et al. Differences in patellofemoral contact mechanics associated with patellofemoral pain syndrome. *Journal of Biomechanics*. 2009;42(16): 2802–2807.
13. Liebensteiner MC, Szubski C, Raschner C, et al. Frontal plane leg alignment and muscular activity during maximum eccentric contractions in individuals with and without patellofemoral pain syndrome. *Knee*. 2008;15(3):180–186.
14. McAlindon TE. The knee. *Baillieres Clin Rheumatol*. 1999; 13(2):329–344.
15. Malone TR, Hazle C, Grey ML. *Imaging in Rehabilitation*. New York, NY: McGraw-Hill; 2008. http://www.accessphysiotherapy.com/resource/613. Accessed March 15, 2013.
16. Dutton M. *Dutton's Orthopedic Survival Guide: Managing Common Conditions*. New York, NY: McGraw-Hill; 2011. http://www.accessphysiotherapy.com/resource/685. Accessed March 15, 2013.
17. Doberstein ST, Romeyn RL, Reineke DM. The diagnostic value of the Clarke sign in assessing chondromalacia patella. *J Athl Train*. 2008;43(2):190–196.
18. Prentice WE. Chapter 7. Biofeedback. In: Prentice WE, Quillen WS, Underwood F, eds. *Therapeutic Modalities in Rehabilitation*.4th ed. New York, NY: McGraw-Hill; 2011. http://www.accessphysiotherapy.com/abstract/8137237. Accessed March 15, 2013.
19. Lowry CD, Cleland JA, Dyke K. Management of patients with patellofemoral pain syndrome using a multimodal approach: a case series. *J Orthop Sports Phys Ther*. 2008;38(11):691–702.
20. Dye SF. Patellofemoral pain current concepts: an overview. *Sports Med Arthrosc*. 2001;9:264–272. Review.
21. Patellofemoral: Rehabilitation. AccessPysiotherapy Multimedia. http://www.accessphysiotherapy.com/abstract/8955131. Accessed March 15, 2013.

ADDITIONAL REFERENCES

- Bolgla LA, Boling MC. An update for the conservative management of patellofemoral pain syndrome: a systematic review of the literature from 2000 to 2010. *Int J Sports Phys Ther*. 2011;6(2): 112–125.
- ICD9DATA web site. http://www.icd9data.com. Accessed March 16, 2013.
- ICD10DATA web site. http://www.icd10data.com. Accessed March 16, 2013.

191 FIBULA FRACTURE

Jennifer Cabrera, DPT, GCS
Eric Shamus, PhD, DPT, PT, CSCS

CONDITION/DISORDER SYNONYMS

- Proximal fibular fracture
- Fibula stress fracture
- Midshaft fibular fracture
- Maisonneuve fracture
- Dupuytren fracture

ICD-9-CM CODES

- 823.0 Fracture of upper end of tibia and fibula closed
- 823.01 Closed fracture of upper end of fibula
- 823.02 Closed fracture of upper end of fibula with tibia
- 823.1 Fracture of upper end of tibia and fibula open
- 823.11 Open fracture of upper end of fibula
- 823.12 Open fracture of upper end of fibula with tibia
- 823.2 Fracture of shaft of tibia and fibula closed
- 823.21 Closed fracture of shaft of fibula
- 823.22 Closed fracture of shaft of fibula with tibia
- 823.3 Fracture of shaft of tibia and fibula open
- 823.31 Open fracture of shaft of fibula
- 823.32 Open fracture of shaft of fibula with tibia
- 823.4 Torus fracture of tibia and fibula
- 823.41 Torus fracture of fibula alone
- 823.42 Torus fracture of fibula with tibia
- 823.8 Fracture of unspecified part of tibia and fibula closed
- 823.81 Closed fracture of unspecified part of fibula
- 823.82 Closed fracture of unspecified part of fibula with tibia
- 823.9 Fracture of unspecified part of tibia and fibula open
- 823.91 Open fracture of unspecified part of fibula
- 823.92 Open fracture of unspecified part of fibula with tibia

ICD-10-CM CODES

- S82.401A Unspecified fracture of shaft of right fibula, initial encounter for closed fracture
- S82.402A Unspecified fracture of shaft of left fibula, initial encounter for closed fracture
- S82.90XA Unspecified fracture of unspecified lower leg, initial encounter for closed fracture

PREFERRED PRACTICE PATTERN

- 4G: Impaired Joint Mobility, Muscle Performance, and Range of Motion Associated with Fracture[1]

PATIENT PRESENTATION

A 55-year-old man was involved in a motor vehicle accident. He reported acute lower leg pain immediately after the accident. He was unable to bear weight on the foot upon exiting his vehicle. He presented with pain, swelling of the lower leg, ankle, and foot with notable hematoma. Radiographs showed a nondisplaced oblique fracture of the distal fibula. Patient referred to physical therapy 3 weeks later wearing a cam walker.

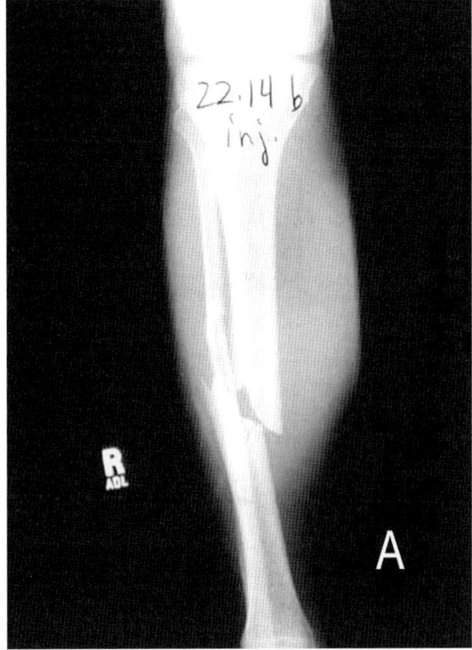

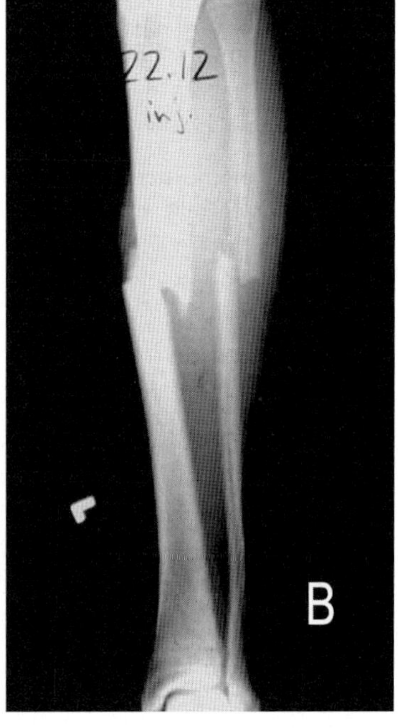

FIGURE 191-1 (**A**) Anteroposterior and (**B**) lateral radiographs of a displaced midshaft tibia fracture. (From Doherty GM. *Current Diagnosis & Treatment: Surgery.* 13th ed.. www.accessmedicine.com. Copyright ©The McGraw-Hill Companies, Inc. All rights reserved.)

KEY FEATURES

Description

- Fracture[2]
- Any defect in continuity of the fibula
- Displaced (fibula is moved on either side of the fracture) or nondisplaced (fibula has not moved)
- Closed (skin is intact) or open (skin is breached)
- Dupuytren fracture: proximal fibular fracture, involves the syndesmosis at the ankle
- Maisonneuve fracture is a proximal fibular fracture from external rotation

Essentials of Diagnosis

- Diagnosis usually made by clinical examination
- May be third degree ankle sprain rather than fracture

General Considerations

- Recent increases in number and severity secondary to an active older population.
- Often associated with tibia fracture or severe ankle sprain.
- Weight bearing and ambulation is possible with isolated fibula fractures.

Demographics

- Affects all ages

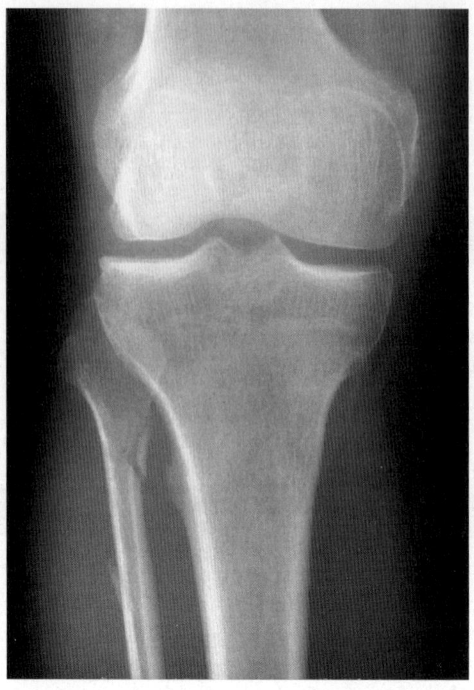

FIGURE 191-2 AP view of the knee. The proximal fibula is fractured. (From Chen MYM, Pope TL, Ott DJ. *Basic Radiology.* 2nd ed. http://www.accessmedicine.com. Copyright © The McGraw-Hill Companies, Inc. All rights reserved.)

CLINICAL FINDINGS

SIGNS AND SYMPTOMS

- Pain, moderate to severe
- Point tenderness and swelling in the calf
- Increased pain on weight bearing
- Inability to bear weight
- Edema
- Ecchymosis
- Bone deformity
- Loss of general function
- Loss of active mobility
- Point tenderness over the fibular head
- Muscle guarding with passive movement
- Numbness or coldness below the fracture, impaired blood supply

Functional Implications

- Pain with standing
- Inability to bear weight on injured lower extremity
- Pain with open-chain ankle movements (e.g., driving)

Possible Contributing Causes

- Impaired standing balance
- History of high-impact activities
- Trauma
- Motor vehicle accident
- Indirect or rotational forces
- Improper footwear
- Chronic ankle injuries
- Osteoporosis
- Cigarette smoking

Differential Diagnosis

- Fibular dislocation
- Ankle sprain
- Achilles tendonitis
- Lateral collateral ligament sprain

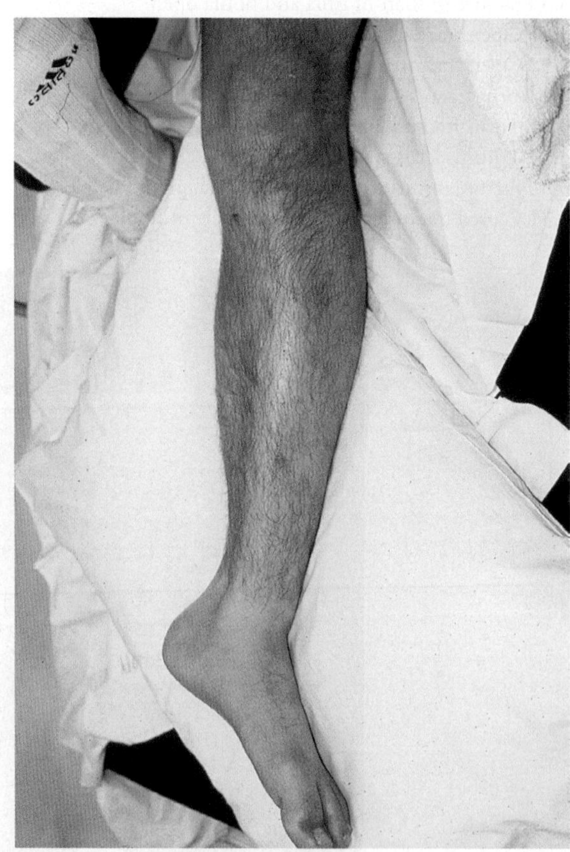

FIGURE 191-3 Tibial–Fibular Fracture. Deformity associated with a midshaft tibial and fibular fracture. (From Knoop KJ, Stack L, Storrow A, et al. *The Atlas of Emergency Medicine.* 3rd ed. http://www.accessmedicine.com. Copyright © The McGraw-Hill Companies, Inc. All rights reserved. Photo contributor: Kevin J. Knoop, MD, MS.)

- Lateral meniscus tear
- Compartment syndrome
- Peripheral vascular injuries

MEANS OF CONFIRMATION OR DIAGNOSIS

Imaging

- X-ray for fracture, often limited view[3]
- CT scan for detailed imaging[2]
- Bone scan if stress fracture suspected[4]
- Ultrasonography

Diagnostic Procedures

- Ottawa foot rules

FINDINGS AND INTERPRETATION

- Hop-to gait sequence or decreased stance-time on injured lower extremity secondary to pain.
- Exposed bone in the case of open and displaced fracture.
- Integumentary deformity over underlying fracture.
- If vascular structures are involved, foot will appear cool and pale.
- If neurologic structures are involved, individual will report numbness and decreased ability to move the foot or toes.

REFERRALS/ADMITTANCE

- To hospital for imaging: X-ray or CT[2]
- To physician for medication: NSAID or opiod for pain management
- To physician for orthopedic consult
  - Fracture reduction
- Surgical intervention: Open reduction and internal fixation (ORIF)
- Immobilization with casting or splinting of the ankle

IMPAIRMENTS

- Antalgic gait secondary to pain, causing inability to push off
- Inability to ambulate long distances secondary to pain or decreased weight-bearing status, which make ambulating difficult
- Decreased stance-time on affected lower extremity during ambulation
- Inability to stand for long periods of time secondary to pain

TESTS AND MEASURES

- Straight-leg raise limited secondary to muscle tightness[3]
- Gait assessment (with appropriate assistive device and/ or prosthesis)
  - Observational analysis
  - Gait speed via the 10-m walk test
  - 2-minute walk test
  - 6-minute walk test
- Balance
  - Static single-leg standing (eyes open, eyes closed)
  - Dynamic standing (with prosthesis)
    - Berg Balance Scale
    - Gait Assessment Rating Score
    - Rancho Los Amigo observational gait analysis
    - Multi-directional reach test (MDRT)
- Pain with resistance
- Palpation of pulses in the foot

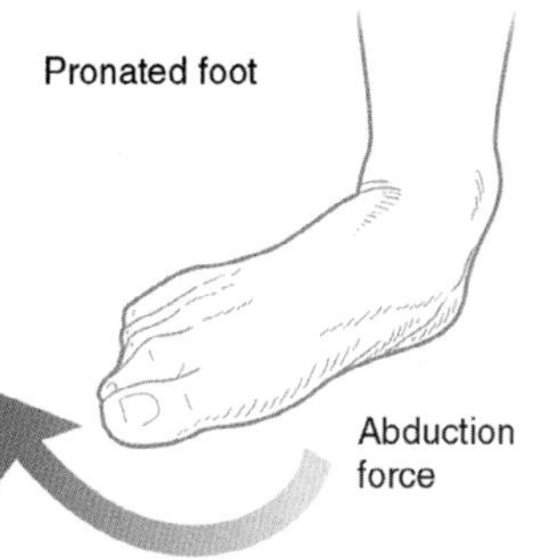

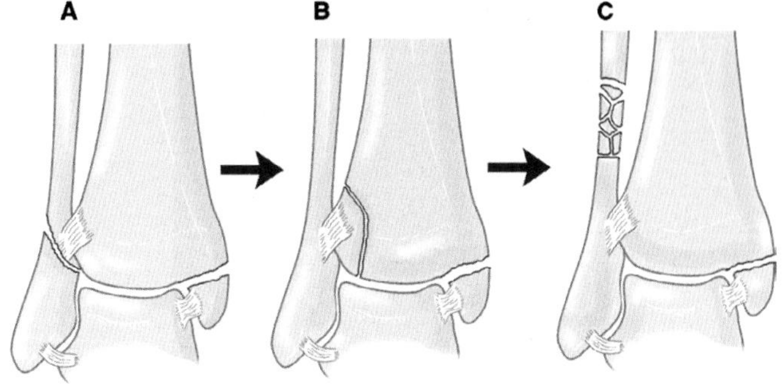

FIGURE 191-4 Schematic representing the progression of injury following forced abduction of the pronated foot. (**A**) Isolated medial malleolus fracture. (**B**) With increasing force, the anterior tibiofibular ligament avulses a portion of the distal tibia. (**C**) Finally, a transverse or comminuted fibula fracture occurs. (From Simon RR, Sherman SC. *Emergency Orthopedics.* 6th ed. http://www.accessemergencymedicine.com. Copyright © The McGraw-Hill Companies, Inc. All rights reserved.)

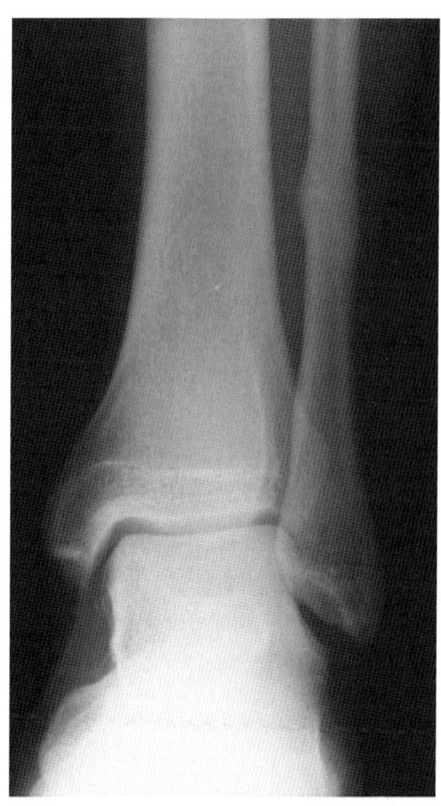

FIGURE 191-5 This AP radiograph reveals periosteal reaction of the distal fibula consistent with a stress fracture. Such injuries are often found in runners. (From Malone TR, Hazle C, Grey ML. *Imaging in Rehabilitation.* http://www.accessphysiotherapy.com. Copyright © The McGraw-Hill Companies, Inc. All rights reserved.)

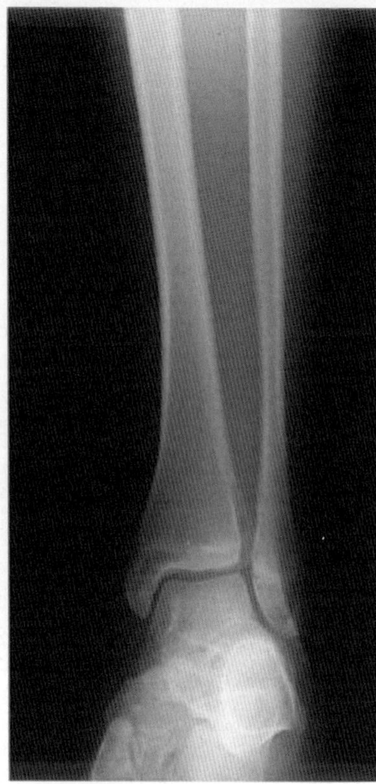

FIGURE 191-6 Radiograph showing grade I Salter–Harris fracture of fibula. (From Dutton M. *Dutton's Orthopaedic Examination, Evaluation, and Intervention*. 3rd ed. http://www.accessphysiotherapy.com. Copyright © The McGraw-Hill Companies, Inc. All rights reserved.)

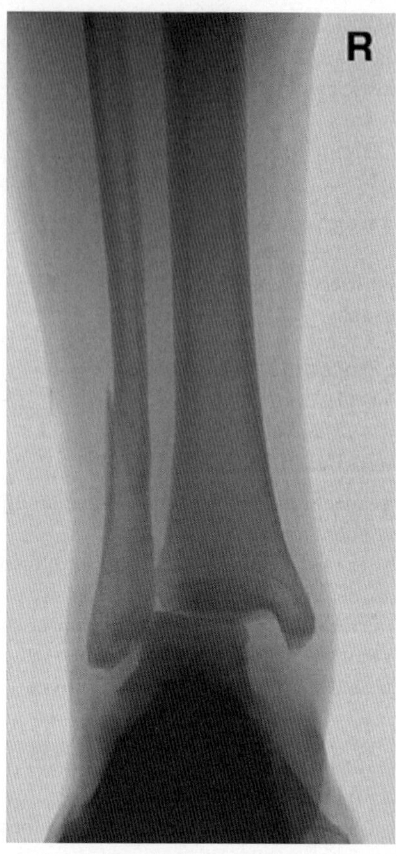

FIGURE 191-7 In this AP radiograph, disruption of the mortise and a fracture of the fibula are apparent. The mechanism of injury is usually due to an external rotation force. So-called Maisonneuve fractures are typically characterized by a proximal fibula fracture, although more distal injuries are sometimes included in this same category. (From Malone TR, Hazle C, Grey ML. *Imaging in Rehabilitation*. http://www.accessphysiotherapy.com. Copyright © The McGraw-Hill Companies, Inc. All rights reserved.)

- Capillary refill
- Strength Functional strength testing
  - Five-times-sit-to-stand test
  - Manual muscle test (MMT)

INTERVENTION

- Depending on the type of fracture, more severe cases require ORIF
- Ultrasound to stimulate fracture-healing in skeletally mature patients[5]
- CAM walker/rocker boot to limit dorsiflexion to neutral, stirrup brace
- Orthotics to provide proper arch support with neutral subtalar positioning in order to avoid stressing injured structures[4]
- Address swelling
  - Ice/Cryotherapy[6]
  - Compression
  - Elevation
  - Electrical stimulation[7]
- Address pain
  - Ice/Cryotherapy[6]
  - Massage
  - Electrical stimulation[7]
- Address mobilization
  - Anterior distal tibiofibular glide to increase plantarflexion
  - Posterior distal tibiofibular glide to increase dorsiflexion
  - Gentle talocrural distraction for pain control
  - Subtalar distraction for general inversion or eversion
  - Medial subtalar glide for eversion
  - Lateral subtalar glide for inversion
- Address lack of flexibility via stretching
  - Gastrocnemius
  - Soleus
- Address weakness via strengthening activities
  - Open-chain ankle movements in all planes with resistance bands
  - Heel raises
  - Toe raises
  - Toe curls, intrinsic flexors
  - Active positioning of foot in subtalar neutral
- Address proprioception[8]
  - Standing balance activities with foam
    - Eyes open
    - Eyes closed
  - Standing balance activities on balance machines
- Gait training[9]
  - Lateral weight shifting to promote stance-time on injured lower extremity
  - Resisted walking to promote proper gait sequence with eccentric/concentric control
  - Promote push-off and heel-strike

FUNCTIONAL GOALS

- Patient will be able to:
  - Achieve 15 degrees of talocrural dorsiflexion in order to enhance push-off phase of gait.
  - Maintain subtalar neutral for 1 minute during single-limb stance with eyes open.
  - Increase speed of gait to 1.2 m/s or greater to promote safe community ambulation.
  - Ascend/descend 12 to 16 steps with unilateral hand rail in order to facilitate mobility while in school.

PROGNOSIS

- Very good, though normal fracture healing time varies individual's age.
  - Children 4 to 6 weeks
  - Adolescents 6 to 8 weeks
  - Adults 10 to 18 weeks
- Most individuals return to normal levels of function, except sports activity, within 3 to 4 months.
- Some individuals will still be recovering up to 2 years after injury.

PATIENT RESOURCE

- American Academy of Orthopaedic Surgeons. *Stress Fractures of the Foot and Ankle.* Available at: http://orthoinfo.aaos.org/topic.cfm?topic=A00379. Accessed April 13, 2013.

REFERENCES

1. American Physical Therapy Association. Pattern 4G: Impaired joint mobility, muscle performance, and range of motion associated with fracture. *Interactive Guide to Physical Therapist Practice.* 2003. doi: 10.2522/ptguide.3.1_7. Online February 28, 2012. Accessed April 1, 2013.
2. Hall SJ. Chapter 4. The biomechanics of human bone growth and development. *Basic Biomechanics.*4th ed. New York, NY: McGraw-Hill; 2007. http://www.accessphysiotherapy.com/abstract/6060836#6060838. Accessed April 8, 2013.
3. Malone TR, Hazle C, Grey ML. Chapter 1. Introduction to musculoskeletal imaging. *Imaging in Rehabilitation.* New York, NY: McGraw-Hill; 2008. http://www.accessphysiotherapy.com/abstract/5940003#5940003. Accessed April 8, 2013.
4. Dutton M. Chapter 19. The ankle and foot. *Orthopaedic Examination, Evaluation, and Intervention.* New York, NY: McGraw-Hill; 2008. http://www.accessphysiotherapy.com/abstract/55586760#55587364. Accessed April 8, 2013.
5. Prentice WE, Blake B. Chapter 1. The basic science of therapeutic modalities. In: Prentice WE, Quillen WS, Underwood F, eds. *Therapeutic Modalities in Rehabilitation.* 4th ed. New York, NY: McGraw-Hill; 2011. http://www.accessphysiotherapy.com/abstract/8135087#8135091. Accessed April 8, 2013.
6. Prentice WE. Chapter 9. Cryotherapy and thermotherapy. In: Prentice WE, Quillen WS, Underwood F, eds. *Therapeutic Modalities in Rehabilitation.*4th ed. New York, NY: McGraw-Hill; 2011. http://www.accessphysiotherapy.com/content/8137995#8137995. Accessed April 8, 2013.
7. Hooker DN, Prentice WE. Chapter 5. Basic principles of electricity and electrical stimulating currents. In: Prentice WE, Quillen WS, Underwood F, eds. *Therapeutic Modalities in Rehabilitation* 4th ed. New York, NY: McGraw-Hill; 2011. http://www.accessphysiotherapy.com/content/8136367#8136367. Accessed April 8, 2013.
8. Dutton M. Chapter 2. The nervous system. *Orthopaedic Examination, Evaluation, and Intervention.* New York, NY: McGraw-Hill; 2008. http://www.accessphysiotherapy.com/abstract/5541168#5541193. Accessed April 8, 2013.
9. Dutton M. Chapter 17. Therapeutic exercise. *NPTE (National Physical Therapy Examination).* 2nd ed. 2012. http://www.accessphysiotherapy.com/abstract/5405700#5405706. Accessed April 8, 2013.

ADDITIONAL REFERENCES

- Goodman CC, Boissonnault WG, Fuller KS. *Pathology: Implications for the Physical Therapist.* 2nd ed. Philadelphia, PA: Saunders; 2003.
- ICD9DATA web site. http://www.icd9data.com. Accessed April 1, 2013.
- ICD10DATA web site. http://www.icd10data.com. Accessed April 1, 2013.
- Kisner C, Colby LA. *Therapeutic Exercise: Foundations and Techniques.* 5th ed. Philadelphia, PA: F.A. Davis Company; 2007.
- Magee DJ. *Orthopedic Physical Assessment.* 5th ed. St. Louis, MO: Saunders Elsevier. 2008.

192 HAMSTRING STRAIN

Josh A. Barabas, MPT, OCS, CSCS
Christina L. Pettie, MHA, PT

CONDITION/DISORDER SYNONYM

- Pulled hamstring

ICD-9-CM CODE

- 848.9 Unspecified site of sprain and strain

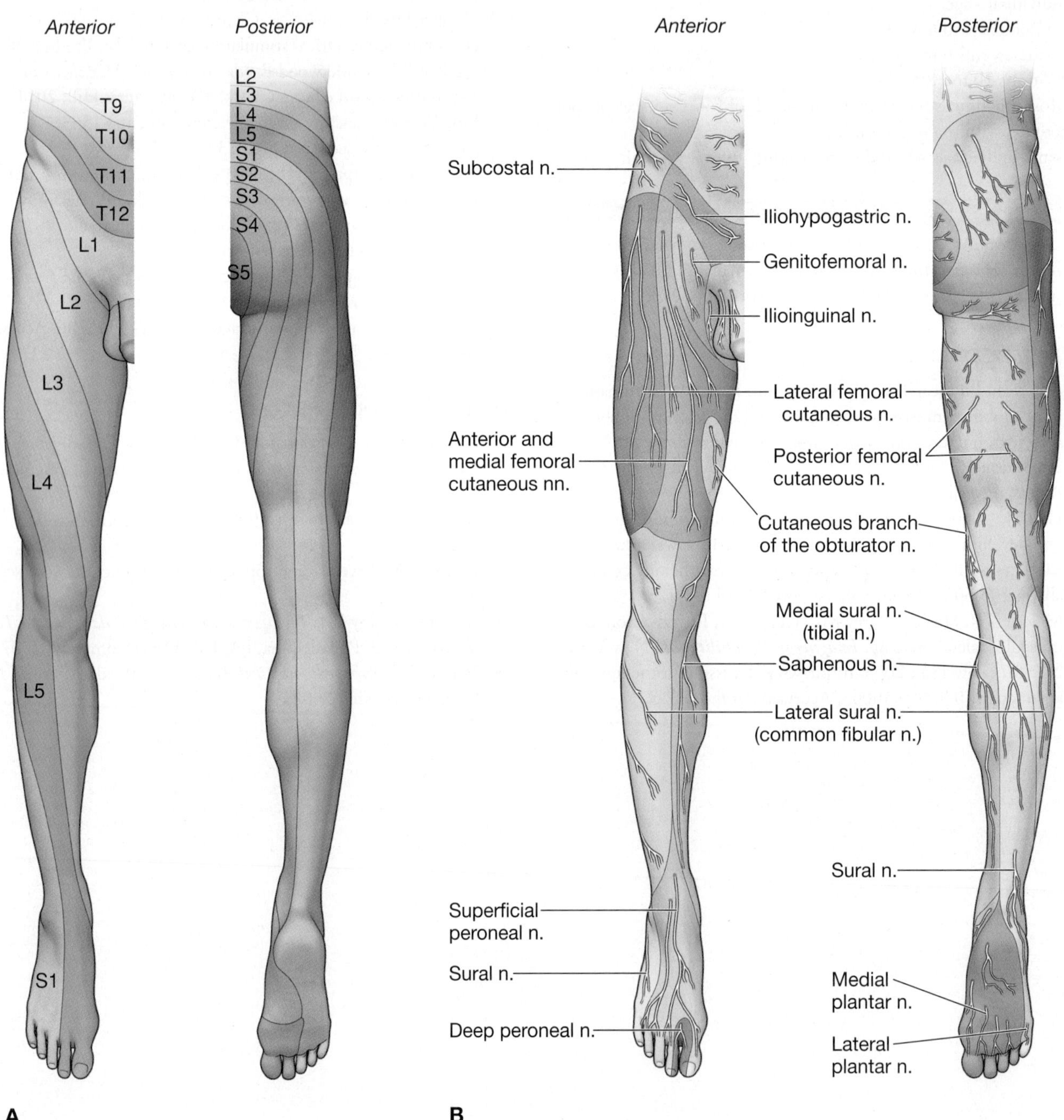

FIGURE 192-1 Dermatomal (**A**) and cutaneous (**B**) innervation of the lower limb. (From Morton DA, Foreman KB, Albertine KH. *The Big Picture: Gross Anatomy*. http://www.accessmedicine.com. Copyright © The McGraw-Hill Companies, Inc. All rights reserved.)

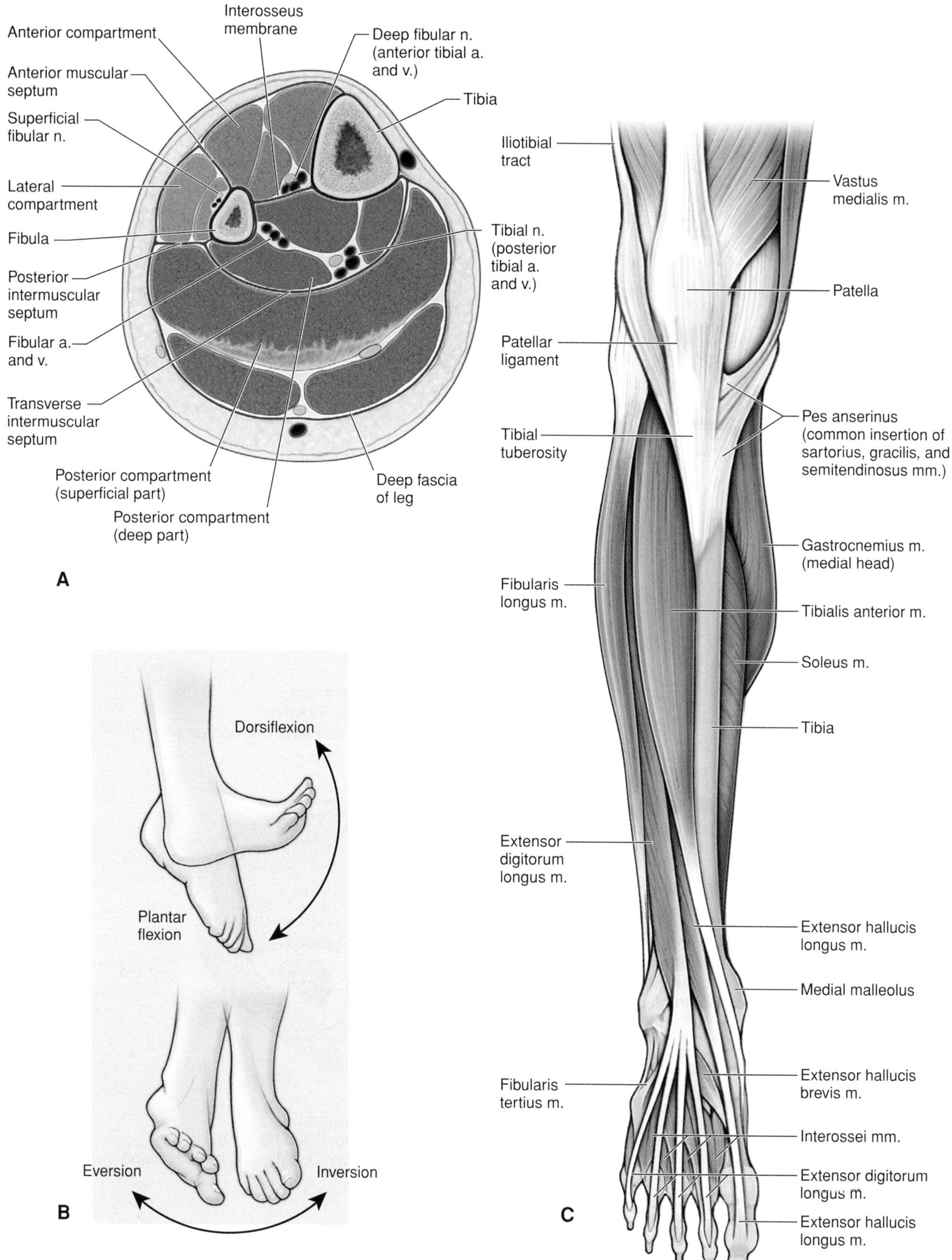

FIGURE 192-2 (**A**) Cross-section of the right leg. (**B**) Movements of the ankle. (**C**) Muscles of the anterior compartment of the leg. (From Morton DA, Foreman KB, Albertine KH. *The Big Picture: Gross Anatomy*. http://www.accessmedicine.com. Copyright © The McGraw-Hill Companies, Inc. All rights reserved.)

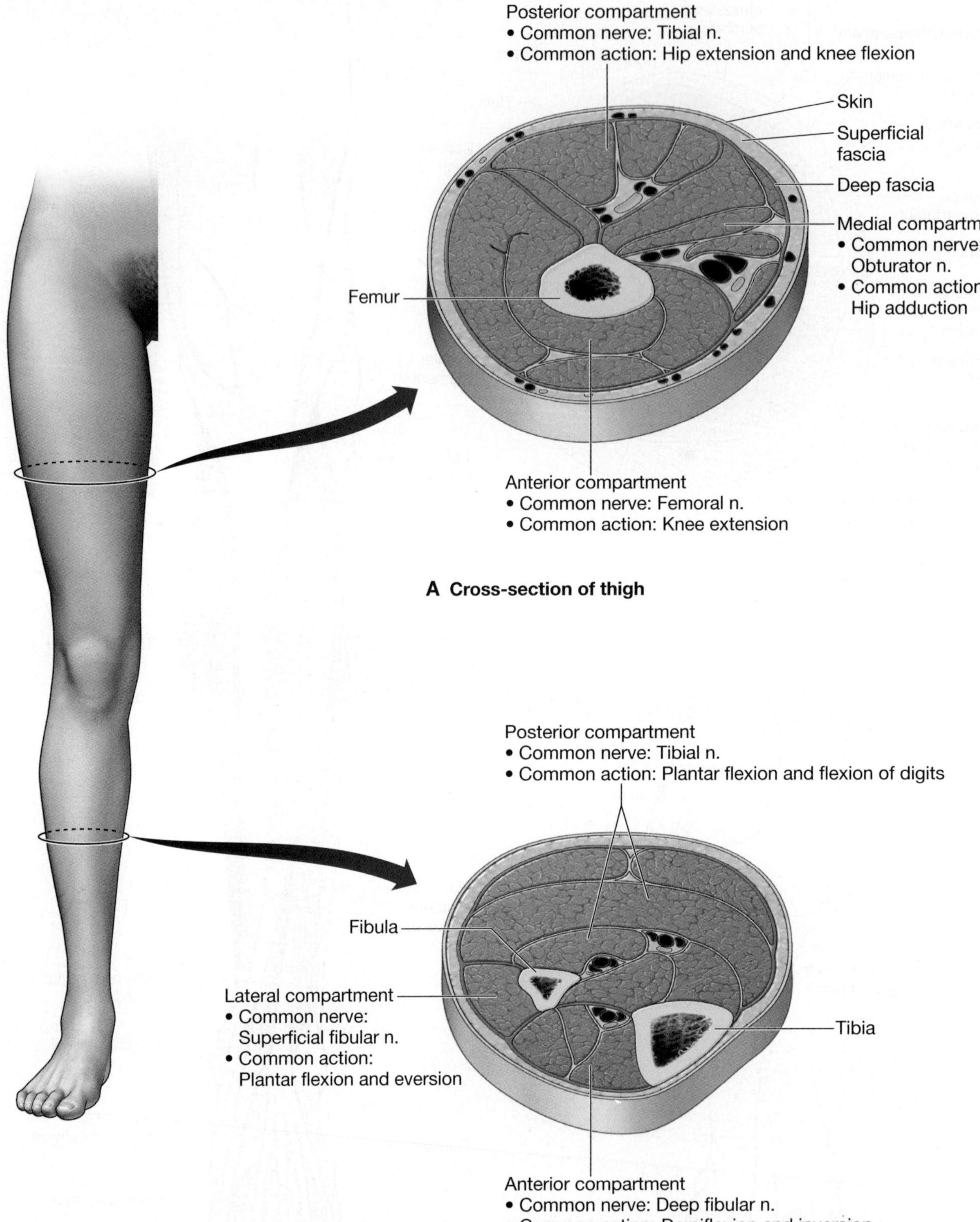

FIGURE 192-3 Cross-section of the thigh (**A**) and leg (**B**). (From Morton DA, Foreman KB, Albertine KH. *The Big Picture: Gross Anatomy.* http://www.accessmedicine.com. Copyright © The McGraw-Hill Companies, Inc. All rights reserved.)

ICD-10-CM CODE

- T14.9 Dislocation, sprain, and strain of unspecified body region

PREFERRED PRACTICE PATTERNS

- 4D: Impaired joint mobility, motor function, muscle performance, and range of motion (ROM) associated with connective tissue dysfunction
- 4E: Impaired joint mobility, motor function, muscle performance, and ROM associated with localized inflammation

PATIENT PRESENTATION

A 21-year-old female presents complaining of right posterior thigh and buttock pain. She indicates the pain began suddenly 3 days ago during the fourth set of high intensity 100-m sprint intervals. She recently added speed work into her distance running regiment. She denies hearing an audible pop. She reports pain is worse with bending forward and running. She presents without ecchymosis or visible edema. Palpation reveals tenderness distal to her right ischial tuberosity. Manual muscle testing reveals significant strength deficits due to pain in both knee flexion and hip extension compared to the uninvolved side. Hamstring flexibility is 65 degrees on right side compared to 90 degrees on left in a straight-leg raise (SLR) position. Testing proves negative for lumbar radiculopathy.

KEY FEATURES

Description

- Stretch injury to biceps femoris or semimembranosus resulting in disruption of muscular or musculotendinous units[1]
  - Grade I: Mild
  - Grade II: Moderate
  - Grader III: Severe to complete tear or rupture

Essentials of Diagnosis

- Diagnosis made with patient history and clinical findings or with imaging
- Pain with resistance
- Location of lesion may influence prognosis

General Considerations

- Mechanisms of injury[2]
  - Deceleration during swing phase while running
    - Typically occurs during high-speed running
    - Involves intramuscular tendon or aponeurosis of biceps femoris (long head), semitendinosus (secondary injury)
  - Excessive stretch while dancing or kicking
    - Typically during extreme hip flexion with full knee extension
    - Injury at proximal tendon of semimembranosus

Demographics

- Previous hamstring injury is a strong predictor of recurrence
- Athletes in high-speed-demand sports (e.g., football, track, rugby, soccer)
- Athletes in sports/competition involving kicking or extreme hip flexion and knee extension (e.g., dancing, water-skiing)

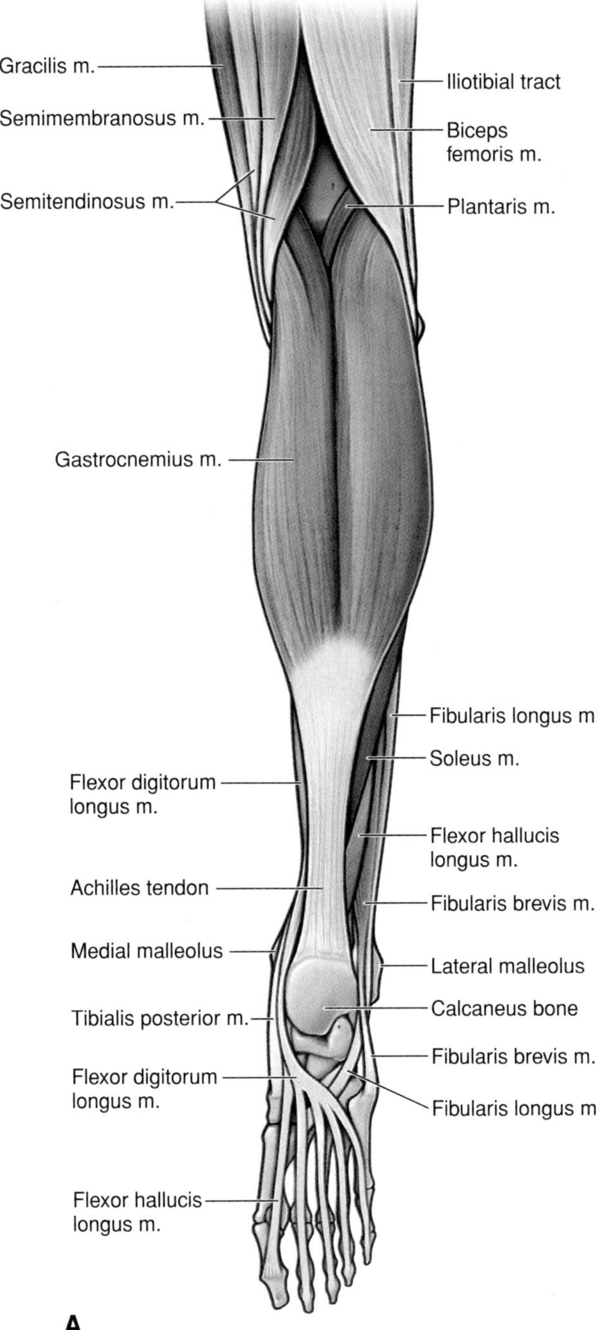

FIGURE 192-4 Muscles of the posterior compartment of the leg: (**A**) superficial dissection, (*continued*)

CLINICAL FINDINGS

SIGNS AND SYMPTOMS

- Acute-onset pain at proximal hamstring during high-speed running, often with audible pop, typically early or late in athletic event
- Pain at ischial tuberosity with sitting[1]
- Decreased ROM in knee and hip

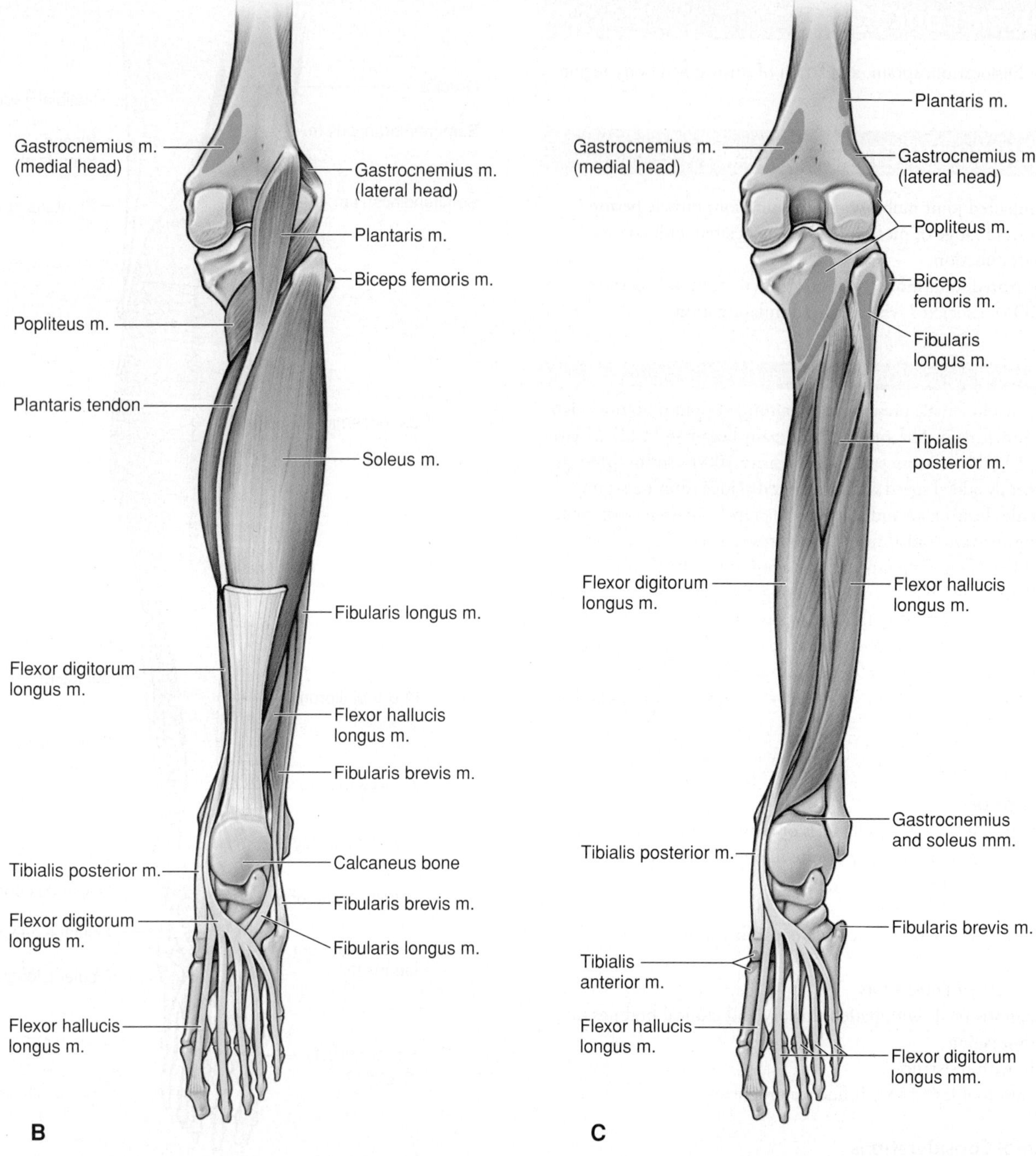

FIGURE 192-4 (*Continued*) (**B**) intermediate dissection, (**C**) deep dissection. (From Morton DA, Foreman KB, Albertine KH. *The Big Picture: Gross Anatomy*. http://www.accessmedicine.com. Copyright © The McGraw-Hill Companies, Inc. All rights reserved.)

- Decreased strength with knee flexion and hip extension
- Tenderness to palpation (possible palpable lesion) at proximal tendon or musculotendinous junction
- Tenderness may occur along muscle belly proximal to ischial tuberosity

Functional Implications

- Inability to run or sprint
- Inability to sit without limitation from pain
- Inability to flex hip with knee fully extended

Possible Contributing Causes

- Previous history of hamstring injury
- Explosion activity without proper warm-up
- Muscle imbalance between quadriceps and hamstring
- Sacroiliac or lumbar spine dysfunction

Differential Diagnosis

- Adverse neural tension
- Adductor muscle strain
- Avulsion fractures at ischial tuberosity
- Lumbar radiculopathy

- Sacroiliac dysfunction
- Sciatica

MEANS OF CONFIRMATION OR DIAGNOSIS

Imaging

- MRI for soft tissue[2]

FINDINGS AND INTERPRETATION

- MRI can reveal area of fluid accumulation and location of lesion

TREATMENT

Medication

- NSAIDs[3]

MEDICAL PROCEDURES

- Surgery to repair grade-III strain or avulsion

REFERRALS/ADMITTANCE

- To hospital for imaging (MRI)
- Surgery (if grade-III strain)

IMPAIRMENTS

- Inability to run or sprint
- Inability to sit without limitation from pain
- Inability to flex hip with knee fully extended

TESTS AND MEASURES

- SLR limited secondary to muscle tightness[3]
- Gait assessment (with appropriate assistive device and/or prosthesis)
  - Observational analysis
  - Gait speed via the 10-m walk test
  - 2-minute walk test
  - 6-minute walk test
- Balance
  - Static single-leg standing (eyes open, eyes closed)
  - Dynamic standing (with prosthesis)
    - Berg Balance Scale
    - Gait Assessment Rating Score
    - Rancho Los Amigo observational gait analysis
    - Multi-directional reach test (MDRT)
- Pain with resistance
- Strength functional strength testing
  - Five-times-sit-to-stand test
  - Manual muscle test (MMT)
    - Hamstrings

INTERVENTION

- Take caution initially not to overstretch and eccentrically load injured muscle
- Early and continued incorporation of core stability and eccentric hamstring loading progressing to full length
- Rehabilitation for grade-I and grade-II strains
  - Phase 1, 1 to 5 days postinjury
    - Reduce edema and pain
    - Ice, NSAIDs
    - Protect tissue remodeling

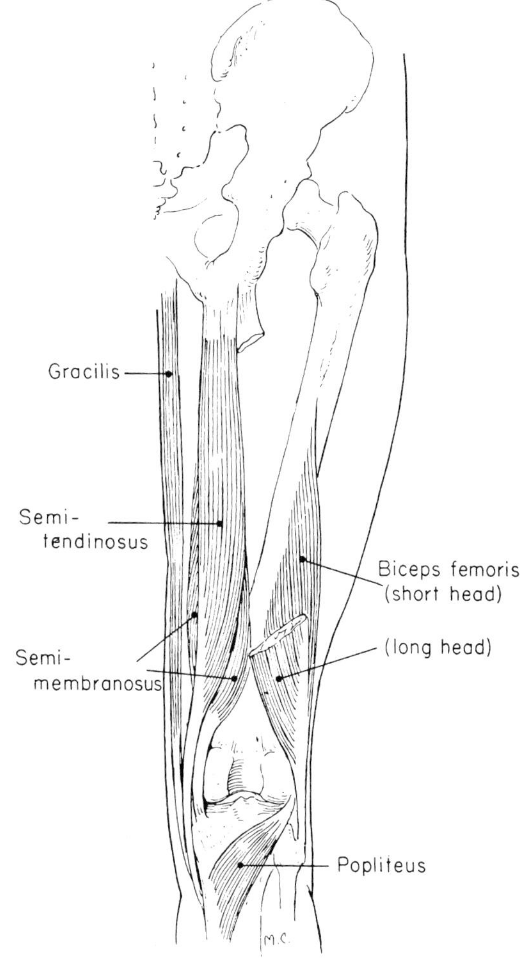

FIGURE 192-5 Posterior muscles of thigh and knee. (From Hamilton N, Weimar W, Luttgens K. *Kinesiology: Scientific Basis of Human Motion*. 11th ed. http://www.accessphysiotherapy.com. Copyright © McGraw-Hill Education. All rights reserved.)

    - Avoid excessive stretching
    - Lower-extremity and lumbar-stabilization exercise
    - Limited and pain-free ROM
    - Progression criteria
      - Pain-free normal stride length with walking
      - Pain-free low-speed jogging
      - Pain-free sub-maximal (<70%) isometric muscle contraction
  - Phase 2
    - Restore full ROM
    - Avoid end-range lengthening if strength deficits persist
    - Avoid strenuous, eccentric strengthening
    - Avoid running at >50% intensity
    - Reduce pain after treatment
      - Ice
      - NSAIDs not recommended, potential negative effects on tissue healing
    - Therapeutic exercises
      - Agility
      - Neuromuscular control
      - Lumbar stabilization
  - Progress from transverse and frontal-plane movements to sagittal

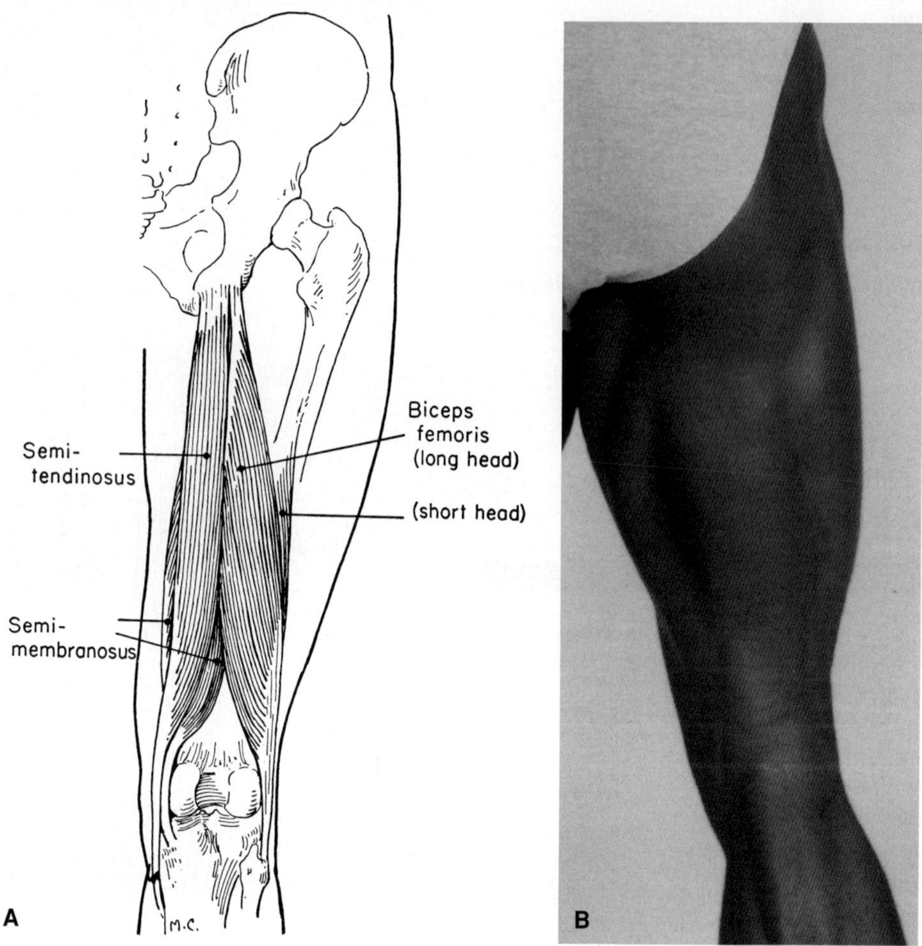

FIGURE 192-6 Hamstring muscles. (**A**) Line drawing, (**B**) patient with contraction of the hamstring muscles. (From Hamilton N, Weimar W, Luttgens K. *Kinesiology: Scientific Basis of Human Motion*. 11th ed. http://www.accessphysiotherapy.com. Copyright © McGraw-Hill Education. All rights reserved.)

- Sub-maximal eccentric strengthening in functional patterns; avoid hamstring isolation
  - Progression criteria
    - Full, pain-free strength at 1 repetition maximum, 5 out of 5 MMT
    - Pain-free forward and backward jogging at 50% intensity
- Phase 3
  - Return to sports
  - Avoid sprinting and explosive acceleration until all return-to-sport criteria are met
  - Therapeutic exercises
    - Progress to single-limb, asymmetrical, multi-planar movements
    - Progress to end-range eccentric activation
  - Return-to-sport criteria
    - Full, pain-free ROM, strength, and functional ability
    - Functional sports-related tasks

- Injury prevention
  - Eccentric strengthening
  - Trunk stability
  - Stretching program

FUNCTIONAL GOALS

- Patient will
  - Demonstrate normal gait as necessary for community and household ambulation without limitation from pain.
  - Score 5 out of 5 for strength in isolated-hamstring MMT without pain so as to climb stairs.
  - Be able to do job at 50% full speed without limitation from pain.
  - Demonstrate full-speed sprinting, cutting, jumping as necessary for return to sports, without limitation from pain.

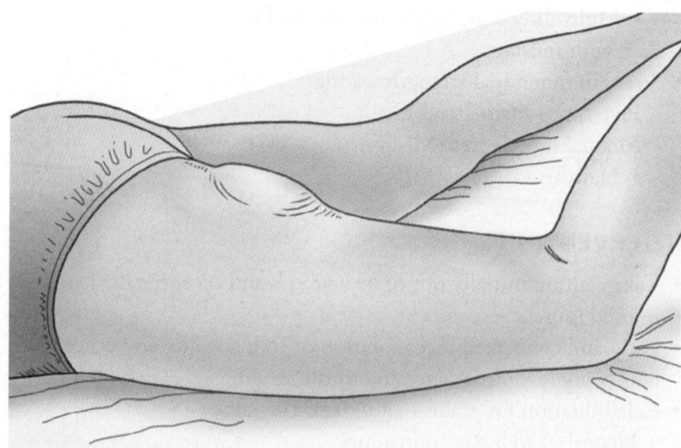

FIGURE 192-7 A large tear in the hamstring muscle group. (From Simon RR, Sherman SC. *Emergency Orthopedics*. 6th ed. http://www.accessemergencymedicine.com. Copyright © The McGraw-Hill Companies, Inc. All rights reserved.)

 - Patient will have full, pain-free knee- and hip-ROM so as to transfer in and out of car.
 - Patient will be able to jog and sprint without limitation from pain.
 - Patient will regain full performance of sports-related activity without limitation from pain.

PROGNOSIS

- Median time to regain pre-injury level of activity/performance
  - Maximum or sub-maximum speed injury: 16 weeks.
  - Extreme hip-flexion/knee-extension injury: 50 weeks.
- May remain a nagging injury until complete rest occurs.
- Closer site of maximum pain to ischial tuberosity predicts proportionally longer rehabilitation time.

PATIENT RESOURCE

- Hamstring Strain. MedlinePlus, NIH National Institutes of Health. http://www.nlm.nih.gov/medlineplus/ency/patientinstructions/000551.htm Accessed July 5, 2013.

REFERENCES

1. American Physical Therapy Association. *Anatomy and Physiology Revealed.* New York, NY: McGraw-Hill; 2007. http://anatomy.mcgraw-hill.com/apt.html?login=1317987200225&system=Muscular§ion=Dissection&topic=Hip%20and%20thigh&topicAbbr=Hip&view=Posterior&viewAbbr=Pos&catAbbr=Oth&grpAbbr=San&structure=Surface%20projection%20of%20hamstring%20tendons. Accessed July 2, 2013.
2. Hamilton N, Weimar W, Luttgens K. *Kinesiology: Scientific Basis of Human Motion.* New York, NY: McGraw-Hill; 2008. http://www.accessphysiotherapy.com/resource/618. Accessed July 5, 2013.
3. Dutton M. *Orthopaedic Examination, Evaluation, and Intervention.* New York, NY: McGraw-Hill; 2008. http://www.accessphysiotherapy.com/resource/612. Accessed July 5, 2013.

ADDITIONAL REFERENCES

- Armfield DR, Kim DH, Towers JD, et al. Sports-related injury in the lower extremity. *Clin Sports Med.* 2006;25(4):803–842.
- Heiderscheit BC, Sherry MA, Slider A, et al. Hamstring Strain Injuries: recommendations for diagnosis, dehabilitation, and injury prevention. *J Orthop Sports Phys Ther.* 2010:40(2):67–81. doi: 10.2519/jospt.2010.3047.
- ICD9DATA web site. http://www.icd9data.com. Accessed July 6, 2013.
- ICD10DATA web site. http://www.icd10data.com. Accessed July 6, 2013.

193 KNEE LATERAL COLLATERAL LIGAMENT SPRAIN

Raine Osborne, DPT, PT, OCS, FAAOMPT

CONDITION/DISORDER SYNONYM

- LCL sprain

ICD-9-CM CODE

- 844.0 Sprain of lateral collateral ligament of knee

ICD-10-CM CODE

- S83.429A Sprain of lateral collateral ligament of unspecified knee, initial encounter

PREFERRED PRACTICE PATTERN

- 4I: Impaired Joint Mobility, Motor Function, Muscle Performance, and Range of Motion Associated with Bony or Soft Tissue Surgery[1]

PATIENT PRESENTATION

A 33-year-old female presents with left lateral knee pain following being kicked in the medial left knee during a karate class 1 week ago. The patient reports the pain is worse with trying to use the left leg as a stance leg during kicks and with trying to get out of the car, especially from the driver's seat. She denies popping, clicking, or giving way in the knee, but does report feeling less stable when performing karate moves that involve standing on the left leg only. There is mild swelling and moderate tenderness in the lateral knee. Range of motion is full with pain at end range extension. There is no pain with resisted knee flexion or extension, but hip abduction in side lying does reproduce pain. Patellar instability testing is negative, but varus stress test is positive for pain with a firm end feel and no apparent laxity.

KEY FEATURES

Description

- Tear of the lateral collateral ligament of the knee
- Graded based on extent of damage
  - Grade I: Localized tenderness with no instability
  - Grade II: Localized tenderness, moderate fiber disruption, slight to moderate abnormal motion
  - Grade III: Complete fiber disruption, noted instability

Essentials of Diagnosis

- Injury is generally traumatic, can occur at any age; trauma usually a high-impact force applied to the medial knee.
- Clinical diagnosis is generally made through history of injury and knee varus stability testing.
- Diagnosis may be confirmed with MRI.[2]

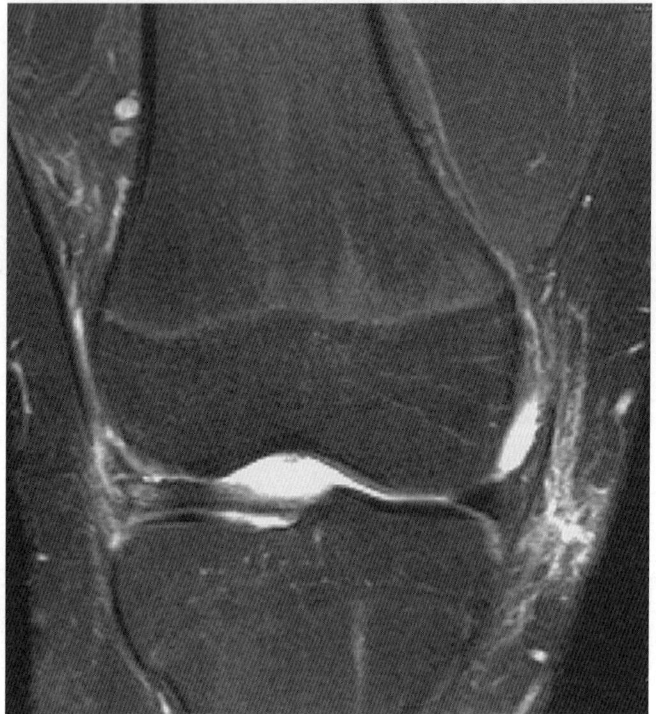

FIGURE 193-1 In this coronal slice MR image, areas of increased signal intensity are noted in the medial and lateral collateral ligaments, suggesting incomplete tears of each. Also note the appearance of the lateral meniscus; the increased signal intensity in the body of the meniscus is consistent with a tear of this structure. (From Malone TR, Hazle C, Grey ML. *Imaging in Rehabilitation.* http://www.accessphysiotherapy.com. Copyright © The McGraw-Hill Companies, Inc. All rights reserved.)

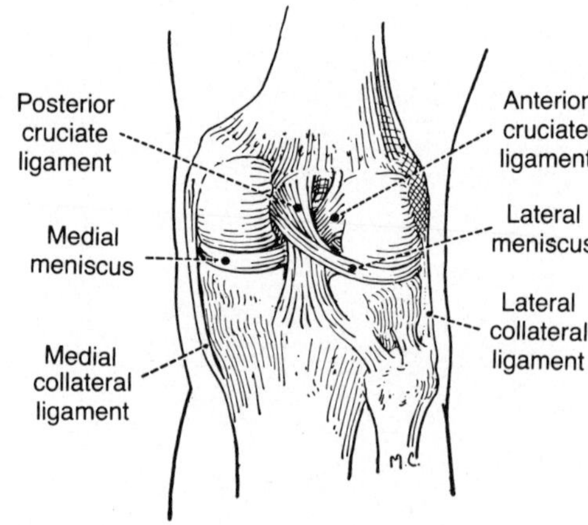

FIGURE 193-2 Posterior view of knee joint showing cruciate ligaments. (From Hamilton N, Weimar W, Luttgens K. *Kinesiology: Scientific Basis of Human Motion.* 11th ed. http://www.accessphysiotherapy.com. Copyright © McGraw-Hill Education. All rights reserved.)

General Considerations

- Lateral collateral ligament is most taught in extended knee position

Demographics

- Injury to lateral collateral ligament less common than to medial collateral
- Most common in young athletic population

CLINICAL FINDINGS

SIGNS AND SYMPTOMS

- Lateral knee pain
- Pain with palpation over lateral knee
- Pain with varus force to knee
- Pain with extension
- Feeling of instability or "giving way" in the knee

Functional Implications

- Pain with swinging legs in/out of car or bed
- Decreased stability while walking on uneven surfaces
- Decreased stability with change of direction

Possible Contributing Causes

- Usually related to traumatic varus stress applied to the knee
    - Sports injury
    - Motor vehicle accident
- May be related to severe, degenerative osteoarthrosis

Differential Diagnosis

- Anterior cruciate ligament sprain or tear
- Arcuate-popliteal complex
- Biceps femoris tendinopathy or strain
- Iliotibial band syndrome
- Joint-line pain related to knee osteoarthrosis
- Posterior cruciate ligament sprain or tear
- Proximal tibiofibular joint pathology
- Referred pain to hip, low back, sacroiliac joint

MEANS OF CONFIRMATION DIAGNOSIS

Imaging

- MRI[2]
- Valgus stress radiograph[3]
    - Isolated injury of LCL
        - Increased lateral joint gap of 2.7 mm
    - Grade-III posterolateral corner injury
        - Increased lateral joint gap of 4.0 mm

FINDINGS AND INTERPRETATION

- Pain, tenderness, swelling in lateral knee from tissue disruption and inflammatory process
- Possible laxity with varus force to knee, depending on extent of tissue disruption
- Reports of "giving way" or instability with walking due to decreased lateral stability of the knee

REFERRALS/ADMITTANCE

- To physician for pain management
- To hospital for MRI if questionable diagnosis or if meniscus injury or tibial plateau fracture suspected[2]
- To physician, orthotist or physical therapist for knee brace

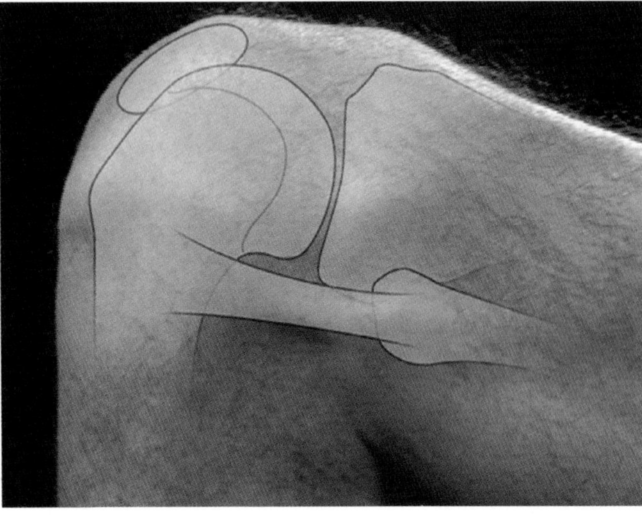

FIGURE 193-3 Anatomical orientation of the lateral collateral ligament. (From Lawry GV. *Systematic Musculoskeletal Examinations*. www.accessmedicine.com. Copyright © The McGraw-Hill Companies, Inc. All rights reserved.)

IMPAIRMENTS

- Decreased range of motion in knee
- Muscle guarding
- Decreased lower-extremity muscle performance related acutely to inhibition or chronically to disuse with immobilization in severe cases
- Impaired lower-extremity proprioception
- Impaired lower-extremity coordination

TESTS AND MEASURES

- Posteriorlateral drawer test
- External rotation recurvatum Test
- Reverse pivot shift test
- Knee varus stress test in 30-degree knee flexion[4]
    - Grading of laxity[5,6]
        - 1+ = 3 to 5 mm laxity
        - 2+ = 6 to 10 mm laxity 3+ = >10 mm laxity

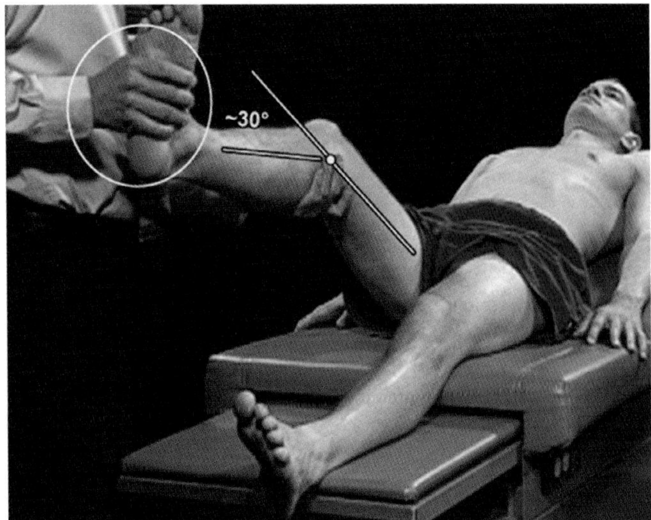

FIGURE 193-4 Knee varus stress test at 30-degree knee flexion. (From Lawry GV. *Systematic Musculoskeletal Examinations*. www.accessmedicine.com. Copyright © The McGraw-Hill Companies, Inc. All rights reserved.)

- Limb strength
  - Functional strength testing
    - Five-times-sit-to-stand test
  - Biodex testing, comparison of bilateral quadriceps and quadricep to hamstring ratio
  - Manual muscle test (MMT)
    - Hamstrings
    - Quadriceps
    - Iliopsoas
    - Gluteus maximus
    - Gluteus medius
    - Gluteus minimus
    - Adductors
- LE contralateral limb strength
- Balance
  - Static single-leg standing (eyes open, eyes closed)
    - Contralateral LE
  - Dynamic standing
    - Berg Balance Scale
    - Functional gait assessment
- Gait assessment
  - Observational analysis
  - Gait speed via the 10-m walk test
  - 2-minute walk test
  - 6-minute walk test
  - Retro running

INTERVENTION

- Education[5]
  - Early education to reduce varus loading to knee (e.g., car transfers, bed mobility)
  - Later education on progressive return to activity
- Bracing[5]
  - Duration and type of bracing related to severity of injury
    - Grade I: Bracing generally not required; may use unlocked hinged brace
    - Grade II: Bracing for approximately 3 weeks with hinged brace locked in full extension, progressing to unlocked hinged brace
    - Grade III: Bracing for approximately 6 weeks with hinged brace locked in full extension, progressing to unlocked hinged brace
  - Prophylactic bracing for sports activity may be considered
- Manual therapy
  - Soft tissue mobilization for muscle guarding
  - Knee PROM to promote ROM and tissue healing[3]
    - Grade I: Should begin immediately
    - Grade II: Performed in pain-free range with greater caution during first 3 weeks in more severe cases
    - Grade III: Avoid for first 3 weeks, then slow progression in pain-free range
  - Joint mobilization
    - Generally not required
    - May be necessary with prolonged immobilization due to arthrofibrosis
- Therapeutic exercises[7]
  - Phase I
    - Elevated knee AROM for edema reduction and to promote tissue healing
    - Modified varus loading to promote tissue healing and collagen alignment

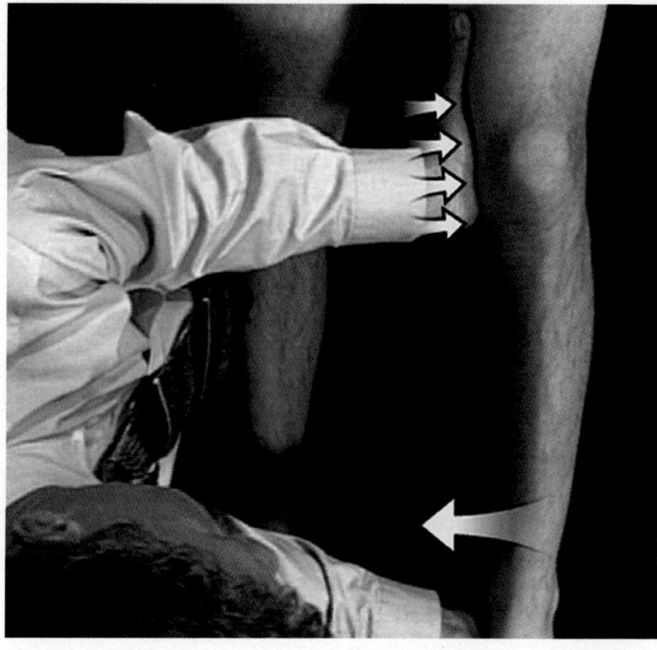

FIGURE 193-5 Knee varus stress test. (From Lawry GV. *Systematic Musculoskeletal Examinations*. www.accessmedicine.com. Copyright © The McGraw-Hill Companies, Inc. All rights reserved.)

  - Phase II
    - Weight-bearing proprioception and coordination exercises with progressively dynamic surface and movement
    - Endurance exercises for muscles that were guarded or immobilized
    - Strengthening exercises for any muscle with identified weakness
  - Phase III
    - Sport or activity-specific performance training

FUNCTIONAL GOALS

- Patient will
  - Demonstrate ability to get in and out of car 5 times without knee pain to demonstrate independence with car transfers.

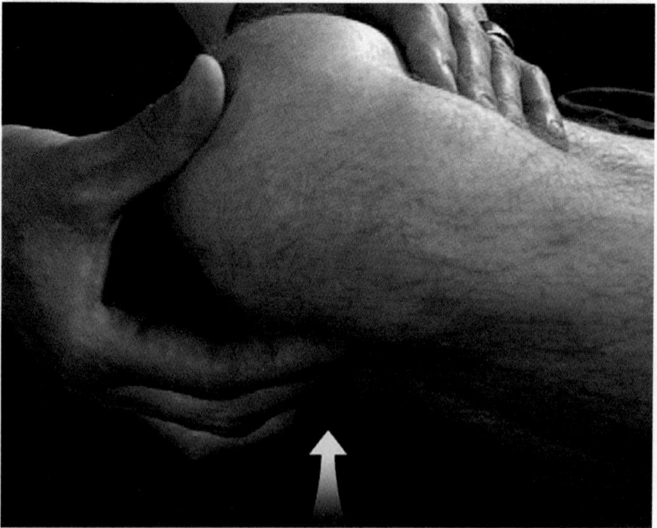

FIGURE 193-6 Palpation of the lateral collateral knee ligament. (From Lawry GV. *Systematic Musculoskeletal Examinations*. www.accessmedicine.com. Copyright © The McGraw-Hill Companies, Inc. All rights reserved.)

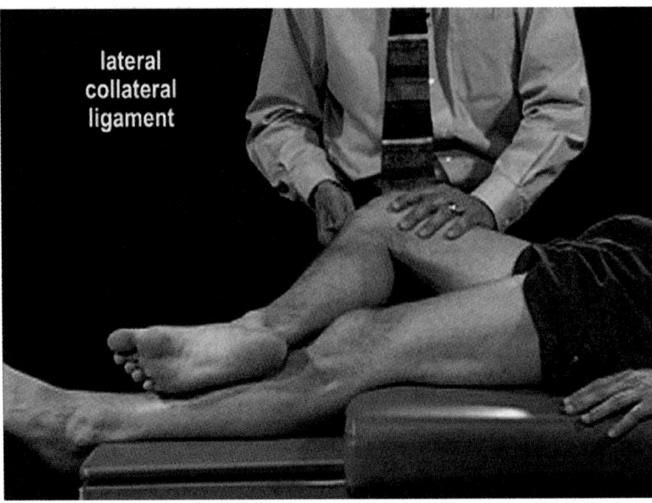

FIGURE 193-7 Palpation for gapping at the lateral collateral ligament. (From Lawry GV. *Systematic Musculoskeletal Examinations*. www.accessmedicine.com.)

- ○ Report improved walking tolerance for usual daily distances without pain.
- ○ Demonstrate walking with quick 90-degree direction changes 5 times in each direction to demonstrate stability with community ambulation.
- ○ Demonstrate straight-ahead running for 100 yards without knee pain.
- ○ Be able to complete box drill 5 times in each direction at full speed without pain to demonstrate knee stability with sports activities.

PROGNOSIS

- Conservative care generally indicated with isolated sprains of all grades.
- Knee bracing may be indicated in moderate to severe sprains.
- Return to sports or normal activity usually expected.

PATIENT RESOURCE

- Medial and Lateral Collateral Ligament Injuries. NIH, National Institute of Arthritis and Musculoskeletal and Skin Diseases. http://www.niams.nih.gov/health_info/knee_problems. Accessed June 1, 2013.

REFERENCES

1. American Physical Therapy Association. Pattern 4I: Impaired joint mobility, motor function, muscle performance, and range of motion associated with bony or soft tissue surgery. *Interactive Guide to Physical Therapist Practice*. 2003. doi: 10.2522/ptguide.3.1_9. Accessed June 5, 2013.
2. Dutton M. *Dutton's Orthopaedic Examination, Evaluation, and Intervention*. 3rd ed. New York, NY: McGraw-Hill; 2012. http://www.accessphysiotherapy.com/resource/612. Accessed June 5, 2013.
3. Wijdicks CA, Griffith CJ, Johansen S, et al. Injuries to the Medial Collateral Ligament and Associated Medial Structures of the Knee. *J Bone Joint Surg Am*. 2010;92(5):1266–1280.
4. Dutton M. *Dutton's Orthopedic Survival Guide: Managing Common Conditions*. New York, NY: McGraw-Hill; 2011. http://www.accessphysiotherapy.com/resource/685. Accessed June 5, 2013.
5. Edson C. Conservative and postoperative rehabilitation of isolated and combined injuries of the medial collateral ligament. *Sports Med Arthrosc Rev*. 2006;14(2):105–110.
6. LaPrade RF, Heikes C, Bakker AJ, et al. The reproducibility and repeatability of varus stress radiographs in the assessment of isolated fibular collateral ligament and grade-iii posterolateral knee injuries: An in vitro biomechanical study. *J Bone Joint Surg*. 2008;90:2069–2076.
7. Rivard J, Grimsby O. Science theory and clinical application in orthopaedic manual physical therapy. *Applied Science and Theory*. Taylorsville, UT: Academy of Graduate Physical Therapy, 2008; Vol. 1.

ADDITIONAL REFERENCES

- APTA Guide to Physical Therapist Practice. http://guidetoptpractice.apta.org./ Accessed June 1, 2013.
- ICD-9-CM. http://www.icd9data.com. Accessed June 1, 2013.
- ICD-10-CM. http://www.icd10data.com. Accessed June 1, 2013.
- Zhong YL, Wang Y, Wang HP, et al. Stress changes of lateral collateral ligament at different knee flexion with or without displaced movements: a 3-dimensional finite element analysis. *Chin J Traumatol*. 2011;14(2):79–83. [PMID 21453572]

194 KNEE MEDIAL COLLATERAL (MCL) LIGAMENT SPRAIN

Raine Osborne, DPT, PT, OCS, FAAOMPT

CONDITION/DISORDER SYNONYM

- Tibial collateral ligament sprain

ICD-9-CM CODE

- 844.1 Sprain of medial collateral ligament of knee

ICD-10-CM CODE

- S83.419A Sprain of medial collateral ligament of unspecified knee, initial encounter

PREFERRED PRACTICE PATTERNS

- 4D: Impaired joint mobility, motor function, muscle performance, and range of motion (ROM) associated with connective tissue dysfunction
- 4E: Impaired joint mobility, motor function, muscle performance, and ROM associated with localized inflammation

PATIENT PRESENTATION

A 24-year-old male presents with right medial knee pain following an injury during a recreational flag football game 2 days ago. The patient reports a player fell on the outside of his right leg while he was blocking another player. He felt immediate knee pain but did not hear an audible pop. Since the injury he reports mild to moderate swelling and pain with fully extending or fully bending his knee, getting his legs out of the car, and going from supine to sit in his bed, especially to the left. The patient denies clicking or popping, but does report a slight feeling of giving away on occasion with changing directions while walking. On physical examination there is tenderness over the medal aspect of the knee. Range of motion is full but painful at end range flexion and extension. Lachman's test is negative and valgus stress testing is positive on the right for pain with 1+ laxity and a firm end feel.

KEY FEATURES

Description

- Tear of the medial collateral ligament of the knee
- May be graded based on extent of damage[1,2]
  - Grade I: Localized tenderness with no instability
  - Grade II: Localized tenderness, moderate fiber disruption; slight to moderate abnormal motion
  - Grade III: Complete fiber disruption; noted instability

Essentials of Diagnosis

- Injury is generally traumatic and can occur at any age.
- Trauma is usually a high impact force applied to the lateral knee.
- The anterior cruciate ligament (ACL) and medial meniscus are commonly injured concurrently.
- Clinical diagnosis is generally made through history of injury and knee valgus stability testing.
- Diagnosis may be confirmed with magnetic resonance imaging (MRI).

General Considerations

- Medial collateral ligament is most taut in knee extension.
- Commonly injured from an outside force hitting the lateral portion of the knee, that is football tackle.
- Anterior fibers of superficial band is taut with flexion.[2]

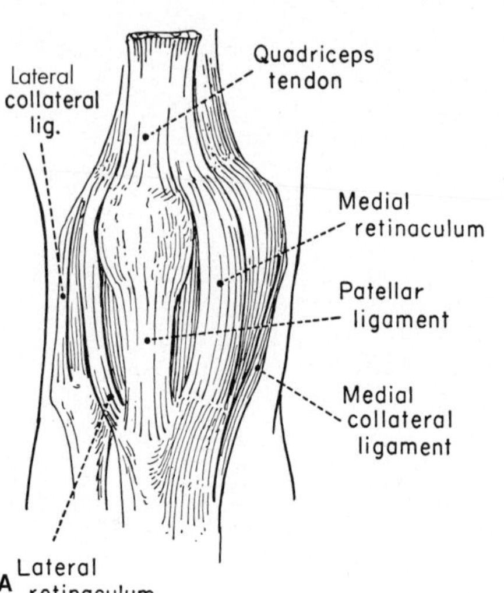

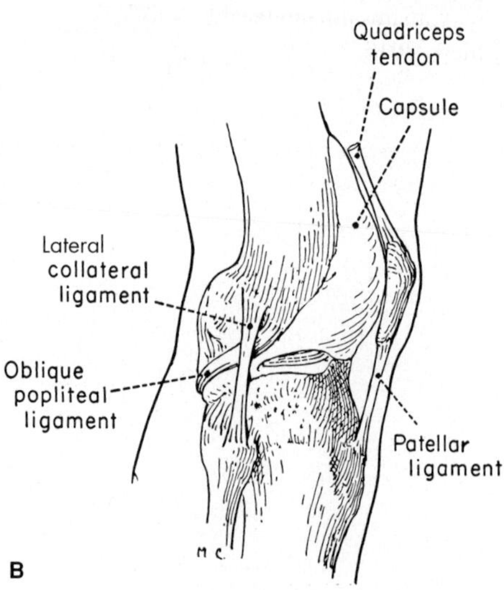

FIGURE 194-1 (**A**) Anterior and (**B**) lateral views of knee joint showing ligaments. (From Hamilton N, Weimar W, Luttgens K. *Kinesiology: Scientific Basis of Human Motion*. 11th ed. http://www.accessphysiotherapy.com. Copyright © McGraw-Hill Education. All rights reserved.)

Demographics
- Most commonly injured knee ligament
- Incidence (United States)[2]
  - Average 0.24 per 1000
  - Male = 0.36 per 1000, female = 0.18 per 1000
- Most common in young athletic population

CLINICAL FINDINGS

SIGNS AND SYMPTOMS
- Medial knee pain
- Pain with palpation over medial knee
- Pain with valgus force to knee
- Pain with extension and deep flexion
- Feeling of instability or "giving way" in the knee

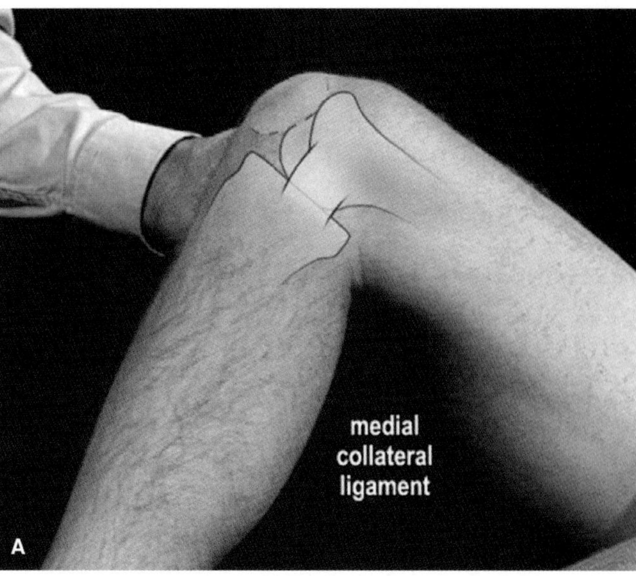

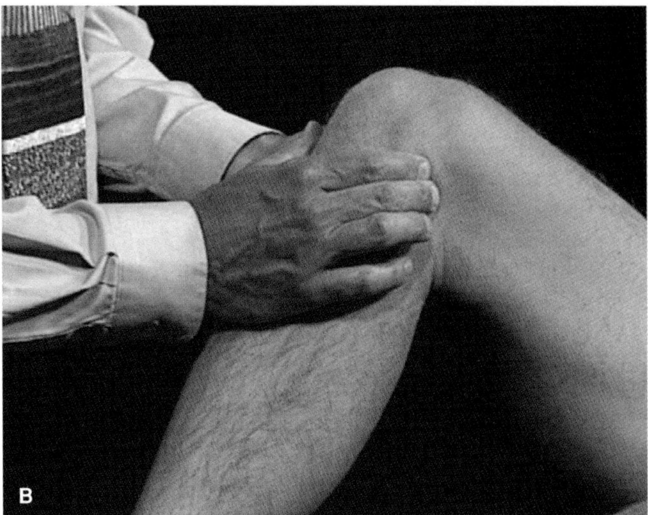

FIGURE 194-2 (**A**) Anatomical alignment of the medial collateral ligament, (**B**) Palpation of the medical collateral ligament. (From Lawry GV. *Systematic Musculoskeletal Examinations*. www.accessmedicine.com. Copyright © The McGraw-Hill Companies, Inc. All rights reserved.)

Functional Implications
- Decreased squatting ability
- Difficulty with transitioning from sit-to-stand or stand-to-sit
- Pain with swinging legs in/out of car and/or bed
- Decreased stability while walking on uneven surfaces
- Decreased stability with change of direction

Possible Contributing Causes
- Usually related to traumatic valgus stress applied to the knee[2]
  - Sports injury
  - Motor vehicle accident
- May be related to severe degenerative osteoarthritis

Differential Diagnoses
- Medial joint line pain related to knee osteoarthritis
- Pes anserine bursitis
- Adductor strain
- Meniscus injury
- Patellofemoral pain syndrome
- Referred hip pain

MEANS OF CONFIRMATION OR DIAGNOSIS

Imaging
- MRI
- Valgus stress radiograph[2]

FINDINGS AND INTERPRETATION
- Valgus stress radiograph[2]
  - Isolated injury of superficial MCL Increased medial gapping of 1.7 mm at 0-degree knee flexion
  - Increased medial gapping of 3.2 mm at 20-degree knee flexion
- Complete injury of MCL
  - Increased medial joint gapping of 6.5 mm at 0-degree knee flexion

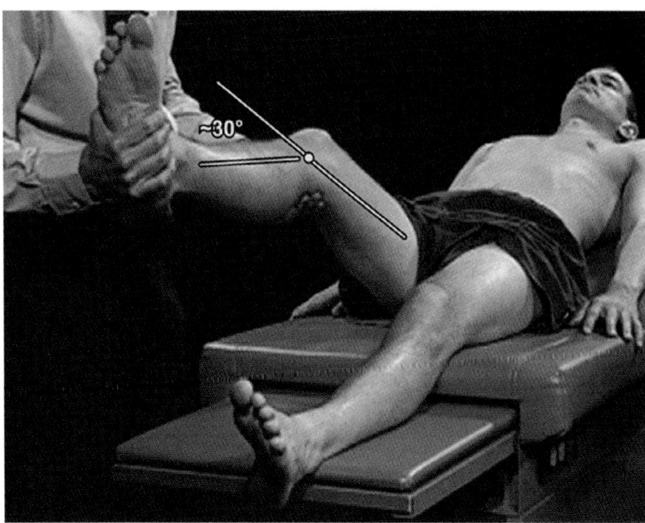

FIGURE 194-3 Valgus stress test at 30-degree of knee flexion. (From Lawry GV. *Systematic Musculoskeletal Examinations*. www.accessmedicine.com. Copyright © The McGraw-Hill Companies, Inc. All rights reserved.)

REFERRALS/ADMITTANCE
- Possible referral to physician for pain management
- Possible referral for MRI if questionable diagnosis or if meniscus injury or tibial plateau fracture is suspected
- Possible referral for knee brace

IMPAIRMENTS

- Decreased knee range of motion
- Muscle guarding
- Acutely decreased lower–extremity (LE) muscle performance related to inhibition or disuse with immobilization in severe cases
- Impaired LE proprioception
- Impaired LE coordination

TESTS AND MEASURES

- Knee valgus stress test in 30° knee flexion
  - Grading of laxity[2]
    - 1+ = 3 to 5 mm laxity
    - 2+ = 6 to 10 mm laxity
    - 3+ = >10 mm laxity
- Limb strength
  - Functional strength testing
    - Five-times-sit-to-stand test
  - Biodex testing, comparison of bilateral quadriceps and quadricep to hamstring ratio
  - Manual muscle test (MMT)
    - Hamstrings
    - Quadriceps
    - Iliopsoas
    - Gluteus maximus
    - Gluteus medius
    - Gluteus minimus
    - Adductors
- LE contralateral limb strength
- Balance
  - Static single-leg standing (eyes open, eyes closed)
    - Contralateral LE
  - Dynamic standing
    - Berg Balance Scale
    - Functional gait assessment
- Gait assessment
  - Observational analysis
  - Gait speed via the 10-m walk test
  - Two-minute walk test
  - Six-minute walk test
  - Retro running

INTERVENTION

- Education[1]
  - Early education to reduce valgus loading to knee (e.g., car transfers, bed mobility)
  - Later education on progressive return to activity
- Bracing[1]
  - Amount of time and type of bracing is related to severity of injury
    - Grade I: Bracing generally not required; may use unlocked hinged brace
    - Grade II: Bracing for around 3 weeks with hinged brace locked in full extension progressing to unlocked hinged brace
    - Grade III: Bracing for around 6 weeks with hinged brace locked in full extension progressing to unlocked hinged brace
  - Prophylactic bracing for sport may be considered
- Manual therapy
  - Soft tissue mobilization for muscle guarding
  - Knee PROM to promote ROM and tissue healing[1]
    - Grade I: Should begin immediately

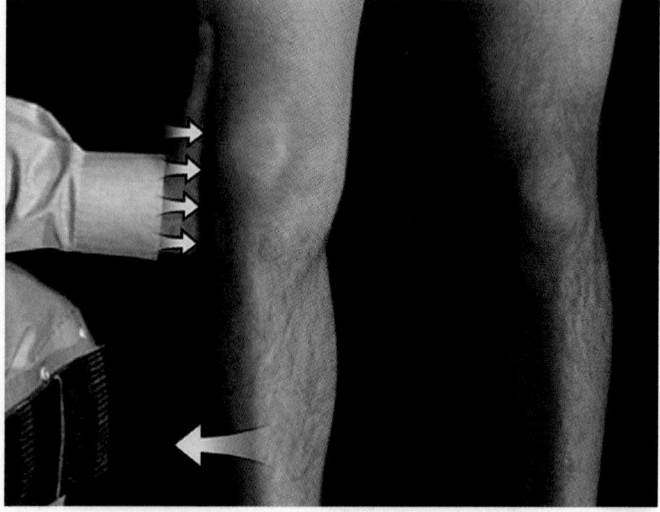

FIGURE 194-4 Valgus stress test from the same side of the patient. (From Lawry GV. *Systematic Musculoskeletal Examinations*. www.accessmedicine.com.)

    - Grade II: Performed in pain-free range with greater caution during the first 3 weeks in more severe cases
    - Grade III: Avoid for first 3 weeks then slow progression in pain-free range
  - Joint mobilizations
    - Generally not required
    - May be necessary with prolonged immobilization due to arthrofibrosis
- Therapeutic exercises[3]
  - Phase I
    - Elevated knee AAROM for edema reduction and to promote tissue healing
    - Modified valgus loading to promote tissue healing and collagen alignment
  - Phase II
    - Weight-bearing proprioception and coordination exercises with progressively dynamic surface and movement

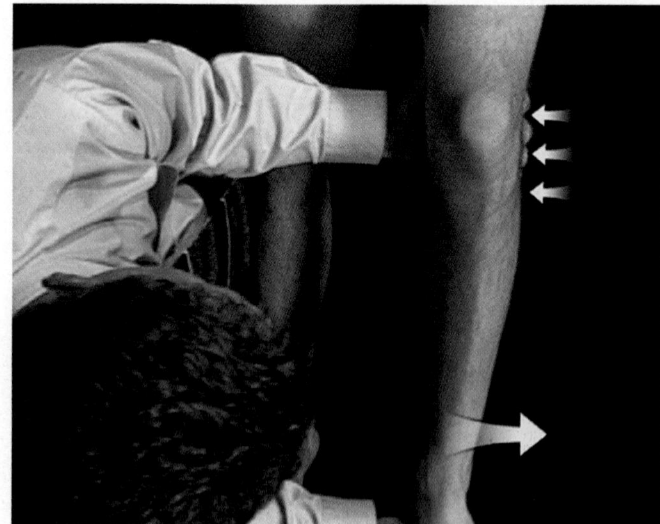

FIGURE 194-5 Valgus stress test from the opposite side of the patient. (From Lawry GV. *Systematic Musculoskeletal Examinations*. www.accessmedicine.com.)

        - Endurance exercises for muscles that were guarded or immobilized
        - Strengthening exercises for any muscle where weakness is identified
    - Phase III
        - Sport- or activity-specific performance training

FUNCTIONAL GOALS

- Patient will be able to
    - Perform 10 sit-to-stands from average height chair without knee pain to demonstrate independence with chair transfers.
    - Get in/out of the car 5× without knee pain to demonstrate independence with car transfers.
    - Perform sit-to-supine and supine-to-sit 5× on low mat table without knee pain to demonstrate independence with bed transfers.
    - Tolerate improved to usual daily distances without pain.
    - Walk with quick 90-degree change of directions 5× in each direction to demonstrate stability with community ambulation.
    - Run straight ahead for 100 yards without knee pain.
    - Complete box drill 5× in each direction at full speed without pain to demonstrate knee stability with sport activities.

PROGNOSIS

- Conservative care is generally indicated with isolated sprains of all grades.
- Knee bracing may be indicated in moderate to severe sprains.
- Return to sport or activity is usually expected.

ADDITIONAL INFORMATION

- Case Study in Therapeutic Modalities in Rehabilitation, 4th ed. at www.accessphysiotherapy.com

PATIENT RESOURCE

- Medial and Lateral Collateral Ligament Injuries. NIH, National Institute of Arthritis and Musculoskeletal and Skin Diseases. http://www.niams.nih.gov/health_info/knee_problems. Accessed July 1, 2013.

REFERENCES

1. Edson CJ. Conservative and postoperative rehabilitation of isolated and combined injuries of the medial collateral ligament. *Sports Med Arthrosc*. 2006;14(2):105–110.
2. Wijdicks CA, Griffith CJ, Johansen S, et al. Injuries to the medial collateral ligament and associated medial structures of the knee. *J Bone Joint Surg Am*. 2010;92(5):1266–1280.
3. Rivard J, Grimsby O, eds. *Science Theory and Clinical Application Orthopaedic Manual Physical Therapy*. Volume 1: Applied Science and Theory. Taylorsville, UT: The Academy of Graduate Physical Therapy; 2008.

ADDITIONAL REFERENCES

- ICD-9-CM. http://www.icd9data.com. Accessed August 9, 2014.
- ICD-10-CM. http://www.icd10data.com. Accessed August 9, 2014.
- APTA Guide to Physical Therapist Practice. http://guidetoptpractice.apta.org./ Accessed July 1, 2013.
- Dutton M. Common orthopedic conditions. In: Dutton M, ed. *Dutton's Orthopedic Survival Guide: Managing Common Conditions*. New York, NY: McGraw-Hill; 2011. http://www.accessphysiotherapy.com/content/8654920. Accessed August 9, 2014.
- Hooker DN, Prentice WE. Chapter 5. Basic principles of electricity and electrical stimulating currents. In: Prentice WE, Quillen WS, Underwood F, eds. *Therapeutic Modalities in Rehabilitation*. 4th ed. New York, NY: McGraw-Hill; 2011. http://www.accessphysiotherapy.com/content/8136027. Accessed August 9, 2014.

195 KNEE OSTEOARTHRITIS

Eric Shamus, PhD, DPT, PT, CSCS
Reuben Escorpizo, DPT, MSc, PT

CONDITION/DISORDER SYNONYMS

- Knee arthritis
- Arthrosis
- Osteoarthrosis
- Degenerative joint disease
- Knee degenerative joint disease

ICD-9-CM CODES

- 715 Osteoarthrosis and allied disorders
- 715.16 Osteoarthrosis localized primary involving lower leg
- 715.26 Osteoarthrosis localized secondary involving lower leg
- 715.36 Osteoarthrosis localized not specified whether primary or secondary involving lower leg
- 715.9 Osteoarthrosis, unspecified whether generalized or localized
- 715.95 Osteoarthrosis, unspecified whether generalized or localized involving pelvic region and thigh

ICD-10-CM CODES

- M17.10 Unilateral primary osteoarthritis, unspecified knee
- M17.5 Other unilateral secondary osteoarthritis of knee
- M17.9 Osteoarthritis of knee, unspecified

PREFERRED PRACTICE PATTERNS

- 4D: Impaired Joint Mobility, Motor Function, Muscle Performance, and Range of Motion (ROM) Associated with Connective Tissue Dysfunction[1]
- 4F: Impaired Joint Mobility, Motor Function, Muscle Performance, Range of Motion, and Reflex Integrity Associated with Spinal Disorders[2]
- 4H: Impaired Joint Mobility, Motor Function, Muscle Performance, and ROM Associated With Joint Arthroplasty[3]
- 4I: Impaired Joint Mobility, Motor Function, Muscle Performance, and ROM Associated with Bony or Soft Tissue Surgery[4]

PATIENT PRESENTATION

Patient is a 70-year-old male that presents with bilateral knee pain. Patient states the pain in both of his knees has been progressively getting worse over the last 10 years. About 5 years ago, he had bilateral knee arthroscopies to clean out the joints. Last year, he had a Synvisc injection with some relief. The patient has limited knee ROM with bilateral genu varum. He states that if he is on his feet for any period of time he needs to sit down. The patient has morning stiffness. If he rides his stationary bike for a few minutes, the knee pain subsides for a little. He finds pool exercises are helping. The x-ray shows bilateral decreased joint space.

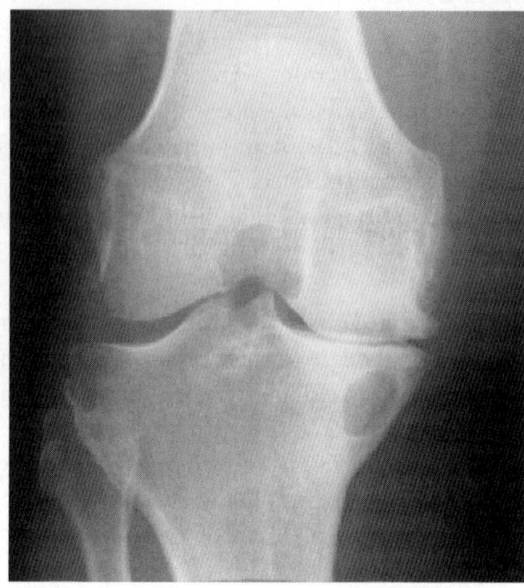

FIGURE 195-1 Frontal view of a 65-year-old man shows the classic features of osteoarthritis of the knee with medial articular space narrowing, subchondral cyst formation, sclerosis, and osteophyte formation. Osteoarthritis of the knee initially involves the medial compartment but may, over time, progress to involve the lateral and patellofemoral compartments. (From Chen MYM, Pope TL, Ott DJ: *Basic Radiology*, 2nd ed. http://www.accessmedicine.com. Copyright © The McGraw-Hill Companies, Inc. All rights reserved.)

KEY FEATURES

Description

- Most common form of arthritis
- Degenerative
- Commonly affects hip and knee joints, weight-bearing joints

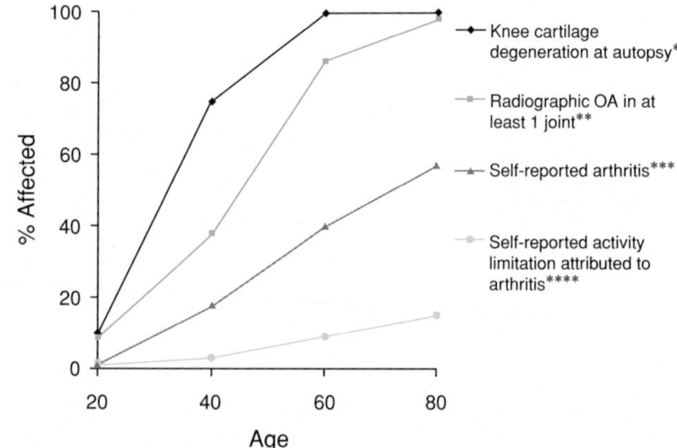

FIGURE 195-2 Effect of age on the prevalence of arthritis. *Knee cartilage degeneration at autopsy is the prevalence of significant histological changes of degeneration. **Radiographic evidence of OA (Kellgren and Lawrence Grade 2 or greater) present in at least one joint site (hands, feet, spine, knees, and hips) in a population survey in northern England. ***Self-reported arthritis and ****activity limitation attributable to arthritis derived from the National Health Interview Survey—US, 1989–1991. (Reproduced with permission from Loeser RF. Aging and the etiopathogenesis and treatment of osteoarthritis. *Rheum Dis Clin North Am*. 2000;26:547.)

- Can also affect spinal facet joints
- Associated with increasing age, obesity, female sex
- Associated with abnormal loading of the joints
- Characterized by joint pain

Essentials of Diagnosis

- Conventional radiograph is most commonly used tool in OA[5]
- Kellgren–Lawrence (KL) Grade ≥2 (definite radiographic OA)[6]
- Osteophytes, joint-space narrowing, sclerosis
- Cartilage lesions, bone marrow lesions, synovitis, effusion, and subchondral bone attrition/sclerosis
- Erosion of articular cartilage
- Synovial hyperplasia
- Fibrosis
- Inflammatory cell infiltration
  - With or without OA symptoms

General Considerations

- Low bone mineral density (BMD)
- Bone or joint morphology
- Calcification (of the knee meniscus)
- Bone formation, cyst formation
- Thickening of subchondral bone plate, osteosclerosis
- Long-term disease
- Secondary problems
  - Muscle atrophy and weakness
  - Bony protrusion/prominence
  - Joint deformity

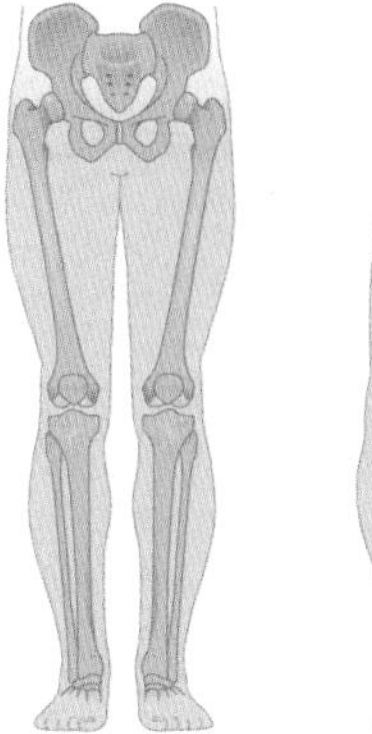

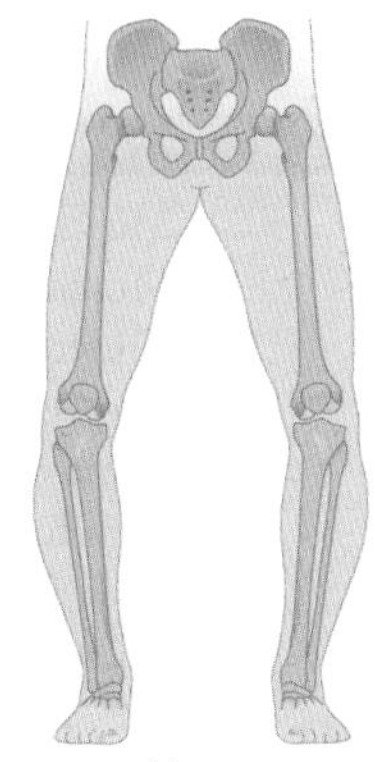

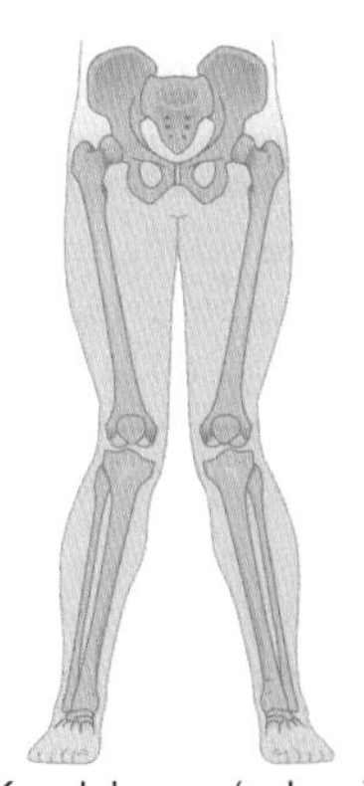

FIGURE 195-3 The two types of limb malalignment in the frontal plane: varus, in which the stress is placed across the medial compartment of the knee joint, and valgus, which places excess stress across the lateral compartment of the knee. (From Longo DL, Fauci A,Kasper D, et al., eds. *Harrison's Principles of Internal Medicine*, 18th ed. New York, NY: McGraw-Hill, 2012.)

Demographics

- Aging (onset middle- to old-age)
- Women more commonly affected than men
- African Americans and Caucasians more commonly affected
- May affect approximately 12% of the population (US and other developed countries)[7]

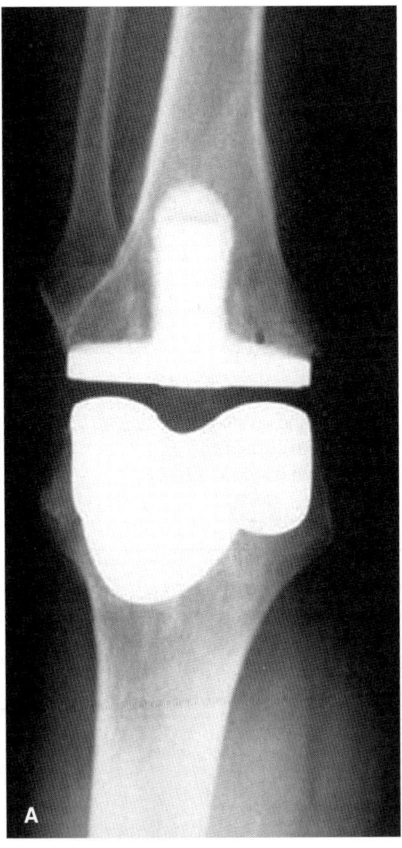

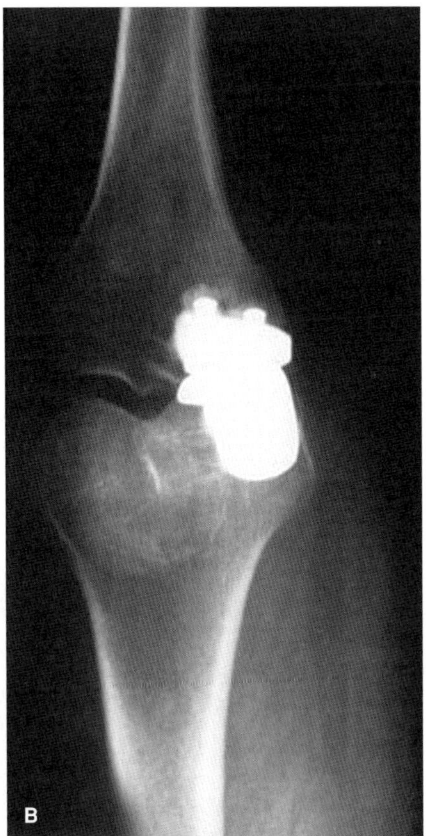

FIGURE 195-4 Total (**A**) and partial (**B**) knee replacement. (From Morgan GE, Mikhail MS, Murray MJ: *Clinical Anesthesiology*, 4th ed. www.accessmedicine.com. Copyright © The McGraw-Hill Companies, Inc. All rights reserved.)

CLINICAL FINDINGS

SIGNS AND SYMPTOMS

- Joint swelling and inflammation (in certain cases, severe cases)
- Joint pain
- Aching joint
- Joint stiffness
- Morning stiffness, pain subsides with movement
- Muscle weakness
- Muscle atrophy
- Crepitus
- Bony enlargement
- Limited joint ROM
- Joint line tenderness
- Joint deformity in severe cases

Functional Implications

- Activity limitation
  - Difficulty walking
  - Difficulty with ADLs
- Limited mobility
- Limited or restricted household and work-related activity
- Decreased activity and participation overall

Possible Contributing Causes

- Chronic factors affecting the joint such as obesity, BMD
- Repetitive joint use or loading
- Joint alignment
- Leg-length discrepancy or inequality (LLD)
- Aging
- Chronic and vigorous joint loading
- Previous chronic joint injury (e.g., accident, trauma); hence secondary OA

Differential Diagnosis

- Ankylosing spondylitis
- Fibromyalgia syndrome

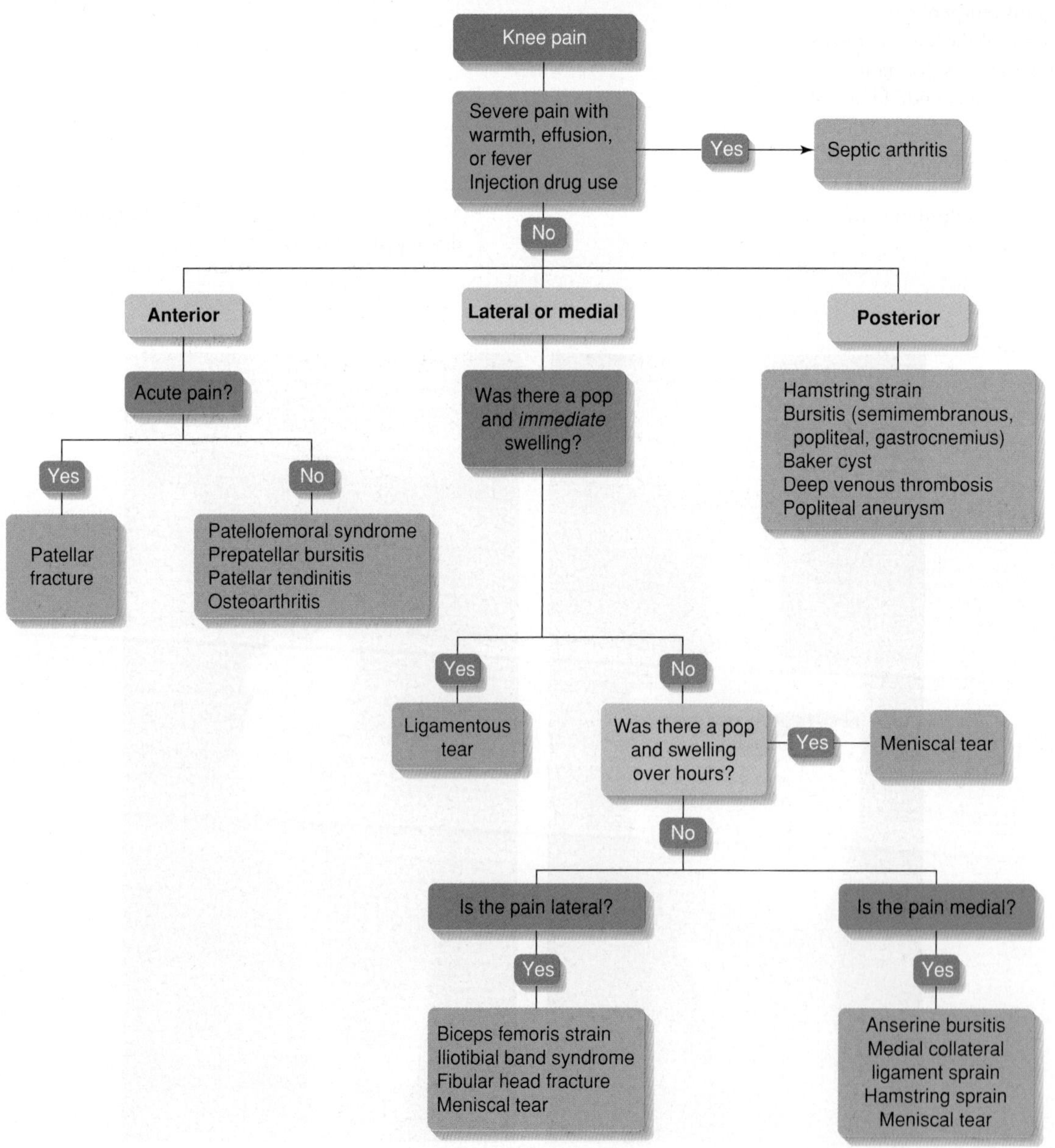

FIGURE 195-5 Diagnostic approach: Knee pain. (From Henderson MC, Tierney LM, Smetana GW. *The Patient History: An Evidence-Based Approach to Differential Diagnosis:* http://www.accessmedicine.com.)

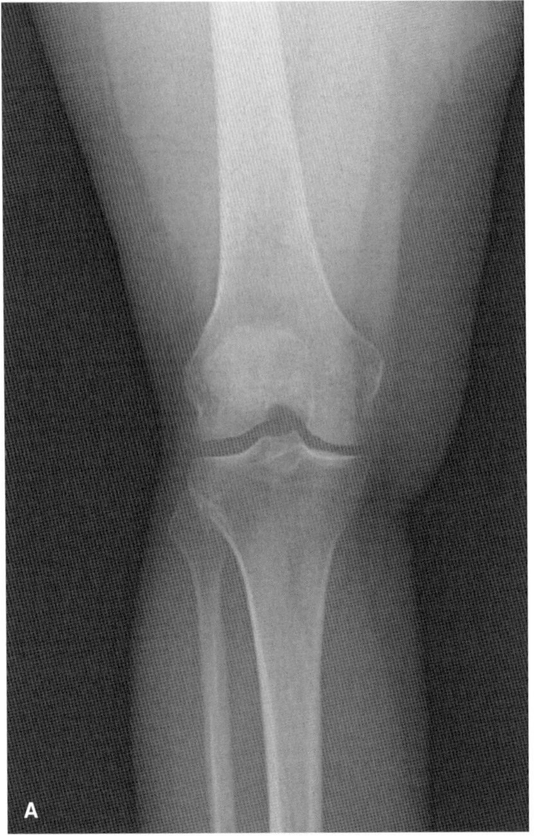

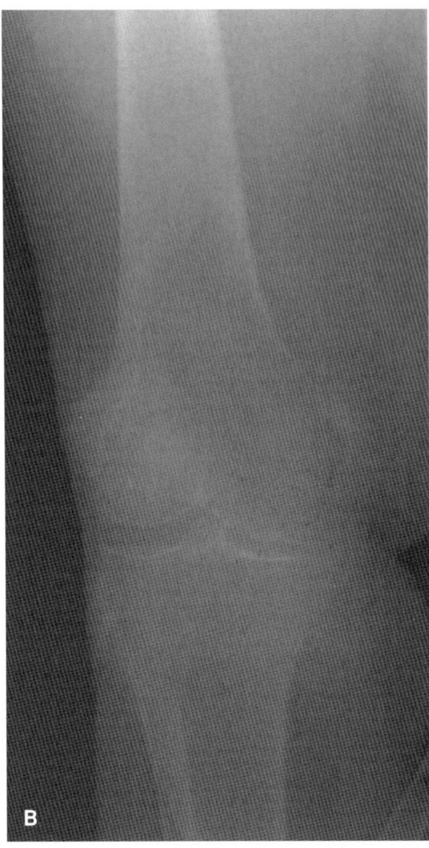

FIGURE 195-6 (**A**) In this AP radiograph, there is very early indication of a loss of medial compartment joint space, which is consistent with early OA. (**B**) In this image, the degenerative disease process is advanced as evidenced by the near complete obliteration of medial joint space, sclerosis of the subchondral bone, flattening of the medial femoral condyle, and osteophyte formation around the margin of the tibia. (From Malone TR, Hazle C, Grey ML. *Imaging in Rehabilitation*. http://www.accessphysiotherapy.com. Copyright © The McGraw-Hill Companies, Inc. All rights reserved.)

- Gout
- Lumbar radiculopathy
- Polyarthrosis
- Rheumatoid arthritis
- Spondyloarthropathy
- Stress fracture
- Tendinitis

MEANS OF CONFIRMATION OR DIAGNOSIS

Laboratory Tests

- Synovial fluid examination (not required)
- Other laboratory tests may be done to rule out other conditions

Imaging

- Conventional radiograph of the joint
- MRI of the joint
- Diagnostic Ultrasound of the joint and synovium[8]

Findings and Interpretation

- OA is a clinical diagnosis, which can be based on
  - Persistent usage-related pain in joint(s)
  - Age ≥45 years[2]
  - Morning stiffness equal or less than 30 minutes[2]
- Imaging studies (radiograph)
  - Osteophytes, joint-space narrowing, sclerosis
  - Cartilage lesions, bone marrow lesions, synovitis, effusion, and subchondral bone attrition/sclerosis
  - Articular cartilage erosion
  - KL Grade ≥2 (definite radiographic OA)

TREATMENT

Medication

- NSAIDs (including topical, capsaicin)[8]
- Acetaminophen
- Opioids
- Glucosamine and chondroitin sulfate
- Glucocorticoids or corticosteroids
- Intra-articular injections (corticosteroids, hyaluronic acid)
- Emerging drug options (e.g., anti-TNF, calcitonin, growth factors, nerve growth factor antibodies
- Homeopathic agents: arnica gel and fish oil

MEDICAL PROCEDURES

- Surgery: Total joint replacement, joint lavage, debridement

REFERRALS/ADMITTANCE

- To rheumatologist, assess underlying complications
- To internal medicine specialist
- To orthopedic specialist
- To physical and rehabilitation medicine specialist
- For surgical consult
- To dietician, nutritional counseling

IMPAIRMENTS

- Mobility
- Self-care
- Roles at home and in the community
- School and work
- Recreation, leisure, sports

TESTS AND MEASURES

- Self-report patient-specific measures of health-related quality of life[3]
  - Patient-specific functional scale (PSFS)
- Pain, visual analog scale (VAS)
  - 24-hour pain
  - Worst average pain
  - Best average pain
- Functional independence measure
  - Bed mobility
  - Transfers
  - Locomotion
- Cardiovascular integrity
  - Blood pressure at rest and after activity
  - Blood pressure in response to position changes
  - Heart rate at rest and after activity
  - Oxygen saturation
  - Presence lower-extremity pulses
- Skin integrity
  - Associated skin assessment
    - Edema (linear girth measurements, palpation)
    - Color
    - Mobility/turgor
    - Temperature
- Neurologic examination
- Sensation
  - Light touch
  - Pin prick
  - Protective sensation
  - Lower-extremity deep tendon reflexes
  - Proprioception at the hip/knee
  - Kinesthetic awareness at the hip/knee
  - Coordination
- Trunk active and passive ROM
- Hip and knee active and Passive ROM
- Flexibility testing
  - Hamstrings
  - Iliopsoas
  - Quadriceps
  - Iliotibial band
  - Abductors
  - Adductors
- Joint integrity of the spine
- Sacroiliac joint integrity
- Hip joint integrity
  - Hip scour
  - Flexion abduction external rotation (FABER) test
  - Flexion induction internal rotation (FAIR) test
  - FADDIR test
- Limb strength
  - Functional strength testing
    - Five-times-sit-to-stand test

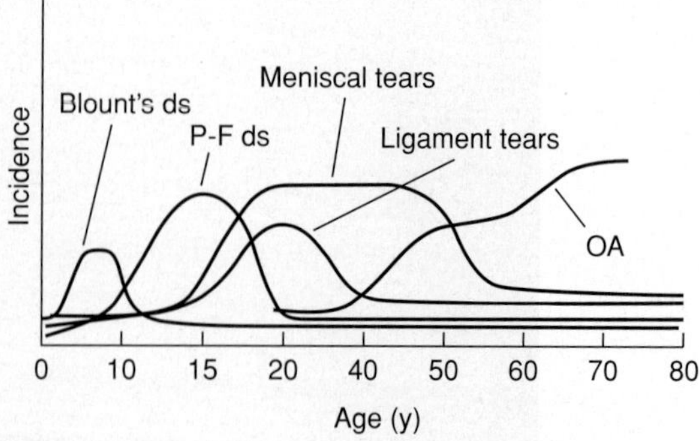

FIGURE 195-7 The age distribution of knee disorders is given schematically as a function of age. Blount's ds, tibia vara; P-F ds, patellofemoral arthralgia; OA, osteoarthrosis. Meniscal tears can be either medial or lateral and are traumatic in the younger age group and degenerative in the older age group. Osteoarthrosis shows an earlier onset with the knee than with the hip because there is an incidence of medial gonarthrosis in the 40s and 50s caused by medial meniscectomy in the late teens and early 20s. (From Skinner HB. *Current Diagnosis & Treatment in Orthopedics*. 4th ed. http://www.accessmedicine.com. Copyright © The McGraw-Hill Companies, Inc. All rights reserved.)

  - Manual muscle test (MMT)
    - Hamstrings
    - Quadriceps
    - Iliopsoas
    - Gluteus maximus
    - Gluteus medius
    - Gluteus minimus
    - Adductors
    - Abdominals
    - Multifidus
- LE contralateral limb strength
- Balance
  - Static single-leg standing (eyes open, eyes closed)
    - Contralateral LE
  - Dynamic standing
    - Berg Balance Scale
    - Functional gait assessment
- Gait assessment
  - Observational analysis
  - Timed up and go test
  - Gait speed via the 10-m walk test
  - 2-minute walk test
  - 6-minute walk test
  - Dual task assessment
    - Timed up and go: Manual, cognitive
    - Walking while talking test: Simple, complex
- Fall risk
  - Dynamic gait assessment
  - Functional gait assessment
- Fear of falling
  - Activities-specific balance confidence scale
  - Falls Efficacy Scale

INTERVENTION

- Exercises (resistance, endurance, flexibility)
  - Aquatic exercises
  - Unweighted
- Training on ADLs

- Assistive or adaptive devices
- Heat therapy
- Weight management
- Rest
- Orthoses, splints
- Walking aids
- Ice[9]
- Diet
- Acupuncture
- Pain management
- Energy conservation techniques
- Joint protection
- Footwear
- Psychosocial support
- Ultrasound[10]
- Electric stimulation[11]
- Patient education

FUNCTIONAL GOALS

- Patient will demonstrate
  - Improved joint mobility and stability; improved balance.
  - Improved muscle strength so as to climb stairs.
  - Improved muscle and aerobic endurance.
  - Improved activity, participation in home, work, and community activities.
  - Ability to walk 0.5 miles pain-free without assistive device.
  - Ability to walk 1 mile pain-free with assistive device.
  - Return to pain-free ADLs (sweeping, mopping, etc.).

PROGNOSIS

- No definite cure.
- Treatment for symptom management, but emerging drugs may modify OA disease mechanism.
- Joint damage is irreversible.
- Recovery or relief from symptoms may depend on disease duration and timely intervention.
- OA is a chronic disease with possible long-term burden.
- Factors that may affect prognosis include.
  - Demographics
  - Severity and natural history of the disease
  - Medical comorbidities
  - Behavioral comorbidities, such as fear avoidance, catastrophization, central sensitization
- General endurance, good muscle strength, and mobile joints are good prognosticating factors.
- Motivation and compliance with physical therapy intervention (e.g., home exercise program) and family/environmental support could improve outcomes.

PATIENT RESOURCES

- Osteoarthritis. Arthritis Today. Arthritis Foundation. http://www.arthritistoday.org/community/expert-q–a/osteoarthritis/index.php. Accessed August 9, 2014.
- Osteoarthritis Research Society International. *OARSI Primer*; 2010. (last updated 2011). http://primer.oarsi.org. Accessed August 9, 2014.

REFERENCES

1. The American Physical Therapy Association. Pattern 4D: Impaired joint mobility, motor function, muscle performance, and range of motion associated with connective tissue dysfunction. *Interactive Guide to Physical Therapist Practice*. 2003. doi: 10.2522/ptguide.3.1_4. Online February 28, 2012. Accessed April 28, 2013.
2. The American Physical Therapy Association. Pattern 4F: Impaired joint mobility, motor function, muscle performance, range of motion, and reflex integrity associated with spinal disorders. *Interactive Guide to Physical Therapist Practice*. 2003. doi: 10.2522/ptguide.3.1_6. Online February 28, 2012. Accessed April 28, 2013.
3. The American Physical Therapy Association. Pattern 4H: Impaired joint mobility, motor function, muscle performance, and range of motion associated with joint arthroplasty. *Interactive Guide to Physical Therapist Practice*. 2003. doi: 10.2522/ptguide.3.1_8. Online February 28, 2012. Accessed April 28, 2013.
4. The American Physical Therapy Association. Pattern 4I: Impaired joint mobility, motor function, muscle performance, and range of motion associated with bony or soft tissue surgery. *Interactive Guide to Physical Therapist Practice*. 2003. doi: 10.2522/ptguide.3.1_9. Online February 28, 2012. Accessed April 28, 2013.
5. McKinnis LN. *Fundamentals of Musculoskeletal Imaging*. F.A. Davis Company: 2005.
6. Kellgren JH, Lawrence JS. *Atlas of Standard Radiographs*. Oxford, UK: Oxford University Press; 1963.
7. National Collaborating Centre for Chronic Conditions (UK). *Osteoarthritis: National Clinical Guideline for Care and Management in Adults*. London: Royal College of Physicians; 2008.
8. Dutton M. *Orthopaedic Examination, Evaluation, and Intervention*. New York, NY: McGraw-Hill; 2008. http://www.accessphysiotherapy.com/resource/612. Accessed April 28, 2013.
9. Prentice WE. Chapter 9. Cryotherapy and thermotherapy. In: Prentice WE, Quillen WS, Underwood F, Eds. *Therapeutic Modalities in Rehabilitation*.4th ed. McGraw-Hill; 2005. http://www.accessphysiotherapy.com/abstract/8138405#8138406. Accessed April 28, 2013.
10. Draper DO, Prentice WE. Chapter 10. Therapeutic ultrasound. In: Prentice WE, Quillen WS, Underwood F, Eds. *Therapeutic Modalities in Rehabilitation*.4th ed. McGraw-Hill; 2005. http://www.accessphysiotherapy.com/abstract/8138405#8138406. Accessed April 28, 2013.
11. Dutton M. Chapter 18. Adjunctive interventions. *McGraw-Hill's NPTE (National Physical Therapy Examination)*. 2nd ed. McGraw-Hill Medical; 2012. http://www.accessphysiotherapy.com/abstract/5406031#5406117. Accessed April 28, 2013.

ADDITIONAL REFERENCES

- ICD9DATA web site. http://www.icd9data.com. Accessed August 9, 2014.
- ICD10DATA web site. http://www.icd10data.com. Accessed August 9, 2014.
- Tanaka R, Ozawa J, Kito N, et al. Efficacy of strengthening or aerobic exercise on pain relief in people with knee osteoarthritis: a systematic review and meta-analysis of randomized controlled trials. *Clin Rehabil.* 2013 Dec;27(12):1059–71.

196 MEDIAL TIBIAL STRESS SYNDROME

Eric Shamus, PhD, DPT, PT, CSCS
Jennifer Shamus, PhD, DPT, COMT, CSCS

CONDITION/DISORDER SYNONYMS

- Medial tibial stress syndrome
- Posterior medial tibial periostitis
- Posterior medial tibial stress fracture

ICD-9-CM CODE[1]

- 733.93 Stress fracture of the tibia

ICD-10-CM CODE[2]

- M84.369A Stress fracture, unspecified tibia and fibula, initial encounter for fracture

PREFERRED PRACTICE PATTERN[3]

- 4E: Impaired Joint Mobility, Motor Function, Muscle Performance, and Range of Motion (ROM) Associated with Localized Inflammation

PATIENT PRESENTATION

A 25-year-old female presents with right medial shin pain. She indicates that 3 weeks earlier she began an exercise program that involves jogging 3 miles per day. The patient just bought new sneakers. The pain starts about mile 2 and has to stop running. The X-ray was positive for a stress fracture. The left lower extremity (LE) measures 2 cm longer. Palpable swelling along the medial tibia.

KEY FEATURES

Description

- Bone pain is localized in the medial aspects of the tibia
- Stress-reaction inflammation of the periosteal and musculotendinous fascial junctions
- Attributed to a loss in bone mineral density
- Recurring dull ache along the posterior medial aspect of the lower tibia

Essentials of Diagnosis

- Diagnosis is usually made by bone scan and x-ray
- Muscle length and strength imbalances, especially a tight gastrocnemius-soleus muscle group

General Considerations

- Looks like tibilais posterior tendinitis, but does not respond to treatment
- Tendinopathy
- Periostitis
- Periosteal remodeling
- Nutritional imbalance
- No relief with conservative treatment

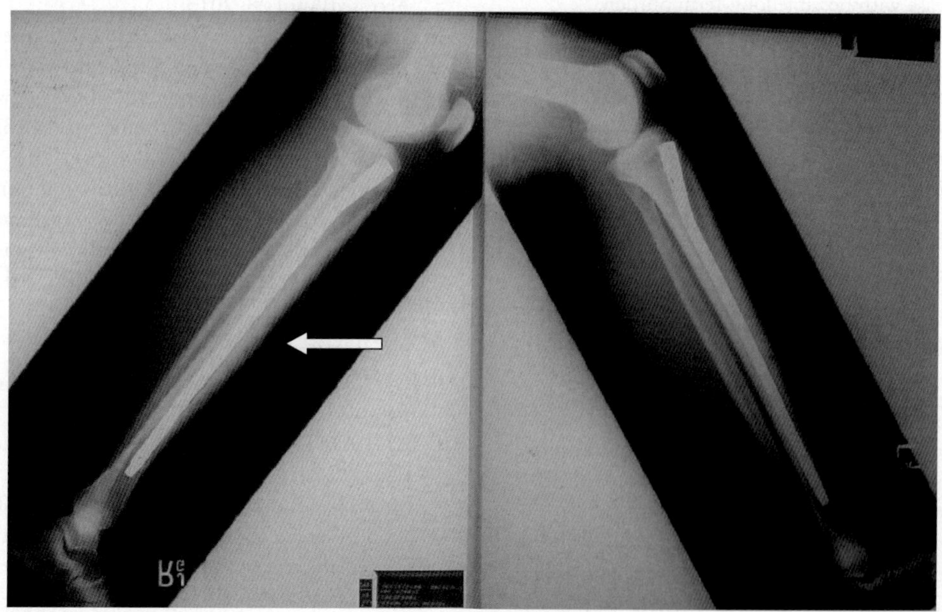

FIGURE 196-1 Intramedullary screw (*white arrow*) fixation of bilateral anterior medial tibial stress fractures. (From South-Paul JE, Matheny SC, Lewis EL. *Current Diagnosis & Treatment in Family Medicine*. 3rd ed. http://www.accessmedicine.com. Copyright © The McGraw-Hill Companies, Inc. All rights reserved.)

Demographics
- College athletes

CLINICAL FINDINGS

SIGNS AND SYMPTOMS
- Pain: Mild to severe with weight-bearing activities and gait
- Described as a dull ache to LEs
- Point tenderness to tibia at posterior medial aspect
- Possible localized swelling

Functional Implications
- Pain with standing or during activity
- Inability of injured LE to bear weight
- Pain with closed chain ankle movements (i.e., driving)

Possible Contributing Causes
- Running/standing on a hard surface
- Leg-length inequality
- Compensation from an injury on the opposite limb
- History of high/repetitive impact activities
- Overtraining

Differential Diagnosis
- Fracture of the tibia or fibula
- Contusion
- Gastrocnemius/soleus muscle strain
- Cellulitis
- Referred pain from sciatic nerve, spinal stenosis, or Baker's cyst
- Deep vein thrombosis (DVT): Homan's test
- Superficial thrombophlebitis
- Peripheral arterial disease
- Venous insufficiency
- Myofascial pain
- Fibromyalgia
- Popliteal artery entrapment
- Soft-tissue tumor or bony metastasis
- Osteomyelitis

MEANS OF CONFIRMATION OR DIAGNOSIS

Imaging
- X-ray for fracture, often limited view
- Triple-phase bone scintigraphy
- Computed tomography (CT) scan for detailed imaging
- Bone scan if stress fracture is suspected
- MRI/MRA
- Arteriograms

Diagnostic Procedures
- Compartmental pressure measurements
- Palpation of pulses in the foot
- Capillary refill

FINDINGS AND INTERPRETATION
- Imaging shows changes in bone density

TREATMENT
- Medication: NSAID for pain management
- Walking boot
- Immobilization, splinting of the lower leg in severe cases

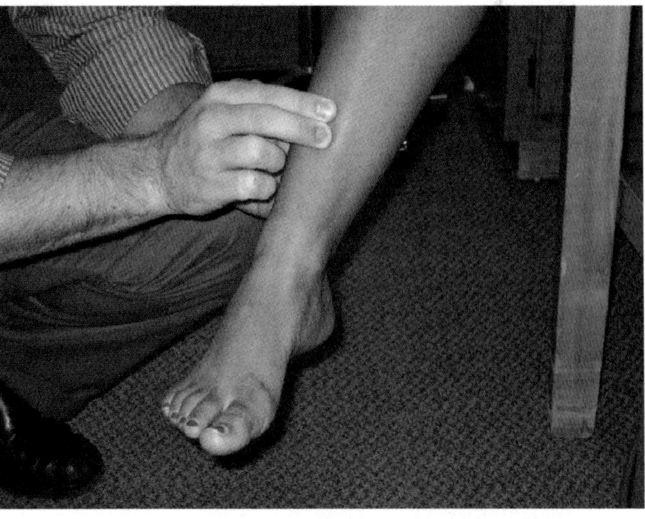

FIGURE 196-2 Site of maximum pain and tenderness in medial tibial stress syndrome. (From Patel DR, Greydanus DE, Baker RJ. *Pediatric Practice: Sports Medicine*. http://www.accesspediatrics.com. Copyright © The McGraw-Hill Companies, Inc. All rights reserved.)

REFERRALS/ADMITTANCE
- For imaging: x-ray or CT
- Orthopedic consult

IMPAIRMENTS
- Antalgic gait secondary to pain, which causes an inability to push off during gait
- Inability to ambulate long distances secondary to pain and/or likelihood of decreased weight-bearing status that makes ambulating a taxing activity
- Decreased stance time on the involved LE during ambulation
- Inability to stand for long periods of time secondary to pain

TESTS AND MEASURES
- Shin palpation test and shin edema test[4]
  - When both positive likelihood ratio of 7.94, 8 times more likely to develop shin splints
  - When both negative likelihood ration <0.001, extremely unlikely to develop shin splints
- Navicular drop test
- Compartment syndrome pressure assessment
- Pain, visual analog scale (VAS)
  - 24-hour pain
  - Worst average pain
  - Best average pain
- Functional independence measure
  - Locomotion
- Cardiovascular integrity
  - Blood pressure at rest and after activity
  - Heart rate at rest and after activity
- Skin Integrity
  - Associated skin assessment
    - Edema (linear girth measurements, palpation)
    - Color
    - Temperature

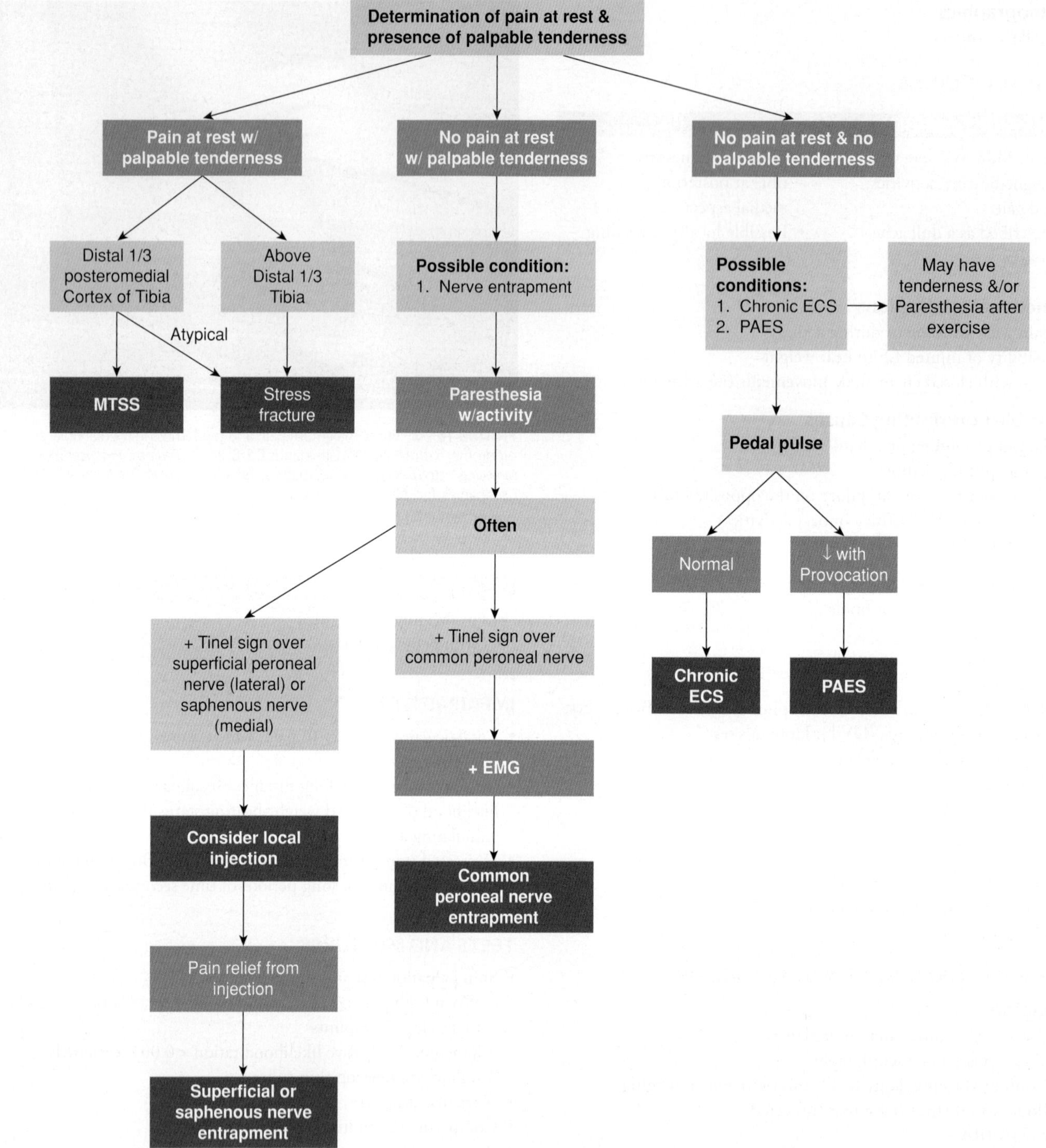

FIGURE 196-3 History and examination algorithm for chronic leg pain. (Adapted and redrawn from Edwards PH, Wright ML, Hartman JF. A practical approach to differential diagnosis of chronic leg pain in the athlete. *Am J Sport Med.* 2005;33(8):1241–1249.)

- Neurologic examination
  - Sensation
    - Light touch
    - Pin prick
  - LE deep tendon reflexes
  - Proprioception at the hip, knee, and ankle
  - Kinesthetic awareness
  - Coordination
- Trunk active and passive ROM
- Hip, knee, ankle active and passive ROM
- Flexibility testing
  - Gastrocnemius
  - Soleus
  - Hamstrings
  - Iliopsoas
  - Quadriceps
  - Iliotibial band
  - Abductors
  - Adductors
- Joint integrity of the spine

- Sacroiliac joint integrity
- Hip joint integrity
  - Flexion abduction external rotation (FABER) test
- Limb strength
  - Manual muscle test (MMT)
    - Anterior tibialis
    - Posterior tibialis
    - Hamstrings
    - Quadriceps
    - Iliopsoas
    - Gluteus maximus
    - Gluteus medius
    - Gluteus minimus
    - Adductors
- LE contralateral limb strength
- Balance
  - Static single-leg standing (eyes open, eyes closed)
    - Contralateral LE
  - Dynamic standing
    - Berg Balance Scale
    - Functional gait assessment
- Gait assessment
  - Observational analysis
  - Gait speed via the 10-m walk test
  - 2-minute walk test
  - 6-minute walk test
  - Retro running

INTERVENTION

- Rest
- Taping
  - Decrease strain on tibialis posterior tendon
  - Arch taping
- Correction of biomechanical defects
- Orthotics: Provide proper arch support with neutral subtalar positioning to avoid stressing injured structures
- Address swelling
  - Ice/cryotherapy
- Address pain
- Laser therapy
- Appropriate shoes for high impact activities

FUNCTIONAL GOALS

- Patient will be able to:
  - Ambulate pain-free for greater than 30 minutes.
  - Return to high impact activity such as running, hiking, and dancing.
  - Demonstrate and maintain neutral calcaneal alignment with heel strike through toe-off phases of gait.
  - Demonstrate 15 degrees of talocrural dorsiflexion during push-off phase of gait.
  - Stand and walk without limitation due to pain after sitting for >1 hour.
  - Demonstrate 5/5 manual muscle testing of involved gastrocnemius without limitation due to pain.
  - Demonstrate 50% speed running for 1 mile without limitation due to pain.
  - Demonstrate single-leg hopping on involved side without limitation due to pain.

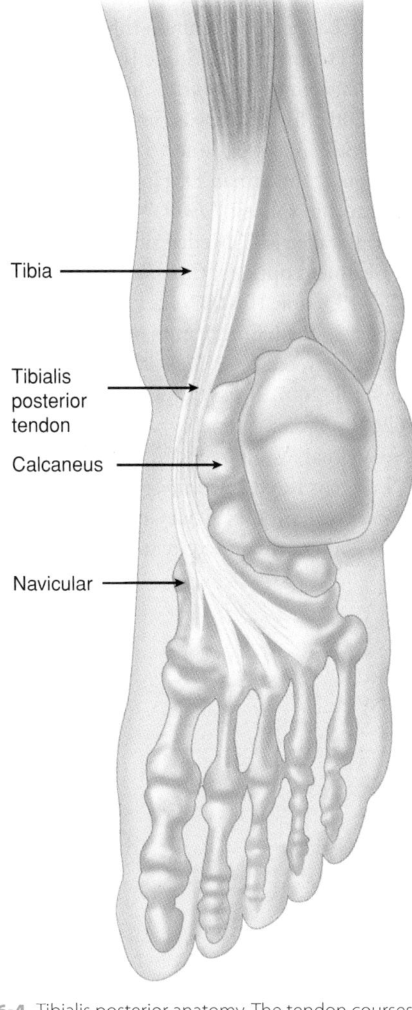

FIGURE 196-4 Tibialis posterior anatomy. The tendon courses behind and below the medial malleolus at it enters the foot, to be inserted at multiple sites on the navicular, cuneiforms, and second, third, and fourth metatarsals. (From Patel DR, Greydanus DE, Baker RJ. *Pediatric Practice: Sports Medicine*. http://www.accesspediatrics.com. Copyright © The McGraw-Hill Companies, Inc. All rights reserved.)

PROGNOSIS

- In most cases, the patient resumes normal functioning and returns to previous workout regimen when bone density has normalized.

PATIENT RESOURCE

- Shin Splints. *Orthogate*. http://www.orthogate.org/patient-education/ankle/shin-splints.html. Accessed June 15, 2013.

REFERENCES

1. ICD-9-CM. http://www.icd9data.com. Accessed June 29, 2013.
2. ICD 10-CM. http://www.icd10data.com. Accessed June 29, 2013.
3. The American Physical Therapy Association. *Guide to Physical Therapist Practice*. Alexandria, VA: The American Physical Therapy Association; 2003. http://guidetoptpractice.apta.org/. Accessed June 29, 2013.
4. Newman P, Adams R, Waddington G. Two simple tests for predicting onset of medial tibial stress syndrome: shin palpation test and shin edema test. *Br J Sports Med*. 2012;46(12):861–864.

ADDITIONAL REFERENCES

- Brown JR, CR. Chapter 62. Common injuries from running. In: Imboden JB, Hellmann DB, Stone JH, eds. *CURRENT Rheumatology Diagnosis & Treatment*. 2nd ed. New York, NY: McGraw-Hill; 2007. http://www.accessmedicine.com/content.aspx?aID=2729862. Accessed June 15, 2013.
- Carr K, Stevetson E, Aukerman D. How can you help athletes prevent and treat shin splints? *J Fam Pract*. 2008;57(6):406–408.
- Galbraith RM, Lavallee ME. Medial tibial stress syndrome: conservative treatment options. *Curr Rev Musculoskelet Med*. 2009;2(3):127–133. doi: 10.1007/s12178-009-9055-6.
- Hall SJ. Chapter 8. The biomechanics of the human lower extremity. In: Hall SJ, ed. *Basic Biomechanics*. 5th ed. New York, NY: McGraw-Hill; 2007. http://www.accessphysiotherapy.com/content/6062676. Accessed June 29, 2013.
- Hamilton N, Weimar W, Luttgens K. The leg. In: Hamilton N, Weimar W, Luttgens K, eds. *Kinesiology: Scientific Basis of Human Motion*. New York, NY: McGraw-Hill; 2008. http://www.accessphysiotherapy.com/content/6153064. Accessed June 29, 2013.
- Houglum PA. *Therapeutic Exercise for Musculoskeletal Injuries*. 2nd ed. Champaign, IL: Human Kinetics; 2005.
- Kisner C, Colby LA. *Therapeutic Exercise: Foundations and Techniques*. 5th ed. Philadelphia, PA: F.A. Davis Company; 2007.
- Patel DR, Lyne ED. Chapter 29. Overuse injuries of the leg, ankle, and foot. In: Patel DR, Greydanus DE, Baker RJ, eds. *Pediatric Practice: Sports Medicine*. New York, NY: McGraw-Hill; 2009. http://www.accessphysiotherapy.com/content/6980676. Accessed June 29, 2013.
- Shin Splints. MedlinePlus, NIH National Institutes of Health. http://www.nlm.nih.gov/medlineplus/ency/article/003177.htm. Accessed June 5, 2013.
- Simon RR, Sherman SC. Leg soft-tissue injury. In: Simon RR, Sherman SC, eds. *Emergency Orthopedics*. 6th ed. New York, NY: McGraw-Hill; 2011. http://www.accessphysiotherapy.com/content/7708294. Accessed June 29, 2013.
- Story J, Cymet TC. Shin splints painful to have and to treat. *Comprehensive Therapy*. 2006;32(3):192–195.

197 MENISCUS TEAR

Tasha Mouton, DPT, MOT, OCS, FAAOMPT, MTC
Eric Shamus, PhD, DPT, PT, CSCS

CONDITION/DISORDER SYNONYMS

- Lateral meniscus tear
- Medial meniscus tear

ICD-9-CM CODES

- 717 Internal derangement of knee
- 717.0 Old bucket handle tear of medial meniscus
- 717.1 Derangement of anterior horn of medial meniscus
- 717.2 Derangement of posterior horn of medial meniscus
- 717.3 Other and unspecified derangement of medial meniscus
- 717.4 Derangement of lateral meniscus
- 717.40 Derangement of lateral meniscus unspecified
- 717.41 Bucket handle tear of lateral meniscus
- 717.42 Derangement of anterior horn of lateral meniscus
- 717.43 Derangement of posterior horn of lateral meniscus
- 717.49 Other derangement of lateral meniscus
- 717.5 Derangement of meniscus not elsewhere classified

ICD-10-CM CODES

- M23.009 Cystic meniscus, unspecified meniscus, unspecified knee
- M23.202 Derangement of unspecified lateral meniscus due to old tear or injury, unspecified knee
- M23.205 Derangement of unspecified medial meniscus due to old tear or injury, unspecified knee
- M23.219 Derangement of anterior horn of medial meniscus due to old tear or injury, unspecified knee
- M23.229 Derangement of posterior horn of medial meniscus due to old tear or injury, unspecified knee
- M23.239 Derangement of other medial meniscus due to old tear or injury, unspecified knee
- M23.249 Derangement of anterior horn of lateral meniscus due to old tear or injury, unspecified knee
- M23.259 Derangement of posterior horn of lateral meniscus due to old tear or injury, unspecified knee
- M23.269 Derangement of other lateral meniscus due to old tear or injury, unspecified knee
- M23.305 Other meniscus derangements, unspecified medial meniscus, unspecified knee
- M23.319 Other meniscus derangements, anterior horn of medial meniscus, unspecified knee
- M23.329 Other meniscus derangements, posterior horn of medial meniscus, unspecified knee
- M23.339 Other meniscus derangements, other medial meniscus, unspecified knee
- M23.349 Other meniscus derangements, anterior horn of lateral meniscus, unspecified knee
- M23.359 Other meniscus derangements, posterior horn of lateral meniscus, unspecified knee

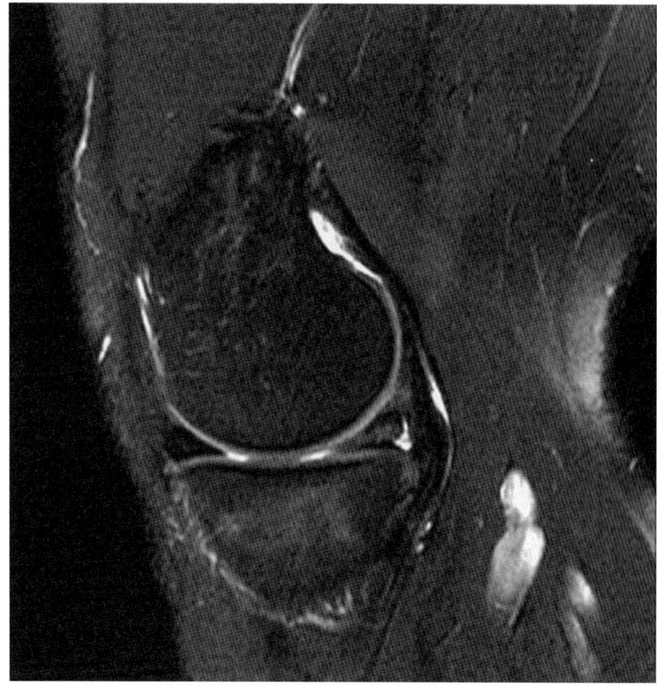

FIGURE 197-1 This sagittal slice MRI reveals increased signal intensity in the posterior horn of the meniscus as well as at the meniscocapsular junction, suggesting a tear of the meniscus and possible separation from the peripheral attachment. (From Malone TR, Hazle C, Grey ML. *Imaging in Rehabilitation*. http://www.accessphysiotherapy.com. Copyright © The McGraw-Hill Companies, Inc. All rights reserved.)

- M23.369 Other meniscus derangements, other lateral meniscus, unspecified knee

PREFERRED PRACTICE PATTERN

- 4I: Impaired Joint Mobility, Motor Function, Muscle Performance, and Range of Motion Associated with Bony or Soft Tissue Surgery

PATIENT PRESENTATION

A 40-year man was out playing in the backyard with his son and twisted his knee when he was running and stepped on a sprinkler head. The patient stated he heard a pop and had difficulty moving the knee. He states it was not very painful but feels like the knee is locked. With traction the therapist was able to regain full range of motion. The patient was referred to a physician who ordered an MRI. The patient has a bucket handle tear and underwent arthroscopic surgery.

KEY FEATURES

Description

- Tear of the fibrocartilage of the meniscus
- Tears commonly occur from a twisting of the knee with knee flexion

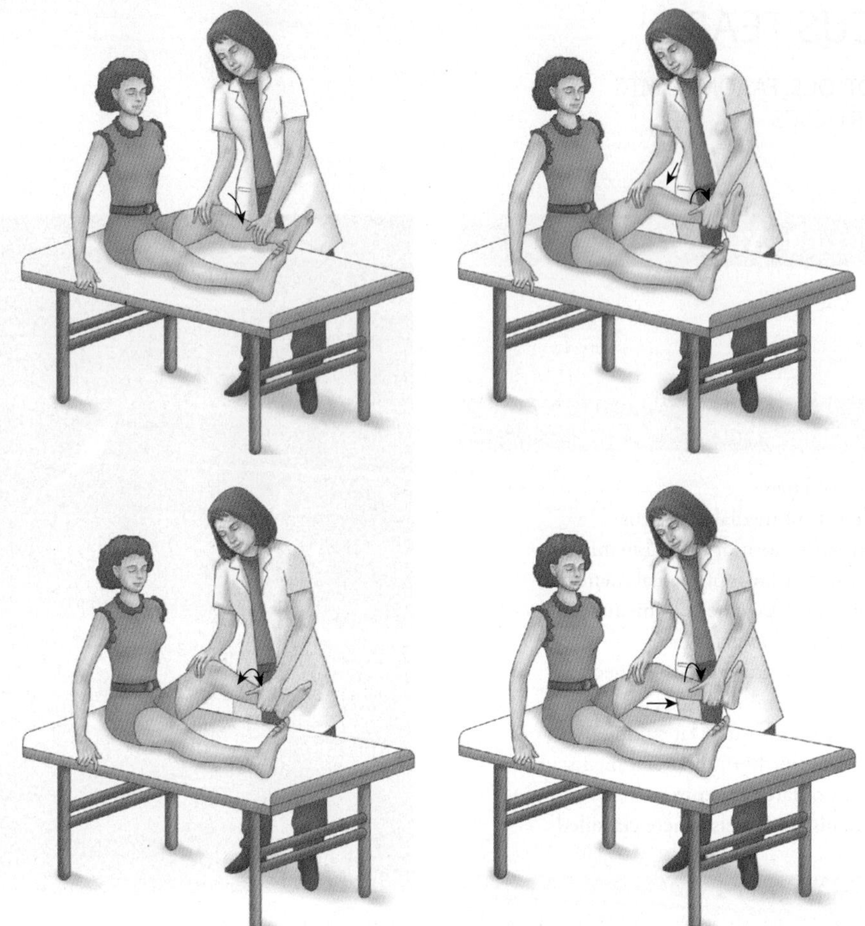

FIGURE 197-2 McMurray test. (From Dutton M. *Dutton's Orthopedic Survival Guide: Managing Common Conditions*. http://www.accessphysiotherapy.com.)

- Can develop because of laxity in the knee
- Complaint of joint locking and inability to straighten the knee

Essentials of Diagnosis

- Frequency
  - No true data on isolated incidence and prevalence of meniscal injury[1]
- Mechanism of injury
  - Activities that include cutting, deceleration, and landing from a jump[2]
- Classification of tear[3]
  - Longitudinal tear: Vertical tear in the meniscus with a longitudinal direction; usually located in the periphery of the meniscus
    - The longer the tear, the more unstable it is, and the end result is the dislocated central part of the meniscus (bucket-handle tear)
  - Horizontal tear: Horizontal cleavage in the meniscal tissue
  - Radial tear: Vertical tear starting in the free (central) margin of the meniscal tissue
  - Flap tear: Oblique vertical cleavage causing a flap tear (parrot beak); a flap tear can also be caused by a horizontal tear
  - Tear in degenerative meniscus: A tear or multiple tears in a degeneratively changed meniscal tissue

General Considerations

- Depending on the zone of the tear (based on blood supply), some maybe able to surgically repair.
- The meniscus is a crescent-shaped fibrocartilaginous structure that lines the articular surface of the tibia.
- Its primary roles include shock absorption, load transmission, proprioception, and improvement of stability and lubrication of the knee joint.[2,4]
- The medial meniscus occupies 50% of the articular surface contact area of the medial compartment.[2]
- The anterior horn is attached firmly to the tibia just anterior to the anterior cruciate ligament, while the posterior horn attaches just anterior to the posterior cruciate ligament.[2]
- The lateral meniscus covers 70% of the lateral tibial plateau.
- The posterior horn is attached to the posterior cruciate ligament and popliteus tendon by ligamentous attachment sites.
- The lateral meniscus is relatively less mobile and less injured relative to the medial meniscus due to its attachments.[2,5]

Demographics

- With increased age and resultant degeneration of the meniscus, minimal insult can cause injury[2,6]
- 5% of meniscal injuries involve patients <15 years of age[6]
- Peak of incidence noted in individuals >55 years of age due to degeneration of the meniscus

CLINICAL FINDINGS

SIGNS AND SYMPTOMS

- Popping or catching[2,5,7]
- Locking occurs at time of injury and prevents terminal knee extension at 20 to 30 degrees of flexion. Subsequent locking and unlocking equally suggestive[6]
- Joint line tenderness to palpation (high false-positives as present in osteoarthritis [OA], fracture, collateral ligament damage)[2,3,6]
- Effusion[5]
- Quadriceps atrophy, especially of the vastus medialis[5]
- Quadriceps weakness via bilateral comparison with asymptomatic extremity[5]

Functional Implications

- Increased intensity and frequency of pain with the following activities: stair climbing, squatting, rising from a low chair, and antalgic gait pattern[2,5,6]

Possible Contributing Causes

- Advanced degeneration in ACL-deficient knee due to increased anterior-posterior shear[3]
- Progressive arthritis[2,3,5]

Differential Diagnoses[7]

- Contusions
- Knee osteochondritis dissecans
- Ligament injuries (anterior or posterior cruciate)
- Lumbosacral radiculopathy
- OA
- Patellofemoral joint dysfunction
- Pes anserine bursitis
- Rheumatoid arthritis
- Tendon inflammation (tendinitis)
- Tibial tubercle avulsion fracture

MEANS OF CONFIRMATION OR DIAGNOSIS

Imaging

- X-rays are routine tests for skeletal injury and may provide insight into loose bodies and degenerative changes.[2]
- MRI
  - Has been shown to have higher false-positive results than false-negative results[8]
  - Equal accuracy of the clinical examination and MRI in diagnosing meniscal and ACL tears
- Arthroscopic evaluation
  - Meniscal injury diagnosed with 90% to 95% accuracy[9]

FINDINGS AND INTERPRETATION

- Combining special tests produced higher sensitivity and specificity for examination-based diagnosis of meniscal tears[8]

REFERRALS/ADMITTANCE

- To referring physician if acute or chronic tear is suspected
- To orthopedist; many repair options exist[5]

IMPAIRMENTS

- Joint effusion
- Impaired joint mobility (potential block end feel)

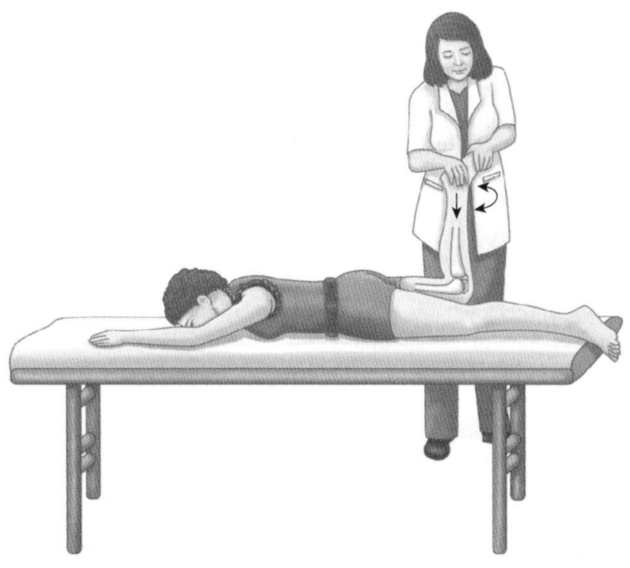

FIGURE 197-3 Apley grind test. (From Dutton M. *Dutton's Orthopedic Survival Guide: Managing Common Conditions*. http://www.accessphysiotherapy.com.)

- Impaired muscle performance
- Impaired strength
- Gait abnormality
- Impaired proprioception

TESTS AND MEASURES

- Anderson Medial–Lateral Grind Test
- Apley test
- Boehler test
- Ege test
- Joint line tenderness[2,5,9]
- McMurray test
- O'Donahue test
- Payr test
- Steinmann tenderness displacement test
- Thessaly test

INTERVENTION

- Therapeutic exercise
- Electrical stimulation
- Early closed-kinetic chain exercise to decrease shear and compression forces[3]
- Neuromuscular-proprioceptive training to address static/dynamic balance training, and coordination[5,9]
- Sport-specific agility training[5]
- Gait training to ensure restoration of normal walking mechanics
- In nonoperative cases, treatment interventions are based on assessment; however, special considerations are listed as follows:
  - In the presence of knee extension deficits, caution must be taken as potential barriers include effusion and displaced meniscus[5]
  - Achieving full extension may come at the cost of further articular or ACL insult[5]
  - Minimize compressive loading on the joint in early rehabilitation, until adequate muscular protection and joint mobility have been developed[5]

FUNCTIONAL GOALS

- Patient will able to
  - Demonstrate increased quadriceps muscle strength to 4+/5 to descend stairs independently.
  - Demonstrate full pain-free AROM/PROM knee flexion and extension to don/doff pants independently.

PROGNOSIS

- In cases of posterior root tear of the medial meniscus, referral to physical therapy has been reported to play an important role in increasing muscular endurance, strength, functional activity, and quality of life for patients with OA.[4]
- Lim et al.[8] reported the following prognostic factors:
  - The overall success rate of meniscal repairs reported was 74%.
  - Meniscal repairs that were performed within 6 weeks of injury had better results (83%) than late repairs (52%).
  - Patients with associated ACL injury had a better chance of a successful outcome, but this was only significant when the ACL was reconstructed at the time of repair.
  - Those patients who had failed meniscal repair had increased radiographic osteoarthritic changes (81%) on long-term follow-up compared with patients with successful repair (14%).

PATIENT RESOURCES

- NIH, National Institute of Arthritis and Musculoskeletal and Skin Diseases. Meniscal Injuries. http://www.niams.nih.gov/health_info/knee_problems. Accessed July 6, 2013.
- American Orthopeadic Society for Sports Medicine. Meniscal Tears in Athletes. http://www.sportsmed.org/uploadedFiles/Content/Patient/Sports_Tips/ST%20Meniscal%20Tears%2008.pdf. Accessed July 6, 2013.

REFERENCES

1. Lobust CA, Stanitski CL. Acute knee injuries. *Clin Sports Med.* 2000;19(4):621–635.
2. Rath E, Richmond JC. The menisci: basic sciences and advantages in treatment. *Br J Sports Med.* 2000;34(4):252–257.
3. Englund M, Roos EM, Lohmander LS. Impact of type of meniscal tear on radiographic and symptomatic knee osteoarthritis: a sixteen-year followup of meniscectomy with matched controls. *Arthritis Rheum.* 2003;48(8):2178–2187.
4. Konan S, Rayan F, Haddad F. Do physical diagnostic tests accurately detect meniscal tears? *Knee Surg Sport Tr A.* 2009;17(7):806–811.
5. Hertling D, Kessler R. *Management of Common Musculoskeletal Disorders: Physical Therapy Principles and Methods.* 4th ed. Philadelphia, PA: Lippincott Williams & Wilkins; 2006.
6. Odgers C, Galinat B. Meniscal injuries in children and adolescents. Clinical case presented at Orthopaedic Department of the Alfred I. Dupont Institute, May 8, 1996; Wilmington, DE. http://gait.aidi.udel.edu/educate/menisc.htm. Accessed January 16, 2013.
7. Calmbach WL, Hutchens M. Evaluation of patient presenting with knee pain: part II. differential diagnosis. *Am Fam Physician.* 2003;68(5):917–922.
8. Lim HC, Bae JH, Wang JH, Seok CW, Kim MK. Non-operative treatment of degenerative posterior root tear of the medial meniscus. *Knee Surg Sport Tr A.* 2010;18(4):535–539.
9. Herrlin S, Hållander M, Wange P, Weidenhielm L, Werner S. Arthroscopic or conservative treatment of degenerative medial meniscal tears: a prospective randomised trial. *Knee Surg Sport Tr A.* 2007;15(4):393–401.

ADDITIONAL REFERENCES

- APTA Guide to Physical Therapist Practice. http://guidetoptpractice.apta.org/. Accessed January 16, 2013.
- Dutton M. Meniscal lesion tests. In: Dutton M, ed. *Orthopaedic Examination, Evaluation, and Intervention.* 2nd ed. New York, NY: McGraw-Hill; 2008. http://www.accessphysiotherapy.com/content/55583754. Accessed July 6, 2013.
- ICD-9-CM. http://www.icd9data.com. Accessed July 6, 2013.
- ICD-10-CM. http://www.icd10data.com. Accessed July 6, 2013.

198 PATELLAR TENDINOPATHY

Eric Shamus, PhD, DPT, PT, CSCS
Patricia M. King, PhD, PT, OCS, MTC
Patricia M. Tripp, PhD, ATC

CONDITION/DISORDER SYNONYMS

- Infrapatellar tendonitis
- Jumper's knee
- Patella tendonitis
- Patellar tendinitis
- Patella tendonopathy
- Patella tendonosis

ICD-9-CM CODE

- 726.64 Patellar tendonitis[1]

ICD-10-CM CODE

- M76.50 Patellar tendinitis, unspecified knee[2]

PREFERRED PRACTICE PATTERN

- 4E: Impaired Joint Mobility, Motor Function, Muscle Performance, and Range of Motion Associated with Localized Inflammation[3]

PATIENT PRESENTATION

A 21-year-old, 6′5″, 190 pound, Division II male collegiate basketball player, with no previous history of knee and/or patellofemoral pathology, reports to the athletic training/sports medicine facility complaining of bilateral anterior knee pain. He states the pain began approximately 2 weeks ago, with the highest incidence of pain occurring in the morning after a weight-training session. About 3 days ago, the pain became constant and has impacted his training. He reported that as part of his off-season conditioning, he has increased strength training (e.g., squats, leg extensions, etc.) and plyometric activities (e.g., box jumps, bounding, etc.) aimed toward increasing power output and vertical jump height. His training over the previous 6 weeks focused on the lower extremity, with 30 to 45 minutes per day of cardiovascular training (e.g., running, cycling) to supplement the 4 days per week of Olympic lifting techniques and plyometric training. He admitted he does not focus on pretraining dynamic warm-ups and performs limited postactivity stretching, but did use ice post activity a few times to manage his pain. The patient presents with no obvious deformity or signs of Osgood–Schlatter disease; no obvious laxity or instability at the patellofemoral joint. Manual muscle testing (eccentric break test) WNL for knee and hip with exception of 4/5 grading: bilateral hip flexion, internal rotation, external rotation, and knee extension. He has a positive Thomas test and positive Ely test, suggesting muscular tightness in his iliopsoas and rectus femoris bilaterally. During gait analysis, he presents with an early heel rise during terminal stance, suggesting tight gastroc-soleus (Achilles tendon). Kinetic chain dysfunction from muscular tightness was further evident during an observed body-weight squat. Radiologic findings include X-rays (negative) and musculoskeletal diagnostic ultrasound (positive for inflammation).

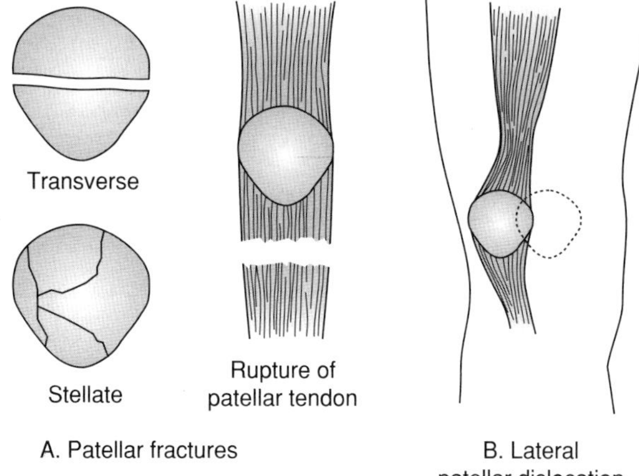

FIGURE 198-1 Traumatic injuries to the anterior knee. (From LeBlond RF, DeGowin RL, Brown DD. *DeGowin's Diagnostic Examination*. 9th ed. www.accessmedicine.com. Copyright © The McGraw-Hill Companies, Inc. All rights reserved.)

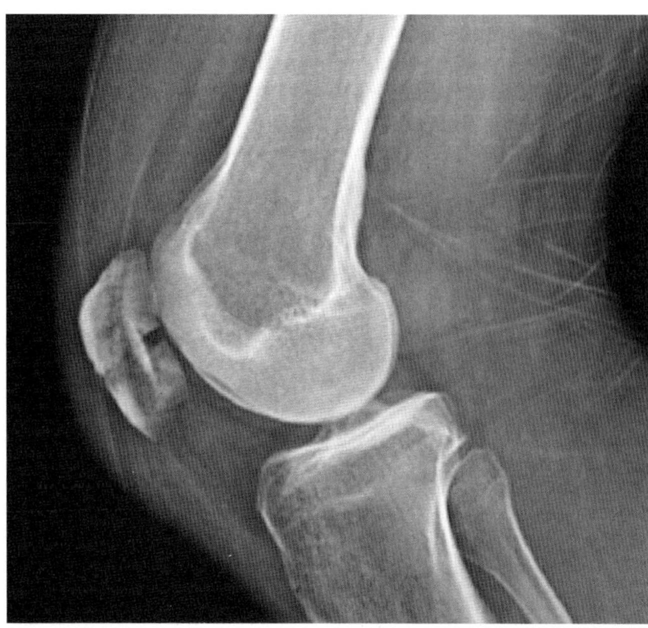

FIGURE 198-2 No displaced patellar fracture seen best on the lateral view. (From Simon RR, Sherman SC, Koenigsknecht SJ. *Emergency Orthopedics: The Extremities*. Fig. 15-26, bottom photo only, p. 405. Copyright 2007. New York, NY: McGraw-Hill.)

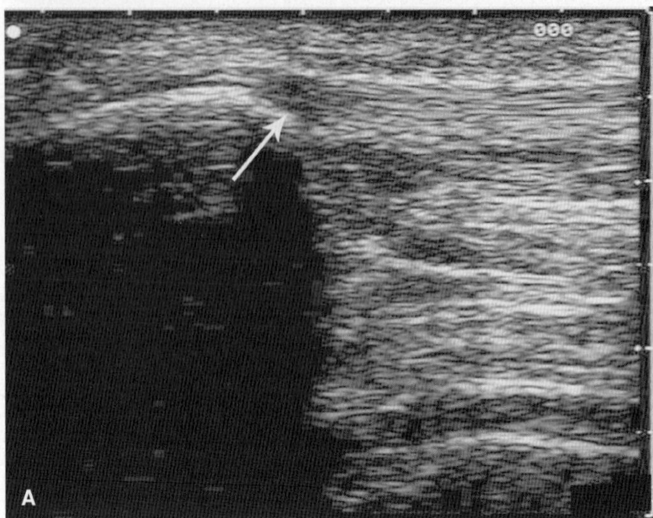

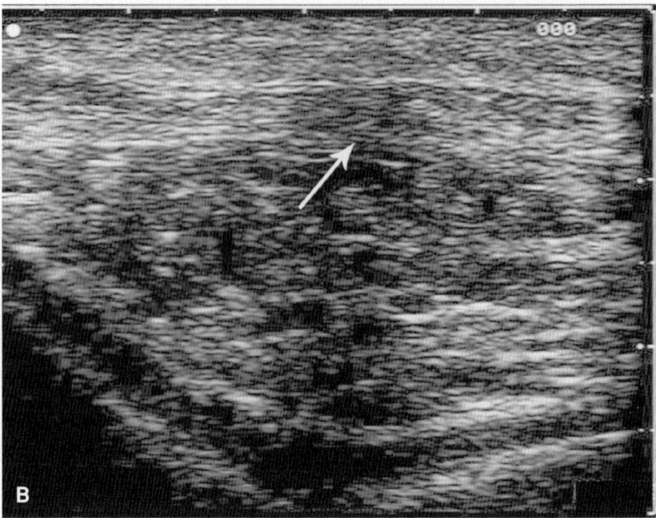

FIGURE 198-3 Patellar tendon defect. (**A**) Long-axis sonogram of the proximal patellar ligament showing a hypoechoic tendon defect near the origin of the patellar tendon (*arrow*). The remainder of the tendon appears fibrillar and echogenic. A heel–toe insonating technique confirmed that a hypoechoic defect was present and that a tendinopathy (jumper's knee) was present. (**B**) Short-axis sonogram of the same patellar ligament. The ligament is seen as a somewhat echogenic horizontal structure approximately 5 mm beneath the skin surface and approximately 4 mm in width. In the central portion of the tendon, there is a focal area of hypoechogenicity that persists with careful imaging (*arrow*). This is the classic location and appearance of a "jumper's knee" or tendinopathy of the proximal patellar tendon. (Reproduced with permission from Ma OJ, Mateer JR, Blaivas M. *Emergency Ultrasound*. 2nd ed. © 2008. New York, NY: McGraw-Hill.)

KEY FEATURES

Description

- Fibers in the middle one-third of the tendon breakdown, degenerate, swell, and thicken
- Pain common over the middle-central tendon
- Overload of eccentric quadriceps muscle action
- Typically lacks the presence of inflammatory cells: Described as tendonosis
  - Terms "tendonitis" or "tendinitis" incorrect
- Typically associated with tissue degeneration
  - Two types
    - Lipoid: Fatty tissue deposited in the tendon
    - Mucoid: Conversion of tendon in softer material with gray or brown appearance
  - Thickening of tendon
  - Neovascularization
  - Increased presence of varicose nerve fibers
    - Most likely source of pain

Essentials of Diagnosis

- Insidious onset
- Symptoms improve initially with movement/warm-up (e.g., increased temperature of tissue, decreases pain and increases elasticity)
- Diagnosis made by patient history and clinical examination
- Posture assessment
- Gait analysis
- Functional movement screening/task assessment
- Musculoskeletal ultrasound or MRI

General Considerations

- Address training errors and kinetic chain (biomechanical) deficits to prevent recurrence
- Poor blood supply limits healing after initial injury insult
- Corticosteroid injections increase risk for tendon degeneration and rupture
- Gender differences in tendon structural and mechanical properties[4]

Demographics

- Physically active individuals participating in running/jumping activities (or workers placed in a poor ergonomic environment for long periods)
- Insidious onset/chronic repetitive activities
- Gender and age correlate[4]

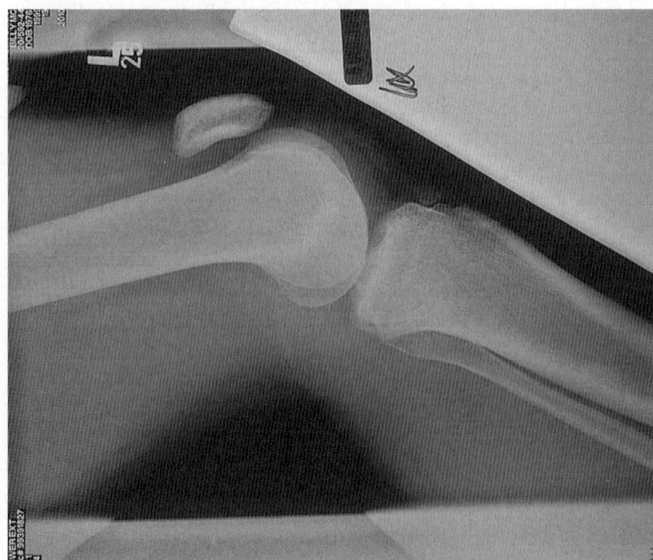

FIGURE 198-4 X-ray of a patella tendon rupture. (From Knoop K, Stack L, Storrow A, Thurman RJ. *Atlas of Emergency Medicine.* 3rd ed. © 2010. New York, NY: McGraw-Hill. Photo contributor: Cathleen M. Vossler, MD.)

CLINICAL FINDINGS

SIGNS AND SYMPTOMS

- No obvious deformity at patellofemoral joint
- Thickening of the tendon (with or without swelling/edema)
- Pain with palpation of the tendon
- Anterior knee pain during activity (increased during eccentric loading)
- Decreased knee flexion ROM
- Decreased knee extension strength (MMT)
- Muscular tightness of iliopsoas (Thomas test), rectus femoris (Ely test)
- Decreased strength of hip muscles (hip internal and external rotators)
- Possible muscular tightness throughout kinetic chain (e.g., Achilles tendon)

Functional Implications

- Inability to climb stairs or ladder
- Inability to push-off during ambulation
- Decreased stride length during ambulation
- Decreased squat depth

Possible Contributing Causes

- Intrinsic risk factors
  - Decreased quadriceps muscle length (passive knee flexion ROM)
  - Decreased eccentric quadriceps strength
  - Abnormal/excessive pronation/calcaneal varus and faster rate of maximum pronation
  - Obesity
  - Patella alta
  - Frog-eyed patella
  - Muscle imbalance along the kinetic chain (quadriceps/hamstrings, hip internal/external rotators, etc.)
  - Hyperlipidemia
  - Hypertension
  - Increased Q angle
- Extrinsic risk factors
  - Training errors
    - Sudden increase in mileage or intensity or incline
    - Increased magnitude of jumping/plyometric activities
    - Return too fast from inactivity
  - Environmental factors
    - High incidence with training in cold weather
  - Faulty equipment
    - Surface too hard
    - Shoes not supportive of foot type

Differential Diagnosis

- ACL instability
- Hoffa fat pad Impingement
- Medial synovial plica syndrome
- Bone spur
- Bursitis
- Chondromalacia patella
- L4 radiculopathy
- Meniscal injury
- Patellar-femoral tracking dysfunction
- Osgood–Schlatter disease
- Osteoarthritis
- Sinding–Larsen–Johansson disease

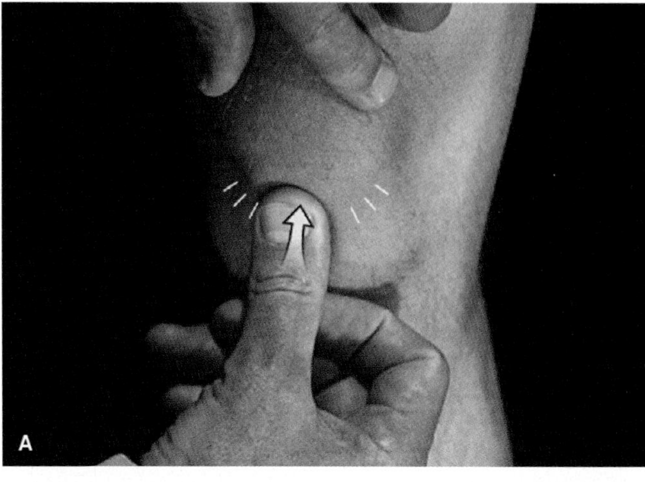

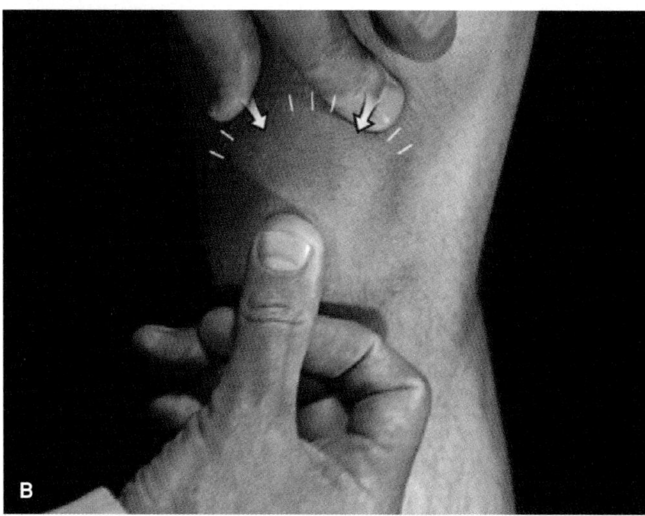

FIGURE 198-5 Patella test for swelling (Ballottement test). (From Lawry GV. *Systematic Musculoskeletal Examinations*. www.accessmedicine.com. Copyright © The McGraw-Hill Companies, Inc. All rights reserved.)

- Tendon partial tear
- Tendon rupture

MEANS OF CONFIRMATION OR DIAGNOSIS

Imaging

- Musculoskeletal ultrasound
- MRI
- X-ray

FINDINGS AND INTERPRETATIONS

- Hypertrophic tendon
- Hyperechoic mass at midtendon
- Irregular tendon structure

TREATMENT

Medication

- NSAIDs
- Prolotherapy: Sclerotic injection (most common dextrose)

MEDICAL PROCEDURES

- Platelet-rich plasma injections
- Tendon debridement
- Extracorpeal shock wave therapy (ESWT)

REFERRALS/ADMITTANCE

- To radiologist for imaging
- To orthopedist for injection

IMPAIRMENTS

- Pain with movement after prolonged immobility with the knee flexed (i.e., after sitting at a desk, driving, movies) that improves with activity
- Pain at beginning of exercise training session that improves with activity, may worsen after activity
- Pain with eccentric quadriceps loading (e.g., stair descending)
- Pain during loading response phase of gait (after initial contact)
- Possible early heel rise during terminal stance (if Achilles tendon tightness)

TESTS AND MEASURES

- Thomas test
- Ely test
- Modified Thomas test
- Ober test
- Anterior draw test
- Gait analysis
- Postural assessment
- Functional movement assessment (Squat)
- Decreased performance of:
  - Hopping
  - Jumping

INTERVENTION

- Eccentric loading (3× 10 to 15 reps; 1 to 2× daily)
  - Decrease pain
  - Improve function
  - Increase strength
  - Superior to concentric training
- Laser therapy
  - Decrease pain/tenderness
  - Decrease tenderness
  - Decrease stiffness
  - Decrease crepitus
- Iontophoresis
  - Decrease pain
  - Improve function
- Stretching
  - Patients with limited flexion
    - Reduce pain
    - Improve function and tissue elongation
- Foot orthoses
  - Reduce pain
  - Altered lower extremity kinematics
- Manual intervention
  - Cross friction fiber massage to tendon and surrounding tissues (chronic tendinosis)
  - Reduce pain
  - Improve mobility and function
- Patella tendon (Cho–Pat) strap
  - Decrease strain on tendon

FUNCTIONAL GOALS

- Patient will be able to
  - Demonstrate and maintain neutral calcaneal alignment with heel strike through toe-off phases of gait.
  - Perform ADLs without pain; especially after prolonged periods of sitting.
  - Stand and walk without limitation due to pain after sitting for >1 hour.
  - Score 5/5 manual muscle testing of quadriceps without limitation due to pain.
  - Squat with proper lower-extremity mechanics.
  - Restore normal biomechanics to prevent reoccurrence.
  - Demonstrate 50% speed running for 1 mile without limitation due to pain.
  - Perform functional assessment tasks (e.g., jogging/running, hopping, bounding, etc.) without pain.

PROGNOSIS

- Acute to subchronic
  - Good, nonsurgical.
  - Significant pain and impairment reduction.
  - Should be able to return pain free.

ADDITIONAL INFORMATION

- For more information, please review Case Study (6-1) on Access-Physiotherapy.com.

PATIENT RESOURCE

- Patellar Tendonitis. About.com. http://orthopedics.about.com/cs/patella disorders/a/patellartendon.htm. Accessed July 7, 2013.

REFERENCES

1. ICD9Data.com. http://www.icd9data.com. Accessed July 7, 2013.
2. ICD10Data.com. http://www.icd10data.com/ICD10CM/Codes. Accessed July 7, 2013.
3. American Physical Therapy Association. Pattern 4E: Impaired joint mobility, motor function, muscle performance, and range of motion associated with localized inflammation. In: *Guide to Physical Therapist Practice*. 2nd ed. Alexandria, VA: American Physical Therapy Association; 2001. Revised 2003.
4. Onambele GN, Burgess K, Pearson SJ. Gender-specific in vivo measurement of the structural properties of the human patella tendon. *J Orthop Res*. 2012;25(12):1635–1642.

ADDITIONAL REFERENCES

- Balasubramaniam P, Prathap K. The effect of injection of hydrocortisone into rabbit calcaneal tendons. *J Bone Joint Surg Br*. 1972;54(4):729–734.
- Diokno E. Appendix A. Introduction to bracing, splinting, and casting. In: Patel DR, Greydanus DE, Baker RJ, eds. *Pediatric Practice: Sports Medicine*. New York, NY: McGraw-Hill; 2009. http://www.accessphysiotherapy.com/content/6983252#6983256. Accessed July 7, 2013.
- Dutton M. Chapter 18. Adjunctive interventions. In: Dutton M, ed. *McGraw-Hill's NPTE (National Physical Therapy Examination).*

2nd ed. New York, NY: McGraw-Hill; 2012. http://www.accessphysiotherapy.com/content/5405918. Accessed July 7, 2013.

- Dutton M, ed. *Orthopaedic Examination, Evaluation, and Intervention*. 2nd ed. New York, NY: McGraw-Hill; 2008. http://www.accessphysiotherapy.com/content/55585614. Accessed July 7, 2013.
- Dutton M. Palpation. In: Dutton M, ed. *Dutton's Orthopedic Survival Guide: Managing Common Conditions*. New York, NY: McGraw-Hill. http://www.accessphysiotherapy.com/content/8655360. Accessed July 7, 2013.
- Hay WW, Levin MJ, Sondheimer JM, Deterding RR. Anterior knee pain. In: Hay WW, Levin MJ, Sondheimer JM, Deterding RR, eds. *CURRENT Diagnosis & Treatment: Pediatrics*. 20th ed. New York, NY: McGraw-Hill; 2011. http://www.accessphysiotherapy.com/content/6586302. Accessed July 7, 2013.
- James SL, Bates BT, Ostering LR. Injuries to runners. *Am J Sports Med*. 1978;6(2):40–50.
- Ohberg L, Alfredson H. Effects on neovascularisation behind the good results with eccentric training in chronic mid-portion Achilles tendinosis? *Knee Surg Sports Traumatol Arthrosc*. 2004;12(5):465–470.
- Prentice WE, Quillen WS, Underwood F, eds. *Therapeutic Modalities in Rehabilitation*. 4th ed. New York, NY: McGraw-Hill; 2011. http://www.accessphysiotherapy.com/content/8136922 . Accessed July 7, 2013.
- Rompe JD, Furia J, Maffulli N. Eccentric loading compared with shock wave therapy for chronic insertional Achilles tendinopathy. A randomized, controlled trial. *J Bone Joint Surg Am*. 2008;90(1):52–61.
- Woodley BL, Newsham-West RJ, Baxter GD. Chronic tendinopathy: effectiveness of eccentric exercise. *Br J Sports Med*. 2007;41(4):188–198.

199 PLICA SYNDROME

Patrick S. Pabian, DPT, PT, SCS, OCS, CSCS

CONDITION/DISORDER SYNONYMS

- Plica syndrome
- Pathologic plica/plicae
- Synovial plica/plicae syndrome

ICD-9-CM CODE

- 727.83 Plica syndrome

ICD-10-CM CODE

- M67.50 Plica syndrome, unspecified knee

PREFERRED PRACTICE PATTERN

- 4E: Impaired Joint Mobility, Motor Function, Muscle Performance, and Range of Motion Associated with Localized Inflammation

PATIENT PRESENTATION

A 20-year-old man presents with anteromedial knee pain that has progressively worsened in the past 3 months. The patient complains of popping and clicking medial to the patella when he flexes and extends his knee. The patient has pain with popping, clicking, and giving away when he ascends and descends stairs or performs squatting activities. Upon palpation, the patient has pain and tenderness in the medial patellofemoral joint, with notable thickened band of soft tissue in this region. The patient has negative McMurray, Apley, Thessaly, and Ege tests for meniscus pathology, and negative patellar apprehension and medial/lateral glides for patellar instability. Patellar bowstring and medial plica shelf tests are positive.

KEY FEATURES

Description

- Plica is a shelf, fold, or pleat in the synovial membrane in the knee
  - Result of incomplete or partial reabsorb during fetal development
  - Can be inferior, medial, or superior to the patella
  - Can vary in size (length or thickness) and clinical relevance
  - Can be thickened and inflamed, usually following acute or chronic trauma
- Medial plica extends from anteromedial aspect of the patella to the suprapatellar pouch
  - Is most implicated
- Suprapatellar plica separates the suprapatellar pouch from the knee joint
- Infrapatellar plica, also termed ligamentum mucosum, runs from the infrapatellar fat pad to the intercondylar notch

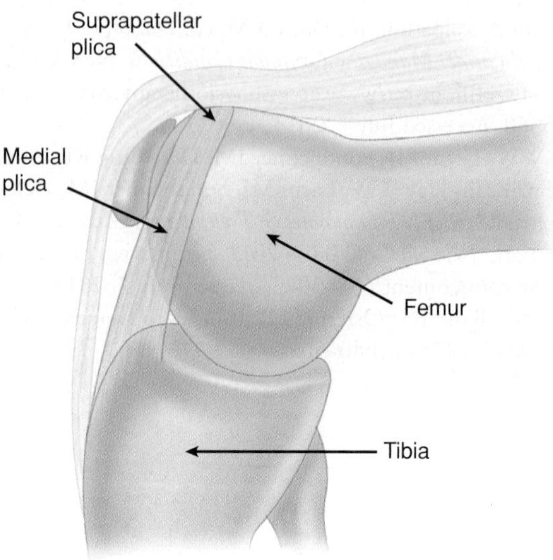

FIGURE 199-1 Plica anatomy. (From Patel DR, Greydanus DE, Baker RJ. *Pediatric Practice: Sports Medicine*. http://www.accesspediatrics.com. Copyright © The McGraw-Hill Companies, Inc. All rights reserved.)

Essentials of Diagnosis

- Diagnosed primarily through symptoms and exclusion of other knee pathologies
- Mechanism of injury can be from either chronic trauma or acute trauma
  - Chronic: Friction or rubbing over the femoral condyle
  - Acute: Pinching under the patella
- Found in concurrence with range of pathologies, both chronic and acute
  - Chronic: Chondromalacia or patellofemoral pain syndrome
  - Acute: ACL or meniscus pathologies or contusion
- Differential diagnosis from other knee pathologies that may warrant a more immediate surgical intervention is essential (meniscus tear)
- Combination of tests/cluster of findings has been reported to have the strongest diagnostic value in terms of sensitivity (1.0) for diagnosis of medial plica syndrome

General Considerations

- Plica are normal unless thickened or inelastic from acute or chronic inflammation.
- Plica syndrome signs and symptoms mimic other knee pathologies.
- Full history of symptoms, medical history screening, and differential knee orthopedic examination will ensure appropriate diagnosis.
- History of anterior knee pain, pain primarily over medial femoral condyle, visible or palpable plica, and exclusion of other anteromedial knee pain.

Demographics

- Plica syndrome most commonly involves the medial plica.[1]
- Presence of a plica has been reported to range from 10% to >50% in normal knees.

- Has been found with much greater frequency in patients who have anterior knee pain.[1]
- No delineation in incidence noted based on gender or age.
- Individuals with Japanese have the highest prevalence of synovial plica in the knee.

CLINICAL FINDINGS

SIGNS AND SYMPTOMS[2]

- Insidious onset of knee pain
- Pain or mechanical symptoms (clicking, catching, giving away) located in the anterior knee
- Symptoms elicited with flexed positions of the knee; transitioning between flexion and extension
- Pain and mechanical symptoms with stairs; squatting
- Tender to palpation over the plica; swelling in plica

Functional Implications

- Pain/Limitation with
  - Ascending or descending stairs
  - Sitting into or rising from chair
- Catching or buckling of knee with
  - Rising from seated positions
  - Walking community distances

Possible Contributing Causes

- Congenital
- Patellofemoral pain syndrome
- Chondromalacia patella (patellofemoral syndrome)
- Patella lateral tilt or tracking

Differential Diagnoses

- Differential diagnosis of common causes of knee pain
- Meniscus tear/pathology
- Septic arthritis
- Osteochondritis dissecans
- Prepatellar bursitis
- Patellofemoral pain syndrome
- Patellar hypermobility
- Patellar subluxation
- Synovitis
- Patellar tendonitis
- Rheumatic disorders
- Infection

MEANS OF CONFIRMATION OR DIAGNOSIS

Imaging

- Radiographs are usually normal.
- MRI will show increased fluid/edema isolated within the synovial plica.

Diagnostic Procedures

- Arthroscopy

FINDINGS AND INTERPRETATION

- MRI will help visualize other potential soft tissue sources of patient symptoms.

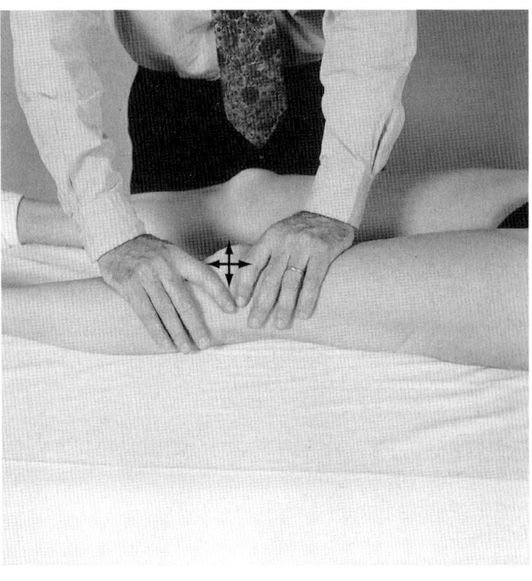

FIGURE 199-2 Patellar mobility testing. (From Dutton M. *Dutton's Orthopedic Survival Guide: Managing Common Conditions*. http://www.accessphysiotherapy.com.)

TREATMENT

Medication

- Non-steroidal anti-inflammatory drugs (NSAIDs)
- Corticosteroid injection
- Antibiotics, if infection confirmed

MEDICAL PROCEDURES

- Arthroscopic examination
  - Recommended if symptoms are chronic and conservative measures have failed
  - Resection of the pathologic plica may be required

REFERRALS/ADMITTANCE

- To radiologist for imaging: X-ray, MRI
- To primary care physician for aspiration and laboratory studies for suspected rheumatic disorder or infection
- To orthopedist for surgical consult for failed conservative treatment

IMPAIRMENTS

- Weakness, pain, or buckling of the knee with squatting down to perform dressing activities or household chores
- Weakness, pain, or buckling of the knee with rising from squat positions or ascending/descending stairs
- Muscle imbalances
  - Quadriceps weakness
  - Iliotibial band or rectus femoris tightness

TESTS AND MEASURES

- Special Tests[3]
  - Apley grind test
  - Hughston plica test
  - Holding test
  - Medial patellar plica syndrome test
  - Medial plica shelf test (Mital–Hayden test)

- Ober test
- Patellar bowstring test
- Patellar shutter test
- Plica shutter test
- Rotation valgus test

INTERVENTION

- Modification/avoidance of activities
  - Immobilization of the knee in extension for a few days, as needed
  - Repetitive flexion and extension
  - Prolonged periods of knee flexion
- Exercise
  - Quadriceps exercises with protection to patellofemoral joint
  - Isometrics; straight leg raises
  - Quadriceps and Iliotibial band flexibility
- Modalities
  - TENS for pain control
  - PRICE: Protection, Rest, Ice Compression, Elevation
  - Ultrasound

FUNCTIONAL GOALS

- Patient will be able to
  - Rise from squatting positions without pain or buckling of the knee (decreasing risk of fall).
  - Squat to don/doff shoes without pain, weakness, or buckling.
  - Ascend and descend stairs in a safe manner, without pain, weakness, or buckling of the knee.

PROGNOSIS

- Fair, depending on the underlying cause of the inflammation and the ability of the patient to
  - Control exacerbating activities.
  - Perform the optimal dosage of therapeutic exercise.
- Often associated with patellofemoral pain syndrome, which can be multifactorial in nature.
- When conservative treatment fails, surgical removal of the plica is usually successful.

PATIENT RESOURCE

- NIH, National Institute of Arthritis and Musculoskeletal and Skin Diseases. Plica Syndrome. http://www.niams.nih.gov/health_info/knee_problems. Accessed July 7, 2013.

REFERENCES

1. Phillips BB. Arthroscopy of the lower extremity. In: Canale ST, Beaty JH, eds. *Campbell's Operative Orthopaedics*. 11th ed. Philadelphia, PA: Mosby Elsevier; 2008:2811–2921.
2. Shetty VD, Vowler SL, Krishnamurthy S, Halliday AE. Clinical diagnosis of medial plica syndrome of the knee: a prospective study. *J Knee Surg*. 2007;20(4):277–280.
3. Stern B, Hegedus EJ, Driesner D. Physical examination tests for the knee. In: Cook CE, Hegedus EJ, eds. *Orthopaedic Physical Examination Tests: An Evidence-Based Approach*. 2nd ed. Boston, MA: Pearson Education; 2013:424–502.

ADDITIONAL REFERENCES

- Al-Hadithy N, Gikas P, Mahapatra AM, Dowd G. Review article: plica syndrome of the knee. *J Orthop Surg (Hong Kong)*. 2011;19(3):354–358.
- Dutton M. Anatomy. In: Dutton M, ed. *Orthopaedic Examination, Evaluation, and Intervention*. 2nd ed. New York, NY: McGraw-Hill; 2008. http://www.accessphysiotherapy.com/content/55582319. Accessed July 7, 2013.
- Dutton M. Special tests for specific diagnoses. In: Dutton M, ed. *Dutton's Orthopedic Survival Guide: Managing Common Conditions*. New York, NY: McGraw-Hill; 2011. http://www.accessphysiotherapy.com/content/8654857. Accessed July 7, 2013.
- Jee WH, Choe BY, Kim JM, Song HH, Choi KH. The plica syndrome: diagnostic value of MRI with arthroscopic correlation. *J Comput Assist Tomogr*. 1998;22(5):814–818.
- Ogata S, Uhthoff HK. The development of synovial plica in human knee joints: An embryologic study. *Arthroscopy*. 1990;6:315–321.
- Standring S. Knee. In: Standring S, ed. *Gray's Anatomy: The Anatomical Basis of Clinical Practice*. 40th ed. Spain: Churchill Livingstone Elsevier; 2008:1393–1410.
- Zanoli S, Piazzai E. The synovial plica syndrome of the knee. Pathology, differential diagnosis and treatment. *Ital J Orthop Traumatol*. 1983;9:241–250.

200 TIBIALIS ANTERIOR TENDINITIS

Dennis Hunt, EdD, CSCS
Eric Shamus, PhD, DPT, PT, CSCS

CONDITION/DISORDER SYNONYMS

- Anterior lateral tibial periostitis
- Anterior lateral tibial stress syndrome
- Anterior lateral stress fracture
- Anterior shin splints
- Anterior tibialis tendonitis

ICD-9-CM CODE[1]

- 844.9 Sprains and strains of unspecified site of knee and leg

ICD-10-CM CODE[2]

- S86.919A Strain of unspecified muscle(s) and tendon(s) at lower leg level, unspecified leg, initial encounter

PREFERRED PRACTICE PATTERN[3]

- 4E: Impaired Joint Mobility, Motor Function, Muscle Performance, and Range of Motion Associated with Localized Inflammation

PATIENT PRESENTATION

A 23-year-old man presents with bilateral anterior shin pain. He indicates that 3 weeks earlier he began an exercise program that involves jogging 3 miles per day. The patient also indicates that his new exercise program increased his activity level considerably from the past year, with a lot more jogging. The patient has been wearing a pair of old sneakers while jogging. The pain starts about mile 2 and he has to stop running. The X-ray was negative for a stress fracture.

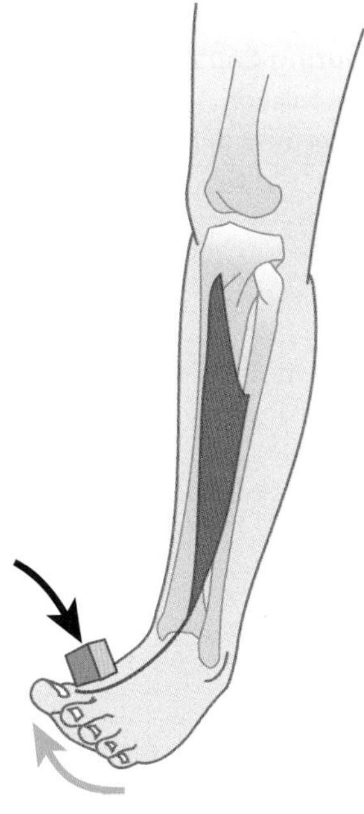

FIGURE 200-1 Tibialis anterior (L4, 5; deep peroneal nerve). The foot is dorsiflexed and inverted against resistance applied by gripping the foot with the examiner's hand. (From Waxman SG. *Clinical Neuroanatomy*. 26th ed. http://www.accessmedicine.com. Copyright © The McGraw-Hill Companies, Inc. All rights reserved.)

KEY FEATURES

Description

- Lower anterior lateral leg pain provoked by activity
- Pain is localized in the anterior lateral aspects of the tibia
- Produced by stress or traction that causes microtrauma to the soleus muscle at the origin point of the shinbone
- Stress-reaction inflammation of the periosteal and musculotendinous fascial junctions
- Results from repeated activity without proper conditioning or allowing enough recovery time between activities
- Attributed to muscles of the lower extremities being overloaded or by biomechanical irregularities
- Recurring dull ache along the anterior lateral aspect of the upper tibia

Essentials of Diagnosis

- Diagnosis usually made by clinical examination
- Pain increases with active dorsiflexion and when the anterior tibialis muscle stretched into plantarflexion
- Muscle length and strength imbalances, especially a tight gastrocnemius-soleus muscle group
- Common to see compartment syndrome associated with shin splints

General Considerations

- Pain with repetitive activity, when the involved musculotendinous unit is stretched

Demographics

- Athletes who increase activity intensity and/or duration along with a lack of appropriate recovery between workouts
- Beginning runners with poor lower-extremity muscle control

CLINICAL FINDINGS

SIGNS AND SYMPTOMS

- Tightness in gastrocnemius, soleus, and plantar muscles
- Pain: Mild to severe with weight-bearing activities and gait

- Described as a dull ache to lower extremities
- Point tenderness to tibia at anterior lateral aspect
- Possible localized swelling
- Muscle guarding with passive movement

Functional Implications

- Pain with standing or during activity
- Inability of injured lower extremity to bear weight
- Pain with closed chain ankle movements (i.e., driving)

Possible Contributing Causes

- Impaired standing balance
- History of high/repetitive impact activities
- Trauma
- Leg length inequality
- Improper footwear
- Chronic ankle injuries
- Overtraining
- Muscle imbalance with ankle dorsiflexors and plantarflexors
  - Tight or strong ankle plantarflexors overpowering the dorsiflexors
- Supinators with decreased shock absorption

Differential Diagnosis

- Achilles tendonitis
- Ankle sprain
- Cellulitis
- Compartment syndrome
- Deep vein thrombosis (DVT): Homan sign
- Entrapment of superficial peroneal nerve
- Fascial hernias
- Fibular dislocation
- Infective or varicose periostitis
- Lateral collateral ligament sprain
- Lateral meniscus tear
- Peripheral vascular injuries
- Popliteal artery entrapment syndromes
- Spinal stenosis
- Tenosynovitis
- Tumor
- Vascular disease

MEANS OF CONFIRMATION OR DIAGNOSIS

Imaging

- X-ray for fracture, often limited view
- Computed tomography (CT) scan for detailed imaging
- Bone scan if stress fracture is suspected
- MRI
- MRA
- Arteriograms

Diagnostic Procedures

- Compartmental pressure measurements
- Palpation of pulses in the foot
- Capillary refill

TREATMENT

- Medication: NSAID for pain management
- Walking boot

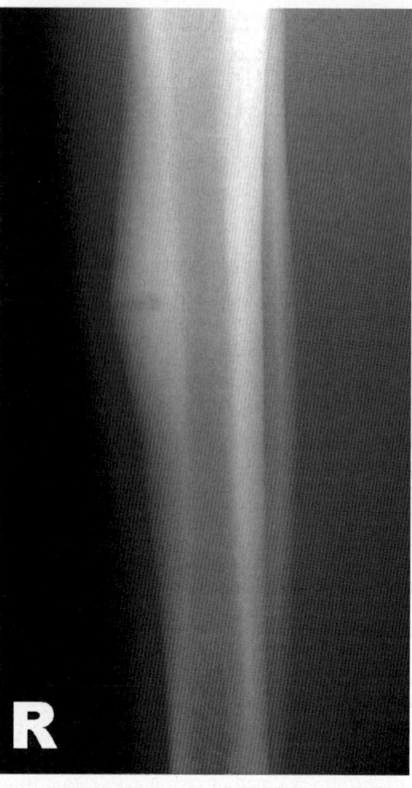

FIGURE 200-2 Dreaded black line at the anterior medial aspect of the tibia. (From South-Paul JE, Matheny SC, Lewis EL. *Current Diagnosis & Treatment in Family Medicine*. 3rd ed. http://www.accessmedicine.com. Copyright © The McGraw-Hill Companies, Inc. All rights reserved.)

FINDINGS AND INTERPRETATION

- Algorithm approach
  - Normal vascular examination
  - Normal neurological examination
  - Normal imaging
  - Palpable tenderness to anterior tibia
  - Occasional localized swelling anterior lateral lower leg
  - Hop-to-gait sequence/decreased stance time on injured lower extremity secondary to pain

REFERRALS/ADMITTANCE

- For imaging: X-ray or computed tomography (CT)
- For orthopedic consult: If no improvement in
  - Rule out stress fracture
    - Surgical intervention: posterior fasciotomy
    - Immobilization with casting or splinting of the lower leg in severe cases

IMPAIRMENTS

- Antalgic gait secondary to pain, which causes an inability to push-off during gait
- Inability to ambulate long distances secondary to pain and/or likelihood of decreased weight-bearing status that makes ambulating a taxing activity
- Decreased stance time on the involved lower extremity during ambulation
- Inability to stand for long periods of time secondary to pain

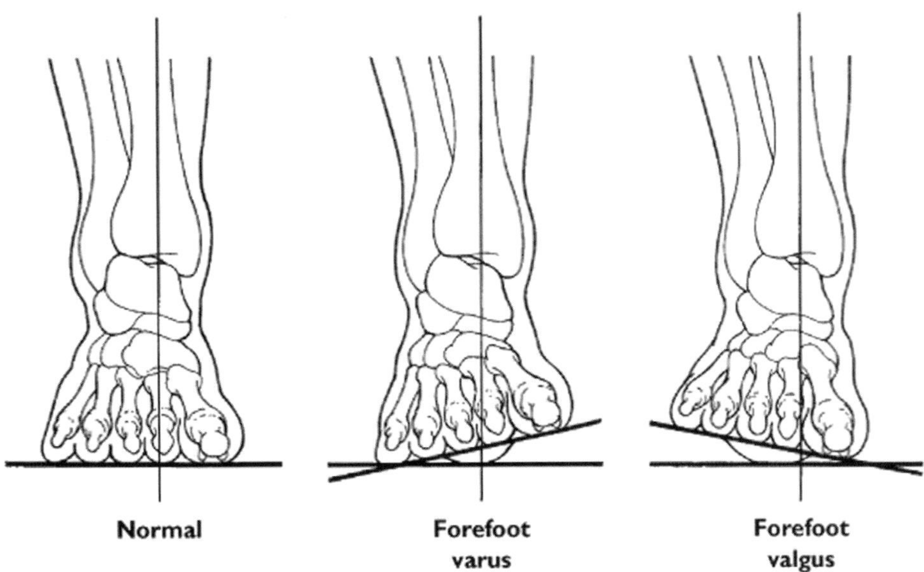

FIGURE 200-3 Varus and valgus conditions of the forefoot. (From Hall SJ. *Basic Biomechanics*. 5th ed. http://www.accessmedicine.com. Copyright © The McGraw-Hill Companies, Inc. All rights reserved.)

TESTS AND MEASURES

- Shin palpation test and shin edema test[4]
  - When both positive likelihood ratio of 7.94, eight times more likely to develop shin splints
  - When both negative likelihood ration <.001, extremely unlikely to develop shin splints
- Navicular drop test
- Compartment syndrome pressure assessment
- Pain, visual analog scale (VAS)
  - 24-hour pain
  - Worst average pain
  - Best average pain
- Functional independence measure
  - Locomotion

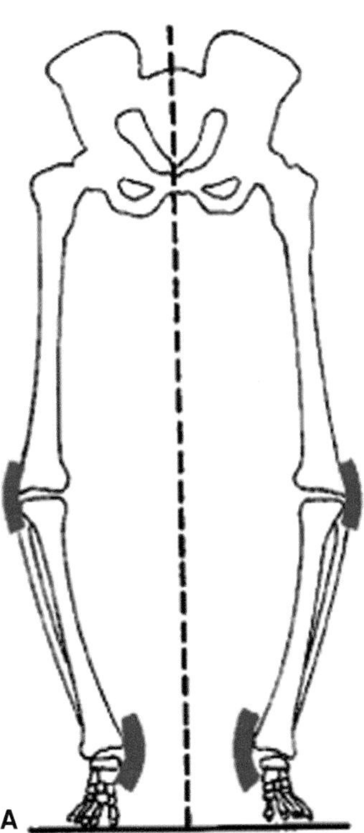

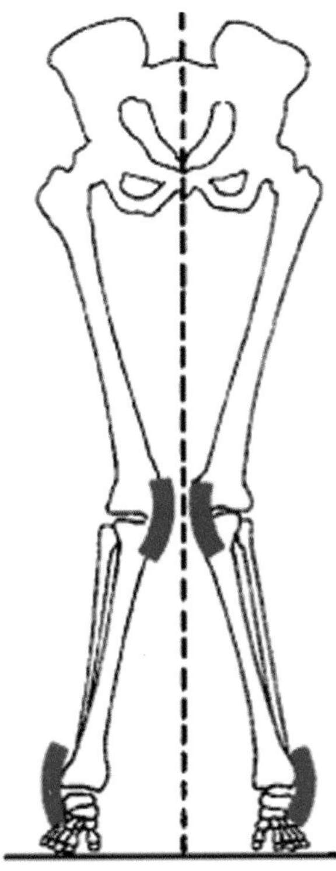

FIGURE 200-4 Areas of strain are highlighted. (**A**) Femoral valgus and tibial varus. (**B**) Femoral varus and tibial valgus. (From Hall SJ. *Basic Biomechanics*. 5th ed. http://www.accessmedicine.com. Copyright © The McGraw-Hill Companies, Inc. All rights reserved.)

TABLE 200-1 The Clinical Characteristics and Imaging Features of Common Causes of Shin Pain in Athletes

Site	Pain	Effect of Exercise	Associated Features	Tenderness	Investigations
Bone stress reaction or stress fracture	Localized, acute or sharp Subcutaneous medial tibial surface or fibula	Constant or increasing Worse with impact	Exacerbated by vibration (tuning fork) and ultrasound	Subcutaneous medial tibial surface or fibula	X-ray may be negative Use magnified views Look for callous or periosteal reaction MRI can stage severity and define prognosis, but is nonspecific
Medial tibial periostitis	Diffuse pain on posterior medial border of tibia; variable intensity	Decreases as athlete warms up and stretches	Worse in the morning and after exercise Pes planus	Posterior medial edge of tibia at muscular insertions	X-rays negative Bone scan shows diffuse uptake MRI shows diffuse edema and periosteal thickening
Chronic exertional compartment syndrome	No pain at rest; ache, tightness, gradually building with exertion	Specific onset variable between athletes, usually 10–15 min into exercise Decreases with rest	Occasional muscle weakness or dysfunction with exercise. Paresthesia of nerve in affected compartment is possible	None at rest Antero and lateral more common with exertion Occasionally related to palpable muscle herniation (superficial peroneal nerve)	X-rays negative Bone scans negative Exertional compartment pressure testing is diagnostic Exertional MRI assessment may also be diagnostic
Popliteal artery entrapment	Pain in calf with exertion not anterolateral "Atypical compartment syndrome"	Worse with exertion, especially active ankle plantarflexion	Pulses may be diminished with palpation or Doppler ultrasound with active plantarflexion	Rarely in proximal calf	X-rays negative MRI may reveal hypertrophic or abnormal insertion of medial gastrocnemius MRA (arteriography) with provocative maneuvers is diagnostic
Muscle–tendon injuries Strains Tendinopathy	Pain at pathologic site with resisted stretch	Pre-exercise stretching usually helps	Good response to NSAIDs and ice	Pain can be at muscle belly, muscle–tendon junction, tendon, or tendon insertion	Rarely required X-rays usually negative MRI gives best view of soft-tissue pathology

Source: From Brukner P, Khan K, Bradshaw C, Hislop M, Hutchinson M. Shin pain. In: Brukner P, Khan K, eds. *Clinical Sports Medicine*. 3rd ed. New York, NY: McGraw Hill Professional; 2007:557.

- Cardiovascular integrity
  - Blood pressure at rest and after activity
  - Heart rate at rest and after activity
- Skin Integrity
  - Associated skin assessment
    - Edema (linear girth measurements, palpation)
    - Color
    - Temperature
- Neurologic Examination
  - Sensation
    - Light touch
    - Pin prick
  - Lower-extremity deep tendon reflexes
  - Proprioception at the hip, knee, and ankle
  - Kinesthetic awareness
  - Coordination
- Trunk active and passive ROM
- Hip, knee, ankle active and passive ROM
- Flexibility testing
  - Gastrocnemius
  - Soleus
  - Hamstrings
  - Iliopsoas
  - Quadriceps
  - Iliotibial band
  - Abductors
  - Adductors
- Joint integrity of the spine
- Sacroiliac joint integrity
- Hip joint integrity
  - Flexion abduction external rotation (FABER) test
- Limb strength

- Manual muscle test (MMT)
  - Anterior tibialis
  - Posterior tibialis
  - Hamstrings
  - Quadriceps
  - Iliopsoas
  - Gluteus maximus
  - Gluteus medius
  - Gluteus minimus
  - Adductors
- LE contralateral limb strength
- Balance
  - Static single-leg standing (eyes open, eyes closed)
    - Contralateral LE
  - Dynamic standing
    - Berg balance scale
    - Functional gait assessment
- Gait assessment
  - Observational analysis
  - Gait speed via the 10-m walk test
  - Two-minute walk test
  - Six-minute walk test
  - Retro running

INTERVENTION

- Prevention: Proper footwear
- Rest
- Muscle stretching and strengthening
- Taping
  - Decrease strain on anterior tibialis tendon
- Correction of biomechanical defects
- Orthotics: Provide proper arch support with neutral subtalar positioning in order to avoid stressing injured structures
- Address swelling
  - Ice/Cryotherapy
- Address pain
- Laser therapy
- Address mobilization of fibular head
- Address lack of flexibility via stretching
- Address weakness via strengthening activities

FUNCTIONAL GOALS

- The patient will be able to
  - Ambulate pain-free for >30 minutes.
  - Return to high-impact activity such as running, hiking, and dancing.
  - Demonstrate and maintain neutral calcaneal alignment with heel strike through toe-off phases of gait.
  - Demonstrate 15 degrees of talocrural dorsiflexion during push-off phase of gait.
  - Stand and walk without limitation due to pain after sitting for >1 hour.
  - Demonstrate 5/5 manual muscle testing of involved gastrocnemius without limitation due to pain.
  - Demonstrate 50% speed running for one mile without limitation due to pain.
  - Demonstrate single-leg hopping on involved side without limitation due to pain.

PROGNOSIS

- In most cases, the patient resumes normal functioning and returns to previous workout regimen within 2 weeks to 3 months.

PATIENT RESOURCES

- Shin Splints. MedlinePlus, NIH National Institutes of Health. http://www.nlm.nih.gov/medlineplus/ency/article/003177.htm. Accessed August 9, 2014.

REFERENCES

1. ICD-9-CM. http://www.icd9data.com. Accessed January 29, 2013.
2. ICD-10-CM. http://www.icd10data.com. Accessed January 29, 2013.
3. The American Physical Therapy Association. *Guide to Physical Therapist Practice*. Alexandria, VA: The American Physical Therapy Association; 2003. http://guidetoptpractice.apta.org/. Accessed January 29, 2013.
4. Newman P, Adams R, Waddington G. Two simple tests for predicting onset of medial tibial stress syndrome: shin palpation test and shin edema test. *Br J Sports Med*. 2012;46(12):861–864.

ADDITIONAL REFERENCES

- Carr K, Stevetson E, Aukerman D. How can you help athletes prevent and treat shin splints? *J Family Pract*. 2008;57(6): 406–408.
- Hall SJ. Chapter 8. The biomechanics of the human lower extremity. In: Hall SJ, ed. *Basic Biomechanics*. 5th ed. New York, NY: McGraw-Hill; 2007. http://www.accessphysiotherapy.com/content/6062676. Accessed August 9, 2014.
- Hamilton N, Weimar W, Luttgens K. The leg. In: Hamilton N, Weimar W, Luttgens K, eds. *Kinesiology: Scientific Basis of Human Motion*. New York, NY: McGraw-Hill; 2008. http://www.accessphysiotherapy.com/content/6153064. Accessed August 9, 2014.
- Houglum PA. *Therapeutic Exercise for Musculoskeletal Injuries*. 2nd ed. Champaign, IL: Human Kinetics; 2005.
- Kisner C, Colby LA. *Therapeutic Exercise: Foundations and Techniques*. 5th ed. Philadelphia, PA: F.A. Davis Company; 2007.
- Patel DR, Lyne ED. Chapter 29. Overuse injuries of the leg, ankle, and foot. In: Patel DR, Greydanus DE, Baker RJ, eds. *Pediatric Practice: Sports Medicine*. New York, NY: McGraw-Hill; 2009. http://www.accessphysiotherapy.com/content/6980676. Accessed August 9, 2014.
- Shin Splints. Orthogate. http://www.orthogate.org/patient-education/ankle/shin-splints.html. Accessed March 15, 2013.
- Simon RR, Sherman SC. Leg soft-tissue injury. In: Simon RR, Sherman SC, eds. *Emergency Orthopedics*. 6th ed. New York, NY: McGraw-Hill; 2011. http://www.accessphysiotherapy.com/content/7708294. Accessed August 9, 2014.

201 TIBIALIS POSTERIOR TENDINITIS

Eric Shamus, PhD, DPT, PT, CSCS
Christina Machuca, DPT, CSCS

CONDITION/DISORDER SYNONYMS

- Medial shin splints
- Tibialis posterior tendonitis

ICD-9-CM CODE[1]

- 844.9 Sprains and strains of unspecified site of knee and leg

ICD-10-CM CODE[2]

- S86.919A Strain of unspecified muscle(s) and tendon(s) at lower leg level, unspecified leg, initial encounter

PREFERRED PRACTICE PATTERN[3]

- 4E: Impaired Joint Mobility, Motor Function, Muscle Performance, and Range of Motion Associated with Localized Inflammation

PATIENT PRESENTATION

A 16-year-old girl presents with right medial shin pain. She indicates that she began running cross country 6 weeks ago on the side walk around her school. The patient is wearing soft flexible sneakers. She complains that it is a little sore when she starts running. She feels fine through the middle of the run and really bothers her when she is done running. The X-ray was negative for a stress fracture. She is a late midstance pronator with a forefoot varus and weak hip external rotators.

KEY FEATURES

Description

- Lower medial leg pain from an overuse activity
- Pain is localized in the posterior medial aspects of the tibia
- Attributed to muscles of the lower extremities being overloaded or by biomechanical irregularities
- Recurring dull ache along the posterior medial aspect of the lower tibia

Essentials of Diagnosis

- Diagnosis is usually made by clinical examination
- Pain increases with active plantar flexion and when the tibialis posterior muscle is stretched into dorsiflexion
- Muscle length and strength imbalances, especially a tight gastrocnemius–soleus muscle group

General Considerations

- Tendinopathy
- Periostitis

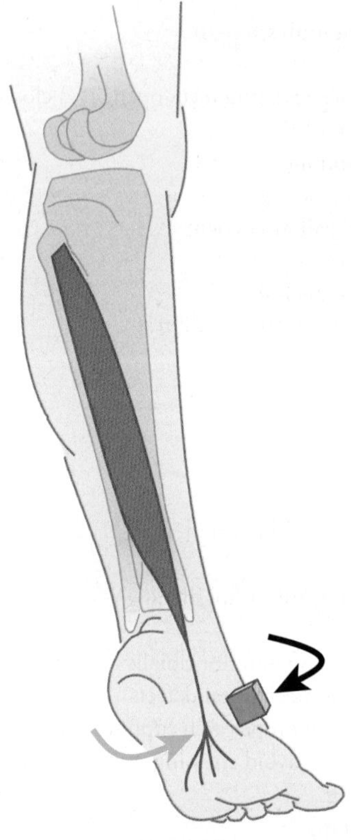

FIGURE 201-1 Tibialis posterior (L5, S1; tibial nerve). The plantar-flexed foot is inverted against resistance applied by gripping the foot with the examiner's hand. (From Waxman SG. *Clinical Neuroanatomy*. 26th ed. http://www.accessmedicine.com. Copyright © The McGraw-Hill Companies, Inc. All rights reserved.)

- Dysfunction of the tibialis posterior and soleus muscles
- Results from repeated activity without proper conditioning or allowing enough recovery time between activities
- Pain with repetitive activity, when the involved musculotendinous unit is stretched

Demographics

- Beginning runners with poor lower-extremity muscle control; increased pronation

CLINICAL FINDINGS

SIGNS AND SYMPTOMS

- Tightness in gastrocnemius, soleus, and plantar muscles
- Pain: Mild to severe with weight-bearing activities and gait
- Described as a dull ache to the lower extremities
- Point tenderness to the tibia at posterior medial aspect
- Muscle guarding with passive movement

Functional Implications

- Pain with standing or during activity
- Inability of injured lower extremity to fully weight bear
- Pain with closed chain ankle movements (i.e., driving)

Possible Contributing Causes

- Impaired standing balance
- Excessive pronation
- Flat feet
- Barefoot walking
- Running on uneven surfaces
- Running in worn out shoes or shoes that do not fit properly
- Running/standing on a hard surface shoes
- Leg length inequality
- Compensation from an injury on the opposite limb
- History of high/repetitive impact activities
- Overtraining
- Muscle imbalance with ankle dorsiflexors and plantar flexors
  - Tight or strong ankle plantar flexors overpowering the dorsiflexors

Differential Diagnosis

- Medial tibial stress syndrome[4]
- Fracture of the tibia or fibula
- Contusion
- Gastrocnemius–soleus muscle strain
- Delayed onset muscle soreness
- Cellulitis
- Nocturnal leg cramps
- Referred pain from sciatic nerve, spinal stenosis, or Baker cyst
- Deep vein thrombosis (DVT): Homan test
- Superficial thrombophlebitis
- Peripheral arterial disease
- Venous insufficiency
- Myofascial pain
- Fibromyalgia
- Popliteal artery entrapment
- Soft-tissue tumor or bony metastasis
- Osteomyelitis

MEANS OF CONFIRMATION OR DIAGNOSIS

Imaging

- X-ray for fracture, often limited view
- Triple-phase bone scintigraphy
- Computed tomography (CT) scan for detailed imaging
- Bone scan if stress fracture is suspected
- MRI/MRA

Diagnostic Procedures

- Palpation of pulses in the foot
- Capillary refill

TREATMENT

- Medication: NSAIDs for pain management
- Walking boot

FINDINGS AND INTERPRETATION

- Algorithm approach
  - Normal vascular examination

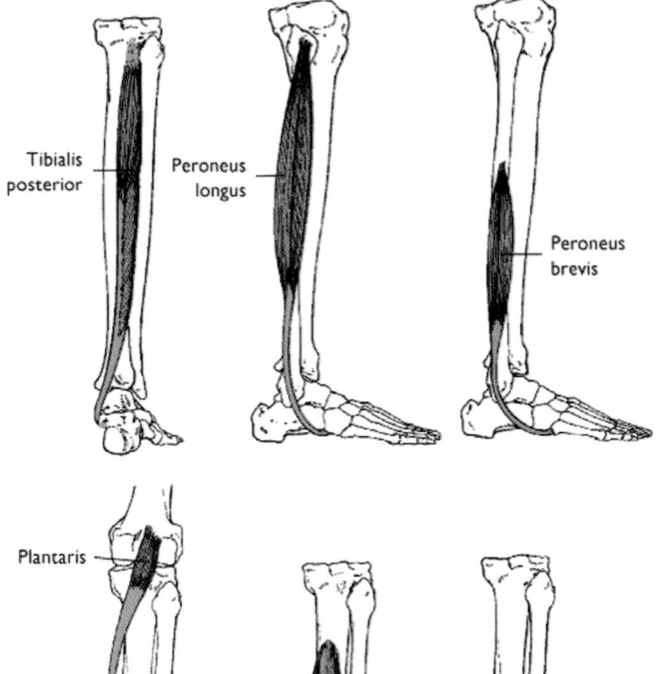

FIGURE 201-2 Muscles with tendons passing posterior to the malleoli assist with plantar flexion of the ankle. (From Hall SJ. *Basic Biomechanics*. 5th ed. http://www.accessmedicine.com. Copyright © The McGraw-Hill Companies, Inc. All rights reserved.)

  - Normal neurological examination
  - Normal imaging
  - Palpable tenderness to posterior medial tibia
  - Occasional localized swelling posterior medial lower leg
  - Hop-to-gait sequence/decreased stance time on injured lower-extremity secondary to pain
  - Commonly associated with biomechanical abnormalities:
    - Genu varus or genu valgus
    - Tibial torsion
    - Femoral anteversion
    - Foot arch abnormalities
    - Leg-length discrepancy

REFERRALS/ADMITTANCE

- For imaging: X-ray or computed tomography (CT)
- For orthopedic consult: If no improvement in
  - Rule out stress fracture
  - Immobilization, splinting of the lower leg in severe cases

IMPAIRMENTS

- Antalgic gait secondary to pain
- Inability to ambulate long distances secondary to pain and/or likelihood of decreased weight bearing status that makes ambulating a taxing activity

TESTS AND MEASURES

- Shin palpation test and shin edema test[4]
  - When both positive likelihood ratio of 7.94, eight times more likely to develop stress fractures
  - When both negative likelihood ration <.001, extremely unlikely to develop stress fractures
- Navicular drop test
- Pain, visual analog scale (VAS)
  - 24-hour pain
  - Worst average pain
  - Best average pain
- Functional independence measure
  - Locomotion
- Skin Integrity
  - Associated skin assessment
    - Edema (linear girth measurements, palpation)
    - Color
    - Temperature
- Neurologic examination
  - Sensation
    - Light touch
    - Pin prick
  - Lower extremity deep tendon reflexes
  - Proprioception at the hip, knee, and ankle
  - Kinesthetic awareness
  - Coordination
- Trunk active and passive ROM
- Hip, knee, ankle active and passive ROM
- Flexibility testing
  - Gastrocnemius
  - Soleus
  - Hamstrings
  - Iliopsoas
  - Quadriceps
  - Iliotibial band
  - Abductors
  - Adductors
- Joint integrity of the spine
- Sacroiliac joint integrity
- Hip joint integrity
  - Flexion abduction external rotation (FABER) test
- Limb strength
  - Manual muscle test (MMT)
    - Anterior Tibialis
    - Posterior Tibialis
    - Hamstrings
    - Quadriceps
    - Iliopsoas
    - Gluteus maximus
    - Gluteus medius
    - Gluteus minimus
    - Adductors
- LE contralateral limb strength

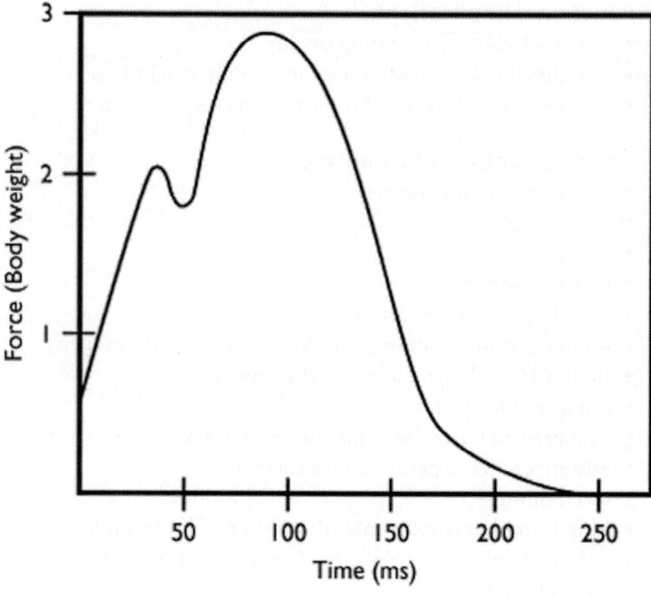

FIGURE 201-3 Vertical ground reaction force during running with an initial impact peak followed almost immediately by a propulsive peak. (From Hall SJ. *Basic Biomechanics*. 5th ed. http://www.accessmedicine.com. Copyright © The McGraw-Hill Companies, Inc. All rights reserved.)

- Balance
  - Static single-leg standing (eyes open, eyes closed)
    - Contralateral LE
  - Dynamic standing
    - Berg Balance Scale
    - Functional gait assessment
- Gait assessment
  - Observational analysis
  - Gait speed via the 10-m walk test
  - Two-minute walk test
  - Six-minute walk test
  - Retro running

INTERVENTION

- Rest
- Ultrasound (depending on age)
- Massage
- Muscle stretching and strengthening
- Taping
  - Decrease strain on tibialis posterior tendon
  - Arch taping
- Correction of biomechanical defects
- Orthotics: Provide proper arch support with neutral subtalar positioning in order to avoid stressing injured structures
- Address swelling
  - Ice/cryotherapy
- Address pain
- Laser therapy
- Address mobilization of the fibular head
- Address lack of flexibility via stretching
- Address weakness via strengthening activities
- Appropriate shoes for high-impact activities

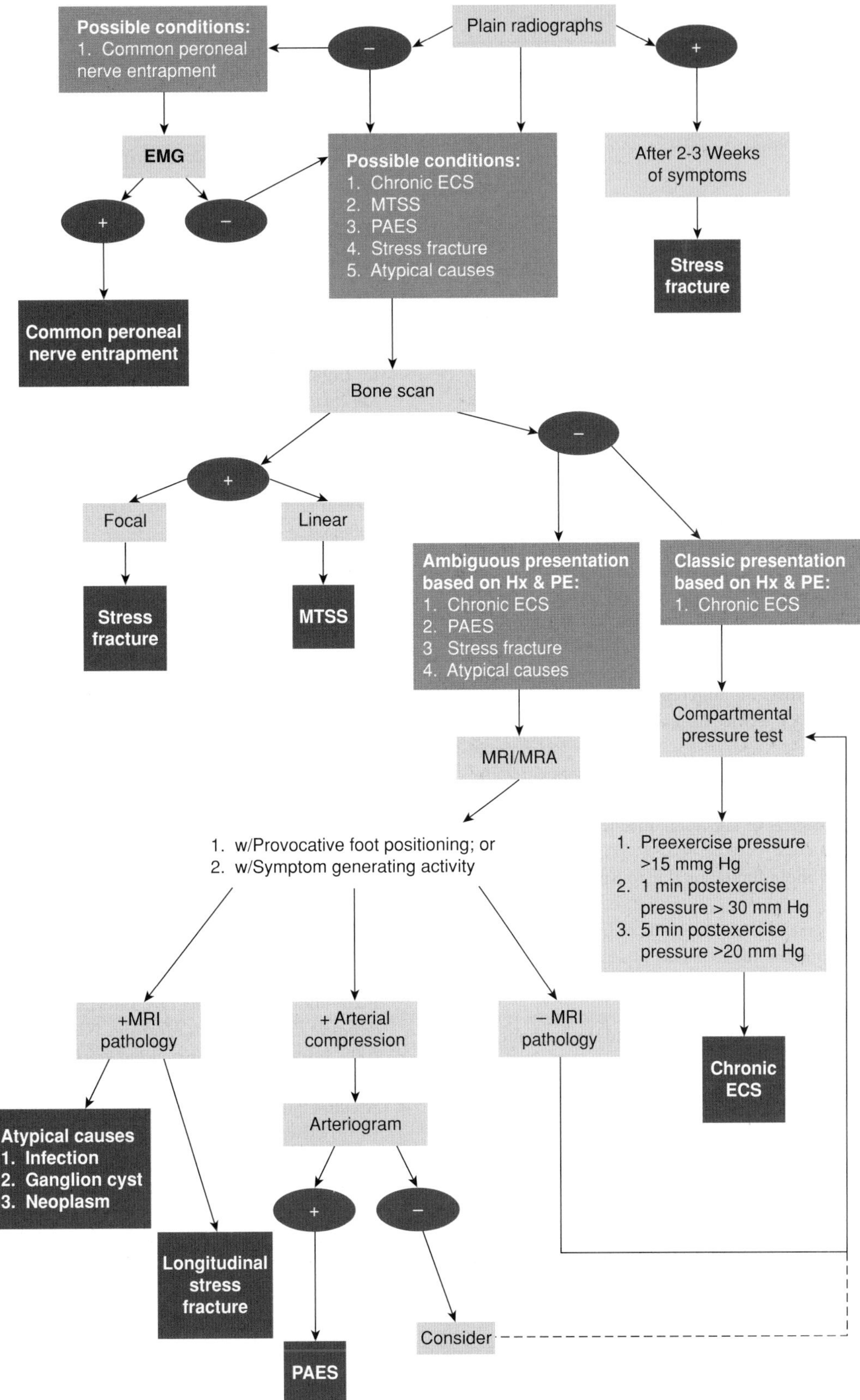

FIGURE 201-4 Diagnostic studies algorithm for chronic leg pain. (Adapted and redrawn from Edwards PH, Wright ML, Hartman JF. A practical approach to differential diagnosis of chronic leg pain in the athlete. *Am J Sport Med*. 2005;33(8):1241–1249.)

TABLE 201-1 Causes of Chronic Leg Pain in Young Athletes

Relatively More Common
Medial tibial stress syndrome
Chronic exertional compartment syndrome
Stress fractures of tibia or fibula
Achilles tendonitis
Muscle strains
Relatively Less Common
Metabolic bone disease
Referred pain from spine, hip, or knee
Rare
Popliteal artery entrapment syndrome
Peripheral entrapment neuropathies
Bone and muscle neoplasms
Osteomyelitis

Source: From Patel DR, Greydanus DE, Baker RJ: Pediatric Practice: Sports Medicine. http://www.accesspediatrics.com.

FUNCTIONAL GOALS

- The patient will be able to
  - Ambulate pain-free for >30 minutes.
  - Return to high-impact activity such as running, hiking, and dancing.
  - Demonstrate and maintain neutral calcaneal alignment with heel strike through toe-off phases of gait.
  - Demonstrate 15 degrees of talocrural dorsiflexion during push-off phase of gait.
  - Stand and walk without limitation due to pain after sitting for >1 hour.
  - Demonstrate 5/5 manual muscle testing of involved gastrocnemius without limitation due to pain.
  - Demonstrate 50% speed running for 1 mile without limitation due to pain.
  - Demonstrate single-leg hopping on involved side without limitation due to pain.

PROGNOSIS

- In most cases, the patient resumes normal functioning and returns to previous workout regimen within 2 weeks to 3 months.

PATIENT RESOURCE

- Shin Splints. *Orthogate*. http://www.orthogate.org/patient-education/ankle/shin-splints.html. Accessed June 15, 2013.

REFERENCES

1. ICD-9-CM. http://www.icd9data.com. Accessed June 29, 2013.
2. ICD-10-CM. http://www.icd10data.com. Accessed June 29, 2013.
3. The American Physical Therapy Association. *Guide to Physical Therapist Practice*. Alexandria, VA: The American Physical Therapy Association; 2003. http://guidetoptpractice.apta.org/. Accessed January 29, 2013.
4. Newman P, Adams R, Waddington G. Two simple tests for predicting onset of medial tibial stress syndrome: shin palpation test and shin edema test. *Br J Sports Med*. 2012;46(12):861–864.

ADDITIONAL REFERENCES

- Brown CR Jr. Chapter 62. Common injuries from running. In: Imboden JB, Hellmann DB, Stone JH, eds. *CURRENT Rheumatology Diagnosis & Treatment*. 2nd ed. New York, NY: McGraw-Hill; 2007. http://www.accessmedicine.com/content.aspx?aID=2729862. Accessed June 15, 2013.
- Carr K, Stevetson E, Aukerman D. How can you help athletes prevent and treat shin splints? *Journal of Family Practice*. 2008;57(6):406–408.
- Galbraith RM, Lavallee ME. Medial tibial stress syndrome: conservative treatment options. *Curr Rev Musculoskeletal Med*. 2009;2(3):127–133.
- Hall SJ. Chapter 8. The biomechanics of the human lower extremity. In: Hall SJ, ed. *Basic Biomechanics*. 5th ed. New York, NY: McGraw-Hill; 2007. http://www.accessphysiotherapy.com/content/6062676. Accessed June 29, 2013.
- Hamilton N, Weimar W, Luttgens K. The leg. In: Hamilton N, Weimar W, Luttgens K, eds. *Kinesiology: Scientific Basis of Human Motion*. New York, NY: McGraw-Hill; 2008. http://www.accessphysiotherapy.com/content/6153064. Accessed June 29, 2013.
- Houglum PA. *Therapeutic Exercise for Musculoskeletal Injuries*. 2nd ed. Champaign, IL: Human Kinetics; 2005.
- Kisner C, Colby LA. *Therapeutic Exercise: Foundations and Techniques*. 5th ed. Philadelphia, PA: F.A. Davis Company; 2007.
- Patel DR, Lyne ED. Chapter 29. Overuse injuries of the leg, ankle, and foot. In: Patel DR, Greydanus DE, Baker RJ, eds. *Pediatric Practice: Sports Medicine*. New York, NY: McGraw-Hill; 2009. http://www.accessphysiotherapy.com/content/6980676. Accessed June 29, 2013.
- MedlinePlus, NIH National Institutes of Health. Shin Splints. http://www.nlm.nih.gov/medlineplus/ency/article/003177.htm. Accessed June 5, 2013.
- Simon RR, Sherman SC. Leg soft-tissue injury. In: Simon RR, Sherman SC, eds. *Emergency Orthopedics*. 6th ed. New York, NY: McGraw-Hill; 2011. http://www.accessphysiotherapy.com/content/7708294. Accessed June 29, 2013.
- Story J, Cymet TC. Shin splints painful to have and to treat. *Compr Ther*. 2006;32(3):192–195.

SECTION I ANKLE AND FOOT DISORDERS

202 ACHILLES TENDINOPATHY

Josh A. Barabas, MPT, OCS, CSCS
Christina L. Pettie, MHA, PT

CONDITION/DISORDER SYNONYMS

- Achilles tendinitis
- Achilles tendonitis
- Achilles tendinosis

ICD-9-CM CODE[1]

- 726.71 Achilles bursitis or tendonitis

ICD-10-CM CODE[2]

- M76.60 Achilles tendinitis, unspecified leg

PREFERRED PRACTICE PATTERN[3]

- 4E: Impaired Joint Mobility, Motor Function, Muscle Performance, and Range of Motion Associated with Localized Inflammation

PATIENT PRESENTATION

A 37-year-old man presents complaining of pain in his left heel. Pain began 3 weeks ago when he increased his total running distance from 20 miles per week to 40 miles per week. He indicates pain worsens with running and stair climbing. Palpation reveals tenderness in the middle portion of his Achilles tendon. Examination reveals he is lacking 15 degrees of passive dorsiflexion compared to his uninvolved side and is unable to perform greater than five single leg calf raises due to pain. The patient tests negative for neural dynamics tests of the lower extremities.

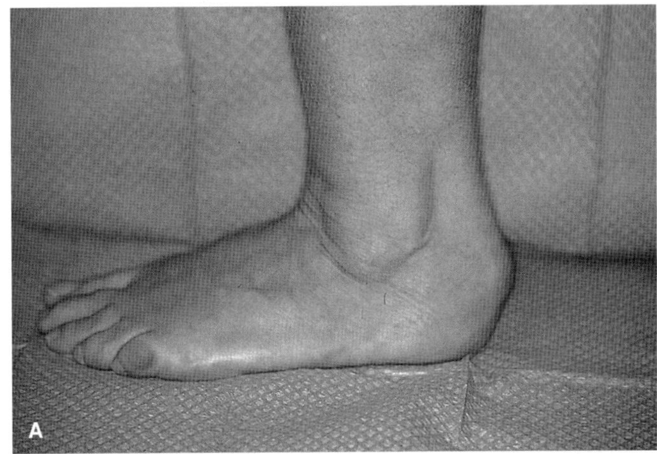

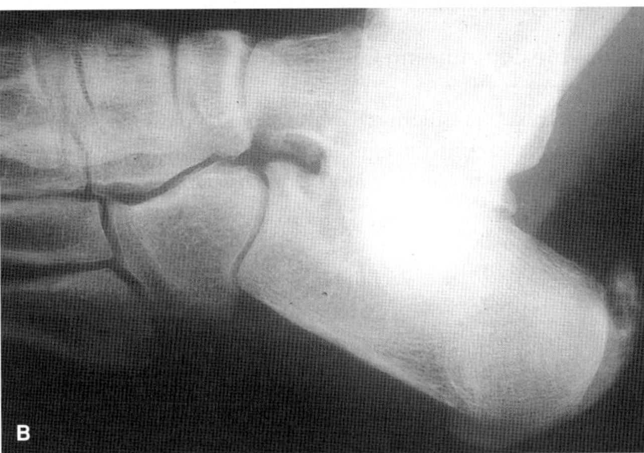

FIGURE 202-1 Achilles tendinitis. (**A**) Photograph of a patient with a prominence in the area of the posterior superior aspect of the calcaneus. (**B**) Lateral view radiograph of same patient demonstrating that an insertional calcific Achilles tendinitis, not Haglund deformity, is the cause of this deformity. (From Imboden J, Hellmann DB, Stone JH. *Current Diagnosis & Treatment in Rheumatology*. 2nd ed. http://www.accessmedicine.com. Copyright © The McGraw-Hill Companies, Inc. All rights reserved.)

KEY FEATURES

Description

- Insertional Achilles tendinitis: Fibers in middle portion of the tendon breakdown, degenerate, swell, thicken
- Noninsertional Achilles tendonitis: Pain in lower portion of heel at tendon attachment
- Pain common at midportion of the Achilles tendon
- Typically lacks presence of inflammatory cells, probably more tendonosis than tendonitis
- Typically associated with tissue degeneration
  - Two types
    - Lipoid: Fatty tissue deposited in the tendon
    - Mucoid: Conversion of the tendon in softer material with gray or brown appearance
  - Thickening of the tendon
  - Neovascularization
  - Increased presence of varicose nerve fibers
    - Most likely source of pain

Essentials of Diagnosis

- Patient history and clinical examination
- Ultrasound or MRI imaging

General Considerations

- Address training errors and biomechanics deficits to prevent recurrence

Demographics

- People participating in athletic activity; condition can also occur in sedentary individuals
  - Runners: 7% to 9% prevalence[4]
- Age: Between 30 and 50 years of age (median)[4]
- Sex: Males more than females[4]
- Onset more common during training versus competitive event

CLINICAL FINDINGS

SIGNS AND SYMPTOMS

- Pain with palpation of tendon 2 to 6 cm proximal to the insertion
- Pain back of the heel
- Tenderness changes position with tendon movement during dorsiflexion and plantar flexion (arc sign)
- Increased swelling throughout the day
- Thickening of the tendon
- Decreased dorsiflexion range of motion (ROM)
- Decreased gastrocnemius strength
- Greater pronation/calcaneal varus and faster rate of maximum pronation
- Decreased plantar flexion strength and endurance verse uninvolved side

Functional Implications

- Inability to climb stairs or ladder
- Inability to push-off during ambulation
- Decreased stride length during ambulation

Possible Contributing Causes

- Intrinsic risk factors
  - Decreased dorsiflexion ROM
  - Decreased gastrocnemius strength
  - Greater pronation/calcaneal varus and faster rate of maximum pronation
  - Comorbidities
  - Obesity (BMI)
  - Diabetes
  - Hyperlipidemia
  - Hypertension
- Extrinsic risk factors
  - Training errors
    - Sudden increase in mileage or intensity or incline
    - Return from inactivity
  - Environmental factors
    - High incidence with training in cold weather
  - Faulty equipment

Differential Diagnosis

- Accessory soleus muscle
- Achilles enthesopathy
- Achilles tendon ossification
- Achilles tendon partial tear
- Achilles tendon rupture
- Bone spur
- Lumbar or S1 radiculopathy
- Os trigonum syndrome
- Posterior ankle impingement
- Retrocalcaneal bursitis
- Sural nerve irritation
- Sural nerve pathology

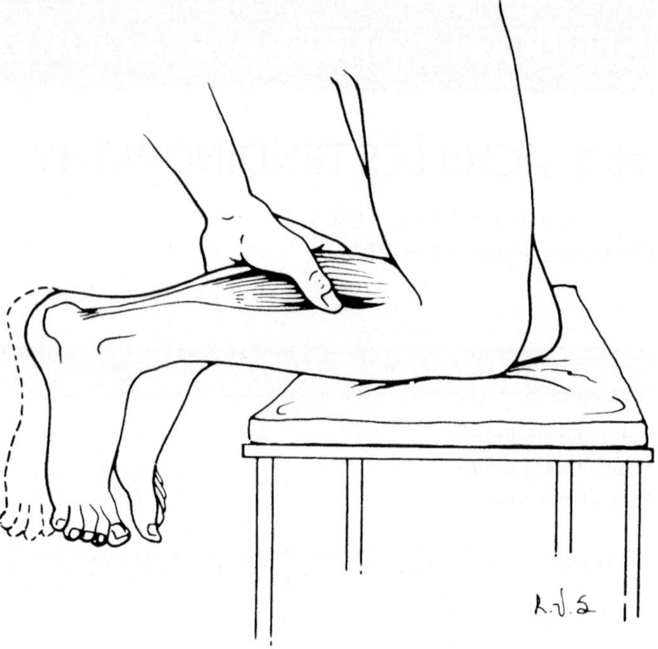

FIGURE 202-2 Test for Achilles tendon continuity. Squeeze the relaxed calf while observing the amount of ankle plantar flexion thus produced. If the tendon is ruptured, less motion occurs compared with that on the uninjured side. (From Stone CK, Humphries RL. *Current Diagnosis & Treatment: Emergency Medicine*. 7th ed. http://www.accessmedicine.com. Copyright © The McGraw-Hill Companies, Inc. All rights reserved.)

- Systemic inflammatory disease
- Xanthoma of the tendon: Accumulation of cholesterol in patients with familial hypercholesterolemia

MEANS OF CONFIRMATION OR DIAGNOSIS

Imaging

- Ultrasonography: Sensitivity of 85% and specificity of 49%[4]

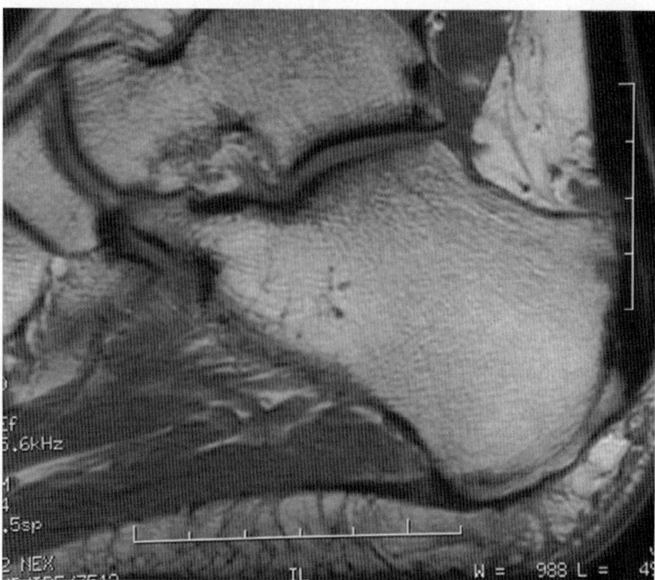

FIGURE 202-3 Magnetic resonance image of the calcaneus (sagittal view) demonstrating Haglund deformity, retrocalcaneal bursitis, cortical erosions, and Achilles tendinitis. (From Imboden J, Hellmann DB, Stone JH. *Current Diagnosis & Treatment in Rheumatology*. 2nd ed. http://www.accessmedicine.com. Copyright © The McGraw-Hill Companies, Inc. All rights reserved.)

- MRI: Sensitivity of 95% and specificity of 50%)[1]
- X-ray

FINDINGS AND INTERPRETATIONS

- Hypertrophic tendon
- Hyperechoic mass at midtendon
- Irregular tendon structure

TREATMENT

Medication

- NSAIDs
- Corticosteroid injection
- Prolotherapy: Sclerosant injection (most common dextrose)

MEDICAL PROCEDURES

- Tendon debridement
- Extracorpeal shock wave therapy (ESWT)

REFERRALS/ADMITTANCE

- To orthopeadic surgeon, family physician, or radiologist, for imaging
- To orthopeadic surgeon, for injection

IMPAIRMENTS

- Pain with movement after prolonged immobility (i.e., after sleeping) that improves with activity
- Pain at beginning of exercise training session that improves with activity, may worsen after activity

TESTS AND MEASURES

- Thompson test for ruptured Achilles tendon
- Matles test for Achilles tendon rupture
- Royal London Hospital test
- Foot and Ankle Ability Measure (FAAM)
- Ankle Joint Functional Assessment Tool (AJFAT)
- Single-limb stance and Star Excursion Balance Test (SEBT)
- Decreased performance of
  - Hopping
  - Jumping
  - Repetitive forceful plantar flexion

INTERVENTION

- Eccentric loading (3 × 10 to 15 reps; one to two times daily)[5–12]
  - Decrease pain
  - Improve function
  - Increase strength
  - Superior to concentric training
- Laser therapy[13–15]
  - Decrease inflammation and pain
  - Decrease tenderness
  - Decrease stiffness
  - Decrease crepitus
- Iontophoresis[16]
  - Decreases pain
  - Improves function
- Stretching[17]
  - Patients with limited dorsiflexion
    - Reduces pain
    - Improves function

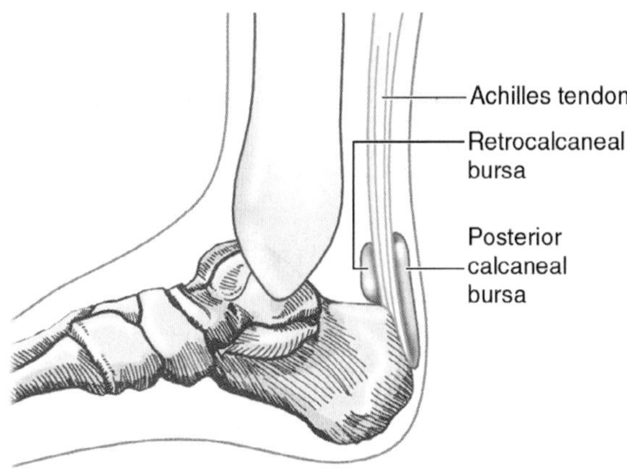

FIGURE 202-4 The posterior calcaneal bursa and the retrocalcaneal bursa. (From Simon RR, Sherman SC. *Emergency Orthopedics*. 6th ed. http://www.accessemergencymedicine.com. Copyright © The McGraw-Hill Companies, Inc. All rights reserved.)

- Foot orthoses[18–20]
  - Reduce pain
  - Alter foot and ankle kinematics while running
- Manual intervention[21]
  - Joint mobilization
  - Soft tissue massage to the Achilles tendon and surrounding tissues
  - Reduce pain
  - Improve mobility and function
- Taping[22]
  - Decrease strain on the tendon
- Heel lifts[23–25]

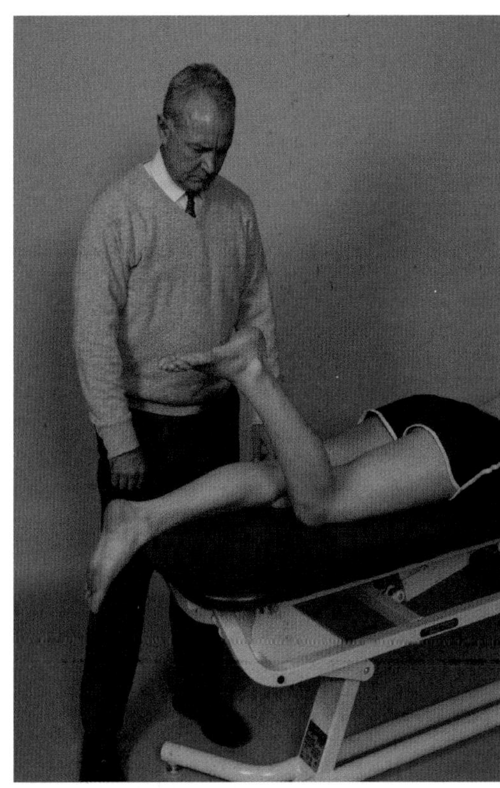

FIGURE 202-5 Matles test for Achilles tendon rupture. (From Dutton M. *Dutton's Orthopaedic Examination, Evaluation, and Intervention*. 3rd ed. http://www.accessphysiotherapy.com. Copyright © The McGraw-Hill Companies, Inc. All rights reserved.)

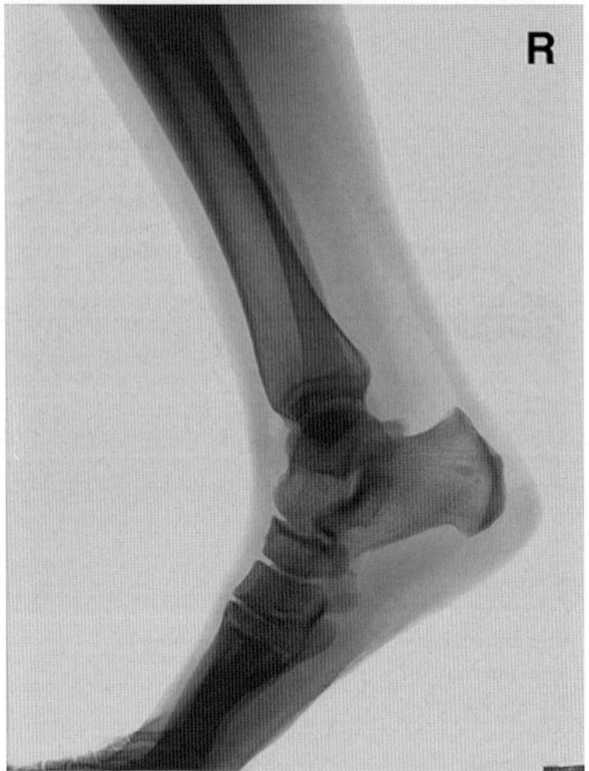

FIGURE 202-6 This plantar flexion view is used to assess for the possibility of posterior impingement at the talocrural joint by the relationship of the distal posterior tibia and posterior talus. (From Malone TR, Hazle C, Grey ML. *Imaging in Rehabilitation*. http://www.accessphysiotherapy.com. Copyright © The McGraw-Hill Companies, Inc. All rights reserved.)

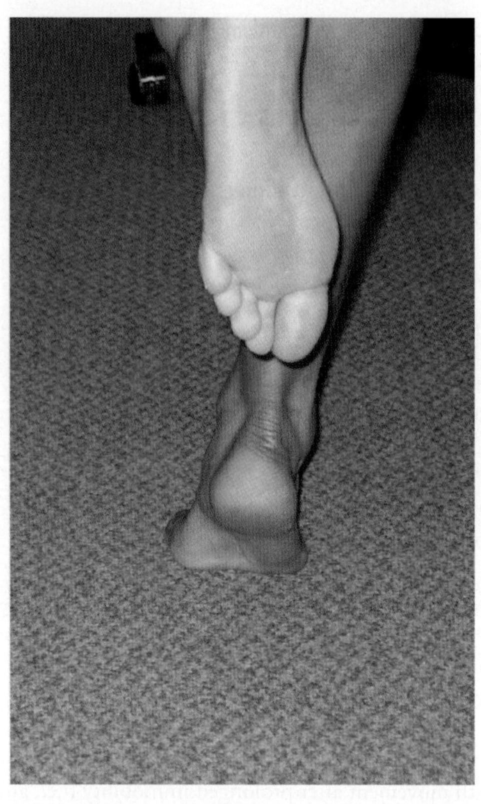

FIGURE 202-7 Single heel raise test. Normally when the athlete is asked to raise the heel of one foot and bear all weight on that leg the heel goes into varus locking the hindfoot as shown. With weakness or dysfunction of the posterior tibialis tendon the athlete is not able to do the heel raise or the foot tends to roll on to the lateral border. (From Patel DR, Greydanus DE, Baker RJ. *Pediatric Practice: Sports Medicine*. http://www.accesspediatrics.com. Copyright © The McGraw-Hill Companies, Inc. All rights reserved.)

- Night splints[10,26]
  - Not beneficial in reducing pain versus eccentric loading

FUNCTIONAL GOALS

- Patient will be able to
  - Demonstrate and maintain neutral calcaneal alignment with heel strike through toe-off phases of gait.
  - Demonstrate 15 degrees of talocrural dorsiflexion during stance phase of gait.
  - Stand and walk without limitation due to pain after sitting for more than 1 hour.
  - Demonstrate 5/5 manual muscle testing of involved gastrocnemius without limitation due to pain.
  - Demonstrate 50% speed running for 1 mile without limitation due to pain.
  - Demonstrate single-leg hopping on involved side without limitation due to pain.

PROGNOSIS

- Acute to subchronic
  - Significant pain and impairment reduction at 6 to 12 weeks[27]
  - 2 to 8 year follow-up 71% to 100% of patients return to prior level of function with minimal or no complaints[27]
  - When conservative management fails (24%–49%), recommend surgery to remove adhesions and nodules[27]
  - Average age responding to therapy—33 years old[27]
  - Average age requiring surgery—48 years old[27]
  - 4 to 6 months recommended conservative management[27]

ADDITIONAL INFORMATION

- Case Study 2 Heel Pain in Orthopaedic Case Studies[28]

PATIENT RESOURCES

- American Academy of Orthopaedic Surgeons. Achilles Tendinitis. http://orthoinfo.aaos.org/topic.cfm?topic=A00147. Accessed August 9, 2014.
- Mayo Clinic. Achilles Tendinitis. http://www.mayoclinic.com/print/achilles-tendinitis/DS00737/DSECTION=all&METHOD=print. Accessed August 9, 2014.

REFERENCES

1. ICD-9-CM. http://www.icd9data.com, Accessed January 20, 2013.
2. ICD-10-CM. http://www.icd10data.com, Accessed January 20, 2013.
3. APTA Guide to Physical Therapist Practice. http://guidetoptpractice.apta.org/. Accessed January 20, 2013.
4. Carcia C, Martin R, Houck J, Wukich D. Achilles pain, stiffness, and muscle power deficits: Achilles tendinitis. *J Orthop Sports Phys Ther*. 2010:40(9):A1–A26.
5. Alfredson H, Pietila T, Jonsson P, Lorentzon R. Heavy-load eccentric calf muscle training for the treatment of chronic Achilles tendinosis. *Am J Sports Med*. 1998;26(3):360–366.

6. Fahlstrom M, Jonsson P, Lorentzon R, Alfredson H. Chronic Achilles tendon pain treated with eccentric calf-muscle training. *Knee Surg Sports Traumatol Arthrosc.* 2003;11(5):327–333.
7. Knobloch K, Kraemer R, Jagodzinski M, et al. Eccentric training decreases paratendon capillary blood flow and pre-serves paratendon oxygen saturation in chronic achilles tendinopathy. *J Orthop Sports Phys Ther.* 2007;37(5):269–276.
8. Mafi N, Lorentzon R, Alfredson H. Superior short-term results with eccentric calf muscle training compared to concentric training in a randomized prospective multicenter study on patients with chronic Achilles tendinosis. *Knee Surg Sports Traumatol Arthrosc.* 2001;9(1):42–47.
9. Rompe JD, Furia J, Maffulli N. Eccentric loading versus eccentric loading plus shock-wave treatment for midportion achilles tendinopathy: a randomized controlled trial. *Am J Sports Med.* 2009;37(3):463–470.
10. Roos EM, Engstrom M, Lagerquist A, Soderberg B. Clinical improvement after 6 weeks of eccentric exercise in patients with mid-portion Achilles tendinopathy—a randomized trial with 1-year follow-up. *Scand J Med Sci Sports.* 2004;14(5): 286–295.
11. Shalabi A, Kristoffersen-Wilberg M, Svensson L, Aspelin P, Movin T. Eccentric training of the gastrocnemius-soleus complex in chronic Achilles tendinopathy results in decreased tendon volume and intratendinous signal as evaluated by MRI. *Am J Sports Med.* 2004;32(5):1286–1296.
12. Silbernagel KG, Thomee R, Thomee P, Karlsson J. Eccentric overload training for patients with chronic Achilles tendon pain—a randomised controlled study with reliability testing of the evaluation methods. *Scand J Med Sci Sports.* 2001;11(4):197–206.
13. Bjordal JM, Lopes-Martins RA, Iversen VV. A randomised, placebo controlled trial of low level laser therapy for activated Achilles tendinitis with microdialysis measurement of peritendinous prostaglandin E2 concentrations. *Br J Sports Med.* 2006;40(1):76–80; discussion 76–80.
14. Stergioulas A, Stergioula M, Aarskog R, Lopes-Martins RA, Bjordal JM. Effects of low-level laser therapy and eccentric exercises in the treatment of recreational athletes with chronic Achilles tendinopathy. *Am J Sports Med.* 2008;36(5):881–887.
15. Tumilty S, Munn J, McDonough S, et al. Low level laser treatment of tendinopathy: a systematic review with meta-analysis. *Photomed Laser Surg.* 2010;28(1):3–16.
16. Neeter C, Thomee R, Silbernagel KG, Thomee P, Karlsson J. Iontophoresis with or without dexamethazone in the treatment of acute Achilles tendon pain. *Scand J Med Sci Sports.* 2003;13(6):376–382.
17. Norregaard J, Larsen CC, Bieler T, Langberg H. Eccentric exercise in treatment of Achilles tendinopathy. *Scand J Med Sci Sports.* 2007;17(2):133–138.
18. Donoghue OA, Harrison AJ, Laxton P, Jones RK. Orthotic control of rear foot and lower limb motion during running in participants with chronic Achilles tendon injury. *Sports Biomech.* 2008;7(2):194–205.
19. Mayer F, Hirschmuller A, Muller S, Schuberth M, Baur H. Effects of short-term treatment strategies over 4 weeks in Achilles tendinopathy. *Br J Sports Med.* 2007;41(7):e6.
20. McCrory JL, Martin DF, Lowery RB, et al. Etiologic factors associated with Achilles tendinitis in runners. *Med Sci Sports Exerc.* 1999;31(10):1374–1381.
21. Christenson RE. Effectiveness of specific soft tissue mobilizations for the management of Achilles tendinosis: single case study—experimental design. *Man Ther.* 2007;12(1):63–71.
22. Martin RL, Paulseth S, Carcia CR. Taping techniques for Achilles tendinopathy. *Orthop Phys Ther Pract.* 2009;20:106–107.
23. Clement DB, Taunton JE, Smart GW. Achilles tendinitis and peritendinitis: etiology and treatment. *Am J Sports Med.* 1984;12(3):179–184.
24. Lee KH, Matteliano A, Medige J, Smiehorowski T. Electromyographic changes of leg muscles with heel lift: therapeutic implications. *Arch Phys Med Rehabil.* 1987;68(5 Pt 1):298–301.
25. Lowdon A, Bader DL, Mowat AG. The effect of heel pads on the treatment of Achilles tendinitis: a double blind trial. *Am J Sports Med.* 1984;12(6):431–435.
26. de Vos RJ, Weir A, Visser RJ, de Winter T, Tol JL. The additional value of a night splint to eccentric exercises in chronic midportion Achilles tendinopathy: a randomised controlled trial. *Br J Sports Med.* 2007;41(7):e5.
27. Maffulli N, Sharma P, Luscombe KL. Achilles tendinopathy: aetiology and management. *J R Soc Med.* 2004;97(10):472–476.
28. Heel Pain. Orthopaedic Case Studies. Accessphysiotherapy.com. http://accessphysiotherapy.mhmedical.com/cases.aspx#tab=4. Accessed August 16, 2014.

ADDITIONAL REFERENCES

- APTA PT Now. Achilles Tendinitis. http://www.ptnow.org/ClinicalSummaries/QuickDetail.aspx?cid=d7303dd5-4557-44f2-b488-62b07bde0d61. Accessed February 20, 2013.
- Balasubramaniam P, Prathap K. The effect of injection of hydrocortisone into rabbit calcaneal tendons. *J Bone Joint Surg Br.* 1972;54(4):729–734.
- Dutton M. Palpation. In: Dutton M, ed. *Dutton's Orthopedic Survival Guide: Managing Common Conditions.* New York, NY: McGraw-Hill; 2011. http://www.accessphysiotherapy.com/content/8655355. Accessed January 20, 2013.
- James SL, Bates BT, Osternig LR. Injuries to runners. *Am J Sports Med.* 1978;6(2):40–45.
- Ohberg L, Alfredson H. Effects on neovascularisation behind the good results with eccentric training in chronic mid-portion Achilles tendinosis? *Knee Surg Sports Traumatol Arthrosc.* 2004; 12:465–470.
- Rompe JD, Furia J, Maffulli N. Eccentric loading compared with shock wave therapy for chronic insertional Achilles tendinopathy. *J Bone Joint Surg Am.* 2008;90(1):52–61.
- Voorn R. Case report: can sacroiliac joint dysfunction cause chronic Achilles tendinitis? *J Orthop Sports Phys Ther.* 1998; 27:436–443.
- Woodley BL, Newsham-West RJ, Baxter GD. Chronic tendinopathy: effectiveness of eccentric exercise. *Br J Sports Med.* 2007; 41(4):188–198.

203 ANTERIOR TALOFIBULAR LIGAMENT SPRAIN

Sean M. Wells, DPT, PT, OCS, ATC, CSCS
Eric Shamus, PhD, DPT, PT, CSCS

CONDITION/DISORDER SYNONYMS

- Inversion ankle sprain
- Lateral ankle sprain
- ATFL sprain
- ATFL tear

ICD-9-CM CODE

- 845.0 Ankle sprain

ICD-10-CM CODE

- S93.409A Sprain of unspecified ligament of unspecified ankle, initial encounter

PREFERRED PRACTICE PATTERN[1]

- 4E: Impaired Joint Mobility, Motor Function, Muscle Performance, and Range of Motion Associated with Connective Tissue Dysfunction

PATIENT PRESENTATION

Patient is a 31-year-old female. She bought a new pair of high heels and was walking in them when she turned her ankle inward and fell. Patient was able to walk home but could not wear the high heels. She saw the physician the next day who took x-rays that were negative. The physician placed her in a walking boot for 2 weeks to try and get some stability. Patient presents swelling, pain, and decreased mobility. She is still having difficulty with ambulation.

KEY FEATURES

Description

- Disruption of anterior lateral ligament of the ankle
  - May be acute or chronic
- The anterior talofibular ligament (ATFL) restricts anterior translation of the talus
- The ATFL also restricts inversion and adduction at the subtalar joint
- Most commonly injured with rapid inversion, adduction, and plantar flexion movements, in either contact or noncontact situations
- Pain and edema at lateral ankle
- Can occur with structure progression to the calcaneofibular (CF) ligament and then posterior talofibular ligament

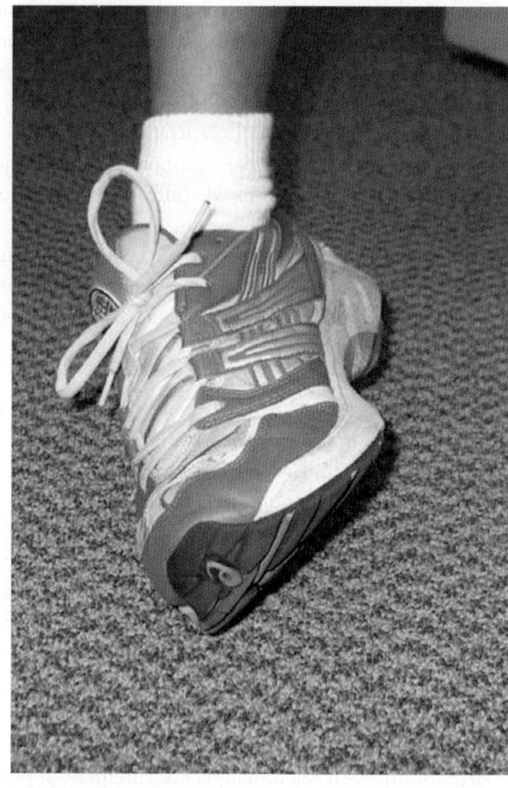

FIGURE 203-1 Mechanism of inversion sprain. (From Patel DR, Greydanus DE, Baker RJ. *Pediatric Practice: Sports Medicine*. http://www.accesspediatrics.com. Copyright © The McGraw-Hill Companies, Inc. All rights reserved.)

Essentials of Diagnosis

- Positive anterior drawer test and talar tilt test
- Ultrasonography (US), radiography, or MRI may be utilized in select cases[2]

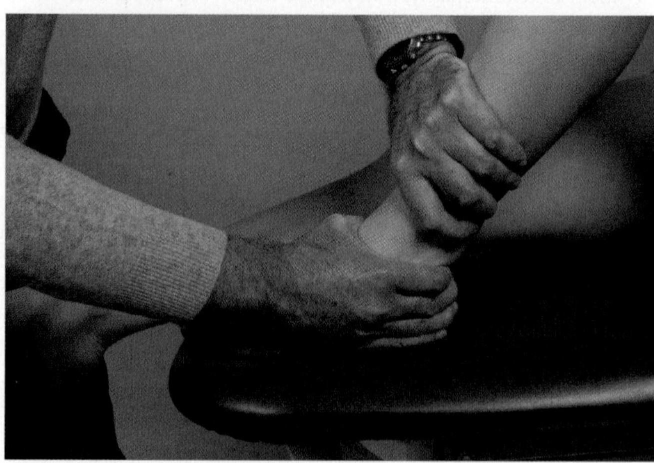

FIGURE 203-2 Anterior drawer test. (From Dutton M. *Dutton's Orthopaedic Examination, Evaluation, and Intervention*. 3rd ed. http://www.accessphysiotherapy.com. Copyright © The McGraw-Hill Companies, Inc. All rights reserved.)

- US or MRI is recommended following an inversion ankle sprain in a patient with chronic ankle instability
- Radiographs utilized within the constraints of Ottawa ankle rules
- ATFL tears are classified based on the anatomical degree of damage or functional stability found on clinical examination
- Anatomical
  - Grade 1: Partial microscopic tearing of the ligament, minimal to no loss of function, mild swelling and pain
  - Grade 2: Partial macroscopic tearing of the ligament, with mild–moderate loss of function, moderate swelling/pain/tenderness
  - Grade 3: Complete rupture with severe loss of function, severe swelling/pain/tenderness
- Functional stability
  - Stable: No laxity with talar tilt or anterior drawer testing (ATFL, Grade 1)
  - Unstable: Laxity with anterior drawer testing (ATFL, Grade 2); laxity with both anterior drawer and talar tilt (ATFL and CF, Grade 3)

General Considerations

- May occur with concomitant CF sprain, posterior talofibular sprain, synovitis, chondral lesion, or fracture
- Most commonly sprained ankle ligament

Demographics

- Prevalent in athletes, though does occur in sedentary individuals
  - Most common in basketball, soccer, and football[3]
- Males between 15 and 24 years of age have higher rates of ankle sprains than female counterparts; females over 30 years of age have higher rates than male counterparts[3]
- A previous ankle sprain is the strongest predictor of a subsequent ankle sprain[4]

CLINICAL FINDINGS

SIGNS AND SYMPTOMS[5]

- Pain in lateral ankle or foot
  - Grade 1: Minimal
  - Grade 2: Moderate
  - Grade 3: Severe
- May posture in greater pronation to avoid plantar flexed/inversion moments
- Edema lateral ankle
  - Grade 1: Minimal
  - Grade 2: Moderate
  - Grade 3: Severe
- Pain with palpation of ATFL
- Possible inability to bear partial or full weight
- Guarded active/passive inversion ROM
- May have increased inversion passive ROM (positive Talar tilt test)
- Decreased active/passive dorsiflexion ROM
- Decreased peroneal/eversion strength
- In moderate to severe cases, increased talar anterior glide on mortise (positive anterior drawer test)

Functional Implications[5]

- Loss of functional ability
  - Grade 1: Minimal
  - Grade 2: Some
  - Grade 3: Great
- Inability to stand secondary to weight bearing
  - Grade 1: None
  - Grade 2: Usually
  - Grade 3: Almost always
- Reduced midstance time during ambulation
- Reduced contralateral step length
- Impaired single-limb balance
- Inability to execute cutting maneuvers

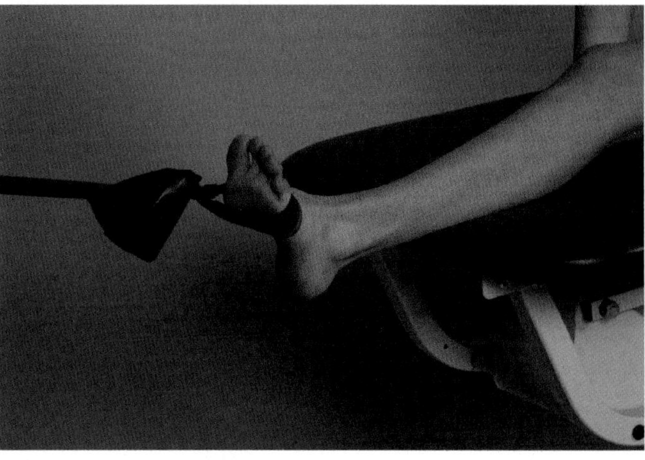

FIGURE 203-3 Eversion PRE with resistive tubing. (From Dutton M. *Dutton's Orthopaedic Examination, Evaluation, and Intervention*. 3rd ed. http://www.accessphysiotherapy.com. Copyright © The McGraw-Hill Companies, Inc. All rights reserved.)

Possible Contributing Causes

- Intrinsic risk factors
  - Prior ankle sprains
  - Decreased dorsiflexion ROM and strength[6]
  - Decreased evertor-to-inverter muscle function ratio[6]
  - Pes cavus
  - Impaired proprioception/balance[6]
  - Obesity[6]
- Extrinsic risk factors
  - Equipment
    - High-heeled shoes
    - Noncompliance with reinjury prevention strategies such as bracing
  - Environmental factors
    - Uneven playing field or surface
    - Artificial turf[6]
- Sport position—participation in sport at the beginning of the season or at the end of game[7]

Differential Diagnosis

- Achilles tendon strain
- CF ligament sprain
- Chondral lesion
- Extensor digitorum brevis strain
- Inverted talus
- Jones fracture
- Osteochondritis dissecans
- Peroneal muscle strain
- Peroneal tendon subluxation
- Peroneus tertius inflammation
- Posterior talofibular ligament sprain
- S1 radiculopathy
- Syndesmotic ankle sprain

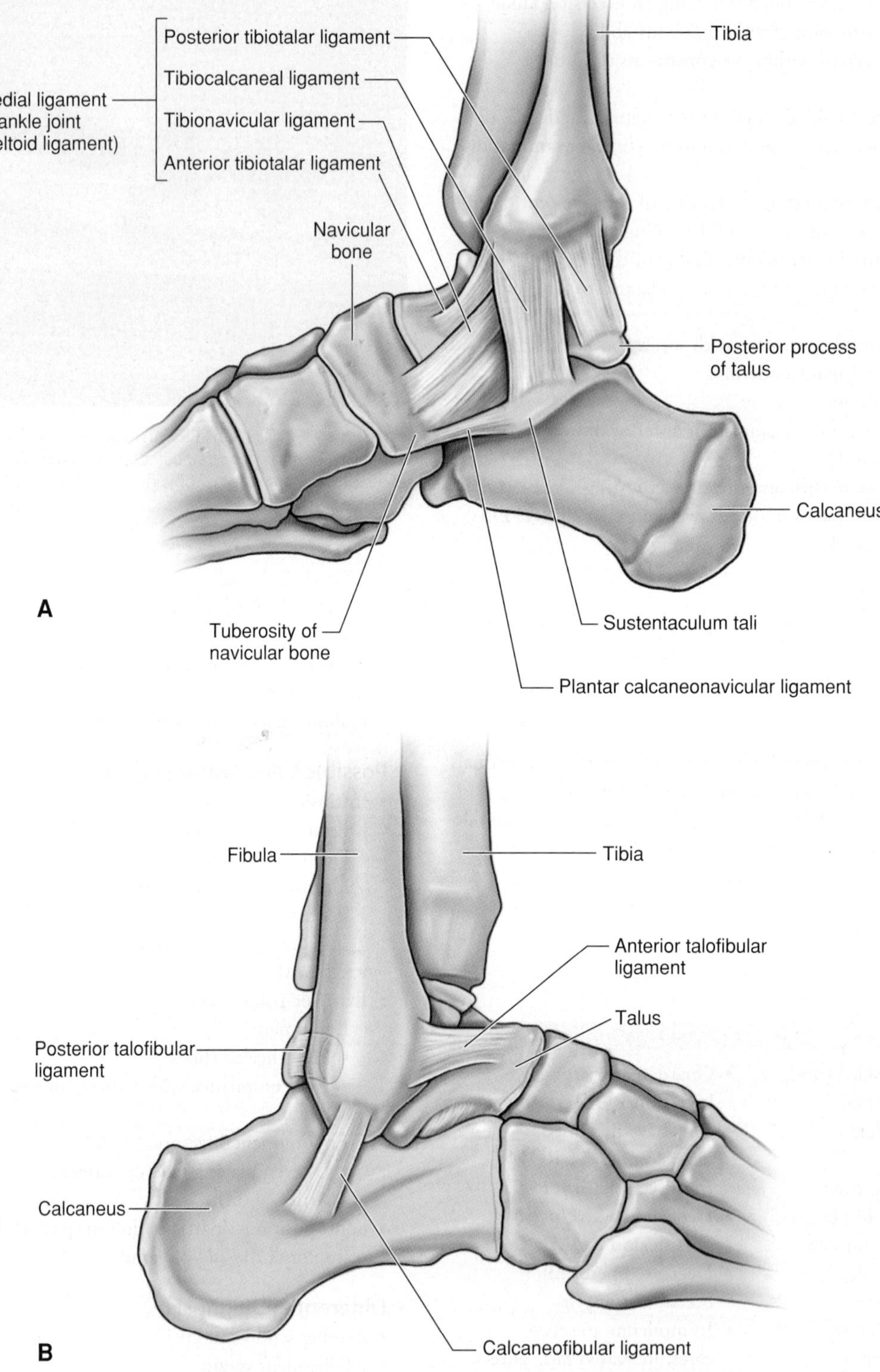

FIGURE 203-4 (**A**) Medial and (**B**) lateral views of the right ankle joint. (From Henderson MC, Tierney LM Jr, Smetana GW. *The Patient History: An Evidence-Based Approach to Differential Diagnosis*. 2nd ed. http://www.accessmedicine.com. Copyright © The McGraw-Hill Companies, Inc. All rights reserved.)

- Synovitis
- Talotibial impingement syndrome
- Talus fracture

MEANS OF CONFIRMATION OR DIAGNOSIS

Imaging[5]

- Procedure
  - Rule out fracture or syndesmotic ankle sprain
    - Additional imaging warranted if patient meets the Ottawa ankle rules, presents with a possible dislocation, or has positive syndesmotic ankle sprain tests[8]
  - If initial examination is limited due to pain and syndesmotic ankle sprain, testing cannot be done
    - Allow patient to protect, rest, ice, compress, elevate, and use crutches (if needed) for 3 to 5 days, followed by re-examination to screen for syndesmotic ankle sprain via ankle MRI[8]

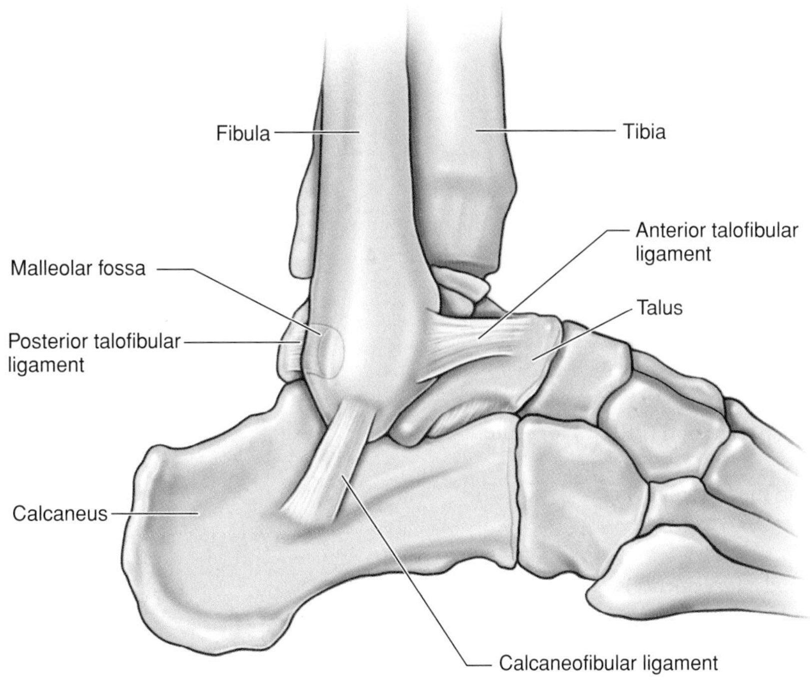

FIGURE 203-5 Lateral ligaments. (Reproduced with permission from Morton DA, Foreman KB, Albertine KH. *The Big Picture: Gross Anatomy*. McGraw-Hill; 2011.)

- US: sn = 92%, sp = 83%
- MRI: Ankle series: (sn = 95%, sp = 50%)
- Arthrogram: sn = 100%
- 3D CT: sp = 94.4%
- Radiographs with use of Ottawa ankle rules, anterior–posterior views with 10 to 20 degrees internal rotation: (sn = 100%, sp = 40%)

FINDINGS AND INTERPRETATION

- Once fracture or syndesmotic ankle sprain has been ruled out, key findings will be the aforementioned functional losses and signs and symptoms.
- Imaging for isolated ATFL sprains will reveal increased signal uptake, wavy or curved contour, or disruption of the ligament's integrity on MRI and CT.
- US presents torn ATFL ligament as discontinuous bundles and hypoechoic lesion.[9]
  - Further studies are needed to confirm routine use of US for isolated ATFL tears.
  - MRIs are implemented in ATFL tears with suspect chondral lesions or chronic instability.[8]

TREATMENT

Medication

- Nonsteroidal anti-inflammatory medications

MEDICAL PROCEDURES

- ATFL reconstruction only in chronic cases not responding to conservative management
- Therapeutic hyaluronic acid injections (limited evidence)

REFERRALS/ADMITTANCE

- For imaging, for concomitant osseous lesions
- For medical management, for concomitant osseous lesions

IMPAIRMENTS

- Edema in lateral ankle
- May have increased inversion passive ROM (positive talar tilt test)
- Decreased active/passive dorsiflexion ROM
- Decreased peroneal strength
- In moderate-to-severe cases: Increased talar anterior glide on mortise (positive anterior drawer test)
- Reduced posterior glide of distal fibula on tibia
- Reduced single-limb balance

TESTS AND MEASURES

- Palpation of ankle
- Eversion ankle strength

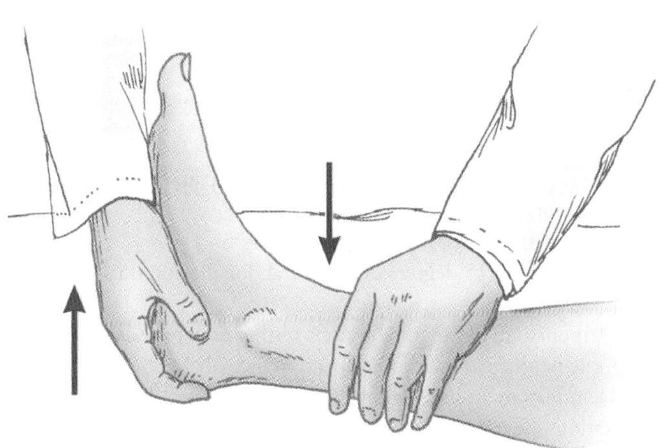

FIGURE 203-6 Technique for performing anterior drawer stress test of the ankle. (From Simon RR, Sherman SC. *Emergency Orthopedics*. 6th ed. http://www.accessemergencymedicine.com. Copyright © The McGraw-Hill Companies, Inc. All rights reserved.)

- Ankle ROM
  - Inversion: Hindfoot 20 degrees
  - Eversion: Pronation 10 degrees
  - Dorsiflexion: 20 degrees
  - Plantar flexion: 30 to 50 degrees
- Anterior drawer test
- Inversion stress test
- Talar tilt test
- Gait assessment
- Foot and Ankle Ability Measure (FAAM)
- Ankle Joint Functional Assessment Tool (AJFAT)
- Single-limb stance and Star Excursion Balance Test (SEBT)

INTERVENTION

- Protection, rest, ice, compression, elevation (PRICE) for acute stage (moderate evidence)
  - Short-term semirigid bracing superior to taping[8]
  - Decreases pain
  - Improves function
- Early functional treatment (moderate evidence)
  - Promotes weight bearing as long as gait pattern is normal
    - Use assistive device if gait deviations exist
    - Implement supervised early active ROM and weight-bearing proprioception/neuromuscular exercises
  - Increases strength
  - Increases ROM, decreases swelling, return to normal gait
- Balance and coordination exercises: 6 to 8 weeks or longer (strong evidence)
  - Improves balance function
  - Increases strength
  - Dynamic and static tasks
  - Can prevent reinjury (not for chronic ankle instability)
- Taping, bracing, and wrapping (moderate evidence)
  - Improves swelling, subjective stability
  - Bracing superior to taping based on cost effectiveness and ease[8]
- Manual intervention (moderate evidence[9])
  - Mobilization with movement to promote posterior talar gliding[10]
  - Posterior mobilization of fibula on tibia
  - Reduces pain, improves ankle dorsiflexion, improves stride speed
- Ultrasound for acute injury (limited evidence)
- Electrotherapy or hyperbaric treatments (limited evidence[11])

FUNCTIONAL GOALS

- Patient will be able to
  - Stand and walk without limitation due to pain or edema for >1 hour.
  - Demonstrate full contralateral step length.
  - Demonstrate 15 degrees of talocrural dorsiflexion during stance phase of gait.
  - Demonstrate 5/5 manual muscle testing of peroneals to promote neutral subtalar joint during stance phase of gait.
  - Demonstrate in-line jogging at 5.0 mph for 1 mile without limitation due to pain.
  - Complete cutting maneuvers for sport or work without compensatory movement patterns or pain.
  - Demonstrate SEBT on involved side without limitation due to pain or instability.

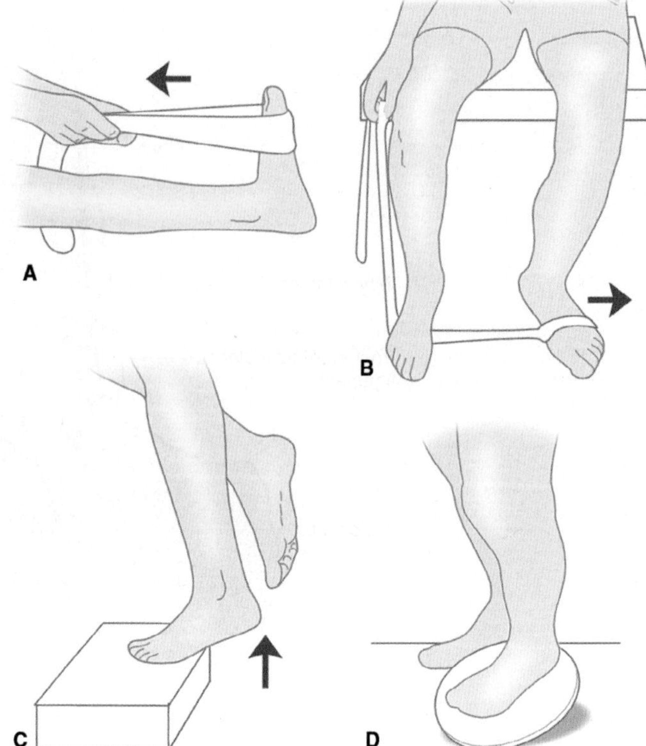

FIGURE 203-7 Functional rehabilitation following an ankle sprain consists of restoring range of motion, muscle strengthening exercises, proprioceptive training, and, finally, gradual return to activity. (**A**) Achilles tendon stretching exercises should begin within 48 hours of injury. Other range of motion exercises include knee bends with the heel on the floor (five repetitions five times/day) and alphabet exercises, in which the patient "draws" the letters of the alphabet with the toes. (**B, C**) Strengthening exercises begin once swelling and pain are controlled. Isometric exercises (plantar flexion, dorsiflexion, inversion, and eversion) against a wall are followed by isotonic exercises. (**D**) Proprioceptive exercises begin once full weight bearing without pain has been achieved. A "wobble board" is used for 5 to 10 minutes two times/day, first while seated, and then while standing. The patient rotates the board clockwise and counterclockwise. (From Simon RR, Sherman SC. *Emergency Orthopedics*. 6th ed. http://www.accessemergencymedicine.com. Copyright © The McGraw-Hill Companies, Inc. All rights reserved.)

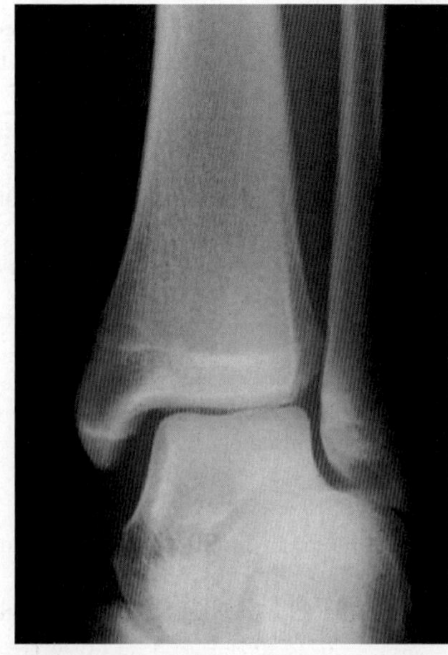

FIGURE 203-8 X-ray of syndesmotic injury. Note widening of the tibiofibular syndesmosis. (From Patel DR, Greydanus DE, Baker RJ. *Pediatric Practice: Sports Medicine*. http://www.accesspediatrics.com. Copyright © The McGraw-Hill Companies, Inc. All rights reserved.)

TABLE 203-1 West Point Grading of Ankle Sprains

Criterion	Grade 1	Grade 2	Grade 3
Location of tenderness	ATFL	ATFL, CFL	ATFL, CFL, PTFL
Edema, ecchymosis	Slight, local	Moderate, local	Significant, diffuse
Weight-bearing ability	Full or partial	Difficult without crutches	Impossible without significant pain
Ligament damage	Stretched	Partial tear	Complete tear
Instability	None	None or slight	Definite

Source: Patel DR, Greydanus DE, Baker RJ. *Pediatric Practice: Sports Medicine.* http://www.accesspediatrics.com.

PROGNOSIS

- Inversely proportional to severity.[5]
- Acute injury
  - Excellent, nonsurgical, active conservative care.
  - No additional benefit of adding surgery to conservative care for ATFL sprains.[10]
  - Significant functional, pain, and impairment reduction at 1 week with grades 1 and 2.
  - 40% of athletes with inversion ankle sprains will develop chronic ankle instability.[4]
  - Prevention of reinjury through semirigid braces.
- Chronic injury/instability
  - May respond to conservative care, such as balance/coordination exercises.
  - Patients that fail conservative care have good outcomes with surgical intervention.[12]

PATIENT RESOURCE

- Physical Therapist's Guide to Ankle Sprain. Ameican Physical Therapy Association. February 28, 2011. Accessed January 11, 2013.

REFERENCES

1. The American Physical Therapy Association. *Interactive Guide to Physical Therapist Practice.* Alexandria, VA: The American Physical Therapy Association; 2003. http://guidetoptpractice.apta.org./ Accessed January 11, 2013.
2. Guillodo Y, Riban P, Guennoc X, Dubrana F, Saraux A. Usefulness of Ultrasonographic detection of talocrural effusion in ankle sprains. *J Ultrasound Med.* 2007;26(6):831–836.
3. Waterman BR, Owens BD, Davey S, Zacchilli MA, Belmont PJ Jr. The epidemiology of ankle sprains in the United States. *J Bone Joint Surg Am.* 2010;92(13):2279–2284.
4. Hubbard TJ, Cordova M. Mechanical instability after an acute lateral ankle sprain. *Arch Phys Med Rehabil.* 2009;90(7):1142–1146.
5. Dutton M. The ankle and foot complex. In: Dutton M, ed. *Dutton's Orthopedic Survival Guide: Managing Common Conditions.* New York, NY: McGraw-Hill; 2011. http://www.accessphysiotherapy.com/content/8655656. Accessed January 11, 2013.
6. Fong DT, Chan YY, Mok KM, Yung PS, Chan KM. Understanding acute ankle ligamentous sprain injury in sports. *Sports Med Arthrosc Rehabil Ther Technol.* 2009;1:1–14.
7. Kofotolis ND, Kellis E, Vlachopoulos S. Ankle sprain injuries and risk factors in amateur soccer players during a 2-year period. *Am J Sports Med.* 2007;35(3):458–466.
8. Polzer H, Kanz KG, Prall WC, et al. Diagnosis and treatment of acute ankle injuries: development of an evidence-based algorithm. *Orthop Rev(Pavia).* 2012;4(1):e5.
9. Oae K, Takao M, Uchio Y, Ochi M. Evaluation of anterior talofibular ligament injury with stress radiography, ultrasonography and MR imaging. *Skeletal Radiol.* 2010;39(1):41–47.
10. Vicenzino B, Branjerdporn M, Teys P, Jordan K. Initial changes in posterior talar glide and dorsiflexion of the ankle after mobilization with movement in individuals with recurrent ankle sprain. *J Orthop Sports Phys Ther.* 2006;36(7):464–471.
11. Bleakley CM, McDonough SM, MacAuley DC. Some conservative strategies are effective when added to controlled mobilisation with external support after acute ankle sprain: a systematic review. *Aust J Physiother.* 2008;54(1):7–20.
12. Kamper SJ, Grootjans SJ. Surgical versus conservative treatment for acute ankle sprains. *Br J Sports Med.* 2012;46(1):77–88.

ADDITIONAL REFERENCES

- Dutton M. The ankle and foot complex. In: Dutton M, ed. *Dutton's Orthopedic Survival Guide: Managing Common Conditions.* New York, NY: McGraw-Hill; 2011. http://www.accessphysiotherapy.com/content/8655397. Accessed January 11, 2013.
- Green T, Refshauge K, Crosbie J, Adams R. A randomized controlled trial of a passive accessory joint mobilization on acute ankle inversion sprains. *Phys Ther.* 2001;81(4):984–994.
- Hamilton N, Weimar W, Luttgens K. The lower extremity: the knee, ankle, and foot. In: Hamilton N, Weimar W, Luttgens K, eds. *Kinesiology: Scientific Basis of Human Motion.* New York, NY: McGraw-Hill; 2008. http://www.accessphysiotherapy.com/content/6153087. Accessed January 11, 2013.
- Hooker DN, Prentice WE. Basic principles of electricity and electrical stimulating currents. In: Prentice WE, Quillen WS, Underwood F, eds. *Therapeutic Modalities in Rehabilitation.* 4th ed. New York, NY: McGraw-Hill; 2011. http://www.accessphysiotherapy.com/content/8136027. Accessed January 11, 2013.
- McKeon PO, Hertel J. Systematic review of postural control and lateral ankle instability, part II: is balance training clinically effective? *J Athl Train.* 2008;43(3):305–315.
- Mulligan B. *Manual therapy, 'NAGs,' 'SNAGs,' and 'MWMs,'* etc. 6th ed. Wellington, NZ: Plane View Services; 2010.

- Seah R, Mani-Babu S. Managing ankle sprains in primary care: what is best practice? A systematic review of the last 10 years of evidence. *Br Med Bull.* 2011;97:105–135.
- Prentice WE, Quillen WS, Underwood F. Basic principles of electricity and electrical stimulating currents. In: Prentice WE, Quillen WS, eds. *Therapeutic Modalities in Rehabilitation.* 4th ed. New York, NY: McGraw-Hill; 2011. http://www.accessphysiotherapy.com/resource/675. Accessed January 11, 2013.
- Simon RR, Sherman SC. Ankle. In: Simon RR, Sherman SC, eds. *Emergency Orthopedics.* 6th ed. New York, NY: McGraw-Hill; 2011. http://www.accessphysiotherapy.com/content/7708597. Accessed January 11, 2013.
- van den Bekerom MP, van der Windt DA, Ter Riet G, van der Heijden GJ, Bouter LM. Therapeutic ultrasound for acute ankle sprains. *Cochrane Database Syst Rev.* 2011;(6):CD001250.
- Vicenzino B, Branjerdporn M, Teys P, Jordan K. Initial changes in posterior talar glide and dorsiflexion of the ankle after mobilization with movement in individuals with recurrent ankle sprain. *J Orthop Sports Phys Ther.* 2006;36(7):464–471.
- Wilson PE, Pengel KB. Sports Medicine. In: Hay WW, Levin MJ, Sondheimer JM, Deterding RR, eds. *CURRENT Diagnosis & Treatment: Pediatrics.* 20th ed. New York, NY: McGraw-Hill; 2011. http://www.accessphysiotherapy.com/content/6586350. Accessed January 11, 2013.
- Zech A, Hubscher M, Vogt L, et al. Neuromuscular training for rehabilitation of sports injuries: a systematic review. *Med Sci Sports Exerc.* 2009;41(10):1831–1841.

204 CALCANEUS FRACTURE

Jennifer Cabrera, DPT, GCS
Eric Shamus, PhD, DPT, PT, CSCS

CONDITION/DISORDER SYNONYMS

- Heel fracture
- Lover's fracture
- Don Juan fracture

ICD-9-CM CODES

- 825.0 Fracture of calcaneus closed
- 825.1 Fracture of calcaneus open

ICD-10-CM CODES

- S92.009A Unspecified fracture of unspecified calcaneus, initial encounter for closed fracture
- S92.009B Unspecified fracture of unspecified calcaneus, initial encounter for open fracture

PREFERRED PRACTICE PATTERN

- 4G: Impaired Joint Mobility, Muscle Performance, and Range of Motion Associated with Fracture[1]

PATIENT PRESENTATION

A 43-year-old man fell off of a ladder from approximately 7 ft high and landed completely on one foot. He reported immediate pain in the foot with inability to bear weight. He presented with constant pain, swelling of the foot and ankle and worsening pain with all ankle/foot movements. Patient presents on the day of injury as a direct access patient. The patient is still unable to bear weight. Patient is positive in the Ottawa ankle rules and referred to the emergency room for an X-ray. Radiographs showed a calcaneus fracture.

KEY FEATURES

Description

- Fracture[2]
- Any defect in continuity of the calcaneus[3]
- Displaced (calcaneus is moved on either side of fracture) or nondisplaced (calcaneus has not moved)
- Closed (skin is intact)
- Open (skin is breached)
- Extra-articular calcaneal fracture
  - Involvement of the calcaneus anterior (Type A), middle (Type B), posterior (Type C)
- Intra-articular calcaneal fracture[4]
  - More common
  - Posterior talar articular facet of the calcaneus
  - Sanders system of classification categorizes into four types based on location at posterior articular surface

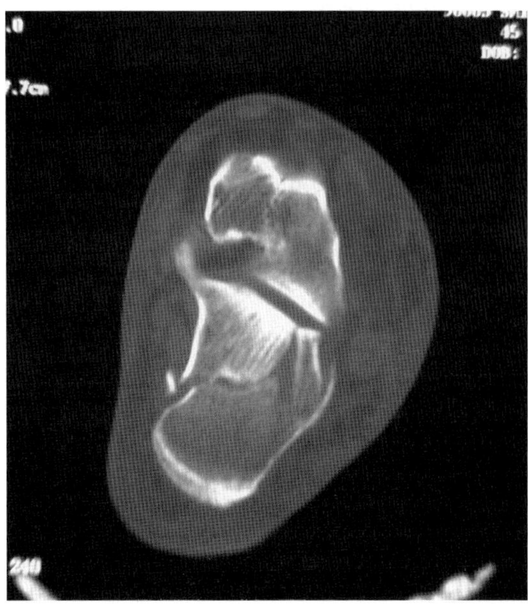

FIGURE 204-1 Axial CT section showing a fracture of the calcaneus caused by an axial loading mechanism. (From Doherty GM. *Current Diagnosis & Treatment: Surgery*. 13th ed. http://www.accessmedicine.com. Copyright © The McGraw-Hill Companies, Inc. All rights reserved.)

Essentials of Diagnosis

- Diagnosis usually made by clinical examination
- May not be fracture, but plantar fasciitis or heel spur
- Böhler angle (Tuber angle)
  - Vertex between a line from the top of the posterior articular facet to the top of the posterior tuberosity and a line from the top of the posterior tuberosity to the top of the anterior articular facet
  - Angle <20 degrees suggests drop of the posterior facet and possible calcaneal fracture
- Angle of Gissane (Critical angle)
  - Downward and upward slope of the calcaneal superior surface
  - Angle >130 degrees suggests fracture of the posterior subtalar joint surface

General Considerations

- Occurs most often during high-energy collisions (fall from height, motor vehicle accident)
- Most frequently fractured tarsal bone
- May affect leg length with compression of the fracture

CLINICAL FINDINGS

SIGNS AND SYMPTOMS

- Pain with weight bearing
- Point tenderness
- Increased pain on weight bearing
- Edema
- Redness
- Ecchymosis
- Fracture blister

- Loss of general function
- Loss of active mobility
- Muscle guarding with passive movement
- Heel deformity
- Mondor sign: Hematoma going to the bottom of the foot

Functional Implications

- Pain with standing
- Antalgic gait
- Inability to bear weight on injured lower extremity
- Pain with open or closed chain ankle movements (driving)

Possible Contributing Causes

- History of high-impact activities
- Trauma
- History of falls
- Osteoporosis

Differential Diagnosis

- Achilles tendinopathy
- Heel spur
- Plantar fasciitis
- Stress fracture

MEANS OF CONFIRMATION OR DIAGNOSIS

Imaging

- X-ray for fracture
    - Ottawa ankle rules
    - Often limited view[5]
- CT scan for detailed imaging[5]
- Bone scan if stress fracture is suspected[4]

FINDINGS AND INTERPRETATION

- Hop-to-gait sequence or decreased stance time on injured lower extremity secondary to pain
- Exposed bone in cases of open and displaced fracture
- Integumentary deformity over underlying fracture
- If vascular structures involved, foot will appear cool and pale
- If neurologic structures involved, patient will report numbness and decreased ability to move the foot and toes

REFERRALS/ADMITTANCE

- To radiology for imaging, X-ray, CT[5]
- To physician for medication: NSAIDs or opioid pain management
- To orthopedist for consult, possible fracture reduction via
    - Surgical intervention: Open reduction internal fixation (ORIF)
    - Immobilization with casting or splinting of ankle and foot

IMPAIRMENTS

- Antalgic gait secondary to pain, causes inability to push off
- Inability to ambulate long distances secondary to pain or decreased weight-bearing status that makes ambulating taxing
- Decreased stance time on involved lower extremity during ambulation
- Inability to stand for long periods of time secondary to pain

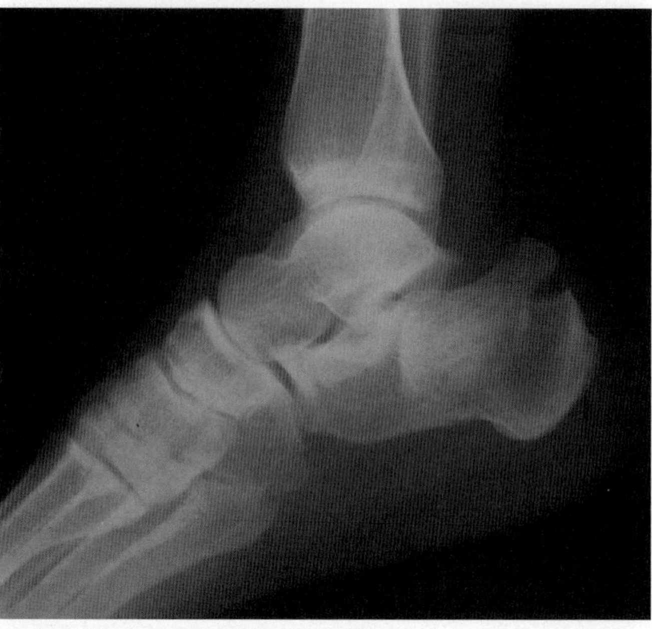

FIGURE 204-2 Tongue-type fracture of the calcaneus showing involvement of the subtalar joint. (From Skinner HB. *Current Diagnosis & Treatment in Orthopedics*. 4th ed. http://www.accessmedicine.com. Copyright © The McGraw-Hill Companies, Inc. All rights reserved.)

TEST AND MEASURES

- Ottawa ankle rules
- Tuning fork
- Calcaneal squeeze test to produce heel pain
- Weight-bearing assessment
- Leg-length assessment, malleolus to floor
- Gait analysis

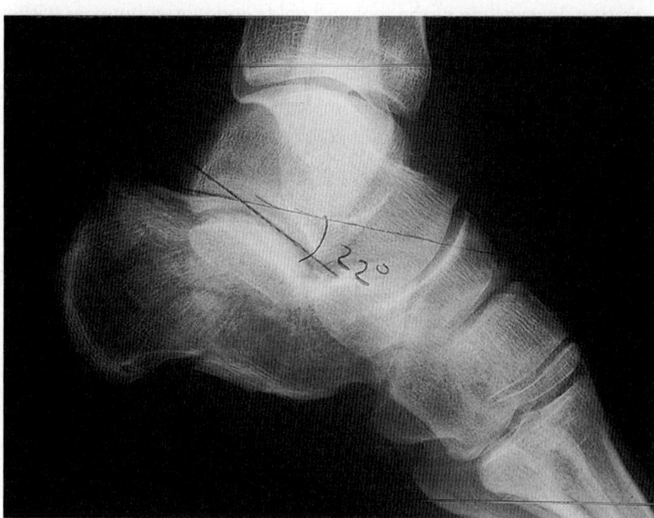

FIGURE 204-3 Calcaneus fracture. This patient fell from a ladder and struck his heel. A cortical step-off is seen on the inferior aspect of the calcaneus. The Böhler angle has been calculated at approximately 22 degrees. (From Knoop KJ, Stack LB, Storrow AB, Thurman RJ. *The Atlas of Emergency Medicine*. 3rd ed. http://www.accessmedicine.com. Copyright © The McGraw-Hill Companies, Inc. All rights reserved. Photo contributor: Alan B. Storrow, MD.)

INTERVENTION

- Depends on type of fracture, more severe cases require ORIF
- Ultrasound to stimulate fracture healing in skeletally mature populations[6]
- CAM Walker or rocker boot to limit dorsiflexion to neutral
- Orthotics to provide proper arch support with neutral subtalar positioning to avoid stressing injured structures[4]
- Address swelling
  - Ice/Cryotherapy[7]
  - Compression
  - Elevation
  - Electrical stimulation[8]
- Address pain
  - Ice/cryotherapy[7]
  - Massage
  - Electrical stimulation
- Address mobilization
  - Anterior distal tibiofibular glide to increase plantar flexion
  - Posterior distal tibiofibular glide to increase dorsiflexion
  - Gentle talocrural distraction for pain control
  - Subtalar distraction for general inversion/eversion
  - Medial subtalar glide for eversion
  - Lateral subtalar glide for inversion
  - Intertarsal and tarsometatarsal plantar glides for supination
  - Intertarsal and tarsometatarsal dorsal glides for pronation
- Address lack of flexibility via stretching
  - Gastrocnemius
  - Soleus
  - Plantar fascia
- Address weakness via strengthening activities
  - Open-chain ankle movements in all planes with resistance bands
  - Heel raises
  - Toe raises
  - Toe curls, intrinsic flexors
  - Active positioning of foot in subtalar neutral
- Address proprioception[4]
  - Standing balance activities with foam
    - Eyes open
    - Eyes closed
  - Standing balance activities on balance machines
- Gait training[9]
  - Lateral weight shifting to promote stance time on injured lower extremity
  - Resisted walking to promote proper gait sequence with eccentric/concentric control
  - Promote push off and heel strike

FUNCTIONAL GOALS

- Patient will be able to
  - Achieve 5 degrees of rear-foot inversion to facilitate pain-free ambulation on uneven surfaces.
  - Maintain subtalar neutral for 1 minute during single-limb stance with eyes open.
  - Increase gait speed to ≥1.2 m per second to promote safe community ambulation.
  - Report ≤3 out of 10 pain rating at worst in order to return to work or school.

PROGNOSIS

- Good, though healing time for normal fracture varies with patient's age.
  - Children: 4 to 6 weeks healing time.
  - Adolescents: 6 to 8 weeks.
  - Adults: 10 to 18 weeks.
- Healing time varies based on the severity of injury.
  - Individuals with minor fracture will return to normal activities within 3 to 4 months.
  - Those with severe fractures may recover within 1 to 2 years.

PATIENT RESOURCE

- American Academy of Orthopaedic Surgeons. *Calcaneus (Heel bone) Fractures.* Available at: http://orthoinfo.aaos.org/topic.cfm?topic=A00524. Accessed August 9, 2014.

REFERENCES

1. The American Physical Therapy Association. Pattern 4G: Impaired joint mobility, muscle performance, and range of motion associated with fracture. *Interactive Guide to Physical Therapist Practice*. 2003. doi: 10.2522/ptguide.3.1_7. Accessed March 20, 2013.
2. Hall SJ. The biomechanics of human bone growth and development. *Basic Biomechanics.* 4th ed. New York, NY: McGraw-Hill; 2007:Chapter 4. http://www.accessphysiotherapy.com/abstract/6060836#6060838. Accessed March 20, 2013.
3. *Anatomy and Physiology Revealed.* McGraw-Hill; 2007. http://anatomy.mcgraw-hill.com/apt.html?login=1320061609064&system=Muscular§ion=Dissection&topic=Ankle%20and%20foot&topicAbbr=Ank&view=Superior%20and%20inferior&viewAbbr=Sin&catAbbr=Oth&grpAbbr=Ske&structure=Calcaneus. Accessed March 20, 2013.
4. Dutton M. *Orthopaedic Examination, Evaluation, and Intervention.* New York, NY: McGraw-Hill; 2008. http://www.accessphysiotherapy.com/resource/612. Accessed March 20, 2013.
5. Malone TR, Hazle C, Grey ML. *Imaging in Rehabilitation.* New York, NY: McGraw-Hill; 2008. http://www.accessphysiotherapy.com/resource/613. Accessed March 20, 2013.
6. Prentice WE, Blake B. The basic science of therapeutic modalities. In: Prentice WE, Quillen WS, Underwood F, eds. *Therapeutic Modalities in Rehabilitation.* 4th ed. New York, NY: McGraw-Hill; 2011:Chapter 1. http://www.accessphysiotherapy.com/abstract/8135087#8135091. Accessed March 20, 2013.
7. Prentice WE. Cryotherapy and thermotherapy. In: Prentice WE, Quillen WS, Underwood F, eds. *Therapeutic Modalities in Rehabilitation.* 4th ed. New York, NY: McGraw-Hill; 2011:Chapter 9. http://www.accessphysiotherapy.com/content/8137995#8137995. Accessed March 20, 2013.
8. Hooker DN, Prentice WE. Basic principles of electricity and electrical stimulating currents. In: Prentice WE, Quillen WS, Underwood F, eds. *Therapeutic Modalities in Rehabilitation.* 4th ed. New York, NY: McGraw-Hill; 2011:Chapter 5. http://www.accessphysiotherapy.com/content/8136367#8136367. Accessed March 20, 2013.
9. Dutton M. *McGraw Hill's NPTE (National Physical Therapy Examination).*2nd ed. New York, NY: McGraw-Hill; 2012. http://www.accessphysiotherapy.com/resource/611. Accessed March 20, 2013.

ADDITIONAL REFERENCES

- Dowling S, Spooner CH, Liang Y, et al. Accuracy of Ottawa Ankle Rules to exclude fractures of the ankle and midfoot in children: a meta-analysis. *Acad Emerg Med.* 2009;16(4): 277–287. doi:10.1111/j.1553-2712.2008.00333.x.
- Goodman CC, Boissonnault WG, Fuller KS. *Pathology: Implications for the Physical Therapist.* 2nd ed. Philadelphia, PA: Saunders; 2003.
- ICD9DATA. http://www.icd9data.com. Accessed August 9, 2014.
- ICD10DATA. http://www.icd10data.com. Accessed August 9, 2014.
- Kisner C, Colby LA. *Therapeutic Exercise: Foundations and Techniques.* 5th ed. Philadelphia, PA: F.A. Davis Company; 2007.
- Magee DJ. *Orthopedic Physical Assessment.* 5th ed. St. Louis, MO: Saunders Elsevier; 2008.

205 CLAW TOE

Eric Shamus, PhD, DPT, PT, CSCS
Colin Brooks, MBA, SPHR

ICD-9-CM CODES

- 735.5 Claw toe (acquired)
- 755.66 Other anomalies of toes

ICD-10-CM CODE

- M20.5X9 Other deformities of toe(s) (acquired), unspecified foot

PREFERRED PRACTICE PATTERN

- 4E: Impaired Joint Mobility, Motor Function, Muscle Performance, and Range of Motion Associated with Localized Inflammation

PATIENT PRESENTATION

A 33-year-old female presents with pain in her right foot. Patient states ever since she was 16 years old she has worn high heels and shoes that come with a point. She said over the last year she has noticed a cramping in her toes and a difficulty straightening out all of her toes. She is having difficulty with closed-toe shoes and standing for long periods of time. Upon examination it was found that she has a shortened flexor digitorum musculature with hyperextension (dorsiflexed) of the MTP joint with flexion (plantar flexed) of the proximal interphalangeal (PIP) joint, and the distal interphalangeal (DIP) joint is plantar flexed.

KEY FEATURES

Description

- Toe is bent into a claw-like position
- Flexor digitorum brevis contraction/shortening
- Hyperextension (dorsiflexed) of the MTP joint with flexion (plantar flexed) of the PIP, DIP is plantar flexed
- Flexor muscles, fascia, tendons shorten
- Most commonly affects the second toe; can also affect the third to fifth

Essentials of Diagnosis

- Diagnosis is usually made by clinical examination or X-ray.
- Can be an independent diagnosis and not associated with a disease process.

General Considerations

- Swelling
- Inflammation around the joint
- Can be associated with medical conditions
- Can be a flexible or fixed deformity

Demographics

- Infants
  - Congenital

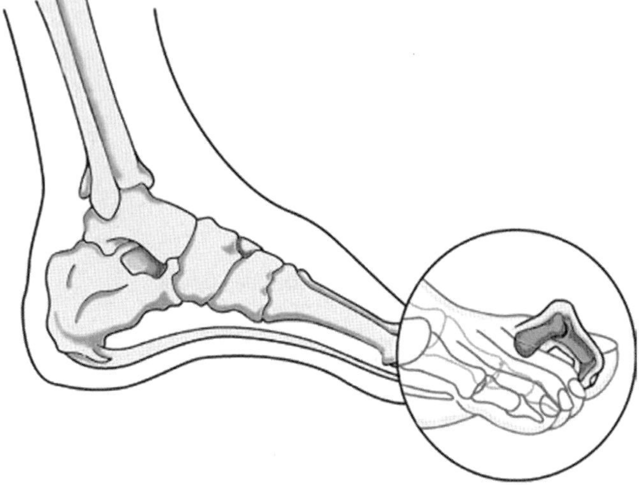

FIGURE 205-1 Claw toe. (From American Society of Orthopaedic Surgeons. http://orthoinfo.aaos.org/topic.cfm?topic=a00156. Accessed April 16, 2013)

- Children
  - Wearing footwear that is too small
- Adults
  - Poor footwear: Improper fit/toe comes to a point/narrow forefoot/high heels
  - Dancers

CLINICAL FINDINGS

SIGNS AND SYMPTOMS

- Pain in metatarsal with walking
- Corn on top of the toe
- Altered joint position
- Decreased extension or dorsiflexion of the toe
- Joint redness and pain
- Callus formation under the metatarsal head
- Difficulty finding shoes that fit properly
- Limited motion of the MTP joint

Functional Implications

- Pain with standing
- Pain with ambulation at the affected toe
- Inability to wear stiff shoes
- Need to wear larger shoes to accommodate bunion, large toe box
- Alteration of gait pattern and mechanical issues of the forefoot
- Altered mechanics during the push-off phase of gait

Possible Contributing Causes

- Muscle imbalance
- Trauma
- Tibia fracture
- Pes planus (flat foot)
- Improper footwear
- Commonly seen in conjunction of bunions

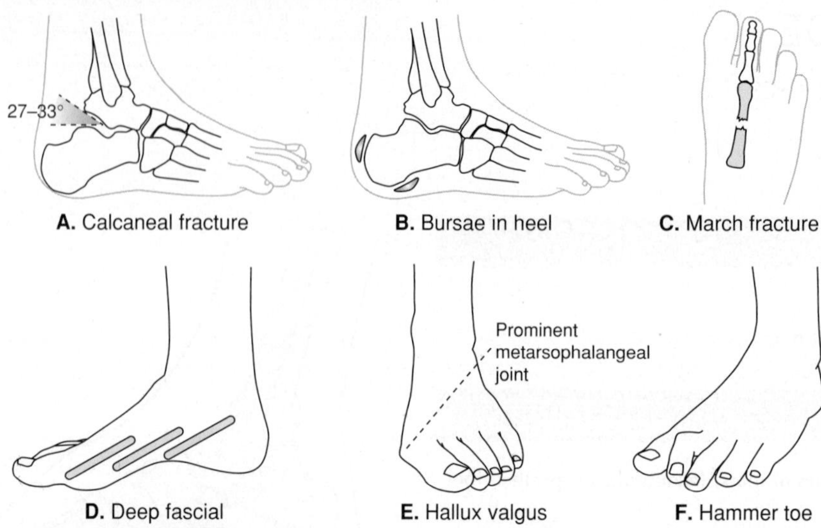

FIGURE 205-2 Lesions of the foot. (**A**) Calcaneal fracture. (**B**) Bursae in the heel. (**C**) March fracture of a metatarsal bone. (**D**) Deep fascial spaces of the foot. (**E**) Hallux valgus: This deformity shows lateral deviation of the great toe, with prominence of the first MTP joint. (**F**) Hammer toe: The second toe is always affected. There is permanent flexion of the PIP joint. (From LeBlond RF, DeGowin RL, Brown DD. *DeGowin's Diagnostic Examination*. 9th ed. http://www.accessmedicine.com. Copyright © The McGraw-Hill Companies, Inc. All rights reserved.)

- Joint arthritis/injury
- Muscle atrophy
- Nerve damage
- Spinal cord injury
- Friedreich ataxia
- Osteoarthritis
- Rheumatoid arthritis
- Stroke
- Charcot–Marie–Tooth disease
- Diabetes mellitus

▸ Differential Diagnosis

- Mallet toe: neutral MTP and PIP joint with flexion (plantar flexion) of only the DIP
- Hammer toe: neutral or dorsiflexed MTP, plantar flexed PIP and neutral or flexed DIP
- Hallux valgus
- Gout
- Osteochondrotic lesion of the first metatarsal head
- Sesamoiditis, turf toe
- Osteochondritis dissecans
- Metatarsalgia
- Metatarsal stress fracture

MEANS OF CONFIRMATION OR DIAGNOSIS

▸ Imaging

- X-ray

FINDINGS AND INTERPRETATION

- Bone spur, location and size

TREATMENT

▸ Surgical

- To straighten out the toe
  - Cut or lengthen tendons and ligaments
  - Fusion of the joint
  - Tendon transfer[1,2]

▸ Medication

- Anti-inflammatory

REFERRALS/ADMITTANCE

- For imaging, X-ray
- For medication, anti-inflammatory or corticosteroid injection
- For surgical consult[1]

IMPAIRMENTS

- Antalgic gait secondary to pain at the toe with push-off
- Hypomobility of the MTP joint
- Inability to ambulate distances of 1 mile secondary to pain

TESTS AND MEASURES

- PIP and DIP ROM
- LE limb strength
- Balance
  - Static single-leg standing (eyes open, eyes closed)
    - Contralateral LE
  - Dynamic standing
    - Berg Balance Scale
    - Functional Gait Assessment
- Gait assessment
  - Observational analysis
  - Gait speed via the 10-m walk test
  - 2-minute walk test
  - 6-minute walk test

INTERVENTION

- Rest, weight off feet will allow for reduction of inflammation
- Orthotics with ray cut out
- Swelling
  - Cryotherapy
- Pain
  - Ice
  - Massage/Myofascial release

- Joint mobilization
- Electrical stimulation
- Iontophoresis
- Infrared
- Weakness, joint instability
  - Strengthening
    - Toe curls and extension, flexor/extensor intrinsic
    - Calf raises to point
    - Active walking
    - Standing arch raises
- Lack of flexibility
  - Stretching
    - Toe intrinsic flexor stretching
    - Gastrocnemius-soleus in cases of Achilles contracture
    - Plantar fascia in patients with pes cavus
    - Fluidotherapy
    - Taping (kinesiotape for inhibition of the flexor tendon to allow for increased length)
- Joint mobilization
  - MTP dorsal/plantar and medial/lateral glides and rotation
  - Posterior talus glides
  - Subtalar joint (STJ) inversion/eversion
  - Navicular/cuboid/cuneiforms
- Soft tissue mobilization
  - Lumbrical/dorsal interossei
  - Plantar fascia
  - Gastrocnemius-soleus
- Patient education in footwear
  - Increased in box space
  - Shoe with a rocker bottom to limit first ray extension

FUNCTIONAL GOALS

- Patient will be able to
  - Recognize and maintain a subtalar neutral position for >2 minutes.
  - Ambulate pain free for >45 minutes.
  - Achieve 15 degrees of talocrural dorsiflexion during stance phase of gait.
  - Achieve pain-free toe extension during push-off phase of gait.
  - Stand in subtalar neutral for 1 minute with eyes open.

PROGNOSIS

- Good with flexible type.
- Surgery may be indicated if the flexion becomes severe and shoes cannot be worn.

PATIENT RESOURCE

- Claw Toe. American Academy of Orthopeadic Surgeons. http://orthoinfo.aaos.org/topic.cfm?topic=A00156. Accessed June 15, 2013.

REFERENCES

1. Errichiello C, Marcarelli M, Pisani PC, Parino E. Treatment of dynamic claw toe deformity flexor digitorum brevis tendon transfer to interosseous and lumbrical muscles: A literature survey. *Foot Ankle Surg*. 2012;18(4):229–232.
2. Fernandez CS, Wagner E, Ortiz C. Lesser toes proximal interphalangeal joint fusion in rigid claw toes. *Foot Ankle Clin*. 2012;17(3):473–480.

ADDITIONAL REFERENCES

- Dutton M. The ankle and foot. In: Dutton M, eds. *Orthopaedic Examination, Evaluation, and Intervention*. 2nd ed. New York, NY: McGraw-Hill; 2012. http://www.accessphysiotherapy.com/content/55586986#55586986. Accessed June 15, 2013.
- Hamilton N, Weimar W, Luttgens K. The kinesiology of fitness and exercise. In: Hamilton N, Weimar W, Luttgens K, eds. *Kinesiology: Scientific Basis of Human Motion*. 11th ed. New York, NY: McGraw-Hill; 2008. http://www.accessphysiotherapy.com/content/6151881#6151881. Accessed June 15, 2013.
- Hooker DN, Prentice WE. Basic principles of electricity and electrical stimulating currents. In: Prentice WE, Quillen WS, Underwood F, eds. *Therapeutic Modalities in Rehabilitation*. 4th ed. New York, NY: McGraw-Hill; 2011. http://www.accessphysiotherapy.com/content/8136028. Accessed June 15, 2013.
- Malone TR, Hazle C, Grey ML. The ankle and foot. In: Malone TR, Hazle C, Grey ML. *Imaging in Rehabilitation*. New York, NY: McGraw-Hill; 2008. http://www.accessphysiotherapy.com/content/5940167. Accessed June 15, 2013.
- Prentice WE. Cryotherapy and thermotherapy. In: Prentice WE, Quillen WS, Underwood F, eds. *Therapeutic Modalities in Rehabilitation*. 4th ed. New York, NY: McGraw-Hill; 2011. http://www.accessphysiotherapy.com/content/8138236#8138236. Accessed June 15, 2013.
- Prentice WE. Cryotherapy and thermotherapy. In: Prentice WE, Quillen WS, Underwood F, eds. *Therapeutic Modalities in Rehabilitation*. 4th ed. New York, NY: McGraw-Hill; 2011. http://www.accessphysiotherapy.com/content/8137946#8137946. Accessed June 15, 2013.
- Schrier JC, Verheyen CC, Louwerens JW. Definitions of hammer toe and claw toe: an evaluation of the literature. *J Am Podiatr Med Assoc*. 2009;99(3):194–197.

206 DELTOID LIGAMENT SPRAIN

Mitchell L. Cordova, PhD, ATC, FNATA, FACSM
Eric Shamus, PhD, DPT, PT, CSCS

CONDITION/DISORDER SYNONYMS

- Deltoid ligament sprain
- Medial ankle sprain
- Eversion ankle sprain

ICD-9-CM CODE

- 845.01 Sprain of deltoid (ligament), ankle

ICD-10-CM CODE

- S93.429A Sprain of deltoid ligament of unspecified ankle, initial encounter

PREFERRED PRACTICE PATTERN

- 4E: Impaired Joint Mobility, Motor Function, Muscle Performance, and Range of Motion Associated with Connective Tissue Dysfunction

PATIENT PRESENTATION

Patient is a 22-year-old collegiate basketball player who landed on another player's foot when coming down with a rebound. The player felt immediate pain and was taken to the locker room for X-rays. The X-rays were negative for fracture. The patient presents with Grade-2 laxity of the deltoid ligament with a positive medial talar tilt test. The patient has difficulty with weight bearing and is wearing a walking boot. There is pain and tenderness along the medial ankle.

KEY FEATURES

Description

- Disruption of deltoid ligament complex of the medial ankle
  - May be acute or chronic.
- Deltoid ligament complex
  - Restricts medial translation of the calcaneus on the talus.
  - Can rupture during forced dorsiflexion of the ankle and eversion of the foot.
  - Can also rupture during excessive external rotation of the talus with or without eversion of the foot.
  - Commonly injured during a lateral malleolus fracture where the talus is rapidly displaced against the fibula during excessive dorsiflexion.
- Severity of the injury will dictate the signs and symptoms that are observed.
- In mild to moderate sprains, pain occurs during passive dorsiflexion and eversion.

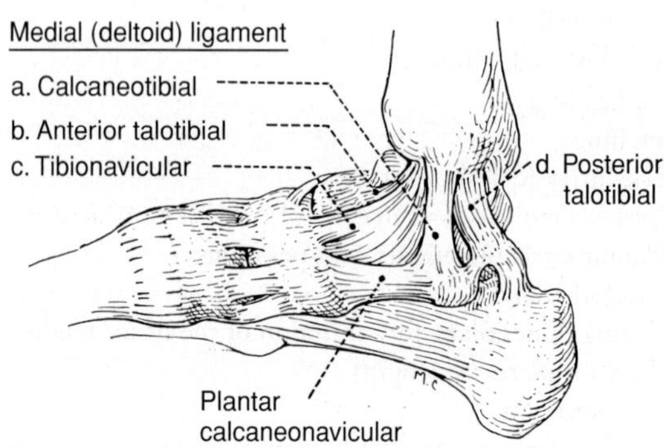

FIGURE 206-1 Medial ligaments of ankle joint. (From Hamilton N, Weimar W, Luttgens K. *Kinesiology: Scientific Basis of Human Motion*. 11th ed. http://www.accessphysiotherapy.com. Copyright © McGraw-Hill Education. All rights reserved.)

- In severe sprains, swelling may be present over the posterior to the lateral malleolus, and deep to the medial in the posteromedial aspect of the distal leg.

Essentials of Diagnosis

- First step being to rule out a fracture or syndesmotic ankle sprain
- Positive Posterior Drawer test and medial talar tilt test
- Positive Kleiger test (external rotation test)
- Ultrasonography (US), radiography, or MRI may be utilized in select cases[1]
  - US or MRI recommended following a medial ankle sprain in a patient with chronic ankle instability[1]
  - Radiographs utilized within the constraints of Ottawa Ankle Rules[2]
- Deltoid ligament complex tears classified based on the anatomical degree of damage or functional stability found on clinical exam[2]
  - Anatomical:
    - Grade 1: Partial microscopic tearing of the ligament, minimal to no loss of function, mild swelling and pain
    - Grade 2: Partial macroscopic tearing of the ligament, with mild–moderate loss of function, moderate swelling/pain/tenderness
    - Grade 3: Complete rupture with severe loss of function, severe swelling/pain/tenderness
  - Functional stability:
    - Stable: No laxity with talar tilt or anterior drawer testing (Grade I)
    - Unstable: Laxity with the anterior drawer testing (ATFL, Grade II); laxity with both the anterior drawer and talar tilt (ATFL and CF, Grade III)

General Considerations

- Deltoid ligament, made up of two short bands of ligaments that run superficial and deep to the medial capsule of the ankle joint

- May occur with concomitant syndemosis sprain, lateral malleolus fracture, or chondral lesion
- Medial ankle sprains are not very common. They account for ~10 to 15% of all ankle sprains.[3,4]
- Medial ankle sprains are usually more severe and result in significantly greater time lost to injury than lateral ankle sprains[3,4]

Demographics

- Prevalent in athletes, though does occur in sedentary individuals
  - Most common in basketball, soccer, and football[5]
- Males between 15 to 24 years of age have higher rates of ankle sprains than female counterparts; females over 30 years old have higher rates than male counterparts[5]
- Male sex, higher level of competition, and exposure to certain sports are the greatest risk factors for a medial ankle sprain[6]

CLINICAL FINDINGS

SIGNS AND SYMPTOMS

- Pain in the medial and/posterior ankle or foot
  - Grade 1: Minimal
  - Grade 2: Moderate
  - Grade 3: Severe
- Pain with palpation of deltoid ligament complex, posteromedial aspect of distal leg
- May posture in greater supination to avoid dorsiflexion eversion moments
- Edema medial ankle and perhaps lateral ankle with lateral malleolus fracture
  - Grade 1: Minimal
  - Grade 2: Moderate
  - Grade 3: Severe
- Possible inability to bear partial or full weight
- Guarded active/passive inversion ROM
- May have increased inversion passive ROM (positive talar tilt test)
- Decreased active/passive ankle dorsiflexion ROM
- Decreased tibialis posterior/foot inversion strength
- In moderate to severe cases, increased talar anterior glide on mortise (positive anterior drawer test)

Functional Implications

- Loss of functional ability
  - Grade 1: Minimal
  - Grade 2: Some
  - Grade 3: Great
- Inability to stand secondary to weight bearing
  - Grade 1: Never
  - Grade 2: Usually
  - Grade 3: Almost always
- Reduced midstance time during ambulation
- Reduced contralateral step length
- Impaired single-limb balance
- Inability to execute cutting maneuvers

Possible Contributing Causes

- Intrinsic risk factors
  - Prior ankle sprains
  - Decreased dorsiflexion ROM and strength[7]
  - Decreased everter-to-inverter muscle function ratio[7]
  - Pes cavus
  - Impaired proprioception/balance[7]
  - Obesity[7]
- Extrinsic risk factors
  - Equipment
    - High-heel shoes
    - Noncompliance with reinjury prevention strategies such as bracing
  - Environmental factors
    - Uneven playing field or surface
    - Artificial turf[7]
  - Sport position; participation in sport at the beginning of the season or at the end of game[8]

Differential Diagnosis

- Deltoid ligament sprain
- Posterior talofibular ligament sprain
- Syndesmotic ankle sprain
- Lateral malleolus fracture
- Navicular fracture
- Talus fracture
- Chondral lesion
- Ostechondritis dissecans
- Talotibial impingement syndrome
- Synovitis
- Avulsion fracture of medial malleolus
- S1 radiculopathy

MEANS OF CONFIRMATION OR DIAGNOSIS

Laboratory Tests

- None

Imaging[9]

- Additional imaging warranted if the patient meets the Ottawa Ankle Rules, presents with a possible dislocation, or has positive syndesmotic ankle sprain tests[2]
- Ultrasonography (US) (sn = 92%, sp = 83%)
- MRI (ankle series) (sn = 95%, sp = 50%)
- Arthrogram (sn = 100%)
- 3D CT (sp = 94.4%)
- Radiographs with use of Ottawa Ankle Rules, taken anterior–posterior with 10 to 20 degrees of internal rotation (sn = 100%, sp = 40%)

FINDINGS AND INTERPRETATION

- Imaging for isolated deltoid sprains will reveal increased signal uptake, wavy or curved contour, or disruption of the ligament's integrity on MRI and CT.
- US presents a torn deltoid ligament as discontinuous bundles and a hypoechoic lesion.[9]
  - Further studies are needed to confirm the routine use of US for deltoid ligament tears.
  - MRIs implemented in deltoid ligament tears with suspected chondral lesions or chronic instability.[2]

TREATMENT

Medication

- Nonsteroidal anti-inflammatory medications

MEDICAL PROCEDURES

- Deltoid ligament reconstruction only in chronic cases not responding to conservative management
- Therapeutic hyaluronic acid injections (limited evidence)

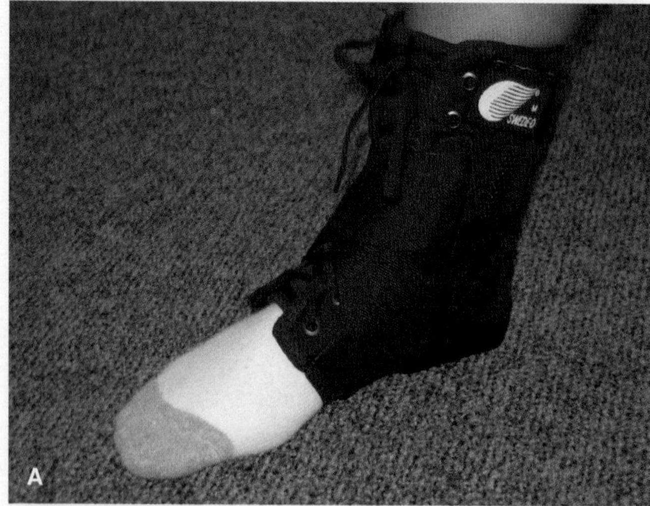

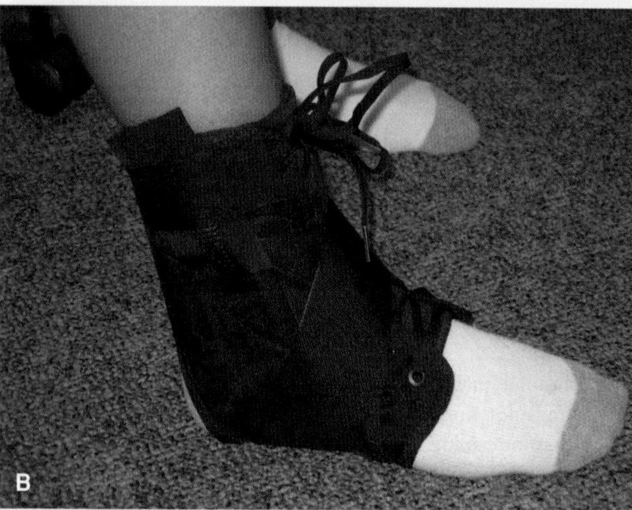

FIGURE 206-2 Lace up braces. (From Patel DR, Greydanus DE, Baker RJ. *Pediatric Practice: Sports Medicine*. http://www.accesspediatrics.com. Copyright © The McGraw-Hill Companies, Inc. All rights reserved.)

REFERRALS/ADMITTANCE

- For MRI[3]
- For surgery
- For injection

IMPAIRMENTS

- Edema medial and lateral ankle
- May have increased eversion passive ROM (positive talar tilt test—medial)
- Decreased active/passive dorsiflexion ROM
- Decreased tibialis posterior strength
- Difficulty weight bearing
- In moderate to severe cases, increased talar anterior glide on mortise (positive anterior drawer test)
- Reduced posterior glide of distal fibula on tibia
- Gait dysfunction
- Reduced single-limb balance

TESTS AND MEASURES

- Self-report patient-specific measures of health-related quality of life[2]
  - Patient-specific functional scale (PSFS)
- Performance-based measures
  - Two-minute walk test
  - Six-minute walk test
- Neurologic examination
  - Sensation
    - Light touch
    - Pin prick
- Palpation of ankle
- Eversion ankle strength
- Ankle ROM
  - Inversion: Hindfoot 20 degrees
  - Eversion: Pronation 10 degrees
  - Dorsiflexion: 20 degrees
  - Plantar flexion: 30 to 50 degrees
- Anterior drawer test
- Eversion stress test
- Talar tilt
- External rotation stress test
- Gait assessment
- Foot and Ankle Ability Measure (FAAM)
- Balance
  - Static and dynamic sitting
    - Sitting functional reach
  - Static single-leg standing (eyes open, eyes closed)
    - Single-limb stance
    - Star Excursion Balance Test (SEBT)
  - Dynamic standing (with prosthesis)
    - Berg Balance Scale
    - Gait Assessment Rating Score
    - Rancho Los Amigo observational gait analysis
    - Multi-directional reach test (MDRT)

INTERVENTION

- If the initial exam is limited due to pain and syndesmotic ankle sprain testing cannot be done.
  - Recommended to allow patient to protect, rest, ice, compress, elevate (PRICE) and use crutches (if needed) for 3 to 5 days; after this period, re-examination is warranted to screen for a syndesmotic ankle sprain, which warrants an ankle MRI series.[2]
- PRICE for acute stage (moderate evidence)
  - Short-term semirigid bracing superior to taping[2]
  - Decreases pain
  - Improves function
- Early functional treatment (moderate evidence)
  - Promote weight bearing as long as gait pattern is normal
  - Use assistive device if gait deviations exist
  - Implement supervised early active ROM and weight-bearing proprioception/neuromuscular exercises
  - Increases strength
  - Increases ROM, decreases swelling, return to normal gait
- Balance and coordination exercises: 6 to 8 weeks or longer (strong evidence)
  - Improves balance function
  - Increases strength
  - Dynamic and static tasks
  - Can prevent reinjury (not for chronic ankle instability)
- Taping, bracing, wrapping (moderate evidence)
  - Improves swelling, subjective stability

- Bracing superior to taping based on costeffectiveness and ease[2]
- Ankle bracing effective in reducing ROM before and after exercise[10]

- Manual intervention (moderate evidence[11])
  - Mobilization with movement to promote posterior talar gliding[12]
  - Posterior mobilization of fibula on tibia
  - Reduces pain, improves ankle dorsiflexion, improves stride speed
- Ultrasound for acute injury (limited evidence)
- Electrotherapy or hyperbaric treatments (limited evidence)[11]

FUNCTIONAL GOALS

- Patient will be able to
  - Ascend/descend a standard height curb.
  - Ambulate over uneven surfaces such as the transition from tile to carpet or up and down a ramp.
  - Ambulate household distances.
  - Stand and walk without limitation due to pain or edema for more than 1 hour.
  - Demonstrate full contralateral step length.
  - Demonstrate 15 degrees of talocrural dorsiflexion during stance phase of gait.
  - Demonstrate 5/5 manual muscle testing of tibialis posterior to promote neutral subtalar joint during stance phase of gait.
  - Demonstrate in-line jogging at 5.0 mph for 1 mile without limitation due to pain.
  - Complete cutting maneuvers for sport or work without compensatory movement patterns or pain.
  - Demonstrate SEBT on involved side without limitation due to pain or instability.

PROGNOSIS

- Inversely proportional to severity.
- Acute injury.
  - Excellent nonsurgical, active conservative care.
  - No additional benefit of adding surgery to conservative care for deltoid ligament sprains.[13]
  - Significant functional, pain, and impairment reduction at 1 week with anatomical Grades I to II.
  - The percent of athletes that develop chronic ankle instability from an eversion ankle sprain is not widely known.
  - Prevention of reinjury through semirigid ankle bracing.
- Chronic injury/instability.
  - May respond to conservative care, such as balance/coordination exercises.
  - Patients that fail conservative care have good outcomes with surgical intervention.

ADDITIONAL INFORMATION

Case study of electrical stimulation for controlling ankle swelling, www.accessphysiotherapy.com

PATIENT RESOURCE

- Ankle Sprain (Medial Ligament). PhysioAdvisor. http://www.physioadvisor.com.au/8047221/physioadvisor-ankle-sprain-ankle-pain-treatmen.htm. Accessed June 20, 2013.

REFERENCES

1. Guillodo Y, Riban P, Guennoc X, Dubrana F, Saraux A. Usefulness of ultrasonographic detection of talocrural effusion in ankle sprains. *J Ultrasound Med*. 2007;26(6):831–836.
2. Polzer H, Kanz KG, Prall WC, et al. Diagnosis and treatment of acute ankle injuries: development of an evidence-based algorithm. *Orthop Rev (Pavia)*. 2012;4(1):e5. doi: 10.4081/or.2012.e5.
3. Fallat L, Grimm DJ, Saracco JA. Sprained ankle syndrome: prevalence and analysis of 639 acute injuries. *J Foot Ankle Surg*. 1998;37:280–285.
4. Gerber JP, Williams GN, Scoville CR, Arciero RA, Taylor DC. Persistent disability with ankle sprains: a prospective examination of an athletic population. *Foot Ankle Int*. 1998;19(10): 653–660.
5. Waterman BR, Owens BD, Davey S, Zacchilli MA, Belmont PJ Jr. The epidemiology of ankle sprains in the United States. *J Bone Joint Surg Am*. 2010;92(13):2279–2284. doi: 10.2106/JBJS.I.01537.
6. Waterman BR, Belmont PJ Jr, Cameron KL, Svoboda SJ, Alitz CJ, Owens BD. Risk factors of syndesmotic and medial ankle sprain: role of sex, sport, and level of competition. *Am J Sports Med*. 2011;39(5):992–998. doi: 10.1177/0363546510391462.
7. Fong DT, Chan YY, Mok KM, Yung PS, Chan KM. Understanding acute ankle ligamentous sprain injury in sports. *Sports Med Arthrosc Rehabil Ther Technol*. 2009;1:14. doi: 10.1186/1758-2555-1-14.
8. Kofotolis ND, Kellis E, Vlachopoulos SP. Ankle Sprain Injuries and Risk Factors in Amateur Soccer Players During a 2-Year Period. *Am J Sports Med*. 2007;35(3):458–466.
9. Oae K, Takao M, Uchio Y, Ochi M. Evaluation of anterior talofibular ligament injury with stress radiography, ultrasonography and MR imaging. *Skeletal Radiol*. 2010;39(1):41–47. doi: 10.1007/s00256-009-0767-x.
10. Cordova ML, Ingersoll CD, LeBlanc MJ. Influence of ankle support on joint range of motion before and after exercise: a meta-analysis. *J Orthop Sports Phys Ther*. 2000;30(4):170–177; discussion 178–82.
11. Bleakley CM, McDonough SM, MacAuley DC. Some conservative strategies are effective when added to controlled mobilisation with external support after acute ankle sprain: a systematic review. *Aust J Physiother*. 2008;54(1):7–20.
12. Vicenzino B, Branjerdporn M, Teys P, Jordan K. Initial changes in posterior talar glide and dorsiflexion of the ankle after mobilization with movement in individuals with recurrent ankle sprain. *J Orthop Sports Phys Ther*. 2006;36(7):464–471.
13. Kamper SJ, Grootjans SJ. Surgical versus conservative treatment for acute ankle sprains. *Br J Sports Med*. 2012;46(1):77–78. doi: 10.1136/bjsports-2011-090722.

ADDITIONAL REFERENCES

- Dutton M. Common Orthopedic Conditions. In: Dutton M, ed. *Dutton's Orthopedic Survival Guide: Managing Common Conditions*. New York, NY: McGraw-Hill; 2011. http://www.accessphysiotherapy.com/content/8655656. Accessed June 20, 2013.
- Hamilton N, Weimar W, Luttgens K. The ankle. In: Hamilton N, Weimar W, Luttgens K, eds. *Kinesiology: Scientific Basis of Human Motion*. New York, NY: McGraw-Hill; 2008. http://www.accessphysiotherapy.com/content/6153087. Accessed June 20, 2013.

- Hay WW, Levin MJ, Sondheimer JM, Deterding RR. Foot & ankle injuries. In: Hay WW, Levin MJ, Sondheimer JM, Deterding RR, eds. *CURRENT Diagnosis & Treatment: Pediatrics*. 20th ed. New York, NY: McGraw-Hill; 2011. http://www.accessphysiotherapy.com/content/6586350. Accessed June 20, 2013.
- Hooker DN, Prentice WE. Chapter 5. Basic principles of electricity and electrical stimulating currents. In: Prentice WE, Quillen WS, Underwood F, eds. *Therapeutic Modalities in Rehabilitation*. 4th ed. New York, NY: McGraw-Hill; 2011. http://www.accessphysiotherapy.com/content/8136027. Accessed June 20, 2013.
- Mulligan B. *Manual therapy, 'NAGs,' 'SNAGs,' and 'MWMs,'* etc. 6th ed. Wellington: Plane View Services; 2010.
- Myerson M. *Foot and Ankle Disorders*. Philadelphia: W.B. Saunders Company; 2000.
- Seah R, Mani-Babu S. Managing ankle sprains in primary care: what is best practice? A systematic review of the last 10 years of evidence. *Br Med Bull*. 2011;97:105–135. doi: 10.1093/bmb/ldq028.
- Simon RR, Sherman SC. Ankle soft-tissue injury and dislocation. In: Simon RR, Sherman SC, eds. *Emergency Orthopedics*. 6th ed. New York, NY: McGraw-Hill; 2011. http://www.accessphysiotherapy.com/content/7708597. Accessed June 20, 2013.
- van den Bekerom MP, van der Windt DA, ter Riet G, van der Heijden GJ, Bouter LM. Therapeutic ultrasound for acute ankle sprains. *Cochrane Database of Systematic Reviews*. 2011;(6):CD001250. doi: 10.1002/14651858.CD001250.pub2.
- Zech A, Hubscher M, Vogt L, Banzer W, Hansel F, Pfeifer K. Neuromuscular training for rehabilitation of sports injuries: a systematic review. *Med Sci Sports Exerc*. 2009;41(10):1831–1841. doi: 10.1249/MSS.0b013e3181a3cf0d.

207 FOOT FRACTURE

Jennifer Cabrera, DPT, GCS
Eric Shamus, PhD, DPT, PT, CSCS

CONDITION/DISORDER SYNONYMS

- Lisfranc fracture (transmetatarsal)
- Fifth metatarsal fracture
- Navicular fracture
- Talar fracture
- Shepard fracture: Posterior process of the talus
- Toe fracture
- Metatarsal fracture

ICD-9-CM CODES

- 825 Fracture of one or more tarsal and metatarsal bones
- 825.0 Fracture of calcaneus closed
- 825.1 Fracture of calcaneus open
- 825.2 Fracture of other tarsal and metatarsal bones closed
- 825.20 Fracture of unspecified bone(s) of foot (except toes) closed
- 825.21 Fracture of astragalus closed
- 825.22 Fracture of navicular (scaphoid) bone of foot closed
- 825.23 Fracture of cuboid bone closed
- 825.24 Fracture of cuneiform bone of foot closed
- 825.25 Fracture of metatarsal bone(s) closed
- 825.29 Other fracture of tarsal and metatarsal bones closed
- 825.3 Fracture of other tarsal and metatarsal bones open
- 825.30 Fracture of unspecified bone(s) of foot (except toes) open
- 825.31 Fracture of astragalus open
- 825.32 Fracture of navicular (scaphoid) bone of foot open
- 825.33 Fracture of cuboid bone open
- 825.34 Fracture of cuneiform bone of foot open
- 825.35 Fracture of metatarsal bone(s) open
- 825.39 Other fractures of tarsal and metatarsal bones open
- 826 Fracture of one or more phalanges of foot
- 826.0 Closed fracture of one or more phalanges of foot
- 826.1 Open fracture of one or more phalanges of foot

ICD-10-CM CODES

- S92.009A Unspecified fracture of unspecified calcaneus, initial encounter for closed fracture
- S92.009B Unspecified fracture of unspecified calcaneus, initial encounter for open fracture
- S92.909A Unspecified fracture of unspecified foot, initial encounter for closed fracture
- S92.109A Unspecified fracture of unspecified talus, initial encounter for closed fracture
- S92.253A Displaced fracture of navicular [scaphoid] of unspecified foot, initial encounter for closed fracture
- S92.256A Nondisplaced fracture of navicular [scaphoid] of unspecified foot, initial encounter for closed fracture
- S92.213A Displaced fracture of cuboid bone of unspecified foot, initial encounter for closed fracture

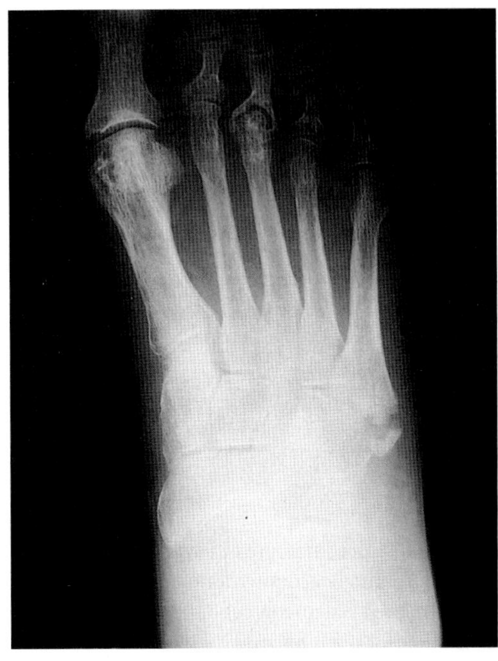

FIGURE 207-1 Fifth metatarsal avulsion fracture. Radiograph illustrating an avulsion-type fracture of the fifth metatarsal base. (From Knoop KJ, Stack LB, Storrow AB, Thurman RJ. *The Atlas of Emergency Medicine*. 3rd ed. http://www.accessmedicine.com. Copyright © The McGraw-Hill Companies, Inc. All rights reserved. Photo contributor: Alan B. Storrow, MD.)

- S92.216A Nondisplaced fracture of cuboid bone of unspecified foot, initial encounter for closed fracture
- S92.223A Displaced fracture of lateral cuneiform of unspecified foot, initial encounter for closed fracture
- S92.226A Nondisplaced fracture of lateral cuneiform of unspecified foot, initial encounter for closed fracture
- S92.233A Displaced fracture of intermediate cuneiform of unspecified foot, initial encounter for closed fracture
- S92.236A Nondisplaced fracture of intermediate cuneiform of unspecified foot, initial encounter for closed fracture
- S92.243A Displaced fracture of medial cuneiform of unspecified foot, initial encounter for closed fracture
- S92.246A Nondisplaced fracture of medial cuneiform of unspecified foot, initial encounter for closed fracture
- S92.309A Fracture of unspecified metatarsal bone(s), unspecified foot, initial encounter for closed fracture
- S92.209A Fracture of unspecified tarsal bone(s) of unspecified foot, initial encounter for closed fracture
- S92.309A Fracture of unspecified metatarsal bone(s), unspecified foot, initial encounter for closed fracture
- S92.909B Unspecified fracture of unspecified foot, initial encounter for open fracture
- S92.109B Unspecified fracture of unspecified talus, initial encounter for open fracture
- S92.253B Displaced fracture of navicular [scaphoid] of unspecified foot, initial encounter for open fracture

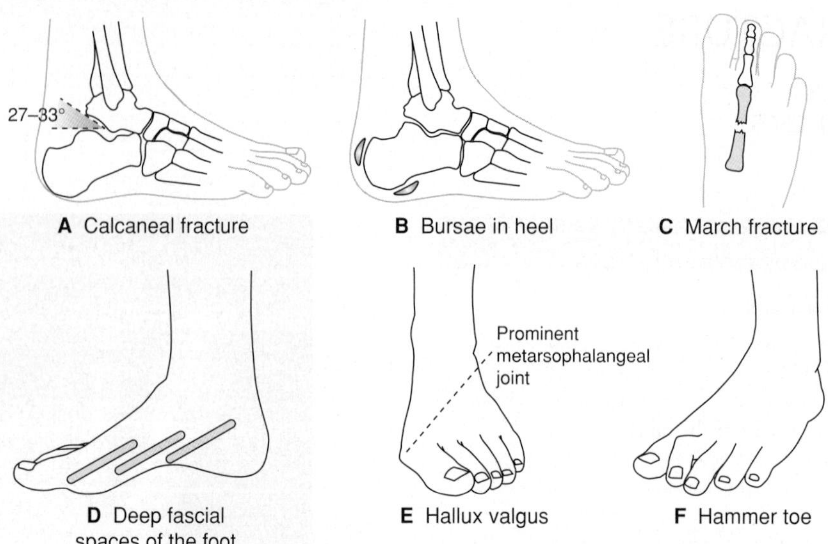

FIGURE 207-2 Lesions of the foot. (**A**) Calcaneal fracture. (**B**) Bursae in the heel. (**C**) March fracture of a metatarsal bone. (**D**) Deep fascial spaces of the foot. (**E**) Hallux valgus: This deformity shows lateral deviation of the great toe with prominence of the first MTP joint. (**F**) Hammer toe: The second toe is always affected. There is permanent flexion of the PIP joint. (From LeBlond RF, DeGowin RL, Brown DD. *DeGowin's Diagnostic Examination*. 9th ed. http://www.accessmedicine.com. Copyright © The McGraw-Hill Companies, Inc. All rights reserved.)

- S92.256B Nondisplaced fracture of navicular [scaphoid] of unspecified foot, initial encounter for open fracture
- S92.213B Displaced fracture of cuboid bone of unspecified foot, initial encounter for open fracture
- S92.216B Nondisplaced fracture of cuboid bone of unspecified foot, initial encounter for open fracture
- S92.223B Displaced fracture of lateral cuneiform of unspecified foot, initial encounter for open fracture
- S92.226B Nondisplaced fracture of lateral cuneiform of unspecified foot, initial encounter for open fracture
- S92.233B Displaced fracture of intermediate cuneiform of unspecified foot, initial encounter for open fracture
- S92.236B Nondisplaced fracture of intermediate cuneiform of unspecified foot, initial encounter for open fracture
- S92.243B Displaced fracture of medial cuneiform of unspecified foot, initial encounter for open fracture
- S92.246B Nondisplaced fracture of medial cuneiform of unspecified foot, initial encounter for open fracture
- S92.309B Fracture of unspecified metatarsal bone(s), unspecified foot, initial encounter for open fracture
- S92.209B Fracture of unspecified tarsal bone(s) of unspecified foot, initial encounter for open fracture
- S92.309B Fracture of unspecified metatarsal bone(s), unspecified foot, initial encounter for open fracture
- S92.403A Displaced unspecified fracture of unspecified great toe, initial encounter for closed fracture
- S92.406A Nondisplaced unspecified fracture of unspecified great toe, initial encounter for closed fracture
- S92.503A Displaced unspecified fracture of unspecified lesser toe(s), initial encounter for closed fracture
- S92.506A Nondisplaced unspecified fracture of unspecified lesser toe(s), initial encounter for closed fracture
- S92.403B Displaced unspecified fracture of unspecified great toe, initial encounter for open fracture
- S92.406B Nondisplaced unspecified fracture of unspecified great toe, initial encounter for open fracture

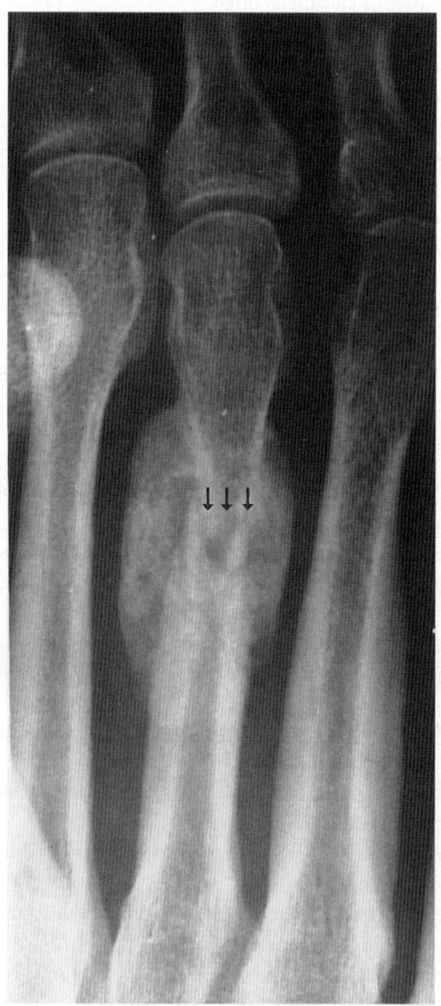

FIGURE 207-3 Stress fracture. Oblique view of the third metatarsal. This typical healing stress fracture demonstrates both a transverse fracture oriented perpendicular to the shaft (arrows), and abundant calus formation. (From Chen MYM, Pope TL, Ott DJ. *Basic Radiology*. 2nd ed. http://www.accessmedicine.com. Copyright © The McGraw-Hill Companies, Inc. All rights reserved.)

- S92.503B Displaced unspecified fracture of unspecified lesser toe(s), initial encounter for open fracture
- S92.506B Nondisplaced unspecified fracture of unspecified lesser toe(s), initial encounter for open fracture

PREFERRED PRACTICE PATTERN

- 4G: Impaired Joint Mobility, Muscle Performance, and Range of Motion Associated with Fracture[1]

PATIENT PRESENTATION

A 78-year-old woman has extensive history of uncontrolled type II diabetes with diabetic neuropathy and bilateral Charcot foot deformity. She receives home health nursing services for insulin administration, but does not regulate her diet. She presented with erythema and swelling of the foot without pain. These symptoms began shortly after she tripped on a curb outside her home 3 days ago. Patient was positive for Ottawa Foot Rules and referred to walk into the clinic for an X-ray. Radiographs showed a navicular fracture.

KEY FEATURES

Description

- Fracture of any of the 26 bones of the foot[2]
- Any defect in continuity of the tarsal or metatarsal bones
- Displaced (tarsal/metatarsal bone is moved on either side of the fracture) or nondisplaced (tarsal/metatarsal bone is not moved)
- Closed (skin intact) or open (skin breached)

Essentials of Diagnosis

- Diagnosis usually made by clinical examination
- May be Morton neuroma, rather than a fracture

General Considerations

- Stress fractures of the foot develop from overuse (e.g., high-impact sports)[3]

Demographics

- Affects all ages

CLINICAL FINDINGS

SIGNS AND SYMPTOMS

- Persistent foot pain
- Instability
- Pain
  - May diminish with rest if individual suffering from stress fracture
- Increased pain on weight bearing
- Edema
- Redness
- Ecchymosis
- Fracture blister
- Loss of general function
- Loss of active mobility
- Muscle guarding with passive movement
- Bone deformity
- Point tenderness over the base of the fifth metatarsal (fifth metatarsal potential fracture)
- Point tenderness over the navicular bone (navicular bone potential fracture)

Functional Implications

- Pain with standing
- Inability to bear weight on injured lower extremity

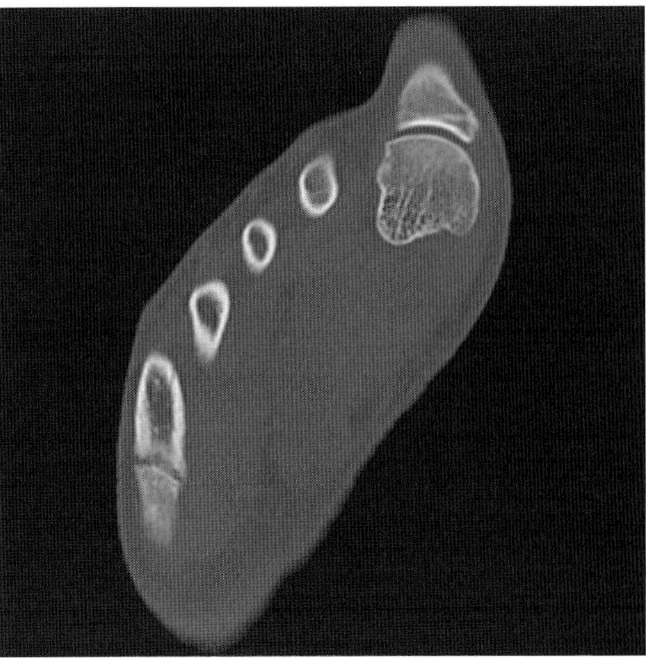

FIGURE 207-4 Greater detail by CT of the fifth metatarsal reveals a more apparent fracture line. Close inspection demonstrates subtle suggestions of sclerosis along the fracture line, which is consistent with nonunion. (From Malone TR, Hazle C, Grey ML. *Imaging in Rehabilitation*. http://www.accessphysiotherapy.com. Copyright © The McGraw-Hill Companies, Inc. All rights reserved.)

Possible Contributing Causes

- History of high-impact activities
- Trauma
- History of falls
- Osteoporosis
- History or chronic overuse (e.g., dancing)

Differential Diagnosis

- Ankle sprain
- Bone dislocation
- Compartment syndrome
- Morton neuroma
- Plantar fasciitis
- Stress fracture
- Heel spur
- Calcaneal fracture
- Metabolic disorder

MEANS OF CONFIRMATION

Imaging

- X-ray for fracture
  - Ottawa Foot Rules
  - Often limited view[4]
- CT scan for detailed imaging[3]
- Bone scan if stress fracture suspected[5]
- Ultrasonography

FINDINGS AND INTERPRETATION

- Antalgic gait sequence
- Decreased stance-time on injured lower extremity secondary to pain

- Exposed bone in the case of open and displaced fracture
- Possible integumentary deformity over underlying fracture
- If vascular structures are involved, foot will appear cool and pale
- If neurologic structures are involved, individual will report numbness and decreased ability to move the foot or toes

REFERRALS/ADMITTANCE

- For imaging: X-ray or CT[4]
- For medication: NSAIDs or opioid for pain management
- For orthopedic consult
  - Fracture reduction
    - Surgical intervention: Open reduction and internal fixation (ORIF)
    - Immobilization with casting/splinting of the foot

IMPAIRMENTS

- Antalgic gait secondary to pain causing inability to push off
- Inability to ambulate long distances secondary to pain or decreased weight-bearing status, which make ambulating difficult
- Decreased stance-time on affected lower extremity during ambulation
- Inability to stand for long periods of time secondary to pain

TESTS AND MEASURES

- Gait assessment (with appropriate assistive device and/or prosthesis)
  - Observational analysis
  - Gait speed via the 10-m walk test
  - 2-minute walk test
  - 6-minute walk test
- Balance
  - Static single-leg standing (eyes open, eyes closed)
  - Dynamic standing (with prosthesis)
    - Berg Balance Scale
    - Gait Assessment Rating Score
    - Rancho Los Amigo observational gait analysis
    - Multidirectional reach test (MDRT)
- Pain with resistance
- Calcaneal squeeze test to produce heel pain
- Palpation of pulses in the foot
- Capillary refill
- Manual muscle test (MMT)
- Functional strength testing
  - Five-times-sit-to-stand test

INTERVENTION

- Depending on the type of fracture, more severe cases require ORIF
- Ultrasound to stimulate fracture healing in skeletally mature individuals[6]
- Med-surg/post-op boot to decrease pressure on forefoot and heel
- Orthotics to provide proper arch support with neutral subtalar positioning so as to avoid stressing injured structures[7]
- Address swelling
  - Ice/Cryotherapy[8]
  - Compression
  - Elevation
  - Electrical stimulation[9]
- Address pain
  - Ice/Cryotherapy[8]
  - Massage
  - Electrical stimulation[9]
- Address mobilization
  - Anterior/Posterior distal tibiofibular glide in order to increase dorsiflexion
  - Dorsal talocrural glide to increase dorsiflexion
  - Ventral talocrural glide to increase plantarflexion
  - Gentle talocrural distraction for pain control
  - Subtalar distraction for general inversion or eversion
  - Medial subtalar glide for eversion
  - Lateral subtalar glide for inversion
  - Intertarsal and tarsometatarsal plantar glides for supination
  - Intertarsal and tarsometatarsal dorsal glides for pronation
- Address lack of flexibility via stretching
  - Gastrocnemius
  - Soleus
  - Plantar fascia
- Address weakness via strengthening activities
  - Open-chain ankle movements in all planes with resistance bands
  - Heel raises
  - Toe raises
  - Toe curls, intrinsic flexors
  - Active positioning of foot in subtalar neutral
- Address proprioception[9]
  - Standing balance activities with foam
    - Eyes open
    - Eyes closed
  - Standing balance activities on balance machines
- Gait training[10]
  - Lateral weight shifting to promote stance-time on injured lower extremity
  - Resisted walking to promote proper gait sequence with eccentric/concentric control
  - Promote push-off and heel strike

FUNCTIONAL GOALS

- Patient will be able to
  - Achieve 15 degrees of forefoot eversion in order to facilitate ambulation on uneven surfaces.
  - Maintain subtalar neutral for 1 minute during single-limb stance with eyes open.
  - Increase speed of gait to 1.2 m/s or greater in order to promote safe community ambulation.
  - Report, at worst, 0 to 3 out of 10 pain rating during high-impact activities (e.g., basketball, gymnastics, dancing, tennis, track and field).

PROGNOSIS

- Good, though normal fracture healing time varies with individual's age.
  - Children: 4 to 6 weeks.
  - Adolescents: 6 to 8 weeks.
  - Adults: 10 to 18 weeks.
- Prognosis for stress fracture varies due to gradual healing nature of the injury and importance of rest on the healing process.

PATIENT RESOURCE

- American Academy of Orthopaedic Surgeons. *Stress Fractures of the Foot and Ankle.* Available at: http://orthoinfo.aaos.org/topic.cfm?topic=A00379. Accessed August 9, 2014.

REFERENCES

1. The American Physical Therapy Association. Pattern 4G: Impaired joint mobility, muscle performance, and range of motion associated with fracture. *Interactive Guide to Physical Therapist Practice.* 2003. doi: 10.2522/ptguide.3.1_7. http://guidetoptpractice.apta.org/content/1/SEC14.extract. Accessed June 3, 2014.
2. Hall SJ. Chapter 4. The Biomechanics of Human Bone Growth and Development. In: *Basic Biomechanics, 4e.* New York, NY: McGraw-Hill; 2007. http://www.accessphysiotherapy.com/abstract/6060836#6060838. Accessed March 1, 2013.
3. Cline S, Patel DR. Chapter 31. Stress fractures. In: Patel DR, Greydanus DE, Baker RJ, eds. *Pediatric Practice: Sports Medicine.* New York, NY: McGraw-Hill; 2009. http://www.accessphysiotherapy.com/abstract/6981470. Accessed March 1, 2013.
4. Malone TR, Hazle C, Grey ML. Chapter 1. Introduction to musculoskeletal imaging. In: *Imaging in Rehabilitation.* New York, NY: McGraw-Hill; 2008. http://www.accessphysiotherapy.com/abstract/5940003#5940003. Accessed March 1, 2013.
5. Dutton M. Chapter 19. The ankle and foot. In: *Orthopaedic Examination, Evaluation, and Intervention.* New York, NY: McGraw-Hill; 2008. http://www.accessphysiotherapy.com/abstract/55586760#55587364. Accessed March 1, 2013.
6. Prentice WE, Blake B. Chapter 1. The basic science of therapeutic modalities. In: Prentice WE, Quillen WS, Underwood F, eds. *Therapeutic Modalities in Rehabilitation.* 4th ed. New York, NY: McGraw-Hill; 2011. http://www.accessphysiotherapy.com/abstract/8135087#8135091. Accessed March 1, 2013.
7. Prentice WE. Chapter 9. Cryotherapy and thermotherapy. In: Prentice WE, Quillen WS, Underwood F, eds. *Therapeutic Modalities in Rehabilitation.* 4th ed. New York, NY: McGraw-Hill; 2011. http://www.accessphysiotherapy.com/content/8137995#8137995. Accessed March 1, 2013.
8. Hooker DN, Prentice WE. Chapter 5. Basic principles of electricity and electrical stimulating currents. In: Prentice WE, Quillen WS, Underwood F, eds. *Therapeutic Modalities in Rehabilitation.* 4th ed. New York, NY: McGraw-Hill; 2011. http://www.accessphysiotherapy.com/content/8136367#8136367. Accessed March 1, 2013.
9. Dutton M. Chapter 2. The nervous system. In: *Orthopaedic Examination, Evaluation, and Intervention.* New York, NY: McGraw-Hill; 2008. http://www.accessphysiotherapy.com/abstract/5541168#5541193. Accessed June 20, 2013.
10. Dutton M. Chapter 17. Therapeutic Exercise. In: *NPTE (National Physical Therapy Examination).* 2nd ed. 2012. http://www.accessphysiotherapy.com/abstract/5405700#5405706. Accessed June 20, 2013.

ADDITIONAL REFERENCES

- Goodman CC, Boissonnault WG, Fuller KS. *Pathology: Implications for the Physical Therapist.* 2nd ed. Philadelphia, PA: Saunders; 2003.
- ICD9DATA web site. http://www.icd9data.com. Accessed August 9, 2014.
- ICD10DATA web site. http://www.icd10data.com. Accessed August 9, 2014.
- Kisner C, Colby LA. *Therapeutic Exercise: Foundations and Techniques.* 5th ed. Philadelphia, PA: F.A. Davis Company; 2007.
- Magee DJ. *Orthopedic Physical Assessment.* 5th ed. St. Louis, MO: Saunders Elsevier; 2008.

208 HALLUX ABDUCTO VALGUS

Christina L. Pettie, MHA, PT
Eric Shamus, PhD, DPT, PT, CSCS

CONDITION/DISORDER SYNONYMS

- Hallux valgus
- Bunion

ICD-9-CM CODE

- 735.0 Hallux valgus (acquired)

ICD-10-CM CODE

- M20.10 Hallux valgus (acquired), unspecified foot

PREFERRED PRACTICE PATTERN

- 4E: Impaired Joint Mobility, Motor Function, Muscle Performance, and ROM Associated with Localized Inflammation[1]

PATIENT PRESENTATION

The patient is a 54-year-old female who presents with complaints of pain at the metatarsophalangeal (MTP) joint of the first toe. She reports that she is a nurse and on her feet all day for 12-hour shifts. She wears flats that are typically more pointed than rounded at the toe. She does have pain with toe-off when walking and redness at the MTP joint toe one after removing her shoes. She has been trying to find a more comfortable pair of shoes to wear but they all seem too tight at the first toe joint. She has noticed that the first toe seems to be drifting inwards toward the other toes.

Evaluation reveals hypermobility of the medial ligaments MTP joint toe one, joint redness and pain, depression of the second metatarsal, and shifting of the big toe laterally toward the other toes on the same foot. X-rays were negative for fracture. Weakness of the flexor hallucis longus (FHL) is also present.

KEY FEATURES

Description

- Valgus deviation (lateral, abduction) of the great toe (hallux) and varus deviation of the first metatarsal.
- Some rotation (valgus rotation) at the first metatarsal is also possible.
- Static subluxation of first MTP.
- Tissue surrounding first metatarsal joint may be inflamed and tender.
- "Bump" on medial side of the first toe is partly due to
  - Inflammation of the bursal sac.
  - Osseous (bony) anomaly on the mesophalangeal joint (where first metatarsal bone and hallux meet).

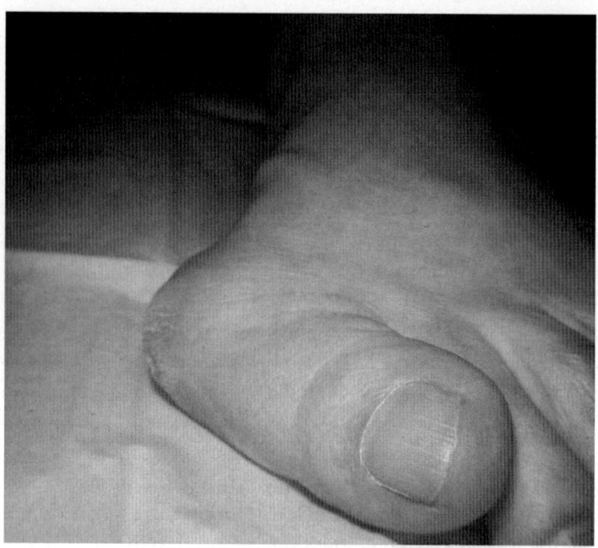

FIGURE 208-1 Severe hallux valgus. (From Imboden J, Hellmann DB, Stone JH. *Current Diagnosis & Treatment in Rheumatology*. 2nd ed. http://www.accessmedicine.com. Copyright © The McGraw-Hill Companies, Inc. All rights reserved.)

  - Large part of the bump tends to be the head of the first metatarsal, as it deviates medially in relation to the phalange.

Essentials of Diagnosis

- Diagnosis usually made by clinical examination or X-ray
- Can be an independent diagnosis, not associated with disease process.

General Considerations

- Important to correct forefoot weight distribution following surgical correction or another bunion will develop
- Need to address barefoot walking or improper footwear

Demographics

- Most common in women: Male–female ratio is 1:9[2]
- 22% to 36% of cases are in adolescents[2]
- Hereditary component
- Poor footwear: Improper fit, pointed toe, narrow forefoot
- Dancers at higher risk

CLINICAL FINDINGS

SIGNS AND SYMPTOMS

- Irritated skin around bunion
- Pain in the first metatarsal with walking
- Paresthesia in the first metatarsal
- Global ligamentous laxity
- Joint redness and pain
- Shift of big toe toward others
- Depression of second metatarsal with possible formation of hammer toe
- Callus and blister formation around bunion
- Difficulty finding shoes with proper fit
- Lateral subluxation of the FHL muscle[2]

Functional Implications

- Pain with standing
- Pain in affected toe with ambulation
- Inability to wear stiff shoes
- Need to wear larger shoes to accommodate bunion
- Altered gait pattern and mechanical issues of the forefoot

Possible Contributing Causes

- Pes planus (flat feet)
- Excessive pronation
- Genu valgus
- Limited dorsiflexion (tight heel cord)
- Abnormal bone structure
- Arthritis
- Leg-length discrepancy
- Congenital Grebe syndrome
- Neurologic conditions, including
  - Cerebral palsy
  - Multiple sclerosis
  - Charcot–Marie–Tooth
  - Marfan syndrome
  - Down syndrome

Differential Diagnosis

- Hallux rigidus
- Sesamoiditis
- Hammer toe
- Metatarsalgia
- Metatarsal stress fracture

MEANS OF CONFIRMATION OR DIAGNOSIS

Imaging

- X-ray[3]

FINDINGS AND INTERPRETATION

- Increased angle between first and second metatarsals

TREATMENT

Medication

- NSAIDs

MEDICAL PROCEDURES

- Surgery to straighten toe, osteotomy
- Botulinum toxin A injection

REFERRALS/ADMITTANCE

- To hospital for imaging, X-ray[3]
- To physician for corticosteroid injection
- To surgeon for surgical consult

IMPAIRMENTS

- Antalgic gait secondary to decreased flexibility with dorsiflexion
- Antalgic gait secondary to pain at first toe with push-off
- Hypomobility of the proximal interphalangeal (PIP) second toe
- Unstable midtarsal joint
- Inability to ambulate 1 mile secondary to pain

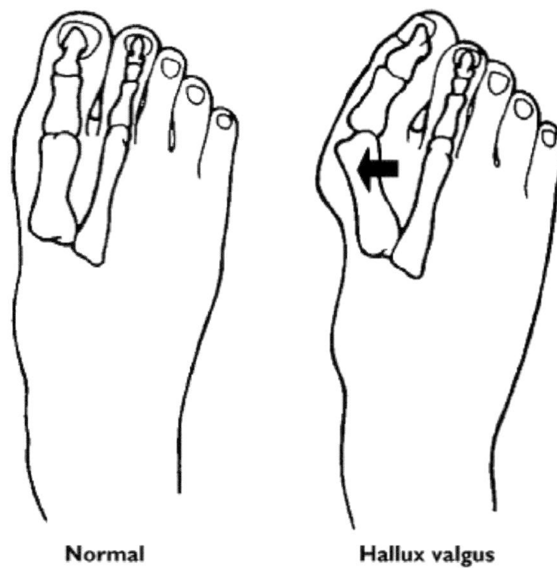

FIGURE 208-2 Wearing shoes with pointed toes can cause hallux valgus. (From Hall SJ. *Basic Biomechanics*, 5th ed. http://www.accessmedicine.com.)

TESTS AND MEASURES

- Intrinsic toe strength
- Pronation assessment
- Gait assessment
- Ankle and foot ROM

INTERVENTION

- Rest: Weight off feet will allow inflammation reduction
- Bunion and arch taping
- Bunion splint for neutral positioning, toe spacer
- Orthotics with a Morton's extension under first MTP[2]

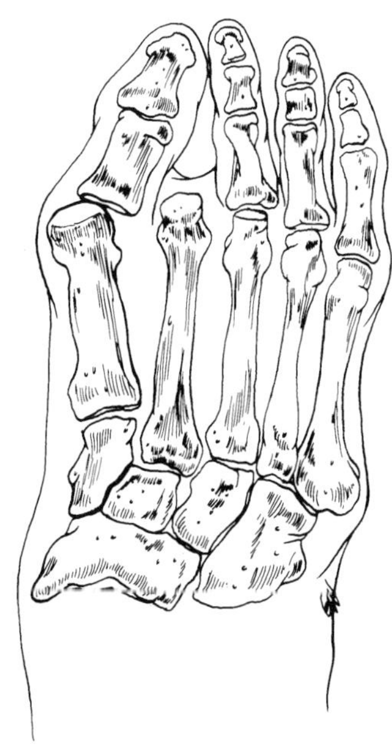

FIGURE 208-3 Severe hallux valgus deformity occurring after isolated second toe amputation. (From Skinner HB. *Current Diagnosis & Treatment in Orthopedics*. 4th ed. http://www.accessmedicine.com.)

- Address swelling
  - Ice[4]
- Address pain
  - Ice
  - Massage
  - Joint mobilization
  - Electric stimulation[5]
  - Iontophoresis
  - Infrared
- Address weakness, joint instability
  - Strengthening[6]
    - Toe curls, flexor intrinsic
    - Great toe abduction
    - Calf raises to point
    - Active walking
    - Standing arch raises
- Address lack of flexibility
  - Stretching
    - Gastrocnemius/Soleus in cases of Achilles contracture[2]
    - Plantar fascia in patients with pes cavus
  - Fluidotherapy[5]
- Address joint mobilization
  - First MTP dorsal/plantar and medial/lateral glides and rotation
  - Second MTP dorsal glides, PIP plantar glides
  - Posterior talus glides
  - Subtalar joint (STJ) inversion/eversion
  - Navicular/Cuboid/cuneiforms
  - Widening of the mortise
    - Distal tibia/fibula mobility
- Address soft-tissue mobilization
  - Abductor hallucis, first and second lumbricals/dorsal interossei
  - Plantar fascia
  - Gastrocnemius/soleus
  - Postsurgical scar
- Patient education regarding appropriate footwear

FUNCTIONAL GOALS

- Patient will be able to
  - Recognize and maintain subtalar neutral position for >2 minutes
  - Ambulate without pain for >45 minutes.
  - Achieve 15 degrees of talocrural dorsiflexion during stance phase of gait.
  - Achieve 70 degrees of great toe extension during push-off phase of gait.
  - Stand unilaterally in subtalar neutral for 1 minute with eyes open.

PROGNOSIS

- Good; patients can expect pain reduction with conservative therapeutic intervention, though structural anomalies will not be changed.
- Patients who undergo bunionectomy can expect restoration of structure.
- Postsurgical recovery may take 6 to12 months.

PATIENT RESOURCE

- Bunion Surgery. American Academy of Orthopeadic Surgeons. http://orthoinfo.aaos.org/topic.cfm?topic=A00140. Accessed March 6, 2013.

REFERENCES

1. The American Physical Therapy Association. Pattern 4E: Impaired joint mobility, motor function, muscle performance, and range of motion associated with localized inflammation. *Interactive Guide to Physical Therapist Practice*. 2003. doi: 10.2522/ptguide.3.1_5. http://guidetoptpractice.apta.org/content/1/SEC12.extract. Accessed June 3, 2014.
2. Dutton M. *Dutton's Orthopaedic Examination, Evaluation, and Intervention*. 3rd ed. New York, NY: McGraw-Hill; 2012. http://www.accessphysiotherapy.com/resource/612. Accessed March 9, 2013.
3. Patel DR, Lyne ED. Chapter 29. Overuse injuries of the leg, ankle, and foot. In: Patel DR, Greydanus DE, Baker RJ, eds. *Pediatric Practice: Sports Medicine*. New York, NY: McGraw-Hill; 2009. http://www.accessphysiotherapy.com/abstract/6981007. Accessed March 8, 2013.
4. Prentice WE. Chapter 9. Cryotherapy and Thermotherapy. In: Prentice WE, Quillen WS, Underwood F, eds. *Therapeutic Modalities in Rehabilitation*. 4th ed. New York, NY: McGraw-Hill; 2011. http://www.accessphysiotherapy.com/content/8137995#8137995. Accessed March 8, 2013.
5. Hooker DN, Prentice WE. Chapter 5. Basic principles of electricity and electrical stimulating currents. In: Prentice WE, Quillen WS, Underwood F, eds. *Therapeutic Modalities in Rehabilitation*. 4th ed. New York, NY: McGraw-Hill; 2011. http://www.accessphysiotherapy.com/content/8136367#8136367. Accessed March 8, 2013.
6. Hamilton N, Weimar W, Luttgens K. Kinesiology: Scientific Basis of Human Motion. New York, NY: McGraw-Hill; 2008. http://www.accessphysiotherapy.com/resource/618. Accessed March 8, 2013.

ADDITIONAL REFERENCES

- Bussewitz BW, Levar T, Hyer CF. Modern Techniques in hallux abducto valgus surgery. *Clin Podiatr Med Surg*. 2011;28(2):287–303, viii.
- Dutton M. *Dutton's Orthopedic Survival Guide: Managing Common Conditions*. New York, NY: McGraw-Hill; 2011. http://www.accessphysiotherapy.com/content/8655656. Accessed January 27, 2013.
- Dutton M. Common orthopedic conditions. In: Dutton M, ed. *McGraw-Hill's NPTE (National Physical Therapy Examination)*. 2nd ed. New York, NY: McGraw-Hill; 2012. http://www.accessphysiotherapy.com/content/5398559. Accessed January 27, 2013.
- Hay WW, Levin MJ, Sondheimer JM, Deterding RR. Common foot problems. In: Hay WW, Levin MJ, Sondheimer JM, Deterding RR, eds. *CURRENT Diagnosis & Treatment: Pediatrics*. 20th ed. New York, NY: McGraw-Hill; 2011. http://www.accessphysiotherapy.com/content/6585912. Accessed January 27, 2013.
- ICD9DATA web site. http://www.icd9data.com. Accessed March 6, 2013.
- ICD10DATA web site. http://www.icd10data.com. Accessed March 6, 2013.
- Radovic PA, Shah E. Nonsurgical treatment for hallux abducto vlagus with botulinum toxin A. *J Am Podiatr Med Assoc*. 2008;98(1):61–65.

209 HALLUX RIGIDUS

Eric Shamus, PhD, DPT, PT, CSCS
Jennifer Shamus, PhD, DPT, COMT, CSCS

CONDITION/DISORDER SYNONYMS

- Stiff big toe
- Hallux limitus

ICD-9-CM CODE

- 735.2 Hallux rigidus

ICD-10-CM CODE

- M20.20 Hallux rigidus, unspecified foot

PREFERRED PRACTICE PATTERN

- 4E: Impaired Joint Mobility, Motor Function, Muscle Performance, and range of motion (ROM) Associated with Localized Inflammation[1]

PATIENT PRESENTATION

A 72-year-old male presents with big toe pain on his right foot. Patient likes to play tennis and said when he reached to hit a ball he started having toe pain. The pain has become so bad he cannot come up on his toes when he tries to serve. X-ray shows degenerative changes at the metatarsophalangeal (MTP) joint along with stiffness with MTP joint mobility.

KEY FEATURES

Description

- Stiff big toe or rigid first ray
- Arthritic degeneration of great toe (hallux)
- Progression to bone spurs at first MTP joint
- Limited MTP joint mobility
- Bump or callus on MTP joint
- Altered mechanics during push-off phase of gait

Essentials of Diagnosis

- Diagnosis usually made by clinical examination or x-ray
- May be independent diagnosis, not associated with disease process
- Classification[2]
  - Grade 0: Dorsiflexion (DF) of 40 to 60 degrees, normal radiograph, no pain
  - Grade 1: DF 30 to 40 degrees, dorsal osteophytes, some loss of ROM of the first MTP joint
  - Grade 2: DF 10 to 30 degrees, greater loss of ROM and cartilage, osteophytes, flattening of the MTP joint
  - Grade 3: DF of less than 10 degrees, significant cartilage loss with irregular sesamoids, constant pain
  - Grade 4: Hallux rigidus, radiograph showing loose bodies and pain throughout the ROM

General Considerations

- Bone spur, osteophyte
- Swelling
- Inflammation around joint

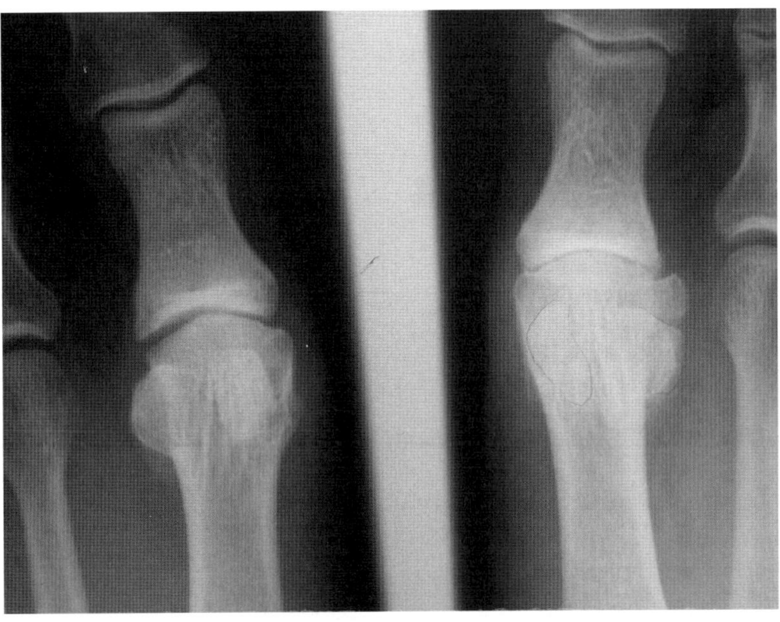

FIGURE 209-1 Radiographs of a patient with bilateral hallux limitus. On the left there is flattening of the metatarsal head and slight joint space narrowing. There is marked joint space narrowing on the more severely affected right first MTP joint. (From Imboden J, Hellmann DB, Stone JH. *Current Diagnosis & Treatment in Rheumatology.* 2nd ed. http://www.accessmedicine.com. Copyright © The McGraw-Hill Companies, Inc. All rights reserved.)

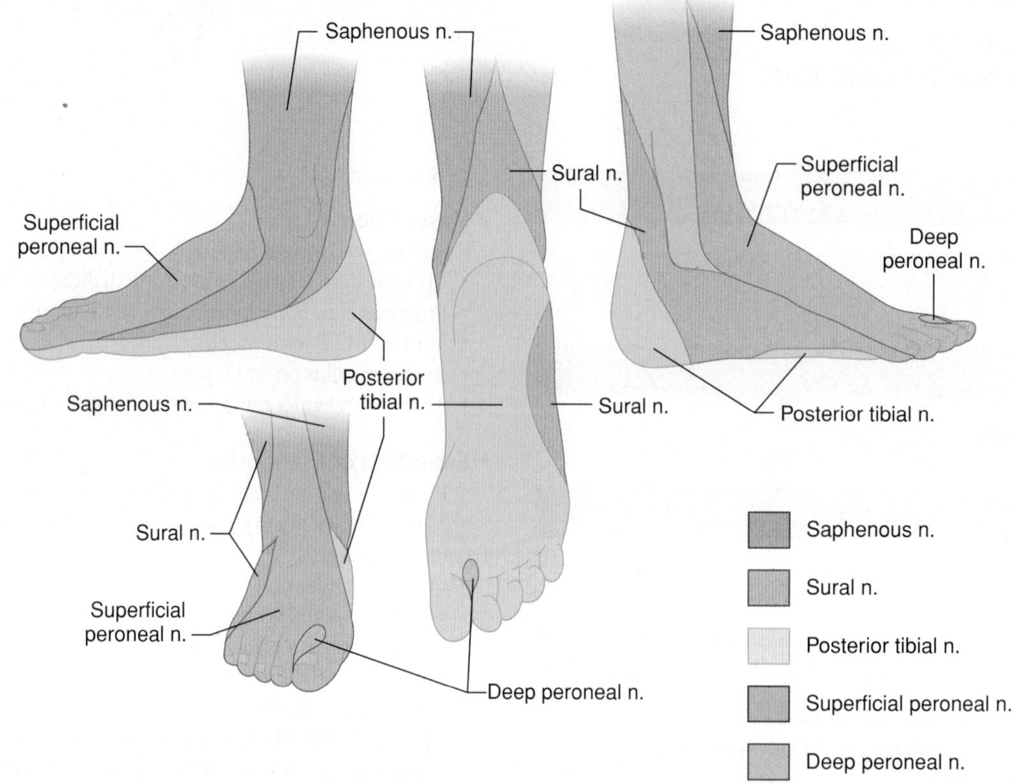

FIGURE 209-2 Sensory innervation of the foot. n., nerve. (From Tintinalli JE, Stapczynski JS, Ma OJ, et al., eds: *Tintinalli's Emergency Medicine: A Comprehensive Study Guide.* 7th ed. http://www.accessmedicine.com. Copyright © The McGraw-Hill Companies, Inc. All rights reserved.)

Demographics

- Adults
  - Generalized degenerative arthritis
  - Poor footwear: Improper fit, pointed toe, narrow forefoot
  - Dancers at higher risk
  - Most common form of arthritis in foot
- Adolescents[3]
  - Osteochondritis dissecans
  - Localized articular disorder

CLINICAL FINDINGS

SIGNS AND SYMPTOMS

- Limited motion of MTP joint
- Pain in first metatarsal with walking
- Decreased extension or dorsiflexion of big toe
- Pain, redness around joint
- Callus bunion on top of foot
- Difficulty finding shoes with proper fit
- Feeling of hard-end during joint motion may indicate bone spur

Functional Implications

- Pain with standing
- Pain in affected toe with ambulation
- Inability to wear high-heeled shoes that create extension at big toe
- Need to wear larger shoes to accommodate bunion
- Altered gait pattern and mechanical issues of the forefoot; increased supination and external rotation of foot for clearance; forefoot abduction with lateral whip

Possible Contributing Causes

- Abnormal bone structure
- Improper footwear
- Cast or immobilized foot
- Osteoarthritis

Differential Diagnosis

- Hallux valgus
- Gout
- Osteochondrotic lesion of the first metatarsal head
- Sesamoiditis, turf toe
- Osteochondritis dissecans
- Metatarsalgia
- Metatarsal stress fracture
- Plantar fasciitis: Patient may initially have more pain at medial arch due to altered mechanics before developing significant toe pain

MEANS OF CONFIRMATION OR DIAGNOSIS

Imaging

- X-ray[4]

FINDINGS AND INTERPRETATION

- Limited joint space
- Location and size of bone spur
- Posterior (dorsal) and lateral osteophytes on metatarsal head

TREATMENT

Medication

- NSAIDs

MEDICAL PROCEDURES

- Surgical correction
- Joint replacement

REFERRALS/ADMITTANCE

- To hospital for imaging, X-ray
- To physician for medication, anti-inflammatory, corticosteroid injection
- To surgeon for surgical consult

IMPAIRMENTS

- Antalgic gait secondary to increased supination; rigid hallux may limit pronation of the foot when lower extremity stays straight.
- Antalgic gait secondary to increased pronation from abduction/external rotation of foot, leads patient to collapse at medial arch and pronate further to avoid toe pain.
- Antalgic gait secondary to pain at first toe with push-off.
- Hypomobility of MTP joint in big toe.
- Inability to ambulate 1 mile secondary to pain.

TEST AND MEASURES

- Joint mobility
- Tendon length
- ROM
- Gait analysis
- Special test for functional hallux limitus[3]

INTERVENTION

- Stage 1: Functional limitus, treated conservatively and with orthotics
- Stage 2: Early joint adaptation, consideration for cheilectomy
- Stage 3: Arthrosis, consideration for osteotomy or hei-implant
- Stage 4: Ankylosis consideration for joint replacement or arthrodesis
- Rest: Weight off feet will allow inflammation reduction
- Orthotics with first ray cut out
- Address pain
  - Ice[5]
  - Massage
  - Joint mobilization
  - Electric stimulation[6]
  - Infrared
- Address weakness, joint instability
  - Strengthening[7]
    - Toe curls, flexor intrinsic
    - Great toe abduction
    - Calf raises to point
    - Active walking
    - Standing arch raises
- Address lack of flexibility
  - Stretching
    - Gastrocnemius/Soleus in cases of Achilles contracture[3]
    - Plantar fascia in patients with pes cavus
  - Fluidotherapy[6]

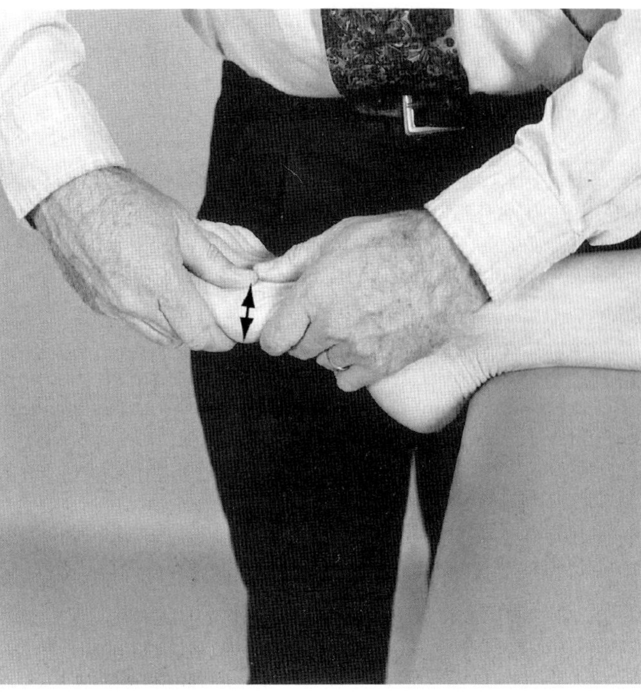

FIGURE 209-3 Testing the first MTP joint motion. (From Dutton M. *Dutton's Orthopedic Survival Guide: Managing Common Conditions.* http://www.accessphysiotherapy.com. Copyright © The McGraw-Hill Companies, Inc. All rights reserved.)

- Address joint mobilization
  - First MTP dorsal/plantar and medial/lateral glides and rotation
  - Second MTP dorsal glides, proximal interphalangeal (PIP) plantar glides
  - Posterior talus glides
  - Subtalar joint (STJ) inversion/eversion
  - Navicular/cuboid/cuneiforms
- Address soft-tissue mobilization
  - Abductor hallucis, first and second lumbricals/dorsal interossei
  - Plantar fascia
  - Gastrocnemius/soleus
- Patient education regarding appropriate footwear
  - Increased size to box space
  - Shoe with a rocker bottom to limit extension of first ray

FUNCTIONAL GOALS

- Patient will be able to:
  - Recognize and maintain subtalar neutral position for >2 minutes.
  - Ambulate pain-free for >45 minutes for grocery shopping.
  - Achieve 15 degrees of talocrural dorsiflexion during stance phase of gait.
  - Achieve 70 degrees of great toe extension during push off phase of gait.
  - Stand unilaterally in subtalar neutral for 1 minute with eyes open.

PROGNOSIS

- Good; patients can expect pain reduction with conservative therapeutic intervention, though structural anomalies will not be changed.

- Patients who undergo surgery (joint replacement) can expect restoration of ROM and structure, though if joint completely degraded, arthrodesis (joint fusion) may be indicated.
- Postsurgical recovery may take 6 months.

PATIENT RESOURCE

- Stiff Big Toe (HALLUX RIGIDUS). American Academy of Orthopaedic Surgeons. http://orthoinfo.aaos.org/topic.cfm?topic=a00168. Accessed June 3, 2014.

REFERENCES

1. The American Physical Therapy Association. Pattern 4E: Impaired joint mobility, motor function, muscle performance, and range of motion associated with localized inflammation. *Interactive Guide to Physical Therapist Practice*. 2003. doi: 10.2522/ptguide.3.1_5. Accessed March 1, 2013.
2. Coughlin MJ, Shurnas PS. Hallux rigidus: demographics, etiology, and radiographic assessment. *Foot Ankle Int.* 2003;24(10):731–743.
3. Dutton M. *Orthopaedic Examination, Evaluation, and Intervention*. New York, NY: McGraw-Hill; 2008. http://www.accessphysiotherapy.com/resource/612. Accessed March 9, 2013.
4. Malone TR, Hazle C, Grey ML. Chapter 1. Introduction to musculoskeletal imaging. In: *Imaging in Rehabilitation*. New York, NY: McGraw-Hill; 2008. http://www.accessphysiotherapy.com/abstract/5940003#5940003. Accessed March 10, 2013.
5. Prentice WE. Chapter 9. Cryotherapy and thermotherapy. In: Prentice WE, Quillen WS, Underwood F, eds. *Therapeutic Modalities in Rehabilitation*.4th ed. New York, NY: McGraw-Hill; 2011. http://www.accessphysiotherapy.com/content/8137995#8137995. Accessed March 8, 2013.
6. Hooker DN, Prentice WE. Chapter 5. Basic principles of electricity and electrical stimulating currents. In: Prentice WE, Quillen WS, Underwood F, eds. *Therapeutic Modalities in Rehabilitation*, .4th ed. New York, NY: McGraw-Hill; 2011. http://www.accessphysiotherapy.com/content/8136367#8136367. Accessed March 8, 2013.
7. Hamilton N, Weimar W, Luttgens K. *Kinesiology: Scientific Basis of Human Motion*. New York, NY: McGraw-Hill; 2008. http://www.accessphysiotherapy.com/resource/618. Accessed March 8, 2013.

ADDITIONAL REFERENCES

- Coughlin MJ, Shurnas PS. Hallus rigidus. Grading and long-term results of operative treatment. *J Bone Joint Surg Am.* 2003;85-A(11):2072–2088.
- Dutton M. Common orthopedic conditions. In: Dutton M, ed. *Dutton's Orthopedic Survival Guide: Managing Common Conditions*. New York, NY: McGraw-Hill; 2011. http://www.accessphysiotherapy.com/content/8655656. Accessed January 27, 2013.
- ICD9DATA web site. http://www.icd9data.com. Accessed March 6, 2013.
- ICD10DATA web site. http://www.icd10data.com. Accessed March 6, 2013.
- Kline AJ, Hasselman CT. Metatarsal head resurfacing for advanced hallus rigidus. *Foot Ankle Int.* 2013;34(5):716–725.
- Roukis TS. Clinical outcomes after isolated periarticular osteotomies of the first metatarsal for hallux rigidus: A systematic review. *J Foot Ankle Surg.* 2010;49(6):553–560. doi: 10.1053/j.jfas.2010.08.014.
- Solan MC, Calder JD, Bendall SP. Manipulation and injection for hallux rigidus. Is it worthwhile? *J Bone Joint Surg Br.* 2001; 83(5):706–708.

210 HAMMER TOE

Eric Shamus, PhD, DPT, PT, CSCS
Jennifer Shamus, PhD, DPT, COMT, CSCS

CONDITION/DISORDER SYNONYM

- Contracted toe

ICD-9-CM CODES

- 735.4 Other hammer toe (acquired)
- 755.66 Other congenital anomalies of toes

ICD-10-CM CODES

- M20.40 Other hammer toe(s) (acquired), unspecified foot
- Q66.89 Other specified congenital deformities of feet

PREFERRED PRACTICE PATTERN

- 4E: Impaired Joint Mobility, Motor Function, Muscle Performance, and Range of Motion (ROM) Associated with Localized Inflammation[1]

PATIENT PRESENTATION

Patient is a 25-year-old soccer player. For fun he was kicking the ball around barefoot and stubbed his toes into the ground when trying to kick the ball. The patient had immediate pain and x-rays were negative for fractures. He presents to the clinic with the third toe bent with flexion of proximal interphalangeal (PIP) and DIP joints. The patient has swelling and cannot wear a closed toe shoe.

KEY FEATURES

Description

- Toe bent with flexion of PIP
- Shortened flexor muscles, fascia, tendons
- Most commonly affects second toe, though may also affect third or fourth
- May alter mechanics during push-off phase of gait

Essentials of Diagnosis

- Diagnosis usually made by clinical examination or X-ray
- May be independent diagnosis, not associated with disease process

General Considerations

- Chronic condition developed over time with callus on top of the joint
- Inflammation around joint
- Altered joint position[2]
- Evaluation of footwear
- Distinguished from claw toe, which includes hyperextension (dorsiflexed) of the MTP joint with flexion (plantarflexed) of the PIP joint, DIP is plantarflexed
- Distinguished from mallet toe, which includes neutral MTP and PIP joint with flexion (plantarflexion) of only the DIP

Demographics

- Infants, congenital
- Children who wear shoes they have outgrown and are too small
- Adults
  - Poor footwear: Improper fit, pointed toe, narrow forefoot, high heels
  - Dancers at higher risk

CLINICAL FINDINGS

SIGNS AND SYMPTOMS

- Pain in metatarsal with walking
- Corn on top of toe
- Decreased extension or dorsiflexion of toe
- Pain, redness around joint
- Callus under metatarsal head
- Difficulty finding shoes with proper fit
- Limited motion of MTP joint

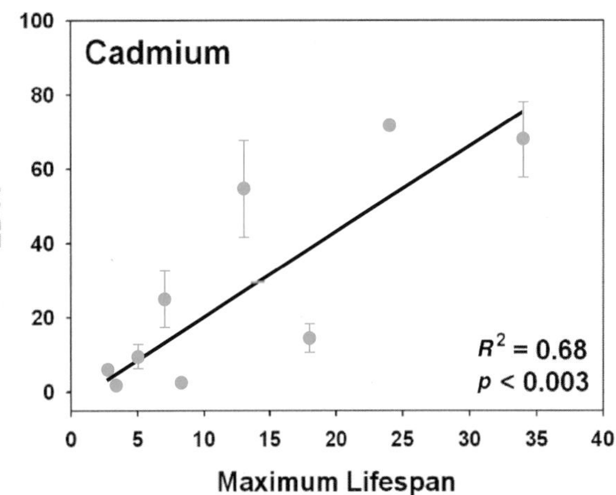

FIGURE 210-1 Multiple hammertoes, hallux flexus, onychauxis, residual of rheumatoid arthritis, and degenerative changes. (From Halter JB et al: *Hazzardís Geriatric Medicine and Gerontology*, 6th edition. www.accessmedicine.com. Copyright © The McGraw-Hill Companies, Inc. All rights reserved.

Functional Implications

- Pain with standing
- Pain in affected toe with ambulation
- Inability to wear stiff shoes
- Need to wear shoes with large toe box to accommodate bunion, corn, flexion, and hypomobile PIP
- Altered gait pattern and mechanical issues of the forefoot

Possible Contributing Causes

- Improper footwear
- Commonly in conjunction with bunions
- Joint arthritis/injury
- Muscle atrophy
- Nerve damage
- Friedrich's ataxia
- Osteoarthritis
- Rheumatoid arthritis
- Stroke
- Charcot–Marie–Tooth disease

Differential Diagnosis

- Mallet toe: Neutral MTP and PIP joints with flexion (plantarflexion) of only the DIP
- Claw toe: Hyperextension (dorsiflexed) of the MTP joint with flexion (plantarflexed) of the PIP joint, DIP is plantarflexed
- Gout
- Osteochondrotic lesion of first metatarsal head
- Osteochondritis dissecans
- Fracture

MEANS OF CONFIRMATION OR DIAGNOSIS

Imaging

- X-ray[2]

FINDINGS AND INTERPRETATION

- Location and size of bone spur on X-ray if there is one

TREATMENT

Medication

- NSAIDs

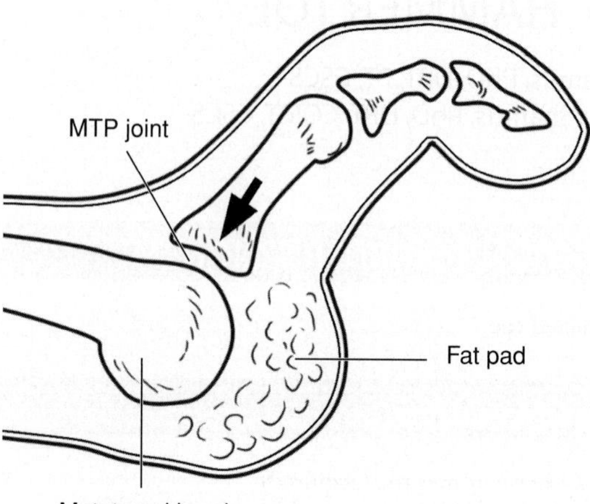

FIGURE 210-2 Diagram of a hammer toe deformity. There is dorsiflexion at the metatarsophalangeal joint and plantarflexion at the proximal interphalangeal joint. The protective fat pad normally beneath the metatarsal head displaces anteriorly. As the toe buckles, the retrograde digital force (*arrow*) places more stress upon the unprotected metatarsal head, creating metatarsalgia. (From Imboden J, Hellmann DB, Stone JH. *Current Diagnosis & Treatment in Rheumatology*. 2nd ed. http://www.accessmedicine.com. Copyright © The McGraw-Hill Companies, Inc. All rights reserved.)

MEDICAL PROCEDURE

- Surgery to straighten toe, involves cutting or lengthening tendons and ligaments, possible fusion of the joint

REFERRALS/ADMITTANCE

- To hospital for imaging, X-ray
- To physician for medication, anti-inflammatory, corticosteroid injection
- To surgeon for surgical consult

IMPAIRMENTS

- Antalgic gait secondary to pain in toe with push-off
- Hypomobility of MTP joint: Dorsally in toe, plantar direction in PIP
- Inability to ambulate 1 mile secondary to pain

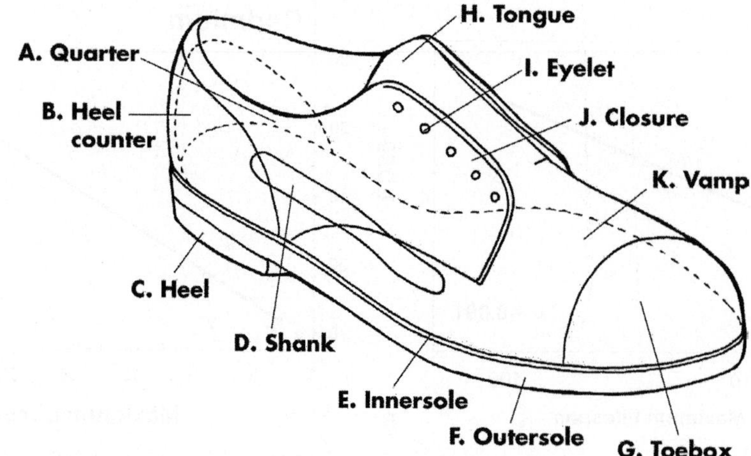

FIGURE 210-3 Anatomy of a shoe. (Reproduced with permission from Prentice, WE, Voight, MI. *Techniques in Musculoskeletal Rehabilitation*. McGraw-Hill. 2001:329.)

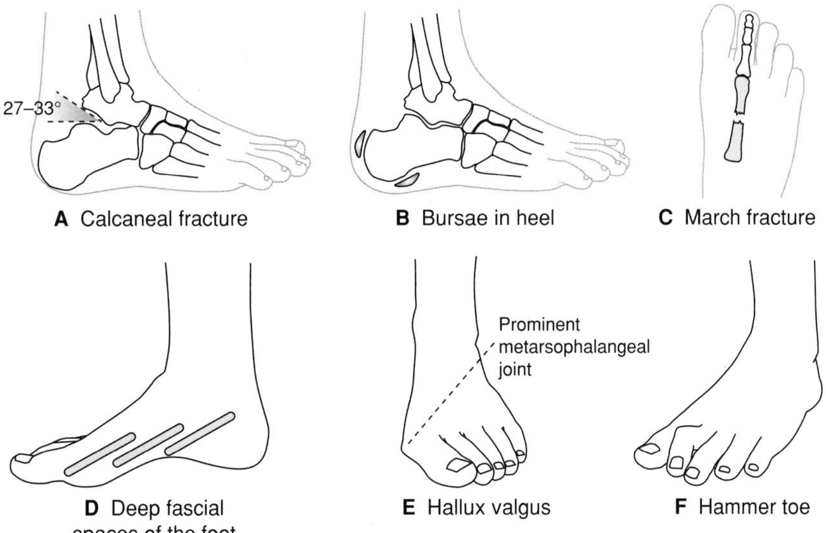

FIGURE 210-4 Lesions of the foot. (**A**) Calcaneal fracture. (**B**) Bursae in the heel. (**C**) March fracture of a metatarsal bone. (**D**) Deep fascial spaces of the foot. (**E**) Hallux valgus: This deformity shows lateral deviation of the great toe, with prominence of the first MTP joint. (**F**) Hammertoe: The second toe is always affected. There is permanent flexion of the PIP joint. (From LeBlond RF, DeGowin RL, Brown DD. *DeGowin's Diagnostic Examination*. 9th ed. http://www.accessmedicine.com. Copyright © The McGraw-Hill Companies, Inc. All rights reserved.)

TEST AND MEASURES

- Gait analysis
- ROM
- Strength
- Joint mobility
- Tendon length

INTERVENTION

- Rest: Weight off feet will allow inflammation reduction
- Orthotics with ray cut out
- Metatarsal pad for MTP support and alignment
- Address swelling
  - Ice[3]
- Address pain
  - Ice
  - Massage
  - Joint mobilization
  - Electric stimulation[4]
  - Infrared
- Address weakness, joint instability
  - Strengthening[5]
    - Toe curls and extension, flexor/extensor intrinsic
    - Calf raises to point
    - Active walking
    - Standing arch raises
- Address lack of flexibility
  - Stretching; prolonged static
    - Toe intrinsic flexor
    - Gastrocnemius/soleus in cases of achilles contracture[2]
    - Plantar fascia in patients with pes cavus
    - Fluidotherapy[4]
- Address joint mobilization
  - MTP and PIP dorsal/plantar and medial/lateral glides and rotation
  - Posterior talus glides
  - Subtalar joint (STJ) inversion/eversion
  - Navicular/cuboid/cuneiforms
- Address soft-tissue mobilization
  - Lumbricals/Dorsal interossei
  - Plantar fascia
  - Gastrocnemius/Soleus
- Patient education regarding proper footwear
  - Increased toe box space
  - Shoe with rocker bottom to limit ray extension

FUNCTIONAL GOALS

- Patient will be able to:
  - Recognize and maintain subtalar neutral position for >2 minutes.
  - Ambulate pain-free for >45 minutes for grocery shopping.
  - Achieve 15 degrees of talocrural dorsiflexion during stance phase of gait.
  - Achieve pain-free toe extension during push-off phase of gait.
  - Stand unilaterally in subtalar neutral for 1 minute with eyes open.

PROGNOSIS

- Good, with therapeutic focus on stretching out toe flexors.
- Surgery may be indicated if flexion becomes severe and shoes cannot be worn.

PATIENT RESOURCE

- Hammer Toe. American Academy of Orthopaedic Surgeons. http://orthoinfo.aaos.org/topic.cfm?topic=A00160. Accessed August 9, 2014.

REFERENCES

1. The American Physical Therapy Association. Pattern 4E: Impaired joint mobility, motor function, muscle performance, and range of motion associated with localized inflammation. *Interactive Guide to Physical Therapist Practice*. 2003. doi: 10.2522/ptguide.3.1_5. Accessed June 16, 2013.

2. Dutton M. *Orthopaedic Examination, Evaluation, and Intervention*. New York, NY: McGraw-Hill; 2008. http://www.accessphysiotherapy.com/resource/612. Accessed June 16, 2013.
3. Prentice WE. Chapter 9. Cryotherapy and thermotherapy. In: Prentice WE, Quillen WS, Underwood F, eds. *Therapeutic Modalities in Rehabilitation*.4th ed. New York, NY: McGraw-Hill; 2011. http://www.accessphysiotherapy.com/content/8137995#8137995. Accessed June 16, 2013.
4. Hooker DN, Prentice WE. Chapter 5. Basic principles of electricity and electrical stimulating currents. In: Prentice WE, Quillen WS, Underwood F, eds. *Therapeutic Modalities in Rehabilitation, 4e*. New York, NY: McGraw-Hill; 2011. http://www.accessphysiotherapy.com/content/8136367#8136367. Accessed June 16, 2013.
5. Hamilton N, Weimar W, Luttgens K. *Kinesiology: Scientific Basis of Human Motion*. New York, NY: McGraw-Hill; 2008. http://www.accessphysiotherapy.com/resource/618. Accessed June 16, 2013.

ADDITIONAL REFERENCES

- ICD9DATA web site. http://www.icd9data.com. Accessed August 9, 2014.
- ICD10DATA web site. http://www.icd10data.com. Accessed August 9, 2014.
- Konkel KF, Sover ER, Menger AG, Halberg JM. Hammer toe correction using an absorbable pin. *Foot Ankle Int*. 2011;32(10):973–978.
- Malone TR, Hazle C, Grey ML. Chapter 10. The ankle and foot. In: Malone TR, Hazle C, Grey ML, eds. *Imaging in Rehabilitation*. New York, NY: McGraw-Hill; 2008. http://www.accessphysiotherapy.com/content/5940084. Accessed August 9, 2014.
- Malone TR, Hazle C, Grey ML. Special plain radiographic views. In: Malone TR, Hazle C, Grey ML, eds. *Imaging in Rehabilitation*. New York, NY: McGraw-Hill; 2008. http://www.accessphysiotherapy.com/content/5940160. Accessed August 9, 2014.
- Schrier JC, Verheyen CC, Louwerens JW. Definitions of hammer toe and claw toe: An evaluation of the literature. *J Am Podiatr Med Assoc*. 2009;99(3):194–197.

211 MALLET TOE

Eric Shamus, PhD, DPT, PT, CSCS

CONDITION/DISORDER SYNONYM

- Claw toe

ICD-9-CM CODES

- 735.4 Other hammer toe (acquired)
- 755.66 Other anomalies of toes

ICD-10-CM CODES

- M20.40 Other hammer toe(s) (acquired), unspecified foot
- Q66.89 Other specified congenital deformities of the feet

PREFERRED PRACTICE PATTERN

- 4E: Impaired Joint Mobility, Motor Function, Muscle Performance, and Range of Motion (ROM) Associated with Localized Inflammation[1]

PATIENT PRESENTATION

A 26-year-old female states she was walking at night in her apartment barefoot to go to the kitchen when she kicked the leg of the sofa which she did not see. Patient states she had severe pain and ecchymosis. She had X-rays which were negative on her second toe. She presents with flexion at the distal interphalangeal (DIP) joint with pain during ambulation. The distal joint of the second toe is bent into a claw like position.

KEY FEATURES

Description

- Distal joint of the toe is bent into a claw like position
- Usually due to trauma from impact on tip of the toe
- Flexor muscles, fascia, tendons shorten
- Flexion of the DIP joint
- Most commonly affects the second toe as it is the longest; can also be third to fifth
- May alter mechanics during the push-off phase of gait

Essentials of Diagnosis

- Diagnosis is usually made by clinical examination or X-ray
- Can be an independent diagnosis and not associated with a disease process
- Can be flexible in the developmental stage
- Rigid toes will have tight tendons and joint capsules

General Considerations

- Swelling
- Inflammation around the joint

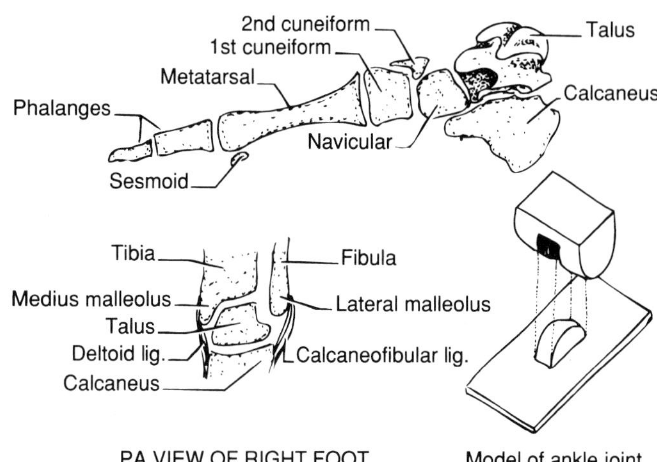

FIGURE 211-1 Structure of the ankle joint and foot. (From LeBlond RF, DeGowin RL, Brown DD. *DeGowin's Diagnostic Evaluation.* 9th ed. http://www.accessmedicine.com. Copyright © The McGraw-Hill Companies, Inc. All rights reserved.)

- Altered joint position
- Tip of the toe can develop a painful corn or ulcer

Demographics

- Infants
  - Congenital
- Children
  - Results from wearing shoes that are too small
- Adults
  - Poor footwear: Too small or narrow, toe comes to a point, high heels
- Dancers
  - Trauma from impact on tip of the toe

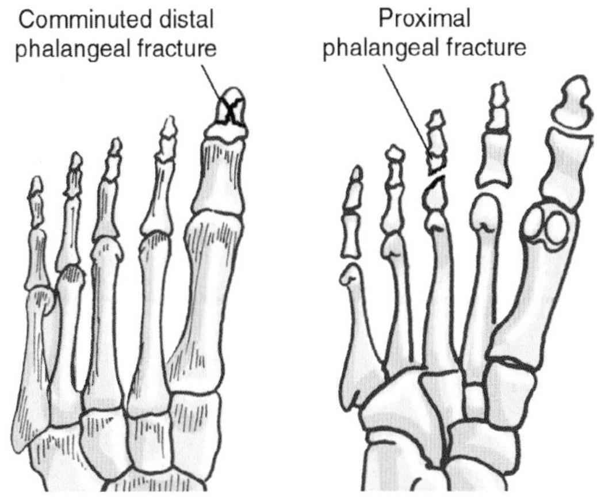

FIGURE 211-2 Toe fractures. (From Simon RR, Sherman SC. *Emergency Orthopedics.* 6th ed. www.accessemergencymedicine.com. Copyright © The McGraw-Hill Companies, Inc. All rights reserved.)

CLINICAL FINDINGS

SIGNS AND SYMPTOMS

- Pain in metatarsal with walking
- Corn on top of the toe above the DIP joint
- Decreased extension or dorsiflexion of the toe
- Joint redness and pain
- Callus formation under the metatarsal head

Functional Implications

- Pain with standing
- Pain with ambulation at the toe
- Inability to wear stiff shoes
- Need to wear larger shoes to accommodate bunion, large toe box
- Alteration of gait pattern (such as no toe off, forefoot abduction, decreased arch height) and mechanical issues of the forefoot
- Difficulty finding shoes

Possible Contributing Causes

- Muscle imbalance
- Trauma
- Pes planus (flat foot)
- Improper show wear
- Commonly seen in conjunction of bunions
- Joint arthritis/injury
- Muscle atrophy
- Nerve damage
- Friedrich's ataxia
- Osteoarthritis
- Rheumatoid arthritis
- Stroke
- Charcot–Marie–Tooth disease
- Diabetes

Differential Diagnosis

- Hammer toe: Different in that it is flexion of the PIP (generally extension/depression of the MTP and DF of PIP)
- Hallux valgus
- Gout
- Osteochondrotic lesion of the first metatarsal head
- Sesamoiditis; turf toe
- Osteochondritis dissecans
- Metatarsalgia
- Metatarsal stress fracture

MEANS OF CONFIRMATION

Imaging

- X-ray

FINDINGS AND INTERPRETATION

- Bone spur, location and size

TREATMENT

Medication

- Anti-inflammatory

MEDICAL PROCEDURES

- Surgery to straighten out the toe and lengthen ligaments/tendons.

REFERRALS/ADMITTANCE

- For imaging, X-ray
- For corticosteroid injection
- For surgical consult to straighten out the toe, which may involve cutting or lengthening tendons and ligaments and possible fusion of the joint

IMPAIRMENTS

- Antalgic gait secondary to pain at the toe with push-off
- Inability to ambulate distances of one mile secondary to pain

TESTS AND MEASURES[2]

- PIP and DIP ROM
- LE limb strength
- Balance
  - Static single-leg standing (eyes open, eyes closed)
    - Contralateral LE
  - Dynamic standing
    - Berg Balance Scale
    - Functional gait assessment
- Gait assessment
  - Observational analysis
  - Gait speed via the 10-m walk test
  - 2-minute walk test
  - 6-minute walk test

INTERVENTION

- Rest, keep weight off feet to reduce inflammation
- Taping to stabilize the great toe and limit extension ROM
  - As pain free ROM increases, allow for more motion with the tape
- Cast Shoe
- Orthotics with firm extension to the toes to limit ROM
  - Once the patient has full pain free ROM, orthotic can be removed
- Address pain
  - Ice[3]
  - Massage
  - Joint mobilization
  - Electric stimulation[4]
- Address weakness and joint instability
  - Strengthening
    - Toe curls and extension, flexor/extensor intrinsic
    - Calf raises to point
    - Active walking
    - Standing arch raises
    - Proximal stability of hip muscle strength
- Address lack of flexibility
  - Stretching
    - Toe intrinsic flexor stretching
    - Gastrocnemius/Soleus in cases of Achilles contracture
    - Plantar fascia in patients with pes cavus
    - Fluidotherapy
- Address joint mobilization
  - PIP dorsal/plantar and medial/lateral glides and rotation[5]
  - Posterior talus glides[5]
  - Navicular/Cuboid/cuneiforms
- Address soft-tissue mobilization
  - Lumbrical/Dorsal interossei

    - Plantar fascia
    - Gastrocnemius/Soleus
- Patient education in shoe wear
    - Increased to box space
    - Shoe with a rocker bottom to limit extension

FUNCTIONAL GOALS

- Patient will be able to:
    - Recognize and maintain a subtalar neutral position for >2 minutes.
    - Ambulate pain-free for >45 minutes.
    - Achieve 15 degrees of talocrural dorsiflexion during stance phase of gait.
    - Achieve pain-free toe extension during push-off phase of gait.
    - Stand unilaterally in subtalar neutral for 1 minute with eyes open.

PROGNOSIS

- Good; focus on stretching out the toe flexors.
- Surgery may be indicated if the flexion becomes severe and shoes cannot be worn.

PATIENT RESOURCE

- Hammertoe and Mallet toe. Mayo Clinic. http://www.mayoclinic.com/health/hammertoe-and-mallet-toe/DS00480. Accessed August 9, 2014.

REFERENCES

1. The American Physical Therapy Association. Pattern 4E: Impaired joint mobility, motor function, muscle performance, and range of motion associated with localized inflammation. Interactive guide to physical therapist practice. *The American Physical Therapy Association*. 2003. http://guidetoptpractice.apta.org/content/1/SEC12.extract?sid=ccb92104-9626-443e-ab17-b2a32a7792b7. doi: 10.2522/ptguide.978-1-931369-64-0. Accessed July 5, 2013.
2. Dutton M. *Dutton's Orthopaedic Examination, Evaluation, and Intervention*. 3rd ed. New York, NY: McGraw-Hill; 2008. http://www.accessphysiotherapy.com/resource/612. Accessed July 5, 2013.
3. Prentice WE. Cryotherapy and thermotherapy. In: Prentice WE, Quillen WS, Underwood F, eds. *Therapeutic Modalities in Rehabilitation*. 4th ed. New York, NY: McGraw-Hill; 2011. http://www.accessphysiotherapy.com/content/8137995#8137995. Accessed July 5, 2013.
4. Hooker DN, Prentice WE. Basic principles of electricity and electrical stimulating currents. In: Prentice WE, Quillen WS, Underwood F, eds. *Therapeutic Modalities in Rehabilitation*. 4th ed. New York, NY: McGraw-Hill; 2011. http://www.accessphysiotherapy.com/content/8136367#8136367. Accessed July 5, 2013.
5. Hamilton N, Weimar W, Luttgens K. *Kinesiology: Scientific Basis of Human Motion*. 11th ed. New York, NY: McGraw-Hill; 2008. http://www.accessphysiotherapy.com/resource/618. Accessed July 5, 2013.

ADDITIONAL REFERENCES

- ICD9Data.com. http://www.icd9data.com. Accessed August 9, 2014.
- ICD10Data.com. http://www.icd10data.com. Accessed August 9, 2014.
- Malone TR, Hazle C, Grey ML. The ankle and foot. In: Malone TR, Hazle C, Grey ML, eds. *Imaging in Rehabilitation*. New York, NY: McGraw-Hill; 2008. http://www.accessphysiotherapy.com/content/5940084. Accessed August 9, 2014.
- Malone TR, Hazle C, Grey ML. The Ankle and Foot. In: Malone TR, Hazle C, Grey ML, eds. *Imaging in Rehabilitation*. New York, NY: McGraw-Hill; 2008. http://www.accessphysiotherapy.com/content/5940160. Accessed August 9, 2014.
- Molloy A, Shariff R. Mallet toe deformity. *Foot Ankle Clin*. 2011; 16(4):537–546.

212 PLANTAR FASCIITIS

Eric Shamus, PhD, DPT, PT, CSCS
Jennifer Shamus, PhD, DPT, COMT, CSCS

CONDITION/DISORDER SYNONYMS

- Plantar fascial fibromatosis
- Plantar fasciopathy

ICD-9-CM CODE

- 728.71 Plantar fascial fibromatosis

ICD-10-CM CODE

- M72.2 Plantar fascial fibromatosis

PREFERRED PRACTICE PATTERN

- 4E: Impaired Joint Mobility, Motor Function, Muscle Performance, and Range of Motion Associated with Localized Inflammation[1]

PATIENT PRESENTATION

Patient reports gradual worsening of heel pain. It is worst with first step of the day and after prolonged sitting. The pain feels better after 2 to 3 minutes of walking. Pain also increases at the end of the day after she has been on her feet at work. Patient states no radicular leg symptoms. When asked, patient states she likes to walk barefoot at home on the tile floors. Patient has had 2 injections into the heel with pain returning. The patient has tried a night splint and continues to have pain.

KEY FEATURES

Description

- Inflammation of fascia on bottom of the foot or at the insertion of the medial calcaneal tubercule
- Overstretching of the fascia can occur via two processes
  - Acute inflammatory process
    - Usually with pes cavus (high arch) foot type[2]
    - Rapid overstretch possible from missing a step or curb
    - May be caused by trauma, as in stepping on hard object or ledge
  - Chronic inflammatory process
    - Usually with a pes planus (flat foot, low arch) foot type[2]
    - Chronic overstretching of the fascia or ligamentous support
    - Degenerative tendinosis of the foot's intrinsic flexors and invertors

Essentials of Diagnosis

- Diagnosis usually made by clinical examination[3]
- Can be an independent diagnosis, not associated with a disease process
- May not be fasciitis, but inflamed flexor digitorum brevis or tibialis posterior[4]
  - May feel better once warmed up
  - Fatigues gradually throughout the day

General Considerations

- Most common orthopedic foot complaint

Demographics

- Most common in middle age
- Men and women equally affected

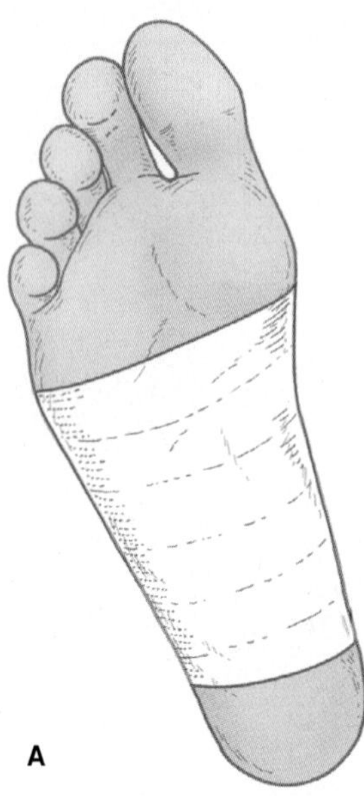

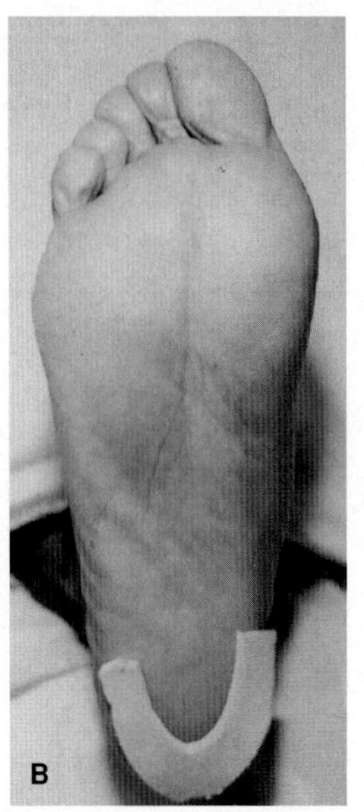

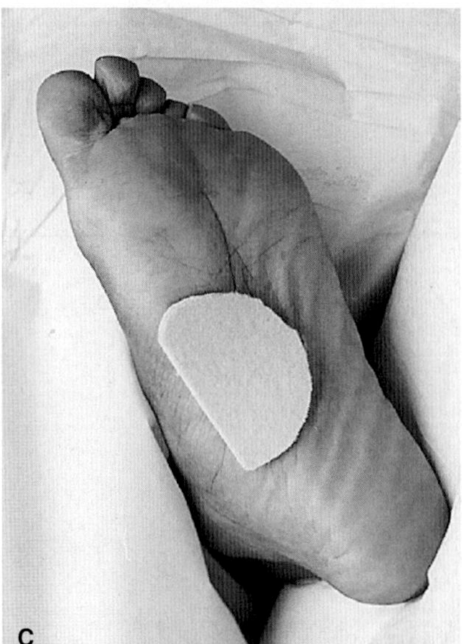

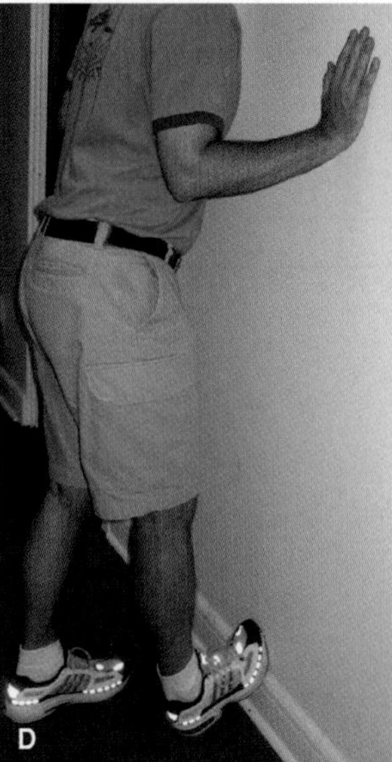

FIGURE 212-1 (**A**) Plantar fascia taping technique. (**B**) Heel pad for treating plantar fasciitis. (**C**) Plantar fascia arch support padding. (**D**) Stretches for plantar fasciitis. (From Simon RR, Sherman SC. *Emergency Orthopedics.* 6th ed. http://www.accessmedicine.com. Copyright © The McGraw-Hill Companies, Inc. All rights reserved.)

- Distance running
- Poor footwear
- Weight gain, pregnancy
- Prolonged standing on hard floors, including cement, tile, hardwood

CLINICAL FINDINGS

SIGNS AND SYMPTOMS

- Stabbing pain in heel with
  - First step of the day[5]
  - First step out of a chair
  - Barefoot walking on a hard surface
- Burning sensation underneath mid arch indicates tibial nerve entrapment[3,5]
- Heel pain with palpation at origin of the fascia where heel spur can occur[5]
- Aching, fatigue, soreness as day progresses may indicate inflamed flexor digitorum brevis or tibialis posterior[5,6]
- Mild swelling along bottom of feet[5]

Functional Implications

- Pain with standing; limitation on standing in one spot
- Pain along bottom of foot and heel with ambulation
- Balance and instability due to altered gait and stance patterns

Possible Contributing Causes

- Pes planus (flat feet) foot type can cause chronic elongation of the fascia
- Pes cavus rigid foot type with acute strain
- Rearfoot and forefoot varus
- Occupation that demands
  - Prolonged standing
  - Steel-toe shoes
  - Shoes with no arch support
  - Standing on hard surfaces
- Sudden weight gain that overloads muscular system
- Pregnancy
  - Ligamentous laxity (hormone relaxin)
  - Excessive weight gain
  - Decreased arch height
  - Barefoot
- Obesity
- Limited dorsiflexion (tight heel cord)
- Lack of talocrural joint mobility
- Jogging or running on cement

Differential Diagnosis

- Heel spur
- Heel pain
- Tibial nerve entrapment
- Flexor digitorum brevis tendonitis
- Tibialis posterior tendonitis
- S1 radiculopathy
- Reiter's syndrome
- Metatarsalgia
- Tarsal tunnel syndrome
- Metatarsal stress fracture

MEANS OF CONFIRMATION OR DIAGNOSIS

Imaging

- X-ray for incidental heel spur[7]

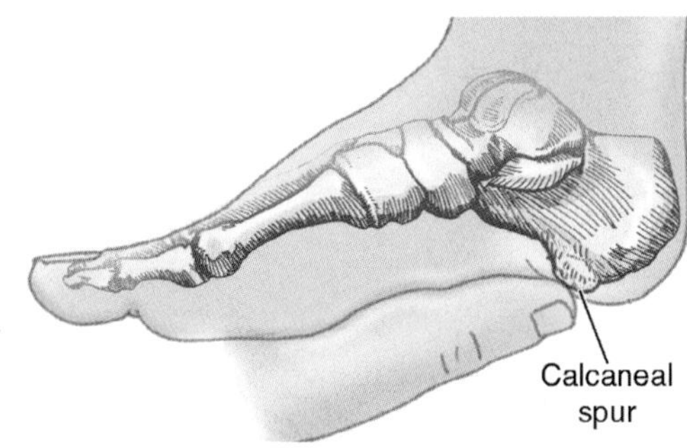

FIGURE 212-2 Palpation in this area is painful in patients with plantar fasciitis. A calcaneal spur is shown which is commonly associated with this condition. (From Simon RR, Sherman SC. *Emergency Orthopedics.* 6th ed. http://www.accessmedicine.com. Copyright © The McGraw-Hill Companies, Inc. All rights reserved.)

- Diagnostic ultrasound for tear or fluid in flexor digitorum or tibialis posterior muscles
- MRI[7]

FINDINGS AND INTERPRETATION

- Heel spur secondary to plantar fascia pulling away from the calcaneus[7]

TREATMENT

Medications

- Corticosteroid injection[8]
- Platelet rich plasma (PRP) injection

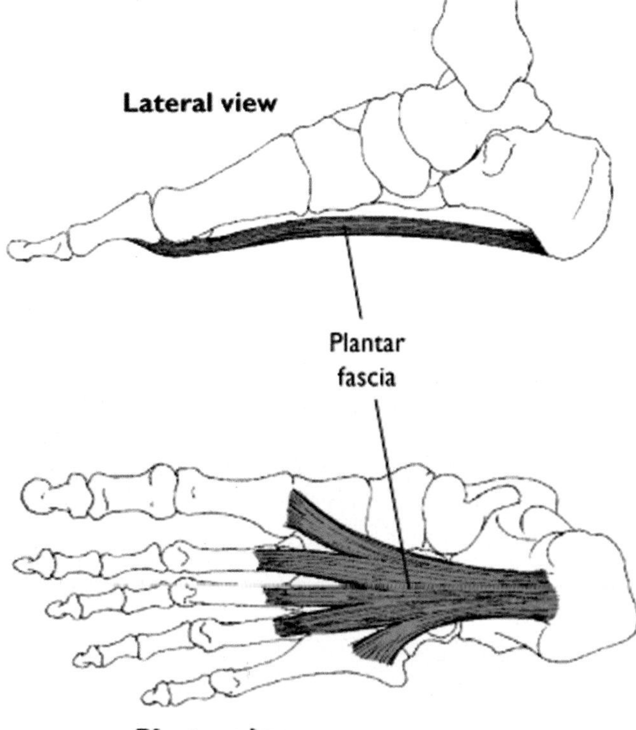

FIGURE 212-3 The plantar fascia. (From Hall SJ. *Basic Biomechanics.* 5th ed. http://www.accessmedicine.com. Copyright © The McGraw-Hill Companies, Inc. All rights reserved.)

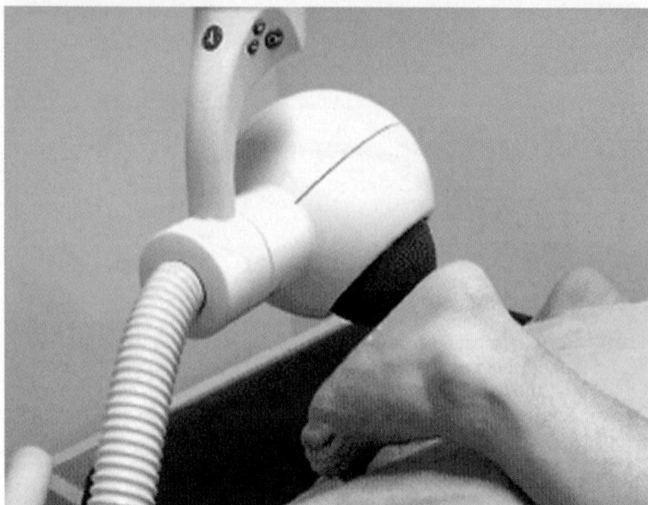

FIGURE 212-4 Patient positioning for treatment of plantar fasciitis. (From Prentice WE, Quillen WS, Underwood F. *Therapeutic Modalities in Rehabilitation.* 4th ed. http://www.accessmedicine.com. Copyright © The McGraw-Hill Companies, Inc. All rights reserved.)

MEDICAL PROCEDURES

- Surgical release
- Extracorporeal shockwave therapy[9]
- Radiofrequency (RF) microtenotomy

REFERRALS/ADMITTANCE

- To hospital for imaging, X-ray[7]
- To physician for medication: Anti-inflammatory or corticosteroid injection[8]
- To orthopedist for extracorporeal shockwave therapy[9]
- To surgeon for surgical consult: Endoscopic plantar fasciotomy

IMPAIRMENTS

- Antalgic gait secondary to weakened intrinsic flexors with push-off
- Unstable midtarsal joint causing overstretching on plantar fascia
- Antalgic gait secondary to decreased flexibility with dorsiflexion
- Inability to ambulate 1 mile secondary to pain
- Inability to stand for greater than 30 minutes secondary to pain

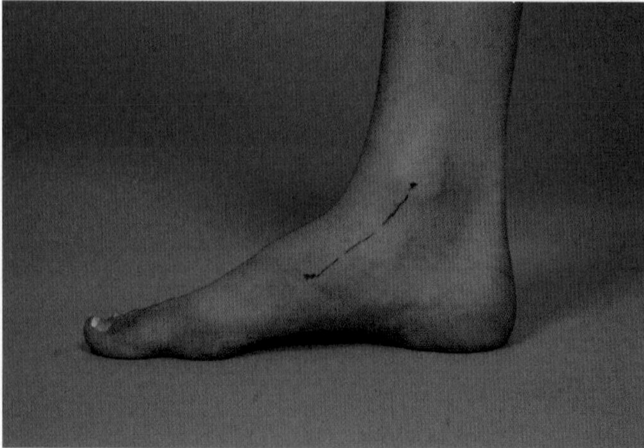

FIGURE 212-5 Feiss line. (From Dutton M: *Dutton's Orthopaedic Examination, Evaluation, and Intervention.* 3rd ed. http://www.accessmedicine.com. Copyright © The McGraw-Hill Companies, Inc. All rights reserved.)

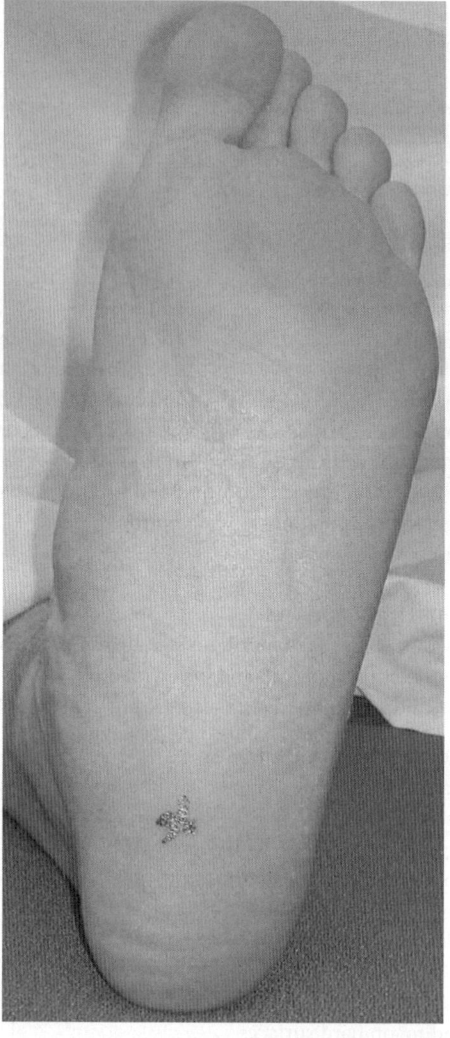

FIGURE 212-6 Plantar fasciitis. Photograph of the plantar aspect of the foot demonstrating the area of maximal tenderness for proximal plantar fasciitis. (From Imboden J, Hellmann DB, Stone JH. *Current Rheumatology Diagnosis & Treatment.* 2nd ed. http://www.accessmedicine.com. Copyright © The McGraw-Hill Companies, Inc. All rights reserved.)

TESTS AND MEASURES

- Dorsiflexion range of motion
- Midtarsal stability
- Navicular drop test: Non–weight-bearing to weight-bearing arch height drop test
- Feiss line test

INTERVENTION

- Rest: Weight off feet will allow tissue healing
- Taping of arch and plantar fascia
- Heel lift
- Orthotics: Heel cup to support arch, limit over stretching[3]
- Controlled ankle motion (CAM) walker or rocker boot to limit pronation
- Proper footwear (arch support) to limit overstretching of fascia[10]
- Night splints for achilles/posterior leg fascia stretch
- Address swelling
  - Ice[11]
  - Elevation[12]

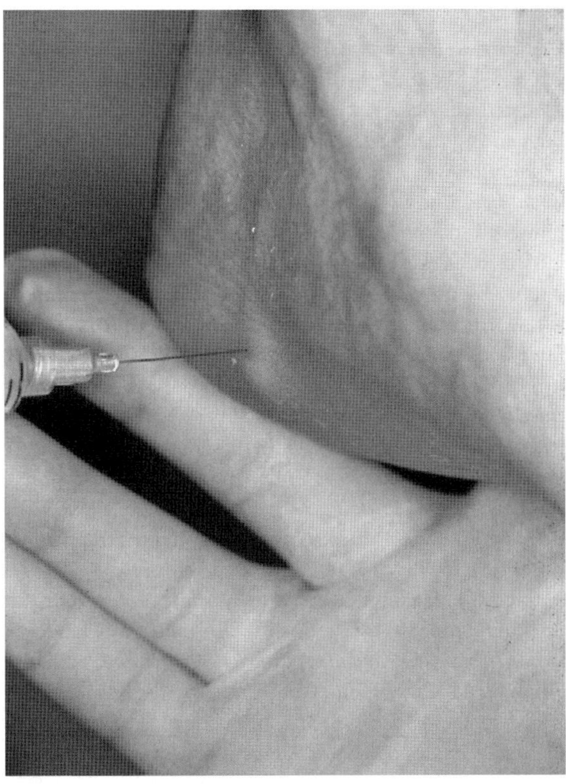

FIGURE 212-7 Therapeutic injection site on the medial heel for plantar fasciitis. (From Imboden J, Hellmann DB, Stone JH. *Current Rheumatology Diagnosis & Treatment.* 2nd ed. http://www.accessmedicine.com. Copyright © The McGraw-Hill Companies, Inc. All rights reserved.)

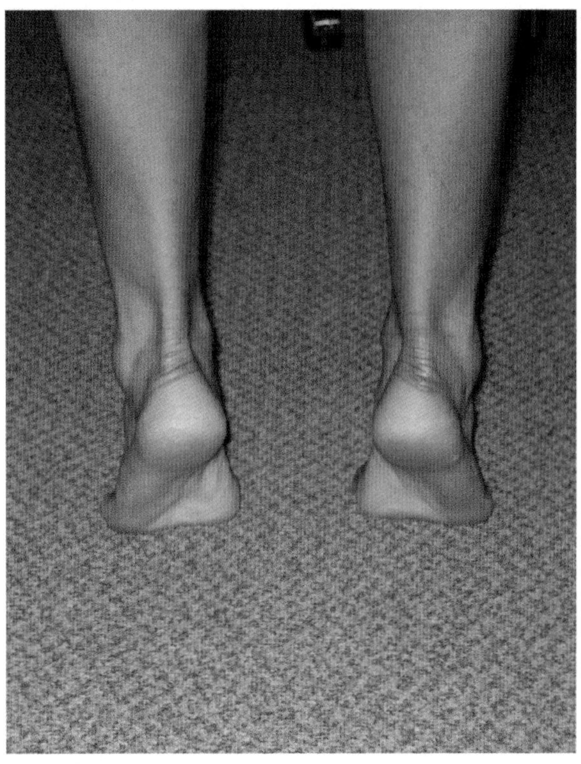

FIGURE 212-8 Toe raise test for pes planus. When the patient is asked to go up on her toes the medial longitudinal arch is normally evident and the heel goes into inversion or varus as shown. (From Patel DR, Greydanus DE, Baker RJ. *Pediatric Practice: Sports Medicine.* http://www.accesspediatrics.com. Copyright © The McGraw-Hill Companies, Inc. All rights reserved.)

- Address pain
  - Ice[11]
  - Massage[13] for trigger points in the calf muscles, plantar fascia and quadratus plantae
  - Electric stimulation[14]
  - Ultrasound[15]
  - Infrared
- Address weakness and joint instability
  - Balance and strengthening[5]
    - Toe curls, flexor intrinsic
    - Calf raises to point
    - Active walking
    - Standing arch raises
    - Single-leg balance
- Address lack of flexibility
  - Fluidotherapy[11]
  - Stretching[16]
    - Gastrocnemius and soleus
    - Fascia if pes cavus foot type
- Address mobilization
  - Posterior talus glides[3]
  - Subtalar mobility
  - Navicular, cuboid, cuneiforms[4]
  - Superior tib-fib joint
  - Widening of the mortise
    - Distal tibia and fibula mobility

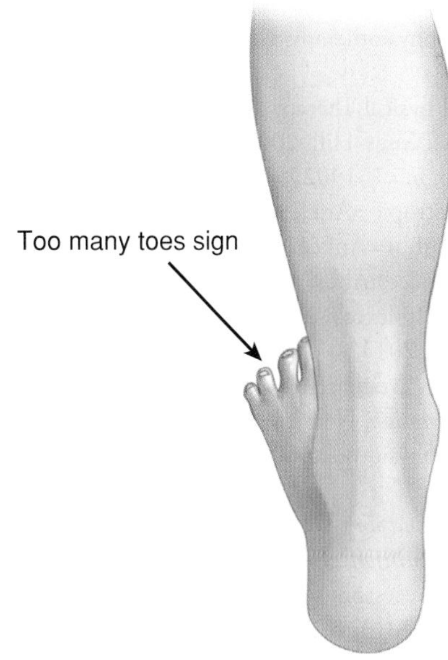

FIGURE 212-9 Too many toes sign. In case of tibialis posterior dysfunction, with the patient standing full weight-bearing the medial longitudinal arch is lost, the foot goes into valgus and hyperpronation, and looking from behind more than one toe are seen lateral to the foot. (From Patel DR, Greydanus DE, Baker RJ. *Pediatric Practice: Sports Medicine.* http://www.accesspediatrics.com. Copyright © The McGraw-Hill Companies, Inc. All rights reserved.)

FUNCTIONAL GOALS

- Patient will be able to:
  - Take the first step of the day pain-free to be able to ambulate to the restroom.
  - Stand maintaining subtalar neutral position for >2 minutes.
  - Ambulate pain-free for >45 minutes for grocery shopping.
  - Achieve 15 degrees of talocrural dorsiflexion during push-off phase of gait.
  - Achieve 70 degrees of great-toe extension during push-off phase of gait.
  - Unilateral stand in subtalar neutral for 1 minute with eyes open.

PROGNOSIS

- Very good, though recovery may take up to 1 year without complete care of modalities and biomechanical changes.

PATIENT RESOURCE

- Plantar Fasciitis. American Orthopaedic Foot and Ankle Society. http://www.aofas.org/footcaremd/conditions/ailments-of-the-heel/Pages/Plantar-Fasciitis.aspx. Accessed February 28, 2013.

REFERENCES

1. The American Physical Therapy Association. Pattern 4E: Impaired joint mobility, motor function, muscle performance, and range of motion associated with localized inflammation. *Interactive Guide to Physical Therapist Practice*. 2003. doi: 10.2522/ptguide.3.1_5. Accessed February 28, 2013.
2. Polousky JD. Chapter 24. Orthopedics. In: Hay W, Levin MJ, Sondheimer JM, Detering RR, eds. *CURRENT Diagnosis & Treatment: Pediatrics*. New York, NY: McGraw-Hill; 2011. http://www.accessphysiotherapy.com/abstract/6585912#6585914. Accessed February 28, 2013.
3. Dutton M. *Dutton's Orthopaedic Examination, Evaluation, and Intervention*. 3rd ed. New York, NY: McGraw-Hill; 2012. http://www.accessphysiotherapy.com/resource/612. Accessed February 28, 2013.
4. American Physical Therapy Association. *Anatomy and Physiology Revealed*. McGraw-Hill. 2007. http://anatomy.mcgraw-hill.com/apt.html?login=1319029535954&system=Muscular§ion=Dissection&topic=Ankle%20and%20foot&topicAbbr=Ank&view=Superior%20and%20inferior&viewAbbr=Sin&catAbbr=Mus&grpAbbr=Mua&structure=Origin%20of%20flexor%20digitorum%20brevis%252. Accessed February 28, 2013.
5. Hamilton N, Weimar W, Luttgens K. *Kinesiology: Scientific Basis of Human Motion*. New York, NY: McGraw-Hill; 2008. http://www.accessphysiotherapy.com/resource/618. Accessed February 28, 2013.
6. Dutton M. *Dutton's Orthopedic Survival Guide: Managing Common Conditions*. New York, NY: McGraw-Hill; 2011. http://www.accessphysiotherapy.com/resource/612. Accessed February 28, 2013.
7. Malone TR, Hazle C, Grey ML. *Imaging in Rehabilitation*. New York, NY: McGraw-Hill; 2008. http://www.accessphysiotherapy.com/resource/613. Accessed February 28, 2013.
8. Panus PC, Jobst EE, Masters SB, Katzung B, Tinsley SL, Trevor AJ. *Pharmacology for the Physical Therapist*. New York, NY: McGraw-Hill; 2009. http://www.accessphysiotherapy.com/resource/615. Accessed February 28, 2013.
9. Thigpen C. Chapter 18. Extracorporeal shock wave therapy. In: Prentice WE, Quillen WS, Underwood F, eds. *Therapeutic Modalities in Rehabilitation*. 4th ed. New York, NY: McGraw-Hill; 2011. http://www.accessphysiotherapy.com/abstract/5385627. Accessed February 28, 2013.
10. Diokno E. Appendix A. Introduction to bracing, splinting, and casting. In: Patel DR, Greydanus DE, Baker RJ, eds. *Pediatric Practice: Sports Medicine*. New York, NY: McGraw-Hill; 2009. http://www.accessphysiotherapy.com/abstract/6983252#6983256. Accessed February 28, 2013.
11. Prentice WE. Chapter 9. Cryotherapy and thermotherapy. In: Prentice WE, Quillen WS, Underwood F, eds. *Therapeutic Modalities in Rehabilitation*. 4th ed. New York, NY: McGraw-Hill; 2011. http://www.accessphysiotherapy.com/content/8137995#8137995. Accessed February 28, 2013.
12. Prentice WE. Chapter 2. Using therapeutic modalities to affect the healing process. In: Prentice WE, Quillen WS, Underwood F, eds. *Therapeutic Modalities in Rehabilitation*. 4th ed. New York, NY: McGraw-Hill; 2011. http://www.accessphysiotherapy.com/abstract/8135233#8135235. Accessed February 28, 2013.
13. Prentice WE. Chapter 16. Therapeutic massage. In: Prentice WE, Quillen WS, Underwood F, eds. *Therapeutic Modalities in Rehabilitation*. 4th ed. New York, NY: McGraw-Hill; 2011. http://www.accessphysiotherapy.com/abstract/8140762. Accessed February 28, 2013.
14. Hooker DN, Prentice WE. Chapter 5. Basic principles of electricity and electrical stimulating currents. In: Prentice WE, Quillen WS, Underwood F, eds. *Therapeutic Modalities in Rehabilitation*. 4th ed. New York, NY: McGraw-Hill; 2011. http://www.accessphysiotherapy.com/content/8136367#8136367. Accessed February 28, 2013.
15. Draper DO, Prentice WE. Chapter 10. Therapeutic ultrasound. In: Prentice WE, Quillen WS, Underwood F, eds. *Therapeutic Modalities in Rehabilitation*.4th ed. New York, NY: McGraw-Hill; 2011. http://www.accessphysiotherapy.com/abstract/8138751. Accessed February 28, 2013.
16. Dutton M. *McGraw Hill's NPTE (National Physical Therapy Examination)*. 2nd ed. New York, NY: McGraw-Hill; 2012. http://www.accessphysiotherapy.com/resource/611. Accessed February 28, 2013.

ADDITIONAL REFERENCES

- Hay WW, Levin MJ, Sondheimer JM, Deterding RR. Common Sports medicine issues & injuries. In: Hay W, Levin MJ, Sondheimer JM, Detering RR, eds. *CURRENT Diagnosis & Treatment: Pediatrics*. New York, NY: McGraw-Hill; 2011. http://www.accessphysiotherapy.com/content/6586350. Accessed February 28, 2013.
- ICD9DATA web site. http://www.icd9data.com. Accessed February 28, 2013.
- ICD10DATA web site. http://www.icd10data.com. Accessed February 28, 2013.

213 SESAMOIDITIS

Christina L. Pettie, MHA, PT
Eric Shamus, PhD, DPT, PT, CSCS

ICD-9-CM CODE

- 733.99 Other disorders of bone and cartilage

ICD-10-CM CODES

- M89.30 Hypertrophy of bone, unspecified site
- M89.8X9 Other specified disorders of bone, unspecified site
- M94.8X9 Other specified disorders of cartilage, unspecified sites

PREFERRED PRACTICE PATTERN

- 4E: Impaired joint mobility, motor function, muscle performance, and ROM associated with localized inflammation

PATIENT PRESENTATION

Patient is a 56-year-old plumber. Two weeks ago he was working in a tight area under the sink and had his ankle dorsiflexed with all of the weight on his forefoot. The toes were all into extension. When he stood up he had pain under his big toe from what he described as an over stretching. He tried to put some ice on his foot. He presents with decreased motion at the first metatarsophalangeal (MTP) joint with swelling. He is having difficulty pushing off on the foot when trying to go up the ladder. Upon palpation he is point tenderness at the flexor hallicus longus and both sesamoids.

KEY FEATURES

Description[1]

- Inflammatory condition of the periosteum of the sesamoid bone
- Inflammation and swelling of the peritendinous structures around the two sesamoid bones under the first metatarsal head, medial (tibial), and lateral (fibular) sesamoid
- If caused by a sudden injury, may have a fracture of one or both sesamoids
- Will alter mechanics during the push-off phase of gait

Essentials of Diagnosis

- Diagnosis is usually made by clinical examination or X-ray
- Can be an independent diagnosis and not associated with a disease process

General Considerations

- Swelling
- Inflammation greatest on the plantar surface of the joint
- Often termed turf toe, but has a different tendinous structure injury[2]

Demographics

- Commonly seen in
  - Dancers
  - People who squat for long periods of time (i.e., baseball players)
  - People who often run/jump on the balls of their feet (i.e., sprinters)
  - Women who wear high heels while standing or walking for long periods of time
  - The elderly, due to age-related changes such as osteoarthritis (OA) and osteoporosis

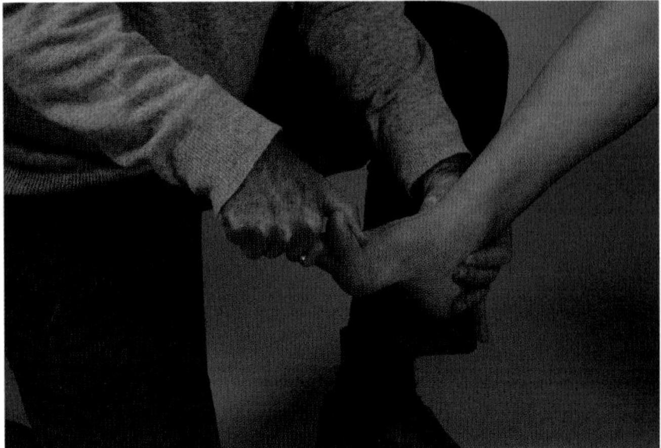

FIGURE 213-1 Resisted great toe extension. (From Dutton M. *Dutton's Orthopaedic Examination, Evaluation, and Intervention.* 3rd ed. http://www.accessphysiotherapy.com. Copyright © The McGraw-Hill Companies, Inc. All rights reserved.)

CLINICAL FINDINGS

SIGNS AND SYMPTOMS

- Early stage
  - Tenderness at the sesamoid bones
  - Mild pain with walking, especially in thin soled shoes
  - Pain with running and jumping
  - Mild swelling of sesamoids that subsides with rest/elevation/ice
- Late stage
  - Constant pain may be present
  - Pain with bending toes up
  - Pain with weight-bearing activity
  - Swelling of the soft tissue that does not subside with rest/elevation
  - Eventually, entire first MTP joint becomes swollen
- Decreased extension or dorsiflexion of the big toe
- Joint redness and pain
- Limited motion of the MTP joint due to pain

Functional Implications

- Pain with standing
- Pain during ambulation at the toe
- Alteration of gait pattern and mechanical issues of the forefoot, can increase supination and external rotation of the foot for clearance; also forefoot abduction, lateral whip

Possible Contributing Causes

- Age-related changes (i.e., OA, which may cause bone spurs, or osteoporosis, which may cause fractures)
- Direct injury (i.e., stepping on something hard)
- Microtrauma: Overuse injury/repetitive stress and high impact
- Hereditary defects
  - High arches; rigid foot causing increased contact of the sesamoids with the ground
  - Plantarflexed first ray
  - Increased pronation
  - Enlarged sesamoids

Differential Diagnosis[3]

- Arthritis
- Bursitis
- Chondromalacia
- Fracture
- Gout
- Hallux rigidus
- Hallux valgus
- Hammer toe
- Metatarsal stress fracture
- Metatarsalgia
- Osteochondritic lesion of the first metatarsal head
- Osteochondritis dissecans
- Rheumatoid arthritis
- Stress fracture
- Synovitis
- Turf toe

MEANS OF CONFIRMATION OR DIAGNOSIS

Imaging

- X-ray
- Bone scan
- CT scan
- MRI

FINDINGS AND INTERPRETATION

- Edema
- Fracture[4]

REFERRALS/ADMITTANCE

- For imaging: X-ray
- For medication: NSAIDs, anti-inflammatory or corticosteroid injection

IMPAIRMENTS

- Antalgic gait secondary to toe pain and inflammation may cause increased supination to avoid pain
- Antalgic gait secondary to toe pain and inflammation may cause more pronation with increased abduction/ER of the foot leading the patient to collapse at the medial arch and pronate further to avoid toe pain
- Antalgic gait secondary to pain at the first toe with push-off
- Hypomobility of the MTP joint big toe
- Inability to ambulate 1-mile distance secondary to pain

TESTS AND MEASURES

- Passive dorsiflexion of the MTP with palpation and stabilization of the sesamoid; Positive Test = pain

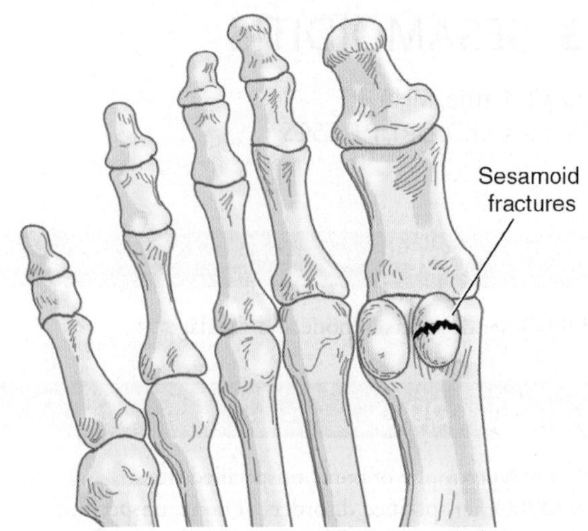

FIGURE 213-2 Sesamoid fractures. (From Simon RR, Sherman SC. *Emergency Orthopedics*. 6th ed. http://www.accessmedicine.com. Copyright © The McGraw-Hill Companies, Inc. All rights reserved.)

- LE limb strength
- Balance
  - Static single-leg standing (eyes open, eyes closed)
    - Contralateral LE
  - Dynamic standing
    - Berg Balance Scale
    - Functional gait assessment
- Gait assessment
  - Observational analysis
  - Gait speed via the 10-m walk test

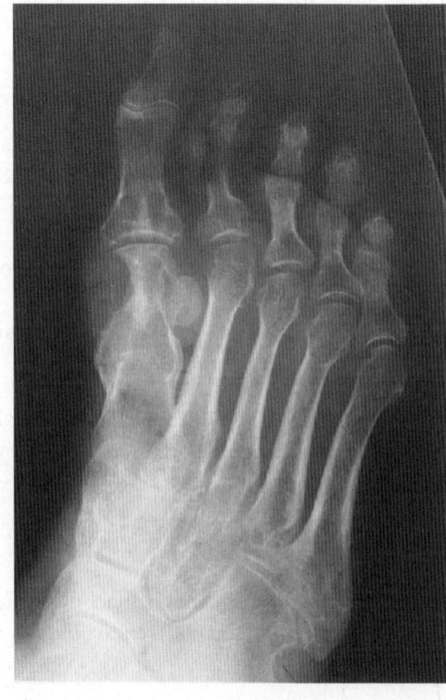

FIGURE 213-3 An oblique view of right foot in a 60-year-old man who presented to the emergency department with intense foot pain. He was a known alcoholic. (From Chen MYM, Pope TL, Ott DJ. *Basic Radiology*. 2nd ed. http://www.accessmedicine.com. Copyright © The McGraw-Hill Companies, Inc. All rights reserved.)

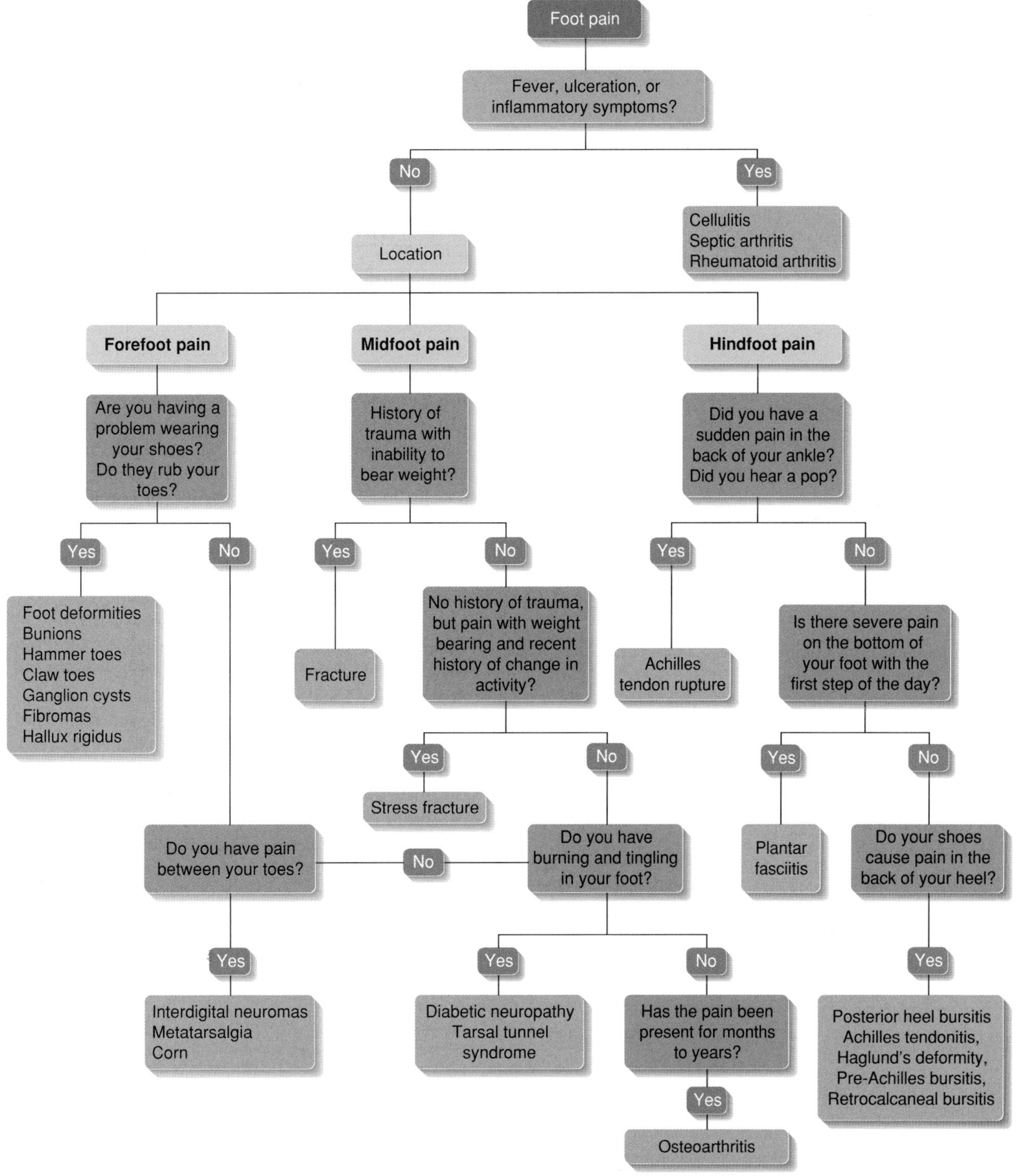

FIGURE 213-4 Diagnostic approach: Foot pain. (From Henderson MC, Tierney LM, Smetana GW. *The Patient History: An Evidence-Based Approach to Differential Diagnosis.* http://www.accessmedicine.com. Copyright © The McGraw-Hill Companies, Inc. All rights reserved.)

- 2-minute walk test
- 6-minute walk test

INTERVENTION

- Rest, keep weight off feet to allow for reduction of inflammation
- Cast or walking boot for fracture
- Stabilize foot with orthotics
- High arch support
- Provide shock absorption for the foot
- Donut pad to offload pressure on the sesamoids or dancer's pad to unweight the sesamoids
- Taping for stabilization
- Address swelling
  - Ice

- Address pain[5–7]
  - Ice
  - Massage
  - Joint mobilization
  - Electric stimulation[6]
  - Iontophoresis
  - Infrared
- Address weakness, joint instability
  - Strengthening
    - Toe curls, flexor hallicus strengthening
    - Great toe abduction
    - Calf raises to point
    - Active walking
    - Standing arch raises
- Address lack of flexibility
  - Stretching
  - Gastrocnemius/Soleus
  - Plantar Fascia
  - Fluidotherapy
  - Heat
- Gastrocnemius/Soleus in cases of Achilles contracture
- Plantar fascia in patients with pes cavus
  - Fluidotherapy
- Address joint mobilization
  - First MTP glides
  - Posterior talus glides
  - Subtalar joint (STJ) inversion/eversion
  - Navicular/Cuboid/Cuneiforms
- Address soft tissue mobilization
  - Abductor hallucis and first and second lumbrical/dorsal interossei
  - Plantar fascia
  - Gastrocnemius/Soleus
- Patient education in footwear
  - Wide and deep toe box
  - Correct length for feet
  - Heel of shoes should be no higher than 1 inch
  - Well-padded innersole, running and jumping in well-padded shoes
  - Orthotic with first ray cut out
- Surgery

FUNCTIONAL GOALS

- Recognize and maintain a subtalar neutral position for >2 minutes.
- Ambulate pain-free for >45 minutes.
  - Achieve 15 degrees of talocrural dorsiflexion during stance phase of gait.
  - Achieve 70 degrees of great toe extension during push-off phase of gait.
  - Stand unilaterally in subtalar neutral position for 1 minute with eyes open.

PROGNOSIS

- Good; patients can expect reduction of pain with conservative therapeutic intervention.

PATIENT RESOURCE

- Sesamoiditis. OrthiInfo: AAOS American Academy of Orthpaedic Surgeons. http://orthoinfo.aaos.org/topic.cfm?topic=A00164&grpwebid=26D4EB. Accessed August 17, 2014.

REFERENCES

1. Dutton M. The ankle and foot. In: *Dutton's Orthopaedic Examination, Evaluation, and Intervention*. 2nd ed. New York, NY: McGraw-Hill; 2008. http://www.accessphysiotherapy.com/content/55587308#55587308. Accessed April 15, 2013.
2. Dutton M. The ankle and foot. In: *Dutton's Orthopaedic Examination, Evaluation, and Intervention*. 2nd ed. New York, NY: McGraw-Hill; 2008. http://www.accessphysiotherapy.com/content/55587003#55587003. Accessed April 15, 2013.
3. Dutton M. The ankle and foot. *Dutton's Orthopaedic Examination, Evaluation, and Intervention*. 2nd ed. New York, NY: McGraw-Hill; 2008. http://www.accessphysiotherapy.com/content/55586986#55586986. Accessed April 15, 2013.
4. Hamilton N, Weimar W, Luttgens K. Kinesiology of fitness and exercise. In: Hamilton N, Weimar W, Luttgens K, eds. *Kinesiology: Scientific Basis of Human Motion*. 11th ed. New York, NY: McGraw-Hill; 2008. http://www.accessphysiotherapy.com/content/6151881#6151881. Accessed April 15, 2013.
5. Prentice WE. Cryotherapy and thermotherapy. In: Prentice WE, Quillen WS, Underwood F, eds. *Therapeutic Modalities in Rehabilitation*. 4th ed. New York, NY: McGraw-Hill; 2011. http://www.accessphysiotherapy.com/content/8138236#8138236. Accessed April 15, 2013.
6. Prentice WE. Basic principles of electricity and electrical stimulating currents. In: Prentice WE, Quillen WS, Underwood F, eds. *Therapeutic Modalities in Rehabilitation*. 4th ed. New York, NY: McGraw-Hill; 2011. http://www.accessphysiotherapy.com/content/8136028. Accessed April 15, 2013.
7. Prentice WE. Cryotherapy and thermotherapy. In: Prentice WE, Quillen WS, Underwood F, eds. *Therapeutic Modalities in Rehabilitation*. 4th ed. New York, NY: McGraw-Hill; 2011. http://www.accessphysiotherapy.com/content/8137946#8137946. Accessed April 15, 2013.

ADDITIONAL REFERENCES

- Hockenbury RT. Forefoot problems in athletes. *Med Sci Sports Exerc*. 1999;31(7 suppl):S448–S458.
- Jahss MH. The sesamoids of the hallux. *Clin Orthop*. 1981;157:88–97.
- McBryde AM Jr, Anderson RB. Sesamoid problems in the athlete. *Clin Sports Med*. 1998;7:51–60.
- Richardson EG. Injuries to the hallucal sesamoids in the athlete. *Foot Ankle*. 1987;7:229–224.
- Sammarco GJ. Turf toe. *Instr Course Lect*. 1993;42:207–212.
- Scranton PE, Rutkowski R. Anatomic variations in the first ray. Part B. Disorders of the sesamoids. *Clin Orthop*. 1980;151: 256–254.
- Van Hal ME, Keeve JS, Lange TA, et al. Stress fractures of the sesamoids. *Am J Sports Med*. 1982;10(2):122–128.
- Weinfeld SB, Schon LC. Hallux metatarsophalangeal arthritis. *Clin Orthop Relat Res*. 1998;349:9–19.

214 TURF TOE

Jennifer Shamus, PhD, DPT, COMT, CSCS
Eric Shamus, PhD, DPT, PT, CSCS

CONDITION/DISORDER SYNONYM

- Metatarsophalangeal (MTP) joint sprain

ICD-9-CM CODE[1]

- 845.12 Sprain of metatarsophalangeal (joint) of foot

ICD-10-CM CODE[2]

- S93.529A Sprain of metatarsophalangeal joint of unspecified toe(s), initial encounter

PREFERRED PRACTICE PATTERN[3]

- 4E: Impaired Joint Mobility, Motor Function, Muscle Performance, and ROM Associated with Localized Inflammation

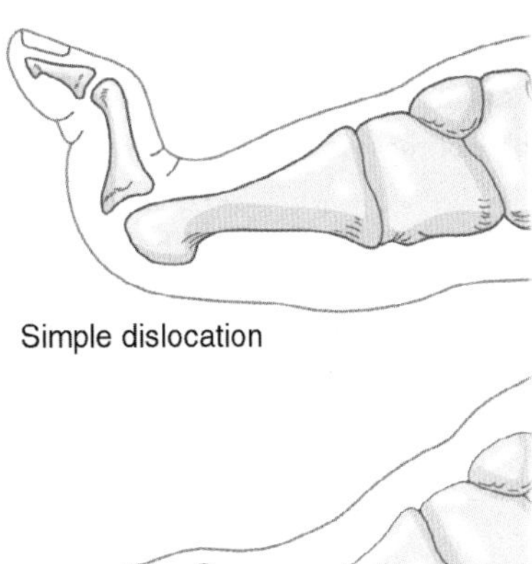

FIGURE 214-1 Metatarsophalangeal dislocations. (From Simon RR, Sherman SC. *Emergency Orthopedics,*. 6th ed. http://www.accessemergencymedicine.com. Copyright © The McGraw-Hill Companies, Inc. All rights reserved.)

PATIENT PRESENTATION

A 20-year-old football player hyperextended the great toe while playing on synthetic turf grass. He thinks his cleat may have gotten stuck in the turf while being tackled. The patient has a painful and swollen MTP joint of the great toe. He cannot walk or run without pain. Patient states the toe hurts the most when he tries to push-off with the toe/foot. The patient has a turf toe orthotic in his shoe.

KEY FEATURES

Description[4]

- Sprain to the ligaments and capsule around the big (great) toe metatarsophalangeal joint (MTP or MTPJ)
- Caused by a hyperextension or hyperflexion injury of the big toe, first MTP joint
- Typically a sudden injury, common to fall (tackled) over a fixed foot overstretching the toe into hyperextension
- Limited joint mobility at the MTP joint
- Can involve the sesamoid bones (two small bones embedded in the flexor hallucis brevis)

Essentials of Diagnosis

- Diagnosis is usually made by clinical examination or x-ray
- Can be an independent diagnosis and not associated with a disease process
- Three grades of severity classification[5]
  - Grade 1 sprain: Minor stretch injury to the soft-tissue restraints with little pain, swelling, or disability
  - Grade 2 sprain: Partial tear of the capsuloligamentous structures with moderate pain, swelling, ecchymosis, and disability
  - Grade 3: Complete tear of the plantar plate with severe swelling, pain, ecchymosis, and an inability to bear weight normally

General Considerations

- Pain and swelling
- Inflammation around the first MTP joint
- Will alter mechanics during the push-off phase of gait
- If not managed properly, arthritis, spurring, and osteophytes can develop

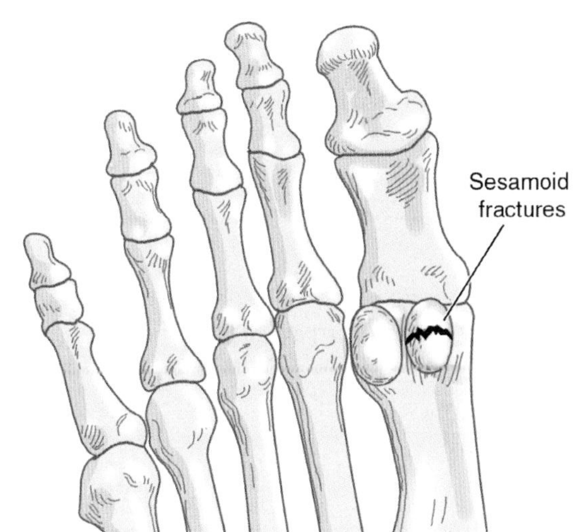

FIGURE 214-2 Sesamoid fractures. (From Simon RR, Sherman SC. *Emergency Orthopedics*. 6th ed. http://www.accessemergencymedicine.com. Copyright © The McGraw-Hill Companies, Inc. All rights reserved.)

Demographics

- Commonly seen in athletes playing on artificial surfaces
- Can happen on grass with a shoe that does not adequately support the foot (such as soccer shoes)
- Dancers, football players, rugby players

CLINICAL FINDINGS

SIGNS AND SYMPTOMS

- Pain at the base of the first toe
- Starts suddenly as a result of injury
- Pain first metatarsal with walking
- Decreased extension or flexion of the big toe
- Joint redness and pain
- Limited motion of the MTP joint due to pain
- Weakness of toe flexion/extension

Functional Implications

- Pain with standing and ambulation
- Lack of push-off with toe and plantar flexion, reducing speed in running
- Pain with ambulation at the toe
- Alteration of gait pattern and mechanical issues of the forefoot can increase supination and external rotation of the foot for clearance, also forefoot abduction, lateral whip

Possible Contributing Causes

- Abnormal bone structure
- Trauma

Differential Diagnosis

- Dislocation of the MTP
- Hallux valgus
- Sesamoiditis
- Hallux rigidus
- Gout
- Osteochondrotic lesion of the first metatarsal head
- Osteochondritis dissecans
- Metatarsalgia
- Metatarsal stress fracture

MEANS OF CONFIRMATION OR DIAGNOSIS

Imaging

- X-ray
- Bone scan
- CT scan
- MRI

FINDINGS AND INTERPRETATION

- Edema
- Ligamentous laxity
- Levels of sprains[5]

TREATMENT

Medication

- Anti-inflammatory
- Corticosteroid injection

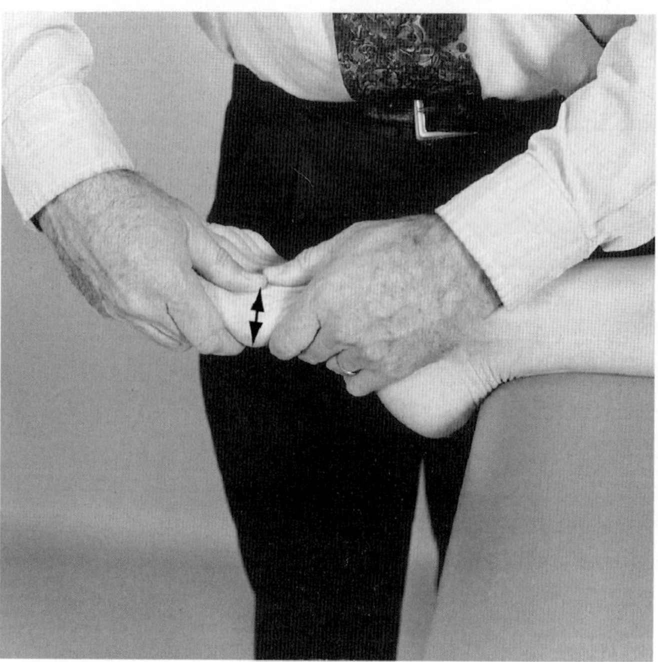

FIGURE 214-3 Testing the first MTP joint motion. (From Dutton M. *Dutton's Orthopedic Survival Guide: Managing Common Conditions:* http://www.accessphysiotherapy.com. Copyright © The McGraw-Hill Companies, Inc. All rights reserved.)

MEDICAL PROCEDURE

- Surgery

REFERRALS/ADMITTANCE

- For imaging
- For medication
- For surgical consult

IMPAIRMENTS

- Antalgic gait secondary to increased supination.
  - The toe pain and inflammation may increase supination to avoid pain or cause more pronation due to abduction/external rotation (ER) of the foot leading the patient to collapse at the medial arch and pronate further as they avoid the toe pain.

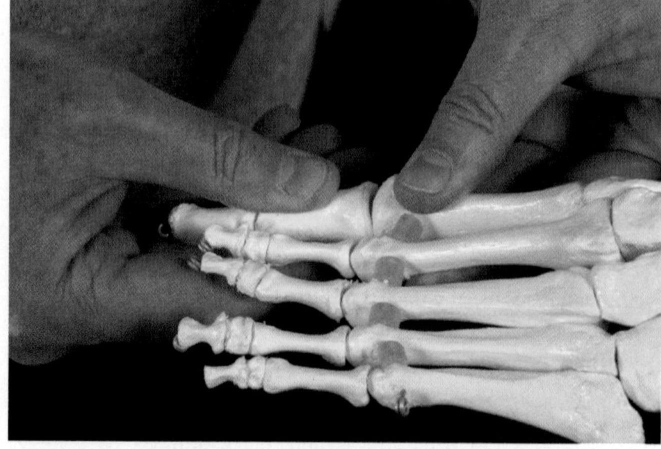

FIGURE 214-4 Long-axis distraction of the MTP joint. (From Dutton M. *Dutton's Orthopedic Survival Guide: Managing Common Conditions:* http://www.accessphysiotherapy.com. Copyright © The McGraw-Hill Companies, Inc. All rights reserved.)

- Antalgic gait secondary to pain at the first toe with push-off.
- Hypermobility of the MTP joint big toe with ligament laxity.
- Inability to ambulate distances of 1 mile secondary to pain.

TESTS AND MEASURES

- Flexor hallicus longus strength
- First metatarsal mobility
- Gait analysis

INTERVENTION

- Rest, weight off feet will allow for reduction of inflammation
- Taping to stabilize the great toe and limit extension ROM
  - As pain free ROM increase, allow more motion with the tape
- Cast shoe
- Orthotics with firm extension to the toes to limit toe ROM
  - Once the patient has full pain free ROM, should be removed
- Rigid foot plate to limit toe extension
- Donut pad to offload pressure on the sesamoids
- Addressing swelling
  - Ice
- Addressing pain
  - Ice or contrast bath
  - Massage
  - Joint mobilization
  - Electric stimulation
  - Iontophoresis
  - Ultrasound
  - Infrared
- Addressing weakness, joint instability
  - Strengthening
    - Toe curls, flexor intrinsics (towel crunches, marble pick-ups)
    - Flexor hallicus longus isotonics
    - Great toe abduction
    - Active walking
    - Standing arch raises
    - Eccentric exercises
    - Calf raises to point
- Addressing lack of flexibility
  - Stretching
    - Gastroc/soleus in cases of Achilles contracture
  - Fluidotherapy
- Addressing joint mobilization
  - MPJ dorsal/plantar/rotational/medial/lateral glides
  - Sesamoid glides superior/inferior
  - Posterior talus glides
  - Subtalar joint (STJ) inversion/eversion
  - Navicular/cuboid/cuneiforms
- Addressing soft-tissue mobilization
  - Abductor hallucis, first and second lumbrical/dorsal interossei, flexor hallicus longus/brevis
  - Plantar fascia
  - Gastroc/soleus
- Patient education in shoewear
  - Shoe with a board last
  - Proper support for activity

FUNCTIONAL GOALS

- Patient will be able to:
  - Recognize and maintain a subtalar neutral position for >2 minutes.
  - Ambulate pain free for >45 minutes.
  - Achieve 15 degrees of talocrural dorsiflexion during stance phase of gait with normal pattern pain free.
  - Achieve 65 degrees of great toe extension during push-off phase of gait with normal pattern pain-free.
  - Stand unilaterally in subtalar neutral position for 1 minute with eyes open.

PROGNOSIS

- Good, patients can expect reduction of pain with conservative therapeutic intervention.
- Grade 1 sprain, return as discomfort allows.
- Grade 2 sprain, 3 to 14 days rest.
- Grade 3 sprain, 2 to 6 weeks.[5]
- Many professional football players' careers ended secondary to turf toe with the inability to push-off with pain and decreased speed.[5]
- Fifty percent of athletes will have persistent symptoms 5 years later.[5]

PATIENT RESOURCE

- Turf Toe. American Academy of Orthopaedic Surgeons. http://orthoinfo.aaos.org/topic.cfm?topic=A00645. Accessed July 14, 2013.

REFERENCES

1. ICD9Data.com. http://www.icd9data.com. Accessed July 14, 2013.
2. ICD10Data.com. http://www.icd10data.com/ICD10CM/Codes. Accessed July 14, 2013.
3. The American Physical Therapy Association. Pattern 4E: Impaired joint mobility, motor function, muscle performance, and range of motion associated with localized inflammation. *Guide to Physical Therapist Practice*. 2nd ed. Alexandria, VA: American Physical Therapy Association; 2001. Revised 2003.
4. Dutton M. Chapter 19. The ankle and foot. In: Dutton M, ed. *Orthopaedic Examination, Evaluation, and Intervention*. 2nd ed. New York, NY: McGraw-Hill; 2008. http://www.accessphysiotherapy.com/content/55585614. Accessed July 14, 2013.
5. Clanton TO, Ford JJ. Turf toe injury. *Clin Sports Med.* 1984;13(4):731–741.

ADDITIONAL REFERENCES

- Glasoe WM, Yack HJ, Saltzman CL. Anatomy and biomechanics of the first ray. *Phys Ther*. 1999;79:854–859.
- Hamilton N, Weimar W, Luttgens K. Chapter 16. Kinesiology of fitness and exercise. In: Hamilton N, Weimar W, Luttgens K, eds. *Kinesiology: Scientific Basis of Human Motion*. New York, NY: McGraw-Hill; 2008. http://www.accessphysiotherapy.com/content/6151836. Accessed July 14, 2013.
- Prentice WE, Quillen WS, Underwood F, eds. *Therapeutic Modalities in Rehabilitation*. 4th ed. New York, NY: McGraw-Hill; 2011. http://www.accessphysiotherapy.com/resource/675. Accessed July 14, 2013.
- Shamus J, Shamus E, Gugel RN, Brucker BS, Skaruppa C. The effect of sesamoid mobilization, flexor hallucis strengthening, and gait training on reducing pain and restoring function in individuals with hallux limitus: a clinical trial. *J Ortho Sports Phys Ther*. 2004;34(7):368–376.

SECTION J NERVE/ENTRAPMENT DISORDERS

215 BELL'S PALSY

Eric Shamus, PhD, DPT, PT, CSCS
Jennie Q. Lou, MD, MSc

CONDITION/DISORDER SYNONYMS

- Facial palsy
- Peripheral facial paralysis

ICD-9-CM CODE

- 351.0 Bell's palsy

ICD-1-CM CODE

- G51.0 Bell's palsy, facial palsy

PREFERRED PRACTICE PATTERN

- 5D: Impaired Motor Function and Sensory Integrity Associated with Nonprogressive Disorders of the Central Nervous System––acquired in adolescence or adulthood

PATIENT PRESENTATION

Patient is a 35-year-old female who woke up with facial nerve paralysis. Patient presents with facial droop (see image 1). On examination it was found that she had absent brow furrowing, weak eye closure and drooping of her mouth angle. She was provided eye lubricants and guidance on keeping her eye moist. Patient is unable to smile or control muscles on the left side of the face. Patient received direct current electric stimulation during exercises.[1]

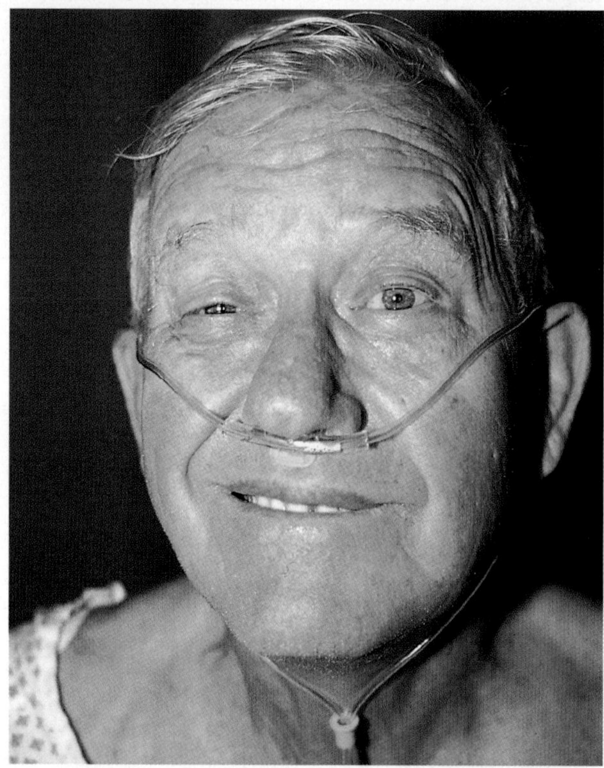

FIGURE 215-1 Peripheral Seventh-Nerve Palsy. A peripheral nerve paralysis involving the entire ipsilateral face, including the forehead, is seen in this patient with Bell palsy. (From Knoop KJ et al: *The Atlas of Emergency Medicine*, 3rd edition. www.accessmedicine.com. Copyright © The McGraw-Hill Companies, Inc. All rights reserved. Photo contributor: Lawrence B. Stack, MD.)

KEY FEATURES

- Paralysis or weakness of muscles on one side of face
- Sudden onset, often overnight
- Damage to the seventh cranial (facial) nerve that controls muscles on one side of the face, causing that side of face to droop[2]
- Nerve damage may affect sense of taste, production of tears and saliva
- Lower motor neuron (LMN) disease
- Diagnosis usually made by history and clinical examination
- Afflicts approximately 40,000 Americans each year
- Equally likely in men and women
- Can present at any age, but less common before age 15 years or after age 60
- More prevalent in people with diabetes or upper respiratory ailments, such as flu or cold
- More likely in pregnant women

CLINICAL FINDINGS

SIGNS AND SYMPTOMS

- Sudden weakness or paralysis on one side of face that causes it to droop (main symptom)
- Difficulty closing eye on affected side
- Drooling
- Dry mouth
- Eye problems, such as excessive tearing or dry eye
- Loss of ability to taste
- Pain in or behind ear
- Facial numbness on affected side
- Increased sensitivity to sound
- Headache
- Facial twitch
- Inability to smile or make facial expressions

▸ Functional Implications

- Dry eyes
- Eating

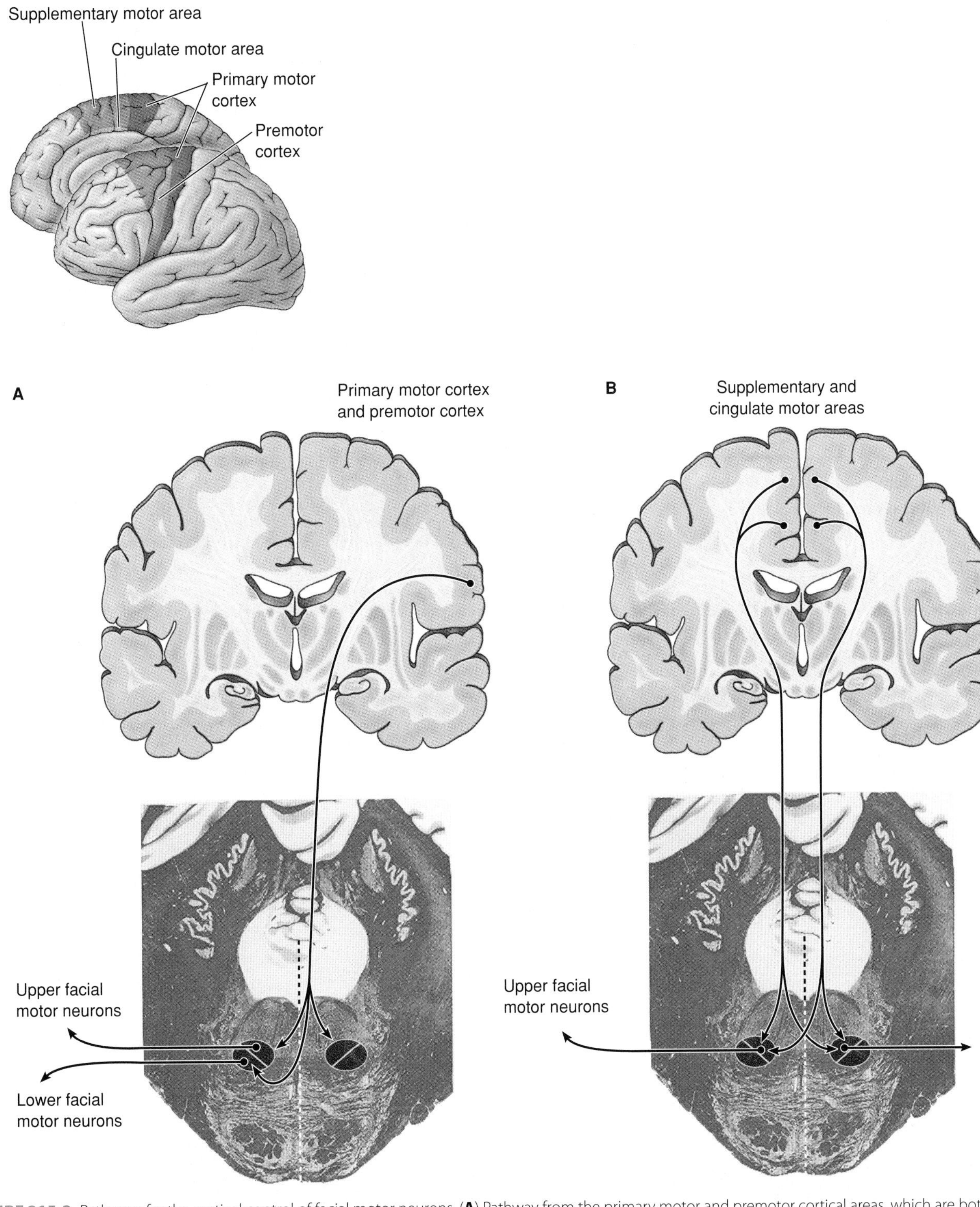

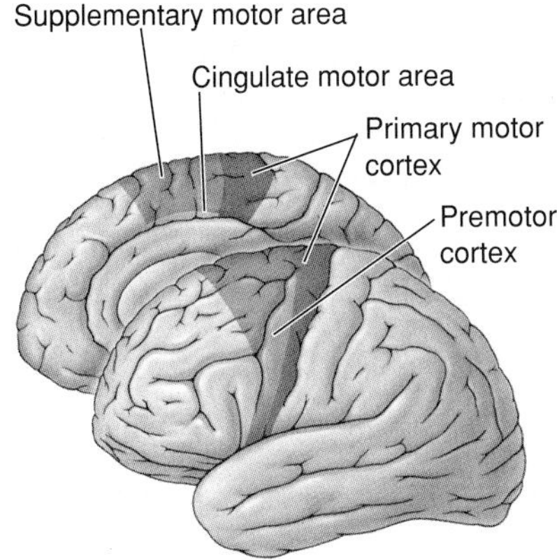

FIGURE 215-2 Pathways for the cortical control of facial motor neurons. (**A**) Pathway from the primary motor and premotor cortical areas, which are both located on the lateral surface of the cortex. (**B**) Pathway from the supplementary (top) and cingulate (bottom) motor areas, which are both located on the medial surface. The inset shows the locations of the primary motor cortex and the three premotor areas: the supplementary motor area, the cingulate motor area, and the premotor cortex. (From Martin JH. *Neuroanatomy Text and Atlas*. 4th ed. New York, NY: McGraw-Hill; 2012.)

- Hearing
- Psychological impact

Possible Contributing Causes

- The nerve that controls muscles on one side of the face is damaged by inflammation in most cases
- Root cause of Bell's palsy is not clear
- Most cases thought to be caused by the herpes virus that causes chickenpox and shingles, or Epstein–Barr virus that causes mononucleosis

Differential Diagnosis

- Brainstem infarct
- Brucellosis

- Diabetes mellitus
- Guillain–Barré syndrome
- Herpes simplex virus
- HIV infection
- Infections
- Lyme disease
- Meningitis
- Middle ear infection
- Ramsay Hunt syndrome[3]
- Sarcoidosis
- Stroke
- Tumors

MEANS OF CONFIRMATION OR DIAGNOSIS

- Blood tests
- MRI of the head to rule out brain tumor
- CT scan of the head to rule out brain tumor
- History and physical and neurological examination to check facial nerve function
- If cause of symptoms is not clear, other tests are needed, such as:
    - Nerve conduction test for facial nerve
    - Electromyography (EMG) for facial nerve

FINDINGS AND INTERPRETATION

- Facial muscle weakness or total paralysis (e.g., unable to frown) due to swollen, inflamed, or compressed facial nerve

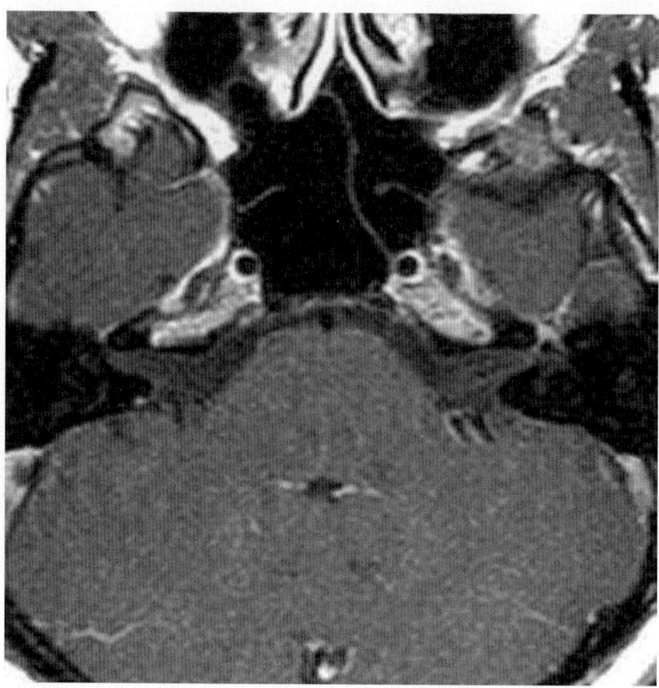

FIGURE 215-3 Facial nerve palsy. Axial postcontrast T1W image demonstrates abnormal enhancement of the genu of the left facial nerve compared with the right. (From Sakai O. *Head and Neck Imaging*. New York, NY: McGraw-Hill; 2011.)

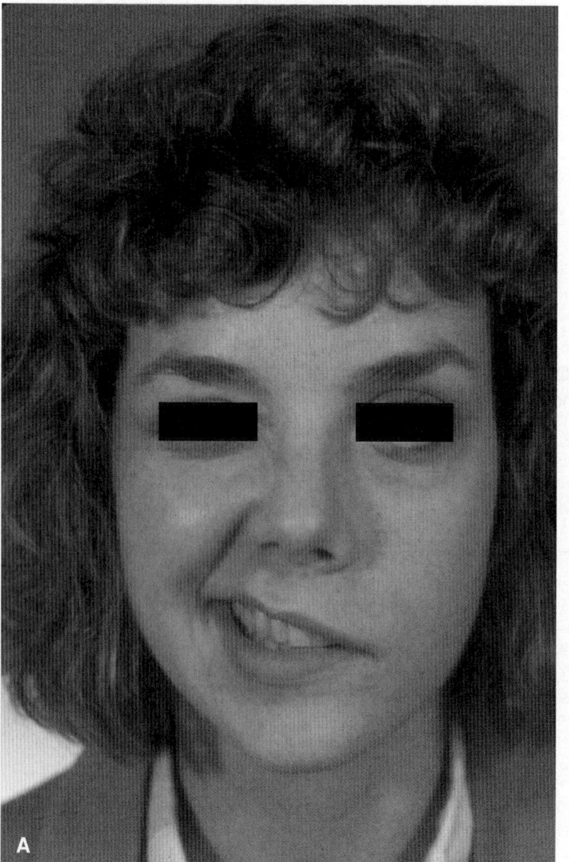

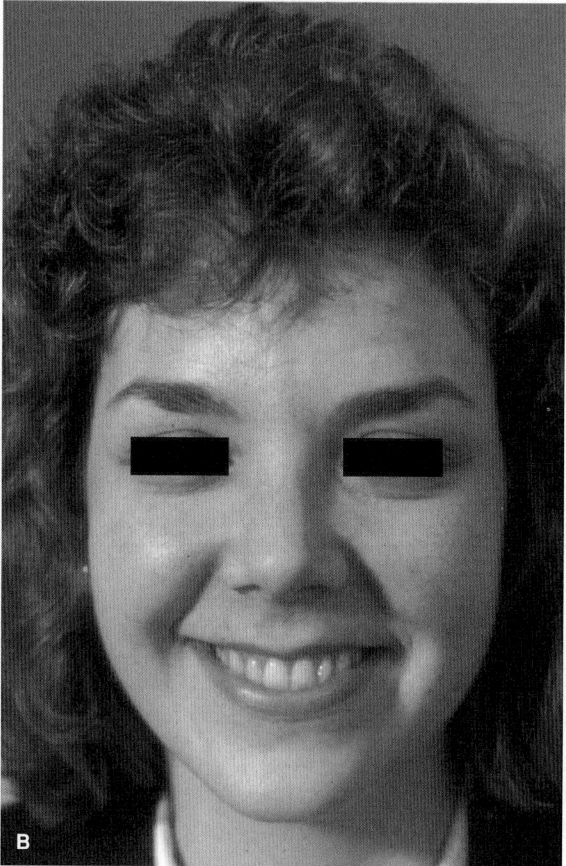

FIGURE 215-4 (**A**) Prototypic case of Bell's palsy. This 28-year-old woman experienced the onset of an acute, left-sided paralysis of the face over a 24-hour period, in a pattern consistent with peripheral nerve dysfunction. Treatment consisted of oral steroid dosing at pharmacological doses for 10 days, followed by a 2-week taper. (**B**) Full recovery of facial motor function 2 months after onset. (From Lalwani AK. *Current Diagnosis & Treatment in Otolaryngology-Head & Neck Surgery*. 3rd ed. www.accesssurgery.com. Copyright © The McGraw-Hill Companies, Inc. All rights reserved.)

- Drooping of eyelid and corner of mouth on the affected side due to muscle weakness or paralysis

REFERRALS/ADMITTANCE

- Ophthalmologists
- Ear, nose, and throat surgeons
- Plastic surgeons
- Psychologists

IMPAIRMENTS

- Impaired facial expression due to paralysis
- Problems eating (food stuck in month or falling out), difficulty swallowing
- Hearing impairment
- Pain

TESTS AND MEASURES

- History
- Physical examination
- Neurological examination to check facial nerve function

INTERVENTION

- Rest and steroids treatment
- Facial exercises
- Electric stimulation[4]
- Eye care
  - Use finger to close and open eyelid often throughout the day
  - Use eye drops (artificial tears) or ointment; use drops during the day and ointment at night while sleeping
  - Wear eye patch while sleeping, wear glasses or goggles the rest of the time
- Mouth care
  - Brush and floss teeth often and well to help prevent gum disease or tooth decay caused by residual food in the month
  - Eat slowly and chew well to prevent swallowing problems
  - Eating soft, smooth foods, such as yogurt

FUNCTIONAL GOALS

- Patient will be able to:
  - Drink without drooling, dripping.
  - Eat and chew independently.

PROGNOSIS

- Generally very good, self-limiting disease, may last several weeks.
- Symptoms may last longer for some.
- Symptoms may never completely disappear in a few cases.
- Disorder may recur in rare cases, either on same or opposite side of the face.

ADDITIONAL INFORMATION

- For additional information, please see Case 8 in the Orthopedic Case Series on AccessPhysiotherapy.com.[5]

PATIENT RESOURCES

- Mayo Clinic. *Bell's Palsy.* http://www.mayoclinic.com/health/bells-palsy/DS00168. Accessed March 1, 2013.
- National Institute of Neurological Disorders and Stroke. *Bell's Palsy.* http://www.ninds.nih.gov/disorders/bells/bells.htm. Accessed March 1, 2013.
- The Bells Palsy Network. http://www.bellspalsy.net. Accessed March 1, 2013.

REFERENCES

1. Chumley H. Chapter 222. Bell's palsy. In: Usatine RP, Smith MA, Chumley H, Mayeaux E Jr, Tysinger J, eds. *The Color Atlas of Family Medicine.* New York, NY: McGraw-Hill; 2009. http://www.accessmedicine.com/content.aspx?aID=8210923. Accessed January 25, 2013.
2. The University of Toledo. *Anatomy and Physiology Revealed.* New York, NY: McGraw-Hill; 2007. http://anatomy.mcgraw-hill.com/apt.html?login=1317985752019&system=Skeletal§ion=Dissection&topic=Temporomandibular%20joint&topicAbbr=Tmj&view=Lateral&viewAbbr=Lat&catAbbr=Oth&grpAbbr=Nrv&structure=Facial%20n.%20(CN%20VII). Accessed March 1, 2013.
3. Dutton M. Chapter 5. Differential diagnosis. In: Dutton M, ed. *Dutton's Orthopaedic Examination, Evaluation, and Intervention.* 3rd ed. New York, NY: McGraw-Hill; 2012. http://www.accessphysiotherapy.com/content/56525010. Accessed January 25, 2013.
4. Dutton M. *McGraw Hill's NPTE (National Physical Therapy Examination).* 2nd ed. New York, NY: McGraw-Hill; 2012. http://www.accessphysiotherapy.com/resource/611. Accessed March 1, 2013.
5. Prentice WE, Quillen WS, Underwood F, Chapter 8. Principles of electrophysiologic evaluation and testing. In: Prentice WE, Quillen WS, Underwood F, eds. *Therapeutic Modalities in Rehabilitation.* 4th ed. http://www.accessphysiotherapy.com/content/8137649#8137649. Accessed March 1, 2013.

ADDITIONAL REFERENCES

- de Almeida JR, Al Khabori M, Guyatt GH, et al. Combined corticosteroid and antiviral treatment for Bell palsy: a systematic review and meta-analysis. *JAMA.* 2009;302(9):985–993. doi: 10.1001/jama.2009.1243.
- Quant EC, Jeste SS, Muni RH, Cape AV, Bhussar MK, Peleg AY. The benefits of steroids versus steroids plus antivirals for treatment of Bell's palsy: a meta-analysis. *BMJ.* 2009;339:b3354. doi: 10.1136/bmj.b3354.
- Rahman I, Sadiq SA. Ophthalmic management of facial nerve palsy: a review. *Surv Ophthalmol.* 2007;52(2):121–144.
- Sassi FC, Mangilli LD, Poluca MC, Bento RF, Andrade CR. Mandibular range of motion in patients with idiopathic peripheral facial palsy. *Brazil Journal of Otorhinolaryngology.* 2011;77(2):237–244.
- Sullivan FM, Swan IR, Donnan PT, et al. A randomised controlled trial of the use of aciclovir and/or prednisolone for the early treatment of Bell's palsy: the BELLS study. *Health Technol Assess.* 2009;13(47):1–130. doi: 10.3310/hta13470
- Waxman SG. Chapter 25. Discussion of cases. In: Waxman SG. *Clinical Neuroanatomy.* 26th ed. http://www.accessphysiotherapy.com/content/5275817#5275817. Accessed March 1, 2013.

216 BRACHIAL PLEXUS INJURY

Eric Shamus, PhD, DPT, PT, CSCS
Jennifer Shamus, PhD, DPT, COMT, CSCS

CONDITION/DISORDER SYNONYMS

- Brachial plexus lesions
- Injury to brachial plexus

ICD-9-CM CODES

- 353.0 Brachial plexus lesions
- 767.6 Injury to brachial plexus due to birth trauma
- 953.4 Injury to brachial plexus

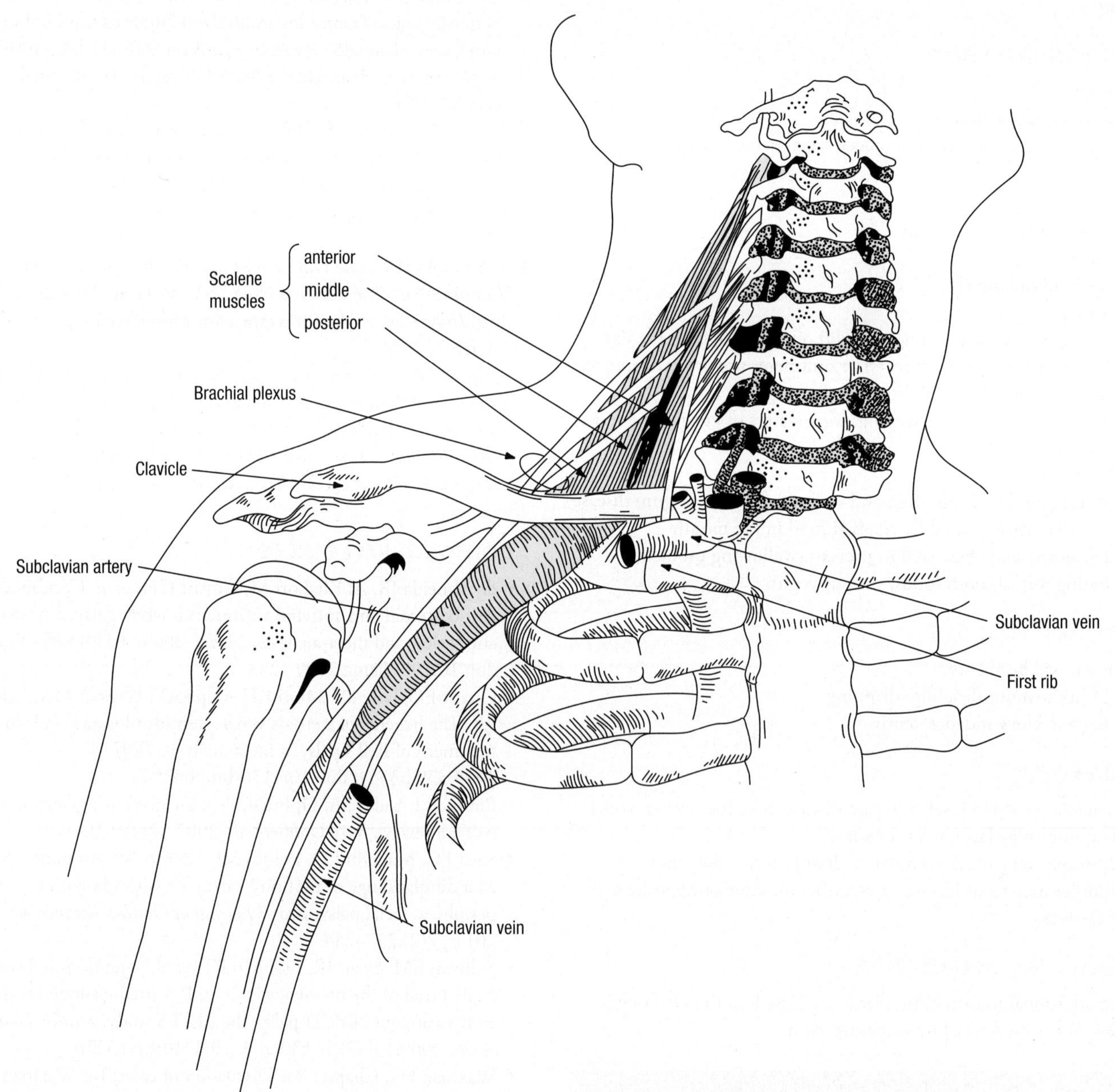

FIGURE 216-1 Course of the brachial plexus and subclavian artery between the anterior scalene and middle scalene muscles. Dilatation of the subclavian artery just distal to the anterior scalene muscle is illustrated. Immediately distal to the anterior and middle scalene muscles is another potential area of constriction, between the clavicle and the first rib. With extension of the neck and turning of the chin to the affected side (Adson maneuver), the tension on the anterior scalene muscle is increased and the subclavian artery compressed, resulting in a supraclavicular bruit and obliteration of the radial pulse. (From Ropper AH, Samuels MA. *Adams & Victor's Principles of Neurology*. 9th ed. New York, NY: McGraw-Hill; 2009.)

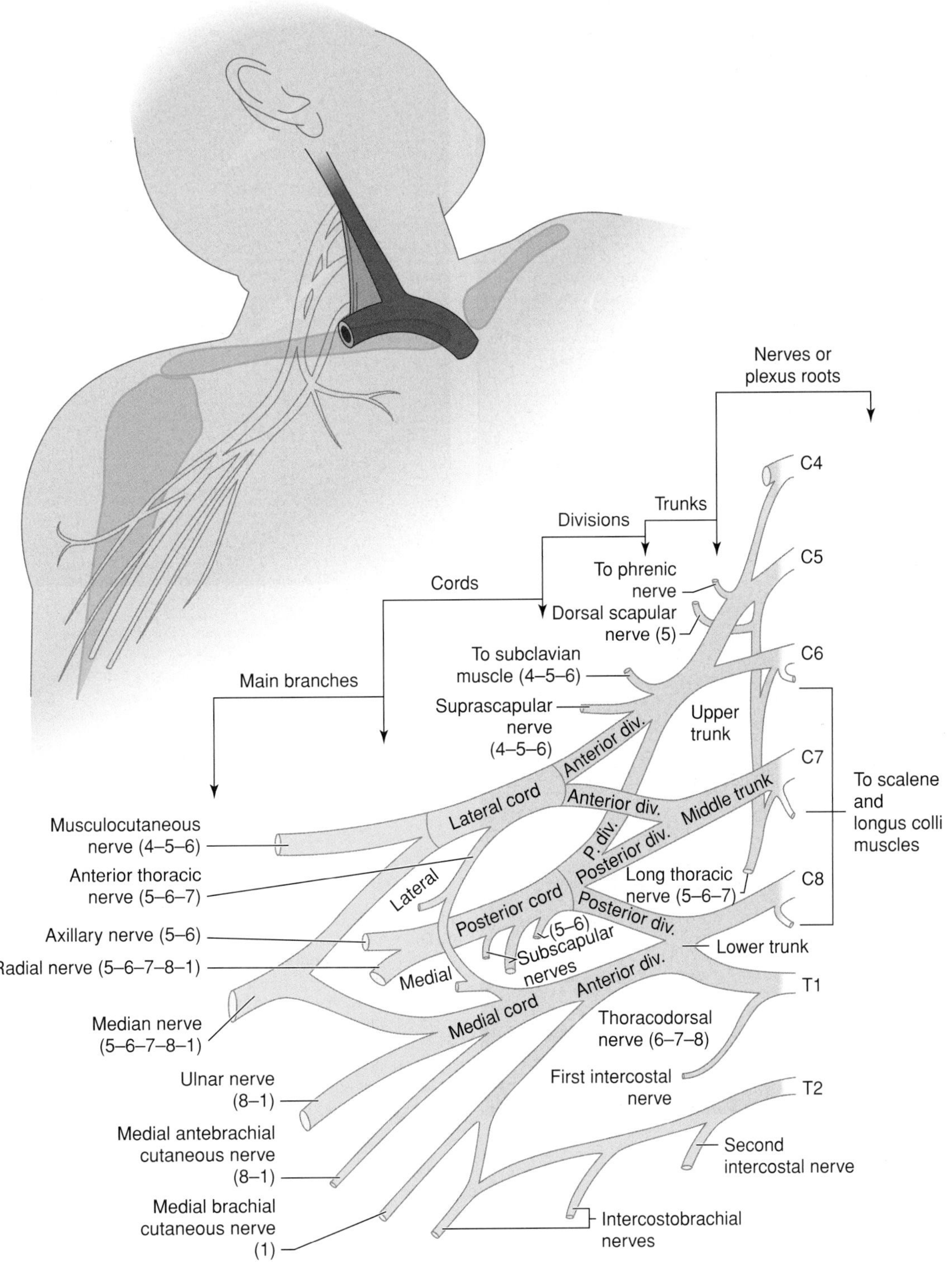

FIGURE 216-2 Brachial plexus. The numbers in parentheses refer to the segmental origin of the nerves depicted. (Reproduced from Waxman SG. *Clinical Neuroanatomy*. 26th ed. New York, NY: McGraw-Hill; 2010.)

ICD-10-CM CODES

- G54.0 Brachial plexus disorders
- P14.0 Erb paralysis due to birth injury
- P14.1 Klumpke paralysis due to birth injury
- P14.3 Other brachial plexus birth injuries
- S14.3XXA Injury of brachial plexus, initial encounter

PREFERRED PRACTICE PATTERNS

- 4F: Impaired Joint Mobility, Motor Function, Muscle Performance, Range of Motion, and Reflex Integrity Associated with Spinal Disorders[1]
- 5F: Impaired Peripheral Nerve Integrity and Muscle Performance Associated with Peripheral Nerve Injury[2]

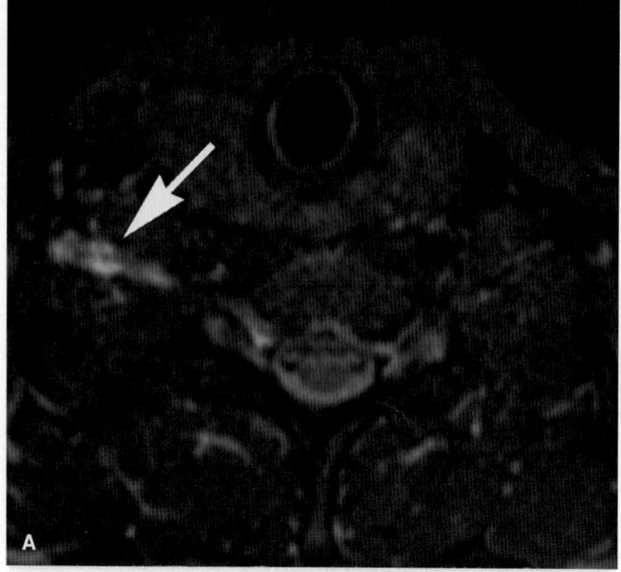

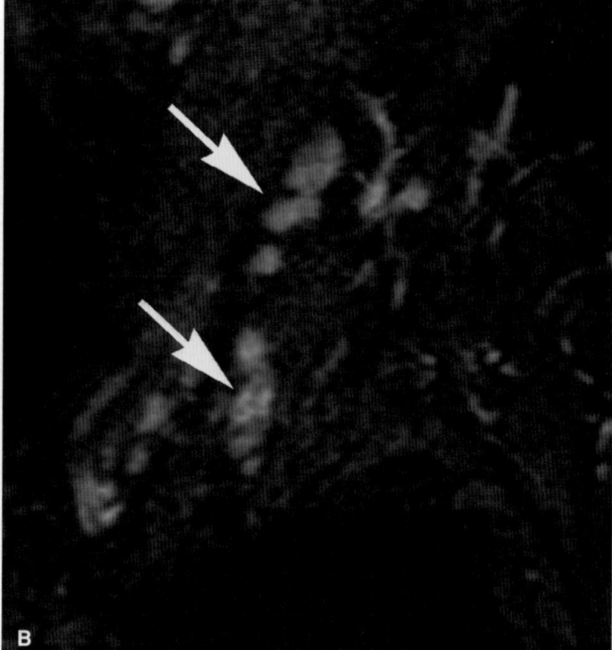

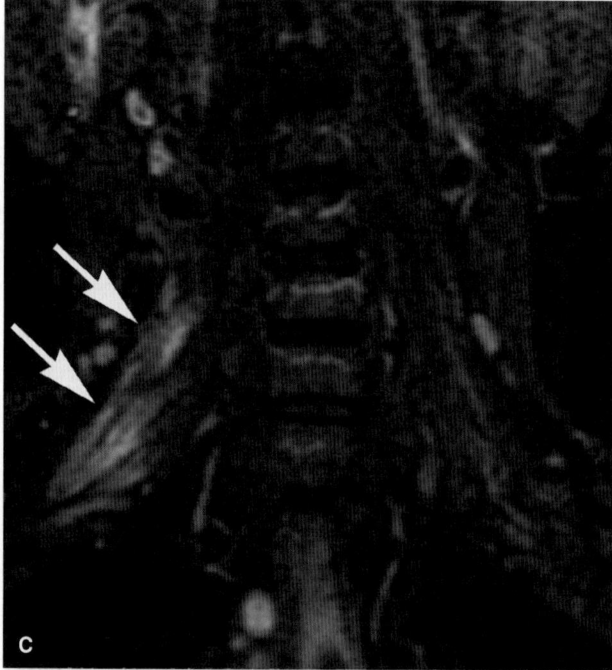

FIGURE 216-3 Brachial plexopathy. Axial (**A**), sagittal (**B**), and coronal (**C, D**) short tau inversion recovery (STIR) MR images demonstrate abnormal enlargement and abnormal high signal involving the right C6, C7, and C8 nerve roots, and the trunks and divisions that originate from these roots (*arrows*). Diffusion-weighted MR imaging (**E**) demonstrates abnormal reduced diffusion within the right C6, C7, C8 nerve roots and their corresponding trunks and divisions (*arrow*). These findings are compatible with radiation-induced brachial plexopathy. (From Longo DL, Fauci A, Kasper D, et al., eds. *Harrison's Principles of Internal Medicine*. 18th ed. New York, NY: McGraw-Hill; 2012.)

PATIENT PRESENTATION

A 22-year-old man presents with weakness and tingling in the right arm after a skiing accident on a trip to Colorado 5 days ago. The patient states he was skiing downhill when his pole got stuck in the snow behind him as he kept moving forward. Since then, the patient reports paresthesias down the right arm, an inability to complete tasks requiring fine motor skills of the right hand, and pain down the right upper extremity at night. The patient exhibits diminished reflexes as well as diminished sensation in the C8-T1 dermatome in the right upper extremity. Manual muscle testing of the right flexor carpi ulnaris is 2/5. Elbow flexion test is positive on the right.

KEY FEATURES

Description

- Weakness in the arm
- Diminished reflexes
- Pain in the upper extremity
- Motor or sensory changes in the ulnar, radial, and median nerve distribution due to pressure from
  - Compression
  - Stretch
  - Friction

Essentials of Diagnosis

- Electromyography
- Hand clumsiness or weakness

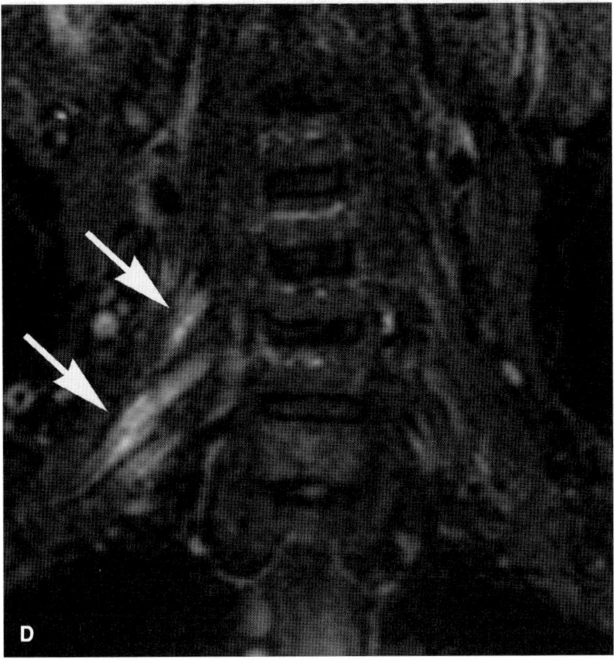

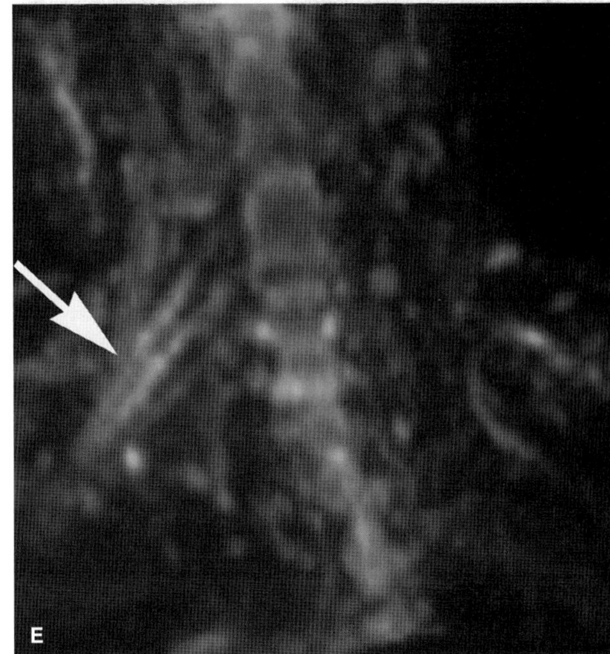

FIGURE 216-3 *(Continued)*

- Symptom changes with cervical spine and elbow positions
- Reproduction of symptoms during clinical examination
- Seddon classification
  - Neurapraxia (Class 1): First degree
  - Axonotmesis (Class 2): Second degree
  - Neurotmesis (Class 3): Third degree nerve fiber interruption, fourth degree epineurium intact, and fifth degree complete transection of the nerve

General Considerations

- Need to differentiate between more proximal and distal ulnar nerve compression, thoracic outlet syndrome (TOS), ulnar tunnel, and cervical radiculopathy
- Nerve compression syndrome in the upper extremity
- Wallerian degeneration occurs below the site of injury
- Patients with mild electrodiagnostic findings, intermittent symptoms, and no atrophy respond well to conservative management

Demographics

- Sports injury landing on the shoulder
- Traction injury
- Individuals who work for sustained periods with power tools or on computers
- Infants, from birth trauma or head traction

CLINICAL FINDINGS

SIGNS AND SYMPTOMS

- Acute or chronic paresthesia
- Pain or burning
- Sensory changes in multiple peripheral nerves of the upper extremity
- Hand clumsiness
- Feeling of arm heaviness
- Hand weakness; decreased grip-power and dexterity
- Intrinsic muscle atrophy
- Erb palsy
  - Waiter's tip sign
  - Caused by excessive lateral neck flexion
  - Loss of lateral rotator, arm flexors, and wrist extensor musculature
- Klumpike paralysis
  - Traction of abducted arm
  - Lower brachial plexus injury
  - Damage to C8 and T1
  - Loss of intrinsic muscles of the hand, wrist, and finger flexors
- Wartenberg sign[3]
- Froment sign for ulnar nerve palsy[4]
- Bishop's deformity
- Positive elbow flexion test[4]

Functional Implications

- Night pain
- Poor sleep habits with arm over head
- Feeling of arm going "dead"
- Limited hand function during ADLs/IADLs due to hand clumsiness and possible loss of strength

Possible Contributing Causes

- Infant head traction during forceps delivery
- Traction to the cervical spine
- Trauma pulling the arm into abduction
- Viral infection
- Ganglion or space-occupying lesion
- Repetitive trauma
- Sustained pressure over the thoracic outlet
- Clavicle fracture
- Glenohumeral dislocation

Differential Diagnosis

- Carpal tunnel syndrome
- Cervical radiculopathy
- Distal ulnar nerve entrapment cubital tunnel (Guyon canal)[3]
- Median neuropathy

- Other potential entrapment sites
  - Medial humeral groove
  - Arcade of Struthers
  - Medial intermuscular septum
  - Flexor digitorum profundus
  - Flexor carpi ulnaris
  - Just proximal to or within Guyon canal
  - Sensory and motor involvement between the abductor digiti minimi and flexor digiti minimi
  - Near hook of hamate: Involves motor only
  - Distal end of Guyon canal: Involves sensory only
- Proximal ulnar nerve entrapment
- Radial neuropathy
- Thoracic outlet syndrome (TOS)
- Wallerian degeneration

MEANS OF CONFIRMATION OR DIAGNOSIS

Imaging

- Allows for dynamic imaging during arm movement
- Enlargement of brachial plexus nerves at entrapment site

Diagnostic Procedures

- Loss of evoked sensory potential
- Decreased electrical velocities across elbow, <50 m/sec
- Electromyographic (EMG): Conduction velocities of ulnar innervated muscles <41 m/sec[5,6]

FINDINGS AND INTERPRETATION

- Muscle weakness of
  - Flexor carpi ulnaris (FCU)
  - Ulnar side of flexor digitorum profundus (FDP)
  - Abductor digiti minimi
  - Palmar and dorsal interossei
  - Intrinsic—interossei and lumbricals[7]
- Sensory changes in mixed ulnar, median, and radial nerve distribution

TREATMENT

Medication

- Lyrica

REFERRALS/ADMITTANCE

- For oral anti-inflammatory
- For steroidal injections
- For diagnostic tests if warranted and depending on physical therapist's (PT's) area of practice

IMPAIRMENTS

- Inability to perform overhead activities, such as swimming, baseball, or tennis
- Inability to perform jobs involving repetitive overhead reaching or lifting

TESTS AND MEASURES

- Disabilities of the Arm, Shoulder, and Hand (DASH) score to assess physical function
- Functional reach test
- Adson or Scalene maneuver
- Elevated arm stress test (EAST) or hand-up test (overhead test)
- Provocative elevation test (passive shoulder shrug)
- Allen pectoralis minor test
- Hallstead maneuver
- Hyperabduction maneuver (Wright test)
- Costoclavicular/military brace
- Roos test
- Upper limb tension test
- Cervical spine compression test
- Pain provocation test
- Shoulder pain and disability index

INTERVENTION

- Myofascial manipulation[4]
- Shoulder sling
- Range of motion exercises to affected areas
- Neural mobilization
- Activity modification/ergonomic intervention
- Soft tissue mobilization
- Postural awareness
- Strengthen as function returns

FUNCTIONAL GOALS

- Patient will
  - Return to full use of affected upper extremity (UE) during activities of daily living (ADLs) and instrumental activities of daily living (IADLs), such as washing dishes and cooking
  - Be able to raise their arm overhead to take a plate out of the cabinet
  - Be able to type for 1 hour at work.

PROGNOSIS

- Prognosis depends on duration of symptoms and motor involvement.
- Nerve regeneration for full motor recovery may take 6 months to 1 year.
- Patients with mild electrodiagnostic findings, intermittent symptoms, and no atrophy respond well to conservative management.

PATIENT RESOURCE

- American academy of orthopeadic surgeons. Burners and Stingers. http://orthoinfo.aaos.org/topic.cfm?topic=A00027. Accessed August 17, 2014.

REFERENCES

1. The American Physical Therapy Association. Pattern 4F: impaired joint mobility, motor function, muscle performance, range of motion, and reflex integrity associated with spinal disorders. *Interactive Guide to Physical Therapist Practice*. 2003. DOI: 10.2522/ptguide.3.1_6. Accessed January 21, 2013.
2. The American Physical Therapy Association. Pattern 5F: Impaired peripheral nerve integrity and muscle performance associated with peripheral nerve injury. *Interactive Guide to Physical Therapist Practice*. 2003. DOI: 10.2522/ptguide.3.2_6. Accessed January 21, 2013.
3. Dutton M. *Dutton's Orthopedic Survival Guide: Managing Common Conditions*. New York, NY: McGraw-Hill; 2011. http://www.accessphysiotherapy.com/resource/685. Accessed January 21, 2013.

4. Dutton M. *Orthopaedic Examination, Evaluation, and Intervention*. New York, NY: McGraw-Hill; 2008. http://www.accessphysiotherapy.com/resource/612. Accessed January 21, 2013.
5. Prentice WE. Chapter 7. Biofeedback. In: Prentice WE, Quillen WS, Underwood F, eds. *Therapeutic Modalities in Rehabilitation*. 4th ed. New York, NY: McGraw-Hill; 2011. http://www.accessphysiotherapy.com/abstract/8137204#8137204. Accessed January 21, 2013.
6. Preston D, Shapiro B. *Electromyography and Neuromuscular Disorders. Clinical Electrophysiologic Correlations*. Boston, MA: Butterworth-Heinemann; 1998.
7. Dutton M. "Integration of practice patterns 4f and 5f: impaired joint mobility, motor function, muscle performance, and range of motion, or reflex integrity secondary to spinal disorders, peripheral nerve entrapments, compartment syndrome, and myofascial pain dysfunction" (Chapter). In: Dutton M, ed. *Orthopaedic Examination, Evaluation, and Intervention*. 2nd ed. http://www.accessphysiotherapy.com/content/55576493. Accessed January 21, 2013.

ADDITIONAL REFERENCES

- Dubuisson AS, Kline DG. Brachial plexus injury: a survey of 100 consecutive cases from a single service. *Neurosurgery*. 2002; 51(3):673–682.
- ICD9DATA web site. http://www.icd9data.com. Accessed August 17, 2014.
- ICD10DATA web site. http://www.icd10data.com. Accessed August 17, 2014.

217 CARPAL TUNNEL SYNDROME

Thomas Bevins, MS, PT
Eric Shamus, PhD, DPT, PT, CSCS

CONDITION/SYNONYM

- Carpal tunnel syndrome (CTS)

ICD-9-CM CODE

- 354.0 Carpal tunnel syndrome

ICD-10-CM CODES

- G56.01 Carpal tunnel syndrome, right upper limb
- G56.02 Carpal tunnel syndrome, left upper limb

PREFERRED PRACTICE PATTERNS

- 4E: Impaired Joint Mobility, Motor Function, Muscle Performance, and Range of Motion Associated with Localized Inflammation[1]
- 5F: Impaired Peripheral Nerve Integrity and Muscle Performance Associated with Peripheral Nerve Injury[2]

PATIENT PRESENTATION

A 42-year-old woman presents with complaints of paresthesias (tingling and lately burning) and occasional pain and numbness in the right thumb, index, and middle fingers. Symptoms were initially intermittent, but becoming more constant, and the pain now often wakes her at night. In addition, recently she has noticed a loss of grip strength and has dropped objects on occasion. Onset was gradual, and symptoms worsening. She first saw her family physician 3 months ago for the numbness and tingling. The patient is a check-out clerk at a local grocery store. She is right-handed; BMI is 40.

On physical examination, sensory testing shows diminished touch and vibration sensation, and decreased two-point discrimination on the palmar surface of the thumb, and index, middle, and radial half of the ring fingers. Phalen and Tinel tests are positive. Thumb abduction, flexion, and opposition strength are only 4/5. Nerve conduction test done last week shows decreased nerve conduction velocity of the median nerve across the right wrist.

KEY FEATURES

Description

- Entrapment neuropathy of the median nerve within the carpal tunnel of the wrist[3,4]
- Signs and symptoms typical of neuropathy, including
  - Pain
  - Paresthesias
  - Loss of sensation
  - Later loss of muscle function

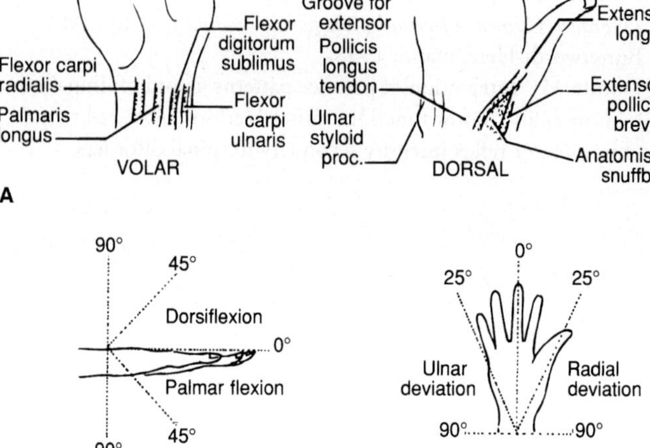

FIGURE 217-1 The wrist. (**A**) Topography of the wrist joint. (**B**) Motions of the wrist joint. (From LeBlond RF, DeGowin RL, Brown DD. *DeGowin's Diagnostic Examination*. 9th ed. http://www.accessmedicine.com. Copyright © The McGraw-Hill Companies, Inc. All rights reserved.)

- Symptoms are seen in the distribution of the median nerve in the hand[3]

Essentials of Diagnosis

- Pain, paresthesias, and sensory loss perceived on the radial side of the palm; the palmar side of the thumb, index, and middle fingers; and the radial side of the ring fingers
- Pain may radiate up to the elbow, shoulder, and neck
- Waking from pain at night is hallmark of this condition[5]
- In advanced cases, motor dysfunction in thenar muscles may occur, characterized by weakness, atrophy, loss of coordination

General Considerations

- In entrapment neuropathy, nerve becomes compressed, causing ischemic damage to the nerve
- The carpal tunnel is a constrained area at the wrist bounded by the carpal bones and the transverse carpal ligament (flexor retinaculum)[3]
- The median nerve and nine flexor tendons pass through the carpal tunnel
- Pathomechanics involve decreased size of the tunnel or increased volume of the contents, causing compression on the median nerve
- Often associated with repetitive motions or sustained position of the wrist and hand
- Unrelieved compression of the nerve results in neurapraxia with segmental demyelination;[6] further ischemic damage results in axonotmesis and Wallerian degeneration[5,6]

Demographics

- Incidence: 3.5 cases per 1,000 in general population[5]
- Prevalence: 2.1%[5]

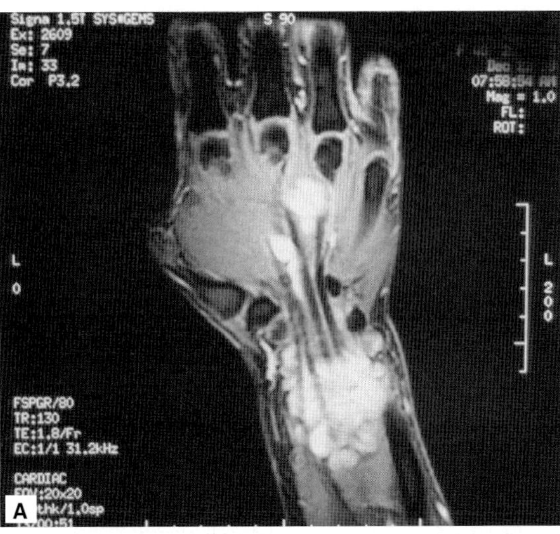
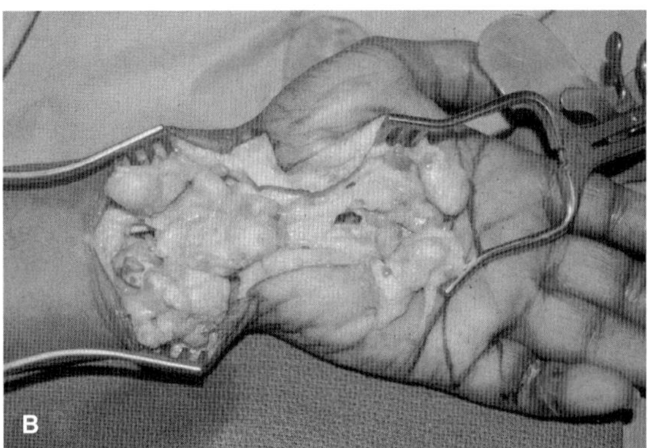
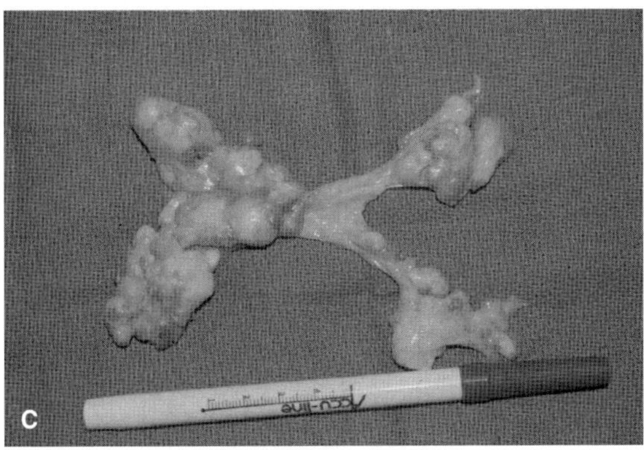

FIGURE 217-2 Median nerve compression due to a giant cell tumor in the carpal tunnel. (**A**) Magnetic resonance image of the giant cell tumor spanning the carpal tunnel. (**B**) Intraoperative view of the tumor within the carpal tunnel. (**C**) The excised giant cell tumor. (From Imboden J, Hellman DB, Stone JH. *Current Rheumatology Diagnosis & Treatment*. 2nd ed. http://www.accessmedicine.com. Copyright © The McGraw-Hill Companies, Inc. All rights reserved.)

- Most common entrapment neuropathy[5]
- More common in women than in men (70% of cases are females)[5]
- 2.5 times more common in obese individuals[5,7]
- Most common among people aged 30 to 60 years[5]
- Nearly one-half of cases will experience bilateral symptoms[5]

CLINICAL FINDINGS

SIGNS AND SYMPTOMS

- First symptom is usually pain or paresthesias;[3] most commonly with gradual onset
- Pain complaints include numbness (most common), tingling, and burning
- Pain or numbness waking the patient at night is very common
- Pain is experienced in distribution of the median nerve in the hand, though may radiate up to the elbow, shoulder, or neck
- Tenderness to percussion or pressure over the carpal tunnel
- Pain may be worse with extreme wrist flexion or extension
- Sensory loss may follow early symptom of pain
- Motor involvement (weakness, loss of coordination, atrophy) may follow in more advanced cases

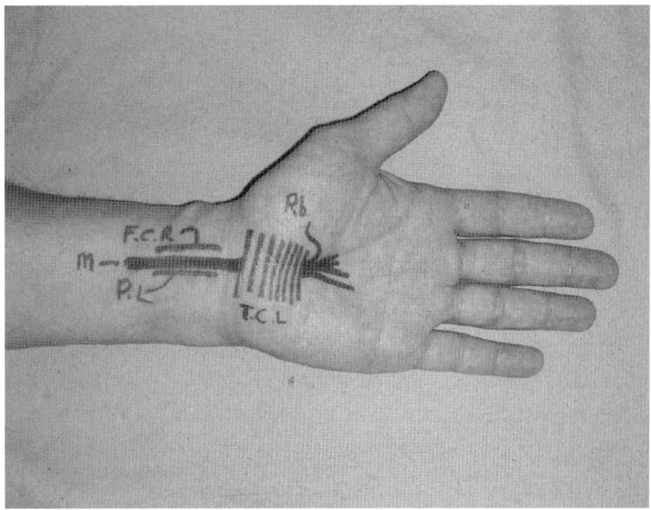

FIGURE 217-3 Surface anatomy of the carpal tunnel. The median nerve (M) becomes more superficial as it approaches the distal one-third of the forearm, but is still deep to both the palmaris longus tendon (P.L.) and the flexor carpi radialis (F.C.R.). As the median nerve continues distally into the hand, it enters the carpal tunnel. The roof of the carpal tunnel is formed by the transverse carpal retinaculum (T.C.L.). The recurrent branch (Rb) generally emerges at the distal edge of the transverse carpal ligament. Occasionally, it will emerge through the fibers of the ligament. The median nerve continues through the proximal hand and then divides into its digital sensory branches. (From Imboden J, Hellman DB, Stone JH. *Current Rheumatology Diagnosis & Treatment*. 2nd ed. http://www.accessmedicine.com. Copyright © The McGraw-Hill Companies, Inc. All rights reserved.)

Functional Implications

- Pain with wrist movements
- Difficulty with grasping and manipulation activities
- Dropping items from the hand

- Impaired sensation
- Loss of strength in advanced cases

▶ Possible Contributing Causes

- Most often idiopathic
- Genetic structural factors
- Swelling of synovial tissues in rheumatoid arthritis
- Swelling from conditions such as infection, congestive heart failure, pregnancy
- Obesity[7]
- Tumors
- Alcoholism
- Kidney failure
- Menopause
- Acromegaly
- Displaced fracture or fracture callus
- Structural abnormalities of carpal bones
- Occupations that require repetitive motion, repetitive stress, sustained positions of the wrist and hand

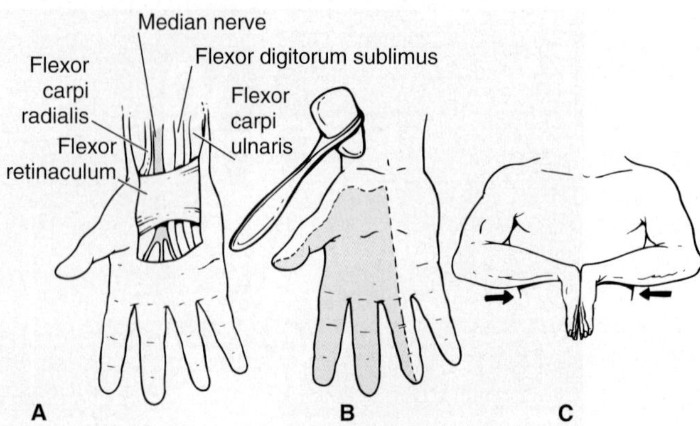

FIGURE 217-4 Carpal tunnel syndrome. (**A**) The carpal tunnel: The flexor retinaculum I the wrist compresses the median nerve to produce hyperesthesia in the radial digits. (**B**) Tinel sign: Percussion on the radial side of the palmaris longus tendon produces tingling in the digital region. (**C**) Phalen Test: Hyperflexion of the wrist for 60 seconds produces pain in the median nerve distribution, which is relieved by extension of the wrist. (From LeBlond RF, DeGowin RL, Brown DD. *DeGowin's Diagnostic Examination*. 9th ed. http://www.accessmedicine.com. Copyright © The McGraw-Hill Companies, Inc. All rights reserved.)

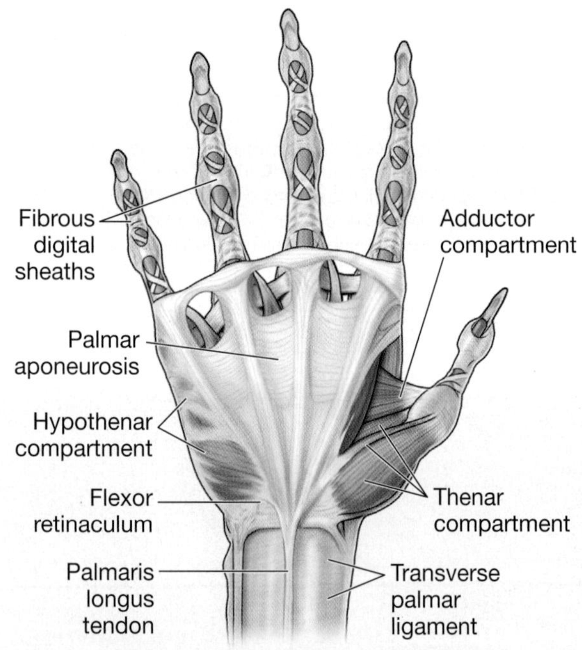

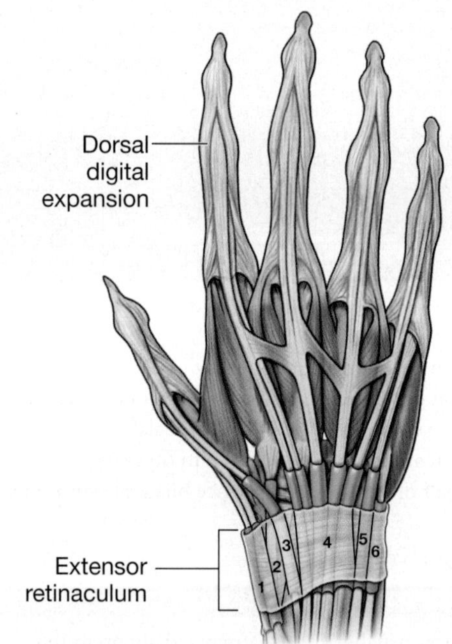

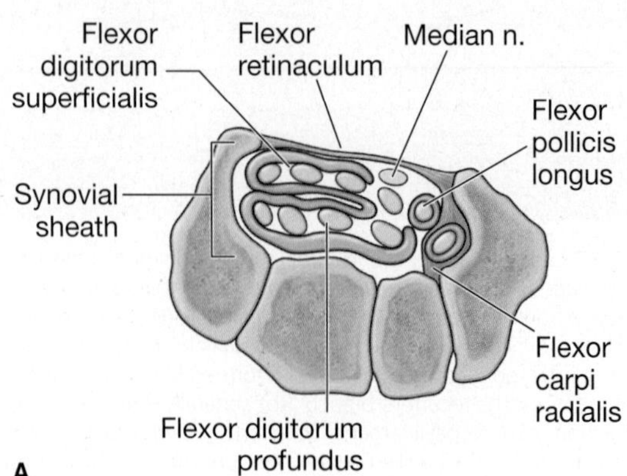

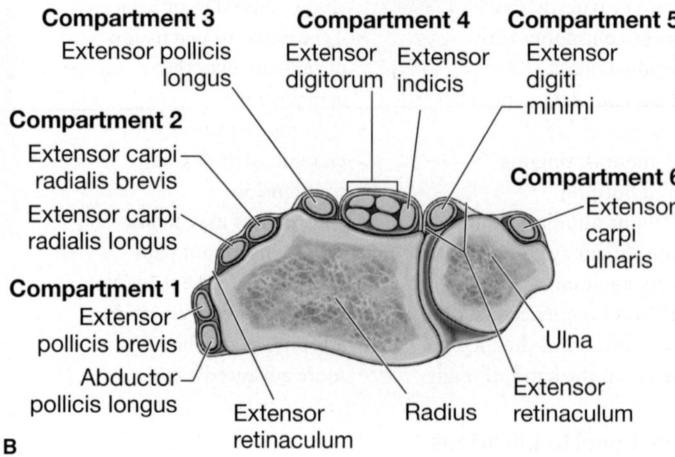

FIGURE 217-5 (**A**) Fascia of the palm of the hand and carpal tunnel. (**B**) Fascia of the posterior hand and extensor compartments. (**C**) Actions of digits 2–4. (**D**) Actions of digit 1 (thumb). (From Morton DA, Foreman KB, Albertine KH. *The Big Picture: Gross Anatomy*. http://www.accessmedicine.com. Copyright © The McGraw-Hill Companies, Inc. All rights reserved.)

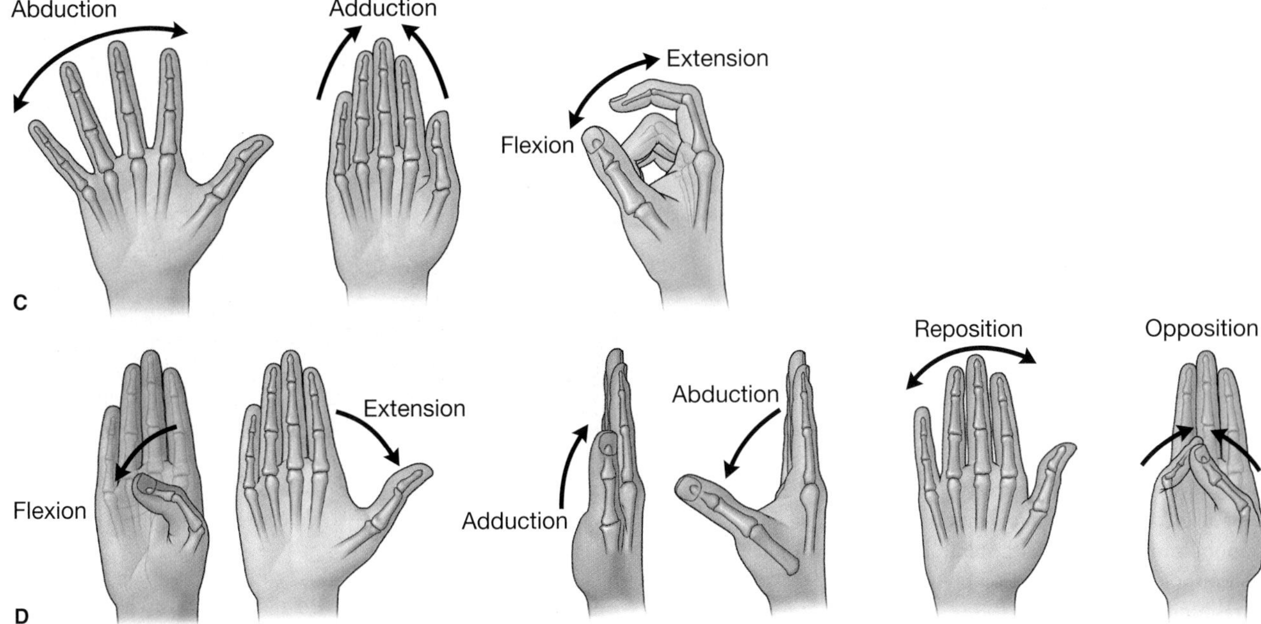

FIGURE 217-5 *(Continued)*

- This point is debated in the literature: Association is seen, but a causal relationship is not clear; genetic structural causes appear more likely.
- Direct trauma to wrist
- Impaired circulation to peripheral nerves, as seen in diabetes, predisposes individuals to nerve compression symptoms

Differential Diagnosis

- Acromegaly
- Cervical radiculopathy
- Hypothyroidism
- Pronator teres syndrome
- Rheumatoid or other arthritis
- Scleroderma
- Thoracic outlet syndrome
- Traumatic nerve lesion

MEANS OF CONFIRMATION OR DIAGNOSIS

Laboratory Tests

- Laboratory studies for suspected rheumatoid disorders

Imaging

- MRI[4]
- Diagnostic ultrasound (ultrasonography)[4]

Diagnostic Procedure

- Nerve conduction

FINDINGS AND INTERPRETATION

- Nerve conduction velocity testing of median nerve across the carpal tunnel is considered gold standard for diagnosis.[5,8]

TREATMENT

Medication

- NSAIDs[4]
- Corticosteroid injection

REFERRALS/ADMITTANCE

- To radiologist for imaging; X-ray for fracture or displacement
- To orthopedist for surgical consult or injection
- To occupational therapist to provide splints and instruct patient in joint protection techniques

IMPAIRMENTS

- Hand weakness with grasping, squeezing, pinching

TESTS AND MEASURES

- Disabilities of the Arm, Shoulder, and Hand (DASH) score to assess physical function

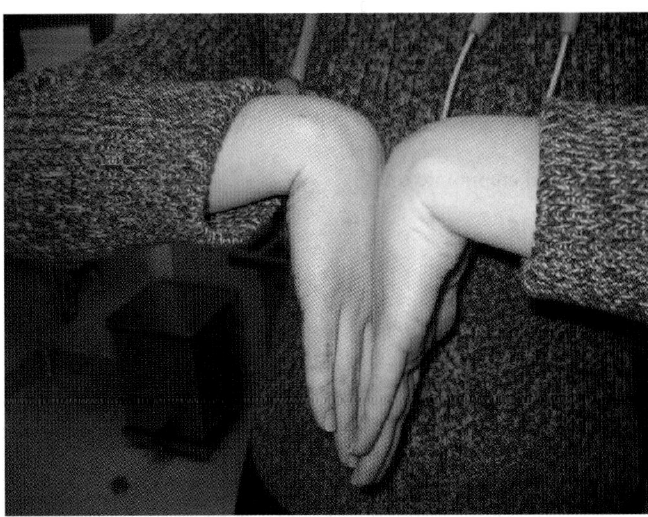

FIGURE 217-6 Phalen test. With the wrist in full flexion for at least 1 minute, tingling or numbness may be elicited in the thumb, index, or middle finger in positive Phalen test. (From Patel DR, Greydanus DE, Baker RJ. *Pediatric Practice: Sports Medicine*. www.accesspediatrics.com. Copyright © The McGraw-Hill Companies, Inc. All rights reserved.)

- Durkan test (carpal compression test)
- Flick sign
- Manipulative ability test (nine-hole peg test)
- Phalen test (sensitivity 0.85, specificity 0.79)[5,9]
- Reverse Phalen test (sensitivity 0.60, specificity 0.67)[5,9]
- Self-reported symptoms on the Katz hand diagram[5]
- Sensory loss may include diminished two-point discrimination, decreased vibration sense, increased threshold in Semmes–Weinstein monofilament test[5]
- Thenar muscle strength test (lateral pinch dynamometry)
- Tinel test for carpal tunnel (sensitivity 0.90, specificity 0.81)[5,9]
- Upper limb tension test 1 (ULTT 1), median nerve dominant[4]

INTERVENTION

- Early conservative intervention
  - Ergonomic analysis and activity modification to reduce repetitive motion or positioning stress
- Second-stage conservative intervention
  - Immobilization of wrist with splint; holding wrist in neutral position to reduce compression pressures[2]
  - Ultrasound[10,11]
  - Median nerve gliding[4]
  - Tendon gliding exercises[11]
  - Manual therapy[11]
    - Carpal bone mobilization plus flexor retinaculum stretch
    - Myofascial release[12]
  - Magnetic therapy[11]
  - Cold low-level laser therapy[10,11]
  - Yoga[4,11]
  - Address swelling
    - Ice[13]
    - Elevation
    - Iontophoresis
- Post-surgical intervention
  - Median nerve gliding[4]
  - Tendon gliding techniques to reduce adhesions
  - Strengthening

FUNCTIONAL GOALS

- Patient will have
  - Improved ability to perform physical tasks, self-care, home management, leisure and occupational activities.
  - Increased tolerance of positions and activities using the hand and wrist.
  - Reduced ergonomic risk.

PROGNOSIS

- Poor: 18% "cure" rate with conservative intervention (anti-inflammatory medication and immobilization).[5]
- Surgical intervention indicated for patients with symptoms lasting >1 year, or those for whom conservative treatment over 3 months has failed.

PATIENT RESOURCES

- American Academy of Orthopaedic Surgeons. Carpal Tunnel Syndrome. http://orthoinfo.aaos.org/topic.cfm?topic=A00005, Accessed March 16, 2013.
- NIH National Institutes of Health. Carpal Tunnel Syndrome. *Medline Plus*. http://www.nlm.nih.gov/medlineplus/ency/article/000433.htm, Accessed March 16, 2013.

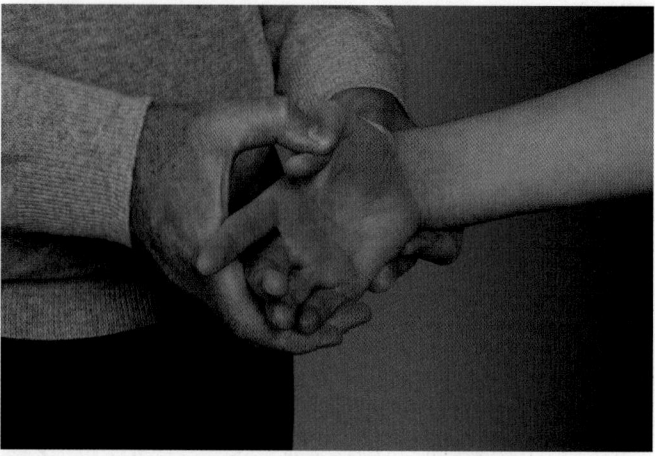

FIGURE 217-7 Single hand Phalen test. (From Dutton D. *Dutton's Orthopaedic Examination, Evaluation, and Intervention*. 3rd ed. www.accessphysiotherapy.com. Copyright © The McGraw-Hill Companies, Inc. All rights reserved.)

REFERENCES

1. The American Physical Therapy Association. Pattern 4E: Impaired joint mobility, motor function, muscle performance, and range of motion associated with localized inflammation. *Interactive Guide to Physical Therapist Practice*. 2003. DOI: 10.2522/ptguide.3.1_5. Accessed March 16, 2013.
2. The American Physical Therapy Association. Pattern 5F: Impaired peripheral nerve integrity and muscle performance associated with peripheral nerve injury. *Interactive Guide to Physical Therapist Practice*. 2003. DOI: 10.2522/ptguide.3.2_6. Accessed March 16, 2013.
3. Dutton M. *Orthopaedic Examination, Evaluation, and Intervention*. New York, NY: McGraw-Hill; 2008. http://www.accessphysiotherapy.com/resource/612. Accessed March 16, 2013.
4. American Physical Therapy Association. *Anatomy and Physiology Revealed*. New York, NY: McGraw-Hill. 2007. http://anatomy.mcgraw-hill.com/apt.html?login=1319880810339&system=Muscular§ion=Dissection&topic=Wrist%20and%20hand&topicAbbr=Wha&view=Anterior&viewAbbr=Ant&catAbbr=Oth&grpAbbr=Ske&structure=Carpal%20tunnel. Accessed March 16, 2013.
5. Goodman CC, Fuller KS. *Pathology: Implications for the Physical Therapist*. 3rd ed. St. Louis, MO: Saunders/Elsevier; 2009.
6. Waxman SG. *Clinical Neuroanatomy*. New York, NY: McGraw-Hill; 2010. http://www.accessphysiotherapy.com/resource/22. Accessed March 16, 2013.
7. Else T, Hammer GD. Chapter 19. Disorders of the hypothalamus & pituitary gland. In: *Pathophysiology of Disease*. New York, NY: McGraw-Hill; 2009. http://www.accessphysiotherapy.com/abstract/5371358#5371358. Accessed March 16, 2013.
8. Halle J, Greathouse D. Chapter 8. Principles of electrophysiologic evaluation and testing. In: Prentice WE, Quillen WS, Underwood F, eds. *Therapeutic Modalities in Rehabilitation*. 4th ed. New York, NY: McGraw-Hill; 2011. http://www.accessphysiotherapy.com/abstract/8137649#8137649. Accessed March 16, 2013.
9. Dutton M. *Dutton's Orthopedic Survival Guide: Managing Common Conditions*. New York, NY: McGraw-Hill; 2011. http://www.accessphysiotherapy.com/resource/685. Accessed March 16, 2013.

10. Houghton PE. Chapter 3. The role of therapeutic modalities in wound healing. In: Prentice WE, Quillen WS, Underwood F, eds. *Therapeutic Modalities in Rehabilitation.* 4th ed. New York, NY: McGraw-Hill; 2011. http://www.accessphysiotherapy.com/abstract/8135453#8135453. Accessed March 16, 2013.
11. Muller M, Tsui D, Schnurr R, et al. Effectiveness of hand therapy interventions in primary management of carpal tunnel syndrome: a systematic review. *J Hand Ther.* 2004;17(2): 210–228.
12. Prentice WE. Chapter 16. Therapeutic massage. In: Prentice WE, Quillen WS, Underwood F, eds. *Therapeutic Modalities in Rehabilitation.* 4th ed. New York, NY: McGraw-Hill; 2011. http://www.accessphysiotherapy.com/abstract/8140838#8140971. Accessed March 16, 2013.
13. Prentice WE. Chapter 9. Cryotherapy and thermotherapy. In: Prentice WE, Quillen WS, Underwood F, eds. *Therapeutic Modalities in Rehabilitation.* 4th ed. New York, NY: McGraw-Hill; 2011. http://www.accessphysiotherapy.com/content/8137995#8137995. Accessed March 16, 2013.

ADDITIONAL REFERENCES

- ICD9DATA web site. http://www.icd9data.com. Accessed March 16, 2013.
- ICD10DATA web site. http://www.icd10data.com. Accessed March 16, 2013.
- Lozano-Calderón S, Anthony S, Ring D. The quality and strength of evidence for etiology: example of carpal tunnel syndrome. *J Hand Surg Am.* 2008;33(4):525–538.

218 COMPARTMENT SYNDROME, FOREARM

Stacey L. Frazee, DPT
Eric Shamus, PhD, DPT, PT, CSCS

CONDITION/DISORDER SYNONYMS

- Chronic compartment syndrome (CCS)
- Chronic exertional compartment syndrome (CECC)
- Limb compartment syndrome
- Myofascial compartment syndrome
- Volar compartment syndrome of forearm (flexors)
- Dorsal compartment syndrome of forearm (extensors)

ICD-9-CM CODES[1]

- 729.71 Nontraumatic compartment syndrome of upper extremity
- 958.91 Traumatic compartment syndrome of upper extremity

ICD-10-CM CODES[2]

- M62.2 Ischemic infarction of muscle (nontraumatic compartment syndrome)
- M79.A1 Nontraumatic compartment syndrome of upper extremity
- T79.6 Traumatic ischemia of muscle

PREFERRED PRACTICE PATTERN[3]

- 4E: Impaired joint mobility, motor function, muscle performance, and range of motion associated with localized inflammation

PATIENT PRESENTATION

A 31-year-old man with a recent forearm crush injury presents with severe unilateral forearm pain that has intensified since his injury. He indicates that his injury was sustained 3 weeks ago. He is currently experiencing tightness in the medial forearm and tingling in the thumb, index and middle fingers. Distal pulses and capillary refill are diminished. He is having weakness throughout the wrist/forearm. There is increased pain with squeezing of the forearm musculature. The patient was referred to the emergency room and his physician was notified.

KEY FEATURES

Description

- Bleeding or edema leads to increased pressure within the fascial compartment and compromises circulation within that space as well as the function of tissues in that area causing ischemia
- Arteriolar compression occurs and causes muscle and nerve ischemia
  - Acute, sensory changes develop after 30 minutes of ischemia
  - Acute, irreversible nerve damage in 12 to 24 hours
  - Acute, irreversible muscle changes (i.e., necrosis) in 3 to 8 hours

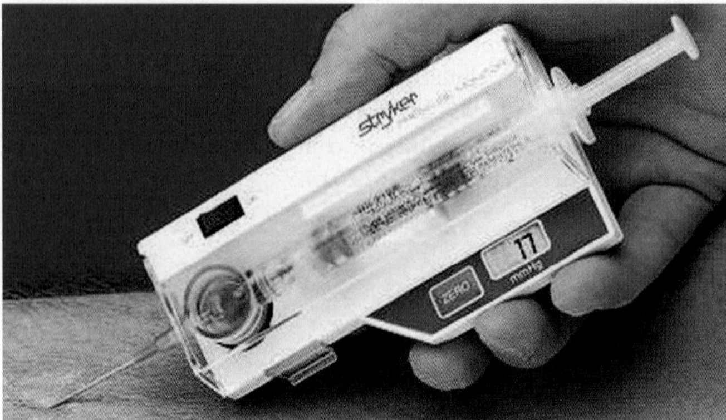

FIGURE 218-1 Stryker STIC device for measuring compartment pressure. (Reprinted with permission from Reichman EF, Simon RR. *Emergency Medicine Procedures*. New York, NY: McGraw-Hill; 2004.)

Essentials of Diagnosis

- Diagnosis is typically made by clinical examination and compartment pressure measurement
- Acute compartment syndrome
  - Medical emergency
  - Immediate surgery, fasciotomy
- Subacute compartment syndrome
  - Less of an emergency, usually surgery, fasciotomy
- Chronic exertional compartment syndrome
  - Conservative treatment first
  - Secondary surgery, fasciotomy
  - Symptoms consistently develop the same point during activity
  - Stops about 30 minutes following exercise
  - Symptoms can become progressively worse to constant
- Severe pain that is not alleviated by elevation or pain medication
  - Pain increases with passive/active range of motion and compression
- Distal pulses are diminished/absent
- Strength and sensation are diminished
- Edema in affected limb

General Considerations

- Require emergency surgery to prevent permanent damage with pressure measurements of 30 mm Hg or higher
- Forearm has two compartments
  - Volar
  - Dorsal
- Classic P's
  - Pain
  - Pallor
  - Pulselessness
  - Paresthesias
  - Paralysis

- Complications
  - Infection
  - Contractures
  - Deformity
  - Amputation
  - Acidosis
  - Hyperkalemia
  - Myoglobinuria
  - Acute renal failure and shock

Demographics

- Younger age, high-energy/high-velocity trauma and systemic hypotension associated with increased risk of traumatic accident
- High risk patients include
  - Males <35 years old with a fracture
  - Soft-tissue injury in males <35 years old with bleeding disorder or receiving anticoagulants
  - Crush injury patients
  - Patients with prolonged limb compression
- Individuals using circumferential wraps, restrictive dressings, casts, or immobilizer are at an increased risk

CLINICAL FINDINGS

SIGNS AND SYMPTOMS

- First signs
  - Decreased sensation, numbness
  - Tingling, parethesias
- Paresis
- Decreased palpable pulses
- Pallor of skin overlying compartment, paleness of skin
- Severe pain that does not go away with pain medicine or raising affected area
- Weakness
- Pain when the area is squeezed
- Extreme pain when moving affected area
  - Deep, throbbing pressure out of proportion to that expected from the injury
- Swelling in affected area

Functional Implications

- Pain out of proportion top to that expected from the injury
- Decreased strength in affected limb
- Loss of sensation and 2-point discrimination deficits
- Inability to use upper extremity
- Fatigue

Possible Contributing Causes

- Traumatic compartment syndrome
  - Car accident
  - Crush injury
  - Surgery
  - Complex fractures
    - Distal radius fracture
    - Ulnar fracture
    - Supracondylar fracture
- Chronic compartment syndrome
  - Repetitive activities
  - Poor upper-extremity biomechanics
- Vascular conditions
  - Arterial or venous injuries with hemorrhage
  - Deep vein thrombosis
  - Tourniquets
  - Bleeding disorders (i.e., hemophilia)

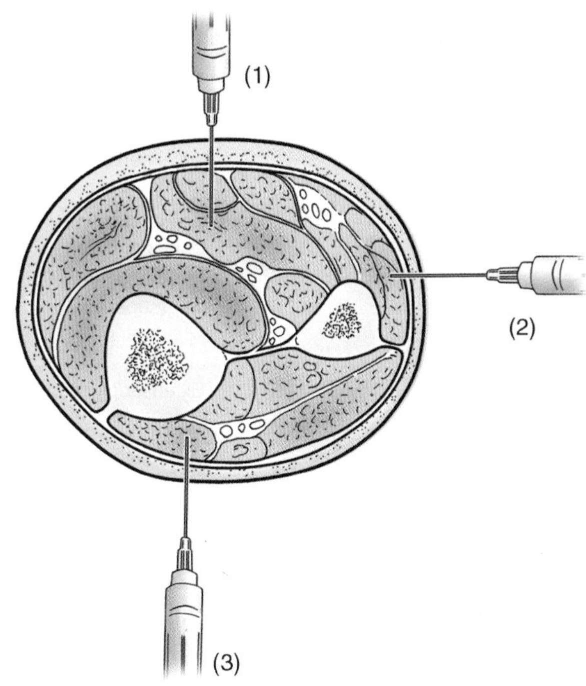

FIGURE 218-2 Cross-sectional view of the three major compartments of the forearm. (1) volar, (2) lateral (mobile wad), (3) dorsal. (Modified, with permission, from Reichman EF, Simon RR. *Emergency Medicine Procedures*. New York, NY: McGraw-Hill; 2004:545.)

- Soft-tissue injuries
  - Burns
  - Crush injury
  - Contusion
  - Snakebite
  - Prolonged limb compression
- Anabolic steroids
- Creatine supplementation[4]

Differential Diagnosis

- Rhabdomyolysis
- Carpal Tunnel syndrome
- Fracture

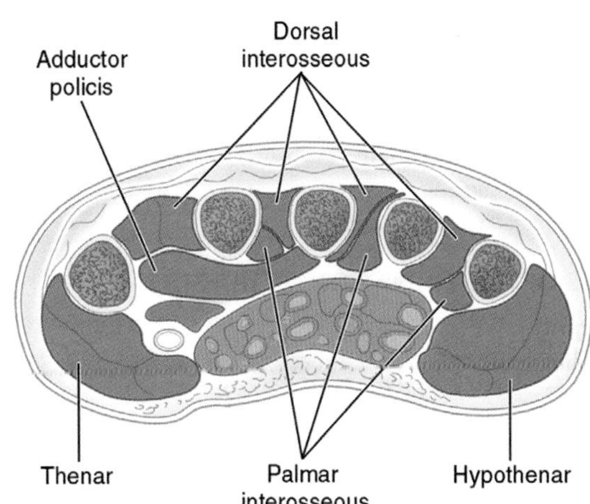

FIGURE 218-3 Cross-section of the palm, through the metatarsal shafts, showing the compartments of the hand. (From Simon RR, Sherman SC. *Emergency Orthopedics*. 6th ed. http://www.accessemergencymedicine.com. Copyright © The McGraw-Hill Companies, Inc. All rights reserved.)

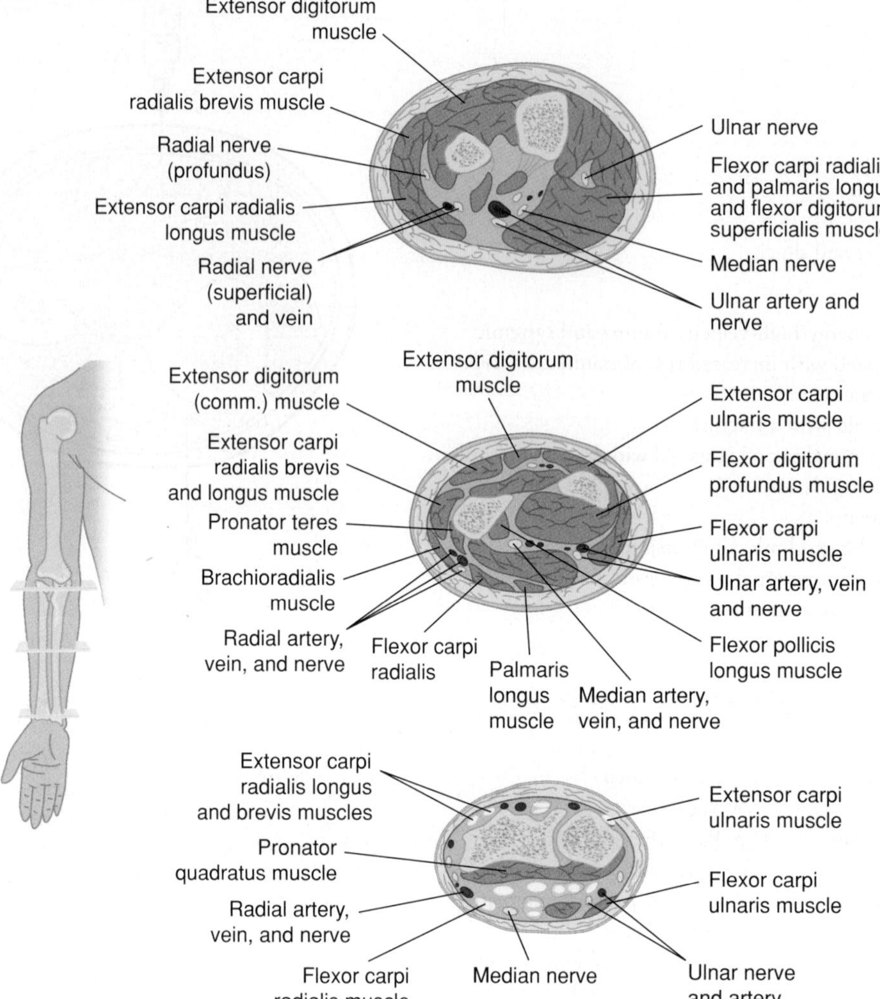

FIGURE 218-4 Forearm compartments: transverse sections through the right forearm at various levels. (From Tintinalli JE, Stephan Stapczynski J, John Ma O, et al., eds. *Tintinalli's Emergency Medicine: A Comprehensive Study Guide*. 7th ed. http://www.accessmedicine.com. Copyright © The McGraw-Hill Companies, Inc. All rights reserved.)

- Periostitis
- Deep vein thrombosis
- Tumor
- Nerve entrapment
- Muscle tear
- Necrotizing fasciitis
- Cellulitis
- Cnidaria Envenomation
- Gas Gangrene
- Peripheral vascular injuries

MEANS OF CONFIRMATION OR DIAGNOSIS

Imaging

- Radiographs
- Bone scans
- CT scans
- MRI
- Doppler ultrasound

Diagnostic Procedure

- Compartmental pressure measurements
- Pulse oximetry to identify limb hypoperfusion

FINDINGS AND INTERPRETATION

- Emergency surgery to prevent permanent damage with pressure measurements of 30 mm Hg or higher
- Radiographs, bone scans, CT scans, or MRI can be used to rule out fractures and/or muscle tears
- Doppler ultrasound used to evaluated arterial flow and rule out Deep vein thrombosis (DVT)

TREATMENT

Medication

- Anti-inflammatory, NSAID

MEDICAL PROCEDURES

- Acute compartment syndrome, immediate open fasciotomy to relieve pressure, and avoid permanent damage
- Subcutaneous fasciotomy
- Hyperbaric oxygen therapy

REFERRALS/ADMITTANCE

- For imaging: x-ray, CT, or MRI
- For surgery if fasciotomy is required

IMPAIRMENTS

- Weakness
- Numbness and tingling
- Severe pain

TESTS AND MEASURES

- Pain, visual analog scale (VAS)
  - 24-hour pain
  - Worst average pain
  - Best average pain
  - Tenderness on palpation
- Functional independence measure
- Cardiovascular integrity
  - Blood pressure at rest and after activity
  - Palpation of distal pulses
  - Capillary refill
- Skin integrity
  - Associated skin assessment
    - Edema (linear girth measurements, palpation)
    - Color
    - Temperature
- Neurologic examination
  - Sensation
    - Light touch
    - Pin prick
    - Limb sensation
    - 2-point discrimination
  - Upper-extremity deep tendon reflexes
  - Proprioception
  - Kinesthetic awareness
  - Coordination
- Limb strength
  - Manual muscle test (MMT)

INTERVENTION

- Avoid external pressure
  - If cast or bandage is causing the problem it should be loosened or removed
  - Avoid splints, tight would dressing
- Rest
- Address swelling
- Address pain
- Wound care
- Laser therapy
  - Decrease pain
  - Decrease tenderness
  - Decrease stiffness

FUNCTIONAL GOALS

- The patient will be able to
  - Use upper-extremity with mild symptoms for 30 minutes
  - Return to activities such as computer use, writing, and driving

PROGNOSIS

- Determined by injury leading to the syndrome
- Permanent injury can occur to nerves or muscles if diagnosis is delayed
- Limb compartment syndrome with absent arterial pulses without a history of arterial trauma is associated with poor prognosis

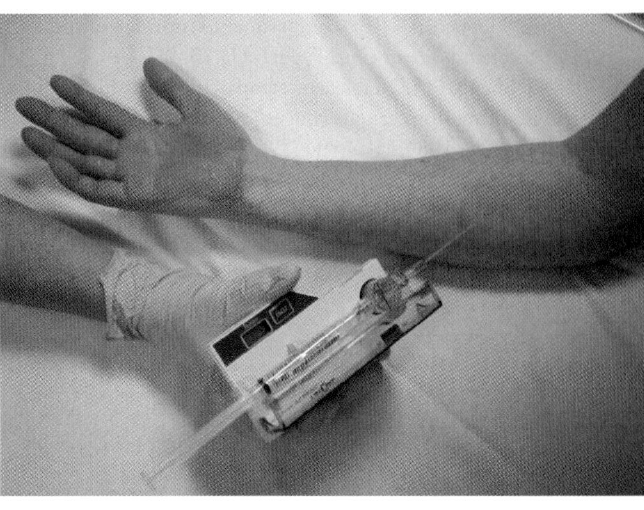

FIGURE 218-5 Pressure measurement of the forearm flexor compartment. (From Tintinalli JE, Stephan Stapczynski J, John Ma O, et al., eds. *Tintinalli's Emergency Medicine: A Comprehensive Study Guide*. 7th ed. http://www.accessmedicine.com. Copyright © The McGraw-Hill Companies, Inc. All rights reserved.)

PATIENT RESOURCE

- MedlinePlus, NIH National Institutes of Health. Compartment Syndrome. http://www.ncbi.nlm.nih.gov/pubmedhealth/PMH0002204/. Accessed June 4, 2013.

REFERENCES

1. ICD-9-CM. http://www.icd9data.com. Accessed June 4, 2013.
2. ICD-10-CM. http://www.icd10data.com. Accessed June 4, 2013.
3. The American Physical Therapy Association. *Guide to Physical Therapist Practice*. Alexandria, VA: The American Physical Therapy Association; 2003. http://guidetoptpractice.apta.org./ Accessed June 4, 2013.
4. Hile AM, Anderson JM, Fiala KA, et al. Creatine supplementation and anterior compartment pressure during exercise in the heat in dehydrated men. *J Athl Train*. 2006;41(1):30–35.

ADDITIONAL REFERENCES

- Botte MJ, Gelberman RH. Acute compartment syndrome of the forearm. *Hand Clin*. 1998;14(3):391–403.
- Fraipont MJ, Adamson GJ. Chronic exertional compartment syndrome. *J Am Acad Orthop Surg*. 2003;11(4):268–276.
- Geiderman JM, Katz D. General principles of orthopedic injuries. In: Marx J, ed. *Emergency Medicine: Concepts and Clinical Practice*. 7th ed. Philadelphia, PA: Mosby Elsevier; 2009: Chapter 46.
- Goodman CC, Fuller KS. *Pathology Implications for the Physical Therapist*. 3rd ed. Philadelphia, PA: Saunders Elsevier; 2009.
- Gourgiotis S, Villias C, Germanos S, Foukas A, Ridolfini MP. Acute limb compartment syndrome: a review. *J Surg Educ*. 2007;64(3):178–186.
- Konstantakos EK, Dalstrom DJ, Nelles ME, Laughlin RT, Prayson MJ. Diagnosis and management of extremity compartment syndromes: an orthopaedic perspective. *Am Surg*. 2007;73(12):1199–1209.
- Marshall ST, Browner BD. Emergency care of musculoskeletal injuries. In: Townsend CM Jr, Beauchamp RD, Evers BM, Mattox KL, eds. *Sabiston Textbook of Surgery*. 19th ed. Philadelphia, PA: Saunders Elsevier; 2012: Chapter 20.

- Naidu SH, Heppenstall RB. Compartment syndrome of the forearm and hand. *Hand Clin*. 1994;10(1):13–27.
- O'Neil D, Sheppard JE. Transient compartment syndrome of the forearm resulting from venous congestion from a tourniquet. *J Hand Surg Am*. 1989;14(5):894–896.
- Otsuka NY, Kasser JR. Supracondylar fractures of the humerus in children. *J Am Acad Orthop Surg*. 1997;5(1):19–26.
- Rasul AT, Lorenzo CT, Agnew S. Acute compartment syndrome. 2001. http://emedicine.medscape.com/article/307668-overview. Accessed June 4, 2013.
- Twaddle BC, Amendola A. Compartment syndrome. In: Browner BD, Jupiter JB, Levine AM, Trafton PG, Krettek C, eds. *Skeletal Trauma*. 4th ed. Philadelphia, PA: Saunders Elsevier; 2008: Chapter 13.
- Wall CJ, Lynch J, Harris IA, et al. Clinical practice guidelines for the management of acute limb compartment syndrome following trauma. *ANZ J Surg*. 2010;80(3):151–156.
- Yamaguchi S, Viegas SF. Causes of upper extremity compartment syndrome. *Hand Clin*. 1998;14(3):365–370, viii.

219 COMPARTMENT SYNDROME, LOWER LEG

Stacey L. Frazee, DPT
Eric Shamus, PhD, DPT, PT, CSCS

CONDITION/DISORDER SYNONYMS

- Chronic compartment syndrome (CCS)
- Chronic exertional compartment syndrome (CECC)
- Limb compartment syndrome
- Myofascial compartment syndrome
- Anterior compartment syndrome of the lower leg
- Lateral/peroneal compartment syndrome of the lower leg
- Deep posterior compartment syndrome of the lower leg
- Superficial posterior compartment syndrome of the lower leg

ICD-9-CM CODES[1]

- 729.72 Nontraumatic compartment syndrome of lower extremity
- 958.92 Traumatic compartment syndrome of lower extremity

ICD-10-CM CODES[2]

- M62.2 Ischemic infarction of muscle (nontraumatic compartment syndrome)
- M79.A2 Nontraumatic compartment syndrome of lower extremity
- T79.6 Traumatic ischemia of muscle

PREFERRED PRACTICE PATTERN[3]

- 4E: Impaired Joint Mobility, Motor Function, Muscle Performance, and Range of Motion Associated with Localized Inflammation

PATIENT PRESENTATION

A 29-year-old man with a recent tibial shaft fracture presents with severe unilateral lower leg pain. He indicates that his fracture was sustained during a crush injury and he is currently experiencing tingling and "tightness" in the area. Distal pulses and capillary refill are diminished. He is having weakness throughout the foot. There is increased pain with squeezing of the calf muscle.

KEY FEATURES

Description

- Bleeding or edema leads to increased pressure within the fascial compartment and compromises circulation within that space as well as the function of tissues in that area causing ischemia
- Arteriolar compression occurs and causes muscle and nerve ischemia
  - Acute, sensory changes develop after 30 minutes of ischemia
  - Acute, irreversible nerve damage in 12 to 24 hours
  - Acute, irreversible muscle changes (i.e., necrosis) in 3 to 8 hours

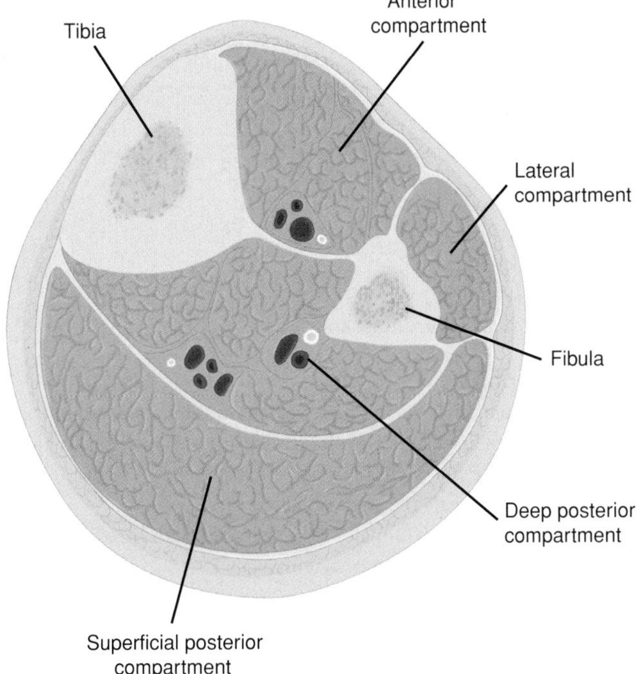

FIGURE 219-1 Schematic illustration of fascial compartments of the lower extremity. (From Brunicardi FC, Andersen D, Billiar T, et al., eds. *Schwartz's Principles of Surgery*. 9th ed. http://www.accessmedicine.com. Copyright © The McGraw-Hill Companies, Inc. All rights reserved.)

Essentials of Diagnosis

- Diagnosis is typically made by clinical examination and compartment pressure measurement
- Acute compartment syndrome
  - Medical emergency
  - Immediate surgery, fasciotomy
- Subacute compartment syndrome
  - Less of an emergency, usually surgery, fasciotomy
- Chronic exertional compartment syndrome
  - Conservative treatment first
  - Secondary surgery, fasciotomy
  - Begins after the start of exercise
  - Stops about 30 minutes following exercise
  - Symptoms can become progressively worse to constant
- Severe pain that is not alleviated by elevation or pain medication
  - Pain increases with passive/active range of motion and compression
- Distal pulses are diminished/absent
- Strength and sensation are diminished
- Edema in affected limb

General Considerations

- Require emergency surgery to prevent permanent damage with pressure measurements of 30 mm Hg or higher

- Lower leg has four compartments
  - Anterior
  - Lateral
  - Deep posterior
  - Superficial posterior
- Classic P's
  - Pain
  - Pallor
  - Pulselessness
  - Paresthesias
  - Paralysis
- Complications
  - Infection
  - Contractures
  - Deformity
  - Amputation
  - Acidosis
  - Hyperkalemia
  - Myoglobinuria
  - Acute renal failure and shock

Demographics

- Younger age, high-energy/high-velocity trauma and systemic hypotension associated with increased risk of traumatic accident.
- High risk patients include
  - Males <35 years old with tibial fracture.
  - Soft-tissue injury in males <35 years old with bleeding disorder or receiving anticoagulants.
  - Crush injury patients.
  - Patients with prolonged limb compression.
- Individuals using circumferential wraps, restrictive dressings, casts, or immobilizer are at an increased risk.

CLINICAL FINDINGS

SIGNS AND SYMPTOMS

- First signs
  - Decreased sensation, numbness
  - Tingling, parethesias
- Paresis
- Decreased palpable pulses
- Pallor of skin overlying compartment, paleness of skin
- Severe pain that does not go away with pain medicine or raising affected area
- Weakness
- Severe cases foot drop is seen
- Pain when the area is squeezed
- Extreme pain when moving affected area
  - Deep, throbbing pressure out of proportion to that expected from the injury
- Swelling in affected area

Functional Implications

- Pain out of proportion top to that expected from the injury
- Decreased strength in affected limb
- Loss of sensation and 2-point discrimination deficits
- Inability to weight bear or use the lower extremity
- Fatigue

Possible Contributing Causes

- Traumatic compartment syndrome
  - Car accident
  - Crush injury
  - Surgery

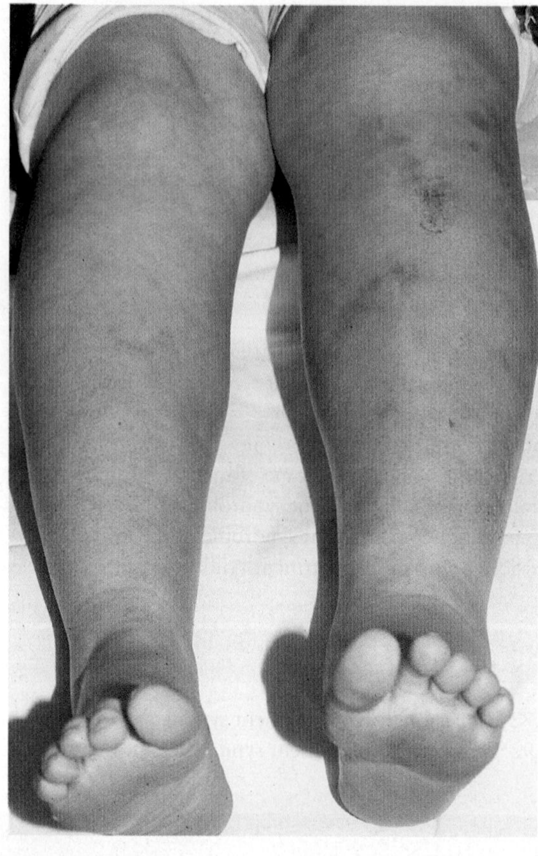

FIGURE 219-2 Compartment pressures. Intracompartmental pressure monitoring can be accomplished with commercially available devices. Normal tissue pressures should be less than 10 mm Hg; orthopedic consultation is recommended when pressures exceed 30 mm Hg. (From Knoop KJ, Stack L, Storrow A, Jason Thurman R. *The Atlas of Emergency Medicine*. 3rd ed. http://www.accessmedicine.com. Copyright © The McGraw-Hill Companies, Inc. All rights reserved. Photo contributor: Selim Suner, MD, MS.)

  - Complex fractures
    - Tibial shaft fracture has the highest risk of lower-extremity compartment syndrome
- Chronic compartment syndrome
  - Repetitive activities such as running and cycling[4]
  - Poor lower extremity biomechanics
- Vascular conditions
  - Arterial or venous injuries with hemorrhage
  - Deep vein thrombosis
  - Tourniquets
  - Bleeding disorders (i.e., hemophilia)
- Soft tissue injuries
  - Burns
  - Crush injury
  - Contusion
  - Snakebite
  - Prolonged limb compression
  - Gastrocnemius rupture
- Anabolic steroids
- Creatine supplementation[5]

Differential Diagnosis

- Rhabdomyolysis
- Shin splints
- Fracture

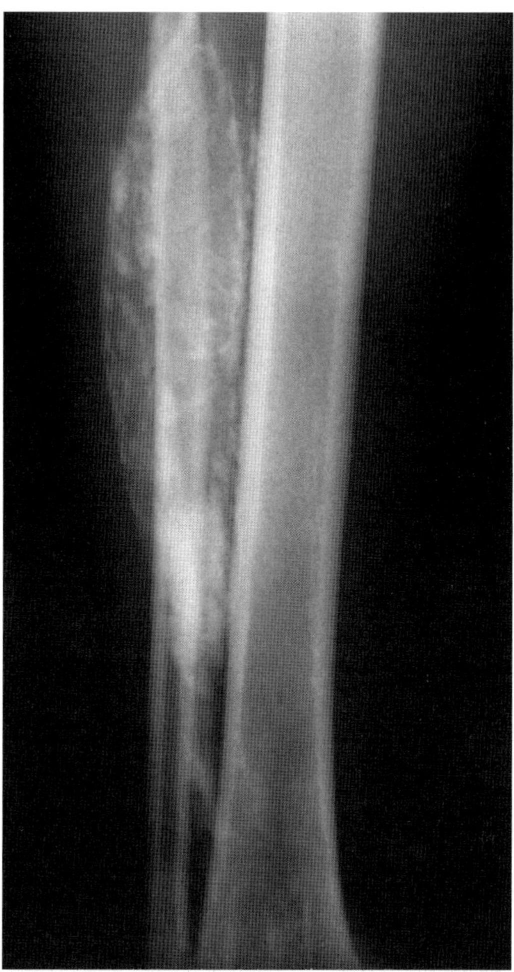

FIGURE 219-3 Radiograph of an old compartment syndrome in the flexor hallucis longus. (From Skinner HB. *Current Diagnosis & Treatment in Orthopedics*. 4th ed. http://www.accessmedicine.com. Copyright © The McGraw-Hill Companies, Inc. All rights reserved.)

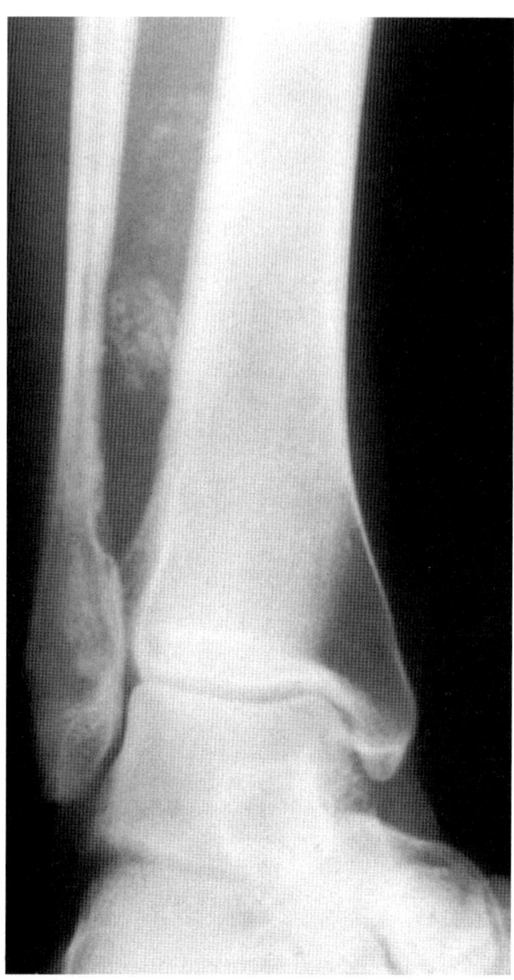

FIGURE 219-4 Radiograph of calcification in synovial sarcoma of the leg. (From Skinner HB. *Current Diagnosis & Treatment in Orthopedics*. 4th ed. http://www.accessmedicine.com. Copyright © The McGraw-Hill Companies, Inc. All rights reserved.)

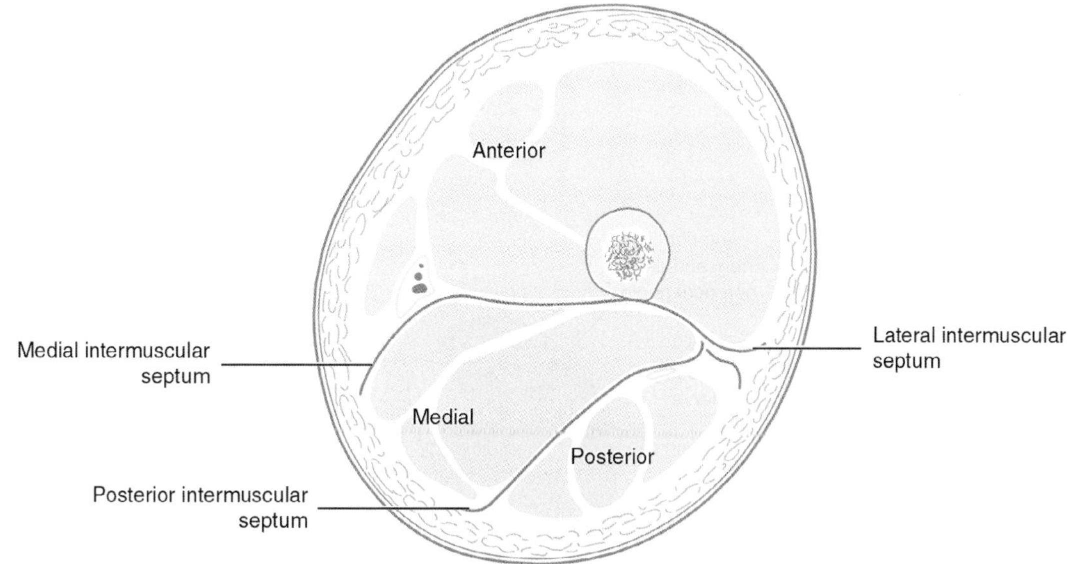

FIGURE 219-5 Compartments of the thigh. (From Simon RR, Sherman SC. *Emergency Orthopedics*. 6th ed. http://www.accessphysiotherapy.com. Copyright © The McGraw-Hill Companies, Inc. All rights reserved.)

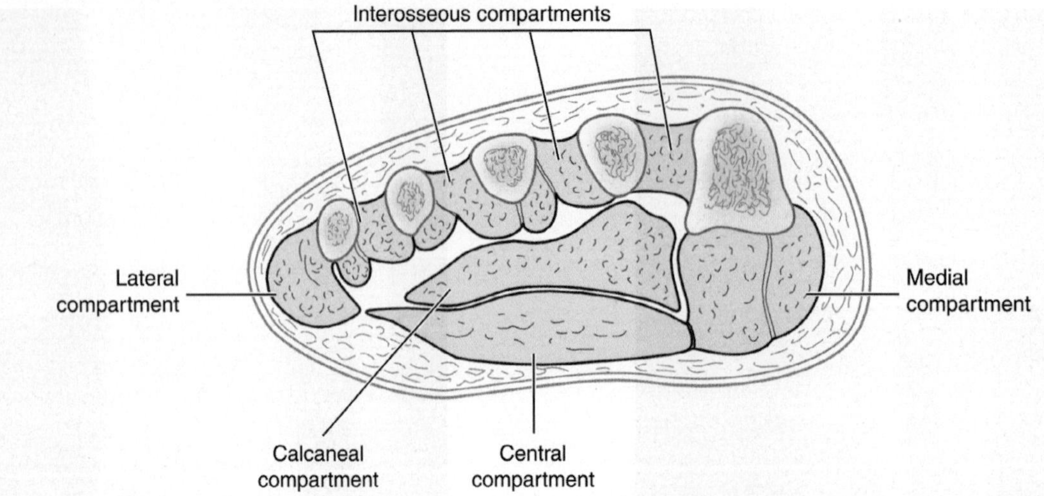

FIGURE 219-6 Cross-section schematic of the compartments of the foot at the level of the proximal metatarsal head. (From Simon RR, Sherman SC. *Emergency Orthopedics*. 6th ed. http://www.accessemergencymedicine.com. Copyright © The McGraw-Hill Companies, Inc. All rights reserved.)

- Periostitis
- Deep vein thrombosis
- Tumor
- Nerve entrapment
- Muscle tear
- Necrotizing fasciitis
- Cellulitis
- Cnidaria Envenomation
- Gas gangrene
- Peripheral vascular injuries

MEANS OF CONFIRMATION OR DIAGNOSIS

Imaging

- Radiographs
- Bone scans
- CT scans
- MRI
- Doppler ultrasound used to evaluated arterial flow and rule out DVT

Diagnostic Procedure

- Compartmental pressure measurements
- Pulse oximetry to identify limb hypoperfusion

FINDINGS AND INTERPRETATION

- Emergency surgery to prevent permanent damage with pressure measurements of 30 mm Hg or higher
- Radiographs, bone scans, CT scans, or MRI can be used to rule out fractures and/or muscle tears

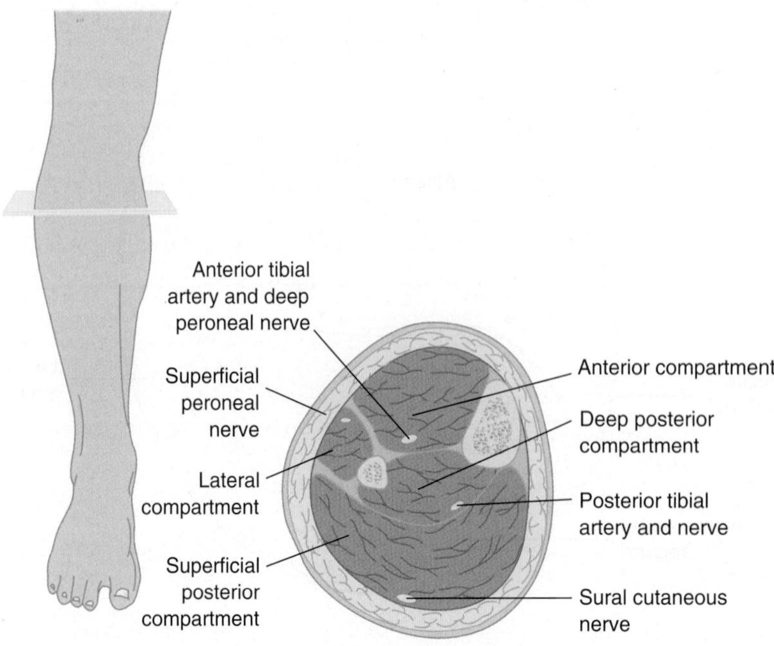

FIGURE 219-7 The four compartments of the leg. (From Tintinalli JE, Stephan Stapczynski J, John Ma O, et al., eds. *Tintinalli's Emergency Medicine: A Comprehensive Study Guide*. 7th ed. http://www.accessmedicine.com. Copyright © The McGraw-Hill Companies, Inc. All rights reserved.)

TABLE 219-1 Symptoms and Signs of Specific Compartment Affected

Compartment	Lateral	Anterior	Superficial Posterior	Deep Posterior
Site of pain	Middle one-third of the anterolateral leg	Anterior leg	Posterior middle third of the leg	Distal one-third of the posteromedial leg
Pain elicited by passive	Inversion and plantar flexion of ankle	Flexion of great toes. Inversion and plantar flexion of the ankle	Dorsiflexion of the ankle	Extension of the toes and dorsiflexion of ankle
Muscles affected	Peroneus longus and brevis	Tibialis anterior, extensor hallucis longus, and extensor digitorum longus	Gastrocnemius and soleus	Flexor hallucis longus, flexor digitorum, and tibialis posterior
Motor weakness elicited with resisted	Eversion of the ankle	Extension of the toes and dorsiflexion of the ankle	Plantar flexion of the ankle	Flexion of the toes and inversion of the ankle
Nerve affected	Superficial peroneal	Deep peroneal	Sural	Tibial
Site of paresthesia and cutaneous sensory loss	Web space between great and second toe	Dorsum of the foot	Lateral aspect of the foot	Plantar aspect of the toes and foot
Arterial pulse that may be diminished		Dorsalis pedis		Posterior tibial

Source: From Patel DR, Greydanus DE, Baker RJ. *Pediatric Practice: Sports Medicine*. New York, NY: McGraw-Hill; 2009.

TREATMENT

▸ Medication

- Anti-inflammatory, NSAID

MEDICAL PROCEDURES

- Acute compartment syndrome, immediate open fasciotomy to relieve pressure and avoid permanent damage
- Subcutaneous fasciotomy
- Hyperbaric oxygen therapy

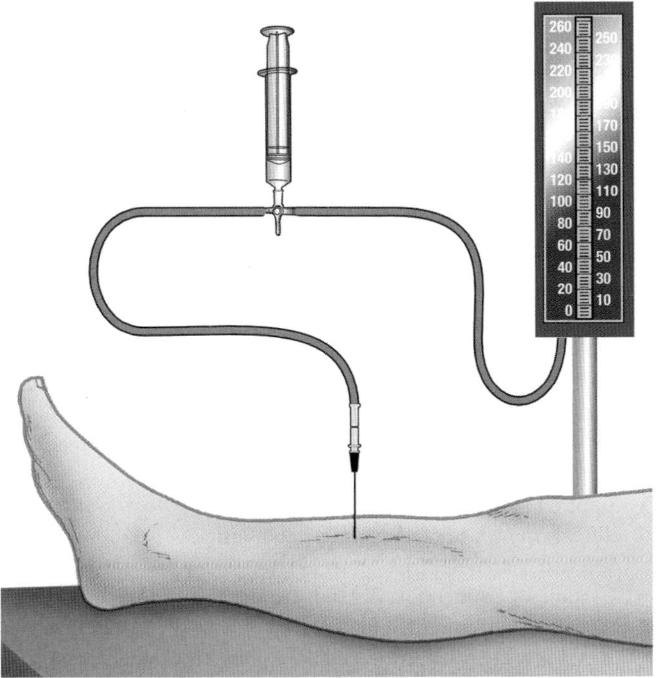

FIGURE 219-8 Infusion technique for measuring compartment pressure. (From Simon RR, Sherman SC. *Emergency Orthopedics*. 6th ed. http://www.accessphysiotherapy.com. Copyright © The McGraw-Hill Companies, Inc. All rights reserved.)

REFERRALS/ADMITTANCE

- For imaging: x-ray, CT, or MRI
- For surgery if fasciotomy is required

IMPAIRMENTS

- Weakness
- Numbness and tingling
- Severe pain

TESTS AND MEASURES

- Homans sign
- Pain, visual analog scale (VAS)
  - 24-hour pain
  - Worst average pain
  - Best average pain
  - Tenderness on palpation
- Functional independence measure
  - Locomotion
- Cardiovascular integrity
  - Blood pressure at rest and after activity
  - Palpation of distal pulses
  - Capillary refill
- Skin integrity

TABLE 219-2 Criteria for Chronic Exertional Compartment Syndrome

Time of Pressure Measurement	Pressure Diagnostic of Compartment Syndrome
Resting or pre-exercise	≥15 mm Hg
1 minute postexercise	≥30 mm Hg
5 minute postexercise	≥20 mm Hg

Source: From Patel DR, Greydanus DE, Baker RJ. *Pediatric Practice: Sports Medicine*. New York, NY: McGraw-Hill; 2009.

TABLE 219-3 Peripheral Nerve Entrapment in the Leg

Nerve	Site of Characteristic Pain	Site of Tingling Sensation on Tinel Test
Common peroneal nerve	Lateral leg and foot	From fibular neck with distal radiation
Superficial peroneal nerve	Lateral calf and dorsum of the foot	Few centimeters proximal to lateral malleolus
Saphenous nerve	Above the medial malleolus	From above the medial malleolus with distal radiation to medial aspect of the foot

Source: From Patel DR, Greydanus DE, Baker RJ. *Pediatric Practice*: Sports Medicine. New York, NY: McGraw-Hill; 2009.

- Associated skin assessment
  - Edema (linear girth measurements, palpation)
  - Color
  - Temperature
- Neurologic examination
  - Sensation
    - Light touch
    - Pin prick limb sensation
    - 2-point discrimination
  - Lower-extremity deep tendon reflexes
  - Proprioception
  - Kinesthetic awareness
  - Coordination
- Limb strength
  - Manual muscle test (MMT)
    - Anterior tibialis
    - Posterior tibialis
    - Foot intrinsics

INTERVENTION

- Avoid external pressure
  - If cast or bandage is causing the problem, it should be loosened or removed
  - Avoid splints, tight would dressing
- Rest
- Address swelling
- Address pain
- Wound care
- Laser therapy
  - Decrease pain
  - Decrease tenderness
  - Decrease stiffness

FUNCTIONAL GOALS

- The patient will be able to
  - Ambulate pain-free for >30 minutes.
  - Return to high-impact activities such as running, hiking, and dancing.
  - Demonstrate and maintain neutral calcaneal alignment with heel strike through toe-off phases of gait.
  - Stand and walk without limitation due to pain after sitting for >1 hour.

PROGNOSIS

- Determined by injury leading to the syndrome.
- Permanent injury can occur to nerves or muscles if diagnosis is delayed.
- Limb compartment syndrome with absent arterial pulses without a history of arterial trauma is associated with poor prognosis.

PATIENT RESOURCE

- MedlinePlus, NIH National Institutes of Health. *Compartment Syndrome.* http://www.ncbi.nlm.nih.gov/pubmedhealth/PMH0002204/ Accessed August 17, 2014.

REFERENCES

1. ICD-9-CM. http://www.icd9data.com. Accessed March 4, 2013.
2. ICD-10-CM. http://www.icd10data.com. Accessed March 4, 2013.
3. The American Physical Therapy Association. *Guide to Physical Therapist Practice*. Alexandria, VA: The American Physical Therapy Association; 2003. http://guidetoptpractice.apta.org./ Accessed March 4, 2013.
4. Wanich T, Hodgkins C, Columbier JA, Muraski E, Kennedy JG. Cycling injuries of the lower extremity. *J Am Acad Orthop Surg.* 2007;15(12):748–756.
5. Hile AM, ANDERSON JM, Fiala KA, et al. Creatine supplementation and anterior compartment pressure during exercise in the heat in dehydrated men. *J Athl Train.* 2006;41(1):30–35.

ADDITIONAL REFERENCES

- Blackman PG. A review of chronic exertional compartment syndrome in the lower leg. *Med Sci Sports Exerc.* 2000;32 (3 Suppl):S4–S10.
- Frink M, Hildebrand F, Krettek C, Brand J, Hankemeier S. Compartment syndrome of the lower leg and foot. *Clin Orthop Relat Res.* 2010;468(4):940–950.
- Geiderman JM, Katz D. General principles of orthopedic injuries. In: Marx J, ed. *Emergency Medicine: Concepts and Clinical Practice.* 7th ed. Philadelphia, PA: Mosby Elsevier; 2009: Chapter 46.
- Goodman CC, Fuller KS. *Pathology Implications for the Physical Therapist.* 3rd ed. Philadelphia, PA: Saunders Elsevier; 2009.
- Gourgiotis S, Villias C, Germanos S, Foukas A, Ridolfini MP. Acute limb compartment syndrome: a review. *J Surg Educ.* 2007;64(3):178–186.
- Marshall ST, Browner BD. Emergency care of musculoskeletal injuries. In: Townsend CM Jr, Beauchamp RD, Evers BM, Mattox KL, eds. *Sabiston Textbook of Surgery.* 19th ed. Philadelphia, PA: Saunders Elsevier; 2012:
- Rasul AT, Lorenzo CT, Agnew S. *Acute compartment syndrome.* 2001. http://emedicine.medscape.com/article/307668-overview. Accessed March 4, 2013.
- Twaddle BC, Amendola A. Compartment syndrome. In: Browner BD, Jupiter JB, Levine AM, Trafton PG, Krettek C, eds. *Skeletal Trauma.* 4th ed. Philadelphia, PA: Saunders Elsevier; 2008: Chapter 13.
- Wall CJ, Lynch J, Harris IA, et al. Clinical practice guidelines for the management of acute limb compartment syndrome following trauma. *ANZ J Surg.* 2010;80(3):151–156.

220 COMPLEX REGIONAL PAIN SYNDROME

Eric Shamus, PhD, DPT, PT, CSCS

CONDITION/DISORDER SYNONYMS

- Reflex sympathetic dystrophy (RSD)
- Sudeck atrophy
- Reflex neurovascular dystrophy (RND)
- Algoneurodystrophy
- Causalgia

ICD-9-CM CODES

- 337.21 Reflex sympathetic dystrophy of the upper limb
- 337.22 Reflex sympathetic dystrophy of the lower limb

ICD-10-CM CODES

- G90.519 Complex regional pain syndrome I of unspecified upper limb
- G90.529 Complex regional pain syndrome I of unspecified lower limb

PREFERRED PRACTICE PATTERN

- 4E: Impaired Joint Mobility, Motor Function, Muscle Performance, and ROM Associated with Localized Inflammation[1]

PATIENT PRESENTATION

A 24-year-old woman presents with increased pain and swelling in her right foot for the past 5 days. The patient is 1 week status post ankle sprain. The patient has an inability to tolerate light touch and has had trouble sleeping due to the sheets brushing against her foot at night. Upon palpation, the patient describes the pain as extreme burning around the foot and ankle. ROM of the right foot is limited with skin color changes. The patient stated she had an x-ray the day after she sprained her ankle and there were no fractures. She is worried because the pain is getting worse each day and she cannot tolerate the ankle brace that was provided to her.

KEY FEATURES

Description

- Autonomic changes
- Severe pain, swelling, skin changes, inability to tolerate light touch
- International Association for the Study of Pain (IASP) classification[2]
  - Type I: No nerve damage
  - Type II: Nerve damage

Essentials of Diagnosis

- Unknown cause
- Electromyography (EMG)
- Usually occurs near the site of injury

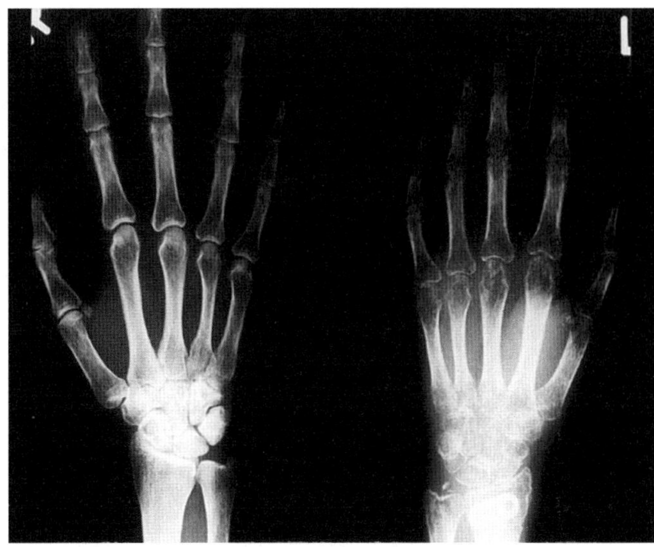

FIGURE 220-1 Radiograph of both hands in a patient with chronic complex regional pain syndrome of the left hand. The radiograph shows a soft-tissue swelling of the dorsum of the hand and around the metacarpophalangeal joints as well as a generalized demineralization, particularly in the distal metacarpal bones. (From Imboden J, Hellmann DB, Stone JH. *Current Rheumatology Diagnosis & Treatment*. 2nd ed. http://www.accessmedicine.com. Copyright © The McGraw-Hill Companies, Inc. All rights reserved.)

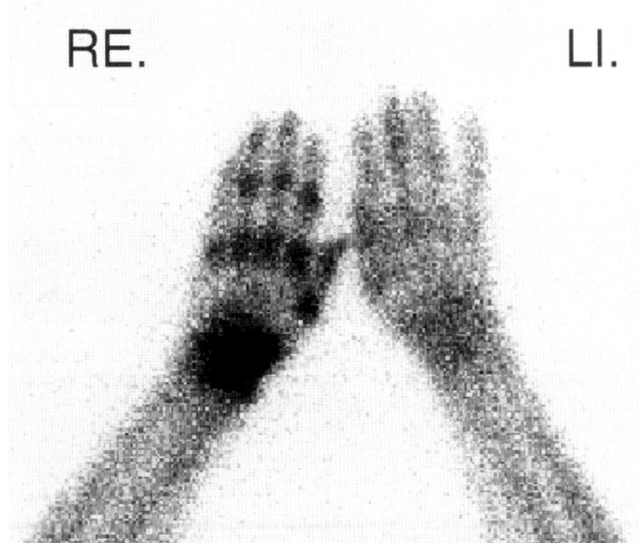

FIGURE 220-2 Three-phase bone scintigraphy of a patient presenting with a complex regional pain syndrome after distal radius fracture of the right hand. The scintigram shows increased bone metabolism in the traumatic wrist area as well as in the metacarpophalangeal and interphalangeal joints, typical findings for complex regional pain syndrome. (From Imboden J, Hellmann DB, Stone JH. *Current Rheumatology Diagnosis & Treatment*. 2nd ed. http://www.accessmedicine.com. Copyright © The McGraw-Hill Companies, Inc. All rights reserved.)

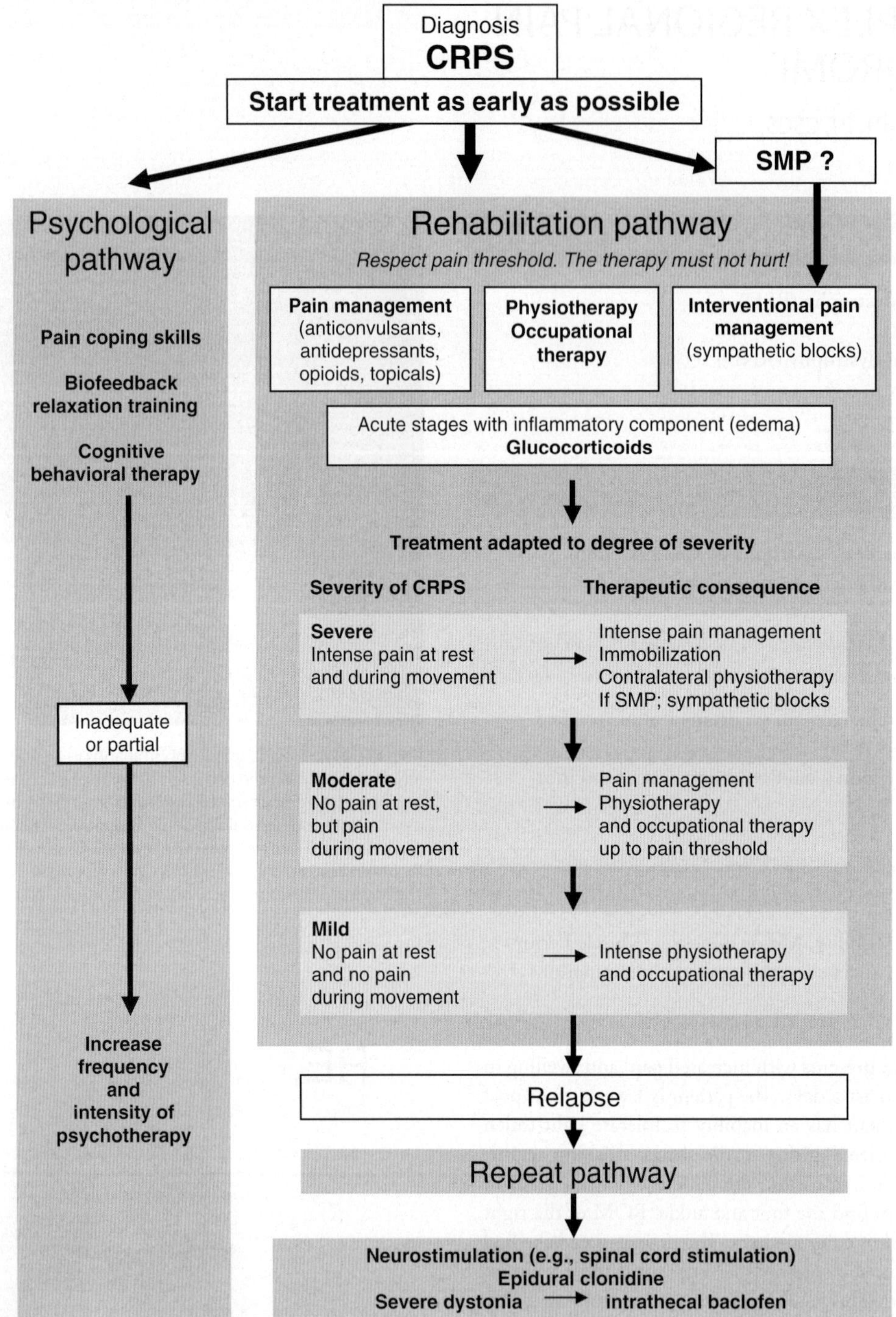

FIGURE 220-3 Treatment algorithm. CRPS, complex regional pain syndrome; SMP, sympathetically maintained pain. (Modified from Stanton-Hicks M, Burton AW, Bruehl SP, et al. An updated interdisciplinary clinical pathway for CRPS: Report of an Expert Panel. *Pain Practice*. 2002;2:1.; modified from Baron R, Binder A, Ulrich W, Maier C. [Complex regional pain syndrome. Reflex sympathetic dystrophy and causalgia.] Nervenarzt. 2002;73:305.; and from McMahon S, Koltzenberg M, eds. *Wall & Melzack's Textbook of Pain*. 5th ed. Churchill Livingstone, 2005:1011.)

- Three stages[3]
  - Stage 1 (inflammatory phase): Severe burning, spasm, stiffness, skin changes, nonfocal pain, decreased ROM
  - Stage 2 (vasomotor phase): Symptoms of stage 1, plus muscle atrophy, osteoporosis, thickening of the dermis, cool skin temperature
  - Stage 3 (end stage): Symptoms of stages 1 and 2, plus irreversible changes in skin and bones, flexor tendon contracture, atrophic stage

General Considerations

- Fatigue, swelling, pain, and sensory changes can cause disability
- Deregulation of the autonomic system

Demographics

- Usually following injury or surgery
- Three times more likely in females than in males[4]

CLINICAL FINDINGS

SIGNS AND SYMPTOMS

- Pain
- Sweating in the area
- Inability to tolerate light touch
- Deregulation of the autonomic system
- Skin-color changes
- Swelling
- Nerve pain
- Cracked nails
- Osteoporosis
- Muscle atrophy
- Flexor tendon contracture
- Skin-temperature change
- Sympathetic hyperactivity
- Associated symptoms may include paresthesias, burning, tingling

Functional Implications

- Pain and stiffness can limit ADLs
- Unable to use the extremity
- Unable to wear socks
- Unable to sleep due to pain from touching the sheets

Possible Contributing Causes

- Unknown etiology
- Surgery
- Injury
- Vascular disease
- Spinal cord injury
- Fracture
- Frostbite
- Amputation
- Psychological components
- Stress
- Anxiety

Differential Diagnosis

- Erythromelalgia
- Myasthenia gravis
- Chronic fatigue syndrome
- Hypothyroidism
- Lyme disease
- Fibromyalgia
- Peripheral nerve injury
- Systemic lupus erythematosus
- Rheumatoid arthritis
- Polymyalgia rheumatica
- Depression
- Chronic neck and back pain

MEANS OF CONFIRMATION OR DIAGNOSIS

Imaging

- X-ray[5]
- Thermography
- MRI[5]

Diagnostic Procedures

- Electromyography (EMG)
- Widespread Pain Index (WPI)
- Symptom severity score
- Sympathetic block
- Skin blood-flow test

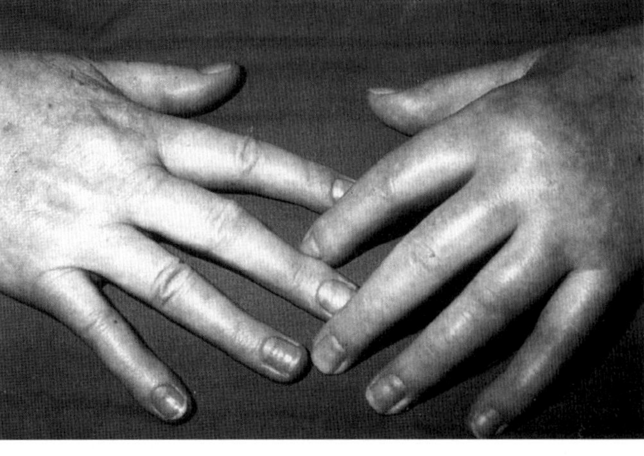

FIGURE 220-4 Complex regional pain syndrome developed in this patient after a radial fracture in the left hand. The marked swelling seen in the left hand started 2 weeks after the initial trauma. (With permission from Baron R, Levine JD, Fields HL. Causalgia and reflex sympathetic dystrophy: does the sympathetic nervous system contribute to the generation of pain? *Muscle Nerve*. 1999;22:678.)

FINDINGS AND INTERPRETATION

- X-ray and MRI negative[5]
- Laboratory tests negative

TREATMENT

Medication

- Sympathetic block
- Cortisone

REFERRALS/ADMITTANCE

- To dietician/nutritionist for nutritional counseling
- To pain clinic for pain management, counseling
- To neurologist for neurologic assessment
- To cognitive-behavioral therapist and psychologist for
  - Counseling
  - Support groups
  - Biofeedback
  - Relaxation techniques

IMPAIRMENTS

- Sleep deprivation
- Limited walking and movement secondary to pain and morning stiffness, which can last throughout the day
- Difficulty standing or sitting in one position for an extended period of time
- Limited aerobic capacity

TESTS AND MEASURES

- Passive physiologic intervertebral mobility testing (PPIVM)
- Disabilities of the Arm, Shoulder, and Hand (DASH) score to assess physical function
- Lower-extremity screening examination
- Postural examination
- Muscle length testing, including the hamstrings, hip flexors, and calf muscles
- Quadrant test
- Straight-leg raise test

- Slump test
- Lower limb nerve tension test
- Prone instability test
- Lower-extremity neurologic screen (dermatome, myotome, reflexes)
- Repeated movement testing
- Fear-Avoidance Beliefs Questionnaire (FABQ)

INTERVENTION

- Cardiovascular training
- Patient education regarding their disease
- Stress relief
- Skin desensitization
- Gentle stretching, flexibility
- Ergonomic education
- Heat
- Massage for relaxation
- Active and passive ROM
- Weight-bearing activities

FUNCTIONAL GOALS

- Patient will be able to
  - Perform 30 minutes of aerobic activity.
  - Perform an 8-hour light-duty job.
  - Tolerate light touch with a sheet on legs at night.
  - Manage stress in order to participate in community activities.

PROGNOSIS

- Good if treated early.
- May go into remission.
- May be severe with poor long-term results.
- Stage 1 lasts 1 to 3 months.
- Stage 2 lasts 3 to 6 months.
- Stage 3 lasts >6 months, often not fully reversible.

ADDITIONAL INFORMATION

- For additional information, please see case 5-5 in chapter 5 of *Therapeutic Modalities in Rehabilitation*, 4e, at www.AccessPhysiotherapy.com.[6]

PATIENT RESOURCES

- American Society for Surgery of the Hand. Complex Regional Pain Syndrome. http://www.assh.org/Public/HandConditions/Pages/Complex-Regional-Pain-Syndrome.aspx. Accessed June 21, 2013.
- Reflex Sympathetic Dystrophy Syndrome Association. http://www.rsds.org/index2.html. Accessed June 21, 2013.

REFERENCES

1. The American Physical Therapy Association. Pattern 4E: Impaired joint mobility, motor function, muscle performance, and range of motion associated with localized inflammation. *Interactive Guide to Physical Therapist Practice*. 2003. DOI: 10.2522/ptguide.3.1_5. Accessed June 21, 2013.
2. Schwarzer A, Maier C. Chapter 33. Complex regional pain syndrome. In: Kopf A, Patel NB, eds. *International Association for the Study of Pain Guide to Pain Management in Low-Resource Settings*. Seattle, WA: IASP; 2010.
3. Dutton M. *Orthopaedic Examination, Evaluation, and Intervention*. New York, NY: McGraw-Hill; 2008. http://www.accessphysiotherapy.com/resource/612. Accessed June 21, 2013.
4. Veldman PH, Reynen HM, Arntz IE, Goris RJ. Signs and symptoms of reflex sympathetic dystrophy: prospective study of 829 patients. *Lancet*. 1993;342(8878):1012–1016.
5. Malone TR, Hazle C, Grey ML. *Imaging in Rehabilitation*. New York, NY: McGraw-Hill; 2008. http://www.accessphysiotherapy.com/resource/613. Accessed June 21, 2013.
6. Hooker DN, Prentice WE. Chapter 5. Basic principles of electricity and electrical stimulating currents. In: Prentice WE, Quillen WS, Underwood F, eds. *Therapeutic Modalities in Rehabilitation*. 4th ed. New York, NY: McGraw-Hill; 2011. http://www.accessphysiotherapy.com/content/8136367#8136367. Accessed June 21, 2013.

ADDITIONAL REFERENCES

- Birklein F, Kunzel W, Sieweke N. Despite clinical similarities there are significant differences between acute limb trauma and complex regional pain syndrome I (CRPS-I). *Pain*. 2001;93:165–171.
- Dutton M. Complex disorders. In: Dutton M, ed. *McGraw-Hill's NPTE (National Physical Therapy Examination)*. 2nd ed. New York, NY: McGraw-Hill; 2012. http://www.accessphysiotherapy.com/content/5402428. Accessed August 17, 2014.
- Dutton M. Integration of Practice Patterns 4F and 5F: Impaired joint mobility, motor function, muscle performance, and range of motion or reflex integrity secondary to referred pain, spinal disorders, peripheral nerve entrapment, myofascial pain syndrome, and complex regional pain syndrome. In: Dutton M, ed. *Orthopaedic Examination, Evaluation, and Intervention*. 2nd ed. New York, NY: McGraw-Hill; 2008. http://www.accessphysiotherapy.com/content/55579236. Accessed August 17, 2014.
- ICD9DATA web site. http://www.icd9data.com. Accessed June 21, 2013.
- ICD10DATA web site. http://www.icd10data.com. Accessed June 21, 2013.
- Gainer MJ. Hypnotherapy for reflex sympathetic dystrophy. *Am J Clin Hypn*. 1992;34(4):227–232.
- Hay WW, Levin MJ, Sondheimer JM, Deterding RR. Noninflammatory pain syndromes. In: Hay WW, Levin MJ, Sondheimer JM, Deterding RR, eds. *CURRENT Diagnosis & Treatment: Pediatrics*. 20th ed. New York, NY: McGraw-Hill; 2011. http://www.accessphysiotherapy.com/content/6586584. Accessed June 21, 2013.
- Hord ED, Oaklander AL. Complex regional pain syndrome: A review of evidence-supported treatment options. *Curr Pain Headache Rep*. 2003;7(3):188–196.
- Quisel A, Gill JM, Witherell P. Complex regional pain syndrome underdiagnosed. *J Fam Pract*. 2005;54(6):524–532.
- Watkins LR, Maier SF. Immune regulation of central nervous system functions: from sickness responses to pathological pain. *J Intern Med*. 2005;257(2):139–155.

221 EHLERS–DANLOS SYNDROME

Martha Henao Bloyer, DPT, PT, PCS

CONDITION/DISORDER SYNONYMS

- EDS
- Cutis hyperelastica

ICD-9-CM CODE

- 756.83 Ehlers–Danlos syndrome

ICD-10-CM CODE

- Q79.6 Ehlers–Danlos syndrome

PREFERRED PRACTICE PATTERN

- 5F: Impaired Peripheral Nerve Integrity and Muscle Performance Associated with Peripheral Nerve Injury[1]

PATIENT PRESENTATION

A 15-year-old female was referred with low back pain and a recent diagnosis of Ehlers–Danlos Syndrome: hypermobility type. She reports pain is 8/10 with activity and 6/10 when seated. During the examination and evaluation, she scores a 6 on the Breighton Scoring System and has severe hypermobility. She also complains of generalized muscular and joint pain limiting her ability to participate in activities with her peers at school and socially. Her affect appears flat and withdrawn during the therapy session. Past medical history is non-contributory. Referral has been made to decrease pain, promote joint stability, and improve overall strength and posture.

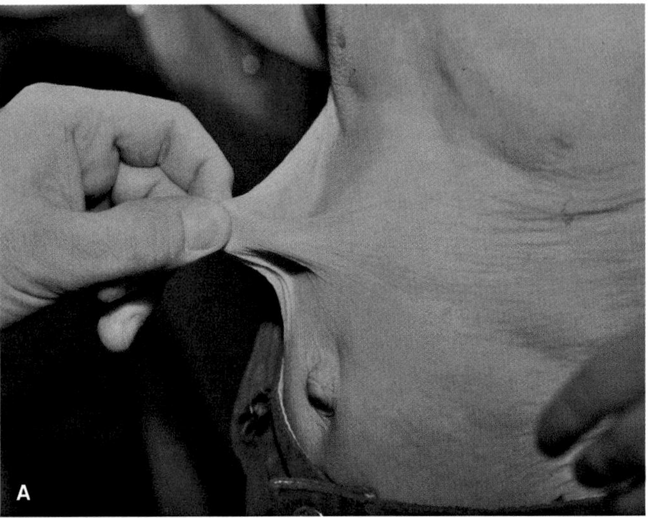

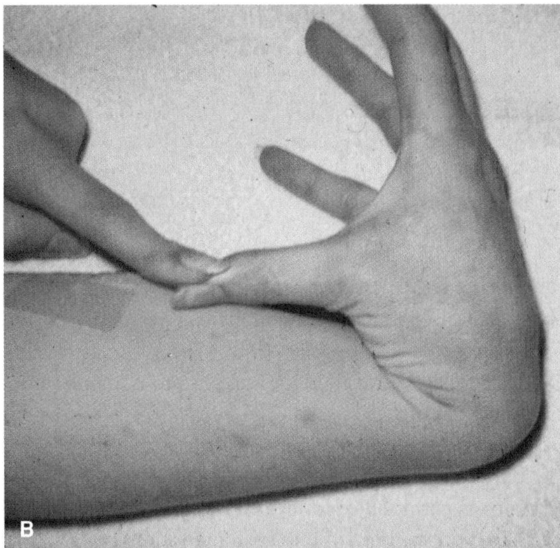

FIGURE 221-1 Ehlers-Danlos syndrome. (**A**) Hyperextensible skin. (**B**) Lax joints. Redundant chordae tendineae and arterial rupture may occur. (From Fuster V, Walsh RA, Harrington RA: *Hurst's The Heart*, 13th Edition. www.accessmedicine.com. Copyright © The McGraw-Hill Companies, Inc. All rights reserved.)

KEY FEATURES

Description

- Group of inherited disorders involving the connective tissue collagen[2,3]
- Major manifestations include[2]
    - Classical: most common form
        - Autosomal dominant heritability
        - Hyperextensible skin with atrophic scars
        - Easy bruising
        - Friability of tissues, which can result in
            - Hiatal hernia
            - Anal prolapse
            - Bleeding and poor wound-healing,
        - Molluscoid pseudo tumors (calcified hematomas)
    - Hypermobility of joints: least severe form
        - Autosomal dominant heritability
        - Affects large and small joints
        - Recurrent joint subluxations and dislocations
            - Shoulder
            - Patella
            - Temporomandibular
    - Vascular: most severe form
        - Autosomal dominant heritability
        - Can lead to organ or arterial rupture
        - Thin, translucent skin

- Facial characteristics
  - Large eyes
  - Thin nose
  - Lobe-less ears
  - Short stature
  - Thin scalp hair
- Kyphoscoliosis
  - Autosomal recessive heritability
  - Scoliosis at birth; progressive throughout life
  - Generalized joint laxity
  - Severe muscle hypotonia at birth
  - Other findings
    - Marfan-like features
    - Microcornea
    - Radiologically considerable osteopenia
- Arthrochalasia
  - Autosomal dominant heritability
  - Congenital bilateral hip dislocation
  - Other manifestations may include
    - Skin hyperextensibility with easy bruising
    - Tissue fragility, including atrophic scars
    - Muscle hypotonia
    - Kyphoscoliosis
    - Radiologically mild osteopenia
- Dermatosparaxis
  - Autosomal recessive heritability
  - Severe skin fragility
  - Sagging, redundant skin
  - Substantial bruising
  - Wound healing not impaired
  - Scars not atrophic

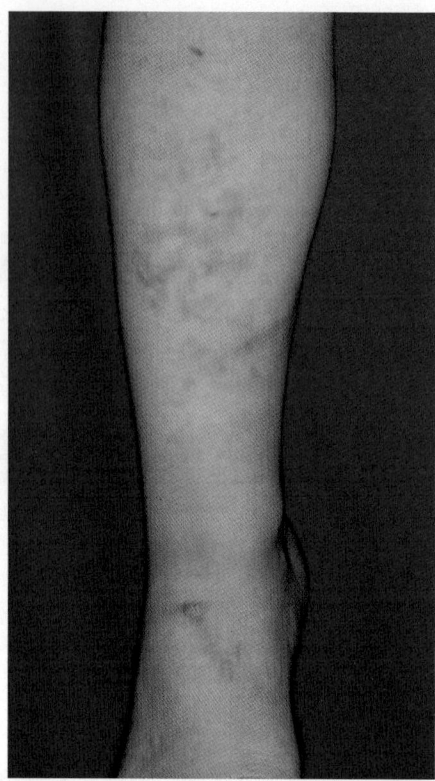

FIGURE 221-2 Classical Ehlers–Danlos syndrome. Chronic discolored scars on the shin and ankle after repeated trauma. This is often associated with firm subcutaneous nodules that can be confused with subcutaneous granuloma annulare. Note the widened scar at the knee area. (From Goldsmith LA et al: *Fitzpatrick's Dermatology in General Medicine*, 8th Edition. www.accessmedicine.com. Copyright © The McGraw-Hill Companies, Inc. All rights reserved.)

Essentials of Diagnosis

- Characterized by joint hypermobility, skin extensibility and tissue fragility[2]
- Six major types, classified according symptom manifestations and family history[2]
  - Clinical evaluation and family history to identify
    - Hypermobile type
    - Joint hypermobility confirmed by a score of five or higher on the nine-point Beighton Scale
  - Skin biopsy to identify the following types
    - Vascular
    - Arthrochalasia
    - Dermatosparaxis
  - Urine test to identify
    - Kyphoscoliosis type

General Considerations

- Hypermobile type is least severe, leads primarily to musculoskeletal complications

Demographics

- Females seek more medical care related to pain and joint complications than males
- Easy bruising may be the primary presenting symptom in early childhood

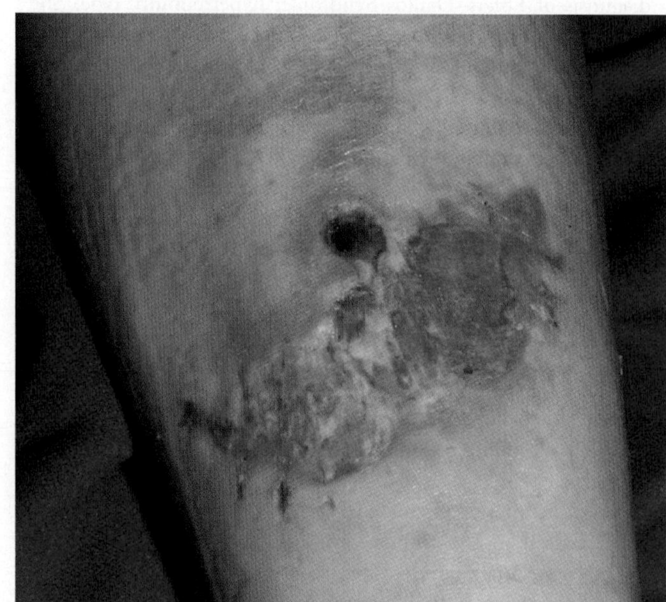

FIGURE 221-3 Classical Ehlers–Danlos syndrome. After suturing for a laceration, the wound dehisced with secondary infection and marked widening. Note the evidence of former sutures at the lower border, now 3 weeks after the injury and treatment with antibiotics. Scars tend to stretch further in the 6 months after closure. (From Goldsmith LA et al: *Fitzpatrick's Dermatology in General Medicine*, 8th Edition. www.accessmedicine.com. Copyright © The McGraw-Hill Companies, Inc. All rights reserved.)

CLINICAL FINDINGS

SIGNS AND SYMPTOMS

- Most often joint and skin related, may include[2, 5]
  - Joints
    - Joint hypermobility: loose, unstable joints; prone to frequent dislocation or subluxation
    - Joint pain
    - Early onset of osteoarthritis
  - Skin
    - Soft, velvety skin
    - Variable skin hyperextensibility
    - Fragile skin that tears or bruises easily
      - Manifests as spontaneous ecchymosis
      - Characteristic brownish discoloration
      - Tendency toward prolonged bleeding despite normal coagulation status
    - Severe scarring
      - Scars found mostly on pressure points (knee, elbow, forehead, chin)
    - Slow and poor wound-healing
    - Development of molluscoid pseudo tumors (fleshy lesions associated with scars over pressure areas)
- Chronic pain
  - Physically and psychosocially disabling
  - Variable age of onset, location, duration, quality, severity, response to therapy
  - Affected individuals may also be diagnosed with
    - Chronic fatigue syndrome
    - Fibromyalgia
    - Depression
    - Hypochondriasis
  - Other pain syndromes
    - Myofascial pain
    - Neuropathic pain
    - Headaches/Migraines
- Hematologic
  - Easy bruising
  - Mildly prolonged bleeding
- Gastrointestinal
  - Gastroesophageal reflux
  - Gastritis
  - Delayed gastric emptying
  - Irritable bowel syndrome
- Cardiovascular
  - Autonomic dysfunction
    - Atypical chest pain
    - Palpitations
    - Orthostatic intolerance
  - Aortic Root Dilatation
    - Occurs in one-quarter to one-third of i ndividuals
  - Mitral valve prolapse
- Oral/dental
  - High, narrow palate; dental crowding
  - Periodontal disease
  - Temporomandibular dysfunction (TMJ)
    - Due to joint degeneration and osteoarthritis
- Obstetric/Gynecologic
  - Pregnancy may be complicated by premature rupture of membranes
  - Rapid labor and delivery
  - Joint laxity and pain increases throughout gestation
- Psychiatric
  - Psychological dysfunction
    - Depression
    - Anxiety
    - Low self-confidence
- Fragility of soft tissues
  - Spontaneous rupture or tear of internal organs
  - Not manifested in hypermobility type

▶ Functional Implications

- Avoid resistance and isometric exercises: can exacerbate joint instability, pain
- Avoid high-impact activity: can increase risk of acute subluxation/dislocation, pain, osteoarthritis
- Cautious use of crutches, canes, walkers: can increase stress on upper extremities

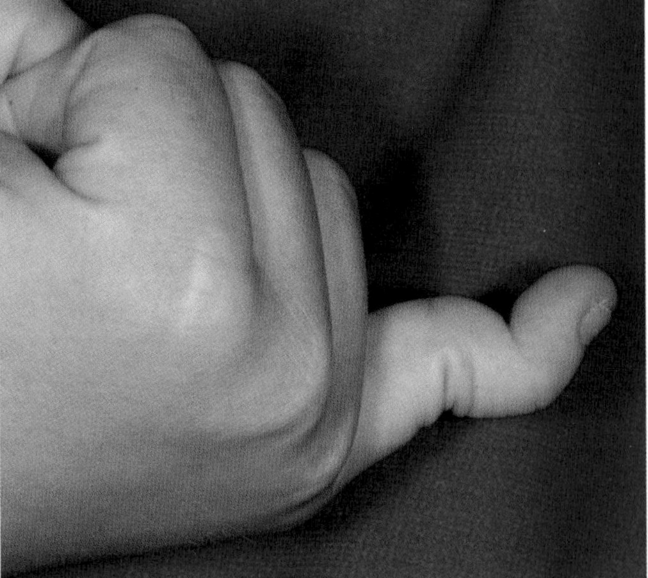

FIGURE 221-4 Classical Ehlers–Danlos syndrome. Hyperextensibility of digits is demonstrated. (From Goldsmith LA et al: *Fitzpatrick's Dermatology in General Medicine*, 8th Edition. www.accessmedicine.com. Copyright © The McGraw-Hill Companies, Inc. All rights reserved.)

▶ Possible Contributing Causes

- Inherited
  - Autosomal dominant (classical, hypermobility, vascular, arthrochalasia types)
  - Autosomal recessive (dermatosparaxis, kyphoscoliosis types)
  - X chromosome-linked

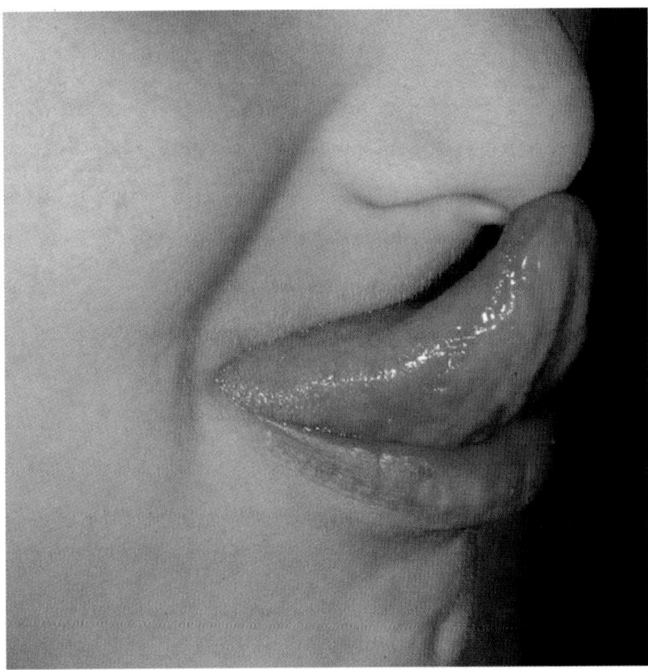

FIGURE 221-5 Classical Ehlers–Danlos syndrome (EDS). Gorlin's sign is the ability to touch the tip of the nose with the tongue and is described in approximately 50% of patients with Ehlers–Danlos, in contrast to 10% of individuals who do not have EDS. (From Goldsmith LA et al: *Fitzpatrick's Dermatology in General Medicine*, 8th Edition. www.accessmedicine.com. Copyright © The McGraw-Hill Companies, Inc. All rights reserved.)

TABLE 221-1 Different Forms of Ehlers–Danlos Syndrome

Type	Typical Features	Inheritance	Gene Defect	Protein Defect
Classic (EDS I—severe and EDS II—mild)	Skin hyperextensibility and fragility, joint hypermobility, tissue fragility manifested by widened atrophic scarring	AD	*COL5A1*	Collagen V
			COL5A2	
		AD	*COL1A1*	Pro α1 (I) and pro α2 (I) chains of procollagen I
		AD, AR	*COL1A2*	
Hypermobile (EDS III)	Joint hypermobility, moderate skin involvement, absence of tissue fragility	AD	*TNXB*	Tenascin X
Vascular (EDS IV)	Markedly reduced life span due to spontaneous rupture of internal organs such as arteries and intestines; skin is thin, translucent, and fragile, with extensive bruising; hypermobile minor joints; characteristic facial appearance	AD	*COL3A1*	Collagen III
X-linked EDS (EDS V)	Similar to classic type	X-linked recessive	Unknown	Unknown
Ocular-scoliotic EDS VI (EDS VIA and EDS VIB)	Features of classic EDS as well as severe muscular hypotonia after birth, progressive kyphoscoliosis, a Marfanoid habitus, osteopenia, occasionally rupture of the eye globe and great arteries	AR	*PLOD1*	Deficiency of procollagen-lysine 5-dioxygenase activity (EDS VIA)
			Unknown for EDS VIB	Unknown for EDS VIB
Arthrochalasic EDS VII (EDS VIIA and EDS VIIB)	Congenital bilateral hip dislocation, hypermobile joints, moderate skin involvement, osteopenia	AD	*COL1A1*	Mutations that prevent cleavage of the N propeptides
			COL1A2	
Dermatosparactic EDS VII C	Redundant and fragile skin, prominent hernias, joint—laxity, dysmorphic features	AR	*ADAMTS2*	Deficiency of procollagen I N-terminal proteinase
Periodontotic EDS VIII	Absorptive periodontosis with premature loss of permanent teeth, fragility of the skin, skin lesions	AD	Unknown	Unknown
EDS due to tenascin X deficiency	Similar to EDS II	AR	*TNXB*	Tenascin X
EDS, progeroid form		AR?	*B4GALT7*	Deficiency of galactosyltransferase 7 (defective synthesis of dermatan sulfate proteoglycans)

Abbreviations: AD = autosomal dominant; AR = autosomal recessive.
Source: Longo DL et al [eds]: *Harrison's Principles of Internal Medicine*, 18th Edition. New York, McGraw-Hill, 2012.

Differential Diagnosis

- Bruising
  - Child abuse should be considered
- Joint laxity is a non-specific manifestation of other diseases and syndromes
- Other diseases and syndromes with characteristic features or involvement of systems other than the joints and skin include
  - Marfan syndrome
  - Loeys–Dietz syndrome
  - Stickler syndrome
  - Williams syndrome
  - Fragile X syndrome (FXS)
  - Achondroplasia and hypochondroplasia
  - Osteogenesis imperfecta (OI)
  - Aneuploidies, such as Down, Turner, Klinefelter syndromes

MEANS OF CONFIRMATION OR DIAGNOSIS

Imaging

- Mitral valve prolapse (MVP) and proximal aortic dilatation diagnosed by echocardiography,[6] CT or MRI[7,8]
- Joint pain
  - Skeletal radiographs may be normal
- Dual-energy X-ray absorptiometry (DEXA)[8]
  - Every two years if bone loss confirmed
- Holter monitoring for cardiovascular: A utonomic dysfunction

Diagnostic Procedures

- Thorough history and physical examination
  - Musculoskeletal
  - Cardiovascular
  - Integumentary
  - Gastrointestinal

FINDINGS AND INTERPRETATION

- Joint hypermobility
  - Assessed using the Beighton Scale
  - Depends on age, gender, family, ethnic background
  - Score 5 out of 9 or greater defines hypermobility
  - Total score obtained by
    - Passive dorsiflexion of each fifth finger greater than 90 degrees: One point for each hand
    - Passive apposition of each thumb to the flexor surface of the forearm: One point for each hand
    - Hyperextension of each elbow greater than 10 degrees: One point for each elbow
    - Hyperextension of each knee greater than 10 degrees: One point for each knee
    - Ability to place palms on the floor with the knees fully extended: One point

REFERRALS/ADMITTANCE

- To orthopedist for joint hypermobility
- To rheumatologist
- To gastroenterologist
- To dentist for periodontal disease and temporomandibular dysfunction
- To occupational therapist for splinting and joint protection
- To hospital for imaging

IMPAIRMENTS

- Joint hypermobility
- Impaired mobility
- Pain
- Psychosocial

TESTS AND MEASURES

- Skin hyperextensibility
  - Test at neutral site, such as volar surface of forearm
  - Measured by pulling up the skin until resistance felt
  - Difficult to assess in young children because abundance of subcutaneous fat
- Joint hypermobility assessed using the Beighton Scale

INTERVENTION

- Management includes genetic counseling to understand the disorder's impact on family and future children
- Treat manifestations
  - Assistive devices for joint stability
    - Braces,and splints
    - Soft neck collars
  - Mobility devices for decreasing stress-load on lower extremities
    - Wheelchairs, scooters
  - Sleeping-surface assistive devices
    - Specialized mattress
  - Pain management
    - Medications (individualized)
    - Acetaminophen
    - NSAIDs
    - Cox-2 inhibitors
    - Topical lidocaine
    - Skeletal muscle relaxants
    - Tricyclic antidepressants
    - Serotonin/Norepinephrine receptor inhibitors (SNRIs)
    - Opioids
    - Glucosamine and chondroitin
    - Supplemental magnesium
    - Psychological and pain-oriented counseling
  - Modalities that reduce spasms
  - Management of gastrointestinal symptoms: gastritis, reflux, irritable bowel syndrome
- Prevention of primary manifestations
  - Low-resistance exercise to increase muscle tone and joint stability
    - Walking, bicycling, swimming, range of motion
    - Progress by increasing repetitions, frequency, duration (not resistance)
  - Assistive devices for hand or finger strain
    - Writing and feeding utensils
- Prevention of secondary complications
  - Maximize bone density
    - Calcium
    - Vitamin D
    - Low impact weight-bearing exercises

FUNCTIONAL GOALS

- Patient will
  - Report decreased level of joint (specify location) pain after 10 minutes of low impact physical activity.
  - Independent in donning and doffing (specific joint) splints.
  - Demonstrate ability to go up and down one flight of stairs using handrail, step-to pattern, energy conservation techniques.
  - Be independent and safe using powered wheelchair mobility, indoor and outdoor.

PROGNOSIS

- First-degree relatives are at 50% risk of having autosomal dominant types.
- Prognosis depends on type.
- Symptoms vary in severity.

PATIENT RESOURCES

- Ehlers–Danlos National Foundation. *What are the Types of EDS?* http://www.ednf.org/index.php?option=com_content&task=view&id=1348&Itemid=88888969. Accessed August 17, 2014.
- Ehlers–Danlos syndrome Network C.A.R.E.S. *A Connective Tissue Disorder*. http://www.ehlersdanlosnetwork.org/causes-symptoms.html. Accessed August 17, 2014.
- Ehlers-Danlos. NIH, National Institute of Arthritis and Musculoskeletal and Skin Diseases. http://www.niams.nih.gov/health_info/Connective_Tissue/default.asp. Accessed August 17, 2014.

REFERENCES

1. The American Physical Therapy Association. Pattern 5F: Impaired peripheral nerve integrity and muscle performance associated with peripheral nerve injury. *Interactive Guide to Physical Therapist Practice*. 2003. DOI: 10.2522/ptguide.3.2_6. Accessed May 24, 2013.
2. Dutton M. *Orthopaedic Examination, Evaluation, and Intervention*. New York, NY: McGraw-Hill; 2008. http://www.accessphysiotherapy.com/resource/612. Accessed May 24, 2013.
3. Levy H. *Ehlers–Danlos Syndrome, Hypermobility Type*. 2004. http://newtons-online.net/documents/EDS%20b.pdf. Accessed May 24, 2013.
4. Miyamoto SD, Sondheimer HM, Fagan TE, Collins KK. Chapter 19. Cardiovascular diseases. In: Hay W, Levin MJ, Sondheimer JM, Detering RR, eds. *CURRENT Diagnosis & Treatment: Pediatrics*. New York, NY: McGraw-Hill; 2011. http://www.accessphysiotherapy.com/abstract/6583154#6583208. Accessed May 24, 2013.
5. Malone TR, Hazle C, Grey ML. *Imaging in Rehabilitation*. New York: McGraw-Hill; 2008. http://www.accessphysiotherapy.com/resource/613. Accessed May 24, 2013.
6. DeTurk WE, Johnson L. Chapter 3. Essentials of exercise physiology. In: DeTurk WE, Cahalin LP, eds. *Cardiovascular and Pulmonary Physical Therapy*. New York, NY: McGraw-Hill: 2011. http://www.accessphysiotherapy.com/abstract/6870690#6870710. Accessed May 24, 2013.

ADDITIONAL REFERENCES

- ICD9DATA web site. http://www.icd9data.com. Accessed August 17, 2014.
- ICD10DATA web site. http://www.icd10data.com. Accessed August 17, 2014.
- Pagon RA, Bird TD, Dolan CR, Stephens K, eds. *Source GeneReviews [Internet]*. Seattle (WA): University of Washington, Seattle; 1993-2004 Oct 22 [updated 2010 Dec 14].

222 ERB PALSY

Eric Shamus, PhD, DPT, PT, CSCS
Mae L. Yahara, MS, PT, ATC

CONDITION/DISORDER SYNONYMS

- Erb–Duchenne palsy
- Erb paralysis
- Brachial plexus injury

ICD-9-CM CODES

- 767.6 Injury to brachial plexus due to birth trauma
- 953.4 Injury to brachial plexus

ICD-10-CM CODES

- G54.0 Brachial plexus disorders
- P14.0 Erb paralysis due to birth injury
- S14.3XXA Injury of brachial plexus, initial encounter

PREFERRED PRACTICE PATTERNS

- 4F: Impaired Joint Mobility, Motor Function, Muscle Performance, Range of Motion, and Reflex Integrity Associated with Spinal Disorders[1]

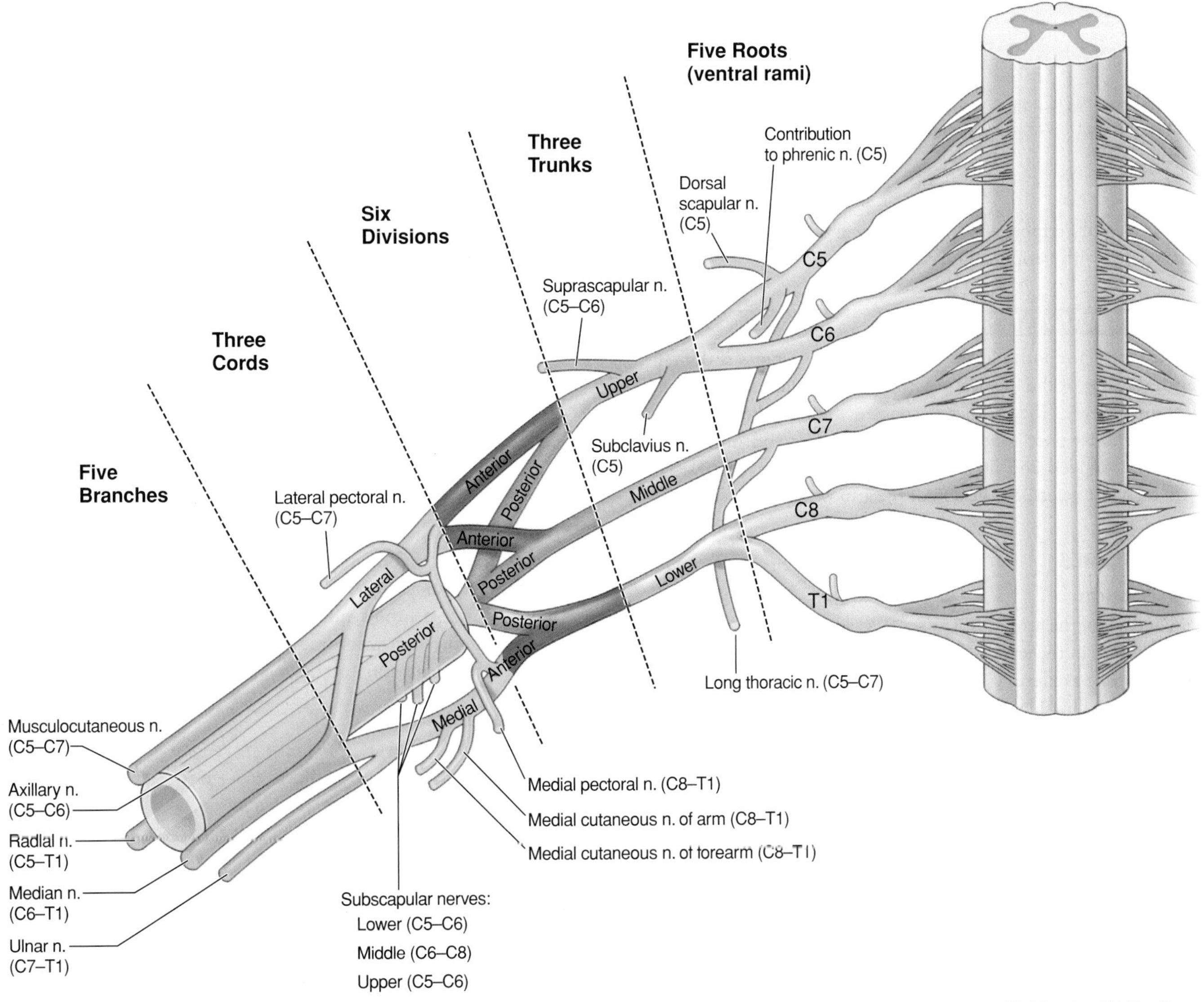

FIGURE 222-1 Schematic of the brachial plexus showing the branches, cords, divisions, trunks, and roots. (From Morton DA, Foreman KB, Albertine KH. *The Big Picture: Gross Anatomy*. www.accessmedicine.com. Copyright © The McGraw-Hill Companies, Inc. All rights reserved.)

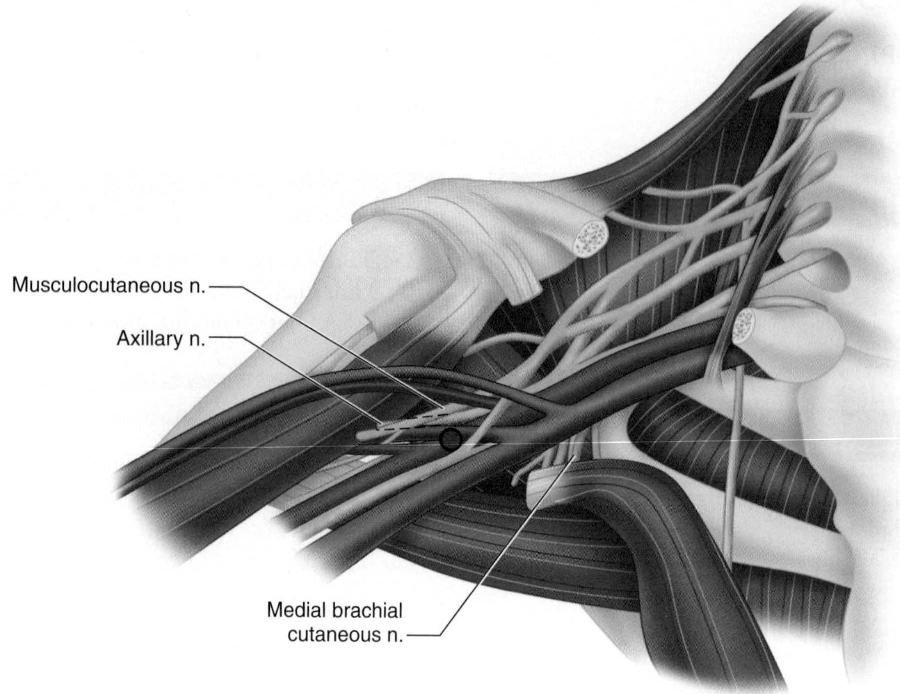

FIGURE 222-2 Axillary block. The axillary, musculocutaneous, and medial brachial cutaneous nerves are usually spared with an axillary approach. (From Butterworth JF, Mackey DC, Wasnick JD. *Morgan & Mikhail's Clinical Anesthesiology*. 5th ed. www.accessmedicine.com. Copyright © The McGraw-Hill Companies, Inc. All rights reserved.)

- 5F: Impaired Peripheral Nerve Integrity and Muscle Performance Associated with Peripheral Nerve Injury[2,3]

PATIENT PRESENTATION

Patient is a 3-month-old infant. His mother reports a difficult birth. Review of the medical record reveals shoulder dystocia and forceps delivery. The mother is concerned about the right arm. Child exhibits poor tone in the right shoulder and upper arm, forearm extended and in pronation. No movement of the right arm on Moro reflex. No flexion of the arm with painful stimulus.

KEY FEATURES

Description

- Paralysis of the arm
- Weakness in the arm
- Diminished reflexes C5–C6 vertebrae
- Arm hangs by side, internally rotated
- Motor or sensory changes in the nerve distribution due to pressure from
  - Compression
  - Stretch

Essentials of Diagnosis

- Electromyography
- Pain
- Numbness
- Sensory changes in multiple peripheral nerves of the upper extremity from C5 and C6 nerve roots
- Hand clumsiness, weakness
- Seddon classification
  - Neuropraxia (Class 1), First degree
  - Axonotmesis (Class 2), Second degree
  - Neurotmesis (Class 3)
    - Third degree, nerve fiber interruption
    - Fourth degree, epineurium intact
    - Fifth degree, complete transection of the nerve

General Considerations

- Involved nerves: Suprascapular nerve, musculocutaneous nerve, axillary nerve
- Must differentiate from more proximal and distal nerve compression, thoracic outlet syndrome (TOS), ulnar tunnel, cervical radiculopathy
- Lower motor-neuron syndrome
- Nerve compression syndrome in the upper extremity
- Wallerian degeneration occurs below the site of injury

Demographics

- Traction injury
- Falls on outstretched arm (affects any age)
- Infants: From birth trauma, head traction

CLINICAL FINDINGS

SIGNS AND SYMPTOMS

- Acute or chronic paresthesia
- Sensory changes: Hypo-sensitivity of hand
- Hand clumsiness
- Feeling of arm heaviness
- Hand weakness, loss of grip-power and dexterity
- Intrinsic muscle atrophy

- Waiter's tip sign
- Caused by excessive lateral neck flexion
- Loss of lateral-rotator, arm-flexor, and wrist-extensor musculature

Functional Implications

- Feeling of arm being dead
- Difficulty with hand function, hand clumsiness, and possible loss of strength during ADLs/IADLs

Possible Contributing Causes

- During forceps delivery, infant has head traction
- Traction to the cervical spine
- Trauma pulling arm into abduction
- Ganglion or space-occupying lesion
- In the womb, sustained pressure over thoracic outlet
- Clavicle fracture
- Glenohumeral dislocation

Differential Diagnosis

- TOS
- Cervical radiculopathy
- Other potential entrapment sites include
  - Medial humeral groove
  - Arcade of Struthers
  - Medial intermuscular septum
  - Flexor digitorum profundus
  - Flexor carpi ulnaris
  - Just proximal to or within Guyon canal
  - Sensory and motor involvement between the abductor digiti minimi and flexor digiti minimi
  - Near hook of hamate: Involves motor function only
  - Distal end of Guyon canal: Involves sensory function only
- Radial neuropathy
- Median neuropathy
- Carpal tunnel syndrome
- Proximal ulnar nerve entrapment
- Distal ulnar nerve entrapment cubital tunnel (Guyon Canal)[4]
- Klumpke paralysis
  - Traction of an abducted arm
  - Lower brachial plexus injury
  - Damage to C8 and T1 vertebrae
  - Loss of intrinsic muscles of the hand, wrist, finger flexors
- Wartenberg sign[4]
- Froment sign; ulnar nerve palsy[5]
- Bishop deformity

MEANS OF CONFIRMATION OR DIAGNOSIS

Imaging

- Diagnostic ultrasound imaging
  - Allows for dynamic imaging during arm movement
  - Enlargement of brachial plexus nerves at entrapment site

Diagnostic Procedures

- Electrodiagnostic testing
  - Loss of evoked sensory potential
  - Electromyographic (EMG): Conduction velocities[6]

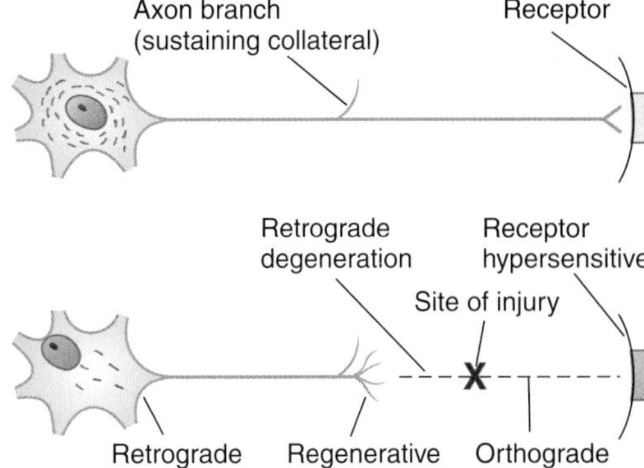

FIGURE 222-3 Summary of changes occurring in a neuron and the structure it innervates when its axon is crushed or cut at the point marked X. (Modified from Ries D. Reproduced with permission, from Ganong WF. *Review of Medical Physiology*. 22nd ed. McGraw-Hill; 2005.)

FINDINGS AND INTERPRETATION

- Muscle weakness of deltoid, biceps, brachialis muscles
- Inability to flex elbow or supinate the arm
- Sensory changes in mixed ulnar, median, and radial nerve distribution

TREATMENT

Medication

- Lyrica

MEDICAL PROCEDURES

- Surgery
  - Nerve transplant
  - Subscapularis release
  - Latissimus dorsi tendon transfer

REFERRALS/ADMITTANCE

- For oral anti-inflammatory, steroidal injections
- For diagnostic tests if warranted and depending on PT's area of practice

IMPAIRMENTS

- Inability to perform overhead activities, such as in swimming, baseball, or tennis
- Inability to perform jobs involving repetitive overhead reaching or lifting

TESTS AND MEASURES

- Neural tension tests
- Disabilities of the Arm, Shoulder and Hand (DASH) score to assess physical function
- Tinel sign at elbow

INTERVENTION

- Myofascial manipulation[5]
- Subscapularis release
- Shoulder sling
- Neural mobilization
- Activity modification, ergonomic intervention

- Stretching of pectoralis
- Postural awareness

FUNCTIONAL GOALS

- Patient will
  - Resume full use of affected upper extremity (arm movement) during ADLs and IADLs.
  - Return to normal ADLs without signs or symptoms.
  - Be able to type for 1 hour at work.

PROGNOSIS

- Patients with mild electrodiagnostic findings, intermittent symptoms, no atrophy may respond well to conservative management.
- Paralysis may resolve on its own; may need therapy or surgery.
- Prognosis depends on duration of symptoms and motor involvement.
- Potential for full motor recovery; may take 6 months to 1 year for nerve regeneration.

PATIENT RESOURCES

- Brachial Plexus Injury. American Society for Surgery of the Hand. http://www.assh.org/Public/HandConditions/Pages/BrachialPlexus.aspx. Accessed August 17, 2014.
- Erbs Palsy. American Academy of Orthopeadic Surgeons. http://orthoinfo.aaos.org/topic.cfm?topic=a00077. Accessed August 17, 2014.
- Erb's Palsy Association of Ireland. http://www.erbspalsy.ie/. Accessed August 17, 2014.
- Erbs Palsy Group. http://www.erbspalsygroup.co.uk. Accessed August 17, 2014.

REFERENCES

1. The American Physical Therapy Association. Pattern 4F: impaired joint mobility, motor function, muscle performance, range of motion, and reflex integrity associated with spinal disorders. *Interactive Guide to Physical Therapist Practice*. 2003. doi: 10.2522/ptguide.3.1_6. http://guidetoptpractice.apta.org/content/1/SEC13.extract. Accessed June 1, 2014.
2. The American Physical Therapy Association. Pattern 5F: impaired peripheral nerve integrity and muscle performance associated with peripheral nerve injury. *Interactive Guide to Physical Therapist Practice*. 2003. doi: 10.2522/ptguide.3.2_6. http://guidetoptpractice.apta.org/content/1/SEC23.extract?sid=4f59a058-1689-4448-bc40-32d9bb9ffaee. Accessed June 1, 2014.
3. Dutton M. Integration of practice patterns 4f and 5f: impaired joint mobility, motor function, muscle performance, and range of motion, or reflex integrity secondary to spinal disorders, peripheral nerve entrapments, compartment syndrome, and myofascial pain dysfunction (Chapter). In: Dutton M, ed. *Orthopaedic Examination, Evaluation, and Intervention*. 2nd ed. http://www.accessphysiotherapy.com/content/55576493. Accessed January 21, 2013.
4. Dutton M. *Dutton's Orthopedic Survival Guide: Managing Common Conditions*. New York, NY: McGraw-Hill; 2011. http://www.accessphysiotherapy.com/resource/685. Accessed January 21, 2013.
5. Dutton M. *Orthopaedic Examination, Evaluation, and Intervention*. New York, NY: McGraw-Hill; 2008. http://www.accessphysiotherapy.com/resource/612. Accessed January 21, 2013.
6. Prentice WE. Biofeedback. In: Prentice WE, Quillen WS, Underwood F, eds. *Therapeutic Modalities in Rehabilitation*. 4th ed. New York, NY: McGraw-Hill; 2011:Chapter 7. http://www.accessphysiotherapy.com/content/8137995#8137995. Accessed January 21, 2013.

ADDITIONAL REFERENCES

- Dutton M. Burn healing and management. In: *McGraw-Hill's NPTE (National Physical Therapy Examination)*. 2nd ed. New York, NY: McGraw-Hill; 2012. http://www.accessphysiotherapy.com/content/5403250. Accessed August 17, 2014.
- ICD9DATA. http://www.icd9data.com. Accessed August 17, 2014.
- ICD10DATA. http://www.icd10data.com. Accessed August 17, 2014.
- Preston D, Shapiro B. Electromyography and neuromuscular disorders. In: *Clinical Electrophysiologic Correlations*. Boston, MA: Butterworth-Heinemann; 1998.

223 FIBROMYALGIA

David Boesler, DO, MS
Eric Shamus, PhD, DPT, PT, CSCS
Marangela Obispo, MSPT, GCS

CONDITION/DISORDER SYNONYMS

- Fibromyalgia syndrome (FM, FMS)
- Chronic fatigue syndrome

ICD-9-CM CODE

- 729.1 Myalgia and myositis unspecified

ICD-10-CM CODE

- M79.7 Fibromyalgia

PREFERRED PRACTICE PATTERNS

- 4E: Impaired Joint Mobility, Motor Function, Muscle Performance, and ROM Associated with Localized Inflammation[1]
- 5F: Impaired Peripheral Nerve Integrity and Muscle Performance Associated with Peripheral Nerve Injury[2]

PATIENT PRESENTATION

A 44-year-old female began complaining of pain in multiple areas including upper back, mid back, low back, and knees for the last 3 months. X-rays and MRI were negative. Laboratory tests including CBC, C-reactive protein, rheumatoid factor, and thyroid profile were also negative. Recently, patient had to stop working as a social worker due to the severity of pain and stiffness, fatigue, difficulty concentrating, and sleep disturbances. She reported difficulty with daily activities mainly due to pain and fatigue. Patient revealed an unremarkable PMH, except for a recent flu virus with no major symptoms. Upon examination, patient was found with multiple tender points with pain radiating to vicinity areas only with palpation. Patient presented with limited ROM in the cervical spine, lumbar spine, and bilateral knee extension. Patient presented with a normal gait pattern, and her 6MWT was abnormal for her age.

KEY FEATURES

Description

- Widespread musculoskeletal pain and fatigue for at least 3 months
- Commonly involves mood disturbances
- Preliminary new criteria from American College of Rheumatology in 2010 include Widespread Pain Index and Symptom Severity Score instead of tender points
- Current criteria: Tender points in at least 11 of 18 areas
    - Arms, chest, buttocks, knees, low back, neck, rib cage, thighs, shoulders

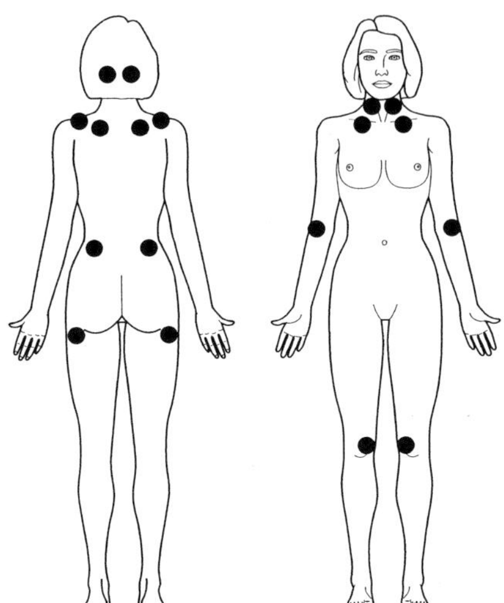

FIGURE 223-1 The tender points of fibromyalgia. There should be tenderness in at least 11 of the 18 points to diagnose fibromyalgia. (From LeBlond RF, DeGowin RL, Brown DD. *DeGowin's Diagnostic Examination*. 9th ed. http://www.accessmedicine.com. Copyright © The McGraw-Hill Companies, Inc. All rights reserved.)

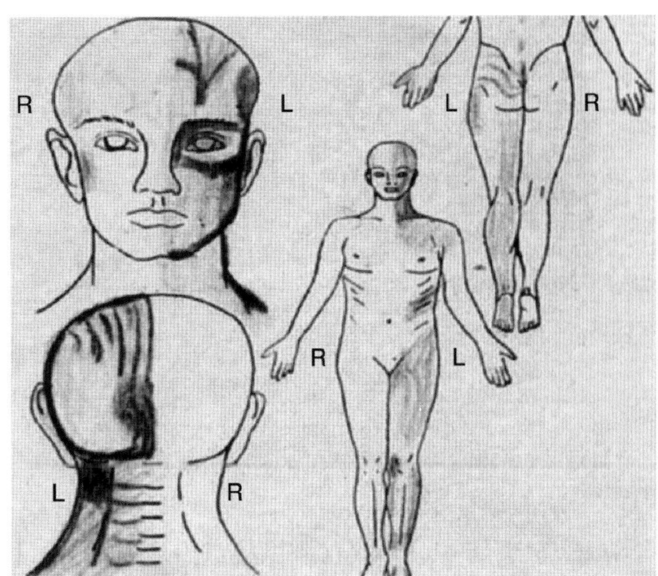

FIGURE 223-2 Typical pain diagram by a patient with fibromyalgia. (From Lalwani AK. *Current Diagnosis & Treatment in Otolaryngology—Head and Neck Surgery*. 3rd ed. http://www.accessmedicine.com. Copyright © The McGraw-Hill Companies, Inc. All rights reserved.)

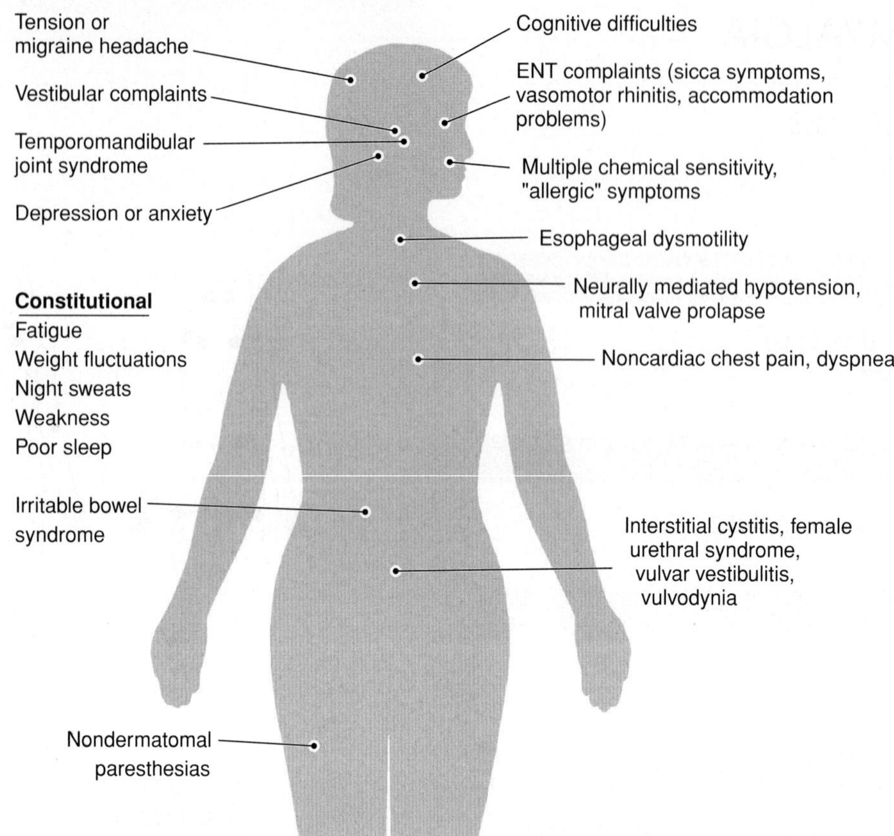

FIGURE 223-3 Symptoms in fibromyalgia in addition to "pain all over" and tender points. ENT, ear, nose, and throat. (From Imboden J, Hellmann DB, Stone JH. *Current Rheumatology Diagnosis & Treatment*. 2nd ed. http://www.accessmedicine.com. Copyright © The McGraw-Hill Companies, Inc. All rights reserved.)

Essentials of Diagnosis

- Diagnosis based primarily on symptoms of widespread pain
- Fatigue, typically begins on rising from sleep
- Morning stiffness, typically lasting all day, does not diminish with activity
- Controversy over diagnosing as psychosomatic disorder
- Tenderness with palpation in at least 11 of 18 areas throughout the body

General Considerations

- Widespread pain throughout the entire body[3]
- Fatigue
- Sleep disturbances
- Memory difficulty
- Morning stiffness

Demographics

- 75% to 90% of cases in females
- Female-to-male ratio 9:1
- Affects 2% to 4% of general population
- Most people develop symptoms between ages 20 and 55 years

CLINICAL FINDINGS

SIGNS AND SYMPTOMS

- Widespread pain and fatigue
- Headaches
- Tenderness in multiple specific anatomic locations
- Mood disturbances, depression, anxiety
- Muscle pain
- Cognitive dysfunction
- Irritable bowel
- Morning stiffness
- Sleep disturbances with constant interruptions of sleep
- Muscle spasm
- Nerve pain
- Sympathetic hyperactivity
- Associated symptoms may include paresthesias, burning, tingling

Functional Implications

- Pain and stiffness may limit daily activities
- Difficulty concentrating and performing tasks

Possible Contributing Causes

- Cold or humid weather
- Nonrestorative sleep
- Stress
- Anxiety
- Physical or mental fatigue/trauma
- Myofascial pain
- Rheumatoid arthritis

Differential Diagnosis

- Chronic fatigue syndrome
- Hypothyroidism
- Lyme disease
- Systemic lupus erythematosus
- Rheumatoid arthritis

Name: ______________________ Date: / /

Directions: For questions 1 through 11, please circle the number that best describes how you did overall for the *past week*. If you don't normally do something that is asked, cross the question out.

Were you able to:	Always	Most	Occasionally	Never
Do shopping?	*0*	*1*	*2*	*3*
Do laundry with a washer and dryer?	*0*	*1*	*2*	*3*
Prepare meals?	*0*	*1*	*2*	*3*
Wash dishes/cooking utensils by hand?	*0*	*1*	*2*	*3*
Vacuum a rug?	*0*	*1*	*2*	*3*
Make beds?	*0*	*1*	*2*	*3*
Walk several blocks?	*0*	*1*	*2*	*3*
Visit friends or relatives?	*0*	*1*	*2*	*3*
Do yard work?	*0*	*1*	*2*	*3*
Drive a car?	*0*	*1*	*2*	*3*
Climb stairs?	*0*	*1*	*2*	*3*

12. Of the 7 days in the past week, how many days did you feel good?

0 1 2 3 4 5 6 7

13. How many days last week did you miss work, including housework, because of fibromyalgia?

0 1 2 3 4 5 6 7

Directions: For the remaining items, mark the point on the line that best indicates how you felt overall for the past week.

14. When you worked, how much did pain or other symptoms of your fibromyalgia interfere with your ability to do your work, including housework?

No problem with work •__|__|__|__|__|__|__|__|__|__|__• Great difficulty with work

15. How bad has your pain been?

No pain •__|__|__|__|__|__|__|__|__|__|__• Very severe pain

16. How tired have you been?

No tiredness •__|__|__|__|__|__|__|__|__|__|__• Very tired

17. How have you felt when you get up in the morning?

Awoke well rested •__|__|__|__|__|__|__|__|__|__|__• Awoke very tired

18. How bad has your stiffness been?

No stiffness •__!__!__!__!__!__!__!__!__!__!__• Very stiff

19. How nervous or anxious have you felt?

Not anxious •__!__!__!__!__!__!__!__!__!__!__• Very anxious

20. How depressed or blue have you felt?

Not depressed •__!__!__!__!__!__!__!__!__!__!__• Very depressed

FIGURE 223-4 Fibromyalgia Impact Questionnaire (FIQ). (Halter JB, Ouslander JG, Tinetti M, Studenski S, High K, Asthana S. *Hazzard's Geriatric Medicine and Gerontology*. 6th ed. http://www.accessmedicine.com. Copyright © The McGraw-Hill Companies, Inc. All rights reserved.)

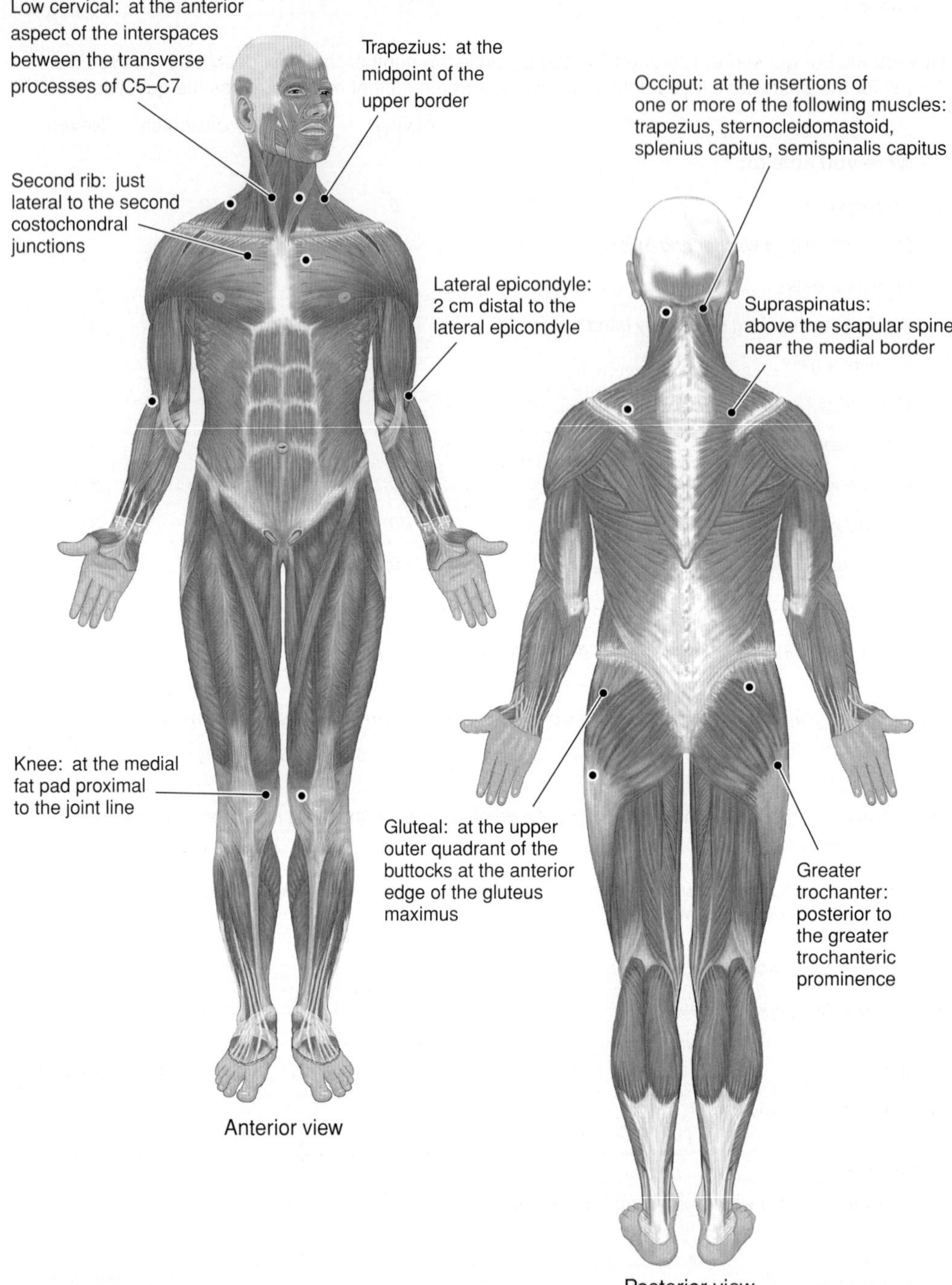

FIGURE 223-5 Eighteen tender points used in the American College of Rheumatology classification criteria for fibromyalgia. (From Imboden J, Hellmann DB, Stone JH. *Current Rheumatology Diagnosis & Treatment*. 2nd ed. http://www.accessmedicine.com. Copyright © The McGraw-Hill Companies, Inc. All rights reserved.)

- Polymyalgia rheumatica
- Sleep disorders
- Depression
- Chronic neck and back pain

MEANS OF CONFIRMATION OR DIAGNOSIS

Laboratory Tests

- CBC
- ESR
- C-reactive protein
- Rheumatoid factor
- Thyroid profile

Imaging

- X-ray[4]
- MRI[5]

Diagnostic Procedures

- Widespread Pain Index (WPI)
- Symptom Severity Score

FINDINGS AND INTERPRETATION

- X-ray: Negative[4]
- MRI: Negative[5]
- Negative laboratory tests, such as CBC, ESR, C-reactive protein, rheumatoid factor, thyroid profile

TREATMENT

Medication

- Analgesics (Tylenol, Ultram)
- Low-dose anti-depressants (tricyclics, SSRI's, SNRI's)
- Lyrica, Cymbalta, Savella[3]

REFERRALS/ADMITTANCE

- To other therapist for gentle osteopathic manipulative treatment
- To dietician for nutritional counseling
- To pain clinic for pain management
- To psychologist for cognitive-behavioral therapy, psychological support
  - Counseling
  - Support groups
  - Biofeedback
  - Relaxation techniques

IMPAIRMENTS

- Limited walking and movement secondary to pain and morning stiffness, can last throughout the day
- Difficulty standing or sitting in one position for extended period of time
- Limited aerobic capacity

TESTS AND MEASURES

- Vascular examination (particularly blood flow to feet)
- Heart rate
- Sensory testing
- Reflex testing
- Manual muscle test
- Active and passive ROM testing, muscle length testing
- Functional assessment (assist, device, environment)
  - Bed mobility
  - Transitions
  - Sitting balance
  - Standing balance
  - Transfers
  - Gait
  - Stairs
- Pain assessment
- Postural assessment
- Cardiovascular endurance

INTERVENTION

- Patient education
- Stress relief
- Therapy
  - Acupuncture
  - Yoga
  - Tai chi
  - Aerobic exercise[6]
  - Heated aquatic therapy
  - Gentle stretching

FUNCTIONAL GOALS

- Patient will be able to
  - Perform 30 minutes of aerobic activity.
  - Perform an 8-hour/day light-duty job.
  - Manage stress so as to participate in community activities.

PROGNOSIS

- Chronic, but not progressive.
- Usually little change in long-term symptoms, but patients can learn to function and manage pain more effectively with treatment.

PATIENT RESOURCES

- American Fibromyalgia Syndrome Association. http://www.afsafund.org. Accessed April 21, 2013.
- National Fribromyalgia Association. http://www.fmaware.org. Accessed April 21, 2013.

REFERENCES

1. The American Physical Therapy Association. Pattern 4E: impaired joint mobility, motor function, muscle performance, and range of motion associated with localized inflammation. *Interactive Guide to Physical Therapist Practice*. 2003. doi: 10.2522/ptguide.978-1-931369-64-0. Accessed April 21, 2013.
2. The American Physical Therapy Association. Pattern 5F: impaired peripheral nerve integrity and muscle performance associated with peripheral nerve injury. *Interactive Guide to Physical Therapist Practice*. 2003. doi: 10.2522/ptguide.3.2_6. Accessed April 21, 2013.
3. Soep JB. Rheumatic diseases. In: Hay WW, Levin MJ, Sondheimer JM, Deterding RR, eds. *CURRENT Diagnosis & Treatment: Pediatrics*. New York, NY: McGraw-Hill; 2011:Chapter 27. http://www.accessphysiotherapy.com/abstract/6586584#6586588. Accessed April 21, 2013.
4. Malone TR, Hazle C, Grey ML. The ankle and foot. In: *Imaging in Rehabilitation*. New York, NY: McGraw-Hill; 2008:Chapter 10. http://www.accessphysiotherapy.com/abstract/5940147. Accessed April 21, 2013.
5. Hamilton N, Weimar W, Luttgens K. The musculoskeletal system: The musculature. In: *Kinesiology: Scientific Basis of Human Motion*. New York, NY: McGraw-Hill 2008:Chapter 3. http://www.accessphysiotherapy.com/abstract/6150358#6150373. Accessed April 21, 2013.
6. Dutton M. *Orthopaedic Examination, Evaluation, and Intervention*. New York, NY: McGraw-Hill; 2004. http://www.accessphysiotherapy.com/abstract/5546970#5546972. Accessed April 21, 2013.

ADDITIONAL REFERENCES

- Buskila D. Pediatric fibromyalgia. *Rheum Dis Clin North Am*. 2009;35(2):253–261.
- Dutton M. Complex disorders. In: Dutton M, ed. *McGraw-Hill's NPTE (National Physical Therapy Examination)*. 2nd ed. New York, NY: McGraw-Hill; 2012. http://www.accessphysiotherapy.com/content/5402428. Accessed April 31, 2013.
- Hay WW, Levin MJ, Sondheimer JM, Deterding RR. Noninflammatory pain syndromes. In: Hay WW, Levin MJ, Sondheimer JM, Deterding RR, eds. *CURRENT Diagnosis & Treatment: Pediatrics*. 20th ed. New York, NY: McGraw-Hill; 2011. http://www.accessphysiotherapy.com/content/6586584. Accessed April 30, 2013.
- ICD9DATA. http://www.icd9data.com. Accessed April 21, 2013.
- ICD10DATA. http://www.icd10data.com. Accessed April 21, 2013.

224 MEDIAN NERVE COMPRESSION

Matthew L. Daugherty, DPT, OTR/L, MOT, MTC, OCS, FAAOMPT
Eric Shamus, PhD, DPT, PT, CSCS

CONDITION/DISORDER SYNONYMS

- Ape-hand deformity
- Median nerve palsy

ICD-9-CM CODES

- 354.1 Other lesion of median nerve
- 955.1 Injury to median nerve

ICD-10-CM CODES

- G56.10 Other lesions of median nerve, unspecified upper limb
- S44.10XA Injury of median nerve at upper arm level, unspecified arm, initial encounter
- S54.10XA Injury of median nerve at forearm level, unspecified arm, initial encounter
- S64.10XA Injury of median nerve at wrist and hand level of unspecified arm, initial encounter

PREFERRED PRACTICE PATTERNS

- 4E: Impaired Joint Mobility, Motor Function, Muscle Performance, and Range of Motion Associated with Localized Inflammation[1]
- 5F: Impaired Peripheral Nerve Integrity and Muscle Performance Associated with Peripheral Nerve Injury[2]

PATIENT PRESENTATION

Patient is a 44-year-old male who works in a new home construction. He spends the majority of his day using power tools, such as a drill and nail gun, in various positions of the elbow and forearm. After a long period of part time work he has returned to work 60+ hours/week and spent the interim lifting weights. Over the past 2 weeks, he has begun to notice a burning/achy pain at his volar/medial forearm. This pain is exacerbated while at work and seems to get worse throughout the day, especially with usage of hand power tools. He also reports a painful tingling that radiates all the way to his thumb and first two fingers when he is really symptomatic. Functionally, he reports that he feels as if his hand fatigues quickly at work.

Clinically, he is a mesomorphic male with hyperalgesia reported across median nerve distribution of hand (thenar eminence, volar surface and tips of digits I, II, and radial side of III. No weakness of pronator teres but overall grip strength is decreased 20 lb on the affected side. Forearm pain is aggravated by sustained forearm pronation, especially with elbow extension. Palpable tenderness deep in the pronator teres with positive pronator compression test and median nerve neurodynamic testing.

KEY FEATURES

Description

- Entrapment neuropathy of the median nerve other than within the carpal tunnel of the wrist[3,4]
- Common entrapment sites include; ligament of Struthers, bicipital aponeurosis, and pronator teres (all generically called pronator syndrome—PN), fibrous arch of flexor digitorum superficialis (anterior interosseous syndrome—AINS)
- Signs and symptoms typical of neuropathy, includes:
  - Pain
  - Paresthesias
  - Loss of sensation
  - Later loss of muscle function
- Symptoms are seen in the distribution of the median nerve in the hand[3], distal upper arm, and volar forearm

Essentials of Diagnosis

- Pain, paresthesias, and sensory loss perceived on radial side of the palm and the palmar side of thumb, index, middle, and radial side of the ring fingers (no sensory loss if AINS)
- Pain may radiate up to the elbow, shoulder, neck
- In advanced cases, motor dysfunction in thenar muscles may occur, characterized by weakness, atrophy, loss of coordination

General Considerations

- In entrapment neuropathy, nerve becomes compressed, causing ischemic damage to the nerve
- Often associated with repetitive motions or sustained position of the elbow
- Unrelieved compression of the nerve results in neurapraxia with segmental demyelination;[6] further ischemic damage results in axonotmesis and wallerian degeneration[5,6]

Demographics

- Four times more common in women (PS)[7]
- AINS is rare, accounting for less than 1% of upper-extremity neuropathies[7]
- Most common among people in their fifth decade of life[7]

CLINICAL FINDINGS

SIGNS AND SYMPTOMS

- Ape-hand deformity
- First symptom is usually pain or paresthesias;[3] most commonly with gradual onset
- Pain at proximal volar forearm exacerbated by repetitive forearm rotation or elbow motion
- Pain complaints include numbness (most common), tingling, burning
- Pain is experienced in distribution of the median nerve in the hand, particularly the palm of hand over the thenar eminence,

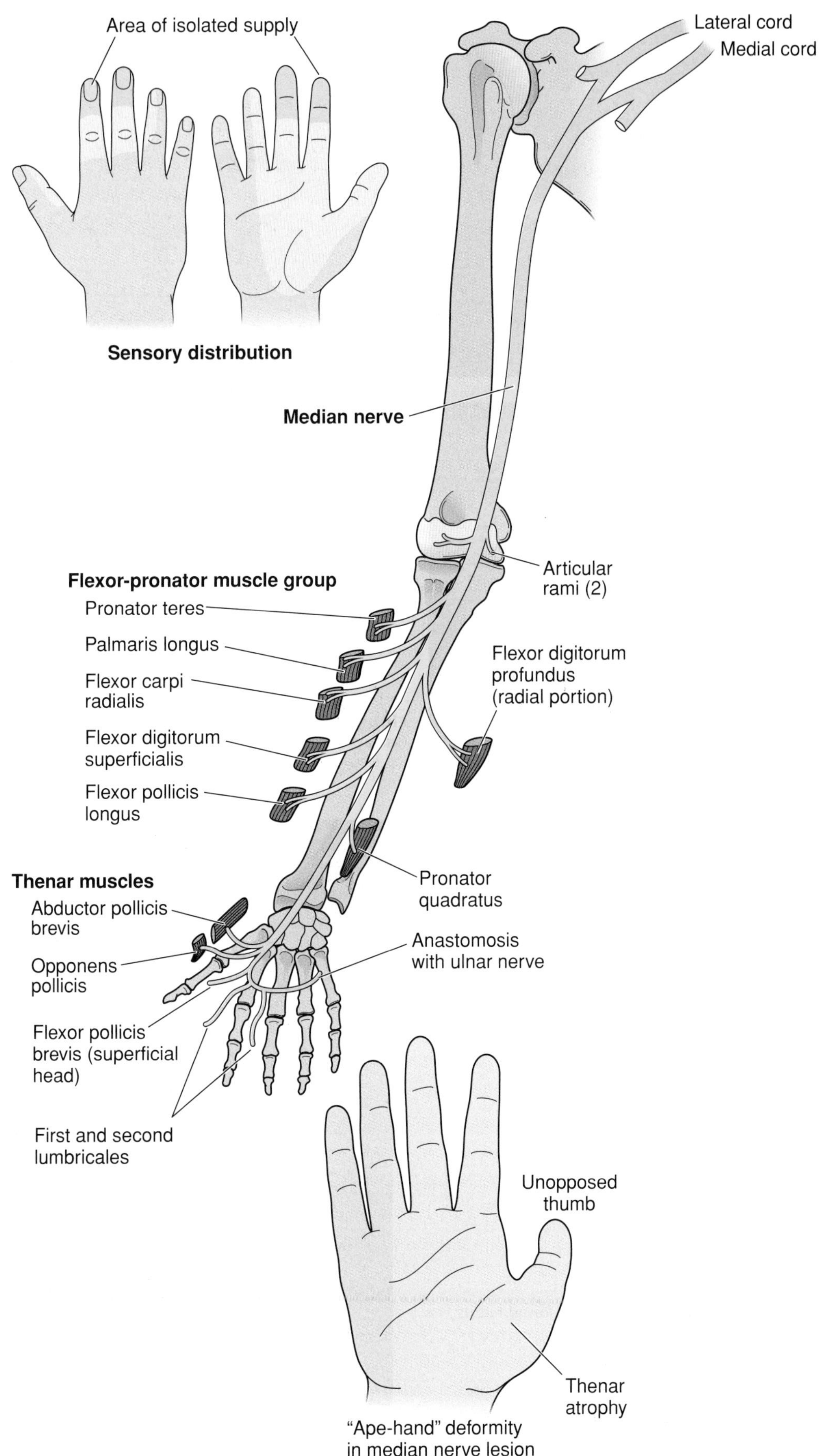

FIGURE 224-1 The median nerve (C6–8, T1). (Reproduced with permission from, Waxman SG: *Clinical Neuroanatomy*. 26th ed. McGraw-Hill; 2010.)

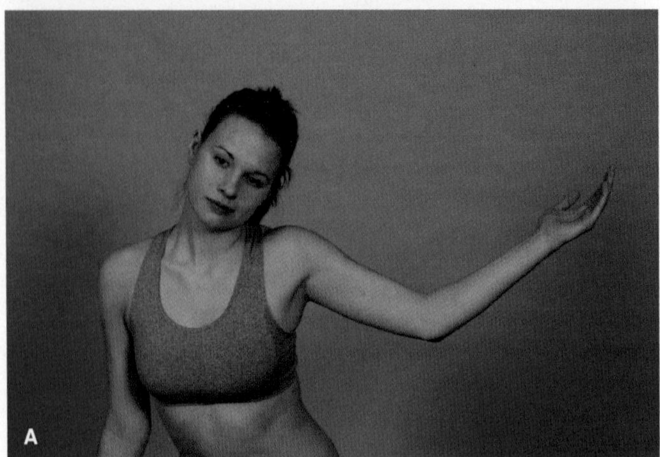

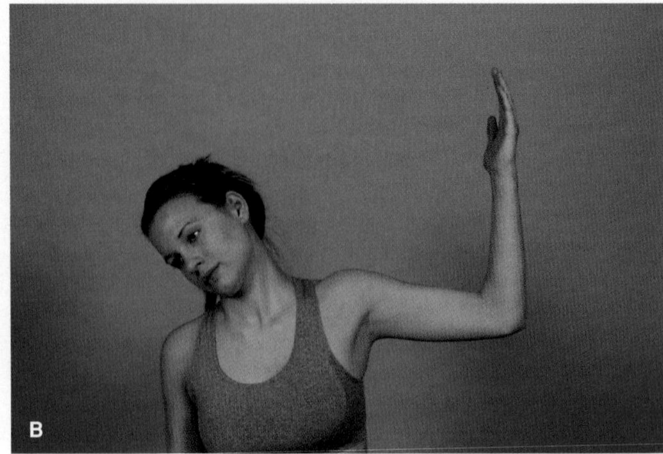

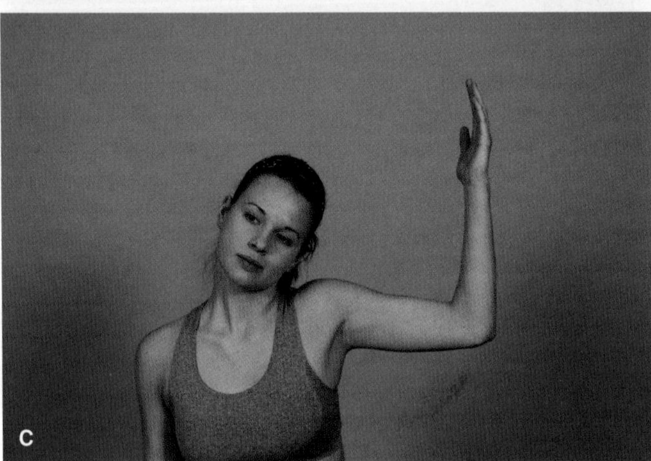

FIGURE 224-2 Upper-extremity nerve mobilization. (From Dutton D. *Dutton's Orthopaedic Examination, Evaluation, and Intervention*. 3rd ed. www.accessphysiotherapy.com. Copyright © The McGraw-Hill Companies, Inc. All rights reserved.)

though may radiate up to elbow, shoulder, or neck
- Tenderness to percussion or deep pressure over the pronator teres, proximal FDS, or distal volar arm above the elbow
- Sensory loss may follow early symptom of pain
- Motor involvement (weakness, loss of coordination, atrophy) may follow in more advanced cases

Functional Implications

- Pain with wrist movements
- Difficulty with grasping and manipulation activities
- Dropping items from the hand
- Impaired sensation
- Loss of strength in advanced cases

Possible Contributing Causes

- Most often idiopathic
- Genetic structural factors
- Tumors
- Displaced fracture or fracture callus, especially of distal radius
- Elbow dislocation
- Structural abnormalities of humerus
- Occupations that require repetitive motion, repetitive stress, sustained positions of elbow and forearm
    - This point is debated in the literature: Association is seen, but a causal relationship is not clear; genetic structural causes appear more likely

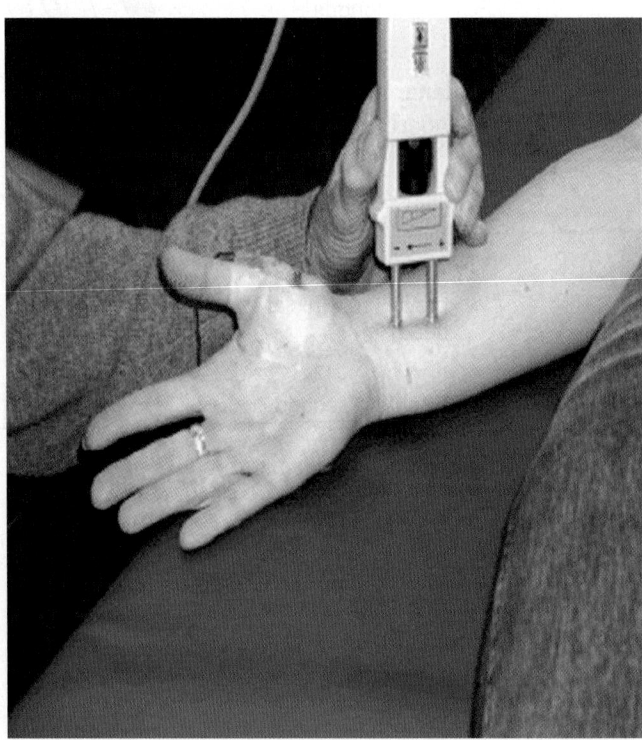

FIGURE 224-3 Setup for a median nerve DML at a distance of 8 cm. (From Prentice WE, Quillen WS, Underwood F. *Therapeutic Modalities in Rehabilitation*. 4th ed. http://www.accessmedicine.com. Copyright © The McGraw-Hill Companies, Inc. All rights reserved.)

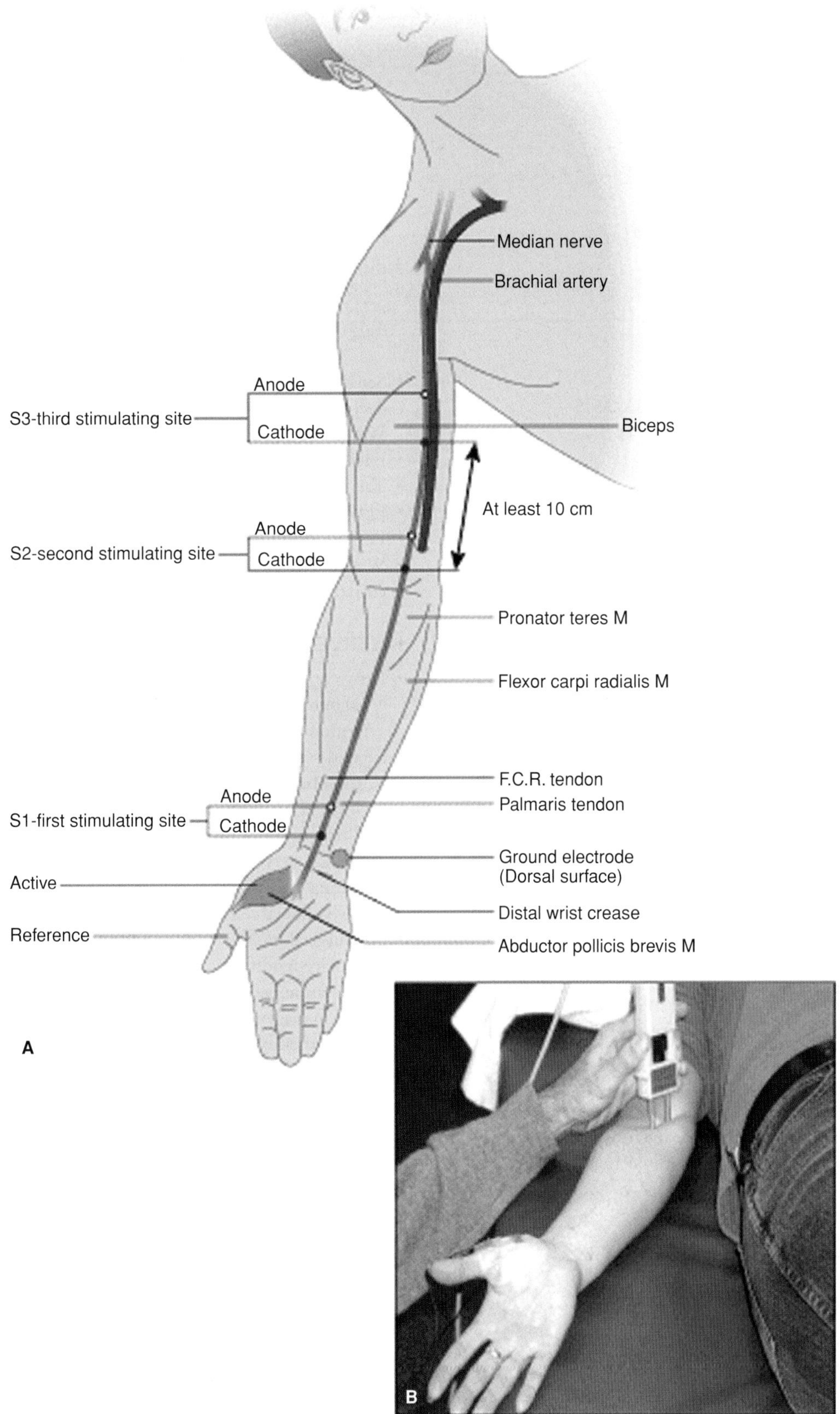

FIGURE 224-4 Setup for a median nerve (motor) with stimulation at the cubital fossa. (**A**) Photograph of the procedure. (**B**) Line illustration with stimulation sites identified. (From Nestor DE, Nelson RM. *Performing Motor and Sensory Neuronal Conduction Studies in Adult Humans—A NIOSH Technical Manual.* DHHS (NIOSH) publication no. 90-113. Morgantown, WV: Division of Safety Research, National Institute for Occupational Safety and Health; 1990.)

- Direct trauma to forearm, elbow or arm
- Impaired circulation to peripheral nerves, as seen in diabetes, predisposes individuals to nerve compression symptoms

▸ Differential Diagnosis

- Cervical radiculopathy
- Thoracic outlet syndrome
- Carpal tunnel syndrome
- Traumatic nerve lesion
- Rheumatoid or other arthritis
- Acromegaly
- Hypothyroidism
- Scleroderma

MEANS OF CONFIRMATION OR DIAGNOSIS

▸ Imaging

- MRI[4]
- Diagnostic ultrasound (ultrasonography)[4]
  - Enlargement of median nerve at entrapment sites

▸ Diagnostic Procedure

- Nerve conduction velocity testing of median nerve across the carpal tunnel is considered gold standard for diagnosis[5,8]

FINDINGS AND INTERPRETATION

- Muscle weakness of[2]
  - Pronator teres
  - Palmaris longus
  - Flexor digitorum superficialis
  - Flexor pollicis longus
  - Flexor digitorum profundus
  - Flexor carpi radialis (FCR)
- Sensory changes in median nerve distribution of the hand

TREATMENT

▸ Medication

- NSAIDs[4]
- Corticosterioid injection

REFERRALS/ADMITTANCE

- To radiologist for imaging; x-ray for fracture or displacement
- To orthopedist for surgical consult or injection

IMPAIRMENTS

- Hand weakness with grasping, squeezing, pinching

TESTS AND MEASURES

- Upper limb tension test
- Cervical spine compression test
- Pain provocation test
- Shoulder pain and disability index
- Resisted motion testing at elbow (forearm pronation with elbow extension, elbow flexion, proximal interphalangeal flexion at the middle finger)[7]
- Pronator compression test[7]
- Tinel sign at proximal forearm

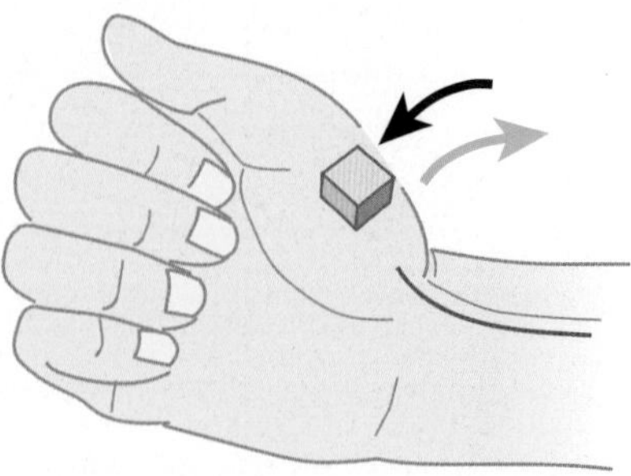

FIGURE 224-5 Flexor carpi radialis (C6, 7; median nerve). The wrist is flexed to the radial side against resistance. (From Waxman SG. *Clinical Neuroanatomy*. 26th ed. http://www.accessmedicine.com. Copyright © The McGraw-Hill Companies, Inc. All rights reserved.)

- Sensory loss may include diminished two-point discrimination, decreased vibration sense, increased threshold in Semmes-Weinstein monofilament test[5]
- Flick sign
- Thenar muscle strength test (lateral pinch dynamometry)
- FDP (index finger) and FPL manual muscle testing if AINS
- Positive pinch grip test (AINS)
- Weakness of pronator teres during manual muscle testing if entrapment at ligament of Struthers or bicipital aponeurosis

INTERVENTION

- Early conservative intervention
  - Ergonomic analysis and activity modification to reduce repetitive motion or positioning stress such as avoiding pronation[9]
- Second-stage conservative intervention
  - Immobilization of elbow with posterior gutter splint; holding elbow at 90 degrees and forearm neutral.[7]
  - Ultrasound[10,11]
  - Median nerve gliding[4]
  - Manual therapy[11–13]
    - Myofascial release[12]
- Postsurgical intervention
  - Activity modification and protected ROM
  - Median nerve gliding
  - Scar management and sensory desensitization
  - Strengthening

FUNCTIONAL GOALS

- Patient will have
  - Improved ability to perform physical tasks, self-care, home management, leisure and occupational activities.

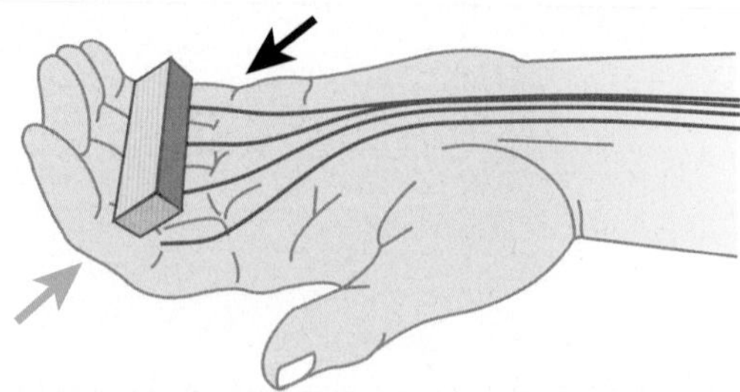

FIGURE 224-6 Flexor digitorum superficialis (C7, 8; T1; median nerve). The fingers are flexed at the first interphalangeal joint against resistance; proximal phalanges remain fixed. (From Waxman SG. *Clinical Neuroanatomy*. 26th ed. http://www.accessmedicine.com. Copyright © The McGraw-Hill Companies, Inc. All rights reserved.)

  - Increased tolerance of positions and activities using elbow, forearm, and wrist.
  - Reduced ergonomic risk.

PROGNOSIS

- Prognosis dependent on duration of symptoms and motor involvement.
- Patients with mild electrodiagnostic findings, intermittent symptoms, and no atrophy may respond well to conservative management.
- Surgical intervention indicated for patients with symptoms lasting more than 1 year, or those for whom conservative treatment over 3 months has failed.

PATIENT RESOURCE

- Wheeless C. Pronator teres compression syndrome - median nerve compression. Manuscript submitted for publication, Department of Orthpaedics, Duke University, Durham, North Carolina. 1996. Retrieved from http://www.wheelessonline.com/ortho/pronator_teres_compression_syndrome. Accessed July 6, 2013.

REFERENCES

1. The American Physical Therapy Association. Pattern 4E: Impaired joint mobility, motor function, muscle performance, and range of motion associated with localized inflammation. *Interactive Guide to Physical Therapist Practice*. 2003. doi: 10.2522/ptguide.3.1_5. Accessed July 6, 2013.
2. The American Physical Therapy Association. Pattern 5F: impaired peripheral nerve integrity and muscle performance associated with peripheral nerve injury. *Interactive Guide to Physical Therapist Practice*. 2003. doi: 10.2522/ptguide.3.2_6. Accessed July 6, 2013.
3. Dutton M. *Orthopaedic Examination, Evaluation, and Intervention*. New York, NY: McGraw-Hill; 2008. http://www.accessphysiotherapy.com/resource/612. Accessed July 6, 2013.
4. American Physical Therapy Association. *Anatomy and Physiology Revealed. McGraw-Hill.* 2007. http://anatomy.mcgraw-hill.com/apt.html?login=1319880810339&system=Muscular§ion=Dissection&topic=Wrist%20and%20hand&topicAbbr=Wha&view=Anterior&viewAbbr=Ant&catAbbr=Oth&grpAbbr=Ske&structure=Carpal%20tunnel. Accessed July 6, 2013.
5. Goodman CC, Fuller KS. *Pathology: Implications for the Physical Therapist*. 3rd ed. St. Louis: Saunders/Elsevier; 2009.
6. Waxman SG. *Clinical Neuroanatomy*. New York, NY: McGraw-Hill; 2010. http://www.accessphysiotherapy.com/resource/22. Accessed July 6, 2013.
7. Skirven TM, Osterman AL, Fedorczyk JM, et al. *Rehabilitation Of The Hand and Upper Extremity*. 6th ed. St. Louis, MO: Mosby Inc; 2011.
8. Halle J, Greathouse D. Principles of electrophysiologic evaluation and testing. In: Prentice WE, Quillen WS, Underwood F, eds. *Therapeutic Modalities in Rehabilitation*. 4th ed. New York, NY: McGraw-Hill; 2011:Chapter 8. http://www.accessphysiotherapy.com/abstract/8137649#8137649. Accessed July 6, 2013.
9. AcSkirven TM, Osterman AL, Fedorczyk JM, et al. *Rehabilitation Of The Hand and Upper Extremity*. 6th ed. St. Louis, MO: Mosby Inc; 2011.
10. Dutton M. *Dutton's Orthopedic Survival Guide: Managing Common Conditions*. New York, NY: McGraw-Hill; 2011. http://www.accessphysiotherapy.com/resource/685. Accessed July 6, 2013.
11. Houghton PE. The role of therapeutic modalities in wound healing. In: Prentice WE, Quillen WS, Underwood F, eds. *Therapeutic Modalities in Rehabilitation*. 4th ed. New York, NY: McGraw-Hill; 2011:Chapter 3. http://www.accessphysiotherapy.com/abstract/8135453#8135453. Accessed July 6, 2013.
12. Muller M, Tsui D, Schnurr R, Biddulph-Deisroth L, Hard J, MacDermid J. Effectiveness of hand therapy interventions in primary management of carpal tunnel syndrome: a systematic review. *J Hand Ther*. 2004;17(2):210–228.
13. Prentice WE. Therapeutic massage. In: Prentice WE, Quillen WS, Underwood F, eds. *Therapeutic Modalities in Rehabilitation*. 4th ed. New York: McGraw-Hill; 2011:Chapter 16. http://www.accessphysiotherapy.com/abstract/8140838#8140971. Accessed July 6, 2013.

ADDITIONAL REFERENCES

- ICD9DATA. http://www.icd9data.com. Accessed July 6, 2013.
- ICD10DATA. http://www.icd10data.com. Accessed July 6, 2013.
- Lozano-Calderón S, Anthony S, Ring D. The quality and strength of evidence for etiology: example of carpal tunnel syndrome. *J Hand Surg Am*. 2008;33(4):525–538.
- NIH National Institutes of Health. Carpal tunnel syndrome. Medline Plus. http://www.nlm.nih.gov/medlineplus/ency/article/000433.htm. Online May 25, 2010. Accessed July 6, 2013.

225 MORTON NEUROMA

Christina L. Pettie, MHA, PT
Eric Shamus, PhD, DPT, PT, CSCS

CONDITION/DISORDER SYNONYMS

- Intermetatarsal disorder
- Morton metatarsalgia
- Plantar nerve lesion

ICD-9-CM-CODE

- 355.6 Lesion of plantar nerve

ICD-10-CM CODES

- G57.6 Lesion of plantar nerve
- G57.60 Lesion of plantar nerve, unspecified lower limb

PREFERRED PRACTICE PATTERN

- 5F: Impaired Peripheral Nerve Integrity and Muscle Performance Associated with Peripheral Nerve Injury

PATIENT PRESENTATION

A 42-year-old female presents with a severe pain in the ball of her right foot that radiates into her second and third toes. She states the pain started about 1 week ago. She describes the pain as being sharp and burning in nature. She does not recall a specific injury but does state that she started barefoot running 6 weeks ago and eliminated her heel strike. She also goes to dance classes for the past 4 weeks. She feels better with a hard soled shoe on but cannot wear her dress shoes, especially heels. Upon palpation there is a thickening of the tissue between toes 2 and 3 right. Tenderness is present in the same region. There is hypomobility of the MTP toes 2 and 3 right and a positive pinch test. The patient's radiograph, which was ordered by the referring physician, is negative for any fractures.

KEY FEATURES

Description

- Painful condition that affects the ball of the foot
- Growth of scar tissue from chronic irritation of compression
- Most common area is between the third and fourth toes, but also can be in between the second and third toes
- Involves a thickening of the tissues (neuroma) around one of the intermetatarsal plantar nerves
- Branches from the medial and lateral plantar nerves
- May alter mechanics during the push-off phase of gait

Essentials of Diagnosis

- Can be an independent diagnosis and not associated with a disease process

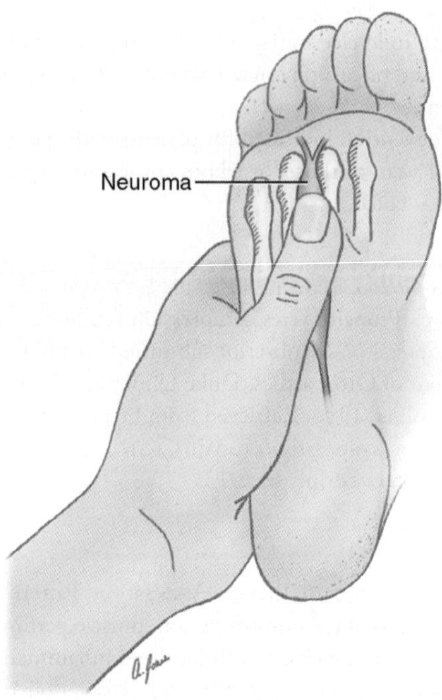

FIGURE 225-1 Morton neuroma. (From Simon RR, Sherman SC. *Emergency Orthopedics*. 6th ed. http://www.accessmedicine.com. Copyright © The McGraw-Hill Companies, Inc. All rights reserved.)

- Characterized by numbness, burning, and pain
- Sometimes relieved by removing shoes
- No visible deformity
- Higher risk for individuals with bunions and flat feet

General Considerations

- Feeling like you are stepping on something like a pebble
- A burning pain in the ball of the foot that radiates to the toes
- Tingling or numbness in the toes
- Titled a neuroma, but is not a tumor formation as "oma"

Demographics

- Ladies wearing high heels
- Rock climbers with repetitive forefoot pressure

CLINICAL FINDINGS

SIGNS AND SYMPTOMS

- Burning pain in the ball of the foot
- Numbness and tingling in the toes, especially between the third and fourth toes
- Difficulty wearing/finding shoes, especially pointed ones
- Limited motion of the MTP joint

Functional Implications

- Pain with standing
- Pain with ambulation at the toe

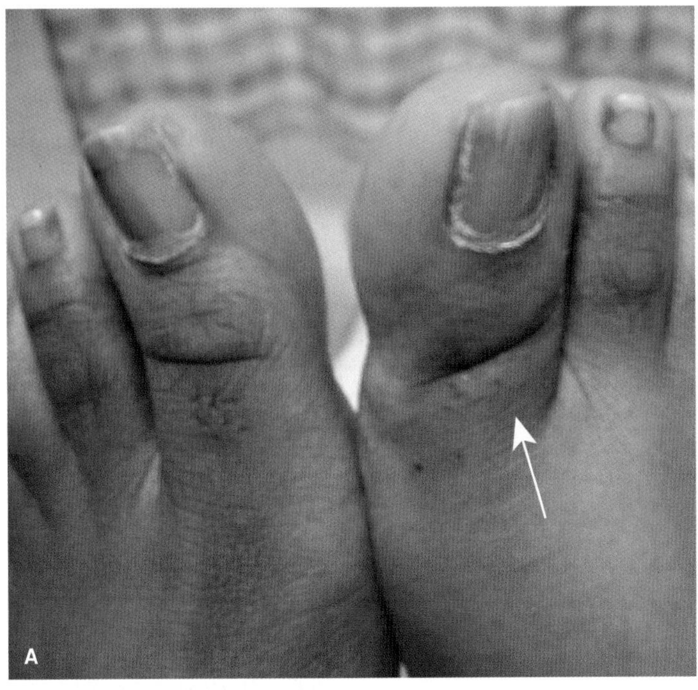

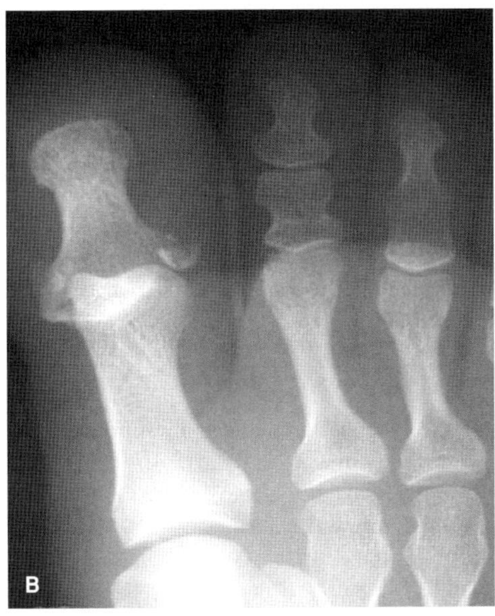

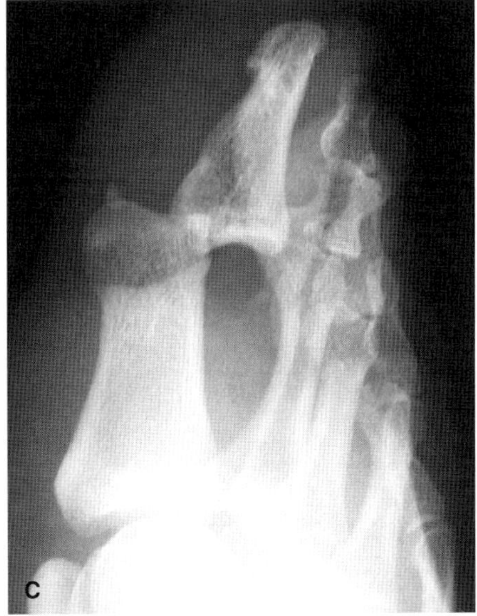

FIGURE 225-2 Dorsal dislocation of the right great toe interphalangeal joint. (**A**) Patient photograph (*arrow*). (**B**) AP radiograph. (**C**) Oblique radiograph. (From Simon RR, Sherman SC. *Emergency Orthopedics*. 6th ed. http://www.accessmedicine.com. Copyright © The McGraw-Hill Companies, Inc. All rights reserved.)

- Inability to wear regular shoes
- Need to wear larger shoes with a larger toe box
- Alteration of gait pattern and mechanical issues of the forefoot

Possible Contributing Causes

- Poor footwear: Improper fit
  - Toe comes to a point (boots)
  - Narrow forefoot (high heels)
- Certain sports
  - Repetitive trauma from high-impact activities, such as jogging or running
  - Those requiring tight shoes, such as snow skiing or rock climbing
- Foot deformities: Bunions, hammer toes, flat feet, excessive flexibility

Differential Diagnoses

- Bursitis
- Capsulitis
- Degenerative arthritis
- Freiburg disease: Osteochondritis of the metatarsal head
- Lumbar radiculopathy
- Metatarsal stress fracture
- Metatarsalgia
- Stress fracture
- Synovitis
- Tendinitis

MEANS OF CONFIRMATION OR DIAGNOSIS

Imaging

- X-ray
- Diagnostic ultrasound
- MRI

Diagnostic Procedures

- Mulder's sign (pinch test)[1]: Lateral squeezing of the forefoot with one hand and the opposite hand pushing up on the nerve

FINDINGS AND INTERPRETATION

- Rule out fracture
- Reveal soft tissue abnormalities

TREATMENT

Medication

- Anti-inflammatories
- Corticosteroid injection

MEDICAL PROCEDURES

- Cryogenic neuroablation
- Decompression surgery
- Removal of the nerve

REFERRALS/ADMITTANCE

- To hospital for imaging: X-ray
- To podiatrist or orthopedic surgeon, for surgical consult

IMPAIRMENTS

- Antalgic gait secondary to pain at the toe with push-off
- Hypomobility of the MTP joint toe
- Inability to ambulate distances of 1 mile, secondary to pain

TESTS AND MEASURES

- Palpation between the metatarsals
- Gait analysis
- Morton test
- Mulder's Sign[1]: A positive test is a click or snap at the nerve with severe pain

INTERVENTION

- Rest with weight off feet reduces inflammation
- Metatarsal pad to increase space between the metatarsal (MT) heads: Taping, padding, or orthotics
- Address swelling
  - Ice
- Address pain
  - Ice
  - Massage
  - Joint mobilization
  - Electric stimulation
  - Iontophoresis
  - Infrared light (IR)
  - Acupuncture
- Address weakness, joint instability
  - Strengthening
    - Toe curls and extension, flexor/extensor intrinsics
    - Calf raises to point
    - Active walking
    - Standing arch raises
- Address lack of flexibility
  - Stretching
    - Toe intrinsic flexor stretching
    - Gastrocnemius/Soleus
    - Plantar fascia, individuals with a high arch
    - Fluidotherapy
- Address joint mobilization
  - MTP dorsal/plantar and medial/lateral glides and rotation
  - Posterior talus glides
  - Subtalar joint (STJ) inversion/eversion
  - Navicular/Cuboid/Cuneiforms
- Address soft tissue mobilization
  - Lumbricale/Dorsal interossei
  - Plantar fascia
  - Gastrocnemius/Soleus
- Patient education in footwear
  - Increased toe box space
  - Avoid high heels or tight shoes
  - Metatarsal bar or dome for the shoes

FUNCTIONAL GOALS

- Patient will be able to
  - Recognize and maintain a subtalar neutral position for >2 minutes.
  - Ambulate pain free for >45 minutes.
  - Achieve 15 degrees of talocrural dorsiflexion during stance phase of gait.
  - Achieve pain-free toe extension during push-off phase of gait.
  - Unilaterally stand in subtalar neutral for 1 minute with eyes open.

PROGNOSIS

- Good. Focus on reducing pressure to the nerve and increasing mobility of the toes.
- Surgery maybe indicated if the nerve pain becomes severe and shoes cannot be worn.

PATIENT RESOURCE

- Morton's Neuroma. American Academy of Orthopeadic Surgeons. http://orthoinfo.aaos.org/topic.cfm?topic=A00158. Accessed July 5, 2013.

REFERENCE

1. Mulder JD. The causative mechanism in Morton's metatarsalgia. *J Bone Joint Surg Br.* 1951;33-B(1):94–95.

ADDITIONAL REFERENCES

- APTA Guide to Physical Therapist Practice. http://guidetoptpractice.apta.org./ Accessed July 1, 2013.
- Bencardino J, Rosenberg ZS, Beltran J, Liu X, Marty-Delfaut E. Morton's Neuroma, Is it Always Symptomatic. *AJR Am J Roentgenol.* 2000;175(3):649–653.
- Hamilton N, Weimar W, Luttgens K. Kinesiology of fitness and exercise. In: Hamilton N, Weimar W, Luttgens K, eds.

Kinesiology: Scientific Basis of Human Motion. New York, NY: McGraw-Hill; 2008:Chapter 16. http://www.accessphysiotherapy.com/content/6151836. Accessed July 5, 2013.
- Hooker DN, Prentice WE. Basic principles of electricity and electrical stimulating currents. In: Prentice WE, Quillen WS, Underwood F, eds. *Therapeutic Modalities in Rehabilitation*. 4th ed. New York, NY: McGraw-Hill; 2011:Chapter 5. http://www.accessphysiotherapy.com/content/8136027. Accessed July 5, 2013.
- ICD-9-CM. http://www.icd9data.com. Accessed July 1, 2013.
- ICD-10-CM. http://www.icd10data.com. Accessed July 1, 2013.
- Malone TR, Hazle C, Grey ML. The ankle and foot. In: Malone TR, Hazle C, Grey ML, eds. *Imaging in Rehabilitation*. New York, NY: McGraw-Hill; 2008:Chapter 10. http://www.accessphysiotherapy.com/content/5940084. Accessed July 5, 2013.
- Prentice WE. Cryotherapy and thermotherapy. In: Prentice WE, Quillen WS, Underwood F, eds. *Therapeutic Modalities in Rehabilitation*. 4th ed. New York, NY: McGraw-Hill; 2011:Chapter 9. http://www.accessphysiotherapy.com/content/8137872. Accessed July 5, 2013.

226 RADIAL NERVE COMPRESSION

Matthew L. Daugherty, DPT, OTR/L, MOT, MTC, OCS, FAAOMPT
Eric Shamus, PhD, DPT, PT, CSCS

CONDITION/DISORDER SYNONYM

- Radial nerve palsy

ICD-9-CM CODE

- 354.3 Radial nerve lesion

ICD-10-CM CODES

- G56.31 Lesion of radial nerve, right upper limb
- G56.32 Lesion of radial nerve, left upper limb

PREFERRED PRACTICE PATTERNS

- 4E: Impaired Joint Mobility, Motor Function, Muscle Performance, and Range of Motion Associated with Localized Inflammation[1]
- 5F: Impaired Peripheral Nerve Integrity and Muscle Performance Associated with Peripheral Nerve Injury[2]

PATIENT PRESENTATION

Patient is a 25-year-old female administrative assistant. She spends a significant amount of time utilizing the computer keyboard. She is reporting a burning pain in her dorsal forearm throughout the day depending on how much typing she has done. The pain is exacerbated by flexing her wrist down, typing, and lifting file folders in pronation. She denies any numbness/tingling into her distal extremity and only reports the local forearm pain. Functionally, she has to take frequent rest breaks throughout the day and when she becomes symptomatic her typing rate decreases as well. She is woken at night approximately 5 days per week especially when her hand drops off the edge of the bed into wrist flexion.

Clinically, she does not present with any sensory deficits. She does have a 10 lb grip strength decrease and reports pain with testing. Palpable tenderness in extensor mass 5 cm distal to lateral epicondyle. Increased symptoms with passive wrist flexion/ulnar deviation/elbow extension combination as well as resisted long finger extension and forearm supination. Positive neurodynamic testing with radial nerve bias.

KEY FEATURES

Description

- Entrapment neuropathy of the radial nerve, particularly the posterior interosseous nerve (PIN) or dorsal radial sensory nerve (DRSN) in the elbow and wrist
  - DRSN compression is synonymous with Wartenberg's syndrome
- Common entrapment sites include[3]:
  - Thickened fascial tissue superficial to radiocapitellar joint
  - Fibrous origin of extensor carpi radialis brevis (ECRB)
  - Radial recurrent vessels-leash of Henry
  - Proximal border of supinator-arcade of Frohse
  - Distal edge of supinator
  - Between tendons of brachioradialis and extensor carpi radialis longus (DRSN)
  - Subcutaneous tissue in distal forearm (DRSN)
- Signs and symptoms typical of neuropathy, includes:
  - Pain
  - Paresthesias
  - Loss of sensation
  - Later loss of muscle function
- Symptoms are seen in the distribution of the radial nerve in the hand[3], dorsal distal upper arm and dorsal forearm 4 to 5 cm distal to the lateral epicondyle

Essentials of Diagnosis

- Burning or aching pain, paresthesias, and sensory loss perceived on dorsum of the forearm, thumb, and digits I–III dorsally; sensory changes only if DRSN syndrome
- Rest pain and night pain are common[3,4]

General Considerations

- In entrapment neuropathy, nerve becomes compressed, causing ischemic damage to the nerve.
- Often associated with repetitive motions or sustained position of the elbow.
- Unrelieved compression of the nerve results in neurapraxia with segmental demyelination[5]; further ischemic damage results in axonotmesis and wallerian degeneration.[6,5]

Demographics

- Coexists with lateral epicondylitis in 5% of patients.[3]
- AINS is rare, accounting for less than 1% of upper-extremity neuropathies.[7]
- Most common among people in their fifth decade of life.[7]

CLINICAL FINDINGS

SIGNS AND SYMPTOMS

- Burning/Aching pain in dorsal forearm exacerbated by repetitive activity in forearm pronation with wrist flexion including:
  - Using a screwdriver, typewriter, computer keyboard, or during handwriting
- Pain reported over anatomical snuff box and dorsal thumb
- Grip strength weakness due to pain

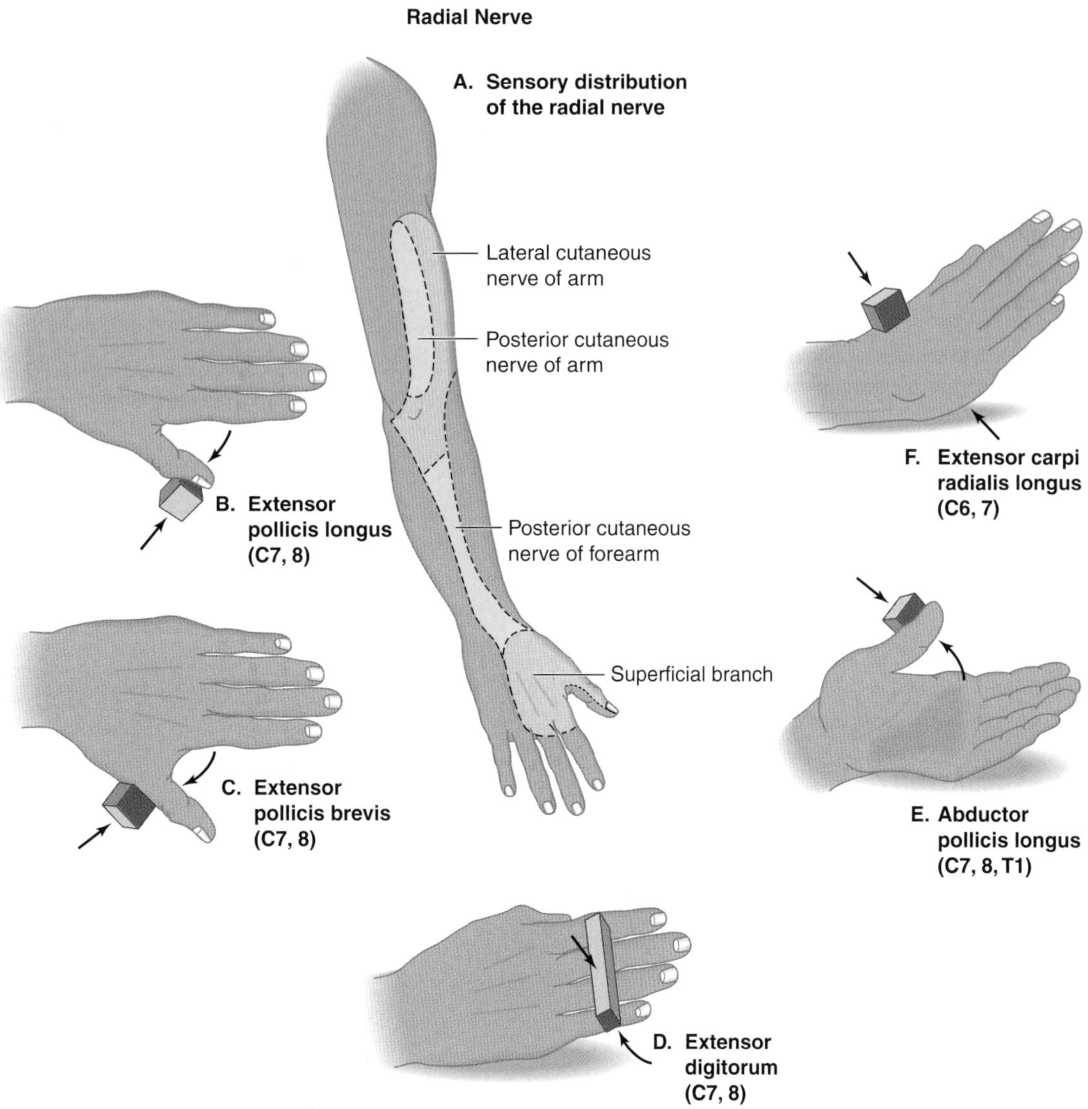

Radial Nerve

A. Sensory distribution of the radial nerve

Lateral cutaneous nerve of arm

Posterior cutaneous nerve of arm

Posterior cutaneous nerve of forearm

Superficial branch

B. Extensor pollicis longus (C7, 8)

C. Extensor pollicis brevis (C7, 8)

D. Extensor digitorum (C7, 8)

E. Abductor pollicis longus (C7, 8, T1)

F. Extensor carpi radialis longus (C6, 7)

FIGURE 226-1 Testing the radial nerve. (**A**) Sensory distribution. The radial nerve supplies the dorsolateral surface of the upper arm, forearm, wrist, and hand; the dorsal surface of the thumb; the dorsal surface of the index and middle fingers above the distal interphalangeal joints; and the lateral half of the dorsal surface of the ring finger above the distal interphalangeal joint. (**B**) Extensor pollicis longus. The thumb is extended at the interphalangeal joint against resistance. (**C**) Extensor pollicis brevis. The thumb is extended at the metacarpophalangeal joint against resistance. (**D**) Extensor digitorum. The fingers are extended at the metacarpophalangeal joints against resistance. (**E**) Abductor pollicis longus. The thumb is abducted (elevated in a plane at 90 degrees to the palm) at the carpometacarpal joint against resistance. (**F**) Extensor carpi radialis longus. The wrist is extended toward the radial (thumb) side against resistance. (From Greenberg DA, Aminoff MJ, Simon RP. *Clinical Neurology*. 8th ed. www.accessmedicine.com. Copyright © The McGraw-Hill Companies, Inc. All rights reserved.)

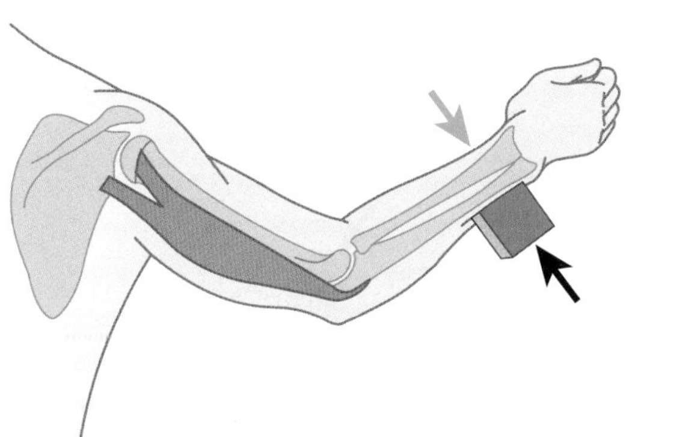

FIGURE 226-2 Triceps (C6–8; radial nerve). The forearm, flexed at the elbow, is extended against resistance. (From Waxman SG. *Clinical Neuroanatomy*. 26th ed. www.accessmedicine.com. Copyright © The McGraw-Hill Companies, Inc. All rights reserved.)

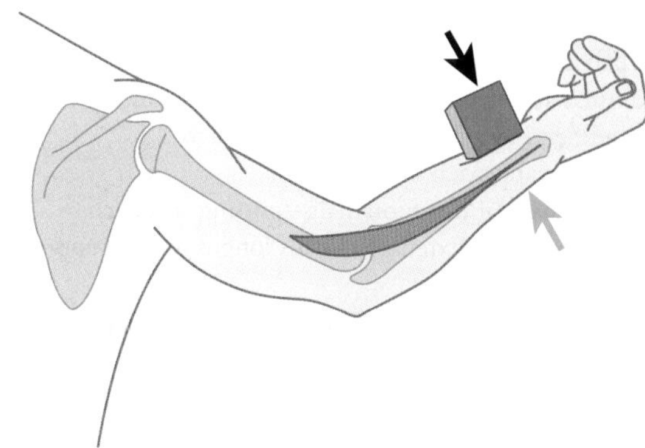

FIGURE 226-3 Brachioradialis (C5, 6; radial nerve). The forearm is flexed against resistance while in a neutral position (neither pronated nor supinated). (From Waxman SG. *Clinical Neuroanatomy*. 26th ed. www.accessmedicine.com. Copyright © The McGraw-Hill Companies, Inc. All rights reserved.)

Functional Implications

- Pain with elbow and wrist movements
- Difficulty with grasping and manipulation activities due to pain
- Impaired sensation
- Loss of grip strength in advanced cases (PIN)

Possible Contributing Causes

- Repeated exposure to severe cold[3]
- Genetic structural factors
- Tumors/lipomas
- Direct trauma
- Impaired circulation to peripheral nerves, as seen in diabetes, predisposes individuals to nerve compression symptoms

Differential Diagnosis

- Cervical radiculopathy
- Thoracic outlet syndrome
- Brachial plexopathy
- Chronic extensor compartment syndrome
- Chronic anconeus compartment syndrome
- Lateral antebrachial neuritis
- Lateral epicondylitis[4]
- Radiocapitellar joint pathology
- De Quervain tenosynovitis, particularly for DRSN compression

MEANS OF CONFIRMATION OR DIAGNOSIS

Imaging

- MRI[4]
- Diagnostic ultrasound (ultrasonography)[4]

Diagnostic Procedure

- Nerve conduction velocity (NCV)
- Electromyography (EMG)

FINDINGS AND INTERPRETATION

- NCV testing of radial nerve across the radial tunnel
- Electromyography (EMG) abnormalities have been reported in extensors in the presence of normal NCVs[8]

TREATMENT

Medication

- NSAIDs[4]
- Corticosteroid injection

Operative Treatment

- Indicated after failure of conservative management
  - Modified Henry approach
  - Posterior approach of Thompson
  - Transmuscular brachioradialis-splitting approach
  - Brachioradialis/Extensor radialis longus interval approach

REFERRALS/ADMITTANCE

- To radiologist for imaging; X-ray for fracture or displacement
- To orthopedist for surgical consult or injection

IMPAIRMENTS

- Hand weakness with grasping, squeezing, pinching, and fine motor manipulation

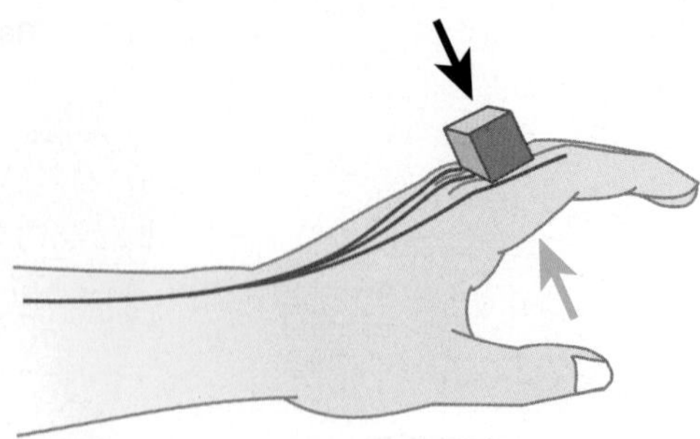

FIGURE 226-4 Extensor digitorum (C7, 8; radial nerve). The fingers are extended at the metacarpophalangeal joints against resistance. (From Waxman SG. *Clinical Neuroanatomy*. 26th ed. www.accessmedicine.com. Copyright © The McGraw-Hill Companies, Inc. All rights reserved.)

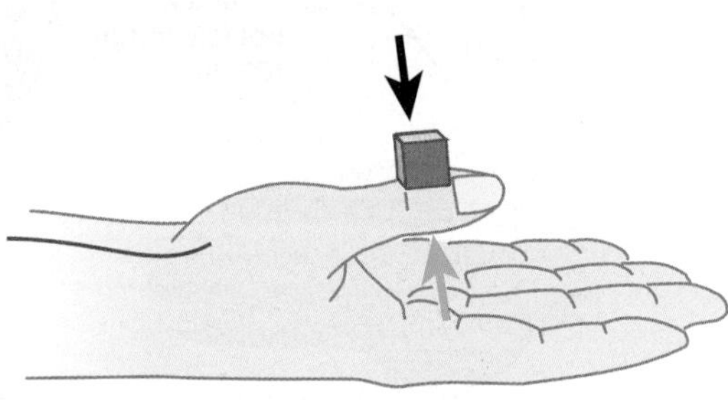

FIGURE 226-5 Abductor pollicis longus (C7, 8; T1; radial nerve). The thumb is abducted against resistance in a plane at a right angle to the palmar surface. (From Waxman SG. *Clinical Neuroanatomy*. 26th ed. www.accessmedicine.com. Copyright © The McGraw-Hill Companies, Inc. All rights reserved.)

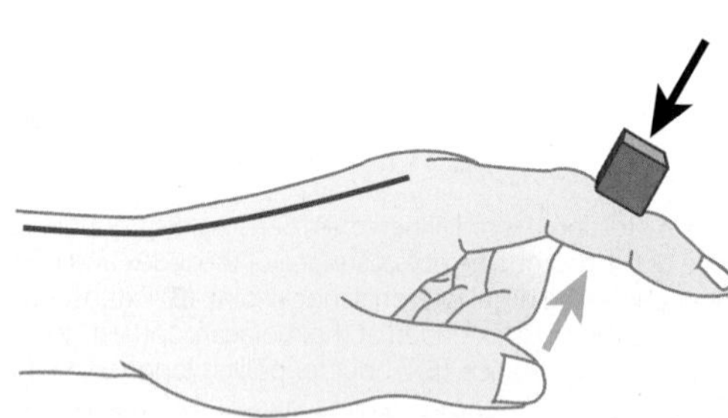

FIGURE 226-6 Extensor indicis proprius (C6–8; radial nerve). The index finger is extended against resistance placed on the dorsal aspect of the finger. (From Waxman SG. *Clinical Neuroanatomy*. 26th ed. www.accessmedicine.com. Copyright © The McGraw-Hill Companies, Inc. All rights reserved.)

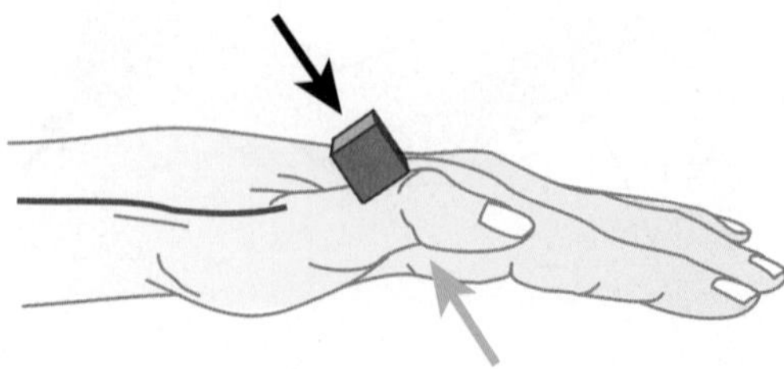

FIGURE 226-7 Extensor pollicis brevis (C7, 8; radial nerve). The thumb is extended at the metacarpophalangeal joint against resistance. (From Waxman SG. *Clinical Neuroanatomy*. 26th ed. www.accessmedicine.com. Copyright © The McGraw-Hill Companies, Inc. All rights reserved.)

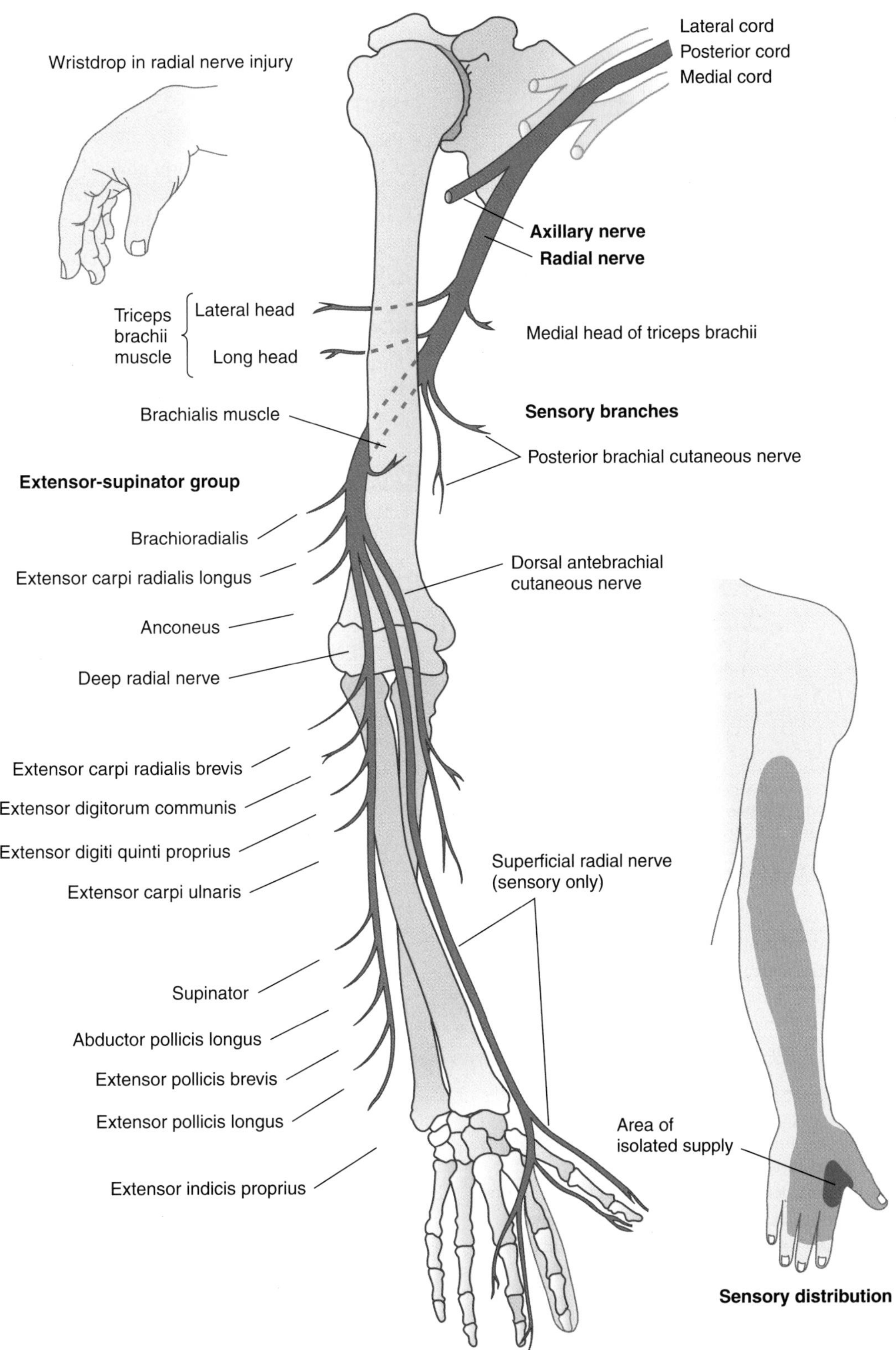

FIGURE 226-8 The radial nerve (C6–8; T1). (From Waxman SG. *Clinical Neuroanatomy*. 26th ed. www.accessmedicine.com. Copyright © The McGraw-Hill Companies, Inc. All rights reserved.)

TESTS AND MEASURES[9]

- Reproduction of symptoms with resisted extension of the long finger with elbow in full extension
- Reproduction of symptoms with resisted supination with the elbow in extension
- Painful palpation within the extensor musculature 4 to 5 cm distal to lateral epicondyle
- Exacerbated symptoms with passive elbow extension, wrist flexion, and ulnar deviation
- Reproduction of symptoms with resisted wrist extension

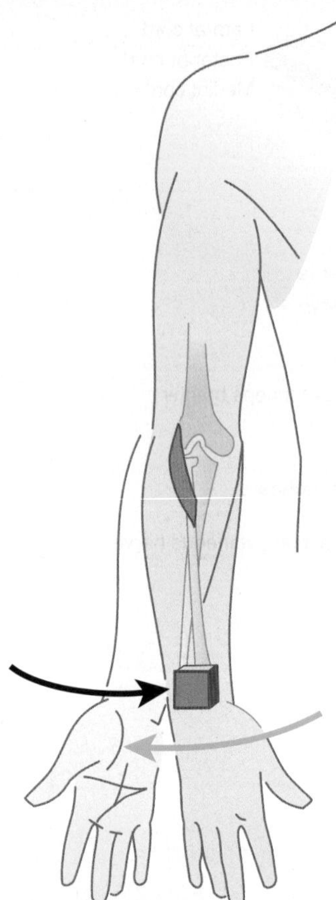

FIGURE 226-9 Supinator (C5–7; radial nerve). The hand is supinated against resistance, with arms extended at the side. Resistance is applied by the grip of the examiner's hand on the patient's forearm near the wrist. (From Waxman SG. *Clinical Neuroanatomy*. 26th ed. www.accessmedicine.com. Copyright © The McGraw-Hill Companies, Inc. All rights reserved.)

- Sensory loss may include diminished two-point discrimination, decreased vibration sense, increased threshold in Semmes-Weinstein monofilament test[6]
- Positive upper limb neurodynamic test with radial nerve bias
- Flexor and thenar muscle strength test (lateral pinch and hand grip dynamometry)

INTERVENTION

- Early conservative intervention
  - Ergonomic analysis and activity modification to reduce repetitive motion or positioning stress such as avoiding pronation, wrist flexion/extension or unloading radial nerve by holding a pen while typing
- Second-stage conservative intervention
  - Wrist hand orthosis in slight wrist extension (PIN, radial tunnel)
  - Volar based thumb orthosis maintaining wrist extension (DRSN)
  - Ultrasound[10,11]
  - Radial nerve gliding[4]
  - Manual therapy[11–13]
    - Myofascial release[12]
- Postsurgical intervention
  - Activity modification and protected ROM
  - Radial nerve gliding[4]
  - Scar management and sensory desensitization
  - Strengthening with focus on improving fine motor skills

FUNCTIONAL GOALS

- Patient will have
  - Improved ability to perform physical tasks, self-care, home management, leisure and occupational activities.
  - Increased tolerance of positions and activities using elbow, forearm, and wrist.
  - Reduced ergonomic risk.

PROGNOSIS

- Surgical intervention indicated for patients with symptoms lasting more than 1 year, or those for whom conservative treatment over 3 months has failed.

PATIENT RESOURCE

- Radial nerve palsy. American Association of Neuromuscular & Electrodiagnostic Medicine (AANEM). http://www.aanem.org/Education/Patient-Resources/Disorders/Radial-Nerve-Palsy.aspx. Accessed August 17, 2014.

REFERENCES

1. The American Physical Therapy Association. Pattern 4E: impaired joint mobility, motor function, muscle performance, and range of motion associated with localized inflammation. *Interactive Guide to Physical Therapist Practice*. 2003. doi: 10.2522/ptguide.3.1_5. Accessed July 8, 2013.
2. The American Physical Therapy Association. Pattern 5F: Impaired peripheral nerve integrity and muscle performance associated with peripheral nerve injury. *Interactive Guide to Physical Therapist Practice*. 2003. doi: 10.2522/ptguide.3.2_6. Accessed July 8, 2013.
3. Skirven TM, Osterman AL, Fedorczyk JM, et al. *Rehabilitation Of The Hand and Upper Extremity*. 6th ed. St. Louis, MO: Mosby Inc; 2011.
4. Dutton M. *Orthopaedic Examination, Evaluation, and Intervention*. New York, NY: McGraw-Hill; 2008. http://www.accessphysiotherapy.com/resource/612. Accessed July 8, 2013.
5. Goodman CC, Fuller KS. *Pathology: Implications for the Physical Therapist*. 3rd ed. St. Louis: Saunders/Elsevier; 2009.
6. American Physical Therapy Association. *Anatomy and Physiology Revealed*. McGraw-Hill. 2007. http://anatomy.mcgraw-hill.com/apt.html?login=1319880810339&system=Muscular§ion=Dissection&topic=Wrist%20and%20hand&topicAbbr=Wha&view=Anterior&viewAbbr=Ant&catAbbr=Oth&grpAbbr=Ske&structure=Carpal%20tunnel. Accessed July 8, 2013.
7. Waxman SG. *Clinical Neuroanatomy*. New York, NY: McGraw-Hill; 2010. http://www.accessphysiotherapy.com/resource/22. Accessed July 8, 2013.
8. Halle J, Greathouse D. Principles of electrophysiologic evaluation and testing. In: Prentice WE, Quillen WS, Underwood F, eds. *Therapeutic Modalities in Rehabilitation*. 4th ed. New York, NY: McGraw-Hill; 2011:Chapter 8. http://www.accessphysiotherapy.com/abstract/8137649#8137649. Accessed July 8, 2013.
9. AcSkirven TM, Osterman AL, Fedorczyk JM, et al. *Rehabilitation Of The Hand and Upper Extremity*. 6th ed. St. Louis, MO: Mosby Inc; 2011.

10. Dutton M. *Dutton's Orthopedic Survival Guide: Managing Common Conditions.* New York, NY: McGraw-Hill; 2011. http://www.accessphysiotherapy.com/resource/685. Accessed July 8, 2013.
11. Houghton PE. The role of therapeutic modalities in wound healing. In: Prentice WE, Quillen WS, Underwood F, eds. *Therapeutic Modalities in Rehabilitation.* 4th ed. New York: McGraw-Hill; 2011:Chapter 3. http://www.accessphysiotherapy.com/abstract/8135453#8135453. Accessed July 8, 2013.
12. Muller M, Tsui D, Schnurr R, Biddulph-Deisroth L, Hard J, MacDermid J. Effectiveness of hand therapy interventions in primary management of carpal tunnel syndrome: a systematic review. *J Hand Ther.* 2004;17(2):210–228.
13. Prentice WE. Therapeutic massage. In: Prentice WE, Quillen WS, Underwood F, eds. *Therapeutic Modalities in Rehabilitation.* 4th ed. New York, NY: McGraw-Hill; 2011:Chapter 16. http://www.accessphysiotherapy.com/abstract/8140838#8140971. Accessed July 8, 2013.

ADDITIONAL REFERENCES

- ICD9DATA. http://www.icd9data.com. Accessed August 17, 2014.
- ICD10DATA. http://www.icd10data.com. Accessed August 17, 2014.
- Lozano-Calderón S, Anthony S, Ring D. The quality and strength of evidence for etiology: example of carpal tunnel syndrome. *J Hand Surg Am.* 2008;33(4):525–538.

227 TARSAL TUNNEL SYNDROME

Kevin Murdoch, DPT, PT, OCS
Eric Shamus, PhD, DPT, PT, CSCS

CONDITION/DISORDER SYNONYMS

- Tarsal tunnel syndrome (TTS)
- Posterior tibial neuralgia

ICD-9-CM CODE

- 355.5 Tarsal tunnel syndrome

ICD-10-CM CODE

- G57.50 Tarsal tunnel syndrome, unspecified lower limb

PREFERRED PRACTICE PATTERNS

- 4E: Impaired Joint Mobility, Motor Function, Muscle Performance, and Range of Motion Associated with Localized Inflammation
- 5F: Impaired Peripheral Nerve Integrity and Muscle Performance Associated with Peripheral Nerve Injury

PATIENT PRESENTATION

A 27-year-old male recreational runner/jogger presents with right ankle and foot pain and numbness of 2 weeks duration. The patient reports spraining his ankle 6 months ago when he turned his ankle inward while jogging on an uneven surface. He sustained a sprain to his medial ankle that resolved uneventfully in 2 to 3 weeks. Upon returning to running/jogging, the patient noted stiffness and generalized right lower-extremity weakness but denied ankle or leg pain. Patient reports that he returned to his typical jogging mileage of more than 35 miles/week with 2 weeks of return to jogging. At this time, he reports medial ankle and foot paresthesia/numbness beneath his medial malleolus that travels into the medial arch and plantar aspect of his foot and heel. Numbness/paresthesia is increased shortly after initiating jogging and is notable with standing and walking, especially if the patient wears sandals or flip-flops. Upon palpation, the patient reports pain and tenderness inferior to his medial malleolus. The patient has a positive Tinel sign with testing inferior to medial malleolus. Weakness noted for flexion of the big toe.

KEY FEATURES

Description

- Tarsal tunnel syndrome is an entrapment syndrome of the tibial nerve behind (posterior to) the medial malleolus and under the flexor retinaculum or laciniate ligament.[1]
- Structures that pass through the tarsal tunnel
  - Flexor hallucis longus muscle
  - Flexor digitorum longus muscle
  - Tibialis posterior muscle
  - Posterior tibial nerve
  - Posterior tibial artery

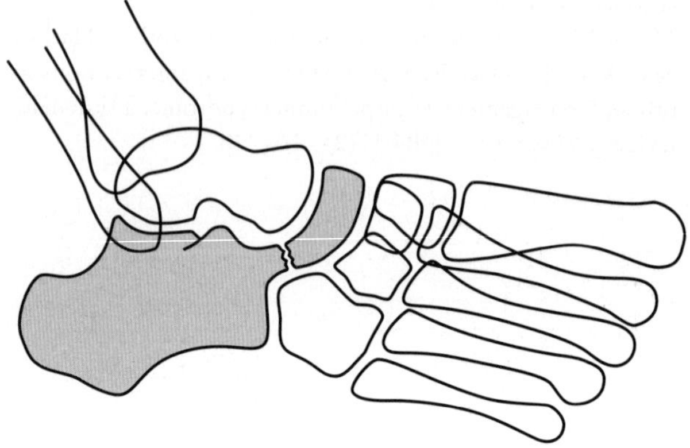

FIGURE 227-1 Calcaneonavicular tarsal coalition is best seen on oblique radiograph projection. (From Skinner HB. *Current Diagnosis & Treatment in Orthopedics*. 4th ed. www.accessmedicine.com. Copyright © The McGraw-Hill Companies, Inc. All rights reserved.)

- The tibial nerve supplies movement and sensation to the calf and foot muscles.
- The deep and superficial aponeuroses of the leg form the laciniate ligament, which is closely attached to the sheath of the three adjacent flexor tendons, the posterior tibial, the flexor digitorum, and flexor hallucis.[1]
- Tarsal tunnel is a peripheral neuropathy that occurs when there is damage to the tibial nerve, one of the lower branches of the sciatic nerve of the leg.
- Nerve entrapment sites, branches of tibial nerve:
  - Lateral plantar nerve (LPN): Supplies most of the foot muscles and the skin of the lateral one-third of the plantar aspect of the fourth and fifth toes.[2]
    - The first branch of the LPN innervates the flexor digitorum brevis, quadratus plantae, and abductor digiti minimi.
  - Medial calcaneal nerve: Sensory innervations to heel fat pad and superficial tissues over the inferior aspect of the calcaneus.
  - Medial plantar nerve: Innervations of abductor hallucis, flexor hallucis brevis, flexor digitorum brevis, first lumbrical, and skin of the medial two-thirds of the plantar aspect of the foot.

Essentials of Diagnosis

- Diagnosis typically made by clinical examination
- Pathophysiology, diagnosis, and management are subject to debate in previous and current literature
- Tarsal tunnel syndrome symptoms may include weakness or loss of sensation in the foot from damage to the tibial nerve

General Considerations

- Often misdiagnosed as plantar fasciitis

Demographics

- Occurs in 15% of adults with foot problems
- Affects males and females
- Athletic and nonathletic populations

CLINICAL FINDINGS

SIGNS AND SYMPTOMS

- Pain with prolonged walking, with gradual onset associated with weight-bearing activities
- Posteromedial ankle and foot pain, tenderness to palpation in posteromedial heel
- Possible positive tinel sign with symptoms radiating from proximal or distal
- Sensory disturbance in medial and plantar aspects of the heel (medial calcaneal nerve)[2]
- Local swelling/edema over and/or beneath the retinaculum
- Nerve tenderness with palpation with symptoms into the longitudinal arch
- There may be tenderness in intertarsal spaces representative of nerve irritability
- Weakness of foot, toes or ankle
- Weakness and/or the inability to curl the toes, push the foot down, or twist the ankle inward

Functional Implications

- Limitations of prolonged walking and standing
- Gait dysfunction
- Severe loss of sensation may lead to toe or foot sores (ulcers) and infections

Possible Contributing Causes

- Alcoholism
- Diabetes
- Ligamentous laxity, pregnancy
- Obesity: Weight gain
- Occupation or activities that demand prolonged standing on hard surfaces
- Pes planus (flat foot, low arch)
- Thyroid disease
- Unsupportive footwear

Differential Diagnosis

- Amyloid neuropathy
- Charcot disease
- Compartment syndrome
- Ganglion cyst: Space occupying lesions including ganglia from subtalar joint or tendon sheaths
- Lipomas
- Plantar fasciitis
- Posterior tibial dysfunction
- Proximal nerve lesions: Injury or disease of structures near the knee may also damage the tibial nerve
- Reactive arthritis
- Rheumatoid arthritis
- Stress fracture
- Subtalar joint bone spurring
- Tenosynovitis of the adjacent flexors
- Tibial nerve may also be affected by diseases that damage many nerves, such as:
  - Diabetes
  - Peripheral neuropathy
  - Radiculopathy
  - Multiple sclerosis

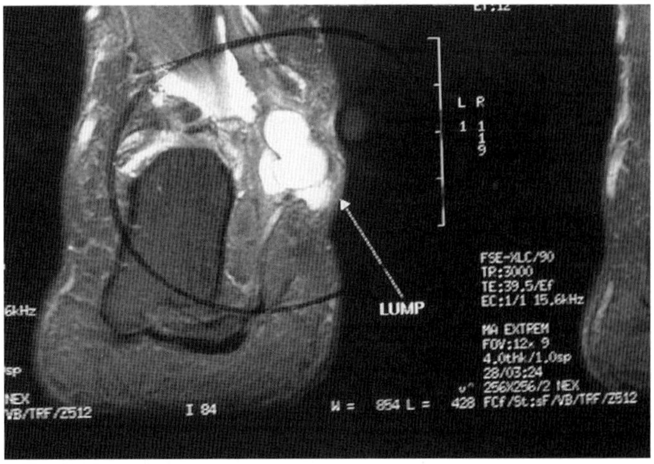

FIGURE 227-2 Coronal plane magnetic resonance image of a ganglion cyst within the tarsal tunnel. The cyst compresses the posterior tibial nerve, leading to symptoms of tarsal tunnel syndrome. (From Imboden J, Hellmann DB, Stone JH. *Current Rheumatology Diagnosis & Treatment*. 2nd ed. www.accessmedicine.com. Copyright © The McGraw-Hill Companies, Inc. All rights reserved.)

MEANS OF CONFIRMATION OR DIAGNOSIS

Imaging

- CT
- X-ray
- MRI
- High-resolution ultrasound

Medical Procedure

- Electromyography (EMG): Positive findings in foot intrinsics, abductor hallucis, abductor digiti quinti, and interossei
- Nerve conduction velocity (NCV) test

FINDINGS AND INTERPRETATION

- Tibial nerve entrapment with paresthesia, associated sensory changes, and muscle weakness
- Nerve conduction tests: May demonstrate reduced tibial nerve conduction
- Associated muscle atrophy may be present

TREATMENT

- Corticosteroid injection
- Surgical release of the posterior tibial nerve

REFERRALS/ADMITTANCE

- To radiologist: Imaging, x-ray, MRI
- To surgical consult if failed conservative measures

IMPAIRMENTS

- Antalgic gait due to weakness of foot intrinsic muscles, lower extremity (LE) weakness
- Antalgic gait due to reduced dorsiflexion
- Restricted/limited talocrural arthrokinematics

TESTS AND MEASURES

- Neurologic examination
  - Sensation
    - Light touch
    - Pin prick

- LE deep tendon reflexes
- Proprioception at the hip
- Kinesthetic awareness at the hip
- Coordination
- Special tests
  - Dorsiflexion-eversion test
  - Neurodynamic tests
  - Plantar flexion-inversion test
  - Tinel sign

INTERVENTION

- Conservative treatment includes:
  - Rest
  - NSAIDs
  - Corticosteroid injections, local anesthetic injections
  - Heel support
  - Night splints to create a stretch on the Achilles
  - Addressing swelling
    - Ice
    - Elevation
  - Addressing pain
    - Ice
    - Massage
    - Electric stimulation
    - Ultrasound
    - Infrared
  - Addressing weakness, joint instability
    - Strengthening
      - Toes curls, flexor intrinsic
      - Calf raises to point
      - Active walking
      - Standing arch raises
  - Addressing lack of flexibility
    - Stretching
      - Gastrocnemius/Soleus
      - Plantar fascia if pes cavus foot type
  - Addressing mobilization
    - Posterior talus glides
    - Navicular/Cuboid/Cuneiforms
    - Widening of the mortise
      - Distal tibia/fibula mobility
  - Medial longitudinal arch support and/or taping
  - Orthotics
  - Supportive footwear
  - Stretching exercises
  - Manual therapy
- Systematic review concluded that the effectiveness of treatment modalities for plantar heel pain has not been established in randomized controlled trials.[3]
- Surgery is considered if at least 6 to 12 months of conservative treatment has failed
- Studies have shown that surgical decompression of the first branch of the LPN relieved symptoms in patients with plantar heel pain
- Primary studies that consider combinations of surgical procedures to enlarge the tarsal tunnel were inconclusive or lacked control interventions
- Job counseling or retraining may be recommended

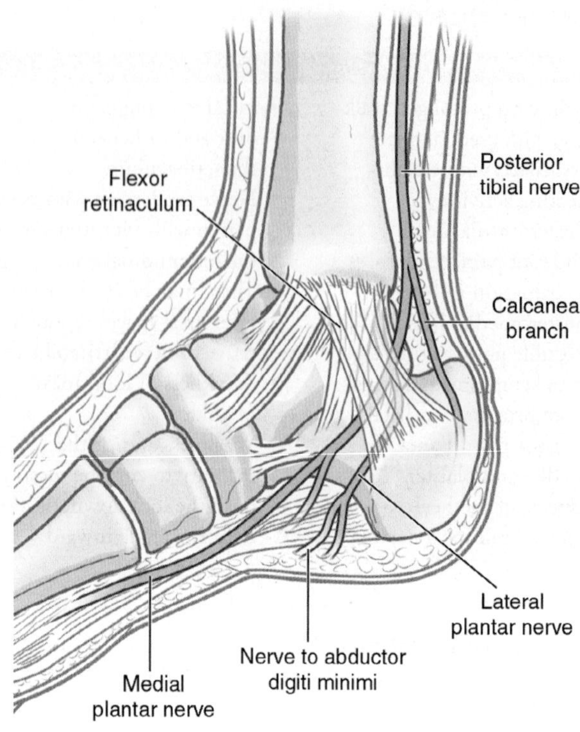

FIGURE 227-3 Medial view of the ankle demonstrating the course of the posterior tibial nerve within the tarsal tunnel. (From Simon RR, Sherman SC. *Emergency Orthopedics*. 6th ed. www.accessemergencymedicine.com Copyright © The McGraw-Hill Companies, Inc. All rights reserved.)

FUNCTIONAL GOALS

- Patient will be able to
  - Stand for self-care, dressing, and grooming without ankle and foot pain in 6 to 8 weeks.
  - Walk for >45 minutes without ankle and foot pain in 6 to 8 weeks.
  - Demonstrate gait with equal step length in 4 to 6 weeks.
  - Travel up and down 10 steps and stairs without ankle and foot pain in 6 to 8 weeks.

PROGNOSIS

- Discrete space occupying lesions with minimal anatomic damage to the tibial nerve should expect full relief and recovery.
- Variable outcomes noted via surgical procedures.
- Cases where there is obvious damage to the nerve via a space occupying lesion, fracture, or osteotomy recover in a variable manner.
- Some patients may have a partial or complete loss of movement or sensation.
- Complications: Deformity of the foot, movement loss in the toes, and sensation loss in the toes or foot.

PATIENT RESOURCE

- *Tarsal Tunnel Syndrome*. American College of Foot and Ankle Surgeons. http://www.heartlandfootandankle.com/docs/TarsalTunnelSyndrome.pdf. Accessed July 11, 2013.

REFERENCES

1. Gould JS. Tarsal tunnel syndrome. *Foot Ankle Clin*. 2011; 16(2):275–286. doi: 10.1016/j.fcl.2011.01.008.

2. Alshami AM, Souvlis T, Coppieters MW. A review of plantar heel pain of neural origin: differential diagnosis and management. *Man Ther.* 2008;13(2):103–111. doi:10.1016/j.math.2007.01.014.
3. Crawford F, Atkins D, Edwards J. Interventions for treating plantar heel pain. *Cochrane Database of Systematic Reviews.* 2003;(3):CD000416. doi: 10.1002/14651858.CD000416.

ADDITIONAL REFERENCES

- Dutton M. The ankle and foot complex. In: Dutton M, ed. *Dutton's Orthopedic Survival Guide: Managing Common Conditions.* New York, NY: McGraw-Hill; 2011:Chapter 10. http://www.accessphysiotherapy.com/content/8655286. Accessed July 11, 2013.
- Dutton M. *Dutton's Orthopaedic Examination, Evaluation, and Intervention.* 3rd ed. New York, NY: McGraw-Hill; 2012. http://www.accessphysiotherapy.com/resource/612. Accessed July 14, 2013.
- Dutton M. Therapeutic exercise. In: Dutton M, ed. *McGraw-Hill's NPTE (National Physical Therapy Examination).* 2nd ed. New York, NY: McGraw-Hill; 2012:Chapter 17. http://www.accessphysiotherapy.com/content/5405417. Accessed July 11, 2013.
- *Guide to Physical Therapist Practice.* 2nd ed. Alexandria, VA: American Physical Therapy Association; 2001. Revised 2003.
- Hay WW, Levin MJ, Sondheimer JM, Deterding RR. Growth disturbances of the musculoskeletal system. In: Hay WW, Levin MJ, Sondheimer JM, Deterding RR, eds. *CURRENT Diagnosis & Treatment: Pediatrics.* 20th ed. New York, NY: McGraw-Hill; 2011. http://www.accessphysiotherapy.com/content/6585882. Accessed July 11, 2013.
- ICD9Data.com. http://www.icd9data.com. Accessed July 13, 2013.
- ICD10Data.com. http://www.icd10data.com. Accessed July 13, 2013.
- Lau JT, Daniels TR. Tarsal tunnel syndrome: a review of the literature. *Foot Ankle Int.* 1999;20(3):201–209.
- Malone TR, Hazle C, Grey ML. The ankle and foot. In: Malone TR, Hazle C, Grey ML, eds. *Imaging in Rehabilitation.* New York, NY: McGraw-Hill; 2008:Chapter 10. http://www.accessphysiotherapy.com/content/5940084. Accessed July 11, 2013.
- Prentice WE, Quillen WS, Underwood F, eds. *Therapeutic Modalities in Rehabilitation.* 4th ed. New York, NY: McGraw-Hill; 2011. http://www.accessphysiotherapy.com/resource/675. Accessed July 4, 2013.

228 THORACIC OUTLET SYNDROME

Yasmin Qureshi, DPT, MPT, MHS (Osteo)
Eric Shamus, PhD, DPT, PT, CSCS

CONDITION/DISORDER SYNDROME

- Neurogenic thoracic outlet syndrome (NTOS)

ICD-9-CM CODE

- 353.0 Brachial plexus lesions

ICD-10-CM CODE

- G54.0 Brachial plexus disorders

PREFERRED PRACTICE PATTERN

- 4E: Impaired Joint Mobility, Motor Function, Muscle Performance, and Rang of Motion Associated with Localized Inflammation

PATIENT PRESENTATION

Patient is a 23-year-old male who is in the army. Patient complains that both of his arms feel heavy. He has a cold sensation in his hands. Patient spent the last 2 weeks in boot camp. He had to hike 5 miles a day while wearing a fully loaded back pack. The heaviness has begun since he started with the hiking. The patient has a positive costoclavicular thoracic outlet test.

KEY FEATURES

Description

- Entrapment of the neurovascular bundle comprising the brachial plexus, subclavian artery and/or subclavian vein, neurogenic or vascular types (venous and arterial)
- Symptomatology and management is different depending on the primary structure compressed
  - Compression on the brachial plexus
    - Direct compression can occur at
      - Scalene triangle
      - Cervical rib/first rib
      - Pectoralis minor
      - Costoclavicular space
      - Unstable humeral head in an anterior/inferior position[1]

Essentials of Diagnosis

- Diagnosis is made by clinical examination and thorough diagnosis of exclusion
- Most common to least common incidence is brachial plexus, subclavian artery, and subclavian vein compression, respectively[2]
- Thoracic outlet syndrome involving the subclavian vein and artery requires immediate medical attention and is often the result of trauma or clot[3]
- Worse with repetitive postural habits, pain at rest, night pain[4]

General Considerations

- Neurological examination and diagnostic imaging is required to rule out the most common differential diagnoses
- Double crush syndrome is a possibility[5]

Demographics

- Young and middle-aged adults most commonly affected[6]
- Females to males 3:1[6]
- Can develop spontaneously, gradual onset due to poor posture or post-trauma
- Teenagers with a cervical rib
- There is increased incidence with participation in sports
- Correlated with a high incidence of forward head carriage and rounded shoulders[7]

CLINICAL FINDINGS

SIGNS AND SYMPTOMS

- Intermittent numbness and tingling in the forearm, wrist and hand
  - Most often in the medial forearm and hand in the distribution of C8/T1 nerve roots but can be whole hand
- Feeling of weakness and fatigue in the upper extremity (UE) especially with arm overhead
- Pain in the arm, neck, shoulders, and upper back
- Aggravated by overhead activities, repetitive activities, and activities that depress the shoulder girdle[4]
- Pain is worse at night.[4,8]
- Pain can be better with rest
- Postural examination may reveal low lying shoulder girdle on affected side, forward head carriage, and anteriorly rounded shoulders[6]
- Isolated venous type of thoracic outlet syndrome presents with unilateral UP edema, pain, cyanosis, paresthesia, fatigue, and heaviness of the UE[4]
- Isolated arterial type of thoracic outlet syndrome presents with cool extremities, absent arterial pulse, possible distal gangrene, muscle cramps in the hand, paresthesia, swelling/heaviness of the UE[4]

Functional Implications

- Difficulty with overhead activities
- Pain with repetitive occupational fine motor tasks such as typing
- Pain/Difficulty with prolonged seated postures
- Difficulty carrying a bag on the ipsilateral side
- Inability to sleep on the affected side

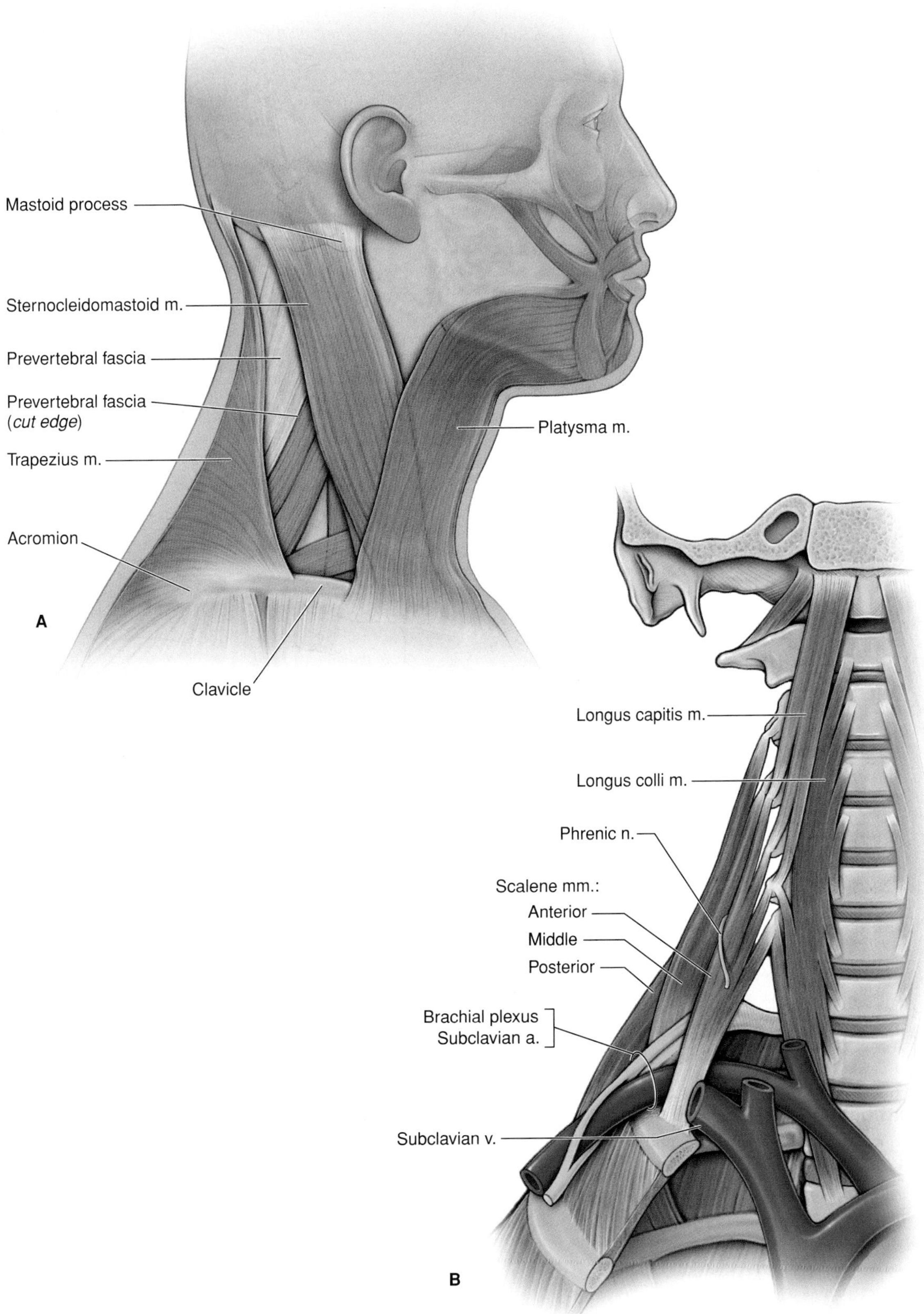

FIGURE 228-1 (**A**) Muscles of the neck. (**B**) Anterior view of the scalene and prevertebral muscles. (From Morton DA, Foreman KB, Albertine KH. *The Big Picture: Gross Anatomy*. www.accessmedicine.com. Copyright © The McGraw-Hill Companies, Inc. All rights reserved.)

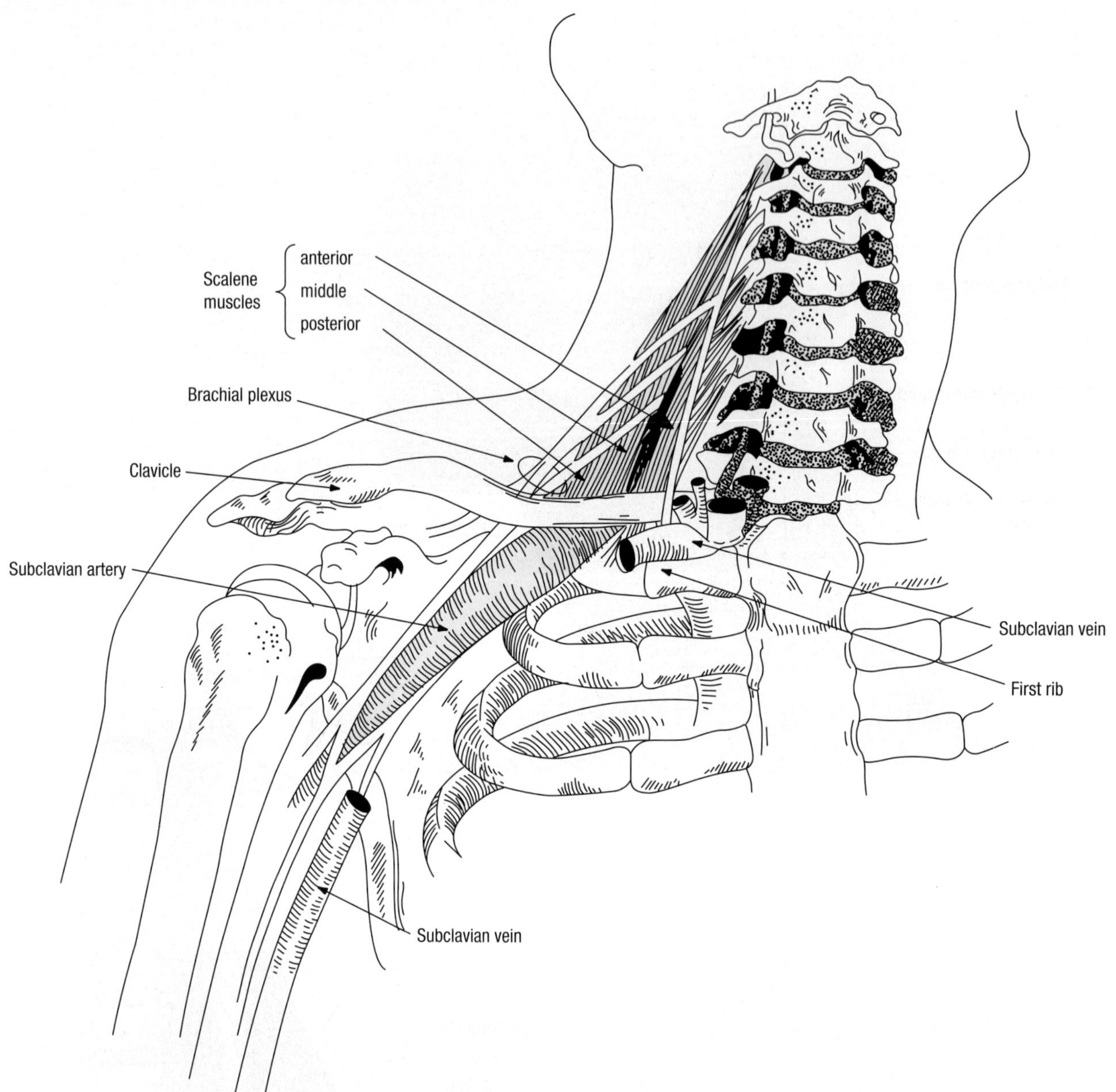

FIGURE 228-2 Course of the brachial plexus and subclavian artery between the anterior scalene and middle scalene muscles. Dilatation of the subclavian artery just distal to the anterior scalene muscle is illustrated. Immediately distal to the anterior and middle scalene muscles is another potential area of constriction, between the clavicle and the first rib. With extension of the neck and turning of the chin to the affected side (Adson maneuver), the tension on the anterior scalene muscle is increased and the subclavian artery compressed, resulting in a supraclavicular bruit and obliteration of the radial pulse. (From Ropper AH, Samuels MA. *Adams & Victor's Principles of Neurology.* 9th ed. www.accessmedicine.com. Copyright © The McGraw-Hill Companies, Inc. All rights reserved.)

Possible Contributing Causes

- Poor posture: Forward rounded posture, military/retracted posture
- Presence of cervical ribs at C7 (incidence 1% general population), seen in early teens as activity increases
- Occupational: Prolonged seated postures and repetitive computer work, those with professions that require overhead work such as electricians or musicians
- Trauma: Whiplash injury, instability of the shoulder, clavicular fracture
- Overhead throwing sports such as volleyball, swimming, and baseball[9]
- Carrying a backpack or heavy bag on one shoulder repetitively

Differential Diagnosis

- Anterior interosseous nerve syndrome
- Carpal tunnel syndrome
- Cervical radiculopathy
- Complex regional pain syndrome
- Cubital tunnel syndrome
- Disc herniation
- Pronator teres syndrome
- T4 syndrome
- Traction injuries of the brachial plexus such as Erb-Duchenne and Dejerine–Klumpke's palsy
- Tumors: Apical pancoast tumor (apex of the lung)[10]
- Tunnel of Guyon entrapment
- Ulnar groove entrapment neuropathy

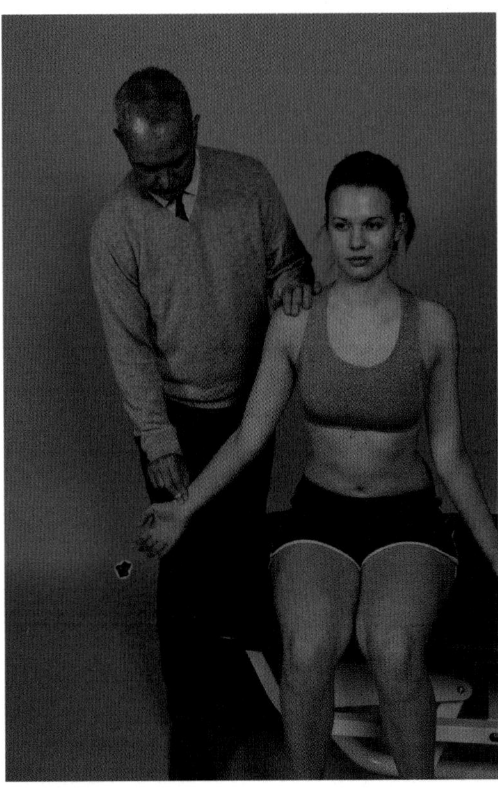

FIGURE 228-3 Adson test. (From Dutton D. *Dutton's Orthopaedic Examination, Evaluation, and Intervention*. 3rd ed. www.accessphysiotherapy.com. Copyright © The McGraw-Hill Companies, Inc. All rights reserved.)

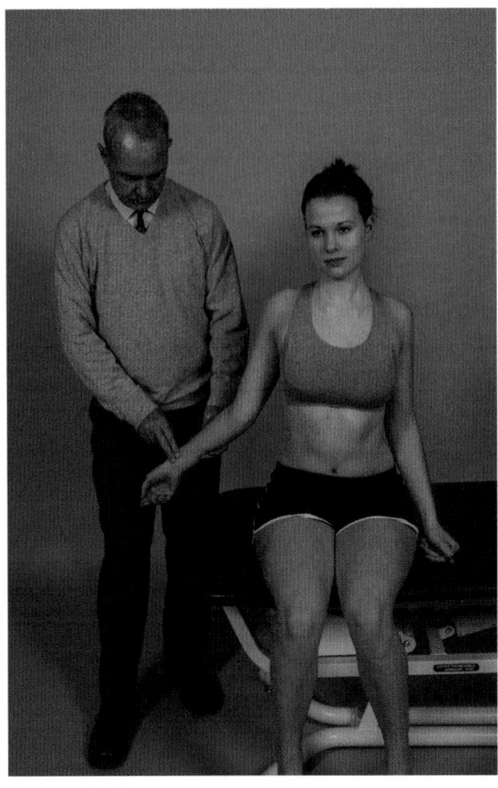

FIGURE 228-4 Costoclavicular test. (From Dutton D. *Dutton's Orthopaedic Examination, Evaluation, and Intervention*. 3rd ed. www.accessphysiotherapy.com. Copyright © The McGraw-Hill Companies, Inc. All rights reserved.)

MEANS OF CONFIRMATION OR DIAGNOSIS

Imaging

- Cervical spine X-rays to diagnose cervical ribs
- CT with contrast (contrast is dye injected into the veins, improved diagnostics for clot or aneurysm)
- Cervical spine MRI with contrast to rule out differential diagnoses
- MRI is the method of choice for neurologic compression
- Doppler ultrasound or angiogram/venogram to diagnose arterial and venous forms, view blood flow and narrowing of vessels[9]
- Electrodiagnostic/nerve conduction testing (often inconclusive)

FINDINGS AND INTERPRETATION

- Positive Adson or Scalene maneuver, Halstead maneuver, hyperabduction maneuver (Wright test) and costoclavicular space/military brace orthopedic tests confirmed by a reduced intensity of the radial pulse[4]
- Positive Roos test[4]
- Upper limb tension tests of the ulnar nerve in particular but also the radial and median
- Apprehension/relocation test for the presence of shoulder instability
- Neurological examination: Reduced sensation, absent/reduced deep tendon reflexes, and weakness in grip strength (C8/T1) or the C5,6 muscle groups if superior trunk of the brachial plexus is involved[4]

REFERRALS/ADMITTANCE

- For diagnostic imaging, X-rays, nerve conduction studies/electromyogram (EMG), MRI
- For medication, oral and topical NSAIDs
- Scalene injections or block: Trigger point into scalene musculature, cortisone to decrease inflammation, botox into the scalenes
- For surgical consult, resection first/cervical rib
- For suspected arterial or venous causes, refer to physician for immediate evaluation

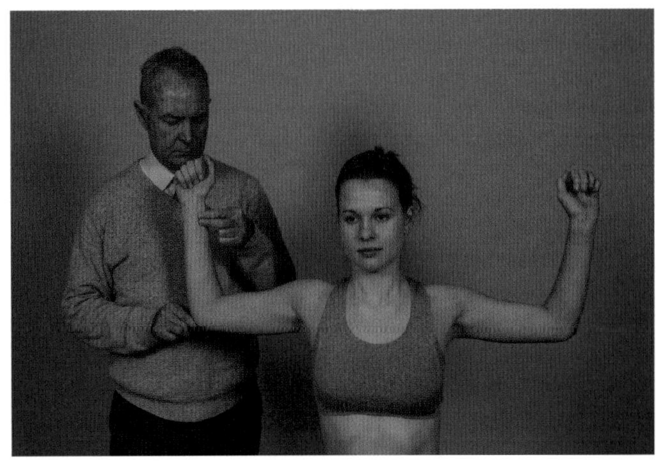

FIGURE 228-5 Roos test. (From Dutton D. *Dutton's Orthopaedic Examination, Evaluation, and Intervention*. 3rd ed. www.accessphysiotherapy.com. Copyright © The McGraw-Hill Companies, Inc. All rights reserved.)

IMPAIRMENTS

- Scapula depressed and downwardly rotated at rest
- Late, insufficient upward rotation of scapula during abduction and flexion of the glenohumeral (GH) joint
- Restricted GH abduction AROM, which inhibits reaching activities
- Decreased concentric strength of the periscapular musculature
- Decreased eccentric control of the periscapular musculature during adduction from a full GH abducted position
- Substitution of shoulder abduction with recruitment of levator scapulae (shrugging) for shoulder flexion greater than 120 degrees+
- Head of the humerus in an anterior position
- Reduced cervical spine AROM into ipsilateral rotation (scalenes are contralateral rotators of the cervical spine)

TEST AND MEASURES

- Adson or Scalene maneuver
- Elevated arm stress test (EAST) or hand-up test (overhead test)
- Provocative elevation test (passive shoulder shrug)
- Allen pectoralis minor test
- Halstead maneuver
- Hyperabduction maneuver (Wright test)
- Costoclavicular/military brace
- Disabilities of the Arm, Shoulder and Hand (DASH) score to assess physical function DASH
- Roos test
- Upper limb tension test
- Cervical spine compression test

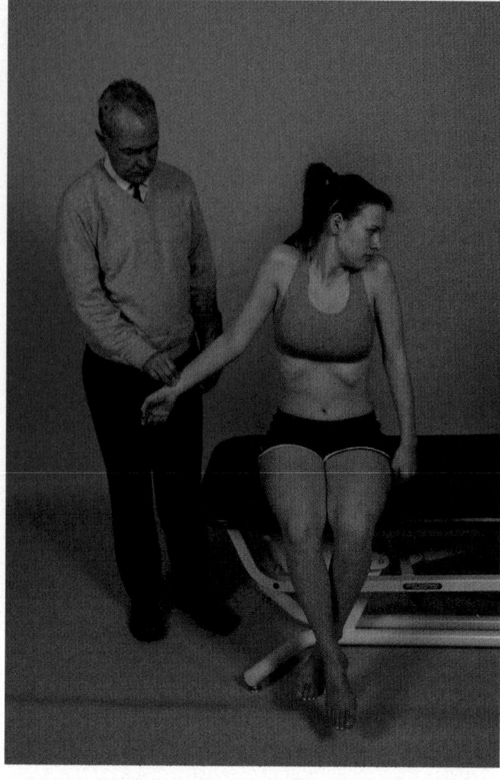

FIGURE 228-6 Hyperabduction maneuver (Wright Test). (From Dutton D. *Dutton's Orthopaedic Examination, Evaluation, and Intervention*. 3rd ed. www.accessphysiotherapy.com. Copyright © The McGraw-Hill Companies, Inc. All rights reserved.)

INTERVENTION

- Postural retraining: Scapula setting exercises, visual cues/postural awareness activities
- Kinesio taping of the shoulder girdle: The axillary sling assists the position of upward rotation of the scapula
- Strengthening of the periscapular musculature, especially the trapezius and serratus anterior
  - Thera-Band punch exercises
  - Open- and closed-chain shoulder stabilization exercises, prone on elbows with perturbation challenges
  - Seated rows, latissimus dorsi isotonic strengthening exercises
- Motor recruitment training of the upward rotators of the scapula—serratus anterior and upper trapezius
- Flexibility exercises: Pectorals and scalene musculature
- Address inflammation and pain: ice, heat, ultrasound, electric stimulation, cold laser
- Address muscle spasm of scalenes or pectoralis minor: Soft tissue
- Address instability of the GH joint if present: Posterior GH glides (to correct for anteriorly located head of the humerus), inferior GH glides (to assist in improvement of shoulder abduction and flexion ROM), and scapulothoracic glides
- Address cervical spine segmental mobility by performing cervical joint mobilizations
- First rib mobilization
- Nerve glides (once the referred pain has centralized)
- Address workplace ergonomics/reduce precipitating factors
- Education on proper sleeping and sitting positions

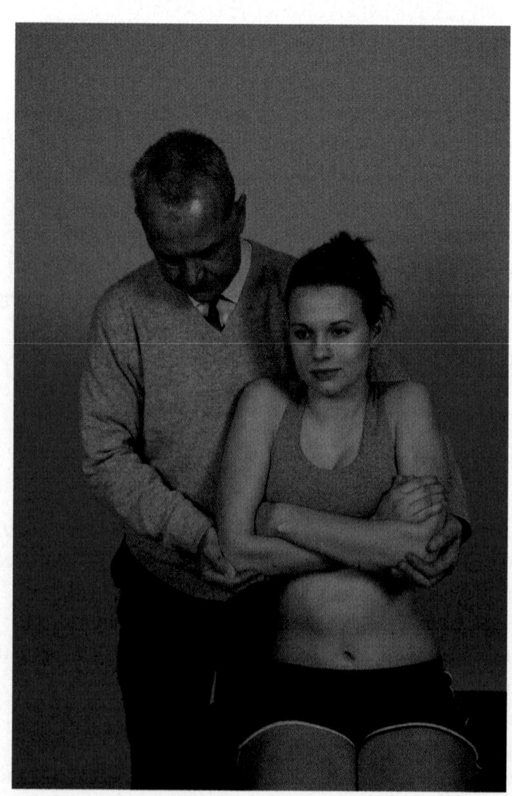

FIGURE 228-7 Passive shoulder shrug. (From Dutton D. *Dutton's Orthopaedic Examination, Evaluation, and Intervention*. 3rd ed. www.accessphysiotherapy.com. Copyright © The McGraw-Hill Companies, Inc. All rights reserved.)

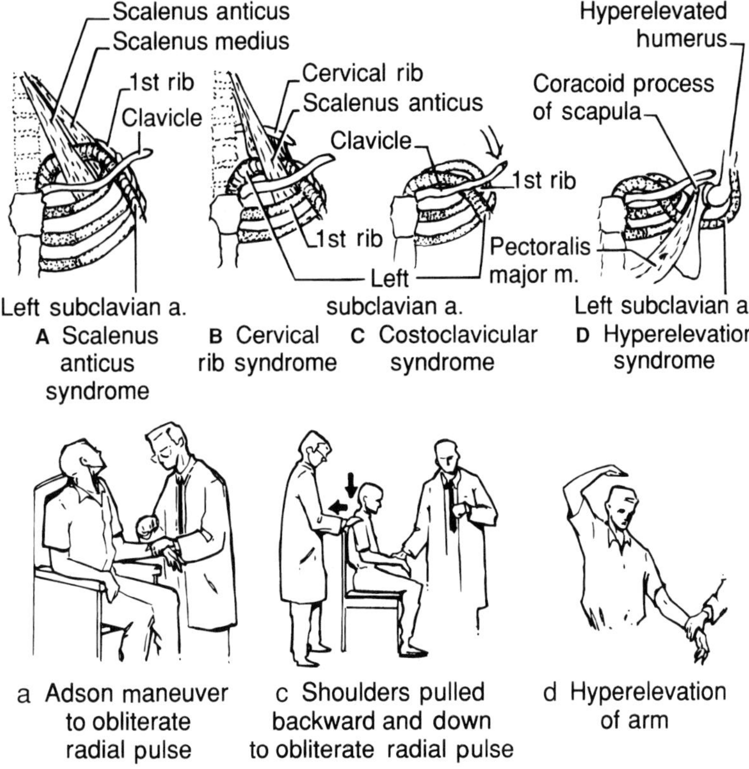

FIGURE 228-8 Compression syndromes of the superior thoracic aperture. (**A**) Scalenus anticus syndrome: The scalenus anticus muscle has attachments to the transverse processes of the cervical vertebrae above and below to the first rib. Posteriorly and behind the subclavian artery, the scalenus medius attaches to the same bones. Hypertrophy of the bellies of the two muscles causes compression of the artery between them, with motions such as turning the head to the ipsilateral side. This is tested by the Adson maneuver (a), where the patient sits with chin raised, head rotated to the left, and chest held in the inspiratory position. A positive test is marked by diminution or disappearance of the left radial pulse. The other side is tested similarly. (**B**) Cervical rib syndrome: The diagram shows a cervical rib compressing the left scalenus anticus muscle and indirectly the subclavian artery. This may produce diminution in the radial pulse or a peripheral neuritis of parts of the brachial plexus. (**C**) Costoclavicular syndrome: The geometry of the aperture may be such that rotation of the clavicles downward and backward compresses the subclavian arteries against the first rib. This is tested (c) by having the patient seated in a chair and the examiner standing behind him. The physician pushes the shoulders downward and backward while an assistant feels for diminution of the radial pulses. (**D**) Hyperelevation of the arm: The geometry of the thorax in some persons is such that hyperelevation of the arm causes the coracoid process of the scapula to impinge and compress the subclavian artery. This is tested by (d) demonstrating that the radial pulse is lost with hyperelevation. (From LeBlond RF, DeGowin RL, Brown DD. *DeGowin's Diagnostic Examination*. 9th ed. www.accessmedicine.com. Copyright © The McGraw-Hill Companies, Inc. All rights reserved.)

FUNCTIONAL GOALS

- Patient will be able to
  - Reach above head to obtain items out of the closet without substituting with shoulder shrugging 100% of the time.
  - Exhibit improved postural awareness while sitting at their workstation 100% of the time.
  - Sit at their computer workstation without precipitation of numbness and tingling down the involved UE for 60 minutes.
  - Dry and style their hair (grooming) without precipitation of numbness and tingling down the involved UE.
  - Sleep throughout the night without being awoken by pain.
  - Alternate holding a bag on either shoulder throughout the day 100% of the time (female).

PROGNOSIS

- Since muscles take approximately 6 to 8 weeks to hypertrophy, improved strength and control of the shoulder motions should be exhibited by this period of time at a minimum.
- Overall, 12 weeks of rehabilitation should be an appropriate amount of time for full strength and ROM gains as well as functional goal attainment.
- Since thoracic outlet syndrome is maintained by poor postural positions, maintenance and recurrence of this condition is possible if ergonomic factors and postural habits are not addressed.[9]

ADDITIONAL INFORMATION

- See Case Study: Neck Pain and Arm Paresthesia on www.AccessPhysiotherapy.com

PATIENT RESOURCE

- Thoracic Outlet Syndrome. American Academy of Orthopaedic Surgeons. http://orthoinfo.aaos.org/topic.cfm?topic=A00336. Accessed July 5, 2013.

REFERENCES

1. Leffert RD, Gumley G. The relationship between dead arm syndrome and thoracic outlet syndrome. *Clin Orthop Relat Res.* 1987;39:1070–1145.
2. Dubuisson AS. Thoracic Outlet Syndrome. Louisiana State University School of Medicine. http://www.medschool.lsuhsc.edu/neurosurgery/nervecenter/TOS.html. Accessed July 12, 2013.

3. Stapleton C, Herrington L, George K. Sonographic evaluation of the subclavian artery during thoracic outlet syndrome shoulder manoeuvres. *Man Ther.* 2009;14(1):19–27. doi:10.1016/j.math.2007.07.010.
4. Watson LA, Pizzari T, Balster S. Thoracic outlet syndrome part 1: clinical manifestations, differentiation and treatment pathways. *Man Ther.* 2009;14(6):586–595. doi:10.1016/j.math.2009.08.007.
5. Watson LA, Pizzari T, Balster S. Thoracic outlet syndrome part 2: conservative management of thoracic outlet. *Man Ther.* 2010;15(4):305–314. doi:10.1016/j.math.2010.03.002.
6. Brantigan CO, Roos DB. Diagnosing thoracic outlet syndrome. *Hand Clin.* 2004;20(1):27–36.
7. Mackinnon SE, Novak CB. Thoracic outlet syndrome. *Curr Probl Surg.* 2002;39:1070–1145. doi:10.1067/msg.2002.127926.
8. Magee DJ. *Orthopedic Physical Assessment.* 5th ed. St. Louis, MO: Saunders Elsevier; 2008:6.
9. Fugate MW, Rotellini-Coltvet L, Freischlag JA. Current management of thoracic outlet syndrome. *Cur Treat Options Cardiovasc Med.* 2009;11(2):176–183.
10. Pitz CC, de la Riviere AB, van Swieten HA, Duurkens VA, Lammers JW, Van den Bosch JM. Surgical treatment of Pancoast tumours. *Eur J Cardiothorac Surg.* 2004;26(1): 202–208. doi:10.1016/j.math.2007.07.010.

ADDITIONAL REFERENCES

- Demondion X, Herbinet P, Van Sint Jan S, Boutry N, Chantelot C, Cotten A. Imaging assessment of thoracic outlet syndrome. *Radiographics.* 2006;26(6):1735–1750. doi: 10.1148/rg.266055079.
- Dutton M, ed. *McGraw-Hill's NPTE (National Physical Therapy Examination).* 2nd ed. New York, NY: McGraw-Hill; 2012. http://www.accessphysiotherapy.com/resource/611. Accessed July 12, 2013.
- Dutton M, ed. *Orthopaedic Examination, Evaluation, and Intervention.* 2nd ed. New York, NY: McGraw-Hill; 2008. http://www.accessphysiotherapy.com/resource/612. Accessed July 12, 2013.
- Dutton M. The Cervical complex. In: Dutton M, ed. *Dutton's Orthopedic Survival Guide: Managing Common Conditions.* New York, NY: McGraw-Hill; 2011:Chapter 11. http://www.accessphysiotherapy.com/content/8656027. Accessed July 12, 2013.
- ICD9Data.com. http://www.icd9data.com. Accessed July 7, 2013.
- ICD10Data.com. http://www.icd10data.com/ICD10CM/Codes. Accessed July 3, 2013.
- Pattern 4E:impaired joint mobility, motor function, muscle performance, and range of motion associated with localized inflammation. In: *Guide to Physical Therapist Practice.* 2nd ed. Alexandria, VA: American Physical Therapy Association; 2001. Revised 2003.
- Prentice WE, Quillen WS, Underwood F, eds. *Therapeutic Modalities in Rehabilitation.* 4th ed. New York, NY: McGraw-Hill; 2011. http://www.accessphysiotherapy.com/resource/675. Accessed July 12, 2013.

229 ULNAR NERVE PATHOLOGY

Matthew L. Daugherty, DPT, OTR/L, MOT, MTC, OCS, FAAOMPT
Eric Shamus, PhD, DPT, PT, CSCS

CONDITION/DISORDER SYNONYMS

- Cubital tunnel syndrome
- Cyclists palsy
- Medial neuritis syndrome
- Tardy ulnar nerve palsy
- Ulnar nerve entrapment
- Ulnar tunnel syndrome (UTS)

ICD-9-CM CODES

- 354.2 Lesion of ulnar nerve
- 354.5 Mononeuritis multiplex
- 955.2 Injury ulnar nerve

ICD-10-CM CODE

- G56.20 Lesion of ulnar nerve, unspecified upper limb

PREFERRED PRACTICE PATTERN

- 5F: Impaired Peripheral Nerve Integrity and Muscle Performance Associated with Peripheral Nerve Injury

PATIENT PRESENTATION

A 14-year-old female comes to clinic reporting sharp and aching pain in the right medial aspect of her elbow, which also radiates to her mid humerus medially and distally. This began 2 weeks ago and appears to be getting worse. She even has symptoms that wake her at night. She reports numbness and tingling that radiates into her little finger and ulnar half of ring finger. Functionally she noticed that her grip is slightly weak especially when it includes her small finger such as opening a jar and feels an overall clumsiness when using her hand.

She believes that this began as a result of her learning to play the acoustic guitar 4 weeks ago. She reports that her symptoms are worse with strumming the guitar or even resting her right arm on the edge of the guitar. Clinically, she presents with hypoalgesia of digit V and ulnar half of IV. Her opponens digiti minimi, flexor digiti minimi and interossei are exhibiting 4-/5 strength. She has a positive percussion test (Tinel's) over the ulnar nerve at the cubital tunnel, positive elbow flexion test, and reproduction of distal symptoms when performing neurodynamic testing.

KEY FEATURES

Description

- Motor and/or sensory changes in the ulnar nerve distribution due to pressure from three possible ways
  - Compression
  - Stretch
  - Friction
- Potential entrapment sites
  - Medial humeral groove
  - Arcade of Struthers
  - Medial intermuscular septum
  - Flexor digitorum profundus (FDP)
  - Flexor carpi ulnaris (FCU)
  - Just proximal to or within Guyon canal
  - Sensory and motor involvement between the abductor digiti minimi and flexor digiti minimi
  - Near hook of hamate, involves motor only
  - Distal end of Guyon canal, involves sensory only

Essentials of Diagnosis

- Night pain
- Sensory changes on volar aspect of digit V and ulnar aspect of digit IV
- Hand clumsiness and/or weakness
- Symptom changes with elbow position and/or pressure over the cubital tunnel
- Reproduction of symptoms during clinical examination

General Considerations

- Need to differentiate from more proximal and distal ulnar nerve compression, thoracic outlet syndrome (TOS), ulnar tunnel, and cervical radiculopathy
- Postoperative therapy depends on surgical procedure performed: Endoscopic release, in situ decompression, medial epicondylectomy, and anterior transposition
- Second-most common nerve compression syndrome in the upper extremity (UE)

Demographics

- Those who work for sustained periods with power tools or on computers

CLINICAL FINDINGS

SIGNS AND SYMPTOMS

- Acute or chronic paresthesia in ulnar nerve distribution (digits IV ulnar half and V) dorsally and volarly
- Sensory changes, hypo- or hypersensitivity of hand
- Night pain especially with elbow flexion and wrist extension
- Inability to separate fingers
- Hand clumsiness
- Hand weakness and loss of grip power and dexterity
- Clawing of the hand (less pronounced than with UTS)[1]
- Intrinsic muscle atrophy and possible guttering
- Wartenberg sign
- Froment sign
- Bishops deformity
- Positive elbow flexion test
- Resting abduction of digit V

Functional Implications

- Night pain/poor sleep habits
- Difficulty with hand function during ADLs/IADLs due to hand clumsiness and possible loss of strength

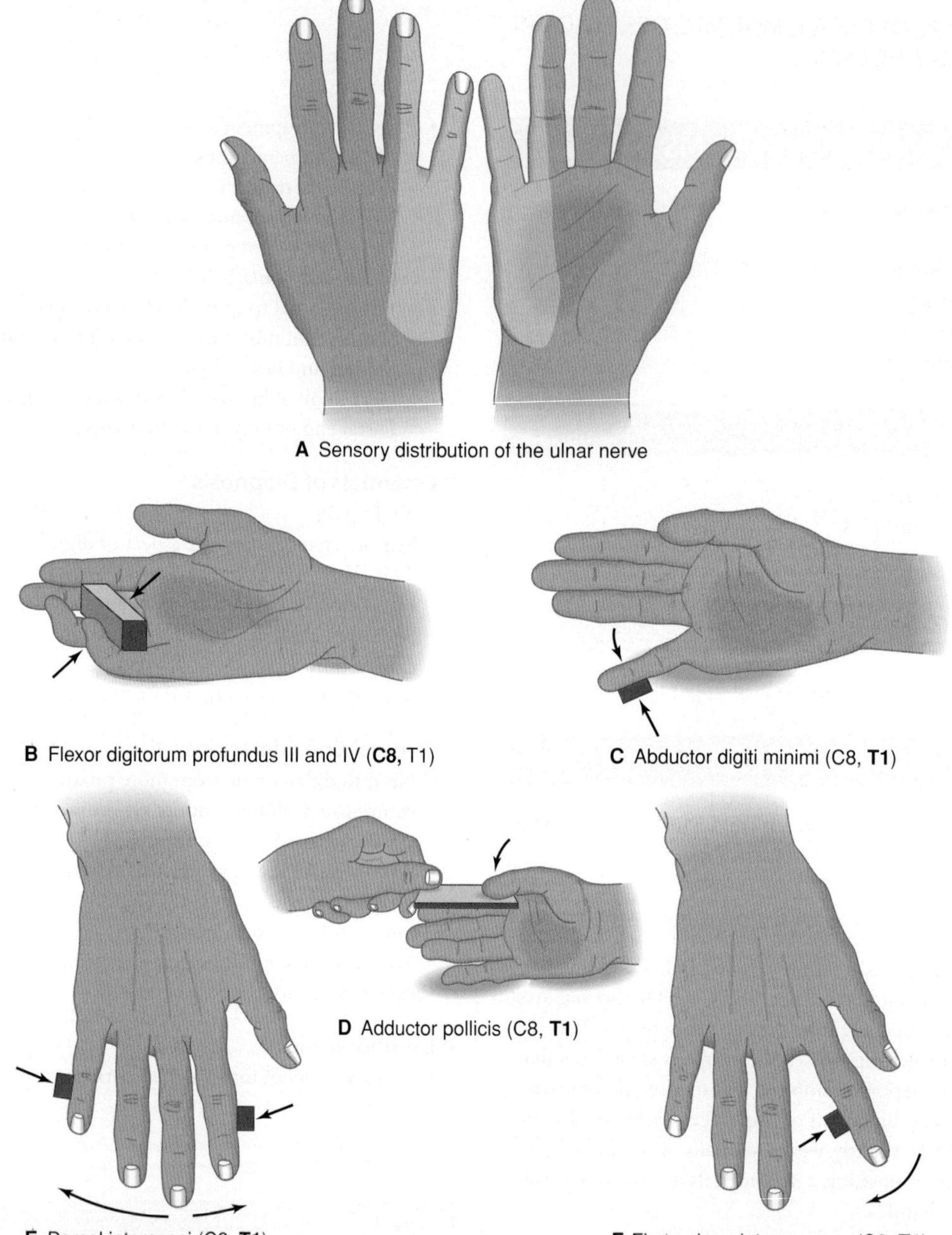

FIGURE 229-1 Testing the ulnar nerve. (**A**) Sensory distribution. The ulnar nerve supplies the dorsal and palmar surfaces of the medial one-third of the hand, the dorsal and palmar surfaces of the little finger, and the dorsal and palmar surfaces of the medial half of the ring finger. (**B**) Flexor digitorum profundus III and IV. The index and middle fingers are flexed at the distal interphalangeal joints against resistance. (**C**) Abductor digiti minimi. The little finger is abducted against resistance. (**D**) Adductor pollicis. A piece of paper is grasped between the thumb and the palm with the thumbnail at 90 degrees to the plane of the palm while the examiner tries to pull the paper away. (**E**) Dorsal interossei. The fingers are abducted against resistance. (**F**) First palmar interosseous. The abducted index finger is adducted against resistance. (From Greenberg DA, Aminoff MJ, Simon RP. *Clinical Neurology*. 8th ed. www.accessmedicine.com. Copyright © The McGraw-Hill Companies, Inc. All rights reserved.)

Possible Contributing Causes

- Prolonged pressure on cubital tunnel, particularly with elbow flexion such as working at a computer[2]
- Laxity of soft tissue structures that hold ulnar nerve in cubital tunnel
- Bony abnormality of the humerus
  - Shallow ulnar groove
  - Small medial condyle
- Tightness of the FCU with distal FCU inflammation
- Viral infection
- Ganglion/space occupying lesion
- Ulnar artery thrombosis
- Ulnar-sided wrist fractures or dislocations
- Anomalous muscles
- Repetitive trauma
- Sustained pressure over Guyon canal such as resting hypothenar eminence on handlebars while long distance cycling

Differential Diagnosis

- TOS
- Cervical radiculopathy
- Radial neuropathy
- Median neuropathy
- Carpal tunnel syndrome
- Proximal ulnar nerve entrapment
- Distal ulnar nerve entrapment cubital tunnel (Guyon canal)

MEANS OF CONFIRMATION OR DIAGNOSIS

Diagnostic Procedure

- Electrodiagnostic testing
  - Loss of evoked sensory potential
  - Decreased electrical velocities across elbow <50 m/sec
  - Electromyographic (EMG): Conduction velocities of ulnar innervated muscles <41 m/sec
- Roentgenographic studies
  - Measure degree of cubitus valgus or assess bony lesions that compromise the cubital tunnel

Imaging

- Diagnostic ultrasound (ultrasonography)
  - Allows for dynamic imaging during elbow flexion
  - Enlargement of ulnar nerve at entrapment site

FINDINGS AND INTERPRETATION

- Muscle weakness of[2]
  - FCU
  - Ulnar side of FDP
  - Abductor digiti minimi
  - Palmar and dorsal interossei
  - Intrinsic-interossei
  - Lumbricles
- Sensory changes in ulnar nerve distribution of the hand, particularly volarly

TREATMENT

Medication

- NSAIDs
- Corticosteroid injection

REFERRALS/ADMITTANCE

- Surgical consult if symptoms include intrinsic muscle atrophy and symptoms occur for longer than 1 year
- Physician or osteopath for oral anti-inflammatory, or steroidal injections
- Physician or osteopath to order diagnostic tests if warranted and depending on PT's area of practice

IMPAIRMENTS

- Inability to perform overhead activities, such as in swimming, baseball, or tennis
- Inability to perform jobs involving repetitive overhead reaching or lifting

TESTS AND MEASURES

- Disabilities of the Arm, Shoulder and Hand (DASH) score to assess physical function

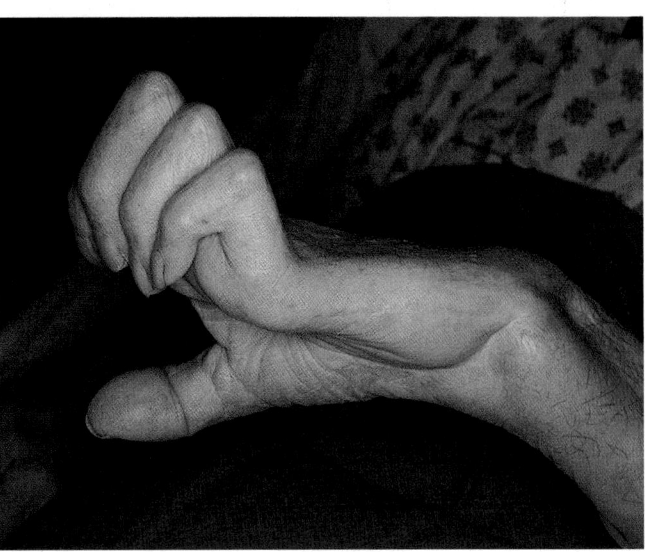

FIGURE 229-2 Claw Hand. Claw-hand appearance resulting from median and ulnar nerve injury. Note metacarpophalangeal joint hyperextension. (From Knoop KJ, Stack LB, Storrow AB, Thurman RJ. *The Atlas of Emergency Medicine*. 3rd ed. http://www.accessmedicine.com. Copyright © The McGraw-Hill Companies, Inc. All rights reserved. Photo contributor: Daniel L. Savitt, MD.)

- Froment sign
- Functional reach test
- Upper limb tension test
- Cervical spine compression test
- Pain provocation test
- Shoulder pain and disability index

INTERVENTION

- Myofascial manipulation
- Elbow orthoses and protection
- Neural mobilization
- Activity modification/ergonomic intervention
- Stretching of FCU
- Postoperative management includes:
  - Protected ROM
  - Neural mobilization
  - Scar management
  - Sensory desensitization
  - Activity modification

FUNCTIONAL GOALS

- Patient will
  - Return to full use of affected UE with ADLs and IADLs, such as washing dishes and cooking.
  - Return to normal activities of daily living (NADLs) without signs/symptoms.
  - Perform typing for 1 hour for work.

PROGNOSIS

- Prognosis is dependent on duration of symptoms and motor involvement.
- Patients with mild electrodiagnostic findings, intermittent symptoms, and no atrophy may respond well to conservative management.
- Potential for full motor recovery after surgery is greatly reduced in patients for whom preoperative symptoms were present for more than 1 year or who have intrinsic muscle atrophy before surgery.

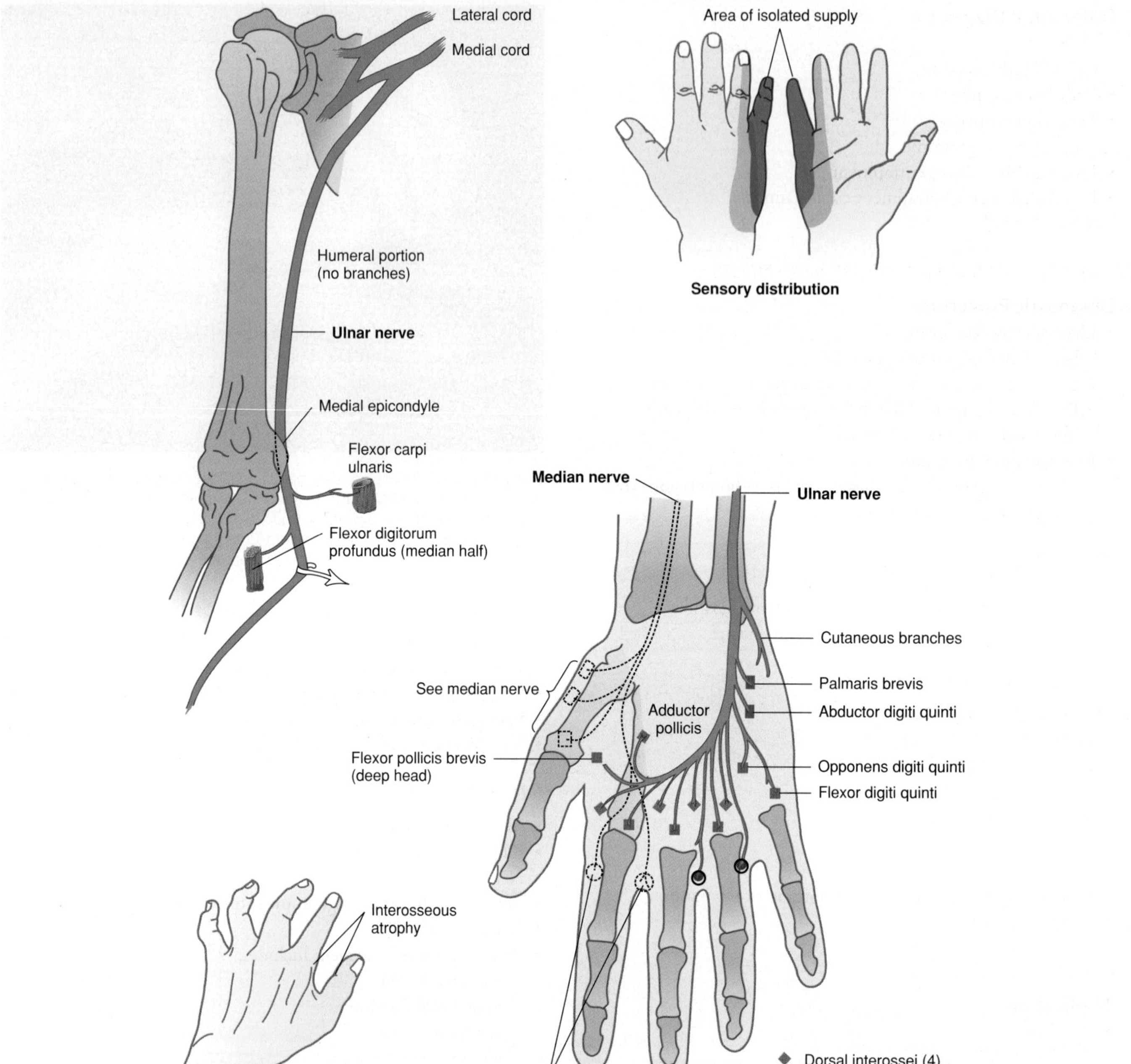

Lateral cord
Medial cord
Humeral portion (no branches)
Ulnar nerve
Medial epicondyle
Flexor carpi ulnaris
Flexor digitorum profundus (median half)
Area of isolated supply
Sensory distribution
Median nerve
Ulnar nerve
Cutaneous branches
Palmaris brevis
Abductor digiti quinti
See median nerve
Adductor pollicis
Flexor pollicis brevis (deep head)
Opponens digiti quinti
Flexor digiti quinti
Interosseous atrophy
Clawhand deformity in ulnar lesions
See median nerve
◆ Dorsal interossei (4)
■ Palmar interossei (3)
● Ulnar lumbricales (2)

FIGURE 229-3 The ulnar nerve (C8, T1). (From Waxman SG. *Clinical Neuroanatomy*. 26th ed. www.accessmedicine.com. Copyright © The McGraw-Hill Companies, Inc. All rights reserved.)

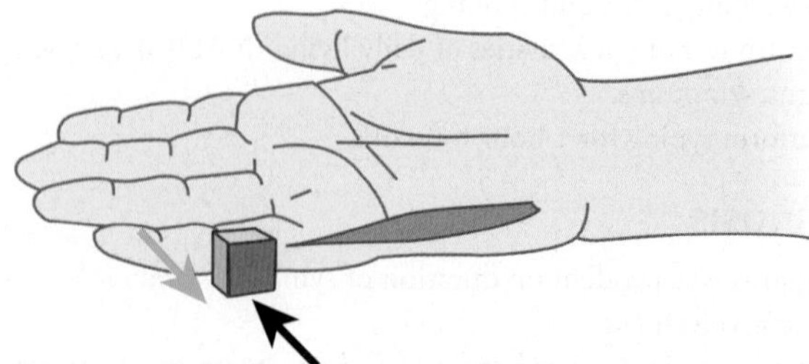

FIGURE 229-4 Abductor digiti quinti (C8, T1; ulnar nerve). The little finger is abducted against resistance as the supinated hand with fingers extended lies on the table. (From Waxman SG. *Clinical Neuroanatomy*. 26th ed. www.accessmedicine.com. Copyright © The McGraw-Hill Companies, Inc. All rights reserved.)

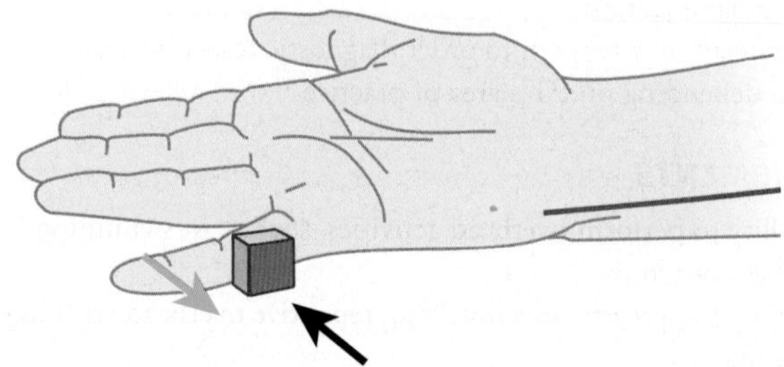

FIGURE 229-5 Flexor carpi ulnaris (C7, 8; T1; ulnar nerve). The little finger is abducted strongly against resistance as the supinated hand lies with fingers extended on the table. (From Waxman SG. *Clinical Neuroanatomy*. 26th ed. www.accessmedicine.com. Copyright © The McGraw-Hill Companies, Inc. All rights reserved.)

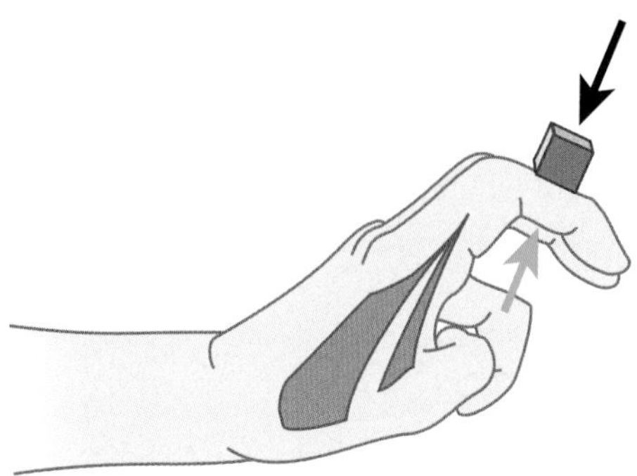

FIGURE 229-6 Lumbricals-interossei, radial half (C8, T1; median and ulnar nerves). The second and third phalanges are extended against resistance; the first phalanx is in full extension. The ulnar has the same innervation and can be tested in the same manner. (From Waxman SG. *Clinical Neuroanatomy*. 26th ed. www.accessmedicine.com. Copyright © The McGraw-Hill Companies, Inc. All rights reserved.)

PATIENT RESOURCE

- Ulnar Nerve Dysfunction. *MedlinePlus*. NIH National Institutes of Health. http://www.nlm.nih.gov/medlineplus/ency/article/000789.htm. Accessed July 14, 2013.

REFERENCES

1. Preston D, Shapiro B. Electromyography and neuromuscular disorders. In: *Clinical Electrophysiologic Correlations*. Boston, MA: Butterworth-Heinemann; 1998.
2. Dutton M. The elbow complex. In: Dutton M, ed. *Orthopaedic Examination, Evaluation, and Intervention*. 2nd ed. New York, NY: McGraw-Hill; 2008:Chapter 15. http://www.accessphysiotherapy.com/content/55575512. Accessed July 14, 2013.

ADDITIONAL REFERENCES

- Dutton M. The forearm, wrist, and hand. In: Dutton M, ed. *Dutton's Orthopedic Survival Guide: Managing Common Conditions*. New York, NY: McGraw-Hill; 2011:Chapter 7. http://www.accessphysiotherapy.com/content/8653078. Accessed August 16, 2014.
- Dutton M. The forearm, wrist, and hand. In: Dutton M, ed. *Orthopaedic Examination, Evaluation, and Intervention*. 2nd ed. New York, NY: McGraw-Hill; 2008:Chapter 16. http://www.accessphysiotherapy.com/content/55577336. Accessed August 16, 2014.
- Dutton M. Integumentary physical therapy. In: Dutton M, ed. *McGraw-Hill's NPTE (National Physical Therapy Examination)*. 2nd ed. New York, NY: McGraw-Hill; 2012:Chapter 13. http://www.accessphysiotherapy.com/content/5402978. Accessed August 16, 2014.

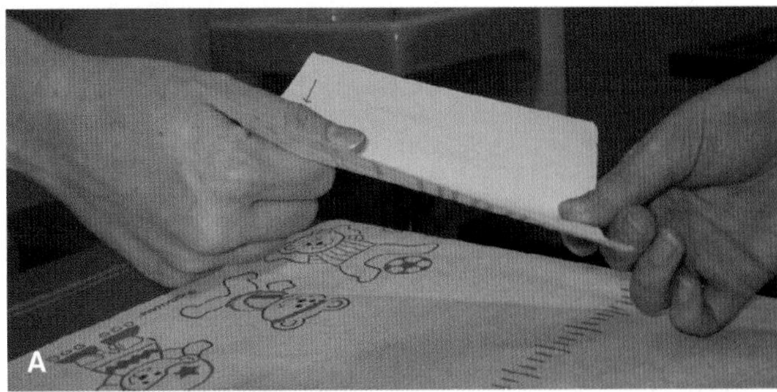

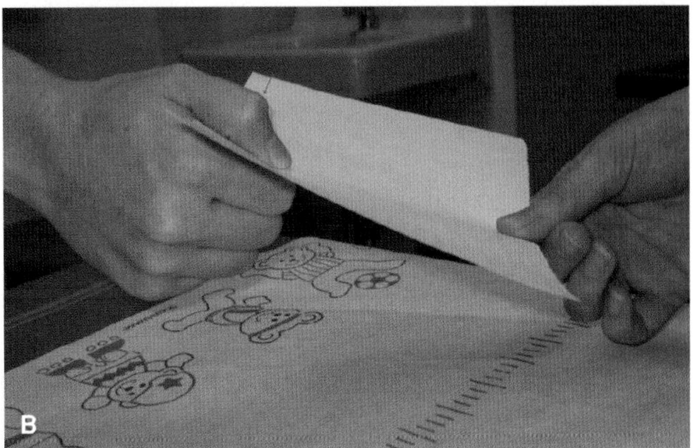

FIGURE 229-7 Froment sign. When the adductors of the thumb are weak, the thumb interphalangeal joint flexes trying to hold on to the paper as shown. (From Patel DR, Greydanus DE, Baker RJ. *Pediatric Practice: Sports Medicine*. www.accesspediatrics.com. Copyright © The McGraw-Hill Companies, Inc. All rights reserved.)

- Giladi AM, Gaston RG, Haase SC, et al; Surgery of the Ulnar Nerve Study Group. Trend of recovery after simple decompression for treatment of ulnar neuropathy at the elbow. *Plast Reconstr Surg*. 2013;131(4):563e–573e. doi: 10.1097/PRS.0b013e318282764f.
- ICD9Data.com. http://www.icd9data.com. Accessed August 16, 2014.
- ICD10Data.com. http://www.icd10data.com/ICD10CM/Codes. Accessed August 16, 2014.
- Landau ME, Campbell WW. Clinical features and electrodiagnosis of ulnar neuropathies. *Phys Med Rehabil Clin N Am*. 2013;24(1):49–66. doi: 10.1016/j.pmr.2012.08.019.
- Prentice WE. Biofeedback. In: Prentice WE, Quillen WS, Underwood F, eds. *Therapeutic Modalities in Rehabilitation*. 4th ed. New York, NY: McGraw-Hill; 2011:Chapter 7. http://www.accessphysiotherapy.com/content/8137179. Accessed August 16, 2014.
- Werner RA. Electrodiagnostic evaluation of carpal tunnel syndrome and ulnar neuropathies. *PMR*. 2013;5(5 Suppl):S14–S21. doi: 10.1016/j.pmrj.2013.03.027. Epub 2013 Mar 28.

PART 5

PEDIATRIC DISORDERS

230 ARTHROGRYPOSIS

Kay Tasso, PhD, PT, PCS
Martha Henao Bloyer, DPT, PT, PCS

CONDITION/DISORDER SYNONYMS

- Arthrogryposis multiplex congenital (AMC)
- Amyoplasia
- Classic arthrogryposis

ICD-9-CM CODES

- 728.3 Other specific muscle disorders
- 754.89 Arthrogryposis multiplex congenita

ICD-10-CM CODE

- Q74.3 Arthrogryposis multiplex congenita

PREFERRED PRACTICE PATTERNS[1]

- 4A: Primary Prevention/Risk Reduction for Skeletal Demineralization
- 5B: Impaired Neuromotor Development

PATIENT PRESENTATION

A 2-year-old female child is referred to outpatient physical therapy with a diagnosis of arthrogryposis multiplex congenital—myopathtic type. The past medical history includes the following: no familial history of arthrogryposis and an uneventful pregnancy of her mother but the mother reports experiencing decreased fetal movements at about 26 weeks gestation. The infant was born via C-section at 36 weeks gestation with bilateral equinovarus, knee extension contractures, dislocated right hip, bilateral shoulder ankylosis, bilateral elbow flexion, wrist flexion contractures, and ulnar deviation. Surgical history includes: club feet corrected at one month of age, knees and hips corrected at 5 months of age, right elbow corrected into extension. The shoulders and wrists have not been surgically corrected and the left elbow remains in flexion.

Upon examination, the child exhibits delays in gross and fine motor areas, and is dependent for transfers in and out of adaptive stroller. She is unable to stand, has decreased strength and endurance in her lower extremities for functional activities, and decreased active range of motion at hips and knees. She has sufficient passive knees and hips range of motion to allow sit independently in a child sized chair. The child can roll from supine to prone and can assume long sitting independently from supine.

The general therapy goal is to facilitate and promote independent function and mobility.

KEY FEATURES

Description

- Term used to describe two or more congenital non-progressive, joint contractures[2]

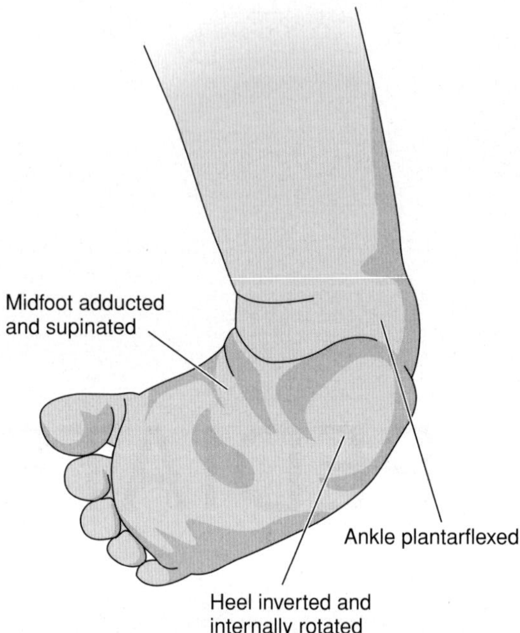

FIGURE 230-1 Clinical appearance of congenital right clubfoot. (From Skinner HB. *Current Diagnosis & Treatment in Orthopedics.* 4th ed. www.accessmedicine.com.)

Essentials of Diagnosis

- Comprises over 300 different disorders

General Considerations

- Types
  - Myopathic: Fixed flexion contractures of joints, chest, and spine
    - Amyoplasia: most common
  - Neuropathic: Fixed contractures
  - Distal
- Categorization based on presence of disorders
  - mainly limb involvement
  - limb involvement plus other body area(s)
  - limb involvement and central nervous system dysfunction
- Affects joints bilaterally
- Distal joints more often involved than proximal joints

Demographics

- 1 in 3000 to 5100 infants[3]
- X-linked recessive origin primarily affects males[3]

CLINICAL FINDINGS

SIGNS AND SYMPTOMS

- Limited range of motion of joints including temporomandibular joint
- Muscle weakness
- Scoliosis
- Craniofacial malformations
- Cardiac, respiratory, or organ anomalies

Functional Implications

- Limits functional mobility
- Developmental delay

Possible Contributing Causes

- Prader–Willi Syndrome[4]
- Amyoplasia (focal arthrogryposis) [4]
- Neonatal neuropathy[4]
- Congenital myopathy[4]
- Congenital muscular dystrophy[4]
- Congenital myasthenia[4]
- Myotonic dystrophy[4]
- Werdnig–Hoffmann motor neuron disease[4]
- Oligohydramnios
- Neuromuscular disorder
- Fetal hyperthermia
- Fetal intrauterine crowding
- Prenatal virus
- Fetal vascular compromise
- Abnormality of connective tissue
- Maternal infection or illness

Differential Diagnosis

- Metabolic disease
- Muscular dystrophy

MEANS OF CONFIRMATION OR DIAGNOSIS

Laboratory Tests

- CPK levels

Imaging

- Computerized tomography (CT)
- Magnetic resonance imaging (MRI)
- Radiograph of bony deformities
- Electromyelogram
- Fetal ultrasound

Diagnostic Procedures

- Muscle biopsy
- Electromyography
- Nerve conduction velocity

FINDINGS AND INTERPRETATION

Medical Procedures

- Osteotomy
- Tenotomy
- Serial casting

REFERRALS/ADMITTANCE

- Admission for surgical correction
- To orthopedist
- To neurologist
- To geneticist
- To orthotist
- To ophthalmologist
- To occupational therapist
- To speech therapist
- To social Worker
- To counseling services

IMPAIRMENTS

- Decreased passive and/or active range of motion
- Decreased strength
- Inability to transfer independently
- Inability to sit independently
- Inability to stand independently
- Inability to roll
- Inability to walk independently
- Decreased independent with ADLs—eating, dressing, toileting

TESTS AND MEASURES

- Goniometer
- Manual muscle test
- Dynamometer
- Bayley Scales of Motor Development or Bayley II
- Peabody Scales of Motor Development

INTERVENTION

- Low load, prolonged stretching[2]
- Positioning
- Strengthening
- Balance and coordination
- Passive range of motion
- Splinting
- Developmental activities
- Assistive devices/technology
- Family education

FUNCTIONAL GOALS

- Patient will be able to
  - Increase passive knee flexion to 90 degrees for play in quadruped position within 3 months.
  - Increase quadriceps knee strength to 4/5 for sit-to-stand transfers within 6 months.
  - Ambulate 25 feet with platform rolling walker with stand-by assistance within 4 months.

PROGNOSIS

- 50% die within first year when central nervous system and extremities involved.[4]

PATIENT RESOURCES

- Arthrogryposis. www.arthrogryposis.net. Accessed June 17, 2013.
- Arthrogryposis Multiplex Congenita. NORD web site. http://rarediseases.org/rare-disease-information/rare-diseases/byID/211/viewAbstract. Accessed June 17, 2013.
- Arthrogryposis. Medscape web site. http://emedicine.medscape.com/article/941917-overview#a0199. Accessed June 17, 2013.

REFERENCES

1. The American Physical Therapy Association. *Interactive Guide to Physical Therapist Practice*. Alexandria, VA: The American Physical Therapy Association; 2003. http://guidetoptpractice.apta.org. Accessed June 17, 2013.
2. Dutton M. Congenital orthopaedic conditions. In: Dutton M, ed. *Dutton's Orthopaedic Examination, Evaluation, and Intervention.*

3rd ed. New York, NY: McGraw-Hill; 2012. http://www.accessphysiotherapy.com/content/56557447. Accessed June 17, 2013.

3. Eriksson M, Gutierrez-Farewik EM, Broström E, Bartonek A. Gait in children with arthrogryposis multiplex congenital. *J Child Orthop*. 2010;4(1):21–31. http://www.ncbi.nlm.nih.gov/pmc/articles/PMC2811679. Accessed June 17, 2013.
4. Ropper AH, Samuels MA. The congenital neuromuscular disorders. In: Ropper AH, Samuels MA, eds. *Adams and Victor's Principles of Neurology*. 9th ed. New York, NY: McGraw-Hill; 2009:Chapter 52. http://www.accessmedicine.com/content.aspx?aID=3642761. Accessed June 17, 2013.

ADDITIONAL REFERENCES

- Bamshad M, Van Heest AE, Pleasure D. Arthrogryposis: a review and update. *J Bone Joint Surg Am*. 2009;91(Suppl 4):40–46. doi: 10.2106/JBJS.I.00281.
- Bernard TJ, Knupp K, Yang ML, Arndt D, Levisohn P, Moe PG. Neurologic & muscular disorders. In: Hay WW, Levin MJ, Sondheimer JM, Deterding RR. eds. *CURRENT Diagnosis & Treatment: Pediatrics*. 20th ed. New York, NY: McGraw-Hill; 2011. http://www.accessphysiotherapy.com/content/6585071. Accessed June 17, 2013.
- Dane B, Dane C, Aksoy F, et al. Arthrogryposis multiplex congenita: analysis of twelve cases. *Clin Exp Obstet Gyneco*. 2009; 36(4):259–262.
- Dutton M. Pediatric physical therapy. In: *McGraw Hill's National Physical Therapy Examination*. 2nd ed. New York, NY: McGraw-Hill; 2012. http://www.accessphysiotherapy.com/content/5404415#5404415. Accessed June 17, 2013.
- Fetal Ultrasound. Mayo Clinic web site. http://www.mayoclinic.com/health/fetal-ultrasound/MY00777. Accessed January 28, 2013.
- ICD9DATA. http://www.icd9data.com/2013/Volume1/710-739/725-729/728/728.3.htm. Accessed June 17, 2013.
- ICD10DATA. http://www.icd10data.com/Search.aspx?search=arthrogryposis&codebook=AllCodes. Accessed June 17, 2013.
- Staheli LT, Hall JG, Jaffe KM, Paholke DO. *Arthrogryposis, A Text Atlas*. Cambridge University Press; 1998. http://www.global-help.org/publications/books/book_arthrogryposis.html. Accessed June 17, 2013.
- Suryawanshi C, Panditrao MM, Rai I. Arthrogryposis multiplex congenita–a rare congenital anomaly. *J Indian Med Assoc*. 2006;104(2):95–96,98.
- Vreeman LI, Long T, Habib ZH. Musculoskeletal developmental disorders. In: Magee DJ, Zachazewski JE, Quillen WS, eds. *Pathology and Intervention in Musculoskeletal Rehabilitation*. St. Louis, MO: Saunders; 2009:750–780.

231 AUTISM SPECTRUM DISORDER

Kay Tasso, PhD, PT, PCS

CONDITION/DISORDER SYNONYMS

- Autism
- Early infantile autism
- Childhood autism
- Kanner's autism
- Pervasive developmental disorder, not otherwise specified (PDD-NOS)

ICD-9-CM CODES[1]

- 299 Pervasive developmental disorders
- 299.0 Autistic disorder
- 299.00 Autistic disorder current or active state
- 299.01 Autistic disorder residual state
- 299.9 Unspecified pervasive developmental disorder
- 299.90 Unspecified pervasive developmental disorder current or active state
- 299.91 Unspecified pervasive developmental disorder residual state

ICD-10-CM CODES[2]

- F84.0 Autistic disorder
- F84.9 Pervasive developmental disorder unspecified
- F84.5 Asperger syndrome
- F84.8 Other pervasive developmental disorders
- F84.9 Pervasive developmental disorder, unspecified

PREFERRED PRACTICE PATTERN

- 5B: Impaired Neuromotor Development[3]

TABLE 231-1 Differential Diagnostic Features of Autism and Nonautistic Pervasive Developmental Disorders

Feature	Autistic Disorder	Asperger's Syndrome	Rett Syndrome	Pervasive Developmental Disorder NOS[a]
Age at recognition (months)	0–36	Usually >36	5–30	Variable
Sex ratio	M > F	M > F	F >> M	M > F
Loss of skills after initial mastery	Variable	Usually not	Marked	Usually not
Social skills	Very poor	Poor	Vary with stage	Variable
Communication skills	Usually poor	Fair	Very poor	Fair to good
Circumscribed interests	Variable (mechanical)	Marked (facts)	NA	Variable
Eye contact	Very poor	Variable	Varies with stage	Variable
Family history of similar problems	Sometimes	Frequent	Not usually	Unknown
Seizure disorder	Common	Uncommon	Frequent	Uncommon
Head growth decelerates	No	No	Yes	No
IQ range	Severe MR to normal	Mild MR to normal	Severe MR	Severe MR to normal
Outcome	Poor to good	Fair to good	Very poor	Fair to good

F, female; IQ, intelligence quotient; M, male; MR, mental retardation; NA, not applicable; NOS, not otherwise specified.
[a]Impairments are not as severe as in autism.
Source: From DiPiro JL, Talbert RL, Yee GC, Matzke GR, Wells BG, Posey LM (eds): *Pharmacotherapy: A Pathophysiologic Approach.* New York, McGraw-Hill Education, 2014. Data from American Psychiatric Association. *Diagnostic and Statistical Manual of Mental Disorders,* 4th ed., Text Revision. Washington, DC, American Psychiatric Association, 2000; Johnson CP, Myers SM. Identification and evaluation of children with autism spectrum disorders. Pediatrics 2007;120:1183-1215; Filipek PA, Accardo PJ, Baranek GT. The screening and diagnosis of autistic spectrum disorders. J Autism Dev Disord 1999;29:439-484; Baird G, Cass H, Slonims V. Diagnosis of autism. BMJ 2003;327:488-493; Chawarska K, Volkmar FR. Autism in infancy and early childhood. In: Volkmar FR, Paul R, Klin A, Cohen DJ, eds. *Handbook of Autism and Pervasive Developmental Disorders.* 3rd ed. Hoboken, N.J.: John Wiley and Sons, Inc.; 2005:223-246.

PATIENT PRESENTATION

A 3-year-old male is referred to physical therapy for poor coordination. His mother reports he was born full term via vaginal delivery with no difficulty with pregnancy or delivery. As an infant, he seldom made eye contact and disliked being held. His mother states "I don't think he likes me." He learned to sit and walk "on time" but now falls often. He prefers to watch the ceiling fan rather than play with toys and doesn't like to play with other children. His mother reports his frequent tantrums make grocery shopping difficult. Upon examination, you note he has difficulty following directions and seldom vocalizes. He exhibits weak abdominals, avoids deep squats, and climbs stairs in a step-to-step pattern.

KEY FEATURES

Description

- Group of disorders, including PDD, autism, and Asperger syndrome,[4,5] each characterized by a variety of features
  - Difficulty with socialization
  - Difficulty with communication
  - Stereotypical movements
  - Developmental delay

Essentials of Diagnosis

- Deficits in socialization
  - Poor or absent eye contact with others
  - Disinterest or difficulty socializing with peers
  - Prefer being alone
  - Difficulty reading social clues[6]
- Deficits in communication
  - Delayed or absent (40%) language[7,8]
  - Echolalia[6]
- Stereotypical or repetitive movements
  - Ritualistic behavior
  - Inflexible behavior, requires predictable routines
  - Self-stimulation behaviors, such as flapping arms or rocking[7]
- Atypical play or interest in toys or objects
  - Preoccupation with ordinary objects, such as door stop or ceiling fan
  - Obsessively arranges objects, such as blocks

General Considerations

- May also have cognitive deficits (30%–51%)[8,9]

Demographics

- 1 in 100 children[8]
- Males three to four times more likely than females[8]
- 2% to 8% greater risk if siblings also have ASD[8]

CLINICAL FINDINGS

SIGNS AND SYMPTOMS

- Generally apparent by 18 months of age
- One of the early signs is child's inability to respond when his or her name is called
- Parents may report infant "does not like them," as child may not like being held
- Developmental delay (e.g., walking)
- Associated disorders
  - Seizures (25%)[8]
  - Sleep disorders
  - Gastrointestinal disorders
  - Sensory integration dysfunction[6]
  - Pica[7]

Functional Implications

- Delayed developmental milestones, including
  - Communication
  - Social–emotional skills
  - Gross motor skills
  - Self-care
  - Cognitive
- Lack of age-appropriate safety skills
- Inability to live independently

Possible Contributing Causes

- Primarily idiopathic
- Possible causes include
  - Genetic[10]
  - Familial
  - Viral[10]
  - Immunologic
  - Abnormality in the brain structure or function
  - Environmental factors

Differential Diagnosis

- Angelman syndrome
- Congenital rubella syndrome
- Cornelia deLange syndrome
- Down syndrome
- Fragile X syndrome
- Rett syndrome[11]
- Tourette syndrome
- Tuberous sclerosis

MEANS OF CONFIRMATION OR DIAGNOSIS

- Diagnostic and Statistical Manual of Mental Disorders-IV (DSM-IV) to confirm diagnosis[12]
- Genetic testing may be indicated to rule out differential diagnoses[13]

FINDINGS AND INTERPRETATION

- Delay in the development of spoken language

TREATMENT

Medication

- Antidepressants, SSRIs (Zoloft or Prozac)[14]
- Anticonvulsants to control seizures (Tegretol, Lamictal, Depakote, or Topamax)[14]
- Risperdal[14]
- Antipsychotic medications (Zyprexa or Haldol)[14]

MEDICAL PROCEDURES

- Applied behavior analysis (ABA)
- Gluten-free, casein-free diet

REFERRALS/ADMITTANCE

- To child psychiatrist for diagnosis and medication
- To child neurologist for developmental progression
- To geneticist to rule out other syndromes
- To early intervention program
- To speech therapist
- To occupational therapist for functional activities

IMPAIRMENTS

- Delayed gross motor skills
- Unable to stand at furniture
- Inability to ambulate with both hands held
- Not cruising
- Ascending stairs in step-to-step pattern (rather than step-over-step pattern)
- Unable to ride tricycle
- Unable to jump using both feet
- Tactile defensiveness (will not wear shoes)

TESTS AND MEASURES

- Bruininks–Oseretsky Test of Motor Proficiency
- Peabody Developmental Motor Scales-2
- Goniometric measurements
- Manual muscle testing

INTERVENTION

- Neurodevelopmental treatment to achieve age-appropriate motor milestones
  - Facilitate sitting balance with and without arm support
  - Facilitate standing at furniture independently by leaning trunk on furniture or using own arm support
  - Facilitate creeping on hands and knees
- Pre-gait training activities or gait training in toddlers and children
- Recommend adaptive equipment or orthotics as needed
- Assist with sensory processing, such as using a swing, for children with gravitational insecurity (e.g., fear of falling, reaching outside of support base when sitting)
- Behavior modification techniques to assist with improving maladaptive behavior
- Patient/family education, including home activities to assist with age-appropriate developmental milestones

FUNCTIONAL GOALS

- Patient will be able to
  - Stand at furniture for 5 minutes with contact guard assistance while playing with toys within 1 month.
  - Walk 5 feet with both hands held within 2 months.
  - Cruise 2 feet at furniture with stand-by assistance to increase mobility, patient will be able to reach toys within 3 months.
  - Ascend stairs in step-over-step pattern while holding the railing with one hand and handheld assistance with the other within 6 months.
  - Ride tricycle 10 feet with assistance 50% of the time within 6 months.
  - Jump on both feet independently from bottom step within 3 months.
  - Wear shoes when outside of home 100% of the time within 1 month.

PROGNOSIS

- Dependent on type and severity of ASD and age of child.
  - If a young child is verbal, ambulatory, and only has difficulties with socialization, the prognosis for independent functioning is good.
  - If a child has PDD-NOS, the prognosis for independent living is fair to poor.

PATIENT RESOURCES

- National Autism Association. http://nationalautismassociation.org. Accessed June 17, 2013.
- Autism Speaks. http://www.autismspeaks.org. Accessed June 17, 2013.
- Autism Society. http://www.autism-society.org. Accessed June 17, 2013.

REFERENCES

1. ICD9DATA web site. http://www.icd9data.com. Accessed June 17, 2013.
2. ICD10DATA web site. http://www.icd10data.com. Accessed June 17, 2013.
3. The American Physical Therapy Association. Pattern 5B: Impaired neuromotor development. *Interactive Guide to Physical Therapist Practice*. 2003. doi: 10.2522/ptguide.3.2_2. http://guidetoptpractice.apta.org/content/1/SEC19.extract?sid=1805f931-dd01-4ea3-ba9a-6c5c1499e62a. Accessed June 4, 2014.
4. National Institute of Child Health and Human Development. Asperger's Syndrome. http://www.nichd.nih.gov/health/topics/asperger_syndrome.cfm. Accessed June 17, 2013.
5. National Institute of Mental Health. What is Autism Spectrum Disorder? A Parent's Guide to Autism Spectrum Disorder. http://www.nimh.nih.gov/health/publications/a-parents-guide-to-autism-spectrum-disorder/what-is-autism-spectrum-disorder-asd.shtml. Accessed June 17, 2013.
6. Centers for Disease Control and Prevention. Autism Spectrum Disorders (ASDs) Signs and Symptoms. http://www.cdc.gov/ncbddd/autism/signs.html. Accessed June 17, 2013.
7. Goldson E, Reynolds A. Child Development & Behavior. In: Hay WW, Levin MJ, Sondheimer JM, Deterding RR, eds. *CURRENT Diagnosis & Treatment: Pediatrics*. 20th ed. New York, NY: McGraw-Hill; 2011. http://www.accessphysiotherapy.com/content/6576866#6576866. Accessed June 17, 2013.
8. Centers for Disease Control and Prevention. Autism Spectrum Disorders (ASDs) Data and Statistics. http://www.cdc.gov/ncbddd/autism/data.html. Accessed June 17, 2013.
9. Autism Speaks. What is Autism: Diagnosis. http://www.autismspeaks.org/what-autism/diagnosis#criteria. Accessed June 17, 2013.
10. Tsai ACH, Manchester DK, Elias ER. Genetics & dysmorphology. In: Hay WW, Levin MJ, Sondheimer JM, Deterding RR, eds. *CURRENT Diagnosis & Treatment: Pediatrics*. 20th ed. New York, NY: McGraw-Hill; 2011. http://www.accessphysiotherapy.com/content/6589176#6589176. Accessed June 17, 2013.
11. National Institute of Mental Health. How is ASD Treated? A Parent's Guide to Autism Spectrum Disorder. http://www.nimh.nih.gov/health/publications/a-parents-guide-to-autism-spectrum-disorder/how-is-asd-treated.shtml. Accessed June 17, 2013.
12. National Institute of Child Health and Human Development. *Autism Overview: What We Know*. NIH publication; 2005. http://www.nichd.nih.gov/publications/pubs/upload/autism_overview_2005.pdf. Accessed June 17, 2013.
13. National Institute of Neurological Disorders and Stroke. Rett Syndrome. http://www.ninds.nih.gov/disorders/rett/detail_rett.htm. Accessed June 17, 2013.
14. Dutton M. *McGraw Hill's National Physical Therapy Examination*. nd ed. New York, NY: McGraw-Hill; 2012. http://www.accessphysiotherapy.com/content/5404424#5404424. Accessed June 17, 2013.

ADDITIONAL REFERENCE

- Web MD. *Autism Spectrum Disorders Health Center*. http://www.webmd.com/brain/autism/autism-spectrum-disorders. Accessed June 17, 2013.

232 CEREBRAL PALSY

Kay Tasso, PhD, PT, PCS

CONDITION/DISORDER SYNONYM

- Cerebral palsy (CP)

ICD-9-CM CODES

- 343 Infantile cerebral palsy
- 343.0 Congenital diplegia
- 343.1 Congenital hemiplegia
- 343.2 Congenital quadriplegia
- 343.3 Congenital monoplegia
- 343.4 Infantile hemiplegia
- 343.8 Other specified cerebral palsy
- 343.9 Infantile cerebral palsy, unspecified

ICD-10-CM CODES

- G80.0 Spastic quadriplegic cerebral palsy
- G80.1 Spastic diplegic cerebral palsy
- G80.2 Spastic hemiplegic cerebral palsy
- G80.3 Athetoid cerebral palsy
- G80.4 Ataxic cerebral palsy
- G80.8 Other cerebral palsy
- G80.9 Cerebral palsy, unspecified

PREFERRED PRACTICE PATTERN

- 5C: Impaired Motor Function and Sensory Integrity Associated with Nonprogressive Disorders of the Central Nervous System—Congenital Origin in Infancy or Childhood[1]

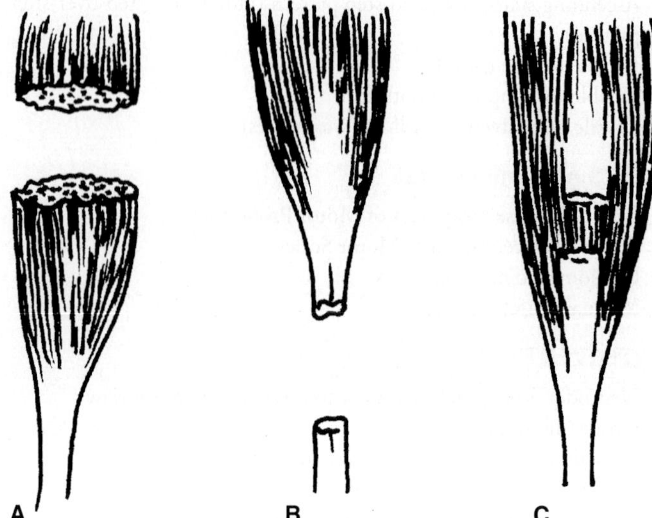

FIGURE 232-1 Schematic representation of surgical options for muscle release or lengthening in cerebral palsy. **A:** Myotomy; **B:** tenotomy; **C:** aponeurotomy. (From Skinner HB. *Current Diagnosis & Treatment in Orthopedics*. 4th ed. www.accessmedicine.com. Copyright © The McGraw-Hill Companies, Inc. All rights reserved.)

PATIENT PRESENTATION

A 3-month-old infant referred to outpatient physical therapy following discharge from neonatal intensive care unit with diagnosis of CP. Infant was born at 27-week gestational age with Apgars of five at 1 minute and seven at 5 minutes. Past medical history includes respiratory distress syndrome, seizure disorder, and gastroesophageal reflux. Upon examination, infant exhibits poor head control, fisted hands, and inability to achieve prone on elbows.

KEY FEATURES

Description

- Nonprogressive damage to cerebral cortex (and other parts of the brain, such as cerebellum) that occurs during prenatal, perinatal, or postnatal period[2]

Essentials of Diagnosis

- Four types of muscle tone (and percentage occurrence in children with CP)[3]
  - Hypotonia
  - Hypertonia (70%–75%)
  - Ataxia (10%–15%)
  - Athetosis (20%)
- Distribution of muscle tone
  - Quadriplegia: All four limbs involved, arms more than legs; cervical area, oral area
  - Diplegia: Primarily legs involved[4]
  - Hemiplegia: Primarily ipsilateral arm and leg involved[4]
  - Monoplegia: Only one limb involved
  - Triplegia: Only three limbs involved
  - In athetosis and ataxia, most often total body distribution: No hemiplegia, diplegia
- Gross motor function classification system[5]
  - Level I (least involved)
  - Level II
  - Level III
  - Level IV (most involved)

General Considerations

- Muscle tone often presents as hypotonia but changes before 12 months of age, most often to hypertonia depending on the type of CP
- Infants (under age 12 months) can also have "transient" muscle tone within first year of life; may initially present as hypertonic but resolves spontaneously without development of CP
- Associated disorders
  - Seizure disorder (in 50% of CP cases)[3]
  - Cognitive impairment (in 53% of CP cases)
  - Orthopedic deformities
  - Sensory integration dysfunction
  - Speech and language deficits

TABLE 232-1 Cerebral Palsy Classifications and Manifestations

	Spastic	Athetoid	Ataxic	Hypotonic
Muscle stiffness	Excessively stiff and taut, especially during attempted movement	Low	Variable	Diminished resting muscle tone and decreased ability to generate voluntary muscle force
Posture	Abnormal postures and movements mass patterns of flexion/extension	Poor functional stability, especially in proximal joint	Low postural tone with poor balance	Variable
Visual tracking	Some deficits	Poor visual tracking	Poor visual tracking, nystagmus	Variable
Muscle tone	Increased in antigravity muscles. Imbalance of tone across joints that can cause contractures and deformities	Fluctuates, but generally decreased—floppy baby syndrome	Slightly decreased	Minimal to none
Initiating movement	Difficult	No problems	No problems	Difficult
Sustaining movement	Able to in some	Unable	No problems	Unable
Terminating movement	Unable	Variable	No problems	Uncontrolled
Muscle coactivation	Abnormal	Poorly timed	No problems	None
ROM limitations	Passive ROM, overall decreased	Hypermobile	In spine	Hypermobile

Source: From Dutton M. McGraw-Hill's NPTE (National Physical Therapy Examination). 2nd ed. www.accessphysiotherapy.com.

- Difficulty feeding
- Microcephaly[3]
- Respiratory distress
- Bronchopulmonary dysplasia[6]
- Hydrocephalus[3]
- Retinopathy of prematurity[7]
- Visual impairment
- Auditory impairment
- Gastroesophageal reflux[8]

Demographics

- Present in 0.2% of the population

CLINICAL FINDINGS

SIGNS AND SYMPTOMS

- Delays in
  - Gross motor skills
  - Fine motor skills
  - Oral motor skills
  - Perceptual motor skills
  - Social–emotional skills
  - Speech and language skills
- Abnormal muscle tone (decreased, increased, fluctuating)
- Arching neck or back into extension
- Scissoring legs (hip adduction) when held in standing
- Describe classic rotary, writhing characteristic of movement in athetosis
- Ataxia: Hypotonia and tremulousness, unsteadiness in gait

Functional Implications

- Abnormal movement postures
  - Capital hyperextension
  - Scapular retraction
  - Fisted hands
  - In supported standing
    - Hip adduction (scissoring)
    - Excessive knee flexion ("crouching")
    - Plantar flexion (standing on toes)
    - Pronation (eversion)
- Refusal to bear weight on feet or hands
- Inability to move against gravity in prone position

TABLE 232-2 Factors That Increase the Risk of Injury and Adversely Affect Ability to Participate in Sports in Athletes With Cerebral Palsy

Decreased musculoskeletal flexibility
Decreased muscle strength and endurance
Muscle strength and flexibility imbalance (i.e., relatively stronger flexors compared to extensors)
Progressively worsening spasticity
Progressively increasing joint contractures
High energy cost of movement (decreased mechanical efficiency)
Decreased anaerobic power and capacity
Decreased aerobic capacity
Increased cost of breathing (decreased lung volume and stiff thoracic cage)
Perceptual motor deficiencies
Visual impairment
Hearing impairment
Impaired hand–eye coordination
Cognitive delay and retardation

Source: From Patel DR, Greydanus DE, Baker RJ. Pediatric Practice: Sports Medicine. http://www.accesspediatrics.com.

- Poor head/trunk control
- Inability to sit independently
- Inability to commando crawl or creep on hands and knees
- Inability to transition from one position to another, such as from prone to sitting
- Inability to ambulate
- Inability to maintain any position because of fluctuating tone in athetosis
- Dependent on help for all ADLs

Possible Contributing Causes

- Hypoxic–ischemic encephalopathy
- Asphyxia[8]
- Intraventricular hemorrhage (IVH)[9]
  - Grade I (mildest)
  - Grade II
  - Grade III
  - Grade IV (worst)
- Periventricular leukomalacia (PVL)[9]
- Germinal matrix hemorrhage (GMH)
- Jaundice, especially due to Rh incompatibility in athetosis
- Perinatal infections[8]
- Teratogens such as[10]
  - Alcohol
  - Illegal drug use
    - Cocaine
    - Heroin
  - Over-the-counter medications
    - Ibuprofen
  - Maternal prescription medications for
    - Seizure disorder
    - Mental illness
    - Hypothyroidism

TABLE 232-3 Gross Motor Function Classification System

Level	Description
I	Walks without restrictions, limitations in more advanced gross motor skills
II	Walks without assistive devices; limitations walking outdoors and in the community
III	Walks with assistive mobility devices; limitations walking outdoors and in the community
IV	Self-mobility with limitations; are transported or use power motor mobility outdoors and in the community
V	Self-mobility is severely limited even with the use of assistive technology

Data from Palisano R, Rosenbaum P, Walter S, Russell D, Wood E, Galuppi B. Development and reliability of a system to classify gross motor function in children with cerebral palsy. *Dev Med Child Neurol.* 1997;39:214–223.

Differential Diagnosis

- Genetic disorders or syndromes
- Metabolic disorders[11]

MEANS OF CONFIRMATION OR DIAGNOSIS

Imaging

- Cranial ultrasound[3]
- CT scan
- MRI

FINDINGS AND INTERPRETATION

- CT shows damage to cerebral cortex (and other parts of the brain, such as cerebellum).

TABLE 232-4 Physical Attributes of Different Types of Cerebral Palsy

Type	Attributes
Spastic (i.e., pyramidal)	Constitutes 75% of patients with cerebral palsy. Patients have signs of upper motor neuron involvement, including hyperreflexia, clonus, extensor Babinski response, persistent primitive reflexes, and overflow reflexes (i.e., crossed adductor). Cognitive impairment is present in approximately 30% of these patients, but most patients with spastic quadriplegia have some cognitive impairment.
Dyskinesia (i.e., extrapyramidal)	Characterized by extrapyramidal movement patterns, abnormal regulation of tone, abnormal postural control, and coordination deficits. Athetosis, chorea, and choreoathetoid or dystonic movements can be seen. Patients often have pseudobulbar involvement with dysarthria, swallowing difficulties, drooling, oromotor difficulties, and abnormal speech patterns. Generally, the child is hypotonic at birth with abnormal movement patterns emerging at 1 to 3 years. The arms are usually more involved than the legs. Abnormal movement patterns may increase with stress or purposeful activity. Muscle tone is normal during sleep. Intelligence is normal in 78% of patients with athetoid cerebral palsy. A high incidence of sensorineural hearing loss is reported.
Spastic diplegia	Patients will often have a period of hypotonia followed by extensor spasticity in the lower extremities with little or no functional limitation of the upper extremities. Patients have a delay in developing gross motor skills. Spastic muscle imbalance often causes persistence of infantile coxa valga and femoral anteversion. Scissoring gait (i.e., hips flexed and adducted, knees flexed with valgus stress, equinus ankles) is observed.
Hemiplegia	Characterized by weak hip flexion and ankle dorsiflexion, overactive posterior tibialis, hip hiking/circumduction, supinated foot in stance, upper extremity posturing (e.g., often held with shoulder adducted, elbow flexed, forearm pronated, wrist flexed, hand clenched in a fist with the thumb in the palm), impaired sensation, impaired 2-point discrimination, and/or impaired position sense. Some cognitive impairment is found in about 28% of these patients.

Source: From Dutton M. McGraw-Hill's NPTE (National Physical Therapy Examination). 2nd ed. www.accessphysiotherapy.com.

TREATMENT

Medication

- Oral baclofen for spasticity[12]

MEDICAL PROCEDURES

- For spasticity
  - Intrathecal baclofen[13]
  - Botox injections targeted at spastic muscles[14]
  - Selective dorsal rhizotomy[15]
  - Constraint induced movement therapy[16]
  - Orthopedic surgeries
    - Osteotomy[17]
    - Tenotomy

REFERRALS/ADMITTANCE

- To orthopedist for bony deformities including scoliosis and developmental dysplasia of hip
- To neurologist for appropriate diagnosis and treatment of seizures
- To occupational therapist for intervention with fine motor, feeding, visual perceptional, and social–emotional deficits
- To speech therapist for oral motor and speech/language deficits
- To orthotist for ankle/foot orthotics
- Admittance for medical procedures, associated disorders, respiratory illnesses

IMPAIRMENTS

- Decreased strength, especially in spastic muscles
- Decreased range of motion or contractures
- Dependent on help for ADLs
- Inability to roll
- Inability to commando crawl or creep on hands and knees
- Inability to sit independently
- Inability to stand
- Inability to transfer without assistance
- Inability to ambulate without assistance
- Poor sitting or standing balance
- Poor head or trunk postural control
- Poor stability in any position
- Gait deviations

TESTS AND MEASURES

- Bayley scales of motor development[9] or Bayley II
- Peabody scales of motor development[9]
- Movement assessment of infants[9]
- Neonatal behavioral assessment scale[18]
- Early intervention developmental profile[19]
- Test of infant motor performance[20]
- Alberta Infant Motor Scale[9]
- Gross motor function measure[9]
- Gross motor function classification system for CP [5]
- Pediatric Evaluation of Disability Inventory[9]
- Functional Independence Measure for Children (WeeFIM)[9]
- Bruininks–Oseretsky test of motor proficiency[9]
- Goniometric measurements

INTERVENTION

- Neurodevelopmental treatment[9]
  - Inhibition of spasticity
  - Facilitation of normal movement patterns
  - Acquisition of motor milestones
- Prevention of muscle contractures
- Therapeutic exercise
  - Strengthening
  - Stretching
- Functional activities
  - Transfers
  - Gait training
  - Stair climbing
- Serial casting or inhibitive casting[9]

FUNCTIONAL GOALS

- The patient will be able to:
  - Stay prone on elbows with 90 degrees cervical extension for 30 to 60 seconds independently within 3 months.
  - Stay quadruped for 5 minutes with minimal assistance while playing with toys within 6 months.
  - Stand at furniture for 2 minutes wearing bilateral ankle–foot orthoses (AFOs) with contact guard assistance within 2 months.
  - Ring sit on the floor propping with hands for 1 minute with stand-by assistance in 1 month.
  - Sit independently on bench with good head control and spinal extension for 10 minutes within 3 months.
  - Creep on hands and knees with minimal assistance for 10 feet in 1 month.
  - Commando crawl independently as primary method of mobility in 3 months.
  - Roll from prone to supine using trunk flexion with moderate assistance in 2 months.
  - Ambulate 25 feet using four-wheeled posterior walker with intermittent assistance for safety in 6 months.
  - Transfer from stand to sitting with moderate assistance in 1 month.

PROGNOSIS

- Dependent on type, distribution, and severity of muscle tone/involvement, and degree of parent support and resources, for example.
  - Children with Level I involvement on the gross motor classification scale have an excellent prognosis for independent mobility and independent ADLs.
  - Children with Level II involvement on the gross motor classification scale have a fair prognosis, will be dependent on help for all mobility and ADLs, and likely have other associated disorders that may result in medical complications.
  - Children with diplegia have a better prognosis than children with quadriplegia.

PATIENT RESOURCE

- United Cerebral Palsy. http://www.ucp.org. Accessed March 17, 2013.

REFERENCES

1. The American Physical Therapy Association. Pattern 5C: Impaired motor function and sensory integrity associated with nonprogressive disorders of the central nervous system - congenital origin or acquired in infancy or childhood. *Interactive Guide*

to Physical Therapist Practice. 2003. doi: 10.2522/ptguide.3.2_3. http://guidetoptpractice.apta.org/content/1/SEC20.extract?sid=2d79565f-9483-42f0-8afc-074fc56c046e. Accessed June 1, 2014.

2. Cerebral Palsy, Case 4. In: Toy EC, ed. *LANGE Case Files*. New York, NY: McGraw-Hill. http://www.accessmedicine.com/caseContent.aspx?aID=510003074&searchStr=cerebral+palsy#510003074. Accessed March 17, 2013.
3. Bernard TJ, Knupp K, Yang ML, Arndt D, Levinson P, Moe PG. Chapter 23. Neurologic & muscular disorders. In: Hay W, Levin MJ, Sondheimer JM, Detering RR, eds. *CURRENT Diagnosis & Treatment: Pediatrics*. New York, NY: McGraw-Hill; 2011. http://www.accessphysiotherapy.com/abstract/6585385#6585406. Accessed March 17, 2013.
4. Chandrasoma P, Taylor CR. Chapter 62. *The Central Nervous System: I. Structure & Function; Congenital Diseases. Concise Pathology*. New York, NY: McGraw-Hill; 1998. http://www.accessphysiotherapy.com/resource/7. Accessed March 17, 2013.
5. Palisano R, Rosenbaum P, Walter S, Russell D, Wood E, Galuppi B. CanChild Centre for Childhood Disability Research web site. *Dev Med Child Neurol*. 1997;39:214–223. http://www.canchild.ca/en/aboutcanchild/resources/GMFCS.pdf. Accessed March 17, 2013.
6. Federico MJ, Kerby GS, Deterding RR, et al. Respiratory tract & mediastinum. In: Hay WW, Levin MJ, Sondheimer JM, Deterding RR, eds. *CURRENT Diagnosis & Treatment: Pediatrics*. 20th ed. New York, NY: McGraw-Hill; 2011. http://www.accessphysiotherapy.com/content/6582352#6582352. Accessed March 17, 2013.
7. Braverman RS. Eye. In: Hay WW, Levin MJ, Sondheimer JM, Deterding RR, eds. *CURRENT Diagnosis & Treatment: Pediatrics*. 20th ed. New York, NY: McGraw-Hill; 2011. http://www.accessphysiotherapy.com/content/6581243#6581243. Accessed March 17, 2013.
8. Thilo EH, Rosenburg AA. The newborn infant. In: Hay WW, Levin MJ, Sondheimer JM, Deterding RR. eds. *CURRENT Diagnosis & Treatment: Pediatrics*. 20th ed. New York, NY: McGraw-Hill; 2011. http://www.accessphysiotherapy.com/content/6576264#6576264. Accessed March 17, 2013.
9. Dutton M. In: *McGraw Hill's National Physical Therapy Examination*. 2nd ed. New York, NY: McGraw-Hill; 2012. http://www.accessphysiotherapy.com/content/5404377#5404377. Accessed March 17, 2013.
10. Tsai ACH, Manchester DK, Elias ER. Genetics & Dysmorphology. In: Hay WW, Levin MJ, Sondheimer JM, Deterding RR, eds. *CURRENT Diagnosis & Treatment: Pediatrics*. 20th ed. New York, NY: McGraw-Hill; 2011. http://www.accessphysiotherapy.com/content/6589287#6589287. Accessed March 17, 2013.
11. Thomas JA, Van Hove JLK. Inborn Errors of Metabolism. In: Hay WW, Levin MJ, Sondheimer JM, Deterding RR, eds. *CURRENT Diagnosis & Treatment: Pediatrics*. 20th ed. New York, NY: McGraw-Hill; 2011. http://www.accessphysiotherapy.com/content/6588543. Accessed March 17, 2013.
12. Panus PC, Jobst EE, Masters SB, Katzung B, Tinsley SL, Trevor AJ. Skeletal muscle relaxants. In: *Pharmacology for the Physical Therapist*. 2009. http://www.accessphysiotherapy.com/content/6095620#6095620. Accessed March 17, 2013.
13. University of Pittsburgh. Intrathecal baclofen treatment for spasticity. http://www.neurosurgery.pitt.edu/pediatric/spasticity/baclofen_spasticity.html. Accessed March 17, 2013.
14. Cincinnati Children's Hospital. Botulin toxin injections. http://www.cincinnatichildrens.org/health/b/botox./ Accessed March 17, 2013.
15. St. Louis Children's Hospital. About Selective Dorsal Rhizotomy. http://www.stlouischildrens.org/content/medservices/aboutselectivedorsalrhizotomy.htm. Accessed March 17, 2013.
16. Cincinnati Children's Hospital Medical Center. Pediatric Constraint Induced Movement Therapy. Published 02-16-2009. http://www.cincinnatichildrens.org/assets/0/78/1067/2709/2777/2793/9199/fa42566b-64d7-4d5b-8c38-62a82d660937.pdf. Accessed March 17, 2013.
17. Polousky JD. Orthopedics. In: Hay WW, Levin MJ, Sondheimer JM, Deterding RR, eds. *CURRENT Diagnosis & Treatment: Pediatrics*. 20th ed. New York, NY: McGraw-Hill; 2011. http://www.accessphysiotherapy.com/content/6586053#6586053. Accessed March 17, 2013.
18. The Brazelton Institute. The neonatal behavioral assessment scale. http://www.brazelton-institute.com/intro.html. Accessed March 17, 2013.
19. Developmental Profile III. Children and adolescents with special needs. http://portal.wpspublish.com/portal/page?_pageid=53,186601&_dad=portal&_schema=PORTAL. Accessed January 14, 2013.
20. The Test of Infant Motor Performance and the Harris Infant Neuromotor Test. IMPS, LLC web site. http://thetimp.com/. Accessed March 17, 2013.

ADDITIONAL REFERENCES

- Brenneman SK, Tecklin JS. Assessment and Testing of Infant and Child Development. In: Tecklin JS, ed. *Pediatric Physical Therapy*. 4th ed. Philadelphia, PA: Lippincott, Williams and Wilkins; 2008.
- Chandrasoma P, Taylor CR. The central nervous system: I. structure & function; congenital diseases. In: *Concise Pathology*. 3rd ed. Stamford, CT: Appleton & Lange; 1998. http://www.accessphysiotherapy.com/content/192909#192909. Accessed March 17, 2013.
- Hay WW, Levin MJ, Sondheimer JM, Deterding RR. Neurologic & muscular disorders. In: Hay WW, Levin MJ, Sondheimer JM, Deterding RR, eds. *CURRENT Diagnosis & Treatment: Pediatrics*. 20th ed. New York, NY: McGraw-Hill; 2011. http://www.accessphysiotherapy.com/content/6585416#6585416. Accessed March 17, 2013.
- Helders PJH, Klepper SE, Takken T, Van Der Net J. Juvenile idiopathic arthritis. In: Campbell SK, Palisano RJ, Orlin MN, eds. *Physical Therapy for Children*. 4th ed. St. Louis, MO: Elsevier Saunders; 2012.
- ICD9DATA web site. http://www.icd9data.com. Accessed March 17, 2013.
- ICD10DATA web site. http://www.icd10data.com. Accessed March 17, 2013.
- Styer-Acevedo J. The infant and child with cerebral palsy. In: Tecklin JS, ed. *Pediatric Physical Therapy*. 4th ed. Philadelphia, PA: Lippincott, Williams and Wilkins; 2008.

233 CHIARI MALFORMATION

Kay Tasso, PhD, PT, PCS

CONDITION/DISORDER SYNONYMS

- Arnold–Chiari II
- Arnold–Chiari malformation
- Chari I malformation
- Chiari II malformation
- Tonsillar ectopia
- Tonsillar herniation

ICD-9-CM CODES

- 348.4 Compression of brain
- 742.2 Congenital reduction for deformities of brain

ICD-10-CM CODES

- G93.5 Compression of brain
- Q04.8 Other specified congenital malformations of brain
- Q07.0 Arnold–Chiari syndrome
- Q07.00 Arnold–Chiari syndrome without spina bifida or hydrocephalus
- Q07.01 Arnold–Chiari syndrome with spina bifida
- Q07.02 Arnold–Chiari syndrome with hydrocephalus
- Q07.03 Arnold–Chiari syndrome with spina bifida and hydrocephalus

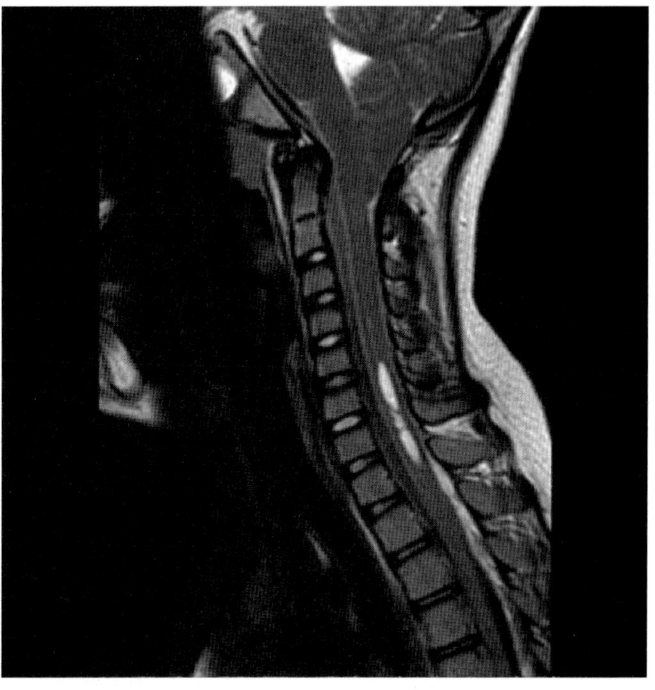

FIGURE 233-1 Sagittal T2-weighted MRI scan of a Chiari showing typical peglike appearance of cerebellar tonsils and associated syringomyelia. (From Doherty GM. *Current Diagnosis & Treatment: Surgery*. 13th ed. www.accessmedicine.com. Copyright © The McGraw-Hill Companies, Inc. All rights reserved.)

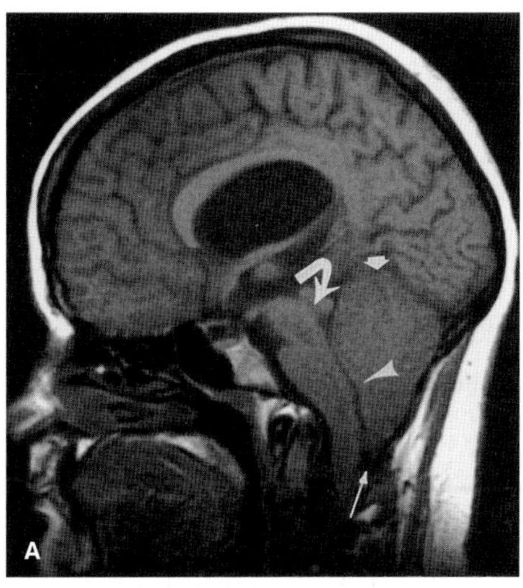

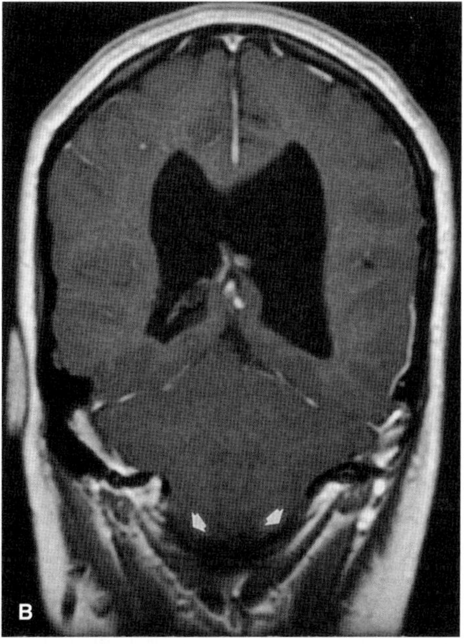

FIGURE 233-2 Uninfused sagittal T1-weighted (**A**) and coronal T1 postcontrast (**B**) imaging in a 30-year-old patient with a Chiari II malformation. (**A**) A small posterior fossa is present, resulting in cerebellar tonsillar ectopia (long arrow), towering of the cerebellum (short arrow), beaking of the tectum (curved arrow), and compression of the fourth ventricle (arrowhead) with resulting hydrocephalus. Partial agenesis of the rostrum and splenium of the corpus callosum is noted. (**B**) Cerebellar tonsillar ectopia into the foramen magnum is demonstrated (arrowheads). (From Chen MYM, Pope TL, Ott DJ. *Basic Radiology*. 2nd ed. www.accessmedicine.com. Copyright © The McGraw-Hill Companies, Inc. All rights reserved.)

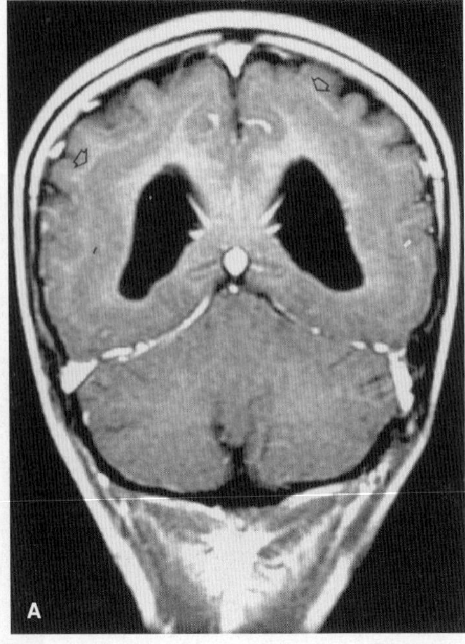

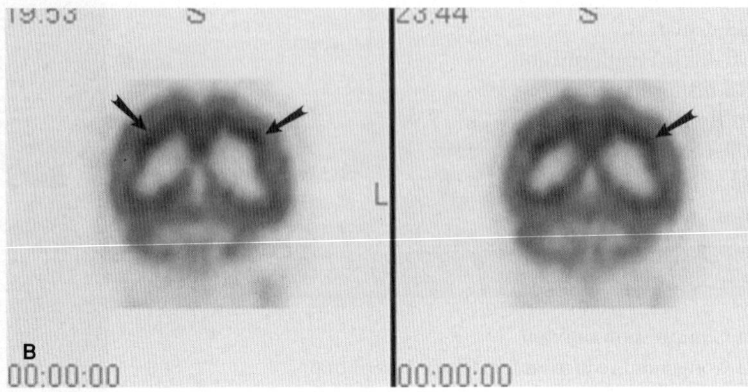

FIGURE 233-3 (**A**) Postcontrast coronal T1-weighted images of the brain in a 32-year-old with intractable seizures. An additional circumferential band of gray matter is seen (arrows) deep to the normal gray matter within the occipital region. This finding was noted to be diffusely present throughout the remaining brain parenchyma (not shown). (**B**) The corresponding PET image in the same patient reveals increased activity of the band heterotopia relative to the adjacent normal cortex (arrows), of unclear significance. (From Chen MYM, Pope TL, Ott DJ. Basic Radiology. 2nd ed. www.accessmedicine.com. Copyright © The McGraw-Hill Companies, Inc. All rights reserved.)

PREFERRED PRACTICE PATTERN

- 5C: Impaired Motor Function and Sensory Integrity Associated with Nonprogressive Disorders of the Central Nervous System—Congenital Origin or Acquired in Infancy or Childhood[1]

PATIENT PRESENTATION

A 5-year-old is referred to physical therapy following decompression surgery for an Arnold–Chiari malformation. Pre-op, the child was complaining of headaches, nausea, vomiting, and had nystagmus and balance difficulties. The child had a history in preschool and kindergarten of poor fine motor and handwriting skills. Upon examination, the therapist notes difficulty walking on a low-balance beam, standing on one leg for more than 2 to 3 seconds, and the need for assistance of the therapist when climbing stairs.

KEY FEATURES

Description

- Defect in cephalad portion of spinal column
- Herniation of portions of the brainstem and spinal cord through the foramen magnum, including the cerebellum, medulla, and cervical spinal cord

Essentials of Diagnosis

- Characteristic signs and symptoms with diagnosis confirmed by MRI[2]

General Consideration

- Most often occurs in presence of spina bifida[3]

Demographics

- 90% of patients with Chiari malformation (CM) also have hydrocephalus[2]
- Three times more common in females than males[2]

CLINICAL FINDINGS

SIGNS AND SYMPTOMS

- Headache is the most common symptom
- Respiratory difficulties
  - Apnea[4]
  - Coughing
  - Stridor[5]
- Vision difficulties
  - Nystagmus[6]
  - Diplopia[7]
  - Blurred vision
  - Esotropia[8]
- Bradycardia[9]
- Cranial nerve palsies
- Ataxia[10]
- Vertigo
- Neck pain worse with coughing or sneezing
- Hydrocephalus
- Decreased balance and coordination
- Spasticity, numbness, or tingling in hands
- Poor fine-motor skills
- Slurred speech
- Developmental delay

Functional Implications

- Delayed motor development
- Difficulty swallowing
- Poor balance

Possible Contributing Causes

- Abnormality during fetal development
- Teratogens[11]
- Possible genetic link
- Infection
- Insufficient maternal vitamins or minerals during gestation

Differential Diagnosis

- Brain tumor
- Syringomyelia[6]

MEANS OF CONFIRMATION OR DIAGNOSIS

Imaging

- MRI[2]

FINDINGS AND INTERPRETATION

- Cerebellar tonsils are normally located above the foramen magnum
- Tonsils hang below the foramen magnum and herniated into the spinal canal
- MRI positive for herniation of neural tissue into foramen magnum[12]

TREATMENT

Medical Procedures

- Tracheostomy[13]
- Gastrostomy[13]
- Posterior fossa decompression[14]
- Cervical laminectomy[15]

REFERRALS/ADMITTANCE

- Geneticist
- Neurologist
- Orthopedic surgeon
- Occupational therapist
- Speech therapist
- Admittance for surgical procedures, such as
  - Tracheostomy
  - Gastrostomy
  - Posterior fossa decompression
  - Cervical laminectomy

IMPAIRMENTS

- Delayed motor milestones
  - Rolling
  - Sitting
- Decreased balance in sitting
- Additional impairments typically associated with spina bifida

TESTS AND MEASURES

- Pediatric Evaluation of Disability Inventory (PEDI)[10]
- Manual muscle test

INTERVENTION

- Therapy
- Child should avoid activities associated with risk for cervical injury
- Developmental activities to facilitate gross motor development
  - Prone on elbows
  - Rolling
  - Sitting
- Balance training

FUNCTIONAL GOALS

- Patient will be able to:
  - Stay prone on elbows for 30 seconds to increase strength in 2 months.

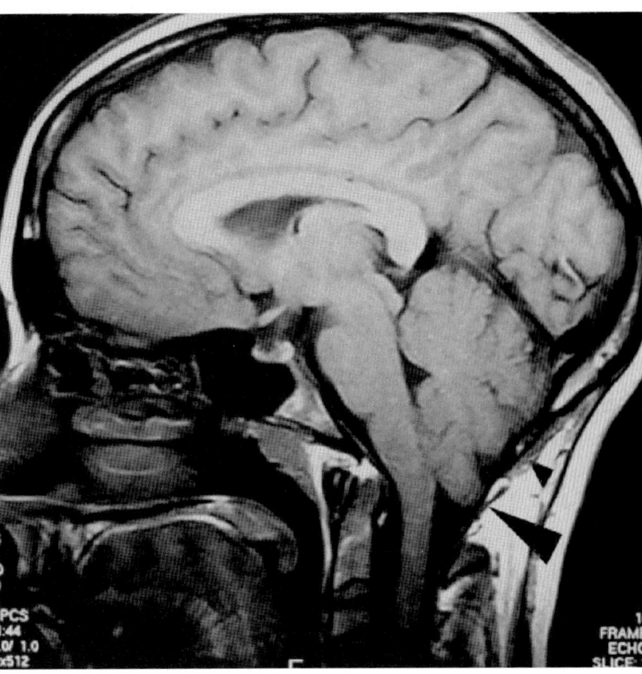

FIGURE 233-4 T1-weighted sagittal magnetic resonance imaging of a patient with a Chiari I malformation. The *large arrowhead* points to the cerebellar tonsils. The *small arrowhead* points to the posterior arch of the foramen magnum. (From Brunicardi FC, Andersen DK, Billiar TR, et al. *Schwartz's Principles of Surgery*. 9th ed. www.accessmedicine.com. Copyright © The McGraw-Hill Companies, Inc. All rights reserved.)

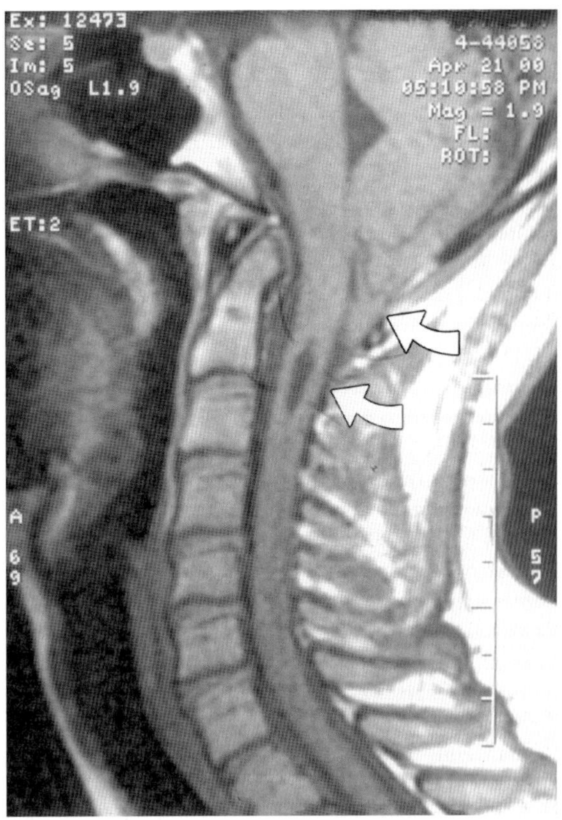

FIGURE 233-5 Chiari-type malformation and developmental syringomyelia. T1-weighted MRI of the low-lying cerebellar tonsils below the foramen magnum and behind the upper cervical cord (*upper arrow*) and the syrinx cavity in the upper cord (*lower arrow*). (From Ropper AH, Samuels MA. *Adams & Victor's Principles of Neurology*. 9th ed. www.accessmedicine.com. Copyright © The McGraw-Hill Companies, Inc. All rights reserved.)

- Roll prone-to-supine and supine-to-prone independently to increase mobility in 3 months.
- Prop self with hands on floor for 30 seconds with stand-by assistance to increase upright activities in 4 months.
- Sit independently for 1 minute with stand-by assistance to improve balance in 1 month.

PROGNOSIS

- No effect on lifespan following surgical repair.

PATIENT RESOURCE

- Chiari Malformation. American Syringomyelia & Chiari Alliance Project. http://www.asap.org/index.php/disorders/chiari-malformation./ Accessed June 17, 2013.

REFERENCES

1. The American Physical Therapy Association. 5C Impaired motor function and sensory integrity associated with nonprogressive disorders of the central nervous system – congenital origin or acquired in infancy or childhood. *Interactive Guide to Physical Therapist Practice*. 2003. doi: 10.2522/ptguide.978-1-931369-64-0. http://guidetoptpractice.apta.org/content/1/SEC20.extract?sid=2d79565f-9483-42f0-8afc-074fc56c046e. Accessed June 1, 2014.
2. Bernard TJ, Knupp K, Yang ML, Arndt D, Levinson P, Moe PG. Chapter 23. Neurologic & muscular disorders. In: Hay W, Levin MJ, Sondheimer JM, Detering RR, eds. *CURRENT Diagnosis & Treatment: Pediatrics*. New York, NY: McGraw-Hill; 2011. http://www.accessphysiotherapy.com/abstract/6585385#6585406. Accessed June 17, 2013.
3. Tsai AC, Manchester DK, Elias ER. Chapter 35. Genetics & Dysmorphology: disorders of multifactorial inhereitance. In: Hay W, Levin MJ, Sondheimer JM, Detering RR, eds. *CURRENT Diagnosis & Treatment: Pediatrics*. New York, NY: McGraw-Hill; 2011. http://www.accessphysiotherapy.com/abstract/6589221#6589221. Accessed June 17, 2013.
4. Thilo EH, Rosenberg AA. Chapter 1. The Newborn Infant: Neonatal intensive care. In: Hay W, Levin MJ, Sondheimer JM, Detering RR, eds. *CURRENT Diagnosis & Treatment: Pediatrics*. New York, NY: McGraw-Hill; 2011. http://www.accessphysiotherapy.com/abstract/6576305#6576336. Accessed June 17, 2013.
5. NIH National Institutes of Health. Stridor. Medline Plus. http://www.nlm.nih.gov/medlineplus/ency/article/003074.htm. Accessed June 17, 2013.
6. Waxman SG. Chapter 17. The Vestibular System. In: *Clinical Neuroanatomy*. New York, NY: McGraw-Hill; 2010. http://www.accessphysiotherapy.com/abstract/5274678#5274679. Accessed June 17, 2013.
7. Dutton M. Chapter 2. The Nervous System. In: *Orthopaedic Examination, Evaluation, and Intervention*. New York, NY: McGraw-Hill; 2008. http://www.accessphysiotherapy.com/abstract/5541218#5541372. Accessed June 17, 2013.
8. Braverman RS. Chapter 15. Eye. In: Hay W, Levin MJ, Sondheimer JM, Detering RR, eds. *CURRENT Diagnosis & Treatment: Pediatrics*. New York, NY: McGraw-Hill; 2011. http://www.accessphysiotherapy.com/abstract/6580635#6580641. Accessed June 17, 2013.
9. Kusumoto FM. Chapter 10. Cardiovascular Disorders: Heart Disease: Pathophysiology of selected cardiovascular disorders. In: *Pathophysiology of Disease*. New York, NY: McGraw-Hill. http://www.accessphysiotherapy.com/abstract/5367685#5367687. Accessed June 17, 2013.
10. Dutton M. *McGraw Hill's NPTE (National Physical Therapy Examination)*. 2nd ed. New York, NY: McGraw-Hill; 2012. http://www.accessphysiotherapy.com/resource/611. Accessed June 17, 2013.
11. Definition of Teratogen. Medicine Net.Com. http://www.medterms.com/script/main/art.asp?articlekey=11315. Accessed June 17, 2013.
12. Incesu L. Imaging in Chiari II Malformation. Medscape Reference. http://emedicine.medscape.com/article/406975-overview. Accessed June 17, 2013.
13. Tracheostomy. Medicine Net.com. http://www.medicinenet.com/tracheostomy/article.htm. Accessed June 17, 2013.
14. Chiari Malformation. Mayo Clinic. http://www.mayoclinic.com/health/chiari-malformation/DS00839. Accessed June 17, 2013.
15. Ullrich PF. Posterior Cervical Laminectomy. Spine Health. http://www.spine-health.com/treatment/back-surgery/posterior-cervical-laminectomy. Accessed June 17, 2013.

ADDITIONAL REFERENCES

- Hinderer KA, Hinderer SR, Shurtleff DB. Myelodysplasia. In: Campbell SK, Palisano RJ, Orlin MN, eds. *Physical Therapy for Children*. 4th ed. St. Louis, MO: Elsevier Saunders; 2012.
- ICD9DATA web site. http://www.icd9data.com. Accessed June 17, 2013.
- ICD10DATA web site. http://www.icd10data.com. Accessed June 17, 2013.
- McPhee SJ, Hammer GD. Arrhythmias. In: McPhee SJ, Hammer GD, eds. *Pathophysiology of Disease*. 6th ed. New York, NY: McGraw-Hill; 2010. http://www.accessphysiotherapy.com/content/5367687#5367687. Accessed June 17, 2013.
- NINDS Chiari Information Page. National Institute of Neurological Disorders and Stroke web site. http://www.ninds.nih.gov/disorders/chiari/chiari.htm. Accessed June 17, 2013.
- Patel DR, Greydanus DE. Physically challenged athletes. In: Patel DR, Greydanus DE, Baker RJ, eds. *Pediatric Practice: Sports Medicine*. New York, NY: McGraw-Hill; 2009. http://www.accessphysiotherapy.com/content/6982289#6982289. Accessed June 17, 2013.
- Stridor. Medline Plus web site. http://www.nlm.nih.gov/medlineplus/ency/article/003074.htm. Accessed June 17, 2013.
- Tappit-Emas E. Spina bifida. In: Tecklin JS, ed. *Pediatric Physical Therapy*. 4th ed. Philadelphia, PA: Lippincott, Williams and Wilkins; 2008: 231–279.
- Waxman SG. Clinical correlations. In: Waxman SG, ed. *Clinical Neuroanatomy*. 26th ed. New York, NY: McGraw-Hill; 2010. http://www.accessphysiotherapy.com/content/5274679#5274679. Accessed June 17, 2013.
- Waxman SG. Examples of specific spinal cord disorders. In: Waxman SG, ed. *Clinical Neuroanatomy*. 26th ed. New York, NY: McGraw-Hill; 2010. http://www.accessphysiotherapy.com/content/5272174#5272174. Accessed June 17, 2013.

234 CLUBFOOT

Kay Tasso, PhD, PT, PCS

CONDITION/DISORDER SYNONYMS

- Congenital talipes equinovarus (CTEV)
- Congenital clubfoot

ICD-9-CM CODE

- 754.51 Congenital talipes equinovarus

ICD-10-CM CODE

- Q66.0 Congenital talipes equinovarus

PREFERRED PRACTICE PATTERN

- 4B: Impaired Joint Mobility, Motor Function, Muscle Performance, and ROM Associated with Impaired Posture[1]

PATIENT PRESENTATION

While hospitalized, a 3-day-old infant is referred to physical therapy with a diagnosis of myelomeningocele. The infant was diagnosed in utero and subsequently, delivered by caesarean section. Surgical reduction of the meningocele occurred within the first 24 hours. Post-op precautions include no positioning in supine. The infant is being monitored to determine if a ventroperitoneal shunt will be needed. Upon examination, the therapist notes bilateral talipes equinovarus with the feet postured in plantar flexion, inversion, and abduction. The physical therapist provides passive range of motion to the feet and ankles and instructs the parents on how to complete this activity as part of the home exercise program.

KEY FEATURES

Description

- Three malformations of the foot/ankle complex seen at birth
  - Plantar flexion (ankle or hindfoot equinus)
  - Inversion (rearfoot varus)[2]
  - Adduction (forefoot varus or metatarsus adductus)[2]

Essentials of Diagnosis

- Idiopathic, though can be hereditary
- Neurogenic
- Associated with syndromes such as arthrogryposis and Larsen syndrome[3]
- Postural or positional; not a true club foot

General Considerations

- Two categories: Flexible or rigid
- Results from abnormally shaped tarsal bones that cause ligament and joint changes

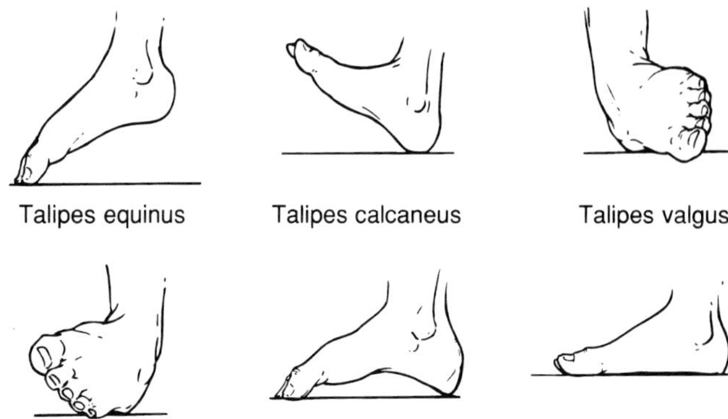

FIGURE 234-1 Deformities of the foot. (From LeBlond RF, DeGowin RL, Brown DD. *DeGowin's Diagnostic Examination*. 9th ed. http://www.accessmedicine.com. Copyright © The McGraw-Hill Companies, Inc. All rights reserved.)

- Often associated with myelomeningocele[4]
- May result from arthrogryposis

Demographics

- Incidence 1 to 2 per 1000 infants
- 2:1 male–female ratio
- Hispanics at greater risk
- Asians at least risk
- 50% bilateral
- Occurs most often in first-born infants

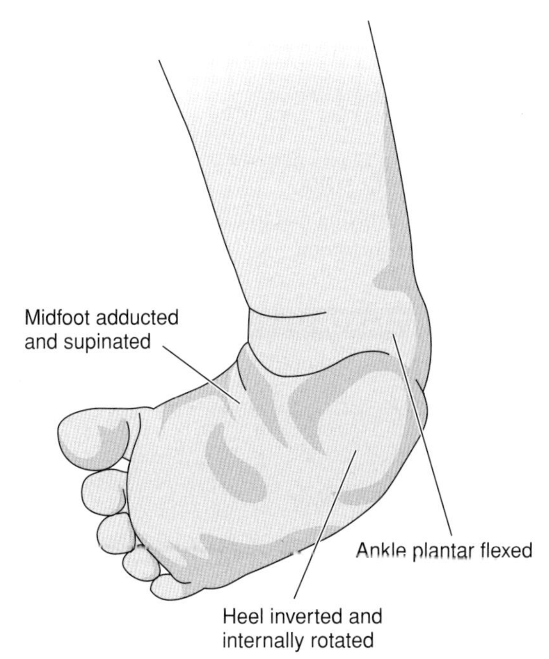

FIGURE 234-2 Clinical appearance of congenital right club foot. (From Skinner HB. *Current Diagnosis & Treatment in Orthopedics*. 4th ed. http://www.accessmedicine.com. Copyright © The McGraw-Hill Companies, Inc. All rights reserved.)

CLINICAL FINDINGS

SIGNS AND SYMPTOMS

- Either flexible or rigid deformities of the foot including plantar flexion, adduction, and inversion
- Contracted intrinsic muscles of the foot
- Vertical talus

▸ Functional Implication

- Unable to stand with flat foot or bear weight on the involved side

▸ Possible Contributing Causes

- Genetic: Siblings 30 times more likely to also have club foot
- Environmental: In utero complications, such as too little amniotic fluid (oligohydramnios) or abnormal fetal positioning
- Dwarfism
- Myelomenigocele
- Polio
- Cerebral palsy

▸ Differential Diagnosis

- Metatarsus adductus
- Postural club foot
- Tarsal coalitions
- Skew foot
- Streeter dysplasia

MEANS OF CONFIRMATION OR DIAGNOSIS

▸ Imaging

- X-ray

FINDINGS AND INTERPRETATION

- Bone misalignment

TREATMENT

- Serial casting[5]
- Surgical
  - Surgical repair (15%–50%)
  - Ponseti method involving manipulation and casting[6]
  - Night splint after correction

REFERRALS/ADMITTANCE

- All patients with CTEV should be referred to an orthopedic surgeon

IMPAIRMENTS

- Unable to stand independently
- Unable to ambulate
- Decreased passive and active ROM for dorsiflexion, abduction, and eversion

TESTS AND MEASURES

- Goniometric measurements
- Joint mobility
- Gait analysis

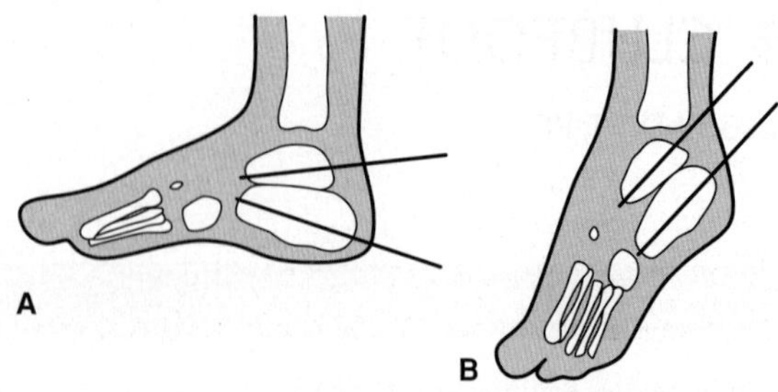

FIGURE 234-3 Diagrammatic appearance of radiograph in club foot. **A.** Normal foot. **B.** Club foot. (From Skinner HB. *Current Diagnosis & Treatment in Orthopedics*. 4th ed. http://www.accessmedicine.com. Copyright © The McGraw-Hill Companies, Inc. All rights reserved.)

INTERVENTION

- Serial casting
- Gentle passive ROM to stretch soft tissue and correct alignment
- Neurodevelopmental treatment to achieve age-appropriate motor milestones in conjunction with serial casting or splinting
  - Facilitate weight bearing while sitting on bench or chair
  - Facilitate weight bearing with supported standing or while standing at furniture
- Pre-gait training activities and gait training
- Manual therapy; mobilize the talonavicular joint by moving the navicular laterally and the head of the talus medially

FUNCTIONAL GOALS

- Patient will be able to:
  - Demonstrate full passive and active ankle and foot ROM to maximize function.
  - Stand at furniture for 5 to 10 minutes while playing.
  - Cruise at furniture to increase mobility.
  - Ambulate with two hands held for household mobility.
  - Ambulate with one hand held as primary method of mobility.
  - Ambulate independently with normal gait pattern for independence with ADLs.
  - Climb stairs (specify ascending or descending) in step-to-step pattern with railing and one hand held to progress to independence.

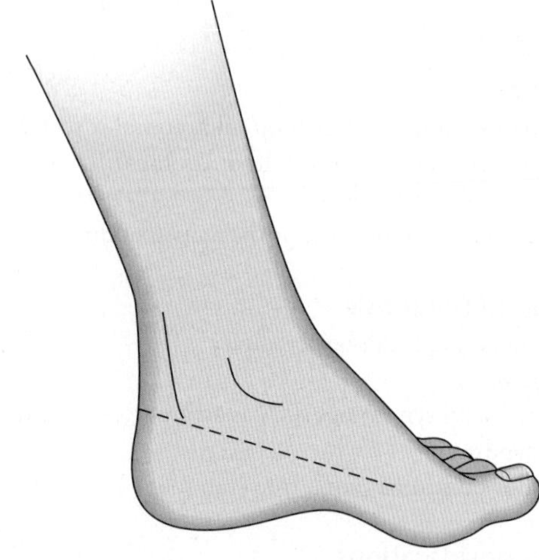

FIGURE 234-4 Cincinnati incision used for surgical correction of club foot. (From Skinner HB. *Current Diagnosis & Treatment in Orthopedics*. 4th ed. http://www.accessmedicine.com. Copyright © The McGraw-Hill Companies, Inc. All rights reserved.

- Climb stairs in step-over-step pattern with railing to progress to independence.

PROGNOSIS

- Good with early intervention (for diagnoses other than myelomeningocele or arthrogryposis).
- Fair with early intervention (<6 months of age) for diagnoses of myelomeningocele (due to recurrence) or arthrogryposis (due to bony limitations).
- If flexible, correctable without surgery.
- If rigid, requires surgical release.

PATIENT RESOURCES

- Clubfoot. American Academy of Orthopeadic Surgeons. http://orthoinfo.aaos.org/topic.cfm?topic=A00255. Accessed February 12, 2013.
- Ponseti International Association. http://www.ponseti.info. Accessed February 12, 2013.

REFERENCES

1. The American Physical Therapy Association. Pattern 4B: Impaired Posture. *Interactive Guide to Physical Therapist Practice.* 2003. doi: 10.2522/ptguide.3.1_2. Online February 29, 2012. http://guidetoptpractice.apta.org/content/1/SEC9.extract?sid=be3f2c03-db2a-44fa-b87f-b9514babca83. Accessed June 1, 2014.
2. Dutton M. *Orthopaedic Examination, Evaluation, and Intervention.* New York, NY: McGraw-Hill; 2008. http://www.accessphysiotherapy.com/resource/612. Accessed March 1, 2013.
3. Polousky JD. Chapter 24. Orthopedics. In: Hay W, Levin MJ, Sondheimer JM, Detering RR, eds. *CURRENT Diagnosis & Treatment: Pediatrics.* New York, NY: McGraw-Hill; 2011. http://www.accessphysiotherapy.com/abstract/6580635#6580641. Accessed March 1, 2013.
4. Waxman SG. *Clinical Neuroanatomy.* New York, NY: McGraw-Hill; 2010. http://www.accessphysiotherapy.com/resource/22. Accessed March 1, 2013.
5. Cincinnati Children's Hospital. Serial casting of the lower extremity. *Evidence-based Care Guideline for Management of Serial Casting in Children.* 2009. http://www.cincinnatichildrens.org/assets/0/78/1067/2709/2777/2793/9199/317d7f8d-943e-42a0-8a65-0bb0c35addb6.pdf. Accessed March 8, 2013.
6. Ponseti International Association. *Ponseti Method.* http://www.ponseti.info/v1/index.php?option=com_content&task=view&id=14&Itemid=28. Accessed March 8, 2013.

ADDITIONAL REFERENCES

- Anatomy and Physiology Revealed. AccessPhysiotherapy Web site. http://www.accessphysiotherapy.com/APR. Accessed March 8, 2013.
- Barnes DV, Wood A. The infant at risk for developmental delay. In: Tecklin JS, ed. *Pediatric Physical Therapy.* 4th ed. Philadelphia, PA: Lippincott, Williams and Wilkins; 2008:101–178.
- Dobbs MB, Gurnett CA. Update on clubfoot: Etiology and treatment. *Clin Orthop Relat Res.* 2009;467(5):1146–1153.
- Hay WW, Levin MJ, Sondheimer JM, Deterding RR. Disturbances of prenatal origin. In: Hay WW, Levin MJ, Sondheimer JM, Deterding RR, eds. *CURRENT Diagnosis & Treatment: Pediatrics.* 20th ed. New York, NY: McGraw-Hill; 2011.
- ICD9DATA web site. http://www.icd9data.com. Accessed January 21, 2013.
- ICD10DATA web site. http://www.icd10data.com. Accessed January 21, 2013.
- Stanger M. Orthopedic management. In: Tecklin JS, ed. *Pediatric Physical Therapy.* 4th ed. Philadelphia, PA: Lippincott, Williams and Wilkins; 2008:417–450.

235 CRI-DU-CHAT SYNDROME

Kay Tasso, PhD, PT, PCS

CONDITION/DISORDER SYNONYMS

- 5p minus
- Deletion of 5p-
- Chromosome 5p deletion syndrome
- 5p minus deletion syndrome[1]
- Cat's cry syndrome[1]

ICD-9-CM CODE

- 758.31 Cri-du-chat syndrome

ICD-10-CM CODE

- Q93.4 Deletion of short arm of chromosome 5

PREFERRED PRACTICE PATTERN

- 5C: Impaired Motor Function and Sensory Integrity Associated with Nonprogressive Disorders of the Central Nervous System—Congenital Origin or Acquired in Infancy or Childhood [2]

PATIENT PRESENTATION

A 3-month-old infant has been referred to physical therapy with a history of atypical facial features and microcephaly. The mother reports no difficulties during pregnancy or delivery. She states the baby has difficulty feeding and has an unusual cry that sounds like a cat. A genetics consult resulted in a diagnosis of cri-du-chat due to an abnormality in chromosome 5. Upon examination, the physical therapist notes hypotonia primarily in the neck and trunk and the infant is not yet able to achieve prone-on-elbows. An evaluation by the local early intervention program is pending.

KEY FEATURES

Description

- Genetic disorder: Deletion of terminal chromosome 5p
  - Cry that sounds like a cat (likely due to abnormal shape of larynx and epiglottis)[3]
  - Characteristic facial features[3]
  - Developmental delay in gross motor skills, oral motor skills, and speech and/or language skills

Essentials of Diagnosis

- Abnormality of chromosome 5 with deletion of short arm

General Considerations

- Associated disorders:
  - Scoliosis[3]
  - Major organ abnormalities

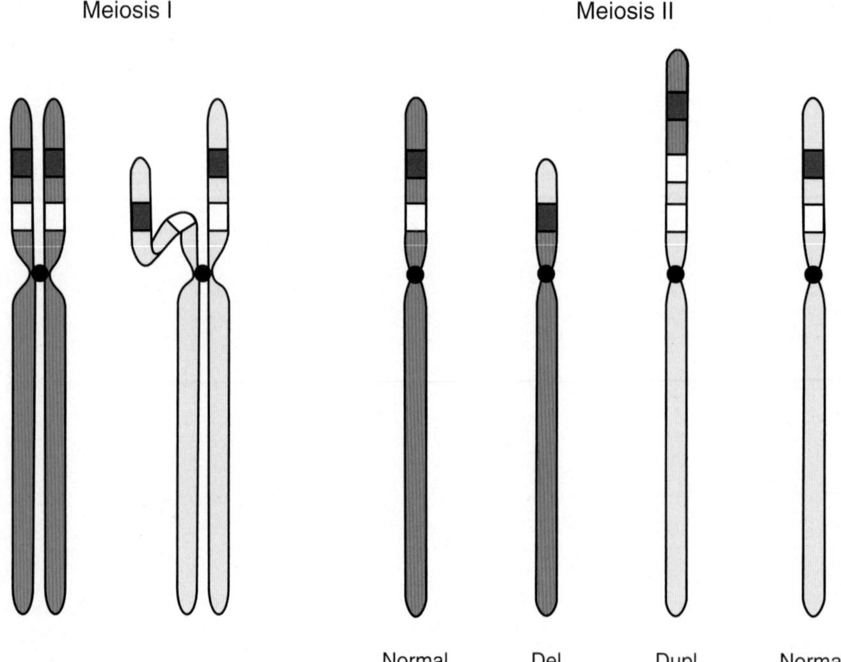

FIGURE 235-1 A mismatch during pairing of homologous chromosomes may lead to a deletion in one chromosome and a duplication in the other. (del = deletion; dup = duplication) (From Spong CY, Cunningham FG, Leveno K, Bloom S, Hauth J, Rouse D. *Williams Obstetrics*. 23rd ed. http://www.accessmedicine.com. Copyright © The McGraw-Hill Companies, Inc. All rights reserved.)

- Diastasis rectii[4]
- Cataracts
- Abnormalities in organs[3]

Demographics

- 1 in 20,000 to 50,000 births[5]
- Females more common than males[6]

CLINICAL FINDINGS

SIGNS AND SYMPTOMS

- High-pitched, cat-like cry
- Moon face
- Antimongoloid slant of palpebral fissures
- Feeding difficulties[6]
- Hypotonia[3]
- Microcephaly[3]
- Hypertelorism
- Epicanthal folds
- Strabismus
- Micrognathia[3]
- Failure to thrive[4]
- Delays in:
  - Gross motor skills
  - Oral motor skills[7]
  - Speech and/or language skills[7]
- Cognitive/intellectual disability
- Stereotypic movements[6]
- Behavioral issues[6]
- Hyperacusis[6]

Possible Contributing Causes

- Defect in either the egg or sperm[1]

Functional Implications

- Poor head control as infant
- Poor trunk control so delayed in sitting independently
- Late walking
- Cognitive impairment[3]
- 50% are hyperactive[3]

Differential Diagnosis

- Patau syndrome[6]
- Wolf–Hischhorn syndrome[6]

MEANS OF CONFIRMATION OR DIAGNOSIS

Laboratory Tests

- DNA analysis[3]

Imaging

- Skeletal radiographs for microcephaly and short metacarpals[6]
- MRI to assess for atrophy[6]
- Echocardiography to rule out cardiac defects[6]
- Barium swallow study[6]

FINDINGS AND INTERPRETATION

- Organ anomalies
  - Ventricular septal defect[8]

TREATMENT

Medication

- None

REFERRALS/ADMITTANCE

- Geneticist
- Ophthalmologist for possible cataracts

TABLE 235-1 Classification and Frequency[a] of Congenital Heart Disease

Without shunt (20%)	
Right-sided	
Pulmonary stenosis	10%
Ebstein anomaly	Rare
Left-sided	
Coarctation of the aorta	10%
Aortic stenosis	Rare
Dextrocardia	Rare
With shunt (80%)	
Acyanotic	
Atrial septal defect	15%
Ventricular septal defect	25%
Patent ductus arteriosus	15%
Cyanotic	
Tetralogy of Fallot	10%
Transposition of great vessels	10%
Truncus arteriosus	Rare
Tricuspid atresia	Rare
Total anomalous pulmonary venous return	Rare
Hypoplastic left heart syndrome	Rare
Eisenmenger syndrome[b]	Rare

[a]Relative frequencies of individual anomalies in children
[b]The term Eisenmenger syndrome is applied to the development of pulmonary hypertension and reversal of shunt direction in patients with atrial septal defect, ventricular septal defect, and patent ductus arteriosus. Surgery to close the defect in the presence of this degree of pulmonary hypertension has a high mortality rate.
Source: From Chandrasoma P, Taylor CR. *Concise Pathology.* 3rd ed. http://www.accessmedicine.com.

- Orthopedics for possible scoliosis or pes planus
- Neurology
- Occupational therapy
- Speech therapy

IMPAIRMENTS

- Decreased strength
- Poor head control
- Poor trunk control

TESTS AND MEASURES

- Bayley Scales of Motor Development or Bayley II
- Peabody Scales of Motor Development
- Movement Assessment of Infants
- Neonatal Behavioral Assessment Scale
- Early Intervention Developmental Profile
- Test of Infant Motor Performance
- Alberta Infant Motor Scale

INTERVENTION

- Behavior modification
- Developmental activities
  - Facilitation of normal movement patterns
  - Acquisition of motor milestones through facilitation

TABLE 235-2 Some Microdeletion Syndromes Detectable by Fluorescence In Situ Hybridization

Syndrome	Features	Location
Alagille	Dysmorphic facies, cholestatic jaundice, pulmonic stenosis, butterfly vertebrae, absent deep-tendon reflexes, poor school performance	20p11.23–20p12.2
Angelman	Dysmorphic facies—"happy puppet" appearance, mental retardation, ataxia, hypotonia, seizures	15q11.2–q13 (maternal genes)
Cri du chat	Growth restriction, hypotonia, severe mental retardation, abnormal laryngeal development with "cat-like" cry	5p15.2–15.3
Kallmann 1	Hypogonadotropic hypogonadism and anosmia	Xp22.3
Miller–Dieker	Severe neuronal migration abnormalities with lissencephaly, microcephaly, failure to thrive, dysmorphic facies	17p13.3
Prader–Willi	Obesity, hypotonia, mental retardation, short stature, hypogonadotropic hypogonadism, small hands and feet	15q11.2–q13 (paternal genes)
Saethre–Chotzen	Acrocephaly, asymmetry of the skull and face, partial syndactyly of fingers and toes	7p21.1
Smith–Magenis	Dysmorphic facies, speech delay, hearing loss, sleep disturbances, self-destructive behaviors	17p11.2
Velocardiofacial/ DiGeorge	May include conotruncal cardiac defects, cleft palate, velopharyngeal incompetence, thymic and parathyroid abnormalities, learning disability, characteristic facial appearance	22q11.2
Williams–Beuren	Aortic stenosis, peripheral pulmonary arterial stenoses, elfin facies, mental retardation, short stature, infantile hypercalcemia	7q11.23
Wolf–Hirschhorn	Dysmorphic facies, severe mental retardation, polydactyly, cutis aplasia, seizures	4p16.3

Source: Adapted from Online Mendelian Inheritance in Man (OMIM). McKusick-Nathans Institute for Genetic Medicine, Johns Hopkins University (Baltimore, MD) and National Center for Biotechnology Information, National Library of Medicine (Bethesda, MD). Available at: http://www.ncbi.nlm.nih.gov/omim/. Accessed April 6, 2009

- Therapeutic exercise
  - Strengthening
  - Balance training
  - Coordination tasks
- Recommendations for adaptive equipment as needed

FUNCTIONAL GOALS

The patient will be able to:

- Sustain prone-on-elbows with 45 degrees cervical extension for 30 to 60 seconds independently within 3 months.
- Brings hands to midline to reach for a toy when in supine within 1 month.
- Sits for 15 to 30 seconds while propping with hands on the floor within 6 months.
- Crawl on hands and knees with minimal assistance for 5 minutes within 4 months.
- Commando crawls independently as primary method of mobility in 3 months.
- Roll from prone to supine using trunk flexion with moderate assistance in 3 months.

PROGNOSIS

- 50% speak by 5 ½ years of age.[3]
- 50% dress selves by 3 ½ years of age.[3]
- 50% walking by 3 years of age.[3]
- Can live to over 50 years of age.[3]

PATIENT RESOURCES

- Cri du chat. www.Criduchat.org. Accessed August 17, 2014.
- Cri du Chate Syndrome Support Group. http://www.cridu-chat.org.uk. Accessed August 17, 2014.
- Five P Minus Society. http://www.fivepminus.org/about.htm director@fivepminus.org Accessed January 14, 2013.

REFERENCES

1. Cri-du-chat. MedlinePlus Web site. http://www.nlm.nih.gov/medlineplus/ency/article/001593.htm. Accessed January 14, 2013.
2. Guide to Physical Therapist Practice. APTA web site. http://guidetoptpractice.apta.org./ Accessed January 14, 2013.
3. Cri du chat syndrome. Orphanet Journal of Rare Diseases web site. http://www.ojrd.com/content/1/1/33. Accessed January 14, 2013.
4. Cri du chat syndrome web site. http://www.criduchatsyndrome.net./ Accessed January 14, 2013.
5. What is Cri-du-chat syndrome? Genetics Home Reference web site. http://ghr.nlm.nih.gov/condition/cri-du-chat-syndrome. Accessed January 14, 2013.
6. Cri-du-chat syndrome. Medscape Reference web site. http://emedicine.medscape.com/article/942897-overview#a0199. Accessed January 14, 2013.
7. Learning about cri du chat syndrome. National Human Genome Research Institute web site. http://www.genome.gov/19517558. Accessed January 14, 2013.
8. Chandrasoma P, Taylor CR. Chapter 21, The Heart: I. Structure & Function; Congenital Diseases. In: Chandrasoma P, Taylor CR, eds. *Concise Pathology*. 3rd ed. New York, NY: McGraw-Hill; 2011. http://www.accessphysiotherapy.com/content/186415/searchStr/cri-du-chat%20syndrome#186415. Accessed January 14, 2013.

ADDITIONAL REFERENCES

- Developmental Profile III. Children and Adolescents with Special Needs. http://portal.wpspublish.com/portal/

page?_pageid=53,186601&_dad=portal&_schema=PORTAL. Accessed January 14, 2013.

- Dutton M. Pediatric Physical Therapy. In: *McGraw Hill's National Physical Therapy Examination.*2nd ed. New York, NY: McGraw-Hill; 2012. http://www.accessphysiotherapy.com/content/5404405#5404405. Accessed January 14, 2013.
- Hay WW, Levin MJ, Sondheimer JM, Deterding RR. Chromosome Deletion Disorders. In: Hay WW, Levin MJ, Sondheimer JM, Deterding RR, eds. *CURRENT Diagnosis & Treatment: Pediatrics*. 20th ed. New York, NY: McGraw-Hill; 2011. http://www.accessphysiotherapy.com/content/6589063. Accessed January 14, 2013.
- ICD9DATA Web Site. http://www.icd9data.com/2012/Volume1/740-759/758/758.31.htm. Accessed January 14, 2013.
- ICD10DATA Web Site. http://www.icd10data.com/Search.aspx?search=cri+du+chat&codebook=AllCodes. Accessed January 14, 2013.
- The Neonatal Behavioral Assessment Scale. The Brazelton Institute web site. http://www.brazelton-institute.com/intro.html. Accessed January 14, 2013.
- The Test of Infant Motor Performance. Infant Motor Performance Scales web site. http://thetimp.com. Accessed January 14, 2013.

236 DEVELOPMENTAL COORDINATION DISORDER

Kay Tasso, PhD, PT, PCS

CONDITION/DISORDER SYNONYMS

- DCD
- Clumsy child syndrome
- Motor dyspraxia
- Developmental dyspraxia
- Sensory integrative dysfunction
- Disorder of attention, motor, and perception
- Minor coordination dysfunction

ICD-9-CM CODE

- 315.4 Developmental coordination disorder

ICD-10-CM CODE

- F82 Specific developmental disorder of motor function

PREFERRED PRACTICE PATTERN

- 5C: Impaired Motor Function and Sensory Integrity Associated with Nonprogressive Disorders of the Central Nervous System—Congenital Origin or Acquired in Infancy or Childhood [1]

PATIENT PRESENTATION

A 5-year-old male is referred for outpatient physical therapy for frequent falling. The parents report he takes Strattera for attention deficit hyperactivity disorder (ADHD) and gets frustrated when trying to play with his 4-year-old sister. Upon examination, the therapist notes the child has mild hypotonia especially in his trunk, has difficulty balancing on one leg, and has poor coordination with kicking or catching a ball. He has fair abdominal strength and descends stairs in a step-to-step pattern.

KEY FEATURES

Description

- Difficulty performing complex gross or fine motor-coordination tasks

Essentials of Diagnosis

- No cognitive or neurological dysfunction

General Considerations

- Four criteria
  - Difficulty performing age-appropriate motor skills
  - Child has had sufficient opportunity to attain motor skills
  - No medical reason for motor difficulty
  - Difficulties impact academics or ADLs

Demographics

- Fifty percent of children with developmental coordination disorder (DCD) also have ADHD[2, 3]
- Affects 5% to 6% of all children[4]
- Affects twice as many males as females[4]

CLINICAL FINDINGS

SIGNS AND SYMPTOMS

- Decreased strength
- Difficulty with coordination
  - Ball skills
    - Catching
    - Throwing
    - Kicking
  - Single-limb stance
  - Jumping
  - Hopping on one foot
  - Skipping
- Ligamentous laxity
- Hypotonia[5]
- Soft neurological signs[6]
- Atypical gait pattern

Functional Implications

- Falls or trips often
- Bumps into objects, other people
- Difficulty using motor skills in new settings

Possible Contributing Causes

- Premature birth[4]

Differential Diagnosis

- Head injury
- Progressive neurological disorder
- Brain tumor
- Autism
- Pervasive developmental disorder[7]
- Cerebral palsy[8,9]
- Visual disturbances

MEANS OF CONFIRMATION OR DIAGNOSIS

Diagnostic Procedures

- Parent–teacher questionnaires: Connors, Burks
- Psychological testing
- IQ testing
- Developmental and Psychosocial evaluation

TREATMENT

Medication

- None for DCD
- Medications available for ADHD
  - Methylphenidate drugs
  - Amphetamines
  - Dexmethylphenidate
  - Dextroamphetamine
  - Lisdexamfetamine

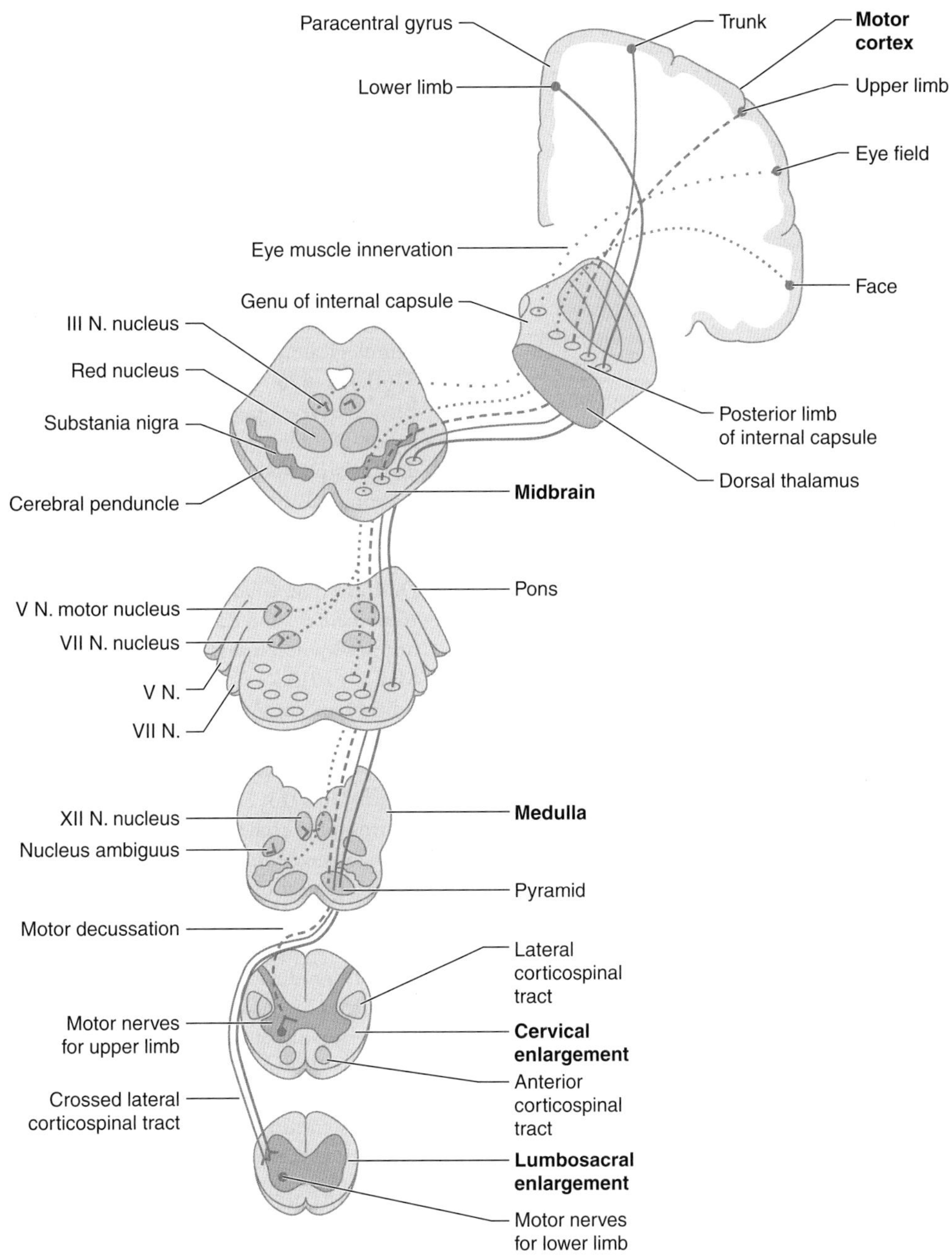

FIGURE 236-1 Upper motor neuron pathways. Tracts at bottom left are shown outside the cord for clarity only. (From McPhee SJ, Hammer GD. *Pathophysiology of Disease: An Introduction to Clinical Medicine*. 6th ed. New York, NY:2009, McGraw Hill.)

REFERRALS/ADMITTANCE

- School psychologist for behavioral therapy
- Neurologist
- Occupational therapist
- Speech therapist

IMPAIRMENTS

- Difficulty climbing stairs without holding railing
- Poor abdominal strength
- Inability to balance on one leg
- Inability to hop on one foot
- Inability to kick a rolling ball
- Inability to catch a ball

TESTS AND MEASURES

- Bruininks–Oseretsky Test of Motor Proficiency[10]
- Peabody Scales of Motor Development, 2nd edition[10]
- School Function Assessment (SFA)[11]
- Vineland Adaptive Behavior Scale, 2nd edition[12]
- Developmental Coordination Disorder Questionnaire[13]
- Movement Assessment Battery for Children, 2nd edition

INTERVENTION

- Strengthening
- Balance training
- Coordination tasks

TABLE 236-1 Subcategories of Developmental Coordination Disorder

Clumsiness: inefficiency in the performance of fine motor movements
Adventitious movements: synkinesis, chorea, tremor, or tics
Dyspraxia: inability to learn or perform serial voluntary movements to complete skilled acts
Material-specific dyspraxia: motor execution below expected for age with regard to writing (dysgraphia), drawing (constructional dyspraxia), or speech (verbal dyspraxia)
Neurologic soft signs: non-normative performance on motor or sensory neurologic tests in the absence of localizable neurologic disease or defect
Pathologic handedness: left-handedness associated with left-hemispheric defect and paresis of the right hand

Source: Ebert MH, Loosen PT, Nurcombe B, Leckman JF eds. *Current Diagnosis & Treatment in Psychiatry*. 2nd ed. www.accessmedicine.com.

- Sensory integration
- Motor learning
- Task-specific intervention

FUNCTIONAL GOALS

- Patient will be able to
  - Complete 10 sit-ups with hands behind head within 3 months to increase abdominal strength.
  - Stand on one leg independently for 5 seconds to improve balance.
  - Jump with both feet off the floor in 6 months to increase quadriceps strength, gluteal strength, coordination.
  - Catch a medium-sized ball from 5 feet away with 75% accuracy in 6 months.
  - Kick a rolling ball with 50% accuracy to increase coordination in 1 month.

PROGNOSIS

- Chronic, but no effect on lifespan.

PATIENT RESOURCE

- Dyspraxia. Developmental Coordination Disorder Association Cork. http://www.dyspraxiadcdcork.ie. Accessed August 17, 2014.

REFERENCES

1. The American Physical Therapy Association. Pattern 5C: Impaired motor function and sensory integrity associated with nonprogressive disorders of the central nervous system - congenital origin or acquired in infancy or childhood. *Interactive Guide to Physical Therapist Practice*. 2003. doi: 10.2522/ptguide.3.2_3. http://guidetoptpractice.apta.org/content/1/SEC20.extract?sid=afbbb374-3c09-49c1-9893-668d2e734706. Accessed June 1, 2014.
2. Goldson E, Reynolds A. Chapter 2. Child Development & Behavior. In: Hay WW, Levin MJ, Sondheimer JM, Deterding RR, eds. *CURRENT Diagnosis & Treatment: Pediatrics*. 20th ed. New York, NY: McGraw-Hill; 2011. http://www.accessphysiotherapy.com/abstract/6576852#6576853. Accessed May 11, 2013.
3. Hay WW, Levin MJ, Sondheimer JM, Deterding RR. Subacute and Chronic Ataxias. In: Hay WW, Levin MJ, Sondheimer JM, Deterding RR, eds. *CURRENT Diagnosis & Treatment: Pediatrics*. 20th ed. New York, NY: McGraw-Hill; 2011. http://www.accessphysiotherapy.com/content/6585540. Accessed May 11, 2013.
4. Rivard L, Missiuna C, Pollock N, David KS. Developmental coordination disorder. In: Campbell SK, Palisano RJ, Orlin MN, eds. *Physical Therapy for Children*. 4th ed. St. Louis, MO: Elsevier Saunders; 2012:498–538.
5. Hypotonia. National Institute of Neurological Disorder and Stroke. http://www.ninds.nih.gov/disorders/hypotonia/hypotonia.htm. Accessed March 11, 2013.
6. Lerer RJ, Lerer MP. The effects of methylphenidate on the soft neurological signs of hyperactive children. *Pediatrics*. 1976; 57(4):521–525.
7. Pervasive Developmental Disorder. National Institute of Neurological Disorder and Stroke. http://www.ninds.nih.gov/disorders/pdd/pdd.htm. Accessed March 11, 2013.
8. Cerebral Palsy. National Institute of Neurological Disorder and Stroke. http://www.ninds.nih.gov/disorders/cerebral_palsy/cerebral_palsy.htm. Accessed May 11, 2013.
9. Dutton M. *McGraw Hill's NPTE (National Physical Therapy Examination)*. 2nd ed. New York, NY: McGraw-Hill; 2012. http://www.accessphysiotherapy.com/resource/611. Accessed May 11, 2013.
10. School Function Assessment Technical Report. http://www.pearsonassessments.com/NR/rdonlyres/D50E4125-86EE-43BE-8001-2A4001B603DF/0/SFA_TR_Web.pdf. Accessed March 11, 2013.
11. Sparrow SS, Cicchetti DV, Balla DA. *Vineland Adaptive Behavior Scales, Second Edition (Vineland-II)*. Pearson; 2005. http://psychcorp.pearsonassessments.com/HAIWEB/Cultures/en-us/Productdetail.htm?Pid=Vineland-II. Accessed March 11, 2013.
12. Developmental Coordination Disorder Questionnaire. Developmental Coordination Disorder Questionnaire web site. http://www.dcdq.ca./ Accessed March 11, 2013.
13. Henderson SE, Sugden DA, Barnett A. *Movement Assessment Battery for Children - Second Edition (Movement ABC-2)*. Pearson; 2007. http://www.pearsonassessments.com/HAIWEB/Cultures/en-us/Productdetail.htm?Pid=015-8541-308&Mode=summary. Accessed March 11, 2013.

ADDITIONAL REFERENCES

- Hay WW, Levin MJ, Sondheimer JM, Deterding RR. Attention-Deficit/Hyperactivity Disorder. In: Hay WW, Levin MJ, Sondheimer JM, Deterding RR, eds. *CURRENT Diagnosis & Treatment: Pediatrics*. 20th ed. New York, NY: McGraw-Hill; 2011. http://www.accessphysiotherapy.com/content/6576853#6576853. Accessed March 11, 2013
- ICD9DATA web site. http://www.icd9data.com/2013/Volume1/290-319/300-316/315/315.4.htm. Accessed May 13, 2013.
- ICD10DATA web site. http://www.icd10data.com/Search.aspx?search=F82&codebook=AllCodes Accessed May 13, 2013.
- Psychiatric Disorders. AllPsych Online. http://allpsych.com/disorders/dsm.html. Accessed March 11, 2013.
- Rivard L, Missiuna C, Pollock N, David KS. Developmental Coordination Disorder. In: Campbell SK, Palisano RJ, Orlin MN, eds. *Physical Therapy for Children*. 4th ed. St. Louis, MO: Elsevier Saunders; 2012.
- Wilson PH. Practitioner review: Approaches to assessment and treatment of children with DCD: An evaluative review. *J Child Psychol Psychiatry*. 2005;46:806–823

237 DEVELOPMENTAL DYSPLASIA OF THE HIP

Kay Tasso, PhD, PT, PCS
Patrick S. Pabian, DPT, PT, SCS, OCS, CSCS

CONDITION/DISORDER SYNONYMS

- Congenital dislocation of the hip (CDH)
- Developmental dislocation of the hip

ICD-9-CM CODES

- 754.3 Congenital dislocation of hip
- 754.30 Congenital dislocation of hip unilateral
- 754.31 Congenital dislocation of hip bilateral
- 754.32 Congenital subluxation of hip unilateral
- 754.33 Congenital subluxation of hip bilateral
- 754.35 Congenital dislocation of one hip with subluxation of other hip
- 756.9 Other and unspecified congenital anomalies of musculoskeletal system

ICD-10-CM CODES

- Q65.00 Congenital dislocation of unspecified hip, unilateral
- Q65.1 Congenital dislocation of hip, bilateral
- Q68.8 Other specified congenital musculoskeletal deformities
- Q79.8 Other congenital malformations of musculoskeletal system
- Q79.9 Congenital malformation of musculoskeletal system, unspecified

PREFERRED PRACTICE PATTERNS

- 4D: Impaired Joint Mobility, Motor Function, Muscle Performance, and Range of Motion Associated with Connective Tissue Dysfunction
- 4F: Impaired Joint Mobility, Motor Function, Muscle Performance, and ROM Associated with Spinal Disorders[1]
- 4I: Impaired Joint Mobility, Motor Function, Muscle Performance, and ROM Associated with Bony or Soft Tissue Surgery[2]

PATIENT PRESENTATION

A 6-month-old infant is referred to physical therapy for congenital muscular torticollis. The mother reports an uneventful pregnancy but difficult delivery requiring forceps. Upon examination, the therapist notes asymmetry of the gluteal folds and limited passive right hip abduction and hip flexion in addition to the typical signs of congenital torticollis and gross motor delay. The therapist contacts the physician to discuss the findings. Subsequently, radiologic studies are completed with a resulting diagnosis of developmental dysplasia of the hip. Following evaluation by a pediatric orthopedist, the infant is placed in a Pavlik harness for 23 hours per day except for bathing and therapy.

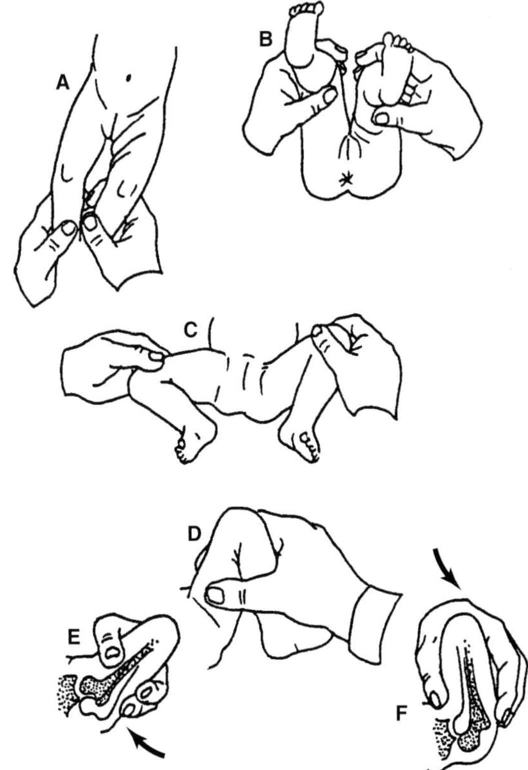

FIGURE 237-1 Clinical examination of developmental dislocation of the hip. In all pictures, the child's left hip is the abnormal side. (**A**) Asymmetric skin folds. (**B**) Galeazzi test. (**C**) Limitation of abduction. (**D– F**) Ortolani and Barlow tests. (From Skinner HB. *Current Diagnosis & Treatment in Orthopedics*. 4th ed. http://www.accessmedicine.com. Copyright © The McGraw-Hill Companies, Inc. All rights reserved.)

KEY FEATURES

Description

- Group of bony abnormalities on hip joint
- Femoral head does not fit tight into the acetabulum
- Femoral head can be manually dislocated from the acetabulum easily[3]
- Congenital or acquired deformation/misalignment of the hip joint[4]
- Hip may be unstable, malformed, dislocated, dislocatable, or subluxated[4]

Essentials of Diagnosis

- Imaging studies could show delayed acetabular development
- Clinical diagnosis from a positive Ortolani sign or Barlow maneuver[4]
- Congenital
  - In utero posture of hip flexion and abduction contributes to disorder
  - Link to relaxin hormone
  - Trait runs in families[5]

- Acquired
  - Result of swaddling, use of a cradle board
  - Breech birth

General Considerations

- More common in infants with congenital muscular torticollis or metatarsus adductus[6]
- Often associated with myelomeningocele[7]
- May occur as a result of arthrogryposis[8]
- Infant dislocation is developmental and associated with osseous development of the acetabulum and proximal femur
  - Observations more evident in infant when approaching ambulatory age

Demographics

- Girl-to-boy ratio: 5:1
- Approximately 1 in 1000 infants
- More common in first-born children
- Three times more common in the left hip than in the right hip
- Developmental dislocation often diagnosed at 3 to 12 months of age
- More common among breech birth position

CLINICAL FINDINGS

SIGNS AND SYMPTOMS

- Developmental prior to ambulatory age
  - The infant's limb may appear shortened, with asymmetry in thigh folds
  - Decreased movement of one leg
- Developmental once ambulatory
  - The child/infant may toe walk on the involved LE
  - If both LEs are involved, the child/infant may have an increased lumbar lordosis and a waddling gait
  - Asymmetry of skin folds in superior, medial thigh or gluteals
  - Trendelenburg gait[6]
- Early development of osteoarthritis

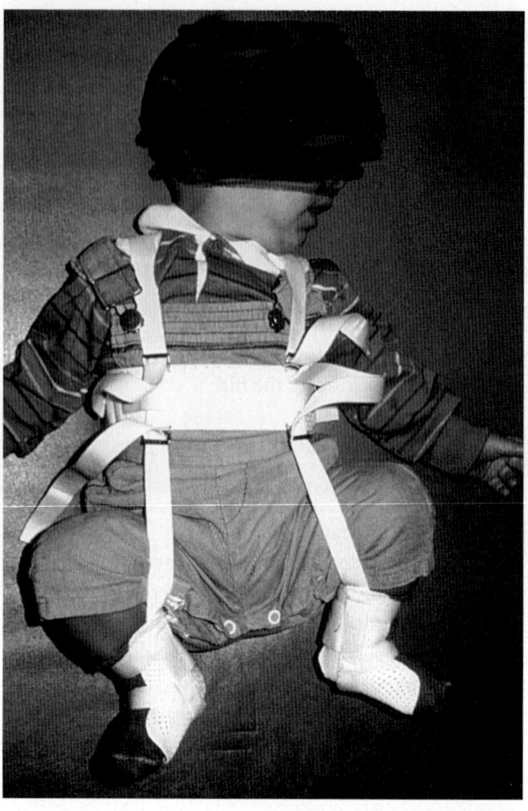

FIGURE 237-2 The Pavlik harness, a device used for treatment of hip dislocation, subluxation, and dysplasia. (From Skinner HB. *Current Diagnosis & Treatment in Orthopedics*. 4th ed. http://www.accessmedicine.com. Copyright © The McGraw-Hill Companies, Inc. All rights reserved.)

Possible Contributing Causes

- Breech presentation or large fetal size
- Abnormal positioning in utero
- Insufficient amniotic fluid (oligohydramnios)
- Hip extension and adduction positioning practiced in some cultures

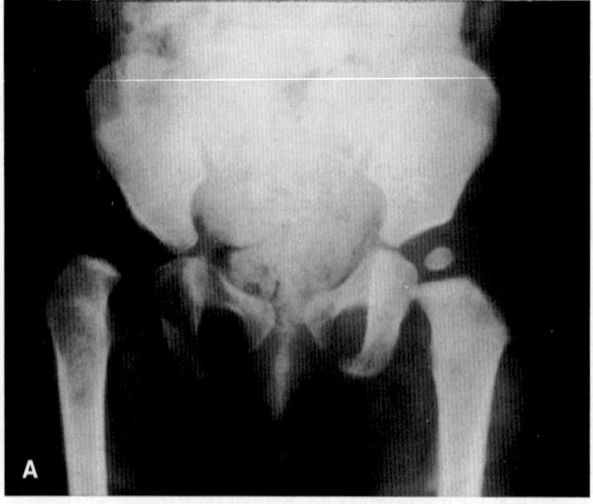

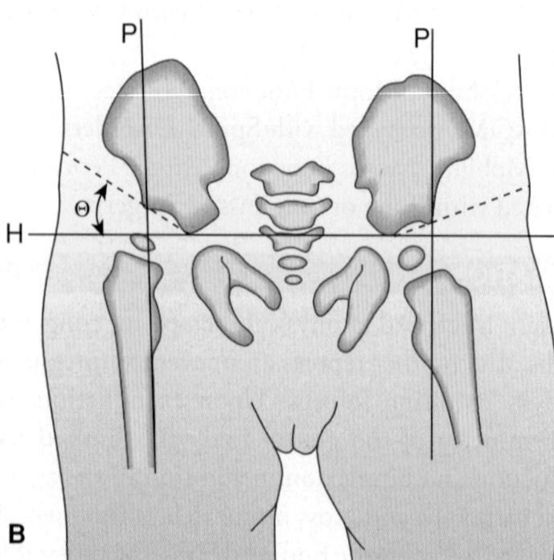

FIGURE 237-3 (**A**) X-ray of congenital dislocation of the right hip. (**B**) Analysis of hip radiographs presupposes adequately exposed films of a properly positioned patient. Hilgenreiner horizontal line is drawn through both triradiate cartilages (H), and Perkins vertical line is drawn through the outer margin of each acetabulum (P). If the hip is located, the proximal femoral epiphysis will lie in the inferomedial quadrant formed by the two intersecting lines. Proximal or lateral displacement indicates dislocation. Abnormal acetabular development is suggested by lack of obvious concavity and by an acetabular index (Θ) greater than 30 degrees. (From Doherty GM. *Current Diagnosis & Treatment: Surgery*. 13th ed. http://www.accessmedicine.com. Copyright © The McGraw-Hill Companies, Inc. All rights reserved.)

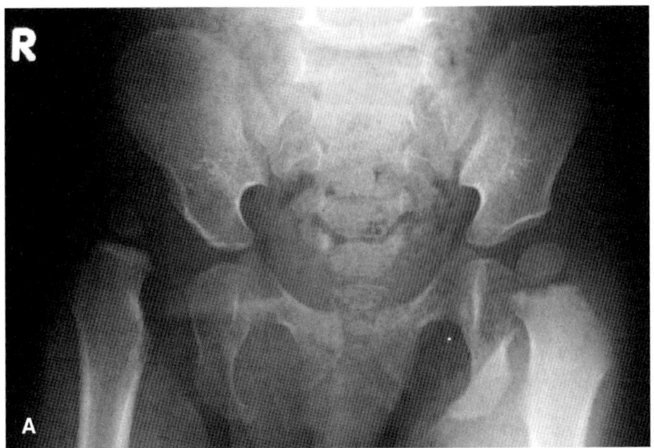

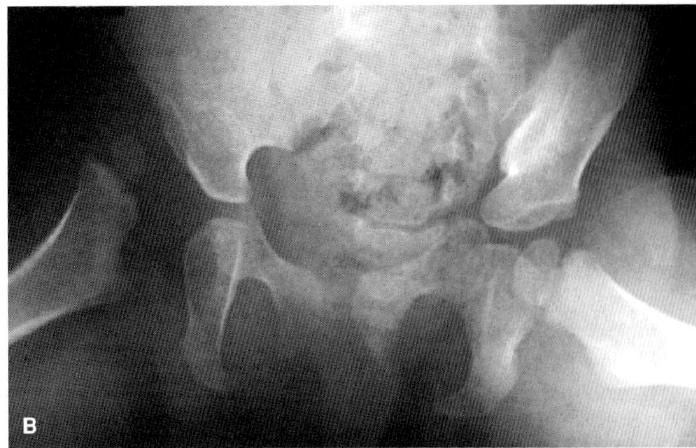

FIGURE 237-4 Developmental hip dislocation of the right hip. (**A**) AP and (**B**) Frog leg lateral. (From Simon RR, Sherman SC. *Emergency Orthopedics*. 6th ed. www.accessemergencymedicine.com. Copyright © The McGraw-Hill Companies, Inc. All rights reserved.)

Functional Implications

- Hip movement
- Standing
- Walking, gait
- Sit-to-stand positional changes

Differential Diagnosis

- Septic hip
- Osteoarthritis
- Rheumatoid arthritis
- Lumbosacral disorder
- Proximal femur or pelvic fracture
- Slipped femoral capital epiphysis
- Legg–Calvé–Perthes disease

MEANS OF CONFIRMATION OR DIAGNOSIS

Imaging

- Diagnostic ultrasound for infants under 6 months of age[9]
- Radiography for older children

FINDINGS AND INTERPRETATION

- Indirect observation in infants aged 3 to 6 months due to lack of visualization of femoral head until that time
- Alignment is determined by analyzing intersecting angles of lines drawn from ossified portions of the pelvis and femoral shaft

TREATMENT

- Developmental
  - Treatments aimed to provide reduction of femoral-acetabular articulation to allow for normal bony development
  - Harness use may be prescribed for up to 3 to 6 months
  - Pavlik harness for infants worn 23 hours per day (except during bathing or physical therapy) from birth to 9 months (over 90% success rate)
  - Frejka pillow
  - Hip abduction orthosis for ambulatory toddlers and children
  - Traction
- Surgery if conservative treatment is not successful
  - Closed reduction, open reduction with or without osteotomy, hip spica cast
  - Casting and possibly open reduction internal fixation may be necessary

REFERRALS/ADMITTANCE

- To hospital for imaging: Radiograph or diagnostic ultrasound of the hip[9]
- To orthopedic/pediatric surgeon for consult

IMPAIRMENTS

- Decreased hip abduction on affected side
- Possible developmental delay due to Pavlik harness
- Gait abnormality in toddlers or older children
- May have decreased active and passive ROM in the hip and knee from hip spica casting following open or closed reduction

TESTS AND MEASURES

- Developmental
  - Ortolani click test
  - Barlow sign
  - Piston sign
  - Galeazzi sign
- Bayley Scales of Motor Development or Bayley II
- Peabody Scales of Motor Development
- Movement Assessment of Infants
- Neonatal Behavioral Assessment Scale
- Early Intervention Developmental Profile
- Test of Infant Motor Performance
- Alberta Infant Motor Scale
- Bruininks–Oseretsky Test of Motor Proficiency
- Neurologic examination
  - Sensation
    - Light touch
    - Pin prick
  - Lower-extremity deep tendon reflexes
  - Proprioception at the hip
  - Kinesthetic awareness at the hip
  - Coordination
- Trunk active and passive ROM
- Hip and knee active and passive ROM

- Flexibility testing
  - Hamstrings
  - Iliopsoas
  - Quadriceps
  - Iliotibial band
  - Abductors
  - Adductors
- Joint integrity of the spine
- Sacroiliac joint integrity
- Hip joint integrity
  - Hip scour
  - Flexion abduction external rotation (FABER) test
  - Flexion induction internal rotation (FAIR) test
- Limb strength
  - Functional strength testing
  - Manual muscle test (MMT)
    - Hamstrings
    - Quadriceps
    - Iliopsoas
    - Gluteus maximus
    - Gluteus medius
    - Gluteus minimus
    - Adductors
- LE contralateral limb strength
- Balance

INTERVENTION

- Passive and active ROM to improve mobility and strength
- Neurodevelopment treatment to achieve age-appropriate motor milestones
  - Facilitate sitting balance with and without arm support
  - Facilitate standing at furniture leaning trunk on furniture for support or supporting self with arms only
  - Facilitate creeping on hands and knees
- Pregait training, gait training in toddlers and children

FUNCTIONAL GOALS

- Patient will be able to
  - Demonstrate full passive and active hip ROM to maximize function.
  - Sit independently for 10 minutes while playing.
  - Creep on hands and knees to explore environment.
  - Stand at furniture for 5 to 10 minutes while playing.
  - Cruise at furniture to increase mobility.
  - Ambulate with both hands held for household mobility.
  - Ambulate with one hand held as primary method of mobility.
  - Ambulate independently with normal gait pattern for independence with ADLs.
  - Climb stairs (specify ascending or descending) in step-to-step pattern with one hand held and holding railing to progress to independence.
  - Climb stairs in step-over-step pattern while holding railing to progress to independence.

PROGNOSIS

- Very good following completion of early orthopedic intervention (for diagnoses other than myelomeningocele or arthrogryposis).
- Fair for diagnoses of myelomeningocele (DDH not always repaired in this population due to recurrence) or arthrogryposis (due to bony limitations).

PATIENT RESOURCES

- Developmental Dislocation (Dysplasia) of the Hip (DDH). http://orthoinfo.aaos.org/topic.cfm?topic=A00347. Accessed June 10, 2013.
- International Hip Dysplasia Institute. http://www.hipdysplasia.org. Accessed June 10, 2013.

REFERENCES

1. The American Physical Therapy Association. Pattern 4F: Impaired joint mobility, motor function, muscle performance, range of motion, and reflex integrity associated with spinal disorders. *Interactive Guide to Physical Therapist Practice*. 2003. DOI: 10.2522/ptguide.3.1_6. Accessed June 10, 2013.
2. The American Physical Therapy Association. Pattern 4I: Impaired joint mobility, motor function, muscle performance, and range of motion associated with bony or soft tissue surgery. *Interactive Guide to Physical Therapist Practice*. 2003. DOI: 10.2522/ptguide.3.1_9. Accessed June 10, 2013.
3. American Physical Therapy Association. Anatomy and physiology revealed. *AccessPhysiotherapy*. http://www.accessphysiotherapy.com/APR. Accessed June 10, 2013.
4. Dutton M. *Orthopaedic Examination, Evaluation, and Intervention*. New York, NY: McGraw-Hill; 2008. http://www.accessphysiotherapy.com/resource/612. Accessed June 10, 2013.
5. Chandrasoma P, Taylor CR. *Concise Pathology*. 3rd ed. Stamford, CT: Appleton & Lang; 1998. http://www.accessphysiotherapy.com/content/187050. Accessed June 10, 2013.
6. Polousky JD. Chapter 24. Orthopedics. In: Hay W, Levin MJ, Sondheimer JM, Detering RR, eds. *CURRENT Diagnosis & Treatment: Pediatrics*. New York, NY: McGraw-Hill; 2011. http://www.accessphysiotherapy.com/abstract/6585834#6585851. Accessed June 10, 2013.
7. Patel DR, Greydanus DE. Chapter 35. Physically challenged athletes. In: Patel DR, Greydanus DE, Baker RJ, eds. *Pediatric Practice: Sports Medicine*. New York, NY: McGraw-Hill; 2009. http://www.accessphysiotherapy.com/abstract/6982260#6982280. Accessed June 10, 2013.
8. Tsai ACH, Manchester DK, Elias ER. Genetics & dysmorphology. In: Hay WW, Levin MJ, Sondheimer JM, Deterding RR, eds. *CURRENT Diagnosis & Treatment: Pediatrics*. 20th ed. McGraw-Hill: New York, NY; 2011. http://www.accessphysiotherapy.com/content/6589246#6589246, Accessed June 10, 2013.
9. Malone TR, Hazle C, Grey ML. Imaging of the Pelvis and Hip. In: Malone TR, Hazle C, Grey ML, eds. *Imaging in Rehabilitation*. New York, NY: McGraw-Hill; 2008. http://www.accessphysiotherapy.com/popup.aspx?aID=5941089. Accessed June 10, 2013.

ADDITIONAL REFERENCES

- Barnes DV, Wood A. The infant at risk for developmental delay. In: Tecklin JS, ed. *Pediatric Physical Therapy*. 4th ed. Philadelphia, PA: Lippincott, Williams and Wilkins; 2008:101–178.
- Dutton M. Chapter 8. The hip joint. In: Dutton M, ed. *Dutton's Orthopedic Survival Guide: Managing Common Conditions*. New

York, NY: McGraw-Hill; 2011. http://www.accessphysiotherapy.com/content/8653838. Accessed June 28, 2013.

- Hay WW, Levin MJ, Sondheimer JM, Deterding RR. Disturbances of prenatal origin. In: Hay WW, Levin MJ, Sondheimer JM, Deterding RR, eds. *CURRENT Diagnosis & Treatment: Pediatrics*. 20th ed. New York, NY: McGraw-Hill; 2011. http://www.accessphysiotherapy.com/content/6585835#6585835, Accessed June 10, 2013.
- ICD9DATA web site. http://www.icd9data.com. Accessed June 10, 2013.
- ICD10DATA Web site. http://www.icd10data.com/ICD10CM/Codes/Q00-Q99/Q65-Q79/Q68-/Q68.8. Accessed June 10, 2013.
- ICD10DATA Web site. http://www.icd10data.com/ICD10CM/Codes/Q00-Q99/Q65-Q79/Q79-/Q79.8. Accessed June 10, 2013.
- Jesse ME, Leach J. Orthopedic conditions. In: Campbell SK, Palisano RJ, Orlin MN, 4th ed. *Physical Therapy for Children*. St. Louis, MO: Elsevier Saunders; 2012:414–452.
- McKinnis L. Radiologic Evaluation of the Pelvis and Hip. In: McKinnis L, ed. *Fundamentals of Musculoskeletal Imaging*. 2nd ed. Philadelphia, PA: F.A. Davis Company; 2005.
- Stanger M. Orthopedic management. In: Tecklin JS, ed. *Pediatric Physical Therapy*. 4th ed. Philadelphia, PA: Lippincott, Williams and Wilkins; 2008:417–450.

238 DOWN SYNDROME

Kay Tasso, PhD, PT, PCS

CONDITION/DISORDER SYNONYMS

- Down syndrome
- Trisomy 21

ICD-9-CM CODE

- 758.0 Down syndrome

ICD-10-CM CODES

- Q90.0 Trisomy 21, nonmosaicism (meiotic nondisjunction)
- Q90.1 Trisomy 21, mosaicism (mitotic nondisjunction)
- Q90.2 Trisomy 21, translocation
- Q90.9 Down syndrome, unspecified

PREFERRED PRACTICE PATTERN

- 4C: Impaired Motor Performance[1]

PATIENT PRESENTATION

A 6-month-old infant is referred to physical therapy from an early intervention program with a diagnosis of Down syndrome. The parents report the infant was diagnosed in utero and was born at full term; otherwise, the pregnancy and delivery were uneventful. Upon examination, the infant is hypotonic and not yet rolling. In prone, the infant can achieve prone on elbows but not yet prone on extended arms. In supine, the infant exhibits decreased activity when reaching against gravity or kicking the legs. There is a mild head lag when pulled into sitting and mild trunk flexion when supported in sitting. The infant does not take weight on the legs when held in supported standing. As a result, direct physical therapy services are recommended.

KEY FEATURES

Description

- Genetic disorder characterized by cognitive impairment and stereotypical physical features
  - Hypotonia
  - Short stature
  - Simian crease
  - Upward-slanting eyes
  - Protruding tongue

Essentials of Diagnosis

- Abnormality of chromosome 21 with three arms rather than two, or translocation
- Can be detected in the early second trimester

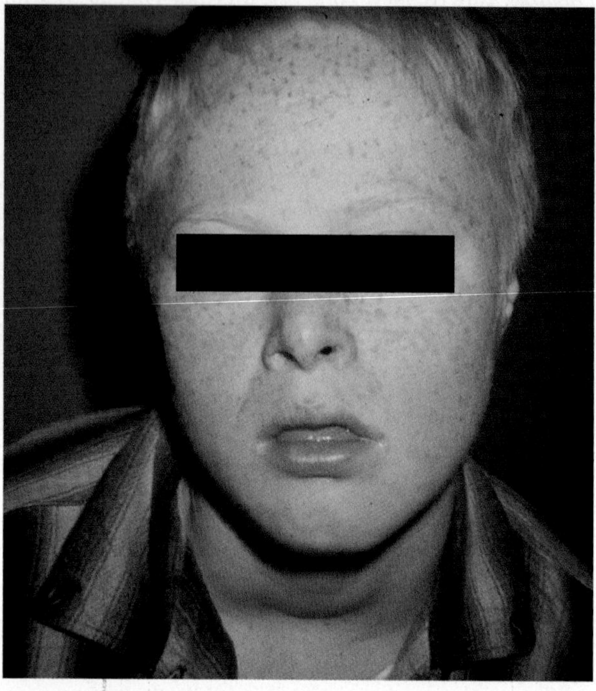

FIGURE 238-1 Down syndrome. (From Fuster V, Walsh RA, Harrington RA. *Hurst's The Heart*. 12th ed. www.accessmedicine.com. Copyright © The McGraw-Hill Companies, Inc. All rights reserved.)

General Considerations

- Associated disorders
  - 50% have heart defects.
  - 52% have scoliosis.[2]
  - 60% to 80% have hearing deficits.[2]
  - 90% have umbilical hernia.[2]
  - 15% have atlantoaxial instability.[3]
  - Leukemia.
  - Hip subluxation.
  - Congenital or adult-onset cataracts or other visual deficits.

Demographics

- Marked rise in risk in mother aged 35 years and over
- At maternal age 45, risk is 1:40
- 1 per 700 births[4]

CLINICAL FINDINGS

SIGNS AND SYMPTOMS

- Facial feature
  - Flat occiput
  - Large tongue
  - Protruding tongue
- Hypotonia
- Single palmar crease
- Hypothyroidism
- Celiac disease
- Ligamentous laxity: Atlanto-axial instability
- Congenital heart disease
- Pes planus
- Obesity
- Delays in
  - Gross motor skills
  - Fine motor skills

- Oral motor skills
- Perceptual motor skills
- Social-emotional skills
- Speech and language skills

Possible Contributing Causes

- Gene deletions
- Chromosome translocation
- Chance mutation
- Angelman syndrome

Functional Implications

- Poor head and trunk control as infant
- Refusal to bear weight on feet
- Learn to sit independently between 12 to15 months of age instead of 6 to 8 months[5]
- Learn to commando crawl or creep on hands and knees between 2.5 to 4 years of age instead of 9 months[5]
- Learn to ambulate between 18 months and 3 years old instead of 12 months[5]
- Excessive motion in acetabulofemoral joint, resulting in use of extreme hip abduction ("a split") to transition between sitting and quadruped

Differential Diagnosis

- Trisomy 18
- Prader–Willi syndrome
- Multiple X chromosomes
- Zellweger syndrome

MEANS OF CONFIRMATION OR DIAGNOSIS

Laboratory Tests

- Amniocentesis[6]
- Chorionic villus sampling[6]
- Fetal sonogram
- "Triple screen" blood test[7]

Imaging

- MRI
- Lateral X-ray

Diagnostic Procedures

- Electrocardiogram for heart defects

FINDINGS AND INTERPRETATION

- MRI or lateral X-ray to assess for atlantoaxial instability

TREATMENT

- Duodenal atresia needs to be treated surgically

REFERRALS/ADMITTANCE

- To geneticist for diagnostic tests
- To cardiologist for cardiac assessment
- To ophthalmologist for visual assessment
- To audiologist for hearing assessment
- To occupational therapist for impaired functional abilities
- To speech therapy for speech/language deficits
- To orthotist for musculoskeletal abnormalities, scoliosis
- Hospital admission for respiratory illness or cardiac repair

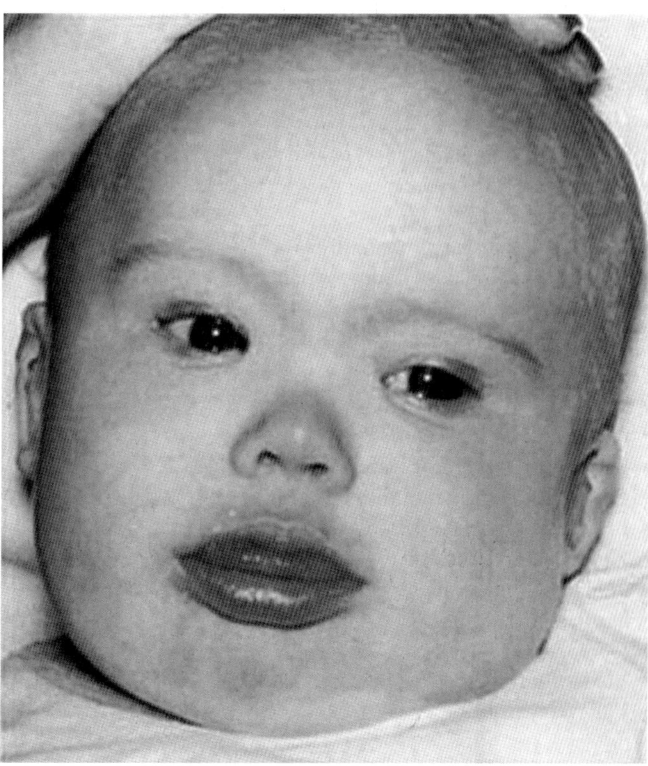

FIGURE 238-2 Down syndrome, showing upward-slanting eyes, a flat profile, and protuberant tongue. (From Chandrasoma P, Taylor CR. *Concise Pathology*. 3rd ed. www.accessmedicine.com. Copyright © The McGraw-Hill Companies, Inc. All rights reserved.)

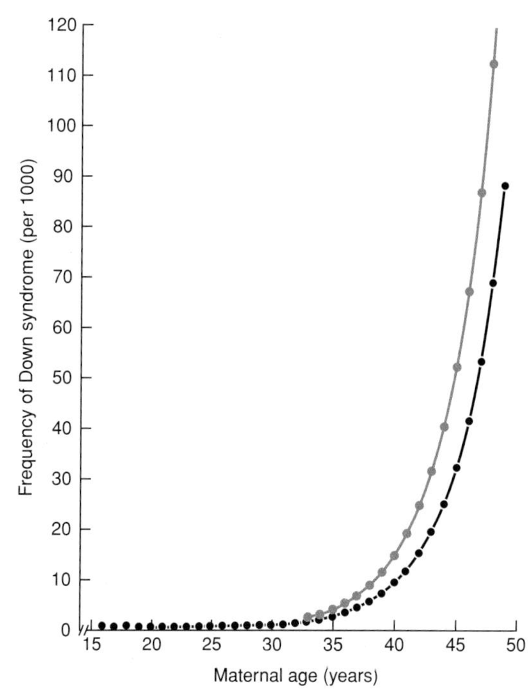

FIGURE 238-3 Relationship of Down syndrome to maternal age. The frequency of Down syndrome rises exponentially with increasing maternal age. The frequency at amniocentesis (blue symbols) is slightly higher than in liveborn infants (black symbols) because miscarriages are more likely in fetuses with Down syndrome. (Data from Scriver CR, Beaudet AL, Sly WS, Valle D. eds. *The Metabolic and Molecular Bases of Inherited Disease*. 8th ed. McGraw-Hill, 2001.)

IMPAIRMENTS

- Decreased strength, especially in trunk muscles
- Dependent for ADLs
- Inability to roll
- Inability to commando crawl or creep on hands and knees
- Inability to sit independently
- Inability to stand
- Inability to transfer without assistance
- Inability to ambulate without assistance
- Poor sitting or standing balance
- Gait deviations, especially wide-based gait

TESTS AND MEASURES

- Gross motor function measure[8]
- Bayley Scales of Motor Development or Bayley II[8]
- Peabody Scales of Motor Development[8]
- Bruininks–Oseretsky Test of Motor Proficiency[8]
- Functional Independence Measure[9]
- Functional Independence Measure for Children (WeeFIM)[8]
- Manual muscle test
- Goniometry
- Blood pressure
- Pulse oximetry[10]

INTERVENTION

- Developmental activities to facilitate normal movement patterns, acquisition of motor milestones
- Therapeutic exercise, including strengthening
- Functional activities
  - Transfers
  - Gait training
  - Stair climbing
- Cardiopulmonary fitness

FUNCTIONAL GOALS

- Patient will be able to
  - Sit independently for 10 minutes while playing with toys to increase independence in 6 months.
  - Creep on hands and knees for 5 feet with minimal assistance to increase mobility in 3 months.
  - Stand at furniture for 2 minutes with moderate assistance to encourage weight bearing in 1 month.
  - Ambulate independently using push-cart 50% of the time to increase mobility in 3 months.
  - Ambulate with both hands held for 25 feet to increase mobility in 6 months.
  - Ambulate with 1 hand held for 10 feet to increase independence in 2 months.
  - Increase quadriceps strength to ascend stairs in step-over-step pattern while holding railing in 4 months.
  - Transfer between standing and squatting to pick up a toy to increase balance and strength in 6 months.

PROGNOSIS

- 100% develop Alzheimer disease before 35 to 40 years of age.
- Level of independence depends on severity of cognitive impairment, but able to live semi-independently.[4]
- 80% live up to 30 years of age.[4]
- Average life expectancy is 50 years.[11]

PATIENT RESOURCES

- National Down Syndrome Society. http://www.ndss.org. Accessed February 26, 2013.
- National Association for Down Syndrome. http://www.nads.org. Accessed February 26, 2013.
- US National Library of Medicine. Down syndrome. *PubMed Health*. http://www.ncbi.nlm.nih.gov/pubmedhealth/PMH0001992/. Accessed February 26, 2013.

REFERENCES

1. The American Physical Therapy Association. Pattern 4C: Impaired muscle performance. *Interactive Guide to Physical Therapist Practice*. 2003. DOI: 10.2522/ptguide.3.1_3. Accessed February 26, 2013.
2. Bertoti DB, Smith DE. Mental Retardation: Focus on down syndrome. In: Tecklin JS, ed. *Pediatric Physical Therapy*. 4th ed. Philadelphia, PA: Lippincott Williams & Wilkins; 2008.
3. Patel DT, Greydanus DE. Physically challenged athletes. In: Patel DT, Greydanus DE, Baker RJ, eds. *Pediatric Practice: Sports Medicine*. China: The McGraw-Hill Companies; 2009. http://www.accessphysiotherapy.com/content/6982414#6982414. Accessed February 26, 2013.
4. Barsh G. Genetics. In: McPhee SJ, Hammer GD, eds. *Pathophysiology of Disease*. 6th ed. China: The McGraw-Hill Companies; 2010. http://www.accessphysiotherapy.com/content/5366638#5366638. Accessed February 26, 2013.
5. Palisano RJ, Walter SD, Russell DJ, et al. Gross motor function of children with Down syndrome: creation of motor growth curves. *Arch Phys Med Rehab*. 2001;82(4):494–500. http://www.archives-pmr.org/article/S0003-9993(01)21252-0/abstract. Accessed February 26, 2013.
6. WebMD. Pregnancy and Amniocentesis. http://www.webmd.com/baby/guide/amniocentesis. Accessed February 26, 2013.
7. American Pregnancy Association. Triple screen test. http://www.americanpregnancy.org/prenataltesting/tripletest.html. Accessed February 26, 2013.
8. Dutton M. *McGraw Hill's NPTE (National Physical Therapy Examination)*. 2nd ed. New York, NY: McGraw-Hill; 2012. http://www.accessphysiotherapy.com/resource/611. Accessed February 26, 2013.
9. Shamus E, Feingold Stern D. *Effective Documentation for Physical Therapy Professionals*. 2nd ed. New York, NY: McGraw-Hill; 2011. http://www.accessphysiotherapy.com/resource/696. Accessed February 26, 2013.
10. Federico MJ, Kerby GS, Deterding RR, et al. Respiratory Tract & Mediastinum. In: Hay WW, Levin MJ, Sondheimer JM, Deterding RR, eds. *CURRENT Diagnosis & Treatment: Pediatrics*. 20th ed. New York, NY: McGraw-Hill; 2011. http://www.accessphysiotherapy.com/content/6582089#6582089. Accessed February 26, 2013.
11. Mayo Clinic. Down syndrome. http://www.mayoclinic.com/health/down-syndrome/DS00182/DSECTION=complications. Accessed February 26, 2013.

ADDITIONAL REFERENCES

- ICD9DATA web site. http://www.icd9data.com. Accessed February 26, 2013.
- ICD10DATA web site. http://www.icd10data.com. Accessed February 26, 2013.
- WebMD. Chorionic Villus Sampling. http://www.webmd.com/baby/guide/amniocentesis. Accessed February 26, 2013.

239 FETAL ALCOHOL SPECTRUM DISORDERS

Kay Tasso, PhD, PT, PCS

CONDITION/DISORDER SYNONYMS

- Fetal alcohol syndrome (FAS)
- Partial fetal alcohol syndrome (pFAS)
- Alcohol-related neurodevelopmental disorder (ARND)
- Alcohol-related birth defects (ARBDs)

ICD-9-CM CODE

- 779.4 Drug reactions and intoxications specific to newborn[1]

ICD-10-CM CODE

- Q86.0 Fetal alcohol syndrome (dysmorphic)[2]

PREFERRED PRACTICE PATTERN

- 5B Impaired Neuromotor Development[3]

PATIENT PRESENTATION

A 9-month-old infant is referred to physical therapy for fetal alcohol syndrome. The infant was recently placed with a local foster family. The foster mother reports no medical history is available regarding the baby but she has noticed the baby is not developing like the other foster children she has had. Upon examination, the therapist notes the infant is mildly hypotonic overall and is exhibiting gross motor delay as evidenced by an inability to roll, crawl, or sit independently.

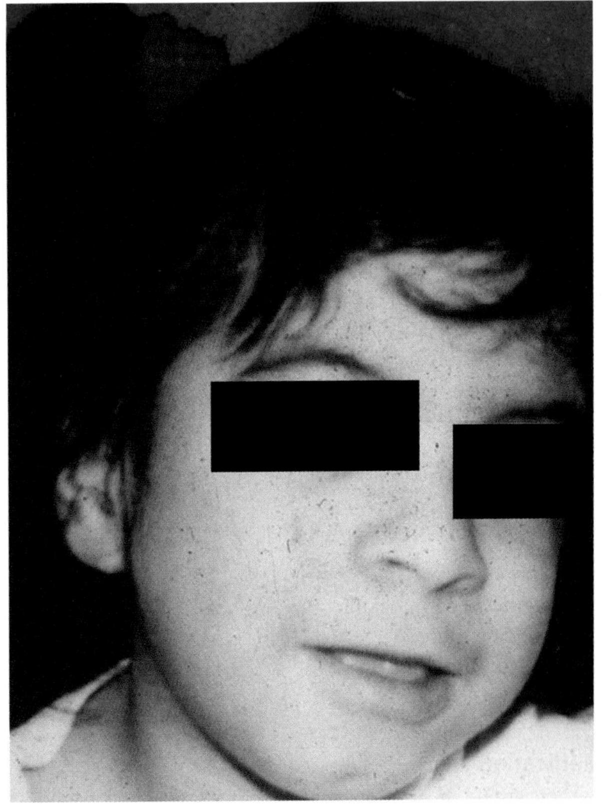

FIGURE 239-1 Characteristic facies associated with fetal alcohol syndrome. (From Tintinalli JE, J. Stephan Stapczynski, O. John Ma, et al., eds. *Tintinalli's Emergency Medicine: A Comprehensive Study Guide*. 7th ed. http://www.accessmedicine.com. Copyright © The McGraw-Hill Companies, Inc. All rights reserved.)

KEY FEATURES

Description

- Includes a range of severity of defects caused by excessive maternal consumption of alcohol during pregnancy[4]
- Fetal alcohol syndrome characterized by[4]
  - Short stature
  - Microcephaly
  - Developmental delay
  - Atypical facial features
  - Cognitive impairment

Essentials of Diagnosis

- Partial fetal alcohol syndrome: Characterized by at least two facial characteristics and at least one of the other typical syndrome characteristics[4]
- Alcohol-related neurologic disorder (ARND): Less severe form[4] that does not involve atypical facial features but does involve at least one of the other typical syndrome characteristics[4]
- ARBDs: Includes at least two facial characteristics, at least one major congenital organ defect, and at least 2 minor defects[2]

General Considerations

- Prenatal exposure to alcohol is the most common preventable cause of mental retardation.
- May also have[4]
  - Cardiac defects.
  - Neural tube defects.
  - Genitourinary defects.
  - Behavioral problems.
    - Stranger anxiety.
    - Inappropriate social interactions.
    - Poor judgment.

Demographics

- 30% to 40% of offspring of mothers whose daily intake of alcohol exceeds 3 ounces[4]
- 0.5 to 2 per 1000 live births[4]

CLINICAL FINDINGS

SIGNS AND SYMPTOMS[4]

- Growth
  - Short stature
  - Developmental delay
  - Failure to thrive
  - Prenatal and postnatal growth deficiency
- Craniofascial
  - Sort palpebral fissures
  - Atypical facial features
  - Flat philtrum
  - Thin vermillion of upper lip
- Central nervous system
  - Microcephaly
  - Optic nerve hypoplasia
  - Hypotonis
  - Partial or complete agenesis of the corpus callosum
  - Cognitive impairment
  - Tremors

Functional Implications

- Difficulty with complex cognitive function[4]
- Short attention span
- Difficulty with short-term memory
- Difficulty with balance and coordination

Possible Contributing Causes

- Consumption of more than 3 ounces of alcohol per day during pregnancy[4]

MEANS OF CONFIRMATION OR DIAGNOSIS

Imaging

- Computerized tomography (CT) scan
- Magnetic resonance imaging (MRI)
- Maternal ultrasound

TREATMENT

Medication

- There are no medications that directly address fetal alcohol spectrum disorders
- Medications may be used to treat symptoms such as
  - Stimulants to treat hyperactivity
  - Antidepressants, antianxiety medication, or neuroleptics to address behavioral difficulties[5]

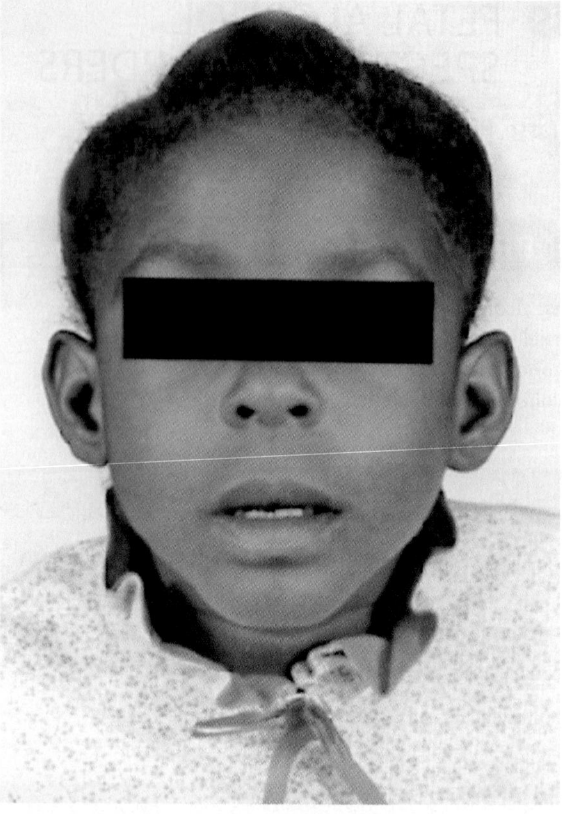

FIGURE 239-2 Fetal alcohol syndrome: midface hypoplasia, absent philtrum, and microcephaly associated with a ventricular septal defect. (From Fuster V, Walsh RA, *Harrigton RA. Hurst's The Heart*. 13th ed.)

REFERRALS/ADMITTANCE

- To neurologist
- To otolaryngologist
- To gastroenterologist
- To occupational therapist
- To speech therapist

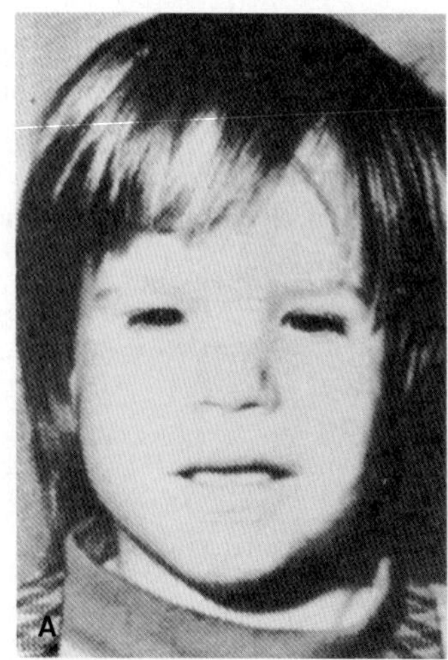

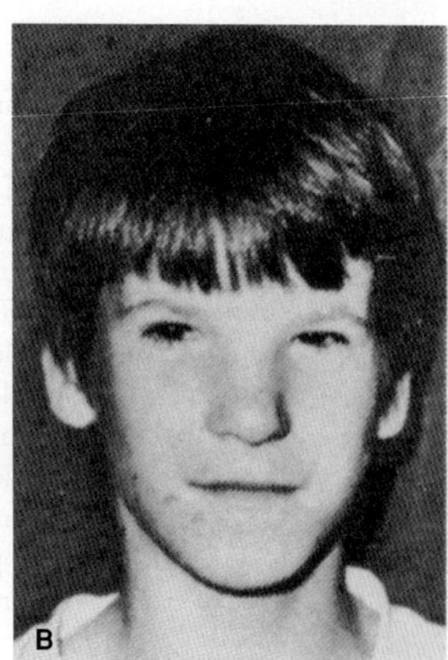

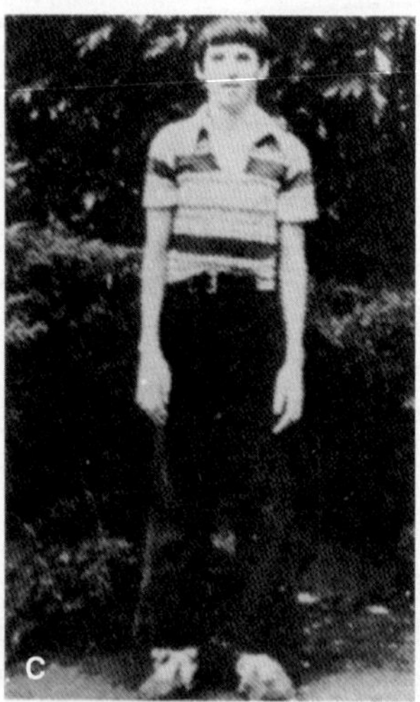

FIGURE 239-3 Fetal alcohol syndrome. (**A**) At 2 1/2 years. (**B, C**) At 12 years. Note persistence of short palpebral fissures, epicanthal folds, flat midface, hypoplastic philtrum, and thin upper vermilion border. This individual also has the short, lean prepubertal stature characteristic of young males with fetal alcohol syndrome. (Reprinted from Streissguth AP, Clarren SK, and Jones KL. *Natural history of the fetal alcohol syndrome: A 10-year-follow-up of eleven patients*. Lancet. 326:85–91. Copyright 1985, with permission from Elsevier.)

TABLE 239-1 Features Observed in Fetal Alcohol Syndrome in the Newborn

Craniofacial
Short palpebral fissures
Thin vermillion of upper lip
Flattened philtrum
Growth
Prenatal and postnatal growth deficiency (small for gestational age, failure to thrive)
Central nervous system
Microcephaly
Partial or complete agenesis of the corpus callosum
Optic nerve hypoplasia
Hypotonia, poor feeding

Source: From Hay WM, Levin MJ, Deterding RR, Abzug MJ, Sondheimer JM. *Current Diagnosis & Treatment: Pediatrics*. 21st ed. www.accessmedicine.com.

IMPAIRMENTS

- Frequently falls when walking
- Decreased coordination

TESTS AND MEASURES

- Bayley Scales of Motor Development or Bayley II
- Peabody Scales of Motor Development
- Neonatal Behavioral Assessment Scale
- Bruininks-Oseretsky Test of Motor Proficiency

INTERVENTION

- Early intervention services[5]
- Behavioral therapy[5]
- Developmental activities
  - Acquisition of motor milestones through facilitation
- Therapeutic exercise
  - Coordination
  - Balance
  - Strengthening

FUNCTIONAL GOALS

The patient will be able to

- Ambulate through an obstacle course without falling within 3 months to increase stability.
- Walk forward on a low balance beam independently without falling in 4 months to increase balance and coordination.
- Stand on one leg for 10 seconds to improve balance skills within 2 months.

PROGNOSIS

- No impact on life expectancy documented.

PATIENT REFERENCES

- CDC Fetal Alcohol Syndrome. http://www.cdc.gov/ncbddd/fas./ Accessed March 13, 2013.
- University of South Dakota. Fetal Alcohol Spectrum Handbook. http://www.usd.edu/medical-school/center-for-disabilities/fetal-alcohol-spectrum-disorders-handbook.cfm. Accessed March 13, 2013.

REFERENCES

1. Guide to Physical Therapist Practice. http://guidetoptpractice.apta.org/content/1/SEC19.body?sid=513e0090-fd45-4f20-bade-1c68e559b285. Accessed March 13, 2013.
2. ICD9DATA Web site. http://www.icd9data.com/2012/Volume1/760-779/764-779/779/779.4.htm. Accessed March 13, 2013.
3. ICD10DATA Web site. http://www.icd10data.com/ICD10CM/Codes/Q00-Q99/Q80-Q89/Q86-/Q86.0. Accessed March 13, 2013.
4. Hay WW, Levin MJ, Sondheimer JM, Deterding RR. Teratogens. In: Hay WW, Levin MJ, Sondheimer JM, Deterding RR, eds. *CURRENT Diagnosis & Treatment: Pediatrics*. 20th ed. New York, NY: McGraw-Hill; 2011. http://www.accessphysiotherapy.com/content/6589287. Accessed March 13, 2013.
5. Center for Disease Control and Prevention. Fetal alcohol spectrum disorders. http://www.cdc.gov/ncbddd/fasd/treatments.html. Accessed March 13, 2013.

ADDITIONAL REFERENCES

- Abel EL. Fetal alcohol syndrome: a cautionary note. *Curr Pharm Des*. 2006;12(12):1521–1529.
- Bernard TJ, Knupp K, Yang ML, et al. Neurologic assessment & neurodiagnostic procedures. In: Hay WW, Levin MJ, Sondheimer JM, Deterding RR, eds. *CURRENT Diagnosis & Treatment: Pediatrics*. 20th ed. New York, NY: McGraw-Hill; 2011. http://www.accessphysiotherapy.com/content/6585049. Accessed March 13, 2013.
- Dutton M. Pediatric physical therapy. In: *McGraw Hill's National Physical Therapy Examination*. 2nd ed. New York, NY: McGraw-Hill; 2012. http://www.accessphysiotherapy.com/content/5404405#5404405. Accessed March 13, 2013.
- Merrick J, Merrick E, Morad M, Kandel I. Fetal alcohol syndrome and its long-term effects. *Minerva Pediatr*. 2006;58(3):211–218.
- O'Leary C, Bower C, Payne J, Elliott E. Fetal alcohol syndrome. *Aust Fam Physician*. 2006;35(4):184.
- Osborn JA, Harris SR, Weinberg J. Fetal alcohol syndrome: Review of the literature with implications for physical therapists. *Phys Ther*. 1993;73(9):599–607. http://physicaltherapyjournal.com/content/73/9/599.full.pdf. Accessed March 13, 2013.
- The Brazelton Institute. The Neonatal Behavioral Assessment Scale. http://www.brazelton-institute.com/intro.html. Accessed March 13, 2013.

240 HEART TRANSPLANT: PEDIATRIC

Kay Tasso, PhD, PT, PCS

CONDITION/DISORDER SYNONYM

- Cardiac transplant

ICD-9-CM CODE

- V42.1 Heart replaced by transplant

ICD-10-CM CODE

- Z94.1 Heart transplant status

PREFERRED PRACTICE PATTERN

- 6C: Impaired Ventilation, Respiration/Gas Exchange, and Aerobic Capacity/Endurance Associated with Airway Clearance Dysfunction

PATIENT PRESENTATION

An 11-month-old infant is referred from an early intervention program for natural environment (home) physical therapy following a heart transplant 6 months ago for hypoplastic left heart syndrome. He has a gastrostomy tube (G-tube) for all feedings due to unwillingness to take food by mouth. The child requires 1 L of oxygen via a nasal cannula and uses an oxygen saturation monitor at night. He takes the following medications: cyclosporine, captopril, zantac, prednisone, heparin, bactrim, and valcyte valganciclovir. Developmentally, he can prop sit but is not yet rolling, creeping on hands and knees, or transferring in or out of sitting or quadruped.

KEY FEATURES

Description

- Diseased or defective heart is partially (heterotopic transplant) or completely (orthotopic transplant) removed due to heart failure
- A healthy donor heart from a deceased person is implanted

Essentials of Diagnosis

- Severity of heart failure classification[1]
  - Stage A: At risk for heart failure
  - Stage B: Abnormal structure or function but no heart failure
  - Stage C: Abnormal structure or function and history of or current heart failure
  - Stage D: Abnormal structure or function resulting in ventilator or cardiac support

General Considerations

- The heart is considered denervated (due to severing of thoracic and vagus nerves[2]) following transplantation
  - Pulse rate can no longer be utilized as the primary method of assessing intensity of exercise
  - Circulating catecholamines regulate the heart's response to exercise
  - As a result, a warm-up period prior to exercise and a cool down period following exercise are crucial to any active exercise program

Demographics

- 5000 heart transplants per year including adults and children

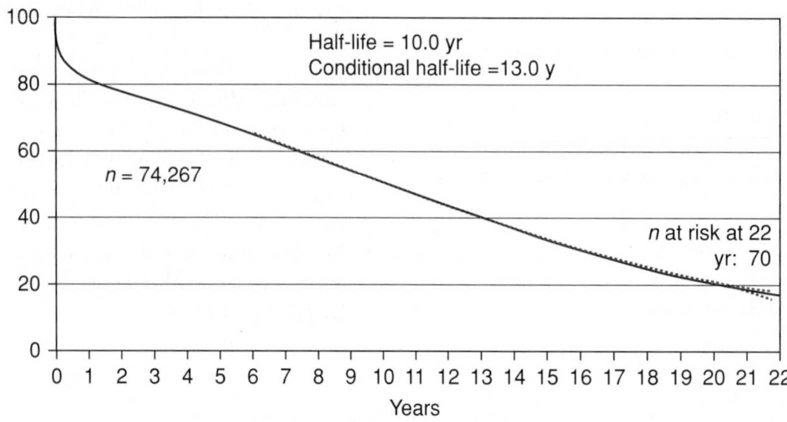

FIGURE 240-1 Actuarial survival for adult and pediatric heart transplant patients performed between January 1982 and June 2004. The half-life is the time at which 50% of those transplanted remain alive, and the conditional half-life is the time at which 50% recipients surviving the first year after transplantation. (Reprinted from Taylor DO, Edwards LB, Aurora P, et al. Registry of the International Society for Heart and Lung Transplantation: twenty-fifth official adult heart transplant report—2008. *J Heart Lung Transplant*. 2008;27(9):943–956. Copyright 2010, with permission from Elsevier.)

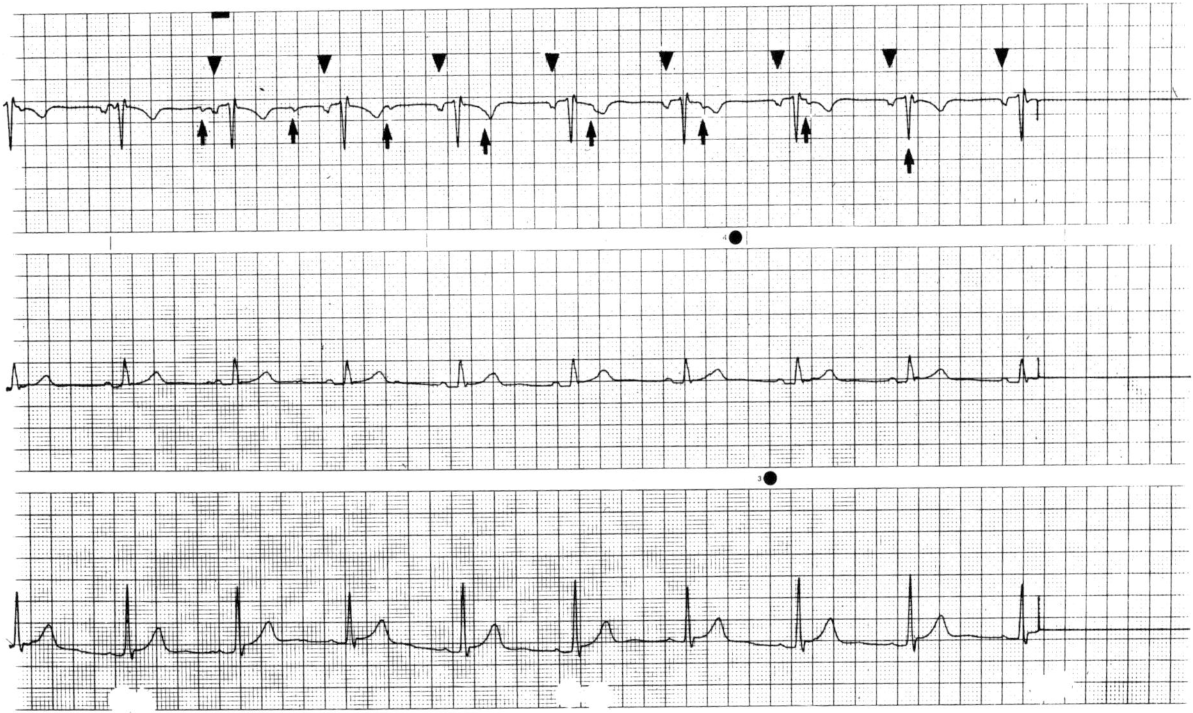

FIGURE 240-2 ECG in a heart transplant patient. ECG demonstrating donor and recipient P waves (*arrowhead*, donor P wave; *arrow*, recipient P wave). (From Tintinalli JE, Stephan Stapczynski J, John Ma O, et al., eds. *Tintinalli's Emergency Medicine: A Comprehensive Study Guide*. 7th ed. http://www.accessmedicine.com. Copyright © The McGraw-Hill Companies, Inc. All rights reserved.)

CLINICAL FINDINGS

SIGNS AND SYMPTOMS

- Cyanosis
- Tachycardia
- Tachypnea
- Syncope

Possible Contributing Causes

- Primarily four reasons[1]:
  - Congenital heart defects such as hypoplastic left heart syndrome or cardiomyopathy
  - Tumors
  - Infections
  - Toxins

Differential Diagnosis

- Cytomegalovirus (CMV)
- Human immunodeficiency virus (HIV)

Functional Implications

- Denervated heart
- Developmental delay
- Deconditioned
- Immunosuppression
- 92% have no functional loss 10 years following transplantation[2]

MEANS OF CONFIRMATION OR DIAGNOSIS

Laboratory Tests

- Complete blood count (CBC)
- Immunosuppressant trough
- CMV test

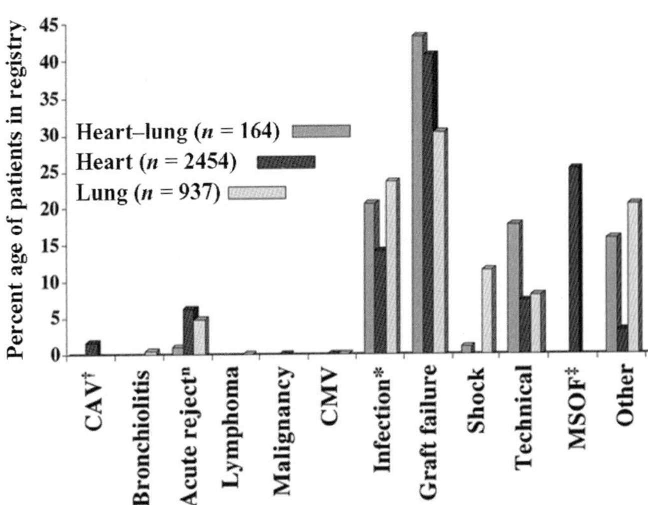

FIGURE 240-3 Graphical presentation of the causes of death in the first 30 days of all patients having had either a heart, heart–lung, or lung transplant who were in the International Society for Heart and Lung Transplantation (ISHLT) registry from the period of January 1992 to June 2002. The graph serves to illustrate the high proportion of deaths from technical problems, infection, and rejection across all types of transplant patients. *Infection relates to non–cytomegalovirus-mediated disease; †cardiac, allograft vasculopathy; ‡multisystem organ failure. Developed using data taken from the ISHLT registry. (Reproduced with permission from Hertz MI, Mohacsi PJ, Taylor DO, et al. The registry of the International Society for Heart and Lung Transplantation: Introduction to the Twentieth Annual Reports—2003. *J Heart Lung Transplant*. 2003;22:610.)

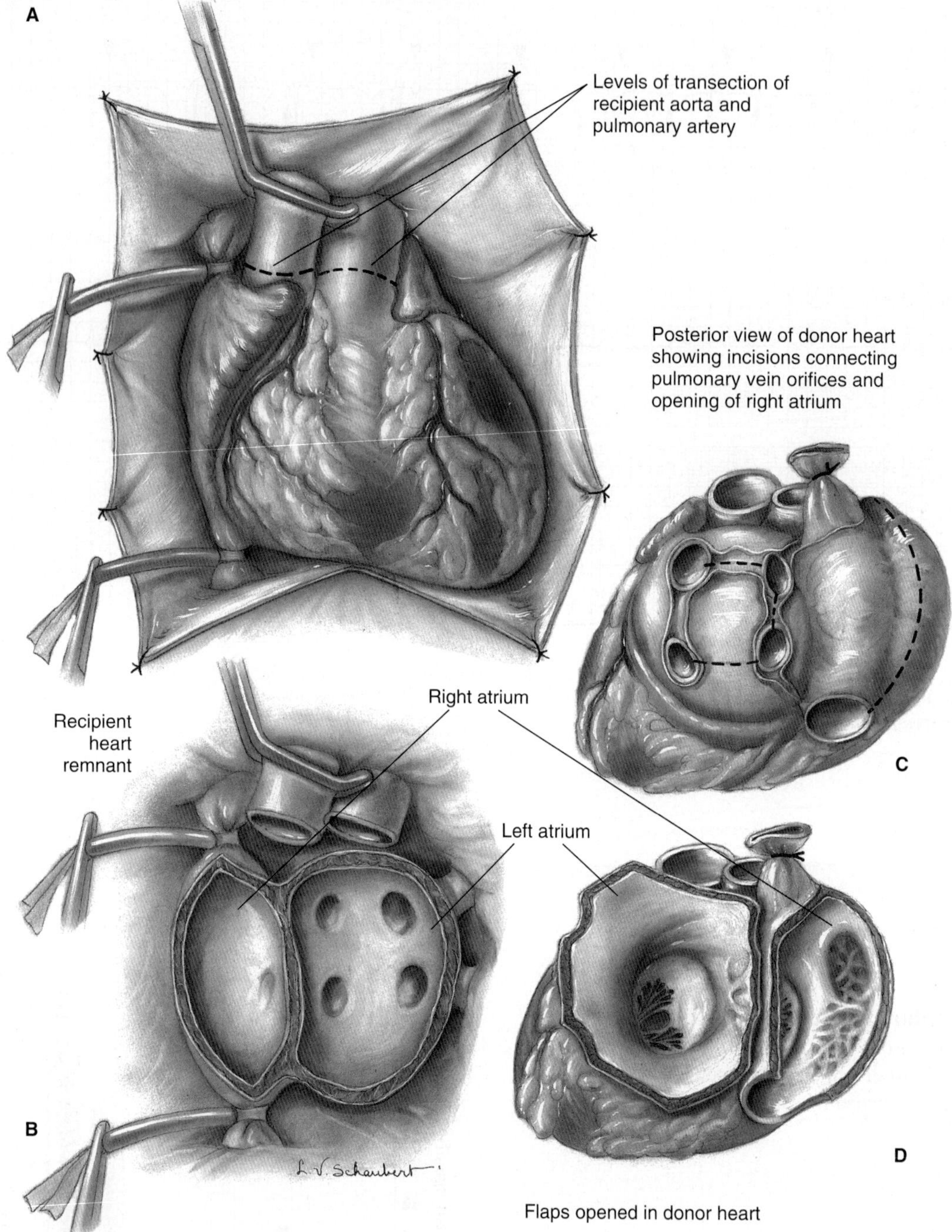

FIGURE 240-4 (**A**) Recipient heart showing levels of transection across aorta and pulmonary artery. (**B**) Implantation site with recipient heart removed. (**C**) Posterior view of donor heart showing lines of incision connecting pulmonary vein orifices and opening the right atrium in preparation for implantation. (**D**) Flaps opened in donor heart in preparation for implantation. (From Doherty GM. *Current Diagnosis & Treatment: Surgery*. 13th ed. http://www.accessmedicine.com. Copyright © The McGraw-Hill Companies, Inc. All rights reserved.)

- HIV test
- Immunoglobulin G levels
- Isotopic glomerular filtration rate

Imaging

- Fetal ultrasound
- Echocardiography
- Renal ultrasound
- Electroencephalogram (EEG)
- Electrocardiogram (EKG)
- CT scan
- MRI
- Chest radiograph
- Kidney radiograph

MEDICAL PROCEDURES

- Cardiac catheterization
- Endomyocardial biopsy
- Coronary angiography
- Sternotomy as part of heart transplant

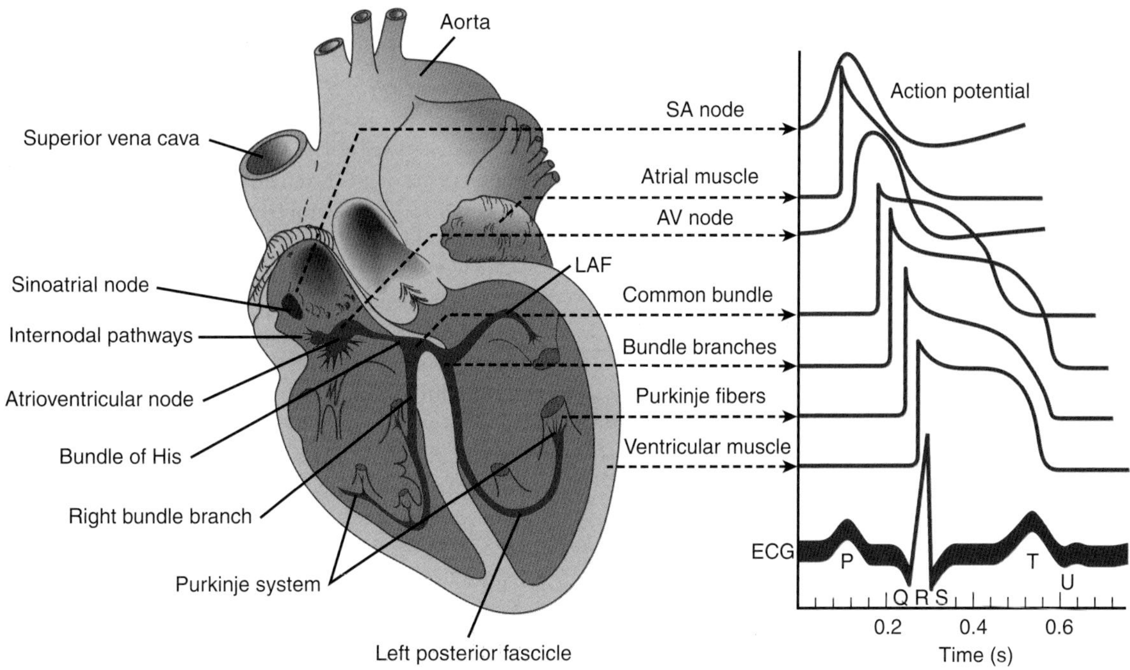

FIGURE 240-5 Conducting system of the heart. Typical transmembrane action potentials for the SA and AV nodes, other parts of the conduction system, and the atrial and ventricular muscles are shown along with the correlation to the extracellularly recorded electrical activity (i.e., the electrocardiogram [ECG]). The action potentials and ECG are plotted on the same time axis but with different zero points on the vertical scale. The PR interval is measured from the beginning of the P wave to the beginning of the QRS. LAF, left anterior fascicle. (Redrawn, with permission, from Ganong WF. *Review of Medical Physiology*. 22nd ed. New York, NY: McGraw-Hill; 2005.)

FINDINGS AND INTERPRETATION

- Electrocardiography (ECG) is performed monthly for the first 3 months, then quarterly until 1 year after transplantation, and then every 6 months thereafter.[1]
- Chest radiography is performed monthly for 3 months, at 12 months, and then annually.[1]

TREATMENT

Medication[3]

- Immunosuppresants (e.g., Cyclosporine)
- Corticosteroids (e.g., Methylprednisolone)
- Vasodilators (e.g., Nitropress)
- Inotropic agents (e.g., dopamine)
- Pulmonary vasodilators (e.g., nitric oxide)
- Immune globulins (e.g., IVIG)

REFERRALS/ADMITTANCE

- May be admitted for infection due to cardiac catheterization, cardiac biopsy, immunosuppression, rejection, or pulmonary hypertension
- To cardiology
- To pulmonology
- To nephrology
- To occupational therapy
- To speech therapy

IMPAIRMENTS

- Decreased strength
- Decreased endurance
- Limited active range of motion
- Unable to ambulate independently
- Dependent for transfers

TESTS AND MEASURES

- Bayley scales of motor development (Bayley II)
- Peabody Developmental Motor Scales (PDMS-2).
- 6-minute walk test
- Goniometric measurements

INTERVENTION

- Borg Rating of Perceived Exertion (RPE) or modified Borg scale to monitor intensity of exercise in adolescents or older children
- Wong-Baker Faces Pain Rating Scale to monitor intensity of exercise in young children
- **AVOID** resistive exercises and limit aerobic activities during periods of rejection[4]
- Must abide by sternal precautions
- Gait training
- Transfer training
- Progressively increase endurance
- Active range of motion
- Stationary bike

FUNCTIONAL GOALS

The patient will be able to

- Sit independently for 10 minutes while playing to increase stability within 2 months.
- Stand at furniture with contact guard assist to increase stability within 4 months.
- Ambulate 50 feet with standby assist to increase mobility within 1 week

- Transfer from supine to sitting with minimal assist of caregiver in 3 days in preparation for discharge.
- Climb one flight of stairs with contact guard assist to increase mobility within 5 days.
- Ride stationary bike for 20 minutes to increase endurance within 1 month.

PROGNOSIS

- 80% to 90% survive 1 year.[1]
- 85% to 90% survive 2 years.[1]
- 70% survival for at least 5 years with many living 20+ years.[1]

PATIENT RESOURCE

- MedlinePlus. Heart Transplant. http://www.nlm.nih.gov/medlineplus/ency/article/003003.htm. Accessed June 8, 2013.

REFERENCES

1. Medscape. Pediatric Heart Transplant. http://emedicine.medscape.com/article/1011927-overview. Accessed April 14, 2013.
2. Howell BA, Tapley C. Chapter 26. Thoracic surgery. In: Campbell SK, Palisano RJ, Orlin MN, eds. *Physical Therapy in Children*. St. Louis, MO: Elsevier Saunders; 2012.
3. Panus PC, Jobst EE, Masters SB, et al. Chapter 32. Immunopharmacology. In: Panus PC, Jobst EE, Masters SB, et al., eds. *Pharmacology for the Physical Therapist*. New York, NY: McGraw-Hill; 2009. http://www.accessphysiotherapy.com/content/6095393. Accessed April 14, 2013.
4. Dutton M. Motor assessments. In: Dutton M, ed. *McGraw-Hill's NPTE (National Physical Therapy Examination)*. 2nd ed. New York, NY: McGraw-Hill; 2012. http://www.accessphysiotherapy.com/content/56513439. Accessed May 9, 2013.

ADDITIONAL REFERENCES

- Adey CK, Nath PH, Soto B, et al. Heterotopic heart transplantation. *RadioGraphics*. 1987;7(I):151–160. http://www.google.com/url?sa=t&rct=j&q=heterotopic%20heart%20transplant&source=web&cd=8&ved=0CHAQFjAH&url=http%3A%2F%2Fradiographics.rsna.org%2Fcontent%2F7%2F1%2F151.full.pdf&ei=Fb6LUaDLKYOs9AToroHIDQ&usg=AFQjCNFFwOE5j0mJqbOH8Jxp3bViM4xX1g&bvm=bv.46226182,d.eWU. Accessed May 9, 2013.
- ATS Statement. Guidelines for the Six-Minute Walk Test. American Thoracic Society web site. www.thoracic.org/statements/resources/pfet/sixminute.pdf. Accessed May 9, 2013.
- Center for Disease Control and Prevention. Perceived Exertion. http://www.cdc.gov/physicalactivity/everyone/measuring/exertion.html. Accessed June 9, 2013.
- Guide to Physical Therapist Practice. APTA web site. http://guidetoptpractice.apta.org/content/1/SEC29.body?sid=b257f74e-89ad-45ae-9eeb-99e01686633b. May 8, 2013.
- Hay WW, Levin MJ, Deterding RR, Abzug MJ, Sondheimer JM. Pediatric neuroradiologic procedures. In: Hay WW, Levin MJ, Deterding RR, Abzug MJ, Sondheimer JM, eds. *CURRENT Diagnosis & Treatment: Pediatrics*. 21st ed. New York, NY: McGraw-Hill; 2012. http://www.accessphysiotherapy.com/content/56823567. Accessed June 9, 2013.
- ICD9DATA Web Site. http://www.icd9data.com/2013/Volume1/V01-V91/V40-V49/V42/V42.1.htm. Accessed June 8, 2013.
- ICD10DATA Web Site. http://www.icd10data.com/ICD10CM/Codes/Z00-Z99/Z77-Z99/Z94-/Z94.1. Accessed June 8, 2013.
- Wong-Baker Faces Foundation. http://www.wongbakerfaces.org./ Accessed June 9, 2013.

241 JUVENILE RHEUMATOID ARTHRITIS

Kay Tasso, PhD, PT, PCS

CONDITION/DISORDER SYNONYMS

- Juvenile idiopathic arthritis (JIA)
- Juvenile rheumatoid arthritis (JRA)

ICD-9-CM CODES

- 714.3 Juvenile chronic polyarthritis
- 714.30 Chronic or unspecified polyarticular juvenile rheumatoid arthritis
- 714.31 Acute polyarticular juvenile rheumatoid arthritis
- 714.32 Pauciarticular juvenile rheumatoid arthritis
- 714.33 Monoarticular juvenile rheumatoid arthritis

ICD-10-CM CODES

- M08.00 Unspecified juvenile rheumatoid arthritis of unspecified site
- M08.3 Juvenile rheumatoid polyarthritis (seronegative)
- M08.40 Pauciarticular juvenile rheumatoid arthritis, unspecified site

PREFERRED PRACTICE PATTERN

- 4D Impaired Joint Mobility, Motor Function, Muscle Performance, and Range of Motion Associated with Connective Tissue Dysfunction[1]

PATIENT PRESENTATION

A 3-year-old is hospitalized due to severe knee pain, unwillingness to weight bear, and daily fevers. Following a medical examination including X-rays and blood work, the child is diagnosed with JRA. Upon examination, the therapist notes erythema, edema, and tenderness to palpation of both knees. The child has decreased active knee flexion and extension but is now able to stand with support.

KEY FEATURES

Description

- Overarching name for multiple disorders
- Chronic inflammation of one or more joints for more than 6 to 12 weeks
- Characterized by acute and chronic episodes, may involve other areas of the body

Essentials of Diagnosis

- International League of Associations for Rheumatology classification
    - Oligoarticular (50% of cases) defined as four or fewer joints involved[2]
        - Persistent
        - Extended
        - Asymmetrical
        - Polyarticular (35% of cases) defined as five or more joints involved, often symmetrical[2]
        - Rheumatoid factor-positive (more destructive, similar to adult form)
        - Rheumatoid factor-negative
    - Systemic, also known as Still's disease, (10%–15% of cases) high fever once or twice a day (often in afternoon) with macular rash on bony prominences during fever spikes; can have hepatosplenomegaly, leukocytosis, lymphadenopathy[2]
    - Enthesitis (<10% of cases) affects mainly legs at tendon insertions in boys greater than 10 years of age [2]
    - Psoriatic arthritis (10% of cases)

General Considerations

- Characterized by periods of acute inflammation followed by chronic residual damage

Demographics

- Onset before 16 years of age
- Oligoarticular and enthesitis in males greater than 8 years of age
- Polyarticular rheumatoid factor-negative
    - 50% of cases occur in children younger than 6 years old
    - Onset often during adolescence
    - More common in females than males
- Polyarticular rheumatoid factor-positive
    - Primarily in females
    - Onset in adolescence or late childhood
- Systemic
    - Onset anytime in childhood
- Psoriatic
    - Onset usually in 2- to 4-year-olds and 9- to 11-year-olds
    - More common in females than males

CLINICAL FINDINGS

SIGNS AND SYMPTOMS

- In one or more joints (unilaterally or bilaterally)
    - Pain
    - Swelling
    - Redness
    - Increased warmth to palpation
- Tenderness
- Morning stiffness
- Rash[3]
- Fever
- Uveitis (inflammation of eye) often asymptomatic
- Serositis (inflammation in the lining of the heart, lungs, abdomen)
- Fatigue
- Anemia

JRA Outcome Study **Form: Haq**

Childhood Health Assessment Questionnaire (CHAQ)

For all children with JRA (all ages)

Patient's Name (print) ______________________ First MI Last

Date of Office Visit: __________

Patient Date of Birth: ______________________

Date this Form Completed: __________

In this section we are interested in learning how your child's illness affects his/her ability to function in daily life. Please feel free to add any comments on the back of this page. In the following questions, please check the one response which best describes your child's usual activities (**averaged over an entire day**) **OVER THE PAST WEEK. ONLY NOTE THOSE DIFFICULTIES OR LIMITATIONS WHICH ARE DUE TO ILLNESS**. If most children at your child's age are not expected to do a certain activity, please mark it as "Not Applicable." For example, if your child has difficulty in doing a certain activity or is unable to do it because he/she is too young but NOT because he/she is RESTRICTED BY ILLNESS, please mark it as "Not Applicable."

Due to JRA Illness Only

	Without ANY Difficulty	With SOME Difficulty	With MUCH Difficulty	UNABLE To Do	Not Applicable
Dressing & Grooming					
Is your child able to:					
1 Dress, including tying shoelaces and doing buttons?	___	___	___	___	___
2 Shampoo his/her hair?	___	___	___	___	___
3 Remove socks?	___	___	___	___	___
4 Cut fingernails?	___	___	___	___	___
Arising					
Is your child able to:					
5 Stand up from a low chair or floor?	___	___	___	___	___
6 Get in and out of bed or stand up in crib?	___	___	___	___	___
Eating					
Is your child able to:					
7 Cut his/her own meat?	___	___	___	___	___
8 Lift a cup or glass to mouth?	___	___	___	___	___
9 Open a new cereal box?	___	___	___	___	___
Walking					
Is your child able to					
10 Walk outdoors on a flat ground?	___	___	___	___	___
11 Climb up five steps?	___	___	___	___	___

Please check any AIDS or DEVICES that your child usually uses for any of the above activities:

______ Cane
______ Walker
______ Crutches
______ Wheelchair
______ Devices used for dressing (button hook, zipper pull, long-handled shoe horn, etc.)
______ Built up pencil or special utensils
______ Special or Built-up chair
______ Other Specify: ______________________

Please check any categories for which your child usually needs help from another person BECAUSE OF ILLNESS:

______ Dressing and Grooming
______ Arising
______ Eating
______ Walking

FIGURE 241-1 Childhood Health Assessment Questionnaire. (Data from JRA Outcome Study Form: Haq Childhood Health Assessment Questionnaire (CHAQ). Copyright © American College of Rheumatology.)

Due to JRA Illness Only

	Without ANY Difficulty	With SOME Difficulty	With MUCH Difficulty	UNABLE To Do	Not Applicable
Hygiene					
Is your child able to:					
12 Wash and dry entire body?	___	___	___	___	___
13 Take a tub bath (get in & out of tub)?	___	___	___	___	___
14 Get on and off the toilet or potty chair?	___	___	___	___	___
15 Brush teeth?	___	___	___	___	___
16 Comb/Brush hair?	___	___	___	___	___
Reach Is your child able to:					
17 Reach and get down a heavy object such as a large game or books from just above his/her head?	___	___	___	___	___
18 Bend down to pick up clothing or a piece of paper from the floor?	___	___	___	___	___
19 Pull on a sweater over his/her head?	___	___	___	___	___
20 Turn neck to look over shoulder?	___	___	___	___	___
Grip					
Is your child able to:					
21 Write or scribble with a pen or pencil?	___	___	___	___	___
22 Open car doors?	___	___	___	___	___
23 Open jars which have been previously opened?	___	___	___	___	___
24 Turn faucets on and off?	___	___	___	___	___
25 Push open a door when he/she has to turn knob?	___	___	___	___	___
Errands, Chores, and Play					
Is your child able to:					
26 Run errands and shop?	___	___	___	___	___
27 Get in and out of car or toy car or school bus?	___	___	___	___	___
28 Ride bike or tricycle?	___	___	___	___	___
29 Do household chores (e.g. wash dishes, take out trash, vacuuming, yardwork, make bed, clean room)?	___	___	___	___	___
30 Run and play?	___	___	___	___	___

Please check any AIDS or DEVICES that your child usually uses for any of the above activities:

______ Raised Toilet Seat
______ Bathtub Seat
______ Bathtub bar
______ Jar Opener (for jars previously opened)
______ Long-Handled Appliances for Reach
______ Long Handled Appliances in Bathroom

Please check any categories for which your child usually needs help from another person BECAUSE OF ILLNESS:

______ Hygiene
______ Reach
______ Gripping and Opening things
______ Errands, Chores, and Play

We are also interested in learning whether or not your child has been affected by pain because of his or her illness. How much pain do you think your child has had because of his/her illness IN THE PAST WEEK?

Place mark on the line below to indicate the severity of the pain.

0 No Pain	--	100 Very Bad Pain

Return to: Researcher Suzanne L. Bowyer, Riley Hospital For Children, Rm 5863, 1 Children's Square, Indianapolis, Indiana 46202

FIGURE 241-1 *(Continued)*

Juvenile Arthritis Functional Assessment Report for Parents (JAFAR)

For children 7 and older with JRA

Patient's Name (print) ______________________________
First MI Last
Patient Date of Birth: ______________________

Date of Office Visit: ____________

Date this Form Completed: ____________

Part 1 **Ability Scale**

On this questionnaire, we are interested in learning how your child's illness affects her/her ability to function in daily life.
Please feel free to add any comments on the back of this page.
Please check the one response which best describes your child's usual abilities **OVER THE PAST WEEK**.

please answer all questions **In the past week, was Patient able to:**		**All the time**	**Sometimes**	**Almost never**
1	Take shirt off hanger	___	___	___
2	Button shirt	___	___	___
3	Pull on sweater over head	___	___	___
4	Turn on water faucet	___	___	___
5	Sit on floor, then stand up	___	___	___
6	Dry back with towel	___	___	___
7	Wash face with wash cloth	___	___	___
8	Tie shoelaces	___	___	___
9	Pull on socks	___	___	___
10	Brush teeth	___	___	___
11	Stand up from chair without using arms	___	___	___
12	Get into bed	___	___	___
13	Cut food with knife and fork	___	___	___
14	Lift empty glass to mouth	___	___	___
15	Reopen previously opened food jar	___	___	___
16	Walk 50 feet without help	___	___	___
17	Walk up 5 steps	___	___	___
18	Stand on tiptoes	___	___	___
19	Reach above head	___	___	___
20	Get out of bed	___	___	___
21	Pick up something from floor from standing position	___	___	___
22	Push open door after turning knob	___	___	___
23	Turn head and look over shoulder	___	___	___

FIGURE 241-2 Juvenile Arthritis Functional Assessment Report for Parents. (Data from JRA Outcome Study Form: Juvenile Arthritis Functional Assessment Report for Parents (JAFAR). Copyright © American College of Rheumatology.)

2 Aids or Devices

Please check any AIDS or DEVICES that your child uses for any of these activities

		Have Used	Have not used
1	Cane	_____	_____
2	Walker	_____	_____
3	Crutches	_____	_____
4	Wheelchair	_____	_____
5	Built-up pencil	_____	_____
6	Button hook	_____	_____
7	Zipper Horn	_____	_____
8	Shoe horn	_____	_____
9	Special eating utensils	_____	_____
10	Special chair	_____	_____
11	A special kind of toilet seat	_____	_____
12	Bathtub seat	_____	_____
13	Jar opener	_____	_____
14	Bathtub bar	_____	_____
15	Reacher	_____	_____

Does your child use any other kind of special tool, appliance, aid or device that helps him or her do things more easily?

IF YES: Could you describe it? ______________________

____

3 Help from Others

Please check any categories for which your child needs HELP FROM ANOTHER PERSON.

		No Help	Some Help
1	Get dressed in the morning	_____	_____
2	Get washed in the morning	_____	_____
3	Get in and out of bed	_____	_____
4	Eat dinner	_____	_____
5	Move around the house	_____	_____
6	Get in and out of chairs	_____	_____
7	Reach and get things for you	_____	_____

4 Pain Scale

We are also interested in learning whether or not your child has been affected by pain because of his/her illness.
How much pain do you think your child has had because of his/her illness IN THE PAST WEEK?
Place a mark on the line below to indicate the severity of the pain.

0 No Pain	100 Very Bad Pain

Comments:____

____

____Jafar1.doc

Return to: Researcher **Suzanne L. Bowyer, Riley Hospital For Children, Rm 5863, 1 Children's Square, Indianapolis, Indiana 46202**

FIGURE 241-2 *(Continued)*

TABLE 241-1 Subgroups of Juvenile Idiopathic Arthritis (JIA)

JIA Subgroup	Oligoarticular	Polyarticular Negative	Polyarticular Positive	Systemic Onset	Juvenile Psoriatic	Enthesitis-Related (ERA)
Percentage of all JIA	40%	20%	15%	10%–20%	≤10%	≤10%
Age at onset and gender	<8 years g > b	8–12 years g = b	Teen years g > b	Any age	Any age	8–12 years b > g
No. of joints involved	<5	Many	Many	Varies	Varies	Varies
Pattern	Asymmetric	Varies	Symmetric	Asymmetric	Asymmetric	Lower extremity joints
Hips involved	Rarely	No	No	Occasionally	Sometimes	Yes
Back pain	No	No	No	Myalgic	Sometimes	Yes
Clinical features	Painless iridocyclitis Requires regular slitlamp examination	Poor weight gain	Aggressive course Nodules Poor weight gain	Fever Evanescent rash Serositis Lymphadenopathy Hepatosplenomegaly MAS Complications can be fatal	DIP joints Nail pitting Psoriatic rash or positive family history Dactylitis Can look like polyarticular JIA or ERA	Enthesitis Heel pain Sausage digits Abnormal Schober test Sacroiliitis Oral ulcers
Distinguishing lab abnormalities	Antinuclear antibody positive	Rheumatoid factor positive	Rheumatoid factor negative	Increased ESR, WBC, CRP, ferritin, platelets Anemia Abnormal LFTs	None	HLA-B27 positive

g, girls; b, boys; CRP, C-reactive protein; ESR, erythrocyte sedimentation rate; HLA, human leukocyte antigen; WBC, white blood cell count; LFTs, liver function tests; DIP, distal interphalangeal; MAS, macrophage activation syndrome.

Source: Imboden J, Hellmann DB, Stone JH. *Current Rheumatology Diagnosis & Treatment*, 2nd ed. http://www.accessmedicine.com.

Functional Implications

- Difficulty with activities of daily living (ADLs)
- Difficulty with transfers, such as rising from furniture
- Difficulty climbing stairs
- Decreased endurance

Possible Contributing Causes

- Unknown etiology
- Autoimmune disease theorized
- Genetic link with viral or bacterial trigger

Differential Diagnosis

- Must rule out
  - Orthopedic conditions (increased pain with activity)
  - Infection of joint or infectious disease
  - Cancer

MEANS OF CONFIRMATION OR DIAGNOSIS

Laboratory Tests

- Patient may or may not have increased
  - Erythrocyte sedimentation rate (ESR)[4]
  - C-reactive protein[5]
  - White blood cell count
  - Platelets
  - Rheumatoid factor[6]
  - Anticyclic citrullinated peptide antibody[7]
  - Antinuclear antibody (ANA)[8]
  - HLA-B27[9]

Imaging

- X-ray to assess joint integrity
- MRI to assess joint and soft-tissue integrity

Diagnostic Procedures

- Joint-fluid analysis (to rule out infection)

FINDINGS AND INTERPRETATION

- Radiographs illustrating
  - Enlarged joint spaces (early in disease)
    - Narrowed joint spaces (late in disease)
    - Osteopenia
    - Osteophytes
    - Soft-tissue swelling
    - Premature closure of epiphyses

TREATMENT

Medication

- Non-steroidal anti-inflammatory drugs (NSAIDs)[10]
  - Naproxen
  - Ibuprofen
  - Voltaren

TABLE 241-2 Recommended Ophthalmologic Screening for Children with Juvenile Idiopathic Arthritis[a]

	Iritis Risk		
JIA Subgroup	**High (Screen Every 3 Months)**	**Moderate (Screen Every 6 Months)**	**Low (Screen Annually)**
Oligoarticular dx at <7 years old; positive ANA	Years 1–3 after dx	Years 4–6 after dx	After year 7 after dx
Extended oligoarticular or oligo- to polyarticular	Years 1–3 after dx	Years 4–6 after dx	After year 7 after dx
Polyarticular dx at <7 years old; positive ANA	Years 1–3 after dx	Years 4–6 after dx	After year 7 after dx
Polyarticular dx at >7 years old; negative ANA		Year 1–6 after dx	After year 7 after dx
Psoriatic arthritis			Low risk: annual screen
Systemic onset			Low risk: annual screen
Enthesitis-related			Low risk: annual screen

[a]Screening should include a slitlamp examination to evaluate the anterior chamber for cells and flare *even in the absence of eye symptoms.*
Source: Imboden J, Hellmann DB, Stone JH. *Current Rheumatology Diagnosis & Treatment,* 2nd ed. http://www.accessmedicine.com.

- Disease-modifying antirheumatic drugs (DMARDs)[10]
  - Methotrexate
- Biologic reagent
  - Enbrel
  - Remicade
  - Humira
- Systemic glucocorticoids[10]
- Leflunomide[10]
- Biologic medications[10]
  - Etanercept
  - Infliximab
  - Adalimumbad
- Biologic agents[11]
  - Anakinra
  - Rituximab
  - Abatacept
- Corticosteroid injections[10]

MEDICAL PROCEDURES

- Soft-tissue release
- Osteotomy
- Arthrotomy
- Synovectomy
- Tenosynovectomy
- Arthrodesis
- Total joint arthoplasty

REFERRALS/ADMITTANCE

- Admittance to hospital primarily for diagnosis or orthopedic surgery
- To pediatric rheumatologist for management of disease
- To pediatric orthopedist for management of joint deformities or soft-tissue contractures
- To ophthalmologist for routine screening of uveitis
- To occupational therapist when ADLs affected

IMPAIRMENTS

- Pain
- Decreased range of motion or joint contractures in extremities, axial skeleton, temporomandibular joint
- Decreased strength or muscle atrophy

TABLE 241-3 Nonsteroidal Anti-Inflammatory Drugs Used in Pediatric Juvenile Idiopathic Arthritis (JIA) Patients[a]

Drug	Dose	Formulation
Naproxen	20 mg/kg/d; 10 mg/kg/dose bid up to 1000 mg/d	Liquid: 125 mg/5 mL Tablet: 220 mg, available over the counter Twice-daily dosing is convenient
Ibuprofen	40 mg/kg/d; 10 mg/kg/dose qid up to 2400 mg/d	Liquid: 100 mg/5 mL Tablet: 200 mg, available over the counter
Tolmetin	30 mg/kg/d; 10 mg/kg/dose tid up to 1800 mg/d	Tablets: 200, 400, and 600 mg
Indomethacin	1–3 mg/kg/d tid or qid up to 200 mg/d	Liquid: 25 mg/5 mL Approved for patients younger than 14 years Used in younger patients with systemic onset JIA or spondylitis
Meloxicam	0.125 mg/kg/d up to 7.5 mg/d	Liquid: 7.5 mg/mL Tablet: 7.5 and 15 mg Once-a-day dosing is convenient

[a]As of this writing, other NSAIDs have not been approved by the Food and Drug Administration for use in the pediatric age group.
Source: Imboden J, Hellmann DB, Stone JH: *Current Rheumatology Diagnosis & Treatment.,* 2nd edition. http://www.accessmedicine.com.

TABLE 241-4 Disease-Modifying Antirheumatic Drugs (DMARDs) Used to Treat Juvenile Idiopathic Arthritis (JIA) in Pediatric Patients[a]

Drug	Dose	Form	Special Considerations
Hydroxychloroquine	6 mg/kg/d qd or bid daily	200-mg pills	• Periodic eye examinations; retinal toxicity rare at these doses
Sulfasalazine	30–50 mg/kg/d tid or bid daily	500-mg tablets	• Contraindicated in sulfa-allergic or aspirin-sensitive patients • Useful in polyarticular or spondylitis subgroups • *Not* for use in systemic onset JIA • Enteric-coated formulation is often better tolerated
Methotrexate	15 mg/m^2 per dose or 0.5–1.0 mg/kg per dose PO, IM, or SC once a week	Pills: 2.5 mg Liquid: 25 mg/mL 2.5 mg = 0.1 mL	• Higher doses well tolerated in children • Poor absorption can cause decreased clinical response; try same dose SC • Avoid concomitant sulfa, tetracycline • Liquid can be taken PO or SC • This is the least expensive DMARD
Cyclosporine	3 mg/kg/d bid	Neoral pills: 25- and 100-mg capsules Liquid: 100 mg/mL	• Neoral has increased bioavailability • Grapefruit juice increases absorption • Most effective in systemic onset JIA • Monitor kidney function and BP frequently • Many drug interactions
Leflunomide	100-mg loading dose + 10 mg PO qod if < 20 kg 100 mg/2 days then 10 mg PO qd if 20–40 kg 100 mg/ 3 days then 20 mg/d if >40 kg	10- and 20-mg pills	• Hair thinning in 1/8 of patients • Loose stools respond to dose adjustment, loperamide • Avoid pregnancy while on treatment until cholestyramine washout completed
Etanercept	0.4 mg/kg/dose SC 2 times/week	Powder to reconstitute with water in prefilled syringe; *refrigerate*	• Avoid live virus immunization during etanercept therapy • Approved and indicated for polyarticular JIA • Combination with methotrexate prolongs effect • Serious infection can occur
Anakinra	1–2 mg/kg/d SC	Prefilled syringe 100 mg; *refrigerate*	• Very effective in systemic onset JIA • Injection-site reaction is common • Infection risk
Infliximab	3–5 mg/kg per infusion given IV at 0, 2, and 6 weeks, then every 8 weeks	IV infusion requires premedication with diphenhydramine and acetaminophen	• Infection risk is high • Chimeric molecule requires concomitant treatment with methotrexate • Avoid live virus immunization • Useful in psoriatic arthritis, inflammatory bowel disease, and spondyloarthropathy
Adalimumab	24 mg/m^2 SC every other week	Prefilled syringe 40 mg; *refrigerate*	• Currently under study for JIA • Early clinical response and ease of administration • Infection risk

[a]Leflunomide, anakinra, infliximab, and adalimumab are currently under investigation regarding their usefulness in the pediatric age group.
Source: Imboden J, Hellmann DB, Stone JH. *Current Rheumatology Diagnosis & Treatment*, 2nd ed. http://www.accessmedicine.com. Copyright © The McGraw-Hill Companies, Inc. All rights reserved.

- Possible leg-length discrepancy
- Decreased function
  - Transfers
  - Stairs
  - ADLs
- Balance
- Coordination

TESTS AND MEASURES

- Childhood Arthritis Health Questionnaire[12]
- Juvenile Arthritis Quality of Life Questionnaire[12]
- Pediatric Quality of Life Questionnaire[12]
- Juvenile Arthritis Functional Assessment Scale[12]
- Juvenile Arthritis Functional Assessment Reports for Parents[12]
- Childhood Health Assessment Questionnaire[12]
- Juvenile Arthritis Functional Assessment Index[12]
- Pediatric Pain Questionnaire[12]
- Visual analog scale (VAS)[13]
- Peabody Developmental Motor Scales-2[12]
- Bruininks-Oseretsky Test of Motor Proficiency[12]
- School function assessment[12]
- Articular severity score

TABLE 241-5 Joint Fluid Analysis

Disorder	Cells/μL	Glucose[a]
Trauma	More red cells than white cells; usually < 2000 white cells	Normal
Reactive arthritis	3000–10,000 white cells, mostly mononuclear cells	Normal
Juvenile idiopathic arthritis and other inflammatory arthritides	5000–60,000 white cells, mostly neutrophils	Usually normal or slightly low
Septic arthritis	>60,000 white cells, >90% neutrophils	Low to normal

[a]Normal value is ≥75% of the serum glucose value.
Source: Hay WM et al. *Current Diagnosis & Treatment: Pediatrics.* 21st ed. www.accessmedicine.com.

- Global range of motion score
- Goniometric measurements
- Manual muscle testing
- Assess for leg-length discrepancy

INTERVENTION

- Heat (during sub-acute or chronic phases)[14]
- Cold[14]
- Paraffin
- Aquatic therapy[15]
- Splinting
- Range of motion (active or active-assisted only, during acute phase)
- Gentle stretching
- Gait training
- Stationary cycling
- Exercise (isometric only during acute phase)
- Patient/family education including joint protection and energy conservation
- Recommendations for adaptive equipment as needed

FUNCTIONAL GOALS

- Patient will be able to:
  - Increase ankle dorsiflexion to 10 degrees for sit-to-stand transfers.
  - Increase shoulder flexion to 120 degrees for patient to brush hair.
  - Decrease pain rating to 3 out of 10 or below on VAS for patient to sleep through the night.
  - Increase quad strength to 3 out of 5 or higher for stair-climbing.
  - Improve dynamic standing balance to "good" for independent ambulation.
  - Increase endurance for child to remain in school for a full day.

PROGNOSIS

- Good; 80% will go into remission, though depends on type and severity of disease.
- Children with severe oligoarticular or polyarticular disease have more damage, as do children with rheumatoid factor-positive, which may develop through adult years.
- Oligoarticular JIA has best prognosis.

PATIENT RESOURCES

- Arthritis in Children. American college of rheumatology. http://www.rheumatology.org/practice/clinical/patients/diseases_and_conditions/juvenilearthritis.asp. Accessed June 17, 2013.
- Juvenile Rheumatoid Arthritis Support Group. http://www.mdjunction.com/arthritis-juvenile-rheumatoid. Accessed June 17, 2013.

REFERENCES

1. The American Physical Therapy Association. Pattern 4D: Impaired joint mobility, motor function, muscle performance, and range of motion associated with connective tissue dysfunction. *Interactive Guide to Physical Therapist Practice.* 2003. doi: 10.2522/ptguide.3.1_4. Accessed June 17, 2013.
2. Soep JB. Chapter 27. Rheumatic diseases. In: Hay W, Levin MJ, Sondheimer JM, Detering RR, eds. *Current Diagnosis & Treatment: Pediatrics.* New York, NY: McGraw-Hill; 2011. http://www.accessphysiotherapy.com/abstract/6586501#6586501. Accessed June 17, 2013.
3. Rheumatology Image Bank. Systemic Juvenile Idiopathic Arthritis: Rash. http://images.rheumatology.org/viewphoto.php?imageId=2862594&albumId=75693. Accessed June 17, 2013.
4. Mayo Clinic. Sed Rate (erythrocyte sedimentation rate). http://www.mayoclinic.com/health/sed-rate/MY00343. Accessed June 17, 2013.
5. Mayo Clinic. C-Reactive Protein. http://www.mayoclinic.com/health/c-reactive-protein/MY01018. Accessed June 17, 2013.
6. Mayo Clinic. Rheumatoid Factor. http://www.mayoclinic.com/health/rheumatoid-factor/MY00241. Accessed June 17, 2013.
7. Wiik AS, van Venrooij WJ. *Hotline: The Use of Anti-cyclic Citrullinated Peptide (anti-CCP) Antibodies in RA.* American College of Rheumatology. http://www.rheumatology.org/publications/hotline/1003anticcp.asp. Accessed January 20, 2013.
8. Mayo Clinic. ANA test. http://www.mayoclinic.com/health/ana-test/MY00787. Accessed June 17, 2013.
9. HLA-B27 antigen. MedlinePlus. http://www.nlm.nih.gov/medlineplus/ency/article/003551.htm. Accessed June 17, 2013.
10. Panus PC, Jobst EE, Masters SB, Katzung B, Tinsley SL, Trevor AJ. *Pharmacology for the Physical Therapist.* New York, NY: McGraw-Hill; 2009. http://www.accessphysiotherapy.com/resource/615. Accessed June 17, 2013.
11. Kalden JR. Expanding role of biologic agents in rheumatoid arthritis. *J Rheumatol.* 2002;29(suppl 66):27–37. http://www.jrheum.com/subscribers/02/11/supplement/27.html. Accessed June 17, 2013.
12. Dutton M. *McGraw Hill's NPTE (National Physical Therapy Examination).* 2nd ed. New York, NY: McGraw-Hill; 2012. http://www.accessphysiotherapy.com/resource/611. Accessed June 17, 2013.

13. Denegar CR, Prentice WE. Managing pain with therapeutic modalities. In: Prentice WE, Quillen WS, Underwood F, eds. *Therapeutic Modalities in Rehabilitation*. 4th ed. New York, NY: McGraw-Hill; 2011. http://www.accessphysiotherapy.com/content/8135806#8135806. Accessed June 17, 2013.
14. Prentice WE. Chapter 9. Cryotherapy and thermotherapy. In: Prentice WE, Quillen WS, Underwood F, eds. *Therapeutic Modalities in Rehabilitation*. 4th ed. New York, NY: McGraw-Hill; 2011. http://www.accessphysiotherapy.com/content/8138157. Accessed June 17, 2013.
15. Dutton M. *Orthopaedic Examination, Evaluation, and Intervention*. New York, NY: McGraw-Hill; 2008. http://www.accessphysiotherapy.com/resource/612. Accessed June 17, 2013.

ADDITIONAL REFERENCES

- Cassidy JT, Petty RE, Laxer RM, Lindsley C. *Textbook of Pediatric Rheumatology*. 6th ed. Philadelphia: WB Saunders & Co, 2010.
- IDC9DATA Web site. http://www.icd9data.com. Accessed June 17, 2013.
- ICD10DATA Web site. http://www.icd10data.com/Convert/714.30. Accessed June 17, 2013.
- Helders PJH, Klepper SE, Takken T, Van Der Net J. Juvenile idiopathic arthritis. In: Campbell SK, Palisano RJ, Orlin MN, eds. *Physical Therapy for Children*. 4th ed. St. Louis, MO: Elsevier Saunders; 2012.
- Klepper SE. Juvenile idiopathic arthritis. In: Tecklin JS, ed *Pediatric Physical Therapy*. 4th ed. Philadelphia, PA: Lippincott, Williams and Wilkins; 2008.
- Schneider R, Passo MH. Juvenile rheumatoid arthritis. *Rheum Dis Clin North Am*. 2002;28(3):503–530.
- Weiss JE, Ilowite NT. Juvenile idiopathic arthritis. *Pediatr Clin North Am*. 2005;52(2):413–442,vi.

242 LEGG–CALVÉ–PERTHES DISEASE

Kay Tasso, PhD, PT, PCS

CONDITION/DISORDER SYNONYMS

- Juvenile osteochondrosis of hip and pelvis
- Avascular necrosis of the proximal femur
- Coxa plana

ICD-9-CM CODE

- 732.1 Juvenile osteochondrosis of hip and pelvis

ICD-10-CM CODE

- M91.1 Juvenile osteochondrosis of head of femur

PREFERRED PRACTICE PATTERN

- 4I: Impaired Joint Mobility, Motor Function, Muscle Performance, and Range of Motion (ROM) Associated with Bony or Soft Tissue Surgery[1]

PATIENT PRESENTATION

An 11-year-old male is referred to physical therapy with a diagnosis of Legg–Calvé–Perthes disease (LCPD). Gait analysis reveals an antalgic gait on the affected side. The child reports 7/10 pain in the hip and groin and difficulty with ambulation and stair climbing. His passive range of motion (RON) is limited in hip internal rotation, abduction, and extension. The parents report use of a Scottish-Rite brace was unsuccessful and the child is scheduled for surgical correction. The therapist instructs the child in crutch training pre-op and then provides gait training, RMO exercises, and strengthening post-op.

KEY FEATURES

Description

- Impairment of blood flow to the hip resulting in destructive changes
- Self-limiting disease of the hip

Essentials of Diagnosis

- Age of onset or detection is best predictor of successful recovery

General Considerations

- Four stages
  - Stage 1. Condensation: bone stops and femoral head becomes necrotic
  - Stage 2. Fragmentation of necrotic bone; femoral head and acetabulum become deformed; revascularization begins
  - Stage 3. Reossification of femoral head
  - Stage 4. Remodeling of femoral head and acetabulum

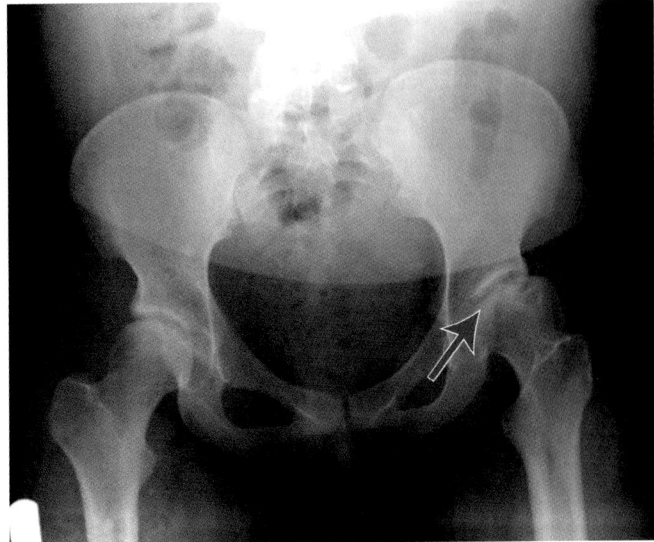

FIGURE 242-1 Legg–Calvé–Perthes disease. Chronic and significant deformity of the left femoral head is apparent (*arrow*). Subcortical cysts are also present. The joint space is normal. (Reproduced with permission from Shah BR, Lucchesi M: *Atlas of Pediatric Emergency Medicine*, © 2006, McGraw-Hill, New York.)

Demographics

- Children aged 3 to 13 years old, especially males aged 5 to 7 years old
- Males 3 to 5 times more likely than females
- Usually unilateral; bilateral 10% to20% of the time
- Uncommon in African Americans

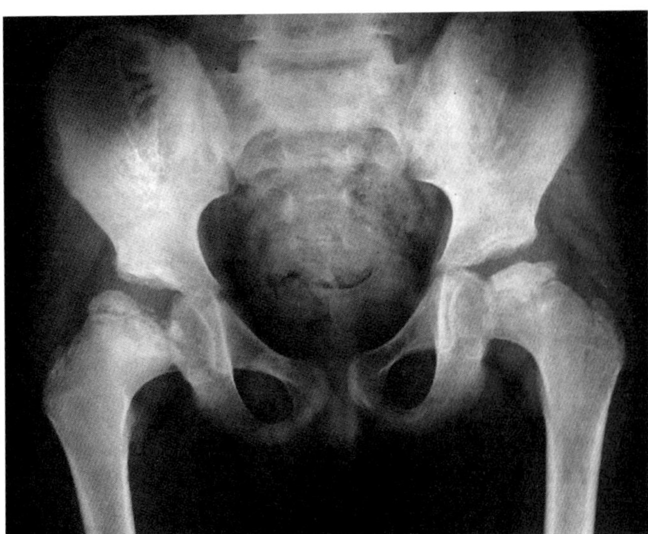

FIGURE 242-2 Legg–Calvé–Perthes disease is present bilaterally. (From Simon RR, Sherman SC *Emergency Orthopedics*. 6th edition. www.accessemergencymedicine.com. Copyright © The McGraw-Hill Companies, Inc. All rights reserved.)

TABLE 242-1 Differentiation of Pediatric Hip Pathologies

	Congenital Hip Dislocation	Septic Arthritis	Legg–Calvé–Perthes Disease	Transient Synovitis	Slipped Femoral Capital Epiphysis
Age	Birth	Less than 2 years; rare in adults	2–13 years	2–12 years	Males: 10–17 years; females: 8–15 years
Incidence	Female > male; left > right; blacks < whites		Male > female; rare in blacks; 15% bilateral	Male > female; unilateral	Male > female; blacks > whites
Observation	Short limb, associated with torticollis	Irritable child, motionless hip, prominent greater trochanter, and mild illness	Short limb, high greater trochanter, quad atrophy, and adductor spasm	Decreased flexion, abduction, and external rotation; thigh atrophy; and muscle spasm	Short limb, obese, quadriceps atrophy, and adductor spasm
Position	Flexed and abducted	Flexed, abducted, and externally rotated			Flexed, abducted, and externally rotated
Pain		Mild pain with palpation and passive motion; often referred to knee	Gradual onset; aching in hip, thigh, and knee	Acute: severe pain in knee; moderate: pain in thigh and knee; tenderness over hip	Vague pain in knee, suprapatellar area, thigh, and hip; pain in extreme motion
History	May be breech birth	Steroid therapy; fever	20–25% familial, low birth weight, and growth delay	Low-grade fever	May be trauma
Range of motion	Limited abduction	Decreased (capsular pattern)	Limited abduction and extension	Decreased flexion, limited extension, and internal rotation	Limited internal rotation, abduction, and flexion, and increased external adductor spasm
Special tests	Galeazzi sign, Ortolani sign, and Barlow sign	Joint aspiration			
Gait		Refuses to walk	Antalgic gait after activity	Refuses to walk; antalgic limp	Acute: antalgic; chronic: Trendelenburg external rotation
Radiologic findings	Upward and lateral displacement and delayed development of acetabulum	CT scan: localized abscess; increased separation of ossification center	In stages: increased density, fragmentation, and flattening of epiphysis	Normal at first; widened medial joint space	Displacement of upper femoral epiphysis, especially in frog position

Source: Richardson JK, Iglarsh ZA. *The Hip, Clinical Orthopaedic Physical Therapy*. Philadelphia, PA: WB Saunders, 1994:367–368.

CLINICAL FINDINGS

SIGNS AND SYMPTOMS

- Pain
- Antalgic gait
- Trendelenburg gait[2]
- Referred pain to groin, thigh, knee
- May have limited hip internal rotation, abduction, extension
- Muscle spasm of hip flexors and adductors

Functional Implications

- Difficulty with ambulation, stairs
- Limited hip mobility
- Antalgic gait

Possible Contributing Causes

- Avascular necrosis of hip (i.e., lack of blood flow to the capital femoral epiphysis) due to:
  - Injury
  - Infection
  - Vascular anomalies (congenital or acquired)
  - Thrombus
  - Synovitis

Differential Diagnosis

- Multiple epiphyseal dysplasia
- Infection
- Septic arthritis
- Hypothyroidism
- Dysplasia
- Synovitis
- Gaucher's disease[3]
- Sickle cell anemia4

MEANS OF CONFIRMATION

Imaging

- X-ray: AP and frog leg-lateral view

FINDINGS AND INTERPRETATION

- X-ray of hip to evaluate for avascular necrosis

REFERRALS/ADMITTANCE

- To orthopedic surgeon for
  - Anti-inflammatory medication
  - Traction
  - Orthotic prescription
    - Petrie cast[5]
    - Scottish–Rite brace[6]
    - Surgical repair including osteotomy

IMPAIRMENTS

- Referred pain from hip
- Muscle spasms of hip flexors and adductors
- Gait deviations
- Decreased mobility due to pain and partial weight-bearing with crutches
- Decreased hip internal rotation, abduction, extension ROM

TESTS AND MEASURES

- 6-minute walk test
- Alberta Infant Motor Scale
- Bayley Scales of Motor Development or Bayley II
- Bruininks Oseretsky Test of Motor Proficiency
- Early Intervention Developmental Profile
- Movement Assessment of Infants
- Neonatal Behavioral Assessment Scale
- Peabody Scales of Motor Development
- Test of Infant Motor Performance

INTERVENTION

- For when patient released by physician for physical therapy after casting or surgical repair
- Modalities to decrease pain
- AROM and PROM of hip
- Strengthening of hip
  - Hip abduction in standing or side-lying
  - Hip extension in standing or prone
    - Bridges
  - Sit-to-stand exercises
  - Wall squats
- Gait training

FUNCTIONAL GOALS

- The patient will be able to:
  - Increase hip AROM and PROM for internal rotation, abduction, extension.
  - Increase strength of hip musculature, especially hip extensors and abductors.
  - Ambulate 150 ft independently with crutches, nonweight bearing on involved leg.
  - Ambulate independently without gait deviations or gait aides for 500 ft.

PROGNOSIS

- Children under 8 years of age with least involvement of femoral head have best outcomes, as bone has time to reshape.
- Children with complete involvement of femoral head have poorest outcomes, as bone may not heal properly.[6]

PATIENT RESOURCES

- Legg-Calve-Perthes disease. Mayo Clinic web site. http://www.mayoclinic.com/health/legg-calve-perthes-disease/DS00654. Accessed July 5, 2013.
- Perthes Disease. American Academy of Orthopedic Surgeons Web site. http://orthoinfo.aaos.org/topic.cfm?topic=A00070. Accessed July 5, 2013.

REFERENCES

1. The American Physical Therapy Association. Pattern 4I: Impaired joint mobility, motor function, muscle performance, and range of motion associated with bony or soft tissue surgery. *Interactive Guide to Physical Therapist Practice*. 2003. doi: 10.2522/ptguide.3.1_9. Accessed July 5, 2013.
2. Dutton M. *Dutton's Orthopaedic Examination, Evaluation, and Intervention*. 3rd ed. New York, NY: McGraw-Hill; 2012. http://www.accessphysiotherapy.com/resource/612. Accessed July 5, 2013.
3. Gaucher disease. PubMed Health. http://www.ncbi.nlm.nih.gov/pubmedhealth/PMH0001590. Accessed July 5, 2013.
4. Chandrasoma P, Taylor CR. *Concise Pathology*. 3rd ed. Stamford, CT: Appleton & Lang; 1998. http://www.accessphysiotherapy.com/content/187050. Accessed July 5, 2013.
5. Perthes Disease. American Academy of Orthopedic Surgeons Web site. http://orthoinfo.aaos.org/topic.cfm?topic=A00070. Accessed July 5, 2013.
6. Conservative Management of Legg-Calve-Perthes Disease. Netter Images Web site. http://www.netterimages.com/image/1205.htm. Accessed July 5, 2013.

ADDITIONAL REFERENCES

- ICD-9-CM. http://www.icd9data.com. Accessed July 5, 2013.
- ICD-10-CM. http://www.icd10data.com. Accessed July 5, 2013.
- Anatomy and Physiology Revealed. AccessPhysiotherapy Web site. http://www.accessphysiotherapy.com/APR. Accessed July 5, 2013.
- Barnes DV, Wood A. The infant at risk for developmental delay. In: Tecklin JS, ed. *Pediatric Physical Therapy*. 4th ed. Philadelphia, PA: Lippincott, Williams and Wilkins; 2008:101–178.
- Dutton M. Gait and posture analysis. In: Dutton M, ed. *Orthopedic Examination, Evaluation, and Intervention*. 2nd ed. New York, NY: McGraw-Hill; 2008. http://www.accessphysiotherapy.com/content/5552001#5552001. Accessed July 5, 2013.
- Dutton M. Imaging studies in orthopedics. In: Dutton M, ed. *Orthopedic Examination, Evaluation, and Intervention*. 2nd ed. New York, NY: McGraw-Hill; 2008. http://www.accessphysiotherapy.com/content/55601112#55601112. Accessed July 5, 2013.
- Dutton M. The hip joint. In: Dutton M, ed. *Dutton's Orthopedic Survival Guide: Managing Common Conditions*. New York, NY: McGraw-Hill; 2011. http://www.accessphysiotherapy.com/content/8654175#8654175. Accessed July 5, 2013.
- Malone TR, Hazle C, Grey ML. Imaging of the Pelvis and Hip. Imaging in Rehabilitation. New York, NY: McGraw-Hill; 2008. http://www.accessphysiotherapy.com/content/5941118#5941118. Accessed July 5, 2013.

- Patel DR, Greydanus DE, Baker RJ. Overuse Injuries of the Hip, Pelvis, and Thigh. In: Patel DR, Greydanus DE, Baker RJ, eds. *Pediatric Practice: Sports Medicine*. http://www.accessphysiotherapy.com/content/6979768. Accessed July 5, 2013.
- Polousky JD. Orthopedics. In: Hay WW, Levin MJ, Sondheimer JM, Deterding RR, eds. *CURRENT Diagnosis & Treatment: Pediatrics*. 20th ed. New York, NY: McGraw-Hill; 2011. http://www.accessphysiotherapy.com/content/6585839#6585839. Accessed July 5, 2013.
- Polousky JD. Orthopedics. In: Hay WW, Levin MJ, Sondheimer JM, Deterding RR, eds. *CURRENT Diagnosis & Treatment: Pediatrics*. 20th ed. New York, NY: McGraw-Hill; 2011. http://www.accessphysiotherapy.com/content/6586029#6586029. Accessed July 5, 2013.
- Stanger M. Orthopedic Management. In: Tecklin JS, ed. *Pediatric Physical Therapy*. 4th ed. Philadelphia, PA: Lippincott, Williams and Wilkins; 2008:417–450.

243 LUNG TRANSPLANT: PEDIATRIC

Kay Tasso, PhD, PT, PCS

CONDITION/DISORDER SYNONYMS

- Single-lung transplant
- Double-lung transplant
- Living donor lobar transplant

ICD-9-CM CODE

- V42.6 Lung replaced by transplant

ICD-10-CM CODE

- Z94.2 Lung transplant status

PREFERRED PRACTICE PATTERN

- 6C: Impaired Ventilation, Respiration/Gas Exchange, and Aerobic Capacity/Endurance Associated With Airway Clearance Dysfunction

PATIENT PRESENTATION

A 16-year-old female is referred to a local outpatient physical therapy clinic 4 months after receiving a double-lung transplant due to cystic fibrosis (CF). She was receiving physical therapy three times a week at the hospital where she received the transplant. Her goal is to progress to swimming as her primary aerobic workout but has been working to progress her exercise tolerance and endurance using a treadmill and stationary bike. She also wants to increase her overall strength.

KEY FEATURES

Description

- Diseased or defective lung (single-lung transplant) or lungs (double-lung transplant) or a portion thereof is removed
- Healthy partial lung from a living donor or complete donor lung(s) from a deceased person is implanted

Essentials of Diagnosis

- Most common causes in children under 1 year of age are congenital heart disease (CHD), peripheral vascular disease (PVD), and CF
- Lung transplant considered when patient death is imminent within 1 to 2 years and all other medical options have been exhausted and/or are ineffective[1]

General Considerations

- Timing of transplant for over 12 years of age depends on their lung allocation score (LAS)
- Long-term outcomes are limited
- Contraindications to lung transplant
  - Malignancy
  - Sepsis
  - Tuberculosis
  - Hepatitis
  - Neuromuscular disease

Demographics[2]

- Forty-four lung transplants in 2011
- Males more common than females
- 0.02% pediatric lung transplants (<18 years old)
- Double-lung transplants 5 to 6 times more common than single-lung transplants

CLINICAL FINDINGS

SIGNS AND SYMPTOMS

- Respiratory failure
- Unable to tolerate exercise
- Hypoxemia
- Carbon dioxide retention
- Failure to thrive
- Abnormal pulmonary function tests (PFTs)
- Syncope
- Cyanosis

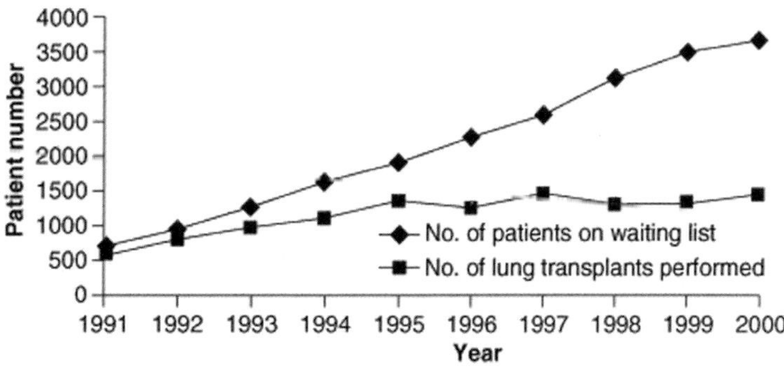

FIGURE 243-1 Number of patients awaiting lung transplants and number of lung transplants performed each year. Data derived from Scientific Registry of Transplant Recipients, 2002 (http://www.ustransplant.org).

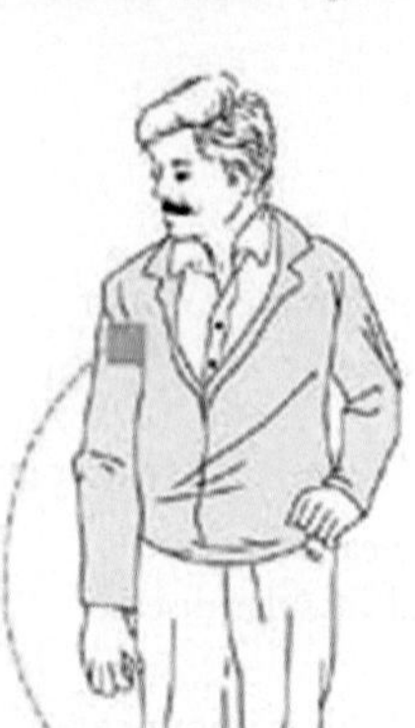

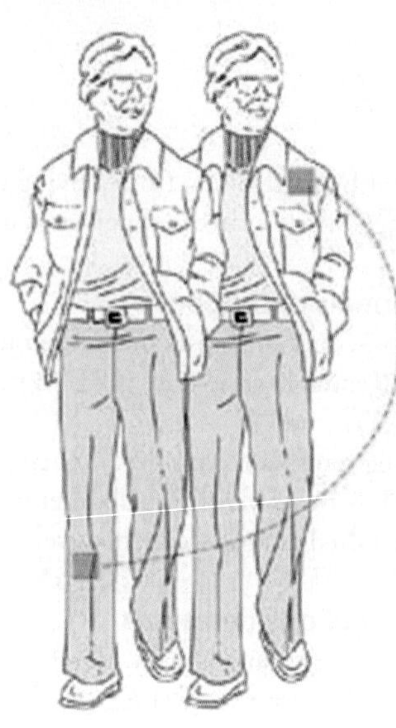

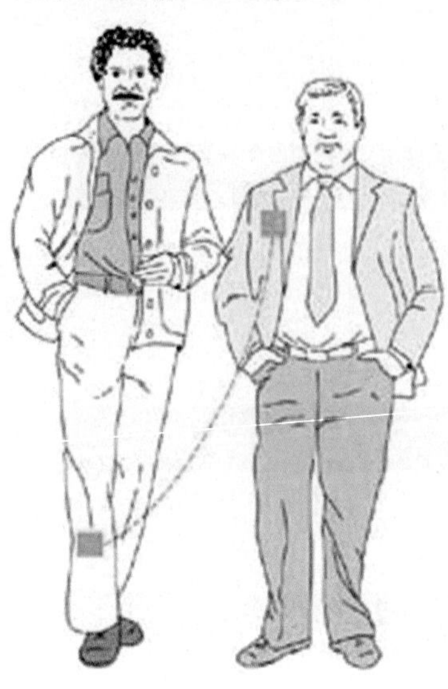

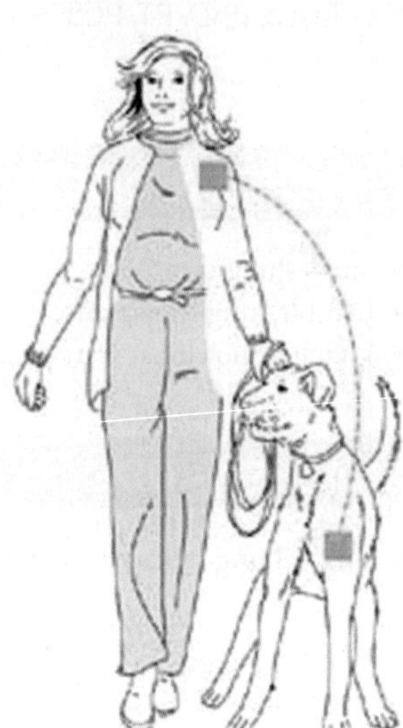

FIGURE 243-2 Different types of tissue transplants (grafts). (From Chandrasoma P, Taylor CR. *Concise Pathology* 3rd ed. www.accessmedicine.com. Copyright © The McGraw-Hill Companies, Inc. All rights reserved.)

Possible Contributing Causes

- Pediatric[3]
  - CHD
  - Surfactant dysfunction
  - Idiopathic pulmonary fibrosis (IPF)
  - Bronchiolitis obliterans (BO)
  - Pulmonary vascular disorder
  - Chronic lung disease of infancy
  - Pulmonary fibrosis/Idiopathic pulmonary fibrosis (IPF)
  - Pulmonary vein anomalies
  - CF
- Adult
  - Pulmonary hypertension
  - Emphysema
  - CF
  - Alpha-1 antitrypsin deficiency[1]
  - IPF[4]
  - Interstitial lung disease[4]
  - Chronic obstructive pulmonary disease[4]

DIFFERENTIAL DIAGNOSIS

Post Surgical Issues

- Rejection
- Infection
- BO

Functional Implications

- Deconditioned
- Developmental delay
- Dependent for ADLs
- Immunosuppression

MEANS OF CONFIRMATION OR DIAGNOSIS

Laboratory Tests

- Complete blood count (CBC)
- Arterial blood gases
- Prothrombin time (PT)
- Liver function test
- Partial thromboplastin time (PTT)
- PFTs
  - Forced expiratory volume in 1 second (FEV_1)
  - Arterial oxygen tension (PaO_2)
  - Arterial carbon dioxide tension ($PaCO_2$)

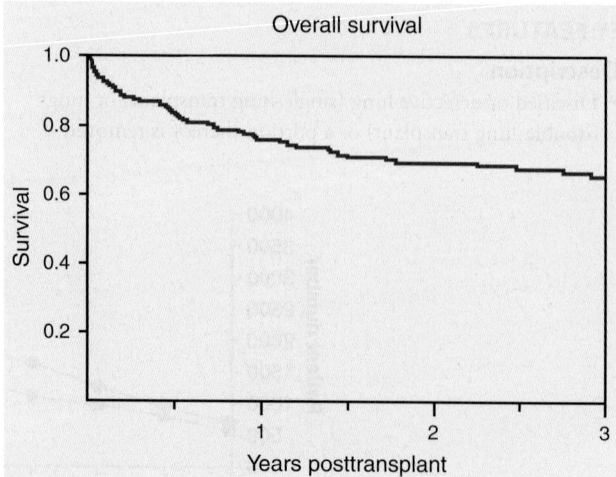

FIGURE 243-3 Overall survival rate after lung transplantation at the University of Minnesota. (From Brunicardi FC, Andersen DK, Billiar TR, et al. *Schwartz's Principles of Surgery.* 9th ed. http://www.accessmedicine.com. Copyright © The McGraw-Hill Companies, Inc. All rights reserved.)

- HIV
- Immunoglobulin G levels (IgG)

Imaging

- X-ray
- Chest CT scan
- Echocardiography

TREATMENT

Medication

- Immunosuppressants[3]
  - Cyclosporin
  - Imuran
  - Cellcept
  - Tacrolimus
  - Corticosteroids
  - Sirolimus

MEDICAL PROCEDURES

- Electrocardiogram (EKG)
- Lung biopsy
- Bronchoscopy
- Transbronchial biopsy to assess for rejection
- Thoracosternotomy[4]
- Cardiac catheterization
- Thoracotomy

REFERRALS/ADMITTANCE

- To hospital for admittance for graft rejection
- To pulmonologist
- To thoracic surgeon
- To cardiologist

IMPAIRMENTS

- Decreased upper extremity (UE) range of motion (ROM)
- Decreased strength
- Decreased endurance

TESTS AND MEASURES

- 6-minute walk test
- Goniometric measurements
- PFT, spirometry, and oximetry
- Strength assessment
- FEV_1

INTERVENTION

- Active ROM only for UE for first 6 weeks post-op
- Aerobic activity
  - Walking
  - Stationary bike
- Breathing: Blowing bubbles, pinwheel
- Squatting
- Developmental activities

FUNCTIONAL GOALS

- The patient will be able to
  - Transfer from supine to sitting with minimal assistance within 3 days to improve bed mobility.

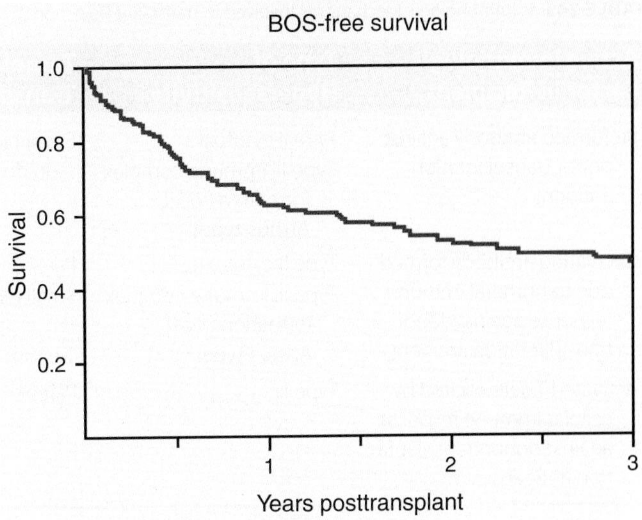

FIGURE 243-4 Survival rate after lung transplantation in the absence of bronchiolitis obliterans syndrome (BOS) at the University of Minnesota. (From Brunicardi FC, Andersen DK, Billiar TR, et al. *Schwartz's Principles of Surgery.* 9th ed. http://www.accessmedicine.com. Copyright © The McGraw-Hill Companies, Inc. All rights reserved.)

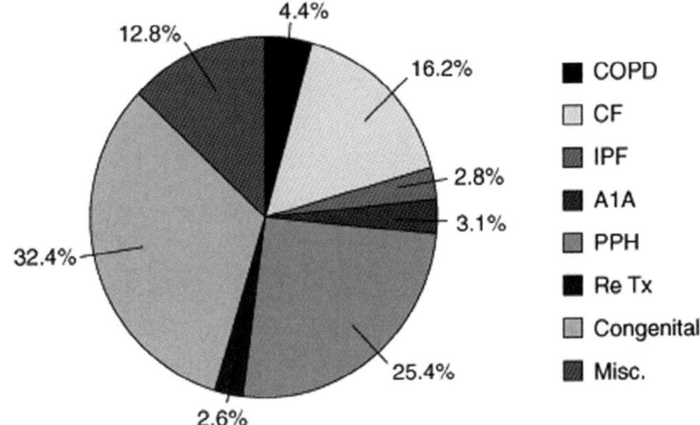

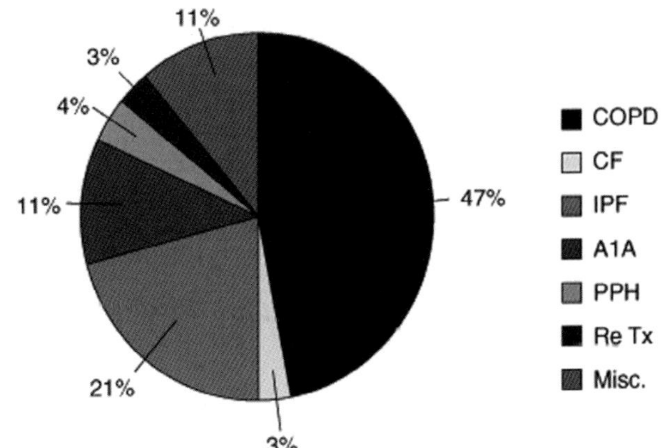

FIGURE 243-5 Pediatric and adult lung transplant recipients. Indications for transplantation. Data derived from ISHLT Registry (http://www.ishlt.org).

TABLE 243-1 Immunologic Mechanisms Involved in Transplant Rejection

Active Immunologic Factor in Recipient	Type of Hypersensitivity	Target Sites in Transplant	Pathologic Effect	Type of Clinical Rejection
Preformed antibody against donor transplantation antigens	Type II cytotoxic Type III immune complex formation (local, Arthus-type)	Small blood vessels in donor tissue	Fibrinoid necrosis and thrombosis of small vessels; ischemic necrosis of parenchymal cells.	Hyperacute rejection
Circulating antibody formed due to humoral immune response against donor transplantation antigens	Type II cytotoxic Type III immune complex formation (local, Arthus-type)	Parenchymal cells Small blood vessels	Acute necrosis of parenchymal cells. Fibrinoid necrosis and thrombosis in acute phase; intimal fibrosis and narrowing in chronic phase.	Acute rejection Acute rejection, chronic rejection
Activated T cells elicited by cellular immune response against donor transplantation antigens	Type IV	Parenchymal cells	Progressive, slow loss of parenchymal cells.	Chronic rejection

Source: Chandrasoma P, Taylor CR. Concise Pathology. 3rd ed. www.accessmedicine.com.

- Ambulate 50 minutes with stand-by assistance within 5 days to increase mobility.
- Ride a stationary bike for 20 minutes within 2 months to increase endurance.
- Brush own hair independently within 3 months to increase active shoulder ROM.
- Cruise at furniture within 3 months to increase mobility.

PROGNOSIS

- Survival rate:[1]
  - 78% for 1st year.
  - 63% for 3rd year.
  - 51% for 5th year.
- 50% develop BO after 3 months and 80% after 5 years.[3]

PATIENT RESOURCE

- *Lung Transplant Handbook*. St Louis: Children's Hospital. http://www.stlouischildrens.org/our-services/lung-transplant-program/lung-transplant-handbook. Accessed July 7, 2013.

REFERENCES

1. What is a Lung Transplant? National Heart, Lung, and Blood Institute web site. http://www.nhlbi.nih.gov/health/health-topics/topics/lungtxp./ Accessed July 7, 2013.
2. Registries - Heart/Lung Registries > Quarterly Data Report. The International Society for Heart & Lung Transplant (ISHLT) web site. http://www.ishlt.org/registries/quarterlyDataReportResults.asp?organ=LU&rptType=all&continent=4. Accessed July 7, 2013.
3. Pediatric Lung Transplantation. Medscape reference web site. http://emedicine.medscape.com/article/1013065-overview#aw2aab6b5. Accessed July 7, 2013.
4. Lung Transplantation. MedlinePlus web site. http://www.nlm.nih.gov/medlineplus/lungtransplantation.html. Accessed July 7, 2013.

ADDITIONAL REFERENCES

- ATS Statement: Guidelines for the Six-Minute Walk Test. American Thoracic Society web site. www.thoracic.org/statements/resources/pfet/sixminute.pdf. Accessed July 7, 2013.
- DeTurk WE, Cahalin LP. Pulmonary hypertension (ICD-9-CM Code: 417). In: DeTurk WE, Cahalin LP, eds. *Cardiovascular and Pulmonary Physical Therapy: An Evidence-Based Approach*. 2nd ed. New York, NY: McGraw-Hill; 2011. http://www.accessphysiotherapy.com/content/6873757. Accessed July 7, 2013.
- DeTurk WE, Cahalin LP. Clinical Correlate. In: DeTurk WE, Cahalin LP, eds. *Cardiovascular and Pulmonary Physical Therapy: An Evidence-Based Approach*. 2nd ed. New York, NY: McGraw-Hill; 2011. http://www.accessphysiotherapy.com/content/6873656. Accessed July 7, 2013.
- Guide to Physical Therapist Practice. APTA web site. http://guidetoptpractice.apta.org/content/1/SEC29.body?sid=b257f74e-89ad-45ae-9eeb-99e01686633b. Accessed July 7, 2013.
- ICD9DATA Web Site. http://www.icd9data.com/2013/Volume1/V01-V91/V40-V49/V42/V42.6.htm. Accessed July 7, 2013.
- ICD10DATA Web Site. http://www.icd10data.com/ICD10CM/Codes/Z00-Z99/Z77-Z99/Z94-/Z94.1. Accessed July 7, 2013.
- Perceived Exertion. Center for Disease Control and Prevention. http://www.cdc.gov/physicalactivity/everyone/measuring/exertion.html. Accessed July 7, 2013.

244 MUSCULAR DYSTROPHY

Kay Tasso, PhD, PT, PCS

CONDITION/DISORDER SYNONYMS

- Adult pseudohypertrophic muscular dystrophy
- Becker muscular dystrophy
- Benign X-linked recessive muscular dystrophy
- Childhood pseudohypertrophic muscular dystrophy
- Duchenne muscular dystrophy

ICD-9-CM CODES[1]

- 359.0 Congenital hereditary muscular dystrophy
- 359.1 Hereditary progressive muscular dystrophy

ICD-10-CM CODES[2]

- G71.0 Muscular dystrophy
- G71.2 Congenital myopathies

PREFERRED PRACTICE PATTERN[3]

- 5E: Impaired Motor Function and Sensory Integrity Associated with Progressive Disorders of the Central Nervous System

PATIENT PRESENTATION

"A 3-year-old boy is brought to his pediatrician to be evaluated for difficulty walking and clumsiness. According to his parents, the patient began walking at the age of 18 months, but in the past year he has begun to fall more frequently and has difficulty getting up from the floor; often supporting himself with his hands along the length of his legs. Birth and developmental history until symptom onset are reportedly normal. There is no contributing family history.

On physical examination the young boy has significant muscle weakness of his hip flexors, knee extensors, deltoids, and biceps muscles. His calves are large, and he walks on his toes during ambulation. Laboratory studies reveal an elevated serum creatine kinase (CK) level of greater than 900 international units per liter (IU/L). Electromyography (EMG) of his muscles reveals a myopathy. Nerve conduction studies reveal relative normal nerve function.[4]

KEY FEATURES

Description

- Group of genetic disorders that result in progressive muscle weakness due to loss of myofibrils[5]
- Causes defects in muscle proteins: Weakens the musculoskeletal system
- Muscle cell and tissue death

Essentials of Diagnosis

- Nine major types of muscular dystrophy (MD)
- Diagnosed through molecular characteristics

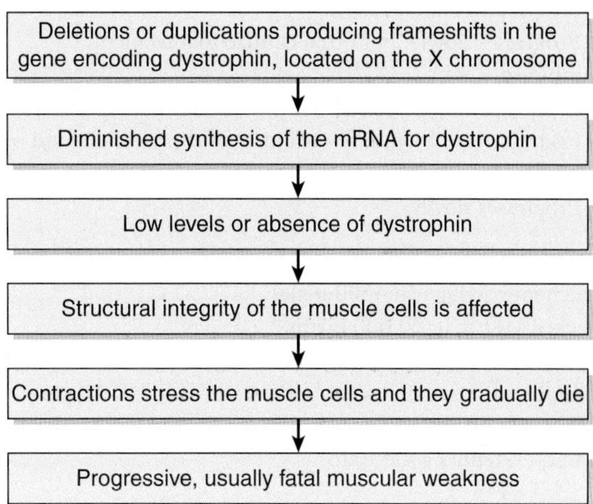

FIGURE 244-1 Summary of mechanisms involved in the causation of Duchenne muscular dystrophy (OMIM 310200). (From Murray RK, Bender D, Botham KM, et al. *Harper's Illustrated Biochemistry.* 29th ed. www.accessmedicine.com. Copyright © The McGraw-Hill Companies, Inc. All rights reserved.)

- Diagnosis is dependent on
  - Age of patient at onset of symptoms
  - Areas of body involved
  - Rate of progression of symptoms

General Considerations

- Duchenne MD (Type I)
  - Symptoms begin around 3 to 5 years of age
  - Characterized by pseudohypertrophy of calves
  - Progresses quickly
- Becker MD (Type II)
  - Symptoms begin around 11 years of age
  - Characterized by muscle weakness of shoulder girdle, trunk, and extremities
  - Progresses slowly
- Congenital MD[5]
  - Congenital MD with central nervous system disease (Fukuyama syndrome, Walker–Warburg syndrome, muscle–eye–brain disease)
  - Integrin-deficient congenital MD
  - Merosin-deficient congenital MD
  - Congenital MD with normal merosin
    - Symptoms begin at birth
    - Characterized by hypotonia and contractures at birth
    - Progresses slowly but varies
- Congenital myotonic MD
  - Symptoms begin at birth
  - Characterized by severe hypotonia and muscle weakness at birth
  - Progresses slowly
  - Cognitive impairment present
- Childhood-onset facioscapulohumeral MD
  - Symptoms begin by 2 to 10 years of age
  - Characterized by muscle weakness of face and shoulder girdle

- Progresses slowly
- Eventually becomes nonambulatory
- Emery–Dreifuss (humeroperoneal) MD
  - Symptoms begin prior to teenage years
  - Characterized by contractures of posterior cervical muscles, biceps, and plantar flexors
  - Progresses slowly, but often cardiac involvement
- Limb-girdle MD
  - Symptoms begin during teen years to adulthood
  - Characterized by muscle weakness of the shoulder and pelvic girdles
  - Progresses slowly

Demographics

- Duchenne MD: 1 in 3500 males
- Becker MD: 1 in 20,000 births
- Congenital myotonic MD: 1 in 8000 births
- Childhood-onset facioscapulohumeral MD: 3 to 10 per 1,000,000 births
- Emery–Dreifuss MD: Rare

CLINICAL FINDINGS

SIGNS AND SYMPTOMS

- Fatigue
- Complaint of muscle cramps (Becker MD)
- Progressive weakness and atrophy of involved muscles
- Fasciculations (of tongue)
- Dysphagia
- Dysarthria
- Contractures at birth (congenital and congenital myotonic forms of MD)
- Scoliosis
- Cognitive impairment
- Learning disabilities (Duchenne and Becker)
- Waddling gait
- Inability to run
- Inability to jump
- Gower sign
- Difficulty stair climbing
- Toe walking
- Falls
- Decreased maximal vital capacity
- Scapular winging
- Club foot (talipes equinovarus)

Functional Implications

- Progressive dependence for assistance with activities of daily living
- Easily fatigued
- Loss of mobility

Possible Contributing Causes[5,6]

- Duchenne, Becker and Emery–Dreifuss MDs are X-linked recessive diseases resulting in an inability to use dystrophin that is important to the sarcolemma
- Congenital MD is autosomal recessive on chromosome 6q22
- Congenital myotonic MD is autosomal dominant for chromosome 3q21
- Childhood-onset facioscapulohumeral MD can occur as autosomal dominant or recessive of chromosome 4q35
- Emery–Dreifuss MD: X-linked recessive on chromosome Xq28 or autosomal dominant or recessive on chromosome 1q21.2
- Limb-girdle MD can result from autosomal dominant or recessive or X-linked involving 15 different genes

Differential Diagnoses

- Spinal muscular atrophy
- Guillain–Barré syndrome

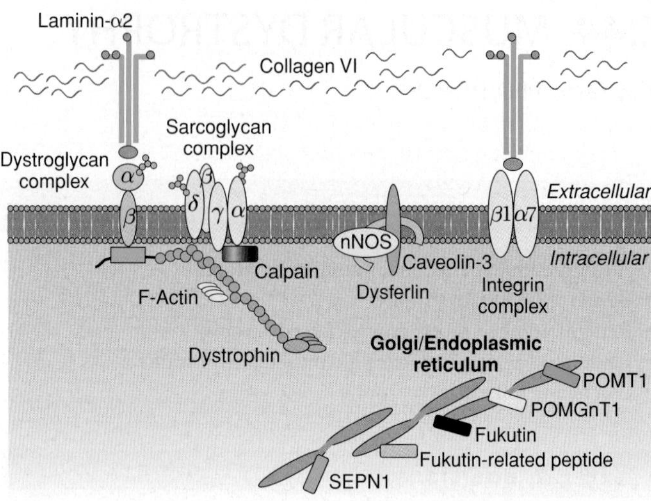

FIGURE 244-2 The molecular organization of the dystrophin–glycoprotein complex in the membrane and sarcolemma and endoplasmic reticulum-Golgi apparatus. These proteins are related to Duchenne, limb-girdle, Miyoshi, and certain congenital dystrophies. (From Ropper AH, Samuels MA. *Adams & Victor's Principles of Neurology.* 9th ed. www.accessmedicine.com. Copyright © The McGraw-Hill Companies, Inc. All rights reserved.)

- Brachial plexus birth injury
- Other genetic syndromes

MEANS OF CONFIRMATION OR DIAGNOSIS

Laboratory Tests

- DNA analysis[5]
- Blood analysis of enzyme levels, such as CK

Imaging

- Plain radiograph for scoliosis

Diagnostic Procedures

- EMG
- Muscle biopsy
- Nerve conduction velocity (NCV)

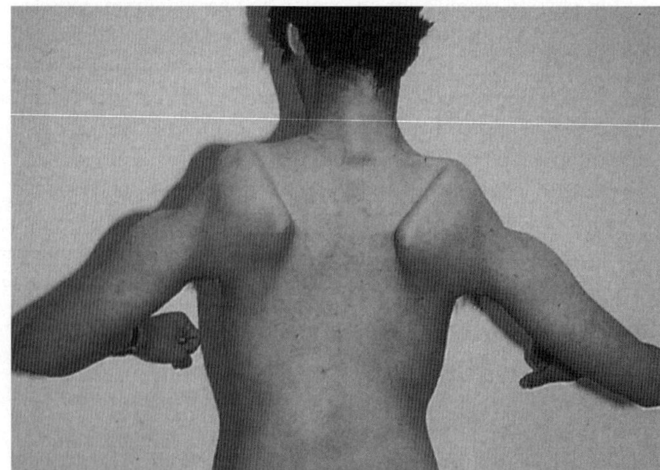

FIGURE 244-3 Facioscapulohumeral dystrophy with prominent scapular winging. (From Longo DL, Fauci A, Kasper D, Hauser S, Jameson J, Loscalzo J eds. *Harrison's Principles of Internal Medicine.* 18th ed. New York, NY: McGraw-Hill, 2012.)

- Echocardiogram for cardiac involvement
- Pulmonary function tests (PFTs)

FINDINGS AND INTERPRETATION

- Increased creatine phosphokinase (CpK3)
- Pseudohypertrophy

TREATMENT

▶ Medication[5]

- Prednisone
- Deflazacort
- Oxandrolone
- Creatine

MEDICAL PROCEDURES

- Tenotomy
- Scoliosis surgical repair
- Fasciotomy
- Tendon transfer

REFERRALS/ADMITTANCE

- Geneticist for counseling
- Occupational therapist for ADL training
- Respiratory therapist for respiratory associated problems
- Orthopedic surgeon for weakness and joint dysfunction
- Speech therapist for voice strengthening and projection

IMPAIRMENTS

- Inability to ambulate
- Decreased strength
- Contractures
- Muscle weakness

TESTS AND MEASURES

- Barthel index
- Dynamometer
- EK (Egen Klassifikation) Scale
- Manual muscle testing
- North Star Ambulatory Assessment
- Pediatric Evaluation of Disability Inventory (PEDI)
- School Function Assessment
- Vignos Functional Rating Scale for Duchenne Muscular Dystrophy[5]

INTERVENTION

- It is important to avoid fatigue, eccentric exercises, or high-resistance exercises
- Strengthening targeting abdominals, gluteus maximus, hip abductors, and quadriceps muscles
- Blowing bubbles or blowing up balloons for pulmonary exercise
- Stretching and range of motion (ROM) to prevent contractures of plantar flexors and tensor fasciae latae
- Bike riding (stationary or standard bicycle)
- Swimming or aquatic therapy
- Standing or walking 2 to 3 hours a day
- Orthotics (knee–ankle–foot, night splints to prevent plantar flexor contractures)
- Standers
- Reciprocating or wheeled walker

FUNCTIONAL GOALS

- The patient will be able to
  - Ambulate independently 25 minutes with rolling walker
  - Increase quadriceps strength to 3+/5 to assist with transfers
  - Utilize night splints (ankle–foot orthotics) to prevent plantar flexor contractures
  - Ride a stationary bike for 20 minutes to prevent loss of aerobic capacity while avoiding fatigue

PROGNOSIS[5]

- Duchenne MD: Nonambulatory by 9 or 10 years of age; death by 20 years of age
- Becker MD: Ambulatory until mean of 27 years of age; death during early forties
- Congenital MD: Life expectancy 15 to 30 years of age
- Congenital myotonic MD: 25% die before 18 months of age, 50% live into their thirties
- Childhood-onset facioscapulohumeral MD: Life expectancy varies
- Emery–Dreifuss MD: Normal life expectancy
- Limb-girdle MD: Most severe cases, life expectancy 20 to early thirties years of age

PATIENT RESOURCES

- Congenital muscular dystrophy overview. NCBI website. http://www.ncbi.nlm.nih.gov/books/NBK1291/. Accessed June 14, 2013.
- Facts about facioscapulohumeral muscular dystrophy. Muscular Dystrophy Association website. http://www.mda.org/publications/PDFs/FA-FSHD.pdf. Accessed June 14, 2013.
- Facts about limb-girdle muscular dystrophy. Muscular Dystrophy Association website. http://www.mda.org/publications/PDFs/FA-LGMD.pdf. Accessed June 14, 2013.
- Facts about rare muscular dystrophies. Muscular Dystrophy Association website. http://www.mda.org/publications/PDFs/FA-RareMD.pdf. Accessed June 14, 2013.

REFERENCES

1. ICD9DATA website. http://www.icd9data.com. Accessed June 13, 2013.
2. ICD10DATA website. http://www.icd10data.com/Convert/359.0. Accessed June 13, 2013.
3. APTA Guide to Physical Therapist Practice. http://guidetoptpractice.apta.org./ Accessed June 1, 2013.
4. Toy EC. Duchenne Muscular Dystrophy, Case 101. LANGE Case Files. http://www.accessmedicine.com/casecontent.aspx?aid=510024564&tabid=1. Accessed June 6, 2013.
5. Stuberg WA. Muscular dystrophy and spinal muscular atrophy. In: Campbell SK, Palisano RJ, Orlin MN, eds. *Physical Therapy for Children*. 4th ed. St. Louis, MO: Elsevier Saunders; 2012: 353–369.
6. Hay WW, Levin MJ, Sondheimer JM, Deterding RR. Neurologic and muscular disorders. In: Hay WW, Levin MJ, Sondheimer JM, Deterding RR, eds. *CURRENT Diagnosis & Treatment: Pediatrics*. 20th ed. New York, NY: McGraw-Hill; 2011. http://www.accessphysiotherapy.com/popup.aspx?aID=6585691. Accessed June 14, 2013.

ADDITIONAL REFERENCES

- Barthel Index. Stroke Center website. http://www.strokecenter.org/wp-content/uploads/2011/08/barthel.pdf. Accessed June 17, 2013.
- Chandrasoma P, Taylor CR. Peripheral neuropathy. In: Chandrasoma P, Taylor CR, eds. *Concise Pathology*. 3rd ed. New York, NY: McGraw-Hill; 2011. http://www.accessphysiotherapy.com/content/193413#193413. Accessed June 16, 2013.
- Deflazacort. Search MedicaRx website. http://www.mims.com/USA/drug/info/deflazacort/?q=corticosteroid%20hormones&type=full. Accessed June 17, 2013.
- Digestive Disorders Health Center. *Web*MD website. http://www.webmd.com/digestive-disorders/tc/difficulty-swallowing-dysphagia-overview. Accessed June 16, 2013.
- Dutton M. Duchenne muscular dystrophy. In: Dutton M, ed. *McGraw-Hill's NPTE (National Physical Therapy Examination)*. 2nd ed. New York, NY: McGraw-Hill; 2012. http://www.accessphysiotherapy.com/content/5404752#5404752. Accessed June 14, 2013.
- Dystrophinopathies. Neuromuscular website. http://neuromuscular.wustl.edu/musdist/dmd.html. Accessed June 16, 2013.
- Fasciotomy. Encyclopedia of Surgery website. http://www.surgeryencyclopedia.com/Ce-Fi/Fasciotomy.html. Accessed June 17, 2013.
- Hall SJ. The biomechanics of human skeletal muscle. In: Hall SJ, ed. *Basic Biomechanics*. 5th ed. New York, NY: McGraw-Hill; 2007. http://www.accessphysiotherapy.com/content/6061338#6061338. Accessed June 16, 2013.
- Hamilton N, Weimar W, Luttgens K. The muscle fiber. In: Hamilton N, Weimar W, Luttgens K, eds. *Kinesiology: Scientific Basis of Human Motion*. New York, NY: McGraw-Hill; 2008. http://www.accessphysiotherapy.com/content/6150251#6150251. Accessed June 15, 2013.
- Hay WW, Levin MJ, Sondheimer JM, Deterding RR. Neurologic and muscular disorders. In: Hay WW, Levin MJ, Sondheimer JM, Deterding RR, eds. *CURRENT Diagnosis & Treatment: Pediatrics*. 20th ed. New York, NY: McGraw-Hill; 2011. http://www.accessphysiotherapy.com/popup.aspx?aID=6585691. Accessed June 13, 2013.
- Malone TR, Hazle C, Grey ML. Radiography. In: Malone TR, Hazle C, Grey ML, eds. Imaging in Rehabilitation. New York, NY: McGraw-Hill; 2008. http://www.accessphysiotherapy.com/content/5940616#5940616. Accessed January 17, 2013.
- North Star Ambulatory Assessment. Muscular Dystrophy website. http://www.muscular-dystrophy.org/assets/0000/6388/NorthStar.pdf. Accessed June 17, 2013.
- Panus PC, Jobst EE, Masters SB, Katzung B, Tinsley SL, Trevor AJ. Corticosteroids and corticosteroid antagonists. In: Panus PC, Jobst EE, Masters SB, Katzung B, Tinsley SL, Trevor AJ, eds. *Pharmacology for the Physical Therapist*. New York, NY: McGraw-Hill; 2009. http://www.accessphysiotherapy.com/content/6093458. Accessed June 17, 2013.
- Prentice WE. Electromyography and biofeedback. In: Prentice WE, Quillen WS, Underwood F, eds. *Therapeutic Modalities in Rehabilitation*. 4th ed. New York, NY: McGraw-Hill; 2011. http://www.accessphysiotherapy.com/content/8137184#8137184. Accessed June 13, 2013.
- Registry of Outcomes Measures. Treat-NMD Neuromuscular Network website. http://www.researchrom.com/masterlist/view/3. Accessed June 17, 2013.
- Tendon transfer. London Foot and Ankle Centre website. http://www.londonfootandanklecentre.co.uk/surgery/tendon_transfer.php. Accessed June 17, 2013.
- Tenotomy. Encyclopedia of Surgery website. http://www.surgery-encyclopedia.com/St-Wr/Tenotomy.html. Accessed June 17, 2013.
- Waxman SG. Language and speech. In: Waxman SG, ed. *Clinical Neuroanatomy*. 26th ed. New York, NY: McGraw-Hill; 2010. http://www.accessphysiotherapy.com/content/5275291#5275291. Accessed June 15, 2013.
- Winging scapula. Shoulderdoc.co.uk website. http://www.shoulderdoc.co.uk/article.asp?section=492, Accessed June 16, 2013.

245 NEUROFIBROMATOSIS

Kay Tasso, PhD, PT, PCS

CONDITION/DISORDER SYNONYMS

- Neurofibromatosis, Type 1 (NF1)
- Von Recklinghausen disease

ICD-9-CM CODES

- 237.70 Neurofibromatosis unspecified
- 237.71 Neurofibromatosis Type 1 von Recklinghausen disease
- 237.72 Neurofibromatosis Type 2 acoustic neurofibromatosis
- 237.73 Schwannomatosis
- 237.7 Neurofibromatosis
- 237.79 Other neurofibromatosis

ICD-10-CM CODES

- Q85.00 Neurofibromatosis, unspecified
- Q85.01 Neurofibromatosis, Type 1
- Q85.02 Neurofibromatosis, Type 2
- Q85.03 Schwannomatosis
- Q85.09 Other neurofibromatosis

PREFERRED PRACTICE PATTERN

- 5E: Impaired Motor Function and Sensory Integrity Associated with Progressive Disorders of the Central Nervous System

PATIENT PRESENTATION

An 18-month-old is referred to physical therapy for frequent falls. The child was diagnosed with neurofibromatosis (NF) at 2 years of age with multiple café-au-lait spots including in the axillary region. The child has an optic nerve tumor on each eye that causes intermittent pain and the latest MRI shows brain tumors that are believed to be the source of the current balance difficulties.

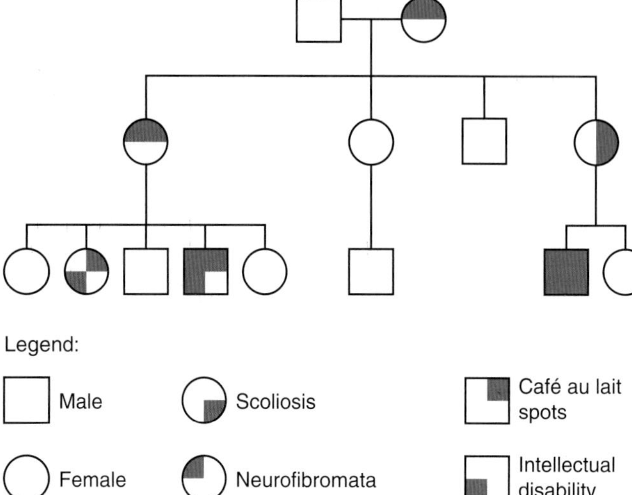

FIGURE 245-1 Autosomal dominant inheritance. Variable expressivity in Neurofibromatosis type 1. (From Hay WM et al: *Current Diagnosis & Treatment: Pediatrics*, 21st edition. www.accessmedicine.com. Copyright © The McGraw-Hill Companies, Inc. All rights reserved.)

KEY FEATURES

Description

- Group of neoplastic disorders resulting from an autosomal dominant genetic disorder or chromosomal mutation
- Type 1 is the most common with hyperpigmentation spots (café-au-lait spots) present at birth, tumors of skin, and progressive decline of nerves, muscle, and bones due to defect of chromosome 17
- Type 2, acoustic neuromas, due to defect of chromosome 22

Essentials of Diagnosis

- At least two of the following needed for diagnosis
  - At least seven café-au-lait spots less than 5 mm prior to puberty and more than 15 mm after puberty
  - More than two neurofibromas
  - Optic glioma
  - More than two Lisch nodules (tumors on the iris)
  - Freckling in axilla or inguinal areas
  - Bony lesions
  - Immediate family member with NF1
- Acoustic neuromas (Type 2) involve tumors on inner ear nerves, brain, skull, spinal cord, including schwannomas, gliomas, and meningiomas

General Considerations

- Type 1 involves dermal and epidermal benign tumors that affect myelin (neurofibromas) of peripheral nerves that can erode bone or cause compression of the nerve including optic nerve gliomas
- Acoustic neuromas result in hearing and balance deficits, as well as difficulty swallowing, and problems with eye movements and speech

Demographics

- NF1 accounts for 95% of all cases[1]
- 1 in 3000 births[2]
- 50% risk in siblings[3]
- 40% of those affected develop complications[3]

CLINICAL FINDINGS

SIGNS AND SYMPTOMS

- Café-au-lait spots (Type 1)
- 62% seizures[3]
- 40% cognitive impairment[3]
- 15% hypertension[3]
- 15% optic glioma[3]
- Skin tumors
- Lisch nodules
- Large head

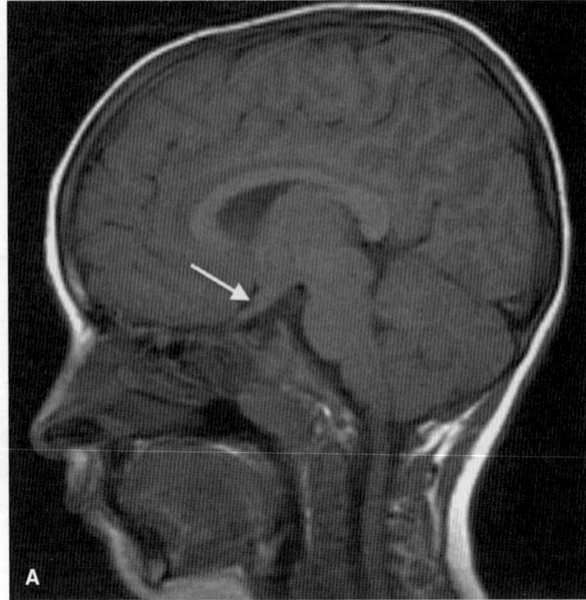

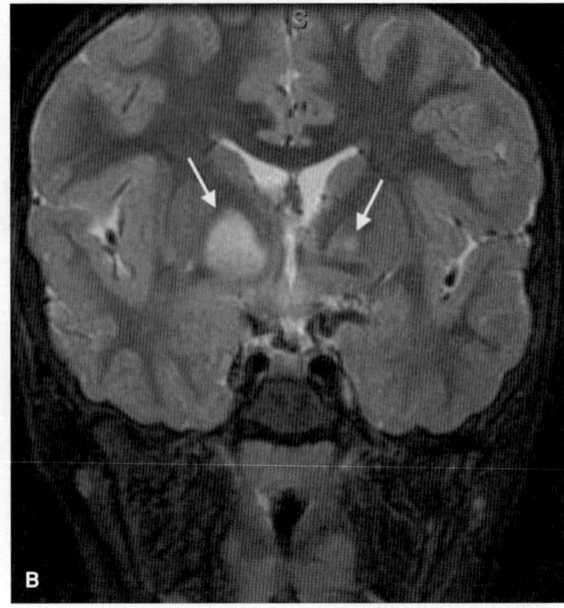

FIGURE 245-2 Noncontrast parasagittal T1-weighted (**A**) and coronal T2-weighted (**B**) images in a 4-year-old male with neurofibromatosis. (**A**) Bulbous enlargement of the optic chiasm is present (arrow), suggesting an optic glioma. (**B**) Foci of increased T2 signal abnormality are demonstrated within the globus palladi (arrows). (From Chen MYM, Pope TL, Ott DJ. *Basic Radiology.* 2nd ed. www.accessmedicine.com. Copyright © The McGraw-Hill Companies, Inc. All rights reserved.)

TABLE 245-1 Phenotype, Inheritance, and Prevalence of Selected Genetic Disorders

Disorder	Phenotype	Genetic Mechanism	Incidence
Down syndrome	Mental and growth retardation, dysmorphic features, internal organ anomalies	Chromosomal imbalance; caused by trisomy 21	≈ 1:800; increased risk with advanced maternal age
Fragile X-associated mental retardation	Mental retardation, characteristic facial features, large testes	X-linked; progressive expansion of unstable DNA causes failure to express gene encoding RNA-binding protein	≈ 1:1500 males; can be manifested in females; multistep mechanism
Sickle cell anemia	Recurrent painful crises, increased susceptibility to infections	Autosomal recessive; caused by a single missense mutation in beta-globin	≈ 1:400 blacks
Cystic fibrosis	Recurrent pulmonary infections, exocrine pancreatic insufficiency, infertility	Autosomal recessive; caused by multiple loss-of-function mutations in a chloride channel	≈ 1:2000 whites; very rare in Asians
Leber hereditary optic neuropathy	Acute or subacute blindness, occasional myopathy or neurodegeneration	Mutation of electron transport chain encoded by mtDNA	≈ 1:50,00–1:10,000
Myoclonic epilepsy with ragged red fibers	Uncontrolled periodic jerking, muscle weakness	Mutation of mitochondrial tRNA in mtDNA	≈ 1:100,000–1:50,000
Neurofibromatosis	Multiple café-au-lait spots, neurofibromas, increased tumor susceptibility	Autosomal dominant; caused by multiple loss-of-function mutations in a signaling molecule	≈ 1:3000; ≈ 50% are new mutations
Duchenne muscular dystrophy	Muscular weakness and degeneration	X-linked recessive; caused by multiple loss-of-function mutations in muscle protein	≈ 1:3000 males; ≈ 33% are new mutations
Osteogenesis imperfecta	Increased susceptibility to fractures, connective tissue fragility, blue scleras	Phenotypically and genetically heterogeneous	≈1:10,000
Phenylketonuria	Mental and growth retardation	Autosomal recessive; caused by multiple loss-of-function mutations in phenylalanine hydroxylase	≈ 1:10,000

Source: McPhee SJ, Hammer GD. *Pathophysiology of Disease: An Introduction to Clinical Medicine.* 6th ed. www.accessmedicine.com. Copyright © The McGraw-Hill Companies, Inc. All rights reserved.

- Scoliosis
- Strabismus (crossed eyes)
- Amblyopia (lazy eye)
- Cranial nerve VIII tumors (Type 2)
- Seizures
- Precocious puberty
- Difficulty with balance
- Tinnitus
- Vertigo
- Pain
- Numbness, tingling, weakness of toes or fingers
- Speech deficits
- Attention deficit hyperactivity disorder (ADHD)

Functional Implications

- Deafness
- Falls due to balance deficits
- Pain resulting in decreased function

Possible Contributing Cause

- Autosomal dominant genetic disorder or mutation of chromosome 17 (Type 1) or chromosome 22 (Type 2)

Differential Diagnoses[2]

- McCune–Albright syndrome
- Noonan syndrome
- LEOPARD (**L**entigines: Reddish-brown to dark brown macules; **E**lectrocardiographic conduction abnormalities: observed on an electrocardiograph as a bundle branch block; **O**cular hypertelorism: Wideset eyes; **P**ulmonary stenosis: Narrowing of the pulmonary artery as it exits the heart; **A**bnormal genitalia: retention of testicles in body or single testicle in males and missing or single ovaries in females; **R**etarded growth: Slow, or stunted growth; **D**eafness: nerve deafness) syndrome
- Bannayan–Riley–Ruvalcaba syndrome (BRRS)

MEANS OF CONFIRMATION OR DIAGNOSIS

Laboratory Tests

- Genetic testing
- Amniocentesis
- Chorionic villus sampling

Imaging

- MRI
- X-ray
- PET scan
- CT scan

TREATMENT

Medical Procedures

- Surgical removal of tumors or cataracts
- Radiation and/or chemotherapy, if tumor malignant

REFERRALS/ADMITTANCE

- Admittance for surgical removal of neurofibromas
- To geneticist; ophthalmologist; dermatologist
- To neurosurgeon; orthopedic surgeon
- To speech therapist; occupational therapist
- To audiologist

IMPAIRMENTS

- Painful joints or soft tissue
- Muscle spasms

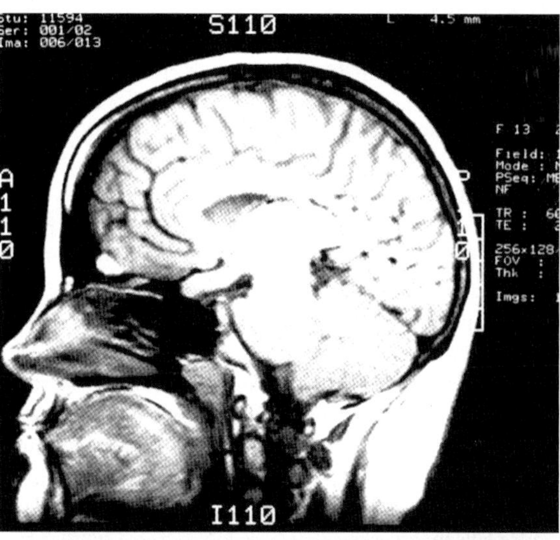

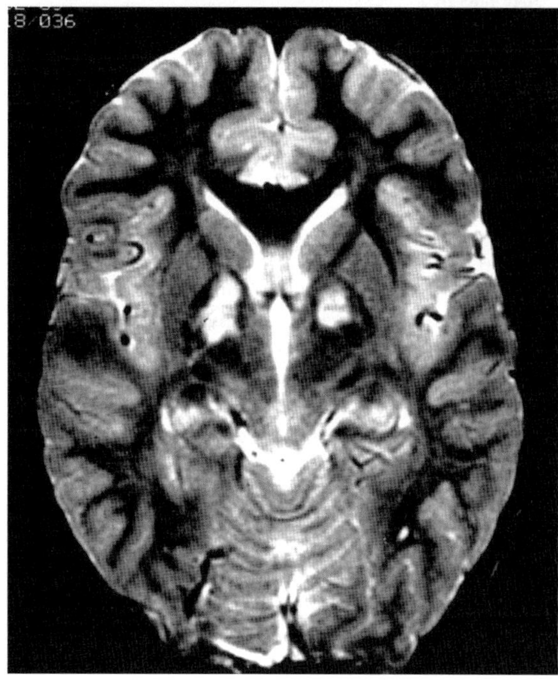

FIGURE 245-3 Neurofibromatosis type 1. T1-weighted MRI in the sagittal plane demonstrating a glioma involving the optic chiasm and brainstem (*above*). T2-weighted axial image showing multiple foci of hyperintensity, presumably hamartomas (*below*). (From Ropper AH, Samuels MA. *Adams & Victor's Principles of Neurology*. 9th ed. www.accessmedicine.com. Copyright © The McGraw-Hill Companies, Inc. All rights reserved.)

- Decreased function
- Decreased strength
- Decreased balance
- Decreased coordination

TESTS AND MEASURES

- Berg Balance Scale (BBS)
- Bruininks–Oseretsky Test of Motor Proficiency
- Manual muscle testing
- Peabody Developmental Motor Scales-2 (PDMS-2)
- Romberg Test
- Scoliosis screening
- Tinetti Balance Assessment Tool

INTERVENTION

- Modalities to decrease pain and/or muscle spasms
- Strengthening
- Coordination exercises
- Balance activities
- Functional activities

FUNCTIONAL GOALS

- The patient will be able to
  - Decrease pain to 2/10 to allow for sleeping through the night within 3 weeks.
  - Increase bilateral quadriceps strength from 3/5 to 5/5 to allow for independent stair climbing within 4 weeks.
  - Gallop 10 feet with either leg leading to increase coordination in 3 months.
  - Stand on one foot for at least 10 seconds to increase balance to reduce falls in 2 weeks.
  - Wash own hair independently within 3 weeks.

PROGNOSIS

- Type 1: Most have normal life span.
- Type 2: If tumors affect brainstem, can cause death.
- Schwannomatosis: Painful, which can result in disability.

PATIENT RESOURCES

- Neurofibromatosis. Minneapolis Clinic of Neurology website. http://www.minneapolisclinic.com/medical-services/121-neurofibromatosis.html. Accessed July 7, 2013.
- NINDS Neurofibromatosis Information Page. National Institute of Neurological Disorders and Stroke website. http://www.ninds.nih.gov/disorders/neurofibromatosis/neurofibromatosis.htm. Accessed July 7, 2013.

REFERENCES

1. ICD9DATA Web site. http://www.icd9data.com. Accessed June 3, 2014.
2. Tsai ACH, Manchester DK, Elias ER. Genetics and dysmorphology. In: Hay WW, Levin MJ, Sondheimer JM, Deterding RR, eds. *CURRENT Diagnosis & Treatment: Pediatrics*. 20th ed. New York, NY: McGraw-Hill; 2011. http://www.accessphysiotherapy.com/content/6589082#6589082. Accessed July 7, 2013.
3. Bernard TJ, Knupp K, Yang ML, Arndt D, Levisohn P, Moe PG. Neurologic and muscular disorders. In: Hay WW, Levin MJ, Sondheimer JM, Deterding RR, eds. *CURRENT Diagnosis & Treatment: Pediatrics*. 20th ed. New York, NY: McGraw-Hill; 2011. http://www.accessphysiotherapy.com/content/6585445#6585445. Accessed July 7, 2013.

ADDITIONAL REFERENCES

- Chorionic Villus Sampling. *Web*MD website. http://www.webmd.com/baby/guide/amniocentesis. Accessed July 7, 2013.
- Dahl AA. Ophthalmologic manifestations of neurofibromatosis type 1. Medscape Reference website. http://emedicine.medscape.com/article/1219222-overview. Accessed July 7, 2013.
- Dutton M. Pediatric physical therapy. In: *McGraw-Hill's National Physical Therapy Examination.* 2nd ed. New York, NY: McGraw-Hill; 2012. http://www.accessphysiotherapy.com/content/5404424#5404424. Accessed July 7, 2013.
- *Guide to Physical Therapist Practice*. Alexandria, VA: American Physical Therapy Association; 2003. http://guidetoptpractice.apta.org/content/1/SEC22.body. Accessed July 7, 2013.
- ICD10DATA Website. http://www.icd10data.com/Convert/237.70. Accessed July 7, 2013.
- Tinetti Balance Assessment Tool. Health Promotion in Berkshire website. http://www.bhps.org.uk/falls/documents/TinettiBalanceAssessment.pdf. Accessed July 7, 2013.

246 OBSTETRIC BRACHIAL PLEXUS INJURY

Kay Tasso, PhD, PT, PCS

CONDITION/DISORDER SYNONYMS

- Erb palsy
- Klumpke palsy
- Brachial plexus injury
- Birth brachial plexus injury

ICD-9-CM CODE[1]

- 767.6 Injury to brachial plexus due to birth trauma

ICD-10-CM CODES[2]

- P13.0 Erb paralysis due to birth injury
- P14.1 Klumpke paralysis due to birth injury
- P14.3 Other brachial plexus birth injuries

PREFERRED PRACTICE PATTERN[3]

- 5F: Impaired Peripheral Nerve Integrity and Muscle Performance Associated with Peripheral Nerve Injury

PATIENT PRESENTATION

A 3-week-old infant is referred to outpatient physical therapy for right Erb palsy. The mother reports an uneventful pregnancy but prolonged and difficult delivery especially in getting the shoulder out of the birth canal. Upon examination, the infant presents with fisting of the left hand and physiologic flexion of the elbow typical of a newborn but the right arm is postured by the baby's side. There is full passive range of motion (ROM) for the elbow, wrist, and hand and at least 90 degrees of right shoulder motions with the therapist deferring assessment above 90 degrees to prevent overstretching of the shoulder. There is active motion of the right upper trapezius but no active shoulder abduction, external rotation, or elbow or wrist extension. The therapist instructs the family on gentle passive ROM, dressing, positioning, and handling of the affected side and recommends weekly physical therapy.

KEY FEATURES

Description

- Traumatic injury to the brachial plexus caused during delivery of an infant

Essentials of Diagnosis

- Stretch or incomplete rupture of the plexus is the most common injury often resulting from vacuum or forceps delivery[4]

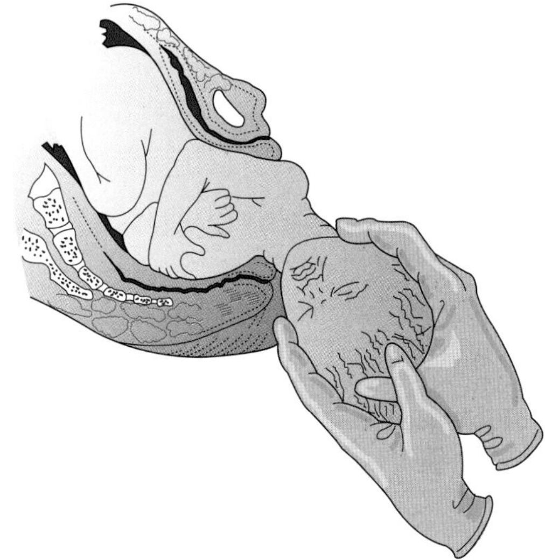

FIGURE 246-1 Delivery of anterior shoulder. (From DeCherney AH, Nathan L. *Current Diagnosis & Treatment Obstetrics & Gynecology.* 11th ed. www.accessmedicine.com. Copyright © The McGraw-Hill Companies, Inc. All rights reserved.)

General Considerations

- Classifications
  - Upper or Erb palsy (C5, C6, and/or C7) is the most common: Arm postured in shoulder adduction, internal rotation, neutral extension; elbow extension; forearm pronation; wrist and finger flexion.
  - Lower or Klumpke palsy (C8, T1) is rare: Hand is flaccid.
  - Total palsy (C5-T1): Arm and hand are involved.

Demographics

- About 1.5 per 1000 infants[4]

CLINICAL FINDINGS

SIGNS AND SYMPTOMS

- Weakness of deltoid, biceps, brachioradialis, brachialis (Erb palsy)
- Weakness of wrist flexors and finger intrinsics (Klumpke palsy)
- All of the above plus sensory loss for total brachial plexus injury

Functional Implications

- Limits ability to use involved arm for reaching, grasping, or participating in ADLs
- Inability to weight bear on involved arm
- Inability to attain quadruped or crawl on hands and knees
- Asymmetrical use of arms
- Neglect of involved side

Possible Contributing Causes

- Compression
- Traction on the shoulder with or without cervical rotation
- Avulsion
- Large birth weight
- Breech presentation[5]
- Shoulder dystocia[5]

Differential Diagnosis

- Spinal cord injury
- Stroke
- Cerebral palsy
- Shoulder dislocation

MEANS OF CONFIRMATION OR DIAGNOSIS

Imaging

- Standard radiograph of arm and chest
- CT scan
- MRI

Diagnostic Procedures

- EMG

FINDINGS AND INTERPRETATION

- Nerve conduction changes

TREATMENT

Medication

- Botox injections to antagonist muscles

MEDICAL PROCEDURE

- Surgery for nerve, tendon, or muscle transfers

REFERRALS/ADMITTANCE

- To neurologist
- To orthopedist
- To occupational therapist

IMPAIRMENTS

- Decreased strength
- Decreased ROM
- Asymmetrical in and/or delay of gross motor skills

TESTS AND MEASURES

- Test of infant motor performance
- Goniometry
- Sensory testing

INTERVENTION

- No ROM for 7 to 10 days old infant[5]
- Avoid lying on affected side
- Avoid picking infant up under axilla
- Splinting
- Gentle, pain-free passive ROM
- Parent/caregiver education
- Serial casting
- Stabilize scapula during ROM and activities
- Facilitate developmental activities

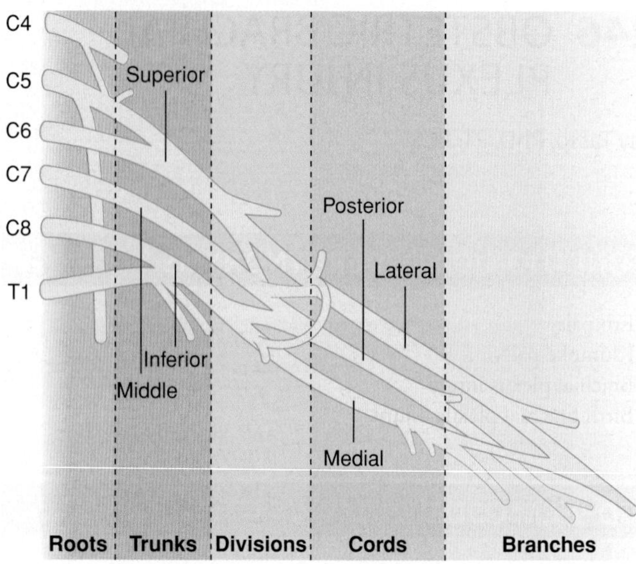

FIGURE 246-2 The anatomy of the brachial plexus. (Reproduced with permission from Reichman EF, Tolson DR. Regional nerve blocks. In: Reichman EF, Simon RR, eds. *Emergency Medicine Procedures*. New York, NY: McGraw-Hill; 2004.)

FUNCTIONAL GOALS

- Patient will be able to
  - Increase strength in right biceps to at least 3/5 to allow for holding bottle with two hands within 6 months.
  - Achieve prone-on-elbows with weight bearing equally on both arms to increase shoulder and scapular stability within 2 months.
  - Reach up against gravity for a toy when in supine to increase shoulder strength within 3 months.

PROGNOSIS

- Best prognosis for Klumpke palsy.[6]
- Deltoid and biceps improvement within 3 months.[7]
- 50% to 90% permanent disability remaining after 3 years of age.[4]
- Most infants never regain full function.[4]
- 86% recovery in infants with Erb palsy.[8]

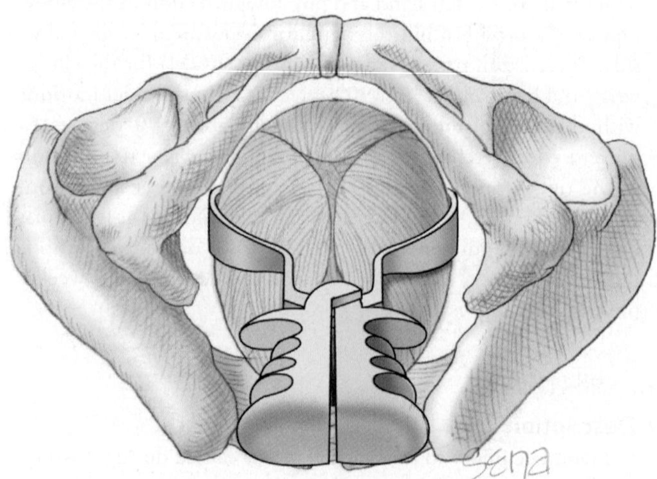

FIGURE 246-3 The vertex is now occiput anterior, and the forceps are symmetrically placed and articulated. (From Cunningham FG, Leveno K, Bloom S, Hauth J, Rouse D, Spong C. *Williams Obstetrics* 23rd ed. http://www.accessmedicine.com. Copyright © The McGraw-Hill Companies, Inc. All rights reserved.)

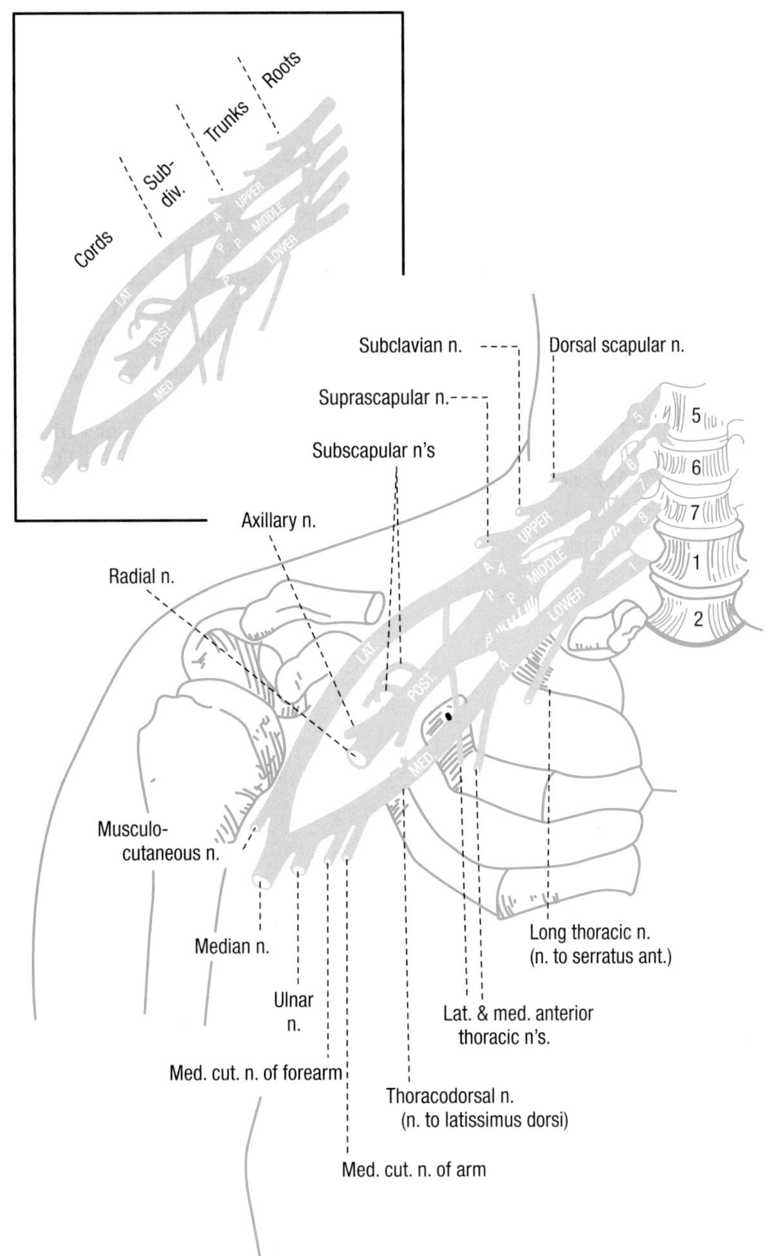

FIGURE 246-4 Diagram of the brachial plexus: the components of the plexus have been separated and drawn out of scale. Note that peripheral nerves arise from various components of the plexus: roots (indicated by cervical roots *5, 6, 7, 8,* and thoracic root *1*); trunks (upper, middle, lower); divisions (anterior and posterior); and cords (lateral, posterior, and medial). The median nerve arises from the heads of the lateral and medial cords. (From Haymaker W, Woodhall B. *Peripheral Nerve Injuries.* 2nd ed. Philadelphia PA; Saunders; 1953, by permission.)

- 36% recovery in infants with Klumpke palsy[8]
- 20% to 30% require surgery[9]
- Related to birth weight
  - Below 7 lbs 11 oz, over 90% had full recovery[5]
  - Above 7 lbs, 11 oz, less than 70% had full recovery[5]
- Recovery up to 4 years post injury although majority of recovery by 9 months of age[5]

PATIENT RESOURCE

- Borrero JL, Gilbert A, Hentz VR. *Obstetrical Brachial Plexus Paralysis.* Self published; 2007. http://www.assh.org/Professionals/ProdsSvcs/Store/Pages/ObstetricalBrachialPlexusParalysis.aspx. Accessed March 10, 2013.

REFERENCES

1. ICD9DATA web site. http://www.icd9data.com/2013/Volume1/760-779/764-779/767/767.6.htm. Accessed February 14, 2013.
2. ICD10ATA web site. http://www.icd10data.com/ICD10CM/Codes/P00-P96/P10-P15/P14. Accessed February 14, 2013.
3. The American Physical Therapy Association. *Interactive Guide to Physical Therapist Practice.* Alexandria, VA: The American Physical Therapy Association; 2003. http://guidetoptpractice.apta.org./ Accessed March 10, 2013.
4. Nath RK, Kumar N, Avila MB, et al. Risk factors at birth for permanent obstetric brachial plexus injury and associated osseous deformities. *ISRN Pediatr.* 2012;2012:307039. doi: 10.5402/2012/307039.

5. Vander Linden DW. Brachial plexus injury. In: Campbell SK, Palisano RJ, Orlin MN, eds. *Physical Therapy for Children*. 4th ed. St. Louis, MO: Elsevier Saunders; 2011:628–643.
6. Dutton M. Basic anatomy. In: Dutton M, ed. *Dutton's Orthopaedic Examination, Evaluation, and Intervention*. 3rd ed. New York, NY: McGraw-Hill; 2012. http://www.accessphysiotherapy.com/content/56521309. Accessed February 16, 2013.
7. Hay WW, Levin MJ, Deterding RR, Abzug MJ, Sondheimer JM. Birth trauma. In: Hay WW, Levin MJ, Deterding RR, Abzug MJ, Sondheimer JM, eds. *CURRENT Diagnosis & Treatment: Pediatrics*. 21st ed. New York, NY: McGraw-Hill; 2012. http://www.accessphysiotherapy.com/content/56807665. Accessed February 16, 2013.
8. Lindqyist PG, Erichs K, Molnar C, Gudmundsson S, Dahlin LB. Characteristics and outcome of brachial plexus birth palsy in neonates. *Acta Paediatr*. 2012;101(6):579–582. doi: 10.1111/j.1651-2227.2012.02620.x
9. Thatte MR, Mehta R. Obstetric brachial plexus injury. *Indian J Plast Surg*. 2011;44(3):380–389. doi: 10.4103/0970-0358.90805.

ADDITIONAL REFERENCES

- Bernard TJ, Knupp K, Yang ML, Arndy D, Levisohn P, Moe PG. Neurologic assessment & neurodiagnostic procedures. In: Hay WW, Levin MJ, Sondheimer JM, Deterding RR, eds. *CURRENT Diagnosis & Treatment: Pediatrics*. 20th ed. New York, NY: McGraw-Hill; 2011. http://accessphysiotherapy.com/content/6585071. Accessed March 10, 2013.
- Cincinnati Children's Hospital. Botulin Toxin Injections. http://www.cincinnatichildrens.org/health/b/botox. Accessed March 10, 2013.
- The Test of Infant Motor Performance and the Harris Infant Neuromotor Test. IMPS, LLC web site. http://thetimp.com/. Accessed March 10, 2013.

247 OSTEOGENESIS IMPERFECTA

Kay Tasso, PhD, PT, PCS

CONDITION/DISORDER SYNONYM

- Brittle bone disease

ICD-9-CM CODE

- 756.51 Osteogenesis imperfecta

ICD-9-CM CODE

- Q78.0 Osteogenesis imperfecta

PREFERRED PRACTICE PATTERN

- 5B: Impaired Neuromotor Development

PATIENT PRESENTATION

A 5-year-old is referred to physical therapy following removal of a cast for a femur fracture and subsequent diagnosis of osteogenesis imperfecta (OI). The child has decreased active and passive knee range of motion (ROM). The child presents with a leg-length difference and decreased strength in the hip, knee, and ankle on the involved side.

KEY FEATURES

Description

- Autosomal dominant genetic disorder that affects Type I collagen resulting in osteopenia and frequent fractures that may be apparent in a newborn infant

Essentials of Diagnosis

- Four types
  - Type I: Mild (most common)
  - Type II: Perinatal lethal
  - Type III: Progressive deforming
  - Type IV: Deforming with normal scleras
- Types I and IV do not have fractures while in utero
- Type II characterized by fractures in utero
- Type III characterized by fractures at birth or as infant

General Considerations

- Disorder results from Type I collagen impairment that affects skin, bone, connective tissue of organs (including GI tract), and vascular system
- Type I: Fewer fractures after puberty; short stature and hearing loss as adult; blue sclera
- Type II: Usually results in death during infancy due to respiratory problems

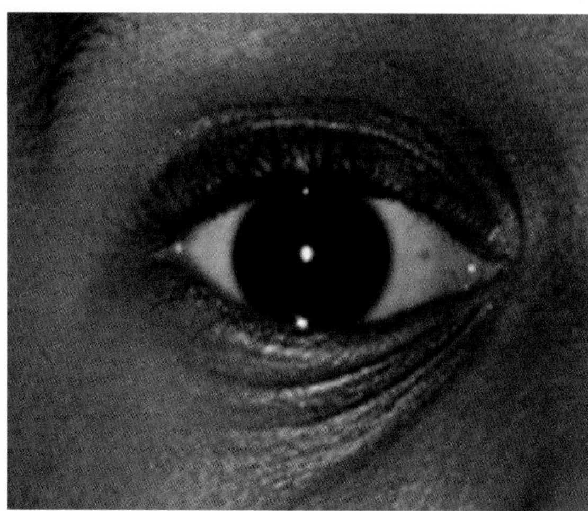

FIGURE 247-1 Osteogenesis imperfecta (OI) Blue sclerae are the most characteristic mucocutaneous feature of patients with mild OI. (From Goldsmith LA, Katz S, Gilchrest B, Paller A, Leffell D, Wolff K, eds. *Fitzpatrick's Dermatology in General Medicine.* 8th ed. http://www.accessmedicine.com. Copyright © The McGraw-Hill Companies, Inc. All rights reserved.)

- Type III: Usually nonambulatory as an adult due to progressive deformities from multiple fractures over time; sclera affected; short stature, scoliosis
- Type IV: Short stature as adult, fractures continue as adult, but remains ambulatory; scoliosis; hearing loss; sclera unaffected

Demographics

- 1 in 20,000 births[1]
- Infants
- Males and females affected equally[1]

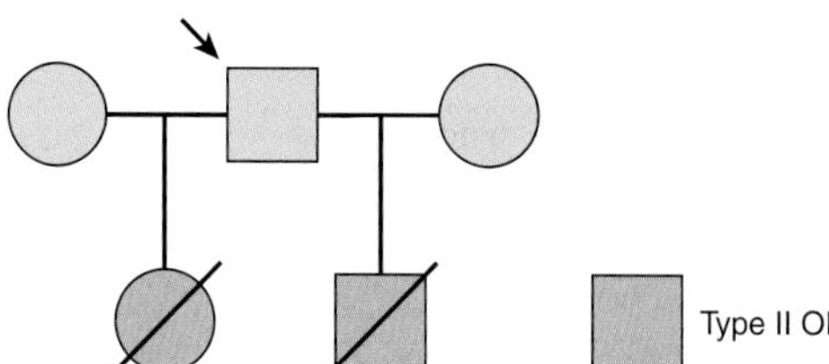

FIGURE 247-2 Gonadal mosaicism for type II osteogenesis imperfecta (OI). In this idealized pedigree, the phenotypically normal father (indicated with the arrow) has had two children by different mates, each of whom is affected with autosomal dominant type II OI. Analysis of the father showed that some of his spermatozoa carried a *COL1A1* mutation, indicating that the explanation for this unusual pedigree is germline mosaicism. (Redrawn from Cohn DH, Starman BJ, Blumberg B, Byers PH,. Recurrence of lethal osteogenesis imperfecta due to parental mosaicism for a dominant mutation in a human type I collagengene [*COL1A1*]. *Am J Hum Genet.* 1990;46:591–601.)

TABLE 247-1 Clinical and Molecular Subtypes of Osteogenesis Imperfecta

Type	Phenotype	Genetics	Molecular Pathophysiology
Type I	Mild: Short stature, postnatal fractures, little or no deformity, blue scleras, premature hearing loss	Autosomal dominant	Loss-of-function mutation in proα1(I) chain resulting in decreased amount of mRNA; quality of collagen is normal; quantity is reduced two-fold
Type II	Perinatal lethal: Severe prenatal fractures, abnormal bone formation, severe deformities, blue scleras, connective tissue fragility	Sporadic (autosomal dominant)	Structural mutation in proα1(I) or proα2(I) chain that has mild effect on heterotrimer assembly; quality of collagen is severely abnormal; quantity often reduced also
Type III	Progressive deforming: Prenatal fractures, deformities usually present at birth, very short stature, usually nonambulatory, blue scleras, hearing loss	Autosomal dominant[a]	Structural mutation in proα1(I) or proα2(I) chain that has mild effect on heterotrimer assembly; quality of collagen is severely abnormal; quantity can be normal
Type IV	Deforming with normal scleras: Postnatal fractures, mild to moderate deformities, premature hearing loss, normal or gray scleras, dental abnormalities	Autosomal dominant	Structural mutation in the proα2(I), or, less frequently, proα1(I) chain that has little or no effect on heterotrimer assembly; quality of collagen is usually abnormal; quantity can be normal

[a]Autosomal recessive in rare cases.

Source: McPhee SJ, Hammer GD. *Pathophysiology of Disease: An Introduction to Clinical Medicine.* 6th ed. http://www.accessmedicine.com.

CLINICAL FINDINGS

SIGNS AND SYMPTOMS

- Fracture(s) at various times throughout lifespan (dependent on type of OI)
- Blue sclera
- Deafness at early age
- Genu varum (bow legged)
- Scoliosis
- Kyphosis
- Muscle weakness
- Joint laxity
- Brittle teeth

Functional Implications

- May cause short stature or joint deformities that can interfere with function
- May cause developmental delay due to immobility or casting associated with fractures
- Weakness may limit function

Possible Contributing Causes

- Inherited disorder

Differential Diagnoses

- Child abuse
- Juvenile osteoporosis
- Temporary brittle-bone syndrome
- Hypophosphatasia
- Menkes syndrome
- Steroid-induced osteoporosis

MEANS OF CONFIRMATION OR DIAGNOSIS

Laboratory Tests

- DNA analysis
- Collagen testing

Imaging

- Prenatal ultrasound
- X-rays

Diagnostic Procedures

- Chorionic villus sampling (CVS)
- Amniocentesis
- Skin punch biopsy

Findings and Interpretation

- CVS is a prenatal test identifying chromosome abnormalities and other inherited disorders.

TREATMENT

Medication

- Pamidronate

MEDICAL PROCEDURES

- Surgical correction of fractures, such as intramedullary rod
- Surgical correction of scoliosis

TABLE 247-2 Osteogenesis Imperfecta: Clinical and Genetic Features

Type	Clinical Features	Inheritance
I	Mild bone fragility, blue sclera	Dominant
II	"Prenatal lethal"; crumpled long bones, thin ribs, dark blue sclera	Dominant
III	Progressively deforming; multiple fractures; early loss of ambulation	Dominant/ recessive
IV	Mild to moderate bone fragility; normal or gray sclera; mild short stature	Dominant

Source: Reproduced with permission from Phillips C, Wenstrup RJ. Biosynthetic and genetic disorders of collagen, in Cohen IK, Diegelmann RF, Linblad WJ eds. *Wound Healing: Biochemical and Clinical Aspects*. Philadelphia, PA: WB Saunders;1992;152.

REFERRALS/ADMITTANCE

- To hospital for surgical repair of fractures as needed
- To geneticist for testing (especially if interested in offspring)
- To occupational therapist
- To orthotist
- To orthopedic surgeon
- To audiologist

IMPAIRMENTS

- Gross motor delay
  - Unable to sit independently
  - Unable to crawl on hands and knees
  - Unable to stand at furniture
- Decreased strength
- Decreased ROM
- Dependent for transfers
- Dependent for ADLs
- Nonambulatory

TESTS AND MEASURES

- Active ROM (but not passive)
- Manual muscle testing (assessed functionally in children)
- Leg-length discrepancy (LLD)

INTERVENTION

- Neurodevelopmental treatment
  - Facilitation techniques to assist with attaining age-appropriate gross motor milestones
- Therapeutic exercise
  - Strengthening
  - Stretching
  - Aerobic
- Functional activities
  - Transfers
  - Gait training
  - Stair climbing
- Aquatic exercise
- Adaptive equipment (may include wheelchair or gait aides)
- Orthotics
- Patient education regarding energy conservation and joint protection
- Family/caregiver education regarding safe handling, positioning, dressing, and bathing

FUNCTIONAL GOALS

- Patient will be able to
  - Tailor sit on the floor with contact guard assistance with good spinal alignment for 2 minutes within 1 month.
  - Pull-to-stand independently with standby assistance within 3 months.
  - Crawl on hands and knees for 5 minutes with moderate assistance in 2 months.
  - Increase quad strength to 5/5 to allow for independence in climbing stairs; holding railing with one hand in 6 weeks.
  - Increase elbow flexion to 110 degrees in 2 weeks to allow patient to brush hair.
  - Transfer from bed to bedside chair with minimal assistance to improve mobility in 2 days.
  - Stand with contact guard assistance to allow for improved independence with hygiene in 1 day.
  - Ambulate 75 minutes with rolling walker and standby assistance in 3 days to improve mobility.

PROGNOSIS

- Type I: Fewer fractures after puberty; short stature and hearing loss as adult; blue sclera; normal life span.
- Type II: Usually results in death during infancy due to respiratory problems.
- Type III: Usually nonambulatory as an adult due to progressive deformities from multiple fractures over time; sclera affected; short stature, scoliosis.
- Type IV: Short stature as adult, fractures continue as adult, but remains ambulatory; scoliosis; hearing loss; sclera unaffected; normal life span.

PATIENT RESOURCES

- Child abuse or osteogenesis imperfecta? Osteogenesis Imperfecta Foundation website. http://www.oif.org/site/DocServer/_Child_Abuse__Child_Abuse_or_Ostegenesis_Imperfecta.pdf?docID=7189. Accessed July 7, 2013.
- Osteogenesis imperfecta. PubMed Health website. http://www.ncbi.nlm.nih.gov/pubmedhealth/PMH0002540. Accessed July 7, 2013.

REFERENCE

1. Osteogenesis imperfecta. Encyclopedia of Children's Health website. http://www.healthofchildren.com/N-O/Osteogenesis-Imperfecta.html. Accessed July 7, 2013.

ADDITIONAL REFERENCES

- Barsh G. Genetic disease. In: McPhee SJ, Hammer GD, eds. *Pathophysiology of Disease: An Introduction to Clinical Medicine*. 6th ed. New York, NY: McGraw-Hill; 2010. http://www.accessphysiotherapy.com/content/5366542#5366542. Accessed July 7, 2013.
- Dutton M. Pediatric physical therapy. In: *McGraw Hill's National Physical Therapy Examination*. New York, NY: McGraw-Hill; 2009. http://www.accessphysiotherapy.com/content/5404584#5404584. Accessed July 7, 2013.
- Guide to Physical Therapist Practice. APTA website. http://guidetoptpractice.apta.org./ Accessed July 7, 2013.
- Handling and care suggestions for infants and toddlers with OI. Osteogenesis Imperfecta Foundation website. http://www.oif.org/site/DocServer/Handling_and_Care_for_Infants__pdf_for_page_12.0_.pdf?docID=7361. Accessed July 7, 2013.
- ICD9DATA website. http://www.icd9data.com. Accessed July 7, 2013.
- ICD10DATA website. http://www.icd10data.com/Convert/756.51. Accessed July 7, 2013.
- Therapeutic strategies for osteogenesis imperfecta: a guide for physical and occupational therapists. NIH Osteoporosis and Related Bone Diseases National Resource Center website. http://www.niams.nih.gov/Health_Info/Bone/Osteogenesis_Imperfecta/therapists_guide.asp. Accessed July 7, 2013.
- Tsai ACH, Manchester DK, Elias ER. Genetics and dysmorphology. In: Hay WW, Levin MJ, Sondheimer JM, Deterding RR, eds. *CURRENT Diagnosis & Treatment: Pediatrics*. 20th ed. New York, NY: McGraw-Hill; 2011. http://www.accessphysiotherapy.com/content/6589116#6589116. Accessed July 7, 2013.

248 PAGET DISEASE

Eric Shamus, PhD, DPT, PT, CSCS
Christopher C. Felton, DO, ATC

CONDITION/DISORDER SYNONYM

- Osteitis deformans

ICD-9-CM CODE[1]

- 731.0 Osteitis deformans without mention of bone tumor

ICD-10-CM CODE[2]

- M88.9 Osteitis deformans of unspecified bone

PREFERRED PRACTICE PATTERNS[3]

- 4A: Primary Prevention/Risk Reduction for Skeletal Demineralization
- 4B: Impaired Posture
- 4C: Impaired Muscle Performance
- 4F: Impaired Joint Mobility, Motor Function, Muscle Performance, ROM and Reflex Integrity Association with Spinal Disorders
- 4G: Impaired Joint Mobility, Muscle Performance, and ROM Associated with Fracture

PATIENT PRESENTATION

A 55-year-old male presents to the office with complaint of worsening low back pain over the last 2 months. He describes the pain as "bone pain" consisting of a deep, dull, constant ache in the region of his lumbar spine. He also has noticed over the last week, short episodes of numbness in his left lower extremity (LE) when he stands for long periods of time. It is relieved with lying supine or sitting. A 14-point review of systems was otherwise negative. Past medical history is unremarkable. His temperature is 98 degrees F, BP is 124/74, HR is 70 bpm, RR is 16 breaths/min, and O_2 sat is 100%. On exam, there is tenderness to palpation over transverse processes of L4 and L5 as well as increased warmth to the skin in the same region. Lumbar spine ROM is limited in flexion and extension secondary to increased pain. Strength is 5/5 in his LE bilaterally, as well as 2+ reflexes at L4 and S1. Overall, lumbar lordosis is decreased. The patient is referred to the physician. Serum alkaline phosphatase (ALP) is mildly elevated, with normal calcium and phosphate. X-ray shows the L4 and L5 vertebrae to be enlarged and an ivory appearance to them.

KEY FEATURES

Description

- Osteometabolic bone disease
- Excessive reabsorption of bone by osteoclasts, followed by vascular and fibrous tissue filling in the bone marrow

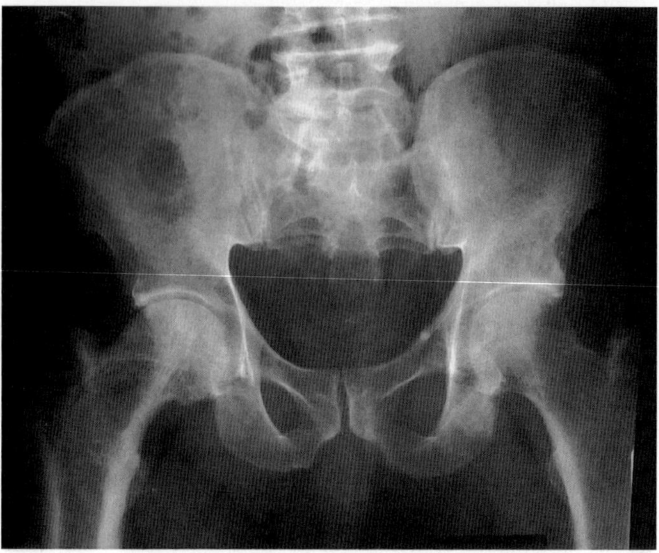

FIGURE 248-1 Radiograph of a 73-year-old man with Paget disease of the right proximal femur. Note the coarsening of the trabecular pattern with marked cortical thickening and narrowing of the joint space consistent with osteoarthritis secondary to pagetic deformity of the right femur. (Reproduced with permission from Fauci AS, Kasper DL, Braunwald E, et al. *Harrison's Principles of Internal Medicine*. 17th ed. © 2008, McGraw-Hill, New York.)

- Weakening of the bones
- Slow progressive enlargement of the bones
- Accelerated bone remodeling

Essentials of Diagnosis[4]

- Phase 1: Osteolytic phase
  - Prominent bone reabsorption and hyper vascularization
- Phase 2: Sclerotic phase
  - Decreased cellular activity and vascularity
- Phase 3: Mixed phased
  - Both active bone reabsorption and bone formation
  - Bones become weakened

General Considerations

- Can be asymptomatic
- Managed with surgery or medicine
- Pathologic fractures
- Can cause paraplegia or stenosis
- Paget disease of the nipple
  - Chronic rash on the nipple

Demographics

- More common with elderly, aging population
- Individuals with absorption issues in the intestines
- Men > women
- Anglo-Saxon descent

CLINICAL FINDINGS

SIGNS AND SYMPTOMS

- Bone growth
- Bone pain
- Bone deformity
- Enlarged head
- Hearing loss
- Headaches
- Joint pain
- Tingling
- Muscle weakness
- Nerve compression
- Joint stiffness
- Genu varus
- Neck pain
- Pathologic fractures
- Osteoarthritis
- Heart failure
- Bone cancer

Functional Implications

- Delayed fracture union
- Hearing problems
- Gait dysfunction

Possible Contributing Causes

- Age (≥50 years)
- Gender (female > male)
- No specific cause
- Several genes maybe related
- Hereditary
- Insufficient calcium and vitamin D

Differential Diagnoses

- Trauma
- Pathologic fracture from neoplasm
- Osteogenesis imperfecta
- Inadequate mineralization of existing bone matrix (osteoid) or poor bone quality
- Osteoporosis
  - Juvenile osteoporosis occurs in children or young adults of both genders with normal gonadal function; onset typically occurs around ages 8 to 14 years and hallmarks include rapid onset of bone pain and/or fracture secondary to trauma.
  - Type I (Postmenopausal osteoporosis) typically occurs in women 50 to 65 years of age and is characterized by accelerated bone loss (trabecular bone).
  - Type II (Age-associated or senile osteoporosis) presents in women and men older than 70 years of age as a result of bone loss associated with the aging process; fractures occur in both cortical and trabecular bone.
- Infections, such as tuberculosis
- Fibrous dysplasia

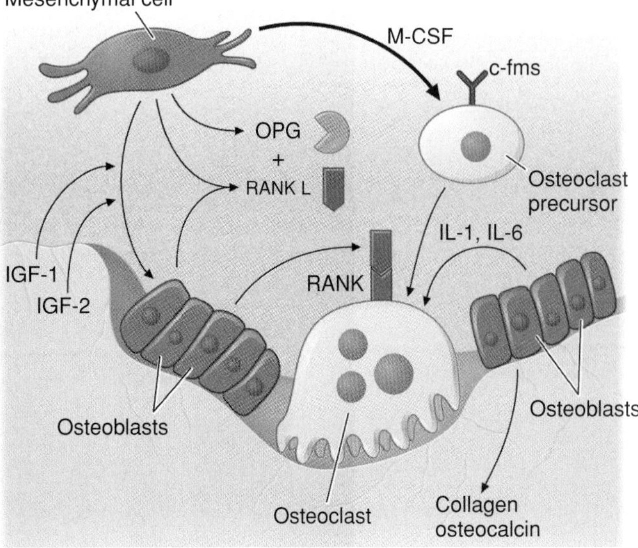

FIGURE 248-2 Diagram illustrating factors that promote differentiation and function of osteoclasts and osteoblasts and the role of the RANK pathway. Stromal bone marrow (mesenchymal) cells and differentiated osteoblasts produce multiple growth factors and cytokines, including macrophage colony-stimulating factor (M-CSF), to modulate osteoclastogenesis. RANKL (receptor activator of NFκB ligand) is produced by osteoblast progenitors and mature osteoblasts and can bind to a soluble decoy receptor known as OPG (osteoprotegerin) to inhibit RANKL action. Alternatively, a cell to cell interaction between osteoblast and osteoclast progenitors allows RANKL to bind to its membrane-bound receptor, RANK, thereby stimulating osteoclast differentiation and function. RANK binds intracellular proteins called TRAFs (tumor necrosis factor receptor-associated factors) that mediate receptor signaling through transcription factors such as NFκB. M-CSF binds to its receptor, c-fms, which is the cellular homologue of the *fms* oncogene. (From Longo DL, Fauci A, Kasper D, Hauser S, Jameson J, Loscalzo J eds. *Harrison's Principles of Internal Medicine.* 18th ed. New York, NY: McGraw-Hill, 2012.)

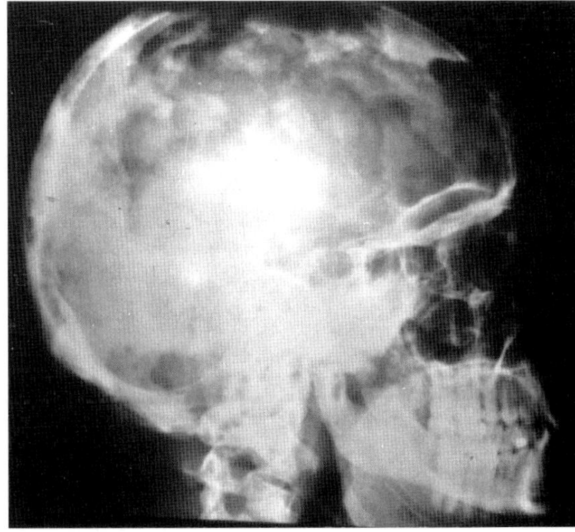

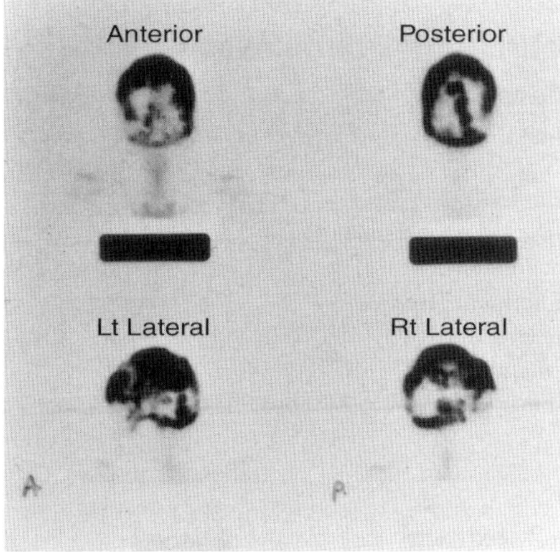

FIGURE 248-3 A 48-year-old woman with Paget disease of the skull. (Left) Lateral radiograph showing areas of both bone resorption and sclerosis. (Right) ^{99m}Tc HDP bone scan with anterior, posterior, and lateral views of the skull showing diffuse isotope uptake by the frontal, parietal, occipital, and petrous bones. (From Longo DL, Fauci A, Kasper D, Hauser S, Jameson J, Loscalzo J eds. Harrison's Principles of Internal Medicine. 18th ed. New York, NY: McGraw-Hill, 2012.)

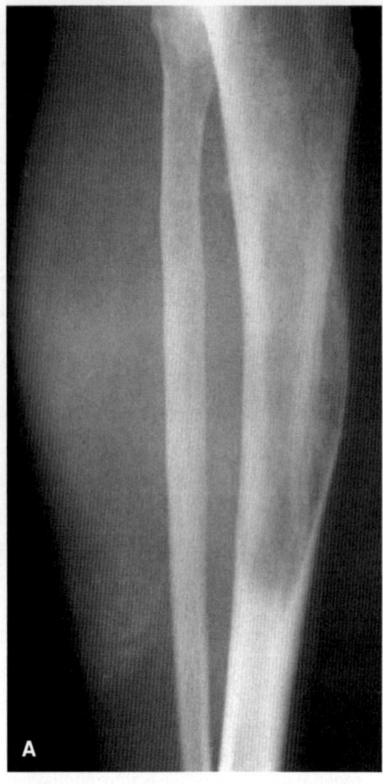

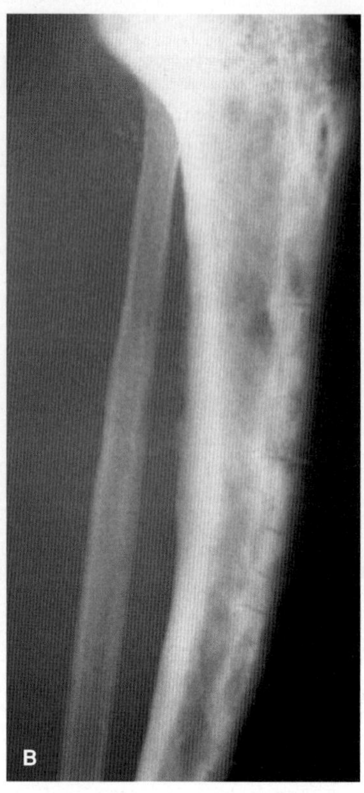

FIGURE 248-4 Early and late radiographs of Paget disease of the tibia, taken when the male patient was 45 years of age (**A**) and when he was 65 years of age (**B**). (From HB Skinner. *Current Diagnosis & Treatment in Orthopedics.* 4th ed. New York, NY: McGraw-Hill, 2007, www.accessmedicine.com.)

- Peripheral neuropathy
- Repetitive stress fractures
- Multiple myeloma, lymphoma, or metastatic cancer
- Leukemia
- Renal osteodystrophy
- Hormone deficiency (estrogen in women; androgen in men)
- Cushing syndrome or glucocorticoid administration
- Hyperthyroidism
- Hyperparathyroidism
- History of drug abuse or misuse (alcohol, tobacco)
- Excessive vitamin D and A

MEANS OF CONFIRMATION OR DIAGNOSIS

▶ Laboratory Tests

- Serum calcium
- ALP
- Blood calcium levels
- 24-hour urine calcium measurement
- Thyroid function test
- Parathyroid hormone levels
- Testosterone level (men)
- 25-hydroxyvitamin D test
- Biochemical markers
- Urine test

▶ Imaging

- Spinal and pelvic X-ray
- Posterior, anterior, and lateral X-rays of affected areas of spine are utilized to identify location and severity of fracture(s)
- Computer assisted tomography (CT)
- Vertebral fracture assessment (VFA)
- Bone scan or radiography
- Diagnostic ultrasound (mobile community-based screening)
- Dual-energy X-ray absorptiometry (DEXA) to diagnose and confirm osteoporosis at both the axial and appendicular skeleton; delivers negligible radiation with a high degree of precision
- Single-energy X-ray (SXA)
- Qualitative/quantitative CT delivers more radiation, but is also accurate in conformation
- Radiographic absorptiometry (RA)

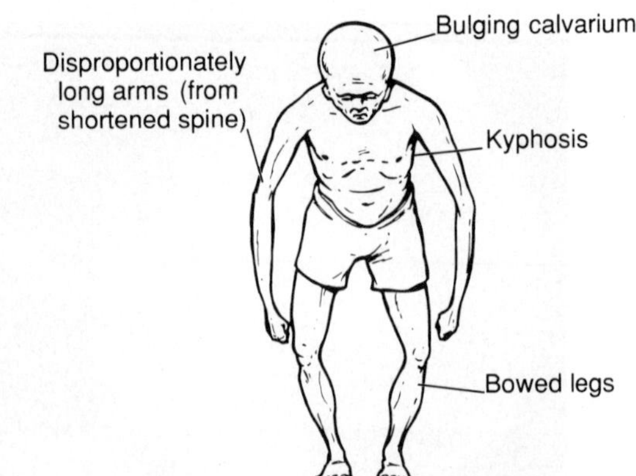

FIGURE 248-5 Bony signs of osteitis deformans (Paget disease of bone). The chief features of Paget disease are the enlarged calvarium (contrasting with the normal-sized face underneath), kyphosis and shortening of the spine, shortening of the spine so the arms look proportionately longer than the trunk, and bowed legs. The figure represents a collection of features, which are unlikely to occur together in the same person. (From LeBlond RF, DeGowin RL, Brown DD. *DeGowin's Diagnostic Examination.* 9th ed. http://www.accessmedicine.com. Copyright © The McGraw-Hill Companies, Inc. All rights reserved.)

Diagnostics Procedure

- Bone biopsy

FINDINGS AND INTERPRETATION

- X-ray may demonstrate demineralization, vertebral compression
- Elevated markers of bone breakdown
- Elevated serum alkaline phosphate
- Improved rates of osteoporosis screenings may help identify persons at increased risk for fracture or low BMD, which enables health care providers to educate the patient on healthy lifestyle changes and preventative strategies to decrease the onset of osteopenia and eventual development osteoporosis

TREATMENT

Medication

- Pain management
  - NSAIDs
  - Narcotics
  - Topical pain relieving agents
  - Nerve blocking injections
- Stimulation of bone formation
  - Bisphosphonates
  - Vitamin D, phosphorus, and calcium supplement
- Reduction of bone resorption
  - Bisphosphonates
  - Estrogens
  - Selective estrogen receptor modulators (SERMs)
  - Calcitonin
  - Calcium
  - Human monoclonal antibody (Denosumab)
  - Thiazide diuretics
  - Anabolic agents (Teriparatide®) if failed bisphosphonate therapy
  - Plicamycin (Mithramycin)

MEDICAL PROCEDURES

- Kyphoplasty
- Vertebroplasty
- Surgical (repair of fracture): Utilized for pain control

REFERRALS/ADMITTANCE

- To endocrinologist
- To general practitioner
- To geriatrician
- To orthopedist for joint assessment
- To rheumatologist
- To pharmacist for bone supplements
- To occupational therapist for ADL training
- To registered dietitian for nutrition education

IMPAIRMENTS

- Physical impairments
  - Chronic or recurrent pain or discomfort
  - Hearing impairment
  - Heart failure
  - Difficulty gripping or holding objects
  - Incomplete use of arms or fingers
  - Incomplete use of feet or legs
  - Disfigurement or deformity
- Activity limitations
  - Self care
  - Mobility
  - Physical transport
  - ADLs
  - Socialization and social activities
  - Work loss or employment restrictions
- Quality of Life (QoL) and Health-Related Quality of Life (HQoL)
- Environment and adjustments
  - Assistive devices
  - Home and occupational modifications
  - Family assistance

TESTS AND MEASURES

- Fall Risk Assessments: FRAS® score (10- year risk assessment)
- Pain, visual analog scale (VAS)
  - 24-hour pain
  - Worst average pain
  - Best average pain
- Functional independence measure
  - Locomotion
- Cardiovascular integrity
  - Blood pressure at rest and after activity
  - Heart rate at rest and after activity
- Neurologic Examination
  - Sensation
    - Light touch
    - Pin prick
  - LE deep tendon reflexes
  - Proprioception at the hip
  - Kinesthetic awareness at the hip
  - Coordination
- Trunk active and passive ROM
- Hip and knee active and passive ROM
- Flexibility testing
  - Hamstrings
  - Iliopsoas
  - Quadriceps
  - Iliotibial band
  - Abductors
  - Adductors
- Limb strength
  - Functional strength testing
    - Five-times-sit-to-stand test
  - Manual muscle test (MMT)
    - Hamstrings
    - Quadriceps
    - Iliopsoas
    - Gluteus maximus
    - Gluteus medius
    - Gluteus minimus
    - Adductors
- LE contralateral limb strength
- Balance
  - Static single-leg standing (eyes open, eyes closed)
    - Contralateral LE
  - Dynamic standing
    - Berg Balance Scale
    - Functional gait assessment

- Gait assessment
    - Observational analysis
    - Gait speed via the 10-m walk test
    - Two-minute walk test
    - Six-minute walk test

INTERVENTION

- Therapeutic exercise
- Progressive weight-bearing exercises (e.g., aquatic therapy)
- Patient education and lifestyle changes
- Transcutaneous electric nerve stimulation (TENS)
- Manual therapy/joint mobilization with precaution of bone density
- Soft-tissue massage
- Orthotics to decrease flexion forces and reduce pain or dysfunction

FUNCTIONAL GOALS

- Prevention of future fractures
- Adequate control of pain
- Prevention of disability
- Improvement strength, flexibility, posture, and balance
- Decrease in risks for falls

PROGNOSIS

- Can be controlled with medication.
- Can develop osteosarcoma.
- Possible need of joint replacement.

PATIENT RESOURCES

- About osteoporosis. International Osteoporosis Foundation website. http://www.iofbonehealth.org/health-professionals/about-osteoporosis.html. Accessed July 7, 2013.
- National Osteoporosis Foundation. *Clinician's Guide to Prevention and Treatment of Osteoporosis.* Washington, DC: National Osteoporosis Foundation; 2010. http://www.nof.org/professionals. Accessed July 7, 2013.
- Osteoporosis Handout on Health (NIH Publication No. 11-5158). NIH Osteoporosis and Related Bone Diseases Resource Center; 2011; Bethesda, MD. http://www.niams.nih.gov/Health_Info/Bone/Osteoporosis/osteoporosis_hoh.asp Accessed July 7, 2013.
- Paget's Disease of Bone. NIH, National Institute of Arthritis and Musculoskeletal and Skin Diseases. http://www.niams.nih.gov/health_info/Pagets/default.asp. Accessed July 7, 2013.

REFERENCES

1. ICD9DATA website. http://www.icd9data.com/2012/Volume1/710-739/730-739/733/733.00.htm. Accessed July 7, 2013.
2. ICD10DATA website. http://www.icd10data.com. Accessed July 7, 2013.
3. Guide to PT Practice. http://guidetoptpractice.apta.org/search?fulltext=osteoporosis&submit=yes&x=0&y=0. Accessed July 7, 2013.
4. Dutton M. Metabolic disease. In: Dutton M, ed. *Orthopaedic Examination, Evaluation, and Intervention.* 2nd ed. New York, NY: McGraw-Hill; 2008. http://www.accessphysiotherapy.com/content/5546939. Accessed July 7, 2013.

ADDITIONAL REFERENCES

- Chandrasoma P, Taylor CR. Metabolic bone disease. In: Chandrasoma P, Taylor CR, eds. *Concise Pathology.* 3rd ed. New York, NY: McGraw-Hill; 2011. http://www.accessphysiotherapy.com/content/193568. Accessed July 7, 2013.
- Jacobs-Kosmin D, Shanmugam S. Osteoporosis. In: Diamond HS, ed. *eMedicine Medscape Reference* website. Published 23 Sep 2011. http://emedicine.medscape.com/article/330598-overview. Accessed July 7, 2013.
- McPhee SJ, Hammer GD. Pathophysiology of selected disorders of calcium metabolism. In: McPhee SJ, Hammer GD, eds. *Pathophysiology of Disease: An Introduction to Clinical Medicine.* 6th ed. New York, NY: McGraw-Hill; 2010. http://www.accessphysiotherapy.com/content/5372181. Accessed July 7, 2013.
- Rahman N, Bhatia K. Impairments and disability associated with arthritis and osteoporosis. Arthritis Series No .4. Cat. no. PHE 90. Canberra: Australian Institute of Health and Welfare (AIHW); 2007 http://www.aihw.gov.au/publication-detail/?id=6442468025. Accessed July 7, 2013.

249 PECTUS EXCAVATUM

Kay Tasso, PhD, PT, PCS

CONDITION/DISORDER SYNONYMS

- Cobbler's chest
- Dent in the chest
- Funnel chest
- Hollowed chest
- Sunken chest

ICD-9-CM CODE[1]

- 754.81 Pectus excavatum

ICD-10-CM CODE[2]

- Q67.6 Pectus excavatum

PREFERRED PRACTICE PATTERN

- 4B: Impaired Posture

PATIENT PRESENTATION

An 18-month-old is referred to physical therapy for developmental delay. Upon examination, the therapist notes the child has hypotonia and pectus excavatum. The mother states she had a viral illness during her first trimester but a normal vaginal delivery. She reports that the orthopedist states no current surgical intervention is necessary for the pectus unless the child's respiratory system becomes compromised as the child ages. The physical therapist plans on treating the gross motor delay with weekly therapeutic activities and strengthening.

KEY FEATURES

Description

- Most common thoracic deformity
- Sternal depression resulting in sunken appearance
- Can cause right sternal rotation resulting in heart to shift to left
- Can cause pain in the back and ribs
- May result in shortening of anterior thoracic muscles and over-lengthening of posterior thoracic muscles

Essentials of Diagnosis

- May be associated with congenital heart disease or murmur due to disrupted blood flow
- Mitral valve prolapse may be present
- Lung capacity can decrease with changed rib cage shape

General Considerations

- Primarily, only of concern for cosmetic or psychological reasons

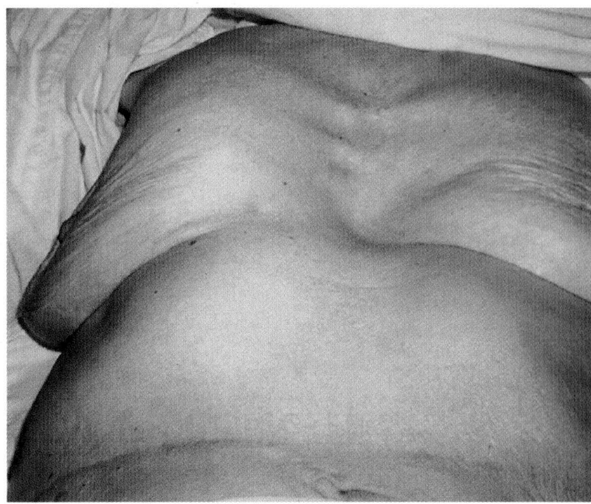

FIGURE 249-1 Marked pectus excavatum. (From Fuster V, Walsh RA, Harrington RA. *Hurst's The Heart*. 13th ed. Copyright © The McGraw-Hill Companies, Inc. All rights reserved.)

- Deformity continues to grow until post-pubescence
- Seen in Marfan syndrome and Ehlers–Danlos syndrome

Demographics

- Males to females, 4:1
- Familial tendency
- Seen at birth or developed at puberty

CLINICAL FINDINGS

SIGNS AND SYMPTOMS

- Present upon clinical observation
- Often asymptomatic
- Cardiovascular limitations[3]
- Adolescents may report fatigue, exercise intolerance, chest or back pain
- Rarely may report dyspnea or palpitations

Functional Implications

- If severe, may result in decreased lung capacity that requires surgical intervention

Possible Contributing Causes

- Celiac disease
- Due to outgrowth of ribs or costal cartilage
- Hypothesized genetic defect
- Marfan syndrome
- Rickets
- Spinal muscular atrophy

Differential Diagnoses

- Scoliosis
- Pectus carinatum
- Kyphoscoliosis

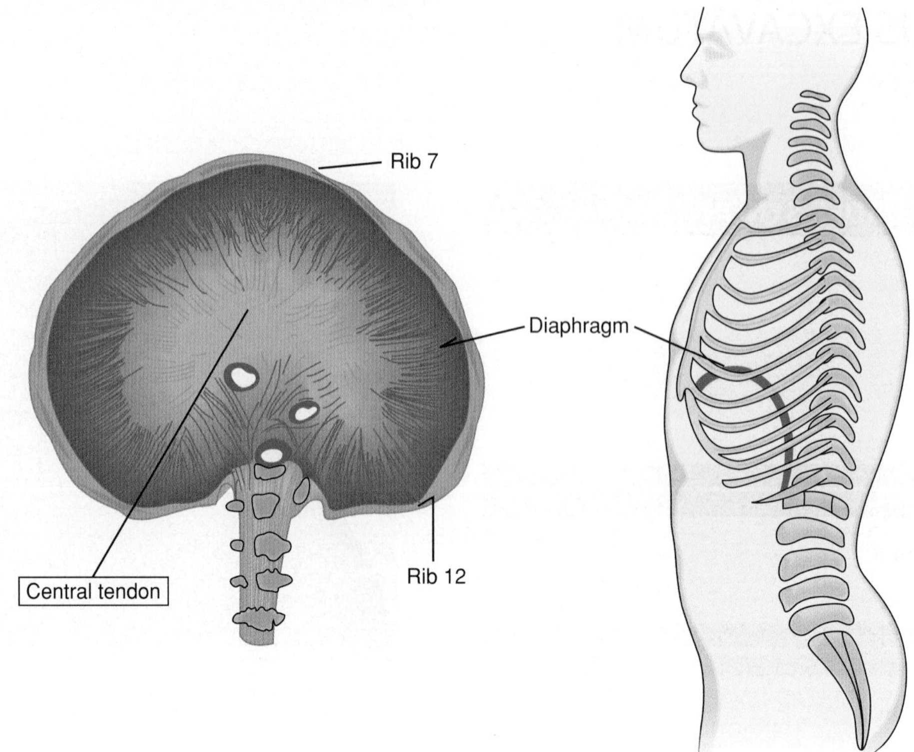

FIGURE 249-2 Transverse and sagittal views of the diaphragm. (From DeTurk WE, Cahalin LP. *Cardiovascular and Pulmonary Physical Therapy: An Evidence-Based Approach.* 2nd ed. http://www.accessphysiotherapy.com. Copyright © The McGraw-Hill Companies, Inc. All rights reserved.)

MEANS OF CONFIRMATION OR DIAGNOSIS

Imaging

- X-ray
- Auscultation
- Haller index
- Pulmonary function test

FINDINGS AND INTERPRETATION

- X-ray and auscultation to confirm severity of deformity or shifting of heart

REFERRALS/ADMITTANCE

- To orthopedic surgeon to determine if surgical intervention warranted

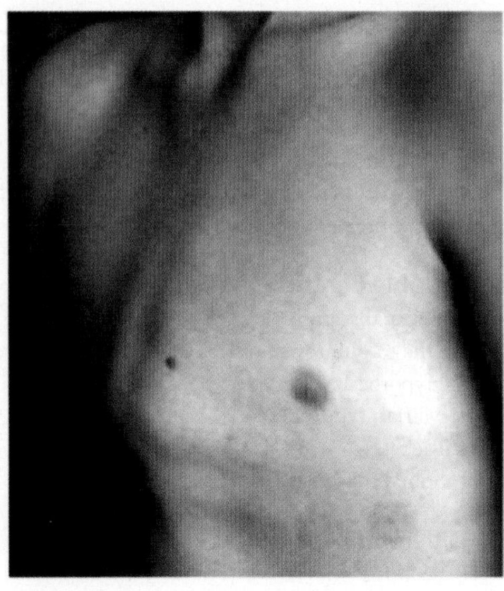

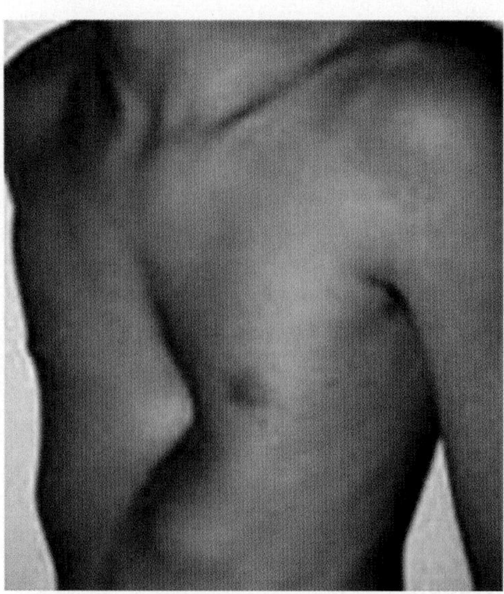

FIGURE 249-3 Pectus carinatum (left) and pectus excavatum. (From Patel DR, Greydanus DE, Baker RJ. *Pediatric Practice: Sports Medicine.* www.accesspediatrics.com. Copyright © The McGraw-Hill Companies, Inc. All rights reserved.)

IMPAIRMENTS

- Exercise intolerance
- Respiratory[3]
- Flexibility
- Strength
- Circulatory
- May result in shortening of anterior thoracic muscles and over-lengthening of posterior thoracic muscles

TESTS AND MEASURES

- Diaphragm and ribcage mobility
- Posture
- Respiration

INTERVENTION

- Surgical if needed
- Postural training and strengthening
- Myofascial release

FUNCTIONAL GOALS

- The patient will be able to
  - Ambulate 75 minutes with rolling walker and standby assistance in 3 days to improve mobility.
  - Regain thoracic mobility to allow for rib expansion during inspiration.

PROGNOSIS

- Excellent, since seldomly requires surgical intervention.

PATIENT RESOURCE

- Pectus Exacavatum. APSA's Complete Parent & Family Resource Center from The American Pediatric Surgical Association. http://www.pediatricsurgerymd.org/AM/Template.cfm?Section=Resources_for_Parents&CONTENTID=1607&TEMPLATE=/CM/ContentDisplay.cfm. Accessed July 7, 2013.

REFERENCES

1. ICD9DATA Website. http://www.icd9data.com/2011/Volume1/740-759/754/754.81.htm. Accessed July 7, 2013.
2. ICD10DATA Website. http://www.icd10data.com/ICD10CM/Codes/Q00-Q99/Q65-Q79/Q67-/Q67.6. Accessed July 7, 2013.
3. Jayaramakrishnan K, Wotton R, Bradley A, Naidu B. Does repair of pectus excavatum improve cardiopulmonary function? *Interact Cardiovasc Thorac Surg*. 2013;16(6):865–870. doi: 10.1093/icvts/ivt045. Epub 2013 Feb 28.

ADDITIONAL REFERENCES

- DeTurk WE, Cahalin LP. Cardiopulmonary concerns in the patient with musculoskeletal and integumentary deficits: an evidence-based approach. In: DeTurk WE, Cahalin LP, eds. *Cardiovascular and Pulmonary Physical Therapy: An Evidence-Based Approach*. 2nd ed. New York, NY: McGraw-Hill; 2011. http://www.accessphysiotherapy.com/content/6879247. Accessed July 7, 2013.
- Dutton M. The thoracic spine and rib cage. In: Dutton M, ed. *Orthopaedic Examination, Evaluation, and Intervention*. 2nd ed. New York, NY: McGraw-Hill; 2008. http://www.accessphysiotherapy.com/content/55594202. Accessed July 7, 2013.
- *Guide to Physical Therapist Practice, APTA*. Alexandria, VA. 2003. http://guidetoptpractice.apta.org./ Accessed July 7, 2013.
- Hay WW, Levin MJ, Sondheimer JM, Deterding RR. Respiratory tract & mediastinum. In: Hay WW, Levin MJ, Sondheimer JM, Deterding RR, eds. *CURRENT Diagnosis & Treatment: Pediatrics*. 20th ed. New York, NY: McGraw-Hill; 2011. http://www.accessphysiotherapy.com/content/6582660. Accessed July 7, 2013.
- Hay WW, Levin MJ, Sondheimer JM, Deterding RR. Mendelian Disorders. In: Hay WW, Levin MJ, Sondheimer JM, Deterding RR, eds. *CURRENT Diagnosis & Treatment: Pediatrics*. 20th ed. New York, NY: McGraw-Hill; 2011. http://www.accessphysiotherapy.com/content/6589079. Accessed July 7, 2013.
- Homnick DN. Chest and pulmonary conditions. In: Patel DR, Greydanus DE, Baker RJ, eds. *Pediatric Practice: Sports Medicine*. New York, NY: McGraw-Hill; 2009. http://www.accessphysiotherapy.com/content/6974862. Accessed July 7, 2013.

250 PIERRE ROBIN SEQUENCE

Kay Tasso, PhD, PT, PCS

CONDITION/DISORDER SYNONYMS

- Cleft Palate, Micrognathia, and Glossoptosis
- Pierre Robin syndrome
- Pierre Robin Malformation Sequence
- Pierre Robin complex
- Pierre Robin anomaly
- Pierre Robin triad
- Robin Anomalad

ICD-9-CM CODE

- 756.0 Anomalies of skull and face bones[1]

ICD-10-CM CODE

- Q87.0 Congenital malformation syndromes predominantly affecting facial appearance[2]

PREFERRED PRACTICE PATTERN

- 5B: Impaired Neuromotor Development

PATIENT PRESENTATION

A 3-month-old infant is referred to physical therapy for hypotonia. The infant was recently diagnosed by the geneticist with Pierre Robin syndrome. His mother reports no difficulty with the pregnancy or delivery. The infant has a history of difficulty feeding due to micrognathia. Upon examination, the therapist notes the infant has poor head control and is unable to achieve prone-on-elbows. The infant is enrolled in an early intervention program and receives physical therapy to assist with gross motor skill acquisition. Therapy is also provided to assist with difficulty feeding.

KEY FEATURES

Description

- Group of congenital malformations usually a triad combination
  - Cleft palate (92%)[3]
  - Micrognathia
    - Small lower jaw
  - Glossoptosis (70%–85%)[3] at birth
    - Tongue tends to fall back toward the throat

Essentials of Diagnosis

- May have failure to thrive or severe respiratory distress[3]

General Considerations

- Present as emergencies in the newborn period because of airway restriction
- May have clubfeet or hearing loss (60%)[3]

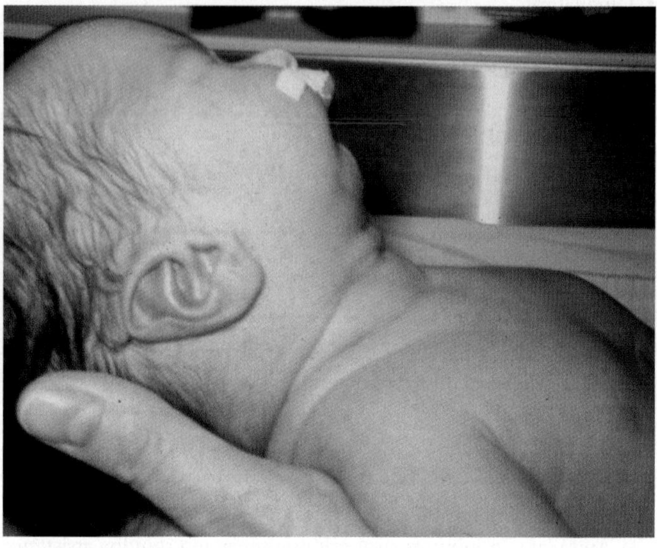

FIGURE 250-1 Pierre Robin syndrome: Hypoplastic mandible associated with a ventricular septal defect. (From Fuster V, Walsh RA, Harrington RA. *Hurst's The Heart*. 13th ed. Copyright © The McGraw-Hill Companies, Inc. All rights reserved.)

- CNS defects (50%)[3]
  - Developmental delay
  - Hypotonia
  - Hydrocephalus
- Infants with Pierre Robin syndrome may have Strickler syndrome and Velocardiofascial syndrome
- Congenital heart disease in 15%[4]

Demographics

- Affects males and females equally unless X-linked[3]
- 1 in 8500 births[5]

CLINICAL FINDINGS

SIGNS AND SYMPTOMS

- Breathing problems
- Cleft soft palate
- Ear infections
- High arched palate
- Large tongue[6]
- Natal teeth
- Small, retracted lower jaw

Functional Implications

- Frequent ear infections[5]
- Difficulty feeding
- Decreased hearing
- Delayed speech

Possible Contributing Causes

- Unknown
- May be a result of positioning of the fetus at the beginning of pregnancy
- May be autosomal recessive[3]

▶ **Differential Diagnosis**[3]
- Stickler syndrome
- Trisomy 11q
- Trisomy 18
- Möbius syndrome
- CHARGE syndrome

MEANS OF CONFIRMATION OR DIAGNOSIS

▶ **Laboratory Tests**
- Genetic testing
- DNA methylation analysis to assess genetic link

▶ **Imaging**
- Radiography to assess craniofacial anatomy

FINDINGS AND INTERPRETATION

- Organ anomalies

TREATMENT

▶ **Medical Procedures**
- Surgery to repair the cleft palate

REFERRALS/ADMITTANCE

- Admittance or continued hospitalization after birth for surgical repair, tracheostomy, gastrostomy, or tympanostomy tubes[3]
- To otolaryngologist
- To geneticist
- To audiologist
- To occupational therapist
- To speech therapist

IMPAIRMENTS

- Inability to achieve or sustain prone-on-elbows
- Inability to roll
- Inability to sit
- Nonambulatory

TESTS AND MEASURES

- Alberta Infant Motor Scale
- Bayley Scales of Motor Development or Bayley II
- Early Intervention Developmental Profile
- Movement Assessment of Infants
- Neonatal Behavioral Assessment Scale
- Peabody Scales of Motor Development
- Test of Infant Motor Performance

INTERVENTION

- Prevent asphyxia until the mandible becomes large enough to accommodate the tongue[7]
- Supine positioning contraindicated until jaw grows or until surgical repair[6]
- Prone positioning is preferred for infants[3, 6]
- Therapeutic exercise
  - Strengthening
  - Stretching
- Functional activities
  - Transfers
  - Gait training
  - Stair climbing

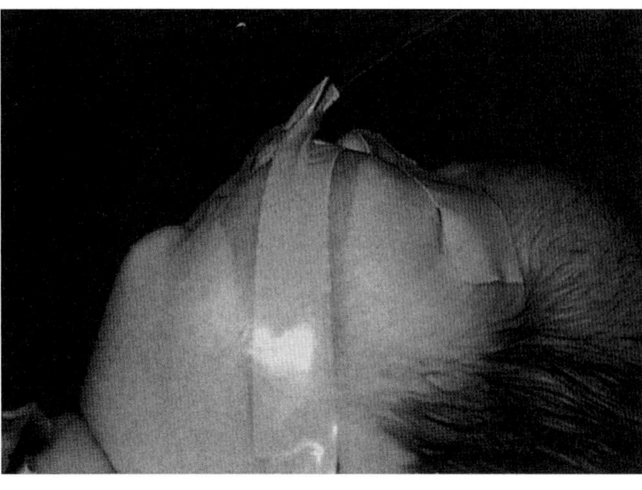

FIGURE 250-2 Pierre Robin sequence. Note the extremely retruded chin in this child, who is being prepared for surgical tongue-lip adhesion. (From Lalwani AK. *Current Diagnosis & Treatment in Otolaryngology-Head & Neck Surgery.* 3rd ed. www.accesssurgery.com. Copyright © The McGraw-Hill Companies, Inc. All rights reserved.)

- Neurodevelopmental treatment
  - Inhibition of spasticity
  - Facilitation of normal movement patterns
  - Acquisition of motor milestones

FUNCTIONAL GOALS

- The patient will be able to
  - Sustains prone-on-elbows for 2 minutes within 3 months.
  - Rolls prone-to-supine with minimal assistance within 4 months.
  - Ring sits for 30 to 60 seconds when placed within 6 months.
  - Ambulates independently ×5 minutes within 5 months.

PROGNOSIS

- No impact on life expectancy documented.

PATIENT RESOURCES

- Pierre Robin Network. www.pierrerobin.org. Accessed July 4, 2013.
- The Cleft Palate Foundation (CPF). www.cleftline.org. Accessed July 4, 2013.

REFERENCES

1. ICD9Data.com. http://www.icd9data.com. Accessed July 4, 2013.
2. ICD10Data.com. http://www.icd10data.com. Accessed July 4, 2013.
3. Pierre Robin Syndrome. Medscape. http://emedicine.medscape.com/article/844143-overview#aw2aab6b3. Accessed July 4, 2013.
4. Tsai AC, Manchester DK, Elias ER. Genetics & Dysmorphology. In: Hay WW, Levin MJ, Sondheimer JM, Deterding RR, eds. *CURRENT Diagnosis & Treatment: Pediatrics*. 20th ed. New York, NY: McGraw-Hill; 2011. http://www.accessphysiotherapy.com/content/6589204. Accessed July 4, 2013.
5. Pierre Robin Sequence. Cleft Palate Foundation. http://www.cleftline.org/what-we-do/publications/fact-sheets/pierre-robin-sequence. Accessed July 4, 2013.

6. Pierre Robin Syndrome. PubMed Health. U.S. National Library of Medicine. http://www.ncbi.nlm.nih.gov/pubmedhealth/PMH0002574. Accessed July 4, 2013.
7. Yoon PJ, Kelley PE, Friedman NR. The throat and oral cavity. In: Hay WW, Levin MJ, Sondheimer JM, Deterding RR, eds. *CURRENT Diagnosis & Treatment: Pediatrics*. 20th ed. New York, NY: McGraw-Hill; 2011. http://www.accessphysiotherapy.com/content/6582052. Accessed July 4, 2013.

ADDITIONAL REFERENCES

- Denny A, Amm C. New technique for airway correction in neonates with severe Pierre Robin sequence. *J Pediatr*. 2005;147(1): 97–101.
- Developmental Profile III. Children and Adolescents with Special Needs. http://portal.wpspublish.com/portal/page?_pageid=53,186601&_dad=portal&_schema=PORTAL. Accessed July 4, 2013.
- Dutton M. Pediatric physical therapy. In: *McGraw Hill's NPTE (National Physical Therapy Examination)*. 2nd ed. New York, NY: McGraw-Hill; 2012. http://www.accessphysiotherapy.com/content/5404405#5404405. Accessed July 4, 2013.
- *Guide to Physical Therapist Practice*. Alexandria, VA: APTA; 2003. http://guidetoptpractice.apta.org. Accessed July 4, 2013.
- The Neonatal Behavioral Assessment Scale. The Brazelton Institute. http://www.brazelton-institute.com/intro.html. Accessed July 4, 2013.
- The Test of Infant Motor Performance and the Harris Infant Neuromotor Test. Infant Motor Performance Scales. http://thetimp.com. Accessed July 4, 2013.

251 PRADER–WILLI SYNDROME

Kay Tasso, PhD, PT, PCS

CONDITION/DISORDER SYNONYM

- Prader-Willi Syndrome (PWS)

ICD-9-CM CODE

- 759.81 Prader–Willi syndrome[1]

ICD-10-CM CODE

- Q87.1 Congenital malformation syndromes predominantly associated with short stature[2]

PREFERRED PRACTICE PATTERN

- 5C: Impaired Motor Function and Sensory Integrity Associated with Nonprogressive Disorders of the Central Nervous System—Congenital Origin or Acquired in Infancy or Childhood

PATIENT PRESENTATION

A 3-month-old infant is referred to physical therapy for examination due to hypotonia. The infant is diagnosed with failure to thrive and difficulty feeding resulting in placement of a gastrostomy tube (G-tube) to assist with weight gain and growth. The mother reports no difficulty with pregnancy and delivery. Upon examination, the infant has poor head control and is unable to achieve prone-on-elbows. After several months, the infant is referred to a geneticist and ultimately, the infant is diagnosed with Prader–Willi syndrome. The infant receives physical therapy through an early intervention program and continues to exhibit developmental delay.

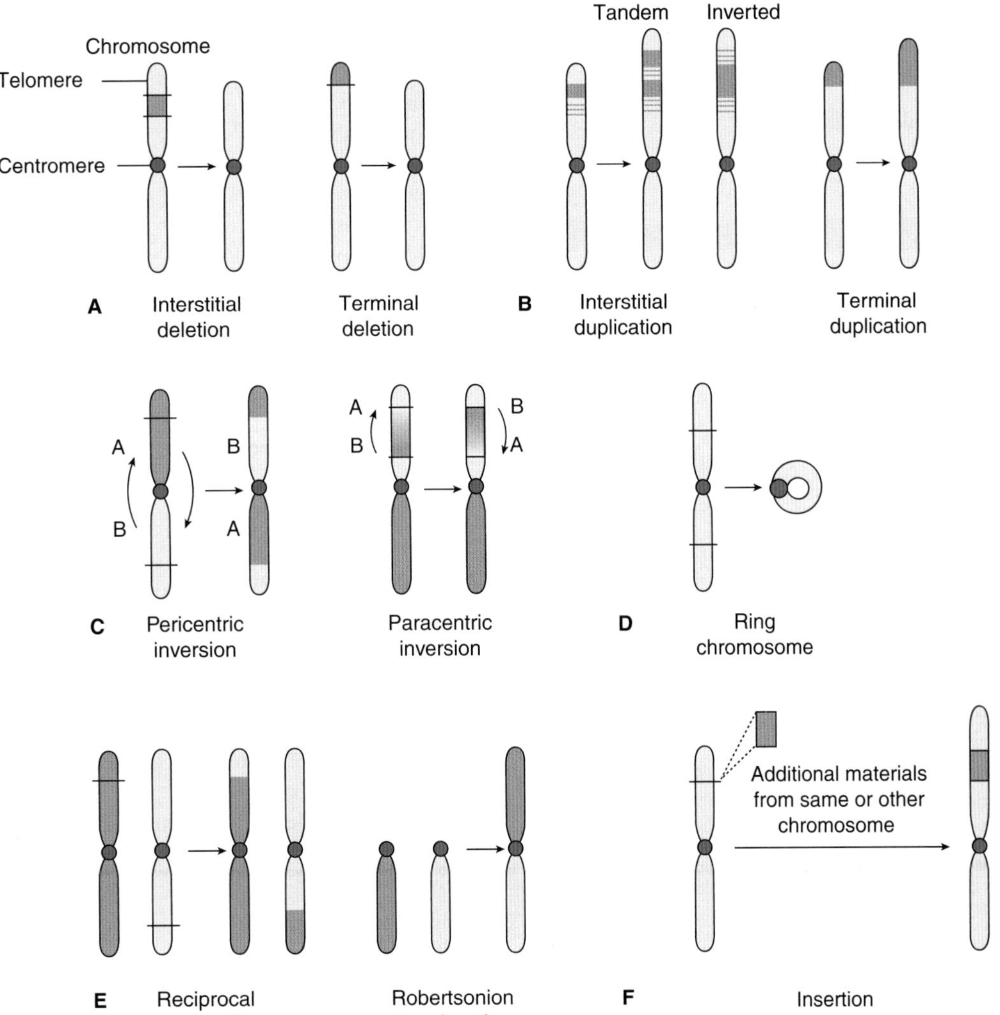

FIGURE 251-1 Examples of structural chromosomal abnormalities: (**A**) Deletion, (**B**) duplication, (**C**) inversion, (**D**) ring chromosome, (**E**) translocation, and (**F**) insertion. (From Hay WW Jr, Levin MJ, Deterding RR, Abzug MJ, Sondheimer JM. *Current Diagnosis & Treatment: Pediatrics.* 21st ed. www.accessmedicine.com. Copyright © The McGraw-Hill Companies, Inc. All rights reserved.)

KEY FEATURES

Description
- Lack of impression from several imprinted genes[3]
- Genetic disorder characterized by
  - Specific facial features such as almond-shaped eyes
  - Hypotonia
  - Hypogonadism
  - Strabismus[4]
  - Short stature
  - Cognitive deficits
  - Inability to regulate appetite
  - Males with undescended testicles[5]
  - Small hands and feet[4,5]

Essentials of Diagnosis
- Two stages[3,6]
  - Stage 1 occurs during infancy with hypotonia and poor suck/swallow reflex that may result in failure to thrive
  - Stage 2 generally begins at about 2 years of age with lack of satiety progressing to obesity

General Considerations
- Growth hormone deficiency[4]
- Often develop complications from obesity and osteoporosis with age[7]

Demographics
- 1 in 15,000[6]
- Affects females and males equally

CLINICAL FINDINGS

SIGNS AND SYMPTOMS
- Poor suck/swallow at birth
- Hypotonia in infancy
- Specific facial features such as almond-shaped eyes
- Hypogonadism
- Strabismus[4]
- Short stature
- Obesity
- Cognitive deficits
- Inability to regulate appetite
- Hypogenitalism/Males with undescended testicles[5]
- Small hands and feet[4,5]
- Developmental delay

Possible Contributing Causes
- Deletion in portion of chromosome 15q11[4]
- Possibly due to dysfunction of hypothalamus[6]

Functional Implications
- May require gastrostomy tube[4]
- Cognitive impairment
- Learning disabilities
- Poor speech articulation
- Behavioral problems[8]
- Obsessive–compulsive disorder[8]
- Scoliosis[8]

Differential Diagnosis[7]
- Obsessive–compulsive disorder
- Failure to thrive
- Fragile X syndrome
- Growth hormone disorder

MEANS OF CONFIRMATION OR DIAGNOSIS

Laboratory Tests
- DNA methylation analysis[6,4]
- Magnetic resonance imaging (MRI) to assess pituitary gland[7]

Imaging
- Fluorescence in situ hybridization (FISH)
- Chromosomal Microarray Analysis (CMA)
- Standard radiograph to screen for scoliosis

FINDINGS AND INTERPRETATION
- Deletion in portion of chromosome 15q11 detected by FISH or microarray[3]

TREATMENT

Medication
- Human growth hormones[7]
  - Saizen
  - Genotropin
  - Humatrope
  - Nutropin
  - Serostim

REFERRALS/ADMITTANCE
- Orthopedist for possible scoliosis
- Endocrinologist
- Geneticist
- Nutritionist
- Ophthalmologist
- Gastroenterologist
- Psychiatrist
- Occupational therapist
- Speech therapist

IMPAIRMENTS
- Poor head control
- Poor trunk control
- Inability to sit independently

TESTS AND MEASURES
- 6-minute walk test
- Alberta Infant Motor Scale
- Bayley Scales of Motor Development or Bayley II
- Bruininks–Oseretsky Test of Motor Proficiency
- Early Intervention Developmental Profile
- Movement Assessment of Infants
- Neonatal Behavioral Assessment Scale
- Peabody Scales of Motor Development
- Skin fold analysis
- Test of Infant Motor Performance

INTERVENTION
- Behavior modification
- Developmental activities
  - Acquisition of motor milestones through facilitation
- Therapeutic exercise
  - Strengthening
  - Aerobics

FUNCTIONAL GOALS

- The patient will be able to
  - Sustain prone-on-elbows for 2 minutes when placed while playing within 2 months.
  - Sit independently for 30 to 60 seconds with standby assistance in 1 month.
  - Stand at furniture with contact guard assistance for 5 minutes while playing.
  - Ambulate 10 minutes with two hands held within 6 months.
  - Ride stationary bike 30 minutes to increase aerobic function within 6 weeks.

PROGNOSIS

- No impact on life expectancy documented.

PATIENT RESOURCE

- Prader–Willi Association. http://www.pwsausa.org. Accessed August 17, 2014.

REFERENCES

1. ICD9DATA Web Site. http://www.icd9data.com/2012/Volume1/740-759/759/759.81.htm. Accessed July 6, 2013.
2. ICD10DATA Web Site. http://www.icd10data.com/ICD10CM/Codes/Q00-Q99/Q80-Q89/Q87-/Q87.1. Accessed July 6, 2013.
3. APTA. *Guide to Physical Therapy Practice*. Alexandria, VA: American Physical Therapy Association; 2003. http://guidetoptpractice.apta.org. Accessed July 6, 2013.
4. Prader-Willi syndrome. PubMed Health web site. http://www.ncbi.nlm.nih.gov/pubmedhealth/PMH0002572. Accessed July 6, 2013.
5. Foundation for Prader-Willi Research Web Site. http://www.fpwr.org/about-prader-willi-syndrome. Accessed July 6, 2013.
6. Hay WW, Levin MJ, Sondheimer JM, Deterding RR. Disorders of Imprinting. In: Hay WW, Levin MJ, Sondheimer JM, Deterding RR, eds. *CURRENT Diagnosis & Treatment: Pediatrics*. 20th ed. New York, NY: McGraw-Hill; 2011. http://www.accessphysiotherapy.com/content/6589169. Accessed July 6, 2013.
7. Prader-Willi syndrome. Mayo Clinic web site. http://www.mayoclinic.com/health/prader-willi-syndrome/DS00922/DSECTION=symptoms. Accessed July 6, 2013.
8. Prader-Willi syndrome. Medscape web site. http://emedicine.medscape.com/article/947954-overview. Accessed July 6, 2013.

ADDITIONAL REFERENCES

- Developmental Profile III. Children and Adolescents with Special Needs. http://portal.wpspublish.com/portal/page?_pageid=53,186601&_dad=portal&_schema=PORTAL. Accessed August 17, 2014.
- Dutton M. Pediatric physical therapy. In: *McGraw Hill's National Physical Therapy Examination,2e*. New York, NY: McGraw-Hill; 2012. http://www.accessphysiotherapy.com/content/5404405#5404405. Accessed August 17, 2014.
- The Neonatal Behavioral Assessment Scale. The Brazelton Institute web site. http://www.brazelton-institute.com/intro.html. Accessed August 17, 2014.
- The Test of Infant Motor Performance. Infant Motor Performance Scales web site. http://thetimp.com. Accessed August 17, 2014.

252 RETT SYNDROME

Kay Tasso, PhD, PT, PCS

CONDITION/DISORDER SYNONYM

- Rett syndrome (RS)

ICD-9-CM CODE[1]

- 299 Pervasive developmental disorders

ICD-10-CM CODE[2]

- F84.2 Rett syndrome

PREFERRED PRACTICE PATTERN

- 5E Impaired Motor Function and Sensory Integrity Associated With Progressive Disorders of the Central Nervous System[3]

PATIENT PRESENTATION

A 2-year-old female child is referred to physical therapy for developmental delay. The mother reports an uneventful pregnancy and delivery. Upon examination, the therapist notes the child is hypotonic, "crawls" on her knees as her primary method of mobility, and sits independently but does not take weight on her legs when

TABLE 252-1 Types of Severe Mental Retardation

I. Dysmorphic defect with somatic developmental abnormalities in non-nervous structures
   A. Those affecting cranioskeletal structures
      1. Microcephaly
      2. Macrocephaly
      3. Hydrocephalus (including myelomeningocele with Chiari malformation and associated cerebral anomalies)
      4. Down syndrome
      5. Cretinism (congenital hypothyroidism)
      6. Mucopolysaccharidoses (Hurler, Hunter, and Sanfilippo types)
      7. Acrocephalosyndactyly (craniostenosis) and other craniosomatic abnormalities
      8. Arthrogryposis multiplex congenita (in certain cases)
      9. Rare specific syndromes: De Lange
      10. Dwarfism, short stature: Russel-Silver dwarf, Seckel bird-headed dwarf, Rubinstein-Taybi dwarf, Cockayne-Neel dwarf, etc.
      11. Hypertelorism, median cleft face syndromes, agenesis of corpus callosum
   B. Those affecting nonskeletal structures
      1. Neurocutaneous syndromes: tuberous sclerosis, Sturge–Weber, neurofibromatosis
      2. Congenital rubella syndrome (deafness, blindness, congenital heart disease, small stature)
      3. Chromosomal disorders: Down syndrome, some cases of Klinefelter syndrome (XXY), XYY, Turner (XO) syndrome (occasionally), and others
      4. Laurence-Moon-Biedl syndrome (retinitis pigmentosa, obesity, polydactyly)
      5. Eye disorders: toxoplasmosis (chorioretinitis), galactosemia (cataract), congenital rubella
      6. Prader–Willi syndrome (obesity, hypogenitalism)

II. Nondysmorphic mental defect without somatic anomalies but with cerebral and other neurologic abnormalities
   A. Cerebral spastic diplegia
   B. Cerebral hemiplegia, unilateral or bilateral
   C. Congenital choreoathetosis or ataxia
      1. Kernicterus
      2. Status marmoratus
   D. Congenital ataxia
   E. Congenital atonic diplegia
   F. Syndromes resulting from hypoglycemia, trauma, meningitis, and encephalitis
   G. Associated with other neuromuscular abnormalities (muscular dystrophy, cerebellar ataxia, etc.)
   H. Cerebral degenerative diseases (lipidoses)
   I. Associated with inborn errors of metabolism (phenylketonuria, other aminoacidurias, organic acidurias, Lesch–Nyhan syndrome)
   J. Congenital infections (some cases of congenital syphilis, cytomegalic inclusion disease)

III. Genetic mental defect with minor or no signs of somatic abnormality or neurologic disorder
   A. Infantile autism, Renpenning, Williams, fragile X, Partington, and Rett syndromes

Source: Ropper AH, Samuels MA. *Adams & Victor's Principles of Neurology*. 9th ed. New York, NY: McGraw-Hill; 2009.

held in standing. She is nonverbal with very few vocalizations and almost constantly wrings her hands at midline. Her mother reports the child has an appointment with geneticist in a few weeks.

KEY FEATURES

Description

- Mutation in the X chromosome gene encoding methyl-CpG-binding protein
- Progressive genetic disorder characterized by
  - Regression of motor skills
  - Wringing of hands
  - Dystonia
  - Hypotonia
  - Bruxism
  - Ataxic gait[4]

Essentials of Diagnosis

- Four stages[5,6]
  - Stage 1: Developmental arrest (6–18 months): lack of eye contact, head growth slows, hypotonia, development plateaus, hand wringing, breath holding
  - Stage 2: Rapid regression (1–4 years old): wringing of hands, no expressive speech, seizures, developmental decline, sleep disorder, strabismus
  - Stage 3: "Pseudostationary period" (2–10 years old): ataxia, rigidity, bruxism, good eye contact, oral motor dysfunction
  - Stage 4: "Late motor deterioration and growth retardation" (over 10 years old): parkinsonism (drooling, bradykinesia,) hypertonia, dystonia, arrest in cognitive decline

General Considerations

- Associated disorders
  - Early onset seizures (60%–90%)[6]
  - Lack of speech
  - Repetitive behaviors
  - Gastrointestinal disorders
  - Swallowing disorders
  - Sleeping during day
  - Sudden death
  - Unusual breathing pattern[5]

Demographics

- Primarily young girls[4]
- 1 in 10,000 to 20,000[5]

CLINICAL FINDINGS

SIGNS AND SYMPTOMS

- Plateau or regression in motor skills
- Wringing of hands
- Delays in
  - Gross motor skills
  - Oral motor skills[7]
  - Speech and/or language skills[7]
- Bruxism[4]
- Ataxia[8]
- Spasticity[8] (late sign)
- Kyphoscoliosis (8–11 year olds)[6,8]
- Foot deformities[8] (late sign)

Possible Contributing Causes

- Genetic mutation of Xq28[5]

TABLE 252-2 Causes of Severe and Mild Mental Retardation in 1,372 Patients at the W.E. Fernald State School in the 1970s

Disease Category	Number of Patients IQ < 50	Number of Patients IQ > 50	% of All Patients
Acquired destructive lesions	278	79	26.0
Chromosomal abnormalities	247	10	18.7
Multiple congenital anomalies	64	16	5.8
Developmental abnormality of brain	49	16	4.7
Metabolic and endocrine diseases	38	5	3.1
Progressive degenerative disease	5	7	0.9
Neurocutaneous diseases	4	0	0.3
Psychosis	7	6	1.0
Cause unknown	385	156	39.5

Source: Ropper AH, Samuels MA. *Adams & Victor's Principles of Neurology.* 9th ed. New York, NY:McGraw-Hill; 2009.

Functional Implications

- Hypotonia
- Poor head control as infant
- Lack of functional hand use
- Inability to communicate
- Unable to follow directions
- Inability to ambulate

Differential Diagnosis

- Autism
- Infantile spasms
- Angelman syndrome[5]

MEANS OF CONFIRMATION OR DIAGNOSIS

Laboratory Tests

- DNA analysis
- Abnormal metabolites in cerebrospinal fluid[4]

Imaging

- Barium swallow[6]

FINDINGS

- Abnormal levels of 5-hydroxyindoleatic acid and catecholamine metabolites are found in the cerebrospinal fluid[4]

TREATMENT

Medication

- Naltrexone for breathing difficulties
- Bromocriptine
- Carnitine
- Lamotrigine
- Carbamazepine
- Valproic acid

MEDICAL PROCEDURES

- Echocardiogram for cardiac defects
- Electroencephalogram for seizures

REFERRALS/ADMITTANCE

- To geneticist
- To neurologist
- To orthopedist for possible scoliosis
- To occupational therapy
- To speech therapy

IMPAIRMENTS

- Decreased strength
- Inability to ambulate
- Difficulty with transfers
- Lack of functional hand use
- Dependent for activities of daily living

TESTS AND MEASURES

- Alberta Infant Motor Scale
- Bayley Scales of motor development or Bayley II
- Early Intervention Developmental Profile
- Movement Assessment of Infants
- Neonatal Behavioral Assessment Scale
- Peabody Scales of Motor Development
- Test of Infant Motor Performance

INTERVENTION

- Developmental activities
  - Acquisition of motor milestones through facilitation
- Therapeutic exercise
  - Strengthening
- Neurodevelopmental treatment
  - Inhibition of spasticity

FUNCTIONAL GOALS

Note: In general, the goal of PT is to retain functional skills and assist child with achieving maximal motor skills.

- The patient will be able to
  - Rock on hands and knees with minimal assistance within 3 months.
  - Stand at furniture for 5 minutes with minimal assistance within 2 months.
  - Cruise along furniture with moderate assistance within 6 months
  - Ambulate 5 feet with moderate assistance within 4 months.
  - Transfer from sitting in child sized chair to standing with hands held within 3 months.

PROGNOSIS

- Average life expectancy varies by reference from 24 years old[6] to 50 years old[7] to 60 or 80 years old.[6]

PATIENT RESOURCE

- Rett syndrome clinical presentation. Medscape web site. Bernstein BE, Pataki C. http://emedicine.medscape.com/article/916377-clinical. Accessed July 7, 2013.

REFERENCES

1. ICD9DATA. http://www.icd9data.com. Accessed July 7, 2013.
2. ICD10DATA. http://www.icd10data.com. Accessed July 7, 2013.
3. *Guide to Physical Therapist Practice*. Alexandria, VA: APTA; 2003. http://guidetoptpractice.apta.org. Accessed July 7, 2013.
4. Watts RL, Standaert D, Obeso JA. Symptomatic dystonias. In: Watts RL, Standaert D, Obeso JA, eds. *Movement Disorders*. 3rd ed. New York, NY: McGraw-Hill; 2012:Chapter 31. http://www.accessphysiotherapy.com/content/55799679. Accessed July 7, 2013.
5. Watts RL, Standaert D, Obeso JA. Rare degenerative syndromes associated with parkinsonism. In: Watts RL, Standaert D, Obeso JA, eds. *Movement Disorders*. 3rd ed. New York, NY: McGraw-Hill; 2012:Chapter 24. http://www.accessphysiotherapy.com/content/55797724. Accessed July 7, 2013.
6. Motor disabilities in Rett syndrome and physical therapy strategies in Brain Development. 1990;12(1):157–161. http://www.sciencedirect.com/science/article/pii/S0387760412802014. Accessed July 7, 2013.
7. Regaining walking ability in individuals with Rett syndrome: a case study. *International Journal on Disability and Human Development*. 11(2):163–169. http://www.degruyter.com/view/j/ijdhd.2012.11.issue-2/ijdhd-2012-0020/ijdhd-2012-0020.xml. Accessed July 7, 2013.
8. Rett syndrome clinical presentation. Medscape web site. Bernstein BE, Pataki C. http://emedicine.medscape.com/article/916377-clinical. Accessed July 7, 2013.

ADDITIONAL REFERENCES

- Developmental Profile III. *Children and Adolescents with Special Needs*. http://portal.wpspublish.com/portal/page?_pageid=53,186601&_dad=portal&_schema=PORTAL. Accessed July 4, 2013.
- Dutton M. Pediatric physical therapy. In: *McGraw Hill's National Physical Therapy Examination*. 2nd ed. New York, NY: McGraw-Hill; 2012. http://www.accessphysiotherapy.com/content/5404405#5404405. Accessed July 7, 2013.
- The Neonatal Behavioral Assessment Scale. The Brazelton Institute web site. http://www.brazelton-institute.com/intro.html. Accessed July 7, 2013.
- The Test of Infant Motor Performance. Infant Motor Performance Scales web site. http://thetimp.com. Accessed July 7, 2013.

253 SPINA BIFIDA

Kay Tasso, PhD, PT, PCS

CONDITION/DISORDER SYNONYMS

- Meningocele
- Meningomyelocele
- Myelocele
- Myelodysplasia
- Myelomeningocele
- Spina bifida aperta
- Spina bifida cystica
- Spina bifida occulta
- Spinal dysraphism

ICD-9-CM CODES

- 741 Spina bifida
- 741.0 Spina bifida with hydrocephalus
- 741.00 Spina bifida unspecified region with hydrocephalus
- 741.01 Spina bifida cervical region with hydrocephalus
- 741.02 Spina bifida dorsal (thoracic) region with hydrocephalus
- 741.03 Spina bifida lumbar region with hydrocephalus
- 741.9 Spina bifida without mention of hydrocephalus
- 741.90 Spina bifida unspecified region without hydrocephalus
- 741.91 Spina bifida cervical region without hydrocephalus
- 741.92 Spina bifida dorsal (thoracic) region without hydrocephalus
- 741.93 Spina bifida lumbar region without hydrocephalus
- 742.0 Encephalocele

ICD-10-CM CODES

- Q01 Encephalocele
- Q01.0 Frontal encephalocele
- Q01.1 Nasofrontal encephalocele
- Q01.2 Occipital encephalocele
- Q01.8 Encephalocele of other sites
- Q05 Spina bifida
- Q01.9 Encephalocele, unspecified
- Q05.0 Cervical spina bifida with hydrocephalus
- Q05.1 Thoracic spina bifida with hydrocephalus
- Q05.2 Lumbar spina bifida with hydrocephalus
- Q05.3 Sacral spina bifida with hydrocephalus
- Q05.4 Unspecified spina bifida with hydrocephalus
- Q05.5 Cervical spina bifida without hydrocephalus
- Q05.6 Thoracic spina bifida without hydrocephalus
- Q05.7 Lumbar spina bifida without hydrocephalus
- Q05.8 Sacral spina bifida without hydrocephalus
- Q05.9 Spina bifida, unspecified
- Q07.01 Arnold–Chiari malformation
- Q07.3 Arnold–Chiari syndrome with spina bifida and hydrocephalus
- Q76.0 Spina bifida occulta

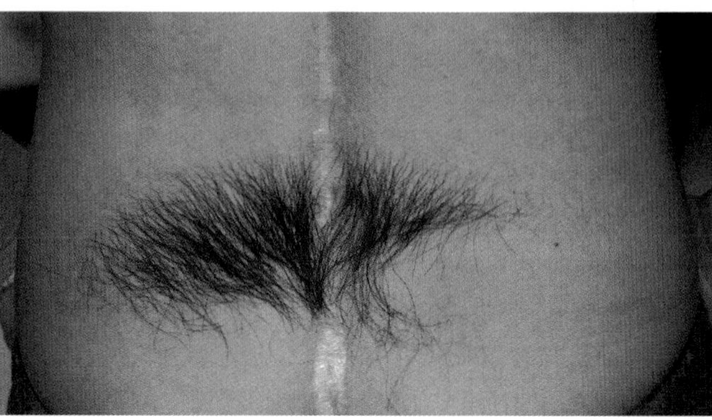

FIGURE 253-1 A large, wide tuft of thick terminal hair on the lumbosacral spine noted at birth. She had underlying tethered cord (note midline scar due to surgical repair). (From Goldsmith LA, Katz SI, Gilchrest BA, Paller A, Leffell DJ, Wolff K, eds. *Fitzpatrick's Dermatology in General Medicine*. 8th ed. http://www.accessmedicine.com. Copyright © The McGraw-Hill Companies, Inc. All rights reserved.)

PREFERRED PRACTICE PATTERN

- 5C: Impaired Motor Function and Sensory Integrity Associated With Nonprogressive Disorders of the Central Nervous System—congenital origin or acquired in infancy or childhood

PATIENT PRESENTATION

A 6-year-old female child with a diagnosis of spina bifida at L2-L3 is referred to physical therapy for evaluation and treatment. The mother reports not being aware of her pregnancy until 9 weeks gestation. At 14 weeks, a fetal ultrasound indicated the presence of myelomeningocele. As a result, the infant was delivered via C-section to prevent rupture of the lumbosacral sac. The infant had surgery to close the sac within 24 hours after birth and placement of a ventroperitoneal shunt within 72 hours after birth. The child received physical therapy as an infant and young child and currently receives services through the public school system. The family requested outpatient physical therapy now to teach the patient how to transfer herself independently as she has grown too large for the mother to transfer her by herself.

KEY FEATURES

Description

- Group of disorders involving failure of closure (split spine) in the caudal end of the spinal column in utero[1]
- Lipomeningocele: Fatty tissue mass without typical neurologic involvement or hydrocephalus
- Anencephaly: Failure of closure of caudal end of neural tube, incompatible with life
- Occipital meningocele: Meningeal sac at the occipital level
- Encephalocele: Meningeal sac containing cerebral tissue
- Spina bifida occulta: Mildest defect characterized by dimple in skin and/or tuft of hair, asymptomatic

- Meningocele: Meningeal sac filled with cerebrospinal fluid without involvement of the spinal elements[1]
- Meningomyelocele: Severe defect characterized by meningeal sac that contains a portion of the spinal cord
- Spina bifida aperta: Rare, most severe type of defect that contains neural plate and rectum in addition to spinal cord

Essentials of Diagnosis

- Often involves the meninges and/or spinal nerves resulting in hydrocephalus and/or Arnold–Chiari malformation
- Open or closed spina bifida

General Considerations

- Extent of neural involvement ranges from anencephaly, sacral agenesis, meningocele, or myelomeningocele

Demographics

- Probability of occurrence in siblings: 1% to 2%[2]
- Probability of occurrence in offspring: 5%[2]
- Meningomyelocele accounts for 94% of all spina bifida occurrences[3]
- Incidence 1:1000 live births
- Highest incidence in Hispanic women
- Irish and Celtic families at increased risk (4.5:1000 live births)
- Japanese families at lowest risk (0.3:1000 live births)

CLINICAL FINDINGS

SIGNS AND SYMPTOMS

- Chiari II malformation: Open lesion on spinal column
- Skin-covered cephalocele
- Hydrocephalus
- Muscle weakness and/or paralysis in lower extremities (LEs)
- Sensory deficits in lower extremities
- Talipes equinovarus (clubfoot)
- Latex allergy
- Visual perceptual deficits
- Cognitive deficits
- Neurogenic bowel and bladder: Speech delay
- Variable paralysis
- Signs and symptoms of tethered cord syndrome
  - Progressive scoliosis
  - Hypertonia in LEs
  - Changes in bladder function
  - Changes in gait pattern
  - Decreased strength
  - Back pain
- Signs and symptoms of shunt malfunction
  - Vomiting
  - Headaches
  - Irritability
  - Lethargy
  - Redness or swelling along shunt

Functional Implications

- Paralysis of LEs
- Insensate LEs
- Neurogenic bladder and bowel
- Hip dislocation or subluxation
- 85% to 90% develop pressure sores[4]
- Obesity
- 10% to 30% have seizures[4]

Possible Contributing Causes

- Insufficient maternal folic acid, early during pregnancy
- Genetic mutation (chromosome 13 or 19)
- Teratogens such as valproic acid

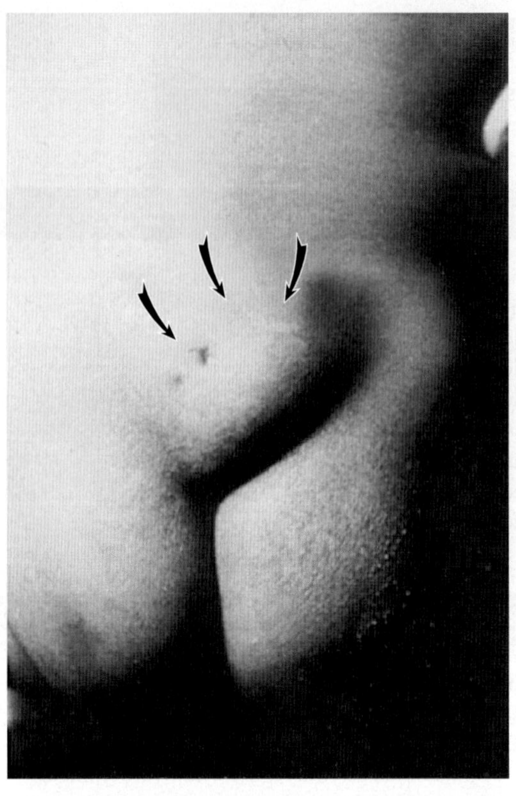

FIGURE 253-2 Spina bifida occulta. The arrows point to a swelling above the buttocks. (From Waxman SG. *Clinical Neuroanatomy*. 26th ed. http://www.accessmedicine.com. Copyright © The McGraw-Hill Companies, Inc. All rights reserved.)

- Maternal obesity
- Family history of spina bifida or other neural tube defects

Differential Diagnosis

- Caudal regression syndrome
- Genetic syndrome
- Spine segmental dysgenesis
- Multiple vertebral segmentation disorder

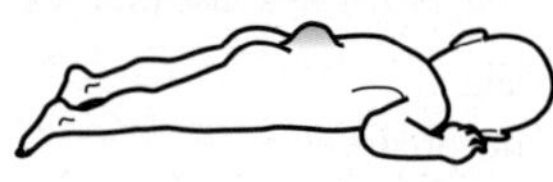

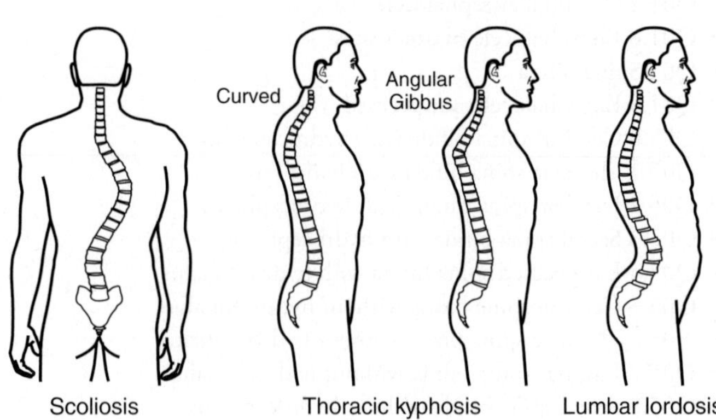

FIGURE 253-3 Spinal Disorders. **A.** Meningocele. **B.** Curvatures of the spine. (From LeBlond RF, DeGowin RL, Brown DD. *DeGowin's Diagnostic Examination*. 9th ed. http://www.accessmedicine.com. Copyright © The McGraw-Hill Companies, Inc. All rights reserved.)

- VACTERL (V - vertebral anomalies, A - anorectal anomalies, C - cardiac anomalies, T - tracheo-, E - oesophageal fisula, R - renal anomalies, L - limb abnormalities) association (60 to 80% have spinal defects)

MEANS OF CONFIRMATION OR DIAGNOSIS

Laboratory Tests

- Prenatal triple or quadruple screen
- Blood test for alpha fetoprotein and acetylcholine esterase between 16 and 18 weeks of gestational age
- Urine culture
- Voiding cystourethrogram (VCUG)

Imaging

- Fetal ultrasound
- Fetal MRI
- Myelogram for suspected tethered cord syndrome
- Renal ultrasound
- Urodynamic study

Diagnostic Procedures

- Amniocentesis
- Chorionic villus sampling

FINDINGS AND INTERPRETATION[4]

- High alpha-fetoprotein in blood
- Presence of acetylcholinesterase in blood
- "Banana" signs on fetal ultrasound

TREATMENT

Medical Procedures

- Intrauterine surgical repair
- Cesarean section for delivery
- Surgical repair of open meningeal sac within first 72 hours of life
- Insertion of shunt to manage hydrocephalus

REFERRALS/ADMITTANCE

- Geneticist
- Neurosurgeon
- Orthopedic surgeon
- Urologist
- Neonatologist
- Orthotist
- Occupational therapist
- Speech therapist
- Admittance immediately after birth for surgical correction of defect in meningeal sac and placement of shunt to correct hydrocephalus
- Admittance for
  - Decompression of Arnold–Chiari malformation
  - Clubfoot repair
  - Repair of tethered cord syndrome
  - Osteotomy due to repair of hip dislocation or subluxation
  - Tenotomy due to contractures
  - Spinal fusion for repair of scoliosis

IMPAIRMENTS

- Abnormal posture
- Clubfoot

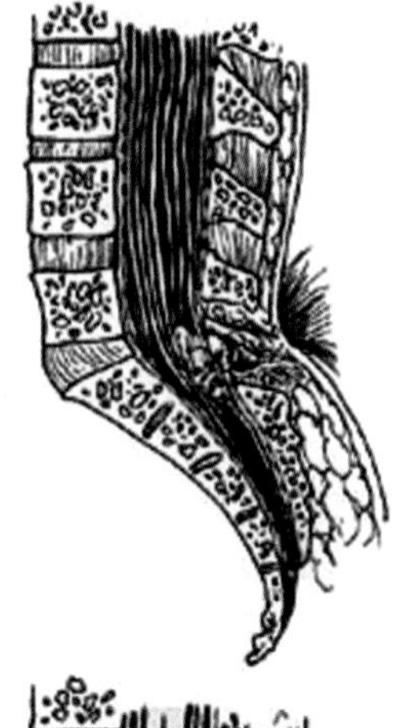

A
Spina bifida occulta
•Vertebral defect
•Normal cord and meninges
•Skin dimple with lipoma, tuft of hair, or sinus

B
Meningocele
•Vertebral defect
•Herniation of menin-geal sac through defect
•Cystic CSF-filled mass covered by skin
•Cord normal
- Minimal neurologic deficits

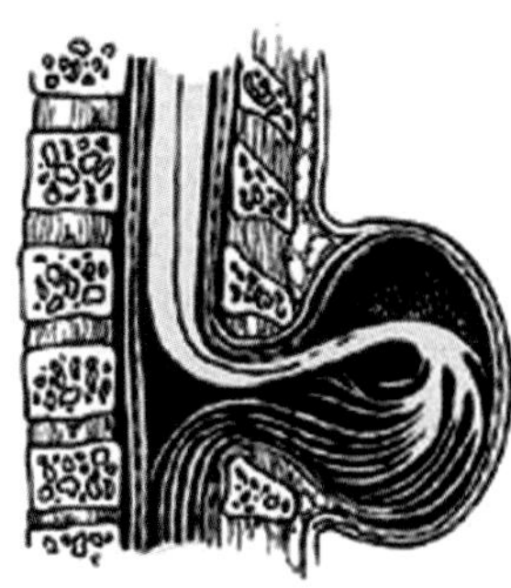

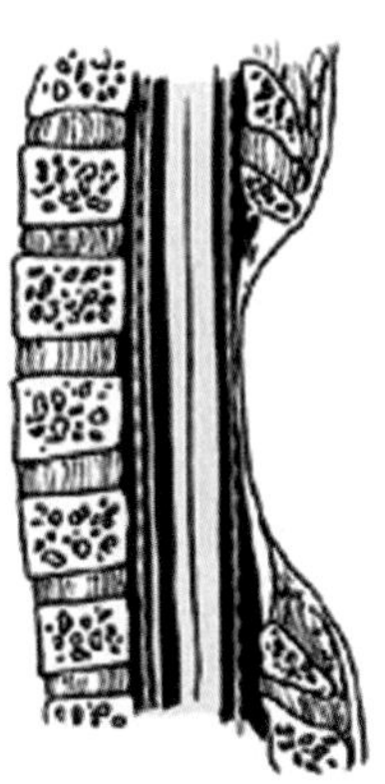

D
Spina bifida aperta
•Complete failure of fusion of caudal neural plate
•Skin and vertebral defect, base of which is undevel-oped neural plate
- Major neurologic deficits

FIGURE 253-4 Spina bifida, showing different degrees of involvement of skin, vertebral column, and neuraxis. (From Chandrasoma P, Taylor CR. *Concise Pathology*. 3rd ed. http://www.accessmedicine.com. Copyright © The McGraw-Hill Companies, Inc. All rights reserved.)

- Contractures
- Hip dislocation or subluxation
- Hyperlordosis
- Hypertonia
- Hypotonia

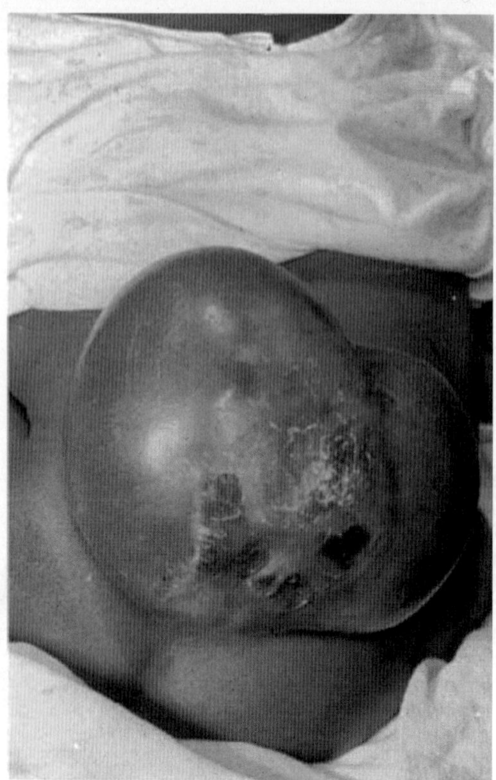

FIGURE 253-5 Meningocele of the lumbar region. (From Chandrasoma P, Taylor CR. *Concise Pathology*. 3rd ed. http://www.accessmedicine.com. Copyright © The McGraw-Hill Companies, Inc. All rights reserved.)

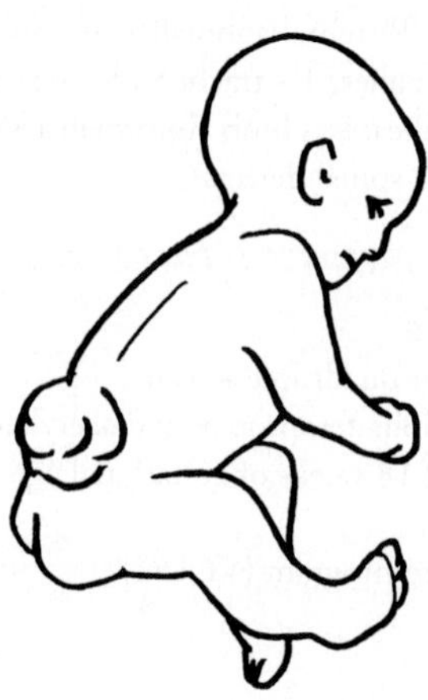

FIGURE 253-6 Spina bifida (myelomeningocele). The sac includes dysplastic spinal cord and membrane elements, and it must be surgically closed in the first days of life. Hydrocephalus and congenital scoliosis are commonly associated. (From Skinner HB. *Current Diagnosis & Treatment in Orthopedics*. 4th ed. http://www.accessmedicine.com. Copyright © The McGraw-Hill Companies, Inc. All rights reserved.)

- Muscle weakness or paralysis
- Osteoporosis
- Pressure sores
- Scoliosis
- Sensory deficits

TESTS AND MEASURES

- Pediatric evaluation of disability inventory
- Manual muscle test
- Range of motion
- Sensory testing

INTERVENTION

- Developmental activities to facilitate gross motor development such as rolling, sitting, crawling
- Strengthening
- Stretching
- Endurance training
- Transfers
- Standers
- Gait training with orthotics and walker
- Donning/doffing orthotics
- Wheelchair propulsion
- Collaboration and recommendations regarding wheelchair, orthotics, and equipment such as a stander

TABLE 253-1 Types of Spina Bifida

Type	Description
Spina bifida occulta	"Occulta" means hidden, thus the defect is not visible. Rarely linked with complications or symptoms. Usually discovered accidentally during an x-ray or MRI for some other reason.
Meningocele (Spina bifida aperta)	The membrane that surrounds the spinal cord may enlarge, creating a lump or "cyst." This is often invisible through the skin and causes no problems. If the spinal canal is cleft, or "bifid," the cyst may expand and come to the surface. In such cases, since the cyst does not enclose the spinal cord, the cord is not exposed. The cyst varies in size, but it can almost always be removed surgically if necessary, leaving no permanent disability.
Myelomeningocele (Spina bifida aperta)	The most complex and severe form of spina bifida. A section of the spinal cord and the nerves that stem from the cord are exposed and visible on the outside of the body; or, if there is a cyst, it encloses part of the cord and the nerves. Usually involves neurological problems that can be very serious or even fatal. This condition accounts for 94% of cases of true spina bifida. The most severe form of spina bifida cystica is myelocele, or myeloschisis, in which the open neural plate is covered secondarily by epithelium and the neural plate has spread out onto the surface.

Source: Dutton M. *McGraw-Hill's NPTE (National Physical Therapy Examination)*. 2nd ed. www.accessphysiotherapy.com. Copyright © The McGraw-Hill Companies, Inc. All rights reserved.

TABLE 253-2 The Neurological Complications Associated with Spina Bifida

Complication	Description
Syringomeningocele	The Greek word syrinx, meaning tube or plate, is combined with meninx (membrane) and kele (tumor); the term thus describes a hollow center with the spinal fluid connecting with the central canal of the cord enclosed by a membrane with very little cord substance.
Syringomyelocele	Protrusion of the membranes and spinal cord lead to increased fluid in the central canal, attenuating the cord tissue against a thin-walled sac.
Diastematomyelia	From the Greek root diastema (interval) and myelon (marrow). Is accompanied by a bony septum in some cases.
Myelodysplasia	From the Greek term myelos, meaning spinal cord, with *dys* for difficult and *plasi* for molding. This is a defective development of any part of the cord.
Arnold–Chiari deformity	Malformation of the cerebellum, with elongation of the cerebellar tonsils. The cerebellum is drawn into the fourth ventricle. The condition also is characterized by smallness of the medulla and pons and internal hydrocephalus. In fact, all patients with spina bifida cystica (failure to close caudally) have some form of Arnold–Chiari malformation (failure to close cranially). The Chiari II malformation is a complex congenital malformation of the brain, nearly always associated with myelomeningocele. This condition includes downward displacement of the medulla, fourth ventricle, and cerebellum into the cervical spinal canal, as well as elongation of the pons and fourth ventricle, probably due to a relatively small posterior fossa. Signs and symptoms include stridor, apnea, irritability, cerebellar ataxia, and hypertonia.
Craniorachischisis (total dysraphism)	A condition in which the brain and spinal cord are exposed. This often results in early spontaneous abortion, often associated with malformations of other organ systems.
Tethered cord	A longitudinal stretch of the spinal cord that occurs with growth resulting in progressive loss of sensory and motor function, long tract signs, and changes in posture and gait. Presence may be signaled by foot deformities previously braced easily, new onset of hip dislocation, or worsening of a spinal deformity, particularly scoliosis. Progressive neurologic defects in growing children may suggest a lack of extensibility of the spine or that it is tethered and low lying in the lumbar canal with the potential for progressive irreversible neurologic damage and requiring surgical release.
Hydrocephalus	Characterized by a tense, bulging fontanel and increased occipital frontal circumference. Signs and symptoms include decreased upper extremity coordination, disturbed balance, strabismus, and ocular problems. Medical intervention involves placement of a shunt between ventricle and heart/abdomen.
Neurogenic bowel and bladder	Incontinence

Source: Shaer CM, Chescheir N, Erickson K, et al. Obstetrician-gynecologists' practice and knowledge regarding spina bifida. *Am J Perinatol.* 2006;23:355–362. Epub Jul 13, 2006; Woodhouse CR. Progress in the management of children born with spina bifida. *Eur Urol.* 2006;49:777–778. Epub Feb 6, 2006; Verhoef M, Barf HA, Post MW, et al. Functional independence among young adults with spina bifida, in relation to hydrocephalus and level of lesion. *Dev Med Child Neurol.* 2006;48:114–119; Ali L, Stocks GM. Spina bifida, tethered cord and regional anaesthesia. *Anaesthesia.* 2005;60:1149–1150; Spina bifida. *Nurs Times.* 2005;101:31; Mitchell LE, Adzick NS, Melchionne J, et al. Spina bifida. *Lancet.* 2004;364:1885–1895; and Dias L. Orthopaedic care in spina bifida: past, present, and future. *Dev Med Child Neurol.* 2004;46:579.

- Parent education for daily passive ROM, daily skin checks, handling, and positioning
- Patient education about pressure reliefs every 2 hours

FUNCTIONAL GOALS

- The patient will be able to
  - Roll prone to supine and supine to prone independently for mobility in 4 months
  - Sit independently propping with arms on floor for upright activities in 3 months
  - Prevent hip flexion and hamstring contractures to optimize positioning in 6 months
  - Increase upper-extremity strength to allow two wheelchair push-ups in 2 months
  - Propel wheelchair 500 ft on sidewalk to increase endurance and independence in 6 months
  - Transfer from floor to wheelchair with minimal assistance to increase independence in 3 months
  - Tolerate use of prone stander for 30 minutes to increase upright activities in 1 month
  - Ambulate with a posterior four-wheeled rolling walker 25 ft with minimal assistance to increase mobility in 6 months
  - Remove ankle-foot orthotics independently to assist with activities of daily living in 2 months

PROGNOSIS

- Meningocele: No severe neurologic involvement
- Spina bifida aperta: Most severe form with significant neurologic involvement
- Thoracic and higher lumbar lesions: Unlikely to ambulate
- Lower lumbar and sacral lesions: Likely to ambulate

PATIENT RESOURCES

- Pregnancy and Amniocentesis. WebMD. http://www.webmd.com/baby/guide/amniocentesis. Accessed July 1, 2013.
- What is Spina Bifida? Spina Bifidia Association. http://www.spinabifidaassociation.org/site/c.evKRI7OXIoJ8H/b.8277225/k.5A79/What_is_Spina_Bifida.htm. Accessed August 14, 2014.

TABLE 253-3 Muscle Function at Neurologic Levels in Myelomeningocoele (Spina Bifida)

Neurologic Level	Functions	Muscles Active
T12	Hip flexion (weak)	Iliopsoas (weak)
L1	Hip flexion	Iliopsoas
L2	Hip adduction (weak)	Adductor longus, brevis (weak)
L3	Hip adduction Knee extension (weak)	Adductors Quadriceps (weak)
L4	Knee extension Ankle dorsiflexion	Quadriceps Anterior tibialis (variable)
L5	Knee flexion Hip abduction	Medial hamstring Tensor fascia lata
S1	Knee flexion Ankle plantar flexion	All hamstrings Gastrocnemius-soleus
S2	Toe flexion	Flexor digitorum longus

Source: Skinner HB. *Current Diagnosis & Treatment in Orthopedics*. 4th ed. http://www.accessmedicine.com.

REFERENCES

1. Chandrasoma P, Taylor CR. Congenital diseases of the nervous system. In: Chandrasoma P, Taylor CR, eds. *Concise Pathology*. 3rd ed. New York, NY: McGraw-Hill; 2011. http://www.accessphysiotherapy.com/content/192887#192887. Accessed July 1, 2013.
2. Hay WW, Levin MJ, Sondheimer JM, Deterding RR. Disorders of multifactorial inheritance. In: Hay WW, Levin MJ, Sondheimer JM, Deterding RR, eds. *CURRENT Diagnosis & Treatment: Pediatrics*. 20th ed. New York, NY: McGraw-Hill; 2011. http://www.accessphysiotherapy.com/content/6589199. Accessed July 1, 2013.
3. Dutton M. Neurologic system. In: Dutton M, ed. *McGraw-Hill's NPTE (National Physical Therapy Examination)*. 2nd ed. New York, NY: McGraw-Hill; 2009. http://www.accessphysiotherapy.com/popup.aspx?aID=5404866. Accessed July 1, 2013.
4. Hinderer KA, Hinderer SR, Shurtleff DB. Myelodysplasia. In: Campbell SK, Palisano RJ, Orlin MN, eds. *Physical Therapy for Children*. 4th ed. St. Louis, MO: Elsevier Saunders; 2012.

ADDITIONAL REFERENCES

- Alpha Fetoprotein. Medline Plus. http://www.nlm.nih.gov/medlineplus/ency/article/003573.htm. Accessed July 1, 2013.
- Barsh G. Genetic disease. In: McPhee SJ, Hammer GD, eds. *Pathophysiology of Disease*. 6th ed. New York, NY: McGraw-Hill; 2010:Chapter 2. http://www.accessphysiotherapy.com/content/5366507. Accessed July 1, 2013.
- Bernard TJ, Knupp K, Yang ML, Arndt D, Levisohn P, Moe PG. Neurologic & muscular disorders. In: Hay WW, Levin MJ, Sondheimer JM, Deterding RR, eds. *CURRENT Diagnosis & Treatment: Pediatrics*. 20th ed. New York, NY: McGraw-Hill; 2011. http://www.accessphysiotherapy.com/content/6585071. Accessed July 1, 2013.
- Definition of Teratogen. MedicineNet.com. http://www.medterms.com/script/main/art.asp?articlekey=11315. Accessed July 1, 2013.
- Fetal Ultrasound. Mayo Clinic. http://www.mayoclinic.com/health/fetal-ultrasound/MY00777. Accessed July 1, 2013.
- Hip Dislocation. *American Academy of Orthopedic Surgeons*. http://orthoinfo.aaos.org/topic.cfm?topic=A00352. Accessed July 1, 2013.
- ICD9Data.com. http://www.icd9data.com/2012/Volume1/default.htm. Accessed July 1, 2013.
- ICD10Data.com. http://www.icd10data.com/ICD10CM/Codes. Accessed July 1, 2013.
- Letts RM, Jawadi AH. Congenital Spinal Deformity. Medscape Reference. http://emedicine.medscape.com/article/1260442-overview#aw2aab6b6. Accessed July 1, 2013.
- Lin VW, Cardenas DD, Cutter NC, et al., eds. *Spinal Cord Medicine: Principles and Practice*. New York, NY: Demos Medical Publishing; 2003.
- McPhee SJ, Hammer GD. Unique pathophysiologic aspects of genetic diseases. In: McPhee SJ, Hammer GD, eds. *Pathophysiology of Disease*. 6th ed. New York: McGraw-Hill; 2010. http://www.accessphysiotherapy.com/content/5366515#5366515. Accessed July 1, 2013.
- Neurogenic Bladder. A.D.A.M Medical Encyclopedia. PubMed Health. http://www.ncbi.nlm.nih.gov/pubmedhealth/PMH0001761/. Accessed July 1, 2013.
- NINDS Encephalocele Information Page. National Institute of Neurological Disorders and Stroke. http://www.ninds.nih.gov/disorders/encephaloceles/encephaloceles.htm. Accessed July 1, 2013.
- NINDS Tethered Spinal Cord Syndrome Information Page. National Institute of Neurological Disorders and Stroke. http://www.ninds.nih.gov/disorders/tethered_cord/tethered_cord.htm. Accessed July 1, 2013.
- Panus PC, Jobst EE, Masters SB, Katzung B, Tinsley SL, Trevor AJ, eds. *Pharmacology for the Physical Therapist*. New York: McGraw-Hill; 2009. http://www.accessphysiotherapy.com/content/6091521#6091521. Accessed July 1, 2013.
- Pattern 5C: impaired motor function and sensory integrity associated with nonprogressive disorders of the central nervous system - congenital origin or acquired in infancy or childhood. In: *Guide to Physical Therapist Practice*. 2nd ed. Alexandria, VA: American Physical Therapy Association; 2001. Revised 2003.
- Shunt Malfunction. National Hydrocephalus Foundation. http://nhfonline.org/signs-of-hydrocephalus-and-shunt-malfunctions.htm. Accessed August 14, 2014.
- Tappit-Emas E. Spina bifida. In: Tecklin JS, ed. *Pediatric Physical Therapy*. 4th ed. Philadelphia, PA: Lippincott, Williams and Wilkins; 2008:231–279.
- Waxman SG. Clinical correlations. In: Waxman SG, ed. *Clinical Neuroanatomy*. 26th ed. New York: McGraw-Hill; 2010. http://www.accessphysiotherapy.com/content/5272268#5272268. Accessed July 1, 2013.

254 SPINAL MUSCULAR ATROPHY

Kay Tasso, PhD, PT, PCS

CONDITION/DISORDER SYNONYMS

- Bulbospinal muscular atrophy
- Hereditary neuronopathy
- Progressive muscular atrophy[1]
- Werdnig-Hoffman disease

ICD-9-CM CODES

- 335.0 Werdnig-Hoffman disease
- 335.1 Spinal muscular atrophy
- 335.10 Spinal muscular atrophy unspecified
- 335.19 Other spinal muscular atrophy

ICD-10-CM CODES

- G12.0 Infantile spinal muscular atrophy, type I [Werdnig-Hoffman]
- G12.8 Other spinal muscular atrophy and related syndromes
- G12.9 Spinal muscular atrophy, unspecified

PREFERRED PRACTICE PATTERN

- 5E: Impaired Motor Function and Sensory Integrity Associated with Progressive Disorders of the Central Nervous System

PATIENT PRESENTATION

A 10-month-old child is referred for physical therapy in the natural environment (at home) through an early intervention program with a diagnosis of infantile spinal muscular atrophy type 1. The child is on a ventilator with an oxygen saturation machine and G-tube for all feeding. There is no active muscle function or head control. Passive dorsiflexion is limited to –10 degrees. The child is dependent for all mobility and ADLs. The family is interested in assistance with obtaining the appropriate equipment for positioning and transportation.

KEY FEATURES

Description

- Group of four subtypes of degeneration of anterior horn cells that results in progressive muscle atrophy
  - Spinal muscular atrophy (SMA I), Werdnig-Hoffman (acute)
  - Spinal muscular atrophy (SMA II), Werdnig-Hoffman (chronic)
  - Spinal muscular atrophy (SMA III), Kugelberg-Welander
  - Spinal muscular atrophy (SMA IV)

Essentials of Diagnosis

- Autosomal recessive genetic disorder that results in a lack of survival motor neuron gene[1] on chromosome 5q11.2-13[2]

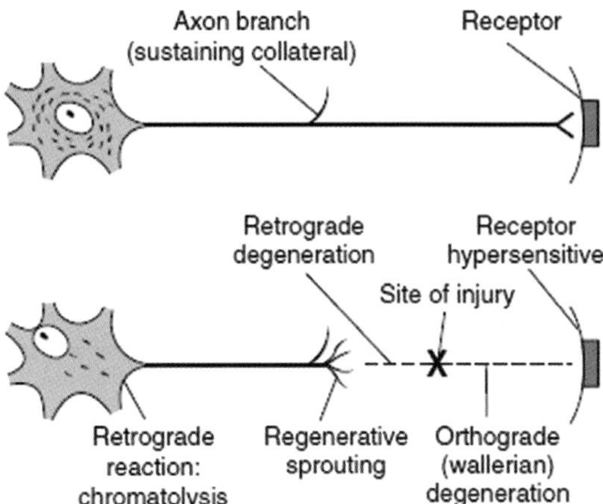

FIGURE 254-1 Summary of changes occurring in a neuron and the structure it innervates when its axon is crushed or cut at the point marked X. Hypersensitivity of the postsynaptic structure to the transmitter previously secreted by the axon occurs largely due to the synthesis or activation of more receptors. There is both orthograde (wallerian) degeneration from the point of damage to the terminal and retrograde degeneration of the axon stump to the nearest collateral (sustaining collateral). Changes also occur in the cell body, including chromatolysis. The nerve starts to regrow, with multiple small branches projecting along the path the axon previously followed (regenerative sprouting). (From Barrett KE, Berman SM, Boitano S, Brooks HL. *Ganong's Review of Medical Physiology*. 24th ed. New York, NY: McGraw-Hill; 2012.)

General Considerations

- SMA type I: Weakness between birth and 3 months of age
- SMA type II: Signs and symptoms by 3 years of age
- SMA type III: Signs and symptoms between 2 and 9 years of age
- SMA type IV: Adult onset

Demographics[2]

- Type I: 27% of all SMA cases
- Types II and III: 46% of all SMA cases
- Type IV: 8% of all SMA cases
- Werdnig-Hoffman: 1:10,000 births
- Kugelberg-Welander: 6:100,000 births

CLINICAL FINDINGS

SIGNS AND SYMPTOMS

- Fasciculations (especially of tongue)
- Muscle weakness
- Hypotonia
- Muscle atrophy
- Decreased or absent deep tendon reflexes
- Difficulty feeding (infant)
- Lack of extension during Landau reflex
- Contractures (type 1)
- Pulmonary infection
- Scoliosis
- Trendelenburg sign during gait

Functional Implications

- Inability to sit independently
- Inability to ambulate
- Require assistance with all activities of daily living

TABLE 254-1 Classification of the Spinal Muscular Atrophies (SMA)

Type	Inheritance	Age of Onset	Clinical Features	Prognosis
SMA I (infantile, Werdnig-Hoffmann)	Autosomal recessive	Preterm to 6 months	Neonatal hypotonia (floppy baby), weakness of sucking and swallowing, may have arthrogryposis, unable to sit	Few survive 1 year
SMA II (intermediate type)	Autosomal recessive	6 to 15 months	Proximal weakness, fasciculation, fine hand tremor, unable to stand	Variable; death from respiratory complications
SMA III (Wohlfahrt- Kugel-berg- Welander)	Autosomal recessive or dominant	1 year to adolescence	Delayed motor development, proximal leg weakness	Slowly progressive, variable outcome
Kennedy syndrome (bulbospinal atrophy)	X-linked (CAG repeat expansion), less often autosomal dominant	Early adulthood	Scapuloperoneal or distal atrophy, oropharyngeal weakness, gynecomastia, oligospermia	Slowly progressive
Fazio–Londe disease	Autosomal recessive, rarely dominant	Childhood to early adolescence	Progressive bulbar and respiratory failure	Survival for years, respiratory failure

Source: Ropper AH, Samuels MA. *Adams & Victor's Principles of Neurology*. 9th ed. New York, NY: McGraw-Hill; 2009.

Possible Contributing Causes

- Autosomal recessive genetic disorder on chromosome 5q11.2-13[2]

Differential Diagnosis

- Congenital myopathies
- Congenital muscular dystrophy
- Guillain–Barré
- Amyotrophic lateral sclerosis
- Brachial plexus birth injury
- Myasthenia graves
- Primary lateral sclerosis
- Other genetic syndromes

MEANS OF CONFIRMATION OR DIAGNOSIS

Laboratory Tests

- Genetic testing

Imaging

- Plain radiograph for scoliosis

Diagnostic Procedures

- Compound motor action potentials (CAMPs) are reduced
- Electromyography (EMG)
- Muscle biopsy

FINDINGS AND INTERPRETATION

- CSF findings are normal
- Homozygous SMN1 gene deletion is 95% sensitive and 100% specific

TREATMENT

Medication

- Albuterol
- Hydroxyurea
- Phenylbutyrate
- Valproic acid

REFERRALS/ADMITTANCE

- To gastroenterologist
- To geneticist
- To occupational therapist
- To pulmonologist
- To speech therapist

IMPAIRMENTS

- Head lag when infant pulled into a sitting position from supine
- Poor head control
- Inability to sit
- Inability to pull to stand
- Inability to walk
- Contractures of biceps and wrist flexors

TESTS AND MEASURES

- Hammersmith Functional Motor Scale for Children[2]
- Dynamometer
- 2-minute walk test
- Manual muscle test
- Forced vital capacity

INTERVENTION

- It is important to avoid fatigue during intervention with patients who have SMA.
- Strengthening
- Stretching to prevent contractures especially of wrist flexors
- Developmental activities
  - Prone on elbows with assistance
  - Supported sitting
  - Supported standing
  - Facilitating pulling up from sitting into standing at furniture
- Pre-gait activities
- Gait training
- Adaptive equipment
  - Manual or power wheelchair
  - Stander
  - Abdominal binder
- Orthotics
  - Thoracic-lumbar-sacral orthotic (TLSO)
  - Knee-ankle-foot orthotics (KAFOs) for SMA II
  - Ankle-foot orthotics (AFOs)

- Chest physical therapy
  - Percussion
  - Postural drainage
- Aquatic therapy
- Swimming
- Switch plate toys

FUNCTIONAL GOALS

- Patient will be able to
  - Tuck their chin when pulling into sitting from supine in 3 months to decrease head lag.
  - Increase quadriceps strength to transfer from sitting to standing with minimal assistance in 3 weeks.
  - Prevent loss of ROM of wrist extension to prevent contractures.
  - Support self prone on elbows for 30 seconds to increase independence during play within 6 months.
  - Sit for 5 minutes while playing with stand-by assistance to increase independent play within 1 month.
  - Pull to standing from sitting with contact guard assistance to increase mobility within 4 months.
  - Drive the power wheelchair into the bathroom with verbal cues within 1 week to increase independent mobility.
  - Stand independently while supporting self with a hand on the wall in the bathroom to assist with hygiene.

PROGNOSIS

- SMA I: Death by age 1 due to respiratory failure.[1]
- SMA II: Mean death age is 10 years old[2]; 75% sit independently until 7 years old and 50% until 14 years old.[3]
- SMA III: Better prognosis if symptoms develop after 2 years of age than prior to that; ambulate throughout life with a wheelchair for long distances[2]

PATIENT RESOURCE

- Modified Hammersmith Functional Motor Scale for Children with Spinal Muscular Atrophy. Project Cure SMA. http://smaoutcomes.org/hammersmith_manual/manual_1.html. Accessed July 3, 2013.

REFERENCES

1. Tsai ACH, Manchester DK, Elias ER. Genetics & dysmorphology. In: Hay WW, Levin MJ, Sondheimer JM, Deterding RR, eds. *CURRENT Diagnosis & Treatment: Pediatrics*. 20th ed. New York, NY: McGraw-Hill; 2011. http://www.accessphysiotherapy.com/content/6589151#6589151. Accessed July 2, 2013.
2. Stuberg WA. Muscular dystrophy and spinal muscular atrophy. In: Campbell SK, Palisano RJ, Orlin MN, eds. *Physical Therapy for Children*. 4th ed. St. Louis, MO: Elsevier Saunders; 2012:369–374.
3. Glanzman AM, Flickinger JM. Neuromuscular disorders in childhood: physical therapy intervention. In: Tecklin JS, ed. *Pediatric Physical Therapy*. 4th ed. Philadelphia, PA. Lippincott, Williams and Wilkins; 2008:354–358.

ADDITIONAL REFERENCES

- 2-Minute Walk Test Instructions. Rehabilitation Measures Database. http://www.rehabmeasures.org/PDF%20Library/2%20Minute%20Walk%20Test%20Instructions.pdf. Accessed July 3, 2013.
- Chandrasoma P, Taylor CR. Peripheral neuropathy. In: Chandrasoma P, Taylor CR, eds. *Concise Pathology*. 3rd ed. New York, NY: McGraw-Hill; 2011. http://www.accessphysiotherapy.com/content/193413#193413. Accessed July 3, 2013.
- Dutton M. The nervous system. In: Dutton M, ed. *Orthopaedic Examination, Evaluation, and Intervention*. 2nd ed. New York, NY: McGraw-Hill; 2008:Chapter 2. http://www.accessphysiotherapy.com/content/5540953#5540953. Accessed July 3, 2013.
- Dutton M. Pediatric physical therapy. In: *McGraw Hill's National Physical Therapy Examination*. 2nd ed. New York, NY: McGraw-Hill; 2012. http://www.accessphysiotherapy.com/resource/611. Accessed July 2, 2013.
- Dutton M. Special tests. In: Dutton M, ed. *Dutton's Orthopedic Survival Guide: Managing Common Conditions*. New York, NY: McGraw-Hill; 2011. http://www.accessphysiotherapy.com/content/8654017#8654017. Accessed July 3, 2013.
- Frugier T, Nicole S, Cifuentes-Diaz C, Melki J. The molecular bases of spinal muscular atrophy. *Curr Opin Genet Dev*. 2002; 12(3):294–298.
- Hamilton N, Weimar W, Luttgens K. Instrumentation for motion analysis. In: Hamilton N, Weimar W, Luttgens K, eds. *Kinesiology: Scientific Basis of Human Motion*. New York, NY: McGraw-Hill; 2008. http://www.accessphysiotherapy.com/content/6152611#6152611. Accessed July 3, 2013.
- Hay WW, Levin MJ, Sondheimer JM, Deterding RR, eds. *CURRENT Diagnosis & Treatment: Pediatrics*. 20th ed. New York, NY: McGraw-Hill; 2011. http://www.accessphysiotherapy.com/resource/14. Accessed July 2, 2013.
- Hydroxyurea. Medline Plus. http://www.nlm.nih.gov/medlineplus/druginfo/meds/a682004.html. Accessed July 3, 2013.
- ICD9Data.com. http://www.icd9data.com. Accessed July 5, 2013.
- ICD10Data.com. http://www.icd10data.com. Accessed July 3, 2013.
- McPhee SJ, Hammer GD. Motor neuron disease. In: McPhee SJ, Hammer GD, eds. *Pathophysiology of Disease*. 6th ed. New York, NY: McGraw-Hill; 2010. http://www.accessphysiotherapy.com/content/5368600#5368600. Accessed July 2, 2013.
- Panus PC, Jobst EE, Masters SB, Katzung B, Tinsley SL, Trevor AJ. Antiseizure Drugs. In: Panus PC, Jobst EE, Masters SB, Katzung B, Tinsley SL, Trevor AJ, eds. *Pharmacology for the Physical Therapist*. New York, NY: McGraw-Hill; 2009:Chapter 14. http://www.accessphysiotherapy.com/content/6091942. Accessed July 10, 2012.
- Pattern 5E: impaired motor function and sensory integrity associated with progressive disorders of the central nervous system. In: *Guide to Physical Therapist Practice*. 2nd ed. Alexandria, VA: American Physical Therapy Association; 2001. Revised 2003.
- Pediatric Neurologic Exam. University of Utah Library. http://library.med.utah.edu/pedineurologicexam/html/06month.html#12. Accessed July 2, 2013.
- Prendergast TJ, Ruoss SJ, Seeley EJ. Pulmonary disease. In: McPhee SJ, Hammer GD, eds. *Pathophysiology of Disease*. 6th ed. New York, NY: McGraw-Hill; 2010. http://www.accessphysiotherapy.com/content/5369068#5369068. Accessed July 3, 2013.
- Prentice WE, Quillen WS, Underwood F. *Therapeutic Modalities in Rehabilitation*. 4th ed. New York, NY: McGraw-Hill; 2011. http://www.accessphysiotherapy.com/resource/675. Accessed July 3, 2013.

255 TAY–SACHS DISEASE

Kay Tasso, PhD, PT, PCS

CONDITION/DISORDER SYNONYMS

- B variant GM2 gangliosidosis
- GM2 gangliosidosis, type 1
- HexA deficiency
- Hexosaminidase A deficiency
- Hexosaminidase alpha-subunit deficiency (variant B)
- Sphingolipidosis, Tay-Sachs
- TSD

ICD-9-CM CODE[1]

- 330.1 Cerebral lipidoses

ICD-10-CM CODE[2]

- E75.02 Tay–Sachs disease

PREFERRED PRACTICE PATTERNS[3]

- 5B Impaired Neuromotor Development
- 5C Impaired Motor Function and Sensory Integrity Associated with Nonprogressive Disorders of the Central Nervous System—congenital origin or acquired in infancy or childhood

PATIENT PRESENTATION

A 9-month-old male child is referred to physical therapy for developmental delay. The parents report an uneventful pregnancy and delivery. The child rolls consecutively as the primary method of mobility and props with his arms for balance when in sitting. Over the next few weeks, the child sees ophthalmologist with a report of cherry red spots on his macula, an MRI indicates cortical atrophy, and geneticist diagnoses him with Tay–Sachs disease. Over the next few months, the infant begins to lose gross motor function such as rolling and prop sitting.

KEY FEATURES

Description

- Progressive autosomal recessive genetic disorder.
- Infant lacks protein, beta-hexosaminidase A (Hex A), that prevents the accumulation of the lipid, ganglioside GM-2, thus, causing damage to brain cells.

Essentials of Diagnosis

- Genetic defect of chromosome 15
- Sandhoff disease: Unable to make (Hexa A or B)

General Considerations

- Categories
    - Infantile: Most common; symptoms appear between 3 to 6 months of age
    - Juvenile: Symptoms begin between 2 and 5 years of age
    - Adult: Symptoms begin during adolescence or as young adult

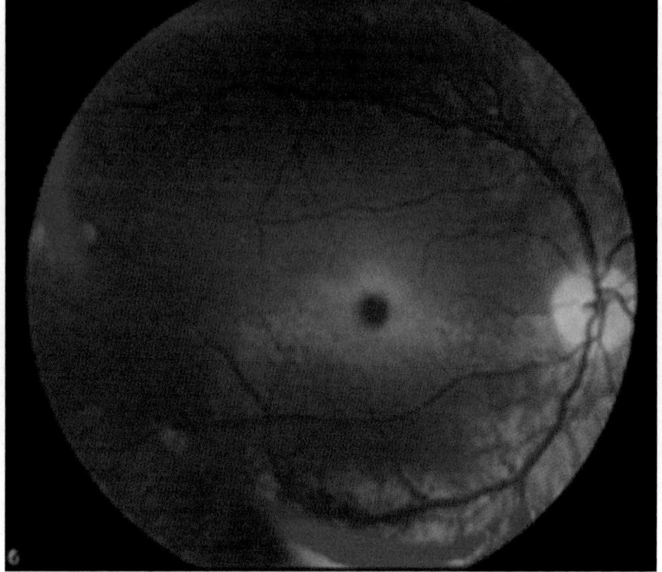

FIGURE 255-1 "Cherry-red" spot in the eye of a Tay–Sachs patient. (From http://www.nei.nih.gov/resources/eyegene.asp.)

Demographics

- 1 in every 27 Ashkenazi Jewish people[4]
- 1 out of 250 people[5]
- 1 in every 27 French Canadian, Louisiana Cajuns, Ashkenazi Jewish people[5]
- 1 in every 50 or 150 British Isles or Irish people[5]
- Equally affects males and females

CLINICAL FINDINGS

SIGNS AND SYMPTOMS

- Deafness
- Blindness
- Loss of gag reflex
- Difficulty swallowing
- Muscle weakness
- Hypotonia
- Seizures
- Paralysis
- Regression in gross motor and fine motor skills
- Cherry-red spot on eyes

Functional Implications

- Progressive muscle weakness resulting in decline in gross motor and fine motor skills such as inability to sit, ambulate or feed self

MEANS OF CONFIRMATION OR DIAGNOSIS

Laboratory Tests

- Performed early in pregnancy by amniocentesis or chorionic villus sampling

- Blood test for hexosaminidase A (hex A) levels
- Blood from the vein of the umbilical cord

Diagnostic Procedure

- DNA analysis, (Hexa) 7 Mutations

FINDINGS AND INTERPRETATION

- Unable to make Hexa A

REFERRALS/ADMITTANCE

- To geneticist
- To neurologist
- To ophthamologist
- To speech pathologist

IMPAIRMENTS

- Inability to roll
- Inability to commando crawl or creep on hands and knees
- Inability to sit
- Inability to ambulate

TESTS AND MEASURES

- Early Intervention Developmental Profile
- Neonatal Behavioral Assessment Scale
- Pediatric Evaluation of Disability Inventory
- Manual muscle test

INTERVENTION

- Developmental activities to
  - Prevent loss of motor milestones
  - Prevent loss of muscle strength
- Therapeutic exercise to
  - Prevent muscle contractures
  - Strengthen
  - Stretch
- Functional activities
  - Transfers
  - Gait training
  - Stair climbing

FUNCTIONAL GOALS

- Patient will be bale to
  - Sit supported in adaptive chair for 15 minutes during play activities in 1 month.
  - Prevent loss of range of motion to allow for optimal positioning within 3 months.
  - Take steps in a gait trainer to allow for independent mobility and upright function within 4 months.
  - Transfer from wheelchair to/from classroom chair with moderate assistance in 6 months.

PROGNOSIS

- Infantile form: Child dies by an age of 4 or 5 years.[4]

PATIENT RESOURCES

- *NINDS Tay-Sachs Information Page*. National Neurological Disorders and Stroke web site. http://www.ninds.nih.gov/disorders/taysachs/taysachs.htm. Accessed July 11, 2013.
- *Tay-Sachs disease*. PubMed Health web site. http://www.ntsad.org/index.php/tay-sachs/causes. Accessed July 11, 2013.

REFERENCES

1. ICD9DATA. http://www.icd9data.com. Accessed July 11, 2013.
2. ICD10DATA. http://www.icd10data.com. Accessed July 11, 2013.
3. *Guide to Physical Therapist Practice*. APTA web site. http://guidetoptpractice.apta.org/. Accessed July 11, 2013.
4. *Tay-Sachs disease*. PubMed Health web site. http://www.ncbi.nlm.nih.gov/pubmedhealth/PMH0002390/. Accessed July 11, 2013.
5. *The Diseases*. National Tay-Sachs & Allied Diseases web site. http://www.ntsad.org/index.php/tay-sachs. Accessed July 11, 2013.

ADDITIONAL REFERENCES

- Developmental Profile III. Children and Adolescents with Special Needs. http://portal.wpspublish.com/portal/page?_pageid=53,186601&_dad=portal&_schema=PORTAL. Accessed July 11, 2013.
- Dutton M. Pediatric physical therapy. In: *McGraw Hill's National Physical Therapy Examination*. 2nd ed. New York, NY: McGraw-Hill; 2012. http://www.accessphysiotherapy.com/content/5404434#5404434. Accessed July 11, 2013.
- *The Neonatal Behavioral Assessment Scale*. The Brazelton Institute web site. http://www.brazelton-institute.com/intro.html. Accessed July 11, 2013.

256 TORCH INFECTIONS

Sharon Irish Bevins, PhD, PT

CONDITION/DISORDER SYNONYMS

- Other: Coxsackievirus, syphilis, varicella-zoster virus, HIV, and parvovirus B19; congenital Lyme disease
- STORCH syndrome
- TORCH
- TORCH
- TORCH complex
- TORCHES
- Toxoplasmosis, Otherother, rubella virus, cytomegalovirus (CMV), herpes simplex virus

ICD-9-CM CODES

- 052.0 Postvaricella encephalitis
- 055.0 Postmeasles encephalitis
- 056.0 Rubella with neurological complications
- 090.4 Juvenile neurosyphilis

ICD-10-CM CODES

- A50.40 Late congenital neurosyphilis, unspecified
- A50.45 Juvenile general paresis
- B01.11 Varicella encephalitis and encephalomyelitis
- B05.0 Measles complicated by encephalitis
- B06.00 Rubella with neurological complication, unspecified

PREFERRED PRACTICE PATTERN

- 5C Impaired Motor Function and Sensory Integrity Associated with Nonprogressive Disorders of the Central Nervous System—congenital origin or acquired in infancy or childhood

PATIENT PRESENTATION

A 7-month-old male child is brought to a physical therapist to be evaluated for a delay in motor skills acquisition. According to parental report, he has been slower to achieve motor milestones than his siblings. He has recently begun rolling from supine to prone and prone to supine and reportedly is beginning to sit momentarily. He was diagnosed with chorioretinitis shortly after birth which was successfully treated with antibiotics and steroids, although he continues to demonstrate mild photosensitivity. Parents report that he had seizures in the first few weeks of life that are well controlled on his current medication. Prenatal maternal history is positive for mild flu-like symptoms in the second trimester that went unreported.

Upon physical examination, the infant plays in supine, while holding a small toy with both hands. He rolls to prone in both directions to secure a toy held out of reach. He is vocally responsive to his parents and the examiner. He smiles and turns toward a musical toy when it is introduced. Minimal redness of his eyes

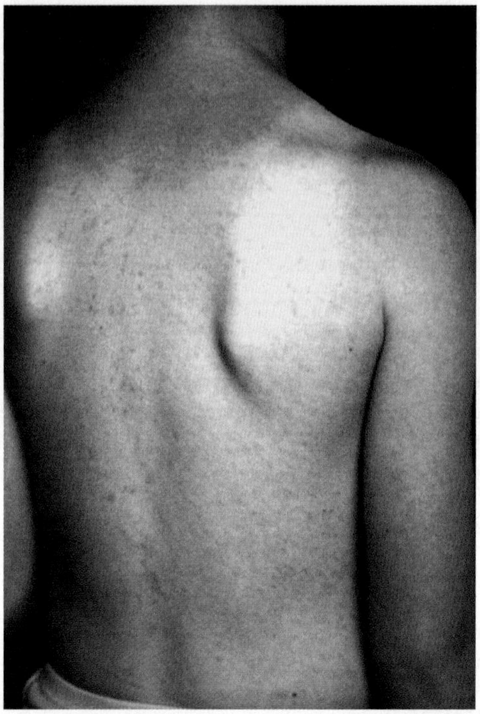

FIGURE 256-1 Mild maculopapular rash of rubella in a child. (From Longo DL, Fauci AS, Kasper DL, Hauser SL, Jameson JL, Loscalzo J, edseds. *Harrison's Principles of Internal Medicine*. 18th ed. New York, NY: McGraw-Hill; 2012.)

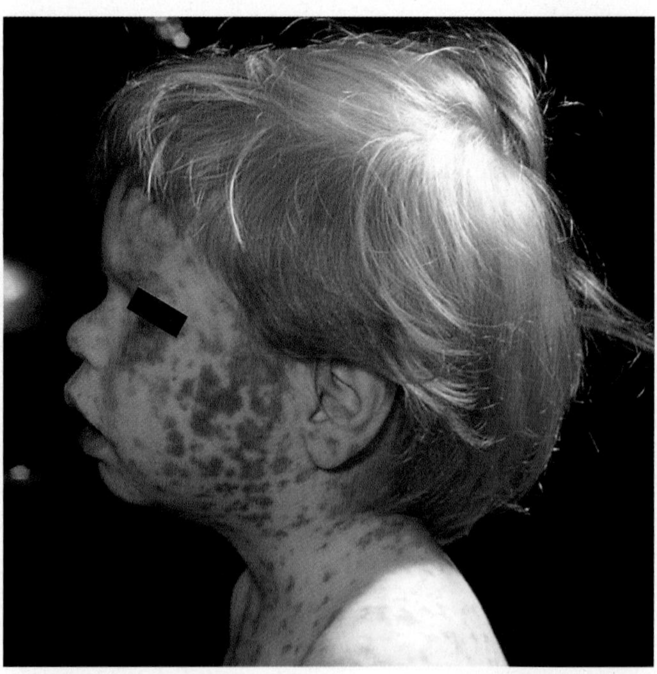

FIGURE 256-2 Rubella. (Courtesy of the Centers for Disease Control and Prevention.)

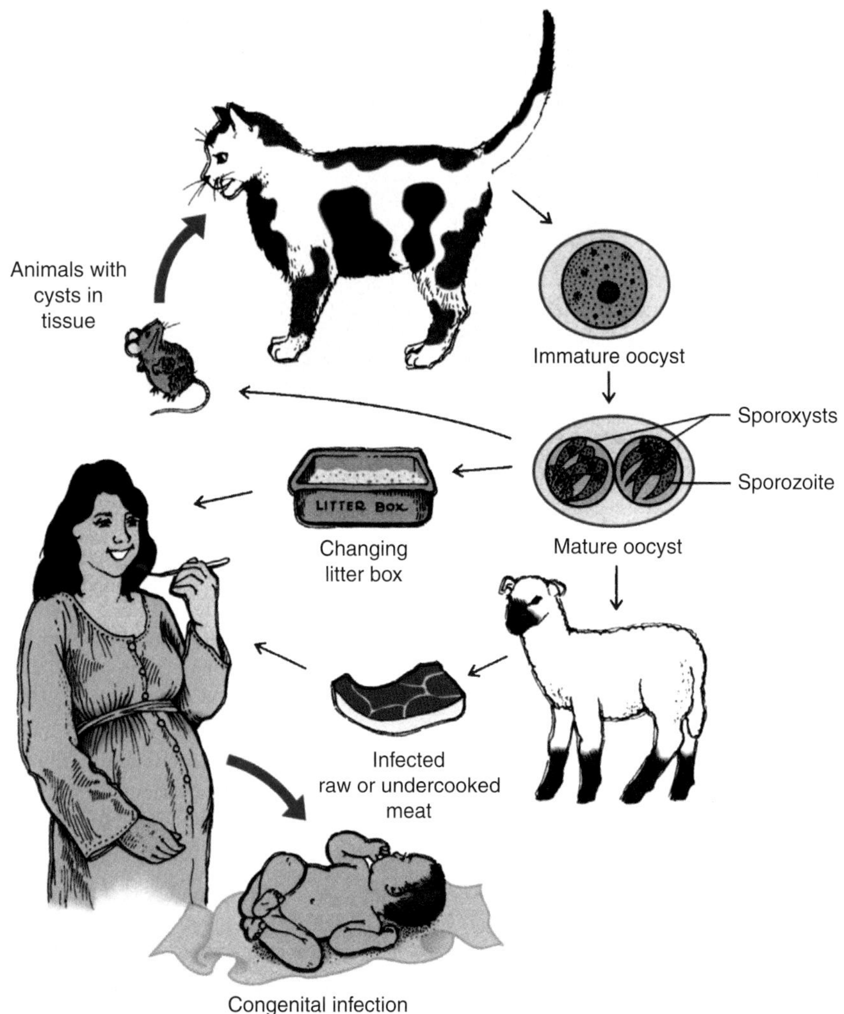

FIGURE 256-3 Toxoplasmosis. *Toxoplasma gondii* life cycle shows oocysts from cat feces or cysts from inadequately cooked meat as infectious to humans and other animals. (Reproduced with permission from Nester EW, Anderson DG, Roberts CE Jr, Nester MT. *Microbiology: A Human Perspective*. 6th ed. New York, NY: McGraw-Hill; 2008.)

with some excess tearing is noted. When placed in sitting, propped forward on extended upper extremities, he is able to maintain the position briefly before falling forward. Laboratory studies revealed antibodies against toxoplasmosis. A recent brain scan revealed cerebral calcifications.

KEY FEATURES

Description

- Acronym for perinatal infections
  - T: Toxoplasmosis
  - O: Other infections
  - R: Rubella
  - C: CMV
  - H(HE): Herpes simplex virus 2
  - S: Syphilis
- Can lead to fetal loss or severe fetal anomalies
- Congenital syndrome characterized by a variety of central nervous system (CNS), growth, cognitive, visual, and auditory deficits
- Hepatitis B: Maternal to fetal during birth, option for caesarean section to avoid contact
- Varicella encephalitis and encephalomyelitis

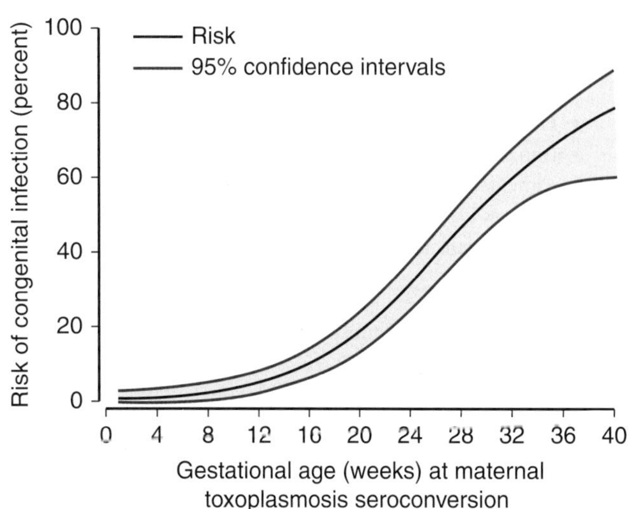

FIGURE 256-4 Risk of congenital toxoplasmosis infection by gestational age at maternal seroconversion. (From D Dunn, M Wallon, F Peyron, et al. Mother-to-child transmission of toxoplasmosis: Risk estimates for clinical counseling. *The Lancet*. Vol. 353, No. 9167, pp. 1829–1833, Copyright 1999, with permission from Elsevier.)

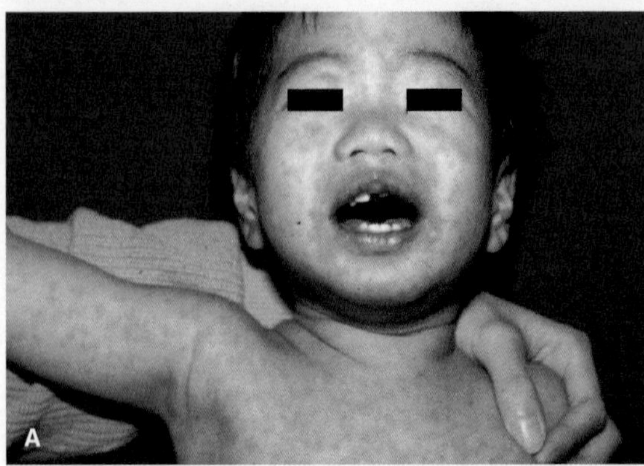

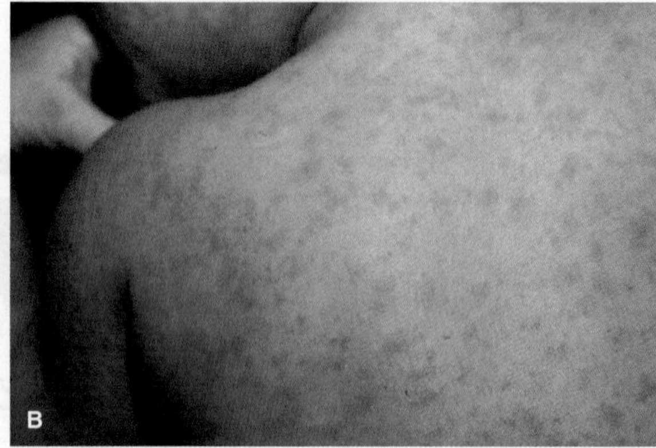

FIGURE 256-5 Toddler with classic morbilliform exanthem of measles. (From Goldsmith LA, Katz SI, Gilchrest BA, Paller A, Leffell DJ, Wolff K. *Fitzpatrick's Dermatology in General Medicine*. 8th ed. www.accessmedicine.com. Copyright © The McGraw-Hill Companies, Inc. All rights reserved.)

Essentials of Diagnosis

- Prenatal viral, bacterial, parasitic infectious exposure resulting in congenital birth defects
- Passed from mother to fetus in the womb across the placenta or during delivery

General Considerations

- Infections that are mild may go unnoticed in a pregnant woman but can have devastating consequences for the unborn child.
- The timing of the prenatal exposure greatly impacts the long-term infant outcome; first trimester exposure is tied to more-severe deficits.
- There is significant variability in newborn outcomes across different infectious organisms.
  - Associated disorders
    - Intrauterine growth retardation resulting in infant being small for gestational age
    - Cognitive impairment ranging from mild deficits to severe mental retardation
    - Visual deficits including chorioretinitis due to CNS involvement of the second cranial nerve
    - Auditory deficits secondary to eighth cranial nerve involvement
    - Skin lesions, eye lesions, and rash
    - Hepatosplenomegaly
    - Impaired motor development due to damage to the brain while developing
    - Seizures
    - Cardiac defects

Demographics

- Overall rate of 17.3 infants per 1000 births receiving antibiotics for suspected neonatal sepsis.[1]
- CMV: 1 in 150 children is born with congenital CMV disease
  - Approximately 1 of every 5 children born with congenital CMV infection will develop permanent problems (such as hearing loss or developmental disabilities) due to the infection.[1]
  - 0.3% to 2% of live-born infants contract CMV, making it the most common intrauterine infection.[2]
- Syphilis: With untreated early syphilis in pregnant women, 25% of pregnancies result in stillbirth and 14% in neonatal death, an overall perinatal mortality is about 40%.[3,4]
- Rubella congenital syndrome is rare, as indicated by an incidence of fewer than 1 person in 2000.[5]
- Toxoplasmosis: Approximately 3500 infected children are born in the United States every year, and the risk of transplacental transmission is greatest during the third trimester of pregnancy; international data varies widely.[6]
- Herpes simplex: Overall, approximately 2% of women acquire herpes simplex virus during pregnancy.[7,8]

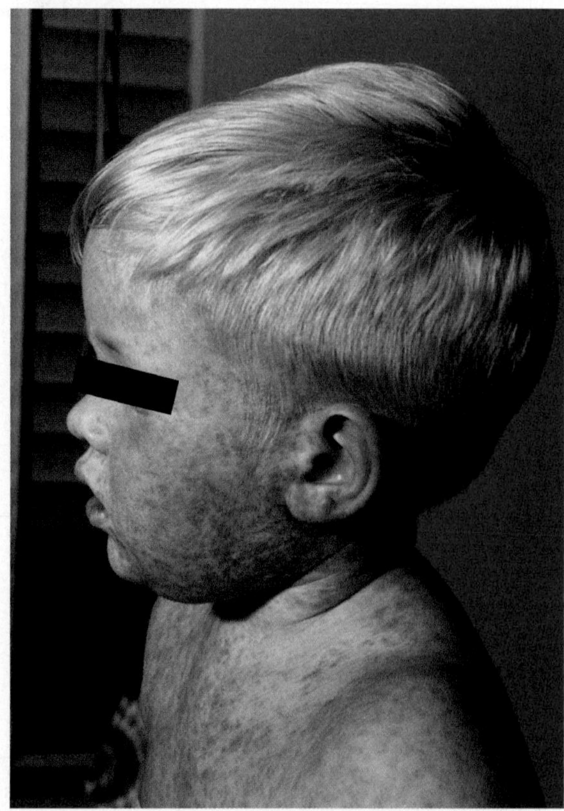

FIGURE 256-6 Measles—Note splotchy "morbilliform" macular-papular rash. (Figure courtesy of Public Health Image Library, Centers for Disease Control and Prevention.)

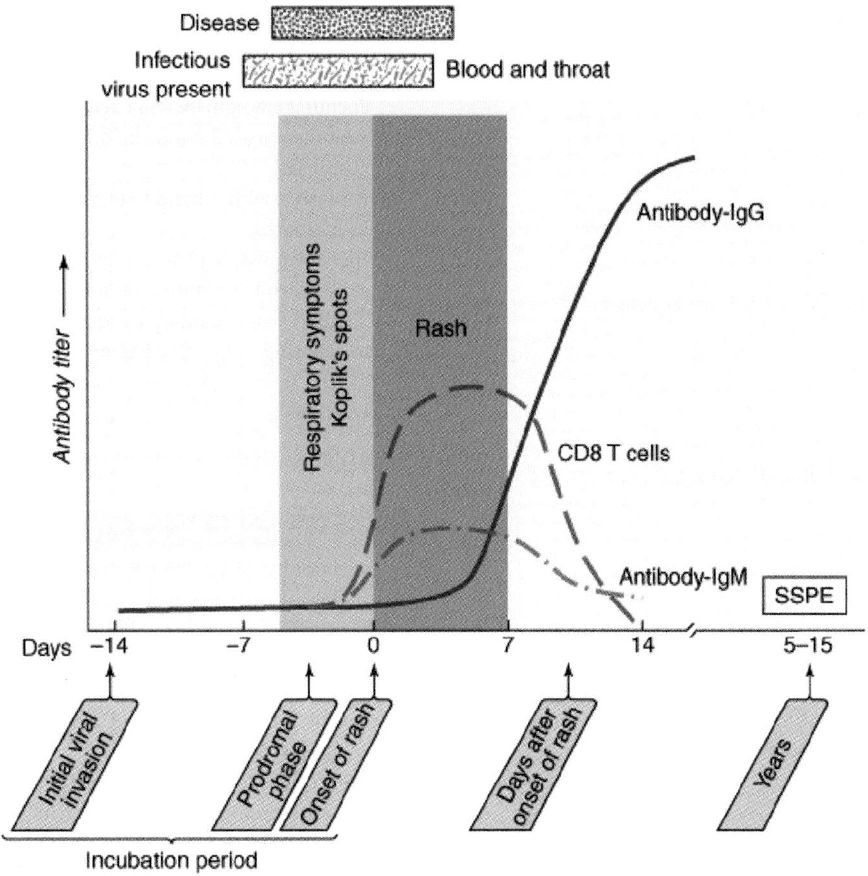

FIGURE 256-7 Natural history of measles infection. Viral replication begins in the respiratory epithelium and spreads to monocyte-macrophages, endothelial cells, and epithelial cells in the blood, spleen, lymph nodes, lung, thymus, liver, and skin and to the mucosal surfaces of the gastrointestinal, respiratory, and genitourinary tracts. The virus-specific immune response is detectable when the rash appears. Clearance of virus is approximately coincident with fading of the rash. (SSPE, subacute sclerosing panencephalitis.) (From Brooks GF, Carroll KC, Butel J, Morse S. *Jawetz, Melnick & Adelberg's Medical Microbiology*. 25th ed. www.accessmedicine.com. Copyright © The McGraw-Hill Companies, Inc. All rights reserved.)

CLINICAL FINDINGS

SIGNS AND SYMPTOMS

- Hypo/hypertonia
- Persistence of developmental reflexes
- Fever
- Poor eating
- Petechial rash
- Jaundice
- Hearing impairment
- Visual impairment

Functional Implications

- Delay or failure to achieve typical milestones in gross and fine motor development
- Difficulties in feeding/eating behaviors with potentially poor weight gain
- Speech and language impairments
- Mental retardation
- Delays in
  - Gross motor skills
  - Fine motor skills
  - Oral motor skills
  - Perceptual motor skills

Possible Contributing Causes

- Compromised maternal immune system

Differential Diagnosis

- Hemolytic disease of the newborn (ABO or Rh incompatibility)
- Other intrauterine growth retardation syndromes
- Cerebral palsy
- Microcephaly/Retardation
- Aicardi–Goutieres syndrome

MEANS OF CONFIRMATION OR DIAGNOSIS

Laboratory Testing

- TORCH panel, also known as the TORCH test,[9] screens blood, urine, spinal fluid for antibodies to infectious agents in mother and newborn
- Pap test for the pregnant mother

Imaging

- Ultrasound to identify brain calcifications

FINDINGS AND INTERPRETATION

- TORCH panel can determine whether there has been recent exposure, past infection, or no exposure.

REFERRALS/ADMITTANCE

- To cardiologist
- To neurologist
- To ophthalmologist
- To audiologist
- To occupational therapy
- To speech therapist
- To nutritionist
- To orthotist
- To educational specialist for vision/hearing deficits [10,11]

IMPAIRMENTS

- Hearing impairment
- Visual impairment
- Can be quite variable depending on timing of exposure and the organism implicated
  - Abnormality of tone
  - Decreased strength
  - Inability to roll
  - Inability to sit
  - Inability to crawl or creep
  - Inability to ambulate
  - Poor static and dynamic sitting or standing balance
  - Gait deviations dependent upon muscle tone

TESTS AND MEASURES

- Alberta Infant Motor Scale
- Bayley Scales of motor development or Bayley II
- Bruininks–Oseretsky test of motor proficiency
- Early Intervention Developmental Profile
- Functional Independence Measure for Children (WeeFIM)
- Gross motor function classification system
- Gross motor function measure
- Hearing test
- Movement assessment of infants
- Neonatal Behavioral Assessment Scale
- Peabody scales of motor development
- Pediatric Evaluation of Disability Inventory
- Test of Infant Motor Performance
- Vision test

INTERVENTION

- Developmental activities to facilitate normal movement patterns and acquisition of motor milestones
- Minimize impact of visual and auditory deficits on motor skill acquisition
- Therapeutic exercise including strengthening
- Functional activities
  - Transfers
  - Gait training
  - Stair climbing

FUNCTIONAL GOALS

- The patient will be able to
  - Sit independently for 10 minutes while playing with toys to increase independence in 6 months.
  - Creep on hands and knees for 5 ft with minimal assistance to increase mobility in 3 months.
  - Stand at furniture for 2 minutes with moderate assistance to encourage weight-bearing activities in 1 month.
  - Ambulate independently using push cart 50% of the time to encourage weight-bearing activities in 3 months.
  - Ambulate with 2 hands held for 25 ft to increase mobility in 6 months.
  - Ambulate with 1 hand held for 10 ft to increase independence in 2 months.
  - Increase quadriceps strength to ascend stairs in a step-over-step pattern while holding railing in 4 months.
  - Transfer from standing to squatting to pick up a toy and return to standing to increase balance and strength in 6 months.

PROGNOSIS

- Variable depending on timing of exposure and type of organism.

PATIENT RESOURCES

- Infections in the Newborn. A Summary of the Curriculum of the First Two Years at the School of Medicine of Case Western Reserve University http://d3jonline.tripod.com/12-Infectious_Disease/Infections_in_the_Newborn.htm. Accessed July 8, 2013.
- Perkins School for the Blind. http://www.Perkins.org. Accessed July 8, 2013.
- The TORCH Panel. Lab Tests Online. http://labtestsonline.org/understanding/analytes/torch/tab/test. Accessed July 8, 2013.

REFERENCES

1. Osterman MJ, Martin JA, Mathews TJ, Hamilton BE. Expanded data from the new birth certificate, 2008. *Natl Vital Stat Rep.* 2011;59(7):1–28.
2. Cytomegalovirus (CMV) and Congenital CMV Infection. Centers for disease control and prevention. http://www.cdc.gov/cmv/overview.html. Accessed July 8, 2013.
3. Guerra B, Simonazzi G, Puccetti C, et al. Ultrasound prediction of symptomatic congenital cytomegalovirus infection. *Am J Obstet Gynecol.* 2008;198(4):380.e1–e7. doi: 10.1016/j.ajog.2007.09.052.
4. Syphilis: CDC Fact Sheet. Centers for disease control and prevention. http://www.cdc.gov/std/syphilis/STDFact-Syphilis.htm. Accessed July 8, 2013.
5. Sexually transmitted infections. World Health Organization. August 2011. http://www.who.int/mediacentre/factsheets/fs110/en/. Accessed July 8, 2013.
6. Congenital Rubella Syndrome. www.orpha.net. http://www.orpha.net/consor/cgi-bin/OC_Exp.php?Lng=GB&Expert=290. Accessed July 8, 2013.
7. Brook I. Pediatric toxoplasmosis. Medscape. http://emedicine.medscape.com/article/1000028-overview#a0156. Accessed July 8, 2013.
8. Brown ZA, Selke S, Zeh J, et al. The acquisition of herpes simplex virus during pregnancy. *N Engl J Med.* 1997;337(8):509–515.
9. Gardella C, Brown Z, Wald A, et al. Risk factors for herpes simplex virus transmission to pregnant women: a couples study. *Am J Obstet Gynecol.* 2005;193(6):1891–1899. doi: 10.1016/j.ajog.2005.07.041.

10. The TORCH Panel. Lab Tests Online. http://labtestsonline.org/understanding/analytes/torch/tab/test. Accessed July 8, 2013.
11. National Consortium on Deaf/Blindness. http://www.nationaldb.org. Accessed July 8, 2013.

ADDITIONAL REFERENCES

- Developmental Profile III. Children and Adolescents with Special Needs. http://portal.wpspublish.com/portal/page?_pageid=53,186601&_dad=portal&_schema=PORTAL. Accessed July 14, 2013.
- Hay WW, Levin MJ, Sondheimer JM, Deterding RR. Protozoal infections. In: Hay WW, Levin MJ, Sondheimer JM, Deterding RR, eds. *CURRENT Diagnosis & Treatment: Pediatrics*. 20th ed. New York, NY: McGraw-Hill; 2011. http://www.accessphysiotherapy.com/content/6591765. Accessed July 12, 2013.
- Pattern 5C: impaired motor function and sensory integrity associated with nonprogressive disorders of the central nervous system—congenital origin or acquired in infancy or childhood. In: *Guide to Physical Therapist Practice*. 2nd ed. Alexandria, VA: American Physical Therapy Association; 2001. Revised 2003.

257 TORTICOLLIS, CONGENITAL

Kay Tasso, PhD, PT, PCS
Eric Shamus, PhD, DPT, PT, CSCS
Ariel Diana Schumer, DPT

CONDITION/DISORDER SYNONYMS

- Congenital contracture of the sternocleidomastoid
- Congenital wry neck
- Congenital sternocleidomastoid torticollis
- Torticollis
- Loxia

ICD-9-CM CODE

- 754.1 Congenital musculoskeletal deformities of sternocleidomastoid muscle

ICD-10-CM CODE

- Q68.0 Congenital deformity of sternocleidomastoid muscle

PREFERRED PRACTICE PATTERNS[1]

- 4B: Impaired Posture
- 4E: Impaired Joint Mobility, Motor Function, Muscle Performance, and ROM Associated with Localized Inflammation

PATIENT PRESENTATION

A 6-month-old is referred to physical therapy with a diagnosis of torticollis. The mother reports she had too little maternal amniotic fluid during the pregnancy and premature rupture of the membranes 2 weeks before the baby was due but no other difficulties during delivery. She reports the infant was born with torticollis but that it is better than at birth. Upon examination, the therapist notes the baby postures into right lateral cervical flexion and left cervical rotation. There is a flattening of the occipital region on the right. The infant will only roll from prone to supine toward the left and supine to prone over the right arm. When placed in prone, the baby puts more weight on the right arm than the left in prone on elbows. When held in supported sitting or standing, the physical therapist notes asymmetry in postural alignment.

KEY FEATURES

Description

- Torticollis is a postural position of the neck with side-bending and opposite rotation.
- Term used to describe asymmetrical posturing of neck due to shortened sternocleidomastoid.
- Contracted state of the cervical muscles with sternocleidomastoid enlargement.

Essentials of Diagnosis

- Congenital torticollis is believed to result from improper position of the fetus in utero with changes in the blood supply or muscles of the neck or trauma during delivery.

General Considerations

- Can have an etiology or can be idiopathic congenital muscular torticollis is the most common type[2]
- Hip dysplasia in 20% of cases
- At risk for scoliosis
- Head tilted to one side and rotated to opposite side typically noted in first 6 to 8 weeks of life

Demographics

- 1 in 250 infants[3]
- Right torticollis most common (75% of the time)
- Most common in first born children[4]

CLINICAL FINDINGS

SIGNS AND SYMPTOMS

- Asymmetrical cervical skin folds
- Asymmetrical posturing of neck with lateral flexion on the affected side and rotation toward the unaffected side
- Decreased passive and/or active range of motion
- Enlargement of the neck muscles
- Facial asymmetries
- Flattened posterior skull
- Pain
- Palpable mass on sternocleidomastoid until 4 to 6 months of age
- Possible difficulty swallowing[5]
- Postural asymmetries
- Shoulder elevation on affected side
- Swelling of neck muscles at birth with congenital

Functional Implications

- Postural control abnormalities
- May have limited active and/or passive movement of the head
- Facial asymmetries
- Cranial asymmetries (deformational plagiocephaly)
- Gross motor asymmetries
- Developmental delay[6]
- Greater reliance on vision for maintaining postural stability[7]

Possible Contributing Causes

- Difficult labor (birth)
- Awkward positioning in utero
- Trauma during delivery resulting in hematoma of sternocleidomastoid that may result in a palpable mass[8]
- Infection
- Gastrointestinal reflux[7]
- Sprengel deformity
- Musculoskeletal anomalies such as hemivertebrae

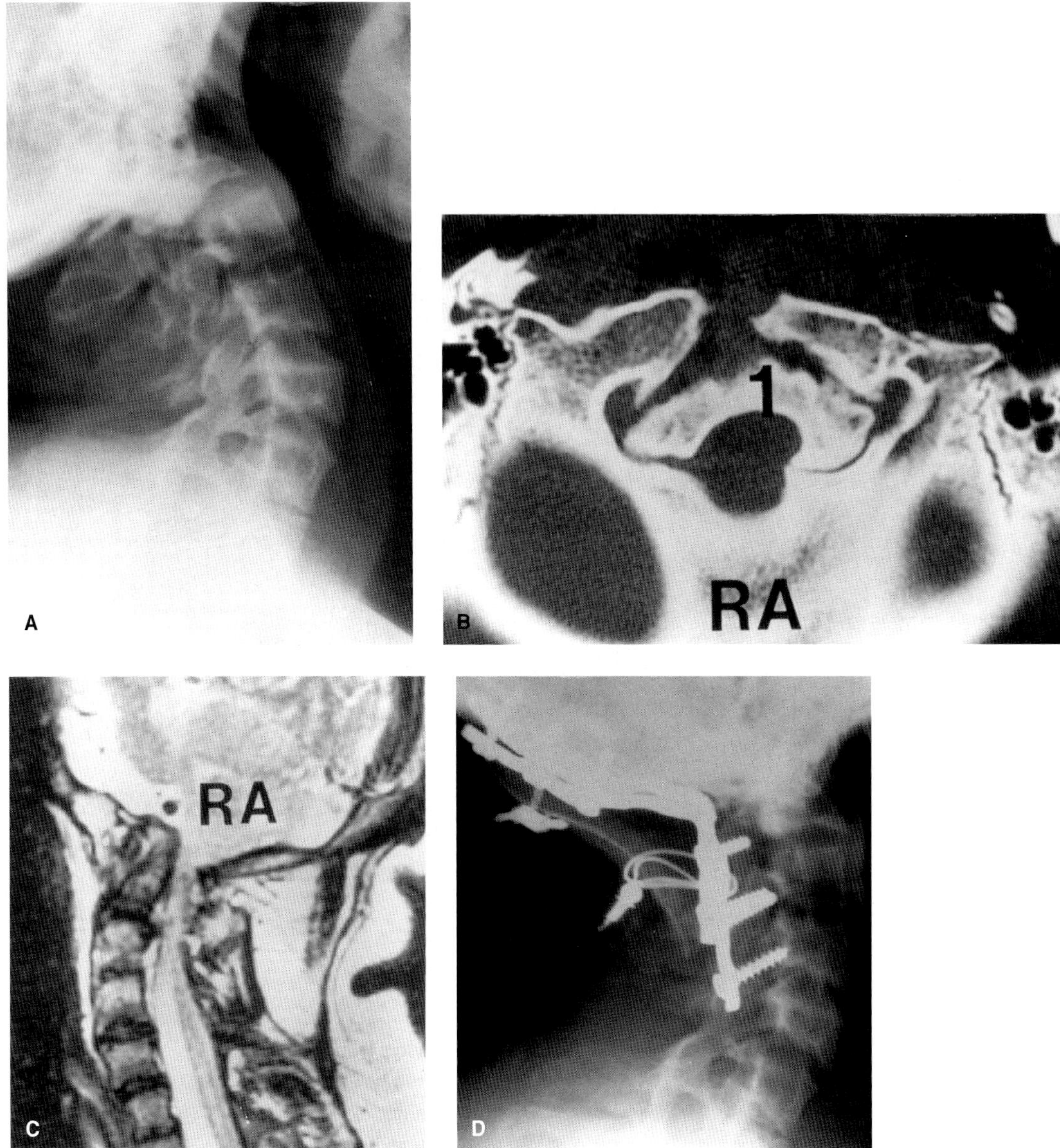

FIGURE 257-1 Imaging studies in a patient with Klippel–Feil syndrome and cervical myelopathy. (**A**) Radiograph showing fusion of the atlas and the occiput and autofusion of the posterior elements of C3 and C4. (**B**) CT scan demonstrates this as well. (**C**) MRI demonstrating severe stenosis of the spinal canal. The odontoid process is above the level of the foramen magnum. (**D**) Radiograph following posterior decompression and fusion between the occiput and C4. (From Skinner HB. *Current Diagnosis & Treatment in Orthopedics*. 4th ed. www.accessmedicine.com. Copyright © The McGraw-Hill Companies, Inc. All rights reserved.)

- Neurological disorder such as Klippel–Feil syndrome
- Ocular abnormalities

Differential Diagnosis

- Inherited torticollis: Change in chromosomes
- Acquired torticollis: Damage to muscle or nerve
- Idiopathic torticollis: Unknown cause
- Ocular torticollis
- Posterior fossa tumor
- Syringomyelia

MEANS OF CONFIRMATION OR DIAGNOSIS

Imaging

- X-ray
- Electromyography (EMG)
- Ultrasound of hips
- Computerized tomography (CT) scan to rule out osseous anomalies
- Magnetic resonance imaging (MRI) if neurological etiology suspected
- Rule out congenital deformities of the cervical spine, ocular anomalies, CNS pathology,[4] neoplasm, thyroiditis, endocrine disease[3]

Diagnostic Procedures

- Diagnosis is made by clinical observation
- Torticollis rating scale of Tsui

FINDINGS AND INTERPRETATION

- Sternocleidomastoid enlargement
- Flattening of the occipital region

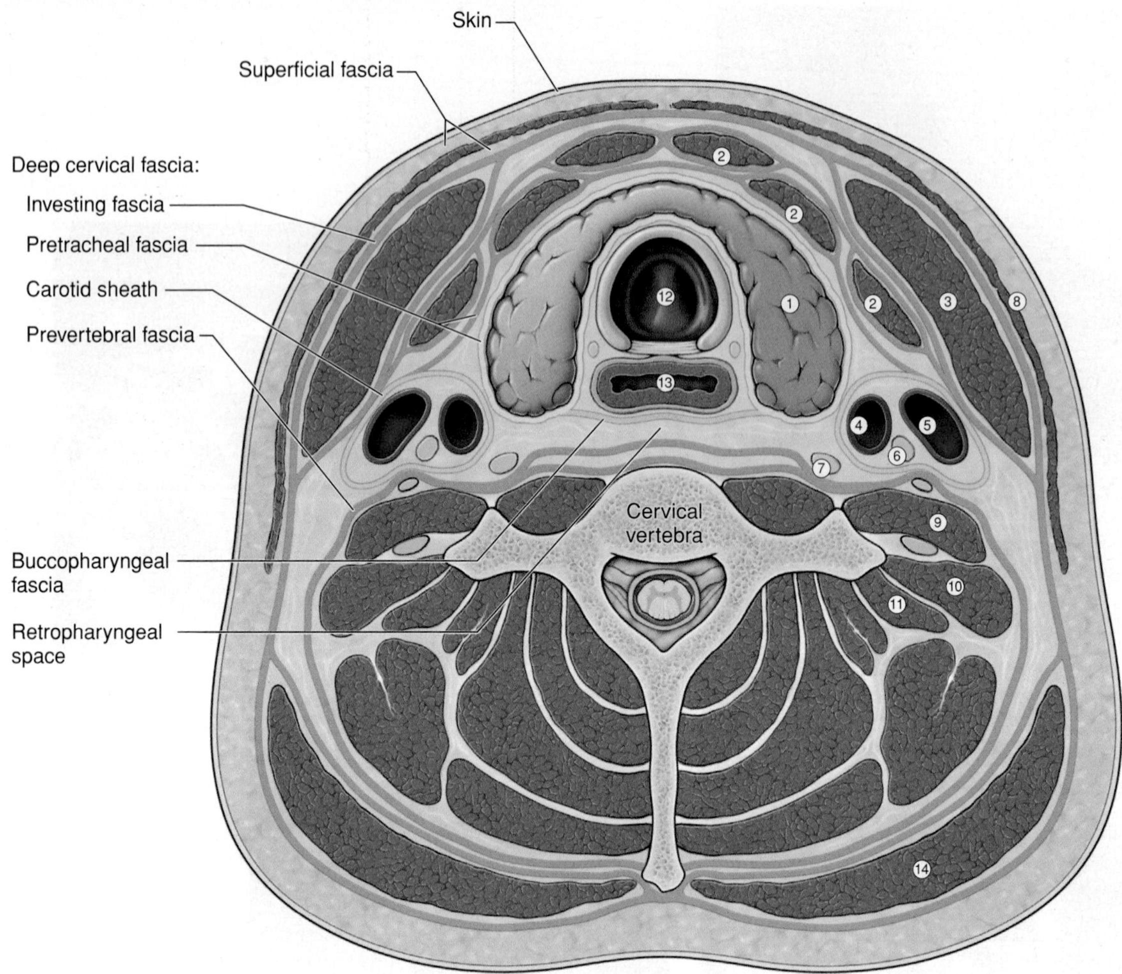

KEY

1. Thyroid gland	8. Platysma m.
2. Infrahyoid mm.	9. Ant. scalene m.
3. Sternocleidomastoid m.	10. Mid. scalene m.
4. Common carotid a.	11. Post. scalene m.
5. Internal jugular v.	12. Trachea
6. Vagus n.	13. Esophagus
7. Sympathetic trunk	14. Trapezius m.

FIGURE 257-2 Cross-section of the neck through the thyroid gland, showing the layers of the cervical fascia. (From Morton DA, Foreman KB, Albertine KH. *The Big Picture: Gross Anatomy*. www.accessmedicine.com. Copyright © The McGraw-Hill Companies, Inc. All rights reserved.)

TREATMENT

Medical Procedures

- Deformational plagiocephaly treated with molded helmet
- Surgical correction if not resolved by 1 year of age or if rotation component remains after 6 months of stretching[3]
  - Selective peripheral denervation
    - For laterocollis, denervation of ipsilateral posterior cervical paraspinals, splenius capitis, and sternocleidomastoid muscles
    - For rotary torticollis, similar to laterocollis with the exception of denervation of the contralateral sternocleidomastoid

REFERRALS/ADMITTANCE

- To orthopedist
- To neurologist
- To gastroenterologist for gastroesophageal reflux
- To orthotist if molded helmet needed
- To physician
  - If cervical subluxation is suspected
  - If patient does not respond to PT
- To occupational and speech therapists as necessary
- To surgeon if alternatives have failed

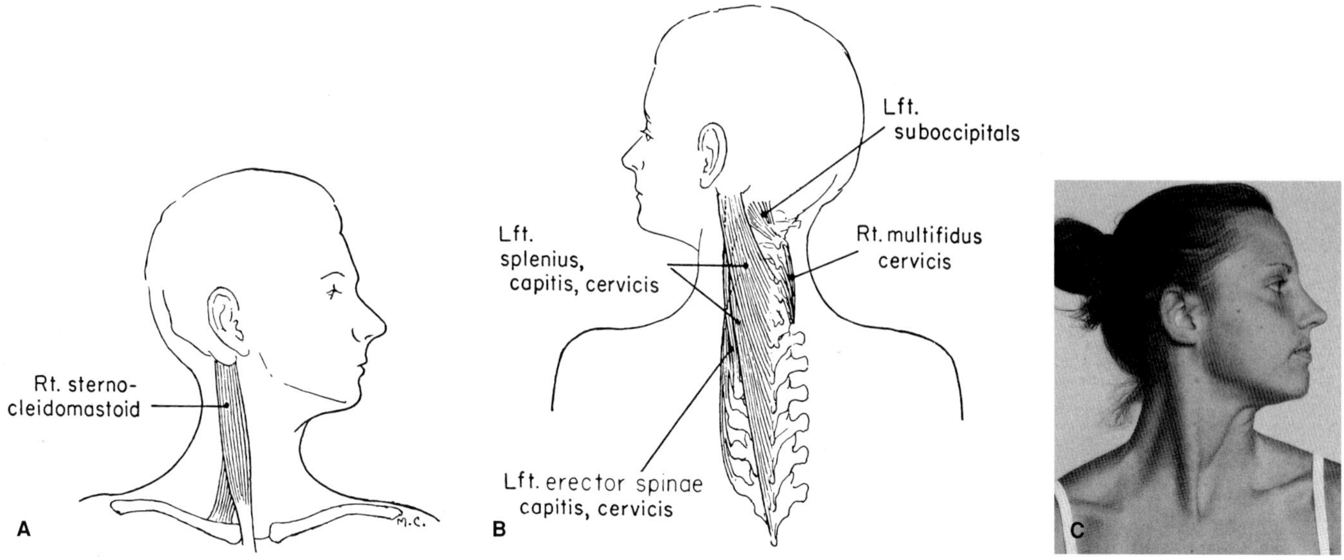

FIGURE 257-3 Muscles that contract to rotate the head and neck to the left. (From Hamilton N, Weimar W, Luttgens K. *Kinesiology: Scientific Basis of Human Motion*. 11th ed. http://www.accessphysiotherapy.com. Copyright © McGraw-Hill Education. All rights reserved.)

IMPAIRMENTS

- Pain
- Decreased cervical ROM
- Decreased cervical strength
- Difficulty maintaining head in midline
- Poor postural alignment
- Balance deficits

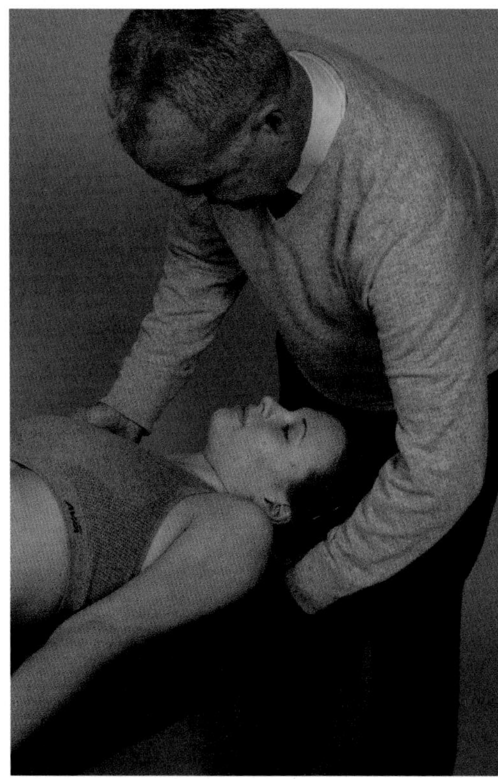

FIGURE 257-4 Muscle length test of the right sternocleidomastoid. (From Dutton M. *Dutton's Orthopaedic Examination, Evaluation, and Intervention*. 3rd ed. http://www.accessphysiotherapy.com. Copyright © The McGraw-Hill Companies, Inc. All rights reserved.)

TESTS AND MEASURES

- Goniometer
- Alberta Infant Motor Scale (AIMS)
- Ortolani
- Barlow maneuver

INTERVENTION

- Stretching of involved sternocleidomastoid
- Strengthening of uninvolved SCM
- Parent education regarding optimal methods for carrying and positioning infant for stretching
- Prone positioning
- Massage
- Taping
- Developmental activities
- Tubular orthosis for torticollis (TOT) collar

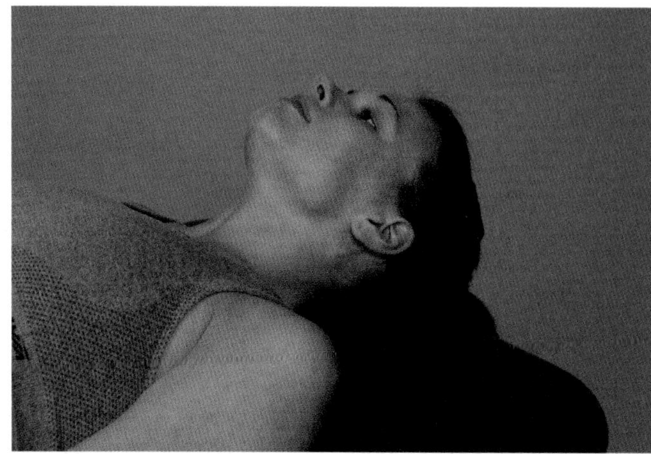

FIGURE 257-5 Patient demonstrating weak neck flexors in the presence of a strong SCM. (From Dutton M. *Dutton's Orthopaedic Examination, Evaluation, and Intervention*. 3rd ed. http://www.accessphysiotherapy.com. Copyright © The McGraw-Hill Companies, Inc. All rights reserved.)

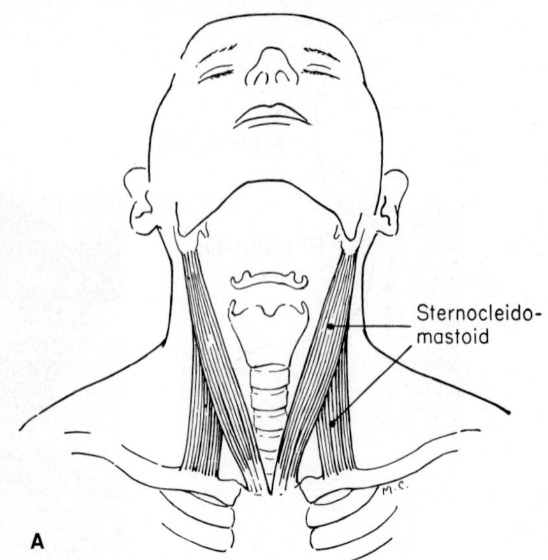

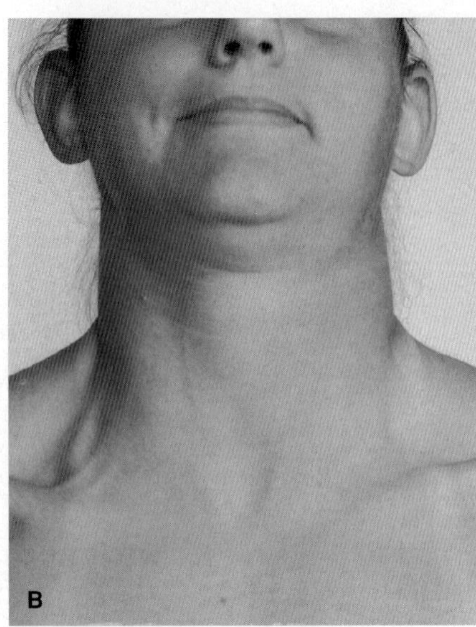

FIGURE 257-6 Sternocleidomastoid muscle. (From Hamilton N, Weimar W, Luttgens K. *Kinesiology: Scientific Basis of Human Motion*. 11th ed. http://www.access-physiotherapy.com. Copyright © McGraw-Hill Education. All rights reserved.)

- A thorough examination includes, but is not limited to
  - Head position, cervical ROM, postural alignment and control, muscle length and strength throughout the spine and shoulder region, tone, and balance.

FUNCTIONAL GOALS

- Patient will be able to
  - Demonstrate full active cervical lateral flexion and rotation bilaterally to track toys during play within 6 months.
  - Weight shift to both directions equally while propping prone on elbows to allow reaching for toys within 3 months.
  - Rolls prone to supine and supine to prone toward both sides to increase mobility within 2 months.
  - Sits independently for 5 minutes with cervical and spinal extension and alignment within 4 months.
  - Creep on hands and knees for 5 feet with minimal assistance to increase mobility within 6 months.

PROGNOSIS

- 80% of infants recover by the age of 1 year.[9]
- Idiopathic usually resolves quickly.
- Persistent torticollis can lead to restricted movements, postural deformity, degenerative osteoarthritis of the cervical spine, and spinal radiculopathies.[10]

PATIENT RESOURCES

- Instructions for Stretching and Positioning Right Sternomastoid Torticollis. Orthopedic Topics web site. http://www.orthoseek.com/articles/ifs-right.html. Accessed July 13, 2013.
- Instructions for Stretching and Positioning Left Sternomastoid Torticollis. Orthopedic Topics web site. http://www.orthoseek.com/articles/ifs-left.html. Accessed July 13, 2013.
- Torticollis. The Pediatric Orthopeadic Society of North America. http://www.posna.org/education/StudyGuide/torticollis.asp. Accessed July 13, 2013.

REFERENCES

1. The American Physical Therapy Association. *Interactive Guide to Physical Therapist Practice*. Alexandria, VA: The American Physical Therapy Association; 2003. http://guidetoptpractice.apta.org. Accessed July 13, 2013.
2. Dutton M. Causes of cervical pain. In: Dutton M, ed. *Dutton's Orthopaedic Examination, Evaluation, and Intervention*. 3rd ed. New York, NY: McGraw-Hill; 2012. http://www.accessphysiotherapy.com/content/56525652. Accessed July 13, 2013.
3. Gray GM, Tasso KH. Differential diagnosis of torticollis: a case study. *Pediatric Physical Therapy*. 2009;21(4):369–374. doi: 10.1097/PEP.0b013e3181beca44.
4. Torticollis. MDGuidelines. http://www.mdguidelines.com/torticollis. Accessed July 13, 2013.
5. Crowner BE. Cervical dystonia: disease profile and clinical management. *Phys Ther*. 2007;87(11):1511–1526. doi: 10.2522/ptj.20060272.
6. Tessmer A, Mooney P, Pelland L. A developmental perspective on congenital muscular torticollis: a critical appraisal of the evidence. *Pediatric Physical Therapy*. 2010;22(4):378–383.
7. Goodman CC, Snyder TEK. Screening the head, neck, and back. In: Goodman CC, Snyder TEK, eds. *Differential Diagnosis for Physical Therapists: Screening for Referral*. St. Louis, MO: Saunders; 2007:640.
8. Goodman CC, Glanzman A, Miedaner J. Genetic and developmental disorders. In: Goodman CC, Boissonnault WG, Fuller KS, eds. *Pathology: Implications for the Physical Therapist*. Philadelphia, PA: Saunders; 2003:858–860.
9. Congenital Muscular Torticolllis. Orthopedic Topics web site. http://www.orthoseek.com/articles/congenmt.html. Accessed July 13, 2013.
10. Fuller KS, Corboy JR, Winkler PS. Degenerative diseases of the central nervous system. In: Goodman CC, Boissonnault WG, Fuller KS, eds. *Pathology: Implications for the Physical Therapist*. Philadelphia, PA: Saunders; 2003:1032–1034.

ADDITIONAL REFERENCES

- Bernard TJ, Knupp K, Yang ML, Arndt D, Levisohn P, Moe PG. Neurologic & muscular disorders. In: Hay WW, Levin MJ, Sondheimer JM, Deterding RR, eds. *CURRENT Diagnosis & Treatment: Pediatrics*. 20th ed. New York, NY: McGraw-Hill; 2011. http://www.accessphysiotherapy.com/content/6585071. Accessed July 13, 2013.
- Binder H, Eng GD, Gaiser JF, Koch B. Congenital muscular torticollis: results of conservative management with long-term follow-up in 85 cases. *Arch Phys Med Rehabil.* 1987;68(4): 222–225.
- Celayir AC. Congenital muscular torticollis: early and intensive treatment is critical. A prospective study. *Pediatr Int.* 2000; 42(5):504–507.
- ICD9Data.com. http://www.icd9data.com. Accessed July 13, 2013.
- ICD10Data.com. http://www.icd10data.com. Accessed July 13, 2013.
- Kiwak KJ. Establishing an etiology for torticollis. *Postgrad Med.* 1984;75(7):126–134.
- Kiesewetter WB, Nelson PK, Pallandino VS, et al. Neonatal torticollis. *JAMA.* 1955;157:1281–1285.
- Martino D, Luizzi D, Macerollo A, Aniello MS, Livrea P, Defazio G. The phenomenology of the geste antagoniste in primary blepharospasm and cervical dystonia. *Mov Disord.* 2010;25(4):407–412. doi: 10.1002/mds.23011.
- Panus PC, Jobst EE, Masters SB, Katzung B, Tinsley SL, Trevor AJ. Skeletal muscle relaxants. In: Panus PC, Jobst EE, Masters SB, Katzung B, Tinsley SL, Trevor AJ, eds. *Pharmacology for the Physical Therapist*. New York, NY: McGraw-Hill; 2009:Chapter 33. http://www.accessphysiotherapy.com/content/6095608. Accessed July 13, 2013.
- Pattern 4E:impaired joint mobility, motor function, muscle performance, and range of motion associated with localized inflammation. In: *Guide to Physical Therapist Practice*. 2nd ed. Alexandria, VA: American Physical Therapy Association; 2001. Revised 2003.
- Sankar WN, Weiss J, Skaggs DL. Orthopaedic conditions in the newborn. *J Am Acad Orthop Surg*. 2009;17(2):112–122.

PART 6

VESTIBULAR DISORDERS

258 ACOUSTIC NEUROMA

Eric Shamus, PhD, DPT, PT, CSCS
Mollie Venglar, DSc, MSPT, NCS

CONDITION/DISORDER SYNONYMS

- Vestibular schwannoma
- Acoustic schwannoma
- Cerebellopontine angle tumor

ICD-9-CM CODE[1]

- 225.1 Benign neoplasm of cranial nerves

ICD-10-CM CODE[2]

- D33.3 Benign neoplasm of cranial nerves

PREFERRED PRACTICE PATTERNS[3]

- 5A: Primary Prevention/Risk Reduction for Loss of Balance and Falling
- 5F: Impaired Peripheral Nerve Integrity and Muscle Performance Associated with Peripheral Nerve Injury

PATIENT PRESENTATION

A 21-year-old college student noticed a ringing in her left ear the day after a big sorority party. She initially thought it was an effect of the loud music at the party, but the ringing persisted and got louder. A couple of weeks later she developed a headache that was reduced but not relieved by acetaminophen. She struggled with studying her textbooks and computerized notes, and began to get dizzy whenever she reached down to the floor or quickly turned her head. She had no limitations in cervical range of motion, strength, or posture. MRI revealed a tumor on the vestibulocochlear nerve.

KEY FEATURES

Description

- Disorder of the vestibulocochlear nerve (eighth cranial nerve) that carries vestibular and auditory input from the inner ear to the central nervous system
- Slow-growing (usually 1–2 mm/yr), benign tumor of the myelin-forming Schwann cells that surround the vestibular portion of the eighth cranial nerve
- Tumor most commonly originates from the inferior vestibular branch
- Tumor forms in the internal auditory canal and can extend into the cerebellopontine angle
- Typically results in a gradual onset of high-frequency sensorineural hearing loss, tinnitus, sense of ear fullness, unsteadiness, dizziness, vertigo

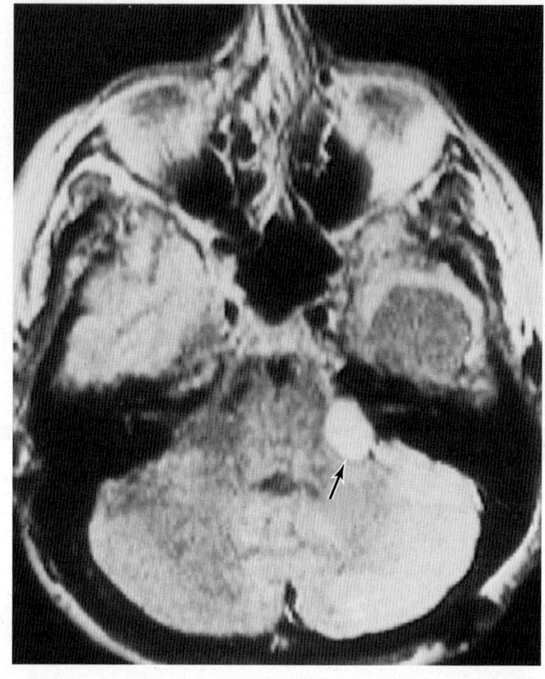

FIGURE 258-1 Magnetic resonance image of a horizontal section through the head at the level of the lower pons and internal auditory meatus. A left acoustic nerve schwannoma with its high intensity is shown in the left cerebellopontine angle (*arrow*). (From Waxman SG. *Clinical Neuroanatomy*. 26th ed. http://www.accessmedicine.com. Copyright © The McGraw-Hill Companies, Inc. All rights reserved.)

- As tumor grows, there may be facial nerve involvement (resulting in facial numbness or weakness), headache, hydrocephalus, incoordination, diplopia, hoarseness, difficulty swallowing, brainstem compression, death
- Tumors classified as sporadic, cystic, or neurofibromatosis type II

Essentials of Diagnosis

- Physical examination normal, unless the cerebellum or brainstem compromised
- Audiogram abnormal
- Imaging studies abnormal
- Neurotologic examination abnormal
- Thorough and detailed history essential to distinguish acoustic neuroma from other vestibular disorders and central pathology

General Considerations

- Patients typically present with complaints of progressive hearing loss and loss of balance worsening gradually over several months
- If tumor growth progresses, may present with other cranial nerve (especially V and VII), brainstem, or cerebellar signs and symptoms

Demographics

- Uncommon in general population, but most common cerebellopontine angle tumor (80% of these tumors)

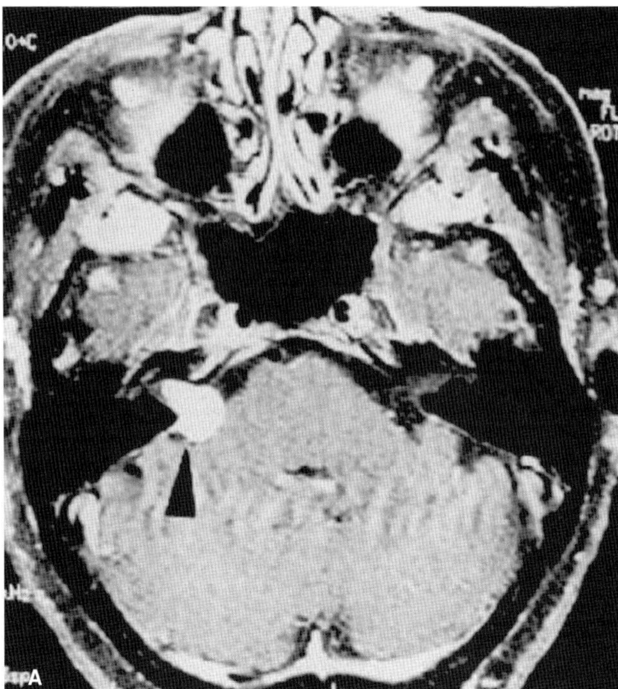

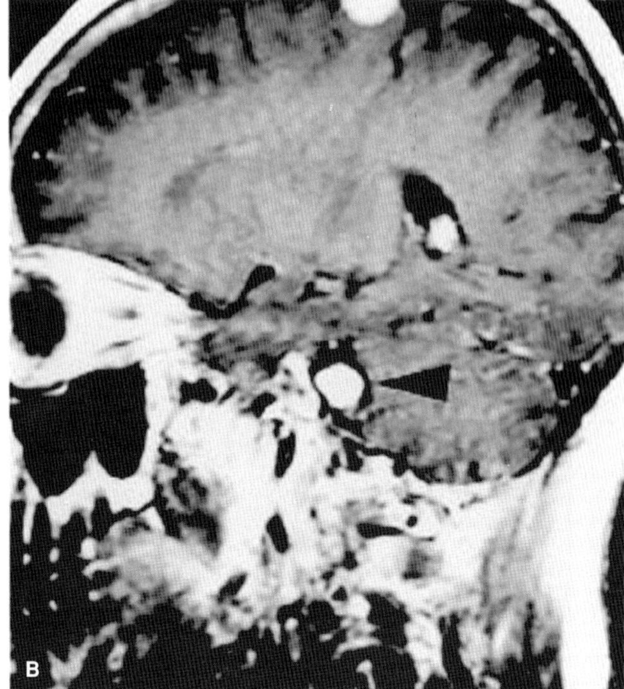

FIGURE 258-2 (**A**) Postcontrast T1-weighted axial magnetic resonance imaging demonstrating a brightly enhancing mass on the right vestibular nerve with an enhancing tail going into the internal auditory canal (*arrowhead*). Pathology demonstrated vestibular schwannoma. (**B**) Postcontrast T1-weighted sagittal magnetic resonance imaging of the same lesion, indicated by the arrowhead. Note small incidental meningioma at the top of the scan. (From Brunicardi FC, Andersen D, Billiar T, et al. *Schwartz's Principles of Surgery*. 9th ed. http://www.accessmedicine.com. Copyright © The McGraw-Hill Companies, Inc. All rights reserved.)

- Unknown etiology
- Typically occurs in fifth or sixth decade of life.
- Mortality has been nearly eliminated; morbidity rates have been significantly reduced due to improved techniques for early diagnosis and improved treatment approaches.

CLINICAL FINDINGS

SIGNS AND SYMPTOMS

- Typical symptoms include tinnitus (ringing or noises in the ear) and sense of ear fullness
- Patients occasionally present with complaints of vertigo or vague report of dizziness
- May complain of blurred vision due to oscillopsia (perceived movement of the environment)
- Unexplained unilateral sensorineural hearing loss with high-frequency loss on audiogram
- Imbalance, as manifested by difficulty standing and walking
- Increased risk of falling
- Vague sense of dizziness; may be constant or increasingly severe with head movement
- Abnormal auditory brainstem response
- Hypoactive or absent caloric response
- May observe nystagmus in room light or with fixation removed
- May present with central symptoms, such as diplopia, dysarthria, dysphagia, dysmetria, numbness, or weakness if tumor has compressed brainstem or cerebellum

Functional Implications

- Impedes balance and contribute to falls
- Provokes dizziness with rapid head movements, such as with turning, bending over, looking up
- Difficulty reading and identifying objects
- Impedes ability to drive and perform everyday tasks

Possible Contributing Causes

- Pathology unknown in majority of cases

Differential Diagnosis

- Arachnoiditis
- Benign paroxysmal positional vertigo
- Bilateral vestibulopathy
- Brainstem stroke or TIA
- Chiari malformation
- Endolymphatic hydrops (Meniere disease)
- Hearing loss of different etiology
- Microvascular compression
- Migraine
- Multiple sclerosis
- Neurofibromatosis type II
- Other posterior fossa tumors
- Perilymphatic fistula
- Superior canal dehiscence
- Thyroid disease
- Vestibular neuritis or labyrinthitis

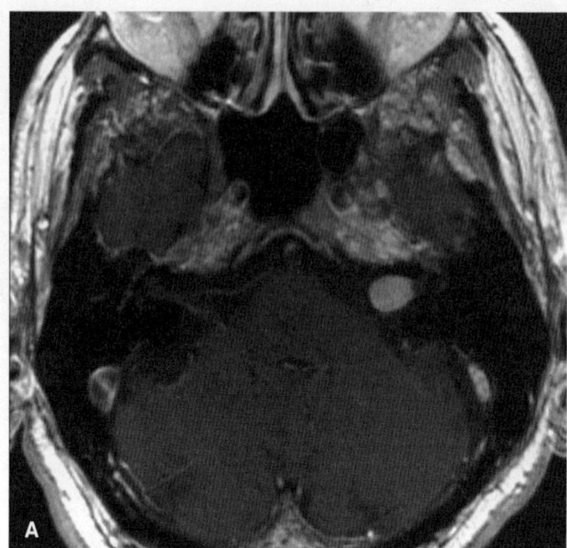

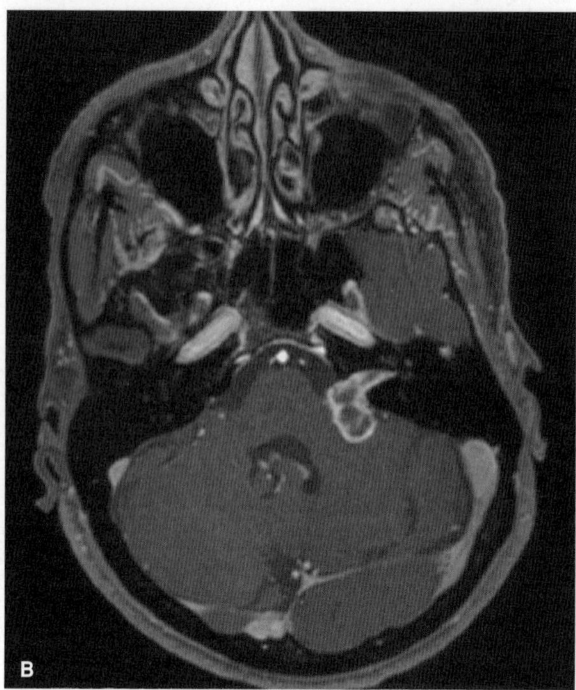

FIGURE 258-3 (**A**) MRI of a small acoustic neuroma emanating from the porus acusticus (canal), showing the typical gadolinium enhancement. (**B**) Larger acoustic neuroma with cystic enhancement and compression of the cerebellopontine angle. (From Ropper AH, Samuels MA. *Adams and Victor's Principles of Neurology.* 9th ed. http://www.accessmedicine.com. Copyright © The McGraw-Hill Companies, Inc. All rights reserved.)

MEANS OF CONFIRMATION OR DIAGNOSIS

Imaging

- MRI with gadolinium-enhanced T1-weighted is gold standard, abnormal
- CT scan of cerebellopontine angle and internal auditory canals within the posterior fossa

Special Tests

- Audiogram
- Auditory brainstem response (ABR; also known as Brainstem auditory evoked responses, BAER)
- Electronystagmography (ENG) or videonystagmography (VNG)
- Rotational chair
- Vestibular evoked myogenic potential (VEMP)
- Subjective visual vertical (SVV; static and dynamic)
- Laboratory testing
- Neurotologic examination (impulse test, headshake test, dynamic visual acuity test, caloric test, VEMP test, or SVV test)

FINDINGS AND INTERPRETATIONS

- Neurotologic examination (impulse test, headshake test, dynamic visual acuity test, caloric test, VEMP test, or SVV test), are all abnormal

TREATMENT

Medical Procedures

- Medical management (indicated for patients with small tumors who are not surgical candidates based on age, health status, hearing status, or patient's choice)
  - "Watch and wait"
  - Periodic serial imaging studies to monitor tumor
  - Corticosteroids to improve acute hearing loss
  - Monitor neurological status
  - Evaluate usefulness of hearing aids
- Microsurgical excision of the vestibular nerve and tumor (most common) to preserve hearing or prevent potentially fatal complications from tumor growth
  - Suboccipital or retrosigmoid approach
    - Can be used with all tumor sizes
    - Hearing preservation is possible
    - Preservation of facial function is favorable
  - Middle cranial fossa approach
    - For small, intracanalicular tumors
    - Preserves hearing
    - Slight increased risk of facial nerve complication
  - Transcranial labyrinthine approach
    - For large tumors
    - Preserves facial nerve
    - Hearing loss expected
- Radiation therapy
  - Stereotactic radiosurgery
  - Fractionated radiation therapy
  - Minimally invasive

REFERRALS/ADMITTANCE

- To hospital emergency department for suspected acute stroke or sudden hearing loss
- To vestibular-trained physical therapist or occupational therapist for rehabilitation
- To neurotologist or neurosurgeon for disease management

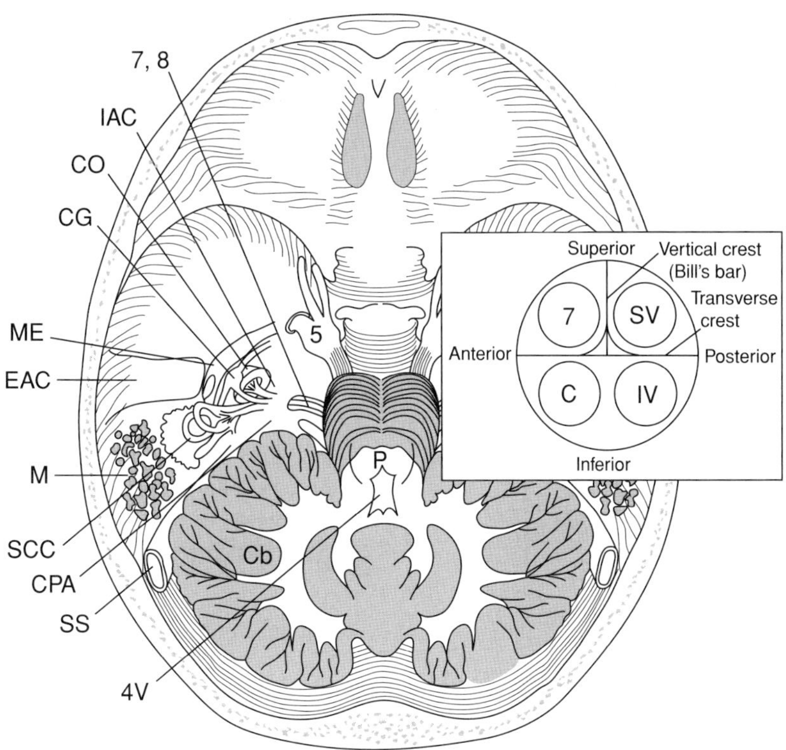

FIGURE 258-4 The anatomy of the CPA and its relationship to the temporal bone within the skull is shown. Inset shows the location of the cranial nerves within the IAC: the facial nerve (7) and the cochlear nerve (C) are in the anterior compartment, whereas the superior and inferior vestibular nerves (SV and IV, respectively) are in the posterior half of the IAC. 5, trigeminal nerve; 7, facial nerve; 8, cochlear nerve; IAC, internal auditory canal; CO, cochlea; GG, geniculate ganglion; ME, middle ear; EAC, external auditory canal; M, mastoid; SCC, semicircular canal; CPA, cerebellopontine angle; SS, sigmoid sinus; 4V, fourth ventricle; Cb, cerebellum; P, pons. (From Lalwani AK. *Current Diagnosis & Treatment in Otolaryngology-Head & Neck Surgery*. 3rd ed. www.accesssurgery.com. Copyright © The McGraw-Hill Companies, Inc. All rights reserved.)

IMPAIRMENTS

- Postural control and balance
- Mobility
- Perceived orientation (dizziness and vertigo)
- Gaze stability
- Facial muscle control, if facial nerve is involved

TESTS AND MEASURES

- Vestibular-ocular reflex (VOR)
  - Dynamic visual acuity
  - Doll's head test
  - Head shaking nystagmus test
  - Head-thrust test
  - The cervico-ocular reflex
- Oculomotor examination (nonvestibular)
  - Ocular motility
  - Pursuit
  - Saccades
  - Optokinetic nystagmus testing (OKN)
  - Vergence
- Oculomotor examination (vestibular)
  - In room light: Spontaneous and gaze-holding nystagmus, head impulse test, dynamic visual acuity
  - Fixation removed: Spontaneous and gaze-holding nystagmus, head shake, pressure-induced nystagmus, hyperventilation-induced nystagmus

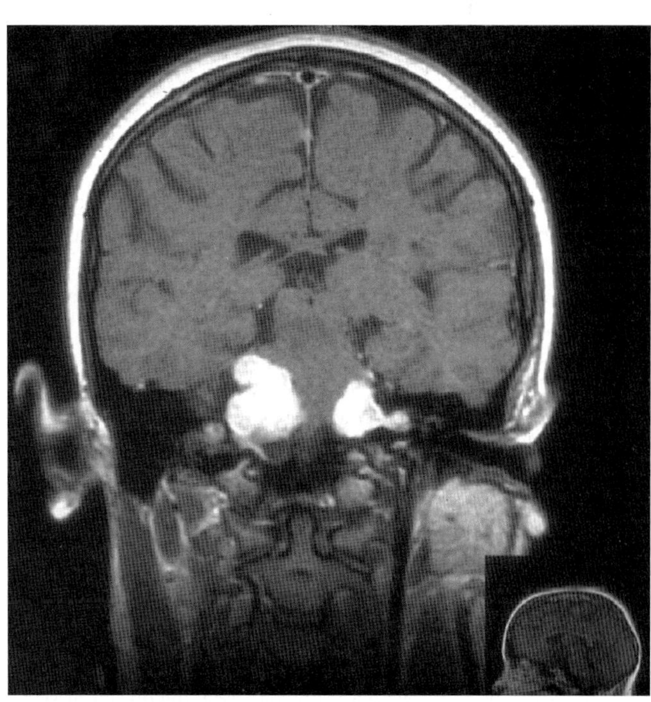

FIGURE 258-5 Coronal MRI of bilateral acoustic neuromas in neurofibromatosis 2. (From Riordan-Eva P, Cunningham E. *Vaughan & Asbury's General Ophthalmology*. 18th ed. http://www.accessmedicine.com. Copyright © The McGraw-Hill Companies, Inc. All rights reserved.)

- Rinne and Weber tests
- Vertebrobasilar insufficiency testing
- Cervical spine special tests
  - Sharp-Purser test
  - Alar ligament test
- Positioning tests
  - Dix–Hallpike maneuver
    - Position
  - Roll test
  - Sidelying test
- Coordination
- Cranial nerve integrity
- Sensation
- Range of motion, including neck
- Strength, including facial muscle testing if cranial nerve VII involved
- Endurance
- Postural alignment
- Postural control and balance
- Gait
- Symptom intensity rating (visual or verbal analog scale, UCLA Dizziness Questionnaire, Motion Sensitivity Quotient)
- Perceived disability
  - Dizziness Handicap Inventory
  - Vestibular Rehabilitation Benefits Questionnaire

INTERVENTION

- Vestibular and balance rehabilitation (promotes central nervous system compensation to reduce dizziness, gaze instability, and imbalance in conservatively managed and postoperatively managed patients)
  - Postural control and balance training
  - Gait training
  - Fall prevention training
  - Vestibular-ocular reflex (VOR) function exercises
  - Habituation exercises
- Facial rehabilitation (for eye protection, promoting normal motor function, and preserving range-of-motion in facial muscles)

FUNCTIONAL GOALS

- The patient will be able to
  - Demonstrate normal standing and walking balance for in-home and work-related tasks.
  - Demonstrate decreased risk of falling during transitions, bending, reaching, standing, and walking.
  - Perform with less than 2 lines difference with dynamic visual acuity testing; ability to read, watch television, and identify objects in the environment while walking.
  - Report reduced frequency and intensity of dizziness (including wooziness, lightheadedness, etc.) during head movements for in-home and work-related tasks.

PROGNOSIS

- Good prognosis for tumor control; slow-growing and nonmetastatic.
- Postsurgical tumor recurrence rate is low.
- Hearing may be preserved with surgery depending on tumor size and surgical approach; hearing loss is permanent if resulting from surgery.
- Facial palsy is usually rare depending on the tumor size and treatment approach.
- Postoperative complications may include headache, CSF leak, meningitis, transient facial nerve weakness, and infrequently, vascular injury.
- Presence of imbalance, dizziness, and gaze instability due to surgically induced damage or complete loss of vestibular function
  - Ranges from minimal impairments similar to those of patients with peripheral vestibular hypofunction.
  - Long-term residual impairments that may occur when the central nervous system is compromised, prohibiting vestibular compensation.
- Vestibular compensation may take weeks or months after surgical resection; use of vestibular rehabilitation, especially in the initial period following surgery, has been shown to improve recovery of postural stability and reduce reports of disequilibrium.

PATIENT RESOURCE

- Acoustic Neuroma. Vestibular Disorders Association. http://vestibular.org/acoustic-neuroma. Accessed January 20, 2013.

REFERENCES

1. ICD-9-CM. http://www.icd9data.com. Accessed January 20, 2013.
2. ICD-10-CM. http://www.icd10data.com. Accessed January 20, 2013.
3. APTA Guide to Physical Therapist Practice. http://guidetoptpractice.apta.org/. Accessed January 20, 2013.

ADDITIONAL REFERENCES

- Fortnum H, O'Neill C, Taylor R, et al. The role of magnetic resonance imaging in the identification of suspected acoustic neuroma: a systematic review of clinical and cost effectiveness and natural history. *Health Technol Assess*. 2009;13(18):iii-iv, ix-xi, 1-154.
- Furman JM, Case SP. *Vestibular Disorders: A Case Study Approach*. Oxford: Oxford University Press; 2003.
- Herdman SJ, Clendaniel RA, Mattox DE, Holliday MJ, Niparko JK. Vestibular adaptation exercises and recovery: acute stage after acoustic neuroma resection. *Otolaryngol Head Neck Surg*. 1995;113(1):77–87.
- Hoistad DL, Melnik G, Mamikoglu B, et al. Update on conservative management of acoustic neuroma. *Otology & Neurotology*. 2001; 22(5):682–685.
- Jacob A, Robinson LL Jr, Bortman JS, Yu L, Dodson EE, Welling DB. Nerve of origin, tumor size, hearing preservation, and facial nerve outcomes in 359 vestibular schwannoma resections at a tertiary care academic center. *Laryngoscope*. 2007;117(12):2087–2092.
- Komatsuzaki A, Tsunoda A. Nerve origin of the acoustic neuroma. *J Laryngol Oto*. 2001;115(5):376–379.
- Pollock BE, Driscoll CL, Foote RL, et al. Patient outcomes after vestibular schwannoma management: a prospective comparison of microsurgical resection and stereotactic radiosurgery. *Neurosurgery*. 2006;59(1):77–85.
- Silk PS, Lane JI, Driscoll CL. Surgical approaches to vestibular schwannomas: what the radiologist needs to know. *Radiographics*. 2009:29(7):1955–1970.

259 BENIGN PAROXYSMAL POSITIONAL VERTIGO

Eric Shamus, PhD, DPT, PT, CSCS
Jennifer Shamus, PhD, DPT, COMT, CSCS

CONDITION/DISORDER SYNONYM

- Benign paroxysmal positional vertigo (BPPV)

ICD-9-CM CODE

- 386.11 Benign paroxysmal positional vertigo

ICD-10-CM CODES

- H81.1 Benign paroxysmal (positional)
- H81.10 Unspecified
- H81.11 Right ear
- H81.12 Left ear
- H81.13 Bilateral

PREFERRED PRACTICE PATTERNS

- 5A: Primary Prevention/Risk Reduction for Loss of Balance and Falling[1]
- 5F: Impaired Peripheral Nerve Integrity and Muscle Performance Associated with Peripheral Nerve Injury[2]

PATIENT PRESENTATION

A 63-year-old man presents with a 3-month history of dizziness. His dizziness comes and goes, but usually lasts for about 10 to 15 seconds. He notices that his dizziness is worse when he rolls over in bed or when he gets out of bed. One time, he became very dizzy while trying to reach for an object on a high shelf. He does not have any nausea or vomiting associated with it. When it occurs, it is severe, and he has tried to avoid sleeping on his left side. He does not have any hearing loss or tinnitus. He denies aural pressure and headache. His past medical history is otherwise unremarkable. He is not on any medications.

On physical examination, he is a healthy appearing 63-year-old man. His temperature is 37.1°C (98.8°F); pulse, 64 beats/min; and blood pressure, 124/74 mm Hg. There are no lesions or masses on his face or head. His voice is normal, and his speech is fluent. His facial nerve function is normal. His ear canals and tympanic membranes are normal appearing. His remaining head and neck examination is normal. The cranial nerve examination is normal. The remaining physical examination is normal."[3]

KEY FEATURES

Description

- Disorder of the inner ear, peripheral vestibular disorder
- Vestibular part of inner ear has three semicircular canals (SCC) and two otolith organs (utricle, saccule) that are interconnected and fluid-filled
- Calcium carbonate crystals (otoconia, otoliths, ear stones) break free from utricular macula and float into one or more of the SCC, making hair cells sensitive to gravity
  - Otoconia can move into the canalithiasis
  - Otoconia can adhere to the cupula
- Causes episodic feelings of rotary vertigo (illusion that the room or oneself is spinning) that occurs with head position changes and usually lasts less than 1 minute
- Usually lasts less than 1 minute

Essentials of Diagnosis

- Physical examination, including neurotologic examination, typically normal
- Thorough and detailed history is essential to distinguish from other vestibular disorders and central pathology
- Positive positioning tests: Dix–Hallpike maneuver, roll test, or side-lying test[4]
- Positioning maneuver results in particular pattern of nystagmus and simultaneous report of vertigo[5]
- Can be spontaneous
- Must rule out central nervous system pathology, which may mimic Benign paroxysmal positional vertigo (BPPV), especially if symptoms associated with head trauma
- Can be classified to which semicircular canal involved: Posterior (most common), Anterior, Horizontal

General Considerations

- Patients feel like either they or the room is spinning.
- Typically triggered by tilting the head backward, rolling over in bed, or bending over.
- Can feel disoriented and off-balance between episodes of spinning.

Demographics

- More common in women than men (2:1 ratio)
- Onset can range from 11 to 84 years of age; most common age of onset between fifth and seventh decades of life
- Uncommon in children
- Can run in families

CLINICAL FINDINGS

SIGNS AND SYMPTOMS

- Patient reports spinning sensation triggered by specific head positions or head position changes
  - Looking down and up
  - Lying down or getting up from bed
- Observe nystagmus and patient reports spinning during positioning test postures
- Reports of dizziness (disorientation, wooziness, lightheadedness) between episodes of vertigo
- Reports of loss of balance and falls

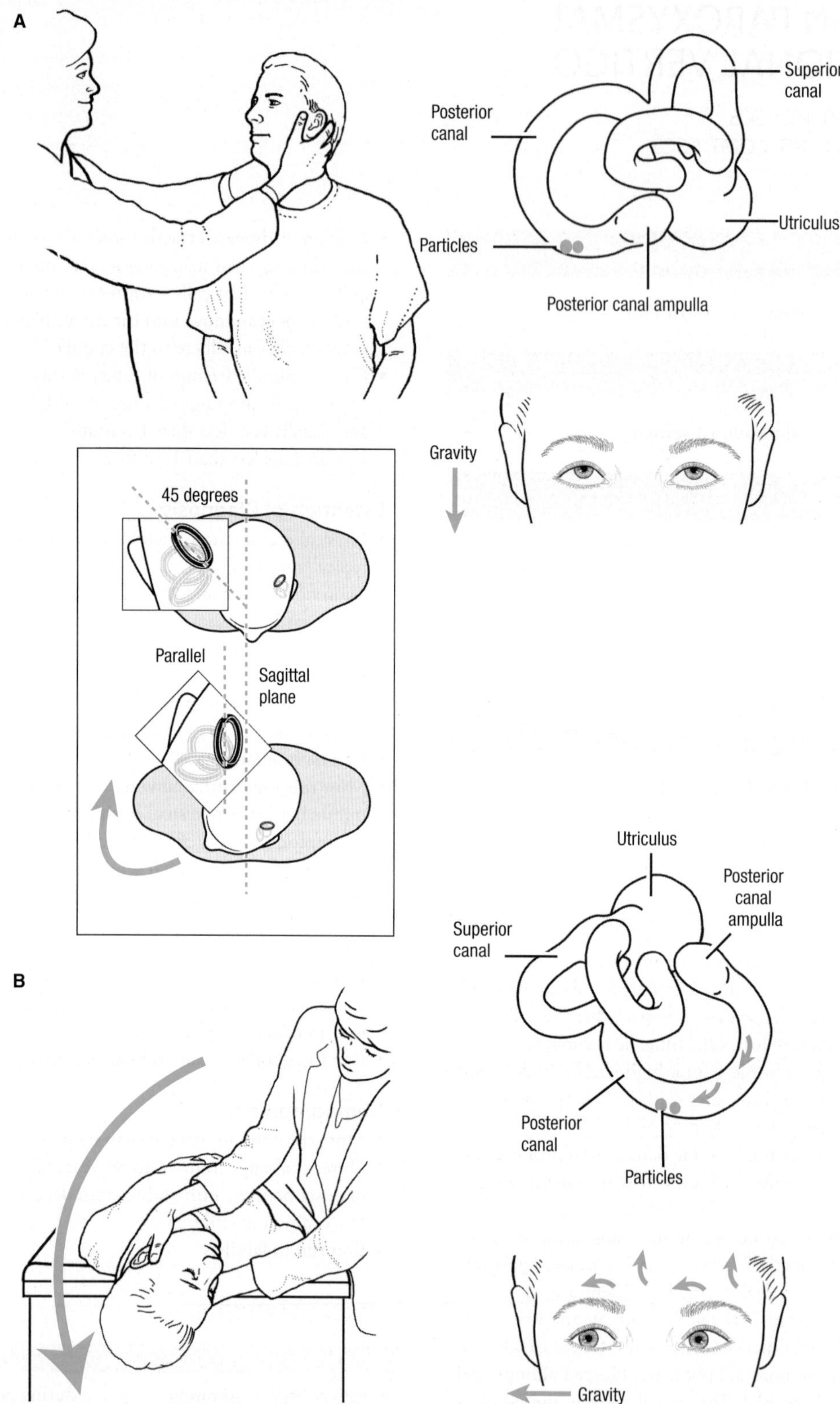

FIGURE 259-1 Dix–Hallpike maneuver to elicit benign positional vertigo (originating in the right ear). The maneuver begins with the patient seated and the head turned to one side at 45 degrees (**A**), which aligns the right posterior semicircular canal with the sagittal plane of the head. The patient is then helped to recline rapidly so that the head hangs over the edge of the table (**B**), still turned 45 degrees from the midline. Within several seconds, this elicits vertigo and nystagmus that is right beating with a rotary (counterclockwise) component. An important feature of this type of "peripheral" vertigo is a change in the direction of nystagmus when the patient sits up again with his head still rotated. If no nystagmus is elicited, the maneuver is repeated after a pause of 30 seconds, with the head turned to the left. Treatment with the canalith repositioning maneuver is shown in Figure 2. (From Ropper AH, Samuels MA. *Adams and Victor's Principles of Neurology*. 9th ed. Copyright ©McGraw-Hill Education. All rights reserved.)

- May also have nausea and vomiting when spinning sensation is provoked
- No central signs (diplopia, dysarthria, dysphagia, dysmetria, numbness, or weakness)

Functional Implications

- Difficulty performing normal head movements (bed mobility, looking up, bending over) because symptoms are provoked
- Impedes balance and contributes to falls
- Reduced or lost ability to perform tasks in home, at work, driving

Possible Contributing Causes

- Primarily idiopathic
- Secondary etiology most commonly head trauma
- Other secondary causes are inner ear pathologies (Ménière disease, post-acute vestibulopathy, migraines)
- Neuritis
- Head trauma
- Ischemia of the anterior vestibular artery
- Vertebrobasilar insufficiency

Differential Diagnosis

- Acoustic neuroma (vestibular schwannoma)
- Acute vestibulopathy (neuritis, labyrinthitis)
- BPPV of childhood
- Brainstem stroke or TIA
- Cervical pain and dysfunction
- Ménière disease
- Meningitis
- Migraine
- Multiple sclerosis
- Necessary when BPPV suspected, but want to rule out other diagnoses because patient does not have classic signs and symptoms or patient does not respond to treatment
- Perilymphatic fistula
- Ramsay Hunt syndrome
- Superior canal dehiscence
- Thyroid disease
- Vertebrobasilar insufficiency
- Vestibular hypofunction

MEANS OF CONFIRMATION OR DIAGNOSIS

Imaging

- MRI[6] or CT[7] of brain, including posterior fossa and internal auditory canals

Diagnostic Procedures

- Electronystagmography (ENG) or videonystagmography (VNG)[4]
- Audiometric testing

FINDINGS AND INTERPRETATION

- ENG or VNG testing can detect abnormal eye movement and determine if dizziness is caused by inner ear disease.
- MRI to rule out acoustic neuroma.

TREATMENT

Medication

- Medication can be used as a vestibular suppressant.
- Medication does not cure the problem.

TABLE 259-1 Symptom Patterns of Vertigo

Benign paroxysmal positional vertigo (benign positional nystagmus, cupulolithiasis): Normal hearing, intermittent episodes of vertigo with head turning, the most common cause of vertigo
Vestibular neuronitis (vestibular neuritis, labyrinthitis): Normal hearing, sudden onset of severe, constant vertigo made worse by head movement that resolves over the course of days to weeks, second in frequency
Recurrent vestibulopathy: Normal hearing, intermittent episodes of constant vertigo lasting minutes or hours
Toxins (drugs such as aminoglycoside toxicity or alcohol): Vertigo with or without hearing loss, bilateral labyrinthine dysfunction
Central causes of vertigo: Vertigo with symptoms of neurologic dysfunction including weakness, impaired speech, diplopia

Source: Furman JM. Dizziness and Vertigo. In: *Principles and Practice of Hospital Medicine.* McKean SC, Ross JJ eds. New York, NY: McGraw-Hill, 2012, p. 577.

- Antihistamine
- Scopolamine
- Sedative

MEDICAL PROCEDURE

- In rare cases, a bone plug maybe placed in the inner ear

REFERRALS/ADMITTANCE

- To emergency department, for suspected acute stroke
- To neurologist, otolaryngologist (ENT), or neurotologist for imaging and diagnosis of central nervous system disease
- To vestibular-trained physical therapist or occupational therapist for BPPV or balance treatment

IMPAIRMENTS

- Perceived orientation (dizziness and vertigo)
- Postural control

TESTS AND MEASURES

- Positioning tests: Dix–Hallpike test/maneuver (gold standard), roll test (horizontal SCC), bow and lean test, and side-lying test (Good if can not tolerate Dix–Hallpike test)[4]
- Activities-specific balance confidence scale (ABC)
- Oculomotor exam
  - Nonvestibular: Ocular motility, pursuit, saccades, OKN, vergence
  - Vestibular
    - In room light: Spontaneous and gaze-holding nystagmus, head thrust, dynamic visual acuity
    - Fixation removed: Spontaneous and gaze-holding nystagmus, head shake, pressure-induced nystagmus, hyperventilation-induced nystagmus
- Dizziness handicap inventory
- Dysequilibrium visual analog scale
- Rinne and Weber tests
- Vertebrobasilar insufficiency testing
- Cervical spine special tests (sharp purser, alar ligament)
- Coordination

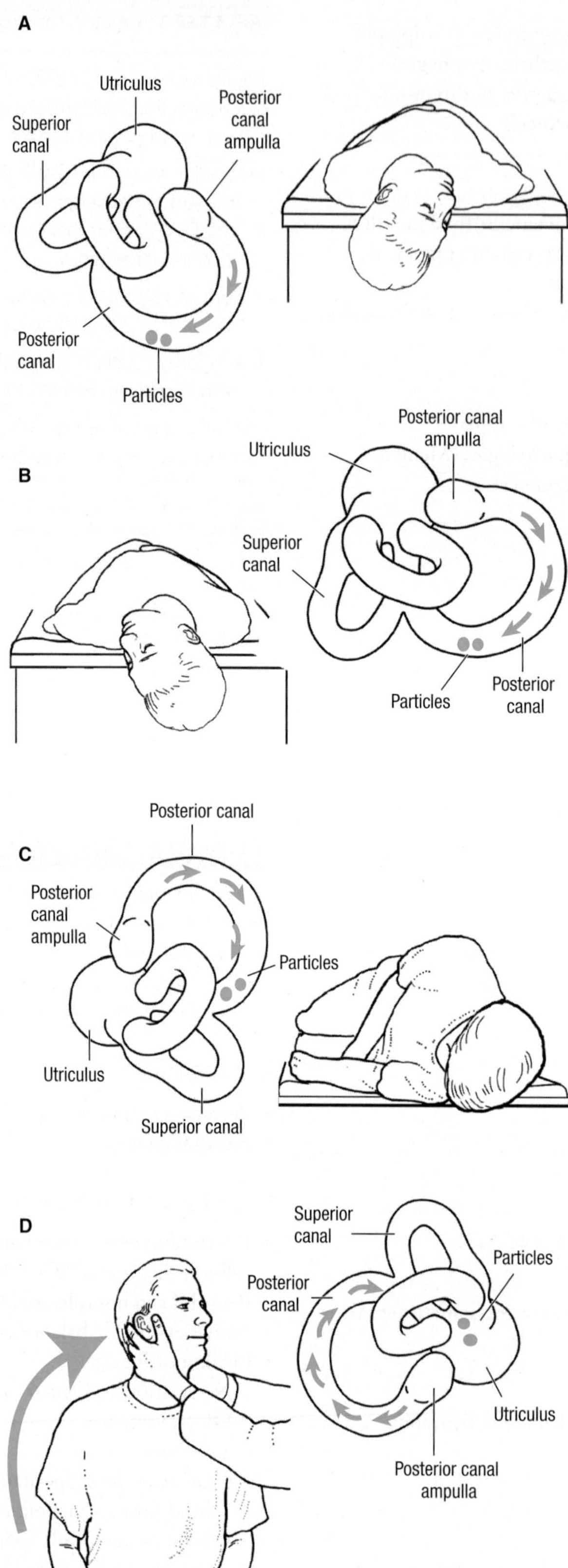

FIGURE 259-2 Bedside maneuver for the treatment of a patient with benign paroxysmal positional vertigo affecting the right ear. The presumed position of the debris within the labyrinth during the maneuver is shown on each panel. The maneuver is a four-step procedure. First, a Dix–Hallpike test is performed with the patient's head rotated 45 degrees toward the (affected) right ear and the neck slightly extended with the chin pointed slightly upward. This position results in the patient's head hanging to the right (**A**). Once the vertigo and nystagmus provoked by this maneuver cease, the patient's head is rotated about the rostral–caudal body axis until the left ear is down (**B**). Then the head and body are further rotated until the head is almost face down (**C**). The vertex of the head is kept tilted upward throughout the rotation. The patient should be kept in the final, facedown position for about 10 to 15 seconds. With the head kept turned toward the left shoulder, the patient is brought into the seated position (**D**). (From Ropper AH, Samuels MA. *Adams and Victor's Principles of Neurology*. 9th ed. Copyright ©McGraw-Hill Education. All rights reserved.)

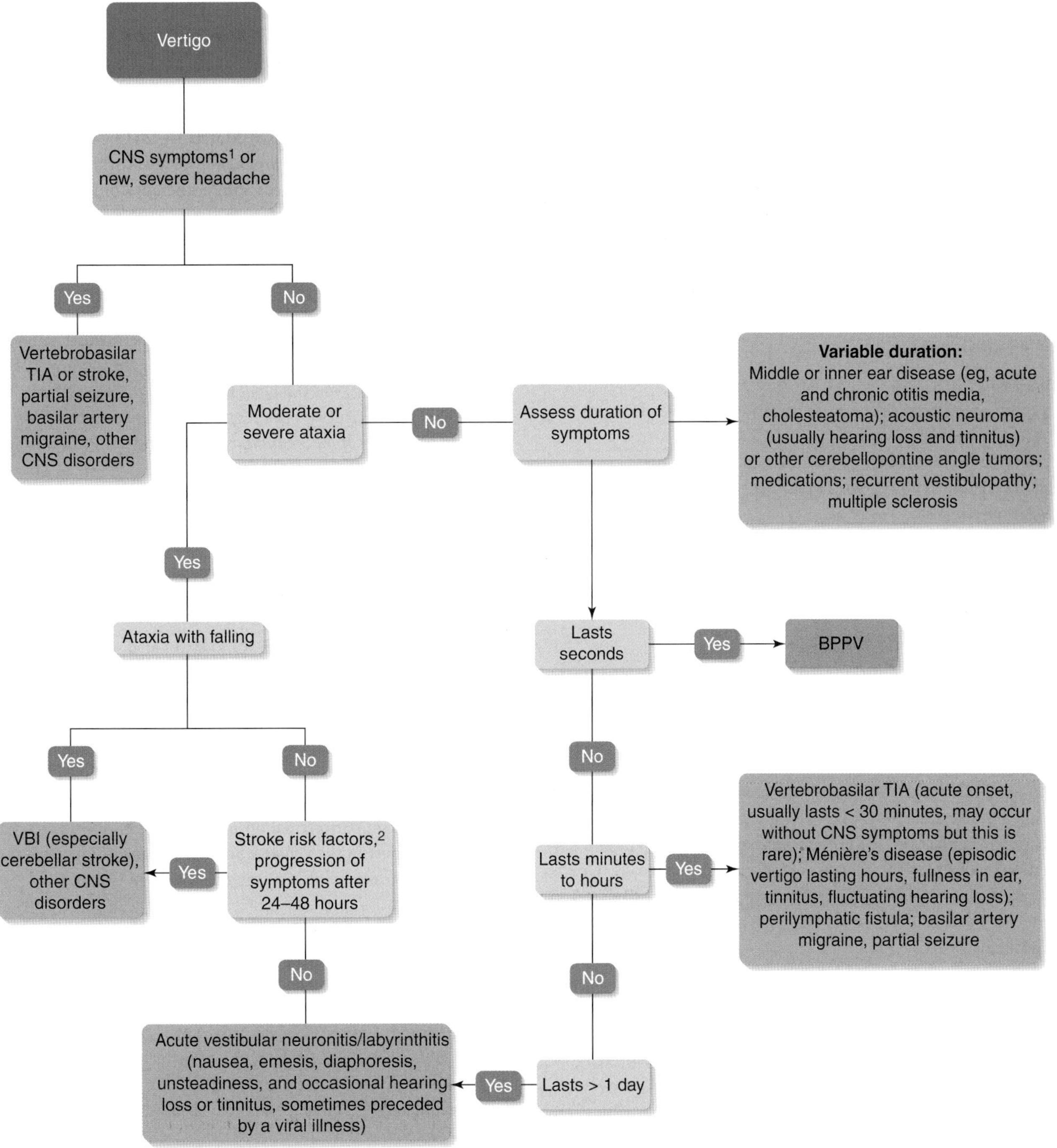

FIGURE 259-3 Diagnostic approach: Vertigo. Benign paroxysmal positional vertigo; CNS, central nervous system; TIA, transient ischemic attack; VBI, vertebrobasilar insufficiency. [1]CNS symptoms: Focal sensory or motor deficits; brainstem findings, e.g., dysarthria, diplopia, dysphagia, hoarseness. [2]Stroke risk factors: Advanced age, smoking, dyslipidemia, family history, diabetes mellitus, hypertension, atrial fibrillation, coronary artery disease, congestive heart failure, peripheral vascular disease. (From Henderson MC, Tierney LM, Smetana GW. *The Patient History: An Evidence-Based Approach to Differential Diagnosis*. 2nd ed. http://www.accessmedicine.com. Copyright © The McGraw-Hill Companies, Inc. All rights reserved.)

- Cranial nerve integrity
- Sensation
- Range of motion, including neck
- Strength
- Endurance
- Postural alignment
- Fall risk assessment
- Postural control and balance
- Gait
- Symptom intensity rating (visual or verbal analog scale, UCLA Dizziness Questionnaire, motion sensitivity quotient)
- Perceived disability (dizziness handicap inventory, vestibular rehabilitation benefits questionnaire)

INTERVENTION

- Epley maneuver
- Canalith repositioning treatment ("modified" Epley)
- Semont maneuver (liberatory)
- Bar-B-Que treatment for horizontal canal canalithiasis
- Appiani maneuver for horizontal canal canalithiasis
- Casani maneuver for horizontal canal canalithiasis
- Brandt–Daroff exercise
- Treatment for residual impairments after successful repositioning
  - Habituation exercises
  - Balance and coordination activities
  - Gait training

FUNCTIONAL GOALS

- Patient will
  - Report no episodes of spinning sensation when head is positioned in specific postures.
  - Report no residual dizziness (disorientation, wooziness, lightheadedness) during head movements for in-home and work-related tasks.
  - Demonstrate normal standing and walking balance for in-home and work-related tasks.
  - Be able to drive without any report of vertigo or dizziness.

PROGNOSIS

- High success rate of remission within a maximum of several treatment sessions using repositioning maneuvers.
- Symptoms usually improve with one or two treatments.

PATIENT RESOURCE

- Benign Paroxysmal Positional Vertigo (BPPV). Vestibular Disorder Association. http://vestibular.org/understanding-vestibular-disorders/types-vestibular-disorders/benign-paroxysmal-positional-vertigo. Accessed January 21, 2013.

REFERENCES

1. The American Physical Therapy Association. Pattern 5A: primary prevention/risk reduction for loss of balance and falling. In: *Interactive Guide to Physical Therapist Practice*. 2003. doi: 10.2522/ptguide.3.2_1. http://guidetoptpractice.apta.org/content/1/SEC18.extract?sid=d8379ef5-e703-4803-bb29-95aa504631c3. Accessed June 6, 2014.
2. The American Physical Therapy Association. Pattern 5F: Impaired peripheral nerve integrity and muscle performance associated with peripheral nerve injury. In: *Interactive Guide to Physical Therapist Practice*. 2003. doi: 10.2522/ptguide.3.2_6. http://guidetoptpractice.apta.org/content/1/SEC23.extract?sid=8ddd7b17-c7d0-44dd-8295-1959cc1546b5. Accessed June 6, 2014.
3. Toy EC. Vertigo, Benign Paroxysmal Positional, Case 98. LANGE Case Files. http://www.accessmedicine.com/casecontent.aspx?aid=510024438&tabid=1 Accessed March 14, 2013.
4. Dutton M. *McGraw Hill's NPTE (National Physical Therapy Examination)*. 2nd ed. New York, NY: McGraw-Hill; 2012. http://www.accessphysiotherapy.com/resource/611. Accessed March 14, 2013.
5. Braverman RS. Eye. In: Hay W, Levin MJ, Sondheimer JM, Detering RR, eds. *CURRENT Diagnosis & Treatment: Pediatrics*. New York, NY: McGraw-Hill; 2011:Chapter 15. http://www.accessphysiotherapy.com/abstract/6580635#6580641. Accessed March 14, 2013.
6. Bernard TJ, Knupp K, Yang ML, Arndt D, Levinson P, Moe PG. Neurologic & Muscular Disorders. In: Hay W, Levin MJ, Sondheimer JM, Detering RR, eds. *CURRENT Diagnosis & Treatment: Pediatrics*. New York, NY: McGraw-Hill; 2011:Chapter 23. http://www.accessphysiotherapy.com/abstract/6585385#6585406. Accessed March 14, 2013.
7. Waxman SG. *Clinical Neuroanatomy*. New York, NY: McGraw-Hill; 2010. http://www.accessphysiotherapy.com/resource/22. Accessed March 14, 2013.

ADDITIONAL REFERENCES

- Aw ST, Halmagyi GM, Curthoys IS, Todd MJ, Yavor RA. Unilateral vestibular deafferentation causes permanent impairment of the human vertical vestibulo-ocular reflex in the pitch plane. *Exp Brain Res*. 1994;102(1):121–130.
- Baloh RW, Honrubia V. Benign Positional Vertigo. In: *Clinical Neurophysiology of the Vestibular System*. 2nd ed. Philadelphia, PA: F.A. Davis Company; 1990;209–213.
- Beasley NJ, Jones NS. Menière's disease: evolution of a definition. *J Laryngol Otol*. 1996;110(12):1107–1113.
- Benign Paroxysmal Positional Vertigo (BPPV). APTA PT Now. http://www.ptnow.org/ClinicalSummaries/QuickDetail.aspx?cid=1fc833bb-ba6d-441f-b809-0765d8b92ca7. Accessed February 21, 2013.
- Bhattacharyya N, Baugh RF, Orvidas L, et al. Clinical practice guideline: benign paroxysmal positional vertigo. *Otolaryngol Head Neck Surg*. 2008;139(5 Suppl 4):S47–S81.
- Devaiah AK, Andreoli S. Postmaneuver restrictions in benign paroxysmal positional vertigo: an individual patient data meta-analysis. *Otolaryngol Head Neck Surg*. 2010;142(2):155–159.
- Fife TD, Iverson DJ, Lempert T, et al. Practice parameter: therapies for benign paroxysmal positional vertigo (an evidence-based review): report of the Quality Standards Subcommittee of the American Academy of Neurology. *Neurology*. 2008;70(22): 2067–2074.
- Froehling DA, Silverstein MD, Mohr DN, Beatty CW, Offoed KP, Ballard DJ. Benign positional vertigo: incidence and prognosis in a population-based study in Olmsted County, Minnesota. *Mayo Clin Proc*. 1991;66(6):596–601.
- Furman JM, Cass SP. Benign paroxysmal positional vertigo. *New Eng J Med*. 1999;341(21):1590–1596.
- Hain TC, Fetter M, Zee DS. Head-shaking nystagmus in patients with unilateral peripheral vestibular lesions. *Am J Otolaryngol*. 1987;8(1):36–47.
- Haybach PJ. *Meniere's Diease: What You Need to Know*. Portland, OR: Vestibular Disorders Association; 1998. ISBN 0-9632611-1-8.
- Helminski JO, Zee DS, Janssen I, Hain TC. Effectiveness of particle repositioning maneuvers in the treatment of benign paroxysmal positional vertigo. *Physical Therapy*. 2010;90(5): 663–678.
- Herdman SJ. Physical therapy in treatment of patients with benign paroxysmal positional vertigo. *Neurology Report*. 1996; 20(6):46–53.
- Hilton M, Pinder D. The Epley (canalith repositioning) manoeuvre for benign paroxysmal positional vertigo. *Cochrane Database Syst Rev*. 2004;2:CD003162.
- Honrubia V, Bell TS, Harris MR, Baloh RW, Fisher LM. Quantitative evaluation of dizziness characteristics and impact of quality of life. *Am J Otology*. 1996;17(4):595–602.

- House MG, Honrubia V. Theoretical models for the mechanisms of benign paroxysmal positional vertigo [erratum in: *Audiol Neurootol.* 2003;8(25:303. *Audiol Neurootol.* 2003;8(2): 91–99.
- ICD9DATA web site. http://www.icd9data.com. Accessed January 21, 2013.
- ICD10DATA web site. http://www.icd10data.com. Accessed January 21, 2013.
- Ishiyama A, Jacobson KM, Baloh RW. Migraine and benign positional vertigo. *Ann Otol Rhinol Laryngol.* 2000;109(4): 377–380.
- Karlberg M, Hall K, Quickert N, Hinson J, Halmagyi GM. What inner ear diseases cause benign paroxysmal positional vertigo? *Acta Otolaryngol.* 2000;120(3):380–385.
- Lempert T, Neuhauser H. Epidemiology of vertigo, migraine and vestibular migraine. *J Neurol.* 2008;256(3):333–338. doi:10.1007/s00415-009-0149-2.
- Li JC, Li CJ, Epley J, Weinberg L. Cost-effective management of benign positional vertigo using canalith repositioning. *Otolaryngol Head Neck Surg.* 2000;122(3):334–339.
- Mandala M, Santoro GP, Awrey J, Nuti D. Vestibular neuritis: recurrence and incidence of secondary benign paroxysmal positional vertigo. *Acta Otolaryngol.* 2010;130:565–567.
- Parnes LS, Agarwal SK, Atlas J. Diagnosis and management of benign paroxysmal positional vertigo (BPPV). *Can Med Assoc J.* 2003;169(7):681–693.
- Semont A, Freyss G, Vitte E. Curing the BPPV with a liberatory maneuver. *Adv Otorhinolaryngol.* 1988;42:290–293.
- von Brevern M, Radtke A, Lezius F, et al. Epidemiology of benign paroxysmal positional vertigo: a population based study. *J Neurol Neurosurg Psychiatry.* 2007;78(7):710–715.
- White J, Savvides P, Cheritan N, Oas J. Canalith Repositioning for Benign Paroxysmal Positional Vertigo. *Otol Neurotol.* 2005; 26(4):704–710.

260 BILATERAL VESTIBULAR HYPOFUNCTION

Eric Shamus, PhD, DPT, PT, CSCS
Jennifer Shamus, PhD, DPT, COMT, CSCS
Mollie Venglar, DSc, MSPT, NCS

CONDITION/DISORDER SYNONYMS

- Bilateral vestibulopathy
- Bilateral vestibular (BVL)

ICD-9-CM CODE

- 386.54 Hypoactive labyrinth, bilateral

ICD-10-CM CODE

- H81.23 Vestibular neuronitis, bilateral

PREFERRED PRACTICE PATTERNS

- 5A: Primary Prevention/Risk Reduction for Loss of Balance and Falling[1]
- 5F: Impaired Peripheral Nerve Integrity and Muscle Performance Associated with Peripheral Nerve Injury[2]

PATIENT PRESENTATION

While working as a relief aide in an underdeveloped country, a 50-year-old woman became extremely ill from a bacterial infection. She was treated with several antibiotics during her hospital stay. Since her discharge from the hospital she has noted several episodes of dizziness throughout the day. Often the feeling of movement doesn't stop when she sits down. She reports losing her balance frequently but more often at night or very early in the morning when she gets out of bed. She displays symptoms of dizziness during vestibulo-ocular reflex (VOR) testing, but no hearing changes or diplopia. CT scan of the head was normal.

KEY FEATURES

Description

- Disorder of the peripheral vestibular system (part of the inner ear).
- The peripheral vestibular system of each ear is made up of the vestibular nerve and five sensory organs (hair cell receptors contained within the superior, posterior, and horizontal semicircular canals, and also within the utricle and saccule).
- Vestibular sensory organs detect head position and head motion to provide input for gaze stability, orientation, and balance.
- Reduction or loss of vestibular function of both systems causes a reduction or loss of neural input, resulting in gaze instability, disorientation, and imbalance.

Essentials of Diagnosis

- Physical examination normal
- Audiogram normal
- Neurotologic examination abnormal
- Thorough, detailed history essential to distinguish bilateral vestibulopathy from other vestibular disorders or central pathology

General Considerations

- Hallmark symptom is gaze instability and imbalance.
- Impairments tend to develop slowly and progressively in most cases, and tend to be more severe than those with unilateral dysfunction.
- Patient complaints may be overlooked as being due to inner ear pathology because reports of vertigo are rare.
- There must be pathological asymmetry of the neural activity between the two inner ears for symptoms of vertigo to occur; with bilateral vestibulopathy, neural impairment or loss is often equal between the two ears and will not create vertigo.
- Patients may or may not report dizziness from head movement
- Patients do not typically report hearing loss, aural fullness, or tinnitus.

Demographics

- Bilateral vestibulopathy is rare among vestibular disorders
- May account for 4% to 9% of diagnoses in clinics specialized in vestibular disorders
- Primarily occurs between ages 61 and 70 years, though can occur at any age

CLINICAL FINDINGS

SIGNS AND SYMPTOMS

- Blurred (bouncing, jumping) vision most noticeable when moving head and walking; due to oscillopsia (apparent movement of the environment) from vestibulo-ocular reflex deficit
- Occasional complaints of vague dizziness
- Postural and gait instability when sensory input challenged
- Increased risk of falling
- Abnormal neurologic examination (impulse test, dynamic visual acuity test, caloric test)
- Usually no report of hearing loss
- No central signs (diplopia, dysarthria, dysphagia, dysmetria, numbness, weakness)

Functional Implications

- Blurred vision while reading signs when walking or driving
- Impeded balance, especially in dimly lit environments or when ground is uneven

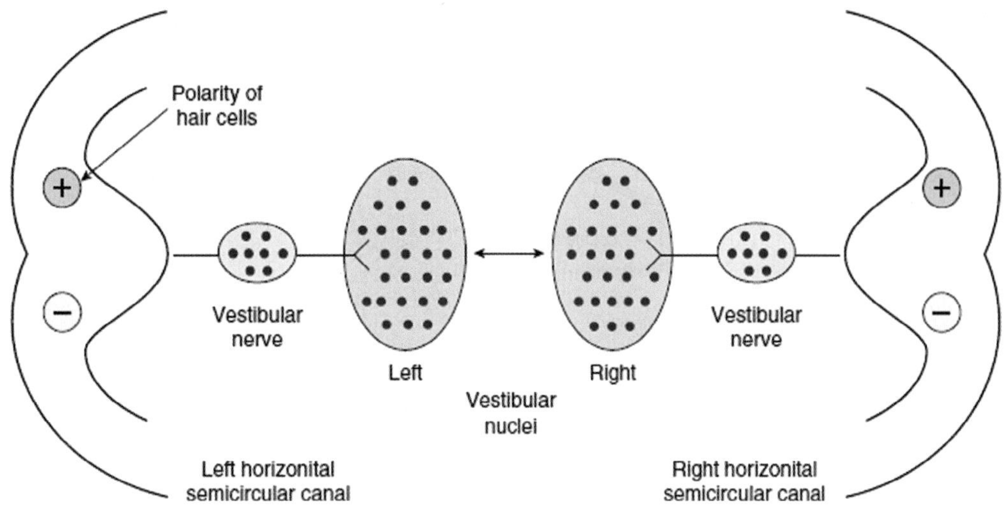

FIGURE 260-1 Push–pull action of the horizontal vestibulo-ocular reflex, with no head movement, left and right vestibular influences are balanced. (From McKean SC, Ross JJ, Dressler DD, Brotman DJ, Ginsberg JS eds. *Principles and Practice of Hospital Medicine*. http://www.accessmedicine.com. Copyright © The McGraw-Hill Companies, Inc. All rights reserved.)

- Reduced or lost ability to perform tasks in home, at work, or driving

Possible Contributing Causes

- Etiology is idiopathic in half of the cases.
- Most common cause is ototoxic drugs (usually aminoglycoside antibiotics; antineoplastic medications, such as vincristine, vinblastine, cisplatinum; or diuretics, such as furosemide, torasemide)
  - Symptoms can be delayed for days, weeks, months following discontinuation of drugs.
- Can occur from sequential dysfunction of the inner ears (Ménière disease, neuritis, labyrinthitis, acoustic neuroma) or from meningitis, otosyphilis.
- May be associated with degenerative cerebellar disease and autoimmune disorders.

Differential Diagnosis

- Acoustic neuroma (vestibular schwannoma)
- Benign paroxysmal positional vertigo
- Brainstem stroke or TIA
- Endolymphatic hydrops (Ménière disease)
- Migraine
- Multiple sclerosis
- Other posterior fossa tumors
- Perilymphatic fistula
- Ramsay Hunt syndrome
- Serous or suppurative labyrinthitis
- Superior canal dehiscence
- Thyroid disease
- Vestibular neuritis

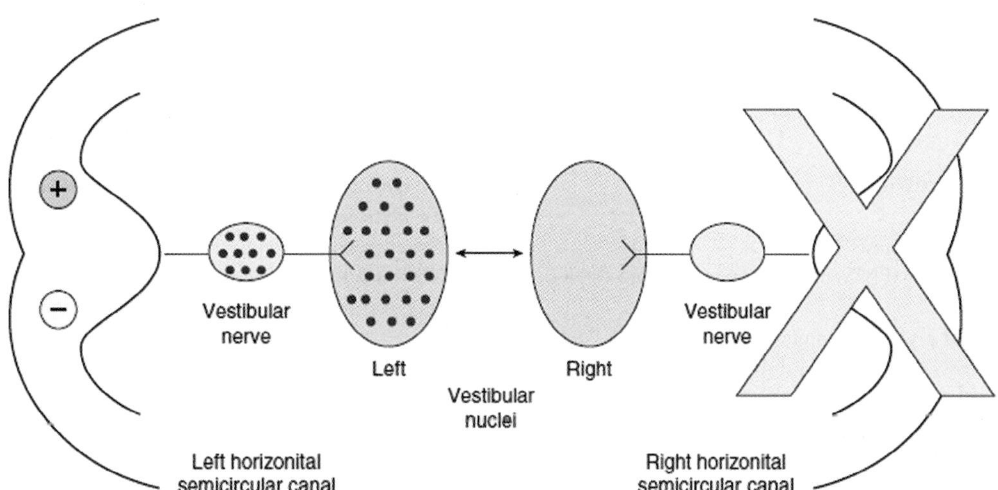

FIGURE 260-2 The reciprocal push–pull interaction of the two labyrinths is disrupted after acute peripheral labyrinthine injury. For example, following the acute loss of right unilateral peripheral vestibular function, there is a loss of resting neural activity in the right vestibular nerve and right vestibular nuclei. Because the brain normally detects differences in activity between the two vestibular nuclear complexes, even when stationary the imbalance in neural activity is interpreted as a rapid head movement, in this case to the left. (From McKean SC, Ross JJ, Dressler DD, Brotman DJ, Ginsberg JSeds. *Principles and Practice of Hospital Medicine*. http://www.accessmedicine.com. Copyright © The McGraw-Hill Companies, Inc. All rights reserved.)

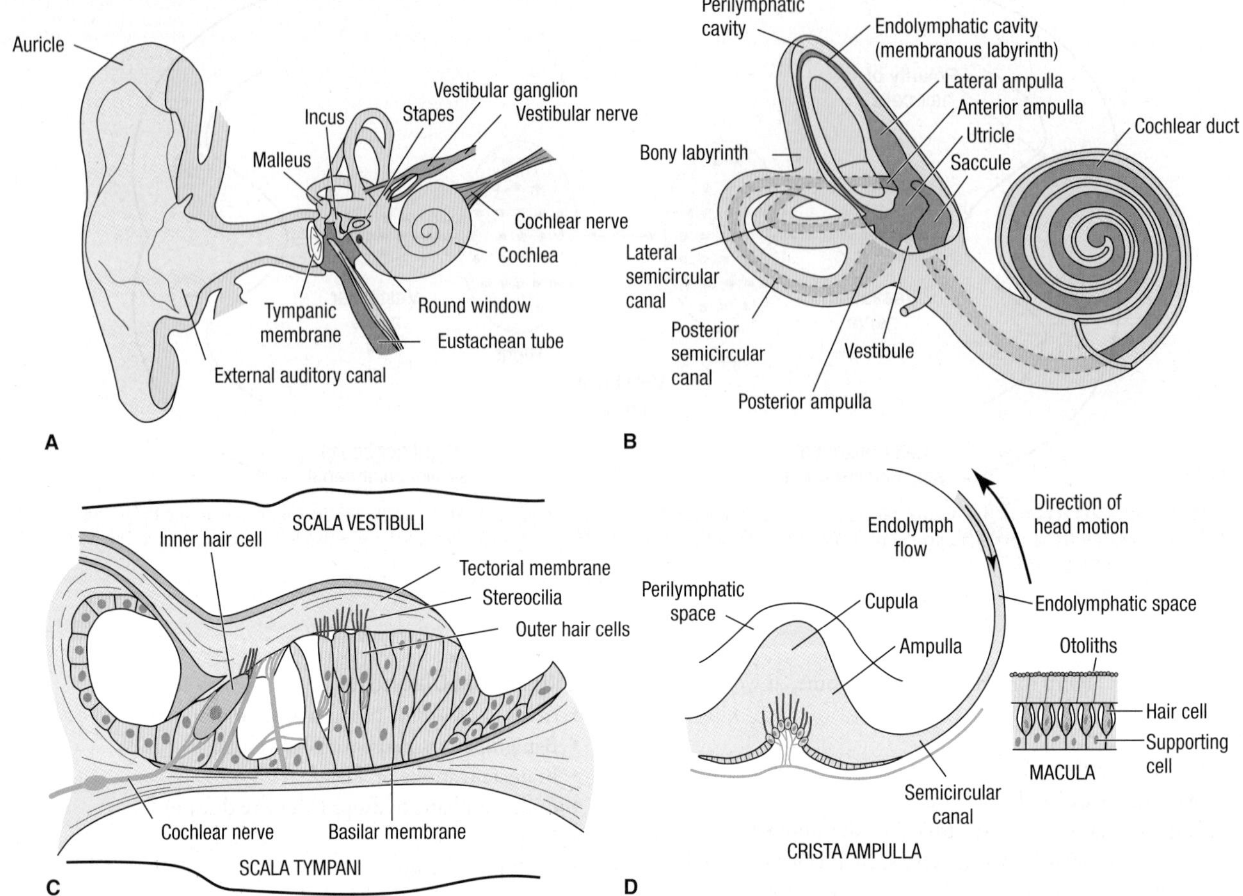

FIGURE 260-3 The auditory and vestibular systems. (**A**) The right ear, viewed from the front, showing the external ear and auditory canal, the middle ear and its ossicles, and the inner ear. (**B**) The main parts of the right inner ear, viewed from the front. The *perilymph* is located between the wall of the bony labyrinth and the membranous labyrinth. In the cochlea, the perilymphatic space takes the form of two coiled tubes—the *scala vestibuli* and *scala tympani*. The *endolymph* is located within the membranous labyrinth, which includes the three semicircular canals, utricle, and saccule. (**C**) The *organ of Corti*. This is the end organ of hearing; it consists of a single row of inner hair cells and three rows of outer hair cells. The stereocilia of the hair cells are embedded in the tectorial membrane. (**D**) Diagram of a crista ampulla, the specialized sensory epithelium of a semicircular canal. The crista senses the displacement of endolymph during head rotation. The direction of head rotation is indicated by the *large arrow*, and endolymph flow by the *small arrow*. The *macula* is the locus of the sensory epithelium in the utricle and saccule. Note that the tips of the hair cells are in contact with the otoliths (calcareous material), which are embedded in a gelatinous mass called the *cupula*. (From Ropper AH, Samuels MA. *Adams & Victor's Principles of Neurology*. 9th ed. http://www.accessmedicine.com. Copyright © The McGraw-Hill Companies, Inc. All rights reserved.)

MEANS OF CONFIRMATION OR DIAGNOSIS

▶ Imaging

- MRI[3] or CT[4] scan of brain, including posterior fossa and internal auditory canals

▶ Diagnostic Procedures

- Serial audiograms
- Serial vestibular function tests
  - Electronystagmography (ENG) or videonystagmography (VNG)[5]
  - Rotational chair
  - Vestibular evoked myogenic potential (VEMP)
  - Subjective visual vertical (static and dynamic SVV)
- Neurologic examinations
  - Impulse test
  - Dynamic visual acuity test
  - Caloric test

FINDINGS AND INTERPRETATION

- Normal audiogram
- Neurotologic examination abnormal

TREATMENT

- Vestibular rehabilitation therapy (VRT)
- Neurotrophin expressing genes as an adjunct to cochlear implantation

REFERRALS/ADMITTANCE

- To emergency department for suspected acute stroke
- To neurologist, otolaryngologist (ENT) or neurotologist for disease management
- To vestibular-trained physical therapist or occupational therapist for rehabilitation

IMPAIRMENTS

- Gaze stability
- Postural control
- Perceived orientation (dizziness)

TESTS AND MEASURES

- Oculomotor examination
  - Nonvestibular: Ocular motility, pursuit, saccades, optokinetic nystagmus testing (OKN), vergence

  - Vestibular
    - In room light: Spontaneous and gaze-holding nystagmus,[6] head impulse test, dynamic visual acuity
    - Fixation removed: Spontaneous and gaze-holding nystagmus, head shake, pressure-induced nystagmus, hyperventilation-induced nystagmus
- Rinne and Weber tests
- Vertebrobasilar insufficiency testing
- Cervical spine special tests (Sharp–Purser, alar ligament)
- Positioning tests: Dix–Hallpike maneuver, roll test, and side-lying test[5]
- Coordination
- Cranial nerve integrity
- Sensation
- Range of motion, including neck
- Strength
- Endurance
- Postural alignment
- Postural control and balance
- Gait[7]
- Symptom intensity rating (visual or verbal analog scale, UCLA Dizziness Questionnaire, Motion Sensitivity Quotient)
- Perceived disability (Dizziness Handicap Inventory, Vestibular Rehabilitation Benefits Questionnaire)

INTERVENTION

- Medical management
  - Monitor ototoxic drugs and restrict or discontinue use if able
  - Prevent attacks of Ménière disease with diuretics and low-salt diet
  - Use of vestibular suppressants not usually appropriate
- Vestibular and balance rehabilitation to reduce impairments
  - Substitution exercises for gaze stability and balance
  - Vestibulo-ocular reflex function exercises (X1 adaptation)
  - Habituation exercises as needed
  - Postural control and balance training
  - Fall prevention and risk factor training
  - Gait training (including assistive device training as needed)

FUNCTIONAL GOALS

- Patient will demonstrate
  - Improved use of sensory input, especially from vision and somatosensation, for standing and walking in home- and work-related tasks.
  - Effective use of assistive device for independent walking in dimly lit environments or uneven ground.
  - Decreased risk of falling when standing and walking.
  - Improved dynamic visual acuity testing so as to read watch television, and identify objects in the environment while walking.
- In those with dizziness symptoms, patient will report reduced frequency and intensity of dizziness (wooziness, lightheadedness) during head movements for home- and work-related tasks.

PROGNOSIS

- Vestibular damage is permanent in most cases; perception of disability can range from slight to moderate in majority of these patients, because of continued gaze instability and imbalance.
- Vestibular and balance rehabilitation can reduce impairments, including risk of falling.

PATIENT RESOURCE

- Causes of Dizziness. Vestibular Disorders Association. http://vestibular.org/node/2 . Accessed January 21, 2013.

REFERENCES

1. The American Physical Therapy Association. Pattern 5A: Primary prevention/risk reduction for loss of balance and falling. *Interactive Guide to Physical Therapist Practice*. 2003. doi: 10.2522/ptguide.3.2_1. http://guidetoptpractice.apta.org/content/1/SEC18.extract?sid=d8379ef5-e703-4803-bb29-95aa504631c3. Accessed June 6, 2014.
2. The American Physical Therapy Association. Pattern 5F: Impaired peripheral nerve integrity and muscle performance associated with peripheral nerve injury. *Interactive Guide to Physical Therapist Practice*. 2003. doi: 10.2522/ptguide.3.2_6. http://guidetoptpractice.apta.org/content/1/SEC23.extract?sid=8ddd7b17-c7d0-44dd-8295-1959cc1546b5. Accessed June 6, 2014.
3. Bernard TJ, Knupp K, Yang ML, Arndt D, Levinson P, Moe PG. Chapter 23. Neurologic & Muscular Disorders. In: Hay W, Levin MJ, Sondheimer JM, Detering RR, eds. *CURRENT Diagnosis & Treatment: Pediatrics*. New York, NY: McGraw-Hill; 2011. http://www.accessphysiotherapy.com/abstract/6585385#6585406. Accessed March 1, 2013.
4. Waxman SG. *Clinical Neuroanatomy*. New York, NY: McGraw-Hill; 2010. http://www.accessphysiotherapy.com/resource/22. Accessed March 1, 2013.
5. Dutton M. *McGraw Hill's NPTE (National Physical Therapy Examination)*. 2nd ed. New York, NY: McGraw-Hill; 2012. http://www.accessphysiotherapy.com/resource/611. Accessed March 1, 2013.
6. Braverman RS. Eye. In: Hay W, Levin MJ, Sondheimer JM, Detering RR, eds. *CURRENT Diagnosis & Treatment: Pediatrics*. New York, NY: McGraw-Hill; 2011:Chapter 15. http://www.accessphysiotherapy.com/abstract/6580635#6580641. Accessed March 1, 2013.
7. Shamus E, Stern D. *Effective Documentation for Physical Therapy Professionals*. 2nd ed. New York, NY: McGraw-Hill; 2011. http://www.accessphysiotherapy.com/resource/696. Accessed March 3, 2013.

ADDITIONAL REFERENCES

- Aw ST, Halmagyi GM, Curthoys IS, Todd MJ, Yavor RA. Unilateral vestibular deafferentation causes permanent impairment of the human vertical vestibulo-ocular reflex in the pitch plane. *Exp Brain Res*. 1994;102(1):121–130.
- Beasley NJ, Jones NS. Menière's disease: evolution of a definition. *J Laryngol Otol*. 1996;110(12):1107–1113.
- Calder JH, Jacobsen GP. Acquired bilateral peripheral vestibular system impairment: rehabilitative options and potential outcomes. *J Am Acad Audiol*. 2000;11(9):514–521.
- Hain TC, Fetter M, Zee DS. Head-shaking nystagmus in patients with unilateral peripheral vestibular lesions. *Am J Otolaryngol*. 1987;8(1):36–47.
- Haybach PJ. *Meniere's Diease: What You Need to Know*. Portland, OR: Vestibular Disorders Association; 1998.
- Herdman SJ, Hall CD, Schubert MC, Das VE, Tusa RJ. Recovery of dynamic visual acuity in bilateral vestibular hypofunction. *Arch Otolaryngol Head Neck Surgery*. 2007;133(4):383–389.
- Honrubia V, Bell TS, Harris MR, Baloh RW, Fisher LM. Quantitative evaluation of dizziness characteristics and impact of quality of life. *Am J Otol*. 1996;17(4):595–602.

- ICD9DATA web site. http://www.icd9data.com. Accessed January 21, 2013.
- ICD10DATA web site. http://www.icd10data.com. Accessed January 21, 2013.
- Isaacson JE, Rubin AM. Taking the history: risk factors for dizziness. In: Goebel JA, ed. *Practical Management of the Dizzy Patient.* Philadelphia: Lippincott, Williams & Wilkins; 2001:Chapter 4.
- Krebs DE, Gill-body KM, Riley PO, Parker SW. Double-blind, placebo-contolled trial of rehabilitation for bilateral vestibular hypofunction: preliminary report. *Otolaryngol Head Neck Surgery.* 1993;109(4):735–741.
- Lee RJ, Thurtell M. Vestibular Areflexia: under the radar. *Ann Neurology.* 2007;61(6):499–500.
- Lempert T, Neuhauser H. Epidemiology of vertigo, migraine and vestibular migraine. *Journal of Neurology.* 2008;256(3):333–338. doi:10.1007/s00415-009-0149-2.
- Zingler VC, Cnyrim C, Jahn K, et al. Causative factors and epidemiology of bilateral vestibulopathy in 255 patients. *Ann Neurol.* 2007;61(6):524–532. [PMID 17393465]
- Zingler VC, Weintz E, Jahn K, et al. Follow-up of vestibular function in bilateral vestibulopathy. *J Neurol Neurosurg Psychiatry.* 2008;79(3):284–288.

261 MÉNIÈRE DISEASE

Eric Shamus, PhD, DPT, PT, CSCS
Jennifer Shamus, PhD, DPT, COMT, CSCS

CONDITION/DISORDER SYNONYM

- Endolymphatic hydrops

ICD-9-CM CODES[1]

- 386.0 Ménière disease
- 386.00 Ménière disease unspecified
- 386.01 Active Ménière disease cochleovestibular
- 386.02 Active Ménière disease cochlear
- 386.03 Active Ménière disease vestibular
- 386.04 Inactive Ménière disease

ICD-10-CM CODES[2]

- H81.01 Ménière disease, right ear
- H81.02 Ménière disease, left ear
- H81.03 Ménière disease, bilateral
- H81.09 Ménière disease, unspecified ear

PREFERRED PRACTICE PATTERNS[3]

- 5A: Primary Prevention/Risk Reduction for Loss of Balance and Falling
- 5F: Impaired Peripheral Nerve Integrity and Muscle Performance Associated with Peripheral Nerve Injury

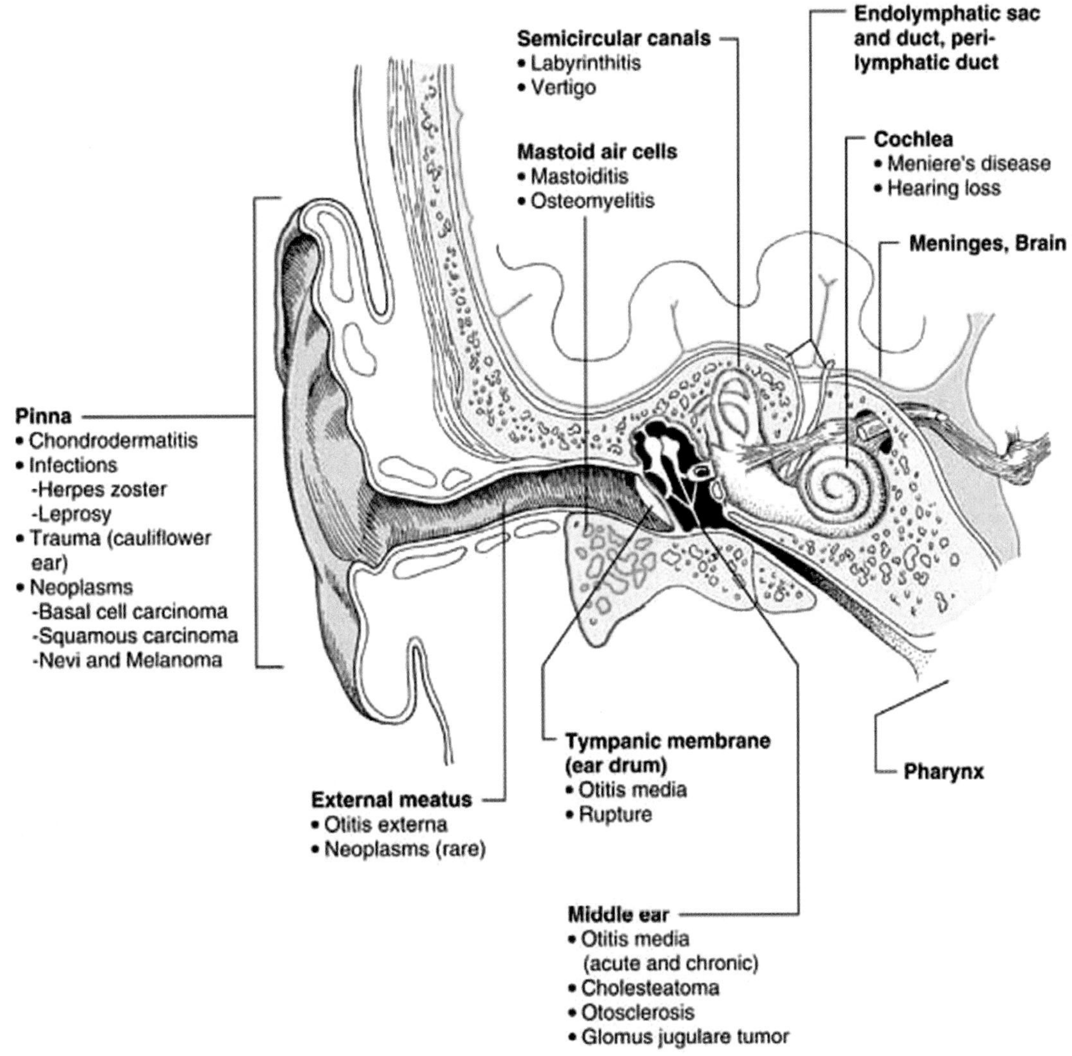

FIGURE 261-1 The structure of the ear and its principal diseases. (From Chandrasoma P, Taylor CR. *Concise Pathology*. 3rd ed. http://www.accessmedicine.com.)

PATIENT PRESENTATION

"A 38-year-old male clerk saw his doctor because of sudden episodes of nausea and dizziness. These attacks had started 3 weeks earlier and seemed to be getting worse. The abnormal episodes at first lasted only a few minutes, during which "the room seemed to spin." Lately, they had been lasting for many hours. A severe attack caused the patient to vomit and to hear abnormal sounds (ringing, buzzing, paper-rolling sounds) in the left ear. He thought that he was becoming deaf on that side.

The neurologic examination was within normal limits except for a slight sensorineural hearing loss in the left ear. Computed tomography (CT) examination of the head was unremarkable."[4]

KEY FEATURES

Description

- Chronic disorder of the peripheral vestibular and auditory systems (inner ear).
- Auditory systems description
  - Complex series of interconnected tubes that are fluid-filled (fluid called endolymph) and form a labyrinth.
  - Peripheral vestibular sensory organs of each ear detect head position and head motion to provide input for gaze stability, orientation, and balance.
  - Peripheral auditory sensory organs of each ear convert sound vibration into a neural impulse to provide input for hearing.
  - Each system sends its respective sensory information, via the vestibulocochlear nerve (cranial nerve VIII), to the central nervous system for processing.
- The pathophysiology of Ménière disease is not completely understood, however it is theorized that it is due to aberrant fluid homeostasis, which leads to overproduction of endolymph and distention of the membranous labyrinth.
- Results in reports of severe relapsing and remitting episodes of rotary vertigo (illusion of spinning motion of the room or self) that can occur for minutes to hours.

TABLE 261-1 Diagnostic Scale for Ménière Disease of the AAO-HNS[a]

Certain Ménière Disease
Definitive Meniere's disease, plus histopathological confirmation
Definitive Ménière Disease
Two or more episodes of vertigo of at least 20 minutes
Audiometrically documented hearing loss on at least one occasion
Tinnitus and aural fullness
Probable Ménière Disease
One definite episode of vertigo
Audiometrically documented hearing loss on at least one occasion
Tinnitus and aural fullness
Possible Ménière Disease
Episodic vertigo without documented hearing loss
Sensorineural hearing loss, fluctuating or fixed, with disequilibrium, but without definitive episodes

[a]In all scales, other causes must be excluded using any technical methods (e.g., imaging, laboratory).

From Lalwani AK. *Current Diagnosis & Treatment in Otolaryngology—Head and Neck Surgery*. 3rd ed. http://www.accessmedicine.com.

- Associated symptoms of fluctuating low-frequency sensory neural hearing loss, ear fullness, and tinnitus (ringing in the ear).

Essentials of Diagnosis

- No definitive objective test for diagnosis is available.
- According to the American Academy of Otolaryngology—head and neck surgery criteria, a definitive diagnosis of Ménière disease requires
  - Two or more episodes of vertigo of at least 20 minutes in length.
  - Audiometrically documented hearing loss on at least one occasion.
  - Tinnitus and aural fullness (ear pressure).
- Thorough and detailed history is essential to distinguish Ménière disease from other vestibular disorders and central pathology.

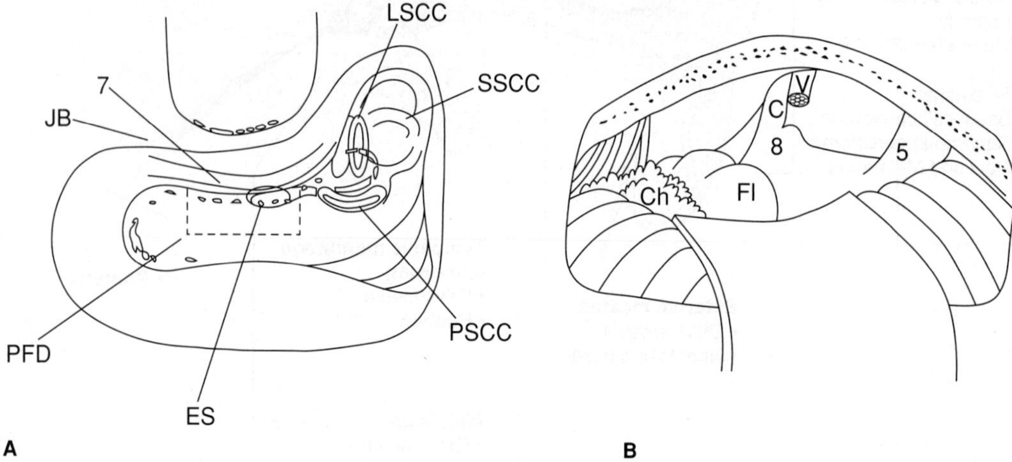

FIGURE 261-2 (**A**) Endolymphatic sac surgery. The sac surgery involves a mastoidectomy and identifying it within the posterior fossa dura. (**B**) Vestibular nerve section. Illustration shows a vestibular neurectomy via the posterior fossa craniotomy. LSCC, lateral semicircular canal; PSCC, posterior semicircular canal; SSCC, superior semicircular canal; ES, endolymphatic sac; PFD, posterior fossa dura; JB, jugular bulb; 7, facial nerve or cranial nerve 7; Fl, flocculus; 8, audiovestibular nerve or cranial nerve 8; C, cochlear division of the audiovestibular nerve; V, vestibular division of the audiovestibular nerve; 5, trigeminal nerve or cranial nerve 5; Ch, choroid plexus. (From Lalwani AK. *Current Diagnosis & Treatment in Otolaryngology—Head and Neck Surgery*. 3rd ed. http://www.accessmedicine.com.)

- Audiogram will fluctuate between normal and abnormal, and in later stages, will demonstrate a fixed loss.
- Neurotologic examination may be normal in early stages and when in remission, however in later stages or when experiencing an episode, can be abnormal.
- Normal physical examination.

General Considerations

- Spontaneous, severe episodes of rotary vertigo that also cause nausea and vomiting and difficulty standing and walking.
- Patients also will have hearing loss, ear fullness, and tinnitus and the symptoms can last from 20 minutes to hours.
- Intervals between these episodes can range from weeks to years.
- In between vertiginous episodes
  - Some patients will recover and not have any symptoms.
  - Other patients can continue to have hearing loss, ear fullness, and tinnitus, however the symptoms may not be as severe.
  - General feeling of dizziness and imbalance that may worsen with quick head movements.
- Frequently occurs only in one ear, however, a range of 20% to 50% of patients will develop it bilaterally.
- Due to the recurrent, unpredictable nature of the episodes, anxiety and depression can be present.

Demographics

- Typically occurs in adults, aged 20 to 50 years

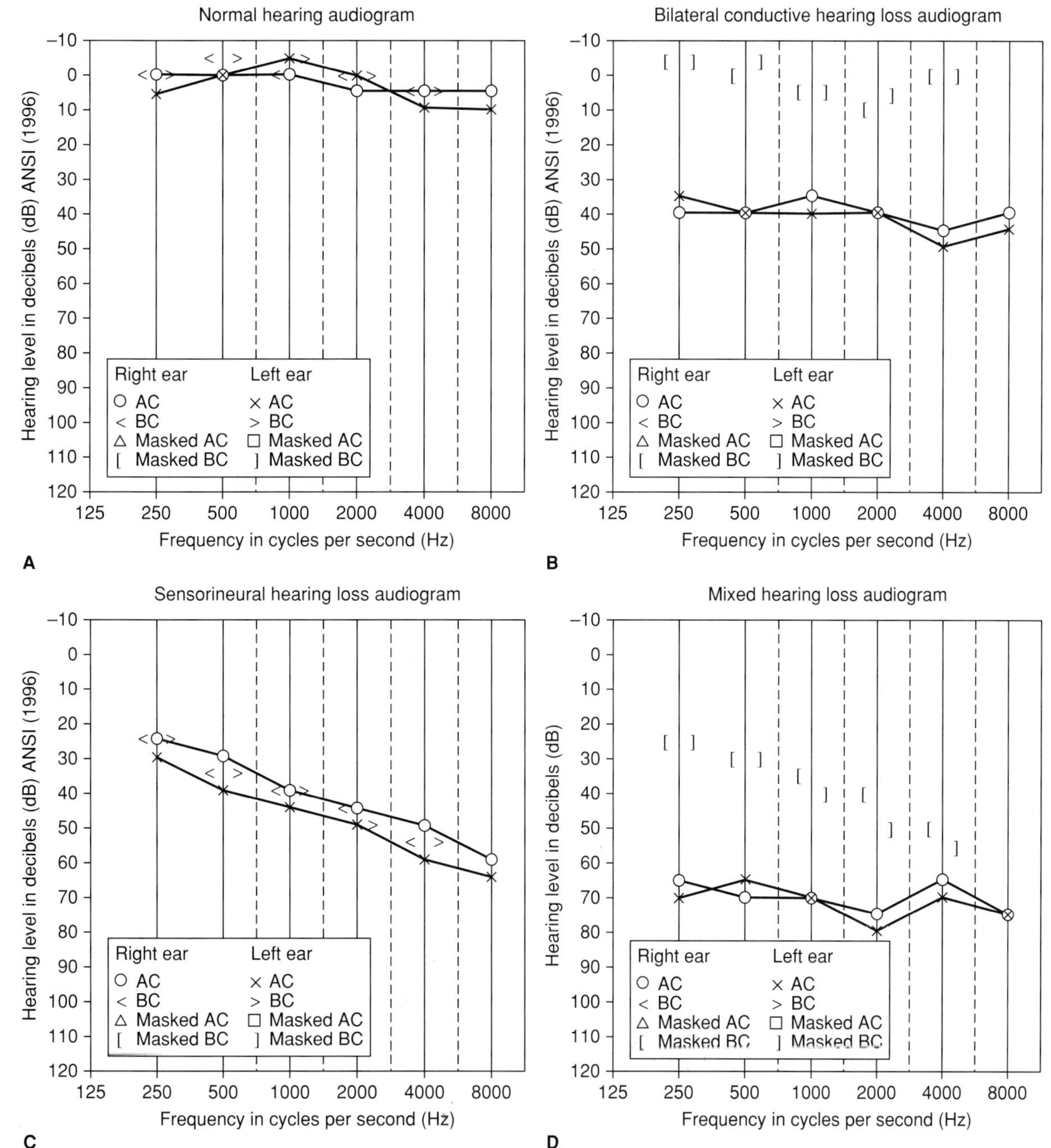

FIGURE 261-3 Examples of audiograms: (**A**) normal hearing thresholds, (**B**) conductive hearing loss, (**C**) sensorineural hearing loss, and (**D**) mixed hearing loss. (From Lalwani AK. *Current Diagnosis & Treatment in Otolaryngology—Head and Neck Surgery*. 3rd ed. http://www.accessmedicine.com. Copyright © The McGraw-Hill Companies, Inc. All rights reserved.)

CLINICAL FINDINGS

SIGNS AND SYMPTOMS

- Episode presentation
  - Report of persistent, episode of severe rotary vertigo, nausea and vomiting, and unsteadiness that lasts for minutes to hours
  - Imbalance manifested by inability to stand and walk without assistance
  - Increased risk of falling
  - Fluctuating hearing loss, tinnitus, and ear fullness
  - Audiological examination abnormal in low frequencies
  - Observe nystagmus in room light and with fixation removed
  - Depending on timing of vertiginous episodes, may or may not have abnormal neurotologic examination
  - No central signs (diplopia, dysarthria, dysphagia, dysmetria, numbness, or weakness)
- Remission presentation
  - Ranges from report of no symptoms of dizziness or unsteadiness to general feelings of dizziness and unsteadiness
  - Variable results with postural and gait instability when sensory input challenged
  - As disease progresses, can demonstrate abnormal neurotologic examination (impulse test, headshake test, caloric test, Vestibular Evoked Myogenic Potential (VEMP) test, and/or Subjective Visual Vertical (SVV) test
  - Hearing loss progressively worsens

▸ Functional Implications

- Difficulty moving head quickly (turning, bending over, looking up) because the action provokes symptoms
- Impedes balance and contributes to falls
- Difficulty identifying objects in environment and reading
- Reduced or lost ability to perform tasks in home, at work, and/or driving, thus reducing quality of life

▸ Possible Contributing Cause

- Unclear etiology, however inflammatory or immunologic-mediated dysfunction is highly suspected.

▸ Differential Diagnoses

- Acoustic neuroma (vestibular schwannoma)
- Benign paroxysmal positional vertigo (BPPV)
- Bilateral vestibulopathy
- Brainstem stroke or Transient Ischemic Attack (TIA)
- Diabetes Mellitus
- Migraine
- Multiple sclerosis
- Other posterior fossa tumors
- Perilymphatic fistula
- Superior canal dehiscence syndrome (SCDS)
- Syphilis
- Thyroid disease
- Vestibular neuritis

MEANS OF CONFIRMATION OR DIAGNOSIS

▸ Laboratory Tests

- Autoimmune serologic tests
- Fluorescent treponemal antibody absorption (FTA-ABS)
- Glycerol testing

▸ Imaging

- MRI with gadolinium contrast to rule out retrocochlear pathology
- CT scan of brain, including posterior fossa and internal auditory canals

▸ Diagnostic Procedures

- Electronystagmography (ENG) or Videonystagmography (VNG)
- Rotational chair test
- VEMP test
- SVV test (static and dynamic)
- Audiogram
- Electrocochleography (ECoG)

FINDINGS AND INTERPRETATIONS

- Audiometrically documented hearing loss

TREATMENT

▸ Medication

- During an episode, the goal is to control symptoms by prescribing vestibular suppressants and antiemetic suppository medications (benzodiazepines, antihistamines, anticholinergics, and antidopaminergics) to help reduce the severe symptoms.
- Sometimes oral or intratympanic steroids are also administered to lessen attack severity and promote earlier recovery of hearing.
- Prescription of diuretics (thiazide, potassium-sparing, loop, and carbonic anhydrase inhibitors) to affect fluid balance in the inner ear.
- Vasodilators (commonly betahistine) to reduce vertigo symptoms.
- Ablation of the vestibular portion of the inner ear using aminoglycosides (intratympanic gentamicin) is a possible treatment when intensity and frequency of symptoms significantly reduce quality of life and normal level of function.

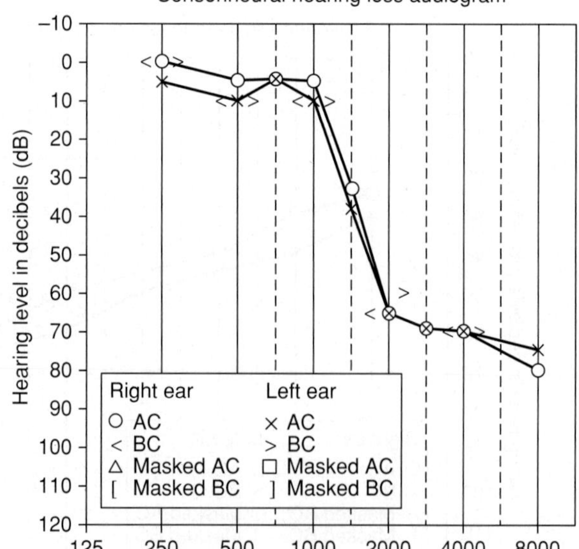

FIGURE 261-4 An example of an audiogram in which the SRT could give misleading information regarding a patient's hearing. Note that the patient has normal hearing to 1000 Hz, which then drops to a moderate hearing loss in the high frequencies. (From Lalwani AK. *Current Diagnosis & Treatment in Otolaryngology—Head and Neck Surgery*. 3rd ed. http://www.accessmedicine.com. Copyright © The McGraw-Hill Companies, Inc. All rights reserved.)

MEDICAL PROCEDURES

- If patient is nonresponsive to traditional treatments, a device that administers low-intensity alternating pressure to external auditory canal (e.g., Meniett® device) may reduce frequency and severity of vertigo.
- Endolymphatic sac surgery.

REFERRALS/ADMITTANCE

- To hospital emergency department for suspected acute stroke or sudden hearing loss
- To audiologist for low and high frequency assessment
- To vestibular-trained physical therapist (PT) or occupational therapist (OT) for rehabilitation
- To neurologist, otolaryngologist, or neurotologist for disease management

IMPAIRMENTS

- As disease progresses, or if has inner ablation to stabilize the vertiginous episodes, may have any or all of the following impairments:
  - Perceived orientation (dizziness)
  - Postural control
  - Gaze stability

TESTS AND MEASURES

- Oculomotor examination
  - Nonvestibular: Ocular motility, pursuit, saccades, optokinetic nystagmus (OKN), and vergence test
  - Vestibular
    - In room light: Spontaneous and gaze-holding nystagmus, head impulse, and dynamic visual acuity tests
    - Fixation removed: Spontaneous and gaze-holding nystagmus, head shake, pressure-induced nystagmus, and hyperventilation-induced nystagmus tests
- Rinne and Weber tests
- Vertebrobasilar insufficiency test
- Cervical spine special tests (Sharp–Purser, Alar Ligament)
- Positioning tests: Dix–Hallpike maneuver,roll test, and side-lying test
- Coordination
- Cranial nerve integrity
- Sensation
- Range of motion (including neck)
- Strength
- Endurance
- Postural alignment
- Postural control and balance
- Gait
- Symptom intensity rating (Visual or verbal analog scale, UCLA Dizziness Questionnaire, motion sensitivity quotient)
- Perceived disability (Dizziness Handicap Inventory, Vestibular Rehabilitation Benefits Questionnaire)

INTERVENTION

- Vestibular and balance rehabilitation
  - While not typically used to treat the attacks of vertigo that have been controlled medically, it may be helpful to treat any residual impairments with the following.
    - Vestibulo-ocular reflect function exercises for gaze instability
    - Habituation exercises for residual dizziness
    - Postural control and balance training for unsteadiness and fall prevention
    - Gait training
- Bed rest and hydration is needed when symptoms are severe.
- Patient education of the disease to avoid triggers (high salt intake, caffeine, alcohol, nicotine, stress, fatigue, monosodium glutamate, and allergy), and adequate hydration is crucial.

FUNCTIONAL GOALS

- Patient will be able to
  - Report reduced frequency and intensity of dizziness during head movements for in-home and work-related tasks.
  - Demonstrate normal standing and walking balance for in-home and work-related tasks.
  - Have decreased risk of falling when standing and walking.
  - Have less than two lines difference with dynamic visual acuity testing, thus able to read, watch TV, and identify objects in the environment while walking.

PROGNOSIS

- There is no cure for Ménière disease.
- Patients with Ménière disease can have severe episodes even after 20 years.
- Generally, vertigo attacks may decline over time.
- Hearing and tinnitus symptoms do not significantly change for most patients.
- The goal of medical management is to control the frequency and severity of episodes of vertigo and reduce the audiological consequences.

PATIENT RESOURCE

- Ménière's Disease. Vestibular Disorders Association. http://vestibular.org/menieres-disease. Accessed July 5, 2013.

REFERENCES

1. ICD-9-CM. http://www.icd9data.com. Accessed July 5, 2013.
2. ICD-10-CM. http://www.icd10data.com. Accessed July 5, 2013.
3. APTA Guide to Physical Therapist Practice. http://guidetoptpractice.apta.org./ Accessed July 5, 2013.
4. Waxman SG. The Vestibular System, case 23. In: Waxman SG, ed. *Clinical Neuroanatomy*. 26th ed. New York, NY: McGraw-Hill; 2010:Chapter 17. http://www.accessmedicine.com/content.aspx?aID=5274652. Accessed July 5, 2013.

ADDITIONAL REFERENCES

- Aw ST, Halmagyi GM, Curthoys IS, Todd MJ, Yavor RA. Unilateral vestibular deafferentation causes permanent impairment of the human vertical vestibulo-ocular reflex in the pitch plane. *Exp Brain Res*. 1994;102(1):121–130.
- Beasley NJ, Jones NS. Ménière's disease: evolution of a definition. *J Laryngol Otol*. 1996;110(12):1107–1113.
- Bennett M. The vertigo case history. In: Jacobson GP, Shepard NT, eds. *Balance Function Assessment and Management*. San Diego, CA: Plural Publishing, Inc.; 2008.

- Clendaniel RA, Tucci Dl. Vestibular rehabilitation strategies in Ménière's disease. *Otolaryngol Head Neck Surg.* 1997;30(6): 1145–1158.
- Coelho DH, Lalwani AK. Medical management of Ménière's disease. *Laryngoscope.* 2008;118(6):1099–1108.
- Dutton M. Diagnostic procedures. In: Dutton M, ed. *McGraw-Hill's NPTE (National Physical Therapy Examination).* 2nd ed. New York, NY: McGraw-Hill; 2012. http://www.accessphysiotherapy.com/content/5399822 . Accessed July 5, 2013.
- Dutton M. Vestibular disorders. In: Dutton M, ed. *McGraw-Hill's NPTE (National Physical Therapy Examination).* 2nd ed. New York, NY: McGraw-Hill; 2012. http://www.accessphysiotherapy.com/content/5400074. Accessed July 5, 2013.
- Furman JM, Cass SP. *Vestibular Disorders: A Case Study Approach.* Oxford: Oxford University Press; 2003.
- Gottshall KR, Hoffer ME, Moore RJ, Balough BJ. The role of vestibular rehabilitation in the treatment of Ménière's disease. *Otolaryngol Head Neck Surg.* 2005;133(3):326–328.
- Hain TC, Fetter M, Zee DS. Head-shaking nystagmus in patients with unilateral peripheral vestibular lesions. *Am J Otolaryngol.* 1987;8(1):36–47.
- Haybach PJ. *Ménière's Disease: What You Need to Know.* Portland, OR: Vestibular Disorders Association; 1998.
- Herraiz C, Plaza G, Aparicio JM, Gallego I, Marcos S, Ruiz C. Transtympanic steroids for Ménière's disease. *Otol Neurotol.* 2010;31(1):162–167.
- Lempert T, Neuhauser H. Epidemiology of vertigo, migraine and vestibular migraine. *J Neurol.* 2008;256(3):333–338. doi:10.1007/s00415-009-0149-2.
- Pullens B, Giard JL, Verschuur HP, van Benthem PP. Surgery for Ménière's disease. *Cochrane Database Syst Rev.* 2010;(1):CD005395. doi: 10.1002/14651858.CD005395.pub2.
- Silverstein H, Wazen J, Van Ess MJ, Daugherty J, Alameda YA. Intratympanic gentamicin treatment of patients with Ménière's disease with normal hearing. *Otolaryngol Head Neck Surg.* 2010;142(4):570–575.
- Van de Heyning PH, Wuyts F, Boudewyns A. Surgical treatment of Ménière's disease. *Curr Opin Neurol.* 2005;18(1):23–28.
- Waxman SG. Chapter 8. Cranial nerves and pathways. In: Waxman SG, ed. *Clinical Neuroanatomy.* 26th ed. New York, NY: McGraw-Hill; 2010. http://www.accessphysiotherapy.com/content/5272646. Accessed July 5, 2013.
- Waxman SG. The vestibular system. In: Waxman SG, ed. *Clinical Neuroanatomy.* 26th ed. New York, NY: McGraw-Hill; 2010. http://www.accessphysiotherapy.com/content/5274652. Accessed July 5, 2013.

262 VESTIBULAR LABYRINTHITIS

Eric Shamus, PhD, DPT, PT, CSCS
Jennifer Shamus, PhD, DPT, COMT, CSCS

CONDITION/DISORDER SYNONYMS

- Serous labyrinthitis
- Circumscribed labyrinthitis
- Suppurative labyrinthitis
- Toxic labyrinthitis
- Viral labyrinthitis

ICD-9-CM CODES[1]

- 386.3 Labyrinthitis
- 386.30 Labyrinthitis unspecified
- 386.31 Serous labyrinthitis
- 386.32 Circumscribed labyrinthitis
- 386.33 Suppurative labyrinthitis
- 386.34 Toxic labyrinthitis
- 386.35 Viral labyrinthitis
- 386.53 Hypoactive labyrinth, unilateral

ICD-10-CM CODES[2]

- H83.09 Labyrinthitis, unspecified ear
- H83.2X1 Labyrinthine dysfunction, right ear
- H83.2X2 Labyrinthine dysfunction, left ear
- H83.2X3 Labyrinthine dysfunction, bilateral
- H83.2X9 Labyrinthine dysfunction, unspecified ear

PREFERRED PRACTICE PATTERNS[3]

- 5A: Primary Prevention/Risk Reduction for Loss of Balance and Falling
- 5F: Impaired Peripheral Nerve Integrity and Muscle Performance Associated with Peripheral Nerve Injury

PATIENT PRESENTATION

A 31-year-old man decided to begin swimming for exercise at his local fitness club. At the end of the first week he noticed that his ear was very red and itched terribly. His doctor diagnosed him with an ear infection and gave him antibiotics. The man noticed increasingly frequent episodes where he felt like the room was spinning. These episodes lasted for a few days then would lessen. He also noticed he struggled to hear accurately in the ear that had been afflicted with the infection. He had no loss of strength or range of motion (ROM) and his reflexes were normal; however, he struggled to keep his balance particularly when he had the sensation of spinning. On testing, he was unable to keep his balance with his eyes closed and he demonstrated nystagmus with head movements.

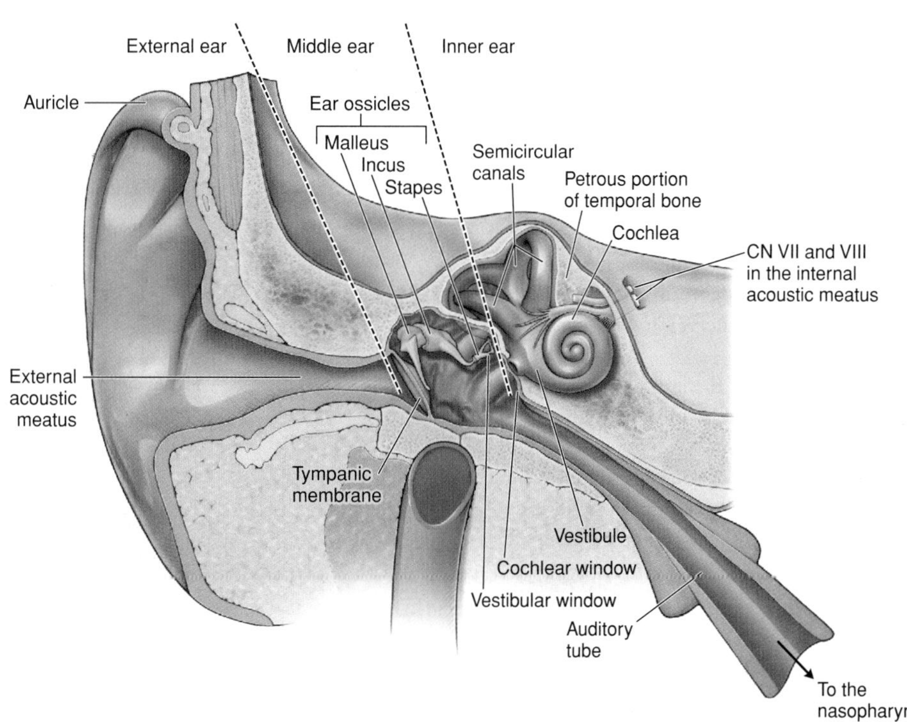

FIGURE 262-1 Coronal section of the temporal bone showing the hearing apparatus. (From Henderson MC, Tierney LM, Smetana GW. *The Patient History: An Evidence-Based Approach to Differential Diagnosis.* http://www.accessmedicine.com. Copyright © The McGraw-Hill Companies, Inc. All rights reserved.)

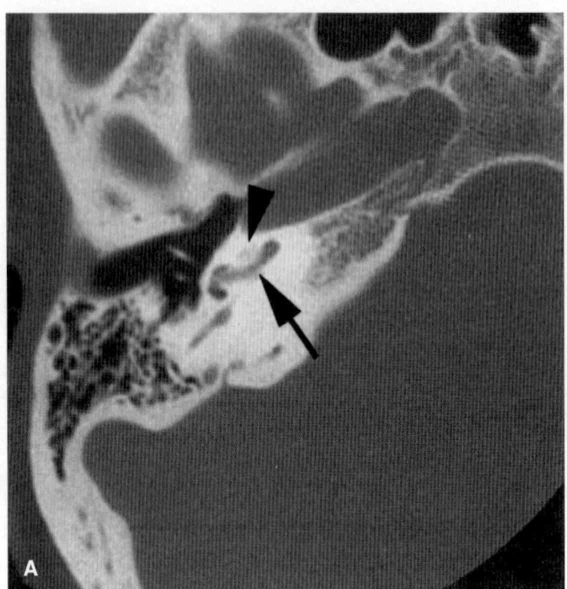

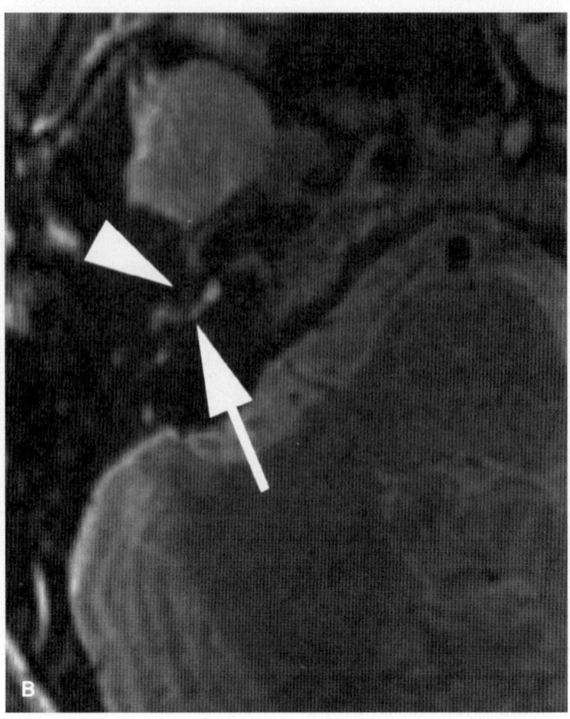

FIGURE 262-2 Labyrinthitis ossificans. (**A**) Axial CT scan viewed in bone window demonstrates ossification and therefore poor visualization of the middle and apical turns of the cochlea (arrowhead) as well as narrowing and subtle sclerosis of the base turn of the cochlea (arrow). (**B**) Axial T2-weighted image in the same patient shows absence of expected fluid signal in the middle and apical turns of the cochlea (expected position indicated by arrowhead), consistent with ossification. The base turn is narrowed, but still has some fluid signal within it (arrow). The information about patency of fluid spaces that is obtained on MRI can be useful to determine if a patient is a candidate for cochlear implantation. (From Lalwani AK. *Current Diagnosis & Treatment in Otolaryngology—Head and Neck Surgery*. 3rd ed. http://www.accessmedicine.com.)

KEY FEATURES

Description

- Disorder of the peripheral vestibular and auditory systems (inner ear).
- These systems consist of a complex series of interconnected tubes that are fluid-filled (fluid called endolymph) and form a labyrinth.
- The peripheral vestibular sensory organs of each ear detect head position and head motion to provide input for gaze stability, orientation, and balance.
- The peripheral auditory sensory organs of each ear convert sound vibration into a neural impulse to provide input for hearing.
- Each system sends its respective sensory information, via the vestibulocochlear nerve (eighth cranial nerve), to the central nervous system for processing.
- Reduction or loss of function of one of the labyrinths due to an infection, which causes an imbalance of neural activity between the two inner ears.
- Results in a spontaneous, severe attack of rotary vertigo (illusion of spinning motion of the room or self) that lasts from 48 to 72 hours as well as sudden hearing loss that can be permanent.

Essentials of Diagnosis

- Physical examination normal
- Audiogram abnormal
- Neurotologic examination abnormal
- Thorough and detailed history is essential to distinguish vestibular labyrinthitis from other vestibular disorders and central pathology.

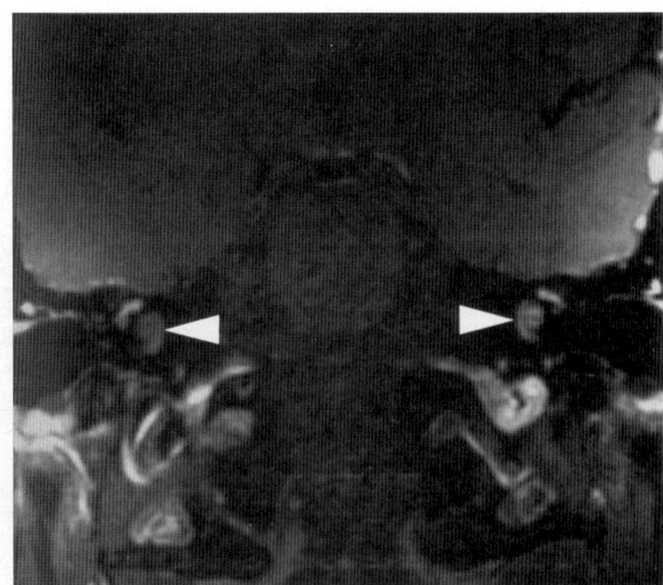

FIGURE 262-3 Radiation-induced labyrinthitis. A patient with bilateral hearing loss who had received radiation therapy 10 years earlier after the resection of a medulloblastoma in the posterior fossa. Postgadolinium T1-weighted image with fat saturation shows mild enhancement in the right cochlea (*notched arrowhead*) and intense enhancement in the left cochlea (*arrowhead*). (From Lalwani AK. *Current Diagnosis & Treatment in Otolaryngology—Head and Neck Surgery*. 3rd ed. http://www.accessmedicine.com.)

General Considerations

- Similar in presentation to vestibular neuritis, however with labyrinthitis, patients also have hearing loss and/or tinnitus (ringing or noises in the ear), which can be permanent.
- Initially, patients report persistent, severe feeling of rotary vertigo that occurs spontaneously but worsens with head movement.
  - Patients complain of nausea and vomiting, difficulty standing and walking without assistance, and blurred vision due to oscillopsia (apparent movement of the environment).
  - Initial symptoms improve over a period of a few days.
- After initial episode, patients typically continue to present with a general feeling of dizziness (disorientation, wooziness, off balance, etc.) and imbalance that mostly occurs with quick head movements and may continue to have difficulty reading.
  - This phase may manifest for up to 6 weeks or longer, until recovery and compensation occur.

Demographics

- More likely to occur after trauma or middle ear infections

CLINICAL FINDINGS

SIGNS AND SYMPTOMS

- Acute presentation
  - Report of persistent, prolonged episode of severe rotary vertigo, nausea and vomiting, unsteadiness, and/or jumping, bouncing vision
  - Imbalance manifested by inability to stand and walk without assistance
  - Increased risk of falling
  - Sudden hearing loss and audiological examination abnormal
  - Observe nystagmus in room light and with fixation removed
  - Abnormal neurotologic examination (impulse test, headshake test, dynamic visual acuity test, caloric test, vestibular evoked myogenic potentials [VEMP] test, and/or subjective visual vertical [SVV test])
  - No central signs (diplopia, dysarthria, dysphagia, dysmetria, numbness or weakness)
- Chronic, or uncompensated presentation
  - Report of general feelings of dizziness, unsteadiness, and/or jumping, bouncing vision
  - Postural and gait instability when sensory input challenged
  - May have continued increased risk of falling
  - May have continued nystagmus with fixation removed
  - May have continued abnormal neurotologic examination (impulse test, headshake test, dynamic visual acuity test caloric test, VEMP test, and/or SVV test)
  - Hearing loss can be permanent

Functional Implications

- Difficulty moving head quickly (turning, bending over, looking up) because of provoking symptoms
- Impedes balance and contributes to falls
- Difficulty identifying objects in environment and reading
- Reduced or lost ability to perform tasks in home, at work, and/or driving

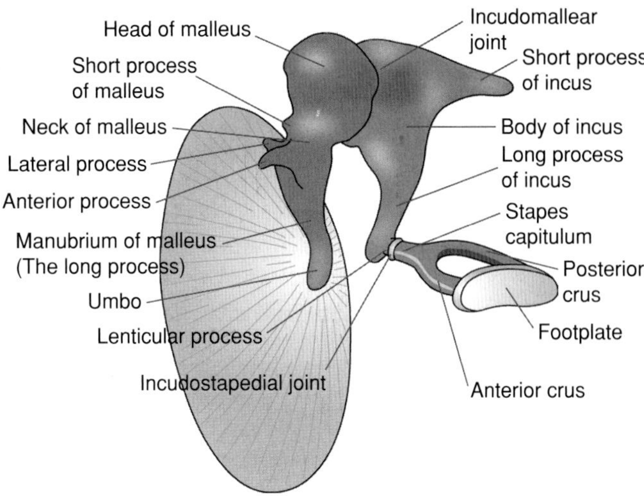

FIGURE 262-4 The middle ear ossicles (a right ear). (From Lalwani AK. *Current Diagnosis & Treatment in Otolaryngology—Head and Neck Surgery*. 3rd ed. http://www.accessmedicine.com. Copyright © The McGraw-Hill Companies, Inc. All rights reserved.)

Possible Contributing Causes

- Generally, due to viral infections
  - Measles
  - Mumps
  - Cytomegalovirus seen in the immune-compromised
  - Ramsay Hunt syndrome
- Bacterial toxins
  - Otitis media
  - Suppuration
  - Meningitis
  - Neurosyphilis
  - Lyme disease

Differential Diagnosis

- Endolymphatic hydrops (Ménière disease)
- Multiple sclerosis
- Acoustic neuroma (vestibular schwannoma)
- Other posterior fossa tumors
- Benign paroxysmal positional vertigo (BPPV)
- Migraine
- Brainstem stroke or transient ischemic attack (TIA)
- Superior canal dehiscence

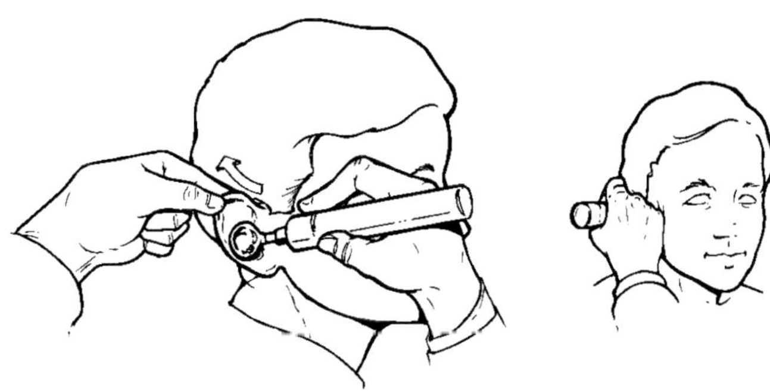

FIGURE 262-5 Use of the otoscope. Insert the ear speculum by pulling the upper edge of the pinna upward and backward to straighten the cartilaginous meatus so that it coincides with the axis of the bony canal. (From LeBlond RF, DeGowin RL, Brown DD. *DeGowin's Diagnostic Examination*. 9th ed. http://www.accessmedicine.com. Copyright © The McGraw-Hill Companies, Inc. All rights reserved.)

TABLE 262-1 Common Vestibular Disorders: Differential Diagnosis Based on Classic Presentations

Duration of Typical Vertiginous Episodes	Auditory Symptoms Present	Auditory Symptoms Absent
Seconds	Perilymphatic fistula	Positioning vertigo (cupulolithiasis), vertebrobasilar insufficiency, migraine-associated vertigo
Hours	Endolymphatic hydrops (Ménière syndrome, syphilis)	Migraine-associated vertigo
Days	Labyrinthitis, labyrinthine concussion, autoimmune inner ear disease	Vestibular neuronitis, migraine-associated vertigo
Months	Acoustic neuroma, ototoxicity	Multiple sclerosis, cerebellar degeneration

Source: Quick Medical Diagnosis & Treatment. New York, NY: McGraw-Hill © 2013.

- Perilymphatic fistula
- Bilateral vestibulopathy
- Vestibular neuritis
- Thyroid disease

MEANS OF CONFIRMATION OR DIAGNOSIS

Diagnostic Procedures

- Imaging tests
  - MRI or CT scan of brain, including posterior fossa and internal auditory canals
- Special tests
  - Electronystagmography (ENG) or videonystagmography (VNG)
  - Rotational chair
  - VEMP
  - Static and dynamic SVV
  - Audiogram
  - Laboratory testing

FINDINGS AND INTERPRETATION

- Abnormal neurotologic examination (impulse test, headshake test, dynamic visual acuity test, caloric test, VEMP test, and/or SVV test)

REFERRALS/ADMITTANCE

- For suspected acute stroke or sudden hearing loss: Emergency department
- For disease management: Neurologist, otolaryngologist (ear, nose, and throat doctor [ENT]) or neurotologist
- For rehabilitation: Vestibular-trained PT or occupational therapist

IMPAIRMENTS

- Perceived orientation (dizziness and vertigo)
- Postural control
- Gaze instability

TESTS AND MEASURES

- Oculomotor examination
  - Nonvestibular: Ocular motility, pursuit, saccades, optokinetic nystagmus testing (OKN), vergence
  - Vestibular
    - In room light: Spontaneous and gaze-holding nystagmus, head impulse test, dynamic visual acuity
    - Fixation removed: Spontaneous and gaze-holding nystagmus, head shake, pressure-induced nystagmus, hyperventilation-induced nystagmus
- Rinne and Weber tests
- Vertebrobasilar insufficiency testing
- Cervical spine special tests (Sharpe–Purser, alar ligament)
- Positioning tests: Dix–Hallpike maneuver, roll test, and side-lying test
- Coordination
- Cranial nerve integrity
- Sensation
- ROM, including neck
- Strength
- Endurance
- Postural alignment
- Postural control and balance
- Gait
- Symptom intensity rating (visual or verbal analog scale, UCLA dizziness questionnaire, motion sensitivity quotient)
- Perceived disability (dizziness handicap inventory, vestibular rehabilitation benefits questionnaire)

INTERVENTION

- Medical management
  - Depending on whether viral or bacterial cause, immediate administration of corticosteroids (methylprednisolone) or antibiotics may improve the rate and extent of recovery.
  - If viral agent is the cause, sometimes antivirals are also prescribed.
  - Vestibular suppressants and antiemetic medications may be prescribed in the acute phase to help reduce the severe symptoms. Only indicated for short term use because can impair vestibular compensation.
  - Bed rest is needed when symptoms are severe.
- Once severe symptoms subside, vestibular and balance rehabilitation is used to promote central nervous system compensation, which reduces dizziness, gaze instability, and imbalance.
  - Vestibular–ocular reflex (VOR) function exercises
  - Habituation exercises
  - Postural control and balance training
  - Gait training

FUNCTIONAL GOALS

- The patient will
  - Report reduced frequency and intensity of dizziness (wooziness, lightheadedness, etc.) during head movements for home- and work-related tasks.

  - Demonstrate normal standing and walking balance for home- and work-related tasks.
  - Have decreased risk of falling when standing and walking.
  - Have less than two lines difference with dynamic visual acuity testing making it possible to read, watch TV, and identify objects in the environment while walking.

PROGNOSIS

- In otherwise healthy individuals, reduction of dizziness, gaze instability, and imbalance and return to normal activities can be expected, especially for those that get adequate physical activity.
- For patients whose symptoms do not improve, vestibular and balance exercises may help promote recovery and compensation.
- Hearing may improve or recover in some patients, especially if they receive immediate medical treatment.

PATIENT RESOURCE

- Labyrinthitis and Vestibular Neuritis. Vestibular Disorder Association. http://vestibular.org/labyrinthitis-and-vestibular-neuritis. Accessed July 5, 2013.

REFERENCES

1. ICD9Data. http://www.icd9data.com. Accessed July 3, 2013.
2. ICD10Data. http://www.icd10data.com. Accessed July 3, 2013.
3. *Guide to Physical Therapist Practice*. 2nd ed. Alexandria, VA: American Physical Therapy Association; 2001. Revised 2003.

ADDITIONAL REFERENCES

- Aw ST, Halmagyi GM, Curthoys IS, Todd MJ, Yavor RA,. Unilateral vestibular deafferentation causes permanent impairment of the human vertical vestibulo-ocular reflex in the pitch plane. *Exp Brain Res*. 1994;102:121–130.
- Beasley NJ, Jones NS. Menière's disease: evolution of a definition. *J Laryngol Otol*. 1996;110(12):1107–1113.
- Dutton M. Vestibular Disorders. In: Dutton M, ed. *McGraw-Hill's NPTE (National Physical Therapy Examination)*. 2nd ed. New York, NY: McGraw-Hill; 2012. http://www.accessphysiotherapy.com/content/5400074. Accessed July 5, 2013.
- Hain, TC, Fetter M, Zee DS. Head-shaking nystagmus in patients with unilateral peripheral vestibular lesions. *Am J Otolaryngol*. 1987;8:36–47.
- Fetter M. Vestibular system disorders. In: Herdman SJ, ed. *Vestibular Rehabilitation*. 2nd ed. Philadelphia, PA: F.A. Davis Company; 2000: Chapter 6;98–107.
- Furman JM, et al. *Vestibular Disorders: A Case Study Approach*. Oxford: Oxford University Press; 2003.
- Gianoli GJ. Chapter 19. DDX: Fixed vestibular deficits. In: Goebel JA, ed. *Practical Management of the Dizzy Patient*. Philadelphia, PA: Lippincott Williams & Wilkins; 2001.
- Hay WW, Levin MJ, Sondheimer JM, Deterding RR, eds. *CURRENT Diagnosis & Treatment: Pediatrics*. 20th ed. New York, NY: McGraw-Hill; 2011. http://www.accessphysiotherapy.com/resource/14. Accessed July 4, 2013.
- Haybach PJ, Underwood J. *Meniere's Disease: What You Need to Know*. Portland, OR: Vestibular Disorders Association; 1998.
- Honrubia V. Quantitative evaluation of dizziness characteristics and impact of quality of life. *Am J of Otology*. 1996;17(4):595–602.
- Lempert T, Neuhauser H. Epidemiology of vertigo, migraine and vestibular migraine. *J Neurol*. 2008;256(3):333–338. doi: 10.1007/s00415-009-0149-2.
- McGraw-Hill's NPTE (National Physical Therapy Examination). http://www.accessphysiotherapy.com/content/5399379. Accessed June 1, 2014.
- Waxman SG, ed. Clinical neuroanatomy. 26th ed. New York, NY: McGraw-Hill; 2010. http://www.accessphysiotherapy.com/resource/22. Accessed July 5, 2013.

263 VESTIBULAR NEURITIS

Eric Shamus, PhD, DPT, PT, CSCS
Jennifer Shamus, PhD, DPT, COMT, CSCS
Mollie Venglar, DSc, MSPT, NCS

CONDITION/DISORDER SYNONYMS

- Acute (or recurrent) peripheral vestibulopathy
- Vestibular hypofunction or loss
- Vestibular neuronitis

ICD-9-CM CODES[1]

- 386.12 Vestibular neuronitis
- 386.53 Hypoactive labyrinth unilateral

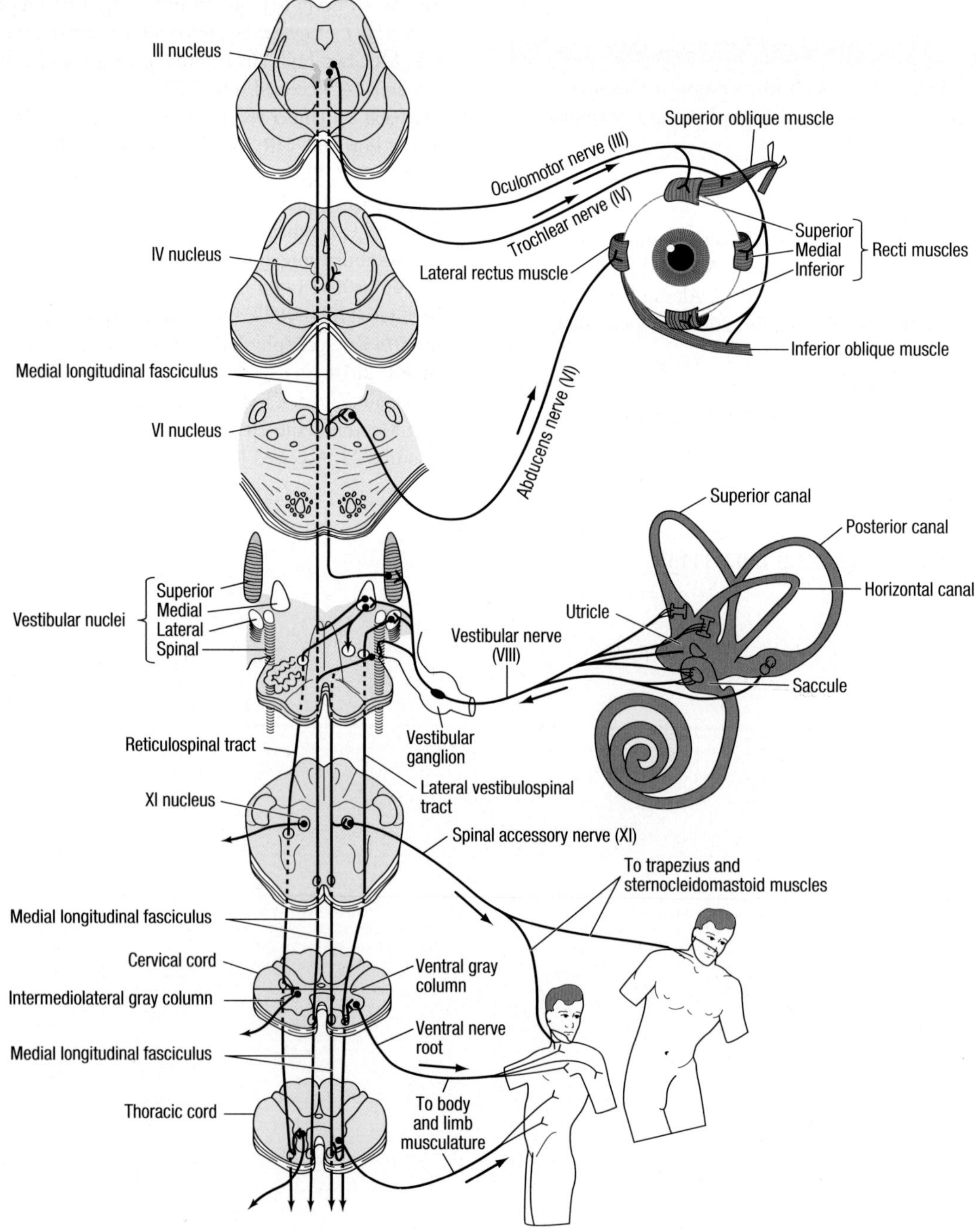

FIGURE 263-1 The vestibular reflex pathways. (Reproduced by permission from House EL. *A Systematic Approach to Neuroscience*. New York, NY: McGraw-Hill, 1979.)

ICD-10-CM CODES[2]

- H81.20 Vestibular neuronitis, unspecified ear
- H81.21 Vestibular neuronitis, right ear
- H81.22 Vestibular neuronitis, left ear
- H81.23 Vestibular neuronitis, bilateral

PREFERRED PRACTICE PATTERNS

- 4F: Impaired Joint Mobility, Motor Function, Muscle Performance, and Range of Motion (ROM), or Reflex Integrity, Secondary to Spinal Disorders
- 5A: Primary Prevention/Risk Reduction for Loss of Balance and Falling
- 5F: Impaired Peripheral Nerve Integrity and Muscle Performance Associated with Peripheral Nerve Injury

PATIENT PRESENTATION

A 44-year-old woman was referred to physical therapy secondary to insidious episodes of severe vestibular symptoms. She reports that she often feels like things in her vision are "jumping up and down" and she feels like she is spinning when she looks up. The symptoms don't subside right away when she stops looking up but rather take several days to lessen. When she doesn't feel like she is spinning, she feels somewhat disoriented and off-balance and has had several episodes of "near falls." She has not been treated with any antibiotics in several years, nor has she experienced any injury to her head. She does not have any change in her hearing. In addition to the sensations of moving and spinning, she has been forced to stop driving because she struggles to read signs and to turn her head quickly enough to drive safely.

KEY FEATURES

Description

- Disorder of the peripheral vestibular system (part of the inner ear)
- The peripheral vestibular system of each ear is made up of five sensory organs (hair-cell receptors contained within the superior, posterior, and horizontal semicircular canals as well as within the utricle and saccule) and the vestibular nerve.
- The vestibular sensory organs detect head position and head motion to provide input for gaze stability, orientation, and balance.
- Reduction or loss of function of one of the systems causes an imbalance of neural activity between the two inner ears, which causes the central nervous system to interpret the aberrant sensory input as head rotation.
- Results in a spontaneous, severe attack of rotary vertigo (the illusion of spinning motion of the room or self) that lasts from 48 to 72 hours.

Essentials of Diagnosis

- Physical examination normal
- Audiogram normal
- Neurotologic examination abnormal
- Thorough and detailed history is essential to distinguish vestibular neuritis from other vestibular disorders and central pathology

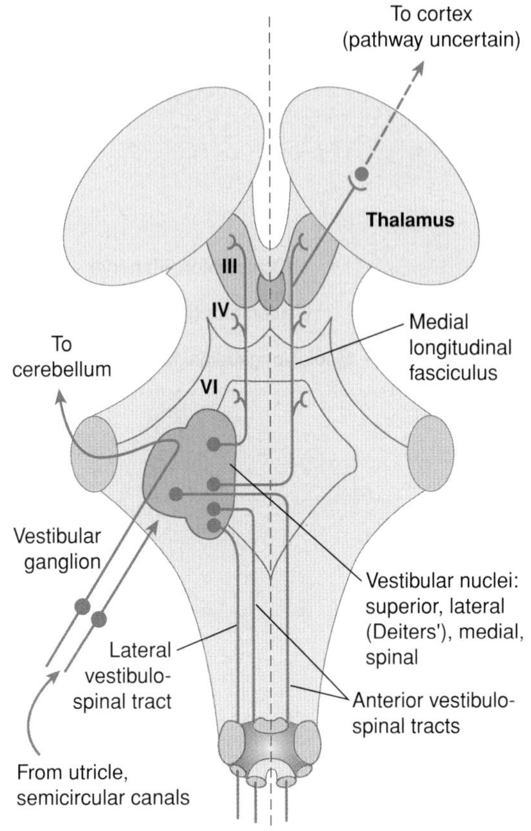

FIGURE 263-2 Principal vestibular pathways superimposed on a dorsal view of the brain stem. Cerebellum and cerebral cortex removed. (Reproduced, with permission, from Ganong WF. *Review of Medical Physiology*. 22nd ed. McGraw-Hill, 2005.)

General Considerations

- Thought to represent a reactivated dormant herpes infection in Scarpa ganglion.[3]
- Initially patients report
  - Persistent, severe feeling of rotary vertigo that occurs spontaneously but worsens with head movement.
  - Nausea and vomiting.
  - Difficulty standing and walking without assistance.
  - Blurred vision due to oscillopsia (apparent movement of the environment).
  - These initial symptoms improve over a period of a few days.
- After initial episode patients
  - Typically continue to present with a general feeling of dizziness (disorientation, wooziness, off balance, etc.).
  - Imbalance that mostly occurs with quick head movements.
  - They may continue to have difficulty reading.
  - This phase may manifest for up to 6 weeks or longer until recovery and compensation occur.
- No audiological symptoms with vestibular neuritis.

Demographics

- Can occur at any age
- Primarily occurs in individuals 30 to 60 years with women having peak occurrence in fourth decade and men in the sixth decade
- In clinics specializing in vestibular disorders, may account for between 3% and 10% of diagnoses

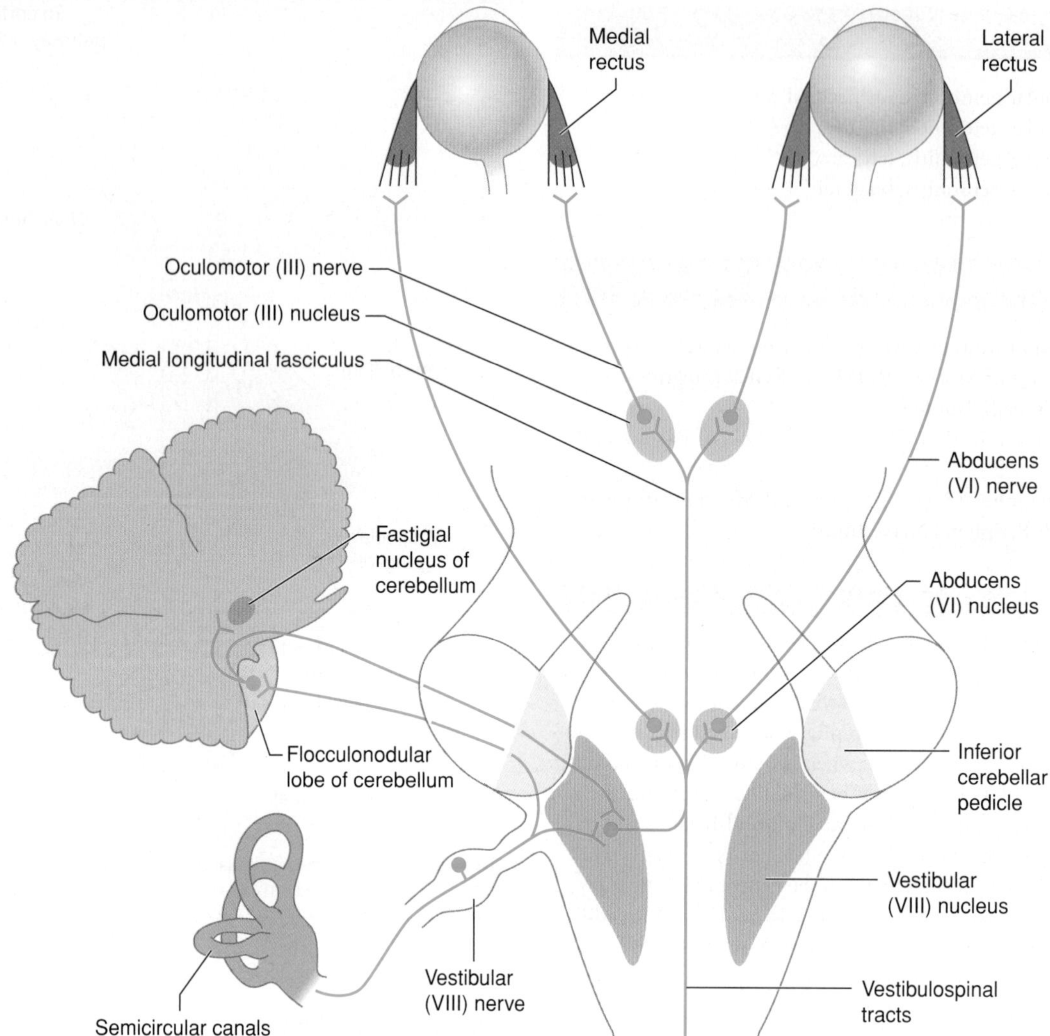

FIGURE 263-3 Peripheral and central vestibular pathways. The vestibular nerve terminates in the vestibular nucleus in the brainstem and midline cerebellar structures that project to the vestibular nucleus. From here, bilateral pathways in the medial longitudinal fasciculus ascend to the abducens (VI) and oculomotor (III) nuclei and descend to the spinal cord (vestibulospinal tracts). (From Greenberg DA, Aminoff MJ, Simon RP. *Clinical Neurology.* 8th ed. http://www.accessmedicine.com. Copyright © The McGraw-Hill Companies, Inc. All rights reserved.)

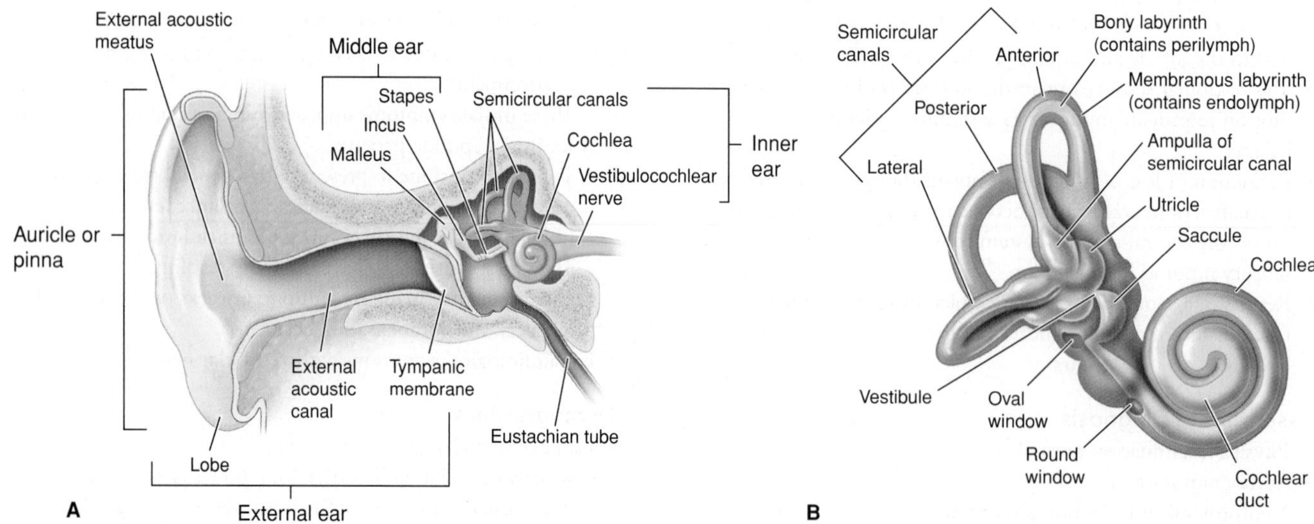

FIGURE 263-4 Ear anatomy. **A.** Drawing of modified coronal section through external ear and temporal bone, with structures of the middle and inner ear demonstrated. **B.** High-resolution view of inner ear. (From Longo DL, Fauci AS, Kasper DL, Hauser SL, Jameson JL, Loscalzo J, eds. *Harrison's Principles of Internal Medicine.* 18th ed. http://www.accessmedicine.com. Copyright © The McGraw-Hill Companies, Inc. All rights reserved.)

CLINICAL FINDINGS

SIGNS AND SYMPTOMS

- Acute presentation
  - Report of persistent, prolonged episode of severe rotary vertigo, nausea and vomiting, unsteadiness, and/or jumping, bouncing vision
  - Imbalance manifested by inability to stand and walk without assistance
  - Increased risk of falling
  - No report of hearing loss, and audiological examination normal
  - Observe nystagmus in room light and with fixation removed
  - Abnormal neurotologic examination (impulse test, headshake test, dynamic visual acuity test, caloric test, vestibular evoked myogenic potential [VEMP] test, and/or subjective visual vertical [SVV] test)
  - No central signs (diplopia, dysarthria, dysphagia, dysmetria, numbness, or weakness)
- Chronic or uncompensated presentation
  - Report of general feelings of dizziness, unsteadiness, and/or jumping, bouncing vision
  - Postural and gait instability when sensory input challenged
  - May have continued increased risk of falling
  - May have continued nystagmus with fixation removed
  - May have continued abnormal neurotologic examination (impulse test, headshake test, dynamic visual acuity test, caloric test, VEMP test, and/or SVV test)

Functional Implications

- Difficulty moving head quickly (turning, bending over, looking up) because doing so provokes symptoms
- Impedes balance and contributes to falls
- Difficulty identifying objects in environment and reading
- Reduced or lost ability to perform tasks in home, at work, and/or while driving

Possible Contributing Causes

- In most cases, cause is idiopathic
- Some cases have proven to be due to an infectious or inflammatory process from the presence of a viral agent (herpes simplex virus type I) or autoimmune etiology
- Onset of symptoms often preceded by upper respiratory or GI tract infection

Differential Diagnosis

- Endolymphatic hydrops (Ménière disease)
- Multiple sclerosis
- Acoustic neuroma (vestibular schwannoma)
- Other posterior fossa tumors
- Benign paroxysmal positional vertigo (BPPV)
- Migraine
- Brainstem stroke or transient ischemic attack (TIA)
- Superior canal dehiscence
- Perilymphatic fistula
- Bilateral vestibulopathy
- Serous or suppurative labyrinthitis
- Ramsay Hunt syndrome
- Meningitis
- Thyroid disease
- Syphilis

MEANS OF CONFIRMATION OR DIAGNOSIS

Imaging

- MRI or CT scan of brain, including posterior fossa and internal auditory canals

TABLE 263-1 Medications Commonly Used to Reduce Dizziness, Vertigo, and Associated Nausea

Drug (Brand Name)	Pharmacologic Class	Dose	Primary Use	Adverse Reactions
Meclizine (Antivert, Bonine)	Anticholinergic Antihistamine	25 mg every 4–6 h orally	Dizziness	Drowsiness
Dimenhydrinate (Dramamine)	Anticholinergic Antihistamine	50 mg every 4–6 h orally	Dizziness	Drowsiness
Cyclizine (Marezine)	Anticholinergic Antihistamine	50 mg every 4–6 h orally or IM	Dizziness	Drowsiness
Diazepam (Valium)	Benzodiazepine	1–2 mg twice daily orally; 2–10 mg (1 dose) given acutely orally, IM or IV	Dizziness	Lethargy
Clonazepam (Klonopin)	Benzodiazepine	0.25–0.5 mg twice daily orally	Dizziness	Lethargy
Prochlorperazine (Compazine)	Phenothiazine	10 mg orally or IM every 6 hours or 25 mg rectally every 12 h	Nausea	Extrapyramidal reactions, drowsiness, anticholinergic effects
Promethazine (Phenergan)	Phenothiazine	25 mg every 6–12 h orally or rectally	Nausea	Extrapyramidal reactions, drowsiness, restlessness
Trimethobenzamine (Tigan)	Substituted ethanolamine	250 mg every 6–8 h or 200 mg rectally or IM	Nausea	Extrapyramidal reaction (unusual)
Diphenhydramine (Benadryl)	Antihistamine	25–100 mg every 8 h orally	Nausea	Drowsiness
Hydroxyzine (Vistaril, Atarax)	Piperazine derivative	25–50 mg every 8 h orally	Nausea	Drowsiness

Source: McKean SC, Ross JJ, DresslerDD, Brotman DJ, Ginsberg JS. *Principles and Practice of Hospital Medicine. www.accessmedicine.com.*

Diagnostic Procedures

- Special tests
  - Electronystagmography (ENG) or videonystagmography (VNG)
  - Rotational chair
  - VEMP
  - Static and dynamic SVV
  - Audiogram
  - Laboratory testing

FINDINGS AND INTERPRETATION

- Physical examination normal
- Audiogram normal
- Neurotologic examination abnormal

REFERRALS/ADMITTANCE

- To emergency department suspected acute stroke
- To neurologist, otolaryngologist (ear, nose, and throat [ENT] doctor) or neurotologist disease management
- To vestibular-trained PT or occupational therapist rehabilitation

IMPAIRMENTS

- Perceived orientation (dizziness and vertigo)
- Postural control
- Gaze stability

TESTS AND MEASURES

- Oculomotor examination
  - Nonvestibular: Ocular motility, pursuit, saccades, optokinetic nystagmus testing (OKN), vergence
  - Vestibular
    - In room light: Spontaneous and gaze-holding nystagmus, head impulse test, dynamic visual acuity
    - Fixation removed: Spontaneous and gaze-holding nystagmus, head shake, pressure-induced nystagmus, hyperventilation-induced nystagmus
- Rinne and Weber tests
- Vertebrobasilar insufficiency testing
- Cervical spine special tests (Sharpe–Purser, alar ligament)
- Positioning tests: Dix–Hallpike maneuver, roll test, and side-lying test
- Side-lying test
- Coordination
- Cranial nerve integrity
- Sensation
- ROM, including neck
- Strength
- Endurance
- Postural alignment
- Postural control and balance
- Gait
- Symptom intensity rating (visual or verbal analog scale, UCLA dizziness questionnaire, motion sensitivity quotient)
- Perceived disability (dizziness handicap inventory, vestibular rehabilitation benefits questionnaire)

INTERVENTION

- Medical management
  - Prescription of corticosteroids (methylprednisolone) within the first week of symptom onset may improve the rate and extent of recovery.
  - Sometimes antivirals are also prescribed.
  - Vestibular suppressants and antiemetic medications may be prescribed in the acute phase to help reduce the severe symptoms.
    - Only indicated for short-term use because they can impair vestibular compensation.
  - Bed rest is needed when symptoms are severe.
- Once severe symptoms subside, vestibular and balance rehabilitation is used to promote central nervous system compensation, which reduces impairments.
  - Vestibulo-ocular reflex function exercises
  - Habituation exercises
  - Postural control and balance training
  - Gait training

FUNCTIONAL GOALS

- Patient will
  - Report reduced frequency and intensity of dizziness (wooziness, lightheadedness, etc.) during head movements for home- and work-related tasks.
  - Demonstrate normal standing and walking balance for home- and work-related tasks.
  - Have decreased risk of falling when standing and walking.
  - Have less than two lines difference with dynamic visual acuity testing and be able to read, watch TV, and identify objects in the environment while walking.

PROGNOSIS

- In otherwise healthy individuals, reduction of symptoms and return to normal activities can be expected, especially for those who get adequate physical activity.
- For patients whose symptoms do not improve, customized vestibular and balance exercises may help promote recovery and compensation.

PATIENT RESOURCE

- Labyrinthitis and Vestibular Neuritis. Vestibular Disorder Association. http://vestibular.org/labyrinthitis-and-vestibular-neuritis. Accessed July 15, 2013.

REFERENCES

1. ICD9Data.com. http://www.icd9data.com. Accessed July 13, 2013.
2. ICD10Data.com. http://www.icd10data.com. Accessed July 13, 2013.
3. Dutton M. The craniovertebral region. In: Dutton M, ed. *Dutton's Orthopaedic Examination, Evaluation, and Intervention*, 3rd ed. New York, NY: McGraw-Hill; 2012:Chapter 23. http://www.accessphysiotherapy.com/content/56549019. Accessed July 17, 2013.

ADDITIONAL REFERENCES

- Aw ST, Halmagyi GM, Curthoys IS, Todd MJ, Yavor RA. Unilateral vestibular deafferentation causes permanent impairment of the human vertical vestibulo-ocular reflex in the pitch plane. *Exp Brain Res.* 1994;102(1):121–130.
- Beasley NJ, Jones NS. Menière's disease: evolution of a definition. *J Laryngol Otol.* 1996;110(12):1107–1113.

- Dutton M, ed. *McGraw-Hill's NPTE (National Physical Therapy Examination).* 2nd ed. New York, NY: McGraw-Hill; 2012. http://www.accessphysiotherapy.com/resource/611. Accessed July 15, 2013.
- Fetter M. Vestibular system disorders. In: Herdman SJ, ed. *Vestibular Rehabilitation.* 2nd ed. Philadelphia, PA: F.A. Davis Company; 2000:Chapter 6;98–107.
- Fetter M, Dichgans J. Vestibular neuritis spares the inferior division of the vestibular nerve. *Brain.* 1996;119(Pt 3):755–763.
- Furman JM, Cass SP. *Vestibular Disorders: A Case Study Approach.* 2nd ed. Oxford: Oxford University Press; 2003.
- *Guide to Physical Therapist Practice.* 2nd ed. Alexandria, VA: American Physical Therapy Association;2001. Revised 2003.
- Hain TC, Fetter M, Zee DS. Head-shaking nystagmus in patients with unilateral peripheral vestibular lesions. *Am J Otolaryngol.* 1987;8(1):36–47.
- Hay WW, Levin MJ, Sondheimer JM, Deterding RR, eds. *CURRENT Diagnosis & Treatment: Pediatrics.* 20th ed. New York, NY: McGraw-Hill; 2011. http://www.accessphysiotherapy.com/resource/14. Accessed July 15, 2013.
- Haybach PJ, Underwood J. *Meniere's Disease: What You Need to Know.* Portland, OR: Vestibular Disorders Association; 1998.
- Lempert T, Neuhauser H. Epidemiology of vertigo, migraine and vestibular migraine. *J Neurol.* 2008;256(3):333–338. doi: 10.1007/s00415-009-0149-2.
- Shamus E, Stern DF. Content Standardization/Component Requirements. In: Shamus E, Stern DF, eds. *Effective Documentation for Physical Therapy Professionals.* 2nd ed. New York, NY: McGraw-Hill; 2011:Chapter 4. http://www.accessphysiotherapy.com/content/55665293. Accessed July 15, 2013.
- Strupp M, Zingler VC, Arbusow V, et al. Methylprednisolone, valacyclovir, or the combination for vestibular neuritis. *N Engl J Med.* 2004;351(4):354–361.
- Waxman SG, ed. *Clinical Neuroanatomy.* 26th ed. New York, NY: McGraw-Hill; 2010. http://www.accessphysiotherapy.com/resource/22. Accessed July 15, 2013.

PART 7

WOMEN'S/MEN'S HEALTH DISORDERS

264 VULVODYNIA

Cynthia E. Neville, DPT, PT, WCS

CONDITION/DISORDER SYNONYMS

- Painful intercourse
- Urogenital pain disorders
- Vaginismus

ICD-9-CM CODES

- 625.0 Dyspareunia
- 625.1 Vaginismus
- 625.7 Vulvodynia
- 625.71 Vulvar vestibulitis
- 728.2 Muscular wasting and disuse atrophy
- 728.85 Spasm of muscle
- 729.1 Myalgia

ICD-10-CM CODES

- M62.83 Muscle spasm
- M79.1 Myalgia
- N94.1 Dyspareunia
- N94.2 Vaginismus
- N94.81 Vulvodynia
- N94.810 Vulvar vestibulitis
- N94.818 Other vulvodynia
- N94.819 Other vulvodynia unspecified
- R10.2 Pelvic and perineal pain

PREFERRED PRACTICE PATTERN

- 4C: Impaired Muscle Performance[1]

PATIENT PRESENTATION

A 34-year-old woman reports that she has been experiencing burning pain at the opening of the vagina during intercourse for the past several months. Prior to this onset, she was able to have pain-free intercourse with her husband of 10 years. The symptoms started after she used an over-the-counter anti-fungal cream to self-treat what she thought was a yeast infection. Lately, when she attempts intercourse the burning pain is severe and she feels that she cannot allow vaginal penetration for intercourse.

KEY FEATURES

Description

- Vulvodynia is chronic pain in the vulvar region without a definable cause.
- Most often described as burning pain; also stinging, stabbing, or rawness.
- Characterized by provoked or constant vulvar pain of varying intensity.

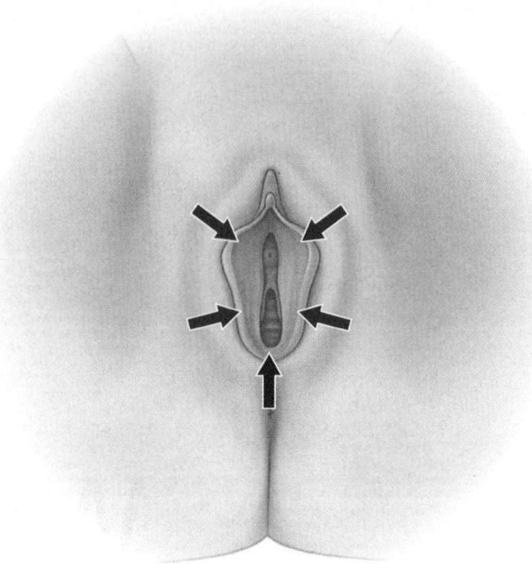

FIGURE 264-1 Hart's line is the outer perimeter of the vestibule. (From DeCherney AH, Nathan L, Laufer N, Roman AS. *Current Diagnosis & Treatment: Obstetrics & Gynecology*. 11th ed. www.accessmedicine.com. Copyright © The McGraw-Hill Companies, Inc. All rights reserved.)

- Vaginismus is persistent difficulty with vaginal insertion despite desire to do so; and a perceived reduction in size of vaginal opening attributed to muscle spasm.

Essentials of Diagnosis

- Any diagnosable gynecological disorder is not vulvodynia; rule out gynecological pathology
  - Infectious: Candidiasis, herpes, etc.
  - Inflammatory: Lichen planus, ummunobullous disorders, etc.
  - Neoplastic: Paget disease, squamous cell carcinoma, etc.
  - Neurologic: Herpes neuralgia, spinal nerve compression, etc.
- Cotton Swab Test: Pain with light palpation of the soft end of a cotton swab at the vaginal introit along Hart's line[2]
- Difficulty with or pain with vaginal insertion during gynecological examination, insertion of tampon, or during and after sexual intercourse

General Considerations

- Female only
- Classified according to site of pain (generalized or localized) and by whether it is provoked, unprovoked, or mixed
- Chronic pain condition often characterized by distress and fear
- Urogenital pain disorders are frequently associated with pain in nearby body areas; especially back, pelvic, hip, groin regions

Demographics

- Lifetime prevalence of vulvodynia is found in 8% of sexually active women of all ages.[3]
- 16% of women (n = 4915) reported chronic unexplained vulvar pain for more than 3 months.[4]

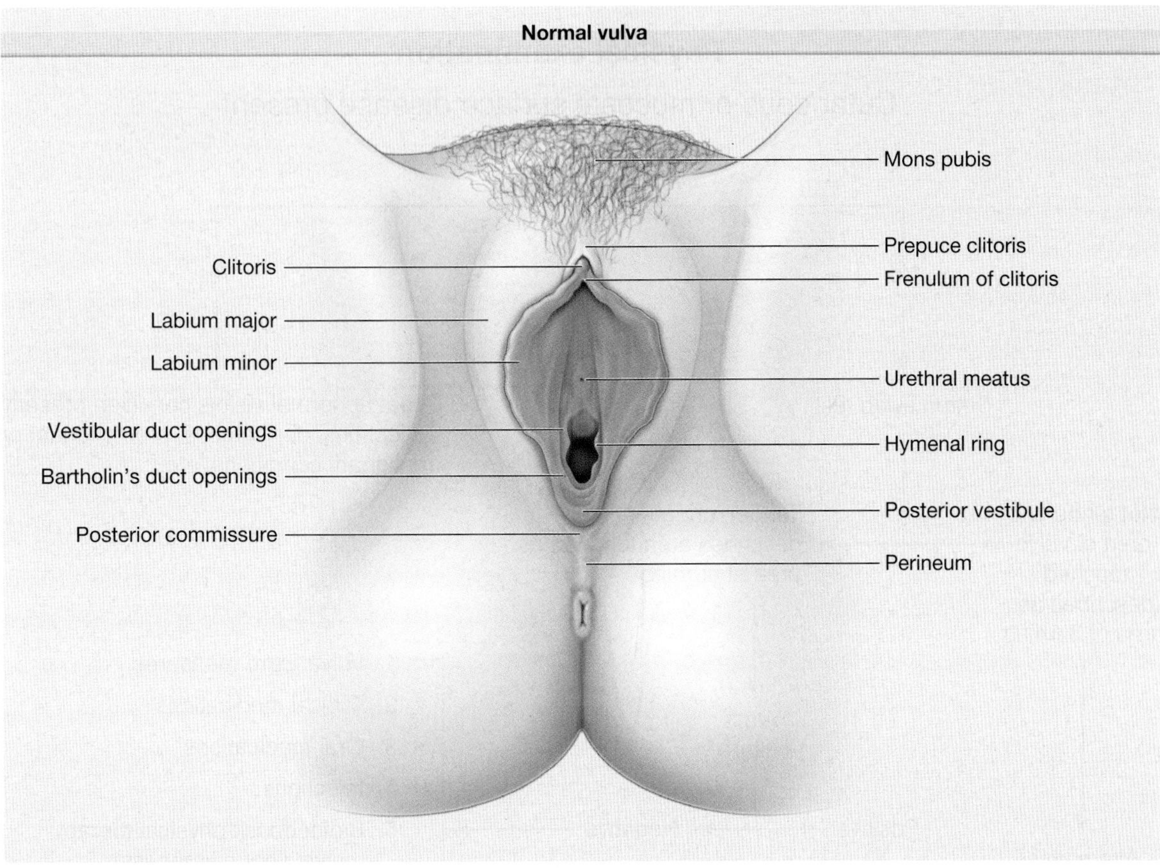

FIGURE 264-2 Normal vulva. (From Goldsmith LA, Katz SI, Gilchrest BA, Paller AS, Leffell DJ, Wolff K. *Fitzpatrick's Dermatology in General Medicine.* 8th ed. www.accessmedicine.com. Copyright © The McGraw-Hill Companies, Inc. All rights reserved.)

- Hispanic women are 80% more likely to report vulvodynia that African American or white women.[4]
- Many patients with pelvic pain will go on to develop chronic pain syndrome with depression, pain out of proportion to pathology, and changing roles in marriage, family, and career.[5]

CLINICAL FINDINGS

SIGNS AND SYMPTOMS

- Generalized vulvodynia involves the whole vulva
  - Provoked: Sexual, nonsexual, both
  - Unprovoked: Always present
  - Mixed: Provoked and unprovoked
- Localized vulvodynia: Involves a portion of the vulva (e.g., vestibulodynia, clitorodynia)
- May complain of lower quadrant abdominal pain during sexual intercourse
- Symptoms may worsen or decrease during and after sexual intercourse

Functional Implications

- Pain during attempted penetration
- Sexual dysfunction
- Women with unprovoked vulvodynia may have pain caused by wearing undergarments or tight-fitting clothing
- May lead to unwanted sexual abstinence
- May lead to decision to not have a subsequent pregnancy

Possible Contributing Causes

- Possible etiologies include:[6]
  - Inflammation
  - Infection
  - Immunologic factors

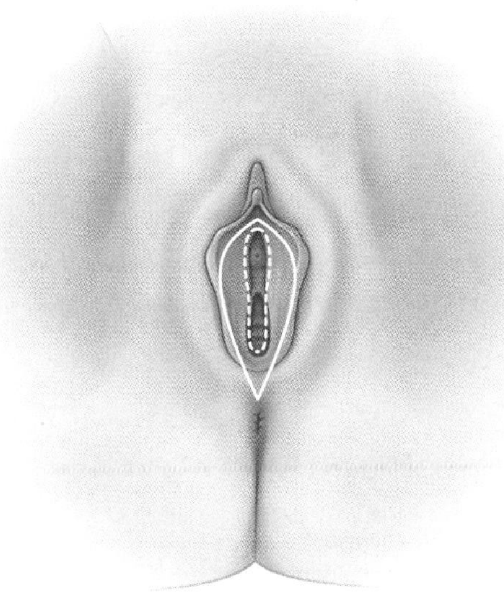

FIGURE 264-3 The outline of vestibulectomy for localized provoked vulvodynia. (From DeCherney AH, Nathan L, Laufer N, Roman AS. *Current Diagnosis & Treatment: Obstetrics & Gynecology.* 11th ed. www.accessmedicine.com. Copyright © The McGraw-Hill Companies, Inc. All rights reserved.)

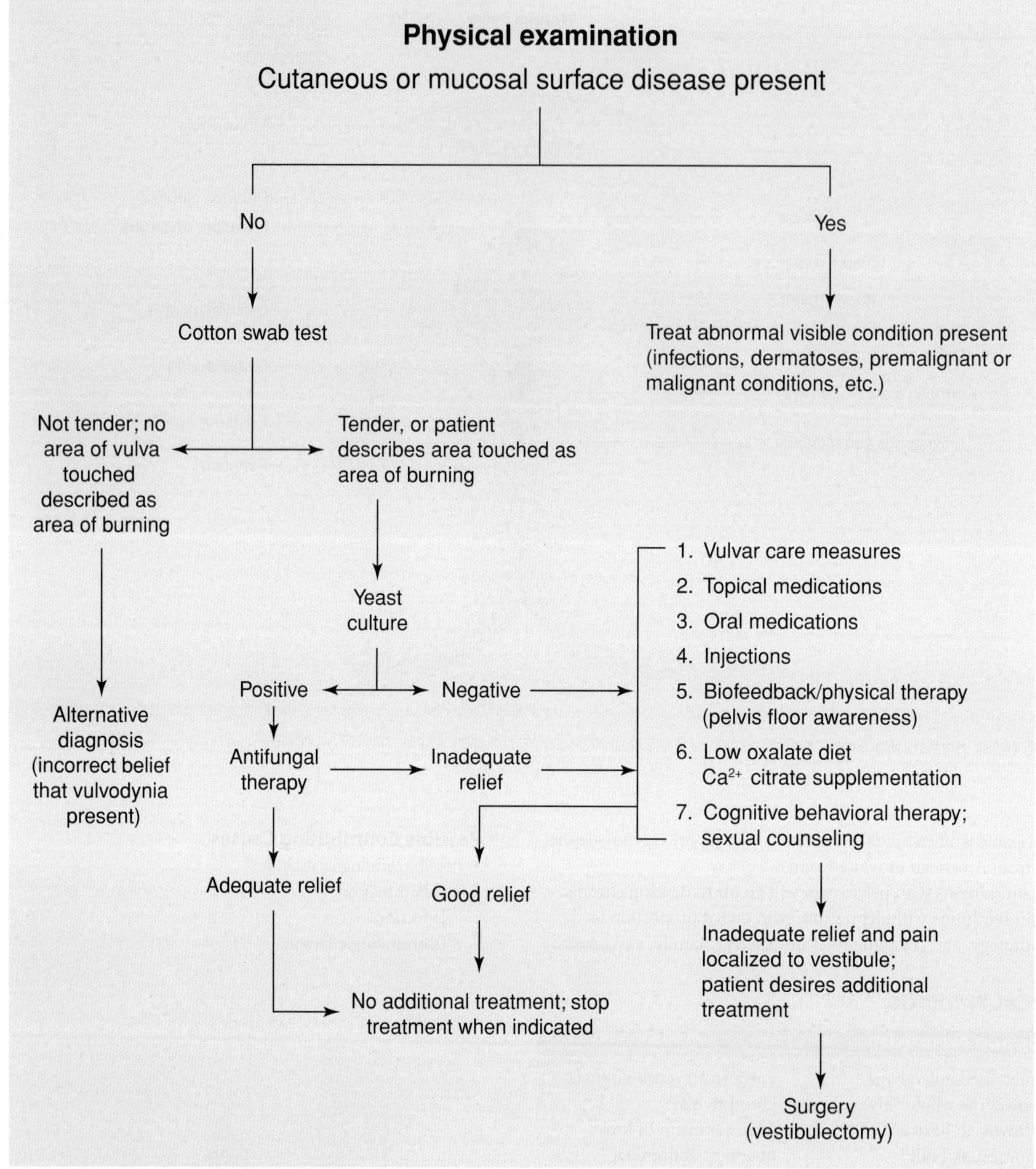

FIGURE 264-4 Algorithm for the diagnosis of vulvodynia. (From Haefner HK, Collins ME, Davis GD, et al. The vulvodynia guideline. *J Low Genit Tract Dis*. 2005;9(1):40–51; *with permission.*)

  - Hormonal influences
  - Genetics
  - Neuropathic changes
  - High levels of urinary oxalates
  - Pelvic floor abnormalities
- History of sexual or physical abuse
- Stress, anxiety
- Fear, catastrophizing

Differential Diagnosis

- Fungal
  - Lichen sclerosis
  - Lichen planus
- Urinary tract infection (UTI)
- Sexually transmitted disease
- Urethritis
- Bladder infection

- Yeast infection
- Bacterial vaginosis
- Organ dysfunction from cancer or malignancy
- Nonmalignant tumor in abdomen or organs
- Gynecologic problems in females
  - Endometriosis
  - Menses
  - Ectopic pregnancy
  - Ovarian cyst
  - Fibroids
  - Menopause
- Appendicitis
- Pelvic inflammatory disease

MEANS OF CONFIRMATION OR DIAGNOSIS

Laboratory Tests

- To rule out other pathology
  - Blood tests to rule out pathology
  - Urine culture/urinalysis to rule out infection
  - H&H for signs of bleeding, anemia, pathogens, immune status, vitamin deficiencies, white blood cell count

Imaging

- All tests to rule out other pathology
  - Cystoscopy
  - Ultrasound
  - CT
  - Bladder scans
  - MRI
  - X-ray

Diagnostic Procedures

- To rule out other pathology
  - Biopsy
  - Bladder biopsy
  - Colonoscopy
  - Cystography
  - Cystometrogram
  - Defecography
  - Postvoid residual
  - Uroflowmetry
  - Video urodynamic testing

FINDINGS AND INTERPRETATION

- sEMG biofeedback assessment of the pelvic floor muscles (PFM) and abdominal muscles

TREATMENT

Medication

- Topical medications
  - Capsaicin
  - EMLA cream
  - Gabapentin
  - Lidocaine ointment 5%
  - Nitroglycerine
- Estraciol and testosterone
- Oral medications
  - Anticonvulsants: Pregabalin
  - Medication for muscle spasms: Flavoxate
  - Tricyclic antidepressants

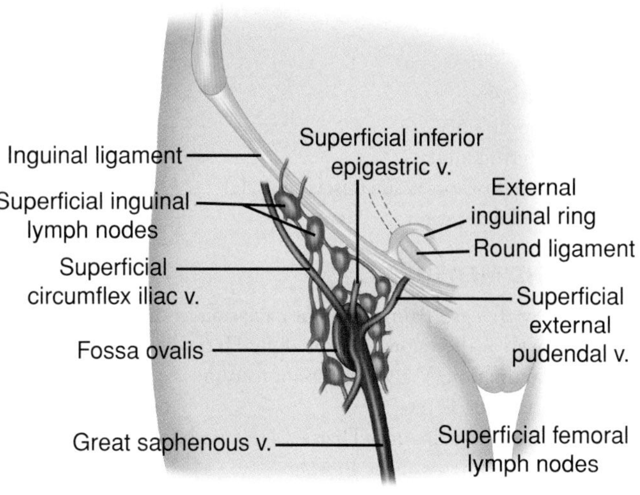

FIGURE 264-5 Lymphatic drainage of the vulva delineated by Stanley Way. v. = vein. (From Brunicardi FC, Andersen DK, Billiar TR, et al. *Schwartz's Principles of Surgery*. 9th ed. www.accessmedicine.com. Copyright © The McGraw-Hill Companies, Inc. All rights reserved.)

MEDICAL PROCEDURES

- Intralesional injections
  - Botulinum toxin injections
  - Trigger point injections
  - Interferon alpha
- Implanted electrical stimulator for neuromodulation (InterStim)
- Surgery
  - Local excision of painful areas
  - Vestibulectomy
  - Perineoplasty

REFERRALS/ADMITTANCE

- To acupuncture
- To biofeedback practitioner
- To certified sex therapist
- To cognitive behavioral pain psychologist
- To dermatologist
- To gynecologists
- To pain medicine
- To pelvic floor physical therapist
- To physical Medicine and rehabilitation physicians
- To primary care physicians
- To urogynecologists
- To urologists
- Interdisciplinary approach is strongly recommended.

IMPAIRMENTS

- PFM dysfunction
  - Overactive
  - Underactive
  - Nonrelaxing
  - Noncontracting
- Incontinence
- Myofascial pelvic pain
- Pelvic organ prolapse

- Decreased sexual appreciation; anorgasmia: Inability to achieve orgasm
- Pain
- Muscle atrophy
- Joint hypomobility
- Posture dysfunction
- Contractures of soft tissue (fascia, muscle)
- Obstructed defecation

TESTS AND MEASURES

- Cotton Swab Test: Pain with light palpation of the soft end of a cotton swab at the vaginal introit along Hart's line[2]
- PFM examination: Via vagina or anorectum
- Abdominal muscle test
- Abdominal wall palpation: Diastalsis rectus abdominis, scar
- Pressure manometry of the PFMs
- Lumbar spine, pelvic girdle, and hip joint examination procedures

INTERVENTION[7]

- PFM exercises/training
  - "Kegel" exercises: Another name for PFM exercises
  - Contraction
  - Relaxation/"Bulging"
  - Motor control
  - Endurance
  - Power
  - sEMG biofeedback
- Progressive vaginal dilation
- TENS
- NMES
- Pressure manometry
- Manual therapy
  - Thiele massage performed vaginally
  - Myofascial release
  - Internal vaginal massage
- Thermal modalities
- Ultrasonography imaging to awareness of muscle contractions
- Posture re-education
- Functional training: "Bulge" or "drop and open" the PFMs prior to vaginal penetration during intercourse, vaginal examination, tampon insertion
- Patient education regarding effects of maladaptive pain cognitions

FUNCTIONAL GOALS

- Patient will be able to
  - Verbalize strategies for independent pain management.
  - Independently perform progressive vaginal dilation to practice vaginal penetration sexual intercourse.
  - Demonstrate independence with long-term PFM exercise program.
  - Identify thoughts and cognitions that may exacerbate symptoms during attempted intercourse.

PROGNOSIS

- Long-term treatment success rate is about 50%.[8]
- Longer duration and greater intensity of pain symptoms negatively impacts prognosis.[5]
- Psychological factors such as pain catastrophizing and fear avoidance negatively impact prognosis.[9]

PATIENT RESOURCES

- International Pelvic Pain Society. http://www.pelvicpain.org./ Accessed April 20, 2013.
- Vaginisums. http://www.vaginismus.com. Accessed July 17, 2013.

REFERENCES

1. The American Physical Therapy Association. Pattern 4C: Impaired muscle performance. In: *Guide to Physical Therapist Practice.* Alexandria, VA: The American Physical Therapy Association; 2003. http://guidetoptpractice.apta.org/content/1/SEC10.extract?sid=9af82a7e-5fc3-41d2-86ab-b8336a9655e9. April 20, 2013.
2. Reed BD, Sen A, Gracely RH. Effect of test order on sensitivity in vulvodynia. *J Reprod Med.* 2007;52(3):199–206.
3. Reed BD, Harlow SD, Sen A, et al. Prevalence and demographic characteristics of vulvodynia in a population-based sample. *Am J Obstet Gynecol.* 2012;206(2):170.e1–170.e9.
4. Harlow BL, Stuart EG. A population-based assessment of chronic unexplained vulvar pan: have we underestimated the prevalence of vulvodynia? *J Am Med Womens Assoc.* 2003;58:82–88.
5. Gyang A, Hartman M, Lamvu G. Musculoskeletal Causes of Chronic Pelvic Pain; What a Gynecologist Should Know. *Obstet Gynecol.* 2013;121:645–650.
6. Cox KJ, Neville CE. Assessment and management options for women with vulvodynia. *J Midwifery Womens Health.* 2012; 57(3):231–240.
7. Strauhal MJ, Frahm J, Morrison P, et al. Vulvar pain: a comprehensive review. *J Womens Health Phys Ther.* 2007;31(3):7–26.
8. Gunter J. Vulvodynia: New thoughts on a devastating condition. *Obstet Gynecol Surv.* 2007;62(12):812–819.
9. Alappattu MJ, Bishop MD. Psychological factors in chronic pelvic pain in women: relevance and application of the fear-avoidance model of pain. *Phys Ther.* 2011;91(10):1542–1550.

ADDITIONAL REFERENCES

- Dutton M. Causes of pelvic pain. In: Dutton M, ed. *Dutton's Orthopaedic Examination, Evaluation, and Intervention.* 3rd ed. New York, NY: McGraw-Hill; 2012. http://www.accessphysiotherapy.com/content/56526028. Accessed July 17, 2013.
- Dutton M. Genitourinary system disorders. In: Dutton M, ed. *McGraw-Hill's NPTE (National Physical Therapy Examination).* 2nd ed. New York, NY: McGraw-Hill; 2012. http://www.accessphysiotherapy.com/content/5402307. Accessed April 20, 2013.
- Fall M, Baranowski AP, Elneil S, et al. EAU guidelines on chronic pelvic pain. *Eur Urol.* 2010;57(1):35–48.
- Hartmann D, Strauhal MJ, Nelson CA. Treatment of women in the United States with localized, provoked vulvodynai: practice survey of women's health physical therapists. *J Reprod Med.* 2007;52(1):48–52.
- Katz D, Tabisel RL. *Private Pain: Understanding Vaginismus and Dyspareunia.* Winnipeg, Canada: Kromar Printing Ltd; 2002. Available at: www.womentc.com. Accessed July 17, 2013
- *Relieving Pain in America.* The National Academies Press. http://www.nap.edu/catalog.php?record_id=13172. Accessed July 17, 2013.

265 ANORGASMIA

Cynthia E. Neville, DPT, PT, WCS
Eric Shamus, PhD, DPT, PT, CSCS

CONDITION/DISORDER SYNONYMS

- Female orgasmic disorder (FOD)
- Inhibited sexual orgasm
- Neurogenic anorgasmia

ICD-9-CM CODES

- 302.73 Female orgasmic disorder
- V41.7 Problems with sexual function

ICD-10-CM CODES

- F54 Sexual dysfunction not due to a substance or known physiological condition
- F52.3 Orgasmic disorder
- F52.31 Female orgasmic disorder

PREFERRED PRACTICE PATTERN

- 4C: Impaired Muscle Performance[1]

PATIENT PRESENTATION

A 56-year-old woman reports that she was sexually inactive for 10 months following treatment for breast cancer. This treatment was 3 years ago. She has attempted to resume sexual relations with her husband: however, now she is unable to achieve an orgasm. They have tried many different approaches include masturbation without success.

KEY FEATURES

Description

- Inability to achieve sexual orgasm during sexual intercourse or other sexual activity despite adequate stimulation and the desire to do so
- Normal libido and sexual excitement
- Primary anorgasmic (preorgasmic): Not yet able to reach organism

TABLE 265-1 Definitions of Sexual Dysfunction

APA Definition[a]	AUA Definition[b]
Hypoactive sexual desire disorder	Sexual desire/interest disorder
Persistent or recurrent deficiency or absence of sexual fantasies and desire for sexual activity. Judgment of deficiency is made by the clinician, taking into account factors that affect sexual functioning	Absent or diminished feelings of sexual interest or desire, absent sexual thoughts or fantasies, and a lack of responsive desire. Motivations for attempting to become sexually aroused are scarce or absent. Lack of interest goes beyond a normal lessening with increasing age and relationship duration
Lack of subjective arousal	Combined arousal disorder
No *DSM-IV* definition addresses the lack of subjective arousal	Absent or markedly reduced feelings of sexual arousal (sexual excitement and sexual pleasure) from any type of stimulation, and absent or impaired genital sexual arousal (vulvar swelling and lubrication)
Lack of subjective arousal	Subjective arousal disorder
No *DSM-IV* definition addresses the lack of subjective arousal	Absent or markedly reduced feelings of sexual arousal (sexual excitement and sexual pleasure) from any type of stimulation. Vaginal lubrication and other signs of physical response still occur
Female sexual arousal disorder	Genital arousal disorder
Persistent or recurrent inability to attain, or to maintain until completion of sexual activity, adequate lubrication, and swelling response of sexual excitement	Absent or impaired genital sexual arousal (minimal vulvar swelling or vaginal lubrication from any type of sexual stimulation, and reduced sexual sensations when genitalia are caressed) Subjective sexual excitement still occurs from nongenital sexual stimuli (e.g., erotica, breast stimulation, kissing)
Female orgasmic disorder	Orgasmic disorder
Persistent or recurrent delay or absence of orgasm after a normal sexual excitement phase	Lack of orgasm, markedly diminished intensity of orgasmic sensations, or marked delay of orgasm from any kind of stimulation, despite self-reported high sexual arousal or excitement

[a]Data from the American Psychiatric Association (APA).
[b]Data from the international committee sponsored by the American Urological Association (AUA).
Source: Tanagho EA, McAninch WJ. *Smith's General Urology*. 17th ed. www.accessmedicine.com.

- Secondary orgasmic disorder: Was previously able to reach orgasm, but is no longer able

Essentials of Diagnosis

- Thorough medical history
- Physical examination to rule out underlying medical cause
- Generalized verse situational
- Lifelong usually more psychogenic
- Acquired can be relationship discord
- Psychological factors

General Considerations

- Orgasm is a complex phenomenon following sexual arousal that depends on a variety of objective and subjective factors.

Demographics

- Wide ranges of prevalence reported in the literature
  - Affected 26.3% of 1,200 Iranian women in a 2010 study[2]
  - 86.6% of married Indian women in a 2009 study[3]

CLINICAL FINDINGS

SIGNS AND SYMPTOMS

- Persistent or recurrent delay in or absence of orgasm following a normal sexual excitement phase

Functional Implications

- May cause dissatisfaction, concerns and/or distress about sexual relationships

Possible Contributing Causes

- General medical condition
- Psychogenic
- Drug induced
- Severe depression
- Social anxiety
- Underactive, overactive, or nonfunctioning pelvic floor muscles
- Pelvic organ prolapse

Differential Diagnosis[4]

- Medical diseases
  - Diabetes
  - Neurological diseases, for example, multiple sclerosis
- Gynecological disorders
- Medications
  - Blood pressure medications
  - Antidepressants, especially SRRIs (selective serotonin reuptake inhibitors)
- Alcohol and drugs

MEANS OF CONFIRMATION OR DIAGNOSIS

Imaging

- Ultrasound imaging to identify abnormalities
  - Bladder
  - Urethra
  - Pelvis
  - Bladder neck position and mobility
  - Pelvic floor function
  - Activity of levator ani
  - Descent of pelvic organs
  - Sphincter integrity
- MRI to examine soft tissue structures of the pelvic support apparatus
- Pelvic/Abdominal ultrasound
  - Rule out other pathologies

Diagnostic Procedures

- Perineal and vaginal examination
- Rule out other medical pathology
- EMG/Nerve conduction

FINDINGS AND INTERPRETATION

- EMG/Nerve conduction can show if the cause is neurogenic anorgasmia.

TREATMENT

Medication

- Systemic or local estrogen therapy
- Testosterone therapy

REFERRALS/ADMITTANCE

- Pelvic floor physical therapist
- Certified sex therapist
- Couples counseling
- Primary care physicians
- Gynecologists
  - Women: Pelvic examination
- Acupuncture

IMPAIRMENTS

- PFM dysfunction
  - Overactive
  - Underactive
  - Nonrelaxing
  - Noncontracting
- Incontinence
- Pelvic pain
- Pelvic organ prolapse

TESTS AND MEASURES

- Changes in sexual functioning questionnaire
- Female sexual function index
- Pelvic floor muscle examination and assessment
- sEMG biofeedback assessment of the pelvic floor muscles
- Pressure manometry of the pelvic floor muscles

INTERVENTION

- Pelvic floor muscle exercises/training
  - "Kegel" exercises: Another name for pelvic floor muscle exercises
  - Contraction
  - Relaxation/"Bulging"
  - Motor control
  - Endurance
  - Power
  - sEMG biofeedback
  - Pressure manometry
  - Weighted vaginal cones to strengthen pelvic floor
    - Hold weighted cone in vagina for up to 15 minutes, two times a day

- Vibrator for self stimulation
- Neuromuscular electrical stimulation for neuromodulation, to facilitate pelvic floor muscle contraction and sensation
  - Frequency of 35 to 50 Hz, pulse width of 200 to 350 usec, asymmetrical biphasic wave form, duty cycle of 5 to 10 seconds on/5 to 10 seconds off
  - Match on time to patients active home exercise program contraction time,
  - Patient may contract pelvic floor muscles while stimulation is on,
  - Duration of 10 to 20 minutes, frequency of treatment 1 to 2 times/day, every other day or daily
  - Anal or vaginal electrode/probe
  - Surface electrodes
    - Sacrum
    - Perineum
    - Suprapubic area
    - Tibial nerve
- Real time ultrasound imaging to facilitate learning of correct performance and coordination of abdominal muscle and pelvic floor muscle co-contraction
- Functional training
  - Contract the pelvic floor muscles during insertion of a vaginal dilator or vibrator
- Patient education

FUNCTIONAL GOALS

- Patient will report improved sexual appreciation to achieve orgasm during sexual stimulation.

PROGNOSIS

- The prognosis is good if a result of psychological factors.[5]
- If substance induced, change of medication may reverse disorder.[5]

PATIENT RESOURCES

- American College of Obstetricians and Gynecologists. ACOG Practice Bulletin No. 119: Female sexual dysfunction. *Obstet Gynecol.* 2011;117(4):96–1007.
- Salonia A, Briganti A, Rigatti P, Montorsi F. Medical conditions associated with female sexual dysfunction. In: Goldstein I, Meston C, Davis S, et al, eds. *Women's Sexual Function and Dysfunction.* New York, NY: Taylor & Francis; 2006:263.

REFERENCES

1. The American Physical Therapy Association. Pattern 4C: impaired muscle performance. *Guide to Physical Therapist Practice.* Alexandria, VA: The American Physical Therapy Association; 2003. http://guidetoptpractice.apta.org/content/1/SEC10.extract?sid=9af82a7e-5fc3-41d2-86ab-b8336a9655e9. Accessed July 2, 2013.
2. Najafabady MT, Salmani Z, Abedi P. Prevalence and related factors for anorgasmia among reproductive aged women in Hesarak, Iran. *Clinics (Sao Paulo).* 2011;66(1):83–86.
3. Amidu N, Owiredu WK, Gyasi-Sarpong CK, Woode E, Quaye L. Sexual dysfunction among married couples living in Kumasi metropolis, Ghana. *BMC Urol.* 2011;11:3.
4. Anorgasmia. http://www.mayoclinic.com/health/anorgasmia/DS01051. Accessed July 2, 2013.
5. Balon R, Segraves RT. Sexual dysfunction and paraphilias. In: Ebert MH, Loosen PT, Nurcombe B, Leckman JF, eds. *CURRENT Diagnosis & Treatment: Psychiatry.* 2nd ed. New York, NY: McGraw-Hill; 2008:Chapter 25. http://www.accessmedicine.com/content.aspx?aID=3287823. Accessed July 2, 2013.

ADDITIONAL REFERENCES

- Anorgasmia. http://www.anorgasmia.com/anorgasmia.htm. Accessed July 2, 2013.
- Caruso S, Intelsano G, Lupo L, Agnello C. Premenopausal women affected by sexual arousal disorder treated with sildenafil: A double-blind, cross-over, placebo-controlled study. *BJOG.* 2001;108(6):623–628.
- Ellison C. Facilitating orgasmic responsiveness. In: Levine S, Risen C, Althof S, eds. *Handbook of Clinical Sexuality for Mental Health Clinicians.* New York, NY: Brunner-Routledge; 2003:167.
- Keller A, McGarvey E, Clayton A. Reliability and construct validity of the changes in sexual functioning questionnaire short form. *J Sex Marital Ther.* 2006;32:43.
- Meston CN, Levine R. Female orgasm dysfunction. In: Balon R, Segraves RT, eds. *Handbook of Sexual Dysfunction.* New York, NY: Taylor & Francis; 2005:193.
- Murtagh J. Female sexual function, dysfunction, and pregnancy: Implications for practice. *J Midwifery Womens Health.* 2010; 55(5):438–446.
- Simon JA. Identifying and treating sexual dysfunction in postmenopausal women: The role of estrogen. *J Womens Health (Larchmt).* 2011;20(10):1453–1465.

266 CHRONIC PELVIC PAIN SYNDROME

Cynthia E. Neville, DPT, PT, WCS

CONDITION/DISORDER SYNONYMS

- Chronic pelvic pain syndrome
- Levator ani syndrome
- Urogenital pain disorders

ICD-9-CM CODES

- 338.4 Chronic pain syndrome
- Associated medical diagnoses
  - 564.6 Anal spasm
  - 569.42 Anal or rectal pain
  - 595.1 Chronic interstitial cystitis
  - 601.1 Chronic prostatitis
  - 617 Endometriosis
  - 625.0 Dyspareunia
  - 625.5 Pelvic congestion syndrome
  - 625.7 Vulvodynia
  - 625.71 Vulvar vestibulitis
- Associated physical therapy diagnoses
  - 719.45 Pain in the hip joint, pelvic region, and thigh
  - 724.7 Disorders of coccyx
  - 728.2 Muscular wasting and disuse atrophy
  - 728.85 Spasm of muscle
  - 728.89 Disorders of muscle, ligament, and fascia
  - 729.1 Myalgia
  - 729.2 Neuralgia/neuritis
  - 729.9 Other disorders of soft tissue
  - 780.7 Malaise and fatigue
  - 782.3 Edema

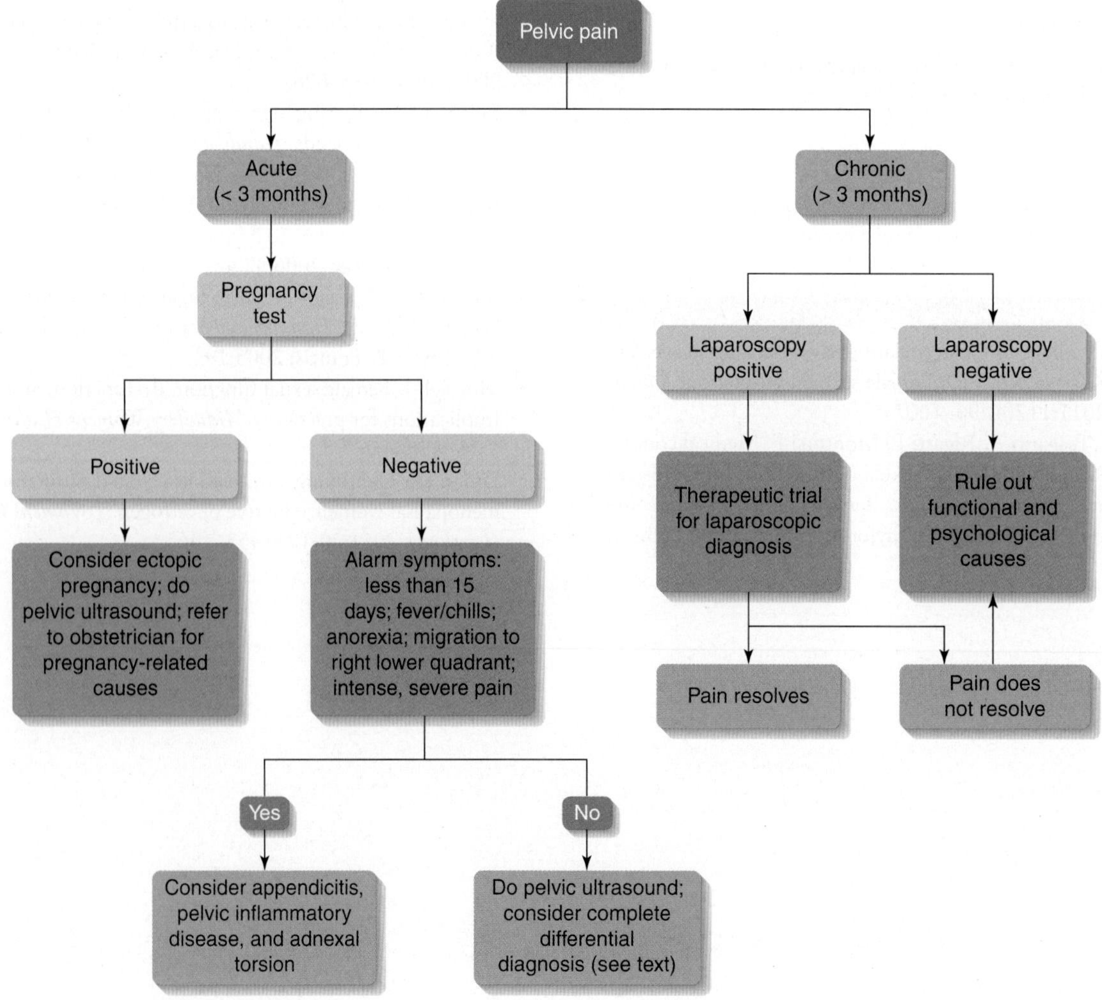

FIGURE 266-1 Diagnostic approach: Pelvic pain. (From Henderson MC, Tierney LM, Smetana GW. *The Patient History: An Evidence-Based Approach to Differential Diagnosis*. www.accessmedicine.com. Copyright © The McGraw-Hill Companies, Inc. All rights reserved.)

ICD-10-CM CODES

- G89.4 Chronic pain syndrome
- N30.10 Interstitial cystitis (chronic) without hematuria
- N30.11 Interstitial cystitis (chronic) with hematuria
- N41.1 Chronic prostatitis
- N80 Endometriosis
- R10.2 Pelvic and perineal pain
- Symptom specific diagnoses
  - K59.5 Anal spasm
  - N53.12 Painful ejaculation
  - N94.1 Dyspareunia
  - N94.81 Vulvodynia
  - N94.810 Vulvar vestibulitis
  - N94.818 Other vulvodynia
  - N94.819 Vulvodynia unspecified
  - N94.89 Other condition associated with female genital organs and menstrual cycle

PREFERRED PRACTICE PATTERN

- As of July 2014, the APTA Guide to Physical Therapist Practice does not include practice patterns for organ system pathology
- Associated or secondary musculoskeletal patterns include:
  - 4C: Impaired Muscle Performance[1]
  - 4D: Impaired Joint Mobility, Motor Function, Muscle Performance, and Range of Motion Associated with Connective Tissue Dysfunction[1]

PATIENT PRESENTATION

A 45-year-old woman reports that 3 years ago she had a urinary tract infection (UTI) that was treated with antibiotics. She had recurrent symptoms of UTIs every 2 to 3 months for the next 2 years until during the last episode, she was told by the physician that the urinalysis was negative. The burning with urination was painful. In the past year she has developed more symptoms. She has noticed that she has to urinate more frequently, at least 10 times per day. She wakes up at least three times at night to urinate. Pain is temporarily relived by urination. She reports that in the last year, she has started having problems with bowel movements. Sometimes she is constipated, and sometimes stools are loose. She never had these problems before. She now is having pain during intercourse, and sometimes feels a throbbing pain in the vaginal regions while she is working at her desk. She has stopped exercising because she is concerned that running is making her symptoms worse. She is afraid to have intercourse because it was very painful the last time.

KEY FEATURES

Description[2]

- Nonspecific, poorly localized pelvic pain or regional pelvic pain syndrome without obvious pathology.
- Defined by a process of exclusion.
- No evidence of infection or inflammation.
- Chronic urogenital pain syndromes are often associated with end-organ pain conditions (such as bladder, vulva) and psychological conditions (such as emotional, sexual, behavioral).

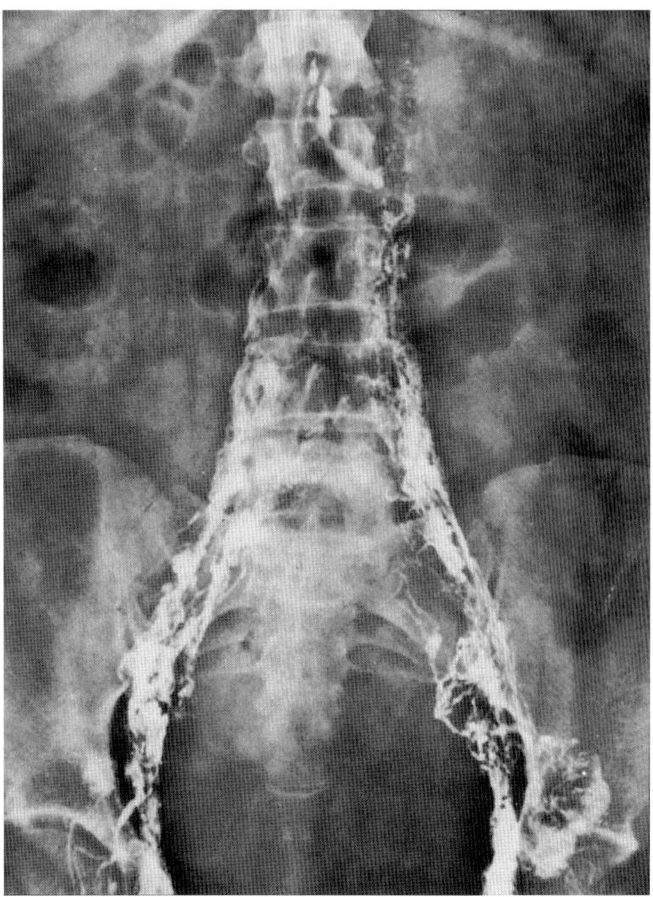

FIGURE 266-2 Lymphangiogram (radiograph) of the lymphatic vessels and lymph nodes of the pelvic region. (Reprinted with permission from, Shier D, Butler J, Lewis R. *Hole's Human Anatomy and Physiology*. 9th ed. Boston, MA: The McGraw-Hill Companies, Inc.; 2002.)

- Genitourinary pain syndromes are all chronic in their nature. Pain is the major complaint but concomitant complaints are of lower urinary tract (UT), bowel, sexual, or gynecological nature.[3]

Essentials of Diagnosis

- Unknown etiology.
- Rule out end-organ pathology.
- Symptoms may be initiated by an acute infection, injury, or inflammation of a pelvic or urogenital organ, however pain persists beyond the duration of the original inciting event or disease.

General Considerations

- Chronic pain condition.
- Often misdiagnosed.
- Physical therapy (PT) intervention is often appropriate for associated musculoskeletal impairments.
- Diagnosis is a process of exclusion and often takes time, requiring intensive diagnostic testing.
- Urogenital pain disorders frequently affect nearby body areas; especially back, pelvic, hip, groin regions and so may be inappropriately referred to PT.
- May mimic other visceral pain conditions including colon cancer or tumor, irritable bowel, colitis.
- May mimic gynecologic problems in females: Endometriosis, uterine fibroids, ectopic pregnancy.

▶ Demographics

- More prevalent in females.
- Exact prevalence of chronic pelvic pain is not known, estimates vary in the literature from 3.8% to 24%.[4]
- Of the estimated 10 million women with chronic pelvic pain, less than 70% will receive proper diagnosis and treatment plans and 61% of patients will remain undiagnosed.[5]
- Many patients with pelvic pain will go on to develop chronic pain syndrome with depression, pain out of proportion to pathology, and changing roles in marriage, family, and career.[6]
- Up to 22% of pelvic pain may have a musculoskeletal cause.

▶ Clinical Findings

- Report of vaginal, rectal, or lower abdominal pain
- Symptoms are usually vague and poorly localized
- Symptoms often worsened by prolonged sitting or standing, anxiety, bowel movements, physical activity, or sexual intercourse
- Pain that starts in the afternoon and becomes progressively worse throughout the day
- Constellation of symptoms that include dyspareunia, lower back pain, bowel symptoms of constipation, diarrhea, excessive flatus, painful defecation, or a sensation of incomplete evacuation, and urinary symptoms of frequency, urgency, or nocturia

FIGURE 266-3 Pelvic compression test (gapping or transverse anterior stress test.) With the athlete supine on the examination table, the examiner stresses the pelvis by pressure over the iliac bones pushing down and out. In case of sprain of sacroiliac ligaments pain in the buttock or posterior thigh is elicited on the injured side. (From Patel DR, Greydanus DE, Baker RJ. *Pediatric Practice: Sports Medicine*. www.accesspediatrics.com Copyright © The McGraw-Hill Companies, Inc. All rights reserved.)

CLINICAL FINDINGS

SIGNS AND SYMPTOMS

- Symptoms are usually vague and poorly localized
- Vaginal, rectal, or lower abdominal pain
- Low back pain, gluteal, groin, or leg pain
- Pain during sexual intercourse
- Irritative voiding secondary to urinary discomfort, frequency, or urgency
- Irritable bowel: Diarrhea and/or constipation
- Pelvic pain
- Bladder pressure and pain
- Burning with urination

▶ Functional Implications

- Pelvic pain
- Painful urination, defecation, and sexual activity
- Incomplete defecation or urination
- Urinary and fecal urgency and frequency
- Sarcopenia resulting in weakness, decreased muscle mass, inability to ambulate, perform self-care
- Decreased exercise tolerance
- Limited physical activity, activities of daily living (ADLs), instrumental activities of daily living (IADLs)
- Fatigue
- Inappropriate self-medication
- Anxiety, depression
- Sexual dysfunction

▶ Possible Contributing Causes

- UT abnormalities
- History of sexual or physical abuse
- Allergy to foods, beverages, or supplements
- Environmental irritant
- Autoimmune reaction
- Poor urogenital hygiene
- Sexual activity
- UT blockage: Kidney stones, enlarged prostate in males
- Immunologic compromise
- Catheter use, especially indwelling
- Infection: Bacterial, viral, food poisoning
- Stress, anxiety
- Fear, catastrophizing

▶ Differential Diagnosis

- UTI
- Sexually transmitted disease (STD)
- Urethritis
- Acute pyelonephritis
- Bladder, rectal, anal cancer
- Bladder infection
- Yeast infection
- Bacterial vaginosis
- Systemic Lupus Erythmyeosis (SLE)
- Fibromyalgia
- Organ dysfunction from cancer or malignancy
- Nonmalignant tumor in abdomen or organs
- Endocrine disorder
- Gynecologic problems in females
  - Endometriosis
  - Menses
  - Ectopic pregnancy
  - Ovarian cyst
  - Fibroids
  - Menopause
- Autoimmune disease affecting upper and lower GI tracts
- Crohn disease
- Irritable bowel syndrome
- Appendicitis
- Peritonitis
- Prostatitis
- Benign prostatic hypertrophy
- Pelvic inflammatory disease

- Gastroenteritis
- Perforated ulcer in GI system
- Kidney pathology
- Abdominal infection
- Bowel disorder
  - Constipation, diarrhea
  - Inflamed abdominal or organ linings
  - Obstruction
  - Torsions
- Referred pain from heart, spine, hip

MEANS OF CONFIRMATION OR DIAGNOSIS

Laboratory Tests

- Blood tests
- Urine culture/urinalysis
- Hemoglobin and hematocrit (H&H)

Imaging

- Cystoscopy
- Ultrasound
- Intravenous urinary pyelogram using dye
- CT
- Bladder scans
- MRI
- X-ray

Diagnostic Procedures

- Postvoid residual
- Bladder biopsy
- Cystography
- Cystometrogram
- Video urodynamic testing
- Colonoscopy
- Defecography
- Biopsy
- Uroflowmetry

FINDINGS AND INTERPRETATION

- H&H for signs of bleeding, anemia, pathogens, immune status, vitamin deficiencies, white blood cell count

TREATMENT

Medication

- Nonsteroidal anti-inflammatory medication (NSAIDs)
- Opioid pain medication
- Medication for muscle spasms: Flavoxate
- Pregabalin
- Tricyclic antidepressants
- Vaginal estrogen if levels low
- Pentosan (Elmiron) for chronic bladder pain
- Anticonvulsants
- Alpha blockers for prostatodynia
- Medication to relax the bladder
  - Anticholinergics: Oxybutynin, tolterodine, darifenacin

MEDICAL PROCEDURES

- Botulism toxin injections
- Trigger point injections
- Implanted electrical stimulator for neuromodulation (InterStim)

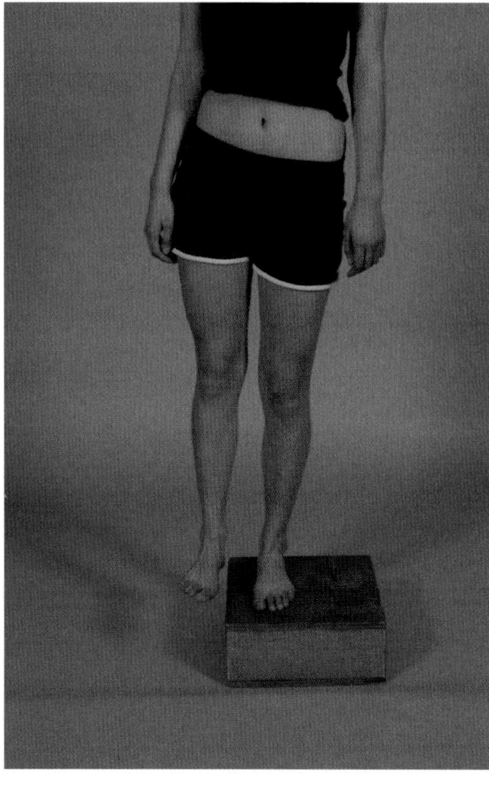

FIGURE 266-4 Pelvic Drop test. (From Dutton M. *Dutton's Orthopaedic Examination, Evaluation, and Intervention.* 3rd ed. http://www.accessphysiotherapy.com. Copyright © The McGraw-Hill Companies, Inc. All rights reserved.)

REFERRALS/ADMITTANCE

- Pelvic floor physical therapist
- Cognitive behavioral pain psychologist
- Primary care physicians
- Physical medicine and rehabilitation physicians
- Gynecologists
- Urologists
- Urogynecologists
- Gastroenterologist
- Colorectal surgeon
- Neurologist
- Pain medicine
- Acupuncture
- Biofeedback practitioner
- Certified sexual therapist

IMPAIRMENTS

- Pelvic floor muscle (PFM) dysfunction
  - Overactive
  - Underactive
  - Nonrelaxing
  - Noncontracting
- Incontinence
- Myofascial pelvic pain
- Pelvic organ prolapse
- Detrusor instability
- Decreased sexual appreciation; anorgasmia: Inability to achieve orgasm
- Muscle atrophy

- Joint hypomobility
- Posture dysfunction
- Gait abnormality, difficulty walking
- Contractures of soft tissue (fascia, muscle)
- Inability to perform self-care
- Obstructed defecation

TESTS AND MEASURES

- PFM examination: Via vagina or anorectum
- Abdominal wall muscle test
- Abdominal wall palpation: Diastalsis rectus abdominis, scar
- Bladder diary
- sEMG biofeedback assessment of the PFM and abdominal muscles
- Pressure manometry of the PFM
- Lumbar spine, pelvic girdle, and hip-joint examination procedures
- Palpation
  - Appendix (McBurney): Apply vertical pressure halfway between right ASIS and umbilicus; −/+ may indicate appendicitis
  - Liver: In supine position, with left hand under trunk parallel to 11th and 12th ribs, lift upward; right hand lateral to rectus, press in and up: +/= reproduction of symptoms with deep breath, indicates liver involvement
  - Ascites: Percuss outward from center with fingers; if sound is dull, ascites may be present
  - Gallbladder (Murphy's): Place fingers right of rectus abdominus below rib cage: +/= sudden pain and muscle tensing with deep breath
  - Kidneys: In supine position, place one hand under client between ribs and iliac crest, other hand on abdomen below ribs and pointing in the opposite direction; +/− tenderness or reproduction of symptoms
  - Bladder: Not usually palpable unless distended and raised above pubic bone; in supine position, place hand above pubis and press down; +/= tenderness, reproduction of pain, ability to feel the bladder: __+ ___ −
- Observation
  - Scars may indicate adhesions or abdominal surgeries causative of diverticula
  - Pink or purplish striae may be indicative of Cushing syndrome
  - Dilated veins may indicate hepatic pathology or inferior vena cava obstruction, not diverticulitis
  - Contour: Roundness, concavity, asymmetry, distension, pregnancy signs
  - Cullen sign: Bluish discoloring around umbilicus may be a sign of retroperitoneal bleeding
  - Bluish discoloration in lower abdomen: Grey Turner's sign, signals hemorrhagic pancreatitis
  - Bulging in groin/abdomen especially apparent with contraction of musculature in area may be hernia
  - Pulsing in navel area may be abdominal aortic aneurysm
  - Left lower quadrant pain, often following a meal
  - Palpable abdominal tenderness: On left side or generalized
  - Psoas sign: Provides resistance over patient's right knee during hip flexion; pain indicates appendicitis, possible inflammation of abdomen
  - Obturator sign: Internal rotation and flexion of right lower extremity (LE) may indicate appendicitis, pelvic inflammation
  - Rovsing sign: Pain on right side of abdomen when pressure applied to left may indicate appendicitis

INTERVENTION

- PFM exercises/training
  - "Kegel" exercises: Another name for PFM exercises
  - Contraction
  - Relaxation/"Bulging"
  - Motor control
  - Endurance
  - Power
  - sEMG biofeedback
- Neuromuscular electrical stimulation to decrease urinary urgency and frequency and detrusor overactivity and to facilitate PFM and anal sphincter contraction
  - Anal or vaginal probe
  - Surface electrodes
    - Sacrum
    - Perineum
    - Suprapubic area
    - Tibial nerve
- TENS
- Pressure manometry
- Manual therapy
- Thermal modalities
- Ultrasonography imaging for awareness of muscle contractions
- Posture re-education
- Bladder retraining including timed voiding schedule and urge suppression technique
- Functional training
  - Precontract the PFM to close the urethra prior to anticipated increase in intra-abdominal pressure
  - "Bulge" or "drop and open" the PFM prior to vaginal penetration during intercourse, vaginal exam, tampon insertion
- Patient education regarding fluid intake and general dietary recommendations for fiber intake

FUNCTIONAL GOALS

- Patient will be able
  - Verbalize strategies for independent pain management.
  - Achieve functional aerobic capacity, gait, and tolerance for ADLs/IADLs.
  - Achieve ≥600 meters in a 6-minute walk test for initiation of safe, functional gait in community without need of bathroom break.
  - Tolerate 30 minutes of continuous, moderate exercise three times per week in ______ weeks, and five times per week in ____________ weeks, depending on disease severity.
  - Demonstrate independence with home exercise program, promoting relaxation and awareness of PFM for long-term self-management.
  - Independently perform vaginal penetration for tampon insertion and/or sexual intercourse.
  - Demonstrate independence with long-term PFM training program.

PROGNOSIS

- Longer duration and greater intensity of pain symptoms negatively impacts prognosis.
- Psychological factors such as pain catastrophizing and fear avoidance negatively impact prognosis.[7]

PATIENT RESOURCE

- International Pelvic Pain Society. http://www.pelvicpain.org/. Accessed April 20, 2013.

REFERENCES

1. The American Physical Therapy Association. Pattern 4C: Impaired muscle performance. In: *guide to physical therapist practice*. Alexandria, VA: The American Physical Therapy Association; 2003. http://guidetoptpractice.apta.org/content/1/SEC10.extract?sid=9af82a7e-5fc3-41d2-86ab-b8336a9655e9. April 20, 2013.
2. Fall M, Baranowski AP, Elneil S, et al; Europe Association of Urology. EAU guidelines on chronic pelvic pain. *Eur Urol.* 2010;57(1):35–48. doi: 10.1016/j.eururo.2009.08.020.
3. Abrams P, Cardozo L, Fall M, et al. The standardization of terminology of lower urinary tract function: report from the Standardization Sub-Committee of the International Continence Society. *Neurourol Urodyn.* 2002;21(2):167–178.
4. Latthe P, Latthe M, Say L, Gulmezoglu M, Khan KS. WHO systematic review of prevalence of chronic pelvic pain: a neglected reproductive health morbidity. *BMC Public Health.* 2006;6:177. doi:10.1186/1471-2458/6/177 [p. 1–7].
5. Zondervan KT, Yudkin PL, Vessey MP, et al. The community prevalence of chronic pelvic pain in women and associated illness behaviour. *Br J Gen Pract.* 2001;51(468):541–547.
6. Gyang A, Hartman M, Lamvu G. Musculoskeletal causes of chronic pelvic pain; What a gynecologist should know. *Obstet Gynecol.* 2013;121:645–650.
7. Alappattu MJ, Bishop MD. Psychological factors in chronic pelvic pain in women: relevance and application of the fear-avoidance model of pain. *Phys Ther.* 2011;91(10):1542–1550.

ADDITIONAL REFERENCES

- Dutton M. Genitourinary system disorders. In: Dutton M, ed. *McGraw-Hill's NPTE (National Physical Therapy Examination).* 2nd ed. New York, NY: McGraw-Hill; 2012. http://www.accessphysiotherapy.com/content/5402307. Accessed April 20, 2013.
- Dutton M. Gynecologic disorders. In: Dutton M, ed. *Dutton's Orthopaedic Examination, Evaluation, and Intervention.* 3rd ed. New York, NY: McGraw-Hill; 2012. http://www.accessphysiotherapy.com/content/5547556. Accessed April 20, 2013.
- Neville C. Pelvic Floor Examination: Standardized Pelvic Floor Examination [Video]. New York, NY: McGraw-Hill; 2014. http://www.accessphysiotherapy.com/. Accessed June 10, 2014.
- "*Relieving Pain in America*" from The National Academies Press. http://www.nap.edu/catalog.php?record_id=13172. Accessed April 20, 2013.

267 INTERSTITIAL CYSTITIS

Eric Shamus, PhD, DPT, PT, CSCS
Debra F. Stern, DPT, DBA, MSM, PT
Cynthia E. Neville, DPT, PT, WCS

CONDITION/DISORDER SYNONYM

- Painful bladder syndrome (PBS)

ICD-9-CM CODES

- 595.1 Chronic interstitial cystitis
- Associated physical therapy (PT) diagnoses
  - 315.4 Coordination disorder (clumsiness, dyspraxia and/or specific motor development disorder)
  - 718.45 Contracture of joint, pelvic region, and thigh
  - 719.70 Difficulty in walking
  - 728.2 Muscular wasting and disuse atrophy
  - 728.89 Disorders of muscle, ligament, and fascia
  - 729.9 Other disorders of soft tissue
  - 780.7 Malaise and fatigue
  - 782.3 Edema
  - 786.0 Dyspnea and respiratory abnormalities

ICD-10-CM CODES

- N30.10 Interstitial cystitis (chronic) without hematuria
- N30.11 Interstitial cystitis (chronic) with hematuria

PREFERRED PRACTICE PATTERN

- As of June 2014, the APTA Guide to Physical Therapist Practice does not include practice patterns for organ system pathology. Therefore, the associated or secondary musculoskeletal, cardiovascular/pulmonary, or potential neuromuscular patterns would be indicated.
- 4C: Impaired Muscle Performance[1]

PATIENT PRESENTATION

A 45-year-old woman reports that 3 years ago she had a urinary tract infection (UTI) that was treated with antibiotics. She had recurrent symptoms of UTIs every 2 to 3 months for the next 2 years until

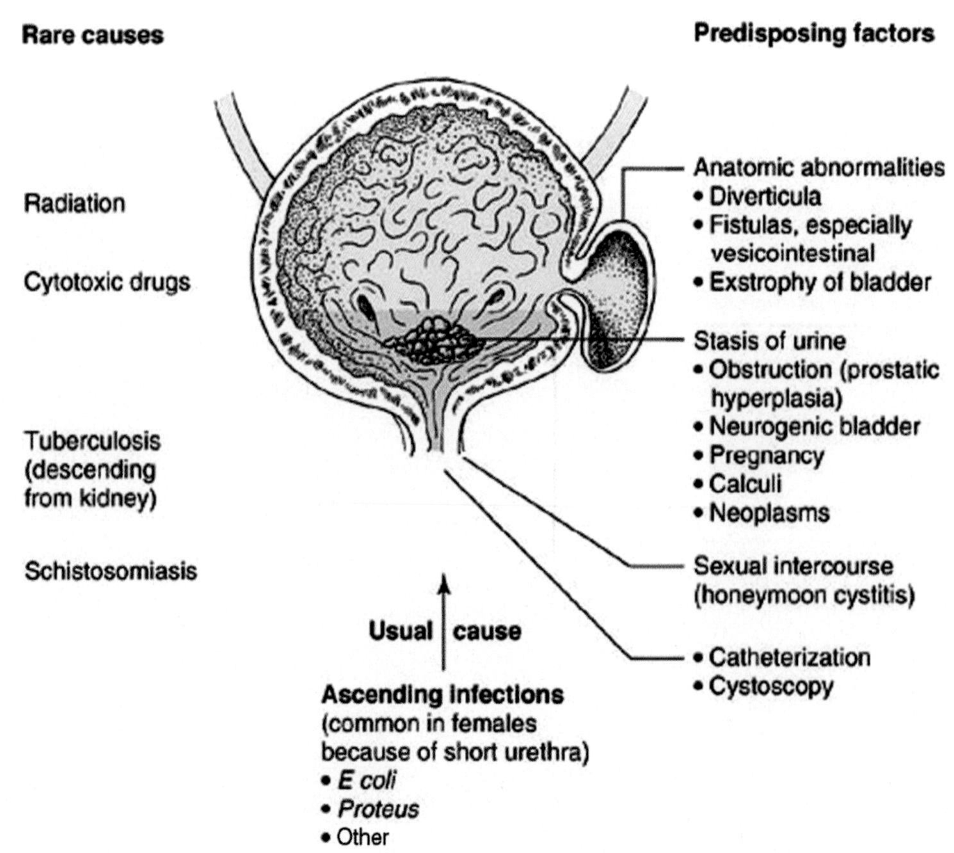

FIGURE 267-1 Causes and predisposing factors of bladder infections. Most cases are due to ascending infections caused by enteric bacteria such as *E coli* and *Proteus* species. (From Chandrasoma P, Taylor CR. *Concise Pathology*. 3rd ed. www.accessmedicine.com. Copyright © The McGraw-Hill Companies, Inc. All rights reserved.)

during the last episode, she was told by the physician that the urinalysis was negative. The burning with urination was painful. In the past year she has developed more symptoms. She has noticed that she has to urinate more frequently, at least 10 times per day. She wakes up at least three times at night to urinate. Pain is temporarily relived by urination.

KEY FEATURES

Description

- Chronic inflammation of the bladder wall
- Frequent, painful urination
- Severe pain with or without attempts at urination, or no pain at all, especially in elderly and children

Essentials of Diagnosis

- Unknown etiology
- Frequent, painful urination
- Difficulty urinating
- Pelvic pressure
- Lower abdomen discomfort
- Pelvic pain in women

General Considerations

- Often misdiagnosed as UTI
- Some urogynecologic (UG) pathologies may be appropriate for PT, though PT does not usually treat UG disorders specifically
- Diagnosis for occult problems may take time, require intensive diagnostic testing
- May refer pain to back, pelvic region
- UG disorders frequently refer pain to other body areas; individuals may be inappropriately referred to PT
- May mimic colon cancer or tumor, irritable bowel, colitis
- May mimic gynecologic problems in females: Endometriosis, uterine fibroids, ectopic pregnancy
- Can have periods of remission

Demographics

- Women more susceptible than men: Female–male ratio 10:1
- Diagnosed in the 40-year-old age group
- Frequently associated with sexual intercourse
- Children also at risk

CLINICAL FINDINGS

SIGNS AND SYMPTOMS

- Bladder pressure and pain
- Pain during sexual intercourse
- Reduced bladder capacity
- Urinary discomfort, frequency, or urgency
- Pelvic pain
- Urethra (urethritis)
  - Burning with urination
- Bladder (cystitis)
  - Pelvic pressure
  - Lower abdomen discomfort
  - Frequent, painful urination
  - Blood in urine
- Kidney (acute pyelonephritis)
  - Upper back and side (flank) pain
  - High fever
  - Shaking, chills
  - Nausea
  - Vomiting

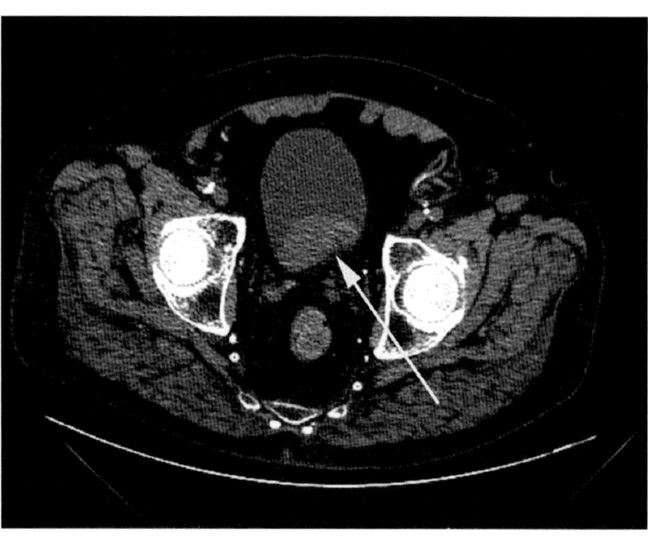

FIGURE 267-2 Noncontrast CT scan showing space-occupying lesion (transitional cell carcinoma) on the posteroinferior of the bladder (arrow). (From Doherty GM. *Current Diagnosis & Treatment: Surgery*. 13th ed. www.accessmedicine.com. Copyright © The McGraw-Hill Companies, Inc. All rights reserved.)

Functional Implications

- Patients often self-confine to house due to fear of not being near a bathroom
- Severe symptoms, such as urgent need to urinate, may be disabling, cause inability to leave home
- Pain
- Urinary retention
- Dehydration secondary to diarrhea, emesis, appetite loss, nausea, inability to swallow
- Sarcopenia resulting in weakness, decreased muscle mass, inability to ambulate, perform self-care
- Presence of catheters (external, indwelling, intermittent) may present problems with stoma retraction associated with abdominal contraction
- Decreased exercise tolerance
- Limited physical activity, activities of daily living (ADLs), instrumental activities of daily living (IADLs)
- Eating disorder, anorexia
- Fatigue
- Inappropriate self-medication
- Anxiety, depression
- Dietary limitations: Reduced caffeine, alcohol, citrus intake

Possible Contributing Causes

- Female sex
- Stress, anxiety
- Urinary tract (UT) abnormalities
- Defect in the epithelium (lining) of the bladder
- Allergy to foods, beverages, or supplements
  - Cranberry juice
  - Fruit juice
  - Tomato products
  - Teas
  - Sodas
  - Multivitamins
- Environmental irritant
- Autoimmune reaction
- Poor UG hygiene

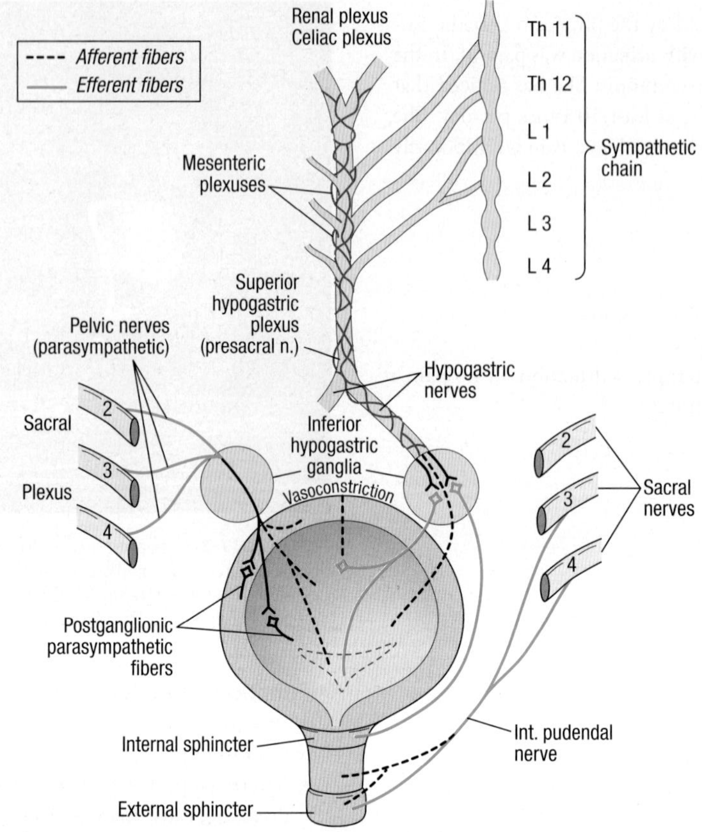

FIGURE 267-3 Innervation of the urinary bladder and its sphincters. (From Ropper AH, Samuels MA. *Adams & Victor's Principles of Neurology*. 9th ed. http://www.accessmedicine.com. Copyright © The McGraw-Hill Companies, Inc. All rights reserved.)

- Sexual activity
- Use of diaphragm and spermicides
- UT blockage: Kidney stones, enlarged prostate in males
- Immunologic compromise
- Catheter use, especially indwelling
- Infection: Bacterial, viral, food poisoning
- Kidney dialysis

Differential Diagnosis

- UTI
- Sexually transmitted disease
- Urethritis
- Acute pyelonephritis
- Bladder cancer
- Bladder infection
- Organ dysfunction from cancer or malignancy
- Nonmalignant tumor in abdomen or organs
- Endocrine disorder
- Gynecologic problems in females
    - Endometriosis
    - Menses
    - Ectopic pregnancy
    - Ovarian cyst
    - Fibroids
    - Menopause
- Autoimmune disease affecting upper and lower GI tracts
- Crohn disease
- Irritable bowel syndrome
- Appendicitis
- Peritonitis
- Prostitis
- Benign prostatic hypertrophy
- Pelvic inflammatory disease
- Gastroenteritis
- Perforated ulcer in GI system
- Kidney pathology
- Abdominal infection
- Bowel disorder
    - Constipation, diarrhea
    - Inflamed abdominal or organ linings
    - Obstruction
    - Torsions
- Referred pain from heart, spine, hip

MEANS OF CONFIRMATION OR DIAGNOSIS

Laboratory Tests

- Blood tests
- Potassium sensitivity test
- Urine culture/urinalysis
- H&H

Imaging

- Cystoscopy
- Ultrasound
- Intravenous urinary pyelogram using dye
- CT
- Bladder scans
- MRI

▶ Diagnostic Procedures

- Bladder biopsy
- Video urodynamic testing
- Manual palpation for tenderness

FINDINGS AND INTERPRETATION

- Urine culture/urinalysis
  - Usually free of bacteria
- H&H for signs of bleeding, anemia, pathogens, immune status, vitamin deficiencies, white blood cell count

TREATMENT

▶ Medication

- Vaginal estrogen if levels low
- Pentosan (Elmiron)
- Antibiotics specific to causative bacteria if infection identified[1]
  - Sulfamethoxazole-trimethoprim
  - Amoxicillin
  - Nitrofurantoin
  - Ampicillin
  - Ciprofloxacin
  - Levofloxacin
  - For sexually active females prone to UTI, instruct to take antibiotic following sexual intercourse
- Opioid pain medication
- Tricyclic antidepressants to relax the bladder

▶ Injections

- Botulism toxin injections
- Trigger point injections

MEDICAL PROCEDURES

- If catheterized, frequent changing, emptying, bladder training to wean off catheter if possible
- Fulguration
- Bladder augmentation
- Instruction on self-testing urine if infections frequent
- Implanted electrical stimulator for neuromodulation (InterStim)

REFERRALS/ADMITTANCE

- If causative problem not considered appropriate for PT intervention, refer to appropriate physician
- To acupuncturist for complementary/alternative medicine option for pain management
- If appropriate for PT, referral or treatment performed by PT specialized in women's and men's health
- To gynecologists
- To urologists
- To urogynecologists

IMPAIRMENTS

- Weakened/impaired pelvic floor muscle
- Muscle atrophy
- Gait abnormality, difficulty walking
- Contractures of soft tissue (fascia, muscle)
- Inability to perform self-care

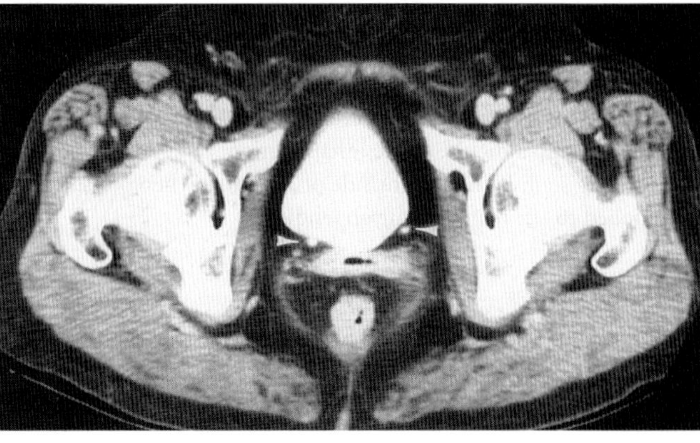

FIGURE 267-4 Normal CT showing the distal ureters and urinary bladder opacified with intravenous (IV) contrast. After a 5-minute delay, the distal ureters (*arrowheads*) and bladder are easily identified. Delayed images may be necessary to evaluate the ureter or bladder in certain circumstances. (From Chen MYM, Pope TL, Ott DJ. *Basic Radiology*. 2nd ed. http://www.accessmedicine.com. Copyright © The McGraw-Hill Companies, Inc. All rights reserved.)

TESTS AND MEASURES

- Palpation
  - Appendix (McBurney's): Apply vertical pressure halfway between right ASIS and umbilicus; −/+ may indicate appendicitis
  - Liver: In supine position, with left hand under trunk parallel to 11th and 12th ribs, lift upward; right hand lateral to rectus, press in and up: +/= reproduction of symptoms with deep breath, indicates liver involvement
  - Ascites: Percuss outward from center with fingers; if sound is dull, ascites may be present
  - Spleen: Not recommended for PT to palpate enlarged spleen secondary to rupture issues (only palpable if enlarged)
  - Gallbladder (Murphy's): Place fingers right of rectus abdominus below rib cage: +/= sudden pain and muscle tensing with deep breath
  - Kidneys: In supine position, place one hand under client between ribs and iliac crest, other hand on abdomen below ribs and pointing in the opposite direction; +/− tenderness or reproduction of symptoms
  - Bladder: Not usually palpable unless distended and raised above pubic bone; in supine position, place hand above pubis and press down; +/= tenderness, reproduction of pain, ability to feel the bladder: __+ ___ −
- Observation
  - Scars may indicate adhesions or abdominal surgeries causative of diverticula
  - Pink or purplish striae may be indicative of Cushing syndrome
  - Dilated veins may indicate hepatic pathology or inferior vena cava obstruction, not diverticulitis
  - Contour: Roundness, concavity, asymmetry, distension, pregnancy signs
  - Cullen sign: Bluish discoloring around umbilicus may be a sign of retroperitoneal bleeding
  - Bluish discoloration in lower abdomen: Grey Turner's sign, signals hemorrhagic pancreatitis
  - Bulging in groin/abdomen especially apparent with contraction of musculature in area may be hernia
  - Pulsing in navel area may be abdominal aortic aneurysm
  - Left lower quadrant pain, often following a meal
  - Palpable abdominal tenderness: On left side or generalized

- Psoas sign: Provide resistance over patient's right knee during hip flexion; pain indicates appendicitis, possible inflammation of abdomen
- Obdurator sign: Internal rotation and flexion of right LE may indicate appendicitis, pelvic inflammation
- Rovsing sign: Pain on right side of abdomen when pressure applied to left may indicate appendicitis

INTERVENTION

- PT intervention consistent with movement-related problems secondary to UG disorder
- Sacral modulation
- Bladder training
- Biofeedback
- Therapeutic exercise
- Pelvic floor retraining
- Self-care training
  - With indwelling catheters, ensure they are not pulled out and drainage clamps are locked
- Neuromuscular re-education
- Heating pads to abdomen for pain management
- Timed voiding should not be used
- Electrical stimulation, TENS device into women's vagina or men's rectum
- Interprofessional
  - Dietary counseling to limit foods/beverages that irritate bladder
    - Alcohol
    - Citrus
    - Onions
    - Monosodium glutamate (MSG)
    - Coffee
    - Cranberry juice
  - Lifestyle modification
  - Smoking cessation
  - Weight management
  - Psychological intervention

FUNCTIONAL GOALS

- Patient will be able to
  - Achieve functional aerobic capacity, gait, and tolerance for ADLs/IADLs without need to go to the bathroom.
  - Achieve ≥600 m in a 6-minute walk test for initiation of safe, functional gait in community without the need of bathroom.
  - Tolerate 30 minutes of continuous, moderate exercise three times per week in ______ weeks, and five times per week in ____________ weeks, depending on disease severity.

PROGNOSIS

- Physician should establish medical prognosis, as pathology is primarily medical in nature.
- For PT prognosis, goals should be established that patient can achieve based on overall condition.
- Patients often respond well to dietary changes.
- Surgery may be required.
- Approximately 40% may be unable to work.[2]
- Approximately 27% may be unable to have sexual intercourse due to pain.[2]

PATIENT RESOURCES

- AUA Foundation: The Official Foundation of the American Urological Association. http://www.urologyhealth.org./ Accessed March 24, 2013.
- Interstitial Cystitis and Overactive Bladder Network. *What is Interstitial Cystitis & Painful Bladder Syndrome?* http://www.ic-network.com/whatisinterstitialcystitis/. Accessed March 22, 2013.

REFERENCES

1. Mayo Clinic. *Interstitial Cystitus.* http://www.mayoclinic.com/health/interstitial-cystitis/DS00497. Accessed April 29, 2013.
2. Webster DC, Brennan T. Self-care effectiveness and health outcomes in women with interstitial cystitis: implications for mental health clinics. *Issues Ment Health Nurs.* 1998;19(5):495–519.

ADDITIONAL REFERENCES

- Dutton M. Genitourinary system disorders. In: Dutton M, ed. *McGraw-Hill's NPTE (National Physical Therapy Examination).* 2nd ed. New York, NY: McGraw-Hill; 2012. http://www.accessphysiotherapy.com/content/5402307. Accessed March 16, 2013.
- Dutton M. Gynecologic disorders. In: Dutton M, ed. *Dutton's Orthopaedic Examination, Evaluation, and Intervention.* 3rd ed. New York, NY: McGraw-Hill; 2012. http://www.accessphysiotherapy.com/content/5547556. Accessed March 16, 2013.
- ICD9DATA web site. http://www.icd9data.com. Accessed March 24, 2013.
- ICD10DATA web site. http://www.icd10data.com. Accessed March 24, 2013.
- Marinkovic SP, Moldwin R, Gillen LM, Stanton SL. The management of interstitial cystitis or painful bladder syndrome in women. *BMJ.* 2009;339:b2707.
- Neville C. Biofeedback and Neuromuscular Electrical Stimulation Treatment for Pelvic Floor Muscle Disorders [Video]. New York, NY:McGraw-Hill; 2014. http://www.accessphysiotherapy.com/. Accessed June 12, 2014.
- Sant GR. Etiology, pathogenesis, and diagnosis of interstitial cystitis. *Rev Urol.* 2002;4(Suppl 1):S9–S15.

268 DYSPAREUNIA

Cynthia E. Neville, DPT, PT, WCS

CONDITION/DISORDER SYNONYMS

- Painful intercourse
- Urogenital pain disorders
- Sexual pain disorder
- Levator ani syndrome
- Vaginismus

ICD-9-CM CODES

- 625.0 Dyspareunia
- Associated Diagnoses
  - 617 Endometriosis
  - 625.1 Vaginismus
  - 625.7 Vulvodynia
  - 625.71 Vulvar vestibulitis
  - 724.7 Disorders of coccyx
  - 728.2 Muscular wasting and disuse atrophy
  - 728.85 Spasm of muscle
  - 729.1 Myalgia

ICD-10-CM CODES

- M62.83 Muscle spasm
- M79.1 Myalgia
- N94.1 Dyspareunia
- N94.2 Vaginismus

PREFERRED PRACTICE PATTERN

- 4C: Impaired Muscle Performance[1]

PATIENT PRESENTATION

A 28-year-old woman delivered her first baby vaginally 12 weeks ago. She sustained a Grade 2 perineal wound during the delivery. The wound became infected. The wound was surgically repaired and revised during a subsequent surgery. The obstetrician (OB) told the patient that some of the perineal scar tissue had to be removed. She was cleared by her OB/gynecologist (Gyn) to have intercourse but experienced severe pain during initial penetration and also with deep penetration during the first attempt at intercourse with her husband.

KEY FEATURES

Description

- Pain during initial or deep penetration during sexual intercourse

Essentials of Diagnosis

- Rule out gynecological pathology
- Pain with vaginal penetration during gynecological examination, insertion of tampon, or during and after sexual intercourse

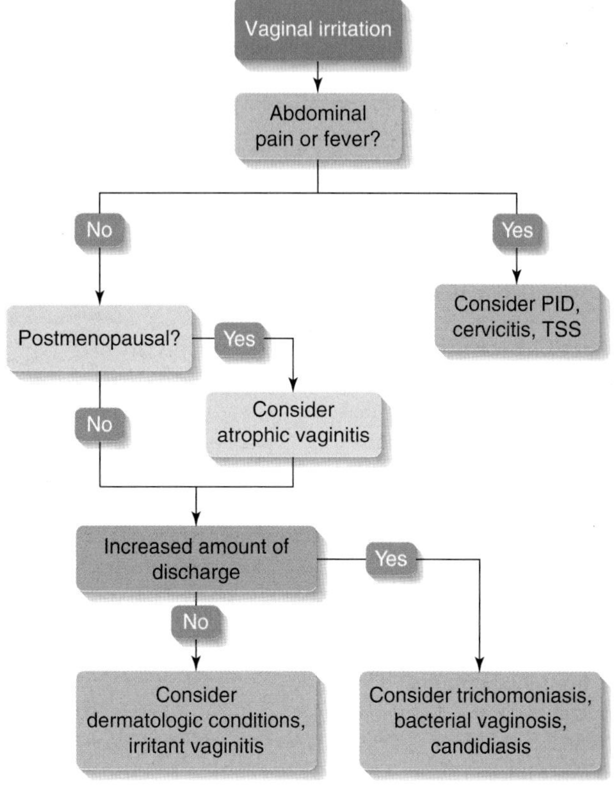

FIGURE 268-1 Diagnostic approach: Vaginitis. PID, pelvic inflammatory disease; TSS, toxic shock syndrome. (From Henderson MC, Tierney LM, Smetana GW. *The Patient History: An Evidence-Based Approach to Differential Diagnosis.* www.accessmedicine.com. Copyright © The McGraw-Hill Companies, Inc. All rights reserved.)

- Pain to palpation of the superficial genital muscles and/or deep levator ani pelvic floor muscles (PFMs)

General Considerations

- Female only
- May be a side effect of vaginal delivery associated with perineal trauma or pelvic joint injury
- Vaginal stenosis and atrophy causing painful intercourse may be secondary to radiation of the pelvis for treatment of cancers
- Urogenital pain disorders are frequently associated with pain in nearby body areas; especially back, pelvic, hip, groin regions

Demographics

- Severe perineal trauma occurs in 0.5% to 10% of vaginal births[2]
- Exact prevalence of pelvic pain is not known, estimates vary in the literature from 3.8% to 24%[3]
- Many patients with pelvic pain will go on to develop chronic pain syndrome with depression, pain out of proportion to pathology, and changing roles in marriage, family, and career[4]

CLINICAL FINDINGS

SIGNS AND SYMPTOMS

- Report of vaginal pain during penetration
- Perceived reduction in size of vaginal opening attributed to muscle spasm
- May complain of lower quadrant abdominal pain during sexual intercourse
- Symptoms may worsen or decrease during and after sexual intercourse

▶ Functional Implications

- Pain during attempted penetration
- Sexual dysfunction
- May lead to unwanted abstinence
- May lead to decision to not have a subsequent pregnancy

▶ Possible Contributing Causes

- Perineal trauma during vaginal delivery
- Coccyx injury or fracture
- Pubic symphysis diastasis
- Urinary tract infection (UTI)
- History of sexual or physical abuse
- Stress, anxiety
- Fear, catastrophizing

▶ Differential Diagnosis

- UTI
- Sexually transmitted disease
- Urethritis
- Bladder infection
- Yeast infection
- Bacterial vaginosis
- Organ dysfunction from cancer or malignancy
- Nonmalignant tumor in abdomen or organs
- Gynecologic problems in females
  - Endometriosis
  - Menses
  - Ectopic pregnancy
  - Ovarian cyst
  - Fibroids
  - Menopause
- Appendicitis
- Pelvic inflammatory disease

MEANS OF CONFIRMATION OR DIAGNOSIS

▶ Laboratory Tests

- To rule out other pathology
  - Blood tests to rule out pathology
  - Urine culture/urinalysis to rule out infection
  - H&H

▶ Imaging

- All tests to rule out other pathology
  - Cystoscopy
  - Ultrasound
  - CT
  - Bladder scans
  - MRI
  - X-ray

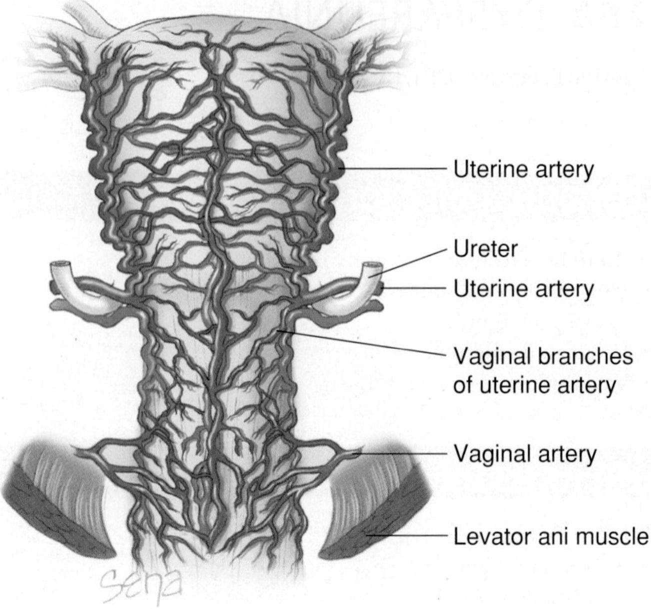

FIGURE 268-2 Uterine and vaginal blood supply. The origin of the vaginal artery varies and may arise from the uterine, inferior vesical, or internal iliac artery. (From Cunningham FG, Leveno KJ, Bloom SL, Hauth JC, Rouse DJ, Spong CY. *Williams Obstetrics*. 23rd ed. www.accessmedicine.com. Copyright © The McGraw-Hill Companies, Inc. All rights reserved.)

▶ Diagnostic Procedures

- To rule out other pathology
  - Postvoid residual
  - Bladder biopsy
  - Cystography
  - Cystometrogram
  - Video urodynamic testing
  - Colonoscopy
  - Defecography
  - Biopsy
  - Uroflowmetry

FINDINGS AND INTERPRETATION

- H&H for signs of bleeding, anemia, pathogens, immune status, vitamin deficiencies, white blood cell count

TREATMENT

▶ Medication

- Nonsteroidal anti-inflammatory medication (NSAIDs)
- Opioid pain medication
- Medication for muscle spasms: Flavoxate
- Pregabalin
- Tricyclic antidepressants
- Vaginal estrogen if levels low
- Anticonvulsants
- Topical lidocaine

MEDICAL PROCEDURES

- Botulinum toxin injections
- Trigger point injections
- Implanted electrical stimulator for neuromodulation (Interstim)

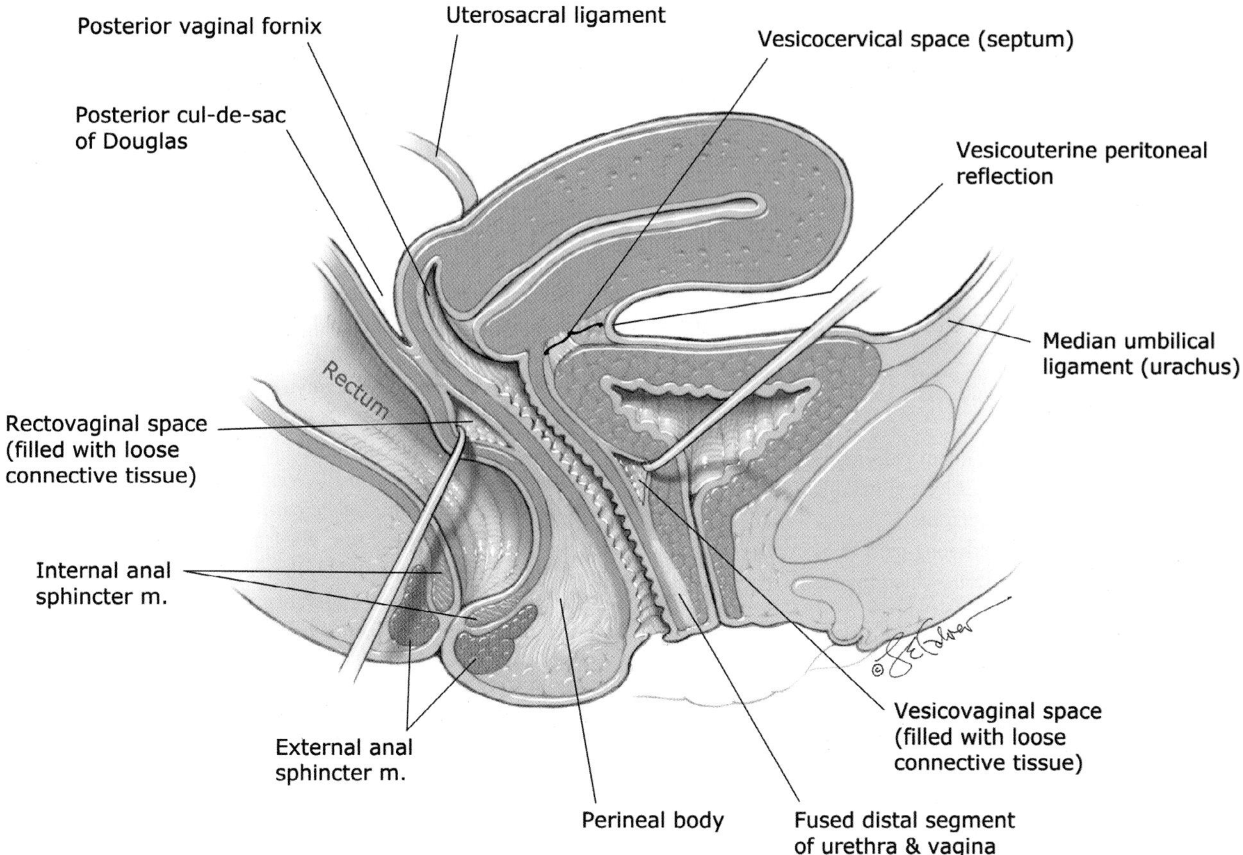

FIGURE 268-3 Surgical cleavage planes and vaginal wall layers. (From Hoffman BL, Schorge JO, Schaffer JI, Halvorson LM, Bradshaw KD, Cunningham, FG. *Williams Gynecology*. 2nd ed. New York, NY: McGraw-Hill, 2012.)

REFERRALS/ADMITTANCE

- Pelvic floor physical therapist
- Cognitive behavioral pain psychologist
- Primary care physicians
- Physical Medicine and Rehabilitation physicians
- Gynecologists
- Urologists
- Urogynecologists
- Pain Medicine
- Acupuncture
- Biofeedback practitioner
- Certified sex therapist

IMPAIRMENTS

- PFM dysfunction
  - Overactive
  - Underactive
  - Nonrelaxing
  - Noncontracting
- Incontinence
- Myofascial pelvic pain
- Pelvic organ prolapse
- Decreased sexual appreciation; anorgasmia: Inability to achieve orgasm
- Pain
- Muscle atrophy
- Joint hypomobility
- Posture dysfunction
- Contractures of soft tissue (fascia, muscle)
- Obstructed defecation

TESTS AND MEASURES

- PFM examination: Via vagina or anorectum
- Abdominal muscle test
- Abdominal wall palpation : Diastalsis rectus abdominis, scar
- sEMG biofeedback assessment of the PFMs and abdominal muscles
- Pressure manometry of the PFMs
- Lumbar spine, pelvic girdle, and hip-joint examination procedures

INTERVENTION

- PFM exercises/training
  - "Kegel" exercises: Another name for PFM exercises
  - Contraction
  - Relaxation/"Bulging"
  - Motor control
  - Endurance
  - Power
  - sEMG biofeedback
- Progressive vaginal dilation
- TENS
- Pressure manometry

- Manual therapy
  - Thiele massage performed vaginally
  - Myofascial release
  - Internal vaginal massage
- Thermal modalities
- US imaging to awareness of muscle contractions
- Posture re-education
- Functional training: "Bulge" or "drop and open" the PFMs prior to vaginal penetration during intercourse, vaginal examination, tampon insertion
- Patient education regarding effects of maladaptive pain cognitions

FUNCTIONAL GOALS

- Patient will be able to
  - Verbalize strategies for independent pain management.
  - Independently perform progressive vaginal dilation to practice vaginal penetration sexual intercourse.
  - Demonstrate independence with long-term PFM exercise program.
  - Identify thoughts and cognitions which may exacerbate symptoms during attempted intercourse.

PROGNOSIS

- Primiparous women who experience severe perineal trauma are less likely to have a subsequent baby, more likely to have a related surgical procedure in the 12 months following the birth and no more likely to have an operative birth or another severe perineal tear in a subsequent birth.
- Longer duration and greater intensity of pain symptoms negatively impacts prognosis.[5]
- Psychological factors such as pain catastophizing and fear avoidance negatively impact prognosis.[6]

PATIENT RESOURCES

- International Pelvic Pain Society at http://www.pelvicpain.org/. Accessed April 20, 2013.
- "*Relieving Pain in America*" from The National Academies Press http://www.nap.edu/catalog.php?record_id=13172. Accessed April 20, 2013.

REFERENCES

1. The American Physical Therapy Association. Pattern 4C: impaired muscle performance. *Guide to Physical Therapist Practice*. Alexandria, VA: The American Physical Therapy Association; 2003. http://guidetoptpractice.apta.org/content/1/SEC10.extract?sid=9af82a7e-5fc3-41d2-86ab-b8336a9655e9. April 20, 2013.
2. Priddis H, Dahlen HG, Schmied V, et al. Risk of recurrence, subsequent mode of birth and morbidity for women who experienced severe perineal trauma in a first birth in New South Wales between 2000–2008: a population based data linkage study. *BMC Pregnancy Childbirth*. 2013;13(1):89.
3. Latthe P, Latthe M, Say L, Gulmezoglu M, Khan KS. WHO systematic review of prevalence of chronic pelvic pain: a neglected reproductive health morbidity. *BMC Public Health*. 2006;6:177. doi:10.1186/1471-2458/6/177 [p. 1–7].
4. Gyang A, Hartman M, Lamvu G. Musculoskeletal Causes of Chronic Pelvic Pain; What a Gynecologist Should Know. *Obstet Gynecol*. 2013;121:645–650.
5. Zondervan KT, Yudkin PL, Vessey MP, et al. The community prevalence of chronic pelvic pain in women and associated illness behaviour. *Br J Gen Pract*. 2001;51(468):541–547.
6. Alappattu MJ, Bishop MD. Psychological factors in chronic pelvic pain in women: Relevance and application of the fear-avoidance model of pain. *Phys Ther*. 2011;91(10):1542–1550.

ADDITIONAL REFERENCES

- Abrams P, Cardozo L, Fall M, et al. The standardization of terminology of lower urinary tract function: report from the Standardization Sub-Committee of the International Continence Society. *Neurourol Urodyn*. 2002;21(2):167–178.
- Dutton M. Genitourinary system disorders. In: Dutton M, ed. *McGraw-Hill's NPTE (National Physical Therapy Examination)*. 2nd ed. New York, NY: McGraw-Hill; 2012. http://www.accessphysiotherapy.com/content/5402307. Accessed April 20, 2013.
- Dutton M. Gynecologic disorders. In: Dutton M, ed. *Dutton's Orthopaedic Examination, Evaluation, and Intervention*. 3rd ed. New York, NY: McGraw-Hill; 2012. http://www.accessphysiotherapy.com/content/5547556. Accessed April 20, 2013.
- Fall M, Baranowski AP, Elneil S, et al. Europe Association of Urology. EAU guidelines on chronic pelvic pain. *Eur Urol*. 2010;57(1):35–48. doi: 10.1016/j.eururo.2009.08.020.
- Neville C. Biofeedback and Neuromuscular Electrical Stimulation Treatment for Pelvic Floor Muscle Disorders [Video]. New York, NY: McGraw-Hill; 2014. http://www.accessphysiotherapy.com. Accessed June 13, 2014.

269 HEMORRHOIDS

Debra F. Stern, DPT, DBA, MSM, PT
Wendy Song, DO

CONDITION/DISORDER SYNONYMS

- External hemorrhoids
- Internal hemorrhoids

ICD-9-CM CODES

- 455.0 Internal hemorrhoids without mention of complication
- 455.1 Internal thrombosed hemorrhoids
- 455.2 Internal hemorrhoids with other complication
- 455.3 External hemorrhoids without mention of complication
- 455.4 External thrombosed hemorrhoids
- 455.5 External hemorrhoids with other complication
- 455.6 Unspecified hemorrhoids without mention of complication
- 455.7 Unspecified thrombosed hemorrhoids
- 455.8 Unspecified hemorrhoids with other complication
- 455.9 Residual hemorrhoidal skin tags
- Associated Diagnoses
  - 315.4 Developmental coordination disorder
  - 718.45 Contracture of joint, pelvic region and thigh
  - 719.70 Difficulty in walking
  - 728.2 Muscular wasting and disuse atrophy
  - 728.89 Other disorders of muscle, ligament, and fascia
  - 729.9 Other disorders of soft tissue
  - 780.7 Malaise and fatigue
  - 781.2 Abnormality of gait
  - 782.3 Edema
  - 786.0 Dyspnea and respiratory abnormalities
  - 786.05 Shortness of breath

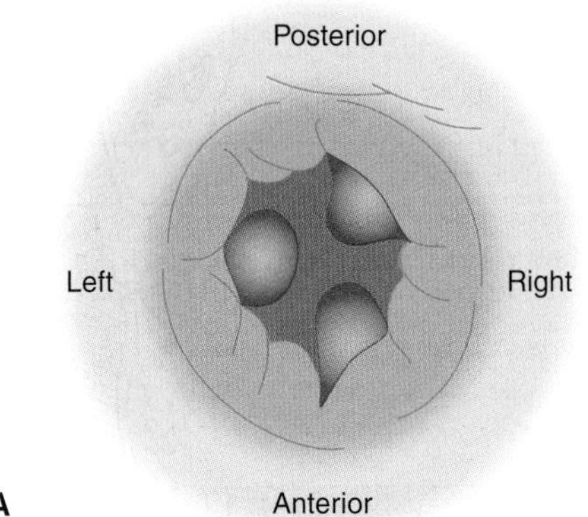

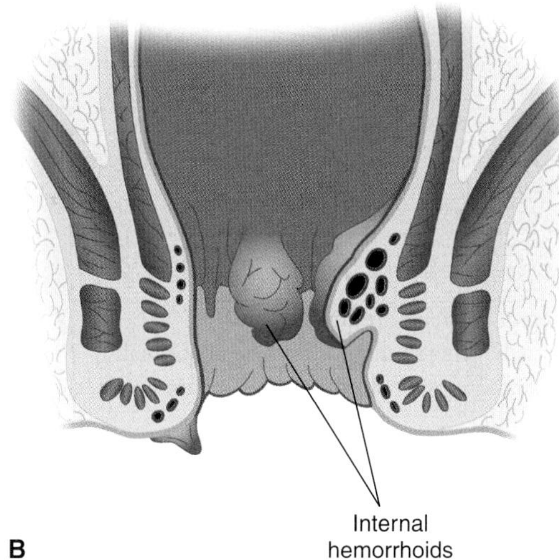

FIGURE 269-1 Common site of hemorrhoids. (**A**) Internal hemorrhoids at 2, 5, and 9 o'clock. (**B**) Protrusion of anal cushions, soft tissue containing vessels. (From Tintinalli JE, Stapczynski JS, John Ma O, et al. eds. *Tintinalli's Emergency Medicine: A Comprehensive Study Guide*. 7th ed. http://www.accessmedicine.com. Copyright © The McGraw-Hill Companies, Inc. All rights reserved.)

ICD-10-CM CODES

- I84 Hemorrhoids
- K64.8 Other hemorrhoids
- K64.9 Unspecified hemorrhoids

PREFERRED PRACTICE PATTERNS

- 4E: Impaired Joint Mobility, Motor Function, Muscle Performance, and Range of Motion (ROM) Associated with Localized Inflammation[1]
- 6B: Impaired Aerobic Capacity/Endurance Associated with Deconditioning[2]

PATIENT PRESENTATION

A 52-year old female presents with tailbone (coccyx) pain. On history, she has noticed drops of bright red blood in the toilet and on tissue paper after bowel movements for 2 months. She admits to constipation with straining and rectal pain on a weekly basis. She reports her bleeding is worse when she is more constipated. Her last colonoscopy was 1 year ago and was normal. Vitals are Temperature: 98.2F, Pulse: 68, Respirations: 16, Blood pressure: 134/85, and SpO_2%: 100%. Physical examination reveals a small purple, tender, hard, protruding swelling of the anal opening at the 7 o'clock position, no anal fissures or blood was found with inspection and digital rectal examination.

KEY FEATURES

Description

- Bright red rectal bleeding, usually associated with bowel movements

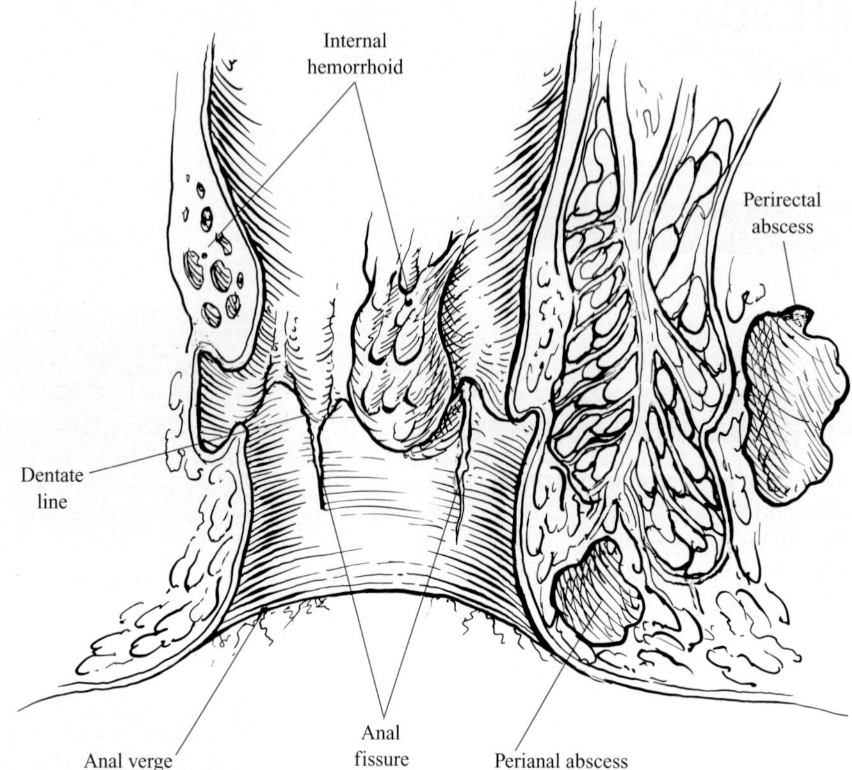

FIGURE 269-2 Perianal–perirectal abscesses. The anatomy of perianal and perirectal abscesses is illustrated. Also shown are anal fissure and internal and external hemorrhoids. (From Knoop KJ, Stack LB, Storrow AB, et al. *The Atlas of Emergency Medicine*. 3rd ed. http://www.accessmedicine.com. Copyright © The McGraw-Hill Companies, Inc. All rights reserved.)

- Bulging of the veins around the anus
  - Internal: Veins swelling inside the anal canal
  - External: Veins swelling near the opening of the anus
  - Protruding
- Superficial pain in rectal area, especially with sitting or attempting to evacuate bowels

Essentials of Diagnosis

- Rectal pain
- Increased rectal pain with attempts at evacuating bowels
- Bright red bleeding

General Considerations

- Diagnosis for more occult problems may take time and require intensive diagnostic testing.
- Rectal bleeding may be indicative of more serious medical problems.
  - Pathology in multiple organ systems
  - GI pathology, especially intestinal, liver
  - Cardiovascular pathology
- May result in secondary problems such as aerobic capacity and muscle endurance impairment, sarcopenia, weakened/impaired muscle performance, musculoskeletal problems, weight gain (secondary to reduced physical activity due to discomfort or bleeding), indicating the need for physical therapy intervention depending on severity.
- As hemorrhoids may refer pain to the back, they should be considered in the differential diagnoses when an individual is referred to physical therapy (PT) for back pain.

Demographics

- Common in pregnancy
- More common with aging, usually over 50 years of age
- Higher occurrence with obesity
- Exact frequency unknown, estimated 4%

CLINICAL FINDINGS

SIGNS AND SYMPTOMS	
• Diarrhea	• Back pain
• Constipation	• Leg pain
• Lump(s) in anal area	• Depression
• Painless bleeding	• Anemia
• Itching	• Fatigue
• Pain in anal/rectal area	• Pallor
• Inflammation	• Rapid heart rate
• Swelling	• Weakness
• Fecal leakage	• Headaches
• Dizziness	• Shortness of breath
• Fainting	• Difficulty concentrating
• Lightheadedness	

Functional Implications

- Severe symptoms including rectal, leg, or back pain
- Swelling in anal area
- Bleeding with need to wear protective pads
- Decreased exercise tolerance
- Sleep disturbance if condition is stressful
- Eating disorders

- Constipation or bowel retention secondary to fear of moving bowels
- Limitations in ADLs or IADLs
- Infection (systemic or local)
- Headaches
- Dizziness
- Fatigue

Possible Contributing Causes

- Bowel straining
- Genetics
- Anal intercourse
- Chronic constipation
- Chronic diarrhea
- Low-fiber diet
- Dehydration
- Pregnancy
- Obesity
- Aging
- Liver disease
- Heart disease

Differential Diagnosis

- Organ dysfunction from cancer or malignancy, especially of the liver
- Anal cancer
- Colorectal cancer
- Nonmalignant tumor in abdomen
- Liver disease
- Heart disease, cardiovascular pathology
- Autoimmune disease with bowel inflammation or dysfunction
- Gastroparesis
- Gynecologic problems in females
  - Endometriosis
  - Irregular menses
  - Ectopic pregnancy
  - Ovarian cysts
  - Fibroids
  - Menopause
- Autoimmune disease affecting upper and lower GI tracts
- Crohn disease
- Irritable bowel syndrome (IBS)
- Systemic lupus erythematosus (SLE)
- Rheumatoid arthritis
- Appendicitis
- Peritonitis
- Prostitis
- Benign prostatic hypertrophy
- Pelvic inflammatory disease
- Gastroenteritis
- Perforated ulcer in GI system
- Diverticulitis
- Bowel disorder
- Post–weight-loss surgery complications

MEANS OF CONFIRMATION OR DIAGNOSIS

Laboratory Tests

- Blood tests
  - Complete blood count (CBC)
  - Stool guaiac

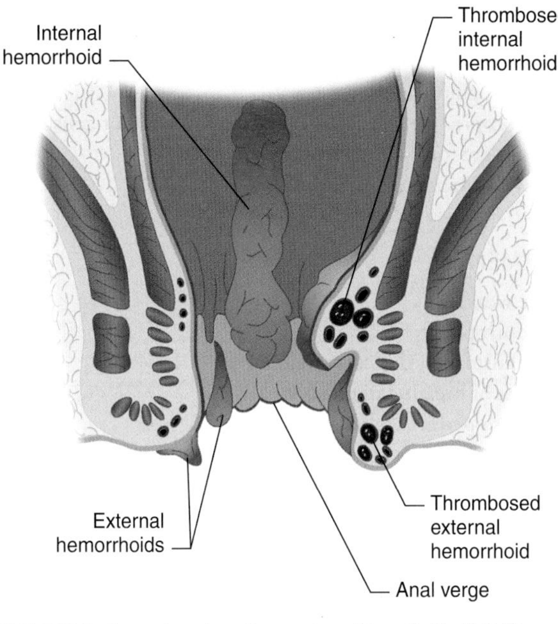

FIGURE 269-3 Coronal section of anorectum. (From Tintinalli JE, Stapczynski JS, John Ma O, et al. eds. *Tintinalli's Emergency Medicine: A Comprehensive Study Guide*. 7th ed. http://www.accessmedicine.com. Copyright © The McGraw-Hill Companies, Inc. All rights reserved.)

Imaging

- Colonoscopy
- CT
- MRI

Diagnostic Procedures

- Biopsy
- Sigmoidoscopy
- Anoscopy
- Visual inspection
- Digital rectal examination

FINDINGS AND INTERPRETATION

- Visual confirmation of internal hemorrhoids with anoscopy or proctoscopy

TREATMENT

Medication

- Topical steroids
- Topical OTC preparations
- Suppositories
- Sclerotherapy
- Oral analgesics for pain

MEDICAL PROCEDURES

- Coagulation using heat or light
- Ligation
- Surgery
  - Stapling
  - Hemorrhoid removal
  - Clot removal

REFERRALS/ADMITTANCE

- To physician if patient history and reactions to PT indicate hemorrhoids
- To appropriate physician if causative problem not considered appropriate for PT intervention
- To ER if emergency identified

IMPAIRMENTS

- Muscle weakness
- Muscle atrophy
- Gait abnormality, difficulty walking
- Shortness of breath, fatigue
- Inability to perform self-care
- Balance impairment, dizziness
- Impaired circulation

TESTS AND MEASURES

- As rectal bleeding may indicate more serious problems, the following should be considered
  - Kidneys: In supine, place one hand under client between ribs and iliac crest, other hand on abdomen below ribs and ribs pointing in opposite direction; +/− tenderness or reproduction of symptoms
  - Bladder: Not usually palpable unless distended and raised above pubic bone; in supine, place hand above pubis and press down; +/= tenderness, reproduction of pain, ability to feel the bladder: +/−
  - Appendix (McBurney's): Apply vertical pressure halfway between right ASIS and umbilicus; −/+ may indicate appendicitis
  - Liver: In supine, with left hand under trunk parallel to 11th and 12th ribs, lift upward; right hand lateral to rectus, press in and up: +/= reproduction of symptoms with deep breath, indicates liver involvement
  - Ascites: Percuss outward from center with fingers; if sound is dull, ascites may be present
  - Spleen: Not recommended for PT to palpate enlarged spleen secondary to ease of rupture (only palpable if enlarged)
  - Gallbladder (Murphy's): Place fingers right of rectus abdominus below rib cage: +/= sudden pain and muscle tensing with deep breath
- Observation
  - Scars: Indicative of adhesions or abdominal surgeries causative of diverticula
  - Pink or purplish striae: May be indicative of Cushing syndrome
  - Dilated veins: May indicate hepatic pathology or inferior vena cava obstruction, not diverticulitis
  - Contour: Roundness, concavity, asymmetry, distension, pregnancy signs
  - Cullen sign: Bluish discoloring around umbilicus may be a sign of retroperitoneal bleeding
  - Bluish discoloration in lower abdomen: Grey Turner's sign, signals hemorrhagic pancreatitis
  - Bulging in groin/abdomen especially apparent with contraction of musculature in area may be hernia
  - Pulsing in navel area may be abdominal aortic aneurysm
  - Palpable abdominal tenderness: On left side or generalized
  - Psoas sign: Provides resistance over patient's right knee as they flex the hip; pain indicates appendicitis, possible inflammation of abdomen
  - Obdurator sign: Internal rotation and flexion of right lower extremity (LE) may indicate appendicitis, pelvic inflammation
  - Rovsing sign: Pain on right side of abdomen when pressure applied to left may indicate appendicitis

INTERVENTION

- Advise patient to
  - Limit time on toilet; use stool softener to decrease straining
  - Soak in warm bath
  - Apply pads with numbing substances, such as witch hazel
  - Avoid dry toilet paper
  - Apply cold compress locally
- Physical therapy intervention is consistent with the movement related problems that occur secondary to diabetes and include as indicated
- Gait training
- Therapeutic exercise: All relevant categories, energy conservation
  - PT should inquire if medication taken. If glucose >300, exercise should be avoided
  - Avoidance of any activity that aggravates hemorrhoids
- Therapeutic activities for bed mobility training, transfer and transitional movement training
- Wheelchair management: Positioning
- Self-care management training
- Neuromuscular re-education; balance and postural training

FUNCTIONAL GOALS

- Patient will be able to
  - Tolerate 30 minutes of continuous seated activity three times a day in ______ weeks, and five times a day in ____________ weeks, depending on severity.
  - Achieve functional aerobic capacity, ability to talk during activity in order to achieve functional gait and activity tolerance for ADLs and IADLs.
  - Achieve functional gait in the home and community (with or without device) to allow for ADLs and IADLs, up to __________ ft based on patient need and prior functional level.
  - Achieve 600 m or greater in a 6-minute walk test for initiation of safe functional gait in the community.
  - Perform active verbalization with increasing taxonomy for safety during gait, including negotiation of even and uneven surfaces, opening and closing doors, and car transfers.

PROGNOSIS

- Hemorrhoids usually resolve.
- In rare cases, anemia may result from severe bleeding or hemorrhoids may strangulate, causing severe pain and requiring surgical intervention.
- Physician should establish medical prognosis, as pathology is primarily medical in nature.
- For PT prognosis, goals should be established that the patient can achieve based on their overall condition.
- Prognosis from a PT perspective should be good, unless medical condition is unstable or goals unrealistic.

PATIENT RESOURCES

- Hemorrhoids. American Society of Colon and Rectal Surgeons. http://www.fascrs.org/patients/conditions/hemorrhoids/. Accessed June 20, 2013.
- Pregnancy and Hemorrhoids. American Pregnancy Association. http://americanpregnancy.org/pregnancyhealth/hemorrhoids.html. Accessed June 20, 2013.
- Living with hemorrhoids. American Gastroenterological Association. http://www.gastro.org/patient-center/digestive-conditions/hemorrhoids. Accessed June 20, 2013.

REFERENCES

1. The American Physical Therapy Association. Pattern 4E: Impaired joint mobility, motor function, muscle performance, and range of motion associated with localized inflammation. *Interactive Guide to Physical Therapist Practice*. 2003. doi: 10.2522/ptguide.3.1_5. Accessed June 20, 2013.
2. The American Physical Therapy Association. Pattern 6B: Impaired aerobic capacity/endurance associated with deconditioning. *Interactive Guide to Physical Therapist Practice*. 2003. doi: 10.2522/ptguide.3.3_2. Accessed June 20, 2013.

ADDITIONAL REFERENCES

- Alonso-Coello P, Castillejo MM. Office evaluation and treatment of hemorrhoids. *J Fam Pract*. 2003;52(5):366–374.
- Chandrasoma P, Taylor CR. The Intestines: I. Structure & Function; Malabsorption Syndrome; Intestinal Obstruction. In: Chandrasoma P, Taylor CR, eds. *Concise Pathology*. 3rd ed. New York, NY: McGraw-Hill; 2011. http://www.accessphysiotherapy.com/content/189207. Accessed June 20, 2013.
- Goodman CC, Fuller KS. *Pathology: Implications for the Physical Therapist*. 3rd ed. Philadelphia, PA: Saunders Elsevier; 2009.
- Hulme-Moir M, Bartolo DC. Hemorrhoids. *Gastroenterol Clin North Am*. 2001;30(1):183–197.

270 MALE CHRONIC PROSTATITIS

Cynthia E. Neville, DPT, PT, WCS

CONDITION/DISORDER SYNONYMS

- Category 3 nonbacterial prostatitis
- Chronic prostatitis/chronic pelvic pain syndrome (CP/CPPS)
- Levator ani syndrome
- Prostatodynia
- Urogenital pain disorders

ICD-9-CM CODES

- 338.4 Chronic pain syndrome
- 601.1 Chronic prostatitis
- Associated physical therapy diagnoses
  - 564.6 Anal spasm
  - 569.42 Anal or rectal pain
  - 719.45 Pain in the hip joint, pelvic region, and thigh
  - 724.7 Disorders of coccyx
  - 728.2 Muscular wasting and disuse atrophy
  - 728.85 Spasm of muscle
  - 728.89 Disorders of muscle, ligament, and fascia
  - 729.1 Myalgia
  - 729.2 Neuralgia/neuritis
  - 729.9 Other disorders of soft tissue

ICD-10-CM CODES

- G89.4 Chronic pain syndrome
- N41.1 Chronic prostatitis
- R10.2 Pelvic and perineal pain
- Symptom-specific diagnoses
  - N53.12 Painful ejaculation
  - N94.1 Dyspareunia
  - K59.5 Anal spasm

PREFERRED PRACTICE PATTERN

- As of July 2014, the APTA Guide to Physical Therapist Practice does not include practice patterns for organ system pathology.
- Associated or secondary musculoskeletal patterns include:
  - 4C: Impaired Muscle Performance[1]
  - 4D: Impaired Joint Mobility, Motor Function, Muscle Performance, and Range of Motion Associated with Connective Tissue Dysfunction[1]

PATIENT PRESENTATION

A 36-year-old man reports pain in the perineum and scrotum which worsens with sitting. He was originally diagnosed with acute bacterial prostatitis, and completed a 6-week course of antibiotics. The pain improved for several weeks, then returned. Testing is now negative for infection. Now, the patient complains that it feels like he is "sitting on a ball." If he has been sitting and having pain for a while, then sexual intercourse and ejaculation are also painful.

KEY FEATURES

Description

- Pelvic pain or regional pelvic pain syndrome (perineal pain, penile pain, testicular pain, suprapubic pain, groin pain) without detectable pathology
- No evidence of infection or inflammation

Essentials of Diagnosis

- Unknown etiology
- Rule out bacterial prostatitis and other organ pathology
- Symptoms may be initiated by an acute infection, injury, or inflammation of a pelvic or urogenital organ, however, pain persists beyond the duration of the original inciting event or disease.[2]

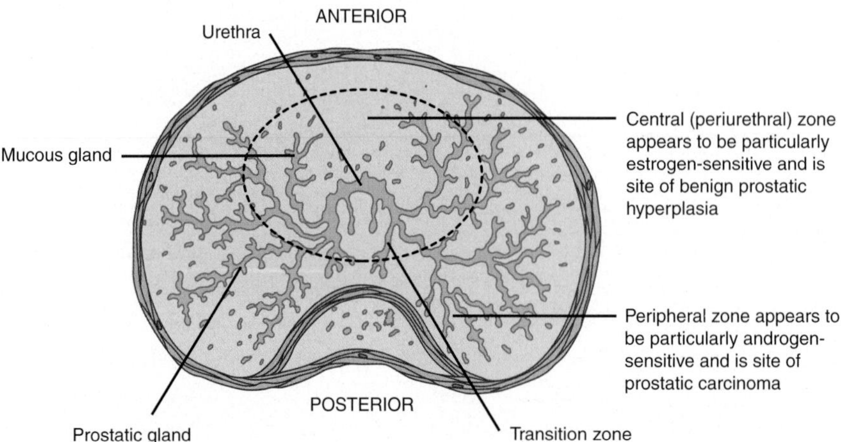

FIGURE 270-1 Structure of the prostate. (Redrawn, with permission, from Chandrasoma P, Taylor CE. *Concise Pathology*. 3rd ed. Originally published by Appleton & Lange. Copyright © 1998 by the McGraw-Hill Companies, Inc.)

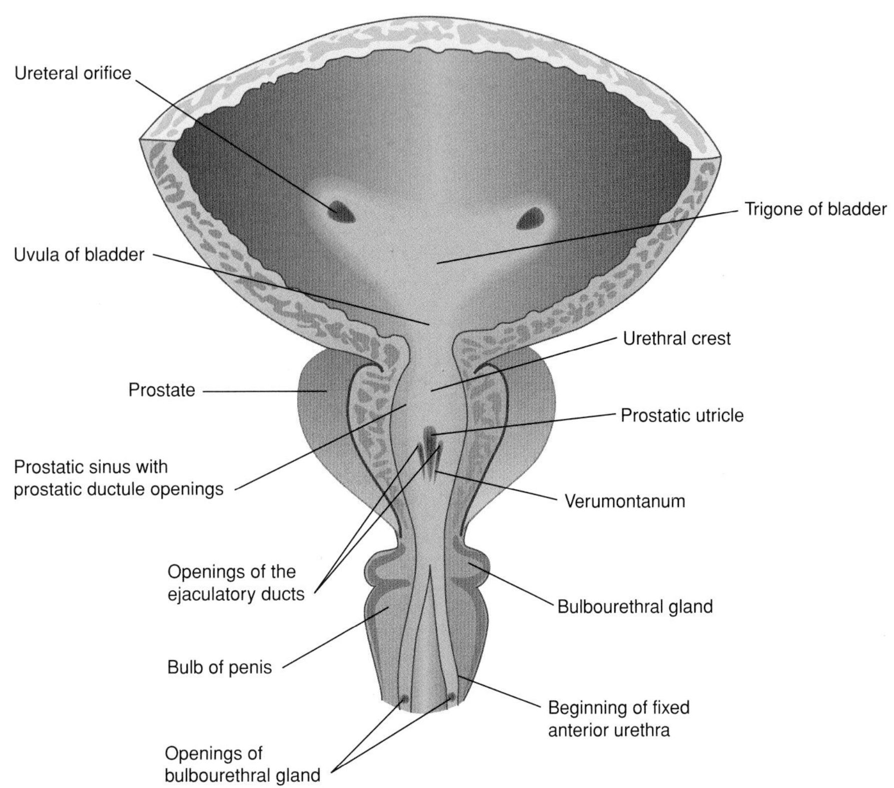

FIGURE 270-2 Anatomic relationships of the prostate. (Redrawn, with permission, from Lindner HH. *Clinical Anatomy*. Originally published by Appleton & Lange. Copyright © 1989 by the McGraw-Hill Companies, Inc.)

General Considerations

- Chronic pain condition.
- Etiology is unknown.
- Diagnosis is a process of exclusion.
- Urogenital pain disorders frequently affect nearby body areas; especially back, pelvic, hip, groin regions.[3]
- PT intervention is often appropriate for associated musculoskeletal impairments.
- May mimic other visceral pain conditions including colon cancer or tumor, irritable bowel, colitis.

Demographics

- 2% to 9% of men report prostatitis like symptoms.
- Exact prevalence of chronic pelvic pain is not known, estimates vary in the literature from 3.8% to 24%.[4]

CLINICAL FINDINGS

- Report of perineal pain, penile pain, testicular pain, suprapubic pain, and/or groin pain.
- Symptoms often worsened by prolonged sitting or standing, anxiety, bowel movements, physical activity, or sexual intercourse.
- Pain that starts in the afternoon and becomes progressively worse throughout the day.
- Constellation of symptoms that include painful ejaculation, low back pain, bowel symptoms of constipation, diarrhea, excessive flatus, painful defecation, or a sensation of incomplete evacuation, and urinary symptoms of frequency, urgency, or nocturia.

SIGNS AND SYMPTOMS

- Perineal pain, penile pain, testicular pain, suprapubic pain, and/or groin pain
- Pain during sexual intercourse
- Irritative voiding secondary to urinary discomfort, frequency, or urgency
- Irritable bowel: Diarrhea and/or constipation
- Pelvic pain
- Bladder pressure and pain
- Burning with urination

Functional Implications

- Pain
- Painful urination, defecation, and sexual activity
- Incomplete defecation or urination
- Urinary and fecal urgency and frequency
- Sarcopenia resulting in weakness, decreased muscle mass, inability to ambulate, perform self-care
- Decreased exercise tolerance
- Limited physical activity, activities of daily living (ADLs), instrumental activities of daily living (IADLs)
- Fatigue
- Inappropriate self-medication
- Anxiety, depression
- Sexual dysfunction

Possible Contributing Causes

- Prostate hyperplasia
- Urinary tract (UT) abnormalities
- History of sexual or physical abuse

- Allergy to foods, beverages, or supplements
- Environmental irritant
- Autoimmune reaction
- Sexual activity
- Upper UT blockage: Kidney stones
- Immunologic compromise
- Infection: Bacterial, viral, food poisoning
- Stress, anxiety
- Fear, catastrophizing
- Neuropathic pain

Differential Diagnosis

- Abdominal infection
- Acute pyelonephritis
- Appendicitis
- Autoimmune disease
- Bacterial prostatitis
- Benign prostatic hypertrophy
- Bladder infection
- Bladder, rectal, anal cancer
- Bowel disorder
    - Constipation, diarrhea
    - Inflamed abdominal or organ linings
    - Obstruction
    - Torsions
- Crohn disease
- Endocrine disorder
- Gastroenteritis
- Irritable bowel syndrome
- Kidney pathology
- Nonmalignant tumor in abdomen or organs
- Organ dysfunction from cancer or malignancy
- Perforated ulcer in GI system
- Peritonitis
- Sexually transmitted disease
- Urethritis
- Urinary tract infection (UTI)

MEANS OF CONFIRMATION OR DIAGNOSIS

Laboratory Tests

- Bacterial count of prostatic fluid
- Blood tests
- H&H
- Urine culture/urinalysis

Imaging

- Cystoscopy
- Ultrasound
- Intravenous urinary pyelogram using dye
- CT
- Bladder scans
- MRI
- X-ray

Diagnostic Procedures

- Uroflowmetry
- Post-void residual
- Bladder biopsy
- Cystography
- Cystometrogram
- Video urodynamic testing
- Colonoscopy
- Defecography
- Biopsy

FINDINGS AND INTERPRETATION

- H&H for signs of bleeding, anemia, pathogens, immune status, vitamin deficiencies, white blood cell count

TREATMENT

Medication

- Nonsteroidal anti-inflammatory medication (NSAID)
- Opioid pain medication
- Medication for muscle spasms: Flavoxate
- Pregabalin
- Tricyclic antidepressants
- Vaginal estrogen if levels low
- Pentosan (Elmiron) for chronic bladder pain
- Anticonvulsants
- Alpha blockers for prostatodynia
- Medication to relax the bladder
    - Anticholinergics: Oxybutynin, tolterodine, darifenacin

MEDICAL PROCEDURES

- Transurethral needle ablation: Prostate tissue heating
- Botulism toxin injections
- Trigger point injections
- Implanted electrical stimulator for neuromodulation (interstim)
- Electromagnetic therapy

REFERRALS/ADMITTANCE

- To pelvic floor physical therapist
- To cognitive behavioral pain psychologist
- To primary care physicians
- To physical medicine and rehabilitation physicians
- To urologists
- To gastroenterologist
- To colorectal surgeon
- To neurologist
- To pain medicine practitioner
- To acupuncture practitioner
- To biofeedback practitioner
- To certified sex therapist

IMPAIRMENTS

- Pelvic floor muscle (PFM) dysfunction
    - Overactive
    - Underactive
    - Nonrelaxing
    - Noncontracting
- Incontinence
- Urinary urgency and frequency
- Myofascial pelvic pain
- Pelvic organ prolapse
- Detrusor instability
- Painful ejaculation
- Muscle atrophy

- Joint hypomobility
- Posture dysfunction
- Gait abnormality, difficulty walking
- Contractures of soft tissue (fascia, muscle)
- Inability to perform self-care
- Obstructed defecation

TESTS AND MEASURES

- PFM examination: Via anorectum
- Abdominal wall muscle test
- Abdominal wall palpation: Diastalsis rectus abdominis, scar
- Bladder diary
- sEMG biofeedback assessment of the PFMs and abdominal muscles
- Pressure manometry of the PFMs
- Lumbar spine, pelvic girdle, and hip-joint examination procedures
- Palpation
  - Appendix (McBurney's): Apply vertical pressure halfway between right ASIS and umbilicus; −/+ may indicate appendicitis
  - Liver: In supine position, with left hand under trunk parallel to 11th and 12th ribs, lift upward; right hand lateral to rectus, press in and up: +/= reproduction of symptoms with deep breath, indicates liver involvement
  - Ascites: Percuss outward from center with fingers; if sound is dull, ascites may be present
  - Gallbladder (Murphy's): place fingers right of rectus abdominis below rib cage: +/= sudden pain and muscle tensing with deep breath
  - Kidneys: In supine position, place one hand under client between ribs and iliac crest, other hand on abdomen below ribs and pointing in the opposite direction; +/− tenderness or reproduction of symptoms
  - Bladder: Not usually palpable unless distended and raised above pubic bone; in supine position, place hand above pubis and press down; +/= tenderness, reproduction of pain, ability to feel the bladder: __+ ___−
- Observation
  - Scars may indicate adhesions or abdominal surgeries causative of diverticula
  - Pink or purplish striae may be indicative of Cushing syndrome
  - Dilated veins may indicate hepatic pathology or inferior vena cava obstruction, not diverticulitis
  - Contour: Roundness, concavity, asymmetry, distension, pregnancy signs
  - Cullen sign: Bluish discoloring around umbilicus may be a sign of retroperitoneal bleeding
  - Bluish discoloration in lower abdomen: Grey Turner sign, signals hemorrhagic pancreatitis
  - Bulging in groin/abdomen especially apparent with contraction of musculature in area may be hernia
  - Pulsing in navel area may be abdominal aortic aneurysm
  - Left lower quadrant pain, often following a meal
  - Palpable abdominal tenderness: On left side or generalized
  - Psoas sign: Provide resistance over patient's right knee during hip flexion; pain indicates appendicitis, possible inflammation of abdomen
  - Obturator sign: Internal rotation and flexion of right lower extremity (LE) may indicate appendicitis, pelvic inflammation
  - Rovsing sign: Pain on right side of abdomen when pressure applied to left may indicate appendicitis

INTERVENTION[6]

- PFM exercises/training
  - "Kegel" exercises: Another name for PFM exercises
  - Contraction
  - Relaxation/"Bulging"
  - Motor control
  - Endurance
  - Power
  - sEMG biofeedback
- Neuromuscular electrical stimulation to decrease urinary urgency and frequency and detrusor overactivity and to facilitate PFM and anal sphincter contraction
  - Anal or vaginal probe
  - Surface electrodes
    - Sacrum
    - Perineum
    - Suprapubic area
    - Tibial nerve
- TENS
- Pressure manometry
- Manual therapy
  - Myofascial treatment of the PFMs
  - Treatment of associated joints in the lumbar spine, pelvic girdle, and hip
- Thermal modalities
- US imaging to awareness of muscle contractions
- Posture reeducation
- Bladder retraining including timed voiding schedule and urge suppression technique
- Functional training
  - "Bulge" or "drop and open" the PFMs for relaxation
- Patient education regarding fluid intake and general dietary recommendations for fiber intake

FUNCTIONAL GOALS

- Patient will be able to
  - Verbalize strategies for independent pain management.
  - Demonstrate independence with home exercise program, promoting relaxation and awareness of PFM for long-term self-management.
  - Reduce urinary urgency and frequency symptoms from _____ to ______ voids per 24 hours.
  - Demonstrate independence with long-term PFM training program.
  - Achieve ≥600 m in a 6-minute walk test for initiation of safe, functional gait in community without need of bathroom.
  - Achieve functional aerobic capacity, gait, and tolerance for ADLs/IADLs.
  - Tolerate 30 minutes of continuous, moderate exercise three times per week in ______weeks, and five times/week in ____________weeks, depending on disease severity.

PROGNOSIS

- Longer duration and greater intensity of pain symptoms negatively impacts prognosis.
- Psychological factors such as pain catastrophizing and fear avoidance negatively impact prognosis.

PATIENT RESOURCE

- Chronic Prostatitis. http://www.chronicprostatits.com. Accessed July 30, 2013.

REFERENCES

1. The American Physical Therapy Association. Pattern 4C: Impaired muscle performance. In: *Guide to Physical Therapist Practice.* Alexandria, VA: The American Physical Therapy Association; 2003. http://guidetoptpractice.apta.org/content/1/SEC10.extract?sid=9af82a7e-5fc3-41d2-86ab-b8336a9655e9. Accessed April 20, 2013.
2. Fall M, Baranowski AP, Elneil S, et al. EAU guidelines on chronic pelvic pain. *Eur Urol.* 2010;57(1):35–48. [PMID 19733958]
3. Abrams P, Cardozo L, Fall M, et al. Lower urinary tract function: standardization of terminology. *Neurourol Urodyn.* 2002;21: 167–178.
4. Latthe P, Latthe M, Say L, Gulmezoglu M, Khan KS. WHO systematic review of prevalence of chronic pelvic pain: a neglected reproductive health morbidity. *BMC Public Health.* 2006;6:177, doi:10.1186/1471-2458/6/177 [pp. 1–7].
5. Nickel JC, Alexander RA, Anderson R, et al. NIH-CPCRN Study Groups. Category III Chronic Prostatitis/Chronic Pelvic Pain Syndrome: Insights from The National Institutes of Health Chronic Prostatitis Collaborative Research Network Studies *Curr Urol Rep.* 2008;9(4):320–327.
6. Wagenlehner F, Naber KG, Bschleipfer T, Brähler E, Weidner W. Prostatitis and Male Pelvic Pain Syndrome: Diagnosis and Treatment. *Dtsch Arztebl Int.* 2009;106(11):175–183.

ADDITIONAL REFERENCE

- "*Relieving Pain in America*" from The National Academies Press. http://www.nap.edu/catalog.php?record_id=13172. Accessed July 30, 2013.

271 MIXED URINARY INCONTINENCE

Stephanie Bush, DPT, MEd, WCS
Cynthia E. Neville, DPT, PT, WCS
Eric Shamus, PhD, DPT, PT, CSCS

CONDITION/DISORDER SYNONYMS

- Unspecified urinary incontinence (UUI)
- None

ICD-9-CM CODES

- 788.3 Urinary incontinence
- 788.30 Urinary incontinence, unspecified
- 788.31 Urge incontinence
- 788.33 Mixed urinary incontinence
- 788.39 Other urinary incontinence

ICD-10-CM CODES

- R32 Unspecified urinary incontinence
- N39.46 Mixed urinary incontinence
- N39.498 Other specified urinary incontinence

PREFERRED PRACTICE PATTERN

- 4C: Impaired Muscle Performance[1]

PATIENT PRESENTATION

A 50-year-old woman reports that she has occasionally leaked urine during coughing, sneezing, and jumping rope over the past 10 years. She thought it was "no big deal" and that it was "normal" after having children. She always wore a panty liner and so she never made her clothes wet. She would just change the liner. Lately, she experiences a sudden strong urge to urinate and cannot make it to the bathroom without leaking. When she leaks, the liner is soaked and sometimes wets her clothes. She has noticed a gradual increase in frequency and urgency of urination over the past few years. Now she wakes up 3 to 4 times per night to urinate. Sometimes in the middle of the night she cannot get to the bathroom and wets her pants.

KEY FEATURES

Description

- Involuntary loss of urine control accompanied by or immediately preceded by urgency combined with involuntary loss of urine control occurring during an increase in intra-abdominal pressure

Essentials of Diagnosis

- High detrusor pressure during leakage episode during urodynamic testing indicative of detrusor overactivity as well as urine leakage during increased intra-abdominal pressure

General Considerations

- Consideration of lower urinary tract infections (UTIs)
  - Sudden onset of symptoms
  - Urinary frequency
  - Urinary urgency
  - Lower back pain
- Myogenic dysfunction of the detrusor
- Urodynamic testing cannot be relied on to diagnose overactive bladder (OAB) but can be used to confirm the diagnosis[2]

Demographics

- Urinary incontinence (UI) affects 30% to 60% of middle-aged and older women.[3,4]
- UI reported by 78% of women with low back pain.[5]
- Severe UI is more prevalent in later years.
- 30% to 52% of homebound elderly suffer from UI.[6]

CLINICAL FINDINGS

SIGNS AND SYMPTOMS

- Combined symptoms of stress and urge UI
- More than seven voids per 24 hours
- Loss of urine without meaning to urinate
- Loss of a moderate-to-large amount of urine preceded by an urge to urinate, often associated with an irritant such as running water, walking by the bathroom, putting a key in a lock, or nervousness
- Increased alpha tone in prostatic and urethral smooth muscle
- Inflammation in the bladder
- Sensitivity to potassium
- Possible triggering of the micturition reflex
- Loss of urine without meaning to urinate during activities where there is an increase in intra-abdominal pressure (including sexual intercourse)
  - Coughing
  - Sneezing
  - Laughing
- Loss of a small amount of urine preceded by an increase in intra-abdominal pressure but without a sensation of urge to urinate

Functional Implications

- Increased risk for falls: 2- to 3.5-fold increase[7–9]
- Increased risk of falls during an inpatient episode of care[9]
- May lead to use of pads and/or wearing of diapers

Possible Contributing Causes

- Benign prostatic hypertrophy (BPH)
- Bladder cancer
- Bladder inflammation
- Bladder obstruction from enlarged prostate
- Bladder stones
- Comorbidities such as diabetes

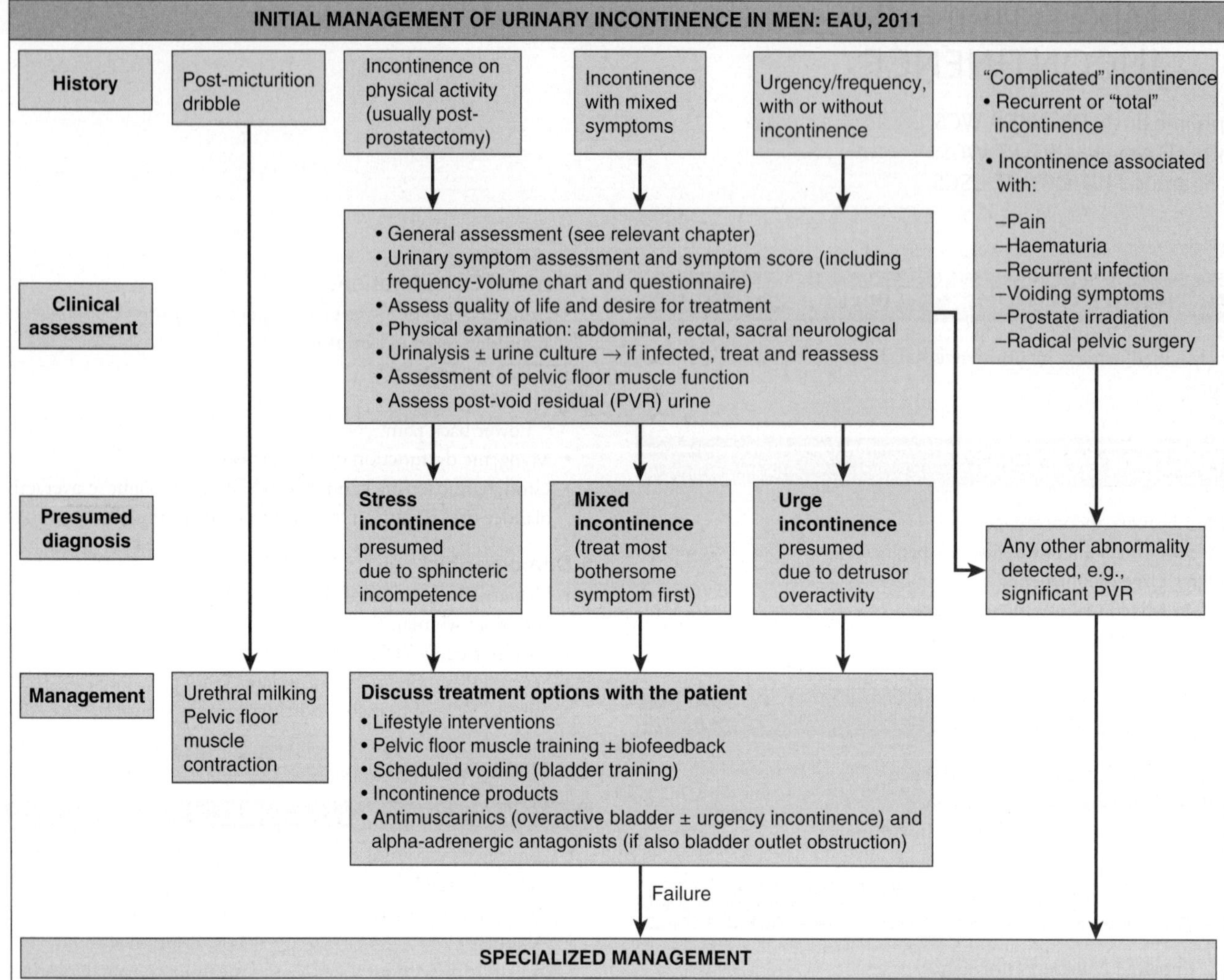

FIGURE 271-1 Initial management of urinary incontinence in men. (From Esherick JS, Clark DS, Slater ED. *Current Practice Guidelines in Primary Care*. 2012. www.accessmedicine.com.)

- Decrease in bladder capacity
- Increase in bladder sensation
- Increase of detrusor overactivity
- Intrinsic sphincter deficiency
- Multiple sclerosis (MS)
- Pelvic organ prolapse
- Reduction of maximal urethral closure pressure
- Spinal cord injury
- Underactive, overactive, or nonfunctioning pelvic floor muscles
- Urethral hypermobility
- UTIs: Bacterial

Differential Diagnosis

- UTI
- Interstitial cystitis
- Detrusor myopathy
- Neuropathy

MEANS OF CONFIRMATION OR DIAGNOSIS

Imaging

- Ultrasound imaging to identify abnormalities
  - Bladder
  - Urethra
  - Pelvis
  - Bladder neck position and mobility
  - Pelvic floor function
  - Activity of levator ani
  - Descent of pelvic organs
  - Sphincter integrity
- MRI to examine soft tissue structures of the pelvic support apparatus
- Pelvic/Abdominal ultrasound
  - Measure bladder capacity
  - Rule out other pathologies

Diagnostic Procedures

- Rule out UTI.
- Postvoid residual volume (PVR): Measures amount of urine left after urinating.
- Urinary stress test
  - Stand with a full bladder and cough.
  - Test does not have good reliability or validity.
  - Test is not specific enough to rule in/out a diagnosis.
  - Urodynamics: Functional study of the lower urinary tract

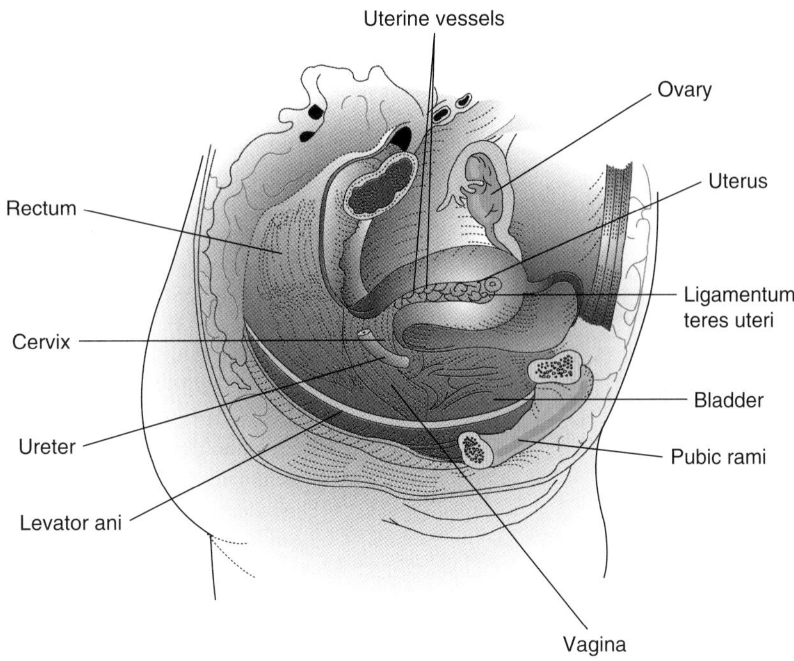

FIGURE 271-2 Pelvic viscera (sagittal view). (From DeCherney AH, Nathan L. *Current Diagnosis & Treatment: Obstetrics & Gynecology*. 10th ed. www.accessmedicine.com. Copyright © The McGraw-Hill Companies, Inc. All rights reserved.)

- Indications: Unclear cause of voiding dysfunction, incontinence unresponsive to conservative treatment, history of hysterectomy, bladder surgeries or pelvic organ prolapse procedures, neurological conditions.
- Assess sphincter competency.
- High detrusor pressure indicates an overactive bladder, detrusor overactivity, urge UI.

- Urethral pressure profile: Study of intraluminal pressure along the length of the urethra via pressure-sensitive catheter.
- Leak point pressure profile: Dynamic study of urethral pressure during activity.

FINDINGS AND INTERPRETATION

- High detrusor pressure during leakage episode during urodynamic testing indicative of detrusor overactivity, contributing to urge UI
- Leak during Valsalva maneuver or cough during urodynamic testing without elevation in detrusor pressure indicative of stress incontinence

TREATMENT

Medication

- Antibiotics if infection exists
- Medication for muscle spasms: Flavoxate
- Tricyclic antidepressants to effect smooth muscles of the bladder
- Medication to relax the bladder
  - Anticholinergics: Oxybutynin, tolterodine, darifenacin
- Estrogen to improve tone of urethral and vaginal tissues

MEDICAL PROCEDURES

- Vaginal sling procedures, tension-free vaginal tape.
  - Sling is placed that supports the urethra.
- Anterior vaginal repair or paravaginal repair procedures.
  - To repair support structures of the bladder.
  - Performed in women when the bladder is bulging into the vagina (called a cystocele).
  - Performed through a surgical cut in the vagina: A paravaginal repair is done through a surgical cut in the vagina or abdomen.
- Artificial urinary sphincter is a surgical device used to treat stress incontinence mainly in men (rarely in women).
- Collagen injections make the area around the urethra thicker, which helps control urine leakage.

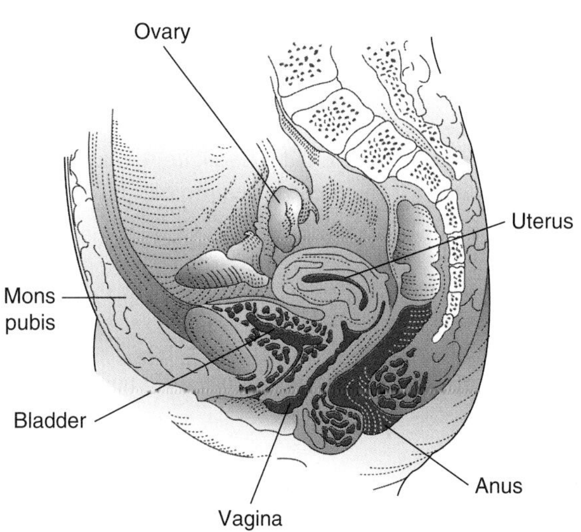

FIGURE 271-3 Pelvic organs (midsagittal view). (Reproduced with permission from, Benson RC. *Handbook of Obstetrics & Gynecology*. 8th ed. Los Altos, CA: Lange; 1983.)

- Male sling is a newer procedure that can be done in certain men.
- Easier to do than placing an artificial urinary sphincter.
- Retropubic suspensions are a group of surgical procedures done to lift the bladder and urethra, performed through a surgical cut in the abdomen.
- Augmentation cystoplasty.
- Performed to create a new bladder when the bladder is removed secondary to cancer or trauma.

REFERRALS/ADMITTANCE

- To primary care physicians
- To gynecologists
  - Women: Pelvic examination
- To urologists
  - Men: Genital examination
- To urogynecologists
- To acupuncture practitioners
- To pelvic floor physical therapist

IMPAIRMENTS

- Pelvic floor muscle dysfunction
  - Overactive
  - Underactive
  - Nonrelaxing
  - Noncontracting
- Incontinence
- Pelvic pain
- Pelvic organ prolapse
- Detrusor instability
- Decreased sexual appreciation
- Anorgasmia
  - Inability to achieve orgasm

TESTS AND MEASURES

- Pelvic floor muscle examination
- Bladder diary to assess patient's behaviors related to
  - Micturition including fluid and food intake
  - Voiding habits
  - Episodes of leakage (activity-related or urge-related)
  - Use of pads
- sEMG biofeedback assessment of the pelvic floor muscles
- Pressure manometry of the pelvic floor muscles
- Inquiry: During last 3 months did you leak urine when you had the urge or feeling that you needed to empty your bladder but could not get to the toilet fast enough?
- Pelvic floor muscle assessment
- Urinary stress test or "cough" test
  - Stand with a full bladder and cough.
  - Test does not have good reliability or validity.
  - Test is not specific enough to rule in/out a diagnosis.

INTERVENTION

- Pelvic floor muscle exercises/training
  - "Kegel" exercises: Another name for pelvic floor muscle exercises
  - Contraction
  - Relaxation/"Bulging"
  - Motor control
  - Endurance
  - Power
  - sEMG biofeedback
  - Weighted vaginal cones to strengthen pelvic floor
    - Hold weighted cone in vagina for up to 15 minutes, two times a day.
- Neuromuscular electrical stimulation to decrease urinary urgency and frequency and detrusor overactivity and to facilitate pelvic floor muscle contraction
  - Stress UI protocol
    - Frequency of 35 to 50 Hz, pulse width of 200 to 350 usec, asymmetrical biphasic wave form, duty cycle of 5 to 10 seconds on/5 to 10 seconds off
    - Match on time to patient's active home exercise program contraction time.
    - Patient may contract pelvic floor muscles while stimulation is on.
    - Duration of 10 to 20 minutes, frequency of treatment 1 to 2 times/day, every other day or daily.
  - Urge protocol: Frequency of 10 to 12 Hz, pulse width of 200 to 350 usec, asymmetrical biphasic wave form, duty cycle of 5 to 10 seconds on/5 to 10 seconds off, duration of 10 to 20 minutes, frequency of treatment 1 to 7 times/week
  - Anal or vaginal probe
  - Surface electrodes
    - Sacrum
    - Perineum
    - Suprapubic area
    - Tibial nerve
- Pressure manometry
- Manual therapy
- US imaging to facilitate pelvic floor muscle training
- Bladder retraining including timed voiding schedule and urge suppression technique
- Functional training: Precontract the pelvic floor muscles to close the urethra prior to anticipated increase in intra-abominal pressure; known as "The Knack"
- Patient education
  - Fluid management strategies
  - Drink enough water: A little bit of fluid throughout the day
  - Minimize consumption of bladder irritants
    - Caffeine
    - Spicy foods
    - Acidic foods including citrus

FUNCTIONAL GOALS

- Patient will be able to
  - Decrease number of episodes of urinary leakage to improve ability to participate in ADLs.
  - Decrease urinary frequency during the day to an average of 5 to 7 times.
  - Decrease total number of nighttime voids.
    - 0–1 per night for individuals <65 years.
    - 1–2 per night for individuals >65 years.
  - Restore average time interval between voiding (ability to store urine) to every 2–5 hours.
  - Reduce/eliminate leaking during increase in intra-abdominal pressure (cough, sneeze, laugh, transfer, intercourse, etc.).
  - Decrease number of episodes of urinary leakage to improve ability to participate in ADLs from ____ to _____.

- Decrease number of pads worn per day from ____ to _____.
- Independence with long-term pelvic floor muscle training program, as appropriate, to manage urinary symptoms.

PROGNOSIS

- Evidence from four randomized clinical trials (RCTs) showed that pelvic muscle training, combined with bladder training, effectively resolved UI in women.[10]
- In a cohort of women with urge incontinence, bladder training was more effective at reducing daytime frequency than use of imipramine.[11,12]
- Overall, electrical stimulation appears to have a 50% improvement/cure rate.[13]
- 83.3% report some improvement in UI symptoms with sacral surface transcutaneous electrical nerve stimulation (TENS).[14]
- A systematic review of eight clinical trials involving 370 women found that women who underwent pelvic floor muscle training for SUI were 17 times more likely to report cure or improvement compared to women who did not undergo supervised pelvic floor muscle training.[8]
- High cure rates for SUI were shown in single-blind RCT's in which women had individual instruction by a trained PT, combined with biofeedback or electrical stimulation, had close follow-up, and high adherence.[9]
- Evidence from four RCTs showed that pelvic muscle training, combined with bladder training, effectively resolved UI in women.[15]
- 45% cure rate for stress incontinence with electrical stimulation treatment: 60% of these patients had continued improvements for 3 to 11 months after treatment.[10,11]
- ICIQ-UI is an outcome measurement tool used to assess the prevalence and frequency of urinary leakage, its impact on everyday life, and the perceived cause of UI.[16]

PATIENT RESOURCE

- Urge Incontinence. MedlinePlus: National Institutes of Health website. http://www.nlm.nih.gov/medlineplus/ency/article/001270.htm. Accessed July 5, 2013.

REFERENCES

1. The American Physical Therapy Association. Pattern 4C: impaired muscle performance. In: *Guide to Physical Therapist Practice*. Alexandria, VA: The American Physical Therapy Association; 2003. http://guidetoptpractice.apta.org/content/1/SEC10.extract?sid=9af82a7e-5fc3-41d2-86ab-b8336a9655e9. Accessed July 3, 2013.
2. Laycock J, Haslam J. *Therapeutic Management of Incontinence and Pelvic Pain*. 2nd ed. London: Springer Publishers; 2008.
3. Herzog AR, Fultz NH. Prevalence and incidence of urinary incontinence in community-dwelling populations. *J Am Geriatr Soc*. 1990;38(3):273–281.
4. Messelink B, Benson T, Berghmans B, et al. Standardization of terminology of pelvic floor muscle function and dysfunction: report from the pelvic floor clinical assessment group of the International Continence Society. *Neurourol Urodyn*. 2005; 24(4):374–380.
5. Dutton M. Pathology, gynecology, and psychology. In: Dutton M, ed. *McGraw-Hill's NPTE (National Physical Therapy Examination)*. 2nd ed. New York, NY: McGraw-Hill; 2012. http://www.accessphysiotherapy.com/content/5402111. Accessed July 3, 2013.
6. Haylen BT, de Ridder D, Freeman RM, et al. An International Urogynecological Association (IUGA)/International Continence Society (ICS) joint report on the terminology for female pelvic floor dysfunction. *Neurourol Urodyn*. 2010;29(1):4–20.
7. Burgio, KL, Lochler JL, Goode PS, et al. Behavioral vs drug treatment for urge urinary incontinence in older women: a randomized controlled trial. *JAMA*. 1998;280(23):1995–2000.
8. Pils K, Neumann F, Meisner W, et al. Predictors of falls in elderly people during rehabilitation after hip fracture—who is at risk of a second one? *Z Gerontol Geriatr*. 2003;36(1):16–22.
9. Takazawa K, Arisawa K. Relationship between the type of urinary incontinence and falls among frail elderly women in Japan. *J Med Invest*. 2005;52(3-4):165–171.
10. Shamliyan TA, Kane RL, Wyman J, Wilt TJ. Systematic review: randomized, controlled trials of nonsurgical treatments for urinary incontinence in women. *Ann Intern Med*. 2008; 148(6):459–473.
11. Brubaker L. Electrical stimulation in overactive bladder. *Urology*. 2000;55(suppl 5A):17–23; discussion 31-2.
12. Landi F, Cesari M, Russo A, et al. Potentially reversible risk factors and urinary incontinence in frail older people living in community. *Age Ageing*. 2003;32(2):194–199.
13. Vecchioli-Scaldazza C, Morosetti C. Effect of aging on urinary incontinence in women. *Arch Ital Urol Androl*. 2010;82(3): 167–171.
14. Yokozuka M, Namima T, Nakagawa H, Ichie M, Handa Y. Effects and indications of sacral surface therapeutic electrical stimulation in refractory urinary incontinence. *Clin Rehabil*. 2004;18(8):899–907.
15. Avery K, Donovan J, Peters TJ, et al. ICIQ: a brief and robust measure for evaluating the symptoms and impact of urinary incontinence. *Neurourol Urodyn*. 2004;23(4):322–330.
16. Abrams P, Cardozo L, Fall M, et al. The standardisation of terminology of lower urinary tract function: report from the Standardisation Sub-committee of the International Continence Society. *Neurourol Urodyn*. 2002;21(2):167–178.

ADDITIONAL REFERENCES

- Abrams P, Cardoza LD, Khoury S, Wein A, eds. *Incontinence Management*. 3rd ed. Plymouth, UK: Health Publications Ltd; 2005.
- Brown JS, Bradley CS, Subak LL, et al. The sensitivity and specificity of a simple test to distinguish between urge and stress urinary incontinence. *Ann Intern Med*. 2006;144(10):715–723.
- Brubaker L, Benson T, Bent A, Clark A, Shott S. Transvaginal electrical stimulation for female urinary incontinence. *Am J Obstet Gynecol*. 1997;177(3):536–540.
- Chiarelli PE, Mackenzie LA, Osmotherly PG. Urinary incontinence is associated with an increase in falls: a systematic review. *Aust J Physiother*. 2009;55(2):89–95.
- Deng DY. Urinary incontinence in women. *Med Clin North Am*. 2011;95(1):101–109.
- Dumoulin C, Bourbonnais D, Morin M, Gravel D, Lemieux MC. Predictors of success for physiotherapy treatment in women with persistent postpartum stress urinary incontinence. *Arch Phys Med Rehabil*. 2010;91:1059–1063.

- Eliasson K, Elfving B, Nordgren B, Mattsson E. Urinary incontinence in women with low back pain. *Man Ther.* 2008;13(3):206–212.
- Godec CJ, Fravel R, Cass AS. Optimal parameters of electrical stimulation in the treatment of urinary incontinence. *Invest Urol.* 1981;18(4):239–241.
- Hunskaar S, Arnold EP, Burgio K, et al. Epidemiology and natural history of urinary incontinence. *Int Urgynecol J Pelvic Floor Dysfunct.* 2000;11(5):301–319.
- Larsson G, Victor A. The frequency/volume chart in genuine stress incontinent women. *Neurourol Urodyn.* 1992;11(1):23–31. http://onlinelibrary.wiley.com/doi/10.1002/nau.1930110103/abstract. Accessed July 5, 2013.
- Lopez R, Smith PC, Therine A. Clinical inquiries. What are the indications for urodynamic testing in older adults with incontinence? *J Fam Pract.* 2002;51(12):1077.
- Minassian VA, Drutz HP, Al-Badr A. Urinary incontinence as a worldwide problem. *Int J Gynaecol Obstet.* 2003;82(3):327–338.
- Neville C. Pelvic floor treatment: urinary incontinence and pelvic floor muscle training [Video]. New York, NY: McGraw-Hill; 2014. http://www.accessphysiotherapy.com. Accessed June 13, 2014.
- Ohlsson BL. Effects of some different pulse parameters on the perception of intravaginal and intra-anal electrical stimulation. *Med Biol Eng Comput.* 1988;26(5):503–508.
- Panus PC, Jobst EE, Masters SB, Katzung B, Tinsley SL, Trevor AJ. Sympathomimetrics and sympatholytics. In: Panus PC, Jobst EE, Masters SB, Katzung B, Tinsley SL, Trevor AJ, eds. *Pharmacology for the Physical Therapist.* New York, NY: McGraw-Hill; 2009. http://www.accessphysiotherapy.com/content/6090704. Accessed July 3, 2013.
- Yamanashi T, Yasuda K, Sakakibara R, Hattori T, Ito H, Muraakami S. Pelvic floor electrical stimulation in the treatment of stress incontinence: an investigational study and placebo controlled double-blind trial. *J Urol.* 1997;158(6):2127–2131.

272 NEUROLOGIC URINARY INCONTINENCE

Cynthia E. Neville, DPT, PT, WCS

CONDITION/DISORDER SYNONYMS

- Detrusor sphincter dyssynergia (DSD)
- Neurogenic detrusor overactivity (NDO)
- Neurogenic dysfunctional voiding
- Neurogenic lower urinary tract dysfunction (NLUTD)

ICD-9-CM CODES

- 344.61 Cauda equine syndrome with neurogenic bladder
- 596.4 Atony of bladder
- 596.5 Other functional disorder of the bladder
- 596.54 Neurogenic bladder NOS
- 596.55 Detrusor sphincter dyssynergia
- 788.3 Urinary incontinence
- 788.30 Urinary incontinence, unspecified
- 788.31 Urge incontinence
- 788.39 Other urinary incontinence

ICD-10-CM CODES

- N31.2 Flaccid neuropathic bladder, not elsewhere classified
- N31.8 Other neuromuscular dysfunction of bladder
- N31.9 Neuromuscular dysfunction of bladder, unspecified
- N36.44 Muscular disorders of urethra
- N39.41 Urge incontinence
- N39.498 Other specified urinary incontinence
- R32 Unspecified urinary incontinence

PREFERRED PRACTICE PATTERNS[1]

- 5D: Impaired Motor Function and Sensory Integrity Associated with Nonprogressive Disorders of the Central Nervous System—acquired in adolescence or adulthood
- 5E Impaired Motor Function and Sensory Integrity Associated with Progressive Disorders of the Central Nervous System
- 5F: Impaired Peripheral Nerve Integrity and Muscle Performance Associated with Peripheral Nerve Injury
- 5G: Impaired Motor Function and Sensory Integrity Associated with Acute or Chronic Polyneuropathies
- 5H: Impaired Motor Function, Peripheral Nerve Integrity, and Sensory Integrity Associated with Nonprogressive Disorders of the Spinal Cord

PATIENT PRESENTATION

A 30-year-old woman with multiple sclerosis (MS) reports having a urinary tract infection (UTI). She also states new onset of bladders symptoms including hesitancy, interrupted urine flow, and failure to empty completely. Urodynamic testing by her urologist reveals simultaneous contraction of the external urinary sphincter (EUS) and the detrusor muscle. Postvoid residual volume is 150 cc. She is scheduled for a 2 week trial of InterStim.

KEY FEATURES

Description

- Involuntary loss of urine control in the presence of a known neurologic condition
- NLUTD may be due to dysfunction of the detrusor (bladder smooth muscle), dysfunction of the EUS, or a combination of both.
- Clinical manifestation encompasses a wide range of symptoms

Essentials of Diagnosis

- Urodynamic testing is valuable in making diagnosis
- NDO
  - High detrusor pressure during leakage episode during urodynamic testing is indicative of detrusor over activity
- DSD
  - Simultaneous contraction of the EUS and detrusor during an attempt to void

General Considerations

- Typical neurological patterns[2]
  - Higher lesions typically lead to a more reflexic LUT.
  - Lower lesions lead to a more areflexic LUT.
    - Lesions between T10 and L2 can be either reflexic or areflexic.
- Severe neurological or non-neurological dysfunctional voiding puts ureteral and renal function at risk.
- Other common urogynecologic conditions, such as pelvic organ prolapse, may also cause bladder symptoms.
- Rule out lower UTIs.
  - Sudden onset of symptoms.
  - Urinary frequency.
  - Urinary urgency.
  - Lower back pain.
- Rule out myogenic dysfunction of the detrusor.

Demographics

- CVA: 28% to 79% after stroke[3]
- Parkinson's: Voiding dysfunction occurs in 35% to 70% of patients.[4]
- Multiple system atrophy (MSA): 73% complain of urinary incontinence (UI).
- MS: 95% of patient with disease over 10 years report urinary complaints[5].
- Prevalence of neurogenic overactive bladder disorders in a US claims database[6]: n = 46, 271 patients.
  - 26.3% had neurogenic bladder not otherwise specified.
  - 17.2% had MS diagnosis.
  - 14.9% had Parkinson disease.

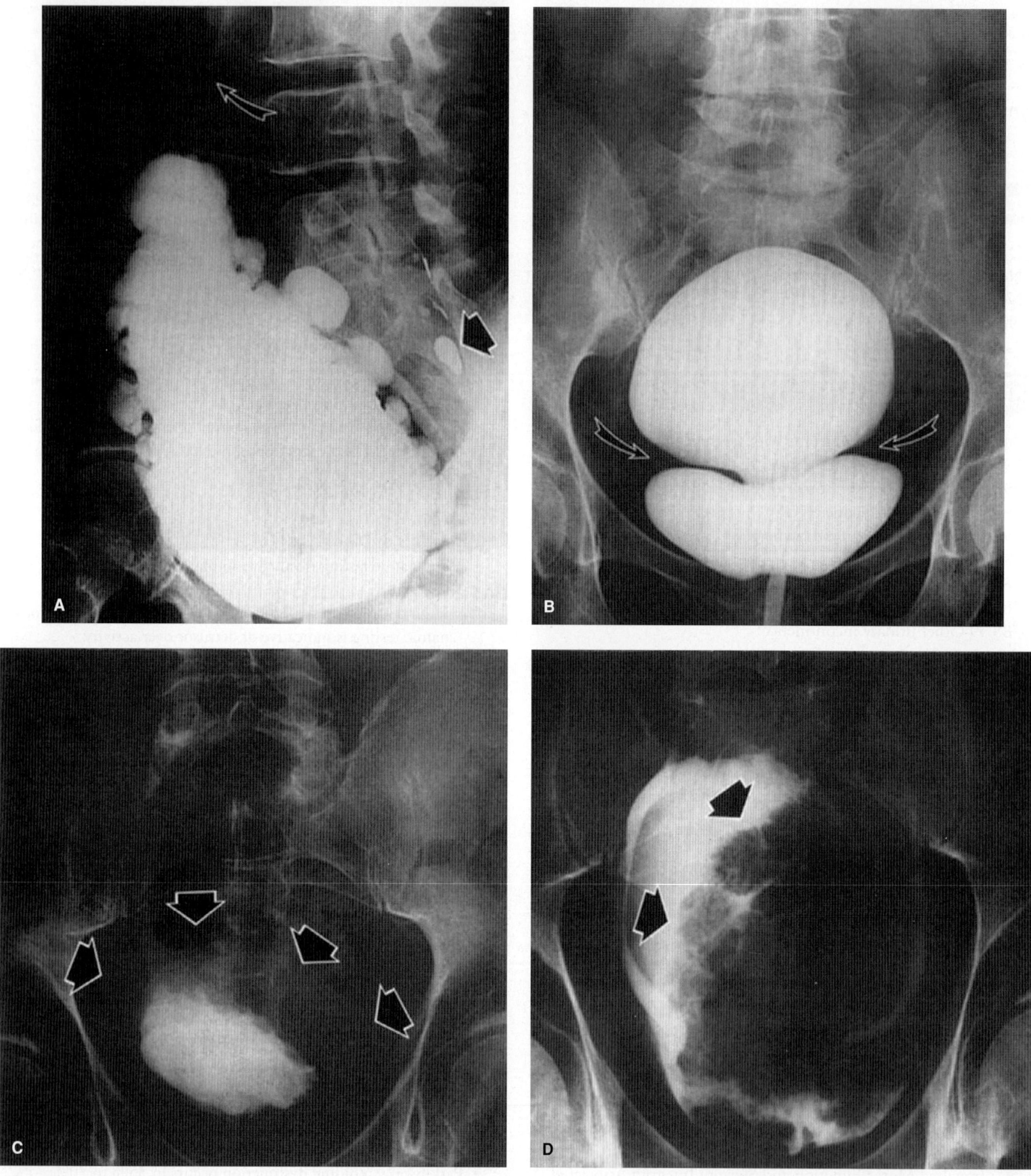

FIGURE 272-1 Abnormal cystograms: retrograde cystograms or "cystograms" as part of excretory urogram studies. (**A**) Neurogenic bladder. This neurogenic bladder has a "Christmas-tree" shape, with gross trabeculation and many diverticula. Residual myelographic contrast medium in spinal canal (*straight arrow*). Right vesicoureteral reflux (*curved arrow*) in a 70-year-old man with urinary incontinence. (**B**) Congenital "hourglass" bladder. Transverse concentric muscular band (*arrows*) separates upper and lower bladder segments, both of which contracted and emptied simultaneously and completely with voiding in a 66-year-old woman with urinary stress incontinence. (**C**) Hodgkin disease of bladder. Global thickening of the bladder wall (*arrows*), more apparent on the left in a 54-year-old man with generalized Hodgkin disease. (**D**) Papillary transitional cell bladder carcinoma. Huge (12 cm) cauliflower-like bladder mass (*arrows*) filling almost the entire bladder. "Cystogram" film of an excretory urogram in a 40-year-old man with recurrent bladder tumor. (From Tanagho EA, McAninch WJ. *Smith's General Urology*. 17th ed. www.accessmedicine.com.)

- 8.9% had cauda equina syndrome.
- 7.8% had paralytic syndrome (quadriplegia, monoplegia; lower extremity).
- 10.6% had stroke.
- 4.3% had spinal cord injury.
- 3% had spina bifida.
- 2.1% had other paralytic syndrome.
- 2% had cerebral palsy diagnosis.
- 1.8% had hemiplagia and hemiparesis.
- 1% had spinal cord neoplasm.
- 0.3% had paralysis of bladder.
- 0.1% had MS plus SCI diagnosis.

CLINICAL FINDINGS

SIGNS AND SYMPTOMS

- Loss of urine without meaning to urinate
- Urinary urgency, frequency, and nocturia
- Slow urine stream
- Small voided volumes
- 60% of patients with NDO also have impaired detrusor contractility resulting in incomplete emptying[7]
- Urinary retention with elevated postvoid residual
- Obstructed voiding: Hesitancy, interrupted urine flow, failure to empty completely
- Elevated intravesical (bladder) pressures: Pressure-driven upper urinary tract damage
- If DSD is left untreated, the resulting high storage pressure can cause
  - Vesicoureteral reflux[7]
  - Hydronephrosis[7]
  - Urolithiasis[7]
  - Urosepsis[7]

Functional Implications/Complications

- Increased risk of UTI[8]
- Increased risk of pressure ulcers[9]
- Urinary urgency, frequency, and incontinence associated with rushing to the bathroom and increased fall risk[10]

Possible Contributing Causes

- Underactive, overactive, or nonfunctioning pelvic floor muscles
- Pelvic organ prolapse
- Urethral hypermobility
- Intrinsic sphincter deficiency
- Bladder cancer
- Bladder inflammation
- Bladder stones
- Spinal cord injury
- MS
- Bladder obstruction from enlarged prostate
- Benign prostatic hypertrophy (BPH)
- Comorbidities such as diabetes
- UTIs: Bacterial
- Increase in bladder sensation
- Decrease in bladder capacity
- Increase of detrusor overactivity
- Reduction of maximal urethral closure pressure

Differential Diagnosis

- UTI
- Detrusor myopathy

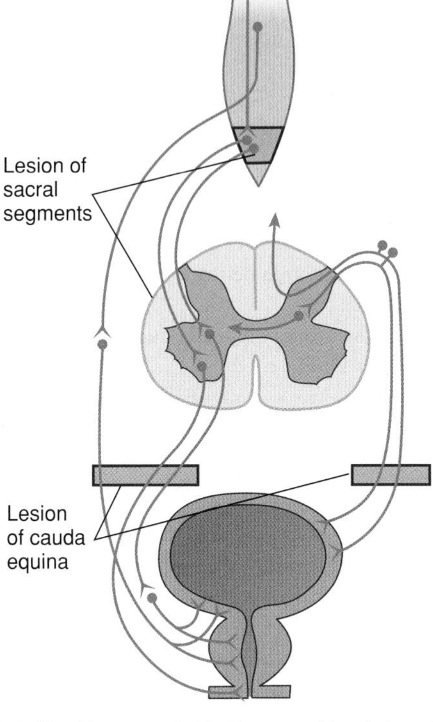

FIGURE 272-2 Flaccid neurogenic bladder, caused by a lesion of either the sacral portion of the spinal cord or the cauda equina. (From Waxman SG. *Clinical Neuroanatomy*. 26th ed. http://www.accessmedicine.com. Copyright © The McGraw-Hill Companies, Inc. All rights reserved.)

MEANS OF CONFIRMATION OR DIAGNOSIS

Imaging

- Ultrasound imaging to identify abnormalities
  - Bladder
  - Urethra
  - Pelvis
  - Bladder neck position and mobility
  - Pelvic floor function
  - Activity of levator ani
  - Descent of pelvic organs
  - Sphincter integrity
- MRI to examine soft tissue structures of the pelvic support apparatus
- Pelvic/Abdominal ultrasound
  - Measure bladder capacity
  - Rule out other pathologies

Diagnostic Procedures

- Rule out UTI.
- Postvoid residual volume (PVR): Measures amount of urine left after urinating.
- Urodynamics: Functional study of the lower urinary tract
  - Indications include: Unclear cause of voiding dysfunction, incontinence unresponsive to conservative treatment, history of hysterectomy, bladder surgeries or pelvic organ prolapse procedures, neurological conditions.
  - Assess sphincter competency.
  - High detrusor pressure indicates an overactive bladder, detrusor overactivity, urge UI.

- Urethral pressure profile: Study of intraluminal pressure along the length of the urethra via pressure sensitive catheter.
- Leak point pressure profile: Dynamic study of urethral pressure during activity.

FINDINGS AND INTERPRETATION

- High detrusor pressure during leakage episode during urodynamic testing indicative of detrusor overactivity, contributing to urge UI
- Leak during Valsalva maneuver or cough during urodynamic testing without elevation in detrusor pressure is indicative of stress incontinence
- Contraction of the urinary sphincter during increase in detrusor pressure indicates DSD

TREATMENT

Medication

- Antibiotics if infection exists
- Medication for muscle spasms: Flavoxate
- Tricyclic antidepressants to affect smooth muscles of the bladder
- Medication to relax the bladder
  - Anticholinergics: Oxybutynin, tolterodine, darifenacin
- Estrogen to improve tone of urethral and vaginal tissues

MEDICAL PROCEDURES

- Botulism toxin injections[11]
- Implanted electrical stimulator for neuromodulation (InterStim)[12]
- Clean intermittent catheterization
  - Augmentation cystoplasty: Performed to create a new bladder when the bladder is removed secondary to cancer or trauma

REFERRALS/ADMITTANCE

- To pelvic floor physical therapist
- To physical medicine and rehabilitation physician
- To primary care physician
- To neurologist
- To gynecologist
  - Women: Pelvic examination
- To urologist
  - Men: Genital examination
- To urogynecologist
- To acupuncture

IMPAIRMENTS

- Pelvic floor muscle dysfunction
  - Overactive
  - Underactive
  - Nonrelaxing
  - Noncontracting
- Incontinence
- Pelvic pain
- Pelvic organ prolapse
- Detrusor instability
- Decreased sexual appreciation
- Anorgasmia
  - Inability to achieve orgasm
  - Erectile dysfunction

TESTS AND MEASURES

- Pelvic floor muscle examination
- Bladder diary to assess patient's behaviors related to
  - Micturition including fluid and food intake
  - Voiding habits
  - Episodes of leakage (activity-related or urge-related)
  - Use of pads
- sEMG biofeedback assessment of the pelvic floor muscles
- Pressure manometry of the pelvic floor muscles

INTERVENTION

- Bladder retraining including timed voiding schedule and urge suppression technique.
- Neuromuscular electrical stimulation to decrease urinary urgency and frequency and detrusor overactivity and to facilitate pelvic floor muscle contraction.
  - Stress UI protocol
    - Frequency of 35 to 50 Hz, pulse width of 200 to 350 usec, asymmetrical biphasic wave form, duty cycle of 5 to 10 seconds on/5 to 10 seconds off.
    - Match on time to patients active home exercise program contraction time.
    - Patient may contract pelvic floor muscles while stimulation is on.
    - Duration of 10 to 20 minutes, frequency of treatment 1 to 2 times/day, every other day or daily.
  - Urge protocol: Frequency of 10 to 12 Hz, pulse width of 200 to 350 usec, asymmetrical biphasic wave form, duty cycle of 5 to 10 seconds on/5 to 10 seconds off, duration of 10 to 20 minutes, frequency of treatment 1 to 7 times/week.
  - Anal or vaginal probe
  - Surface electrodes
    - Sacrum
    - Perineum
    - Suprapubic area
    - Tibial nerve
- Pelvic floor muscle exercises/training
  - "Kegel" exercises: Another name for pelvic floor muscle exercises
  - Contraction
  - Relaxation/"bulging"
  - Motor control
  - Endurance
  - Power
  - sEMG biofeedback
  - Weighted vaginal cones to strengthen pelvic floor
    - Hold weighted cone in vagina for up to 15 minutes, two times a day.
- Pressure manometry
- Manual therapy
- US imaging to facilitate pelvic floor muscle training.
- Functional training: Precontract the pelvic floor muscles to close the urethra prior to anticipated increase in intra-abominal pressure; known as "The Knack."
- Patient education
  - Fluid management strategies.
    - Drink enough water: A little bit of fluid throughout the day.
    - Minimize consumption of bladder irritants.
      - Caffeine
      - Spicy foods
      - Acidic foods including citrus

FUNCTIONAL GOALS

- Patient will be able to
  - Decrease number of episodes of urinary leakage to improve ability to participate in ADLs.
  - Decrease urinary frequency during the day to an average of five to seven times.
  - Decrease total number of nighttime voids.
    - 0 to 1 per night for individuals under 65 years.
    - 1 to 2 per night for individuals over 65 years.
  - Restore average time interval between voiding (ability to store urine) to every 2 to 5 hours.
  - Reduce/eliminate leaking during increase in intra-abdominal pressure (cough, sneeze, laugh, transfer, intercourse, etc.).
  - Decrease number of episodes of urinary leakage to improve ability to participate in ADLs from ____ to _____.
  - Decrease number of pads worn per day from ____ to _____.
  - Independence with long-term pelvic floor muscle training program, as appropriate, to manage urinary symptoms.

PROGNOSIS

- Rehabilitation based interventions, including biofeedback, pelvic floor muscle exercise training, and electrical stimulation, result in better outcomes for stroke patients with UI.[13]
- Incontinent individuals with underlying neurologic conditions also typically report worse health related quality of life (HRQoL) compared with their continent counterparts and the general population.[14]
  - UI in individuals with MS, SCI, Parkinson disease, and stroke has a substantial negative impact on patients' HRQoL.
  - Physical, mental and psychological impairments were consistently observed, with patients reporting detriments in physical function, emotional well being, and social relationships.
  - UI also had a negative effect on the sexual lives of patients with neurologic conditions, and may adversely affect long-term outcomes.

PATIENT RESOURCE

- Guidelines on neurogenic lower urinary tract dysfunction. National Guideline Clearing House. http://www.guideline.gov/content.aspx?id=34062. Accessed July 6, 2013.

REFERENCES

1. The American Physical Therapy Association. Pattern 4C: impaired muscle performance. In: *Guide to Physical Therapist Practice*. Alexandria, VA: The American Physical Therapy Association; 2003. http://guidetoptpractice.apta.org/content/1/SEC10.extract?sid=9af82a7e-5fc3-41d2-86ab-b8336a9655e9. Accessed July 7, 2013.
2. Abrams P, Cardoza L, Khoury S, Wein A. *Incontinence: 3rd International Consultation on Incontinence*. Vols 1 & 2. Plymouth, UK: Health Publication Ltd; 2005.
3. McKenzie P, Badlani GH. The incidence and etiology of overactive bladder in patients after cerebrovascular accident. *Curr Urol Rep*. 2012;13(5):402–406. doi: 10.1007/s11934-012-0269-6.
4. Wein AJ. Neuromuscular dysfunction of the lower urinary tract and its management. In: Walsh PC, Retik AB, Vaughan ED, Wein AJ, eds. *Campbell's Urology*. Philadelphia, PA: WB Saunders; 2002:931–1026.
5. Haensch CA, Jörg J. Autonomic dysfunction in multiple sclerosis. *J Neurol*. 2006;253(Suppl 1):I3–I9.
6. Manack A, Motsko SP, Jones JK, Ravelo A, Haag-Molkenteller C, Dmochowskl. Epidemilogy of neurogeneic bladder patients in a US claims database. *American Urology Association Conference*. 2009. http://www.deggegroup.com/2009-AUA%20-%20Epi%20of%20NOAB%2056478.pdf. Accessed July 7, 2013.
7. Weber LeBrun EEW, Adelowo A, Young SB. Neurogenic bladder. *J Pelvic Med Surg*. 2009;15:123–137.
8. Edokpolo LU, Stavris KB, Foster HE. Intermittent Catheterization and Recurrent Urinary Tract Infection in Spinal Cord Injury. *Top Spinal Cord Inj Rehabil*. 2012;18(2):187–192.
9. Doughty D, Junkin J, Kurz P, et al. Incontinence-associated dermatitis: consensus statements, evidence-based guidelines for prevention and treatment, and current challenges. *J Wound Ostomy Continence Nurs*. 2012;39(3):303–315; quiz 316-7. doi: 10.1097/WON.0b013e3182549118.
10. Chiarelli PE, Mackenzie LA, Osmotherly PG. Urinary incontinence is associated with an increase in falls: a systematic review. *Aust J Physiother*. 2009;55(2):89–95.
11. Wein AJ. Re: Interstim sacral neuromodulation and botox botulinum-a toxin intradetrusor injections for refractory urge urinary incontinence: a decision analysis comparing outcomes including efficacy and complications. *J Urol*. 2012;188(1):223. doi: 10.1016/j.juro.2012.03.066.
12. Medtronic InterStim Therapy System P080025. http://www.fda.gov/MedicalDevices/ProductsandMedicalProcedures/DeviceApprovalsandClearances/Recently-ApprovedDevices/ucm249208.htm. Accessed July 7, 2013.
13. Thomas LH, Cross S, Barrett J, et al. Treatment of urinary incontinence after stroke in adults. *Cochrane Database of Systematic Reviews*. 2008;(1):CD004462.
14. Tapia CI, Khalaf K, Berenson K, Globe D, Chancellor M, Carr LK. Health-related quality of life and economic impact of urinary incontinence due to detrusor overactivity associated with a neurologic condition: a systematic review. *Health Qual Life Outcomes*. 2013;11(1):13. doi: 10.1186/1477-7525-11-13.

ADDITIONAL REFERENCE

- Neville C. Pelvic floor treatment: urinary incontinence and pelvic floor muscle training [Video]. New York, NY: McGraw-Hill; 2014. http://www.accessphysiotherapy.com. Accessed June 13, 2014.

273 PEDIATRIC URINARY INCONTINENCE

Cynthia E. Neville, DPT, PT, WCS

CONDITION/DISORDER SYNONYMS

- Urinary incontinence
  - Enuresis
  - Urge urinary incontinence
  - Overactive bladder
  - Giggle incontinence
  - Nocturnal enuresis
- Dysfunctional voiding, dysfunctional elimination syndrome

ICD-9-CM CODES

- 596.5 Other functional disorder of the bladder
- 788.3 Urinary incontinence
- 788.31 Urge incontinence
- 788.32 Incontinence without sensory awareness
- 788.36 Nocturnal enuresis
- 788.39 Other urinary incontinence

ICD-10-CM CODES

- N33 Bladder disorders in diseases classified elsewhere
- N39.41 Urge urinary incontinence
- N39.42 Incontinence without sensory awareness
- N39.44 Nocturnal enuresis
- N39.498 Other specified urinary incontinence
- R32 Unspecified urinary incontinence

PREFERRED PRACTICE PATTERNS[1]

- 4C Impaired Muscle Performance[1]
- 5C Impaired Motor Function and Sensory Integrity Associated with Nonprogressive Disorders of the Central Nervous System—congenital origin or acquired in infancy or childhood

PATIENT PRESENTATION

A 9-year-old girl who is undergoing physical therapy treatment for gait training and strengthening after hospitalization for meningitis frequently interrupts therapy sessions with urgent requests to go to the bathroom, and then stays in the bathroom for 10 minutes or more. Her school teacher recently reported to her mother this same behavior at school.

KEY FEATURES

Description

- Involuntary loss of urine control during the daytime in a child older than 5 years (or mental age of 5) and/or during the nighttime in a child older than 6[2]
- Involuntary loss of urine control accompanied by or immediately preceded by urgency
- Complete voiding during or immediately after laughing[3]
- Inability to relax the external sphincter during voiding in children with no evidence of neurologic abnormality[4]

Essentials of Diagnosis

- Voiding record observed and recorded by an adult.
- Urodynamic testing
  - Detrusor (smooth muscle of the bladder) overactivity: High detrusor pressure during leakage episode during urodynamic testing is indicative of detrusor overactivity.
  - Detrusor sphincter dyssynergia (DSD): Simultaneous contraction of the external urinary sphincter and detrusor during an attempt to void.

General Considerations

- The fully toilet-trained child has the ability to stop and start the flow of urine, initiate voiding by relaxing external urethral sphincter, and cortically inhibit a bladder contraction.[5]
- Rule out lower urinary tract infections (UTIs).
  - Sudden onset of symptoms
  - Urinary frequency
  - Urinary urgency
  - Lower back pain
- Rule out myogenic dysfunction of the detrusor.

Demographics

- 21.8% of school aged children had lower urinary tract dysfunction.
- Symptoms were most frequent in girls ($p < 0.001$), children aged 6 to 8 years ($p < 0.028$), and attended the school with the lowest social level ($p < 0.001$).
- 30.7% had diurnal urinary incontinence.
  - 19.1% had holding maneuvers; strategies to postpone voiding
  - 13.7% had urinary urgency.[6]
- Enuresis: At age 5, 15% to 25% of children wet the bed.
  - With each year of maturity, the percentage of bed-wetters declines by 15%: 8% of 12-year-old boys and 4% of 12-year-old girls are enuretic, only 1% to 3 % of adolescents are still wetting their bed.[7]

CLINICAL FINDINGS

SIGNS AND SYMPTOMS[8]

- Bed wetting
- Hesitancy: Slow initiation of void after age 5
- Holding maneuvers: Strategies to postpone voiding, after age 5
- Intermittency: Bursts of urine during voiding, physiological up to age 3 if no straining, after 3 is always considered dysfunctional
- Loss of urine without meaning to urinate
- Nocturia: Nighttime voids after age 5, normal = 0
- Straining: Abdominal pressure during void
- Urgency: Sudden unexpected need to urinate, after age 5
- Weak stream: Decreased force of flow

Functional Implications/Complications[9]

- Increased risk of UTI
- Vesicoureteral reflux (VUR): Abnormal flow of urine backward from the bladder to the ureter

Possible Contributing Causes

- Developmental delay
- Underactive, overactive, or nonfunctioning pelvic floor muscles
- Comorbidities such as diabetes
- UTIs: Bacterial
- Detrusor overactivity

Differential Diagnosis

- UTI
- Dysfunctional voiding
- Detrusor myopathy

MEANS OF CONFIRMATION OR DIAGNOSIS

Imaging

- Ultrasound imaging of anatomy
  - Bladder
  - Urethra
  - Pelvis
  - Bladder neck position and mobility
  - Pelvic floor function
- MRI to examine soft tissue structures of the pelvis
- Pelvic/abdominal ultrasound
  - Measure bladder capacity
  - Rule out other pathologies
- Video cystourethrogram (VCUG): Urodynamics with X-ray imaging, usually not done in children under 8 to 10 years of age (may be performed in 3 to 7 year olds with sedation)

Diagnostic Procedures

- Urinalysis to rule out UTI
- Postvoid residual volume (PVR): Measures amount of urine left after urinating
- Urodynamics: Functional study of the lower urinary tract
- Sleep study
- Glucose testing for diabetes

FINDINGS AND INTERPRETATION

- High detrusor pressure during leakage episode during urodynamic testing indicative of detrusor overactivity, contributing to urge urinary incontinence

TREATMENT

Medication

- Antibiotics if infection exists
- Medication for muscle spasms: Flavoxate
- Tricyclic antidepressants to affect smooth muscles of the bladder
- Medication to relax the bladder
  - Anticholinergics
    - Oxybutynin
    - Tolterodine
    - Darifenacin

MEDICAL PROCEDURE

- None

REFERRALS/ADMITTANCE

- To pelvic floor physical therapist
- To primary care physicians
- To pediatricians
- To neurologist
- To urologists
- To acupuncture practitioner

IMPAIRMENTS

- Pelvic floor muscle dysfunction
  - Overactive
  - Underactive
  - Nonrelaxing
  - Noncontracting
- Incontinence
- Detrusor instability

TESTS AND MEASURES

- External palpation examination of pelvic floor muscle contraction
- Bladder diary completed by caregiver to assess patient's behaviors related to
  - Micturition including fluid and food intake
  - Voiding habits
  - Episodes of leakage (activity-related or urge-related)
  - Use of pads
- sEMG biofeedback assessment of the pelvic floor and abdominal muscles

INTERVENTION

- Bladder retraining including timed voiding schedule and urge suppression technique
- Neuromuscular electrical stimulation to decrease urinary urgency and frequency and detrusor overactivity
  - 10 to 12 Hz frequency, pulse width of 200 to 350 μsec, asymmetrical biphasic wave form, duty cycle of 5 to 10 seconds on/5 to 10 seconds off, duration of 10 to 20 minutes, frequency of treatment 1 to 7 times/week
  - Surface electrodes
    - Sacrum
    - Tibial nerve
- Pelvic floor muscle exercises/training
  - "Kegel" exercises: Another name for pelvic floor muscle exercises
  - Contraction
  - Relaxation/"bulging"
  - Motor control
  - Endurance
  - Power
  - sEMG biofeedback
- US imaging to facilitate pelvic floor muscle training
- Diaphragmatic breathing
- Patient education
  - Fluid management strategies
  - Toilet posture
- Behavioral strategies for nocturnal enuresis, for example, wet alarm

FUNCTIONAL GOALS

- Patient will be able to
  - Decrease number of episodes of urinary leakage to improve ability to participate in school (or therapy sessions).
  - Decrease urinary frequency during the day to an average of 5 to 7 times.
  - Eliminate bed wetting.
  - Restore average time interval between voiding (ability to store urine) to every 2 to 5 hours.
  - Decrease number of episodes of urinary leakage to improve ability to participate in school from ____ to _____.

PROGNOSIS

- With motivated parent/caregiver and patient, rehabilitation-based interventions, including biofeedback, pelvic floor muscle exercise training, and diaphragmatic breathing, and patient/family education result in significant improvement in dysfunctional voiding symptoms including decreased episodes of incontinence and enuresis.[4]

PATIENT RESOURCE

- International Children's Continence Society. www.i-c-c-s.org. Accessed July 7, 2013.

REFERENCES

1. The American Physical Therapy Association. Pattern 4C: impaired muscle performance. In: *Guide to Physical Therapist Practice*. Alexandria, VA: The American Physical Therapy Association; 2003. http://guidetoptpractice.apta.org/content/1/SEC10.extract?sid=9af82a7e-5fc3-41d2-86ab-b8336a9655e9. Accessed July 7, 2013.
2. Mikkelson EJ. Enuresis and encopresis: ten years of progress. *J Am Acad Child Adolesc Psychiatry*. 2001;40(10):1146–1158.
3. Chandra M, Saharia R, Shi Q, Hill V. Goggle incontinence in children: a manifestation of detrusor instability. *J Urol.* 2002;168(5):2184–2187.
4. Desantis DJ, Leonard MP, Preston MA, Barrowman NJ, Guerra LA. Effectiveness of biofeedback for dysfunctional elimination syndrome in pediatrics: a systematic review. *J Pediatr Urol.* 2011;7(3):342–348. doi: 10.1016/j.jpurol.2011.02.019.
5. Berry A. A child with daytime wetting: three case studies. *Urol Nurs*. 2005;25(3):202–205.
6. Vaz GT, Vasconcelos MM, Oliveira EA, et al. Prevalence of lower urinary tract symptoms in school-age children. *Pediatr Nephrol.* 2012;27(4):597–603.
7. Wan J, Greenfield S. Enuresis and common voiding abnormalities. *Pediatr Clin North Am*. 1997;44(5):1117–1131.
8. Berry A. Helping children with dysfunctional voiding. *Urol Nurs*. 2005;25(3):193–201.
9. Hellerstein S, Linebarger JS. Voiding dysfunction in pediatric patients. *Clin Pediatr*. 2003;42(1):43–49.

ADDITIONAL REFERENCE

- Neville C. Pelvic floor treatment: urinary incontinence and pelvic floor muscle training [Video]. New York, NY: McGraw-Hill; 2014. http://www.accessphysiotherapy.com. Accessed June 13, 2014.
- Thiedke CC. Nocturnal enuresis. *Am Fam Physician*. 2003;67(7): 1499–1506. http://www.aafp.org/afp/2003/0401/p1499.html. Accessed July 7, 2013.

274 PELVIC CONGESTION SYNDROME

Cynthia E. Neville, DPT, PT, WCS
Eric Shamus, PhD, DPT, PT, CSCS

CONDITION/DISORDER SYNONYMS

- Ovarian vein and pelvic varicosities
- Pelvic venous incompetence

ICD-9-CM CODES

- 625.5 Pelvic congestion syndrome
- Associated Physical Therapy Diagnoses
  - 729.1 Myalgia
  - 782.3 Edema

ICD-10-CM CODES

- G89.4 Chronic pain syndrome
- R10.2 Pelvic and perineal pain
- N94.89 Other conditions associated with female genital organs and menstrual cycle

PREFERRED PRACTICE PATTERN

- As of July 2014, the APTA Guide to Physical Therapist Practice does not include practice patterns for organ system pathology.
- Associated or secondary musculoskeletal patterns include:
  - 4C Impaired Muscle Performance[1]
  - 4D: Impaired Joint Mobility, Motor Function, Muscle Performance, and Range of Motion Associated with Connective Tissue Dysfunction[1]

PATIENT PRESENTATION

A 32-year-old woman reports a gradual onset of pain and swelling in the vaginal area, upper thigh, and labia which worsens when she is sitting. In the past year, she has developed more symptoms. She has noticed that she has to urinate more frequently, at least 10 times per day. She now is having pain during intercourse, and sometimes feels a throbbing pain in the vaginal regions at the end of the day.

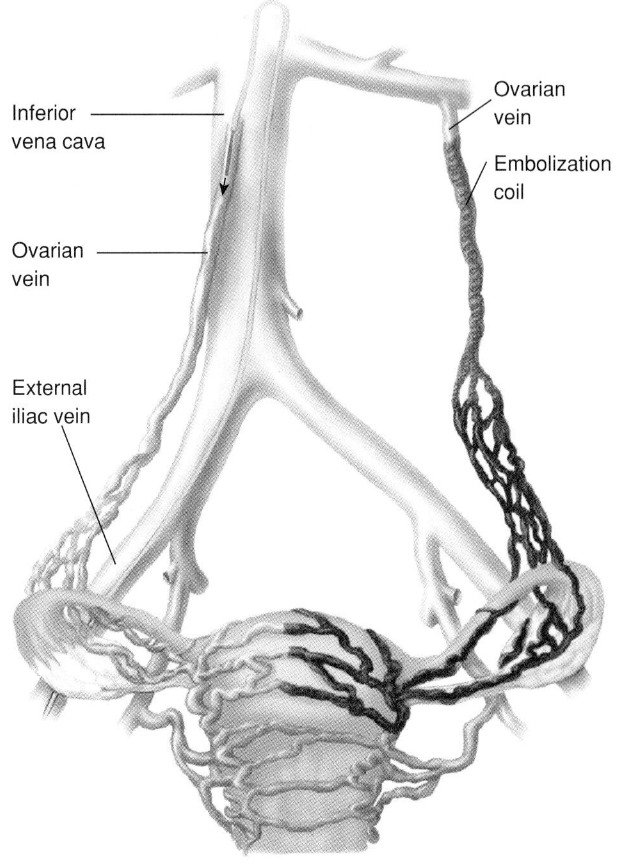

FIGURE 274-1 On the image's right, pelvic varices have already been treated with sclerosant and coils in the left ovarian vein. On the image's left, a guiding catheter is threaded into the right ovarian vein to perform ovarian venography and embolization. (From Kim HS, Malhotra AD, Rowe PC, et al. Embolotherapy for pelvic congestion syndrome: long-term results. *J Vasc Intervent Radiol*. 2006; 17:289, with permission.)

KEY FEATURES

Description[2]

- Noncyclical poorly localized pelvic pain
- Pain worsened by sitting, standing, at the end of the day, during or after intercourse
- Blood pooling in the pelvic and ovarian veins
- Pain associated with varicose veins in the thigh, buttock regions, vaginal area

Essentials of Diagnosis

- Initially is a diagnosis of exclusion
- Multidisciplinary approach to rule out other end-organ pathology
- Standard workup includes abdominal and pelvic examination, Pap smear, routine blood work, cross-sectional imaging

General Considerations

- Chronic pain condition
- Often misdiagnosed
- PT intervention is often appropriate for associated musculoskeletal impairments.
- Diagnosis is a process of exclusion and often takes time, require intensive diagnostic testing.
- Urogenital pain disorders frequently affect nearby body areas; especially back, pelvic, hip, groin regions and so may be inappropriately referred to PT.

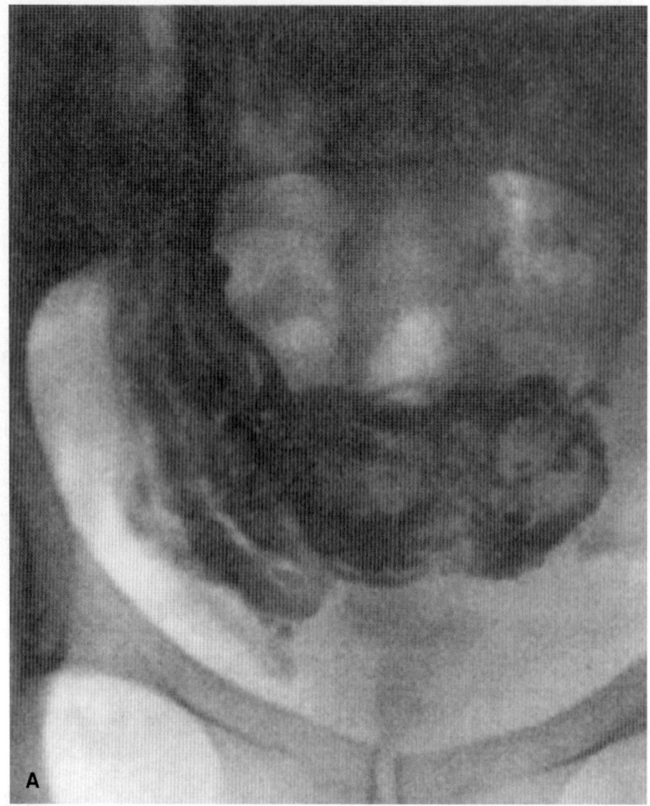

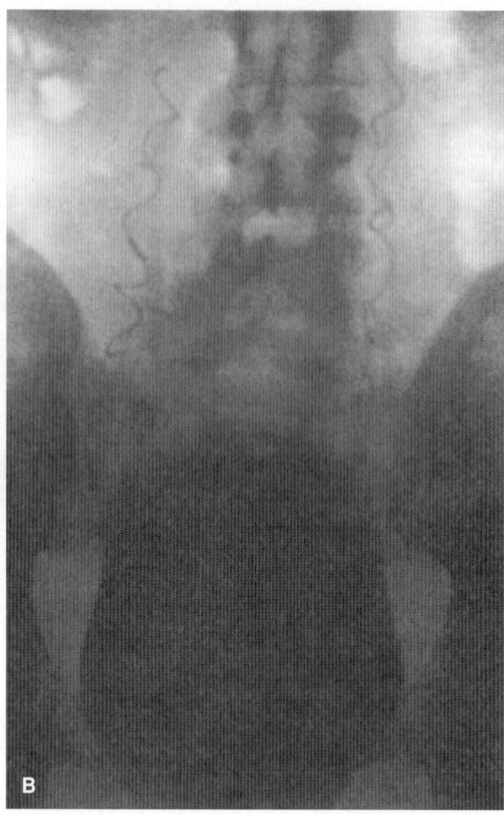

FIGURE 274-2 Embolization of ovarian vein varices in a 30-year-old multiparous woman with pelvic congestion syndrome. She complained of increasing pelvic pain and dyspareunia. On examination there were prominent vulval varicosities. (**A**) Transjugular right ovarian venography demonstrates multiple large ovarian vein varices. (**B**) Radiograph taken after coil embolization of both ovarian veins and tributaries of the internal iliac veins. The varices have been occluded. The patient's symptoms resolved after the procedure. (From Tanagho EA, McAninch WJ. *Smith's General Urology*. 17th ed. www.accessmedicine.com. Copyright © The McGraw-Hill Companies, Inc. All rights reserved.)

- May mimic other visceral pain conditions including colon cancer or tumor, irritable bowel, colitis.
- May mimic gynecologic problems in females: Endometriosis, uterine fibroids, ectopic pregnancy.

Demographics
- Only in females, typically between ages of 20 and 45[2]
- More prevalent in multiparous women
- Exact prevalence of pelvic congestion syndrome unknown.

CLINICAL FINDINGS
- Report of vaginal, rectal, or lower abdominal pain
- Symptoms usually vague and poorly localized

SIGNS AND SYMPTOMS[2]

- Symptoms often worsened by prolonged sitting or standing, anxiety, bowel movements, physical activity, or sexual intercourse
- Pain becomes progressively worse throughout the day
- Generalized lethargy, depression
- Abdominal or pelvic tenderness
- Vaginal discharge
- Dysmenorrhea
- Swollen vulva
- Lumbosacral neuropathy
- Rectal discomfort
- Urinary frequency
- May have tenderness of the uterine cervix, ovaries, or uterus
- Pain during sexual intercourse

Functional Implications
- Pain
- Painful urination, defecation, and sexual activity
- Urinary urgency and frequency
- Fatigue, lethargy

Possible Contributing Causes
- Pregnancy and vaginal childbirth

Differential Diagnosis
- Bowel pathology
- Cancer
- Neurologic pathology
- Musculoskeletal pathology or impairment
- Gynecologic problems in females
  - Endometriosis
  - Menses
  - Ectopic pregnancy
  - Ovarian cyst
  - Fibroids
  - Menopause
  - Uterine prolapse

- Fibromyalgia
- Urologic pathology
- Pelvic inflammatory disease

MEANS OF CONFIRMATION OR DIAGNOSIS

Laboratory Tests

- Blood tests
- Pap smear
- Urine culture/urinalysis
- H&H for signs of bleeding, anemia, pathogens, immune status, vitamin deficiencies, white blood cell count

Imaging

- CT: Greater sensitivity for showing varicosities throughout the lower pelvis[2]
- Pelvic ultrasound: Dynamic information about the visualized venous blood flow[2]
- Venography: Diagnostic venogram
- Cystoscopy
- Intravenous urinary pyelogram using dye
- Bladder scans
- MRI/MRV (MR venogram)
- X-ray

Diagnostic Procedures

- Doppler examination
- Postvoid residual
- Bladder biopsy
- Cystography
- Cystometrogram
- Video urodynamic testing
- Colonoscopy
- Biopsy
- Uroflowmetry
- Laparoscopy

FINDINGS AND INTERPRETATION

- Criteria for sonographic diagnosis of varices
  - Visualization of dilated ovarian veins >4 mm in diameter[2,3]
  - Dilated tortuous arcuate veins in the myometrium that communicate with bilateral pelvic varicose veins[2,3]
  - Slow blood flow (<3 cm/s[2,3])
  - Reversed caudal or retrograde venous blood flow particularly in the left ovarian vein[2,3]

TREATMENT[4]

Medications

- Progestins
- Danazol
- Phlebotonics
- GnRH agonists with HRT
- Nonsteroidal anti-inflammatory medication (NSAID)
- MPA medroxyprogesterone acetate

MEDICAL PROCEDURES

- Vein resection of ovarian vein(s)
- Laparoscopic ligation of veins
- Pelvic vein embolization
- Ovarian vein embolization
- Transcatheter embolotherapy
- Hysterectomy

REFERRALS/ADMITTANCE

- To pelvic floor physical therapist
- To psychotherapist
- To primary care physicians
- To gynecologists
- To oncologists
- To urologists
- To urogynecologists
- To gastroenterologist
- To colorectal surgeon
- To neurologist
- To pain medicine
- To acupuncture practitioner

IMPAIRMENTS

- Pelvic floor muscle (PFM) dysfunction
  - Overactive
  - Underactive
  - Nonrelaxing
  - Noncontracting
- Incontinence
- Myofascial pelvic pain
- Pelvic organ prolapse
- Detrusor instability
- Decreased sexual appreciation; anorgasmia: Inability to achieve orgasm
- Muscle atrophy
- Joint hypomobility
- Posture dysfunction
- Gait abnormality, difficulty walking
- Contractures of soft tissue (fascia, muscle)
- Inability to perform self-care
- Obstructed defecation

TESTS AND MEASURES

- PFM examination: Via vagina or anorectum
- Abdominal wall muscle test
- Abdominal wall palpation: Diastalsis rectus abdominis, scar
- Bladder diary
- sEMG biofeedback assessment of the PFMs and abdominal muscles
- Pressure manometry of the PFMs
- Lumbar spine, pelvic girdle, and hip joint examination procedures

INTERVENTION

- PFM exercises/training
  - "Kegel" exercises: Another name for PFM exercises
  - Contraction
  - Relaxation/"bulging"
  - Motor control
  - Endurance
  - Power
  - sEMG biofeedback

- TENS
- Pressure manometry
- Manual therapy
- Thermal modalities
- US imaging to awareness of muscle contractions
- Posture reeducation
- Functional training: PFM contraction during symptoms to activate skeletal muscle pump and impact arterio venous blood flow
- Patient education regarding pain, self-care

FUNCTIONAL GOALS

- Patient will be able to
  - Verbalize strategies for independent pain management.
  - Achieve functional aerobic capacity, gait, and tolerance for ADLs/IADLs.
  - Tolerate 30 minutes of continuous, moderate exercise three times per week in ______weeks, and 5 times per week in ____________ weeks, depending on disease severity.
  - Demonstrate independence with home exercise program, promoting relaxation and awareness of PFM for long-term self-management.
  - Demonstrate independence with long-term PFM training program.

PROGNOSIS

- 83% of women undergoing embolotherapy reported a positive symptom response at with 48-month follow-up.[5]
- Longer duration and greater intensity of pain symptoms negatively impacts prognosis.
- Psychological factors such as pain catastrophizing and fear avoidance negatively impact prognosis in chronic pelvic pain syndromes.[6]

PATIENT RESOURCE

- International Pelvic Pain Society. http://www.pelvicpain.org/. Accessed April 20, 2013.

REFERENCES

1. The American Physical Therapy Association. Pattern 4C: impaired muscle performance. In: *Guide to Physical Therapist Practice*. Alexandria, VA: The American Physical Therapy Association; 2003. http://guidetoptpractice.apta.org/content/1/SEC10.extract?sid=9af82a7e-5fc3-41d2-86ab-b8336a9655e9. Accessed June 25, 2013.
2. Ignacio EA, Dua R, Sarin S, et al. Pelvic congestion syndrome: diagnosis and treatment. *Semin Intervent Radiol*. 2008;25(4):361–368.
3. Beard RW, Highman JH, Pearce S, Reginald PW. Diagnosis of pelvic varicosities in women with chronic pelvic pain. *Lancet*. 1984;2(8409):946–949.
4. Chung MH, Huh CY. Comparison of treatments for pelvic congestion syndrome. *Tohoku J Exp Med*. 2003;201(13):131–138.
5. Kim HS, Malhotra AD, Rowe PC, Lee JM, Venbrux AC. Embolotherapy for pelvic congestion syndrome: long-term results. *J Vasc Interv Radiol*. 2006;17(2 Pt 1):289–297.
6. Alappattu MJ, Bishop MD. Psychological factors in chronic pelvic pain in women: relevance and application of the fear-avoidance model of pain. *Phys Ther*. 2011;91(10):1542–1550.

ADDITIONAL REFERENCES

- Dutton M. Gynecologic disorders. In: Dutton M, ed. *Dutton's Orthopaedic Examination, Evaluation, and Intervention*. 3rd ed. New York, NY: McGraw-Hill; 2012. http://www.accessphysiotherapy.com/content/5547556. Accessed April 20, 2013.
- Maleux G, Stockx L, Wilms G, et al. Ovarian vein embolization for the treatment of pelvic congestion syndrome: long term technical and clinical results. *J Vasc Interv Radiol*. 2000;11(7):859–864.
- Neville C. Pelvic floor treatment: urinary incontinence and pelvic floor muscle training [Video]. New York, NY: McGraw-Hill; 2014. http://www.accessphysiotherapy.com. Accessed June 13, 2014.
- Venbrux A C, Lambert D L. Embolization of the ovarian veins as a treatment for patients with chronic pelvic pain caused by pelvic venous incompetence (pelvic congestion syndrome). *Curr Opin Obstet Gynecol*. 1999;11:395–399.

275 PELVIC GIRDLE PAIN IN PREGNANCY

Cynthia E. Neville, DPT, PT, WCS

CONDITION/DISORDER SYNONYMS

- Pubic symphysis pain
- Pubic symphysis diastasis
- Sacroiliac joint pain
- Sacroiliac joint dysfunction
- Symphysis pubis dysfunction

ICD-9-CM CODES

- 648.7 Bone and joint disorders of back pelvis and lower limbs of mother complicating pregnancy childbirth or the puerperium
- 719.45 Pain in joint, pelvic region and thigh
- 724.6 Disorders of sacrum
- 846 Sprains and strains of sacroiliac region
- 846.1 Sprain of sacroiliac ligament
- 846.8 Sprain of other specified sites of sacroiliac region
- 846.9 Sprain of unspecified site of sacroiliac region

ICD-10-CM CODES

- CM 026.7 Subluxation of symphysis pubis in pregnancy, childbirth, and the puerperium
- CM 026.71 Subluxation of the symphysis pubis in pregnancy
- CM 026.711 Subluxation of the symphysis pubis in pregnancy, first trimester
- M25.559 Pain in unspecified hip
- S33.2 Dislocation of sacroiliac and sacrococcygeal joint

PREFERRED PRACTICE PATTERN

- 4D: Impaired Joint Mobility, Motor Function, Muscle Performance, and Range of Motion Associated with Connective Tissue Dysfunction

PATIENT PRESENTATION

A 31-year-old female currently 23 weeks pregnant in her second pregnancy reports to her obstetrician/gynecologist that she is experiencing increasing pain in her "butt or her hip." The symptoms have gradually become worse over the past few weeks. She feels sharp pain while rolling in bed, moving from sit to stand position, and when she starts to walk after sitting. She is having difficulty lifting and carrying her 2-year-old.

KEY FEATURES

Description

- Pain experienced between the posterior iliac crest and the gluteal fold, particularly in the vicinity of the sacroiliac joints (SIJ) and/or the pubic symphysis.[1]

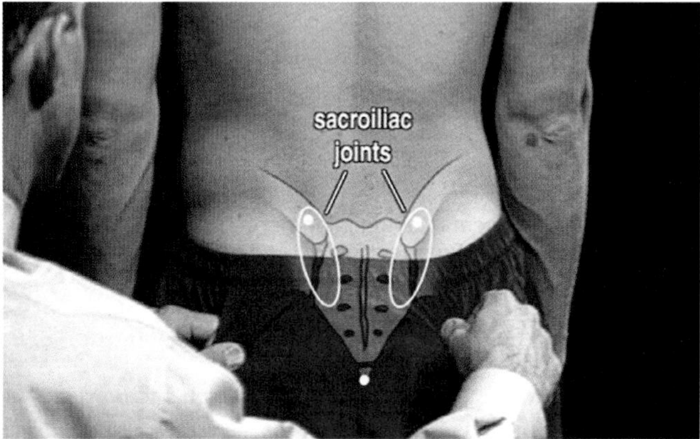

FIGURE 275-1 Palpation and location of the sacroiliac joints. (From Lawry GV. *Systematic Musculoskeletal Examinations*. www.accessmedicine.com. Copyright © The McGraw-Hill Companies, Inc. All rights reserved.)

- Pain may radiate in the posterior thigh and can also occur in conjunction with/or separately in the symphysis.[1]
- Endurance capacity for standing, walking, and sitting is diminished.
- Generally arises in relation to pregnancy, trauma, or reactive arthritis.
- Gradual or acute onset secondary to strain and impairment of load transfer at SIJ or symphysis pubis.

Essentials of Diagnosis

- Diagnosis made by clinical examination including provocation tests and load transfer tests
- Lumbar spine involvement and hip joint involvement must be ruled in or out
- Reproduction of symptoms with clinical examination

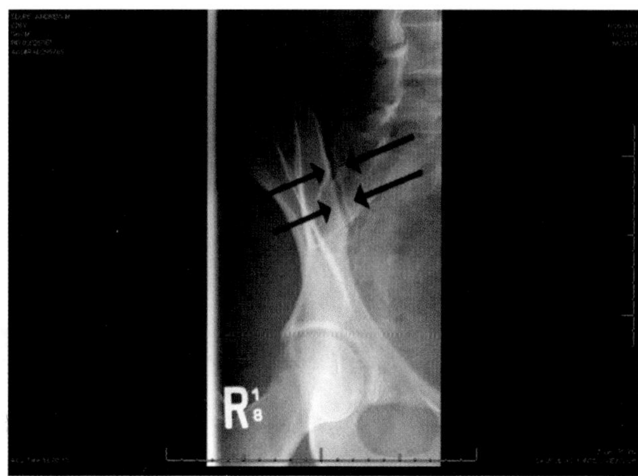

FIGURE 275-2 Sacroiliac joint space on x-ray. (From Lawry GV. *Systematic Musculoskeletal Examinations*. www.accessmedicine.com. Copyright © The McGraw-Hill Companies, Inc. All rights reserved.)

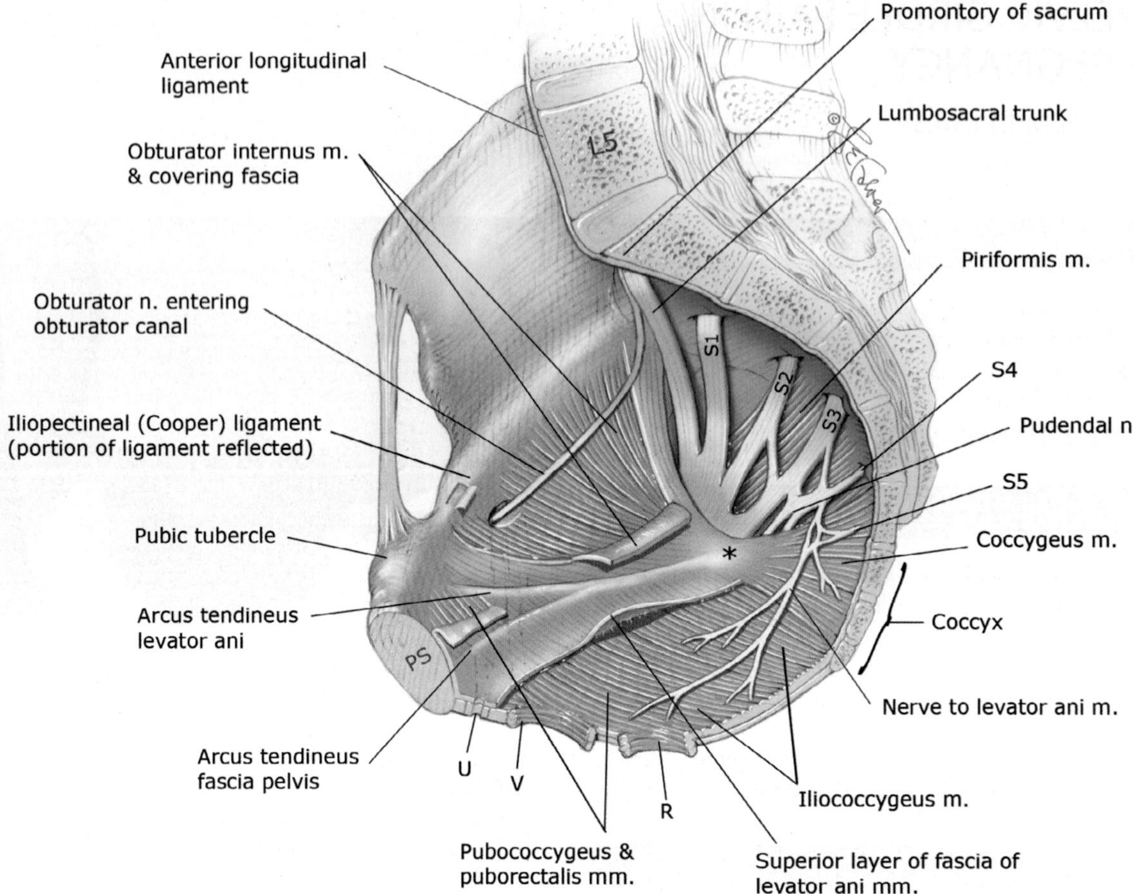

FIGURE 275-3 Muscles and fascia of the pelvic walls and pelvic floor innervation. Ischial spine is marked by an asterisk. L5, fifth lumbar vertebra; PS, pubic symphysis; R, rectum; S1–S5, first through fifth sacral nerves; U, urethra; V, vagina. (From Hoffman BL, Schorge J, Schaffer J, et al. *Williams Gynecology*. 2nd ed. New York, NY: McGraw-Hill; 2012.)

- No imaging performed on pregnant women unless pain associated with acute trauma such as motor vehicle accident

General Considerations

- Pelvic girdle pain (PGP) in pregnancy is related to impaired functional stability of the pelvic girdle joints resulting in impairment of the transfer of load[2]
- Pregnancy predisposes women to PGP because of reduced force closure of the pelvic girdle joints
- May present with or without lumbar spine pain, radicular symptoms

Demographics

- Commonly occurs in women during pregnancy

CLINICAL FINDINGS

SIGNS AND SYMPTOMS

- Pain experienced between the posterior iliac crest and the gluteal fold, particularly in the vicinity of the SIJ and/or the pubic symphysis and/or hips.[1]
- Pain can be unilateral, bilateral in the symphysis, or in all three joints.[3]
- Symphysis pubis pain may be extremely tender to the touch.
- Pain may radiate in the posterior thigh and/or groin/inner thigh.
- Pain can occur in conjunction with/or separately in the lumbar spine and pubic symphysis.
- Asymmetrical appearance of bony landmarks of the pelvis and malalignment of pelvic and/or back joints.
- Audible clicking sound coming from the pelvis.

Functional Implications

- A feeling of the symphysis pubis giving way
- Difficulty lifting legs and pain pulling legs apart
- Difficulty performing transitional movements such as standing up from a sitting position, going up and down stairs, rolling in bed, and going in and out of a car
- Difficulty with movements secondary to pain; driving, twisting
- Endurance capacity for standing, walking, and sitting is diminished[1]
- Inability to sleep because of pain
- Restriction of hip movement
- Unable to stand on one leg
- Unable to transfer weight through pelvis and legs
- Urinary incontinence
- Urinary urgency and/or frequency

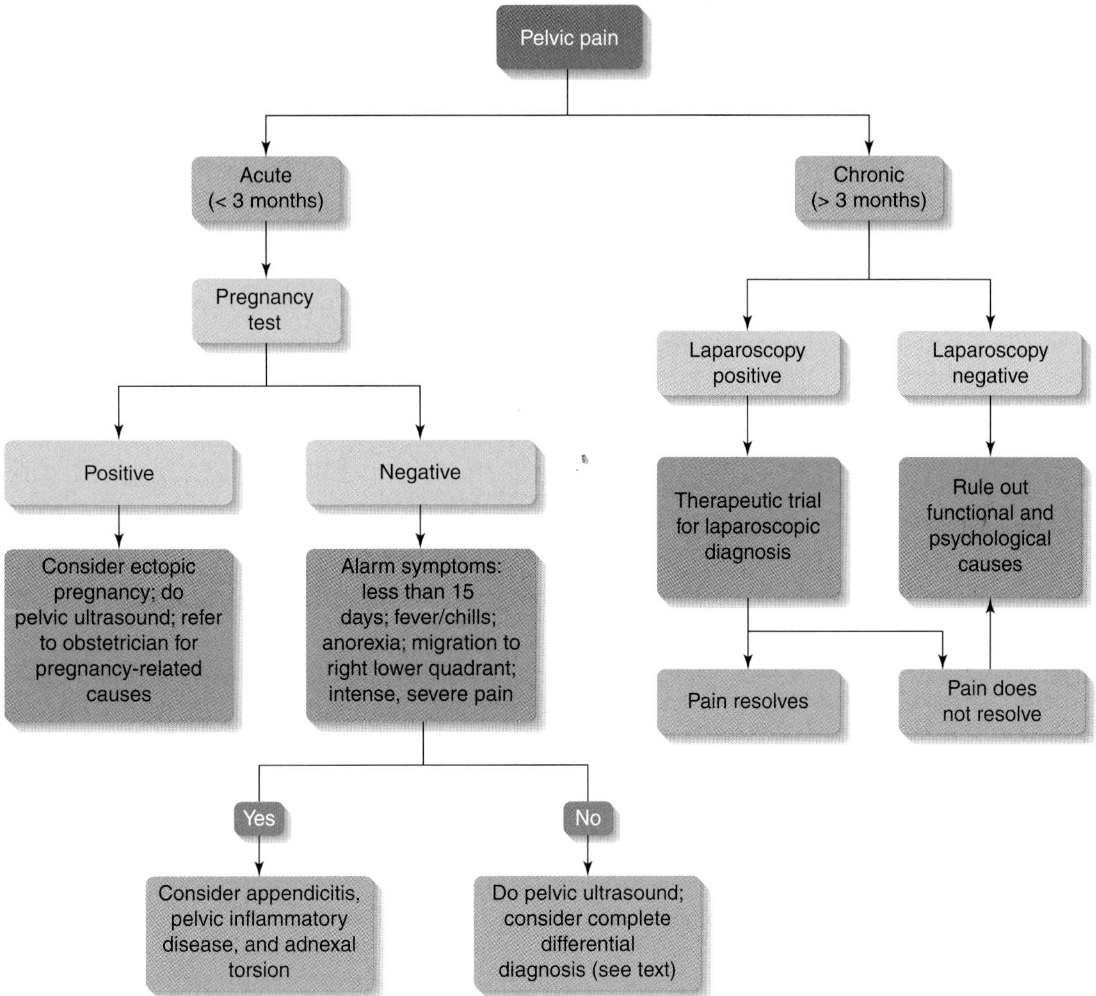

FIGURE 275-4 Diagnostic approach: Pelvic pain. (From Henderson MC, Tierney LM, Smetana GW. *The Patient History: An Evidence-Based Approach to Differential Diagnosis*. www.accessmedicine.com. Copyright © The McGraw-Hill Companies, Inc. All rights reserved.)

- Waddle or shuffle during gait
- Weakness with lifting, prolonged standing

Possible Contributing Causes

- Effect of hormone relaxin on pelvic girdle joints
- Increased width of pubic symphysis as pregnancy progresses[5]
- Asymmetrical laxity of SIJ[3]
- Prior history of pelvic girdle and/or low back pain
- Weak underactive pelvic floor and transverses abdominis muscles

Differential Diagnosis

- Ankylosing spondylitis
- Degenerative disc disease
- Hip pathology with radiating pain pattern
- Lumbar facet joint pain
- Lumbar radiculopathy
- Peripheral nerve impairment
- Piriformis syndrome
- Placenta abruptio
- Preterm labor
- Sciatica

MEANS OF CONFIRMATION OR DIAGNOSIS

Imaging

- If conservative intervention fails, magnetic resonance imaging (MRI) to diagnose lumbar herniated disc or ankylosing spondylitis

Diagnostic Procedures

- Diagnostic injection
  - SIJ injection; performed only in nonpregnant state

FINDINGS AND INTERPRETATION

- Diagnostic injection
  - SIJ injection as a means to confirm the joint as source of pain[4]

REFERRALS/ADMITTANCE

- To orthopedist or physiatrist
  - Corticosteroid injection if condition does not improve
- To primary care or obstetrician/gynecologist
  - Anti-inflammatory medication

IMPAIRMENTS

- Ineffective transfer of load across pelvic joints during weight shifting
- Restricted mobility of the lumbar spine and/or hip

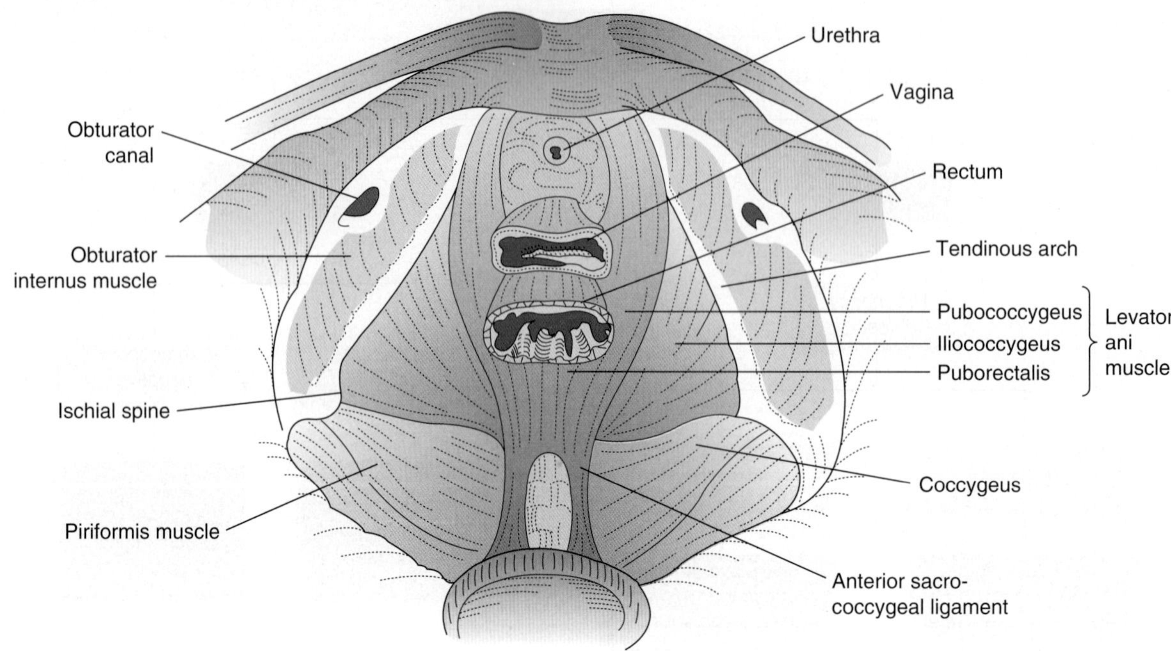

FIGURE 275-5 Pelvic diaphragm from above. (From DeCherney AH Nathan L, Laufer N, Roman AS. *Current Diagnosis & Treatment: Obstetrics & Gynecology.* 11th ed. www.accessmedicine.com. Copyright © The McGraw-Hill Companies, Inc. All rights reserved.)

- Weakness of abdominals, pelvic floor, and core stability
- Weakness of spinal muscles and hip muscles

TESTS AND MEASURES

- Physical examination: Positive provocation tests to confirm pelvic girdle joints as source of pain
  - Posterior pelvic pain provocation test (P4)
  - Patrick (Faber) test
  - Palpation of the long dorsal SIJ ligament
  - Gaenslen test
  - Palpation of the symphysis: Pubic stress test
  - Modified Trendelenburg test of the pelvic girdle
- Load transfer tests
  - ASLR test
  - Stork test[6]
- Abdominal wall assessment
  - Diastasis rectus abdominis
  - Transversus abdominis contraction
- Pelvic floor external palpation examination for confirmation of contraction
- Posture examination: Assess for symmetry of pelvic bony landmarks
- Physical examination to rule in or rule out lumbar radiculopathy
  - Algorithm for examination of the lumbar spine
  - Quadrant test
  - Patrick (FABER) test
  - Rotation limited to ipsilateral side
  - Straight-leg raise test
  - Slump test
  - Lower limb nerve tension test
  - Patella, Achilles, hamstring reflex
  - Radicular pattern
- Passive physiological intervertebral mobility testing (PPIVM)

INTERVENTIONS

- Activation and contraction of pelvic floor muscles and transversus abdominis muscles
- Manual therapy
  - Joint mobilization
  - Muscle energy techniques
  - Self-mobilization techniques performed by patient
- Acute and functional strategies for the SIJ
- Joint mobilizations to the lumbar spine and/or hip
- Sacroiliac belt
- Addressing pain
  - Heat/ice
- Addressing hypertonicity
  - Revascularization exercises
  - Soft tissue massage
  - Moist heat
- Addressing muscle weakness
  - Core stability exercises
  - Spine muscle exercises
  - Abdominal muscle exercises
  - Hip muscle exercises
- Addressing posture
  - Neutral postures during sustained activities such as sitting and sleeping
  - Neutral postures during transitional movements
  - Avoid asymmetrical movements and postures
- Body mechanics training
  - Transfer training
  - Lifting
  - Housework and ADLs

FUNCTIONAL GOALS

- Patient will be able to
  - Perform techniques to improve transfer of body weight across pelvic joints.

- Contract pelvic floor and abdominal muscles to increase force closure of pelvic girdle joints.
- Perform transitional movements such as sit to stand transfers with a neutral lumbar spine posture.
- Avoid asymmetrical postures and movements to reduce strain to the pelvic joints.
- Demonstrate body mechanics for household chores using a neutral lumbar spine posture and with activation of core muscles.
- Be able to sit at work station and perform computer work for 45 minutes with 0/10 pain.
- Be able to rotate lumbar spine 25 degrees with 0/10 lower-extremity pain in order to reach into the back seat in a car.

PROGNOSIS

- Fair to good to very good, dependent upon
  - Duration of symptoms.
  - Severity of symptoms.
  - Participation and adherence to intervention.

PATIENT RESOURCES

- The International Pelvic Pain Society. http://www.pelvicpain.org. Accessed July 7, 2013.
- Pregnancy related pelvic girdle pain. Association of Chartered Physiotherapists in Women's Health. www.csp.org.uk/sites/files/csp/secure/acpwh-pgppat_0.pdf. Accessed July 7, 2013.

REFERENCES

1. Vleeming A, Albert HB, Ostgaard HC, Sturesson B, Stuge B. European guidelines for the diagnosis and treatment of pelvic girdle pain. *Eur Spine J.* 2008;17(6):794–819.
2. O'Sullivan PB, Beales DJ. Diagnosis and classification of pelvic girdle pain disorders—Part 1: a mechanism based approach within a biopsychosocial framework. *Man Ther.* 2007;12(2):86–97.
3. Albert H, Godskesen M, Westergaard J. Evaluation of clinical tests used in classification procedures in pregnancy-related pelvic joint pain. *Eur Spine J.* 2000;9(2):161–166.
4. Damen L, Buyruk HM, Güler-Uysal F, Lotgering FK, Snijders CJ, Stam HJ. The prognostic value of asymmetric laxity of the sacroiliac joints in pregnancy-related pelvic pain. *Spine (Phila Pa 1976).* 2002;27(24):2820–2824.
5. Björklund K, Nordström ML, Bergström S. Sonographic assessment of symphyseal joint distention during pregnancy and post partum with special reference to pelvic pain. *Acta Obstet Gynecol Scand.* 1999;78(2):125–130.
6. Hungerford BA, Gilleard W, Moran M, Emmerson C. Evaluation of the ability of physical therapists to palpate intrapelvic motion with the stork test on the support side. *Phys Ther.* 2007;87(7):879–887.

ADDITIONAL REFERENCES

- Fitzgerald CM, Santos LR, Mallinson T. The association between pelvic girdle pain and urinary incontinence among pregnant women in the second trimester. *Int J Gynaecol Obstet.* 2012;117(3):248–250. doi: 10.1016/j.ijgo.2012.01.014.
- Laslett M, Aprill CN, McDonald B, Young SB. Diagnosis of sacroiliac joint pain: validity of individual provocation tests and composites of tests. *Man Ther.* 2005;10(3):207–218.
- Neville C. Pelvic floor treatment: urinary incontinence and pelvic floor muscle training [Video]. New York, NY: McGraw-Hill; 2014. http://www.accessphysiotherapy.com. Accessed June 13, 2014.

276 PELVIC ORGAN PROLAPSE

Cynthia E. Neville, DPT, PT, WCS

CONDITION/DISORDER SYNONYMS

- Cystocele
- Pelvic organ prolapse
- Rectocele
- Uterine prolapse

ICD-9-CM CODES

- 618.01 Cystocele midline
- 618.02 Cystocele lateral
- 618.04 Rectocele
- 618.1 Uterine prolapsed
- 618.2 Uterovaginal prolapse incomplete
- 618.3 Uterovaginal prolapse complete
- 618.4 Uterovaginal prolapse unspecified
- 867.6 Pelvic organ injury

ICD-10-CM CODES

- N81.10 Cystocele unspecified
- N81.11 Cystocele midline
- N81.12 Cystocele lateral
- N81.6 Rectocele
- N81.2 Incomplete uterovaginal prolapse
- N81.3 Complete uterovaginal prolapsed
- N81.4 Uterovaginal prolapsed unspecified

PREFERRED PRACTICE PATTERN

- 4C: Impaired Muscle Performance[1]

PATIENT PRESENTATION

A 68-year-old female was cleaning her rental apartment after the renters had moved out. She was moving furniture and lifting boxes. Later that day, after urinating and while wiping, she felt something bulging into her vagina. When she stood up, she noticed a feeling of pressure in her vagina.

KEY FEATURES

Description

- Abnormal descent or herniation of pelvic organ from normal attachment sites in the pelvis secondary to damage to connective tissue support structures and/or weakening or muscles of the pelvic floor
  - Bladder
  - Uterus
  - Rectum

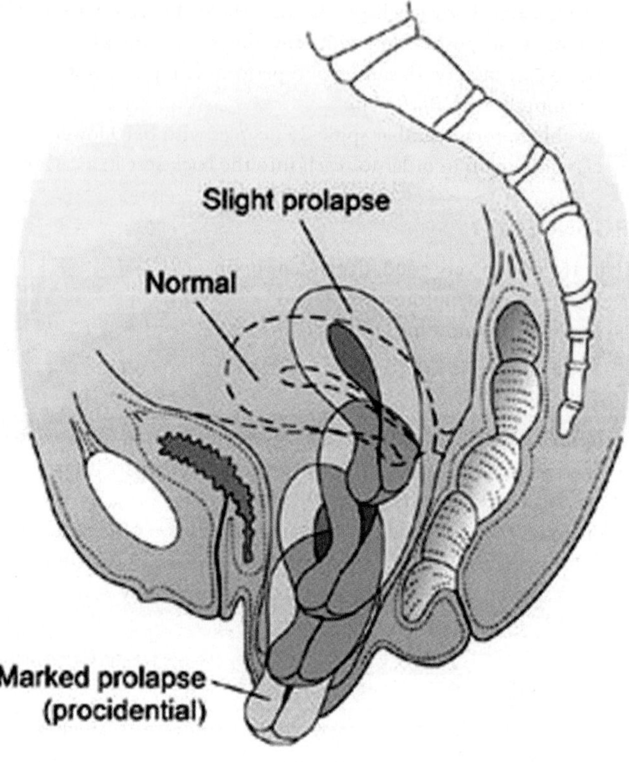

FIGURE 276-1 Prolapse of the uterus. (Reproduced with permission from, DeCherney AH, Pernoll ML eds. *Current Obstetrics & Gynecology Diagnosis & Treatment.* 8th ed. Originally published by Appleton & Lange. Copyright © 1994 by The McGraw-Hill Companies, Inc.)

- May or may not be accompanied by
  - Feelings of pressure or pain
  - Urinary tract infection
  - Urinary incontinence
  - Bladder obstruction
  - Bowel dysfunction
  - Constipation
  - Fecal incontinence

Essentials of Diagnosis

- Physical examination with or without a speculum for palpation and visualization of the position of the pelvic organs relative to the anterior and posterior vaginal walls

General Considerations

- May be asymptomatic.
- If symptomatic, then symptoms are often nonspecific.
- Symptoms of pressure in the vagina and rectum, self palpation of a mass in the vagina, or visualization of the prolapse may be the first indication to the patient of its presence.
- Any complaints or changes in bowel and bladder function should be investigated by a physician.
- Degree of prolapse does not correlate with severity of symptoms.

Demographics[2,3]

- Does not occur in men.
- Some degree of prolpase may be seen in 50% of women in a clinical setting.
  - In women with a uterus, the rate of uterine prolapse was 14.2%; the rate of cystocele was 34.3%; and the rate of rectocele was 18.6%.
  - For women who have undergone hysterectomy, the prevalence of cystocele was 32.9% and of rectocele was 18.3%.
- African American women demonstrated the lowest risk for prolapse.
- Hispanic women had the highest risk for uterine prolapse.
- Parity and obesity were strongly associated with increased risk for uterine prolapse, cystocele, and rectocele.

CLINICAL FINDINGS

SIGNS AND SYMPTOMS[4]

- Many have no symptoms
- May see or feel a bulge in the vagina
- Sensation of protrusion or bulging
- 62% of women with pelvic organ prolapse (POP) also have urinary stress incontinence[5]
- Obstructive bladder symptoms: Difficulty initiating and completing urination
- Obstructive defecation symptoms: Constipation

Functional Implications

- Feelings of pressure during lifting[6]
- Obstructive bladder symptoms: Difficulty initiating and completing urination
- Obstructive defecation symptoms: Constipation

Possible Contributing Causes

- Pregnancy
- Childbirth
- Ligamentous and connective tissue damage
  - Pubocervical fascia
  - Arcus tendineus levator ani
  - Arcus tendineus fascia pelvis
- Underactive, overactive, or nonfunctioning pelvic floor muscles (PFMs)
- Obesity
- Systemic hypermobility

Differential Diagnosis

- Neoplasm

MEANS OF CONFIRMATION OR DIAGNOSIS

- Visualization of the position of the pelvic organs relative to the anterior and posterior vaginal walls via physical examination

Imaging

- Ultrasound imaging to identify abnormalities
  - Bladder and urethra
  - Bladder neck position and mobility
  - Descent of pelvic organs
    - Uterus, rectum
- MRI

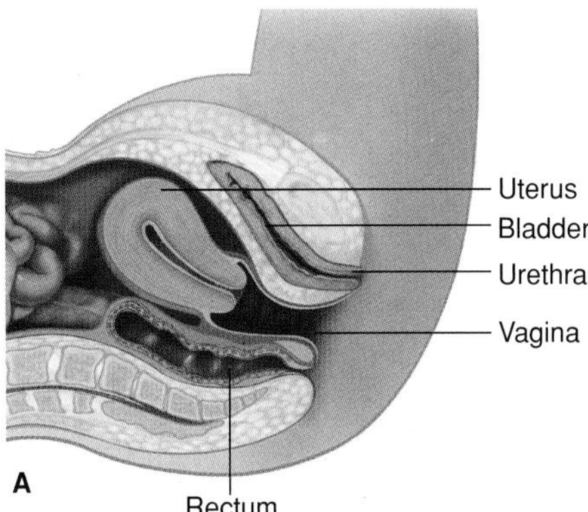

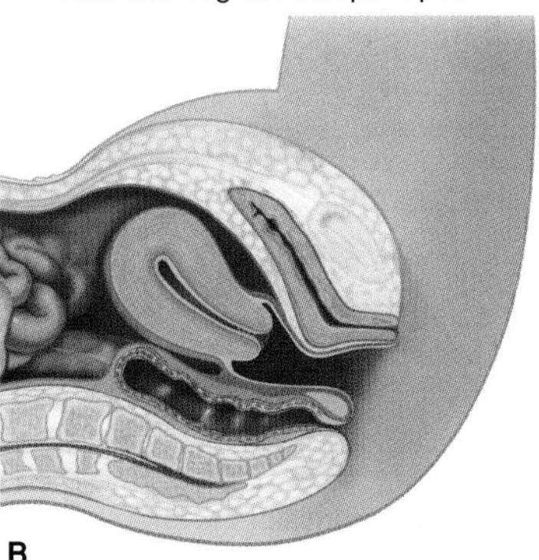

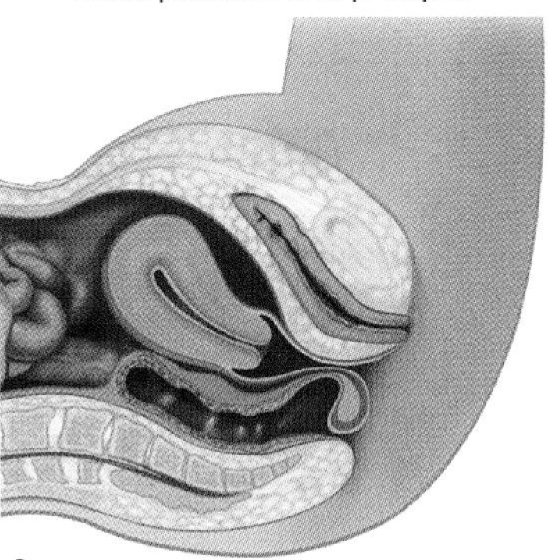

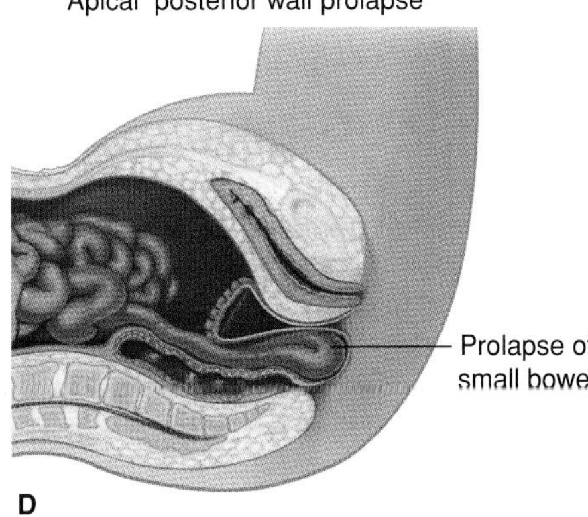

FIGURE 276-2 Sagittal view of pelvic anatomy. (**A**) Normal pelvic anatomy. (**B**) Anterior vaginal wall prolapse or cystocele. (**C**) Distal posterior wall prolapse or rectocele. (**D**) Apical posterior wall prolapse or enterocele. (From Hoffman BL, Schorge JO, Schaffer JI, et al. *Williams Gynecology*. 2nd ed. New York, NY: McGraw-Hill; 2012.)

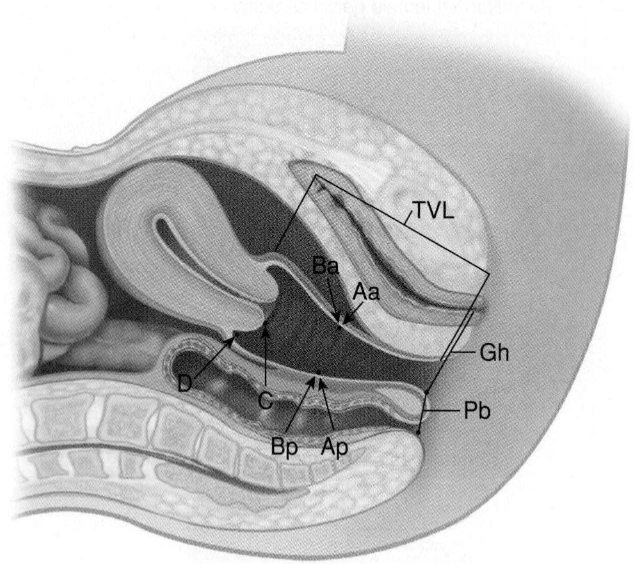

anterior wall Aa	anterior wall Ba	cervix or cuff C
genital hiatus gh	perineal body pb	total vaginal length tvl
posterior wall Ap	posterior wall Bp	posterior fornix D

FIGURE 276-3 Drawing displays the anatomic landmarks used during pelvic organ prolapse quantification (POP-Q). (From Hoffman BL, Schorge JO, Schaffer JI, et al. *Williams Gynecology*. 2nd ed. New York, NY: McGraw-Hill; 2012.)

Diagnostic Procedures[7,8]

- Pelvic Organ Prolapse Quantification (POP-Q)
- Pelvic ultrasound

FINDINGS AND INTERPRETATION

- POP-Q is performed by a physician[9]
  - Stage I: Leading edge of the prolapse is >1 cm above the hymen
  - Stage II: Leading edge of the prolapse is ≤1 cm proximal or distal to the plane of the hymen
  - Stage III: Leading edge of the prolapse is >1 cm below the plane of the hymen but protrudes no further than 2 cm, less than the total vaginal length
  - Stage IV: Essentially complete eversion of the total lower genital tract
- Grading the degree for POP for PTs[10]
  - Grade 1: Not visible at the introitus
  - Grade 2: Bearing down results in tissue at the introitus
  - Grade 3: Bearing down results in tissue outside the introitus

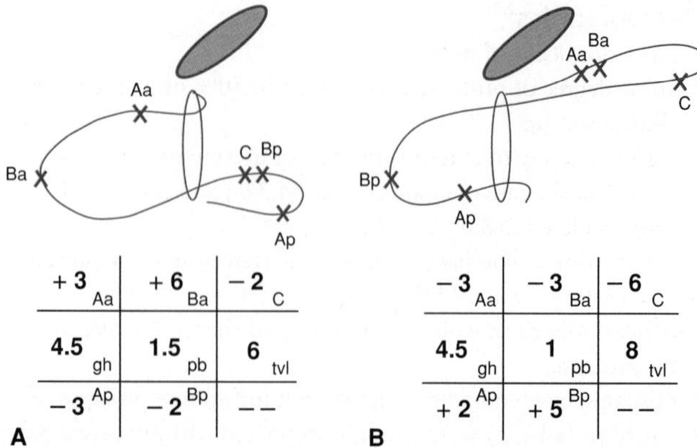

FIGURE 276-5 Grid and drawing of an anterior support defect (**A**) and posterior support defect (**B**) in patients with prior hysterectomy. (From Bump RC, Mattiasson A, Bo K, et al. The standardization of terminology of female pelvic organ prolapse and pelvic floor dysfunction. *Am J Obstet Gynecol.* 1996;175:10, with permission.)

TREATMENT

- Pessary[11]
  - Removable device placed in the vagina to support the prolapsed organ
  - Usually in the shape of a firm ring

Medication

- Estrogen replacement therapy

MEDICAL PROCEDURES

- Surgery[12]
  - Laparoscopic
  - Robotic assisted surgery
  - Mesh repairs

REFERRALS/ADMITTANCE

- Pelvic floor physical therapists
- Primary care physicians
- Gynecologists
  - Women: Pelvic examination
- Urologists
  - Men: Genital examination
- Urogynecologists
- Nurse practitioners

IMPAIRMENTS

- PFM dysfunction
  - Overactive
  - Underactive
  - Nonrelaxing
  - Noncontracting
- Incontinence
- Pelvic pain
- Dyspareunia (painful intercourse)
- Anorgasmia
  - Inability to achieve orgasm
- Constipation/obstructed defecation
- Obstructed urination

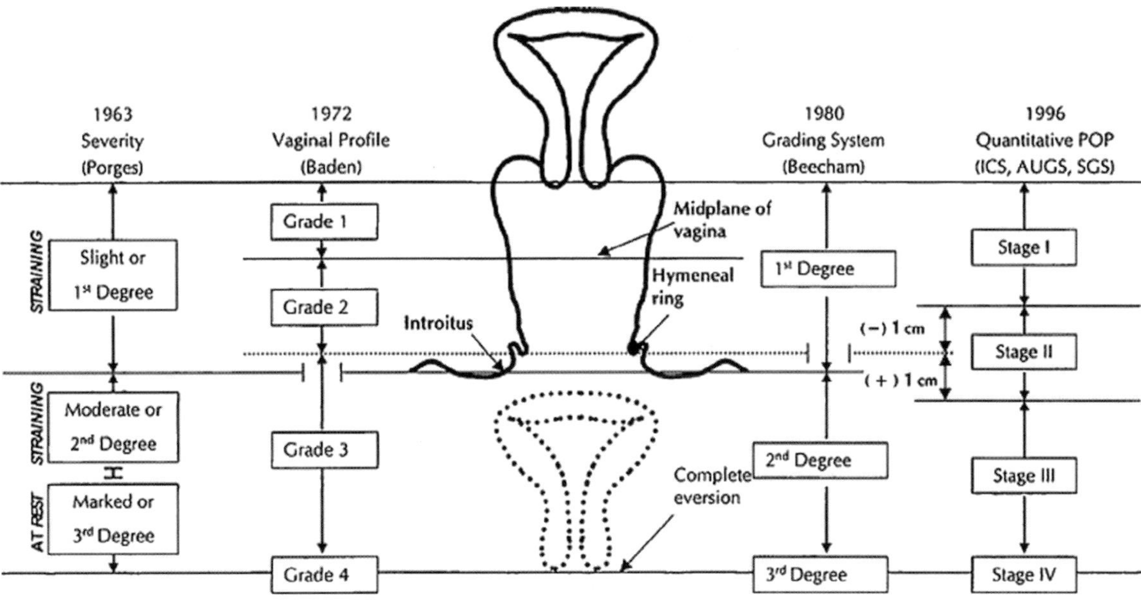

FIGURE 276-6 Comparison of various classification systems of pelvic organ prolapse. (Reproduced with permission from, Theofrastous JP, Swift SE. The clinical evaluation of pelvic floor dysfunction. *Obstet Gynecol Clin North Am.* 1998;25:783.)

TESTS AND MEASURES

- Pelvic Organ Prolapse Simple Screening Inventory (POPSSI)[6]
  - Short questionnaire for identification of POP in the general population; sensitivity 0.455 and specificity 0.874
- PFM examination and assessment
- sEMG biofeedback assessment of the PFM
- Pressure manometry of the PFM

INTERVENTION

- PFM exercises/training: Contraction effectively "closes" the pelvic floor.[13,14]
  - Reduces the size of vaginal opening.
  - Elevates the bladder neck.
  - "Kegel" exercises are another name for PFM exercises.
  - Contraction
    - Motor control
    - Endurance
    - Power
  - sEMG biofeedback
- Motor control/coordination training of abdominal muscles to avoid overuse
- Neuromuscular electrical stimulation to facilitate PFM contraction

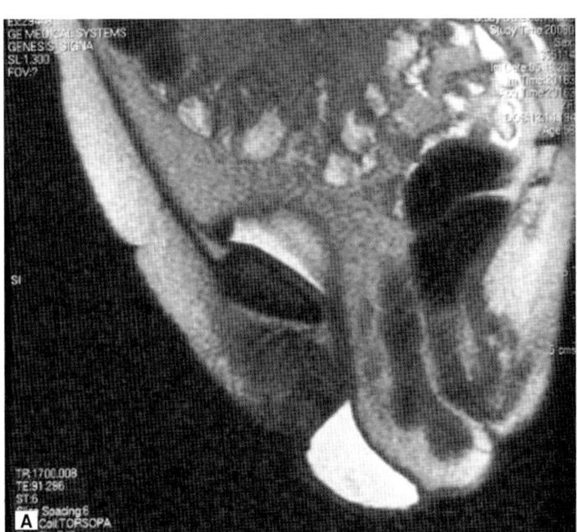

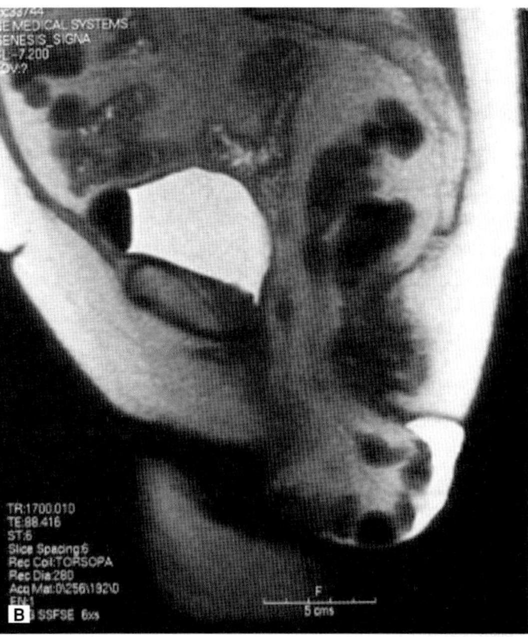

FIGURE 276-7 **A.** Sagittal MRI image of cystocele and enterocele. Small intestine protrudes posterior to the prolapsed bladder (*white*). **B.** Sagittal MRI image of an enterocele only. Bladder does not prolapse past the pubococcygeal line. (From Tanagho EA, McAninch WJ. *Smith's General Urology*. 17th ed. www.accessmedicine.com. Copyright © The McGraw-Hill Companies, Inc. All rights reserved.)

- Protocol for underactive/weak PFMs
  - Frequency of 35 to 50 Hz, pulse width of 200 to 350 usec, asymmetrical biphasic wave form, duty cycle of 5 to 10 seconds on/5 to 10 seconds off
  - Match on time to patient's active home exercise program contraction time
  - Patient may contract PFMs while stimulation is on
  - Duration of 10 to 20 minutes, frequency of treatment 1 to 2 times/day, every other day or daily
- Anal or vaginal electrode /probe
  - Vaginal probe may not be effective with moderate-to-severe prolapse
- Surface electrodes
  - Perineum

- Realtime ultrasound imaging to facilitate learning of correct performance and coordination of abdominal muscle and PFM co-contraction
- Functional training
  - Precontraction of the PFMs to close the urethra prior to anticipated increase in intra-abdominal pressure
  - Known as "The Knack"
- Patient education
  - Instructions and benefits of use of pessary
  - Precontraction of PFM prior to increase in intra-abdominal pressure to reduce risk of exacerbation of prolapse
- Pressure manometry

FUNCTIONAL GOALS

- Patient will be able to
  - Reduce/Eliminate feelings of pressure in the vagina during increase in intra-abdominal pressure.
  - Perform contraction of the PFM prior to increase in intra-abdominal pressure.
  - Independence in the management of symptoms of POP.

PROGNOSIS

- PFM training improves symptoms of POP[13,14]
- Surgery using mesh at the time of anterior vaginal wall repair for POP reduced the risk of recurrent anterior vaginal wall prolapse on examination; however, this was not translated into improved functional or quality-of-life outcomes[12]

PATIENT RESOURCE

- Pelvic Organ Prolapse. http://www.mayoclinic.org/pelvic-organ-prolapse/diagnosis.html. Accessed July 2, 2013.

REFERENCES

1. The American Physical Therapy Association. Pattern 4C: impaired muscle performance. In: *Guide to Physical Therapist Practice*. Alexandria, VA: The American Physical Therapy Association; 2003. http://guidetoptpractice.apta.org/content/1/SEC10.extract?sid=9af82a7e-5fc3-41d2-86ab-b8336a9655e9. Accessed July 1, 2013.
2. Hendrix SL, Clark A, Nygaard I, Aragaki A, Barnabei V, McTiernan A. Pelvic organ prolapse in the Women's Health Initiative: gravity and gravidity. *Am J Obstet Gynecol.* 2002; 186(6):1160–1166.
3. Rortveit G, Brown JS, Thom DH, Van Den Eeden SK, Creasman JM, Subak LL. Symptomatic pelvic organ prolapse: prevalence and risk factors in a population-based, racially diverse cohort. *Obstet Gynecol.* 2007;109(6):1396–1403.
4. Bradley CS, Zimmerman MB, Wang Q, Nygaard IE; Women's Health Initiative. Vaginal descent and pelvic floor symptoms in postmenopausal women: a longitudinal study. *Obstet Gynecol.* 2008;111(5):1148–1153.
5. Luber KM, Boero S, Choe JY. The demographics of pelvic floor disorders: current observations and future projections. *Am J Obstet Gynecol.* 2001;184:1496–1503.
6. Tehrani FR, Hashemi S, Simbar M, Shiva N. Screening of the pelvic organ prolapse without a physical examination; (a community based study). *BMC Womens Health.* 2011;11:48. doi:10.1186/1472-6874-11-48.
7. Shek KL, Dietz HP. Pelvic floor ultrasonography: an update. *Minerva Ginecol.* 2013;65(1):1–20.
8. Dietz HP. Pelvic floor trauma in childbirth. *Aust N Z J Obstet Gynaecol.* 2013;53(3):220–230. doi: 10.1111/ajo.12059.
9. Bump RC, Mattiasson A, Bo K, et al. The standardization of terminology of female pelvic organ prolapse and pelvic floor dysfunction. *Am J Obstet Gynecol.* 1996;175(1):10–17.
10. Laycock J, Haslem J. *Therapeutic Management of Incontinence and Pelvic Pain.* 2nd ed London: Springer Publishers; 2008.
11. Bugge C, Adams EJ, Gopinath D, Reid F. Pessaries (mechanical devices) for pelvic organ prolapse in women. *Cochrane Database Syst Rev.* 2013;2:CD004010.
12. Maher CM, Feiner B, Baessler K, Glazener CM. Surgical management of pelvic organ prolapse in women: the updated summary version Cochrane review. *Int Urogynecol J.* 2011; 22(11):1445–1457.
13. Braekken IH, Majida M, Ellstrom EM, Holme IM, Bo K. Pelvic floor function is independently associated with pelvic organ prolapse. *BJOG.* 2009;116(13):1706–1714.
14. Braekken IH, Majida M, Engh ME, Bo K. Can pelvic floor muscle training reverse pelvic organ prolapse and reduce prolapse symptoms? An assessor-blinded, randomized, controlled trial. *Am J Obstet Gynecol.* 2010;203(2):170.e1–170.e7. doi: 10.1016/j.ajog.2010.02.037.

ADDITIONAL REFERENCES

- Dutton M. Pathology, gynecology, and psychology. In: Dutton M, ed. *McGraw-Hill's NPTE (National Physical Therapy Examination).* 2nd ed. New York, NY: McGraw-Hill; 2012 http://www.accessphysiotherapy.com/content/5402111. Accessed July 2, 2013.
- Neville C. Pelvic floor treatment: urinary incontinence and pelvic floor muscle training [Video]. New York, NY: McGraw-Hill; 2014. http://www.accessphysiotherapy.com. Accessed June 13, 2014.
- Pelvic Organ Prolapse. http://emedicine.medscape.com/article/276259-overview#aw2aab6b2b1aa. Accessed July 2, 2013.
- Pelvic Organ Prolapse. http://cw.tandf.co.uk/obsgynaeby-tenteachers/sample-material/Gynae/02-Gynaecologyby TenTeachers_Ch17.pdf. Accessed July 2, 2013.
- Surgical Management of Anterior Vaginal Wall Prolapse. http://emedicine.medscape.com/article/276259-treatment#aw2aab6b4b3. Accessed July 2, 2013.

277 PUBIC SYMPHYSIS DYSFUNCTION

Cynthia E. Neville, DPT, PT, WCS

CONDITION/DISORDER SYNONYMS

- Diastasis pubic symphysis
- Pelvic girdle pain (PGP)

ICD-9-CM CODES

- 665.6 Damage to pelvic joints and ligaments
- 719.45 Joint pain—pelvis
- 848.5 Sprain of pelvis

ICD-10-CM CODES

- 026.7 Subluxation of symphysis pubis in pregnancy, childbirth, or puerperium
- O26.71 Sublux of symphysis (pubis) in pregnancy
- O26.711 Sublux of symphysis (pubis) in pregnancy, first trimester
- O26.712 Sublux of symphysis (pubis) in pregnancy, second trimester
- O26.713 Sublux of symphysis (pubis) in pregnancy, third trimester
- S33.4 Traumatic rupture of symphysis pubis
- 071.6 Obstetric damage to pelvic joints and ligaments

PREFERRED PRACTICE PATTERNS[1]

- 4B: Impaired Posture
- 4D: Impaired Joint Mobility, Motor Function, Muscle Performance, and Range of Motion Associated with Connective Tissue Dysfunction
- 4E: Impaired Joint Mobility, Motor Function, Muscle Performance, and Range of Motion Associated with Localized Inflammation
- 4G: Impaired Joint Mobility, Muscle Performance, and Range of Motion Associated with Fracture

PATIENT PRESENTATION

A 32-year-old woman who was 24 weeks pregnant was performing Pilates exercises with a trainer using the reformer apparatus. During an exercise, she had one leg kneeling on the reformer and the other leg off of the reformer. She was pushing the leg on the reformer behind her against resistance in a lunge movement. After the exercise session, she started having difficulty walking. She tried to open a heavy door in an office building and had sharp severe pain in her groin. She fell to the ground and could not get up to walk.

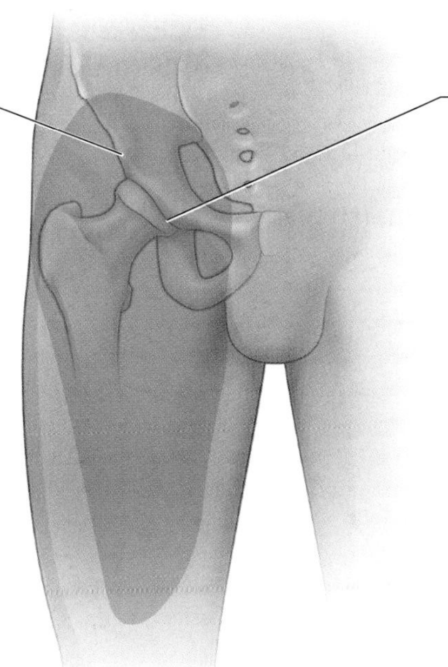

FIGURE 277-1 Potential causes of trochanteric, pubic, and thigh pain. (From Dutton D. *Dutton's Orthopaedic Examination, Evaluation, and Intervention*. 3rd ed. www.accessphysiotherapy.com. Copyright © The McGraw-Hill Companies, Inc. All rights reserved.)

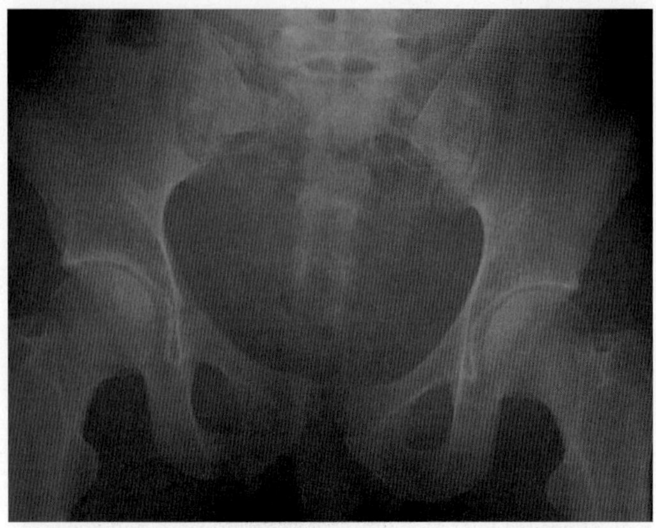

FIGURE 277-2 This AP radiograph in a 20-year-old male following trauma reveals diastasis of the pubic symphysis. (From Malone TR, Hazle C, Grey ML. *Imaging in Rehabilitation*. http://accessphysiotherapy.com. Copyright © The McGraw-Hill Companies, Inc. All rights reserved.)

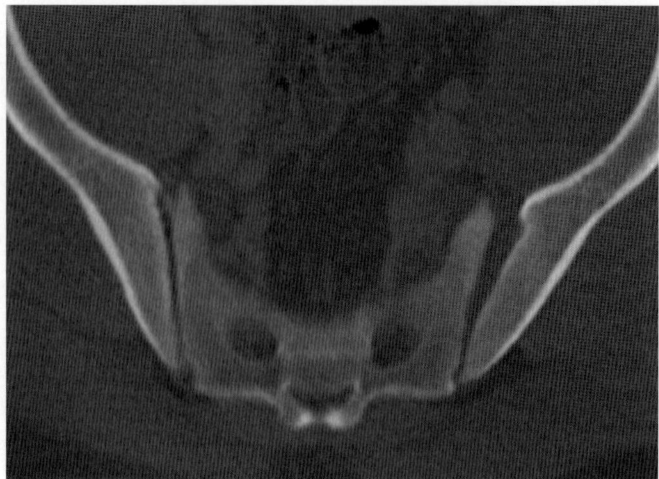

FIGURE 277-3 This axial CT image reveals diastasis of a sacroiliac joint subsequent to trauma. (From Malone TR, Hazle C, Grey ML. *Imaging in Rehabilitation*. http://accessphysiotherapy.com. Copyright © The McGraw-Hill Companies, Inc. All rights reserved.)

KEY FEATURES

Description

- Pubic symphysis pain
- Pain in the groin
- Pain in the perineum
- Pain often increases with weight bearing, sitting, sidelying, transitional movements, and palpation of pubic symphysis
- Pain may radiate to the anterior or upper thigh

Essentials of Diagnosis

- Usually associated with excessive movement of the pubic symphysis
- Difficulty with hip adduction and hip abduction
- Waddling gait
- MRI, X-ray, ultrasound

General Considerations

- Pubic symphysis joint capable of undergoing anatomical changes during pregnancy[2]
- Consider other pelvic girdle joints including sacroiliac (SI) joint involvement, sacrococcygeal joint
- Athletic injuries
- Rule out injury to hip including labral tear
- Chronic condition may result in osteitis pubis: Arthritis of the pubic symphysis joint

Demographics

- May occur during pregnancy, during delivery, or postpartum.
- 1 women in 569 deliveries[3] sustained a pubic symphysis injury.
- Estimated incidence of pubic symphysis separation during delivery is 1 in 300 to 1 in 30,000 pregnancies.

CLINICAL FINDINGS

SIGNS AND SYMPTOMS

- Pain in the groin
- Pain with weight bearing especially on one leg
- Pain in the sitting position
- Pain with transition from sitting to standing
- Pain with standing, walking, forward flexion
- Pain may radiate to the anterior or upper thigh
- Increased pain during menstruation

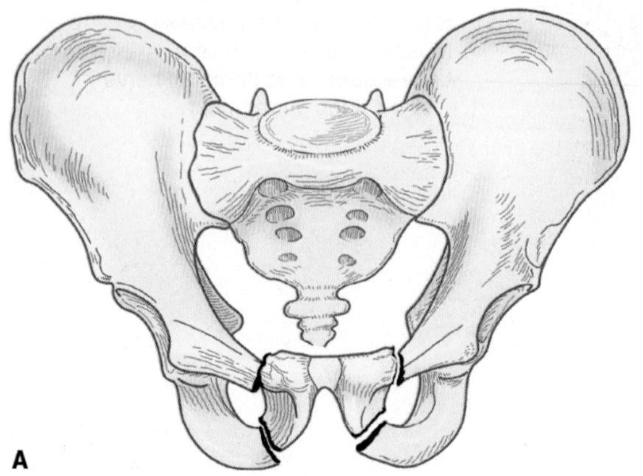

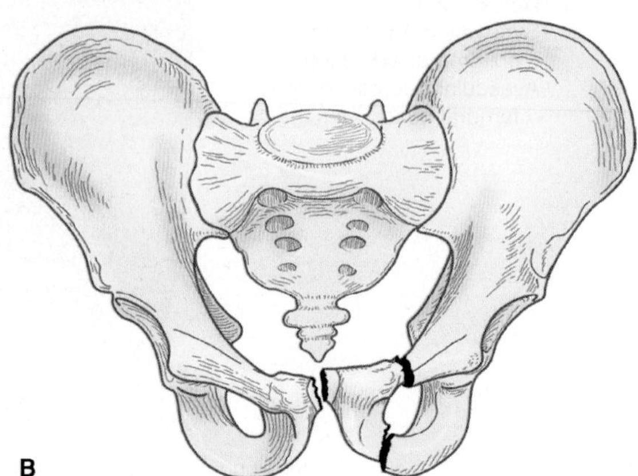

FIGURE 277-4 Straddle injuries. (**A**) Bilateral pubic rami fractures. (**B**) Pubic rami fractures and symphysis pubis disruption. (From Simon RR, Sherman SC. *Emergency Orthopedics*. 6th ed. www.accessemergencymedicine.com. Copyright © The McGraw-Hill Companies, Inc. All rights reserved.)

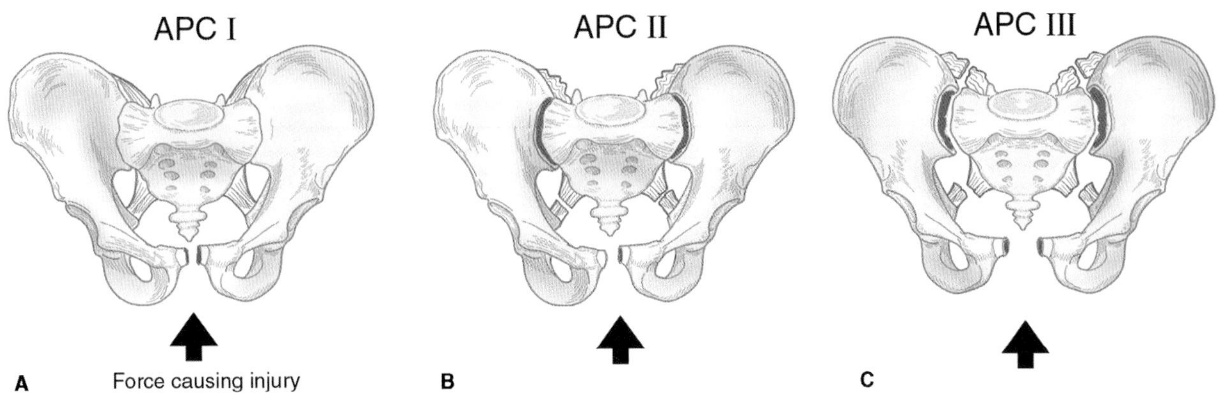

FIGURE 277-5 Anteroposterior compression injuries. (**A**) APC I injury pattern. The ligaments of the pelvic floor and SI joint remain intact while the symphysis pubis ligaments are injured. Separation of the pubic bones >2.5 cm on imaging suggests more significant injury. (**B**) APC II injury pattern. Ligaments of the symphysis pubis and anterior SI joint are disrupted. This injury will result in a pelvis that "opens like a book." (**C**) APC III injury pattern. In this injury, the pelvis is both rotationally and vertically unstable due to rupture of all of the ligaments of the symphysis pubis and SI joint. (From Simon RR, Sherman SC. *Emergency Orthopedics*. 6th ed. www.accessemergencymedicine.com. Copyright © The McGraw-Hill Companies, Inc. All rights reserved.)

- Inflammation
- Poor sitting posture
- Frequent shifts in sitting position, sitting down carefully
- Symptoms are more likely if there is more than 10 mm horizontal and 5 mm vertical separation of the pubic bones[4]

Functional Implications

- Pubic pain with single leg stance
- Difficulty sitting, side lying
- Impacting ability to walk, perform work and daily activities
- Painful sexual intercourse

Possible Contributing Causes

- Stretch or rupture of pubic symphysis ligaments
- Vaginal delivery
  - Forceps delivery
  - Fetal shoulder dystocia; McRoberts maneuver during vaginal delivery[5]
- Postpartum
- Maternal hip dysplasia
- Direct trauma from fracture, fall, childbirth
- Athletic injury
- Neoplasm
- Pelvic asymmetry
- Soft tissue damage

Differential Diagnosis

- Hip labral injury or tear
- SI joint pain
- Urinary tract infection
- Braxton Hicks contractions
- Herniated disc
- Osteitis pubis: Arthritis of the joint

MEANS OF CONFIRMATION OR DIAGNOSIS

Imaging

- X-ray of pelvis
- MRI
- Ultrasound imaging to measure joint separation

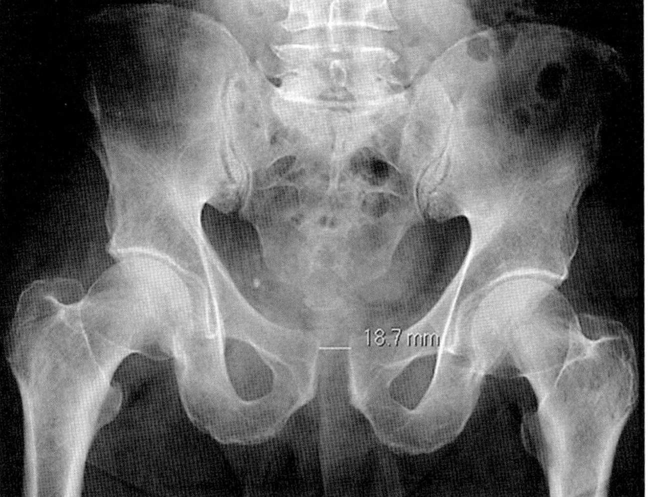

A

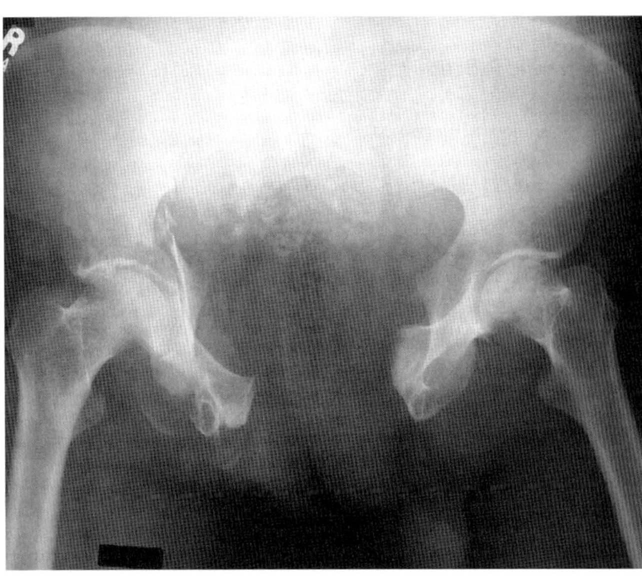

B

FIGURE 277-6 (**A**) Symphysis pubis diastasis (APC I injury). (**B**) "Open book" injury. (From Simon RR, Sherman SC. *Emergency Orthopedics*. 6th ed. www.accessemergencymedicine.com. Copyright © The McGraw-Hill Companies, Inc. All rights reserved.)

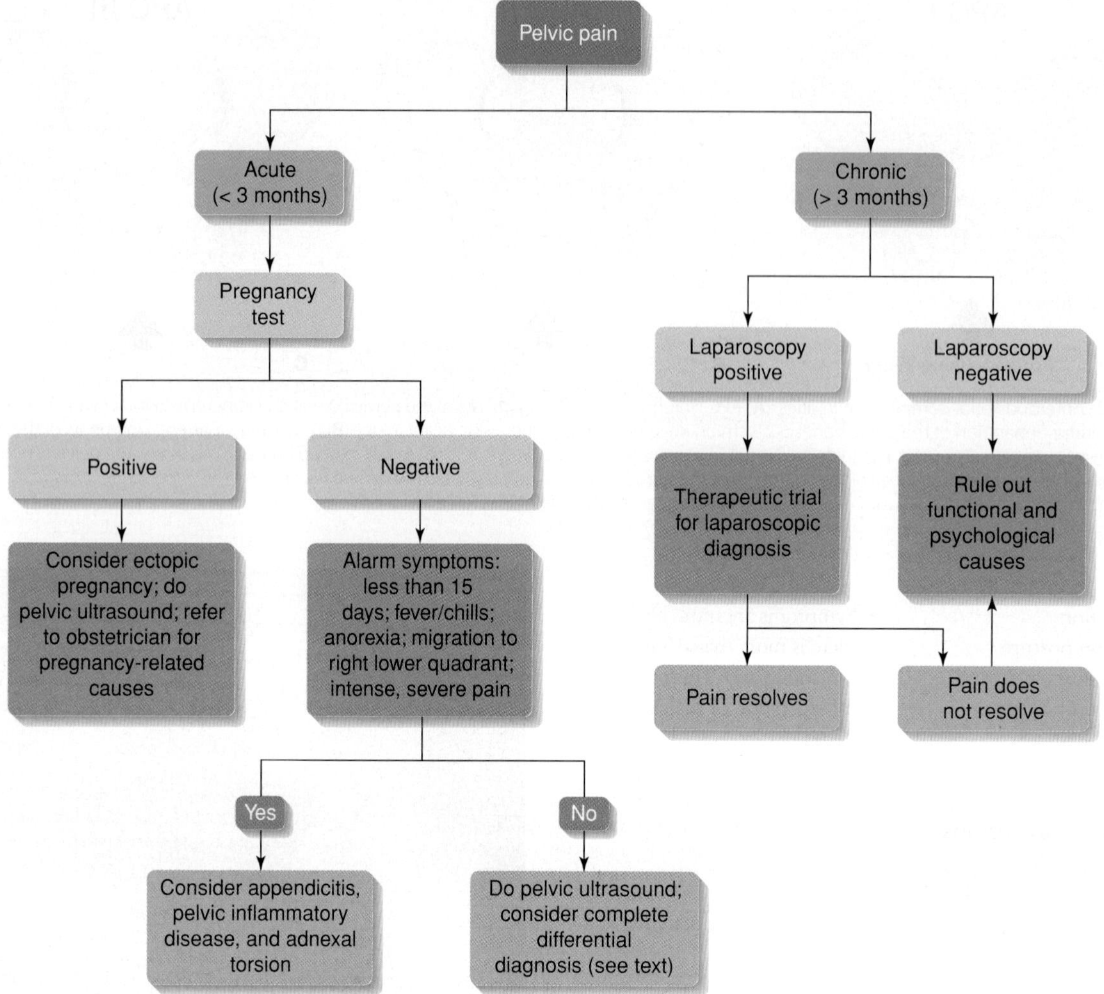

FIGURE 277-7 Diagnostic approach: Pelvic pain. (From Henderson MC, Tierney LM, Smetana GW. *The Patient History: An Evidence-Based Approach to Differential Diagnosis*. www.accessmedicine.com. Copyright © The McGraw-Hill Companies, Inc. All rights reserved.)

Diagnostic Procedures

- Physical examination
- Diagnostic joint injection

FINDINGS AND INTERPRETATION

- Pubic symphysis joint is capable of undergoing anatomical changes during pregnancy including widening of the interpubic gap, increased mobility, thickening of ligaments, and the appearance of gas in the joint.[2]

TREATMENT

Conservative

- Binder or sacroiliac belt

Medications

- Muscle relaxants
- Oral analgesics
- Oral corticosteroids

MEDICAL PROCEDURES

- Surgical: External fixation
- Corticosteroid injection
- Local anesthetic injection
- Trigger point injections

REFERRALS/ADMITTANCE

- To pelvic floor physical therapist; Women's Health Certified Specialist
- To orthopedist
- To physical medicine and rehabilitation
- To pain management
- To acupuncturist
- To pain psychologist

IMPAIRMENTS

- Pain; pubic symphysis, groin, adductor muscles, anterior thigh
- Gait disturbance
- Pelvic floor muscle dysfunction
- Poor posture
- Abnormal joint mobility
- Urinary symptoms: Urgency, frequency, incontinence

TESTS AND MEASURES

- Posture assessment
- Pubic symphysis palpation test
- Active straight-leg raise test for load transfer
- Assessment of pelvic girdle with pain provocation test
- Assessment of hip joint
- Assessment of pelvic floor muscle function
- Assessment of gait

INTERVENTION

- Postural instruction
- Pelvic belt, sacroiliac belt
- Manual therapy
  - Joint mobilizations
  - Connective tissue, myofascial treatment
- Gait training
  - Reduce step length, minimize hip flexion
  - Assistive devices: Crutches, walker
- Pelvic floor muscle exercise and training
  - Contraction
  - Relaxation, "bulging"
  - Motor control: Timing, coordination
  - Endurance
  - Power
- Surface electromyography (sEMG) biofeedback for training pelvic floor muscles
- Exercises to improve biomechanical loading of pelvic girdle joints
- Core stabilization exercises
- Symmetrical lower-extremity positioning during body mechanics

FUNCTIONAL GOALS

- Patient will be able to
  - Demonstrate proper posture to reduce pain and prevent reinjury perform sit-to-stand transfers independently without increased pain.
  - Increase sitting tolerance to ____ minutes to be able to drive, ride in car, perform desk work.
  - Demonstrate independence with home exercise program, promoting strength, relaxation, and awareness of pelvic floor muscle for long-term self-management.

PROGNOSIS

- Pubic symphysis injury is associated with sacroiliac joint pain.
- Pregnant women with a symphyseal width or more than 9.5 mm experience pain.[4]
- Pubic symphysis injury may increase the risk of development of osteitis pubis[6] and adductor tendinopathy.

PATIENT RESOURCE

- Pelvic Instability Network Scotland (PINS). http://www.pelvicinstability.org.uk/. Accessed July 9, 2013.

REFERENCES

1. The American Physical Therapy Association. *Interactive Guide to Physical Therapist Practice*. Alexandria, VA: The American Physical Therapy Association; 2003. http://guidetoptpractice.apta.org/. Accessed July 6, 2013.
2. Becker I, Woodley SJ, Stringer Mark D. The Adult Human pubic symphysis: a systematic review. *J Anat*. 2010;217(5):475–487.
3. Snow RE, Neubert AG. Peripartum pubic symphysis separation: a case series and review of the literature. *Obstet Gynecol Surv*. 1997;52(7):438–443.
4. Björklund K, Nordström M-L, Bergström S. Sonographic assessment of symphyseal joint distention during pregnancy and post partum with special reference to pelvic pain. *Acta Obstet Gynecol Scand*. 1999;78:125–130.
5. Kharrazi FD, Rodgers WB, Kennedy JG, Lhowe DS. Parturition induced pelvic dislocation: a report of four cases. *J Orthop Trauma*. 1997;11(4):277–281.
6. Webb CA, Jiminez ML. What is your diagnosis? Osteitis pubis. *JAAPA*. 2008;21(12):68.

ADDITIONAL REFERENCES

- Dutton M. Pathology, gynecology, and psychology. In: Dutton M, ed. *McGraw-Hill's NPTE (National Physical Therapy Examination)*. 2nd ed. New York, NY: McGraw-Hill; 2012. http://www.accessphysiotherapy.com/content/5402528. Accessed July 9, 2013.
- Dutton M. The sacroiliac joint. In: Dutton M, ed. *Dutton's Orthopaedic Examination, Evaluation, and Intervention*. 3rd ed. New York, NY: McGraw-Hill; 2012. http://www.accessphysiotherapy.com/content/55598142. Accessed July 9, 2013.
- ICD9Data.com. http://www.icd9data.com. Accessed July 9, 2013.
- ICD10Data.com. http://www.icd10data.com. Accessed July 9, 2013.
- Simon RR, Sherman SC. Pelvis. In: Simon RR, Sherman SC, eds. *Emergency Orthopedics*. 6th ed. New York, NY: McGraw-Hill; 2011. http://www.accessphysiotherapy.com/content/7706610. Accessed July 9, 2013.

278 PUDENDAL NEURALGIA

Cynthia E. Neville, DPT, PT, WCS

CONDITION/DISORDER SYNONYMS

- Pelvic pain
- Pudendal neuropathy (PN)
- Pudendal nerve entrapment (PNE)

ICD-9-CM CODE

- 353.8 Other nerve root and plexus disorder

ICD-10-CM CODES

- G54.8 Other nerve root and plexus disorders
- R10.2 Pelvic and perineal pain

PREFERRED PRACTICE PATTERN

- 5F: Impaired Peripheral Nerve Integrity and Muscle Performance Associated With Peripheral Nerve Injury[1]

PATIENT PRESENTATION

A 56-year-old woman reports that she has been experiencing burning pain, tingling, and vibration sensations in the vaginal area. Pain is worse when she is sitting. Sometimes it feels like her tailbone hurts. Symptoms began after she completed a150 mile bicycle ride for charity.

KEY FEATURES

Description

- Pain, burning, numbness, paresthesia in the gluteal, perineal, and/or genital area
- Entrapment and injury to the pudendal nerve in Alcock canal
- Alcock canal (musculo-osteo-aponeurotic tunnel) between sacrotuberous and sacrospinous ligaments, in the absence of organic disease

Essentials of Diagnosis

- "Nantes Criteria"[2]
  - Pain should be limited to the innervation territory of the pudendal nerve.
  - Excludes any pain that is limited to the coccygeal, pelvic, or gluteal areas.
  - Pain is predominantly experienced while sitting.
  - Pain rarely awakens the patient at night.
  - No objective sensory impairment can be found even in the presence of paresthesia on clinical examination.
    - Presence of a sensory defect should prompt investigations to exclude diseases of the sacral nerve roots and the cauda equina.

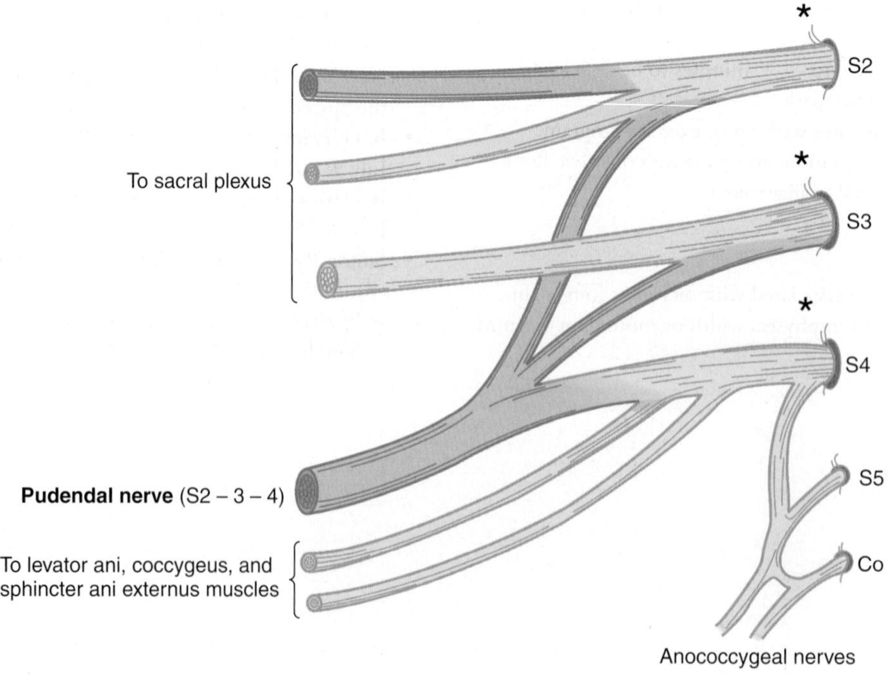

FIGURE 278-1 The pudendal and coccygeal plexuses. (From Waxman SG. *Clinical Neuroanatomy*. 26th ed. www.accessmedicine.com. Copyright © The McGraw-Hill Companies, Inc. All rights reserved.)

   - Pain should be relieved by anesthetic infiltration of the pudendal nerve.
     - This is an essential criterion, but it lacks specificity as pain related to any perineal disease may be relieved by pudendal nerve block.

General Considerations

- Frequently misdiagnosed
- Chronic pain condition
- Urogenital pain disorders are frequently associated with pain and other musculoskeletal impairments in nearby body areas; especially back, pelvic, hip, groin regions

Demographics[3]

- Few epidemiologic data found in the literature
- Mean time to diagnosis is 4 years, ranging from 1 to 15 years
- More prevalent in women; 7 of 10 patients are women

CLINICAL FINDINGS

SIGNS AND SYMPTOMS[3]

- Pain along pudendal nerve distribution
  - Perineal
  - Scrotal/testicular
  - Perianal
  - Suprapubic
  - Pain with ejaculation
  - Pain elicited with pressing along the course of the nerve
- Pain aggravated by sitting, stair climbing
- Pain relieved by standing or lying and with sitting on toilet
- Associated symptoms
  - Voiding dysfunction: Urinary hesitancy, frequency, urgency, obstructive voiding, painful voiding
  - Obstructive defecation: Difficult and painful bowel movements
  - Sexual dysfunction: Painful orgasms, persistent sexual arousal, erectile dysfunction
    - Autonomic dysfunction : Sensation of dryness, itching, sweating

Functional Implications

- Difficulty sitting for prolonged periods
- Sexual dysfunction
  - May lead to unwanted sexual abstinence
- Difficulty with urination and defecation
- Pain during voiding
- Decreased tolerance for exercise
- Inability to work or attend school
- Inability to maintain relationships

Possible Contributing Causes

- Mechanical pudendal nerve: Compression, tension, direct trauma
  - Identifiable trauma in athletes 15 to 25 years old
    - Cycling, weight lifting
    - Sitting: Job, long travel
- PFM dysfunction: TrP, connective tissue restriction
  - Myofascial entrapment along the course of the nerve
    - Sacrospinous and sacrotuberous ligaments
    - Alcock/pudendal canal
- Surgery: Multiple case reports in the literature of new onset ("de-novo") PN following surgeries for urinary incontinence
- Sacral iliac dysfunction
- Pelvic radiation
- Visceral: Noxious stimuli from viscera bombard peripheral nociceptors leading to central sensitization
  - Visceral disease: Endometriosis, gastrointestinal disease
  - Neurological: Sacral nerve root compression may fixate the pudendal nerve causing stretch

Differential Diagnosis

- Urinary tract infection (UTI)
- Sexually transmitted disease
- Urethritis
- Bladder infection
- Yeast infection
- Bacterial vaginosis
- Fungal infection
  - Lichen sclerosis
  - Lichen planus
- Organ dysfunction from cancer or malignancy
- Nonmalignant tumor in abdomen or organs
- Gynecologic problems in females
  - Endometriosis
  - Menses
  - Ectopic pregnancy
  - Ovarian cyst
  - Fibroids
  - Menopause
- Prostatitis
- Pelvic inflammatory disease

MEANS OF CONFIRMATION OR DIAGNOSIS

- See Nantes Criteria above

Laboratory Tests

- To rule out other pathology
  - Blood tests to rule out pathology
  - Urine culture/urinalysis to rule out infection
  - H&H for signs of bleeding, anemia, pathogens, immune status, vitamin deficiencies, white blood cell count

Imaging

- MRI

Diagnostic Procedures

- Pudendal nerve latency testing: Reliability is questionable
- Staged sacral reflex testing
- Diagnostic block: Pudendal nerve block

FINDINGS AND INTERPRETATION

- MRI and other imaging tests are usually normal
- Abnormal electrophysiological test

TREATMENT

Medication

- NSAIDs
- Opiods
- Topical medications
  - Gabapentin

    - Lidocaine ointment 5%
    - Nitroglycerine
  - Oral medications
    - Anticonvulsants: Pregabalin
    - Tricyclic antidepressants: Amitriptyline

MEDICAL PROCEDURES

- Nerve blocks
- Injections
  - Botulism toxin injections
  - Trigger point injections
- Implanted electrical stimulator for neuromodulation (InterStim)
- Surgery
  - Decompression surgery
    - Trans-perineal
    - Trans-ischial-rectal
    - Trans-gluteal

REFERRALS/ADMITTANCE

- Acupuncture
- Biofeedback practitioner
- Certified sex therapist
- Cognitive behavioral pain psychologist
- Gynecologists
- Gastroenterologist
- Pain medicine
- Pelvic floor physical therapist
- Physical medicine and rehabilitation physicians
- Primary care physicians
- Urogynecologists
- Urologists

IMPAIRMENTS

- Adverse neural tension
- Pelvic floor muscle (PFM) dysfunction
  - Overactive
  - Underactive
  - Nonrelaxing
  - Noncontracting
- Depression and anxiety
- Incontinence
- Myofascial pelvic pain
- Decreased sexual appreciation; anorgasmia: Inability to achieve orgasm
- Pain
- Muscle atrophy
- Muscle hypertonicity
- Joint hypomobility
- Posture dysfunction
- Contractures of soft tissue (fascia, muscle), connective tissue restrictions
- Obstructed defecation

TESTS AND MEASURES

- Positive (+) Tinel sign on palpation of the nerve: Distal parasthesia in the distribution of a nerve that is elicited by percussion over the site of compression
- Skin assessments: Subcutaneous panniculus—skin changes associated with autonomic dysfunction: Red blotchy, peau d'orange
- PFM examination: Via vagina or anorectum
- Abdominal muscle test
- Abdominal wall palpation: Diastalsis rectus abdominis, scar
- sEMG biofeedback assessment of the PFMs and abdominal muscles
- Pressure manometry of the PFMs
- Lumbar spine, pelvic girdle, and hip joint examination procedures

INTERVENTION

- PFM exercises/training
  - "Kegel" exercises: Another name for PFM exercises
  - Contraction
  - Relaxation/"Bulging"
  - Motor control
  - Endurance
  - Power
  - sEMG biofeedback
- Progressive vaginal dilation
- TENS
- NMES
- Pressure manometry
- Manual therapy
  - Thiele's massage performed vaginally
  - Myofascial release
  - Internal vaginal massage
- Thermal modalities
- US imaging to awareness of muscle contractions
- Posture reeducation
- Patient education regarding effects of maladaptive pain cognitions

FUNCTIONAL GOALS

- Patient will be able to
  - Verbalize strategies for independent pain management.
  - Increase tolerance to sitting from ___ minutes to ___ minutes.
  - Demonstrate independence with long-term therapeutic exercise program.

PROGNOSIS

- Long-term treatment success is about 50%.[4]
- Longer duration and greater intensity of pain symptoms negatively impacts prognosis.
- Psychological factors such as pain catastrophizing and fear avoidance negatively impact prognosis.

PATIENT RESOURCES

- International Pelvic Pain Society. http://www.pelvicpain.org. Accessed July 3, 2013.
- The role of physical therapy in the treatment of pudendal neuralgia. The International Pelvic Pain Society. http://www.pelvicpain.org/news/pdfs/vol15_no2.pdf. Accessed July 3, 2013.

REFERENCES

1. The American Physical Therapy Association. Pattern 4C: impaired muscle performance. In: *Guide to Physical Therapist Practice*. Alexandria, VA: The American Physical Therapy Association; 2003. http://guidetoptpractice.apta.org/content/1/SEC10.extract?sid=9af82a7e-5fc3-41d2-86ab-b8336a9655e9. Accessed July 3, 2013.

2. Labat JJ, Riant T, Robert R, Amarenco G, Lefaucheur JP, Rigaud J. Diagnostic criteria for pudendal neuralgia by pudendal nerve entrapment (Nantes criteria). *Neurourol Urodyn*. 2008;27:306–310.
3. Itza Santos F, Salinas J, Zarza D, Gómez Sancha F, Allona Almagro A. [Update in pudendal nerve entrapment syndrome: an approach anatomic-surgical, diagnostic and therapeutic]. *Actas Urol Esp*. 2010;34(6):500–509.
4. Benson JT, Griffis K. Pudendal neuralgia: a severe pain syndrome. *Am J Obstet Gynecol*. 2005;192:1663–1668.

ADDITIONAL REFERENCES

- Alappattu MJ, Bishop MD. Psychological factors in chronic pelvic pain in women: relevance and application of the fear-avoidance model of pain. *Phys Ther*. 2011;91(10):1542–1550.
- Dutton M. Genitourinary system disorders. In: Dutton M, ed. *McGraw-Hill's NPTE (National Physical Therapy Examination)*. 2nd ed. New York, NY: McGraw-Hill; 2012. http://www.accessphysiotherapy.com/content/5402307. Accessed July 3, 2013.
- Dutton M. Gynecologic disorders. In: Dutton M, ed. *Dutton's Orthopaedic Examination, Evaluation, and Intervention*. 3rd ed. New York, NY: McGraw-Hill; 2012. http://www.accessphysiotherapy.com/content/5547556. Accessed July 3, 2013.
- Fall M, Baranowski AP, Elneil S, et al. EAU guidelines on chronic pelvic pain. *Eur Urol*. 2010;57(1):35–48.
- Neville C. Pelvic floor treatment: urinary incontinence and pelvic floor muscle training [Video]. New York, NY: McGraw-Hill; 2014. http://www.accessphysiotherapy.com. Accessed June 13, 2014.
- *Relieving Pain in America*. The National Academies Press. http://www.nap.edu/catalog.php?record_id=13172. Accessed July 3, 2013.

279 STRESS URINARY INCONTINENCE

Cynthia E. Neville, DPT, PT, WCS

CONDITION/DISORDER SYNONYM

- Genuine stress incontinence (GSI)

ICD-9-CM CODES

- 623.9 Female stress urinary incontinence
- 788.30 Urinary incontinence, unspecified
- 788.32 Incontinence without sensory awareness
- 788.39 Other urinary incontinence

ICD-10-CM CODES

- N39.3 Stress incontinence (female) (male)
- N39.42 Incontinence without sensory awareness
- N39.49 Other specified urinary incontinence
- R32 Unspecified urinary incontinence

PREFERRED PRACTICE PATTERN

- 4C: Impaired Muscle Performance[1]

PATIENT PRESENTATION

A 30-year-old woman had her third baby by vaginal delivery 2 years ago. She has recently started exercising again. She used to run 5 miles, 3 days per week. She notices now that after running 1 mile she leaks urine and wets her underpants. The other day, she was laughing with her friend and wet her underpants. The worse symptom was last week when she leaked urine during intercourse with her husband.

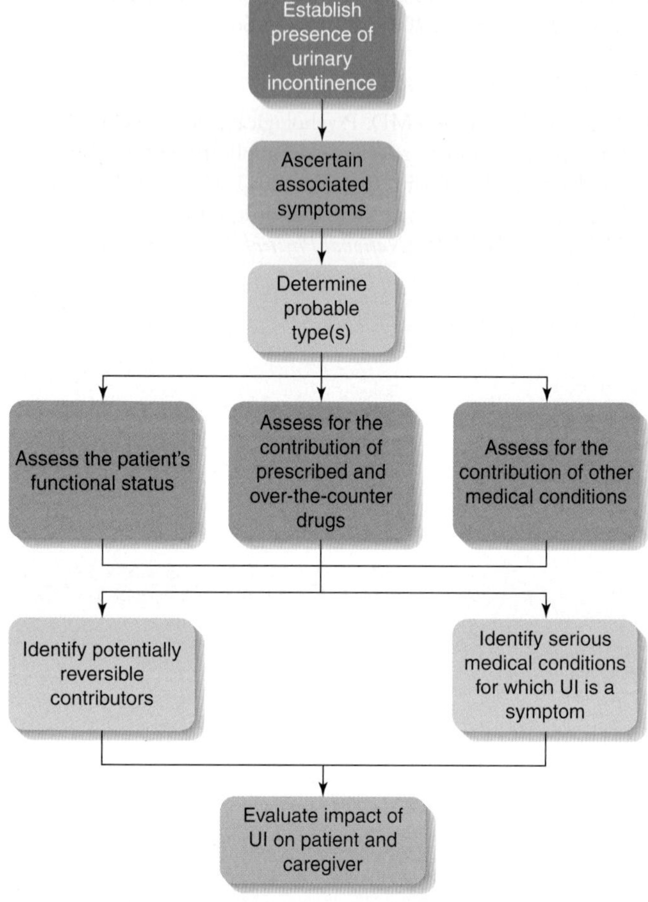

FIGURE 279-1 Diagnostic approach to the patient with urinary incontinence (UI). (From Henderson MC, Tierney LM, Smetana GW. *The Patient History: An Evidence-Based Approach to Differential Diagnosis*. www.accessmedicine.com. Copyright © The McGraw-Hill Companies, Inc. All rights reserved.)

KEY FEATURES

Description

- Involuntary loss of urine control occurring during an increase in intra-abdominal pressure
- Urinary sphincter muscles are not able to prevent urine flow during an episode of intra-abdominal pressure

Essentials of Diagnosis

- Urinary stress test or "cough" test

General Considerations

- Consideration of lower urinary tract infections (UTIs)
  - Sudden onset of symptoms
  - Urinary frequency
  - Urinary urgency
  - Lower back pain
- Myogenic dysfunction of the detrusor

Demographics

- Urinary incontinence affects 30% to 60% of middle-aged and older women and 22% of men.[2–4]
- Urinary incontinence reported by 78% of women with low back pain.[5]
- Severe urinary incontinence is more prevalent in later years.
- 30% to 52% of homebound elderly suffer from urinary incontinence.[6]

CLINICAL FINDINGS

SIGNS AND SYMPTOMS

- Loss of urine without meaning to urinate during activities where there is an increase in intra-abdominal pressure (including sexual intercourse)
  - Coughing
  - Sneezing
  - Laughing

- Loss of a small amount of urine preceded by an increase in intra-abdominal pressure but without a sensation of urge to urinate

Functional Implications

- May lead to use of pads and/or wearing of diapers

Possible Contributing Causes

- Underactive, overactive, or nonfunctioning pelvic floor muscles (PFMs)
- Pelvic organ prolapse
- Urethral hypermobility
- Intrinsic sphincter deficiency
- Bladder cancer
- Bladder inflammation
- Bladder stones
- Benign prostatic hypertrophy (BPH)
- Comorbidities such as diabetes, stroke, hip replacement
- UTIs: Bacterial
- Reduction of maximal urethral closure pressure

Differential Diagnosis

- Spinal cord injury
- Multiple sclerosis
- Prostatitis
- UTI

MEANS OF CONFIRMATION OR DIAGNOSIS

Imaging

- Ultrasound imaging to identify abnormalities
  - Bladder
  - Urethra
  - Pelvis
  - Bladder neck position and mobility
  - Pelvic floor function
  - Activity of levator ani
  - Descent of pelvic organs
  - Sphincter integrity
- MRI to examine soft tissue structures of the pelvic support apparatus
- Pelvic/abdominal ultrasound
  - Measure bladder capacity
  - Rule out other pathologies

Diagnostic Procedures

- Rule out UTI
- Postvoid residual volume (PVR): Measures the amount of urine left after urinating
- Urodynamics: Functional study of the lower urinary tract
  - Indications include: Unclear cause of voiding dysfunction, incontinence unresponsive to conservative treatment, history of hysterectomy, bladder surgeries or pelvic organ prolapse procedures, neurological conditions
  - Assess sphincter competency
- Three Incontinence Questions (3IQ)
  - Sensitivity of 0.86
  - Specificity of 0.60[7]
- Urethral Pressure Profile: Study of intraluminal pressure along the length of the urethra via pressure sensitive catheter

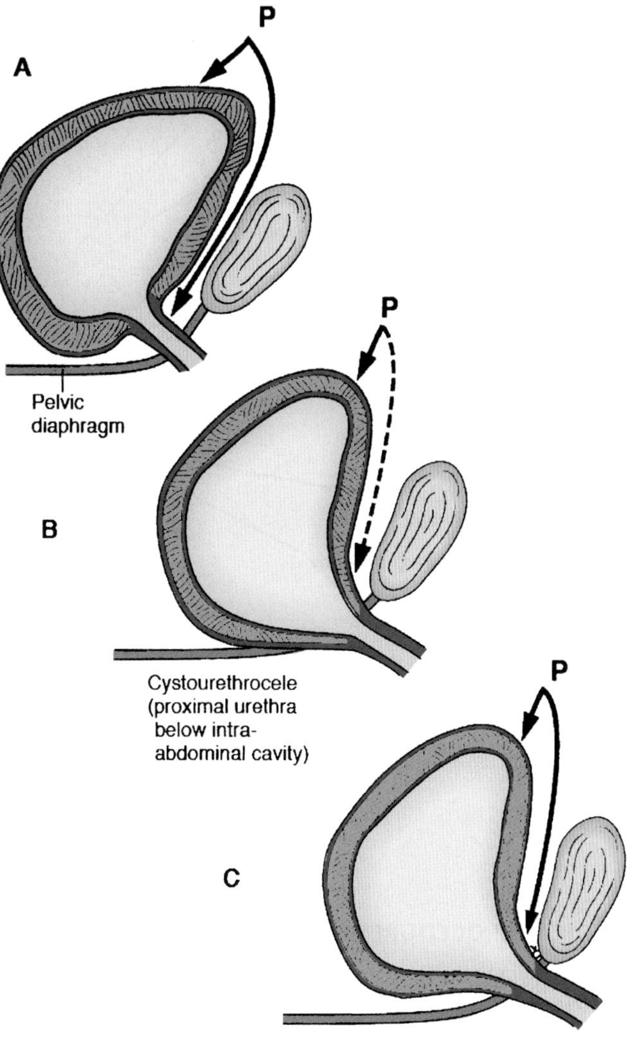

FIGURE 279-2 Bladder position: normal, genuine stress urinary incontinence, and after urethropexy**.** Normally, a Valsalva maneuver causes the increased intra-abdominal pressure *(P)* to be transmitted equally to the bladder and urethra (**A**). With genuine stress urinary incontinence, the proximal urethra has fallen outside the abdominal cavity (**B**) so that the intra-abdominal pressure no longer is transferred to the proximal urethra, leading to incontinence. After urethropexy (**C**), pressure is again transmitted to the urethra. (From Toy EC, Baker B, Ross PJ, Jennings JC.. *Case Files: Obstetrics and Gynecology*. 3rd ed. www.accessmedicine.com. Copyright © The McGraw-Hill Companies, Inc. All rights reserved.)

- Leak point pressure profile: Dynamic study of urethral pressure during activity

FINDINGS AND INTERPRETATION

- Leak during Valsalva maneuver or cough during urodynamic testing without elevation in detrusor pressure is indicative of stress incontinence
- On the 3IQ, a positive likelihood ratio of 2.13 for the classification of stress urinary incontinence (SUI)[7]

TREATMENT

Medication

- Antibiotics if infection exists
- Tricyclic antidepressants to affect smooth muscles of the bladder
- Estrogen to improve tone of urethral and vaginal tissues

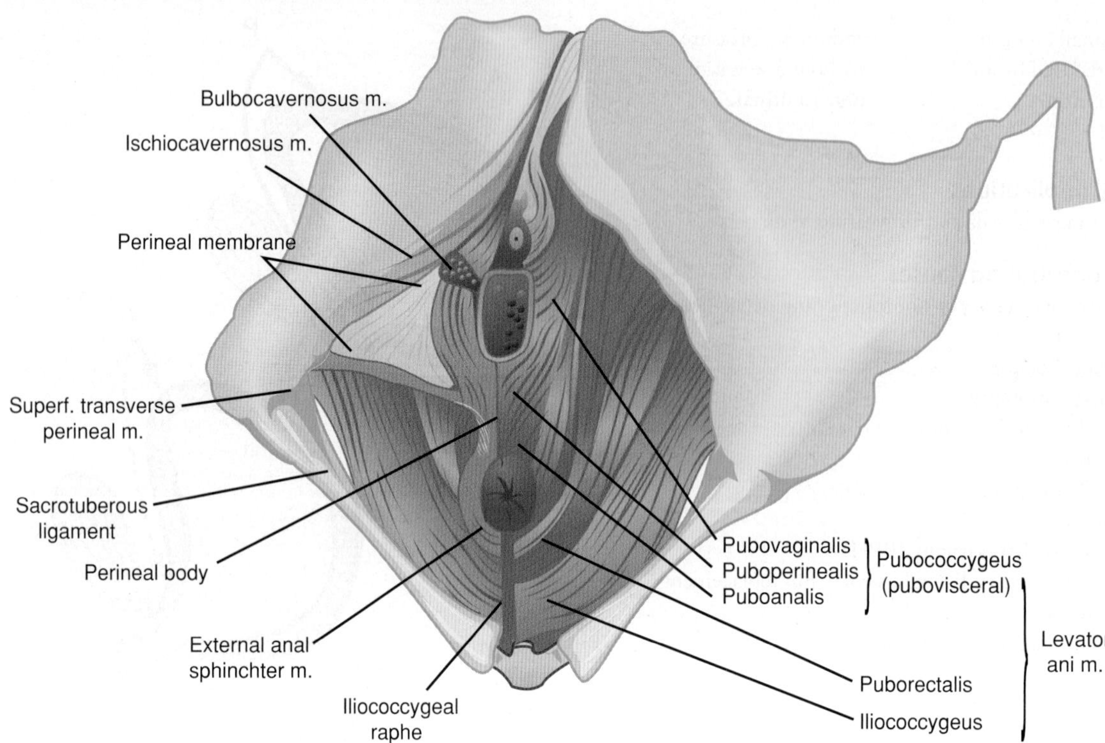

FIGURE 279-3 Anatomy of pelvic support. (From Schorge JO, Williams JW. *Williams Gynecology*. McGraw-Hill Medical; 2008:Figure 38-8.)

MEDICAL PROCEDURES

- Vaginal sling procedures, tension-free vaginal tape
  - Sling is placed that supports the urethra
- Anterior vaginal repair or paravaginal repair procedures
  - To repair support structures of the bladder
  - Performed in women when the bladder is bulging into the vagina (called a cystocele)
  - Performed through a surgical cut in the vagina
  - A paravaginal repair is done through a surgical cut in the vagina or abdomen
- Artificial urinary sphincter is a surgical device used to treat stress incontinence mainly in men (rarely in women)
- Collagen injections make the area around the urethra thicker, which helps control urine leakage
- Male sling is a newer procedure that can be done in certain men
  - Easier to do than placing an artificial urinary sphincter
- Retropubic suspensions are a group of surgical procedures done to lift the bladder and urethra, performed through a surgical cut in the abdomen

REFERRALS/ADMITTANCE

- Primary care physicians
- Gynecologists
  - Women: Pelvic examination
- Urologists
  - Men: Genital examination
- Urogynecologists
- Acupuncture
- Pelvic floor physical therapist

IMPAIRMENTS

- PFM dysfunction
  - Overactive
  - Underactive
  - Nonrelaxing
  - Noncontracting
- Incontinence
- Pelvic pain
- Pelvic organ prolapse
- Decreased sexual appreciation
- Anorgasmia
  - Inability to achieve orgasm

TESTS AND MEASURES

- Urinary stress test or "cough" test
  - Stand with a full bladder and cough
  - Test does not have good reliability or validity
  - Test is not specific enough to rule in/out a diagnosis
- PFM examination and assessment
- Bladder diary to assess patient's behaviors related to
  - Micturition including fluid and food intake
  - Voiding habits
  - Episodes of leakage (activity-related or urge-related)
  - Use of pads
- sEMG biofeedback assessment of the PFMs
- Pressure manometry of the PFMs
- Inquiry: During last 3 months did you leak urine during coughing, sneezing, or physical activity?

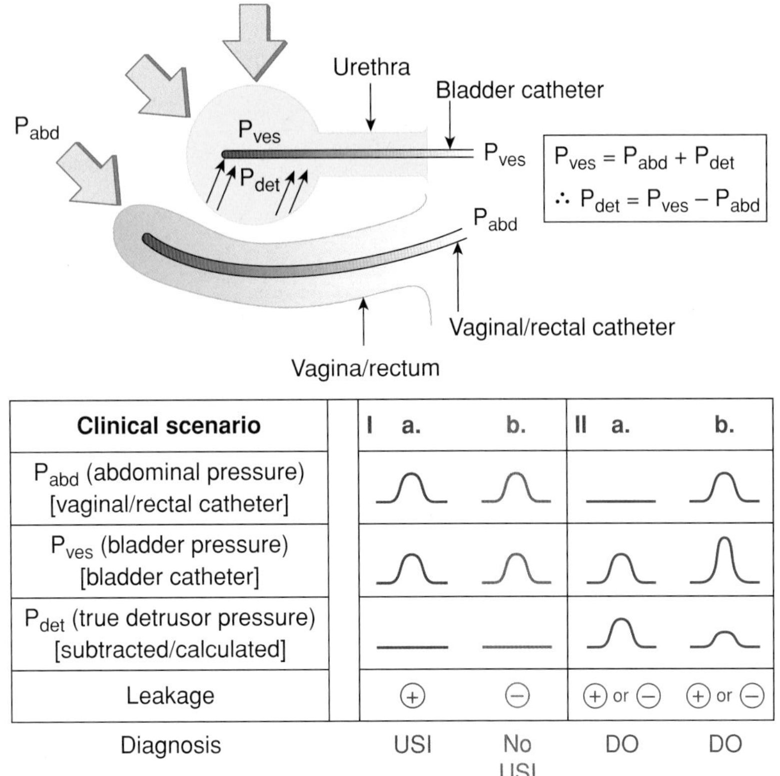

Clinical scenario	I a.	b.	II a.	b.
P_{abd} (abdominal pressure) [vaginal/rectal catheter]				
P_{ves} (bladder pressure) [bladder catheter]				
P_{det} (true detrusor pressure) [subtracted/calculated]				
Leakage	⊕	⊖	⊕ or ⊖	⊕ or ⊖
Diagnosis	USI	No USI	DO	DO

FIGURE 279-4 Interpretation of multichannel urodynamic evaluation: cystometrogram. A catheter is placed in the bladder to determine the pressure generated within it (P_{ves}). The pressure in the bladder is produced from a combination of the pressure from the abdominal cavity and the pressure generated by the detrusor muscle of the bladder. Bladder pressure (P_{ves}) = pressure in abdominal cavity (P_{abd}) + detrusor pressure (P_{det}). A second catheter is placed in the vagina (or rectum if advanced-stage prolapse is present) to determine the pressure in the abdominal cavity (P_{abd}). As room-temperature saline is instilled into the bladder, the patient is asked to cough every 50 mL and the external urethral meatus is observed for leakage of urine around the catheter. The volume at first desire to void and the bladder capacity is recorded. Additionally, the detrusor pressure (P_{det}) channel is observed for positive deflections to determine if there is detrusor activity during testing. The detrusor pressure (P_{det}) cannot be measured directly by any of the catheters. However, from the first equation, we can calculate the detrusor pressure (P_{det}) by subtracting the abdominal pressure (P_{abd}) from the bladder pressure (P_{ves}): Detrusor pressure (P_{det}) = bladder pressure (P_{ves}) – pressure in abdominal cavity (P_{abd}) **I. Urodynamic Stress Incontinence (USI)** Urodynamic stress incontinence is diagnosed when urethral leakage is seen with increased abdominal pressure, in the *absence* of detrusor pressure. **a.** +USI (Column 1): Abdominal pressure is generated with Valsalva maneuver or cough. This pressure is transmitted to the bladder, and a bladder pressure (P_{ves}) is noted. The calculated detrusor pressure is zero. Leakage is observed, and diagnosis of USI is assigned. **b.** No USI (Column 2): Abdominal pressure is generated with Valsalva maneuver or cough. This pressure is transmitted to the bladder, and a bladder pressure (P_{ves}) is noted. The calculated detrusor pressure is zero. Leakage is *not* observed. The patient is *not* diagnosed as having USI. **II. Detrusor Overactivity (DO)** Detrusor overactivity is diagnosed when the patient has involuntary detrusor contractions during testing with or without leakage. **a.** +DO (Column 3): Although no abdominal pressure is observed, a vesicular pressure is noted. A calculated detrusor pressure is recorded and noted to be present. A diagnosis of DO is made regardless of whether leakage is seen. **b.** +DO (Column 4): In this example, an abdominal pressure is observed as well as a vesicular pressure. Using only the P_{abd} and the P_{ves} channels, it is difficult to tell whether or not the detrusor muscle contributed to the pressure generated in the bladder. On subtraction, a calculated detrusor pressure is recorded. Thus, a diagnosis of DO is made, again regardless of whether leakage is seen. In addition to these channels, occasionally a channel to detect electromyographic activity is used. P_{abd}, pressure in abdominal cavity; P_{det}, detrusor pressure (calculated); P_{ves}, bladder pressure. (From Hoffman BL, Schorge J, Schffer J. *Williams Gynecology*. 2nd ed. New York, NY: McGraw-Hill; 2012.)

INTERVENTION

- PFM exercises/training
  - "Kegel" exercises: Another name for PFM exercises
  - Contraction
  - Relaxation/"Bulging"
  - Motor control
  - Endurance
  - Power
  - sEMG biofeedback
  - Weighted vaginal cones to strengthen pelvic floor
    - Hold weighted cone in vagina for up to 15 minutes, 2 times a day
- Neuromuscular electrical stimulation to facilitate PFM contraction
  - SUI protocol
    - Frequency of 35 to 50 Hz, pulse width of 200 to 350 usec, asymmetrical biphasic wave form, duty cycle of 5 to 10 seconds on/5 to 10 seconds off
    - Match on time to patients active home exercise program contraction time
    - Patient may contract PFM while stimulation is on
    - Duration of 10 to 20 minutes, frequency of treatment 1 to 2 times/day, every other day or daily
  - Anal or vaginal electrode/probe
  - Surface electrodes
    - Sacrum
    - Perineum
    - Suprapubic area
    - Tibial nerve

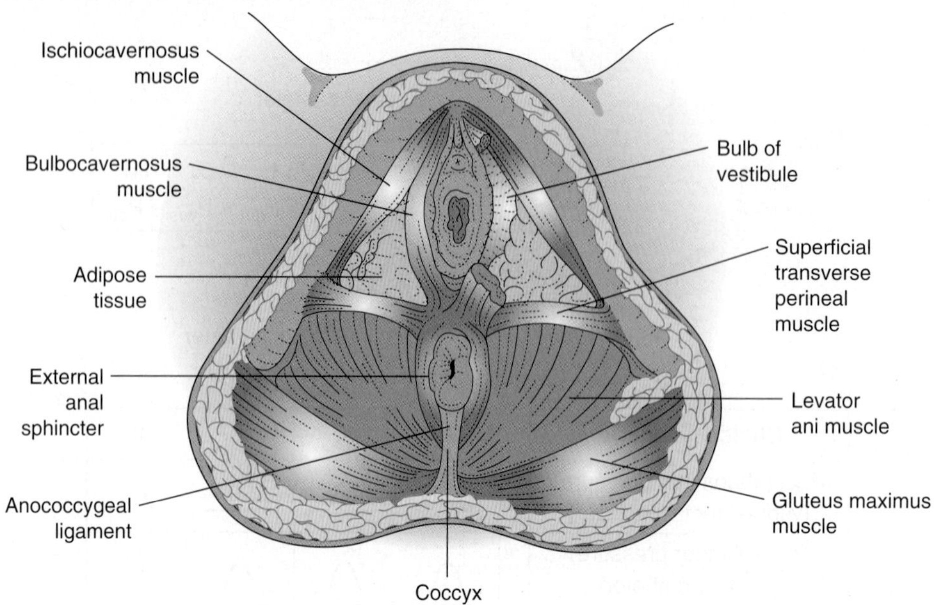

FIGURE 279-5 Pelvic musculature (inferior view). (From DeCherney AH, Nathan L, Goodwin TM, Laufer N, Roman AS. *Current Diagnosis & Treatment: Obstetrics & Gynecology*. 11th ed. www.accessmedicine.com. Copyright © The McGraw-Hill Companies, Inc. All rights reserved.)

- Realtime ultrasound imaging to facilitate learning of correct performance and coordination of abdominal muscle and PFM co-contraction
- Bladder retraining including timed voiding schedule
- Functional training: Precontract the PFM to close the urethra prior to anticipated increase in intra-abdominal pressure; known as "The Knack"
- Patient education
  - Fluid management strategies
  - Drink enough water
    - A little bit of fluid throughout the day
    - 6 to 8 oz glasses of water per day
    - ½ oz fluid per pound of body weight for aging adults
  - Minimize consumption of bladder irritants
    - Caffeine
    - Spicy foods
    - Acidic foods including citrus
- Pressure manometry
- Manual therapy

FUNCTIONAL GOALS

- Patient will be able to
  - Reduce/eliminate leaking during increase in intra-abdominal pressure (cough, sneeze, laugh, transfer, intercourse, etc.).
  - Decrease number of episodes of urinary leakage to improve ability to participate in ADLs from ____ to _____.
  - Decrease number of pads worn per day from ____ to _____.
  - Independence with long-term PFM training program, as appropriate, to manage urinary symptoms.

PROGNOSIS

- A systematic review of 8 clinical trials involving 370 women found that women who underwent PFM training for SUI were 17 times more likely to report cure or improvement compared to women who did not undergo supervised PFM training.[8]
- High cure rates for SUI were shown in single-blind RCT's in which women had individual instruction by a trained PT, combined with biofeedback or electrical stimulation, had close follow-up, and high adherence.[9]
- Evidence from four RCTs showed that pelvic muscle training, combined with bladder training, effectively resolved urinary incontinence in women.[10]
- 45% cure rate for stress incontinence with electrical stimulation treatment; 60% of these patients had continued improvements for 3 to 11 months after treatment.[11,12]
- ICIQ-UI is an outcome measurement tool used to assess the prevalence and frequency of urinary leakage, its impact on everyday life, and the perceived cause of urinary incontinence.[13]
- A systematic review of 24 trials found that women who received biofeedback were significantly more likely to report that their urinary incontinence was cured or improved compared to those who received PFM training alone.[14]

PATIENT RESOURCE

- Stress Urinary Incontinence. MedlinePlus: National Institutes of Health website. http://www.nlm.nih.gov/medlineplus/ency/article/000891.htm. Accessed July 10, 2013.

REFERENCES

1. The American Physical Therapy Association. Pattern 4C: impaired muscle performance. In: *Guide to Physical Therapist Practice*. Alexandria, VA: The American Physical Therapy Association; 2003. http://guidetoptpractice.apta.org/content/1/SEC10.extract?sid=9af82a7e-5fc3-41d2-86ab-b8336a9655e9. July 10, 2013.
2. Hunskaar S, Arnold EP, Burgio K, et al. Epidemiology and natural history of urinary incontinence. *Int Urgynecol J Pelvic Floor Dysfunct*. 2000;11(5):301–319.
3. Landi F, Cesari M, Russo A, et al. Potentially reversible risk factors and urinary incontinence in frail older people living in

community. *Age Ageing*. 2003;32(2):194–199.
4. Minassian VA, Drutz HP, Al-Badr A. Urinary incontinence as a worldwide problem. *Int J Gynaecol Obstet*. 2003;82(3):327–338.
5. Eliasson K, Elfving B, Nordgren B, Mattsson E. Urinary incontinence in women with low back pain. *Man Ther*. 2008; 13(3):206–212.
6. Herzog AR, Fultz NH. Prevalence and incidence of urinary incontinence in community-dwelling populations. *J Am Geriatr Soc*. 1990;38(3):273–281.
7. Avery K, Donovan J, Peters TJ, et al. ICIQ: a brief and robust measure for evaluating the symptoms and impact of urinary incontinence. *Neurourol Urodyn*. 2004;23(4):322–330.
8. Dumoulin C, Bourbonnais D, Morin M, Gravel D, Lemieux MC. Predictors of success for physiotherapy treatment in women with persistent postpartum stress urinary incontinence. *Arch Phys Med Rehabil*. 2010;91:1059–1063.
9. Dumoulin C, Hay-Smith J. Pelvic floor muscle training versus no treatment, or inactive control treatments, for urinary incontinence in women. *Cochrane Database Syst Rev*. 2010;(1): CD005654. doi:10.1002/14651858.CD005654.pub2. Review.
10. Shamliyan TA, Kane RL, Wyman J, Wilt TJ. Systematic review: randomized, controlled trials of nonsurgical treatments for urinary incontinence in women. *Ann Intern Med*. 2008;148(6):459–473.
11. Brubaker L, Benson T, Bent A, Clark A, Shott S. Transvaginal electrical stimulation for female urinary incontinence. *Am J Obstet Gynecol*. 1997;177(3):536–540.
12. Yamanashi T, Yasuda K, Sakakibara R, Hattori T, Ito H, Muraakami S. Pelvic floor electrical stimulation in the treatment of stress incontinence: an investigational study and placebo controlled double-blind trial. *J Urol*. 1997;158(6):2127–2131.
13. Abrams P, Cardozo L, Fall M, et al. The standardisation of terminology of lower urinary tract function: report from the Standardisation Sub-committee of the International Continence Society. *Neurourol Urodyn*. 2002;21(2):167–178.
14. Herderschee R, Hay-Smith EJ, Herbison GP, Roovers JP, Heineman MJ. Feedback or biofeedback to augment pelvic floor muscle training for urinary incontinence in women. *Cochrane Database Syst Rev*. 2011;(7):CD009252.

ADDITIONAL REFERENCES

- Abrams P, Cardoza LD, Khoury S, Wein A, eds. *Incontinence Management*. 3rd ed. Plymouth, UK: Health Publications Ltd; 2005.
- Brown JS, Bradley CS, Subak LL, et al. The sensitivity and specificity of a simple test to distinguish between urge and stress urinary incontinence. *Ann Intern Med*. 2006;144(10):715–723.
- Deng DY. Urinary incontinence in women. *Med Clin North Am*. 2011;95(1):101–109.
- Dutton M. Pathology, gynecology, and psychology. In: Dutton M, ed. *McGraw-Hill's NPTE (National Physical Therapy Examination)*. 2nd ed. New York, NY: McGraw-Hill; 2012.
- Godec CJ, Fravel R, Cass AS. Optimal parameters of electrical stimulation in the treatment of urinary incontinence. *Invest Urol*. 1981;18(4):239–241.
- Haylen BT, de Ridder D, Freeman RM, et al. An International Urogynecological Association (IUGA)/International Continence Society (ICS) joint report on the terminology for female pelvic floor dysfunction. *Neurourol Urodyn*. 2010;29(1):4–20.
- Larsson G, Victor A. The frequency/volume chart in genuine stress incontinent women. *Neurourol Urodyn*. 1992;11(1):23–31.
- Laycock J, Haslam J. *Therapeutic Management of Incontinence and Pelvic Pain*. 2nd ed. London: Springer Publishers; 2008.
- Lopez R, Smith PC, Therine A. Clinical inquiries. What are the indications for urodynamic testing in older adults with incontinence? *J Fam Pract*. 2002;51(12):1077.
- Messelink B, Benson T, Berghmans B, et al. Standardization of terminology of pelvic floor muscle function and dysfunction: report from the pelvic floor clinical assessment group of the International Continence Society. *Neurourol Urodyn*. 2005; 24(4):374–380.
- Neville C. Pelvic floor treatment: urinary incontinence and pelvic floor muscle training [Video]. New York, NY: McGraw-Hill; 2014. http://www.accessphysiotherapy.com. Accessed June 13, 2014.
- Ohlsson BL. Effects of some different pulse parameters on the perception of intravaginal and intra-anal electrical stimulation. *Med Biol Eng Comput*. 1988;26(5):503–508.
- Panus PC, Jobst EE, Masters SB, Katzung B, Tinsley SL, Trevor AJ. Sympathomimetrics and sympatholytics. In: Panus PC, Jobst EE, Masters SB, Katzung B, Tinsley SL, Trevor AJ, eds. *Pharmacology for the Physical Therapist*. New York, NY: McGraw-Hill; 2009. http://www.accessphysiotherapy.com/content/6090704. Accessed Feb 23, 2013.
- Ramsay IN, Hilton P, Cox TF. Time-series analysis of urethral electrical conductance measurements in the assessment of unstable urethal pressure: results in normal patients and those with genuine stress incontinence. *Neurourol Urodyn*. 1993; 12(1):23–31.
- Vecchioli-Scaldazza C, Morosetti C. Effect of aging on urinary incontinence in women. *Arch Ital Urol Androl*. 2010;82(3): 167–171.

280 URGE URINARY INCONTINENCE

Stephanie Bush, DPT, MEd, WCS
Cynthia E. Neville, DPT, PT, WCS
Eric Shamus, PhD, DPT, PT, CSCS

CONDITION/DISORDER SYNONYMS

- Detrusor instability (DI)
- Detrusor overactivity incontinence
- Overactive bladder (OAB)
- Overactive bladder syndrome
- Urge syndrome
- Urgency-frequency syndrome

ICD-9-CM CODES

- 788.3 Urinary incontinence
- 788.30 Urinary incontinence, unspecified
- 788.31 Urge Incontinence

ICD-10-CM CODES

- N39.41 Urge incontinence
- R32 Unspecified urinary incontinence

PREFERRED PRACTICE PATTERN

- 4C: Impaired Muscle Performance[1]

PATIENT PRESENTATION

A 45-year-old woman reports that several times per day she experiences a sudden strong urge to urinate and cannot make it to the bathroom without leaking. She has noticed the gradual increase in frequency and urgency of urination over the past few years. Now she is also waking up three to four times per night to urinate. She is wearing three pads per day and sometimes wets through the pad and her clothes are wet. She has stopped participating in the cross-fit classes that she enjoys, because she is leaking. She is afraid to go to the symphony with her husband because of these symptoms.

KEY FEATURES

Description

- Involuntary loss of urine control accompanied by or immediately preceded by urgency

Essentials of Diagnosis

- High detrusor pressure during urodynamic testing indicative of detrusor overactivity contributing to urge urinary incontinence (UUI)
- 3 Incontinence Questions (3IQ): Sensitivity of 0.75, specificity of 0.77, and a positive likelihood ratio of 3.29 for the classification of UUI

General Considerations

- Consideration of lower urinary tract infections (UTIs): Urinary frequency, urinary urgency, lower back pain
- Myogenic dysfunction of the detrusor
- Urodynamic testing cannot be relied on to diagnose OAB but can be used to confirm the diagnosis[2]

Demographics

- Urinary incontinence affects 30% to 60% of middle-aged and older women[3,4]
- Urinary incontinence reported by 78% of women with low back pain[5]
- Severe urinary incontinence is more prevalent in later years
- 30% to 52% of homebound elderly suffer from urinary incontinence[6]

CLINICAL FINDINGS

SIGNS AND SYMPTOMS

- More than seven voids per 24 hours
- Loss of urine without meaning to urinate
- Loss of a moderate to large amount of urine preceded by an urge to urinate, often associated with an irritant such as running water, walking by the bathroom, putting a key in a lock, or nervousness
- Increased alpha tone in prostatic and urethral smooth muscle
- Inflammation in the bladder
- Sensitivity to potassium
- Possible triggering of the micturition reflex

Functional Implications

- Increased risk for falls: 2- to 3.5-fold increase[7–9]
- Increased risk of falls during an inpatient episode of care[9]

Possible Contributing Causes

- Underactive, overactive, or nonfunctioning pelvic floor muscles
- Bladder cancer
- Bladder inflammation
- Bladder stones
- Spinal cord injury
- Multiple sclerosis (MS)
- Bladder obstruction from enlarged prostate
- Benign prostatic hypertrophy (BPH)
- Comorbidities such as diabetes
- UTIs: Bacterial
- Increase in bladder sensation
- Decrease in bladder capacity
- Increase of detrusor overactivity
- Reduction of maximal urethral closure pressure

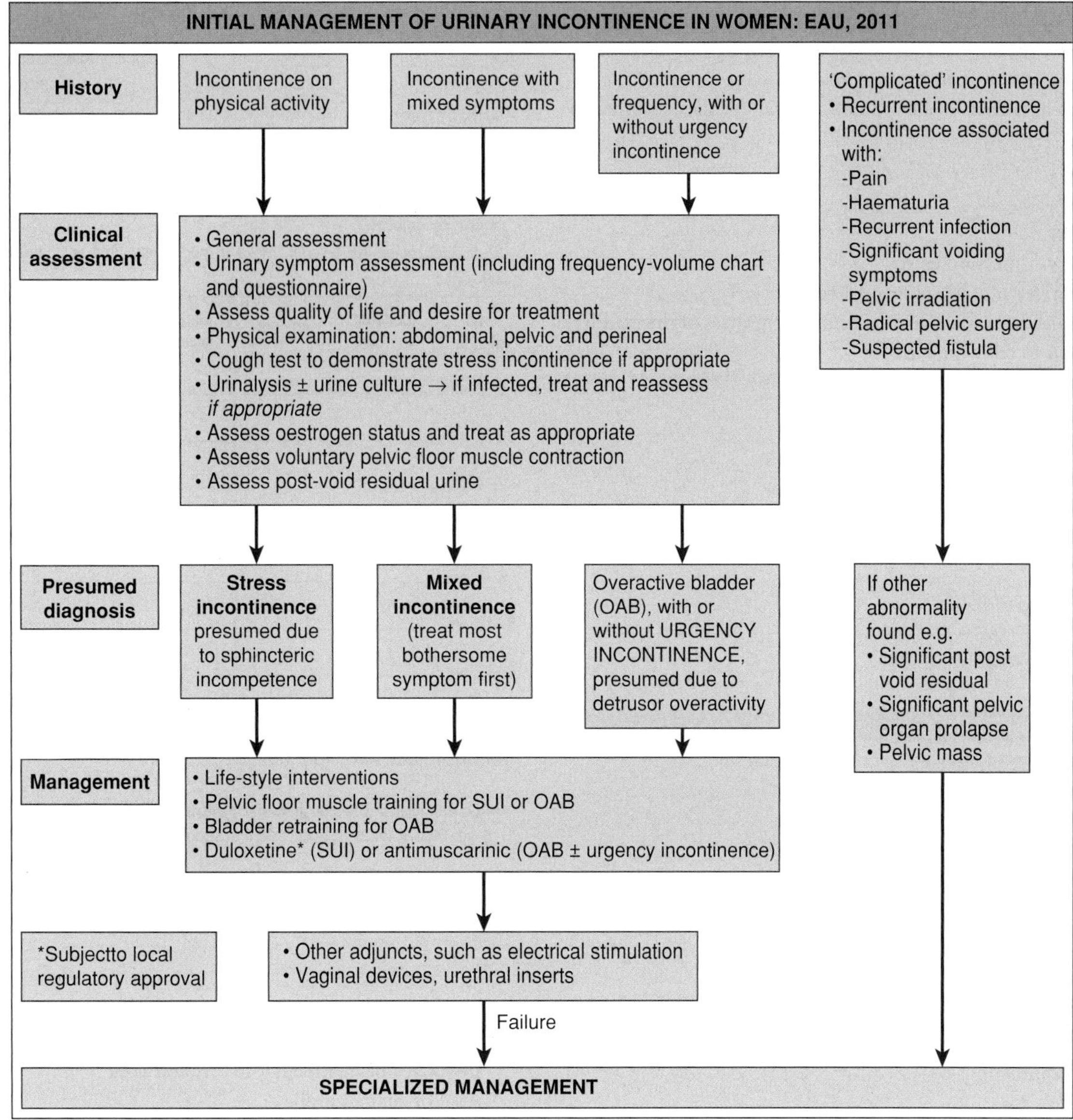

FIGURE 280-1 Initial management of urinary incontinence in women: EAU, 2011. (From Esherick JS, Clark DS, Slater ED. *Current Practice Guidelines in Primary Care 2012*. http://www.accessmedicine.com. Copyright © The McGraw-Hill Companies, Inc. All rights reserved.)

▶ Differential Diagnosis

- UTI
- Interstitial cystitis
- Detrusor myopathy
- Neuropathy

MEANS OF CONFIRMATION OR DIAGNOSIS

▶ Imaging

- Ultrasound imaging to identify abnormalities of the bladder, urethra or pelvis, bladder neck position and mobility, pelvic floor function, activity of levator ani, descent of pelvic organs, and sphincter integrity
- MRI to examine soft tissue structures of the pelvic support apparatus
- Pelvic/abdominal ultrasound
  - Measure bladder capacity
  - Rule out other pathologies

▶ Diagnostic Procedures

- Rule out UTI
- Postvoid residual volume (PVR): Measures the amount of urine left after urinating
- Urinary stress test
  - Stand with a full bladder and cough
  - Test does not have good reliability or validity
  - Test is not specific enough to rule in/out a diagnosis
- Urodynamics: Functional study of the lower urinary tract
  - Indications include: Unclear cause of voiding dysfunction, incontinence unresponsive to conservative treatment, history of hysterectomy, bladder surgeries or pelvic organ prolapse procedures, neurological conditions
  - Assess sphincter competency
  - High detrusor pressure indicates an OAB, detrusor overactivity, UUI
- Three incontinence questions (3IQ): Sensitivity of 0.75, specificity of 0.77[10]

FINDINGS AND INTERPRETATION

- High detrusor pressure during urodynamic testing indicative of detrusor over activity, contributing to UUI
- On the 3IQ, a positive likelihood ratio of 3.29 for the classification of UUI[10]

TREATMENT

Medication

- Antibiotics if infection exists
- Medication for muscle spasms: Flavoxate
- Tricyclic antidepressants to affect smooth muscles of the bladder
- Medication to relax the bladder
  - Anticholinergics: Oxybutynin, tolterodine, darifenacin

MEDICAL PROCEDURES

- No specific surgical options
  - Surgery to treat stress urinary incontinence (SUI) can improve symptoms of urge incontinence, but not performed only for UUI
- Augmentation cystoplasty
  - Performed to create a new bladder when the bladder is removed secondary to cancer or trauma

REFERRALS/ADMITTANCE

- To primary care physicians
- To gynecologists
  - Women: Pelvic examination
- To urologists
  - Men: Genital examination
- To urogynecologists
- To acupuncturist

BLADDER RECORD

Day:________ Date:____/____ (month / day)

INSTRUCTIONS:

1) In the 1st column make a mark every time during the 2-hour period you urinate into the toilet
2) Use the 2nd column to record the amount you urinate (if you are measuring amounts)
3) In the 3rd or 4th column, make a mark every time you accidentally leak urine

Time Interval	Urinated in Toilet	Amount	Leaking Accident	or Large Accident	Reason for Accident*
6–8 am					
8–10 am					
2–4 pm					
4–6 pm					
6–8 pm					
8–10 pm					
10–12 pm					
Overnight					

Number of pads used today:________

*For example, if you coughed and have a leaking accident, write "cough". If you had a large accident after a strong urge to urinate, write "urge".

FIGURE 280-2 Example of a bladder record for ambulatory care settings. (Reprinted with permission from Kane RL, Ouslander JG, Itamar B, et al. *Essentials of Clinical Geriatrics*. 5th ed. New York, NY: McGraw-Hill; 2004.)

IMPAIRMENTS

- Pelvic floor muscle dysfunction: Overactive, underactive, nonrelaxing, noncontracting
- Incontinence
- Pelvic pain
- Pelvic organ prolapse
- DI

TESTS AND MEASURES

- Pelvic floor muscle examination
- Bladder diary to assess patient's behaviors related to micturition including fluid and food intake, voiding habits, episodes of leakage (activity-related or urge-related), and use of pads
- sEMG biofeedback assessment of the pelvic floor muscles
- Pressure manometry of the pelvic floor muscles
- Inquiry: During last 3 months did you leak urine when you had the urge or feeling that you needed to empty your bladder but could not get to the toilet fast enough?
- Pelvic floor muscle assessment

INTERVENTION

- Neuromuscular electrical stimulation to decrease urinary urgency and frequency and detrusor overactivity
  - Urge protocol: Frequency of 10 to 12 Hz, pulse width of 200 to 350 usec, asymmetrical biphasic wave form, duty cycle of 5 to 10 seconds on/5 to 10 seconds off, duration of 10 to 20 minutes, frequency of treatment 1 to 7 times/week
  - Anal or vaginal probe
  - Surface electrodes
    - Sacrum
    - Perineum
    - Suprapubic area
    - Tibial nerve
- Pelvic floor muscle exercises/training
  - Contraction
  - Relaxation/"bulging"
  - Motor control
  - Endurance
  - Power
  - sEMG biofeedback
  - Weighted vaginal cones to strengthen pelvic floor
    - Hold weighted cone in vagina for up to 15 minutes, 2 times a day
    - No literature to support use in urge incontinence
    - Some believe strengthening the pelvic floor will decrease pelvic floor muscle tone
- Kegel exercises
- Pressure manometry
- Manual therapy
- US imaging to facilitate pelvic floor muscle training

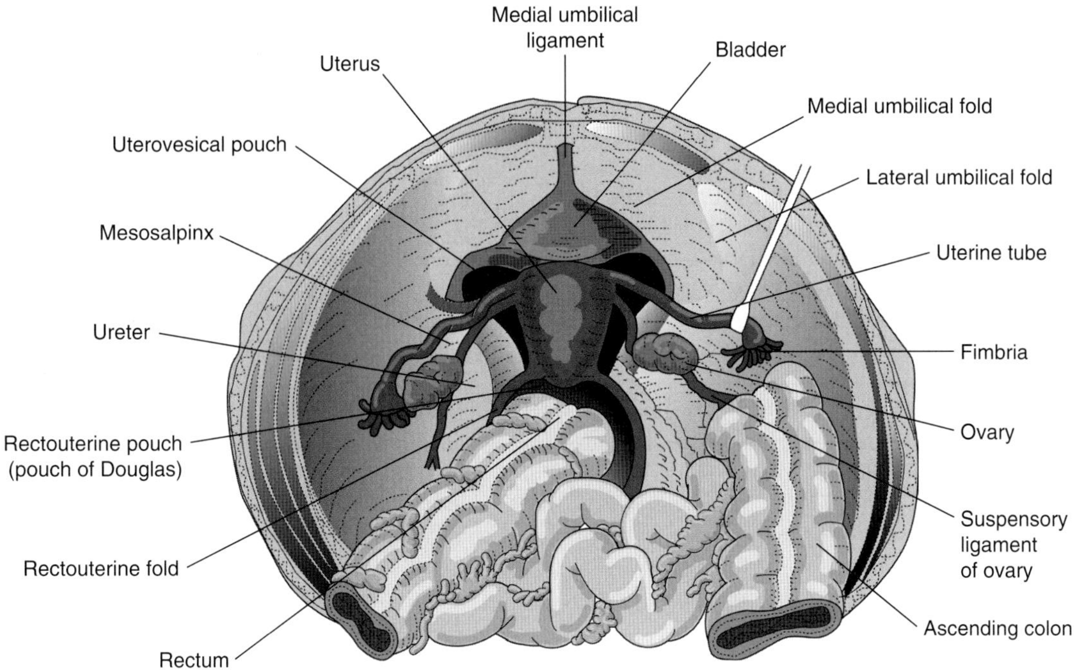

FIGURE 280-3 Female pelvic contents from above. (From DeCherney AH, Nathan L, Goodwin TM, Laufer N, Roman AS. *Current Diagnosis & Treatment: Obstetrics & Gynecology*. 11th ed. www.accessmedicine.com. Copyright © The McGraw-Hill Companies, Inc. All rights reserved.)

- Bladder retraining including timed voiding schedule and urge suppression technique
- Patient education
  - Fluid management strategies
  - Drink enough water: A little bit of fluid throughout the day
  - Minimize consumption of bladder irritants
    - Caffeine
    - Spicy foods
    - Acidic foods including citrus

FUNCTIONAL GOALS

- Patient will be able to
  - Decrease number of episodes of urinary leakage to improve ability to participate in ADLs.
  - Decrease urinary frequency during the day to an average of 5 to 7 times.
  - Decrease total number of nighttime voids.
    - 0 to 1 per night for individuals under 65 years.
    - 1 to 2 per night for individuals over 65 years.
  - Restore average time interval between voiding (ability to store urine) to every 2 to 5 hours.
  - Independence with long-term pelvic floor muscle training program, as appropriate, to manage urinary symptoms.

PROGNOSIS

- Evidence from four RCTs showed that pelvic muscle training, combined with bladder training, effectively resolved urinary incontinence in women.[11]
- In a cohort of women with urge incontinence, bladder training was more effective at reducing daytime frequency than use of Imipramine (Tofranil).[12,13]
- Overall, electrical stimulation appears to have a 50% improvement/cure rate.[14]
- 83.3% report some improvement in urinary incontinence symptoms with sacral surface TENS.[15]
- ICIQ-UI is an outcome measurement tool used to assess the prevalence and frequency of urinary leakage, its impact on everyday life, and the perceived cause of urinary incontinence.[16]

PATIENT RESOURCE

- Urge Incontinence. MedlinePlus: National Institutes of Health website. http://www.nlm.nih.gov/medlineplus/ency/article/001270.htm. Accessed July 1, 2013.

REFERENCES

1. The American Physical Therapy Association. Pattern 4C: impaired muscle performance. In: *Guide to Physical Therapist Practice*. Alexandria, VA: The American Physical Therapy Association; 2003. http://guidetoptpractice.apta.org/content/1/SEC10.extract?sid=9af82a7e-5fc3-41d2-86ab-b8336a9655e9. Accessed July 1, 2013.
2. Laycock J, Haslam J. *Therapeutic Management of Incontinence and Pelvic Pain*. 2nd ed. London: Springer Publishers; 2008.
3. Herzog AR, Fultz NH. Prevalence and incidence of urinary incontinence in community-dwelling populations. *J Am Geriatr Soc*. 1990;38(3):273–281.
4. Messelink B, Benson T, Berghmans B, et al. Standardization of terminology of pelvic floor muscle function and dysfunction: report from the pelvic floor clinical assessment group of the International Continence Society. *Neurourol Urodyn*. 2005;24(4):374–380.
5. Dutton M. Pathology, gynecology, and psychology. In: Dutton M, ed. *McGraw-Hill's NPTE (National Physical Therapy Examination)*. 2nd ed. New York, NY: McGraw-Hill; 2012. http://www.accessphysiotherapy.com/content/5402111. Accessed July e1, 2013.

6. Haylen BT, de Ridder D, Freeman RM, et al. An International Urogynecological Association (IUGA)/International Continence Society (ICS) joint report on the terminology for female pelvic floor dysfunction. *Neurourol Urodyn.* 2010;29(1):4–20.
7. Burgio, KL, Lochler JL, Goode PS, et al. Behavioral vs drug treatment for urge urinary incontinence in older women: a randomized controlled trial. *JAMA.* 1998;280(23):1995–2000.
8. Pils K, Neumann F, Meisner W, et al. Predictors of falls in elderly people during rehabilitation after hip fracture—who is at risk of a second one? *Z Gerontol Geriatr.* 2003;36(1):16–22.
9. Takazawa K, Arisawa K. Relationship between the type of urinary incontinence and falls among frail elderly women in Japan. *J Med Invest.* 2005;52(3-4):165–171.
10. Avery K, Donovan J, Peters TJ, et al. ICIQ: a brief and robust measure for evaluating the symptoms and impact of urinary incontinence. *Neurourol Urodyn.* 2004;23(4):322–330.
11. Shamliyan TA, Kane RL, Wyman J, Wilt TJ. Systematic review: randomized, controlled trials of nonsurgical treatments for urinary incontinence in women. *Ann Intern Med.* 2008;148(6):459–473.
12. Brubaker L. Electrical stimulation in overactive bladder. *Urology.* 2000;55(suppl 5A):17–23; discussion 31-2.
13. Landi F, Cesari M, Russo A, et al. Potentially reversible risk factors and urinary incontinence in frail older people living in community. *Age Ageing.* 2003;32(2):194–199.
14. Vecchioli-Scaldazza C, Morosetti C. Effect of aging on urinary incontinence in women. *Arch Ital Urol Androl.* 2010;82(3): 167–171.
15. Yokozuka M, Namima T, Nakagawa H, Ichie M, Handa Y. Effects and indications of sacral surface therapeutic electrical stimulation in refractory urinary incontinence. *Clin Rehabil.* 2004;18(8):899–907.
16. Abrams P, Cardozo L, Fall M, et al. The standardisation of terminology of lower urinary tract function: report from the Standardisation Sub-committee of the International Continence Society. *Neurourol Urodyn.* 2002;21(2):167–178.

ADDITIONAL REFERENCES

- Abrams P, Cardoza LD, Khoury S, Wein A, eds. *Incontinence Management.* 3rd ed. Plymouth, UK: Health Publications Ltd; 2005.
- Brown JS, Bradley CS, Subak LL, et al. The sensitivity and specificity of a simple test to distinguish between urge and stress urinary incontinence. *Ann Intern Med.* 2006;144(10):715–723
- Brubaker L, Benson T, Bent A, Clark A, Shott S. Transvaginal electrical stimulation for female urinary incontinence. *Am J Obstet Gynecol.* 1997;177(3):536–540.
- Chiarelli PE, Mackenzie LA, Osmotherly PG. Urinary incontinence is associated with an increase in falls: a systematic review. *Aust J Physiother.* 2009;55(2):89–95.
- Deng DY. Urinary incontinence in women. *Med Clin North Am.* 2011;95(1):101–109.
- Dutton M. Pathology, gynecology, and psychology. In: Dutton M, ed. *McGraw-Hill's NPTE (National Physical Therapy Examination).* 2nd ed. New York, NY: McGraw-Hill; 2012. http://www.accessphysiotherapy.com/content/5402334. Accessed July 1, 2013.
- Eliasson K, Elfving B, Nordgren B, Mattsson E. Urinary incontinence in women with low back pain. *Man Ther.* 2008;13(3): 206–212.
- Godec CJ, Fravel R, Cass AS. Optimal parameters of electrical stimulation in the treatment of urinary incontinence. *Invest Urol.* 1981;18(4):239–241.
- Hunskaar S, Arnold EP, Burgio K, et al. Epidemiology and natural history of urinary incontinence. *Int Urgynecol J Pelvic Floor Dysfunct.* 2000;11(5):301–319.
- Larsson G, Victor A. The frequency/volume chart in genuine stress incontinent women. *Neurourol Urodyn.* 1992;11(1):23–31.
- Lopez R, Smith PC, Therine A. Clinical inquiries. What are the indications for urodynamic testing in older adults with incontinence? *J Fam Pract.* 2002;51(12):1077.
- Minassian VA, Drutz HP, Al-Badr A. Urinary incontinence as a worldwide problem. *Int J Gynaecol Obstet.* 2003;82(3):327–338.
- Neville C. Pelvic floor treatment: urinary incontinence and pelvic floor muscle training [Video]. New York, NY: McGraw-Hill; 2014. http://www.accessphysiotherapy.com. Accessed June 13, 2014.
- Ohlsson BL. Effects of some different pulse parameters on the perception of intravaginal and intra-anal electrical stimulation. *Med Biol Eng Comput.* 1988;26(5):503–508.
- Panus PC, Jobst EE, Masters SB, Katzung B, Tinsley SL, Trevor AJ. Sympathomimetrics and sympatholytics. In: Panus PC, Jobst EE, Masters SB, Katzung B, Tinsley SL, Trevor AJ, eds. *Pharmacology for the Physical Therapist.* New York, NY: McGraw-Hill; 2009. http://www.accessphysiotherapy.com/content/6090704. Accessed July 1, 2013.

Note: Page number followed by f and t indicates figure and table respectively.

C

D

E

H

J

K

L

N

U

V

W

Y